DRUG FACTS AND COMPARISONS®

2012

POCKET VERSION

Wolters Kluwer Health | Facts & Comparisons®

YOUR ANSWER FOR DRUG ANSWERS

Drug Facts and Comparisons® Pocket Version, Sixteenth Edition, 2012

Adapted from *Drug Facts and Comparisons®* loose-leaf drug information service through the February 2011 update.

ISBN 1-57439-329-4
ISBN 978-1-57439-329-3

Printed in the United States of America

The information contained in *Drug Facts and Comparisons®* pocket version is available for licensing as source data. For more information on data licensing, please call 1-800-223-0554.

Wolters Kluwer Health
77 Westport Plaza Drive, Suite 450
St. Louis, Missouri 63146-3125
Phone 314/216-2100 • 800/223-0554
Fax 314/878-5563
www.factsandcomparisons.com

FACTS & COMPARISONS® EDITORIAL ADVISORY PANEL

BURGUNDA (GUNDY) V. SWEET, PharmD, FASHP
Director, Drug Information and Medication Use Policy
Clinical Associate Professor of Pharmacy
University of Michigan Health System and College of Pharmacy
Ann Arbor, Michigan

DAVID S. TATRO, PharmD
Drug Information Analyst
San Carlos, California

THOMAS L. WHITSETT, MD
Professor of Medicine and Pharmacology
Vascular Medicine Program
OU Regents Professor
University of Oklahoma Health Sciences Center
Oklahoma City, Oklahoma

Table of Contents

HOW TO USE

Drug monographs in *Drug Facts and Comparisons®*, *Pocket Version* are arranged by use. Drugs with similar therapeutic or pharmacologic characteristics have been grouped together to allow the health care provider to compare these drugs easily and determine the most appropriate drug therapy. Standard sections within the monographs occur in a consistent format. Once the user is familiar with the organization of the data, the desired information can be located quickly.

Monograph Organization

1. *Therapeutic class:* Drugs that share the same therapeutic class will share a common title that appears on the right-hand pages. The monograph title appears on the left-hand pages. If there is no shared class, the monograph title will repeat on the right-hand page.
2. *Drug name:* Generic names and any common synonyms appear in a horizontal bar that introduces a new monograph. Synonyms follow the generic name in parentheses and are separated by semicolons.
3. *Product table:* Doseforms and strengths of generic drugs are listed in the left column with their schedules (eg, *Rx*, *otc*, *c-ii*). If more than one generic entity is included in the monograph (eg, beta blockers), the drugs appear in all caps with specific information underneath it. The more common trade names, with their specific manufacturers/distributors, are listed in the right-hand column. If the drug is available generically, the word "Various" appears at the beginning of the trade name listing.
4. *Warning box:* Potentially life-threatening reactions specified in the product labeling will appear in a box.
5. *Indications:* All FDA-approved indications are included.
6. *Administration and Dosage:* Appropriate dosage, dosage range, and administration information is included. When available, specific information for administration in situations such as in renal impairment and elderly patients is included.
7. *Actions:* This section includes a brief discussion of significant pharmacologic and pharmacokinetic information.
8. *Contraindications:* All known contraindications are included.
9. *Warnings/Precautions:* This section includes a brief description of major warnings and other significant situations where caution is warranted with the drug. The Pregnancy section generally only lists the Standard Pregnancy Category (A, B, C, D, or X). A description of these categories can be found in the Appendix.
10. *Drug Interactions:* Drugs that may interact (affect or be affected by the interacting agent) are listed. Lab test and drug/food interactions also are included.
11. *Adverse Reactions:* Where possible, reactions that occur in 3% or more of patients have been listed. When percentages are not available, significant reactions not discussed in Warnings/Precautions are included.

❶ **ANTIPLATELET AGENTS**

❷ CILOSTAZOL

❸ **Tablets: 50 and 100 mg (Rx)** *Various, Pletal* (Otsuka America Pharmaceutical)

❹ **Warning:**

Cilostazol and several of its metabolites are inhibitors of phosphodiesterase (PDE) 3. Several drugs with this pharmacologic effect have caused decreased survival compared with placebo in patients with class III to IV congestive heart failure. Cilostazol is contraindicated in patients with congestive heart failure of any severity.

❺ Indications

Intermittent claudication: For the reduction of symptoms of intermittent claudication, as indicated by an increased walking distance.

❻ Administration and Dosage

Recommended dosage: 100 mg twice daily taken at least 30 minutes before or 2 hours after breakfast and dinner.

Concomitant medications: Consider 50 mg twice daily during coadministration of inhibitors of CYP3A4 (eg, diltiazem, erythromycin, itraconazole, ketoconazole) and during coadministration of inhibitors of CYP2C19 (eg, omeprazole).

❼ Actions

Pharmacology: The mechanism of the effects of cilostazol on the symptoms of intermitent claudication is not fully understood. Cilostazol and metabolites are cyclic adenosine monophosphate (cAMP) PDE 3 inhibitors, leading to inhibition of platelet aggregation and vasodilation, respectively.

Pharmacokinetics:

Absorption – Cilostazol is absorbed after oral administration. A high-fat meal increases absorption.

Distribution – Cilostazol is 95% to 98% protein bound.

Metabolism/Excretion – Cilostazol is extensively metabolized by hepatic cytochrome P-450 enzymes, mainly 3A4, and 2C19. Cilostazol and its active metabolites have apparent elimination half-lives of about 11 to 13 hours.

❽ Contraindications

Congestive heart failure; hemostatic disorders or active pathologic bleeding, such as bleeding peptic ulcer and intracranial bleeding; known or suspected hypersensitivity to any of its components.

❾ Warnings/Precautions

Hematologic effects: Rare cases of thrombocytopenia or leukopenia progressing to agranulocytosis have been reported when cilostazol was not immediately discontinued.

Pregnancy: Category C.

Lactation: Because of the potential risk to breast-feeding infants, decide whether to discontinue breast-feeding or cilostazol.

Children: The safety and efficacy of cilostazol in children have not been established.

❿ Drug Interactions

Drugs that may affect cilostazol include clopidogrel, CYP3A4 inhibitors, CYP2C19 inhibitors, diltiazem, and lovastatin.

Drugs that may be affected by cilostazol include lovastatin.

Drug/Food interactions: A high-fat meal increases absorption with an approximately 90% increase in C_{max} and a 25% increase in AUC.

⓫ Adverse Reactions

Adverse reactions occurring in at least 3% of patients include the following: abdominal pain, abnormal stools, back pain, cough increased, diarrhea, dizziness, dyspepsia, flatulence, headache, infection, myalgia, nausea, palpitation, peripheral edema, pharyngitis, rhinitis, tachycardia, vertigo.

PREFACE

The Pocket Version of *Drug Facts and Comparisons®* (*DFC*) is an abridged version of the full *DFC* publication designed for quick reference by the health care professional. The purpose of the *DFC Pocket Version* is to provide an easy-to-use, concise, portable reference that can be utilized in daily practice. It is not intended to replace the complete information found in *DFC*; however, it provides the same reliable source of drug information.

In addition to the extensive review panel for *DFC*, a separate panel of drug information specialists and hospital pharmacists was established to determine which drug monographs would be most valuable to the health care professional along with the data for each drug needed most. The book is arranged therapeutically in 12 chapters in a consistent format. Single-agent monographs have been pared down to provide the essential information that a health care provider needs to aid in drug therapy decisions. Product tables that list trade names, doseforms, strengths, and manufacturers are included at the beginning of each monograph. Group monographs contain product information and dosing instructions for each of the drugs in a specific class (eg, beta blockers). Indications, administration and dosage, actions, contraindications, warnings, drug interactions, and significant adverse reactions (those occurring in at least 3% of patients) also are included for all monographs. The useful tables that are so common to *DFC* have, for the most part, been retained in the Pocket Version.

Appendix material (eg, Management of Overdosage, FDA Pregnancy Categories) also is available for reference. A comprehensive index helps the reader reach the desired information quickly and easily.

Wolters Kluwer Health hopes health care providers find *Drug Facts and Comparisons® Pocket Version* a valuable tool in daily practice. As always, comments and suggestions are appreciated.

Cathy H. Reilly
Vice President and Publisher

Chapter 1

NUTRIENTS AND NUTRITIONAL AGENTS

RECOMMENDED DIETARY ALLOWANCES OF VITAMINS AND MINERALS

In 1941, the Food and Nutrition Board (FNB) of the Institute of Medicine, National Academy of Sciences, published the first edition of the Recommended Dietary Allowances (RDAs) to be used to evaluate the nutritional intakes of large populations. The primary purpose for the RDAs was to prevent diseases caused by nutritional deficiencies. Over the years, these guidelines were periodically updated and revised based on cumulative scientific evidence, and the tenth edition was published in 1989. In response to the growth of scientific knowledge regarding the roles of nutrients in human health, the FNB in partnership with Health Canada revised the RDAs and developed the Dietary Reference Intakes (DRIs).

The DRIs were published as a series of 8 reports from 1997 to 2005 and include the following nutrient reference values: Estimated Average Requirement (EAR), RDAs, Adequate Intake (AI), and Tolerable Upper Intake Level (UL). EAR refers to the intake value of a nutrient that is estimated to meet the nutritional needs by a specified indicator of adequacy in 50% of an age- and gender-specific group. RDAs are based on EARs and are estimated to meet the needs of most individuals (97% to 98%). AIs are used when an RDA cannot be determined. UL is the maximum amount of daily nutrient intake (from food, water, and supplements) that is likely to pose no risk of adverse reactions.

In the following DRI tables, the RDAs are in bold type and the AIs are in ordinary type followed by an asterisk (*). These values may be used as goals for individual intake. For healthy breast-fed infants, the AI represents mean intake. For all other life-stage groups, the AI is believed to cover the needs of all individuals, but a lack of data or uncertainty in the data prevent specifying with confidence the percentage of individuals covered by this intake.

DRIs: Recommended Intakes for Individuals (Vitamins)

Life-stage group	Vitamin A (mcg/d)[a]	Vitamin C (mg/d)	Vitamin D (mcg/d)[b,c]	Vitamin E (mg/d)[d]	Vitamin K (mcg/d)	Thiamine (mg/d)	Riboflavin (mg/d)	Niacin (mg/d)[e]	Vitamin B_6 (mg/d)	Folate (mcg/d)[f]	Vitamin B_{12} (mcg/d)	Pantothenic acid (mg/d)	Biotin (mcg/d)	Choline (mg/d)[g]
Infants														
0 to 6 mo	400*	40*	5*	4*	2*	0.2*	0.3*	2*	0.1*	65*	0.4*	1.7*	5*	125*
7 to 12 mo	500*	50*	5*	5*	2.5*	0.3*	0.4*	4*	0.3*	80*	0.5*	1.8*	6*	150*
Children														
1 to 3 y	300	15	5*	6	30*	0.5	0.5	6	0.5	150	0.9	2*	8*	200*
4 to 8 y	400	25	5*	7	55*	0.6	0.6	8	0.6	200	1.2	3*	12*	250*
Men														
9 to 13 y	600	45	5*	11	60*	0.9	0.9	12	1	300	1.8	4*	20*	375*
14 to 18 y	900	75	5*	15	75*	1.2	1.3	16	1.3	400	2.4	5*	25*	550*
19 to 30 y	900	90	5*	15	120*	1.2	1.3	16	1.3	400	2.4	5*	30*	550*
31 to 50 y	900	90	5*	15	120*	1.2	1.3	16	1.3	400	2.4	5*	30*	550*
51 to 70 y	900	90	10*	15	120*	1.2	1.3	16	1.7	400	2.4[h]	5*	30*	550*
> 70 y	900	90	15*	15	120*	1.2	1.3	16	1.7	400	2.4[h]	5*	30*	550*
Women														
9 to 13 y	600	45	5*	11	60*	0.9	0.9	12	1	300	1.8	4*	20*	375*
14 to 18 y	700	65	5*	15	75*	1	1	14	1.2	400[i]	2.4	5*	25*	400*
19 to 30 y	700	75	5*	15	90*	1.1	1.1	14	1.3	400[i]	2.4	5*	30*	425*
31 to 50 y	700	75	5*	15	90*	1.1	1.1	14	1.3	400[i]	2.4	5*	30*	425*
51 to 70 y	700	75	10*	15	90*	1.1	1.1	14	1.5	400	2.4[h]	5*	30*	425*
> 70 y	700	75	15*	15	90*	1.1	1.1	14	1.5	400	2.4[h]	5*	30*	425*
Pregnancy														
14 to 18 y	750	80	5*	15	75*	1.4	1.4	18	1.9	600[j]	2.6	6*	30*	450*
19 to 30 y	770	85	5*	15	90*	1.4	1.4	18	1.9	600[j]	2.6	6*	30*	450*
31 to 50 y	770	85	5*	15	90*	1.4	1.4	18	1.9	600[j]	2.6	6*	30*	450*

DRIs: Recommended Intakes for Individuals (Vitamins)

Life-stage group	Vitamin A (mcg/d)[a]	Vitamin C (mg/d)	Vitamin D (mcg/d)[b,c]	Vitamin E (mg/d)[d]	Vitamin K (mcg/d)	Thiamine (mg/d)	Riboflavin (mg/d)	Niacin (mg/d)[e]	Vitamin B_6 (mg/d)	Folate (mcg/d)[f]	Vitamin B_{12} (mcg/d)	Pantothenic acid (mg/d)	Biotin (mcg/d)	Choline (mg/d)[g]
Lactation														
14 to 18 y	**1,200**	**115**	5*	**19**	75*	**1.4**	**1.6**	**17**	**2**	**500**	**2.8**	7*	35*	550*
19 to 30 y	**1,300**	**120**	5*	**19**	90*	**1.4**	**1.6**	**17**	**2**	**500**	**2.8**	7*	35*	550*
31 to 50 y	**1,300**	**120**	5*	**19**	90*	**1.4**	**1.6**	**17**	**2**	**500**	**2.8**	7*	35*	550*

NOTE: AIs are in ordinary type followed by an asterisk (*), and RDAs are in bold type.

[a] As retinol activity equivalents (RAEs). 1 RAE = retinol 1 mcg, β-carotene 12 mcg, α-carotene 24 mcg, or β-cryptoxanthin 24 mcg. The RAE for dietary provitamin A carotenoids is 2-fold greater than retinol equivalents (RE), whereas the RAE for preformed vitamin A is the same as RE.

[b] As cholecalciferol. Cholecalciferol 1 mcg = vitamin D 40 units.

[c] Values based on the absence of adequate exposure to sunlight.

[d] As α-tocopherol. α-Tocopherol includes *RRR*-α-tocopherol, the only form of α-tocopherol that occurs naturally in foods, and the 2*R*-stereoisomeric forms of α-tocopherol (*RRR*-, *RSR*-, *RRS*-, and *RSS*-α-tocopherol) that occur in fortified foods and supplements. It does not include the 2*S*-stereoisomeric forms of α-tocopherol (*SRR*-, *SSR*-, *SRS*-, and *SSS*-α-tocopherol), also found in fortified foods and supplements.

[e] Includes nicotinic acid amide, nicotinic acid (pyridine-3-carboxylic acid), and derivatives that exhibit the biological activity of nicotinamide. As niacin equivalents (NE). Niacin 1 mg = tryptophan 60 mg; 0 to 6 months = preformed niacin (not NE).

[f] As dietary folate equivalents (DFE). One DFE = food folate 1 mcg = folic acid 0.6 mcg from fortified food or as a supplement consumed with food = 0.5 mcg of a supplement taken on an empty stomach.

[g] Although AIs have been set for choline, there are few data to assess whether a dietary supply of choline is needed at all stages of the life-cycle, and it may be that the choline requirement can be met by endogenous synthesis at some of these stages.

[h] Because 10% to 30% of older people may malabsorb food-bound B_{12}, it is advisable for individuals older than 50 years of age to meet their RDA mainly by consuming foods fortified with B_{12} or a supplement containing B_{12}.

[i] In view of evidence linking folate intake with neural tube defects in the fetus, it is recommended that all women capable of becoming pregnant consume 400 mcg from supplements or fortified foods in addition to intake of food folate from a varied diet.

[j] It is assumed that women will continue consuming 400 mcg from supplements or fortified food until their pregnancy is confirmed and they enter prenatal care, which ordinarily occurs after the end of the periconceptional period—the critical time for formation of the neural tube.

DRIs: Recommended Intakes for Individuals (Elements)

Life-stage group	Calcium (mg/d)	Chromium (mcg/d)	Copper (mcg/d)	Fluoride (mg/d)	Iodine (mcg/d)	Iron (mg/d)[a]	Magnesium (mg/d)	Manganese (mg/d)	Molybdenum (mcg/d)	Phosphorus (mg/d)	Selenium (mcg/d)	Zinc (mg/d)[b]	Potassium (g/d)	Sodium (g/d)	Chloride (g/d)
Infants															
0 to 6 mo	210*	0.2*	200*	0.01*	110*	0.27*	30*	0.003*	2*	100*	15*	2*	0.4*	0.12*	0.18*
7 to 12 mo	270*	5.5*	220*	0.5*	130*	**11**	75*	0.6*	3*	275*	20*	**3**	0.7*	0.37*	0.57*
Children															
1 to 3 y	500*	11*	**340**	0.7*	**90**	**7**	**80**	1.2*	**17**	**460**	**20**	**3**	3*	1*	1.5*
4 to 8 y	800*	15*	**440**	1*	**90**	**10**	**130**	1.5*	**22**	**500**	**30**	**5**	3.8*	1.2*	1.9*
Men															
9 to 13 y	1,300*	25*	**700**	2*	**120**	**8**	**240**	1.9*	**34**	**1,250**	**40**	**8**	4.5*	1.5*	2.3*
14 to 18 y	1,300*	35*	**890**	3*	**150**	**11**	**410**	2.2*	**43**	**1,250**	**55**	**11**	4.7*	1.5*	2.3*
19 to 30 y	1,000*	35*	**900**	4*	**150**	**8**	**400**	2.3*	**45**	**700**	**55**	**11**	4.7*	1.5*	2.3*
31 to 50 y	1,000*	35*	**900**	4*	**150**	**8**	**420**	2.3*	**45**	**700**	**55**	**11**	4.7*	1.5*	2.3*
51 to 70 y	1,200*	30*	**900**	4*	**150**	**8**	**420**	2.3*	**45**	**700**	**55**	**11**	4.7*	1.3*	2*
> 70 y	1,200*	30*	**900**	4*	**150**	**8**	**420**	2.3*	**45**	**700**	**55**	**11**	4.7*	1.2*	1.8*
Women															
9 to 13 y	1,300*	21*	**700**	2*	**120**	**8**	**240**	1.6*	**34**	**1,250**	**40**	**8**	4.5*	1.5*	2.3*
14 to 18 y	1,300*	24*	**890**	3*	**150**	**15**	**360**	1.6*	**43**	**1,250**	**55**	**9**	4.7*	1.5*	2.3*
19 to 30 y	1,000*	25*	**900**	3*	**150**	**18**	**310**	1.8*	**45**	**700**	**55**	**8**	4.7*	1.5*	2.3*
31 to 50 y	1,000*	25*	**900**	3*	**150**	**18**	**320**	1.8*	**45**	**700**	**55**	**8**	4.7*	1.5*	2.3*
51 to 70 y	1,200*	20*	**900**	3*	**150**	**8**	**320**	1.8*	**45**	**700**	**55**	**8**	4.7*	1.3*	2*
> 70 y	1,200*	20*	**900**	3*	**150**	**8**	**320**	1.8*	**45**	**700**	**55**	**8**	4.7*	1.2*	1.8*
Pregnancy															
14 to 18 y	1,300*	29*	**1,000**	3*	**220**	**27**	**400**	2*	**50**	**1,250**	**60**	**12**	4.7*	1.5*	2.3*
19 to 30 y	1,000*	30*	**1,000**	3*	**220**	**27**	**350**	2*	**50**	**700**	**60**	**11**	4.7*	1.5*	2.3*
31 to 50 y	1,000*	30*	**1,000**	3*	**220**	**27**	**360**	2*	**50**	**700**	**60**	**11**	4.7*	1.5*	2.3*
Lactation															
14 to 18 y	1,300*	44*	**1,300**	3*	**290**	**10**	**360**	2.6*	**50**	**1,250**	**70**	**13**	5.1*	1.5*	2.3*
19 to 30 y	1,000*	45*	**1,300**	3*	**290**	**9**	**310**	2.6*	**50**	**700**	**70**	**12**	5.1*	1.5*	2.3*
31 to 50 y	1,000*	45*	**1,300**	3*	**290**	**9**	**320**	2.6*	**50**	**700**	**70**	**12**	5.1*	1.5*	2.3*

NOTE: AIs are in ordinary type followed by an asterisk (*) and RDAs are in bold type.

[a] Non-heme iron absorption is lower for those consuming vegetarian diets than for those eating nonvegetarian diets. Therefore, it has been suggested that the iron requirement for individuals consuming a vegetarian diet is approximately 2-fold greater than for individuals consuming a nonvegetarian diet.

[b] Zinc absorption is lower for those consuming vegetarian diets than for those eating nonvegetarian diets. Therefore, it has been suggested that the zinc requirement for individuals consuming a vegetarian diet is approximately 2-fold greater than for individuals consuming a nonvegetarian diet.

VITAMIN C (Ascorbic Acid)

ASCORBIC ACID	
Tablets: 25, 50, 100, 250, 500, and 1,000 mg (*otc*)	Various, *One A Day Extras Vitamin* C (Miles)
Tablets, chewable: 60, 100, 250, and 500 mg (*otc*)	Various
Tablets and caplets, timed-release: 500, 1,000, and 1,500 mg (*otc*)	Various
Caplets: 500 mg (*otc*)	*SunKist Vitamin* C (Ciba)
Capsules, timed-release: 500 mg (*otc*)	Various, *Ascorbicap* (ICN), *Cevi-Bid* (Geriatric)
Lozenges: 60 mg (*otc*)	*N'ice Vitamin C Drops* (SmithKline Beecham Consumer), *N'ice* (Insight)
Crystals: 4 g/teaspoonful (*otc*)	*Vita-C* (Freeda)
Powder: 4 g/teaspoonful (*otc*)	*Dull-C* (Freeda)
Liquid: 35 mg/0.6 mL (*otc*)	*Ce-Vi-Sol* (Mead Johnson Nutritional)
Solution: 100 mg/mL (*otc*)	*Cecon* (Abbott)
Syrup: 500 mg/5 mL (*otc*)	Various
Injection: 250 and 500 mg/mL (*Rx*)	Various
CALCIUM ASCORBATE	
Tablets: 610 mg (equiv. to 500 mg ascorbic acid) (*otc*)	Various
Powder: 1 g (equiv. to 826 mg ascorbic acid)/ ¼ teaspoonful (*otc*)	Various
SODIUM ASCORBATE	
Tablets: 585 mg (equiv. to 500 mg ascorbic acid) (*otc*)	Various
Crystals: 1,020 mg (equiv. to 900 mg ascorbic acid)/ ¼ teaspoonful (*otc*)	Various
Injection: 250 mg/mL (equiv. to 222 mg/mL ascorbic acid) (*Rx*)	Various
562.5 mg/mL (equiv. to 500 mg/mL ascorbic acid) (*Rx*)	*Cenolate* (Hospira)

Indications

Prevention and treatment of scurvy. Parenteral administration is desirable in an acute deficiency or when absorption of oral ascorbic acid is uncertain.

Unlabeled uses: Vitamin C (at least 2 g/day) may be used as a urinary acidifier in conjunction with methenamine therapy.

Vitamin C in doses of at least 150 mg has been used to control idiopathic methemoglobinemia (less effective than methylene blue).

Administration and Dosage

Parenteral: Administer IV, IM, or subcutaneously. Avoid too rapid IV injection. Absorption and utilization are somewhat more efficient with the IM route, which is usually preferred.

Infants: Average daily protective requirement is 30 mg. The usual curative dose is 100 to 300 mg daily, continued as long as clinical symptoms persist or until saturation, as indicated by excretion tests, has been attained.

Premature infants: May require 75 to 100 mg/day.

Adults: The average protective dose is 70 to 150 mg/day. For scurvy, 300 mg to 1 g daily is recommended. However, up to 6 g/day has been administered parenterally to normal adults without evidence of toxicity.

Enhanced wound healing – Doses of 300 to 500 mg daily for 7 to 10 days both preoperatively and postoperatively are adequate, although considerably larger amounts have been recommended.

Burns – For severe burns, daily doses of 1 to 2 g are recommended.

In other conditions in which the need for vitamin C is increased, 3 to 5 times the daily optimum allowances appears adequate.

Actions

Pharmacology: Vitamin C, a water-soluble vitamin, is an essential vitamin in man; however, its exact biological functions are not fully understood. It is essential for the formation and the maintenance of intercellular ground substance and collagen, for catecholamine biosynthesis, for synthesis of carnitine and steroids, for conversion of folic acid to folinic acid and for tyrosine metabolism.

The deficiency state scurvy is characterized by degenerative changes in the capillaries, bone, and connective tissues. Mild vitamin C deficiency symptoms may include faulty bone and tooth development, gingivitis, bleeding gums, and loosened teeth.

Absorption of dietary ascorbate from the intestines is nearly complete. Vitamin C is readily available in citrus fruit, tomatoes, potatoes, and leafy vegetables.

Warnings/Precautions

Excessive vitamin C doses: Diabetics, patients prone to recurrent renal calculi, those undergoing stool occult blood tests and those on sodium restricted diets or anticoagulant therapy should not take excessive doses of vitamin C over an extended time period.

Pregnancy: Category C. Do not administer ascorbic acid to pregnant women in excess of the amount needed for treatment. The possibility of the fetus adapting to high levels of the vitamin could result in a scorbutic condition after birth when the intake drops to normal levels. This action is controversial.

Lactation: Ascorbic acid is excreted in breast milk.

Drug Interactions

Contraceptives (oral) and estrogens: Ascorbic acid increases serum levels of estrogen and estrogen contained in oral contraceptives, possibly resulting in adverse reactions.

Warfarin: The anticoagulant action of warfarin may be reduced.

Drug/Lab test interactions: Large doses (more than 500 mg) of vitamin C may cause false-negative urine glucose determinations.

No exogenous vitamin C should be ingested for 48 to 72 hours before amine-dependent stool occult blood tests are conducted because possible false-negative results may occur.

Adverse Reactions

Large doses may cause diarrhea and precipitation of cystine, oxalate, or urate renal stones if the urine becomes acidic during therapy.

Transient mild soreness may occur at the site of IM or subcutaneous injection. Too rapid IV administration may cause temporary faintness or dizziness.

NIACIN

Tablets; oral: 50, 100, 250, and 500 mg (*otc*[a])	Various
Tablets; oral: 500 mg (*Rx*)	*Niacor* (Upsher-Smith)
Tablets, extended-release; oral: 500, 750, and 1,000 mg (*Rx*)	*Niaspan* (Kos Pharmaceutical)
Tablets, timed-release; oral: 250 and 500 mg (*otc*[a])	Various
Tablets, sustained-release; oral: 500 mg (*otc*[a])	Various
Tablets, controlled-release; oral: 250, 500, and 750 mg (*otc/sf*[a])	*Slo-Niacin* (Upsher-Smith)
Capsules, extended-release; oral: 250 and 400 mg (*otc*[a])	Various
Capsules, timed-release; oral: 250 and 500 mg (*otc*[a])	Various
Capsules, sustained-release; oral: 125 and 500 mg (*otc*[a])	Various

[a] Some products may be available *Rx*, according to distributor discretion. Most of these products are marketed as nutritional supplements.

Indications

Dietary supplement: For the treatment of niacin deficiency.

Pellagra: Prevention and treatment of pellagra.

Hypercholesterolemia: Adjunct to diet for the reduction of elevated total and low-density lipoprotein (LDL) levels in patients with primary hypercholesterolemia.

Hypertriglyceridemia (Types IV and V): Adjunctive therapy for treatment in adult patients with very high serum triglyceride levels (Type IV and V hyperlipidemia) who present a risk of pancreatitis and who do not respond adequately to dietary control.

Niacor:

Hypercholesterolemia – Alone or in combination with a bile-acid binding resin, is indicated as an adjunct to diet for the reduction of elevated total and LDL cholesterol levels in patients with primary hypercholesterolemia (Types IIa and IIb).

Hypertriglyceridemia – Adjunctive therapy for treatment of adult patients with very high serum triglyceride levels (Type IV and V hyperlipidemia) who present a risk of pancreatitis and who do not respond to dietary effort.

Niaspan:

Hypercholesterolemia – Indicated as an adjunct to diet for reduction of elevated TC, (low-density lipoprotein-cholesterol) LDL-C, Apo B and TG levels, and to increase high-density lipoprotein-cholesterol (in patients with primary hypercholesterolemia (heterozygous familial and nonfamilial) and mixed dyslipidemia (Frederickson Types IIa and IIb), when the response to an appropriate diet has been inadequate.

In combination with lovastatin for the treatment of primary hypercholesterolemia (heterozygous familial and nonfamilial) and mixed dyslipidemia (Fredrickson Types IIa and IIb) when treatment with both *Niaspan* and lovastatin is appropriate and as an adjunct to diet.

Niacin extended-release tablets in combination with a bile acid binding resin are indicated as an adjunct to diet for reduction of elevated TC and LDL-C levels in adult patients with primary hypercholesterolemia (Type IIa), when the response to an appropriate diet, or diet plus monotherapy, has been inadequate.

Combination therapy is not indicated as initial therapy.

Hypertriglyceridemia (Types IV and V) – Adjunctive therapy for treatment in adult patients with very high serum triglyceride levels (Type IV and V hyperlipidemia) who present a risk of pancreatitis and who do not respond adequately to dietary control.

Prevention of recurring myocardial infarction (MI) – In patients with a history of MI and hypercholesterolemia, niacin is indicated to reduce the risk of recurrent nonfatal MI.

Atherosclerotic disease – In patients with a history of coronary artery disease and hypercholesterolemia, niacin, in combination with a bile acid binding resin, is indicated to slow progression or promote regression of atherosclerotic disease.

Administration and Dosage

To reduce flushing, begin therapy by slowly increasing the dose (100 mg 3 times a day each week).

Recommended dietary allowances (RDAs): Adult men, 15 to 20 mg; adult women, 13 to 15 mg. Niacin is recommended at 6.6 mg per 1,000 Kcal intake.

OTC *sustained-release formulations:* Do not substitute sustained-release (modified-release, timed-release) nicotinic acid preparations for equivalent doses of immediate-release (crystalline) nicotinic acid.

Tablet interchangeability – Equivalent doses of *Niaspan* extended-release tablets should not be substituted for sustained-release (modified-release, timed-release) niacin preparations or immediate-release (crystalline) niacin. Patients previously receiving other niacin products should be started with the recommended *Niaspan* extended-release tablet titration schedule, and the dose should subsequently be individualized based on patient response. Single-dose bioavailability studies have demonstrated that *Niaspan* extended-release tablet strengths are not interchangeable.

Pellagra: Up to 500 mg/day.

Hyperlipidemia: 1 to 2 g 2 or 3 times daily. Do not exceed 6 g/day.

OTC:

Slo-Niacin controlled-release tablets –

Adults:

250 or 500 mg – 1 niacin tablet morning or evening, or as directed by a health care provider.

750 mg – One-half niacin tablet morning or evening, or as directed by a health care provider. Before using more than 500 mg daily, consult a health care provider.

Niacin tablets may be broken, but should not be crushed or chewed. The inactive matrix of the tablet may be excreted intact in the stool.

Niacin timed-release capsules – Take 1 capsule daily, or as directed by a health care provider.

Niacin 500 mg flush-free capsules, Niacin 100 mg tablets – For adults, take 1 capsule or tablet daily, preferably with a meal.

Niaspan: Niaspan extended-release tablets should be taken at bedtime, after a low-fat snack, initiated at 500 mg every bedtime in order to reduce the incidence and severity of adverse reactions.

***Niaspan* Recommended Dosing**			
	Weeks	Daily dose	*Niaspan* dosing
Initial titration schedule	1 to 4	500 mg	1 *Niaspan* 500 mg tablet at bedtime
	5 to 8	1000 mg	2 *Niaspan* 500 mg tablets at bedtime
	[a]	1500 mg	2 *Niaspan* 750 mg tablets or 3 *Niaspan* 500 mg tablets at bedtime
	[a]	2000 mg	2 *Niaspan* 1000 mg tablets or 4 *Niaspan* 500 mg tablets at bedtime

[a] After week 8, titrate to patient response and tolerance. If response to 1,000 mg daily is inadequate, increase dose to 1,500 mg daily; may subsequently increase dose to 2,000 mg daily. Daily dose should not be increased more than 500 mg in a 4-week period, and doses above 2,000 mg daily are not recommended. Women may respond at lower doses than men.

If therapy is discontinued for an extended period, reinstitution of therapy should include a titration phase.

Maintenance dose – The daily dosage should not be increased by more than 500 mg in any 4-week period.

The recommended maintenance dose is 1,000 mg to 2,000 mg once daily at bedtime. Doses greater than 2,000 mg daily are not recommended.

To reduce flushing: Flushing of the skin may be reduced in frequency or severity by pretreatment with aspirin (taken 30 minutes prior to *Niaspan* extended-release tablet dose) or nonsteroidal anti-inflammatory drugs. Tolerance to this flushing develops rapidly over the course of several weeks. Flushing, pruritus, and GI distress are also greatly reduced by slowly increasing the dose of niacin and avoiding administration on an empty stomach.

Niaspan extended-release tablets should be taken whole and should not be broken, crushed or chewed before swallowing.

Combination therapy: If lipid response to *Niaspan* extended-release tablets alone is insufficient, or if higher doses of *Niaspan* extended-release tablets are not well tolerated, some patients may benefit from combination therapy with a bile-acid binding resin or an HMG-CoA reductase inhibitor.

Concomitant therapy with lovastatin – The usual recommended starting dose of lovastatin is 20 mg once a day. Dose adjustments should be made at intervals of 4 weeks or more. Combination therapy with *Niaspan* and lovastatin should not exceed doses of 2,000 mg and 40 mg daily, respectively.

Renal/hepatic function impairment – Use of *Niaspan* extended-release tablets in patients with renal or hepatic function impairment has not been studied. *Niaspan* extended-release tablets are contraindicated in patients with significant or unexplained hepatic dysfunction. *Niaspan* extended-release tablets should be used with caution in patients with renal insufficiency.

Niacor: The usual adult dosage of nicotinic acid is 1 to 2 g 2 or 3 times a day. Start with one-half tablet (250 mg) as a single daily dose following the evening meal. The frequency of dosing and total daily dose can be increased every 4 to 7 days until the desired LDL cholesterol or triglyceride level is achieved or the first-level therapeutic dose of 1.5 to 2 g/day is reached. If the patient's hyperlipidemia is not adequately controlled after 2 months at this level, the dosage can then be increased at 2- to 4-week intervals to 3 g/day (1 g 3 times per day). In patients with marked lipid abnormalities, a higher dose is occasionally required, but generally should not exceed 6 g/day.

Tablet interchangeability – Sustained-release (modified-release, timed-release) nicotinic acid preparations should not be substituted for equivalent doses of immediate-release (crystalline) nicotinic acid.

Actions

Pharmacology: Niacin, vitamin B_3, is the common name for nicotinic acid and niacinamide (nicotinamide). Nicotinic acid is present in the body as its active form, nicotinamide (niacinamide).

Niacin decreases the rate of hepatic synthesis of very low density lipoprotein (VLDL) and low-density lipoprotein (LDL).

Nicotinic acid (but not nicotinamide) in gram doses produces an average 10% to 20% reduction in total and LDL cholesterol, a 30% to 70% reduction in triglycerides, and an average 20% to 35% increase in HDL cholesterol. Nicotinic acid also decreases serum levels of apolipoprotein B-100, the major component of VLDL and LDL fractions. The mechanism by which nicotinic acid exerts these effects is not entirely understood but may involve several actions, including a decrease in esterification of hepatic triglycerides.

Pharmacokinetics:

Absorption –

Niaspan extended-release tablets: Niacin is rapidly and extensively absorbed when administered orally. To maximize bioavailability and reduce the risk of gastrointestinal (GI) upset, administer with a low-fat meal or snack.

Niacor tablets: Nicotinic acid is characterized by rapid absorption from the GI tract and a short plasma elimination half-life. Peak plasma concentrations are reached within 30 to 60 minutes.

Distribution –

Niaspan extended-release tablets: Studies using radiolabeled niacin in mice show that niacin and its metabolites concentrate in the liver, kidney and adipose tissue.

Metabolism – The pharmacokinetic profile of niacin is complicated due to rapid and extensive first-pass metabolism, which is species and dose-rate specific.

Excretion – Niacin and its metabolites are rapidly eliminated in the urine.

The plasma elimination half-life of nicotinic acid ranges from 20 to 45 minutes.

Contraindications

Do not administer niacin unless recommended by and taken under the supervision of a health care provider if any of the following conditions exist: gallbladder disease, gout, arterial bleeding, glaucoma, diabetes, impaired liver function, peptic ulcer, pregnancy, or lactation.

Known hypersensitivity to niacin or any component of this medication; significant or unexplained hepatic function impairment; active peptic ulcer disease; arterial bleeding.

Warnings/Precautions

Alcohol: Use with caution in patients who consume substantial quantities of alcohol or have a history of liver disease.

Schizophrenia: There is no evidence to support the use of nicotinic acid in the treatment of schizophrenia as part of what is referred to as "orthomolecular psychiatry."

Heart disease: People with heart disease, particularly those who have recurrent chest pain (angina) or who recently suffered a heart attack, should take niacin only under the supervision of a health care provider.

Skeletal muscle effects: Rare cases of rhabdomyolysis have been associated with concomitant administration of lipid-altering doses (1 g/day or more) of niacin and HMG-CoA reductase inhibitors. Monitor patients for signs and symptoms of muscle pain, tenderness, or weakness. Consider periodic serum creatine phosphokinase (CPK) and potassium determinations, although there is no assurance that such monitoring will prevent the occurrence of severe myopathy.

Extended-release preparations: Niacin extended-release tablet preparations should not be substituted for equivalent doses of immediate-release (crystalline) niacin. For patients switching from immediate-release niacin to niacin extended-release tablets, therapy with niacin extended-release tablets should be initiated with low doses (ie, 500 mg every night) and the niacin extended-release tablet dose should then be titrated to the desired therapeutic response.

Hepatic effects: Cases of severe hepatic toxicity, including fulminant hepatic necrosis, have occurred in patients who have substituted sustained-release (modified-release, timed-release) niacin products for immediate-release (crystalline) niacin at equivalent doses. Discontinue the drug if the transaminase levels show evidence of progression, particularly if they rise to 3 times the upper limit of normal and are persistent or if they are associated with symptoms of nausea, fever, or malaise. Consider liver biopsy if elevations persist beyond discontinuation.

Diabetes: Observe diabetic or borderline diabetic patients closely for decreased glucose tolerance.

Gout: Elevated uric acid levels have occurred.

Flushing: Flushing generally begins 20 minutes after ingestion and lasts 30 to 60 minutes. Flushing will usually subside after 3 to 6 weeks of continued therapy. The flush response can be attenuated by slowly increasing the niacin dose (100 mg 3 times/day each week), administering with food or milk, or administering either a prostaglandin inhibitor (eg, aspirin 325 mg) 60 minutes prior to niacin administration, or administering sustained-release niacin preparations.

Hyperlipidemia: Before instituting therapy with niacin, make an attempt to control hyperlipidemia with appropriate diet, exercise, and weight reduction in obese patients, and to treat other underlying medical problems.

Renal/Hepatic function impairment: Use nicotinic acid with caution in patients who have a history of liver disease. Active liver diseases or unexplained transaminase elevations are contraindications to the use of nicotinic acid.

Niaspan – *Niaspan* extended-release tablets are contraindicated in patients with significant or unexplained hepatic function impairment; use with caution in patients with renal function impairment.

Special risk: Use caution when nicotinic acid is used in patients with unstable angina or in the acute phase of MI, particularly when such patients are also receiving vasoactive drugs such as nitrates, calcium channel blockers, or adrenergic blocking agents.

Pregnancy: *Category* A. (*Category* C if used in doses above the RDA). If a woman receiving nicotinic acid for primary hypercholesterolemia (types IIa or IIb) becomes pregnant, discontinue the drug. If a woman being treated with nicotinic acid for hypertriglyceridemia (types IV or V) becomes pregnant, assess the benefits and risks of continued drug therapy on an individual basis.

Lactation: Niacin is actively excreted in breast milk.

Children: Safety and efficacy in children have not been established in doses that exceed the RDA.

Lab test abnormalities: Monitor phosphorus levels periodically in patients at risk for hypophosphatemia.

Monitoring: Frequently monitor liver function and blood glucose. Serum transaminase levels, including AST and ALT, should be monitored before treatment begins, every 6 to 12 weeks for the first year, and periodically thereafter (eg, at approximately 6-month intervals).

Drug Interactions

Drugs that may be affected by niacin include HMG-CoA reductase inhibitors, anticoagulants, antihypertensive agents (ganglionic agents and vasoactive agents).

Drugs that may affect niacin include aspirin, alcohol or hot drinks, bile acid sequestrants, and other sources of niacin.

Adverse Reactions

Adverse reactions occurring in at least 3% of patients include the following: abdominal pain, diarrhea, dyspepsia, headache, nausea, pain, pruritus, rash, rhinitis, and vomiting.

NIACINAMIDE

Tablets: 100 and 500 mg (*otc*[a])	Various

[a] Some products may be available *Rx*, according to distributor discretion.

Indications

Pellagra: Prophylaxis and treatment of pellagra.

Administration and Dosage

100 to 500 mg/day.

Actions

Pharmacology: Niacinamide is synonymous with nicotinamide, 3-pyridine carboxamide, and nicotinic acid amide. Niacinamide is the amide of nicotinic acid (niacin, vitamin B_3). Although nicotinic acid and nicotinamide function identically as vitamins, their pharmacologic effects differ. Nicotinamide does not have the hypolipidemic or vasodilating effects characteristic of niacin (nicotinic acid).

Adverse Reactions

Liver dysfunction in high doses.

VITAMIN B_{12}

Tablets: 100, 500 and 1,000 mcg (*otc*)	Various, *Twelve Resin-K* (Key Company)
Tablets, extended-release: 1,500 mcg (*otc*)	*B-12* (Mason Natural)
Tablets, sublingual: 1,000, 1,500, and 5,000 mcg (*otc*)	Various
Lozenges: 50, 100, 250, and 500 mcg (*otc*)	Various
Injection: 1,000 mcg/mL (*Rx*)	Various
Spray, intranasal: 25 mcg per 0.1 mL (*Rx*)	*Calomist* (Fleming)
500 mcg per 0.1 mL (500 mcg/actuation) (*Rx*)	*Nascobal* (Questcor)

Indications

B_{12} deficiency: Nutritional vitamin B_{12} deficiency.

Administration and Dosage

Recommended dietary allowances (RDAs): Adults, 2 mcg/day. For a complete listing of RDAs by age, sex, or condition, refer to the RDA table.

CaloMist: Initial dose is 1 spray in each nostril once daily (25 mcg per nostril, total daily dose 50 mcg) increased to 1 spray in each nostril twice daily (total daily dose 100 mcg) for patients with an inadequate response to once-daily dosing.

The dosing of *CaloMist* and other intranasal medications should be separated by several hours. Patients should have more frequent monitoring of vitamin B_{12} concentrations because of the potential for erratic absorption.

Nascobal: Initial dose is 1 spray (500 mcg) administered in 1 nostril once weekly.

Nascobal nasal spray should be administered at least 1 hour before or 1 hour after ingestion of hot foods or liquids.

Actions

Pharmacology: Vitamin B_{12} is essential to growth, cell reproduction, hematopoiesis, nucleic acid, and myelin synthesis. Sources of vitamin B_{12} include liver, meat, fish, and dairy products (eg, milk and cheese). Deficiency results in megaloblastic anemia, GI lesions, and neurologic damage.

Pharmacokinetics: The parietal cells of the stomach secrete intrinsic factor, which regulates the amount of vitamin B_{12} absorbed in the terminal ileum. The peak concentrations after administration of intranasal spray were reached in 1.25 ± 1.9 hours.

Bioavailability of oral preparations is approximately 25%. The bioavailability of the B_{12} nasal spray was found to be 10% less than the B_{12} nasal gel. Vitamin B_{12} is primarily stored in the liver. Enterohepatic circulation plays a key role in recycling vitamin B_{12} from mainly bile. If plasma-binding proteins are saturated, excess free vitamin B_{12} will be excreted in the kidney.

Contraindications

Hypersensitivity to cyanocobalamin.

Warnings/Precautions

Leber disease: Patients with early Leber disease (hereditary optic nerve atrophy) treated with vitamin B_{12} suffered severe and swift optic atrophy. Cyanocobalamin should not be used in these patients.

Megaloblastic anemia:

Nascobal – Hypokalemia and sudden death may occur in severe megaloblastic anemia that is treated intensely with vitamin B_{12}. Folic acid is not a substitute for vitamin B_{12}, although it may improve vitamin B_{12}–deficient megaloblastic anemia.

CaloMist – Folic acid may result in a hematological response in patients with vitamin B_{12} deficiency, but will not prevent irreversible neurological manifestations. Vitamin B_{12} is not an appropriate treatment for folate deficiency.

Blunted response to vitamin B_{12} therapy: Blunted or impeded therapeutic response to vitamin B_{12} may be caused by such conditions as infection, uremia, drugs having bone marrow suppressant properties (eg, chloramphenicol), and concurrent iron or folic acid deficiency.

Vitamin B_{12} deficiency: Vitamin B_{12} deficiency that is allowed to progress for longer than 3 months may produce permanent degenerative lesions of the spinal cord. Dosages of folic acid of more than 0.1 mg/day may result in hematologic remission in patients with vitamin B_{12} deficiency.

If a patient is not properly maintained with intranasal vitamin B_{12}, IM vitamin B_{12} is necessary for adequate treatment of the patient.

Folate deficiency: Dosages of vitamin B_{12} exceeding 10 mcg/day may produce a hematologic response in patients with folate deficiency.

Vitamin B_{12} is not a substitute for folic acid, and because it might improve folic acid deficient megaloblastic anemia, indiscriminate use of vitamin B_{12} could mask the true diagnosis.

Hypokalemia and thrombocytosis: Hypokalemia and thrombocytosis could occur upon conversion of severe megaloblastic to normal erythropoiesis with vitamin B_{12} therapy. Carefully monitor serum potassium levels and platelet count during therapy.

Polycythemia vera: Vitamin B_{12} deficiency may suppress the signs of polycythemia vera. Treatment with vitamin B_{12} may unmask this condition.

Nasal symptoms: The effectiveness of intranasal cyanocobalamin in patients with nasal congestion, allergic rhinitis, and upper respiratory tract infections has not been determined. Defer treatment until symptoms have subsided. Patients with chronic nasal symptoms or significant nasal pathology are not ideal candidates for intranasal vitamin B_{12} therapy. If therapy is attempted, monitor vitamin B_{12} concentrations more frequently because of the potential for erratic or blunted absorption.

Hypersensitivity reactions: Anaphylactic shock, death, and angioedema have been reported after parenteral vitamin B_{12} administration. No such reactions have been reported in clinical trials with *Nascobal* nasal spray, *Nascobal* nasal gel, or *CaloMist* nasal spray.

Test dose – An intradermal test dose of parenteral vitamin B_{12} is recommended before intranasal administration to patients suspected of cyanocobalamin sensitivity.

Renal/Hepatic function impairment: Patients with vitamin B_{12} deficiency and concurrent renal or hepatic disease may require increased doses or more frequent administration of vitamin B_{12} therapy.

Pregnancy: Category C.

Lactation: Vitamin B_{12} is excreted into breast milk. Vitamin B_{12} is considered to be compatible with breast-feeding according to the American Academy of Pediatrics.

Children:

Nascobal – Intake in pediatric patients should be in the amount recommended by the Food and Nutrition Board, NAS-NRC.

CaloMist – Because *CaloMist* nasal spray has not been studied in children, safety and effectiveness have not been established.

Monitoring: Obtain hematocrit, reticulocyte count, vitamin B_{12}, folate, and iron levels prior to treatment.

Nascobal – If folate levels are low, also administer folic acid. All hematologic parameters should be normal when beginning treatment.

Monitor vitamin B_{12} blood levels and peripheral blood counts 1 month after the start of treatment and then at 3- to 6-month intervals.

Carefully monitor serum potassium levels and platelet count during therapy.

CaloMist – All hematologic parameters, including vitamin B_{12} concentrations, should be normal before initiating treatment with *CaloMist* nasal spray. Periodic monitoring of serum vitamin B_{12} concentrations must be obtained to confirm adequacy of therapy. Monitor vitamin B_{12} concentrations and complete blood counts 1 month after starting *CaloMist* nasal spray and then at 3- to 6-month intervals thereafter. Patients with boderline-low vitamin B_{12} concentrations (less than 300 ng/L) should also undergo measurement of methylmalonic acid and homocysteine concentrations. Patients with declining or abnormally low vitamin B_{12} concentrations, despite maximal doses of *CaloMist* nasal spray, should be switched back to IM vitamin B_{12} injections.

Drug Interactions

Bone marrow suppressants: Bone marrow suppressants (eg, chloramphenicol) may blunt the therapeutic response to vitamin B_{12}.

Drug/Lab test interactions: Most antibiotics, methotrexate, or pyrimethamine invalidate folic acid and vitamin B_{12} diagnostic blood assays.

The validity of diagnostic vitamin B_{12} or folic acid blood assays could be compromised by medications.

Adverse Reactions

Adverse reactions occurring in at least 3% of patients taking *CaloMist* include the following: arthralgia, asthma, back pain, bronchitis, cough, dizziness, epistaxis, headache, hypersomnia, influenza-like illness, malaise, nasal discomfort, nasopharyngitis, pain, pharyngolaryngeal pain, postnasal drip, procedural pain, pyrexia, rash, rhinorrhea, scab, sinus headache, sinusitis, tooth abscess.

CALCIUM

CALCIUM ACETATE	
Tablets: 667 elemental mg (169 mg elemental calcium) (*Rx*)	*Calphron* (Nephro-Tech)
Capsules: 667 mg (169 mg elemental calcium) (*Rx*)	*PhosLo* (Fresenius Medical Care)
Gelcaps: 667 mg (169 mg elemental calcium) (*Rx*)	
CALCIUM CARBONATE	
Tablets: 500 mg (200 mg elemental calcium) (*otc*)	Various
600 mg (240 mg elemental calcium) (*otc*)	Various
648 to 650 mg (260 mg elemental calcium) (*otc*)	Various
1,250 mg (500 mg elemental calcium) (*otc*)	Various, *Cal-Carb Forte* (Vitaline), *Oyster Shell Calcium* (Various), *Oysco 500* (Rugby), *Oyst-Cal 500* (Goldline), *Os-Cal 500* (GlaxoSmithKline Consumer)
1,500 mg (600 mg elemental calcium) (*otc*)	Various, *Calcium 600* (Various), *Caltrate 600* (Whitehall Robins), *Nephro-Calci* (Watson)
Tablets, chewable: 400 mg (160 mg elemental calcium) (*otc*)	*Maalox Children's* (Novartis Consumer Health), *Mylanta Children's* (J&J/Merck) *Pepto Children's* (Procter & Gamble)
420 mg (168 mg elemental calcium) (*otc*)	*Trial Antacid* (Zee Medical)
500 mg (200 mg elemental calcium) (*otc*)	Various, *Cal•Gest* (Rugby), *Dicarbosil* (BIRA), *Equilet* (Mission), *Maalox Antacid Barrier Maximum Strength* (Novartis)
750 mg (300 mg elemental calcium (*otc*)	Various, *Tums E-X*, *Tums Calcium for Life PMS*, *Tums Kids*, *Tums Smooth Dissolve* (GlaxoSmithKline Consumer)
850 mg (340 mg elemental calcium) (*otc*)	*Alka-Mints* (Bayer)
1,000 mg (400 mg elemental calcium) (*otc*)	*Tums Ultra* (GlaxoSmithKline Consumer)
1,177 mg (470.8 mg elemental calcium) (*otc*)	*Rolaids Extra Strength Softchews* (Pfizer Consumer Health)
1,250 mg (500 mg elemental calcium) (*otc*)	Various, *Cal-Carb Forte* (Vitaline), *Calci-Chew* (Watson), *Os-Cal 500*, *Tums Calcium for Life Bone Health* (GlaxoSmithKline Consumer)
Capsules: 1,250 mg (500 mg elemental calcium) (*otc*)	*Calci-Mix* (Watson)
Capsules and tablets: 364 mg calcium carbonate (145.6 mg elemental calcium) and 8.3 mg sodium fluoride (*otc*)	*Florical* (Mericon)
Gum: 300 mg (120 mg elemental calcium) (*otc*)	*Surpass* (Wrigley)
450 mg (180 mg elemental calcium) (*otc*)	*Surpass Extra Strength* (Wrigley)
500 mg (200 mg elemental calcium) (*otc*)	*Chooz* (Schering-Plough)
Oral suspension: 1,250 mg (500 mg elemental calcium)/5 mL (*otc*)	Various
Powder (*otc*)	Various, *Tums Quik Pak* (GlaxoSmithKline Consumer)
CALCIUM CHLORIDE	
Injection: 10% (*Rx*)	Various
CALCIUM CITRATE	
Tablets: 200 mg elemental calcium (*otc*)	*Citracal* (Mission)
200 mg calcium citrate (*otc*)	*Citrus Calcium* (Rugby)
250 mg elemental calcium (*otc*)	Various, *Cal-Cee* (Key Company), *Cal-Citrate* (Bio-Tech)
950 mg (*otc*)	Various
Capsules: 180 mg elemental calcium (*otc*)	*Cal-C-Caps* (Key Company)
225 mg elemental calcium (*otc*)	*Cal-Citrate-225* (Bio-Tech)
Powder for oral suspension: 760 mg elemental calcium/5 mL (*otc*)	Various
CALCIUM GLUBIONATE	
Syrup: 1.8 g/5 mL (*otc*)	Various, *Calciquid* (Breckenridge)
CALCIUM GLUCEPTATE	
Injection: 1.1 g/5 mL (*Rx*)	Various
CALCIUM GLUCONATE	
Capsules: 500 mg (*otc*)	*Calcium Gluconate* (Bio-Tech)
700 mg (*otc*)	*Cal-G* (Key)

Tablets: 500 mg (45 mg elemental calcium), 50 mg elemental calcium, 648 to 650 mg (58.5 to 60 mg elemental calcium), 972 to 975 mg (87.75 to 90 mg elemental calcium) (*otc*)	Various
Tablets, chewable: 650 mg (*otc*)	Various
Powder for oral suspension: 346.7 mg elemental calcium/15 mL (*otc*)	Various
Injection: 10% (*Rx*)	Various
CALCIUM LACTATE	
Tablets: 648 to 650 mg (84.5 mg elemental calcium), 100 mg elemental calcium (*otc*)	Various
Capsules: 500 mg (96 mg elemental calcium) (*otc*)	*Cal-Lac* (Bio-Tech)
CALCIUM SALT COMBINATIONS	
Injection: 50 mg calcium glycerophosphate and 50 mg calcium lactate per 10 mL in sodium chloride solution (0.08 mEq Ca/mL) (*Rx*)	*Calphosan* (Glenwood)
TRICALCIUM PHOSPHATE	
Tablets: 600 mg elemental calcium (*otc*)	*Posture* (Iverness Medical)

Indications

Oral: As a dietary supplement when calcium intake may be inadequate.

Oral calcium may also be used in the treatment of osteoporosis, osteomalacia, rickets, and latent tetany.

Calcium taken daily may help reduce typical premenstrual syndrome (PMS) symptoms such as bloating, cramps, fatigue, and moodiness.

Calcium acetate (PhosLo) – Control of hyperphosphatemia in end-stage renal failure; does not promote aluminum absorption.

Parenteral:

Hypocalcemia – To correct plasma calcium levels (eg, neonatal tetany and tetany due to parathyroid deficiency, vitamin D deficiency, alkalosis); prevention of hypocalcemia during exchange transfusions; conditions associated with intestinal malabsorption.

Calcium chloride and gluconate – Adjunctive therapy in the treatment of insect bites or stings, such as Black Widow spider bites to relieve muscle cramping; sensitivity reactions, particularly when characterized by urticaria; depression due to overdosage of magnesium sulfate; acute symptoms of lead colic; rickets; osteomalacia.

Calcium chloride – To combat severe hyperkalemia pending correction of increased potassium in the extracellular fluid.

Cardiac resuscitation: After open heart surgery, when epinephrine fails to improve weak or ineffective myocardial contractions.

Calcium gluconate – To decrease capillary permeability in allergic conditions, nonthrombocytopenic purpura and exudative dermatoses such as dermatitis herpetiformis; for pruritus of eruptions caused by certain drugs; in hyperkalemia, calcium gluconate may aid in antagonizing the cardiac toxicity, provided the patient is not receiving digitalis therapy.

Administration and Dosage

Oral:

Dietary supplement – The usual daily dose is 500 mg to 2 g, 2 to 4 times/day.

Calcium is recommended in doses of 1,500 mg/day for men older than 65 years of age and for postmenopausal women not taking estrogen replacement therapy.

PhosLo – For adult dialysis patients, the initial dose is 2 tablets/capsules/gelcaps with each meal. The dosage may be increased gradually to bring the serum phosphate value less than 6 mg/dL, as long as hypercalcemia does not develop. Most patients require 3 to 4 tablets with each meal.

The recommended initial dose of the half-size (333.5 mg) *PhosLo* for the adult dialysis patient is 4 capsules with each meal. The dosage may be increased gradually to bring the serum phosphate value below 6 mg/dL, as long as hypercalcemia does not develop. Most patients require 6 to 8 capsules with each meal.

Florical – 1 capsule or tablet daily.

Parenteral: Calcium gluconate is generally preferred over calcium chloride as it is less irritating.

IV – Warm solutions to body temperature and give slowly (0.5 to 2 mL/min); stop if patient complains of discomfort. Resume when symptoms disappear. Following injection, patient should remain recumbent for a short time. Repeated injections may be needed because of the rapid calcium excretion. Inject **calcium chloride** and **gluconate** through a small needle into a large vein to minimize venous irritation.

IM administration – IM administration of **calcium gluceptate** and **gluconate** should be reserved for emergencies when technical difficulty makes IV injection impossible. Administer **calcium gluconate** only by the IV route and **calcium chloride** by the IV or intraventricular route.

CALCIUM CARBONATE –

Antacid:

Tablets – Swallow or chew 2 to 4 tablets as symptoms occur. Repeat hourly if symptoms return or as directed by a health care provider.

Gum – Chew 1 or 2 tablets (calcium carbonate 500 to 1,000 mg) every 2 to 4 hours.

CALCIUM CHLORIDE –

For IV use only: Injection is irritating to veins and must not be injected into tissues. Avoid extravasation. Administer slowly (not to exceed 0.5 to 1 mL/min).

Intraventricular administration – In cardiac resuscitation, injection may be made into the ventricular cavity; do not inject into the myocardium. Replace the IV needle with a suitable intracardiac needle.

The intraventricular dose usually ranges from 200 to 800 mg (2 to 8 mL).

Hypocalcemic disorders:

Adults – 500 mg to 1 g at intervals of 1 to 3 days, depending on response of patient or serum calcium determinations.

Children – 0.2 mL/kg up to 1 to 10 mL/day.

Magnesium intoxication: Give 500 mg promptly; observe patient for signs of recovery before further doses are given.

Hyperkalemic ECG disturbances of cardiac function: Adjust dosage by constant monitoring of ECG changes during administration.

Cardiac resuscitation:

Adults – Dose ranges from 500 mg to 1 g IV or 200 to 800 mg injected into the ventricular cavity.

Children – 0.2 mL/kg

CALCIUM GLUBIONATE –

Infants younger than 12 months of age: 1 teaspoon 5 times daily (may be given alone or mixed with juice or formula).

Children younger than 4 years of age: 2 teaspoons 3 times daily.

Adults and children 4 years of age and older: 1 tablespoon 3 times daily.

Pregnant or breast-feeding women: 1 tablespoon 3 times daily.

CALCIUM GLUCEPTATE –

IM: 2 to 5 mL (0.44 to 1.1 g). Inject 5 mL (1.1 g) doses in the gluteal region or, in infants, in the lateral thigh.

IV: 5 to 20 mL (1.1 to 4.4 g). Warm solution to body temperature and administer slowly (no more than 2 mL/min).

Exchange transfusions in newborns: 0.5 mL (0.11 g) after every 100 mL of blood exchanged.

CALCIUM GLUCONATE – For IV use only, either directly or by infusion. Do not exceed a rate of 0.5 to 2 mL/min. Calcium gluconate may also be administered by intermittent infusion at a rate not exceeding 200 mg/min, or by continuous infusion. Discontinue injection if the patient complains of discomfort.

Adults: 500 mg to 2 g (5 to 20 mL) as required.

Children: 200 to 500 mg IV (2 to 5 mL), well diluted; give slowly in divided doses.

Infants: Not more than 200 mg IV (2 mL).

Admixture incompatibilities: Calcium salts should not generally be mixed with carbonates, phosphates, sulfates, or tartrates in parenteral admixtures; they are conditionally compatible with potassium phosphates, depending on concentration. Calcium ions will chelate tetracycline.

CALCIUM LACTATE –

Tablets:

Adults – Take 600 mg calcium lactate, preferably with food and liquid.

Capsules: As a dietary supplement, 100 or 200 mg calcium lactate 3 times daily, or as directed by a health care provider.

Actions

Pharmacology: Calcium is essential for the functional integrity of the nervous and muscular systems, for normal cardiac contractility and the coagulation of blood. It also functions as an enzyme cofactor and affects the secretory activity of endocrine and exocrine glands.

Patients with advanced renal insufficiency (CrCl less than 30 mL/min) exhibit phosphate retention and some degree of hyperphosphatemia. The retention of phosphate plays a role in causing secondary hyperparathyroidism associated with osteodystrophy and soft-tissue calcification. Calcium acetate, when taken with meals, combines with dietary phosphate to form insoluble calcium phosphate, which is excreted in the feces.

Elemental Calcium Content of Calcium Salts[a]

Calcium salt	% Calcium	mEq Ca^{++}/g
Calcium glubionate	6.5	3.3
Calcium gluconate	9	4.5
Calcium lactate	13	6.5
Calcium citrate	21	10.6
Calcium acetate	25	12.6
Tricalcium phosphate	39	19.3
Calcium carbonate	40	20

[a] 1 mEq of elemental calcium = 20 mg

Pharmacokinetics:

Absorption – Calcium is absorbed from the GI tract by passive diffusion and active transport. Calcium must be in a soluble, ionized form for absorption to occur. Vitamin D is required for calcium absorption and increases the absorptive mechanisms. Calcium absorption is increased in the presence of food. Oral bioavailability in adults ranges from 25% to 35% when given with a standardized breakfast. Absorption from milk was approximately 29% under the same conditions.

Distribution – Calcium is rapidly incorporated into skeletal tissue. Normal serum calcium concentrations range from 9 to 10.4 mg/dL (4.5 to 5.2 mEq/L), but only ionized calcium is active. Calcium crosses the placenta and reaches higher concentrations in fetal blood than maternal blood. Calcium also is distributed in milk.

Excretion – Calcium is mainly excreted in the feces. Urinary excretion does not exceed 150 mg/day in patients on low calcium diets. Urinary excretion decreases with age, in early renal failure, and during pregnancy. Calcium also is excreted by the sweat glands.

Contraindications

Oral: Hypercalcemia, ventricular fibrillation.

Parenteral: Hypercalcemia; ventricular fibrillation; digitalized patients.

Warnings/Precautions

Extravasation: **Calcium chloride** and **gluconate** can cause severe necrosis, sloughing, and abscess formation with IM or subcutaneous administration.

PhosLo: End-stage renal failure patients may develop hypercalcemia when given calcium with meals. Do not give other calcium supplements concurrently with *PhosLo*. Monitor serum calcium levels twice weekly during the early dose adjustment period. Do not allow serum calcium times phosphate product to exceed 66.

GI effects: Oral calcium salts may be irritating to the GI tract and also may cause constipation.

Hypercalcemia: Hypercalcemia may occur when large doses of calcium are administered to patients with chronic renal failure. Mild hypercalcemia may exhibit as nausea, vomiting, anorexia, or constipation, with mental changes such as stupor, delirium, coma, or confusion.

Renal calculi: Recent studies show that high dietary intake of calcium decreases the risk of symptomatic renal calculi, while intake of supplemental calcium may increase the risk of symptomatic stones. This conflicts with the previous theory that high calcium intake contributes to the risk of renal calculi.

Oral:

Monitoring – Monitor serum calcium concentrations and maintain at 9 to 10.4 mg/dL (4.5 to 5.2 mEq/L). Do not allow levels to exceed 12 mg/dL.

Special risk patients – Use calcium salts cautiously in patients with sarcoidosis, cardiac or renal disease, and in patients receiving cardiac glycosides.

Phenylketonurics – Inform phenylketonuric patients that some of these products contain phenylalanine.

Parenteral:

Cardiovascular effects – High concentrations of calcium may cause cardiac syncope.

Pregnancy: Category C. (*PhosLo* and parenteral).

Children: Safety and efficacy in children have not been established (*PhosLo*).

Drug Interactions

Drugs that may be affected by calcium include sodium polystyrene sulfonate, tetracyclines, verapamil. Iron salts and quinolones (oral only); digitalis glycosides (parenteral only).

Calcium citrate: Avoid concurrent aluminum-containing antacids.

Drug/Lab test interactions: Transient elevations of plasma 11-hydroxy-corticosteroid levels (Glenn-Nelson technique) may occur when IV calcium is administered, but levels return to control values after 1 hour. In addition, IV calcium gluconate can produce false-negative values for serum and urinary magnesium.

Drug/Food interactions: Diets high in dietary fiber have been shown to decrease absorption of calcium because of decreased transit time in the GI tract and complexing of fiber with the calcium.

Calcium acetate, when taken with meals, combines with dietary phosphate to form insoluble calcium phosphate which is excreted in the feces.

Adverse Reactions

Oral – May cause constipation and headache. Mild hypercalcemia (Ca^{++} greater than 10.5 mg/dL) may be asymptomatic or manifest itself as anorexia, nausea, and vomiting. More severe hypercalcemia (Ca^{++} 12 mg/dL) is associated with confusion, delirium, stupor, and coma.

IM administration – Mild local reactions may occur (calcium gluceptate). Local necrosis and abscess formation may occur with **calcium gluconate**. Severe necrosis and sloughing may occur with IM or subcutaneous administration of **calcium chloride**.

IV administration – Rapid IV administration may cause bradycardia, sense of oppression, tingling, metallic, calcium, or chalky taste, or "heat waves". Rapid IV **calcium gluconate** may cause vasodilation, decreased blood pressure, cardiac arrhythmias, syncope, and cardiac arrest. **Calcium chloride** injections cause peripheral vasodilation and a local burning sensation; blood pressure may fall moderately.

MAGNESIUM

Tablets: 27.5 mg elemental magnesium, 30 mg elemental magnesium, 80 mg elemental magnesium, 100 mg elemental magnesium (*otc*)	Various
200 mg elemental magnesium (as oxide) (*otc*)	*Mag-200* (Optimox)
250 mg elemental magnesium (as oxide) (*otc*)	Various
400 mg magnesium oxide (241.3 mg elemental magnesium) (*otc*)	Various, *Mag-Ox 400* (Blaine)
420 mg magnesium oxide (253 mg elemental magnesium) (*otc*)	*Maox 420* (Manne Co.)
500 mg magnesium gluconate dihydrate (27 mg elemental magnesium) (*otc*)	*Mag-G* (Cypress), *Magonate* (Fleming)
500 mg magnesium gluconate (29 mg elemental magnesium) (*otc*)	*Magtrate* (Mission)
500 mg magnesium oxide (302 mg elemental magnesium) (*otc*)	Various
Tablets, enteric-coated: 64 mg elemental magnesium (as chloride hexahydrate) (*otc*)	*Slow-Mag* (Purdue)
615 mg magnesium-L-aspartate hydrochloride (61 mg elemental magnesium) (*otc*)	*Maginex* (Logan Pharm)
Tablets, sustained-release: 84 mg elemental magnesium (as L-lactate dihydrate) (*otc*)	*Mag-Tab SR* (Niche)
Capsules: 140 mg magnesium oxide (84.5 mg elemental magnesium) (*otc*)	*Uro-Mag* (Blaine)
Capsules: ≈ 140 mg magnesium oxide (85 mg elemental magnesium) (*otc*)	*Mag-Caps* (Genesis)
Liquid: 3.52 mg elemental magnesium/mL (as gluconate) (*otc*)	*Magonate Natal* (Fleming)
1,000 mg magnesium gluconate dihydrate/5 mL (54 mg elemental magnesium/5 mL) (*otc*)	*Magonate* (Fleming)
Powder: 1,230 mg magnesium-L-aspartate hydrochloride (122 mg elemental magnesium)/packet (*otc*)	*Maginex DS* (Geist)
Injection: 20% magnesium chloride (1.97 mEq/mL) (*Rx*)	Various, *Chloromag* (Merit)
4% magnesium sulfate (0.325 mEq/mL), 8% magnesium sulfate (0.65 mEq/mL), 10% magnesium sulfate (0.8 mEq/mL), 12.5% magnesium sulfate (1 mEq/mL), 50% magnesium sulfate (4 mEq/mL) (*Rx*)	Various

Indications

Oral: As a dietary supplement.

Parenteral:

Hypomagnesemia – Magnesium sulfate is used as replacement therapy in magnesium deficiency especially in acute hypomagnesemia accompanied by signs of tetany similar to those observed in hypocalcemia. In such cases, the serum magnesium (Mg++) level is usually below the lower limit of normal (1.5 to 2.5 or 3 mEq/L) and the serum calcium (Ca++) level is normal (4.3 to 5.3 mEq/L) or elevated.

Total parenteral nutrition: Total parenteral nutrition patients may develop hypomagnesemia (less than 1.5 mEq/L) without supplementation. Magnesium is added to correct or prevent hypomagnesemia.

Preeclampsia/eclampsia/nephritis (magnesium sulfate) – Prevention and control of convulsions of severe preeclampsia and eclampsia and for control of hypertension, encephalopathy, and convulsions associated with acute nephritis in children.

Administration and Dosage

Oral: 1 g magnesium = 83.3 mEq (41.1 mmol).

Dietary supplement – 40 to 400 mg/day in divided doses. Refer to product labeling. Magnesium-containing antacids may also be used.

Recommended dietary allowances (RDAs):

Adults – Males, 270 to 400 mg; females, 280 to 300 mg.

Parenteral: Individualize dosage. Monitor the patient's clinical status to avoid toxicity. Discontinue as soon as the desired effect is obtained. Repeat doses are dependent on the continuing presence of the patellar reflex and adequate respiratory function.

IV administration – Do not exceed 1.5 mL/min of a 10% concentration (or its equivalent), except in cases of severe eclampsia with seizures. Dilute IV infusion solutions to a concentration of 20% or less prior to IV administration. The most commonly used diluents are dextrose 5% injection and sodium chloride 0.9% injection.

IM administration – Deep IM injection of the undiluted (50%) solution is appropriate for adults, but dilute to 20% or less concentration prior to IM injection in children.

Admixture incompatibilities – Magnesium sulfate in solution may result in a precipitate formation when mixed with solutions containing: Alcohol (in high concentrations); alkali carbonates and bicarbonates; alkali hydroxides; arsenates; barium; calcium; clindamycin phosphate; heavy metals; hydrocortisone sodium succinate; phosphates; polymyxin B sulfate; procaine hydrochloride; salicylates; strontium; tartrates.

Hyperalimentation – Maintenance requirements are not precisely known. Maintenance dose range:

Adults: 8 to 24 mEq/day.

Infants: 2 to 10 mEq/day.

Mild magnesium deficiency –

Adults: 1 g (8.12 mEq; 2 mL of 50% solution) IM every 6 hours for 4 doses (total of 32.5 mEq/24 hours).

Severe hypomagnesemia –

IM: As much as 2 mEq/kg (0.5 mL of 50% solution) within 4 hours if necessary.

IV: 5 g (approximately 40 mEq)/L of dextrose 5% injection or sodium chloride 0.9% solution, infused over 3 hours. In treatment of deficiency states, observe caution to prevent exceeding renal excretory capacity.

Acute nephritis in children – 20 to 40 mg/kg IM as needed to control seizures. Dilute the 50% concentration to a 20% solution and give 0.1 to 0.2 mL/kg.

Severe pre-elampsia or eclampsia – Initial dose is 10 to 14 g magnesium sulfate. To initiate therapy, 4 g magnesium sulfate in water for injection (premixed) or 4 to 5 g in 250 mL of dextrose 5% injection or sodium chloride 0.9% injection administered IV. Simultaneously, 4 to 5 g magnesium sulfate administered IM into each buttock using undiluted 50% magnesium sulfate injection.

Alternatively, the initial IV dose of 4 g may be given by diluting the 50% solution to a 10% or 20% concentration; then give IV over a period of 3 to 4 minutes.

After the initial IV dose, some clinicians administer 1 to 2 g/h by constant IV infusion. Subsequent IM doses of 4 to 5 g magnesium sulfate may be injected into alternate buttocks every 4 hours, depending on the presence of the patellar reflex, adequate respiratory function, and absence of signs of magnesium toxicity. Continue therapy until paroxysms cease.

A serum magnesium level of 3 to 6 mg/dL (2.5 to 5 mEq/L) is considered optimal for control of seizures. Do not exceed a total daily dose of 30 to 40 g magnesium sulfate.

Renal function impairment – Obtain serum magnesium concentrations frequently. Maximum dose is 20 g/48 hours.

Actions

Pharmacology: Magnesium is the fourth most abundant mineral in the body and the second most abundant in muscles and other organs. Potassium cannot be retained in soft tissues if magnesium is deficient. An adequate amount of magnesium also is required for the absorption and utilization of calcium, favoring the deposition of calcium in bone and preventing deposition of calcium in the soft tissues and kidneys. Magnesium is required for the normal activity of 300 enzymes.

Magnesium prevents or controls convulsions by blocking neuromuscular transmission and decreasing the amount of acetylcholine liberated by the motor nerve impulse.

Pharmacokinetics: IM injection results in therapeutic plasma levels within 60 minutes and persists for 3 to 4 hours. IV doses provide immediate effects that last for 30 minutes. Effective anticonvulsant serum levels range from 2.5 to 7.5 mEq/L. Magnesium is excreted by the kidneys at a rate proportional to the plasma concentration and glomerular filtration.

Contraindications

Magnesium sulfate: Heart block or myocardial damage; IV magnesium to patients with preeclampsia during the 2 hours preceding delivery.

Magnesium chloride: Renal function impairment; marked myocardial disease; coma.

Warnings/Precautions

IV use: IV use in eclampsia is reserved for immediate control of life-threatening convulsions. Administer slowly to avoid producing hypermagnesemia.

Flushing/Sweating: Administer with caution if flushing or sweating occurs.

Excessive dosage: Excessive dosage may cause diarrhea and GI irritation.

Heart disease: Magnesium supplements may make this condition worse.

Renal function impairment: Use with caution. Parenteral use in the presence of renal function impairment may lead to magnesium intoxication. In patients with severe impairment, dosage should not exceed 20 g in 48 hours. Monitor serum magnesium in such patients.

Pregnancy: Category A (parenteral only). It is unknown whether magnesium supplementation will harm an unborn child or a breast-feeding child. Do not take this mineral without speaking to a health care provider if pregnant, planning a pregnancy, or breast-feeding.

Lactation: Because magnesium is distributed into milk, exercise caution when administering to a breast-feeding mother. The American Academy of Pediatrics considers magnesium sulfate compatible with breast-feeding.

Children: Safety and efficacy of oral magnesium supplementation in children have not been established.

When administered by continuous IV infusion (especially for more than 24 hours preceding delivery) to control convulsions in toxemic mothers, the newborn may show signs of magnesium toxicity, including neuromuscular or respiratory depression.

Elderly: Elderly patients often require reduced dosage because of impaired renal function.

Monitoring: Maintain urine output at a level of at least 100 mL every 4 hours. Monitor serum magnesium levels and clinical status to avoid overdosage in preeclampsia.

Serum magnesium levels usually sufficient to control convulsions range from 3 to 6 mg/dL (2.5 to 5 mEq/L). Keep an injectable calcium salt immediately available to counteract potential hazards of magnesium intoxication in eclampsia.

Drug Interactions

Drugs that may be affected by magnesium salts include aminoquinolines, cellulose sodium phosphate, nitrofurantoin, penicillamine, and tetracyclines.

Drugs that may affect magnesium include sodium polystyrene sulfonate.

CNS depressants: When barbiturates, narcotics, other hypnotics (or systemic anesthetics), or other CNS depressants are to be given in conjunction with parenteral magnesium, adjust their dosage with caution because of additive CNS depressant effects of magnesium.

Neuromuscular blockers: Magnesium sulfate potentiates the neuromuscular blockade produced by neuromuscular blocking agents.

Adverse Reactions

Adverse reactions are usually the result of magnesium intoxication and include flushing; sweating; hypotension; stupor; depressed reflexes; flaccid paralysis; hypothermia; circulatory collapse; cardiac and CNS depression proceeding to respiratory paralysis (the most life-threatening effect).

Hypocalcemia with signs of tetany secondary to magnesium sulfate therapy for eclampsia has occurred.

POTASSIUM REPLACEMENT PRODUCTS

POTASSIUM REPLACEMENT PRODUCTS	
Tablets, controlled-release: 8 and 10 mEq (600 and 750 mg) potassium chloride in a wax matrix (*Rx*)	Various, *K+10* (Alra), *Klor-Con 8* (Upsher-Smith), *Kaon Cl-10* (Savage), *Klor-Con 10* (Upsher-Smith), *Klotrix* (Bristol), *K-Tab* (Abbott)
Tablets, extended-release: 8 mEq potassium chloride (*Rx*)	Various, K^+8 (Alra)
10 mEq potassium (from 750 mg potassium chloride) (*Rx*)	*Klor-Con M10* (Upsher-Smith)
15 mEq potassium (from 1,125 mg potassium chloride) (*Rx*)	*Klor-Con M15* (Upsher-Smith)
20 mEq potassium (from 1,500 mg potassium chloride) (*Rx*)	*Klor-Con M20* (Upsher-Smith)
750 mg potassium chloride equivalent to 10 mEq potassium in a wax matrix (*Rx*)	Various
Tablets, controlled-release: 750 mg microencapsulated potassium chloride equivalent to 10 mEq potassium (*Rx*)	*K-Dur 10* (Key)
1,500 mg microencapsulated potassium chloride (equivalent to 20 mEq potassium) (*Rx*)	Various, *K-Dur 20* (Key)
Tablets: 99 mg potassium (as potassium gluconate) (*Rx*)	Various
500 mg potassium gluconate (83.45 mg potassium) (*Rx*)	Various
595 mg potassium gluconate (99 mg potassium) (*Rx*)	Various
Tablets, effervescent: 20 mEq potassium (from potassium bicarbonate) (*Rx*)	*K + Care ET* (Alra)
20 mEq potassium (from potassium chloride and bicarbonate and lysine hydrochloride) (*Rx*)	*Klorvess* (Sandoz)
25 mEq potassium (from potassium chloride and bicarbonate and l-lysine monohydrochloride and citric acid) (*Rx*)	*K•Lyte/Cl* (Bristol)
50 mEq potassium (from potassium chloride and bicarbonate, l-lysine monohydrochloride and citric acid) (*Rx*)	*K•Lyte/Cl 50* (Bristol)
25 mEq potassium (from potassium bicarbonate) (*Rx*)	*K + Care ET* (Alra)
25 mEq potassium (as bicarbonate and citrate) (*Rx*)	Various, *Effer-K* (Nomax), *Klor-Con/EF* (Upsher-Smith), *K•Lyte* (Bristol)
25 mEq potassium and chloride (from 1.5 g potassium chloride, 0.5 g potassium bicarbonate, 0.91 g l-lysine monohydrochloride, 0.55 g citric acid) (*Rx*)	Various
50 mEq potassium (from potassium bicarbonate and citrate and citric acid) (*Rx*)	*K•Lyte DS* (Bristol)
Capsules, controlled-release: 600 mg potassium chloride equivalent to 8 mEq potassium. Microencapsulated particles (*Rx*)	*Micro-K Extencaps* (Robins)
10 mEq (750 mg) potassium chloride. Microencapsulated particles (*Rx*)	Various, *Micro-K 10 Extencaps* (Thera-Rx)
Liquid: 20 mEq/15 mL potassium and chloride (10% KCl) (*Rx*)	Various, *Cena-K* (Century), *Potasalan* (Lannett)
40 mEq/15 mL potassium and chloride (20% KCl) (*Rx*)	Various, *Kaon-Cl 20%* (Adria)
20 mEq/15 mL potassium (as potassium gluconate) (*Rx*)	Various, *Kaon* (Adria), *Kaylixir* (Lannett)
20 mEq/15 mL potassium (as potassium gluconate and potassium citrate) (*Rx*)	*Twin-K* (Boots)
Powder: 15 mEq potassium chloride per packet (*Rx*)	*K + Care* (Alra)
20 mEq potassium chloride per packet (*Rx*)	Various, *Gen-K* (Goldline), *K + Care* (Alta), *K-Lor* (Abbott), *Klor-Con* (Upsher-Smith)
25 mEq potassium chloride per packet (*Rx*)	*K + Care* (Alra), *Klor-Con/25* (Upsher-Smith)
20 mEq potassium and chloride from 1.5 g potassium chloride (*Rx*)	*K-vescent Potassium Chloride* (Major)
POTASSIUM ACETATE	
Injection: 2 and 4 mEq/mL (*Rx*)	Various
POTASSIUM CHLORIDE CONCENTRATE	
Injection: 2 mEq/mL and 10, 20, 30, 40, 60, and 90 mEq (*Rx*)	Various

Indications

Oral: Treatment of hypokalemia in the following conditions: With or without metabolic alkalosis; digitalis intoxication; familial periodic paralysis; diabetic acidosis; diarrhea and vomiting; surgical conditions accompanied by nitrogen loss, vomiting, suction drainage, diarrhea, and increased urinary excretion of potassium; certain cases of uremia; hyperadrenalism; starvation and debilitation; corticosteroid or diuretic therapy.

Prevention of potassium depletion when dietary intake is inadequate in the following conditions: Patients receiving digitalis and diuretics for CHF; significant cardiac arrhythmias; hepatic cirrhosis with ascites; states of aldosterone excess with normal renal function; potassium-losing nephropathy; certain diarrheal states.

When hypokalemia is associated with alkalosis, use potassium chloride. When acidosis is present, use the bicarbonate, citrate, acetate, or gluconate potassium salts.

IV:

Potassium acetate – Potassium acetate is useful as an additive for preparing specific IV fluid formulas when patient needs cannot be met by standard electrolyte or nutrient solutions.

Also indicated for marked loss of GI secretions by vomiting, diarrhea, GI intubation, or fistulas; prolonged diuresis; prolonged parenteral use of potassium-free fluids; diabetic acidosis, especially during vigorous insulin and dextrose treatment; metabolic alkalosis; attacks of hereditary or familial periodic paralysis; hyperadrenocorticism; primary aldosteronism; overmedication with adrenocortical steroids, testosterone, or corticotropin; healing phase of scalds or burns; cardiac arrhythmias, especially due to digitalis glycosides.

Administration and Dosage

Oral: The usual dietary intake of potassium ranges between 40 to 150 mEq/day.

Individualize dosage. Usual range is 16 to 24 mEq/day for the prevention of hypokalemia to 40 to 100 mEq/day or more for the treatment of potassium depletion.

Reserve slow release potassium chloride preparations for patients who cannot tolerate liquids or effervescent potassium preparations, or for patients in whom there is a problem of compliance with these preparations.

Some studies suggest the "microencapsulated" preparations are less likely to cause GI damage; however, evidence conflicts and a specific recommendation of one solid oral product over another cannot be made. Avoid enteric coated products.

Potassium intoxication may result from any therapeutic dosage.

IV:

Do not administer undiluted potassium – Potassium preparations must be diluted with suitable large volume parenteral solutions, mixed well and given by slow IV infusion.

Too rapid infusion of hypertonic solutions may cause local pain and, rarely, vein irritation. Adjust rate of administration according to tolerance. Use of the largest peripheral vein and a small bore needle is recommended.

The usual additive dilution of potassium chloride is 40 mEq/L of IV fluid. The maximum desirable concentration is 80 mEq/L, although extreme emergencies may dictate greater concentrations.

In critical states, potassium chloride may be administered in saline (unless saline is contraindicated) because dextrose may lower serum potassium levels by producing an intracellular shift.

Avoid "layering" of potassium by proper agitation of the prepared IV solution. Do not add potassium to an IV bottle in the hanging position.

Individualize dosage. Guide dosage and rate of infusion by ECG and serum electrolyte determinations. The following may be used as a guide:

Potassium Dosage/Rate of Infusion Guidelines

Serum K+	Maximum infusion rate	Maximum concentration	Maximum 24 hour dose
> 2.5 mEq/L	10 mEq/h	40 mEq/L	200 mEq
< 2 mEq/L	40 mEq/h	80 mEq/L	400 mEq

Add electrolytes to the mixed solutions only after considering electrolytes already present and potential incompatibilities such as calcium and phosphate or sulfate.

Children – IV infusion up to 3 mEq/kg or 40 mEq/m^2/day. Adjust volume of administered fluids to body size.

Actions

Pharmacology: Potassium participates in a number of essential physiological processes, such as maintenance of intracellular tonicity and a proper relationship with sodium across cell membranes, cellular metabolism, transmission of nerve impulses, contraction of cardiac, skeletal, and smooth muscle, acid-base balance, and maintenance of healthy renal function. Normal potassium serum levels range from 3.5 to 5 mEq/L.

mEq/g of Various Potassium Salts

Potassium salt	mEq/g
Potassium gluconate	4.3
Potassium citrate	9.8
Potassium bicarbonate	10
Potassium acetate	10.2
Potassium chloride	13.4
Dibasic potassium phosphate[a]	11.5
Monobasic potassium phosphate[a]	7.3

[a] Commercial preparations of potassium phosphate injection contain a mixture of both mono- and dibasic salts.

Potassium participates in carbohydrate utilization and protein synthesis and is critical in regulating nerve conduction and muscle contraction, particularly in the heart.

Pharmacokinetics: Normally about 80% to 90% of potassium intake is excreted in urine with the remainder voided in stool and, to a small extent, in perspiration. Kidneys do not conserve potassium well; during fasting or in patients on a potassium-free diet, potassium loss from the body continues, resulting in potassium depletion. A deficiency of either potassium or chloride will lead to a deficit of the other.

Contraindications

Oral: Severe renal function impairment with oliguria or azotemia; untreated Addison disease; hyperkalemia from any cause; adynamia episodica hereditaria; acute dehydration; heat cramps; patients receiving potassium-sparing diuretics or aldosterone-inhibiting agents.

IV: Diseases where high potassium levels may be encountered; hyperkalemia; renal failure and conditions in which potassium retention is present; oliguria or azotemia; anuria; crush syndrome; severe hemolytic reactions; adrenocortical insufficiency (untreated Addison disease); adynamica episodica hereditaria; acute dehydration; heat cramps; hyperkalemia from any cause; early postoperative oliguria except during GI drainage.

Warnings/Precautions

Hyperkalemia: This occurs most commonly in patients given IV potassium, but also may occur in patients given oral potassium. Potentially fatal hyperkalemia can develop rapidly and may be asymptomatic.

GI lesions: Potassium chloride tablets have caused stenotic or ulcerative lesions of the small bowel and death. These lesions are caused by a concentration of potassium ion in the region of a rapidly dissolving tablet, which injures the bowel wall and produces obstruction, hemorrhage, or perforation. The reported frequency of small bowel lesions is much less with wax matrix tablets and microencapsulated tablets than with enteric coated tablets. Immediately discontinue either type of tablet and consider the possibility of bowel obstruction or perforation if severe vomiting, abdominal pain or distention, or GI bleeding occurs.

Patients at greatest risk for developing potassium chloride-induced GI lesions include: The elderly, the immobile and those with scleroderma, diabetes mellitus, mitral valve replacement, cardiomegaly, or esophageal stricture/compression.

Metabolic acidosis and hyperchloremia: Potassium depletion is rarely associated with metabolic acidosis and hyperchloremia. Replace with potassium bicarbonate, citrate, acetate, or gluconate.

Potassium intoxication: Do not infuse rapidly. High plasma concentrations of potassium may cause death through cardiac depression, arrhythmias, or arrest. Monitor potassium replacement therapy whenever possible by continuous or serial ECG. In addition to ECG effects, local pain, and phlebitis may result when a more than 40 mEq/L concentration is infused.

Renal function impairment or adrenal insufficiency – Renal function impairment or adrenal insufficiency may cause potassium intoxication. Potassium salts can produce hyperkalemia and cardiac arrest. Potentially fatal hyperkalemia can develop rapidly and be asymptomatic. Use with great caution, if at all.

Concentrated: Concentrated potassium solutions are for IV admixtures only; do not use undiluted. Direct injection may be instantaneously fatal.

Metabolic alkalosis: Potassium depletion is usually accompanied by an obligatory loss of chloride resulting in hypochloremic metabolic alkalosis. Treat the underlying cause of potassium depletion and administer IV potassium chloride.

Use solutions containing acetate ion carefully in metabolic or respiratory alkalosis, and when there is an increased level or impairment of utilization of this ion.

Musculoskeletal/Cardiac effects: When serum sodium or calcium concentration is reduced, moderate elevation of serum potassium may cause toxic effects on the heart and skeletal muscle. Weakness and later paralysis of voluntary muscles, with consequent respiratory distress and dysphagia, are generally late signs, sometimes significantly preceding dangerous or fatal cardiac toxicity.

Fluid/Solute overload: IV administration can cause fluid or solute overloading resulting in dilution of serum electrolyte concentrations, overhydration, congested states, or pulmonary edema.

Renal function impairment: Renal function impairment requires careful monitoring of the serum potassium concentration and appropriate dosage adjustment.

Special risk: Use with caution in the presence of cardiac disease, particularly in digitalized patients or in the presence of renal disease, metabolic acidosis, Addison disease, acute dehydration, prolonged or severe diarrhea, familial periodic paralysis, hypoadrenalism, hyperkalemia, hyponatremia, and myotonia congenita.

Pregnancy: Category C.

Children: Safety and efficacy for use in children have not been established.

Monitoring: Close medical supervision with frequent ECGs and serum potassium determinations. Plasma levels are not necessarily indicative of tissue levels.

Drug Interactions

Drugs that may interact include ACE inhibitors, potassium-sparing diuretics, digitalis, and potassium-containing salt substitutes.

Adverse Reactions

Oral: Adverse reactions may include nausea, vomiting, diarrhea, flatulence, and abdominal discomfort due to GI irritation. They are best managed by diluting the preparation further, by taking with meals, or by dose reduction. Severe reactions may include hyperkalemia; GI obstruction, bleeding, ulceration, or perforation.

Parenteral:

Hyperkalemia: Adverse reactions involve the possibility of potassium intoxication. Signs and symptoms include paresthesias of extremities; flaccid paralysis; muscle or respiratory paralysis; areflexia; weakness; listlessness; mental confusion; weakness and heaviness of legs; hypotension; cardiac arrhythmias; heart block; ECG abnormalities such as disappearance of P waves, spreading and slurring of the QRS complex with development of a biphasic curve and cardiac arrest.

SODIUM CHLORIDE

Solution: 0.45% (77 mEq/L sodium, 77 mEq/L chloride) (*Rx*)	Various
0.45% sodium chloride (*otc*)	Dey
0.9% (154 mEq/L sodium, 154 mEq/L chloride) (*Rx*)	Various
0.9% sodium chloride (*otc*)	Dey
3% (513 mEq/L sodium, 513 mEq/L chloride) (*Rx*)	Various
5% (855 mEq/L sodium, 855 mEq/L chloride) (*Rx*)	Various
Concentrated solution: 14.6% and 23.4% sodium chloride (*Rx*)	Various
Injection: 0.9% sodium chloride (*Rx*)	Various

Indications

0.45% and 0.9% flexible plastic containers: Parenteral replenishment of fluid and sodium chloride.

0.9% syringe: For use in flushing the indwelling venipuncture device where the medication to be administered is incompatible with heparin.

0.45% and 0.9% vial: For diluting or dissolving drugs for intramuscular, intravenous (IV), or subcutaneous injection, or for inhalation according to instructions of the manufacturer of the drug to be administered.

Also flushing of intravenous catheters and for tracheal lavage.

3% and 5% concentrates: Sources of electrolytes and water.

Hyponatremia and hypochloremia.

14.6% concentrate: Electrolyte replenisher in parenteral fluid therapy; IV sodium supplement in hyponatremia; additive for total parenteral nutrition (TPN); additive for carbohydrate-containing IV fluids.

23.4% concentrate: As an additive in parenteral fluid therapy.

Administration and Dosage

IV: In the average adult, daily requirements of sodium and chloride are met by the infusion of 1 L of sodium chloride 0.9% (154 mEq each of sodium and chloride). Base fluid administration on calculated maintenance or replacement fluid requirements.

IV catheters (0.9%) – Prior to and after administration of the medication, entirely flush with preservative-free 0.9% sodium chloride for injection.

Calculation of sodium deficit – To calculate the amount of sodium that must be administered to raise serum sodium to the desired level, use the following equation (TBW = total body water): Na deficit (mEq) = TBW (desired – observed plasma Na).

Base the repletion rate on the degree of urgency in the patient. Use of hypertonic saline (eg, 3% or 5%) will correct the deficit more rapidly.

3% and 5% concentrates: Do not use plastic container in series connection.

Discontinue pumping action before the container runs dry or air embolism may result.

When administered peripherally, it should be slowly infused through a small bore needle, placed well within the lumen of a large vein to minimize venous irritation. Carefully avoid infiltration.

Maximum IV dosage should be 100 mL given over a period of 1 hour. Before additional amount is given, evaluate the need for more sodium chloride.

IV administration of these solutions should not exceed 100 mL/hour or 400 mL/24 hours.

14.6% concentrate: Administer IV, after dilution in a larger volume of fluid.

23.4% concentrate: Concentrated sodium chloride injection is strongly hypertonic and must be diluted prior to administration.

Actions

Pharmacology: Solutions which provide combinations of hypotonic or isotonic concentrations of sodium chloride are suitable for parenteral maintenance or replacement of water and electrolyte requirements.

Sodium, the major cation of the extracellular fluid, functions primarily in the control of water distribution, fluid balance, and osmotic pressure of body fluids. Sodium is also associated with chloride and bicarbonate in the regulation of the acid-base equilibrium of body fluid.

Chloride, the major extracellular anion, closely follows the metabolism of sodium, and changes in the acid-base balance of the body are reflected by changes in the chloride concentration.

Contraindications

Hypernatremic and fluid retention syndromes. Elevated, normal, or only slightly decreased plasma electrolyte concentrations, or when additives of sodium and chloride could be clinically detrimental.

Warnings/Precautions

Fluid/Solute overload: Excessive amounts of sodium chloride by any route may cause hypokalemia and acidosis. Excessive amounts by the parenteral route may precipitate congestive heart failure and acute pulmonary edema, especially in patients with cardiovascular disease and in patients receiving corticosteroids or corticotropin or drugs that may give rise to sodium retention.

Excessive infusion of hypertonic sodium chloride may supply more sodium and chloride than normally found in serum, resulting in hypernatremia; this may cause a loss of bicarbonate ions, resulting in an acidifying effect.

Sodium retention: Use solutions containing sodium ions with great care, if at all, in congestive heart failure, severe renal insufficiency, and in clinical states where edema with sodium retention exists.

14.6% and 23.4% concentrates: Sodium chloride injection is hypertonic and must be diluted prior to administration. Inadvertent direct injection or absorption of concentrated sodium chloride injection may give rise to sudden hypernatremia and such complications as cardiovascular shock, CNS disorders, extensive hemolysis, cortical necrosis of the kidneys, and severe local tissue necrosis (if administered extravascularly).

Aluminum toxicity (23.4% concentrate) – This product contains aluminum that may be toxic. Aluminum may reach toxic levels with prolonged parenteral administration if kidney function is impaired. Premature neonates are particularly at risk.

Surgical patients: Surgical patients should seldom receive salt-containing solutions immediately following surgery unless factors producing salt depletion are present. Because of renal retention of salt during surgery, additional electrolytes given IV may result in fluid retention, edema, and overloading of the circulation.

Hypokalemia: Hypokalemia may result from excessive administration of potassium-free solutions.

3% and 5% sodium chloride solutions: Infuse very slowly and use with caution to avoid pulmonary edema; observe patients constantly.

Electrolyte losses: Extraordinary electrolyte losses may occur during protracted nasogastric suction, vomiting, diarrhea, or gastrointestinal fistula drainage and may necessitate additional electrolyte supplementation.

Renal function impairment: In patients with diminished renal function, administration of solutions containing sodium may result in sodium retention. The IV administration of this solution can cause fluid or solute overloading resulting in dilution of other serum electrolyte concentrations, overhydration, congested states, or pulmonary edema.

Special risk:

3% and 5% concentrates – Use these solutions with care in patients with hypervolemia, renal insufficiency, urinary tract obstruction, or impending or frank cardiac decompensation.

Exercise care in administering solutions containing sodium to patients with renal or cardiovascular insufficiency, with or without congestive heart failure. Use special caution in administering sodium-containing solutions to patients with severe renal function impairment, cirrhosis of the liver, or other edematous or sodium-retaining states.

Pregnancy: Category C.

Lactation: It is not known whether sodium chloride injection is excreted in human milk.

Children: Safety and efficacy have not been established.

For use in newborns, use only preservative-free sodium chloride injection 0.9%.

0.45% and 0.9% flexible plastic containers – The safety and efficacy in the pediatric population are based on the similarity of the clinical conditions of the pediatric and adult populations. In neonates or very small infants, the volume of fluid may affect fluid and electrolyte balance.

Monitoring: Monitor changes in fluid balance, electrolyte concentrations, and acid-base balance during prolonged parenteral therapy or whenever the condition of the patient warrants such evaluation.

Drug Interactions

Corticosteroids and corticotropin.

Adverse Reactions

Reactions due to solution or technique of administration: Febrile response, infection at the site of injection, venous thrombosis or phlebitis, extravasation, and hypervolemia.

Too rapid infusion: Too rapid infusion of hypertonic solutions may cause local pain and venous irritation and hypernatremia.

14.6% concentrate: Postoperative salt intolerance.

SODIUM BICARBONATE

Injection: 4.2% (0.5 mEq/mL), 5% (0.6 mEq/mL), 7.5% (0.9 mEq/mL), 8.4% (1 mEq/mL) (*Rx*)	Various
Neutralizing additive solution: 4% (0.48 mEq/mL) (*Rx*)	*Neut* (Abbott)
4.2% (0.5 mEq/mL) (*Rx*)	Various

Indications

Metabolic acidosis: In severe renal disease; uncontrolled diabetes; circulatory insufficiency due to shock, anoxia, or severe dehydration; extracorporeal circulation of blood; cardiac arrest; and severe primary lactic acidosis where a rapid increase in plasma total CO_2 content is crucial. Treat metabolic acidosis in addition to measures designed to control the cause of the acidosis. Because an appreciable time interval may elapse before all ancillary effects occur, bicarbonate therapy is indicated to minimize risks inherent to acidosis itself.

At one time it was suggested to administer bicarbonate during cardiopulmonary resuscitation following cardiac arrest; however, recent evidence suggests that little benefit is provided and its use may be detrimental. For treatment of acidosis in this clinical situation, concentrate efforts on restoring ventilation and blood flow. According to the American Heart Association guidelines, use as a last resort after other standard measures have been utilized.

Urinary alkalinization: In the treatment of certain drug intoxications (eg, salicylates, lithium) and in hemolytic reactions requiring alkalinization of the urine to diminish nephrotoxicity of blood pigments.

Severe diarrhea: Severe diarrhea that is often accompanied by a significant loss of bicarbonate.

Neutralizing additive solution: To reduce the incidence of chemical phlebitis and patient discomfort due to vein irritation at or near the infusion site by raising the pH of IV acid solutions.

Administration and Dosage

One g sodium bicarbonate provides 11.9 mEq each of sodium and bicarbonate.

Cardiac arrest: Bicarbonate administration in this situation may be detrimental. Administer according to results of arterial blood pH and $PaCO_2$ and calculation of base deficit. Flush IV lines before and after use.

Adults – A rapid IV dose of 200 to 300 mEq of bicarbonate, given as a 7.5% or 8.4% solution.

Infants (2 years of age or younger) – 4.2% solution for IV administration at a rate not to exceed 8 mEq/kg/day to guard against the possibility of producing hypernatremia, decreasing CSF pressure, and inducing intracranial hemorrhage.

Initial dose – 1 to 2 mEq/kg/min given over 1 to 2 minutes followed by 1 mEq/kg every 10 minutes of arrest. If base deficit is known, give calculated dose of 0.3 × kg × base deficit. If only 7.5% or 8.4% sodium bicarbonate is available, dilute 1:1 with 5% dextrose in water before administration.

Severe metabolic acidosis – Administer 90 to 180 mEq/L (approximately 7.5 to 15 g) at a rate of 1 to 1.5 L during the first hour. Adjust to patient's needs for further management.

Less urgent forms of metabolic acidosis – Sodium bicarbonate injection may be added to other IV fluids. The amount of bicarbonate to be given to older children and adults over a 4- to 8-hour period is approximately 2 to 5 mEq/kg, depending on the severity of the acidosis as judged by the lowering of total CO_2 content, blood pH, and clinical condition. Initially, an infusion of 2 to 5 mEq/kg over 4 to 8 hours will produce improvement in the acid-base status of the blood.

Alternatively, estimates of the initial dose of sodium bicarbonate may be based on the following equation:

$$0.5\ (\text{L/kg}) \times \text{body weight (kg)} \times \text{desired increase in serum } HCO_3^- \text{ (mEq/L)} = \text{bicarbonate dose (mEq)}$$

or

$$0.5\ (\text{L/kg}) \times \text{body weight (kg)} \times \text{base deficit (mEq/L)} = \text{bicarbonate dose (mEq)}.$$

The next step of therapy is dependent on the clinical response of the patient. If severe symptoms have abated, reduce frequency of administration and dose.

If the CO_2 plasma content is unknown, a safe average dose of sodium bicarbonate is 5 mEq (420 mg)/kg.

It is unwise to attempt full correction of a low total CO_2 content during the first 24 hours, because this may accompany an unrecognized alkalosis due to delayed readjustment of ventilation to normal. Thus, achieving total CO_2 content of about 20 mEq/L at the end of the first day will usually be associated with a normal blood pH.

Neutralizing additive solution – One vial of neutralizing additive solution added to 1 L of any of the commonly used parenteral solutions including dextrose, sodium chloride, Ringer's, etc, will increase the pH to a more physiologic range (specific pH may vary slightly).

Note – Some products such as amino acid solutions and multiple electrolyte solutions containing dextrose will not be brought to near physiologic pH by the addition of sodium bicarbonate neutralizing additive solution. This is due to the relatively high buffer capacity of these fluids.

Admixture incompatibilities – Avoid adding sodium bicarbonate to parenteral solutions containing calcium, except where compatibility is established; precipitation or haze may result. Norepinephrine, dopamine, and dobutamine are incompatible.

Actions

Pharmacology: Increases plasma bicarbonate; buffers excess hydrogen ion concentration; raises blood pH; reverses the clinical manifestations of acidosis.

Pharmacokinetics: Sodium bicarbonate in water dissociates to provide sodium and bicarbonate ions. Sodium is the principal cation of extracellular fluid. Bicarbonate is a normal constituent of body fluids and normal plasma level ranges from 24 to 31 mEq/L. Plasma concentration is regulated by the kidney. Bicarbonate anion is considered "labile" because, at a proper concentration of hydrogen ion, it may be converted to carbonic acid, then to its volatile form, carbon dioxide, excreted by lungs. Normally, a ratio of 1:20 (carbonic acid: bicarbonate) is present in extracellular fluid. In a healthy adult with normal kidney function, almost all the glomerular filtered bicarbonate ion is reabsorbed; less than 1% is excreted in urine.

Contraindications

Losing chloride by vomiting or from continuous GI suction; receiving diuretics known to produce a hypochloremic alkalosis; metabolic and respiratory alkalosis; hypocalcemia in which alkalosis may produce tetany, hypertension, convulsions, or congestive heart failure (CHF); when sodium use could be clinically detrimental.

Neutralizing additive solution: Do not use as a systemic alkalinizer.

Warnings/Precautions

Cardiac effects:

Cardiac arrest – The risk of rapid infusion must be weighed against the potential for fatality due to acidosis.

CHF – Because sodium accompanies bicarbonate, use cautiously in patients with CHF or other edematous or sodium-retaining states.

Fluid/Solute overload: IV administration can cause fluid or solute overloading resulting in dilution of serum electrolyte concentrations, overhydration, congested states, or pulmonary edema.

Extravasation: Extravasation of IV hypertonic solutions of sodium bicarbonate may cause chemical cellulitis (because of their alkalinity), with tissue necrosis, ulceration, or sloughing at the site of infiltration. Prompt elevation of the part, warmth, and local injection of lidocaine or hyaluronidase are recommended to prevent sloughing.

Too rapid infusion: Too rapid infusion of hypertonic solutions may cause local pain and venous irritation. Adjust the rate of administration according to tolerance. Use of the largest peripheral vein and a well placed small bore needle is recommended.

Too rapid or excessive administration may result in hypernatremia and alkalosis accompanied by hyperirritability or tetany. Hypernatremia may be associated with edema and exacerbation of CHF due to the retention of water, resulting in an expanded extracellular fluid volume.

Avoid overdosage and alkalosis: Avoid overdosage and alkalosis by giving repeated small doses and periodic monitoring by appropriate laboratory tests.

Potassium depletion: Potassium depletion may predispose to metabolic alkalosis, and coexistent hypocalcemia may be associated with carpopedal spasm as the plasma pH rises. Minimize by treating electrolyte imbalances prior to or concomitantly with bicarbonate.

Chloride loss: Patients losing chloride by vomiting or GI intubation are more susceptible to developing severe alkalosis if given alkalinizing agents.

Neutralizing additive solution: Administer this solution promptly. When introducing additives, mix thoroughly, and do not store. Raising pH of IV fluids with neutralizing additive solution will reduce incidence of chemical irritation caused by infusate.

Renal function impairment: Administration of solutions containing sodium ions may result in sodium retention. Use with caution. Also use cautiously in oliguria or anuria.

Pregnancy: Category C.

Children:

Neonates and children (younger than 2 years of age) – Rapid injection (10 mL/min) of hypertonic sodium bicarbonate solutions may produce hypernatremia, a decrease in cerebrospinal fluid pressure and possible intracranial hemorrhage. Do not administer more than 8 mEq/kg/day. A 4.2% solution is preferred for such slow administration.

Elderly: Exercise particular care when administering sodium-containing solutions to elderly or postoperative patients with renal or cardiovascular insufficiency, with or without CHF.

Monitoring: Adverse reactions may result from an excess or deficit of one or more of the ions in the solution; frequent monitoring of electrolyte levels is essential.

Drug Interactions

Drugs that may interact include chlorpropamide, lithium, methotrexate, salicylates, tetracyclines, anorexiants, flecainide, mecamylamide, quinidine, and sympathomimetics.

Adverse Reactions

Adverse reactions may include extravasation; local pain; venous irritation; hypernatremia; alkalosis.

Chapter 2

HEMATOLOGICAL AGENTS

IRON-CONTAINING PRODUCTS, ORAL

FERROUS SULFATE	
Tablets: 27 mg (*otc*), 200 mg (65 mg iron), 300 mg (60 mg iron), 325 mg (65 mg iron) (*otc*)	Various, *Feosol* (GlaxoSmithKline), *FeroSul* (Major)
Tablets, slow release; oral: 160 mg (50 mg iron) (*otc*)	Various, *Slow Release Iron* (Cardinal Health)
Tablets, extended release; oral: 142 mg (42 mg iron) (*otc*)	*Slow Fe* (Novartis Consumer)
Drops, oral: 15 mg iron per mL (*otc*)	Various, *Enfamil Fer-In-Sol (Mead Johnson Nutritionals)*, *Fer-Iron* (Rugby)
Liquid, oral: 300 mg per 5 mL (60 mg iron per 5 mL)	Various
Elixir: 220 mg per 5 mL (iron 44 mg per 5 mL) (*otc*)	Various
FERROUS ASPARTATE	
Tablets: 112 mg (elemental iron 18 mg)/aspartic acid 85 mg) (*otc*)	*FE Aspartate* (Miller)
FERROUS SULFATE EXSICCATED (DRIED)	
Tablets: 200 mg (iron 65 mg) (*otc*)	*Feosol* (GlaxoSmithKline)
300 mg (iron 60 mg) (*otc*)	*Feratab* (Upsher-Smith)
Tablets, slow-release: 160 mg (iron 50 mg) (*otc*)	Various, *Slow FE* (Ciba)
FERROUS GLUCONATE	
Tablets: 225 mg (iron 27 mg) (*otc*)	Various, *Fergon* (Bayer)
324 mg (iron 38 mg), 325 mg (iron 36 mg) (*otc*)	Various
FERROUS FUMARATE	
Tablets: 90 mg (iron 29.5 mg) (*otc*)	Various
324 mg (iron 106 mg) (*otc*)	Various, *Hemocyte* (US Pharmaceutical Corp.)
325 mg (iron 106 mg) (*otc*)	*Ferretts* (Pharmics)
Tablets, timed-release: 150 mg (iron 50 mg) (*otc*)	*Ferro-Sequels* (Iverness Medical Innovations)
CARBONYL IRON	
Tablets: 45 mg iron (*otc*)	*Feosol* (GlaxoSmithKline)
66 mg iron (*otc*)	*Ircon* (Kenwood)
Tablets, chewable: 15 mg carbonyl iron (*otc*)	*Icar* (Hawthorn), *Iron Chews* (Midlothian)
Suspension: 15 mg carbonyl iron per 1.25 mL (*otc*)	
POLYSACCHARIDE-IRON COMPLEX	
Capsules: iron 60 mg (*otc*)	*Niferex* (Ther-Rx)
iron 150 mg (*otc*)	Various, *Ferrex 150* (Breckenridge), *Nu-Iron 150* (Merz)
iron 200 mg (*otc*)	*EZFE 200* (McNeil)
Elixir: iron 100 mg per 5 mL (*otc*)	*Niferex* (Ther-Rx)
IRON WITH VITAMIN C	
Tablets: iron 66 mg, ascorbic acid 125 mg (*otc*)	*Vitron-C* (Heritage Consumer Products)
Tablets, controlled-release: iron 105 mg, sodium ascorbate 500 mg (*otc*)	*Fero-Grad-500* (Abbott)
Capsules: iron 150 mg, ascorbic acid 50 mg (*otc*)	*Ferrex 150 Plus* (Breckenridge)
iron 150 mg, calcium ascorbate and calcium threonate 50 mg (*otc*)	*Niferex-150* (Ther-Rx)
iron 65 mg, ascorbic acid 150 mg (*otc*)	*Vitelle Irospan* (Fielding)

Warning:

Accidental overdose of iron-containing products is a leading cause of fatal poisoning in children younger than 6 years of age. Keep products out of the reach of children. In case of accidental overdose, call a doctor or a poison control center immediately.

Indications

Iron deficiency: For the prevention and treatment of iron deficiency and iron deficiency anemias.

Iron supplement: As a dietary supplement for iron.

Unlabeled uses: Iron supplementation may be required by most patients receiving epoetin therapy. Failure to administer iron supplements (oral or intravenous) during epoetin therapy can impair the hematologic response to epoetin.

Administration and Dosage

Because of the availability of multiple salt forms, close attention is warranted when administering iron. Substitution of 1 salt for another without proper adjustment may result in serious over or under dosing.

Carbonyl iron and polysaccharide-iron complex are reported to be associated with fewer GI effects and are less toxic than other forms of iron.

The length of iron therapy depends upon the cause and severity of the iron deficiency. In general, approximately 4 to 6 months of oral iron therapy is required to reverse uncomplicated iron deficiency anemias. Iron therapy should increase hemoglobin levels by 1 g/week.

Iron replacement therapy in deficiency states: Iron doses are given as elemental iron.

Premature infants – 2 to 4 mg/kg/day given in 1 to 2 divided doses. Maximum dosage is 15 mg/day.

Children – 3 to 6 mg/kg/day given in 1 to 3 divided doses.

Adults – 150 to 300 mg/day given in 3 divided doses. Alternatively, 60 mg given 2 to 4 times per day may help lessen GI effects.

Prevention of iron deficiency:

Premature infants – 2 mg/kg/day given in 1 to 3 divided doses. Maximum dosage is 15 mg/day.

Children – 1 to 2 mg/kg/day given in 1 to 3 divided doses. Maximum dosage is 15 mg/day.

Adults – 60 mg/day given in 1 to 2 divided doses.

Recommended dietary allowances: For a complete listing of recommended dietary allowances (RDAs), refer to the RDAs section of the Nutrients and Nutritionals chapter.

RDAs for Iron

Patients	RDA for iron (mg/day)
Children	
7 to 12 months of age	11
1 to 3 years of age	7
4 to 8 years of age	10
Males	
9 to 13 years of age	8
14 to 18 years of age	11
≥ 19 years of age	8
Females	
9 to 13 years of age	8
14 to 18 years of age	15
19 to 50 years of age	18
> 50 years of age	8
Pregnancy	27
Lactation	
≤ 18 years of age	10
≥ 19 years of age	9

Iron supplementation:

Pregnancy – Elemental iron 15 to 30 mg/day should be adequate to meet the daily requirement of the last 2 trimesters.

Actions

Pharmacology: Iron, an essential mineral, is a component of hemoglobin, myoglobin, and a number of enzymes. Approximately two-thirds of total body iron is in the circulating red blood cell mass in hemoglobin, the major factor in oxygen transport.

Pharmacokinetics:

Absorption/Distribution – The average dietary intake of iron is 12 to 20 mg/day for males and 8 to 15 mg/day for females; however, only about 10% of this iron is absorbed (1 to 2 mg/day) in individuals with adequate iron stores. Absorption is enhanced (20% to 30%) when storage iron is depleted or when erythropoiesis occurs at an increased rate. Iron is primarily absorbed from the duodenum and jejunum.

The ferrous salt form is absorbed 3 times more readily than the ferric form. The common ferrous salts (ie, sulfate, gluconate, fumarate) are absorbed almost on a milligram-for-milligram basis but differ in the content of elemental iron. Sustained-release or enteric-coated preparations reduce the amount of available iron; absorption from these doseforms is reduced because iron is transported beyond the duodenum. Dose also influences the amount of iron absorbed. The amount of iron absorbed increases progressively with larger doses; however, the percentage absorbed decreases. Food can decrease the absorption of iron by 40% to 66%; however, gastric intolerance may often necessitate administering the drug with food.

Excretion – The daily loss of iron from urine, sweat, and sloughing of intestinal mucosal cells amounts to approximately 0.5 to 1 mg in healthy men. In menstruating women, approximately 1 to 2 mg is the normal daily loss.

Elemental Iron Content of Iron Salts

Iron salt	% Iron
Ferrous fumarate	≈ 33
Ferrous gluconate	≈ 12
Ferrous sulfate	≈ 20
Ferrous sulfate, exsiccated	≈ 32

Contraindications

Hemochromatosis; hemosiderosis; hemolytic anemias; known hypersensitivity to any ingredients.

Warnings/Precautions

Chronic iron intake: Individuals with normal iron balance should not take iron chronically.

Accidental overdose: Accidental overdose of iron-containing products is a leading cause of fatal poisoning in children younger than 6 years of age. Keep this product out of reach of children.

Intolerance: Discontinue use if symptoms of intolerance appear.

GI effects: Occasional GI discomfort, such as nausea, may be minimized by taking with meals and by slowly increasing to the recommended dosage.

Tartrazine/Sulfite sensitivity: Some of these products contain tartrazine or sulfites, which may cause allergic-type reactions.

Pregnancy: Category A.

Drug Interactions

Iron salts may be affected by the following agents: AHA, antacids, ascorbic acid, calcium salts, chloramphenicol, digestive enzymes, H_2 antagonists, proton pump inhibitors, tetracyclines, and trientine.

Agents that may be affected by iron salts include: captopril, cephalosporins, levodopa, levothyroxine, methyldopa, mycophenolate mofetil, penicillamine, quinolones, tetracyclines, thyroid hormones, and trientine.

Drug/Food interactions: Administration of iron with food decreases iron absorption by at least 50%. Administration of calcium and iron supplements with food can reduce ferrous sulfate absorption by 33%. If combined iron and calcium supplementation is required, iron absorption is not decreased if calcium carbonate is used and the supplements are taken between meals.

Adverse Reactions

Anorexia, constipation, diarrhea, GI irritation, nausea; vomiting . Stools may appear darker in color. Iron-containing liquids may cause temporary staining of the teeth.

IRON DEXTRAN

Injection: 50 mg iron/mL (as dextran) (*Rx*) — *InFeD* (Schein), *DexFerrum* (American Regent)

Warning:

The parenteral use of complexes of iron and carbohydrates has resulted in anaphylactic-type reactions. Deaths associated with such administration have been reported; therefore, use iron dextran injection only in those patients in whom the indications have been clearly established and laboratory investigations confirm an iron-deficient state not amenable to oral iron therapy. Because fatal anaphylactic reactions have been reported after administration of iron dextran injection, administer the drug only when resuscitation techniques and treatment of anaphylactic and anaphylactoid shock are readily available.

Indications

For treatment of patients with documented iron deficiency in whom oral administration is unsatisfactory or impossible.

Unlabeled uses: Iron supplementation may be required by most patients receiving epoetin therapy. Failure to administer iron supplements (oral or IV) during epoetin therapy can impair the hematologic response to epoetin.

Administration and Dosage

Maximum dose: 2 mL of undiluted iron dextran daily.

Iron deficiency anemia: The accompanying formula and table are applicable for dosage determinations only in patients with iron deficiency anemia; they are not to be used for dosage determinations in patients requiring iron replacement for blood loss.

The total amount of iron (in mL) required to restore hemoglobin to normal levels and to replenish iron stores may be approximated from the following formula:

$$\text{Dose (mL)} = 0.0442\,(\text{desired Hb} - \text{observed Hb}) \times \text{Weight}^* + (0.26 \times \text{Weight}^*)$$

*For adults and children more than 15 kg (33 lbs), use the lesser of lean body weight or actual body weight in kilograms. Lean body weight is 50 kg (for males) or 45.5 kg (for females) plus 2.3 kg for each inch over 5 feet. For children 5 to 15 kg (11 to 33 lbs), use actual weight in kilograms. Do not give iron dextran during the first 4 months of life.

Total Amount of Iron Dextran Required (to the nearest mL) for Hemoglobin and Iron Stores Replacement[a]

Lean body weight[b]		Amount required (mL) based on observed hemoglobin							
kg	lb	3 g/dL	4 g/dL	5 g/dL	6 g/dL	7 g/dL	8 g/dL	9 g/dL	10 g/dL
5	11	3	3	3	3	2	2	2	2
10	22	7	6	6	5	5	4	4	3
15	33	10	9	9	8	7	7	6	5
20	44	16	15	14	13	12	11	10	9
25	55	20	18	17	16	15	14	13	12
30	66	23	22	21	19	18	17	15	14
35	77	27	26	24	23	21	20	18	17
40	88	31	29	28	26	24	22	21	19
45	99	35	33	31	29	27	25	23	21
50	110	39	37	35	32	30	28	26	24
55	121	43	41	38	36	33	31	28	26
60	132	47	44	42	39	36	34	31	28
65	143	51	48	45	42	39	36	34	31
70	154	55	52	49	45	42	39	36	33
75	165	59	55	52	49	45	42	39	35
80	176	63	59	55	52	48	45	41	38
85	187	66	63	59	55	51	48	44	40

Total Amount of Iron Dextran Required (to the nearest mL) for Hemoglobin and Iron Stores Replacement[a]

Lean body weight[b]		Amount required (mL) based on observed hemoglobin							
kg	lb	3 g/dL	4 g/dL	5 g/dL	6 g/dL	7 g/dL	8 g/dL	9 g/dL	10 g/dL
90	198	70	66	62	58	54	50	46	42
95	209	74	70	66	62	57	53	49	45
100	220	78	74	69	65	60	56	52	47
105	231	82	77	73	68	63	59	54	50
110	242	86	81	76	71	67	62	57	52
115	253	90	85	80	75	70	65	59	54
120	264	94	88	83	78	73	67	62	57

[a] Table values were calculated based on a normal adult hemoglobin of 14.8 g/dL for weights greater than 15 kg (33 lbs) and a hemoglobin of 12 g/dL for weights 15 kg (33 lbs) or less.

[b] For adults and children older than 15 kg (33 lbs), use the lesser of lean body weight or actual body weight in kilograms. See above equation.

Administration –

IV injection: Individual doses of 2 mL or less may be given on a daily basis until the calculated total amount required has been reached. After administration, evidence of a therapeutic response can be seen in a few days as an increase in reticulocyte count.

Give undiluted and slowly (not to exceed 1 mL/min).

Test dose – Prior to administering the first therapeutic dose, give all patients an IV test dose of 0.5 mL. Administer the test dose at a gradual rate over at least 30 seconds (*InFeD*) or at least 5 minutes (*DexFerrum*). Although anaphylactic reactions known to occur following administration are usually evident within a few minutes or sooner, it is recommended that a period of at least 1 hour elapse before the remainder of the initial therapeutic dose is given.

Individual doses of 2 mL or less may be given on a daily basis until the calculated total amount required has been reached.

Give undiluted and slowly, not to exceed 50 mg/min (1 mL/min).

IM injection:

Test dose – Prior to administering the first therapeutic dose, give all patients an IM test dose of 0.5 mL. If no adverse reactions are observed, the injection can be given according to the following schedule until the calculated total amount required has been reached. Each day's dose should ordinarily not exceed 0.5 mL (25 mg iron) for infants less than 5 kg (11 lb), 1 mL (50 mg iron) for children less than 10 kg (22 lb) and 2 mL (100 mg iron) for other patients.

Inject only into the muscle mass of the upper outer quadrant of the buttock (never into the arm or other exposed areas) and inject deeply with a 2- or 3-inch 19- or 20-gauge needle. If the patient is standing, have them bear their weight on the leg opposite the injection site, or if in bed, have them in a lateral position with injection site uppermost. To avoid injection or leakage into the subcutaneous tissue, a Z-track technique (displacement of the skin laterally prior to injection) is recommended.

Iron replacement for blood loss: Direct iron therapy in these patients toward replacement of the equivalent amount of iron represented in the blood loss. The table and formula described under *Iron deficiency anemia* are not applicable for simple iron replacement values.

The following formula is based on the approximation that 1 mL of normocytic, normochromic red cells contains 1 mg elemental iron:

$$\text{Replacement iron (in mg)} = \text{Blood loss (in mL)} \times \text{hematocrit}$$

Actions

Pharmacology: Iron dextran, a hematinic agent, is a complex of ferric hydroxide and dextran for IM or IV use. The iron dextran complex is dissociated by the reticuloendothelial system, and the ferric iron is transported by transferrin and incorporated into hemoglobin and storage sites.

Pharmacokinetics:

Absorption/Distribution – The major portion of IM injections of iron dextran is absorbed within 72 hours; most of the remaining iron is absorbed over the ensuing 3 to 4 weeks. Various studies have yielded half-life values ranging from 5 hours (circulating iron dextran) to more than 20 hours (total iron, both circulating and bound).

Metabolism/Excretion – Dextran, a polyglucose, is either metabolized or excreted. Negligible amounts of iron are lost via the urinary or alimentary pathways after administration of dextran.

Contraindications

Hypersensitivity to the product; all anemias not associated with iron deficiency; acute phase of infectious kidney disease.

Warnings/Precautions

Maximum dose: 2 mL of undiluted iron dextran is the maximum recommended daily dose.

Total dose infusion: Large IV doses, such as those used with total dose infusions (TDI), have been associated with an increased incidence of adverse reactions. The adverse reactions frequently are delayed (1 to 2 days). Reactions are typified by one or more of the following symptoms: arthralgia, backache, chills, dizziness, moderate to high fever, headache, malaise, myalgia, nausea, vomiting.

Accidental overdose: Accidental overdose of iron-containing products is a leading cause of fatal poisoning in children younger than 6 years of age. Keep this product out of reach of children.

Iron overload: Unwarranted therapy with parenteral iron will cause excess storage of iron with the consequent possibility of exogenous hemosiderosis.

Cardiovascular disease: Adverse reactions of iron dextran may exacerbate cardiovascular complications in patients with preexisting cardiovascular disease.

Chronic renal dialysis: Although serum ferritin is usually a good guide to body iron stores, the correlation of body iron stores and serum ferritin may not be valid in patients on chronic renal dialysis who are also receiving iron dextran complex.

Allergies/Asthma: Use with caution in patients with history of significant allergies/asthma.

Arthritis: Patients with rheumatoid arthritis may have an acute exacerbation of joint pain and swelling following administration of iron dextran.

Hypersensitivity reactions: Anaphylaxis and other hypersensitivity reactions have been reported after uneventful test doses as well as therapeutic doses of iron dextran injection. Therefore, consider administration of subsequent test doses during therapy. Have epinephrine immediately available in the event of acute hypersensitivity reactions.

Hepatic function impairment: Use this preparation with extreme caution in the presence of serious hepatic function impairment.

Carcinogenesis: A risk of carcinogenesis may attend the IM injection of iron-carbohydrate complexes.

Pregnancy: Category C.

Lactation: Traces of unmetabolized iron dextran are excreted in breast milk. Exercise caution when administering to a breast-feeding woman.

Children: Not recommended for use in infants younger than 4 months of age.

Monitoring: Serum iron determinations (especially by colorimetric assays) may not be meaningful for 3 weeks; serum ferritin peaks after about 7 to 9 days and slowly returns to baseline after about 3 weeks.

Drug Interactions

Chloramphenicol: Serum iron levels may be increased because of decreased iron clearance and erythropoiesis due to direct bone marrow toxicity from chloramphenicol.

Drug/Lab test interactions: Large doses of iron dextran (5 mL or more) give a brown color to serum from a blood sample drawn 4 hours after administration; they may cause falsely elevated values of serum bilirubin and falsely decreased values of serum calcium.

Adverse Reactions

Anaphylactic reactions including fatal anaphylaxis; other hypersensitivity reactions including dyspnea, urticaria, other rashes, and febrile episodes; inflammation at or near injection site, including sterile abscesses (IM); brown skin discoloration at injection site (IM); flushing and hypotension with overly rapid IV administration; hypotensive reaction; arthralgia.

The following pattern of signs/symptoms has been reported as a delayed (1 to 2 days) reaction at recommended doses: Fever; chills; backache; headache; myalgia; malaise; nausea; vomiting; dizziness.

FERUMOXYTOL

Injection, solution: elemental iron 30 mg/mL (*Rx*)	*Feraheme* (AMAG Pharmaceuticals)

Indications

Iron deficiency anemia: For the treatment of iron deficiency anemia in adults with chronic kidney disease (CKD).

Administration and Dosage

Adults:

Iron deficiency anemia – 510 mg intravenously (IV) followed by a second 510 mg IV injection 3 to 8 days later. The recommended dose may be readministered to patients with persistent or recurrent iron deficiency anemia.

Renal function impairment:

Hemodialysis – Administer ferumoxytol once the blood pressure is stable and the patient has completed at least 1 hour of hemodialysis.

Administration: Administer as an undiluted IV injection delivered at a rate of up to 1 mL/sec (30 mg/sec).

Actions

Pharmacology: Ferumoxytol consists of a superparamagnetic iron oxide that is coated with a carbohydrate shell. The iron is released from the iron-carbohydrate complex within vesicles in the macrophages. Iron then enters the intracellular storage iron pool (eg, ferritin) or is transferred to plasma transferrin for transport to erythroid precursor cells for incorporation into hemoglobin.

Pharmacokinetics:

Absorption – The mean maximum observed plasma concentration (C_{max}) and time of maximum concentration (T_{max}) were 206 mcg/mL and 0.32 h, respectively.

Distribution – The estimated value of volume of distribution following 2 doses of ferumoxytol 510 mg administered IV within 24 hours was 3.16 L.

Excretion – The half-life of ferumoxytol is approximately 15 hours in humans. The estimated value of clearance following 2 doses of ferumoxytol 510 mg administered IV within 24 hours was 69.1 mL/h.

Contraindications

Evidence of iron overload; hypersensitivity to ferumoxytol or any of its components; anemia not caused by iron deficiency.

Warnings/Precautions

Hypotension: Hypotension may follow ferumoxytol administration.

Iron overload: Excessive therapy with parenteral iron can lead to excess storage of iron with the possibility of iatrogenic hemosiderosis. Do not administer ferumoxytol to patients with iron overload.

In the 24 hours following administration of ferumoxytol, laboratory assays may overestimate serum iron and transferrin-bound iron by also measuring the iron in the ferumoxytol complex.

Magnetic resonance imaging: Administration of ferumoxytol may transiently affect the diagnostic ability of magnetic resonance imaging (MRI). Conduct anticipated MRI studies prior to the administration of ferumoxytol. Alteration of MRI studies may persist for up to 3 months following the last ferumoxytol dose.

Hypersensitivity reactions: Ferumoxytol may cause serious hypersensitivity reactions, including anaphylaxis and/or anaphylactoid reactions.

Pregnancy: Category C.

Lactation: It is not known whether ferumoxytol is present in human milk. Because many drugs are excreted in human milk and because of the potential for adverse reactions in breast-feeding infants, decide whether to discontinue breast-feeding or to avoid ferumoxytol.

Children: The safety and effectiveness of ferumoxytol in children have not been established.

Elderly: In general, be cautious in dose administration to elderly patients, reflecting the greater frequency of decreased hepatic, renal, or cardiac function, and of concomitant disease or other drug therapy.

Monitoring: Observe patients for signs and symptoms of hypersensitivity for at least 30 minutes following ferumoxytol injection and only administer the drug when personnel and therapies are readily available for the treatment of hypersensitivity reactions. Monitor patients for signs and symptoms of hypotension following ferumoxytol administration. Regularly monitor the hematologic response during parenteral iron therapy.

Drug Interactions

Oral iron: Ferumoxytol may reduce the absorption of concomitantly administered oral iron.

Adverse Reactions

Adverse reactions occurring in 3% or more of patients include diarrhea, hypotension, and nausea.

IRON SUCROSE

Injection: 20 mg elemental iron/mL (*Rx*)	*Venofer* (Fresenius)

Indications

Iron-deficiency anemia: For the treatment of iron-deficiency anemia in the following patients:

- non-dialysis-dependent chronic kidney disease (NDD-CKD) patients receiving an erythropoietin
- NDD-CKD patients not receiving an erythropoietin
- hemodialysis-dependent chronic kidney disease (HDD-CKD) patients receiving an erythropoietin
- peritoneal dialysis-dependent chronic kidney disease (PDD-CKD) patients receiving an erythropoietin

Administration and Dosage

The dosage of iron sucrose is expressed in terms of milligrams of elemental iron. Each 5 mL vial contains 100 mg of elemental iron (20 mg/mL).

Iron deficiency anemia: Most patients will require a minimum cumulative dose of 1,000 mg of elemental iron to achieve a favorable hemoglobin or hematocrit response. Patients may continue to require therapy with iron sucrose or other IV iron preparations at the lowest dose necessary to maintain target levels of hemoglobin, hematocrit, and laboratory parameters of iron storage within acceptable limits.

Adult dosage –

HDD-CKD patients: Iron sucrose may be administered undiluted as a 100 mg slow IV injection over 2 to 5 minutes or as an infusion of 100 mg, diluted in a maximum of 100 mL of sodium chloride (NaCl) 0.9% over a period of at least 15 minutes per consecutive hemodialysis session for a total cumulative dose of 1,000 mg.

NDD-CKD patients: Iron sucrose is administered as a total cumulative dose of 1,000 mg over a 14-day period as a 200 mg slow IV injection undiluted over 2 to 5 minutes on 5 different occasions within the 14-day period. There is limited experience with administration of an infusion of iron sucrose 500 mg, diluted in a maximum of 250 mL of NaCl 0.9% over a period of 3.5 to 4 hours on day 1 and day 14; hypotension occurred in 2 of 30 patients treated.

PDD-CKD patients: Iron sucrose is administered as a total cumulative dose of 1,000 mg in 3 divided doses, given by slow IV infusion, within a 28-day period; 2 infusions of 300 mg over 1.5 hours 14 days apart, followed by one 400 mg infusion over 2.5 hours 14 days later. The iron sucrose dose should be diluted in a maximum of 250 mL of NaCl 0.9%.

Actions

Pharmacology: Iron is essential to the synthesis of hemoglobin to maintain oxygen transport and to the function and formation of other physiologically important heme and nonheme compounds.

Pharmacokinetics: In healthy adults treated with IV doses of iron sucrose, its iron component exhibits first order kinetics with an elimination half-life of 6 hours, total clearance of 1.2 L/h, non-steady-state apparent volume of distribution of 10 L, and steady-state apparent volume of distribution of 7.9 L.

Following IV administration of iron sucrose, it is dissociated into iron and sucrose by the reticuloendothelial system. The sucrose component is eliminated mainly by urinary excretion. Some iron also is eliminated in the urine.

Contraindications

Evidence of iron overload; known hypersensitivity to iron sucrose or any of its inactive components; anemia not caused by iron deficiency.

Warnings/Precautions

Iron overload: Exercise caution to withhold iron administration in the presence of evidence of tissue iron overload. Dosages of iron sucrose in excess of iron needs may lead to accumulation of iron in storage sites, leading to hemosiderosis. Do not administer iron sucrose to patients with iron overload.

Hypotension: Hypotension following administration of iron sucrose may be related to rate of administration and total dose administered. Cautiously administer iron sucrose according to recommended guidelines.

Hypersensitivity reactions: In clinical studies, several patients experienced hypersensitivity reactions presenting with wheezing, dyspnea, hypotension, rashes, or pruritus. Serious episodes of hypotension occurred in 2 patients treated with iron sucrose 500 mg.

From the postmarketing spontaneous reporting system, there were 104 reports of anaphylactoid reactions, including patients who experienced serious or life-threatening reactions (anaphylactic shock, loss of consciousness or collapse, bronchospasm with dyspnea, or convulsion) associated with iron sucrose administration.

Pregnancy: Category B.

Lactation: It is not known whether this drug is excreted in human breast milk.

Children: Safety and efficacy of iron sucrose in children have not been established.

Elderly: No overall differences in safety were observed between these subjects and younger subjects, and other reported clinical experience has not identified differences in responses between the elderly and younger patients, but greater sensitivity of some older individuals cannot be ruled out.

Monitoring: Exercise caution to withhold iron administration in the presence of evidence of tissue iron overload. Periodically monitor hematologic and hematinic parameters (hemoglobin, hematocrit, serum ferritin, and transferrin saturation). Withhold iron therapy in patients with evidence of iron overload. Transferrin saturation values increase rapidly after IV administration of iron sucrose; thus, serum iron values may be reliably obtained 48 hours after IV dosing.

Drug Interactions

Drug interactions involving iron sucrose have not been studied. However, like other parenteral iron preparations, iron sucrose may be expected to reduce the absorption of concomitantly administered oral iron preparations.

Adverse Reactions Adverse reactions occurring in 3% or more of patients include the following: abdominal pain, arthralgia, back pain, catheter-site infection, chest pain, constipation, cough, diarrhea, dizziness, dysgeusia, dyspnea, edema, fatigue, fecal occult blood positive, fluid overload, graft complications, headache, hypertension, hypesthesia, hypotension, infusion-site burning, muscle cramp, myalgia, nausea, pain in extremity, peripheral edema, peritoneal infection, pharyngitis, pruritus, urinary tract infection NOS, vomiting.

HDD-CKD patients: Adverse reactions reported in more than 5% of treated patients were as follows: hypotension (39.4%); muscle cramps (29.4%); nausea (14.7%); headache (12.6%); graft complications (9.5%); vomiting (9.1%); dizziness, hypertension (6.5%); chest pain (6.1%); diarrhea (5.2%).

NDD-CKD patients: Adverse reactions, whether or not related to iron sucrose, reported by at least 5% of the iron sucrose exposed patients were as follows: dysgeusia, peripheral edema (7.7%); constipation, diarrhea, dizziness, hypertension, nausea (5.5%).

In an additional study of iron sucrose with varying erythropoietin doses reported by at least 5% of iron sucrose–exposed patients, adverse reactions are as follows: diarrhea, edema (16.5%); nausea (13.2%); vomiting (12.1%); arthralgia, back pain, dysgeusia, headache, hypertension (7.7%); dizziness (6.6%); extremity pain, injection-site burning (5.5%).

PDD-CKD patients: Adverse reactions reported by at least 5% of these patients are as follows: diarrhea, hypertension, nausea, peripheral edema, peritoneal infection, pharyngitis, and vomiting.

SODIUM FERRIC GLUCONATE COMPLEX

Injection: 62.5 mg/5 mL (12.5 mg/mL) elemental iron (*Rx*) *Ferrlecit* (Watson Pharma)

Indications

Iron deficiency: For the treatment of iron deficiency anemia in patients 6 years of age and older undergoing chronic hemodialysis who are receiving supplemental epoetin therapy.

Administration and Dosage

The dosage of sodium ferric gluconate complex is expressed in milligrams of elemental iron. Each 5 mL ampule contains 62.5 mg elemental iron (12.5 mg/mL).

Iron deficiency:

Adults – 10 mL (elemental iron 125 mg), may be diluted in 100 mL of sodium chloride 0.9% administered by intravenous (IV) infusion over 1 hour. It may also be administered undiluted as a slow IV injection (at a rate up to 12.5 mg/min). Most patients will require a minimum cumulative dose of 1 g elemental iron administered over 8 sessions at sequential dialysis treatments to achieve a favorable hemoglobin or hematocrit response. Patients may continue to require therapy with IV iron at the lowest dose necessary to maintain the target levels of hemoglobin, hematocrit, and laboratory parameters of iron storage within acceptable limits.

Sodium ferric gluconate complex has been administered at sequential dialysis sessions by infusion or by slow IV injection during the dialysis session itself.

Children – 0.12 mL/kg (1.5 mg/kg of elemental iron) diluted in 25 mL of sodium chloride 0.9% and administered by IV infusion over 1 hour at 8 sequential dialysis sessions. The maximum dosage should not exceed 125 mg/dose.

Admixture incompatibility: The compatibility of sodium ferric gluconate complex with IV infusion vehicles other than sodium chloride 0.9% has not been evaluated.

Actions

Pharmacology: Sodium ferric gluconate complex in sucrose injection is a stable macromolecular complex used to replete the total body content of iron.

Pharmacokinetics:

Absorption/Distribution – In multiple, sequential single-dose IV studies, peak drug levels (C_{max}) varied significantly by dosage and by rate of administration with the highest C_{max} observed in the regimen in which 125 mg was administered in 7 minutes (19 mg/L). The initial volume of distribution of 6 L corresponds well to calculated blood volume. The AUC for bound iron varied by dose from 17.5 mg•h/L (62.5 mg) to 35.6 mg•h/L (125 mg). Approximately 80% of drug bound iron was delivered to transferrin as a mononuclear ionic iron species within 24 hours of administration in each dosage regimen. Mean peak transferrin saturation did not exceed 100% and returned to near baseline by 40 hours after administration of each dosage regimen.

Metabolism/Excretion – The terminal elimination half-life for drug bound iron was approximately 1 hour, varying by dose but not by rate of administration. Total clearance was 3.02 to 5.35 L/h. In vitro, less than 1% of the iron species within sodium ferric gluconate complex can be dialyzed through membranes with pore sizes corresponding to 12,000 to 14,000 daltons over a period of up to 270 minutes.

Contraindications

All anemias not associated with iron deficiency; hypersensitivity to sodium ferric gluconate complex or any of its inactive components; evidence of iron overload.

Warnings/Precautions

Hypotension: Hypotension associated with lightheadedness, malaise, fatigue, weakness, or severe pain in the chest, back, flanks, or groin has been associated with administration of IV iron. These hypotensive reactions are not associated with signs of hypersensitivity and have usually resolved within 1 or 2 hours.

Benzyl alcohol: This product contains benzyl alcohol, which has been associated with a fatal "gasping syndrome" in premature infants.

Iron overload: Unnecessary therapy with parenteral iron will cause excess storage of iron with consequent possibility of iatrogenic hemosiderosis. Do not administer sodium ferric gluconate complex to patients with iron overload.

Hypersensitivity reactions: Serious hypersensitivity reactions have been rarely reported. One case of a life-threatening hypersensitivity reaction has been observed in a patient who received a single dose of sodium ferric gluconate complex in a postmarketing study. Three serious hypersensitivity reactions have been reported from the spontaneous reporting system.

Mutagenesis: A clastogenic effect was produced in an in vitro chromosomal aberration assay in Chinese hamster ovary cells.

Pregnancy: *Category B.*

Lactation: It is not known whether this drug is excreted in breast milk.

Children: Safety and efficacy have not been established in children younger than 6 years of age. Sodium ferric gluconate complex contains benzyl alcohol; therefore, do not use in neonates.

Elderly: Cautiously select dose for an elderly patient, usually starting at the low end of the dosing range, reflecting the greater frequency of decreased hepatic, renal, or cardiac function and of concomitant disease or other drug therapy.

Drug Interactions

Oral iron preparations: Coadministration of parenteral iron preparations may reduce absorption of oral iron preparations.

Adverse Reactions

Sodium ferric gluconate complex administered to patients during dialysis may cause transient hypotension. Administration may augment hypotension caused by dialysis.

Many chronic renal failure patients experience cramps, pain, nausea, rash, flushing, and pruritus.

Adults – Adverse reactions experienced by at least 5% of patients receiving sodium ferric gluconate complex include the following: abdominal pain, abnormal erythrocytes, asthenia, chest pain, cramps, diarrhea, dizziness, dyspnea, fatigue, fever, generalized edema, headache, hyperkalemia, hypertension, hypotension, injection-site reaction, leg cramps, nausea, pain, paresthesias, pruritus, syncope, tachycardia, upper respiratory tract infection, vomiting.

Children – Adverse reactions experienced by at least 3% of patients include the following: abdominal pain, diarrhea, fever, headache, hypertension, hypotension, infection, nausea, pharyngitis, rhinitis, tachycardia, thrombosis, vomiting.

FOLIC ACID (Folacin; Pteroylglutamic Acid; Folate)

Tablets: 0.4, 0.8, and 1 mg (*Rx*[a])	Various
Injection: 5 mg/mL (*Rx*)	Various, *Folvite* (Lederle)

[a] Although most folic acid products carry the *Rx* legend, products that provide no more than 0.4 mg (or 0.8 mg for pregnant or lactating women) may be *otc* items.

Indications

Megaloblastic anemia: Treatment of megaloblastic anemias due to a deficiency of folic acid as seen in tropical or nontropical sprue, anemias of nutritional origin, pregnancy, infancy, or childhood.

Administration and Dosage

Give orally, except in severe intestinal malabsorption. Although most patients with malabsorption cannot absorb food folates, they are able to absorb folic acid given orally.

Parenteral administration is not advocated but may be necessary in some individuals (eg, patients receiving parenteral or enteral alimentation). Give IM, IV, or subcutaneously if disease is very severe or GI absorption is very severely impaired. Doses greater than 0.1 mg should not be used unless anemia due to vitamin B_{12} deficiency has been ruled out or is being adequately treated with cobalamin.

Usual therapeutic dosage: Up to 1 mg daily. Resistant cases may require larger doses.

Maintenance: When clinical symptoms have subsided and the blood picture has normalized, use the dosage below. Never give less than 0.1 mg/day. Keep patients under close supervision and adjust maintenance dose if relapse appears imminent. In the presence of alcoholism, hemolytic anemia, anticonvulsant therapy, or chronic infection, the maintenance level may need to be increased.

Infants – 0.1 mg/day.

Children (younger than 4 years of age) – Up to 0.3 mg/day.

Adults and children (older than 4 years of age) – 0.4 mg/day.

Pregnant and lactating women – 0.8 mg/day.

Recommended Dietary Allowances (RDAs): Adult males, 0.15 to 0.2 mg/day; females, 0.15 to 0.18 mg/day.

For a complete listing of RDAs by age and sex, refer to the RDA table in the Nutritionals chapter.

Actions

Pharmacology: Exogenous folate is required for nucleoprotein synthesis and maintenance of normal erythropoiesis. Folic acid stimulates production of red and white blood cells and platelets in certain megaloblastic anemias.

Pharmacokinetics: Oral synthetic folic acid is a monoglutamate and is completely absorbed following administration, even in the presence of malabsorption syndromes.

Folic acid appears in the plasma approximately 15 to 30 minutes after an oral dose; peak levels are generally reached within 1 hour. After IV administration, the drug is rapidly cleared from the plasma. Folic acid is metabolized in the liver. Normal serum levels of total folate have been reported to be 5 to 15 ng/mL; normal CSF levels are approximately 16 to 21 ng/mL. In general, folate serum levels less than 5 ng/mL indicate folate deficiency, and levels less than 2 ng/mL usually result in megaloblastic anemia. A majority of the metabolic products appeared in the urine after 6 hours; excretion was generally complete within 24 hours.

Contraindications

Treatment of pernicious anemia and other megaloblastic anemias where vitamin B_{12} is deficient (not effective).

Warnings/Precautions

Pernicious anemia: Folic acid in doses greater than 0.1 mg/day may obscure pernicious anemia in that hematologic remission can occur while neurologic manifestations remain progressive.

Except during pregnancy and lactation, do not give folic acid in therapeutic doses greater than 0.4 mg/day until pernicious anemia has been ruled out. Do not include daily doses exceeding the Recommended Dietary Allowance in multivitamin preparations; if therapeutic amounts are necessary, give folic acid separately.

Pregnancy: Category A.

Lactation: Folic acid is excreted in breast milk.

Elderly: It may be prudent to consider the status of folate in people older than 65 years of age.

Drug Interactions

Drugs that may interact with folic acid include aminosalicylic acid, oral contraceptives, dihydrofolate reductase inhibitors (eg, methotrexate, trimethoprim), sulfasalazine, hydantoins.

Adverse Reactions

Adverse reactions may include erythema, skin rash, nausea, abdominal distention, altered sleep patterns, irritability, mental depression, confusion, and impaired judgement.

LEUCOVORIN CALCIUM (Folinic Acid; Citrovorum Factor)

Tablets: 5, 15, and 25 mg (*Rx*)	Various
Injection: 3 mg/mL (*Rx*)	Various
Powder for injection: 50, 100, and 350 mg/vial (*Rx*)	Various

Indications

Oral and parenteral: Leucovorin "rescue" after high-dose methotrexate therapy in osteosarcoma.

Parenteral: Treatment of megaloblastic anemias due to folic acid deficiency when oral therapy is not feasible.

In combination with 5-fluorouracil (5-FU) to prolong survival in the palliative treatment of patients with advanced colorectal cancer.

Administration and Dosage

Oral administration of doses greater than 25 mg is not recommended.

Advanced colorectal cancer: Either of the following 2 regimens is recommended:

1.) Leucovorin 200 mg/m^2 by slow IV injection over a minimum of 3 minutes, followed by 5-FU 370 mg/m^2 by IV injection.
2.) Leucovorin 20 mg/m^2 by IV injection followed by 5-FU 425 mg/m^2 by IV injection.

Treatment is repeated daily for 5 days. This 5-day treatment course may be repeated at 4-week (28-day) intervals for 2 courses and then repeated at 4- to 5-week (28- to 35-day) intervals provided that the patient has completely recovered from the toxic effects of the prior treatment course.

Institute dosage modifications of 5-FU as follows, based on the most severe toxicities: If diarrhea or stomatitis are moderate, WBC/mm^3 nadir is 1,000 to 1,900 or platelets/mm^3 are 25,000 to 75,000, reduce the 5-FU dose by 20%; if diarrhea or stomatitis are severe, WBC/mm^3 nadir is less than 1,000, or platelets/mm^3 are less than 25,000, reduce the 5-FU dose by 30%.

If no toxicity occurs, the 5-FU dose may increase 10%.

Defer treatment until WBCs are 4,000/mm^3 and platelets are 130,000/mm^3. If blood counts do not reach these levels within 2 weeks, discontinue treatment.

Leucovorin rescue after high-dose methotrexate therapy: The recommendations for leucovorin rescue are based on a methotrexate dose of 12 to 15 g/m^2 administered by IV infusion over 4 hours. Leucovorin rescue at a dose of 15 mg (approximately 10 mg/m^2) every 6 hours for 10 doses starts 24 hours after the beginning of the methotrexate infusion. In the presence of GI toxicity, nausea, or vomiting, administer leucovorin parenterally.

Determine serum creatinine and methotrexate levels at least once daily. Continue leucovorin administration, hydration, and urinary alkalinization (pH of at least 7) until the methotrexate level is less than 5×10^{-8}M (0.05 mcM).

If significant clinical toxicity is observed, extend leucovorin rescue for an additional 24 hours (total of 14 doses over 84 hours) in subsequent courses of therapy.

Impaired methotrexate elimination or inadvertent overdosage: Begin leucovorin rescue as soon as possible after an inadvertent overdosage and within 24 hours of methotrexate administration when there is delayed excretion. Administer leucovorin 10 mg/m^2 IV, IM, or orally every 6 hours until the serum methotrexate level is less than 10^{-8}M. In the presence of GI toxicity, nausea, or vomiting, administer leucovorin parenterally.

Determine serum creatinine and methotrexate levels at 24-hour intervals. If the 24-hour serum creatinine has increased 50% over baseline or if the 24- or 48-hour methotrexate level is greater than 5×10^{-6}M or greater than 9×10^{-7}M, respectively, increase the dose of leucovorin to 100 mg/m^2 IV every 3 hours until the methotrexate level is less than 10^{-8}M.

Megaloblastic anemia due to folic acid deficiency: No more than 1 mg leucovorin/day. There is no evidence that doses greater than 1 mg/day have greater efficacy than 1 mg doses.

Actions

Pharmacology: Leucovorin is one of several active, chemically reduced derivatives of folic acid. It is useful as an antidote to drugs that act as folic acid antagonists. Administration of leucovorin can counteract the therapeutic and toxic effects of folic acid antagonists such as methotrexate, which act by inhibiting dihydrofolate reductase.

Pharmacokinetics:

Leucovorin Pharmacokinetics[a]

Parameter	IV	IM	Oral
Total reduced folates:			
Mean peak conc. (ng/mL)	1,259 (range, 897 to 1,625)	436 (range, 240 to 725)	393 (range, 160 to 550)
Mean time to peak	10 min	52 min	2.3 h
Terminal half-life	6.2 h	6.2 h	5.7 h
5-Methyl-THF[b]			
Mean peak conc. (ng/mL)	258	226	367
Mean time to peak	1.3 h	2.8 h	2.4 h
5-Formyl-THF[c]			
Mean peak conc. (ng/mL)	1,206	360	51
Mean time to peak	10 min	28 min	1.2 h

[a] Following administration of a 25 mg dose.
[b] The major metabolite to which leucovorin is primarily converted in the intestinal mucosa and which becomes the predominant circulating form of the drug.
[c] The parent compound.

Following oral administration, leucovorin is rapidly absorbed and expands the serum pool of reduced folates. Oral absorption of leucovorin is saturable at doses greater than 25 mg. The apparent bioavailability of leucovorin was 97% for 25 mg, 75% for 50 mg, and 37% for 100 mg.

Contraindications

Pernicious anemia and other megaloblastic anemias secondary to lack of vitamin B_{12}.

Warnings/Precautions

Anemias: Leucovorin is improper therapy for pernicious anemia and other megaloblastic anemias secondary to the lack of vitamin B_{12}.

5-FU dosage/toxicity: Leucovorin enhances the toxicity of 5-FU.

Therapy with leucovorin/5-FU must not be initiated or continued in patients who have symptoms of GI toxicity of any severity, until those symptoms have completely resolved. Patients with diarrhea must be monitored with particular care until the diarrhea has resolved, as rapid clinical deterioration leading to death can occur.

Methotrexate concentrations: Monitoring of the serum methotrexate concentration is essential in determining the optimal dose and duration of treatment with leucovorin. Delayed methotrexate excretion may be caused by a third space fluid accumulation, renal insufficiency, or inadequate hydration. Under such circumstances, higher doses of leucovorin or prolonged administration may be indicated. Doses higher than those recommended for oral use must be given IV.

Calcium content: Because of the calcium content of the leucovorin solution, inject no more than 160 mg/min IV.

Folic acid antagonist overdosage: In the treatment of accidental overdosages of folic acid antagonists, administer leucovorin as promptly as possible. As the time interval between antifolate administration (eg, methotrexate) and leucovorin rescue increases, leucovorin's effectiveness in counteracting toxicity decreases.

Pregnancy: *Category C.*

Lactation: It is not known whether this drug is excreted in breast milk.

Elderly: Take particular care in the treatment of elderly or debilitated colorectal cancer patients, as these patients may be at increased risk of severe toxicity.

Drug Interactions

Drugs that may be affected by leucovorin include anticonvulsants.

Adverse Reactions

Allergic sensitization, including anaphylactoid reactions and urticaria, following administration of both oral and parenteral leucovorin.

The following adverse reactions occurred when leucovorin was administered at both high (200 mg/m^2) and low (20 mg/m^2) doses in combination with 5-FU: Leukopenia, thrombocytopenia, infection, nausea, vomiting, diarrhea, stomatitis, constipation, lethargy/malaise/fatigue, alopecia, dermatitis, anorexia.

VITAMIN B_{12}

CYANOCOBALAMIN	
Tablets; oral: 50, 100, 250, 500, and 1,000 mcg (*otc*)	Various
500 and 1,000 mcg (as crystalline cyanocobalamin) (*otc*)	Various
1,000 mcg on resin (*otc*)	*Twelve Resin-K* (Key Co.)
Tablets, extended-release: 1,000 and 1,500 mcg (*otc*)	*B-12* (Mason Natural)
Tablets, sublingual: 500, 1,000, 2,500, 5,000, and 6,000 mcg (*otc*)	Various, *B-12 Microlozenge* (Natures Bounty)
Liquid; oral: 200 mcg/spray (otc)	*Rapid B-12 Energy* (Mason Vitamins)
Lozenges: 50 and 500 mcg (*otc*)	Various
Spray, intranasal: 500 mcg per 0.1 mL (500 mcg/actuation) (*Rx*)	*Nascobal* (Par)
Injection: 1,000 mcg/mL (*Rx*)	Various

Indications

Vitamin B_{12} deficiency: Vitamin B_{12} deficiency due to malabsorption syndrome as seen in pernicious anemia; GI pathology, dysfunction or surgery; fish tapeworm infestation; malignancy of pancreas or bowel; gluten enteropathy; sprue; small bowel bacterial overgrowth; total or partial gastrectomy; accompanying folic acid deficiency.

Increased vitamin B_{12} requirements: Increased vitamin B_{12} requirements associated with pregnancy, thyrotoxicosis, hemolytic anemia, hemorrhage, malignancy, and hepatic and renal disease.

Vitamin B_{12} absorption test: Vitamin B_{12} absorption test (Schilling test).

Administration and Dosage

CYANOCOBALAMIN, CRYSTALLINE:

Addisonian pernicious anemia – Parenteral therapy is required for life; oral therapy is not dependable. Administer 100 mcg daily for 6 or 7 days by IM or deep subcutaneous injection. If there is clinical improvement and a reticulocyte response, give the same amount on alternate days for 7 doses, then every 3 to 4 days for another 2 to 3 weeks. By this time, hematologic values should have become normal. Follow this regimen with 100 mcg monthly for life. Administer folic acid concomitantly if needed.

Other patients with vitamin B_{12} deficiency – In seriously ill patients, administer both vitamin B_{12} and folic acid. It is not necessary to withhold therapy until the precise cause of B_{12} deficiency is established. For hematologic signs, children may be given 10 to 50 mcg/day for 5 to 10 days followed by 100 to 250 mcg/dose every 2 to 4 weeks; for neurologic signs, 100 mcg/day for 10 to 15 days, then once or twice weekly for several months, possibly tapering to 250 to 1,000 mcg/month by 1 year.

Oral – Up to 1000 mcg/day. Oral vitamin B_{12} therapy is not usually recommended for vitamin B_{12} deficiency. The maximum amount of vitamin B_{12} that can be absorbed from a single oral dose is 1 to 5 mcg. The percent absorbed decreases with increasing doses.

IM or subcutaneous – 30 mcg/day for 5 to 10 days followed by 100 to 200 mcg/month. Larger doses (eg, 1,000 mcg) have been recommended, even though a larger amount is lost through excretion. However, it is possible that a greater amount is retained, allowing for fewer injections.

CYANOCOBALAMIN, INTRANASAL: Prime prior to initial use. Repriming between doses is not necessary if the unit is upright. Administer at least 1 hour before or 1 hour after ingestion of hot foods or liquids.

Vitamin B_{12} malabsorption in remission following injectable vitamin B_{12} therapy – 500 mcg intranasally once weekly.

Vitamin B_{12} deficiency (CaloMist) – For maintenance of vitamin B_{12} concentrations after normalization with IM vitamin B_{12} therapy in patients with vitamin B_{12} deficiency who have no nervous system involvement, give one spray in each nostril once daily (25 mcg per nostril, total daily dose of 50 mcg). The dose should be increased to one spray in each nostril twice daily (total daily dose 100 mcg) in patients with an inadequate response to once-daily dosing.

The dosing of *CaloMist* and other intranasal medications should be separated by several hours, and these patients should have more frequent monitoring of vitamin B_{12} concentrations because of the potential for erratic absorption.

Actions

Pharmacology: Vitamin B_{12} is essential to growth, cell reproduction, hematopoiesis, and nucleoprotein and myelin synthesis. Its physiologic role is associated with methylation, participating in nucleic acid and protein synthesis. Cyanocobalamin participates in red blood cell formation through activation of folic acid coenzymes.

Pharmacokinetics: Absorption of vitamin B_{12} depends on the presence of sufficient intrinsic factor and calcium. In general, absorption of oral B_{12} is inadequate in malabsorptive states and in pernicious anemia (unless intrinsic factor is simultaneously administered).

Cyanocobalamin – Cyanocobalamin is rapidly absorbed from IM and subcutaneous injection sites; the plasma level peaks within 1 hour. Once absorbed, it is bound to plasma proteins, stored mainly in the liver and is slowly released when needed to carry out normal cellular metabolic functions. Within 48 hours after injection of 100 to 1,000 mcg of vitamin B_{12}, 50% to 98% of the dose appears in the urine. The major portion is excreted within the first 8 hours. More rapid excretion occurs with IV administration; there is little opportunity for liver storage.

Peak concentration of B_{12} after intranasal administration is 1 to 2 hours; Bioavailability is 8.9%.

Contraindications

Hypersensitivity to cobalt, vitamin B_{12}, or any component of these products.

Warnings/Precautions

Inadequate response: A blunted or impeded therapeutic response may be due to infection, uremia, bone marrow suppressant drugs, concurrent iron or folic acid deficiency, or misdiagnosis.

Vitamin B_{12} deficiency: Vitamin B_{12} deficiency allowed to progress for more than 3 months may produce permanent degenerative lesions of the spinal cord.

Optic nerve atrophy: Patients with early Leber disease (hereditary optic nerve atrophy) treated with cyanocobalamin suffer severe and swift optic atrophy.

Hypokalemia: Hypokalemia and sudden death may occur in severe megaloblastic anemia which is treated intensely.

Test dose: Anaphylactic shock and death have occurred after parenteral vitamin B_{12} administration. Give an intradermal test dose in patients sensitive to the cobalamins.

Folate: Doses greater than 10 mcg/day may produce hematologic response in patients with folate deficiency. Indiscriminate use may mask the true diagnosis of pernicious anemia.

Doses of folic acid greater than 0.1 mg/day may result in hematologic remission in patients with vitamin B_{12} deficiency. Neurologic manifestations will not be prevented with folic acid, and if not treated with vitamin B_{12}, irreversible damage will result.

Polycythemia vera: Vitamin B_{12} deficiency may suppress the signs of polycythemia vera.

Vegetarian diets: Vegetarian diets containing no animal products (including milk products or eggs) do not supply any vitamin B_{12}.

Immunodeficient patients: Vitamin B_{12} malabsorption may occur in patients with AIDS or HIV infection. Consider monitoring levels.

Nasal symptoms: The effectiveness of intranasal cyanocobalamin in patients with nasal congestion, allergic rhinitis, and upper respiratory tract infections has not been determined. Defer treatment until symptoms have subsided.

Pregnancy: Category C (parenteral).

Lactation: Vitamin B_{12} is excreted in breast milk in concentrations that approximate the mother's vitamin B_{12} blood level. Amounts of B_{12} recommended by the Food and Nutrition Board, National Academy of Sciences-National Research Council (2.6 mcg/day) should be consumed during lactation.

Children: The Food and Nutrition Board, National Academy of Sciences-National Research Council recommends a daily intake of 0.3 to 0.5 mcg/day for infants younger than 1 year of age and 0.7 to 1.4 mcg/day for children 1 to 10 years of age.

Monitoring: During treatment of severe megaloblastic anemia, monitor serum potassium levels closely for the first 48 hours and replace potassium if necessary. Obtain reticulocyte counts, hematocrit and vitamin B_{12}, iron and folic acid plasma levels prior to treatment and between the fifth and seventh days of therapy, and then frequently until the hematocrit is normal. If folate levels are low, also administer folic acid.

Drug Interactions

Drugs that may affect vitamin B_{12} include aminosalicylic acid, chloramphenicol, colchicine, and alcohol.

Drug/Lab test interactions: Methotrexate, pyrimethamine, and most antibiotics invalidate folic acid and vitamin B_{12} diagnostic microbiological blood assays.

Adverse Reactions

The following reactions are associated with parenteral vitamin B_{12}: Anaphylactic shock, death, pulmonary edema, congestive heart failure early in treatment, severe and swift optic nerve atrophy.

PHYTONADIONE (K_1, Phylloquinone, Methylphytyl Naphthoquinone)

Tablets: 5 mg (*Rx*)	*Mephyton* (Merck)
Injection, emulsion: 2, 10 mg/mL (*Rx*)	(Hospira)

Warning:

IV or IM use: Severe reactions, including fatalities, have occurred during and immediately after intravenous (IV) injection, even with precautions to dilute the injection and to avoid rapid infusion. Severe reactions, including fatalities, also have been reported following intramuscular (IM) administration. Typically, these severe reactions have resembled hypersensitivity or anaphylaxis, including shock and cardiac or respiratory arrest. Some patients have exhibited these severe reactions on receiving phytonadione for the first time. Therefore, restrict the IV and IM routes to those situations where the subcutaneous route is not feasible and the serious risk involved is considered justified.

Indications

Coagulation disorders: Coagulation disorders due to faulty formation of factors II, VII, IX, and X when caused by vitamin K deficiency or interference with vitamin K activity.

Oral: Anticoagulant-induced prothrombin deficiency caused by coumarin or indandione derivatives; hypoprothrombinemia secondary to antibacterial therapy; hypoprothrombinemia secondary to administration of salicylates; hypoprothrombinemia secondary to obstructive jaundice or biliary fistulas, but only if bile salts are administered concurrently since otherwise the oral vitamin K will not be absorbed.

Parenteral: Phytonadione injection is indicated in anticoagulant-induced prothrombin deficiency caused by coumarin or indandione derivatives, prophylaxis and therapy of hemorrhagic disease of the newborn, hypoprothrombinemia secondary to factors limiting absorption or synthesis of vitamin K, and other drug-induced hypoprothrombinemia where it is definitely shown that the result is due to interference with vitamin K metabolism.

Administration and Dosage

Oral Phytonadione Summary of Dosage Guidelines	
Adults	Initial dosage
Anticoagulant-induced prothrombin deficiency (caused by coumarin or indandione derivatives)	2.5 to 10 mg or up to 25 mg (rarely 50 mg)
Hypoprothrombinemia due to other causes (antibiotics; salicylates or other drugs; factors limiting absorption or synthesis)	2.5 to 25 mg or more (rarely up to 50 mg)

Phytonadione Injection Summary of Dosage Guidelines	
Newborns	Dosage
Hemorrhagic disease of the newborn	
Prophylaxis	0.5 to 1 mg IM within 1 hour of birth
Treatment	1 mg subcutaneously or IM (higher doses may be necessary if the mother has been receiving oral anticoagulants)
Adults	**Initial dosage**
Anticoagulant-induced prothrombin deficiency (caused by coumarin or indandione derivatives)	2.5 to 10 mg or up to 25 mg (rarely 50 mg)
Hypoprothrombinemia due to other causes (antibiotics; salicylates or other drugs; factors limiting absorption or synthesis)	2.5 to 25 mg or more (rarely up to 50 mg)

Hypoprothrombinemia due to other causes in adults: If possible, discontinue or reduce the dosage of drugs interfering with coagulation mechanisms (eg, salicylates, antibiotics) as an alternative to phytonadione. The severity of the coagulation disorder should determine whether the immediate administration of phytonadione is required.

The oral route should be avoided when the clinical disorder would prevent proper absorption. Bile salts must be given with the tablets when the endogenous supply of bile to the GI tract is deficient.

Anticoagulant-induced prothrombin deficiency in adults: Determine subsequent doses by prothrombin time (PT) response or clinical condition. If in 6 to 8 hours after parenteral administration (or 12 to 48 hours after oral administration), the PT has not been shortened satisfactorily, repeat dose. If shock or excessive blood loss occurs, transfusion of blood or fresh frozen plasma may be required.

Treatment of hemorrhagic disease of the newborn: Whole blood or component therapy may be indicated if bleeding is excessive. Give phytonadione concurrently.

Administration of injection: Whenever possible, give phytonadione by the subcutaneous route. When IV administration is considered unavoidable, inject the drug very slowly, not exceeding 1 mg per minute.

Actions

Pharmacology: Phytonadione tablets and phytonadione aqueous colloidal solution of vitamin K_1 for parenteral injection posses the same type and degree of activity as does naturally-occurring vitamin K, which is necessary for the production via the liver of active prothrombin (factor II), proconvertin (factor VII), plasma thromboplastin component (factor IX), and Stuart factor (factor X). The pharmacological action of vitamin K is related to its normal physiological function; that is, to promote the hepatic biosynthesis of vitamin K–dependent clotting factors.

Pharmacokinetics: Phytonadione is only absorbed from the GI tract via intestinal lymphatics in the presence of bile salts. Although initially concentrated in the liver, vitamin K is rapidly metabolized, and very little tissue accumulation occurs.

Contraindications

Hypersensitivity to any component of this medication.

Warnings/Precautions

Oral anticoagulant-induced hypoprothrombinemia: Vitamin K will not counteract the anticoagulant action of heparin.

Immediate coagulant effect should not be expected. It takes a minimum of 1 to 2 hours for a measurable improvement in the PT.

The prothrombin test is sensitive to the levels of factors II, VII, and X. Whole blood or component therapy may also be necessary if bleeding is severe.

With phytonadione use and anticoagulant therapy indicated, the patient is faced with the same clotting hazards prior to starting anticoagulant therapy. Phytonadione is not a clotting agent, but overzealous therapy may restore original thromboembolic phenomena conditions. Keep dosage as low as possible and check PT regularly.

Benzyl alcohol: Benzyl alcohol as a preservative in bacteriostatic sodium chloride injection has been associated with toxicity in newborns.

Renal function impairment: Patients with impaired kidney function, including premature neonates, who receive parenteral levels of aluminum at more than 4 to 5 mcg/kg/day accumulate aluminum at levels associated with CNS and bone toxicity. Tissue loading may occur at even lower rates of administration.

Hepatic function impairment: Repeated large doses of vitamin K are not warranted in liver disease if the initial response is unsatisfactory. Failure to respond to vitamin K may indicate a coagulation defect or a condition unresponsive to vitamin K.

Paradoxically, giving excessive doses of vitamin K or its analogs in an attempt to correct hypoprothrombinemia associated with severe hepatitis or cirrhosis may actually result in further depression of the prothrombin concentration.

Pregnancy: Category C.

Lactation: It is not known whether this drug is excreted in human milk.

Children: Safety and efficacy in children have not been established. Hemolysis, jaundice, and hyperbilirubinemia in newborns, particularly in premature infants, have been reported with vitamin K. These effects may be dose related. Therefore, do not exceed recommended dose.

Benzyl alcohol has been reported to be associated with a fatal "gasping syndrome" in premature infants.

Monitoring: Prothrombin time should be checked regularly as clinical conditions indicate.

Drug Interactions

Drugs that may interact include anticoagulants and mineral oil.

Adverse Reactions

Adverse reactions from parenteral administration may include transient "flushing sensations" and "peculiar" sensations of taste. Deaths have occurred after IV administration. Hyperbilirubinemia has been observed in the newborn following administration of phytonadione. Anaphylactoid reactions may occur with either dose form.

Severe reactions, including fatalities also have been reported following IM administration. Typically, these severe reactions have resembled hypersensitivity or anaphylaxis, including shock and cardiac or respiratory arrest. Pain, swelling, and tenderness at the injection site may occur.

EPOETIN ALFA (Erythropoietin; EPO)

Injection; solution: 2,000, 3,000, 4,000, 10,000, 20,000, and 40,000 units per mL (*Rx*)	*Epogen* (Amgen), *Procrit* (Centocor Ortho Biotech)

Warning:

Renal failure: Patients experienced greater risks for death and serious CV events when administered erythropoiesis-stimulating agents (ESAs) to target higher versus lower hemoglobin levels (13.5 vs 11.3 g/dL; 14 vs 10 g/dL) in 2 clinical studies. Individualize dosing to achieve and maintain hemoglobin levels within the range of 10 to 12 g/dL.

Cancer:

- ESAs shortened overall survival and/or increased the risk of tumor progression or recurrence in some clinical studies in patients with breast, non–small cell lung, head and neck, lymphoid, and cervical cancers.
- To decrease these risks, as well as the risk of serious cardio- and thrombovascular events, use the lowest dose needed to avoid red blood cell transfusions.
- Use ESAs only for treatment of anemia caused by concomitant myelosuppressive chemotherapy.
- ESAs are not indicated for patients receiving myelosuppressive therapy when the anticipated outcome is cure.
- Discontinue following the completion of a chemotherapy course.

Perisurgery: Epoetin alfa increased the rate of deep venous thromboses in patients not receiving prophylactic anticoagulation. Consider deep venous thrombosis prophylaxis.

See also Warnings/Precautions, Indications, and Administration and Dosage for more information.

Indications

Anemia associated with chronic renal failure (CRF): Treatment of anemia associated with CRF, including patients on dialysis (end-stage renal disease) and patients not on dialysis, to elevate or maintain the red blood cell level (as manifested by the hematocrit or hemoglobin determinations) and to decrease the need for transfusions. Nondialysis patients with symptomatic anemia considered for therapy should have a hemoglobin less than 10 g/dL. Not intended for patients who require immediate correction of severe anemia.

Anemia related to zidovudine therapy in HIV-infected patients: To elevate or maintain the red blood cell level (as manifested by the hematocrit or hemoglobin determinations) and to decrease the need for transfusions in these patients.

Anemia in cancer patients on chemotherapy: Treatment of anemia in patients with nonmyeloid malignancies where anemia is due to the effect of concomitantly administered chemotherapy. It is intended to decrease the need for transfusions in patients who will be receiving chemotherapy for a minimum of 2 months.

Reduction of allogeneic transfusion in surgery patients: For the treatment of anemic patients (hemoglobin greater than 10 to 13 g/dL or less) scheduled to undergo elective, noncardiac, nonvascular surgery to reduce the need for allogeneic blood transfusions.

Administration and Dosage

CRF patients:

Starting dosage –

Adults: 50 to 100 units/kg 3 times per week IV or subcutaneously.

Children on dialysis: 50 units/kg 3 times per week IV or subcutaneously.

Dose reduction – If the hemoglobin is increasing and approaching 12 g/dL or increases by more than 1 g/dL in any 2-week period, reduce the dose by approximately 25%. If the hemoglobin continues to increase, the dose should be temporarily withheld until the hemoglobin begins to decrease, at which point therapy should be reinitiated at a dose approximately 25% below the previous dose.

Dose increase – Increases in dose should not be made more frequently than once a month.

If the hemoglobin is less than 10 g/dL, the increase in hemoglobin is less than 1 g/dL over 4 weeks, and iron stores are adequate, the dose of epoetin alfa may be increased by approximately 25% of the previous dose. Further increases may be made at 4-week intervals until the specified hemoglobin is obtained.

If the transferrin saturation is more than 20%, the dose of epoetin alfa may be increased. Such dose increases should not be made more frequently than once a month, unless clinically indicated, because the response time of the hemoglobin to a dose increase can be 2 to 6 weeks. Hemoglobin should be measured twice weekly for 2 to 6 weeks following dose increases.

Maintenance –

Adults not on dialysis: The dose should be individualized to maintain hemoglobin levels between 10 and 12 g/dL. A dose of 75 to 150 units/kg/week has been shown to maintain hematocrit of 36% to 38% for up to 6 months. The maintenance dose must also be individualized.

Adults on hemodialysis: Median dose is 75 units/kg 3 times/week (range, 12.5 to 525 units/kg 3 times/week).

Children on hemodialysis: Median dose of 167 units/kg/week (range, 49 to 477 units/kg/week) in divided doses, 2 to 3 times/week.

Children on peritoneal dialysis: Median dose of 76 units/kg/week (range, 24 to 323 units/kg/week) in divided doses of 2 to 3 times per week to achieve the target hematocrit range of 30% to 36%.

Lack or loss of response – If a patient fails to respond or maintain a response, an evaluation for causative factors should be undertaken. If the transferrin saturation is less than 20%, supplemental iron should be administered.

For patients whose hemoglobin dose not attain a level within the range of 10 to 12 g/dL despite the use of appropriate epoetin alfa dose titrations over a 12-week period:

- do not administer higher epoetin alfa doses and use the lowest dose that will maintain a hemoglobin level sufficient to avoid the need for recurrent RBC transfusions,
- evaluate and treat for other causes of anemia, and
- thereafter, hemoglobin should continue to be monitored and, if responsiveness improves, epoetin alfa dose adjustments should be made as described; discontinue epoetin alfa if responsiveness does not improve and the patient needs recurrent RBC transfusions.

Pretherapy iron evaluation – Prior to and during epoetin therapy, the patient's iron stores, including transferrin saturation (serum iron divided by iron binding capacity) and serum ferritin, should be evaluated. Transferrin saturation should be at least 20%, and ferritin should be at least 100 ng/mL. Virtually all patients will eventually require supplemental iron to increase or maintain transferrin saturation to levels that will adequately support erythropoiesis stimulated by epoetin alfa.

Zidovudine-treated, HIV-infected patients: Available evidence suggests that patients receiving zidovudine with endogenous serum erythropoietin levels greater than 500 milliunits/mL are unlikely to respond to therapy. The dose of epoetin alfa should be titrated for each patient to achieve and maintain the lowest hemoglobin level sufficient to avoid the need for blood transfusion, not to exceed 12 g/dL.

Adults, initial dose – For patients with serum erythropoietin levels 500 milliunits/mL or less who are receiving a dose of zidovudine 4,200 mg/week or less, the recommended starting dose is 100 units/kg as an IV or subcutaneous injection 3 times/week for 8 weeks.

Children, dose range – Published literature has reported the use of epoetin alfa in zidovudine-treated, anemic, HIV-infected children 8 months to 17 years of age treated with 50 to 400 units/kg subcutaneously or IV 2 to 3 times per week.

If the response is not satisfactory in terms of reducing transfusion requirements or increasing hematocrit after 8 weeks of therapy, the dose can be increased by 50 to 100 units/kg 3 times/week. Evaluate response every 4 to 8 weeks thereafter and adjust the dose accordingly by 50 to 100 units/kg increments 3 times/week. If patients have not responded satisfactorily to a 300 units/kg dose 3 times/week, it is unlikely that they will respond to higher doses.

Maintenance dose – When the desired response is attained, titrate the dose to maintain the response based on factors such as variations in zidovudine dose and the presence of intercurrent infectious or inflammatory episodes. If hemoglobin exceeds 12 g/dL, stop the dose until hemoglobin drops to 11 g/dL. When resuming treatment, reduce the dose by 25%, then titrate to maintain desired hemoglobin.

Cancer patients on chemotherapy: Individually titrate to achieve and maintain hemoglobin levels between 10 and 12 g/dL.

Three Times Weekly Dosing for Cancer Patients on Chemotherapy

	Starting dose
Adults	150 units/kg 3 times/week subcutaneously or 40,000 units subcutaneously weekly.
Children	600 units/kg (maximum of 40,000 units) IV once per week
Reduce dose by 25% when:	1) Hemoglobin reaches a level needed to avoid transfusion or 2) Hemoglobin increases by more than 1 g/dL in any 2-week period.
Withhold dose when:	Hemoglobin exceeds 12 g/dL, until the hemoglobin falls to 11 g/dL, and then restart dose at 25% below the previous dose.
Discontinue:	Following the completion of a chemotherapy course.
Increase dose if:	Response is not satisfactory (no reduction in transfusion requirements or rise in hemoglobin) after 8 weeks; increase dose to 300 units/kg 3 times/week. or If response is not satisfactory (no increase in hemoglobin by 1 g/dL or more after 4 weeks of therapy), increase dose to 60,000 units subcutaneously weekly for adults and 900 units/kg IV (max, 60,000 units) for children.
Suggested target hemoglobin range	10 to 12 g/dL

Weekly Dosing for Cancer Patients on Chemotherapy

	Starting dose
Adults	40,000 units subcutaneously weekly
Increase dose if:	After 4 weeks of therapy, the hemoglobin has not increased by 1 g/dL or more, in the absence of RBC transfusion; increase the dose to 60,000 units weekly for adults and 900 units/kg IV (max, 60,000 units) in children.
Withhold dose if:	Hemoglobin exceeds 12 g/dL, and when the hemoglobin falls to less than 11 g/dL, then restart dose at 25% below the previous dose.
Reduce dose by 25% when:	Treatment produces a very rapid hemoglobin response (eg, hemoglobin increases by more than 1 g/dL in any 2-week period).

Surgery – Prior to initiating treatment with epoetin alfa, a hemoglobin should be obtained to establish that it is more than 10 g/dL to less than or equal to 13 g/dL. The recommended dose is 300 units/kg/day subcutaneously for 10 days before surgery, on the day of surgery and for 4 days after surgery.

An alternate dose schedule is 600 units/kg subcutaneously in once-weekly doses (21, 14, and 7 days before surgery) plus a fourth dose on the day of surgery.

All patients should receive adequate iron supplementation. Initiate iron supplementation no later than the beginning of treatment with epoetin alfa and continue throughout the course of therapy. Strongly consider deep vein thrombosis prophylaxis.

Actions

Pharmacology: Erythropoietin is a glycoprotein that stimulates red blood cell production. It is produced in the kidney and stimulates the division and differentiation of erythroid progenitors in bone marrow. Hypoxia and anemia generally increase the production of erythropoietin, which in turn stimulates erythropoiesis. In patients with CRF, erythropoietin production is impaired; this deficiency is the primary cause of their anemia. Epoetin alfa stimulates erythropoiesis in anemic patients on dialysis and those who do not require regular dialysis.

Pharmacokinetics:

Absorption/Distribution – Within the therapeutic dosage range, detectable levels of plasma erythropoietin are maintained for at least 24 hours. After subcutaneous administration of epoetin alfa to patients with CRF, peak serum levels are achieved within 5 to 24 hours after administration and decline slowly thereafter. The half-life is similar between adult patients not on dialysis with a serum creatinine level of more than 3 and those maintained on dialysis. The half-life in healthy volunteers is approximately 20% shorter than in CRF patients.

Metabolism/Excretion – Epoetin alfa IV is eliminated via first-order kinetics with a circulating half-life of 4 to 13 hours in patients with CRF. In anemic cancer patients, the average elimination half-life was similar (40 hours; range, 16 to 67 hours) after both dosing regimens.

Special populations –

Children: Limited data are available in neonates. A study of 7 preterm, very low birth weight neonates and 10 healthy adults given IV erythropoietin suggested that distribution volume was approximately 1.5 to 2 times higher in preterm neonates than in healthy adults, and clearance was approximately 3 times higher in preterm neonates than in healthy adults.

Contraindications

Uncontrolled hypertension; hypersensitivity to mammalian cell-derived products or to human albumin.

Warnings/Precautions

Increased mortality, serious cardiovascular (CV) and thromboembolic events: Epoetin alfa and other ESAs increased the risk for death and serious CV events in controlled clinical trials when administered to target a hemoglobin of more than 12 g/dL. There was an increased risk of serious arterial and venous thromboembolic reactions, including myocardial infarction (MI), stroke, CHF, and hemodialysis graft occlusion. A rate of hemoglobin rise of more than 1 g/dL over 2 weeks may also contribute to these risks.

Cancer patients: An increased incidence of thrombotic events has also been observed in patients with cancer treated with erythropoietic agents.

Increased mortality and/or tumor progression: ESAs, when administered to target a hemoglobin of more than 12 g/dL, shortened the time to tumor progression in patients with advanced head and neck cancer receiving radiation therapy. ESAs also shortened survival in patients with metastatic breast cancer receiving chemotherapy when administered to target a hemoglobin of more than 12 g/dL.

Surgery patients: An increased incidence of deep vein thrombosis in patients receiving epoetin alfa undergoing surgical orthopedic procedures has been observed.

Pure red cell aplasia (PRCA): PRCA has been reported in a limited number of patients exposed to epoetin alfa. This has been reported predominantly in patients with CRF receiving epoetin alfa by subcutaneous administration. Evaluate any patient with loss of response to epoetin alfa for the etiology of loss of effect. Discontinue epoetin alfa in any patient with evidence of PRCA and evaluate the patient for the presence of binding and neutralizing antibodies to epoetin alfa, native erythropoietin, and any other recombinant erythropoietin administered to the patient. In patients with PRCA secondary to neutralizing antibodies to erythropoietin, do not administer epoetin alfa, and do not switch such patients to another product as anti-erythropoietin antibodies cross-react with other erythropoietins.

Albumin (human): Epoetin alfa contains albumin, a derivative of human blood. Based on effective donor screening and product manufacturing processes, it carries an extremely remote risk for transmission of viral diseases. No cases of transmission of viral diseases or Creutzfeldt-Jakob disease have ever been identified for albumin.

Hypertension: Do not treat patients with uncontrolled hypertension with epoetin alfa; control blood pressure adequately before initiation of therapy. Up to 80% of patients with CRF have a history of hypertension. Although there does not appear to be any direct pressor effects of epoetin alfa, blood pressure may rise during epoetin alfa therapy. During the early phase of treatment when the hematocrit is increasing, approximately 25% of patients on dialysis may require initiation of, or increases in, antihypertensive therapy. Hypertensive encephalopathy and seizures have been observed in patients with CRF treated with epoetin alfa.

Seizures: Seizures have occurred in patients with CRF participating in epoetin alfa clinical trials. Given the potential for an increased risk of seizure during the first 90 days of therapy, closely monitor blood pressure and the presence of premonitory neurologic symptoms. While the relationship between seizures and the rate of rise in hemoglobin is uncertain, it is recommended that the dose be decreased if the hemoglobin increase exceeds 1 g/dL in any 2-week period.

Hematology: Exacerbation of porphyria has been observed rarely in patients with CRF treated with epoetin alfa. However, epoetin alfa has not caused increased urinary excretion of porphyrin metabolites in healthy volunteers, even in the presence of a rapid erythropoietic response. Nevertheless, use epoetin alfa with caution in patients with known porphyria.

The elevated bleeding time characteristic of CRF decreases toward normal after correction of anemia in patients treated with epoetin alfa. Reduction of bleeding time also occurs after correction of anemia by transfusion.

Iron evaluation: During epoetin alfa therapy, absolute or functional iron deficiency may develop. Functional iron deficiency, with normal ferritin levels but low transferrin saturation, is presumably because of the inability to mobilize iron stores rapidly enough to support increased erythropoiesis. Transferrin saturation should be at least 20%, and ferritin should be at least 100 ng/mL.

Prior to and during epoetin alfa therapy, evaluate the patient's iron status, including transferrin saturation (serum iron divided by iron-binding capacity) and serum ferritin. Virtually all patients will eventually require supplemental iron to increase or maintain transferrin saturation to levels that will adequately support erythropoiesis stimulated by epoetin alfa. Provide all surgery patients being treated with epoetin alfa with adequate iron supplementation throughout the course of therapy in order to support erythropoiesis and avoid depletion of iron stores.

Bone marrow fibrosis: Bone marrow fibrosis is a complication of CRF and may be related to secondary hyperparathyroidism or unknown factors.

Lack or loss of response: If the patient fails to respond or to maintain a response to doses within the recommended range, consider and evaluate the following etiologies:

1.) Iron deficiency. Virtually all patients will eventually require supplemental iron therapy.
2.) Underlying infectious, inflammatory, or malignant processes.
3.) Occult blood loss.
4.) Underlying hematologic diseases (ie, refractory anemia, thalassemia, other myelodysplastic disorders).
5.) Vitamin deficiencies: folic acid or vitamin B_{12}.
6.) Hemolysis.
7.) Aluminum intoxication.
8.) Osteitis fibrosa cystica.

9.) Pure red cell aplasia or antierythropoietin antibody-associated anemia. In the absence of another etiology, evaluate the patient for evidence of pure red cell aplasia and test sera for the presence of antibodies to erythropoietin.

Diet: Reinforce the importance of compliance with dietary and dialysis prescriptions.

Hyperkalemia: Hyperkalemia is not uncommon in patients with CRF.

Dialysis management: Therapy with epoetin alfa results in an increase in hematocrit and a decrease in plasma volume that could affect dialysis efficiency.

Benzyl alcohol: Benzyl alcohol, which is contained in some of these products as a preservative, has been associated with an increased incidence of neurological and other complications in premature infants that are sometimes fatal.

Hypersensitivity reactions: Skin rashes and urticaria are rare, mild, and transient. If an anaphylactoid reaction occurs, immediately discontinue the drug and initiate appropriate therapy.

Renal function impairment: In adult patients with CRF not on dialysis, closely monitor renal function and fluid and electrolyte balance.

Fertility impairment: In female rats treated IV with epoetin alfa, there was a trend for slightly increased fetal wastage at doses of 100 and 500 units/kg.

Pregnancy: Category C.

Lactation: It is not known whether epoetin alfa is excreted in breast milk.

Children: Safety and efficacy have not been established in patients younger than 1 month of age.

Monitoring:

Patients with CRF not requiring dialysis – Monitor blood pressure and hematocrit no less frequently than for patients maintained on dialysis. Closely monitor renal function and fluid and electrolyte balance, as an improved sense of well-being may obscure the need to initiate dialysis in some patients.

Determine the hemoglobin twice a week until it has stabilized in the target range and the maintenance dose has been established. After any dose adjustment, determine the hemoglobin twice weekly for at least 2 to 6 weeks until the hemoglobin has stabilized; then monitor at regular intervals.

Perform complete blood count with differential and platelet counts regularly. Modest increases have occurred in platelets and white blood cell counts, but values remained within normal ranges.

Monitor serum chemistry values (including blood urea nitrogen, uric acid, creatinine, phosphorus, and potassium) regularly.

Zidovudine-treated, HIV-infected and cancer patients – Measure hemoglobin once a week until it is stabilized; measure periodically thereafter.

Iron evaluation – During therapy, absolute or functional iron deficiency may develop. Transferrin saturation should be at least 20%, and ferritin should be at least 100 ng/mL. Prior to and during therapy, evaluate the patient's iron status, including transferrin saturation (serum iron divided by iron binding capacity) and serum ferritin. Virtually all patients will eventually require supplemental iron to increase or maintain transferrin saturation to levels that will adequately support epoetin alfa-stimulated erythropoiesis.

Adverse Reactions

CRF patients – Epoetin alfa is generally well tolerated. The following adverse reactions are frequent (greater than 3%) sequelae of CRF and are not necessarily due to epoetin alfa therapy: hypertension, headache, arthralgia, nausea, edema, fatigue, diarrhea, vomiting, chest pain, asthenia, dizziness, skin reaction, and clotted vascular access.

Zidovudine-treated HIV-infected patients – Adverse experiences greater than 3% were consistent with the progression of HIV infection: pyrexia, fatigue, headache, cough, diarrhea, rash, nausea, respiratory congestion, shortness of breath, asthenia, skin reaction, and dizziness.

Surgery patients – Adverse reactions 3% or more include the following: pyrexia, nausea, constipation, skin reactions at injection site, vomiting, itching, insomnia, headache, dizziness, urinary tract infection, hypertension, anxiety, diarrhea, dyspepsia, edema, deep venous thrombosis.

Cancer patients in chemotherapy – Adverse reactions greater than 3% were consistent with the underlying disease state: pyrexia, diarrhea, nausea, vomiting, edema, asthenia, fatigue, shortness of breath, paresthesia, upper respiratory infection, dizziness, and trunk pain.

Children with CRF – In children with CRF on dialysis, the pattern of most adverse reactions was similar to that found in adults. Additional adverse reactions reported during the double-blind phase in more than 10% of children in either treatment group were the following: abdominal pain; constipation; cough; dialysis access complications, including access infections and peritonitis in those receiving peritoneal dialysis; fever; pharyngitis; and upper respiratory tract infection.

DARBEPOETIN ALFA

Injection, solution[a]: 25 mcg per 0.42 mL, 25 mcg/mL, 40 mcg per 0.4 mL, 40 mcg/mL, 60 per 0.3 mL, 60 mcg/mL, 100 mcg per 0.5 mL, 100 mcg/mL, 150 mcg per 0.3 mL, 150 mcg per 0.75 mL, 200 mcg per 0.4 mL, 200 mcg/mL, 300 mcg per 0.6 mL, 300 mcg/mL, and 500 mcg/mL (*Rx*)	*Aranesp* (Amgen)

[a] The polysorbate solution contains 0.05 mg of polysorbate 80, sodium phosphate monobasic monohydrate 2.12 mg, sodium phosphate dibasic anhydrous 0.66 mg, and sodium chloride 8.18 mg. The albumin solution contains albumin 2.5 mg (human), sodium phosphate monobasic monohydrate 2.23 mg, sodium phosphate dibasic anhydrous 0.53 mg, and sodium chloride 8.18 mg.

Warning:

Increased mortality, serious cardiovascular and thromboembolic reactions, and increased risk of tumor progression or recurrence:

Renal failure – Patients experienced greater risks for death and serious cardiovascular reactions when administered erythropoiesis-stimulating agents (ESAs) to target higher versus lower hemoglobin levels (13.5 vs 11.3 g/dL; 14 vs 10 g/dL) in 2 clinical studies. Individualize dosing to achieve and maintain hemoglobin levels within the range of 10 to 12 g/dL.

Cancer –

- ESAs shortened overall survival and/or increased the risk of tumor progression or recurrence in some clinical studies in patients with breast, non–small cell lung, head and neck, lymphoid, and cervical cancers.
- To decrease these risks, as well as the risk of serious cardiovascular and thrombovascular events, use the lowest dose needed to avoid red blood cell (RBC) transfusion.
- Use ESAs only for treatment of anemia caused by concomitant myelosuppressive chemotherapy.
- ESAs are not indicated for patients receiving myelosuppressive therapy when the anticipated outcome is cure.
- Discontinue following the completion of a chemotherapy course.

Indications

Anemia: For the treatment of anemia associated with chronic renal failure, including patients on dialysis and patients not on dialysis, and for the treatment of anemia in patients with nonmyeloid malignancies in which anemia is caused by the effect of coadministered chemotherapy.

Administration and Dosage

Chronic renal failure patients: In patients not receiving dialysis, an initial dose of 0.75 mcg/kg may be administered subcutaneously as a single injection once every 2 weeks.

The dose should be individualized to achieve and maintain hemoglobin levels within the range of 10 to 12 g/dL.

Starting dose –

Correction of anemia: In patients on hemodialysis, the IV route is recommended, 0.45 mcg/kg body weight, administered as a single IV or subcutaneous injection once weekly. Titrate doses to not exceed a target hemoglobin concentration of 10 to 12 g/dL.

Discontinue darbepoetin alfa following the completion of a chemotherapy course.

Conversion from epoetin alfa to darbepoetin: Estimate the starting weekly dose of darbepoetin based on the weekly epoetin alfa dose at the time of substitution. Administer once a week if the patient was receiving epoetin alfa 2 to 3 times/week. Administer darbepoetin once every 2 weeks if the patient was receiving epoetin alfa once per week. Maintain the route of administration (IV or subcutaneously). For children receiving a weekly epoetin alfa dose of less than 1,500 units/week, the available data are insufficient to determine a darbepoetin alfa conversion dose.

Estimated Darbepoetin Alfa Starting Doses (mcg/week) Based on Previous Epoetin Alfa Dose (units/week)

Previous weekly epoetin alfa dose (units/week)	Weekly starting darbepoetin alfa dose (mcg/week)	
	Adults	Children
< 1,500	6.25	[a]
1,500 to 2,499	6.25	6.25
2,500 to 4,999	12.5	10
5,000 to 10,999	25	20
11,000 to 17,999	40	40
18,000 to 33,999	60	60
34,000 to 89,999	100	100
≥ 90,000	200	200

[a] For children receiving a weekly epoetin alfa dose < 1,500 units/week, the available data are insufficient to determine a darbepoetin alfa conversion dose.

Dose adjustment – Increases in dose should not be made more frequently than once a month.

If the hemoglobin is approaching 12 g/dL, the dose should be reduced by approximately 25%. If the hemoglobin continues to increases, withhold doses until the hemoglobin decreases. Reinitiate therapy at a dose approximately 25% below the previous dose. If the hemoglobin increases by more than 1 g/dL in a 2-week period, decrease dose by approximately 25%.

If the increase in hemoglobin is less than 1 g/dL over 4 weeks and iron stores are adequate, the dose of darbepoetin may be increased by approximately 25% of the previous dose. Further increases may be made at 4-week intervals until the specified hemoglobin is obtained.

Maintenance dose – Adjust darbepoetin dosage to maintain a target hemoglobin not to exceed 12 g/dL. If the hemoglobin exceeds 12 g/dL, the dose may be adjusted as previously described.

For patients whose hemoglobin does not attain a level within the range of 10 to 12 g/dL despite the use of appropriate darbepoetin alfa dose titrations over a 12-week period:

- do not administer higher darbepoetin alfa doses and use the lowest dose that will maintain a hemoglobin level sufficient to avoid the need for recurrent red blood cell transfusions,
- evaluate and treat for other causes of anemia, and
- thereafter, hemoglobin should continue to be monitored and, if responsiveness improves, darbepoetin alfa dose adjustments should be made as previously described; discontinue darbepoetin alfa if responsiveness does not improve and the patient needs recurrent RBC transfusions.

Cancer patients receiving chemotherapy: The recommended starting dose for darbepoetin alfa is 2.25 mcg/kg administered as a weekly subcutaneous injection. The recommended starting dosage for darbepoetin alfa administered once every 3 weeks is 500 mcg as a subcutaneous injection.

Therapy should not be initiated at hemoglobin levels 10 g/dL or more.

For patients receiving weekly administration, if there is less than a 1 g/dL increase in hemoglobin after 6 weeks of therapy, increase the dose of darbepoetin alfa up to 4.5 mcg/kg.

If hemoglobin increases by more than 1 g/dL in a 2-week period, or when the hemoglobin reaches a level needed to avoid transfusion, reduce the dose by approximately 40%. Reinitiate therapy at a dose approximately 40% below the previous dose. If the hemoglobin exceeds a level needed to avoid transfusion, darbepoetin alfa should be temporarily withheld until the hemoglobin approaches a level where transfusions may be required.

Preparation: Do not shake. Do not dilute. Do not administer darbepoetin in conjunction with other drug solutions. Darbepoetin is packaged in single-use vials and contains no preservatives. Discard any unused portion. Do not pool unused portions.

Actions

Pharmacology: Darbepoetin alfa is an erythropoiesis-stimulating protein produced by recombinant DNA technology. Darbepoetin stimulates erythropoiesis by the same mechanism as endogenous erythropoietin.

Pharmacokinetics:

Absorption/Distribution – Postsubcutaneous administration, chronic renal failure patients' peak concentrations occur at 48 hours, whereas cancer patients' peak concentrations are at 90 hours.

The bioavailability of darbepoetin alfa as measured in chronic renal failure patients after subcutaneous administration is 37%.

Metabolism/Excretion – Following IV administration to these patients, darbepoetin alfa serum concentration-time profiles are biphasic, with a distribution half-life of approximately 1.4 hours and a mean terminal half-life of 21 hours.

When administered IV, the terminal half-life of darbepoetin alfa is approximately 3-fold longer than epoetin alfa.

In chronic renal failure patients receiving dialysis, the average half-life was 46 hours and, in chronic renal failure patients not receiving dialysis, the average half-life was 70 hours.

Contraindications

Uncontrolled hypertension; known hypersensitivity to the active substance or any of the excipients.

Warnings/Precautions

Increased mortality, serious cardiovascular and thromboembolic reactions: Patients with chronic renal failure experienced greater risks for death and serious cardiovascular events when administered ESAs to target higher versus lower hemoglobin levels (13.5 vs 11.3 g/dL; 14 vs 10 g/dL) in 2 clinical studies. Patients with chronic renal failure and an insufficient hemoglobin response to ESA therapy may be at an even greater risk for cardiovascular events and mortality than other patients. Darbepoetin alfa and other ESAs increased the risks for death and serious cardiovascular events in controlled clinical trials of patients with cancer. These events included MI, stroke, CHF, and hemodialysis vascular access thrombosis. A rate of hemoglobin rise of more than 1 g/dL over 2 weeks may contribute to these risks.

Increased mortality and/or tumor progression: ESAs, when administered to target a hemoglobin of more than 12 g/dL, shortened the time to tumor progression in patients with advanced head and neck cancer receiving radiation therapy. ESAs also shortened survival in patients with metastatic breast cancer receiving chemotherapy when administered to target a hemoglobin of more than 12 g/dL.

Hypertension: Do not treat patients with uncontrolled hypertension with darbepoetin; control blood pressure before initiation of therapy. Blood pressure may rise during treatment of anemia with darbepoetin or epoetin alfa.

Seizures: Seizures have occurred in patients with chronic renal failure participating in clinical trials of darbepoetin and epoetin alfa. During the first several months of therapy, closely monitor blood pressure and the presence of premonitory neurologic symptoms.

Pure red cell aplasia: Pure red cell aplasia, in association with neutralizing antibodies to native erythropoietin, has been observed in patients treated with recombinant erythropoietins. This has been reported predominantly in patients with chronic renal failure.

Compromised erythropoietic response: A lack of response or failure to maintain a hemoglobin response with darbepoetin doses within recommended dosing range should prompt a search for causative factors.

The safety and efficacy of darbepoetin therapy have not been established in patients with underlying hematologic diseases (eg, hemolytic anemia, sickle cell anemia, thalassemia, porphyria).

Hematology: Allow sufficient time to determine a patient's responsiveness to a dose of darbepoetin alfa before adjusting the dose. Because of the time required for erythropoiesis and the RBC half-life, an interval of 2 to 6 weeks may occur between the time of a dose adjustment (ie, initiation, increase, decrease, discontinuation) and a significant change in hemoglobin.

Patients with chronic renal failure not requiring dialysis: Patients with chronic renal failure not yet requiring dialysis may require lower maintenance doses of darbepoetin than patients receiving dialysis. Predialysis patients may be more responsive to the effects of darbepoetin and require judicious monitoring of blood pressure and hemoglobin.

Patients transitioning to dialysis: During the transition period onto dialysis, carefully monitor hemoglobin and blood pressure; patients may need to have their maintenance doses adjusted to maintain hemoglobin levels within the range of 10 to 12 g/dL.

Dialysis management: Therapy with darbepoetin results in an increase in red blood cells and a decrease in plasma volume, which could reduce dialysis efficiency; patients who are marginally dialyzed may require adjustments in their dialysis prescription.

Immunogenicity: As with all therapeutic proteins, there is a potential for immunogenicity. Neutralizing antibodies to erythropoietin, in association with pure red cell aplasia or severe anemia (with or without other cytopenias), have been reported in patients receiving darbepoetin alfa during postmarketing experience.

Latex allergy: The needle cover of the prefilled syringe contains dry natural rubber (a derivative of latex), which may cause allergic reactions in individuals sensitive to latex.

Hypersensitivity reactions: There have been rare reports of potentially serious allergic reactions, including skin rash and urticaria, associated with darbepoetin alfa.

Pregnancy: Category C.

Lactation: It is not known whether darbepoetin is excreted in human milk.

Children:

Children with chronic renal failure – A study of the conversion from epoetin alfa to darbepoetin alfa among children with chronic renal failure older than 1 year of age showed similar safety and efficacy to the findings from adult conversion studies. Safety and efficacy in the initial treatment of anemic children with chronic renal failure or in the conversion from another erythropoietin to darbepoetin alfa in children with chronic renal failure younger than 1 year of age have not been established.

Children with cancer – The safety and efficacy of darbepoetin alfa in children with cancer have not been established.

Monitoring: After initiating therapy, determine the hemoglobin weekly until stabilized and the maintenance dose is established. After a dose adjustment, determine the hemoglobin weekly for at least 4 weeks until the hemoglobin has stabilized in response to the dose change. Then monitor the hemoglobin at regular intervals.

Evaluate iron status for all patients before and during treatment. Supplemental iron therapy is recommended for all patients whose serum ferritin is below 100 mcg/L or whose serum transferrin saturation is below 20%.

Closely monitor blood pressure and the presence of premonitory neurologic symptoms during the first several months of therapy. Closely monitor renal function and electrolyte balance in patients with chronic renal failure not requiring dialysis.

Adverse Reactions

Adverse reactions occurring in at least 3% of patients include the following: abdominal pain, access hemorrhage, access infection, acute MI, angina pectoris/cardiac chest pain, arthralgia, asthenia, back pain, bronchitis, cardiac arrhythmias/cardiac arrest, congestive heart failure, constipation, cough, death, dehydration, diarrhea, dizziness, dyspnea, edema, fatigue, fever, fluid overload, headache, hypertension, hypotension, infection (eg, abscess, bacteremia, peritonitis, pneumonia, sepsis), influenza-like symptoms, injection-site pain, limb pain, muscle spasm, myalgia, nausea, peripheral edema, pruritus, pulmonary embolism, rash, seizure, stroke, thrombosis, thrombosis vascular access, thrombotic events, transient ischemic attack, upper respiratory tract infection, vomiting.

ANAGRELIDE

Capsules: 0.5 and 1 mg (*Rx*)	Various, *Agrylin* (Shire)

Indications

Thrombocythemia: For the treatment of patients with thrombocythemia, secondary to myeloproliferative disorders, to reduce the elevated platelet count and the risk of thrombosis and to ameliorate associated symptoms including thrombo-hemorrhagic events.

Administration and Dosage

Adults: The recommended starting dosage of anagrelide for adult patients is 0.5 mg 4 times daily or 1 mg 2 times daily, which should be maintained for at least 1 week.

Children: Starting dosages in pediatric patients have ranged from 0.5 mg/day to 0.5 mg 4 times daily. Because there are limited data on the appropriate starting dosage for pediatric patients, an initial dosage of 0.5 mg/day is recommended.

Dosage adjustments: In both adult and pediatric patients, dosage should then be adjusted to the lowest effective dosage required to reduce and maintain platelet count below 600,000/mcL, and ideally to the normal range. The dosage should be increased by not more than 0.5 mg/day in any 1 week. Maintenance dosing is not expected to be different between adult and pediatric patients. Dosage should not exceed 10 mg/day or 2.5 mg in a single dose.

Hepatic function impairment: It is recommended that patients with moderate hepatic function impairment start anagrelide therapy at a dosage of 0.5 mg/day and be maintained for a minimum of 1 week with careful monitoring of cardiovascular effects. The dosage increment must not exceed more than 0.5 mg/day in any 1 week. The potential risks and benefits of anagrelide therapy in a patient with mild and moderate impairment of hepatic function should be assessed before treatment is commenced. Use of anagrelide in patients with severe hepatic function impairment has not been studied. Use of anagrelide in patients with severe hepatic function impairment is contraindicated.

Response to therapy: Typically, platelet count begins to respond within 7 to 14 days at the proper dosage. The time to complete response, defined as platelet count less than or equal to 600,000/mcL, ranged from 4 to 12 weeks. Most patients will experience an adequate response at a dosage of 1.5 to 3 mg/day. Patients with known or suspected heart disease, renal insufficiency, or hepatic dysfunction should be monitored closely.

Actions

Pharmacology: The mechanism by which anagrelide reduces blood platelet count is under investigation. Studies support a hypothesis of dose-related reduction in platelet production resulting from a decrease in megakaryocyte hypermaturation. Anagrelide inhibits cyclic AMP phosphodiesterase, which can also inhibit platelet aggregation.

Pharmacokinetics:

Absorption/Distribution – The available plasma concentration time data at steady state in patients showed that anagrelide does not accumulate in plasma after repeated administration.

Metabolism/Excretion – Following oral administration of 14^{C}-anagrelide in people, more than 70% of radioactivity was recovered in urine.

Warnings/Precautions

Cardiovascular: Use with caution in patients with known or suspected heart disease. Because of the positive inotropic effects and side effects of anagrelide, a pretreatment cardiovascular examination is recommended along with careful monitoring during treatment.

Hepatic function impairment: Exposure to anagrelide is increased 8-fold in patients with moderate hepatic function impairment. Use of anagrelide in patients with severe hepatic function impairment has not been studied. In patients with moderate hepatic function impairment, dose reduction is required; carefully monitor patients for cardiovascular effects.

Pregnancy: Category C.

Lactation: It is not known whether this drug is excreted in breast milk.

Children: Myeloproliferative disorders are uncommon in children and limited data are available in this population.

Monitoring: Anagrelide therapy requires close clinical supervision of the patient. While the platelet count is being lowered (usually during the first 2 weeks of treatment), monitor blood counts (hemoglobin, white blood cells), liver function (AST, ALT), and renal function (serum creatinine, serum urea nitrogen [BUN]).

Blood pressure – In 9 subjects receiving a single 5 mg dose of anagrelide, standing blood pressure fell an average of 22/15 mm Hg, usually accompanied by dizziness. Only minimal changes in blood pressure were observed following a 2 mg dose.

Interruption of therapy – In general, interruption of anagrelide treatment is followed by an increase in platelet count. After sudden discontinuation of therapy, the increase in platelet count can be observed within 4 days.

Drug Interactions

CYP-450 system: Anagrelide enhanced the inhibition of platelet aggregation by aspirin and is an inhibitor of cyclic AMP PDE III (may exaggerate the properties of milrinone, enoximone, amrinone, olprinone, and cilostazol).

Drug/Food interactions: Bioavailability is reduced by food.

Adverse Reactions

Adverse reactions occurring in at least 5% of patients include the following: abdominal pain, anorexia, asthenia, back pain, chest pain, cough, diarrhea, dizziness, dyspepsia, dyspnea, edema, fever, flatulence, headache, malaise, nausea, pain, palpitations, paresthesia, peripheral edema, pharyngitis, pruritus, rash (eg, urticaria), tachycardia, vomiting.

DIPYRIDAMOLE

Tablets: 25, 50, and 75 mg (*Rx*)	Various, *Persantine* (Boehringer Ingelheim)

Indications

Thromboembolic complications: Adjunct to coumarin anticoagulants in the prevention of postoperative thromboembolic complications of cardiac valve replacement.

Administration and Dosage

Adjunctive use in prophylaxis of thromboembolism after cardiac valve replacement: The recommended dose is 75 to 100 mg 4 times/day as an adjunct to the usual warfarin therapy.

Actions

Pharmacology: Dipyridamole lengthens abnormally shortened platelet survival time in a dose-dependent manner.

Dipyridamole is a platelet adhesion inhibitor, although the mechanism of action has not been fully elucidated. The mechanism may relate to: 1) Inhibition of red blood cell uptake of adenosine, itself an inhibitor of platelet reactivity, 2) phosphodiesterase inhibition leading to increased cyclic-3′, 5′-adenosine monophosphate within platelets and, 3) inhibition of thromboxane A_2 formation, which is a potent stimulator of platelet activation.

Pharmacokinetics:

Metabolism – Following an oral dose of dipyridamole, the average time to peak concentration is approximately 75 minutes. The decline in plasma concentration fits a two-compartment model. The α half-life (the initial decline following peak concentration) is approximately 40 minutes. The β half-life (the terminal decline in plasma concentration) is approximately 10 hours. Dipyridamole is highly bound to plasma proteins. It is metabolized in the liver where it is conjugated as a glucuronide and excreted with the bile.

Warnings/Precautions

Hypotension: Use with caution in patients with hypotension because it can produce peripheral vasodilation.

Fertility impairment: A significant reduction in number of corpora lutea with consequent reduction in implantations and live fetuses was observed at 155 times the maximum recommended human dose.

Pregnancy: Category B.

Lactation: Dipyridamole is excreted in breast milk.

Children: Safety and efficacy in children younger than 12 years of age have not been established.

Adverse Reactions

Adverse reactions at therapeutic doses are usually minimal and transient. With long-term use, initial adverse reactions usually disappear. The following reactions were reported in 2 heart valve replacement trials comparing dipyridamole and warfarin therapy to either warfarin alone or warfarin and placebo: dizziness, abdominal distress, headache, and rash.

On those uncommon occasions when adverse reactions have been persistent or intolerable, they have ceased on withdrawal of the medication.

DIPYRIDAMOLE AND ASPIRIN

Capsules: 200 mg extended-release dipyridamole/25 mg aspirin (*Rx*)	*Aggrenox* (Boehringer Ingelheim)

Indications

Stroke: To reduce the risk of stroke in patients who have had transient ischemia of the brain or complete ischemic stroke due to thrombosis.

Administration and Dosage

The recommended dose of dipyridamole and aspirin combination therapy is 1 capsule given orally twice daily, 1 in the morning and 1 in the evening. Swallow whole; do not crush or chew.

Do not interchange with individual components of aspirin and dipyridamole tablets.

Actions

Pharmacology: Antithrombotic action is the result of the additive antiplatelet effects of dipyridamole and aspirin.

Pharmacokinetics:

Absorption –

Dipyridamole: Peak plasma levels of dipyridamole are achieved approximately 2 hours after administration of a daily dose of 400 mg dipyridamole and aspirin combination (given as 200 mg twice daily). The peak plasma concentration at steady-state is approximately 1.98 mcg/mL and the steady-state trough concentration is approximately 0.53 mcg/mL.

Aspirin: Peak plasma levels of aspirin are achieved approximately 0.63 hours after administration of a 50 mg/day aspirin dose from dipyridamole and aspirin combination (given as 25 mg twice/day). The peak plasma concentration at steady-state is approximately 319 ng/mL. Aspirin undergoes moderate hydrolysis to salicylic acid in the liver and the GI wall, with 50% to 75% of an administered dose reaching the systemic circulation as intact aspirin.

Distribution –

Dipyridamole: Dipyridamole is highly lipophilic; however, it has been shown that the drug does not cross the blood-brain barrier to any significant extent in animals. The steady-state volume of distribution of dipyridamole is approximately 92 L. Approximately 99% of dipyridamole is bound to plasma proteins, predominantly to α1-acid glycoprotein and albumin.

Aspirin: Aspirin is poorly bound to plasma proteins and its apparent volume of distribution is low (10 L). Its metabolite, salicylic acid, is highly bound to plasma proteins, but its binding is concentration-dependent (nonlinear). At low concentrations (less than 100 mcg/mL), approximately 90% of salicylic acid is bound to albumin. Salicylic acid is widely distributed to all tissues and fluids in the body, including the CNS, breast milk, and fetal tissues.

Metabolism/Excretion –

Dipyridamole: Dipyridamole is metabolized in the liver, primarily by conjugation with glucuronic acid, of which monoglucuronide, which has low pharmacodynamic activity, is the primary metabolite. In plasma, approximately 80% of the total amount is present as parent compound and 20% as monoglucuronide. Most of the glucuronide metabolite (approximately 95%) is excreted via bile into the feces, with some evidence of enterohepatic circulation. Renal excretion of parent compound is negligible and urinary excretion of the glucuronide metabolite is low (approximately 5%).

Aspirin: Aspirin is rapidly hydrolyzed in plasma to salicylic acid with a half-life of 20 minutes. Plasma levels of aspirin are essentially undetectable 2 to 2.5 hours after dosing, and peak salicylic acid concentration occurs 1 hour (range, 0.5 to 2 hours) after aspirin administration. Salicylic acid is primarily conjugated in the liver to form a number of minor metabolites. Salicylate metabolism is saturable and the total body clearance decreases at higher serum concentrations.

The elimination of acetylsalicylic acid follows first-order kinetics with the dipyridamole and aspirin combination and has a half-life of 0.33 hours. The half-life of salicylic acid is 1.71 hours.

Contraindications

Hypersensitivity to dipyridamole, aspirin, or any of the other product components.

Allergy: Aspirin is contraindicated in patients with a known allergy to NSAIDs and in patients with asthma, rhinitis, and nasal polyps. Aspirin may cause severe urticaria, angioedema, or bronchospasms (asthma).

Reye syndrome: Do not use in children or teenagers with viral infections with or without fever. There is a risk of Reye syndrome with concomitant use of aspirin in certain viral illnesses.

Warnings/Precautions

Alcohol: Counsel patients who consume 3 or more alcoholic drinks every day about the bleeding risks involved with chronic, heavy alcohol use while taking aspirin.

Coagulation abnormalities: Even low doses of aspirin can inhibit platelet function leading to an increase in bleeding time. This can adversely affect patients with inherited or acquired bleeding disorders (eg, liver disease, vitamin K deficiency).

Peptic ulcer disease: Avoid using aspirin, which can cause gastric mucosal irritation and bleeding in patients with a history of active peptic ulcer disease.

Dipyridamole and aspirin combination is not interchangeable with the individual components of aspirin and dipyridamole tablets.

Coronary artery disease: Due to the vasodilatory effect of dipyridamole, use with caution in patients with severe coronary artery disease (eg, unstable angina, recently sustained MI). Chest pain may be aggravated in patients with underlying coronary artery disease who are receiving dipyridamole. For stroke or transient ischemic attack patients for whom aspirin is indicated to prevent recurrent MI or angina pectoris, the aspirin in this product may not provide adequate treatment for the cardiac indications.

Hypotension: Dipyridamole can produce peripheral vasodilation; use with caution in patients with hypotension.

Renal function impairment: No changes were observed in the pharmacokinetics of dipyridamole or its glucuronide metabolite with creatinine clearances ranging from approximately 15 mL/min to more than 100 mL/min if data were corrected for differences in age. Avoid aspirin in patients with severe renal failure (glomerular filtration rate less than 10 mL/min).

Hepatic function impairment: Elevations of hepatic enzymes and hepatic failure have been reported in association with dipyridamole administration. Dipyridamole can be dosed without restriction as long as there is no evidence of hepatic failure. Avoid aspirin in patients with severe hepatic function impairment.

Mutagenesis: Aspirin induced chromosome aberrations in cultured human fibroblasts.

Fertility impairment: Aspirin inhibits ovulation in rats.

Pregnancy: *Category B* (dipyridamole); *Category D* (aspirin).

Lactation: Dipyridamole and aspirin are excreted in human breast milk in low concentrations.

Children: Safety and efficacy of dipyridamole and aspirin combination capsules in children have not been studied. Because of the aspirin component, use of this product in the pediatric population is not recommended.

Elderly: Plasma concentrations (determined as AUC) of dipyridamole in healthy elderly subjects older than 65 years of age were approximately 40% higher than in subjects younger than 55 years of age receiving treatment with the dipyridamole and aspirin combination.

Lab test abnormalities: Aspirin has been associated with elevated hepatic enzymes, blood urea nitrogen and serum creatinine, hyperkalemia, proteinuria, and prolonged bleeding time. Dipyridamole has been associated with elevated hepatic enzymes.

Drug Interactions

Drugs that may be affected by dipyridamole are adenosine and cholinesterase inhibitors.

Drugs that may be affected by aspirin include ACE inhibitors, acetazolamide, anticoagulants, anticonvulsants (hydantoins, valproic acid), beta blockers, diuretics, methotrexate, NSAIDs, oral hypoglycemics, and uricosuric agents (probenecid, sulfinpyrazone).

Drug/Lab test interactions: Over the course of 24 months, patients treated with dipyridamole and aspirin combination therapy showed a decline (mean change from baseline) in hemoglobin of 0.25 g/dL, hematocrit of 0.75%, and erythrocyte count of $0.13 \times 10^6/mm^3$.

Adverse Reactions

Adverse reactions that occurred in at least 3% of patients included the following: headache; abdominal pain; dyspepsia; nausea; vomiting; diarrhea; hemorrhage; arthralgia; pain; fatigue; back pain.

TICLOPIDINE HYDROCHLORIDE

Tablets: 250 mg (*Rx*)	*Ticlid* (Syntex)

Warning:

Ticlopidine can cause life-threatening hematological adverse reactions, including neutropenia/agranulocytosis and thrombotic thrombocytopenic purpura (TTP).

Neutropenia/agranulocytosis: Neutropenia defined as an absolute neutrophil count (ANC) less than 1,200 neutrophils/mm^3 occurred in 50 of 2048 (2.4%) stroke patients who received ticlopidine in clinical trials. Neutropenia is calculated as follows: ANC = WBC × % neutrophils. In 17 patients (0.8%) the neutrophil count was less than 450/mm^3.

TTP: TTP was not seen during clinical trials, but US physicians reported about 100 cases between 1992 and 1997. Based on an estimated patient exposure of 2 to 4 million, and assuming an event reporting rate of 10% (the true rate is not known), the incidence of ticlopidine-associated TTP may be as high as 1 case in every 2,000 to 4,000 patients exposed.

Monitoring clinical and hematologic status: Severe hematological adverse reactions may occur within a few days of initiating therapy. The incidence of TTP peaks after approximately 3 to 4 weeks of therapy and neutropenia peaks at approximately 4 to 6 weeks with both declining thereafter. Only a few cases have arisen after more than 3 months of treatment. Hematological adverse reactions cannot be reliably predicted by any identified demographic or clinical characteristics. During the first 3 months of treatment, hematologically and clinically monitor patients receiving ticlopidine for evidence of neutropenia or TTP. Immediately discontinue ticlopidine if there is any evidence of neutropenia or TTP.

Indications

Thrombotic stroke: To reduce the risk of thrombotic stroke (fatal or nonfatal) in patients who have experienced stroke precursors, and in patients who have had a completed thrombotic stroke.

Because ticlopidine is associated with a risk of life-threatening blood dyscrasias including TTP and neutropenia/agranulocytosis, reserve for patients who are intolerant or allergic to aspirin therapy or who have failed aspirin therapy.

Administration and Dosage

Recommended dose: 250 mg twice daily taken with food.

Actions

Pharmacology: Ticlopidine is a platelet aggregation inhibitor. When taken orally, ticlopidine causes a time and dose-dependent inhibition of both platelet aggregation and release of platelet granule constituents, as well as a prolongation of bleeding time. Ticlopidine interferes with platelet membrane function by inhibiting ADP-induced platelet-fibrinogen binding and subsequent platelet-platelet interactions. The effect on platelet function is irreversible for the life of the platelet.

After discontinuation of ticlopidine, bleeding time and other platelet function tests return to normal within 2 weeks in the majority of patients.

Pharmacokinetics: Ticlopidine is rapidly absorbed (more than 80%), with peak plasma levels occurring at approximately 2 hours after dosing, and is extensively metabolized. Administration after meals results in a 20% increase in the area under the plasma concentration-time curve (AUC). Ticlopidine displays nonlinear pharmacokinetics and clearance decreases markedly on repeated dosing.

Ticlopidine binds reversibly (98%) to plasma proteins, mainly to serum albumin and lipoproteins. The binding to albumin and lipoproteins is nonsaturable over a wide concentration range. Ticlopidine also binds to alpha-1 acid glycoprotein; at concentrations attained with the recommended dose, 15% or less in plasma is bound to this protein.

Ticlopidine is metabolized extensively by the liver; only trace amounts of intact drug are detected in the urine. Following an oral dose, 60% is recovered in the urine and 23% in the feces. Approximately, 33% of the dose excreted in the feces is intact ticlopidine, possibly excreted in the bile. Approximately 40% to 50% of the metabolites circulating in plasma are covalently bound to plasma proteins, probably by acylation. Although analysis of urine and plasma indicates 20 metabolites or more, no metabolite that accounts for the activity of ticlopidine has been isolated.

Contraindications

Hypersensitivity to the drug; presence of hematopoietic disorders such as neutropenia and thrombocytopenia or a history of TTP; presence of a hemostatic disorder or active pathological bleeding; severe liver impairment.

Warnings/Precautions

Neutropenia: Neutropenia may occur suddenly. Bone-marrow examination typically shows a reduction in myeloid precursors. After withdrawal of ticlopidine, the neutrophil count usually rises to more than 1,200/mm^3 within 1 to 3 weeks.

Thrombocytopenia: Rarely, thrombocytopenia may occur in isolation or together with neutropenia. If clinical evaluation and repeat laboratory testing confirm the presence of thrombocytopenia, discontinue the drug.

TTP: Clinically, fever might suggest neutropenia or TTP. Weakness, pallor, petechiae or purpura, dark urine (because of blood, bile pigments, or hemoglobin) or jaundice, or neurological changes might also suggest TTP. Have the patient discontinue ticlopidine and contact the physician immediately upon the occurrence of these findings.

Monitoring – Monitor patients for neutropenia, thrombocytopenia, and TTP prior to initiating ticlopidine and every 2 weeks through the third month of therapy. If therapy is stopped during this 3-month period, continue to monitor for 2 weeks after discontinuation. More frequent monitoring and monitoring after the first 3 months of therapy are necessary only in patients exhibiting clinical signs or hematological laboratory signs (eg, neutrophil count less than 70% of baseline count, decrease in hematocrit or platelet count).

Laboratory monitoring includes complete blood count, especially the absolute neutrophil count, platelet count, and the appearance of the peripheral smear. Thrombocytopenia induced by ticlopidine is occasionally unrelated to TTP. Further investigate for a diagnosis of TTP with the occurrence of any acute, unexplained reduction in hemoglobin or platelet count. Discontinue ticlopidine if there are laboratory signs of TTP or the neutrophil count is less than 1200/mm^3.

Cholesterol elevation: Ticlopidine therapy causes increased serum cholesterol and triglycerides. Serum total cholesterol levels are increased 8% to 10% within 1 month of therapy and persist at that level. The ratios of lipoprotein subfractions are unchanged.

Hematological effects: Rare cases of pancytopenia and TTP, some of which have been fatal, have occurred.

Anticoagulant drugs: If a patient is switched from an anticoagulant or fibrinolytic drug to ticlopidine, discontinue the former drug prior to ticlopidine administration.

Increased bleeding risk: Use with caution in patients who may be at risk of increased bleeding from trauma, surgery, or pathological conditions. If it is desired to eliminate the antiplatelet effects of ticlopidine prior to elective surgery, discontinue the drug 10 to 14 days prior to surgery. Increased surgical blood loss has occurred in patients undergoing surgery during treatment with ticlopidine.

Prolonged bleeding time is normalized within 2 hours after administration of 20 mg methylprednisolone IV. Platelet transfusions also may be used to reverse the effect of ticlopidine on bleeding. If possible, avoid platelet transfusions because they may accelerate thrombosis in patients with TTP on ticlopidine.

GI bleeding: Ticlopidine prolongs template bleeding time. Use with caution in patients who have lesions with a propensity to bleed (such as ulcers). Use drugs that might induce such lesions with caution in patients on ticlopidine.

Renal function impairment: There is limited experience in patients with renal function impairment. No unexpected problems have been encountered in patients having mild renal function impairment, and there is no experience with dosage adjustment in patients with greater degrees of renal function impairment. Nevertheless, for renally impaired patients, it may be necessary to reduce ticlopidine dosage or discontinue it altogether if hemorrhagic or hematopoietic problems are encountered.

Hepatic function impairment: The average plasma concentration in patients with advanced cirrhosis was slightly higher than that seen in older subjects. Because of limited experience in patients with severe hepatic disease who may have bleeding diatheses, the use of ticlopidine is not recommended.

Pregnancy: Category B.

Lactation: It is not known whether this drug is excreted in human breast milk.

Children: Safety and efficacy in patients younger than 18 years of age have not been established.

Elderly: Clearance of ticlopidine is somewhat lower in elderly patients and trough levels are increased. No overall differences in safety or efficacy were observed between elderly patients and younger patients, but greater sensitivity of some older individuals cannot be ruled out.

Drug Interactions

The dose of drugs metabolized by hepatic microsomal enzymes with low therapeutic ratios, or being given to patients with hepatic function impairment, may require adjustment to maintain optimal therapeutic blood levels when starting or stopping concomitant therapy with ticlopidine.

Drugs that may interact include antacids, cimetidine, aspirin, digoxin, phenytoin, and theophylline.

Drug/Food interactions: The oral bioavailability of ticlopidine is increased by 20% when taken after a meal. Administration with food is recommended to maximize GI tolerance.

Adverse Reactions

Adverse reactions were relatively frequent, with more than 50% of patients reporting at least one. Most involved the GI tract. Most adverse effects are mild, but 21% of patients discontinued therapy because of an adverse event, principally diarrhea, rash, nausea, vomiting, GI pain, and neutropenia. Most adverse effects occur early in the course of treatment, but a new onset of adverse effects can occur after several months. Ticlopidine has been associated with a number of bleeding complications such as ecchymosis, epistaxis, hematuria, conjunctival hemorrhage, GI bleeding, posttraumatic bleeding, and perioperative bleeding. The incidence of elevated alkaline phosphatase (more than 2 times upper limit of normal) was 7.6% in ticlopidine patients. The incidence of elevated AST (more than 2 times upper limit of normal) was 3.1% in ticlopidine patients.

CILOSTAZOL

Tablets: 50 and 100 mg (*Rx*) — *Pletal* (Otsuka America Pharmaceutical)

Warning:

Cilostazol and several of its metabolites are inhibitors of phosphodiesterase (PDE) 3. Several drugs with this pharmacologic effect have caused decreased survival compared with placebo in patients with class III to IV congestive heart failure. Cilostazol is contraindicated in patients with congestive heart failure of any severity.

Indications

Intermittent claudication: For the reduction of symptoms of intermittent claudication, as indicated by an increased walking distance.

Administration and Dosage

Recommended dosage: 100 mg twice daily taken at least 30 minutes before or 2 hours after breakfast and dinner.

Concomitant medications: Consider 50 mg twice daily during coadministration of inhibitors of CYP3A4 (eg, diltiazem, erythromycin, itraconazole, ketoconazole) and during coadministration of inhibitors of CYP2C19 (eg, omeprazole).

Actions

Pharmacology: The mechanism of the effects of cilostazol on the symptoms of intermittent claudication is not fully understood. Cilostazol and metabolites are cyclic adenosine monophosphate (cAMP) PDE 3 inhibitors, leading to inhibition of platelet aggregation and vasodilation, respectively.

Pharmacokinetics:

Absorption – Cilostazol is absorbed after oral administration. A high-fat meal increases absorption.

Distribution – Cilostazol is 95% to 98% protein bound.

Metabolism/Excretion – Cilostazol is extensively metabolized by hepatic CYP-450 enzymes, mainly 3A4, and 2C19. Cilostazol and its active metabolites have apparent elimination half-lives of about 11 to 13 hours.

Contraindications

Congestive heart failure; hemostatic disorders or active pathologic bleeding, such as bleeding peptic ulcer and intracranial bleeding; known or suspected hypersensitivity to any of its components.

Warnings/Precautions

Hematologic effects: Rare cases of thrombocytopenia or leukopenia progressing to agranulocytosis have been reported when cilostazol was not immediately discontinued.

Pregnancy: Category C.

Lactation: Because of the potential risk to breast-feeding infants, decide whether to discontinue breast-feeding or cilostazol.

Children: The safety and efficacy of cilostazol in children have not been established.

Drug Interactions

Drugs that may affect cilostazol include clopidogrel, CYP3A4 inhibitors, CYP2C19 inhibitors, diltiazem, and lovastatin.

Drugs that may be affected by cilostazol include lovastatin.

Drug/Food interactions: A high-fat meal increases absorption with an approximately 90% increase in C_{max} and a 25% increase in AUC.

Adverse Reactions

Adverse reactions occurring in at least 3% of patients include the following: abdominal pain, abnormal stools, back pain, cough increased, diarrhea, dizziness, dyspepsia, flatulence, headache, infection, myalgia, nausea, palpitation, peripheral edema, pharyngitis, rhinitis, tachycardia, vertigo.

CLOPIDOGREL

Tablets: 75 and 300 mg (as base) (*Rx*) — *Plavix* (Bristol-Myers Squibb)

Warning:

Diminished effectiveness in poor metabolizers: The effectiveness of clopidogrel is dependent on its activation to an active metabolite by the cytochrome P450 (CYP-450) system, principally CYP2C19. Poor metabolizers treated with clopidogrel at recommended doses exhibit higher cardiovascular event rates following acute coronary syndrome or percutaneous coronary intervention (PCI) than patients with normal CYP2C19 function. Tests are available to identify a patient's CYP2C19 genotype and can be used as an aid in determining therapeutic strategy. Consider alternative treatment or treatment strategies in patients identified as CYP2C19 poor metabolizers.

Indications

Acute coronary syndrome:

Unstable angina/Non–ST-segment elevation – For patients with non–ST-segment elevation acute coronary syndrome (unstable angina/non–Q-wave myocardial infarction [MI]), including patients who are to be managed medically and who are to be managed with coronary revascularization, clopidogrel has been shown to decrease the rate of a combined end point of cardiovascular death, MI, or stroke, as well as the rate of a combined end point of cardiovascular death, MI, stroke, or refractory ischemia.

ST-segment elevation acute myocardial infarction – For patients with ST-segment elevation acute MI, clopidogrel has been shown to reduce the rate of death from any cause and the rate of a combined end point of death, reinfarction, or stroke. This benefit is not known to pertain to patients who receive primary PCI.

Recent myocardial infarction or stroke, or established peripheral arterial disease: For patients with a history of recent MI, recent stroke, or established peripheral arterial disease, clopidogrel has been shown to reduce the rate of a combined end point of new ischemic stroke (fatal or not), new MI (fatal or not), and other vascular death.

Administration and Dosage

Clopidogrel can be administered with or without food.

Acute coronary syndrome:

Non–ST-segment elevation – Initiate with a single 300 mg loading dose and then continue at 75 mg once daily. Aspirin (75 to 325 mg once daily) should be initiated and continued in combination with clopidogrel.

ST-segment elevation acute myocardial infarction – 75 mg once daily, administered in combination with aspirin (75 to 325 mg once daily), with or without thrombolytics. Clopidogrel may be initiated with or without a loading dose

Recent myocardial infarction, recent stroke, or established peripheral arterial disease: 75 mg once daily.

CYP2C19 poor metabolizers: CYP2C19 poor metabolizer status is associated with diminished antiplatelet response to clopidogrel. Although a higher dose regimen (600 mg loading dose followed by 150 mg once daily) in poor metabolizers increases antiplatelet response, an appropriate dose regimen for this patient population has not been established in clinical outcome trials.

Discontinuation of therapy: If a patient is to undergo surgery and an antiplatelet effect is not desired, discontinue clopidogrel 5 days prior to surgery.

Avoid lapses in therapy and restart as soon as possible. Premature discontinuation of clopidogrel may increase the risk of cardiovascular events.

Actions

Pharmacology: Clopidogrel is a thienopyridine derivative, chemically related to ticlopidine, that inhibits platelet aggregation. It acts by irreversibly modifying the platelet ADP receptor. Consequently, platelets exposed to clopidogrel are affected for the remainder of their lifespan.

Pharmacokinetics:

Absorption/Distribution – Clopidogrel absorption is 50% or more and is rapid after oral administration. Both the parent compound (98%) and the main metabolite (94%) bind reversibly in vitro to plasma protein.

Metabolism/Excretion – Clopidogrel is extensively metabolized by the liver and by a metabolic pathway mediated by multiple CYP-450 enzymes. It undergoes rapid hydrolysis into its carboxylic acid derivative; glucuronidation also occurs.

Approximately 50% of total radioactivity was excreted in the urine and 46% in the feces 5 days after dosing. After a single oral dose of 75 mg, clopidogrel has a half-life of approximately 6 hours.

Contraindications

Hypersensitivity to the drug or any component of the product; active pathological bleeding such as peptic ulcer or intracranial hemorrhage.

Warnings/Precautions

CYP2C19 poor metabolizers: The metabolism of clopidogrel to its active metabolite can be impaired by genetic variations in CYP2C19 and by concomitant medications that interfere with CYP2C19. Avoid concomitant use of clopidogrel and drugs that inhibit CYP2C19 activity.

Bleeding risk: If a patient is to undergo surgery and an antiplatelet effect is not desired, discontinue clopidogrel 5 days prior to surgery. Withholding a dose will not be useful in managing a bleeding event or the risk of bleeding associated with an invasive procedure. It may be possible to restore hemostasis by administering exogenous platelets; however, platelet transfusions within 4 hours of the loading dose or 2 hours of the maintenance dose may be less effective.

Ischemic events: In patients with recent transient ischemic attack or stroke who are at high risk for recurrent ischemic reactions, the combination of aspirin and clopidogrel has not been shown to be more effective than clopidogrel alone, but the combination has been shown to increase major bleeding.

Thrombotic thrombocytopenic purpura: Thrombotic thrombocytopenic purpura, sometimes fatal, has been reported following use of clopidogrel, sometimes after a short exposure (less than 2 weeks). It is characterized by thrombocytopenia, microangiopathic hemolytic anemia, neurological findings, renal dysfunction, and fever.

Renal function impairment: Experience is limited in patients with moderate and severe renal function impairment.

Hepatic function impairment: No dosage adjustment is necessary in patients with hepatic impairment.

Pregnancy: Category B.

Lactation: It is not known whether this drug is excreted in human breast milk. Because many drugs are excreted in human milk and because of the potential for serious adverse reactions in breast-feeding infants, decided whether to discontinue breast-feeding or the drug, taking into account the importance of the drug to the mother.

Children: Safety and efficacy have not been established.

Monitoring: Because of the risk of bleeding and undesirable hematological effects, promptly consider blood cell count determination and/or other appropriate testing whenever such suspected clinical symptoms arise during the course of treatment.

Drug Interactions

CYP-450 system: Clopidogrel is metabolized to its active metabolite in part by CYP2C19. Concurrent use of drugs that inhibit the activity of this enzyme reduce plasma concentrations of the active metabolite of clopidogrel and reduce platelet inhibition. Avoid drugs that inhibit CYP2C19 (eg, omeprazole).

Drugs that may affect clopidogrel include aspirin, CYP2C19 inhibitors, macrolide antibiotics, nonsteroidal anti-inflammatory drugs, proton pump inhibitors, rifamycins, and warfarin. Drugs that may be affected by clopidogrel include bupropion and warfarin.

Adverse Reactions

Adverse reactions occurring in at least 3% of patients include the following: major bleeding, minor bleeding, noncerebral bleeding (any), and other noncerebral bleeding (nonmajor).

PRASUGREL

Tablets; oral: 5 and 10 mg (*Rx*) — *Effient* (Eli Lilly and Company)

Warning:

Bleeding risk: Prasugrel can cause significant, sometimes fatal, bleeding.

Do not use prasugrel in patients with active pathological bleeding or a history of transient ischemic attack (TIA) or stroke.

In patients 75 years of age and older, prasugrel is generally not recommended because of the increased risk of fatal and intracranial bleeding and uncertain benefit, except in high-risk situations (patients with diabetes or a history of prior myocardial infarction [MI]) in which its effect appears to be greater and its use may be considered.

Do not start prasugrel in patients likely to undergo urgent coronary artery bypass graft surgery (CABG). When possible, discontinue prasugrel at least 7 days prior to any surgery.

Additional risk factors for bleeding include body weight less than 60 kg, propensity to bleed, and concomitant use of medications that increase the risk of bleeding (eg, warfarin, heparin, fibrinolytic therapy, chronic use of nonsteroidal anti-inflammatory drugs [NSAIDs]).

Suspect bleeding in any patient who is hypotensive and has recently undergone coronary angiography, percutaneous coronary intervention (PCI), CABG, or other surgical procedures in the setting of prasugrel.

If possible, manage bleeding without discontinuing prasugrel. Discontinuing prasugrel, particularly in the first few weeks after acute coronary syndrome, increases the risk of subsequent cardiovascular (CV) events.

Indications

Acute coronary syndrome: To reduce the rate of thrombotic CV events (including stent thrombosis) in patients with acute coronary syndrome (ACS) who are to be managed with PCI as follows: patients with unstable angina or non–ST elevation MI (NSTEMI); patients with ST elevation MI (STEMI) when managed with primary or delayed PCI.

Administration and Dosage

Adults:

Acute coronary syndrome – Prasugrel should be taken with aspirin 75 to 325 mg daily. May be administered with or without food. Do not break the tablet.

Weighing 60 kg or more: 10 mg orally once daily.

Weighing less than 60 kg: 5 mg orally once daily should be considered.

Loading dose: 60 mg orally.

Discontinuation of therapy: Discontinue prasugrel for active bleeding, elective surgery, stroke, or TIA. Avoid lapses in therapy, and if thienopyridines must be temporarily discontinued because of an adverse event(s), restart therapy as soon as possible.

Actions

Pharmacology: Prasugrel is a thienopyridine class inhibitor of platelet activation and aggregation through the irreversible binding of its active metabolite to the $P2Y_{12}$ class of adenosine diphosphate (ADP) receptors on platelets.

Pharmacokinetics:

Absorption – Following oral administration, at least 79% of the dose is absorbed. The absorption is rapid, with peak plasma concentrations (C_{max}) of the active metabolite occurring approximately 30 minutes after dosing. The active metabolite is bound about 98% to human serum albumin. The major inactive metabolites are highly bound to human plasma proteins.

Metabolism/Excretion – Prasugrel is a prodrug and is rapidly metabolized to a pharmacologically active metabolite and inactive metabolites. The active metabolite has an elimination half-life of about 7 hours (range, 2 to 15 hours).

Prasugrel is not detected in plasma following oral administration. It is rapidly hydrolyzed in the intestine to a thiolactone, which is then converted to the active metabolite by a single step, primarily by CYP3A4 and CYP2B6, and to a lesser extent by CYP2C9 and CYP2C19. Approximately 68% of the prasugrel dose is excreted in the urine and 27% in the feces as inactive metabolites.

Contraindications

Active pathological bleeding such as peptic ulcer or intracranial hemorrhage; prior transient ischemic attack or stroke.

Warnings/Precautions

Risk of bleeding: Thienopyridines, including prasugrel, increase the risk of bleeding. The bleeding risk is highest initially.

Other risk factors for bleeding are the following: 75 years of age and older (because of the risk of bleeding, including fatal bleeding, and uncertain effectiveness in patients 75 years of age and older, use of prasugrel is generally not recommended in these patients, except in high-risk situations [patients with diabetes or history of MI] in which its effect appears to be greater and its use may be considered); CABG or other surgical procedure; body weight less than 60 kg; propensity to bleed (eg, recent trauma, recent surgery, recent or recurrent GI bleeding, active peptic ulcer disease, or severe hepatic impairment); medications that increase the risk of bleeding (eg, oral anticoagulants, chronic use of NSAIDs, fibrinolytic agents).

Thienopyridines inhibit platelet aggregation for the lifetime of the platelet (7 to 10 days).

Coronary artery bypass graft surgery–related bleeding: Do not start prasugrel in patients likely to undergo urgent CABG. CABG-related bleeding may be treated with transfusion of blood products, including packed red blood cells and platelets; however, platelet transfusions within 6 hours of the loading dose or 4 hours of the maintenance dose may be less effective.

Prior transient ischemic attack or stroke: Prasugrel is contraindicated in patients with a history of prior TIA or stroke. Patients who experience a stroke or TIA while on prasugrel generally should have therapy discontinued.

Thrombotic thrombocytopenic purpura: Thrombotic thrombocytopenic purpura (TTP) has been reported with the use of other thienopyridines, sometimes after a brief exposure (less than 2 weeks).

Renal function impairment: In patients with end-stage renal disease, exposure to the active metabolite was approximately half that in healthy controls and patients with moderate renal impairment.

Hepatic function impairment: Patients with severe hepatic impairment are generally at higher risk of bleeding.

Pregnancy: Category B.

Lactation: It is not known whether prasugrel is excreted in human milk.

Children: Safety and effectiveness in children have not been established.

Elderly: Patients 75 years of age and older who received prasugrel had an increased risk of fatal bleeding events (1%) compared with patients who received clopidogrel (0.1%). Because of the risk of bleeding and because effectiveness is uncertain in patients 75 years of age and older, use of prasugrel is generally not recommended in these patients, except in high-risk situations (diabetes and history of MI) where its effect appears to be greater and its use may be considered.

Drug Interactions

Warfarin: Coadministration of prasugrel and warfarin increases the risk of bleeding.

NSAIDs: Coadministration of prasugrel and NSAIDs (used chronically) may increase the risk of bleeding.

Adverse Reactions

Adverse reactions occurring in 3% or more of patients include major or minor bleeding, reoperation, transfusion of 5 units or more, epistaxis, hypertension, hypotension, dizziness, fatigue, headache, nausea, cough, dyspnea, back pain, hypercholesterolemia/hyperlipidemia, noncardiac chest pain.

ANTICOAGULANTS

Blood coagulation resulting in the formation of a stable fibrin clot involves a cascade of proteolytic reactions involving the interaction of clotting factors, platelets, and tissue materials. Clotting factors (see table) exist in the blood in inactive form and must be converted to an enzymatic or activated form before the next step in the clotting mechanism can be stimulated. Each factor is stimulated in turn until an insoluble fibrin clot is formed.

Two separate pathways, intrinsic and extrinsic, lead to the formation of a fibrin clot. Both pathways must function for hemostasis.

Intrinsic pathway: All the protein factors necessary for coagulation are present in circulating blood. Clot formation may take several minutes and is initiated by activation of factor XII.

Extrinsic pathway: Coagulation is activated by release of tissue thromboplastin, a factor not found in circulating blood. Clotting occurs in seconds because factor III bypasses the early reactions.

Refer to the next page for the complete coagulation pathway.

Anticoagulants used therapeutically include heparin, warfarin (a coumarin derivative), and anisindione (an indandione derivative).

Blood Clotting Factors

Factor	Synonym	Vitamin K-dependent
I	Fibrinogen	no
II	Prothrombin	yes
III	Tissue thromboplastin, tissue factor	no
IV	Calcium	no
V	Labile factor, proaccelerin	no
VII	Proconvertin	yes
VIII	Antihemophilic factor, AHF	no
IX	Christmas factor, plasma thromboplastin component, PTC	yes
X	Stuart factor, Stuart-Prower factor	yes
XI	Plasma thromboplastin antecedent, PTA	no
XII	Hageman factor	no
XIII	Fibrin stabilizing factor, FSF	no
HMW-K	High molecular weight Kininogen, Fitzgerald factor	no
PL	Platelets or phospholipids	no
PK	Prekallikrein, Fletcher factor	no
Protein C[a]		yes
Protein S[b]		yes

[a] Partially responsible for inhibition of the extrinsic pathway. Inactivates factors V and VIII and promotes fibrinolysis. Activity declines following warfarin administration.

[b] A cofactor to accelerate the anticoagulant activity of protein C. Decreased levels occur following warfarin administration.

COAGULATION PATHWAY

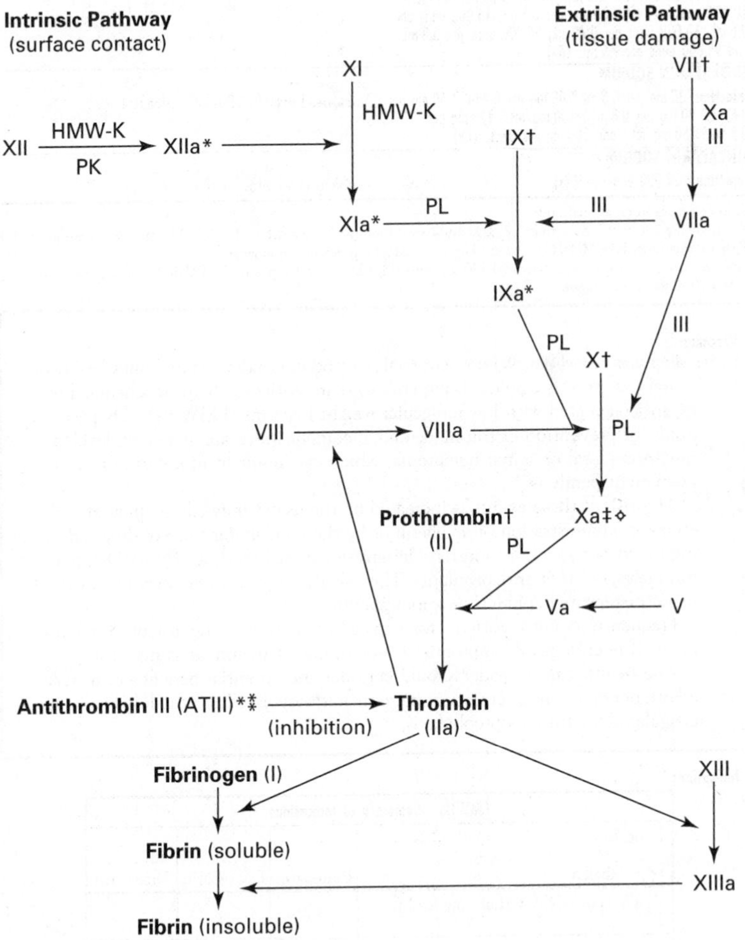

* Major site of activity for unfractionated heparin
† Site of activity for warfarin and anisindione
‡ Major site of activity for fractionated heparin
⁑ Minor site of activity for fractionated heparin
◇ Minor site of activity for unfractionated heparin

LOW MOLECULAR WEIGHT HEPARINS

DALTEPARIN SODIUM	
Injection, solution[a]: 2,500 units per 0.2 mL, 5,000 units per 0.2 mL, 7,500 units per 0.3 mL, 10,000 units per 0.4 mL, 10,000 units/mL, 12,500 units per 0.5 mL, 15,000 units per 0.6 mL, 18,000 units per 0.72 mL, 95,000 units per 3.8 mL, and 95,000 units per 9.5 mL. (*Rx*)	*Fragmin* (Pfizer)
ENOXAPARIN SODIUM	
Injection: 30 mg per 0.3 mL,[b] 40 mg per 0.4 mL,[b] 60 mg per 0.6 mL,[b] 80 mg per 0.8 mL,[b] 100 mg/mL,[b] 120 mg per 0.8 mL,[c] 150 mg/mL,[c] and 300 mg per 3 mL[b] (*Rx*)	Various, *Lovenox* (Sanofi-Aventis)
TINZAPARIN SODIUM	
Injection[a]: 20,000 units/mL (*Rx*)	*Innohep* (Celgene Corp)

[a] Anti-factor Xa international units.
[b] Approximate anti-factor Xa activity of 1,000 units per 0.1 mL (with reference to the World Health Organization [WHO] First International Low Molecular Weight Heparin [LMWH] Reference Standard).
[c] Approximate anti-factor Xa activity of 1,500 units per 0.1 mL (with reference to the [WHO] First International [LMWH] Reference Standard).

Warning:

Spinal/Epidural hematomas: When neuraxial anesthesia (epidural/spinal anesthesia) or spinal puncture is employed, patients who are anticoagulated or scheduled to be anticoagulated with low molecular weight heparins (LMWHs) or heparinoids for prevention of thromboembolic complications are at risk of developing an epidural or spinal hematoma, which can result in long-term or permanent paralysis.

The risk of these events is increased by the use of indwelling epidural catheters for administration of analgesia or by the concomitant use of drugs affecting hemostasis, such as nonsteroidal anti-inflammatory drugs (NSAIDs), platelet inhibitors, or other anticoagulants. The risk also appears to be increased by traumatic or repeated epidural or spinal puncture.

Frequently monitor patients for signs and symptoms of neurological impairment. If neurological compromise is noted, urgent treatment is necessary.

The health care provider should consider the potential benefit versus risk before neuraxial intervention in patients anticoagulated or scheduled to be anticoagulated for thromboprophylaxis.

Indications

LMWHs - Summary of Indications

Indications ✔ = labeled	Dalteparin	Enoxaparin	Tinzaparin
Prophylaxis of DVT that may lead to PE[a]			
In patients undergoing abdominal surgery	✔	✔	—
In patients undergoing hip replacement surgery	✔	✔	—
In patients undergoing knee replacement surgery	—	✔	—
In patients with severely restricted mobility during acute illness	✔	✔	—
Treatment of DVT[b] with or without PE[c,d]	—	✔	✔
Prophylaxis of ischemic complications in unstable angina and non–Q-wave MI[e]	✔	✔	—

LMWHs - Summary of Indications			
Indications ✔ = labeled	Dalteparin	Enoxaparin	Tinzaparin
Extended treatment of symptomatic VTE[f] (proximal DVT and/or PE), to reduce the recurrence of VTE in patients with cancer.	✔	—	—
Acute STEMI[g] receiving thrombolysis and being managed medically or with PCI[h]	—	✔	—

[a] In patients at risk for thromboembolic complications.
[b] DVT = Deep vein thrombosis.
[c] In conjunction with warfarin therapy.
[d] PE = Pulmonary embolism.
[e] In conjunction with aspirin therapy.
[f] VTE = Venous thromboembolism.
[g] STEMI = ST-segment elevation myocardial infarction.
[h] PCI = Percutaneous coronary intervention.

Administration and Dosage

DALTEPARIN:

Unstable angina/Non–Q-wave MI – 120 units/kg of body weight (but not more than 10,000 units) subcutaneously every 12 hours with concurrent oral aspirin (75 to 165 mg/day) therapy. Continue treatment until the patient is clinically stabilized. The usual duration of treatment is 5 to 8 days.

Volume of Dalteparin to be Administered by Patient Weight						
Patient weight (lb)	< 110	110 to 131	132 to 153	154 to 175	176 to 197	≥ 198
Patient weight (kg)	< 50	50 to 59	60 to 69	70 to 79	80 to 89	≥ 90
Volume of dalteparin (mL)[a]	0.55	0.65	0.75	0.9	1	1

[a] Calculated volume based on the 9.5 mL multiple-dose vial (10,000 anti-Factor Xa units/mL).

DVT, prophylaxis –

Abdominal surgery: Administer 2,500 units subcutaneously once daily, starting 1 to 2 hours prior to surgery and repeat once daily for 5 to 10 days postoperatively.

High-risk patients – In abdominal surgery at high risk for thromboembolic complications (eg, malignancy), administer 5,000 units subcutaneously the evening before surgery and repeat once daily for 5 to 10 days postoperatively. Alternatively, in patients with malignancy, administer 2,500 units subcutaneously 1 to 2 hours prior to surgery with an additional 2,500 unit dose 12 hours later and then 5,000 units once daily for 5 to 10 days postoperatively.

Hip replacement surgery: The usual duration of administration is 5 to 10 days after surgery; up to 14 days was well tolerated in controlled clinical trials.

Dalteparin Subcutaneous Dosing for Patients Undergoing Hip Replacement Surgery				
Timing of first dose of dalteparin	10 to 14 h before surgery	≤ 2 h before surgery	4 to 8 h after surgery[a]	Postoperative period[b]
Postoperative start	—	—	2,500 units[c]	5,000 units once daily
Preoperative start: day of surgery	—	2,500 units	2,500 units[c]	5,000 units once daily
Preoperative start: evening before surgery[d]	5,000 units	—	5,000 units	5,000 units once daily

[a] Or later, if hemostasis has not been achieved.
[b] Up to 14 days of treatment were well tolerated in controlled clinical trials, where the usual duration of treatment was 5 to 10 days postoperatively.
[c] Allow a minimum of 6 hours between this dose and the dose to be given on postoperative day 1. Adjust the timing of the dose on postoperative day 1 accordingly.
[d] Allow approximately 24 hours between doses.

Patients with severely restricted mobility during acute illness: 5,000 units administered by subcutaneous injection once daily. In clinical trials, the usual duration of administration was 12 to 14 days.

Symptomatic VTE: In patients with cancer and symptomatic VTE, for the first 30 days of treatment, administer dalteparin 200 units/kg total body weight subcutaneously once daily. The total daily dose should not exceed 18,000 units.

Month 1 –

Dalteparin Dose to be Administered Subcutaneously by Patient Weight During the First Month		
Body weight (lbs)	Body weight (kg)	Dalteparin dose (units) (prefilled syringe) once daily
≤ 124	≤ 56	10,000
125 to 150	57 to 68	12,500
151 to 181	69 to 82	15,000
182 to 216	83 to 98	18,000
≥ 217	≥ 99	18,000

Months 2 to 6 – Administer dalteparin at a dose of approximately 150 units/kg subcutaneously once daily during months 2 through 6. The total daily dose should not exceed 18,000 units.

Dalteparin Dose to be Administered Subcutaneously by Patient Weight During Months 2 to 6		
Body weight (lbs)	Body weight (kg)	Dalteparin dose (units) (prefilled syringe) once daily
≤ 124	≤ 56	7,500
125 to 150	57 to 68	10,000
151 to 181	69 to 82	12,500
182 to 216	83 to 98	15,000
≥ 217	≥ 99	18,000

Safety and efficacy beyond 6 months have not been evaluated in patients with cancer and acute symptomatic VTE.

Unstable angina/non–Q-wave myocardial infarction: 120 units/kg of body weight, but not more than 10,000 units, subcutaneously every 12 hours with concurrent oral aspirin (75 to 165 mg/day) therapy.

Maximum dose – Not more than 10,000 units, subcutaneously every 12 hours.

Volume of Dalteparin Sodium Injection to Be Administered by Patient Weight		
Body weight (lb)	Body weight (kg)	Volume of dalteparin (mL)[a]
< 110	< 50	0.55
110 to 131	50 to 59	0.65
132 to 153	60 to 69	0.75
154 to 175	70 to 79	0.9
176 to 197	80 to 89	1
≥ 198	≥ 90	1

[a] Calculated volume based on the 9.5 mL (10,000 units/mL) multidose vial.

Treatment should be continued until the patient is clinically stabilized. The usual duration of administration is 5 to 8 days. Concurrent aspirin therapy is recommended except when contraindicated.

Dose reductions:

Thrombocytopenia – In patients who experience platelet counts between 50,000 and 100,000/mm^3, reduce the daily dose by 2,500 units until the platelet count recovers to at least 100,000/mm³. In patients who experience platelet counts less than 50,000/mm³, discontinue dalteparin until the platelet count recovers above 50,000/mm³.

Renal function impairment in extended treatment of acute symptomatic VTE in patients with cancer: In patients with severe renal function impairment (creatinine clearance [CrCl] less than 30 mL/min), monitoring for anti-Xa levels is recommended to determine the appropriate dalteparin dose. Target anti-Xa range is 0.5 to 1.5 units/mL. Sampling should be performed 4 to 6 hours after dalteparin dosing and only after the patient has received 3 to 4 doses.

Administration: Dalteparin is administered by subcutaneous injection. It must not be administered by intramuscular (IM) injection.

Subcutaneous injection technique – Administer by deep subcutaneous injection while patient is sitting or lying down. Dalteparin may be injected in a U-shaped area around the navel, the upper outer side of the thigh, or the upper outer quadrangle of the buttock. Vary the injection site daily. When the area around the navel or the thigh is used, use the thumb and forefinger to lift up a fold of skin while giving the injection. Insert the entire length of the needle at a 45° to 90° angle.

ENOXAPARIN:

Administration – For subcutaneous use or IV bolus injection. Enoxaparin must not be administered by IM injection.

Acute STEMI – Single IV bolus of 30 mg plus a 1 mg/kg subcutaneous dose followed by 1 mg/kg administered subcutaneously every 12 hours (maximum 100 mg for the first 2 doses only, followed by 1 mg/kg dosing for the remaining doses). Dosage adjustments are recommended in patients 75 years of age and older.

When administered in conjunction with a thrombolytic (fibrin-specific or nonfibrin-specific), enoxaparin should be given between 15 minutes before and 30 minutes after the start of fibrinolytic therapy.

For patients managed with PCI: If the last subcutaneous administration was given less than 8 hours before balloon inflation, no additional dosing is needed. If the last subcutaneous administration was given more than 8 hours before balloon inflation, an IV bolus of enoxaparin 0.3 mg/kg should be administered.

Elderly patients with acute STEMI: For the treatment of acute STEMI in patients 75 years of age and older, do not use an initial IV bolus. Initiate dosing with 0.75 mg/kg subcutaneously every 12 hours (maximum 75 mg for the first 2 doses only, followed by 0.75 mg/kg dosing for the remaining doses).

DVT, prophylaxis –

Hip or knee replacement surgery: 30 mg every 12 hours by subcutaneous injection, with the initial dose given within 12 to 24 hours postoperatively provided hemostasis has been established. The average duration of administration is 7 to 10 days; up to 14 days have been well tolerated.

For hip replacement surgery, consider a dose of 40 mg once daily subcutaneously, given initially 9 to 15 hours prior to surgery. Continue prophylaxis for 3 weeks.

Abdominal surgery: Administer 40 mg once daily subcutaneously with the initial dose given 2 hours prior to surgery. The usual duration of administration is 7 to 10 days, up to 12 days.

Medical patients during acute illness: In medical patients at risk for thromboembolic complications due to severely restricted mobility during acute illness, the recommended dose is 40 mg once daily subcutaneously. The usual duration of administration is 6 to 11 days; up to 14 days have been well tolerated.

DVT with or without PE –

Outpatient treatment: 1 mg/kg subcutaneously every 12 hours.

Inpatient treatment: 1 mg/kg subcutaneously every 12 hours or 1.5 mg/kg subcutaneously once daily (same time each day).

Outpatient and inpatient treatment: Initiate warfarin therapy when appropriate (usually within 72 hours of enoxaparin). Continue enoxaparin for a minimum of 5 days and until a therapeutic anticoagulant effect has been achieved (international normalized ratio [INR] 2 to 3). The average duration is 7 days; up to 17 days have been well tolerated.

Unstable angina/Non-Q-wave MI – 1 mg/kg subcutaneously every 12 hours in conjunction with oral aspirin therapy (100 to 325 mg once daily). Treat with enoxaparin for at least 2 days and continue until clinical stabilization. The usual duration of treatment is 2 to 8 days; up to 12.5 days have been well tolerated. Leave the vascular access sheath for instrumentation in place for 6 to 8 hours following a dose of enoxaparin. Give the next scheduled dose at least 6 to 8 hours after sheath removal. Observe site for signs of bleeding or hematoma formation.

Subcutaneous injection technique – Do not expel the air bubble from the syringe before the injection. Administer by deep subcutaneous injection while patients are lying down. Alternate administration between the left and right anterolateral and left and right posterolateral abdominal wall. Introduce the whole length of the needle into a skin fold held between the thumb and forefinger; hold the skin fold throughout the injection. To minimize bruising, do not rub the injection site. Prefilled syringes and graduated prefilled syringes are available with a system that shields the needle after injection.

Renal function impairment – Although no dose adjustment is recommended in patients with mild (CrCl 50 to 80 mL/min) and moderate (CrCl 30 to 50 mL/min) renal function impairment, observe all such patients carefully for signs and symptoms of bleeding.

The recommended prophylaxis and treatment dosage regimens for patients with severe renal function impairment (CrCl less than 30 mL/min) are described in the following table.

Enoxaparin Sodium Injection Dosage Regimens for Patients With Severe Renal Impairment (CrCl < 30 mL/min)

Indication	Dosage regimen
Acute STEMI in patients < 75 years of age, when administered in conjunction with aspirin	30 mg single IV bolus plus a 1 mg/kg dose subcutaneously followed by 1 mg/kg subcutaneously once daily
Acute STEMI in patients ≥ 75 years of age, when administered in conjunction with aspirin	1 mg/kg subcutaneously once daily (no initial bolus)
Prophylaxis of DVT: abdominal surgery, hip or knee replacement surgery, medical patients during acute illness	30 mg subcutaneously once daily
Prophylaxis of ischemic complications of unstable angina/non–Q-wave MI, when coadministered with aspirin	1 mg/kg subcutaneously once daily
Treatment of acute DVT with or without pulmonary embolism, when administered in conjunction with warfarin (inpatient)	1 mg/kg subcutaneously once daily
Treatment of acute DVT without pulmonary embolism, when administered in conjunction with warfarin (outpatient)	1 mg/kg subcutaneously once daily

TINZAPARIN: Evaluate all patients for bleeding disorders before administration of tinzaparin.

Adults – 175 anti-Xa units/kg of body weight, administered subcutaneously once daily for at least 6 days and until the patient is adequately anticoagulated with warfarin (INR at least 2 for 2 consecutive days). Initiate warfarin sodium therapy when appropriate (usually within 1 to 3 days of tinzaparin initiation).

As tinzaparin may theoretically affect the prothrombin time (PT)/INR, draw blood for PT/INR determination just prior to the next scheduled dose of tinzaparin for patients receiving tinzaparin and warfarin.

Tinzaparin Weight-Based Dosing for Treatment of DVT With or Without Symptomatic PE			
		DVT treatment	
		175 units/kg subcutaneously once daily 20,000 units/mL	
Body weight (lbs)	Body weight (kg)	Dose (units)	Amount (mL)
68 to 80	31 to 36	6,000	0.3
81 to 94	37 to 42	7,000	0.35
95 to 107	43 to 48	8,000	0.4
108 to 118	49 to 53	9,000	0.45
119 to 131	54 to 59	10,000	0.5
132 to 144	60 to 65	11,000	0.55
145 to 155	66 to 70	12,000	0.6
156 to 168	71 to 76	13,000	0.65
169 to 182	77 to 82	14,000	0.7
183 to 195	83 to 88	15,000	0.75
196 to 206	89 to 93	16,000	0.8
207 to 219	94 to 99	17,000	0.85
220 to 232	100 to 105	18,000	0.9
233 to 243	106 to 110	19,000	0.95
244 to 256	111 to 116	20,000	1
257 to 270	117 to 122	21,000	1.05
271 to 283	123 to 128	22,000	1.1
284 to 294	129 to 133	23,000	1.15
295 to 307	134 to 139	24,000	1.2
308 to 320	140 to 145	25,000	1.25
321 to 331	146 to 150	26,000	1.3
332 to 344	151 to 156	27,000	1.35
345 to 358	157 to 162	28,000	1.4

Use the following equation to calculate the volume (mL) of tinzaparin 175 anti-Xa units/kg subcutaneous dose for treatment of DVT:

Patient weight (kg) × 0.00875 mL/kg = volume to be given (mL) subcutaneously.

Administration – Administer by subcutaneous injection. Do not administer by IM or IV injection. Do not mix tinzaparin with other injections or infusions.

Subcutaneous injection technique – Position patients either lying down or sitting, and administer by deep subcutaneous injection. Alternate administration between left and right anterolateral and left and right posterolateral abdominal wall. Vary the injection site daily. Introduce the whole length of the needle into a skin fold held between the thumb and forefinger; hold the skin fold throughout the injection. To minimize bruising, do not rub the injection site after completion of the injection.

Actions

Pharmacology: **Enoxaparin, tinzaparin,** and **dalteparin** are LMWHs. These agents enhance the inhibition of Factor Xa and thrombin by binding to and accelerating antithrombin activity. They preferentially potentiate the inhibition of Factor Xa, while only slightly affecting thrombin and clotting time (activated partial thromboplastin time [APTT] or PT).

Pharmacokinetics:

LMWHs Pharmacokinetics Based on Anti-Xa Activity[a]						
LMWH	Max activity (h)	Duration (h)	Bioavailability	T_{max} (h)	Vd	Terminal t½ (h)
Dalteparin	—	—	≈ 87%	4	40 to 60 mL/kg	3 to 5
Enoxaparin	3 to 5[b]	12 (40 mg daily dose)	≈ 100%	3 to 4.5	4.3 L	4.5 (single dose) 7 (repeated doses)
Tinzaparin	—	—	86.7%	3.7 (single dose)	3.1 to 5 L	3 to 4

[a] Information listed without regard to dosage or indication.
[b] Maximum anti-Factor Xa and antithrombin activities.

Contraindications

Hypersensitivity to LMWHs, heparin, or pork products; hypersensitivity to sulfites or benzyl alcohol (multidose vials); history of heparin-induced thrombocytopenia (**dalteparin, tinzaparin**); active major bleeding; thrombocytopenia associated with positive in vitro tests for antiplatelet antibody in the presence of a LMWH.

Do not give dalteparin to patients undergoing regional anesthesia for unstable angina or non–Q-wave MI because of an increased risk of bleeding associated with the dosage of dalteparin recommended for unstable angina and non–Q-wave MI.

Warnings/Precautions

Route of administration: For subcutaneous administration only; do not administer IM.

Interchangeability with heparin: LMWHs cannot be used interchangeably (unit for unit) with unfractionated heparin or other LMWHs.

Spinal/Epidural anesthesia: As with other anticoagulants, there have been rare cases of neuraxial, spinal, or epidural hematomas reported with the concurrent use of LMWHs and spinal/epidural anesthesia or spinal puncture resulting in long-term or permanent paralysis. The risk of these events may be higher with the use of postoperative indwelling epidural catheters or by the concomitant use of additional drugs affecting hemostasis such as NSAIDs (see Warning Box).

Hemorrhage: Use LMWHs, like other anticoagulants, with extreme caution in patients who have an increased risk of hemorrhage, such as those with severe uncontrolled hypertension, bleeding diathesis, diabetic retinopathy, bacterial endocarditis, congenital or acquired bleeding disorders (including hepatic failure and amyloidosis), active ulceration and angiodysplastic GI disease, hemorrhagic stroke, or shortly after brain, spinal, or ophthalmological surgery, or in patients treated concomitantly with platelet inhibitors.

Thrombocytopenia: The incidence of thrombocytopenia with platelet counts between 50,000/mm^3 and 100,000/mm^3 was 1.3% in patients treated with **enoxaparin**, 1% with **tinzaparin**, and less than 1% with **dalteparin**.

Priapism: Priapism has been reported from postmarketing surveillance of **tinzaparin** as a rare occurrence. In some cases, surgical intervention was required.

Benzyl alcohol: The multiple-dose vials of **dalteparin, enoxaparin**, and **tinzaparin** contain benzyl alcohol as a preservative. Benzyl alcohol has been associated with a fatal "gasping syndrome" in premature infants. Because benzyl alcohol may cross the placenta, do not use LMWHs preserved with benzyl alcohol in pregnant women.

Thromboembolic events: If thromboembolic events occur despite LMWH prophylaxis, discontinue and initiate appropriate therapy.

Mechanical prosthetic heart valves: The use of **enoxaparin** injection has not been adequately studied for thromboprophylaxis or long-term use in patients with mechanical prosthetic heart valves. Isolated cases of prosthetic heart valve thrombosis have been reported in patients with mechanical prosthetic heart valves who have received enoxaparin for thromboprophylaxis.

Low-weight patients: An increase in exposure of **enoxaparin** with prophylactic dosages (less than 45 kg) and low-weight men (less than 57 kg) has been observed. Observe all such patients carefully for signs and symptoms of bleeding.

Sulfite sensitivity: **Tinzaparin** contains metabisulfite, a sulfite that may cause allergic-type reactions, including anaphylactic symptoms and life-threatening asthmatic episodes, in certain susceptible people.

Renal/Hepatic function impairment: Delayed elimination of LMWHs may occur with severe liver or kidney insufficiency. Use with caution.

Because exposure of **enoxaparin** is significantly increased in patients with severe renal function impairment (CrCl less than 30 mL/min), a dosage adjustment is recommended for therapeutic and prophylactic dosage ranges.

Special risk: Use with care in patients with a bleeding diathesis, uncontrolled arterial hypertension, or a history of recent GI ulceration or bleeding, diabetic retinopathy, hemorrhage, or severe liver or kidney insufficiency.

Pregnancy: Category B.

Lactation: It is not known whether these drugs are excreted in breast milk.

Children: Safety and efficacy have not been established.

Elderly: Delayed elimination of **enoxaparin** and **tinzaparin** may occur.

Monitoring: Periodic complete blood counts, including platelet count, and stool occult blood tests are recommended during treatment. If platelet count falls below 100,000/mm^3, discontinue the LMWH. Anti-Factor Xa may be used to monitor the anticoagulant effect in patients with significant renal function impairment or if abnormal coagulation parameters or bleeding should occur. Consider monitoring of elderly patients with low body weight (less than 45 kg) and those predisposed to renal function impairment.

Drug Interactions

Antithrombin: The risk of severe bleeding may be increased when coadministered with **dalteparin**, **enoxaparin**, or **tinzaparin**.

Anticoagulants and platelet inhibitors: Use LMWHs with care in patients receiving oral anticoagulants or platelet inhibitors (eg, aspirin, salicylates, NSAIDs including ketorolac tromethamine, dipyridamole, sulfinpyrazone, dextran, ticlopidine, clopidogrel) and thrombolytics because of increased risk of bleeding. Unless needed, discontinue agents that may enhance the risk of hemorrhage prior to initiation of **enoxaparin** therapy. Aspirin, unless contraindicated, is recommended in patients treated for unstable angina or non–Q-wave MI.

Selective serotonin reuptake inhibitors (fluoxetine): The risk of severe bleeding may be increased when coadministered with **dalteparin**, **enoxaparin**, or **tinzaparin**.

Drug/Lab test interactions: Asymptomatic reversible increases in AST and ALT aminotransferase levels have occurred in patients treated with LMWHs and heparin. Because aminotransferase determinations are important in the differential diagnosis of MI, liver disease, and PE, interpret elevations that might be caused by LMWHs with caution.

Adverse Reactions

Adverse reactions associated with LMWHs include anemia, clinically significant bleeding, dyspnea, hematuria, hemorrhage, injection-site hematoma, injection-site hemorrhage, nausea, pain at injection site, peripheral edema, urinary tract infection, and wound hematoma. Approximately 10% of pregnant women receiving **tinzaparin** experienced significant vaginal bleeding.

HEPARIN

HEPARIN SODIUM	
Injection: 1,000, 2,000, 2,500, 5,000, 10,000, 20,000, and 40,000 units/mL (multiple-dose vials) (*Rx*)	Various
1,000, 5,000, 10,000, 20,000, and 40,000 units/mL (single-dose amps and vials) (*Rx*)	Various
1,000, 2,500, 5,000, 7,500, 10,000, and 20,000 units/dose (unit-dose vials) (*Rx*)	Various
HEPARIN SODIUM AND SODIUM CHLORIDE	
Injection: 1,000 and 2,000 units (*Rx*)	*Heparin Sodium and 0.9% Sodium Chloride* (Baxter Healthcare)
12,500 and 25,000 units (*Rx*)	*Heparin Sodium and 0.45% Sodium Chloride* (Abbott)
HEPARIN SODIUM LOCK FLUSH	
Injection: 1 unit/mL (*Rx*)	*Heparin I.V. Flush* (Medefil)
10 and 100 units/mL (*Rx*)	Various, *Hep-Lock* (Various), *Hepflush-10* (American Pharmaceutical Partners)

Indications

Prophylaxis and treatment: Prophylaxis and treatment of venous thrombosis and its extension; pulmonary embolism; peripheral arterial embolism; for prevention of clotting in arterial and cardiac surgery; atrial fibrillation with embolization.

Diagnosis and treatment: Diagnosis and treatment of acute and chronic consumption coagulopathies (disseminated intravascular coagulation [DIC]).

Postoperative: Low dose regimen for prevention of postoperative deep venous thrombosis (DVT) and pulmonary embolism in patients undergoing major abdominothoracic surgery or patients who are at risk of developing thromboembolic disease.

Anticoagulant: Blood transfusions, extracorporeal circulation, dialysis procedures, and blood samples for laboratory purposes.

Clotting prevention: Heparin lock flush solution is intended to maintain patency of an indwelling intravenous catheter.

Administration and Dosage

Potency changes: According to the FDA, heparin manufactured after October 1, 2009 will be approximately 10% less potent than heparin manufactured prior to that date.

The change in heparin potency may have clinical significance in some situations, such as when heparin is administered as a bolus IV dose and an immediate anticoagulant effect is clinically important.

The potency change may require more frequent or intensive aPTT or ACT monitoring.

Health care providers should be aware that larger doses of heparin will be required to achieve therapeutic levels of anticoagulation

For heparin products made according to the new standard, most manufacturers will include an "N" in the lot number or following the expiration date.

Give by intermittent IV injection, continuous IV infusion or deep subcutaneous (ie, above the iliac crest of abdominal fat layer) injection. Avoid IM injection because of the danger of hematoma formation.

Adjust dosage according to coagulation test results prior to each injection. Dosage is adequate when WBCT is approximately 2.5 to 3 times control value, or when aPTT is 1.5 to 2 times normal.

General heparin dosage guidelines: Although dosage must be individualized, the following may be used as guidelines:

Heparin Dosage Guidelines

Method of administration	Frequency	Recommended dose[a]
Subcutaneous[b]	Initial dose	10,000 – 20,000 units[c]
	Every 8 hours	8,000 – 10,000 units
	Every 12 hours	15,000 – 20,000 units

Heparin Dosage Guidelines		
Method of administration	Frequency	Recommended dose[a]
Intermittent IV	Initial dose	10,000 units[d]
	Every 4 to 6 hours	5,000 – 10,000 units[d]
IV Infusion	Continuous	20,000 – 40,000 units/day[c]

[a] Based on a 68 kg (150 lb) patient.
[b] Use a concentrated solution.
[c] Immediately preceded by IV loading dose of 5000 units.
[d] Administer undiluted or in 50 to 100 mL 0.9% NaCl.

Children: In general, the following dosage schedule may be used as a guideline:

Initial dose – 50 units/kg IV bolus.

Maintenance dose – 100 units/kg/dose IV drip every 4 hours, or 20,000 units/m²/24 hours continuous IV infusion.

Clotting prevention in blood transfusion: Addition of heparin 400 to 600 units per 100 mL of whole blood is usually employed to prevent coagulation.

Low-dose prophylaxis of postoperative thromboembolism: Give 5,000 units subcutaneously 2 hours before surgery and 5,000 units every 8 to 12 hours thereafter for 7 days or until the patient is fully ambulatory, whichever is longer. Administer by deep subcutaneous injection above the iliac crest or abdominal fat layer, arm, or thigh using a concentrated solution.

Surgery of the heart and blood vessels: Give an initial dose of not less than 150 units/kg to patients undergoing total body perfusion for open heart surgery. Often, 300 units/kg is used for procedures less than 60 minutes and 400 units/kg is used for procedures more than 60 minutes.

Extracorporeal dialysis: Follow equipment manufacturers' operating directions.

Laboratory samples: Add 70 to 150 units per 10 to 20 mL sample of whole blood to prevent coagulation of sample.

Converting to oral anticoagulant therapy: Perform baseline coagulation tests to determine prothrombin activity when heparin activity is too low to affect PT or INR. When the results of the initial prothrombin determinations are known, initiate the oral anticoagulant in the usual amount. Thereafter, perform coagulation tests and prothrombin activity at appropriate intervals. When the prothrombin activity reaches the desired therapeutic range, discontinue heparin and continue oral anticoagulants.

Compatibility: Sodium chloride 0.9% injection.

Incompatibility: Heparin injection should not be mixed with doxorubicin, droperidol, ciprofloxacin, or mitoxantrone because it has been reported that these drugs are incompatible with heparin and a precipitate may form.

Heparin lock flush:

Maintenance of potency of IV devices – Heparin lock flush solution is injected via the injection hub in a quantity sufficient to fill the entire device. Replace solution each time the device is used. Aspirate before administering any solution in order to confirm patency and location of needle or catheter tip. If the drug to be administered is incompatible with heparin, flush with sterile water or normal saline before and after the medication is administered; following the second flush, reinstill the heparin lock flush solution into the set.

Usually this dilute heparin solution will maintain anticoagulation within the device for up to 4 hours.

Withdrawal of blood samples – When heparin (or sodium chloride) would interfere or alter the results of blood tests, the heparin solution should be cleared by aspirating and discarding it before withdrawing the blood sample.

Actions

Pharmacology: Small amounts of heparin in combination with antithrombin III (heparin cofactor) inhibit thrombosis by inactivating factor Xa and inhibiting the conversion of prothrombin to thrombin. Once active thrombosis has developed, larger amounts of heparin can inhibit further coagulation by inactivating thrombin and preventing the conversion of fibrinogen to fibrin. In combination with antithrombin III, heparin inactivates factors IX, X, Xa, XI, XII, and thrombin, inhibiting conversion of fibrinogen to fibrin. Heparin also prevents the formation of a stable fibrin clot by inhibiting the activation of factor XIII (the fibrin stabilizing factor). Other effects include the inhibition of thrombin-induced activation of factors V and VIII.

Heparin inhibits reactions that lead to clotting, but does not significantly alter the concentration of the normal clotting factors of blood. Although clotting time is prolonged by full therapeutic doses, in most cases it is not measurably affected by low doses of heparin. Bleeding time is usually unaffected.

Pharmacokinetics:

Absorption/Distribution – Heparin is not adsorbed from the GI tract. An IV bolus results in immediate anticoagulant effects. The duration of action is dose-dependent. Peak plasma levels of heparin are achieved 2 to 4 hours following subcutaneous use. Once absorbed, heparin is distributed in plasma and is extensively protein bound.

Metabolism/Excretion – Following administration, heparin demonstrates a biphasic elimination curve. The lack of relationship between plasma and pharmacologic half-lives may reflect factors such as protein binding. Heparin is rapidly cleared from plasma with an average half-life of 30 to 180 minutes. Half-life is dose-dependent and may be significantly prolonged at higher doses. Heparin is partially metabolized by liver heparinase and the reticuloendothelial system. There may be a secondary site of metabolism in the kidneys. In patients with deep venous thrombosis, plasma clearance is more rapid and half-life is shorter than in patients with pulmonary embolism. Heparin is excreted in urine as unchanged drug (50% or less) particularly after large doses. Some urinary degradation products have anticoagulant activity.

Contraindications

Hypersensitivity to heparin; severe thrombocytopenia; uncontrolled bleeding (except when it is due to DIC); any patient for whom suitable blood coagulation tests cannot be performed at the appropriate intervals (there is usually no need to monitor coagulation parameters in patients receiving low-dose heparin).

Warnings/Precautions

Hemorrhage: Hemorrhage can occur at virtually any site in patients receiving heparin. An unexplained fall in hematocrit, fall in blood pressure or any other unexplained symptom should lead to serious consideration of a hemorrhagic event. An overly prolonged coagulation test or bleeding can usually be controlled by withdrawing the drug. Signs and symptoms will vary according to the location and extent of bleeding and may present as paralysis, headache, chest, abdomen, joint or other pain, shortness of breath, difficulty breathing or swallowing, unexplained swelling, or unexplained shock. GI or urinary tract bleeding may indicate an underlying occult lesion. Certain hemorrhagic complications may be difficult to detect.

Use heparin with extreme caution in disease states in which there is increased danger of hemorrhage. These include:

Cardiovascular – Subacute bacterial endocarditis; arterial sclerosis; dissecting aneurysm; increased capillary permeability; severe hypertension.

CNS – During and immediately following spinal tap, spinal anesthesia, or major surgery, especially of the brain, spinal cord, or eye.

Hematologic – Hemophilia; some vascular purpuras; thrombocytopenia.

GI – Ulcerative lesions, diverticulitis or ulcerative colitis; continuous tube drainage of the stomach or small intestine.

Obstetric – Threatened abortion; menstruation.

Other – Liver disease with impaired hemostasis; severe renal disease.

Hyperlipidemia: Heparin may increase free fatty acid serum levels by induction of lipoprotein lipase.

Resistance: Increased resistance to the drug is frequently encountered in fever, thrombosis, thrombophlebitis, infections with thrombosing tendencies, MI, cancer, and postoperative states.

Thrombocytopenia: Thrombocytopenia has occurred in patients receiving heparin. The incidence of heparin-associated thrombocytopenia is higher with bovine than with porcine heparin. The severity also appears to be related to heparin dose.

Early thrombocytopenia – Early thrombocytopenia (Type I) develops 2 to 3 days after starting heparin, tends to be mild and is due to a direct action of heparin on platelets.

Delayed thrombocytopenia – Delayed thrombocytopenia (Type II) develops 7 to 12 days after either low-dose or full-dose heparin, can have serious consequences and may reflect the presence of an immunoglobulin that induces platelet aggregation.

Mild thrombocytopenia – Mild thrombocytopenia may remain stable or reverse even if heparin is continued. However, closely monitor thrombocytopenia of any degree. If a count falls below 100,000/mm^3 or if recurrent thrombosis develops, discontinue heparin. If continued heparin therapy is essential, administration of heparin from a different organ source can be reinstituted with caution.

White clot syndrome – Rarely, patients may develop new thrombus formation in association with thrombocytopenia resulting from irreversible aggregation of platelets induced by heparin, the so-called "white clot syndrome." The process may lead to severe thromboembolic complications.

Hyperkalemia: Hyperkalemia may develop, probably due to induced hypoaldosteronism. Use with caution in patients with diabetes or renal insufficiency. Monitor patient closely.

Hypersensitivity reactions: Heparin is derived from animal tissue; use with caution in patients with a history of allergy. Before a therapeutic dose is given, a trial dose may be advisable. Have epinephrine 1:1000 immediately available.

Vasospastic reactions – Vasospastic reactions may develop 6 to 10 days after starting therapy and last 4 to 6 hours. The affected limb is painful, ischemic, and cyanotic. After repeated injections, the reaction may gradually increase to generalized vasospasm with cyanosis, tachypnea, feeling of oppression, and headache.

Hepatic function impairment: Heparin half-life may be prolonged in liver disease.

Pregnancy: Category C.

Lactation: Heparin is not excreted in breast milk.

Children: Safety and efficacy have not been determined in newborns; germinal matrix intraventricular hemorrhage occurs more often in low-birth-weight infants receiving heparin.

Use heparin lock-flush solution with caution in infants with disease states in which there is an increased danger of hemorrhage. The use of the 100 unit/mL concentration is not advised because of bleeding risk, especially in low-birth-weight infants.

Elderly: A higher incidence of bleeding has occurred in women older than 60 years of age.

Monitoring: The most common test used to monitor heparin's effect is aPTT. Other tests used include Activated Coagulation Time (ACT) and Lee White-Whole Blood Clotting Time (WBCT). If the coagulation test is unduly prolonged or if hemorrhage occurs, discontinue the drug promptly. Perform periodic platelet counts, hematocrit and tests for occult blood in stool during the entire course of therapy, regardless of route of administration.

Drug Interactions

Drugs that may interact include cephalosporins, nitroglycerin, penicillins, and salicylates.

Drug/Lab test interactions: Significant elevations of aminotransferase (AST and ALT) levels have occurred in a high percentage of patients. Cautiously interpret aminotransferase increases that might be caused by heparin.

If heparin comprises 10% or more of the total volume of a sample for blood gas analysis, errors in measurements of carbon dioxide pressure, bicarbonate concentration, and base excess may occur.

Adverse Reactions

Adverse reactions associated with heparin include hemorrhage, chills, fever, urticaria, and thrombocytopenia.

COUMARIN AND INDANDIONE DERIVATIVES

WARFARIN SODIUM

Tablets, oral: 1, 2, 2.5, 3, 4, 5, 6, 7.5, and 10 mg (*Rx*)	Various, *Coumadin* (DuPont)
Powder for injection, lyophilized: 5.4 mg (2 mg/mL when reconstituted) (*Rx*)	

Warning:

Bleeding risk: Warfarin can cause major or fatal bleeding. Bleeding is more likely to occur during the starting period and with a higher dose (resulting in a higher international normalized ratio [INR]). Risk factors for bleeding include high intensity of anticoagulation (INR of more than 4), 65 years of age and older, highly variable INRs, history of GI bleeding, hypertension, cerebrovascular disease, serious heart disease, anemia, malignancy, trauma, renal function impairment, concomitant drugs, and long duration of warfarin therapy. Regular monitoring of INR should be performed on all treated patients. Those at high risk of bleeding may benefit from more frequent INR monitoring, careful dose adjustment to desired INR, and a shorter duration of therapy. Patients should be instructed about prevention measures to minimize risk of bleeding and to report immediately to health care provider signs and symptoms of bleeding.

Indications

Prophylaxis and/or treatment of venous thrombosis and its extension and pulmonary embolism.

Prophylaxis and/or treatment of the thromboembolic complications associated with atrial fibrillation and/or cardiac valve replacement.

To reduce the risk of death, recurrent myocardial infarction (MI), and thromboembolic events such as stroke or systemic embolization after MI.

Administration and Dosage

Dosage: Individualize dosage.

Initial dosage – The dosing must be individualized according to patient's sensitivity to the drug as indicated by the prothrombin time (PT)/INR. Adjust dosage based on the patient's PT/INR. Use of a large loading dose may increase the incidence of hemorrhagic and other complications, does not offer more rapid protection against thrombi formation, and is not recommended. It is recommended that warfarin therapy be initiated with a dose of 2 to 5 mg per day with dosage adjustments based on the results of PT/INR determinations.

Maintenance – Most patients are satisfactorily maintained at a dose of 2 to 10 mg/day. Gauge the individual dose and interval by the patient's prothrombin response. An INR of more than 4 appears to provide no additional therapeutic benefit in most patients and is associated with a higher risk of bleeding.

Duration of therapy – Individualize the duration of therapy. Continue anticoagulant therapy until the danger of thrombosis and embolism has passed.

Missed dose – The anticoagulant effect of warfarin persists beyond 24 hours. If the patient forgets to take the prescribed dose of warfarin at the scheduled time, the dose should be taken as soon as possible on the same day. The patient should not take the missed dose by doubling the daily dose to make up for missed doses.

IV route of administration – Warfarin injection provides an alternative administration route for patients who cannot receive oral drugs. The IV dosages would be the same as those that would be used orally if the patient could take the drug by the oral route. Administer as a slow bolus injection over 1 to 2 minutes into a peripheral vein. Warfarin is not recommended for IM administration.

The following are the recommended therapeutic ranges for oral anticoagulation therapy from the American College of Chest Physicians (7th ACCP).

ACCP Recommended Therapeutic Range for Oral Anticoagulant Therapy

Condition	PT Ratio[a]	INR
Acute MI[b]	1.3 to 1.5	2 to 3
MI, prevent recurrent	1.4 to 1.6	2.5 to 3.5
Atrial fibrillation[b]	1.3 to 1.5	2 to 3
Mechanical prosthetic valves	1.4 to 1.6	2.5 to 3.5
Bileaflet mechanical valve in aortic position	1.3 to 1.5	2 to 3
Pulmonary embolism, treatment	1.3 to 1.5	2 to 3
Tissue heart valves[b]	1.3 to 1.5	2 to 3
Valvular heart disease[b]	1.3 to 1.5	2 to 3
Venous thrombosis		
Prophylaxis (high-risk surgery)	1.3 to 1.5	2 to 3
Treatment	1.3 to 1.5	2 to 3

[a] International Sensitivity Index (ISI) of 2.8.
[b] To prevent systemic embolism.

Management of nontherapeutic INRs: The following is a suggested approach for treatment of overanticoagulated patients:

Management of Nontherapeutic INRs

INR	Significant bleeding	Rapid reversal	Intervention
< 5	No	No	Lower or omit a dose; resume therapy at lower dose when INR is in therapeutic range. If the INR is only minimally greater than the therapeutic range, no dose reduction may be required.
> 5 but < 9	No	No	Omit next few doses, monitor INR more frequently, resume therapy at lower dose when INR is in therapeutic range.
	Yes	No	Omit dose, give ≤ 5 mg vitamin K_1 orally.
	Yes	Yes	Give 2 to 4 mg vitamin K_1 orally, decrease in INR within 24 h. If INR still high, give additional dose of 1 to 2 mg vitamin K_1 orally.
≥ 9	No	No	Hold warfarin therapy, administer 5 to 10 mg vitamin K_1 orally; decrease in INR within 24 to 48 h; monitor INR frequently, repeat dose if necessary. Resume therapy at lower dose when INR is in therapeutic range.
Serious bleeding at any elevation of INR	Yes	Yes	Hold warfarin therapy. Give 10 mg vitamin K_1 slow IV infusion, may repeat dose every 12 h, supplement with plasma or prothrombin complex concentrate (PCC).
Life-threatening bleeding	Yes	Yes	Hold warfarin therapy. Give PCC supplemented with 10 mg vitamin K_1 slow IV. Repeat if necessary.

Treatment during dentistry and surgery: In patients who must be anticoagulated prior to, during, or immediately following dental or surgical procedures, adjusting the dosage to maintain the PT at the low end of the therapeutic range (or maintain the corresponding INR value) may safely allow for continued anticoagulation. Limit the operative site to permit effective use of local measures for hemostasis. Under these conditions, dental and surgical procedures may be performed without undue risk of hemorrhage.

Conversion from heparin therapy: Because the anticoagulant effect of warfarin is delayed, heparin is preferred initially for rapid anticoagulation. Conversion to warfarin therapy may begin concomitantly with heparin therapy or may be delayed 3 to 6 days. To ensure continuous anticoagulation, it is advisable to continue full dose heparin therapy and that warfarin therapy be overlapped with heparin for 4 to 5 days until warfarin therapy has produced the desired therapeutic response as determined by PT/INR. When warfarin has produced the desired PT/INR or prothrombin activity, heparin may be discontinued.

Actions

Pharmacology: Anticoagulants interfere with the hepatic synthesis of vitamin K-dependent clotting factors, which results in an in vivo depletion of clotting factors VII, IX, X, and II (prothrombin). Half-lives of these clotting factors are as follows: factor II, 60 hours; VII, 4 to 6 hours; IX, 24 hours; X, 48 to 72 hours. The half-lives of proteins C and S are approximately 8 and 30 hours, respectively. Hence, the reduction in the rate of synthesis of the clotting factors determines the clinical response. Although factor VII is quickly depleted and an initial prolongation of the PT is seen in 8 to 12 hours, maximum anticoagulation (thus, antithrombotic effects) is not approached for 3 to 5 days as the other factors are depleted and the drug achieves steady-state.

Warfarin is available as a racemic mixture containing the R(+) and S(–) enantiomers in equal proportions; however, the S-isomer is 3 to 6 times more potent as an anticoagulant than the R-isomer.

Pharmacokinetics:

Absorption – Warfarin is completely absorbed after oral administration with peak concentration generally attained within the first 4 hours.

Distribution – Oral anticoagulants are highly bound to plasma proteins (97% to more than 99%), primarily albumin.

Metabolism/Excretion – Warfarin is metabolized by hepatic microsomal enzymes and are excreted primarily in the urine and feces as inactive metabolites. The terminal half-life of warfarin after a single dose is approximately 1 week; however, the effective half-life ranges from 20 to 60 hours, with a mean of about 40 hours.

Contraindications

Women who are pregnant or may become pregnant; hemorrhagic tendencies or blood dyscrasias; recent or contemplated surgery of the CNS or eye, or traumatic surgery resulting in large, open surfaces; bleeding tendencies associated with active ulceration or overt bleeding of the GI, respiratory, or GU tracts, cerebrovascular hemorrhage, aneurysm (cerebral, dissecting aorta), pericarditis and pericardial effusion, or bacterial endocarditis; threatened abortion, eclampsia and preeclampsia; inadequate laboratory facilities; unsupervised patients with senility, alcoholism, or psychosis or other lack of patient cooperation; spinal puncture and other diagnostic or therapeutic procedures with potential for uncontrollable bleeding; major regional, lumbar block anesthesia; malignant hypertension; known hypersensitivity to warfarin or any other components of the product.

Warnings/Precautions

Hemorrhage/Necrosis: The most serious risks associated with anticoagulant therapy with warfarin are hemorrhage in any tissue or organ and, less frequently, necrosis or gangrene of skin and other tissues. Observe increased caution when warfarin is administered in the presence of any predisposing condition for which added risk of hemorrhage, necrosis, and/or gangrene is present. Hemorrhage and necrosis have in some cases been reported to result in death or permanent disability. Necrosis appears to be associated with local thrombosis and usually appears within a few days of the start of anticoagulant therapy.

Atheroemboli/Microemboli: Anticoagulation therapy with warfarin may enhance the release of atheromatous plaque emboli, thereby increasing the risk of complications from systemic cholesterol microembolization, including "purple toes syndrome." Discontinuation of warfarin therapy is recommended when such phenomena are observed.

Systemic atheroemboli and cholesterol microemboli can present with a variety of signs and symptoms, including purple toes syndrome; livedo reticularis; rash; gangrene; abrupt and intense pain in the leg, foot, or toes; foot ulcers; myalgia; penile gangrene; abdominal pain; flank or back pain; hematuria; renal function impairment; hypertension; cerebral ischemia; spinal cord infarction; pancreatitis; symptoms simulating polyarteritis; or any other sequelae of vascular compromise caused by embolic occlusion. The most commonly involved visceral organs are the kidneys, followed by the pancreas, spleen, and liver. Some cases have progressed to necrosis or death.

Purple toes syndrome: Purple toes syndrome is a complication of oral anticoagulation characterized by a dark, purplish or mottled color of the toes, usually occurring between 3 to 10 weeks, or later, after the initiation of therapy with warfarin or related compounds. Major features of this syndrome include purple color of the planter surfaces and sides of the toes that blanches on moderate pressure and fades with elevation of the leg, pain and tenderness of the toes, and waxing and waning of the color over time. When the purple toes syndrome is reported to be reversible, some cases progress to gangrene or necrosis, which may require debridement of the affected area or may lead to amputation.

Heparin-induced thrombocytopenia: Warfarin should be used with caution in patients with heparin-induced thrombocytopenia and deep venous thrombosis.

Special risk patients: Exercise caution in the presence of any predisposing condition where added risk of hemorrhage, necrosis, and/or gangrene is present, as well as in the following: severe to moderate hepatic or renal function impairment; infectious diseases or disturbances of intestinal flora (eg, sprue, antibiotic therapy); trauma that may result in internal bleeding; surgery or trauma resulting in large exposed raw surfaces; indwelling catheters; severe to moderate hypertension; polycythemia vera; vasculitis; severe diabetes; minor and severe allergic/hypersensitivity reactions and anaphylactic reactions.

Patients with congestive heart failure (CHF) may exhibit greater than expected PT/INR response to warfarin.

Protein C deficiency: Known or suspected hereditary, familial, or clinical deficiency in protein C has been associated with necrosis following warfarin therapy.

Enhanced anticoagulant effects: Endogenous factors that may be responsible for increased PT/INR response include blood dyscrasias; cancer; collagen vascular disease; CHF; diarrhea; elevated temperature; hepatic disorders (eg, infectious hepatitis, jaundice); hyperthyroidism; poor nutritional state; steatorrhea; vitamin K deficiency.

Patient selection: Use care in the selection of patients to ensure cooperation, especially from alcoholic, senile, or psychotic patients.

Decreased anticoagulant effects: Endogenous factors that may reduce the response to the oral anticoagulants or decrease the PT or INR include edema; hyperlipidemia; hypothyroidism; hereditary resistance to oral anticoagulants; nephrotic syndrome.

Hypersensitivity reactions: Minor and severe allergic/hypersensitivity reactions and anaphylactic reactions have been reported.

Pregnancy: Category X.

Lactation: Warfarin appears in breast milk in an inactive form. Infants breast-fed by warfarin-treated mothers had no change in PT.

Anisindione and dicumarol or their metabolites may be excreted in breast milk in amounts sufficient to cause a prothrombopenic state and bleeding in the newborn.

Children: Safety and efficacy in children younger than 18 years of age have not been established. Oral anticoagulants may be beneficial in children with rare thromboembolic disorder secondary to other disease states such as the nephrotic syndrome or congenital heart lesions. Heparin is probably the initial anticoagulant of choice because of its immediate onset of action.

Elderly: Older patients may be more sensitive to these agents. Lower doses are recommended.

Monitoring:

PT – Treatment is highly individualized. Control dosage by periodic determination of PT or other suitable coagulation tests (eg, INR). Monitor PT daily during the initiation of therapy and whenever any other drug is added to or discontinued from therapy that may alter the patient's response. Concurrent heparin therapy will elevate the PT 10% to 20%; if target PT levels are not increased by the same percentage during concurrent therapy, the patient could be inadequately anticoagulated when the heparin therapy is discontinued. Once stabilized, monitor PT every 4 to 6 weeks.

INR – INR is based on the determination of an International Normalized Ratio that provides a common basis for PT results and interpretations of therapeutic ranges.

Drug Interactions

Oral anticoagulants have a great potential for clinically significant drug interactions. Warn all patients about potential hazards and instruct against taking **any** drug, including nonprescription products and herbal medications, without the advice of a health care provider or pharmacist.

Careful monitoring and appropriate dosage adjustments usually will permit safe administration of combined therapy. Critical times during therapy occur when an interacting drug is added to or discontinued from a patient stabilized on anticoagulants.

Coumarin and indandione derivatives are affected by many drugs. Those that may significantly affect coumarin and indandione derivatives include acetaminophen; alcohol; allopurinol; aminoglycosides, oral; amiodarone; anabolic steroids (eg, danazol, oxandrolone, oxymethalone, stanozol); anticoagulants (eg, argatroban, bivalirudin, dicumarol, lepirudin); antineoplastic agents (eg, capecitabine, cyclophosphamide, fluorouracil, gefitinib); azole antifungals (eg, fluconazole, itraconazole, miconazole); beta-blockers (eg, atenolol, propranolol); cephalosporins, parenteral (eg, cefamandole, cefazolin, cefoperazone, cefotetan, cefoxitin, ceftriaxone); chenodiol; chloramphenicol; chlorpropamide; cimetidine; cyclosporine; dextran; dextrothyroxine; diazoxide; disulfiram; estrogens; felbamate; fenofibrate; fish oil; flutamide; gemfibrozil; glucagon; griseofulvin; haloperidol; heparin; HMG-CoA reductase inhibitors (ie, fluvastatin, lovastatin, simvastatin); influenza virus vaccine; isofamide; isoniazid; leflunomide; levamisole; loop diuretics (ie, ethacrynic acid, furosemide); macrolide antibiotics (eg, azithromycin, clarithromycin, erythromycin); mefloquine; methyldopa; methylphenidate; metronidazole; mineral oil; nalidixic acid; neomycin; NSAIDs, COX-2 selective; omeprazole; orlistat; pentoxifylline; phenylbutazone; propafenone; propoxyphene; proton pump inhibitors (eg, esomeprazole, lansoprazole, omeprazole, pentoprazole, rabeprazole); quinidine; quinine; quinolones (eg, ciprofloxacin, levofloxacin, norfloxacin, ofloxacin); ropinirole; selective COX-2 inhibitors (eg, celecoxib, rofecoxib, valdecoxib); SSRIs (ie, fluoxetine, fluvoxamine, paroxetine, sertraline); sulfonamides (eg, sulfamethazole, sulfisoxazole, trimethoprim, sulfamethoxazole); sulfinpyrazone; tamoxifen; tetracyclines (eg, doxycycline, tetracycline); thrombolytics (eg, streptokinase, tissue plasminogen activator, urokinase); thyroid hormones (eg, levothyroxine, liothyonine, thyroid); tolbutamide; tolterodine; tramadol; trastuzumab; valproate; vitamin E; zafirlukast; zileuton.

Herbal medicines: Exercise caution when herbal medicine are taken concomitantly with warfarin. Specific herbals reported to affect warfarin therapy include the following:

- Bromelains, danshen, dong quai (*Angelica sinensis*), garlic, *Ginkgo biloba*, ginseng, and cranberry products are associated most often with an increase in the effects of warfarin.

- Coenzyme Q_{10} (ubidecarenone) and St. John's wort are associated most often with a decrease in the effects of warfarin. Conversely, other herbals may have coagulant properties when taken alone or may decrease the effects of warfarin.

Drug/Food interactions: Vitamin K–rich vegetables may decrease the anticoagulant effects of warfarin by interfering with absorption. Minimize consumption of vitamin K–rich foods (eg, spinach, seaweed, broccoli, turnip greens) or nutritional supplements. Mango has been shown to increase warfarin's effect.

Adverse Reactions

Hemorrhage – Hemorrhage is the principal adverse reaction of warfarin.

Other adverse reactions include nausea; diarrhea; pyrexia; dermatitis; exfoliative dermatitis; urticaria; alopecia; sore mouth; mouth ulcers; fever; abdominal cramping; leukopenia; red-orange urine; priapism (causal relationship not established); paralytic ileus and intestinal obstruction from submucosal or intramural hemorrhage.

DESIRUDIN

Powder for injection, lyophilized: 15 mg (*Rx*)	*Iprivask* (Aventis)

Warning:

Spinal/Epidural hematomas: When neuraxial anesthesia (epidural/spinal anesthesia) or spinal puncture is employed, patients anticoagulated or scheduled to be anticoagulated with selective inhibitors of thrombin such as desirudin may be at risk of developing an epidural or spinal hematoma which can result in long-term or permanent paralysis.

The risk of these events may be increased by the use of indwelling spinal catheters for administration of analgesia or by the concomitant use of drugs affecting hemostasis such as nonsteroidal anti-inflammatory drugs (NSAIDs), platelet inhibitors, or other anticoagulants. Likewise with such agents, the risk appears to be increased by traumatic or repeated epidural or spinal puncture.

Patients should be frequently monitored for signs and symptoms of neurological impairment. If neurological compromise is noted, urgent treatment is necessary.

The physician should consider the potential benefit versus risk before neuraxial intervention, in patients anticoagulated or to be anticoagulated for thromboprophylaxis.

Indications

Deep vein thrombosis, prophylaxis: For the prophylaxis of deep vein thrombosis in patients undergoing elective hip-replacement surgery.

Administration and Dosage

Initial dosage: 15 mg every 12 hours administered by subcutaneous injection, with the initial dose given up to 5 to 15 minutes prior to surgery, but after induction of regional block anesthesia, if used. Up to 12 days administration (average duration 9 to 12 days) has been well tolerated in controlled clinical trials.

Renal function impairment:

Desirudin Use in Renal Function Impairment

Degree of renal insufficiency	Creatinine clearance (mL/min/1.73 m^2 body surface area)	aPTT monitoring and dosing instructions
Moderate	≥ 31 to 60	Initiate therapy at 5 mg every 12 hours by subcutaneous injection. Monitor aPTT and serum creatinine at least daily. If aPTT exceeds 2 times control: 1) interrupt therapy until the value returns to less than 2 times control; 2) resume therapy at a reduced dose guided by the initial degree of aPTT abnormality.
Severe	< 31	Initiate therapy at 1.7 mg every 12 hours. Monitor aPTT and serum creatinine at least daily. If aPTT exceeds 2 times control: 1) interrupt therapy until the value returns to less than 2 times control; 2) consider further dose reductions guided by the initial degree of aPTT abnormality.

Admixture incompatibilities: Desirudin should not be mixed with other injections, solvents, or infusions.

Actions

Pharmacology: Desirudin is a selective inhibitor of free circulating and clot-bound thrombin.

Pharmacokinetics:

Absorption – The absorption of desirudin is complete when administered subcutaneous at doses of 0.3 mg/kg or 0.5 mg/kg. Following subcutaneous administration of single doses of 0.1 to 0.75 mg/kg, plasma concentrations of desirudin increased to a maximum level (C_{max}) between 1 and 3 hours. Both C_{max} and area-under-the-curve (AUC) values are dose proportional.

Distribution – The pharmacokinetic properties of desirudin following IV administration are well described by a 2- or 3- compartment disposition model. Desirudin is distributed in the extracellular space with a volume of distribution at steady state of 0.25 L/kg, independent of the dose. Desirudin binds specifically and directly to thrombin, forming an extremely tight, noncovalent complex.

Metabolism – Desirudin is primarily eliminated and metabolized by the kidney. The total urinary excretion of unchanged desirudin amounts to 40% to 50% of the administered dose. Total clearance of desirudin is approximately 1.5 to 2.7 mL/min/kg following either subcutaneous or IV administration and is independent of dose. This clearance value is close to the glomerular filtration rate.

Excretion – The elimination of desirudin from plasma is rapid after IV administration, with approximately 90% of the dose disappearing from the plasma within 2 hours of the injection. Plasma concentrations of desirudin then decline with a mean terminal elimination half-life of 2 to 3 hours. After subcutaneous administration, the mean terminal elimination half-life is also approximately 2 hours.

Renal function impairment – In a pharmacokinetic study of renally impaired subjects, subjects with mild, moderate, and severe renal insufficiency, were administered a single IV dose of 0.5, 0.25, or 0.125 mg/kg desirudin, respectively. This resulted in mean dose-normalized AUC_{effect} ($AUC_{0\text{-}60th}$ for aPTT prolongation) increases of approximately 3-, and 9-fold for the moderate and severe renally impaired subjects, respectively, compared with healthy individuals. In subjects with severe renal insufficiency, terminal elimination half-lives were prolonged up to 12 hours compared with 2 to 4 hours in healthy volunteers or subjects with mild-to-moderate renal insufficiency.

Contraindications

Hypersensitivity to natural or recombinant hirudins; active bleeding or irreversible coagulation disorders.

Warnings/Precautions

Hemorrhagic events: Desirudin is not intended for IM injection, as local hematoma formation may result.

Use with caution in patients with increased risks of hemorrhage such as those with recent major surgery, organ biopsy or puncture of a noncompressible vessel within the last month; a history of hemorrhagic stroke, intracranial or intraocular bleeding including diabetic (hemorrhagic) retinopathy; recent ischemic stroke, severe uncontrolled hypertension, bacterial endocarditis, a known hemostatic disorder (congenital or acquired [eg, hemophilia, liver disease]) or a history of GI or pulmonary bleeding within the past 3 months.

Bleeding can occur at any site during therapy with desirudin. An unexplained fall in hematocrit or blood pressure should lead to a search for a bleeding site.

Spinal/Epidural anesthesia: See Warning Box.

Interchangeability: Desirudin cannot be used interchangeably with other hirudins as they differ in manufacturing process and specific biological activity (ATUs). Each of these medicines has its own instructions for use.

Antibodies/reexposure: Antibodies have been reported in patients treated with hirudins. Potential for cross-sensitivity to hirudin products cannot be excluded.

Renal function impairment: Use with caution in patients with renal function impairment, particularly in those with moderate and severe renal function impairment (creatinine clearance less than or equal to 60 mL/min/1.73 m^2 body surface area). Daily aPTT and serum creatinine monitoring are recommended for patients with moderate or severe renal function impairment. See Administration and Dosage.

Pregnancy: Category C.

Lactation: It is not known whether desirudin is excreted in human milk. Exercise caution when desirudin is administered to a breast-feeding woman.

Children: Safety and efficacy in children have not been established.

Elderly: Serious adverse reactions occurred more frequently in patients 75 years of age or older as compared with those younger than 65 years of age.

Monitoring: Activated partial thromboplastin time (aPTT) should be monitored daily in patients with increased risk of bleeding or renal function impairment. Serum creatinine should be monitored daily in patients with renal function impairment. Peak aPTT should not exceed 2 times control. Should peak aPTT exceed this level, dose reduction is advised, based on the degree of aPTT abnormality. If necessary, therapy with desirudin should be interrupted until aPTT falls to less than 2 times control, at which time treatment with desirudin can be resumed at a reduced dose).

Drug Interactions

Drugs that may interact with desirudin and increase the risk of bleeding include thrombolytics (eg, alteplase), glucocorticoids, dextran, anticoagulants (eg, heparin), antiplatelets, and glycoprotein IIb/IIIa antagonists (eg, abciximab).

Adverse Reactions

Adverse reactions occurring in at least 3% of patients include the following: Anemia, hemorrhage, injection site mass, wound secretion.

LEPIRUDIN

Powder for injection: 50 mg (*Rx*)	*Refludan* (Hoechst-Marion Roussel)

Indications

Thrombocytopenia, heparin-induced: For anticoagulation in patients with heparin-induced thrombocytopenia (HIT) and associated thromboembolic disease in order to prevent further thromboembolic complications.

Administration and Dosage

Initial dosage: 0.4 mg/kg (110 kg or less) slowly IV (ie, over 15 to 20 seconds) as a bolus dose followed by 0.15 mg/kg (110 kg/h or less) as a continuous IV infusion for 2 to 10 days or longer if clinically needed.

Normally the initial dosage depends on the patient's body weight; this is valid for patients 110 kg or less. In patients with a body weight over 110 kg, the initial dosage should not be increased beyond the 110 kg body weight dose (maximal initial bolus dose of 44 mg, maximal initial infusion dose of 16.5 mg/h).

Determine patient baseline activated partial thromboplastin time (aPTT) prior to initiation of therapy with lepirudin, because lepirudin should not be started in patients presenting with a baseline aPTT ratio of 2.5 or more in order to avoid initial overdosing.

Monitoring: Adjust the dosage (infusion rate) according to the aPTT ratio.

The target range for the aPTT ratio during treatment (therapeutic window) should be 1.5 to 2.5.

The first aPTT determination for monitoring treatment should be done 4 hours after start of the lepirudin infusion. Follow-up aPTT determinations are recommended at least once daily, as long as treatment is ongoing.

More frequent aPTT monitoring is highly recommended in patients with renal function impairment or serious liver injury or with an increased risk of bleeding.

Dose modifications: Any aPTT ratio out of the target range is to be confirmed at once before drawing conclusions with respect to dose modifications, unless there is a clinical need to react immediately.

If the confirmed aPTT ratio is above the target range, stop the infusion for 2 hours. At restart, decrease the infusion rate by 50% (no additional IV bolus should be administered). Determine the aPTT ratio again 4 hours later.

If the confirmed aPTT ratio is below the target range, increase the infusion rate in steps of 20%. Determine the aPTT ratio again 4 hours later.

Do not exceed an infusion rate of 0.21 mg/kg/h without checking for coagulation abnormalities, which might be preventive of an appropriate aPTT response.

Renal function impairment: As lepirudin is almost exclusively excreted in the kidneys, consider individual renal function prior to administration. In case of renal function impairment, relative overdose might occur even with the standard dosing regimen. Therefore, the bolus dose and infusion rate must be reduced in case of known or suspected renal insufficiency (CrCl less than 60 mL/min or serum creatinine more than 1.5 mg/dL).

There is only limited information on the therapeutic use of lepirudin in HIT patients with significant renal function impairment. The following dosage recommendations are mainly based on single-dose studies in a small number of patients with renal function impairment. Therefore, these recommendations are only tentative.

In all patients with renal insufficiency, reduce the bolus dose to 0.2 mg/kg.

The standard initial infusion rate must be reduced according to the recommendations given in the following table. Additional aPTT monitoring is highly recommended.

Reduction of Lepirudin Infusion Rate in Patients with Renal Function Impairment

CrCl (mL/min)	Serum creatinine (mg/dL)	Adjusted infusion rate	
		% of standard initial infusion rate	mg/kg/h
45 to 60	1.6 to 2	50%	0.075
30 to 44	2.1 to 3	30%	0.045
15 to 29	3.1 to 6	15%	0.0225
< 15[a]	> 6[a]	avoid or stop infusion[a]	

[a] In hemodialysis patients or in case of acute renal failure (CrCl less than 15 mL/min or serum creatinine more than 6 mg/dL), avoid or stop infusion of lepirudin. Consider additional IV bolus doses of 0.1 mg/kg every other day only if the aPTT ratio falls below the lower therapeutic limit of 1.5.

Concomitant use with thrombolytic therapy: Clinical trials in HIT patients have provided only limited information on the combined use of lepirudin and thrombolytic agents. The following dosage regimen of lepirudin was used in 9 HIT patients in the studies who presented with TECs at baseline and were started on both lepirudin and thrombolytic therapy (alteplase, urokinase, or streptokinase).

Pay special attention to the fact that thrombolytic agents per se may increase the aPTT ratio. Therefore, aPTT ratios with a given plasma level of lepirudin are usually higher in patients who receive concomitant thrombolysis than in those who do not.

Initial IV bolus – 0.2 mg/kg.

Continuous IV infusion – 0.1 mg/kg/h.

Patients scheduled to switch to oral anticoagulation: If a patient is scheduled to receive coumarin for oral anticoagulation after lepirudin therapy, the dose of lepirudin should first be gradually reduced in order to reach an aPTT ratio just above 1.5 before initiating oral anticoagulation. As soon as an international normalized ratio (INR) of 2 is reached, stop lepirudin therapy.

Initial IV bolus: IV injection of the bolus is to be carried out slowly (ie, over 15 to 20 seconds).

Standard Bolus Injection Volumes of Lepirudin According to Body Weight for a 5 mg/mL Concentration

Body weight (kg)	Injection Volume	
	Dosage 0.4 mg/kg	Dosage 0.2 mg/kg[a]
50	4 mL	2 mL
60	4.8 mL	2.4 mL
70	5.6 mL	2.8 mL
80	6.4 mL	3.2 mL
90	7.2 mL	3.6 mL
100	8 mL	4 mL

Standard Bolus Injection Volumes of Lepirudin According to Body Weight for a 5 mg/mL Concentration		
Body weight (kg)	Injection Volume	
	Dosage 0.4 mg/kg	Dosage 0.2 mg/kg[a]
≥ 110	8.8 mL	4.4 mL

[a] Dosage recommended for all patients with renal insufficiency.

IV infusion: For continuous IV infusion, solutions with concentration of 0.2 or 0.4 mg/mL may be used.

The infusion rate (mL/h) is to be set according to body weight (see following table).

Standard Infusion Rates of Lepirudin According to Body Weight		
Body weight (kg)	Infusion rate at 0.15 mg/kg/h	
	500 mL infusion bag 0.2 mg/mL	250 mL infusion bag 0.4 mg/mL
50	38 mL/h	19 mL/h
60	45 mL/h	23 mL/h
70	53 mL/h	26 mL/h
80	60 mL/h	30 mL/h
90	68 mL/h	34 mL/h
100	75 mL/h	38 mL/h
≥ 110	83 mL/h	41 mL/h

Actions

Pharmacology: Lepirudin (rDNA), a recombinant hirudin derived from yeast cells, is a highly specific direct inhibitor of thrombin.

One molecule of lepirudin binds to one molecule of thrombin and thereby blocks the thrombogenic activity of thrombin. As a result, all thrombin-dependent coagulation assays are affected (eg, aPTT values increase in a dose-dependent fashion).

Pharmacokinetics:

Absorption/Distribution – Following IV administration, distribution is essentially confined to extracellular fluids and is characterized by an initial half-life of about 10 minutes. Elimination follows a first-order process and is characterized by a terminal half-life of about 1.3 hours in young healthy volunteers. As the IV dose is increased over the range of 0.1 to 0.4 mg/kg, the maximum plasma concentration and the AUC increase proportionally.

Metabolism/Excretion – Lepirudin is thought to be metabolized by release of amino acids via catabolic hydrolysis of the parent drug; however, conclusive data are not available. Approximately 48% of the administered dose is excreted in the urine, which consists of unchanged drug (35%) and other fragments of the parent drug.

The systemic clearance of lepirudin is proportional to the glomerular filtration rate or creatinine clearance. Dose adjustment based on creatinine clearance is recommended (see Administration and Dosage). In patients with marked renal insufficiency (creatinine clearance less than 15 mL/min) and on hemodialysis, elimination half-lives are prolonged 2 days or less.

Special populations: The systemic clearance of lepirudin in women is about 25% lower than in men. In elderly patients, the systemic clearance of lepirudin is 20% lower than in younger patients. This may be explained by the lower creatinine clearance in elderly patients compared with younger patients.

Contraindications

Hypersensitivity to hirudins.

Warnings/Precautions

Intracranial bleeding: Following concomitant thrombolytic therapy with alteplase (tPA) or streptokinase may be life-threatening. Carefully assess the risk of lepirudin administration vs its anticipated benefit in patients with increased risk of bleeding. In particular, this includes the following conditions:

- Recent puncture of large vessels or organ biopsy
- Anomaly of vessels or organs
- Recent cerebrovascular accident, stroke, intracerebral surgery, or other neuraxial procedures
- Severe uncontrolled hypertension
- Bacterial endocarditis
- Advanced renal function impairment
- Hemorrhagic diathesis
- Recent major surgery
- Recent major bleeding (eg, intracranial, GI, intraocular, pulmonary)

Antibodies: Formation of antihirudin antibodies was observed in approximately 40% of HIT patients treated with lepirudin. This may increase the anticoagulant effect of lepirudin possibly because of delayed renal elimination of active lepirudin-antihirudin complexes. Therefore, strict monitoring of aPTT is necessary also during prolonged therapy. No evidence of neutralization of lepirudin or of allergic reactions associated with positive antibody test results was found.

Hepatic injury: Serious liver injury (eg, cirrhosis) may enhance the anticoagulant effect of lepirudin caused by coagulation defects secondary to reduced generation of vitamin K-dependent coagulation factors.

Reexposure: There is limited information to support any recommendations for reexposure to lepirudin. Of 13 patients reexposed in 2 studies, one experienced a mild allergic skin reaction during the second treatment cycle.

Allergic reactions: Approximately 53% of all allergic reactions or suspected allergic reactions occurred in patients who concomitantly received thrombolytic therapy (eg, streptokinase) for acute MI or contrast media for coronary angiography (see Adverse Reactions).

Renal function impairment: With renal function impairment, relative overdose might occur even with a standard dosage regimen. In patients with marked renal insufficiency (creatinine clearance less than 15 mL/min) and on hemodialysis, elimination half-lives are prolonged 2 days or less. Reduce the bolus dose and rate of infusion in patients with known or suspected renal insufficiency (see Administration and Dosage).

Pregnancy: *Category B.* Use during pregnancy only if clearly needed.

Lactation: It is not known whether lepirudin is excreted in breast milk. Because of the potential for serious adverse reactions in breast-feeding infants, decide whether to discontinue breast-feeding or to discontinue the drug, taking into account the importance of the drug to the mother.

Children: Safety and efficacy have not been established.

Lab test abnormalities: In general, adjust the dosage (infusion rate) according to the aPTT ratio (patient aPTT at a given time over an aPTT reference value, usually the median of the laboratory normal range for aPTT; see Administration and Dosage). Other thrombin- dependent coagulation assays are affected by lepirudin.

Drug Interactions

Drugs that may interact with lepirudin and increase the risk of bleeding include thrombolytics (eg, tPA, streptokinase) and coumarin derivatives (vitamin K antagonists).

Adverse Reactions

Adverse events occurring in at least 3% of patients include the following: Abnormal liver function; allergic skin reactions; anemia or isolated drop in hemoglobin; bleeding from puncture sites and wounds; epistaxis; fever; GI and rectal bleeding; other hematoma and unclassified bleeding; hematuria; multiorgan failure; pneumonia; sepsis.

ARGATROBAN

Injection, solution, concentrate: 100 mg/mL (*Rx*) *Argatroban* (GlaxoSmithKline)

Indications

Heparin-induced thrombocytopenia/heparin-induced thrombosis-thrombocytopenia syndrome: As an anticoagulant for prophylaxis or treatment of thrombosis in patients with heparin-induced thrombocytopenia (HIT)/heparin-induced thrombosis-thrombocytopenia syndrome (HITTS).

Percutaneous coronary intervention in heparin-induced thrombocytopenia/thrombosis-thrombocytopenia syndrome: As an anticoagulant in patients with or at risk for HIT undergoing percutaneous coronary intervention (PCI).

Administration and Dosage

Argatroban, as supplied, is a concentrated drug (100 mg/mL) that must be diluted 100-fold prior to infusion. Do not mix with other drugs prior to dilution.

Initial dosage in heparin-induced thrombocytopenia or heparin-induced thrombocytopenia and thrombosis syndrome: Before administering argatroban, discontinue heparin therapy and obtain a baseline activated partial thromboplastin time (aPTT). The recommended initial dose of argatroban for adults without hepatic function impairment is 2 mcg/kg/min administered as a continuous infusion.

Standard Infusion Rates for 2 mcg/kg/min Dose of Argatroban (1 mg/mL Final Concentration)

Body weight (kg)	Dose (mcg/min)	Infusion rate (mL/h)
50	100	6
60	120	7
70	140	8
80	160	10
90	180	11
100	200	12
110	220	13
120	240	14
130	260	16
140	280	17

Monitoring therapy – In general, argatroban therapy is monitored using aPTT. Tests of anticoagulant effects (including aPTT) typically attain steady-state levels within 1 to 3 hours following initiation of argatroban. Check the aPTT 2 hours after initiation of therapy to confirm the aPTT is within the desired therapeutic range.

Dosage adjustment – After the initial dose of argatroban, the dose can be adjusted as clinically indicated (not to exceed 10 mcg/kg/min), until the steady-state aPTT is 1.5 to 3 times the initial baseline value (not to exceed 100 seconds).

Percutaneous coronary intervention in heparin-induced thrombosis-thrombocytopenia syndrome patients:

Initial dosage – Start an infusion of argatroban at 25 mcg/kg/min and a bolus of 350 mcg/kg administered via a large bore intravenous (IV) line over 3 to 5 minutes. Check activated clotting time (ACT) 5 to 10 minutes after the bolus dose is completed. Proceed with PCI if the ACT is more than 300 seconds.

Dosage adjustment – If the ACT is less than 300 seconds, administer an additional IV bolus dose of 150 mcg/kg, increase the infusion dose to 30 mcg/kg/min, and check the ACT 5 to 10 minutes later. If the ACT is more than 450 seconds, decrease the infusion rate to 15 mcg/kg/min and check the ACT 5 to 10 minutes later. Once a therapeutic ACT (between 300 and 450 seconds) has been achieved, continue this infusion dose for the duration of the procedure.

Recommended Doses and Infusion Rates of Argatroban for Patients Undergoing PCI (1 mg/mL Final Concentration)[a]

	For ACT 300 to 450 seconds: initial dosage[b] 25 mcg/kg/min			If ACT < 300 seconds: dosage adjustment[c] 30 mcg/kg/min			If ACT > 450 seconds: dosage adjustment 15 mcg/kg/min	
Body weight (kg)	Bolus dose (mcg)	Infusion dose (mcg/min)	Infusion rate (mL/h)	Bolus dose (mcg)	Infusion dose (mcg/min)	Infusion rate (mL/h)	Infusion dose (mcg/min)	Infusion rate (mL/h)
50	17,500	1,250	75	7,500	1,500	90	750	45
60	21,000	1,500	90	9000	1,800	108	900	54
70	24,500	1,750	105	10,500	2,100	126	1,050	63
80	28,000	2,000	120	12,000	2,400	144	1,200	72
90	31,500	2,250	135	13,500	2,700	162	1,350	81
100	35,000	2,500	150	15,000	3,000	180	1,500	90
110	38,500	2,750	165	16,500	3,300	198	1,650	99
120	42,000	3,000	180	18,000	3,600	216	1,800	108
130	45,500	3,250	195	19,500	3,900	234	1,950	117
140	49,000	3,500	210	21,000	4,200	252	2,100	126

[a] Note: 1 mg = 1,000 mcg; 1 kg = 2.2 lbs.
[b] Initial IV bolus dose of 350 mcg/kg should be administered.
[c] Administer additional IV bolus dose of 150 mcg/kg if ACT is < 300 seconds.

In case of dissection, impending abrupt closure, thrombus formation during the procedure, or inability to achieve or maintain an ACT over 300 seconds, additional bolus doses of 150 mcg/kg may be administered and the infusion dose increased to 40 mcg/kg/min. Check the ACT after each additional bolus or change in the rate of infusion.

Monitoring therapy – Obtain ACTs before dosing, 5 to 10 minutes after bolus dosing, after change in infusion rate, and at the end of the PCI procedure. Draw additional ACTs about every 20 to 30 minutes during a prolonged procedure.

Continued anticoagulation after percutaneous coronary intervention – If a patient requires anticoagulation after the procedure, argatroban may be continued at a lower infusion dose.

Hepatically impaired patients: For patients with moderate hepatic function impairment, an initial dose of 0.5 mcg/kg/min is recommended, based on the approximate 4-fold decrease in argatroban clearance relative to those with normal hepatic function. Monitor the aPTT closely and adjust the dosage as clinically indicated.

Children: Initial argatroban infusion doses are lower for seriously ill children compared with adults with healthy hepatic function.

Conversion to oral anticoagulant therapy:

Initiating oral anticoagulant therapy – Recognize the potential for combined effects on international normalized ratio (INR) with coadministration of argatroban and warfarin. Do not use a loading dose of warfarin. Initiate therapy using the expected daily dose of warfarin. To ensure continuous anticoagulation when initiating warfarin, it is recommended to overlap argatroban and warfarin therapy.

Use of argatroban with warfarin results in prolongation of INR beyond that produced by warfarin alone.

Measure INR daily while argatroban and warfarin are coadministered.

Coadministration of warfarin and argatroban at doses of up to 2 mcg/kg/min – In general, with doses of argatroban of up to 2 mcg/kg/min, argatroban can be discontinued when the INR is greater than 4 on combined therapy. After argatroban is discontinued, repeat the INR measurement in 4 to 6 hours. If the repeat INR is below the desired therapeutic range, resume the infusion of argatroban and repeat the procedure daily until the desired therapeutic range on warfarin alone is reached.

Coadministration of warfarin and argatroban at doses greater than 2 mcg/kg/min – For doses greater than 2 mcg/kg/min, the relationship of INR on warfarin alone to the INR on warfarin plus argatroban is less predictable. In this case, in order to predict the INR on warfarin alone, temporarily reduce the dose of argatroban to a dose of 2 mcg/kg/min. Repeat the INR on argatroban and warfarin 4 to 6 hours after reduction of the argatroban dose and follow the process outlined previously for administering argatroban at doses of up to 2 mcg/kg/min.

Actions

Pharmacology:

Mechanism of action – Argatroban is a direct thrombin inhibitor that reversibly binds to the thrombin active site. It inhibits thrombin-catalyzed or induced reactions, including fibrin formation; activation of coagulation factors V, VIII, and XIII; protein C; and platelet aggregation.

Argatroban can inhibit the action of free and clot-associated thrombin. Argatroban does not interact with heparin-induced antibodies.

Pharmacokinetics:

Distribution – Argatroban has an apparent steady-state volume of distribution of 174 mL/kg. It is 54% bound to human serum proteins.

Metabolism – The main route of argatroban metabolism is in the liver by the microsomal CYP-450 enzymes CYP3A4/5. Data suggest that CYP3A4/5 mediated metabolism is not an important elimination pathway in vivo.

Excretion – The terminal elimination half-life of argatroban ranges between 39 and 51 minutes. Argatroban is excreted primarily in the feces, presumably through biliary secretion.

Pharmacokinetic/Pharmacodynamic relationship – Steady-state levels of drug and anticoagulant effect are typically attained within 1 to 3 hours and are maintained until the infusion is discontinued or the dosage is adjusted.

Contraindications

Overt major bleeding; hypersensitivity to this product or any of its components.

Warnings/Precautions

Argatroban is intended for IV administration. Discontinue all parenteral anticoagulants before administration of argatroban.

Hemorrhage: Hemorrhage can occur at any site in the body in patients receiving argatroban. An unexplained fall in hematocrit or blood pressure, or any other unexplained symptom, should lead to consideration of a hemorrhagic event. Use argatroban with extreme caution in disease states and other circumstances in which there is an increased danger of hemorrhage.

Hepatic function impairment: Exercise caution when administering argatroban to patients with hepatic disease by starting with a lower dose and carefully titrating until the desired level of anticoagulation is achieved. Also, upon cessation of argatroban infusion in the hepatically impaired patient, full reversal of anticoagulant effects may require more than 4 hours because of decreased clearance and increased elimination half-life of argatroban.

Avoid use of high doses of argatroban in PCI patients with clinically significant hepatic disease or AST/ALT levels of at least 3 times the upper limit of normal.

Pregnancy: *Category B.*

Lactation: Discontinue breast-feeding or discontinue the drug.

Children: The safety and effectiveness of argatroban, including the appropriate anticoagulation goals and duration of therapy, have not been established in children.

Monitoring: Check aPTT 2 hours after initiation of therapy.

In clinical trials in PCI, the ACT was used for monitoring argatroban activity during the procedure. Obtain ACTs before dosing, 5 to 10 minutes after bolus dosing, after change in infusion rate, and at the end of the PCI procedure. Draw additional ACTs approximately every 20 minutes to 30 minutes during a prolonged procedure.

Drug Interactions

Drugs that may interact with argatroban include heparin and warfarin, antiplatelet agents, glycoprotein IIb/IIIa antagonists, and thrombolytics (eg, alteplase, streptokinase).

Adverse Reactions

Adverse reactions occurring in at least 3% of patients include the following: abdominal pain, atrial fibrillation, back pain, bradycardia, cardiac arrest, chest pain, diarrhea, dyspnea, fever, headache, hypotension, infection, myocardial infarction, nausea, pain, pneumonia, sepsis, urinary tract infection, ventricular tachycardia, vomiting.

Major hemorrhagic events: Overall bleeding.

Minor hemorrhagic events: GI; hematuria/GU; decreased hemoglobin, hematocrit; groin; groin (bleeding or hematoma).

DABIGATRAN ETEXILATE

Capsules; oral: 75 and 150 mg (*Rx*) — *Pradaxa* (Boehringer Ingelheim Pharmaceuticals)

Indications

Stroke/Systemic embolism prevention: To reduce the risk of stroke and systemic embolism in patients with nonvalvular atrial fibrillation.

Administration and Dosage

Stroke/systemic embolism prevention (adults): 150 mg twice daily. If a dose is missed, the dose should be taken as soon as possible on the same day; the missed dose should be skipped if it cannot be taken at least 6 hours before the next scheduled dose. The dose should not be doubled to make up for a missed dose.

Renal function impairment:

Creatinine clearance 15 to 30 mL/min – 75 mg twice daily.

Creatinine clearance less than 15 mL/min or dialysis – Dosing recommendations cannot be provided.

Conversion:

Warfarin – Discontinue warfarin and start dabigatran when the international normalized ratio (INR) is below 2.

For creatinine clearance (CrCl) greater than 50 mL/min, start warfarin 3 days before discontinuing dabigatran; for CrCl 31 to 50 mL/min, start warfarin 2 days before discontinuing dabigatran; for CrCl 15 to 30 mL/min, start warfarin 1 day before discontinuing dabigatran; and for CrCl less than 15 mL/min, no recommendations can be made.

Parenteral anticoagulants – Start dabigatran 0 to 2 hours before the time that the next dose of the parenteral drug was due or at the time of discontinuation of a continuously administered parenteral drug (eg, intravenous [IV] unfractionated heparin).

For patients currently taking dabigatran, wait 12 hours (CrCl 30 mL/min or more) or 24 hours (CrCl less than 30 mL/min) after the last dose of dabigatran before initiating treatment with a parenteral anticoagulant.

Invasive or surgical procedures: If possible, discontinue dabigatran 1 to 2 days (CrCl 50 mL/min or more) or 3 to 5 days (CrCl less than 50 mL/min) before invasive or surgical procedures. Consider longer times for patients undergoing major surgery, spinal puncture, or placement of a spinal or epidural catheter or port, in whom complete hemostasis may be required.

Administration: Swallow the capsules whole. Take with or without food.

Actions

Pharmacology: Dabigatran is a competitive, direct thrombin inhibitor. Thrombin inhibition prevents the development of a thrombus. Free and clot-bound thrombin and thrombin-induced platelet aggregation are inhibited by the active moieties.

Pharmacokinetics:

Absorption – The absolute bioavailability of dabigatran is approximately 3% to 7%. Maximum plasma concentrations occur at 1 hour postadministration in the fasted state.

Distribution – Dabigatran is approximately 35% bound to human plasma proteins.

Metabolism – Dabigatran is not a substrate, inhibitor, or inducer of cytochrome P450 enzymes.

Excretion – Dabigatran is eliminated primarily in the urine. The half-life of dabigatran in healthy subjects is 12 to 17 hours.

Contraindications

Active pathological bleeding; history of a serious hypersensitivity reaction to dabigatran (eg, anaphylactic reaction, anaphylactic shock).

Warnings/Precautions

Bleeding: Dabigatran increases the risk of bleeding and can cause significant and sometimes fatal bleeding. Risk factors for bleeding include the use of drugs that increase the risk of bleeding in general (eg, antiplatelet agents, heparin, fibrinolytic therapy, chronic use of nonsteroidal anti-inflammatory drugs [NSAIDs]), and labor and delivery.

Discontinuation: Discontinuing anticoagulants, including dabigatran, for active bleeding, elective surgery, or invasive procedures places patients at an increased risk of stroke. Avoid lapses in therapy.

Pregnancy: *Category* C.

Lactation: It is not known whether dabigatran is excreted in human milk.

Children: Safety and effectiveness of dabigatran in children have not been established.

Elderly: The risk of stroke and bleeding increase with age, but the risk-benefit profile is favorable in all age groups.

Monitoring: Monitor for signs of bleeding throughout therapy.

Drug Interactions

Drugs that may affect dabigatran include amiodarone, clopidogrel, drugs that increase the risk of bleeding (eg, antiplatelet agents [eg, clopidogrel], fibrinolytic therapy [alteplase], heparin, chronic use of NSAIDs [eg, ibuprofen]), ketoconazole, quinidine, rifamycins, and verapamil.

Adverse Reactions

Adverse reactions occurring in 3% of patients or more include bleeding (any), bleeding (major), dyspepsia, gastritis-like symptoms, and GI bleeds.

BIVALIRUDIN

Powder for injection, lyophilized: 250 mg (*Rx*)	*Angiomax* (Medicines Co.)

Indications

Concomitant aspirin therapy: Bivalirudin is intended for use with aspirin and has been studied only in patients receiving concomitant aspirin.

The safety and efficacy of bivalirudin have not been established in patients with acute coronary syndromes who are not undergoing percutaneous transluminal coronary angioplasty (PTCA) or percutaneous coronary intervention (PCI).

PCI: Bivalirudin with provisional use of glycoprotein IIb/IIIa inhibitor (GPIIb/IIIa inhibitor) is indicated for use as an anticoagulant in patients undergoing PCI.

PTCA: Bivalirudin is indicated for use as an anticoagulant in patients with unstable angina undergoing PTCA.

Heparin-induced thrombocytopenia/heparin-induced thrombocytopenia and thrombosis syndrome (HIT/HITTS): For patients with, or at risk of, HIT/HITTS undergoing PCI.

Administration and Dosage

PCI/PTCA: The recommended dosage is an intravenous (IV) bolus dose of 0.75 mg/kg. Follow by an infusion of 1.75 mg/kg/h for the duration of the PCI procedure. Five minutes after the bolus dose has been administered, an activated clotting time (ACT) should be performed and an additional bolus of 0.3 mg/kg should be given if needed. GPIIb/IIIa inhibitor administration should be considered in the event that any of the following conditions are present:

- decreased thrombosis in myocardial infarction (TIMI) flow (0 to 2) or slow reflow;
- dissection with decreased flow;
- new or suspected thrombus;
- persistent residual stenosis;
- distal embolization;
- unplanned stent;
- suboptimal stenting;
- side branch closure;
- abrupt closure;
- clinical instability;
- prolonged ischemia.

HIT/HITTS: The recommended dose is an IV bolus dose of 0.75 mg/kg. Follow by a continuous infusion at a rate of 1.75 mg/kg/h for the duration of the procedure.

Continuation of therapy: Continuation of the infusion following PCI for up to 4 hours post-procedure is optional, at the discretion of the treating health care provider. After 4 hours, an additional IV infusion of bivalirudin may be initiated at a rate of 0.2 mg/kg/h for up to 20 hours, if needed.

Concomitant aspirin therapy: Bivalirudin is intended for use with aspirin (300 to 325 mg daily) and has been studied only in patients receiving concomitant aspirin.

Administration: The dose to be administered is adjusted according to the patient's weight (see the following table).

Bivalirudin Dosing

	Using 5 mg/mL concentration		Using 0.5 mg/mL concentration
Weight (kg)	Bolus 0.75 mg/kg (mL)	Infusion 1.75 mg/kg/h (mL/h)	Subsequent low-rate infusion 0.2 mg/kg/h (mL/h)
43 to 47	7	16	18
48 to 52	7.5	17.5	20
53 to 57	8	19	22
58 to 62	9	21	24
63 to 67	10	23	26
68 to 72	10.5	24.5	28
73 to 77	11	26	30
78 to 82	12	28	32
83 to 87	13	30	34
88 to 92	13.5	31.5	36
93 to 97	14	33	38
98 to 102	15	35	40
103 to 107	16	37	42
108 to 112	16.5	38.5	44
113 to 117	17	40	46
118 to 122	18	42	48
123 to 127	19	44	50
128 to 132	19.5	45.5	52
133 to 137	20	47	54
138 to 142	21	49	56
143 to 147	22	51	58
148 to 152	22.5	52.5	60

Administer bivalirudin via an IV line. No incompatibilities have been observed with glass bottles or polyvinyl chloride bags and administration sets. The following drugs should not be administered in the same IV line with bivalirudin because they resulted in haze formation, microparticulate formation, or gross precipitation when mixed with bivalirudin: alteplase, amiodarone, amphotericin B, chlorpromazine, diazepam, prochlorperazine edisylate, reteplase, streptokinase, and vancomycin.

Inspect parenteral drug products visually for particulate matter and discoloration prior to administration. Do not use preparations of bivalirudin containing particulate matter.

Actions

Pharmacology: Bivalirudin directly inhibits thrombin by specifically binding to the catalytic site and to the anion-binding exosite of circulating and clot-bound thrombin. The binding of bivalirudin to thrombin is reversible.

Pharmacokinetics: Bivalirudin exhibits linear pharmacokinetics following IV administration to patients undergoing routine angioplasty. In these patients, a mean steady-state bivalirudin concentration of about 12.3 mcg/mL is achieved following an IV bolus of 1 mg/kg and a 4-hour 2.5 mg/kg/h IV infusion. Bivalirudin is cleared from plasma by a combination of renal mechanisms and proteolytic cleavage, with a half-life in patients with normal renal function of 25 minutes. Drug elimination is related to glomerular filtration rate (GFR). Total body clearance is similar for patients with normal renal function and with mild renal function impairment (60 to 89 mL/min). Clearance is reduced about 20% in patients with moderate and severe renal function impairment and reduced about 80% in dialysis-dependent patients. For patients with renal function impairment, monitor the activated clotting time (ACT). Bivalirudin is hemodialyzable. Approximately 25% is cleared by hemodialysis.

Bivalirudin does not bind to plasma proteins (other than thrombin) or to red blood cells.

Special populations –

Renal function impairment:

Bivalirudin Pharmacokinetic Parameters in Renal Function Impairment		
Renal function (GFR, mL/min)	Clearance (mL/min/kg)	Half-life (minutes)
Normal renal function (≥ 90 mL/min)	3.4	25
Mild renal function impairment (60 to 90 mL/min)	3.4	22
Moderate renal function impairment (30 to 59 mL/min)	2.7	34
Severe renal function impairment (10 to 29 mL/min)	2.8	57
Dialysis-dependent patients (off dialysis)	1	3.5 hours

Contraindications

Active major bleeding or hypersensitivity to bivalirudin or any of its components.

Warnings/Precautions

Hematologic effects: Bivalirudin is not intended for intramuscular administration. Although most bleeding associated with the use of bivalirudin in PCI occurs at the site of arterial puncture, hemorrhage can occur at any site.

Brachytherapy: An increased risk of thrombus formation has been associated with the use of bivalirudin in gamma brachytherapy, including fatal outcomes.

Immunogenicity/Reexposure: Among 494 subjects who received bivalirudin in clinical trials and were tested for antibodies, 2 subjects had treatment-emergent positive bivalirudin antibody tests. Neither subject demonstrated clinical evidence of allergic or anaphylactic reactions and repeat testing was not performed. Nine additional patients who had initial positive tests were negative on repeat testing.

Renal function impairment: Drug elimination was related to GFR. Clearance was reduced approximately 20% in patients with moderate and severe renal function impairment and was reduced approximately 80% in dialysis-dependent patients.

Special risk: Use bivalirudin with caution in patients with disease states associated with an increased risk of bleeding.

Pregnancy: Category B.

Lactation: It is not known whether bivalirudin is excreted in breast milk. Exercise caution when bivalirudin is administered to a breast-feeding woman.

Children: The safety and efficacy in pediatric patients have not been established.

Elderly: In studies of patients undergoing PCI, 44% were 65 years of age and older, and 12% were older than 75 years of age. Elderly patients experienced more bleeding events than younger patients. Patients treated with bivalirudin experienced fewer bleeding events in each age stratum, compared with heparin.

Drug Interactions

Hematological agents: In clinical trials in patients undergoing PTCA/PCI, coadministration of bivalirudin with heparin, warfarin, thrombolytics, or GPIIb/IIIa inhibitors was associated with increased risks of major bleeding events compared with patients not receiving these concomitant medications. There is no experience with coadministration of bivalirudin and plasma expanders such as dextran.

Adverse Reactions

The most frequent adverse reactions reported were back pain, pain, nausea, headache, and hypotension. Percent of patients with major hemorrhage was 3.7%.

Adverse Reactions Other Than Bleeding Occurring in ≥ 5% of Patients in Either Treatment Group in Randomized Clinical Trials

Adverse reaction	Treatment group: Bivalirudin (n = 2,161)	Treatment group: Heparin (n = 2,151)
Cardiovascular		
Hypotension	12	17
Hypertension	6	5
Bradycardia	5	8
CNS		
Headache	12	10
Insomnia	7	6
Anxiety	6	7
Nervousness	5	4
GI		
Nausea	15	16
Vomiting	6	8
Abdominal pain	5	5
Dyspepsia	5	5
Miscellaneous		
Back pain	42	44
Pain	15	17
Injection site pain	8	13
Pelvic pain	6	8
Fever	5	5
Urinary retention	4	5

FONDAPARINUX SODIUM

Injection: 2.5 mg per 0.5 mL, 5 mg per 0.4 mL, 7.5 mg per 0.6 mL, 10 mg per 0.8 mL (*Rx*)	*Arixtra* (GlaxoSmithKline)

Warning:

Spinal/Epidural hematomas: When neuraxial anesthesia (epidural/spinal anesthesia) or spinal puncture is employed, patients anticoagulated or scheduled to be anticoagulated with low molecular weight heparins (LMWHs), heparinoids, or fondaparinux for prevention of thromboembolic complications are at risk of developing an epidural or spinal hematoma that can result in long-term or permanent paralysis.

The risk of these events is increased by the use of indwelling epidural catheters for administration of analgesia or by the concomitant use of drugs affecting hemostasis, such as NSAIDs, platelet inhibitors, or other anticoagulants. The risk also appears to be increased by traumatic or repeated epidural or spinal puncture.

Frequently monitor patients for signs and symptoms of neurological impairment. If neurologic compromise is noted, urgent treatment is necessary.

Consider the potential benefit vs risk before neuraxial intervention in patients anticoagulated or to be anticoagulated for thromboprophylaxis. Fondaparinux, like other anticoagulants, should be used with extreme caution in conditions with increased risk of hemorrhage, such as congenital or acquired bleeding disorders, active ulcerative and angiodysplastic GI disease, hemorrhagic stroke, or shortly after brain, spinal, or ophthalmological surgery, or in patients treated concomitantly with platelet inhibitors.

Indications

Prophylaxis of deep vein thrombosis (DVT): For the prophylaxis of deep vein thrombosis, which may lead to pulmonary embolism (PE) in patients undergoing the following: hip fracture surgery, including extended prophylaxis; hip replacement surgery; knee replacement surgery; abdominal surgery in those at risk for thromboembolic complications.

Treatment of acute DVT: For the treatment of acute DVT when administered in conjunction with warfarin.

Treatment of acute PE: For the treatment of acute PE when administered in conjunction with warfarin when initial therapy is administered in the hospital.

Administration and Dosage

Administration: Administer by subcutaneous injection. Do not administer by IM injection. Do not expel the air bubble from the syringe before the injection. Administer in the fatty tissue, alternating injection sites (eg, between the left and right anterolateral or the left and right posterolateral abdominal wall).

Acute DVT and PE treatment: In patients with acute symptomatic DVT and in patients with acute symptomatic PE, the recommended dosage of fondaparinux is 5 mg (body weight less than 50 kg), 7.5 mg (body weight 50 to 100 kg), or 10 mg (body weight greater than 100 kg) by subcutaneous injection once daily. Continue fondaparinux treatment for at least 5 days until a therapeutic oral anticoagulant effect is established (international normalized ratio [INR] 2 to 3). Initiate concomitant treatment with warfarin as soon as possible, usually within 72 hours. The usual duration of administration of fondaparinux is 5 to 9 days.

DVT prophylaxis: In patients undergoing hip fracture surgery, hip replacement surgery, or knee replacement surgery, the recommended dose is 2.5 mg subcutaneously once daily. After hemostasis has been established, give the initial dose 6 to 8 hours after surgery. The usual duration of administration is 5 to 9 days.

Admixture incompatibilities: Do not mix fondaparinux with other injections or infusions.

Actions

Pharmacology: The antithrombotic activity is the result of antithrombin III (ATIII)-mediated selective inhibition of Factor Xa. Neutralization of Factor Xa interrupts the blood coagulation cascade and thus inhibits thrombin formation and thrombus development.

Fondaparinux does not inactivate thrombin (activated Factor II) and has no known effect on platelet function, fibrinolytic activity, or bleeding time.

Pharmacokinetics:

Absorption – Subcutaneous injection is rapidly and completely absorbed (absolute bioavailability is 100%). Steady-state plasma concentration is reached approximately 3 hours postdose.

Distribution – Fondaparinux is highly (at least 94%) and specifically bound to ATIII.

Metabolism/Excretion – The majority of the administered dose is eliminated unchanged in urine in individuals with normal kidney function. The elimination half-life is 17 to 21 hours.

Contraindications

Severe renal function impairment (CrCl less than 30 mL/min); fondaparinux as prophylactic therapy in patients with body weight less than 50 kg undergoing hip fracture, hip replacement, knee replacement surgery, or abdominal surgery; active major bleeding; bacterial endocarditis; thrombocytopenia associated with a positive in vitro test for antiplatelet antibody in the presence of fondaparinux; known hypersensitivity to fondaparinux.

Warnings/Precautions

Injection: Not intended for IM injection.

Interchangeability: Do not use interchangeably (unit for unit) with heparin, LMWHs, or heparinoids, as they differ in manufacturing process, anti-Xa and anti-IIa activity, units, and dosage.

Hemorrhage: See Warning Box.

Neuraxial anesthesia and postoperative indwelling epidural catheter use: See Warning Box.

Thrombocytopenia: Moderate thrombocytopenia (platelet counts between 100,000/mm^3 and 50,000/mm^3) occurred at a rate of 3% in patients in orthopedic clinical trials. Severe thrombocytopenia (platelet counts less than 50,000/mm^3) occurred at a rate of 0.2% in patients in orthopedic clinical trials. Moderate thrombocytopenia occurred at a rate of 0.5% in patients given the fondaparinux treatment regimen in the DVT and PE treatment clinical trials. Severe thrombocytopenia occurred at a rate of 0.04% in patients given the fondaparinux treatment regimen in the DVT and PE treatment clinical trials.

Closely monitor thrombocytopenia of any degree. Discontinue if the platelet count falls below 100,000/mm^3.

Special populations: Use fondaparinux with care in patients with a bleeding diathesis, uncontrolled arterial hypertension, or a history of recent GI ulceration, diabetic retinopathy, and hemorrhage.

Renal function impairment: Use fondaparinux with caution in patients with moderate renal function impairment (CrCl 30 to 50 mL/min). Periodically assess renal function in patients receiving fondaparinux. Immediately discontinue the drug in patients who develop severe renal function impairment while on therapy. After discontinuation of fondaparinux, its anticoagulant effects may persist for 2 to 4 days in patients with normal renal function. The anticoagulant effects of fondaparinux may persist even longer in patients with renal function impairment.

Pregnancy: *Category B.*

Lactation: It is not known whether this drug is excreted in human milk. Exercise caution when administered to a breast-feeding mother.

Children: Safety and efficacy of fondaparinux in children have not been established.

Elderly: Serious adverse reactions increased with age for patients receiving fondaparinux. Careful attention to dosing directions and concomitant medications (especially antiplatelet medication) is advised.

Because elderly patients are more likely to have decreased renal function, it may be useful to monitor renal function.

Monitoring: Periodic routine CBCs (including platelet count), serum creatinine level, and stool occult blood tests are recommended during the course of treatment.

The anti-Factor Xa activity of fondaparinux can be measured by anti-Xa assay using the appropriate calibrator.

If during fondaparinux therapy unexpected changes in coagulation parameters or major bleeding occurs, discontinue fondaparinux.

If thrombotic events occur despite fondaparinux prophylaxis, initiate appropriate therapy.

Drug Interactions

Discontinue agents that may enhance the risk of hemorrhage prior to initiation of fondaparinux therapy. If coadministration is essential, close monitoring may be appropriate. Coumarin may be affected by fondaparinux.

Adverse Reactions

Adverse reactions occurring in 3% or more of patients include anemia, bullous eruption, confusion, constipation, dizziness, edema, fever, headache, hypokalemia, hypotension, increased wound drainage, insomnia, major/minor bleeding, nausea, postoperative hemorrhage, purpura, rash, surgical site reaction, urinary tract infection, vomiting.

Local: Mild local irritation (eg, injection-site bleeding, rash, pruritus) may occur following subcutaneous injection.

Chapter 3

ENDOCRINE AND METABOLIC AGENTS

ESTROGENS

ESTRADIOL TRANSDERMAL SYSTEM	
Transdermal patch: 0.014 mg per 24 hours (*Rx*)	*Menostar* (Berlex)
0.025 mg per 24 hours (*Rx*)	Various, *Alora* (Watson), *Climara* (Berlex), *Vivelle-Dot* (Novartis)
0.0375 mg per 24 hours (*Rx*)	Various, *Climara* (Berlex), *Vivelle*, *Vivelle-Dot* (Novartis)
0.05 and 0.1 mg per 24 hours (*Rx*)	*Estradiol Transdermal System* (Mylan), *Alora* (Watson), *Climara* (Berlex), *Estraderm*, *Vivelle*, *Vivelle-Dot* (Novartis)
0.06 mg per 24 hours (*Rx*)	Various, *Climara* (Berlex)
0.075 mg per 24 hours (*Rx*)	Various, *Alora* (Watson), *Climara* (Berlex), *Vivelle*, *Vivelle-Dot* (Novartis)
0.1 mg per 24 hours (*Rx*)	*Estradiol Transdermal System* (Mylan), *Alora* (Watson), *Climara* (Berlex), *Vivelle*, *Vivelle-Dot* (Novartis)
ESTRADIOL, ORAL	
Tablets; oral 2 mg micronized estradiol (*Rx*)	Various, *Estrace* (Warner Chilcott), *Gynodiol* (Novavax Inc.)
ESTRADIOL VALERATE IN OIL	
Injection: 10, 20, and 40 mg/mL (*Rx*)	*Delestrogen* (JHP), *Estradiol Valerate* (Sandoz)
CONJUGATED ESTROGENS, ORAL	
Tablets; oral: 0.3, 0.45, 0.625, 0.9, and 1.25 mg (*Rx*)	*Premarin* (Wyeth-Ayerst)
CONJUGATED ESTROGENS, PARENTERAL	
Injection, powder for solution: 25 mg (*Rx*)	*Premarin Intravenous* (Wyeth-Ayerst)
ESTERIFIED ESTROGENS	
Tablets; oral: 0.3, 0.625, 1.25, and 2.5 mg (*Rx*)	*Menest* (Monarch)
ESTROPIPATE	
Tablets; oral: 0.75 and 1.5 mg estropipate (*Rx*)	Various, *Ortho-Est 0.625* (Women First Healthcare)
3 mg estropipate (*Rx*)	Various, *Ortho-Est 1.25* (Women First Healthcare)
6 mg estropipate (*Rx*)	Various
SYNTHETIC CONJUGATED ESTROGENS, A	
Tablets; oral: 0.3, 0.45, 0.625, 0.9, and 1.25 mg (*Rx*)	*Cenestin* (Barr/Duramed)
SYNTHETIC CONJUGATED ESTROGENS, B	
Tablets; oral: 0.3, 0.45, 0.625, 0.9, and 1.25 mg (*Rx*)	*Enjuvia* (Barr/Duramed)
ESTRADIOL CYPIONATE IN OIL	
Injection: 5 mg/mL (*Rx*)	*Depo-Estradiol* (Pfizer US)
MISCELLANEOUS ESTROGENS, TOPICAL	
Emulsion; topical: 2.5 mg estradiol hemihydrate/g (*Rx*)	*Estrasorb* (Graceway)
Gel; topical: 0.06% estradiol (0.52 mg estradiol per 0.87 g unit dose) (*Rx*)	*Elestrin* (Kenwood Therapeutics)
0.06% estradiol (0.75 mg estradiol per 1.25 g unit dose) (*Rx*)	*Estrogel* (Unimed)
0.1% estradiol (*Rx*)	*Divigel* (Upsher-Smith)
Spray, solution; topical: 1.53 mg estradiol (*Rx*)	*Evamist* (Ther-Rx)

Warning:

Estrogens increase the risk of endometrial cancer: Close clinical surveillance of all women taking estrogens is important. Use adequate diagnostic measures, including endometrial sampling when indicated, to rule out malignancy in all cases of undiagnosed persistent or recurring abnormal vaginal bleeding. There is currently no evidence that "natural" estrogens results in a different endometrial risk profile than synthetic estrogens at equivalent estrogen dose(s).

Do not use estrogens during pregnancy: Estrogen therapy during pregnancy is associated with an increased risk of congenital defects in the reproductive organs of the fetus and possibly other birth defects. Studies of women who received diethylstilbestrol during pregnancy have shown that female offspring have an increased risk of vaginal adenosis, squamous cell dysplasia of the uterine cervix, and clear cell vaginal cancer later in life; male offspring have an increased risk of urogenital abnormalities and possibly testicular cancer later in life.

There is no indication for estrogen therapy during pregnancy or during the immediate postpartum period. Estrogens are ineffective for the prevention or treatment of threatened or habitual abortion. Estrogens are not indicated for the prevention of postpartum breast engorgement.

If estrogens are used during pregnancy, or if the patient becomes pregnant while taking estrogens, inform her of the potential risks to the fetus.

Cardiovascular and other risks: Do not use estrogens with or without progestins for the prevention of cardiovascular disease.

The Women's Health Initiative (WHI) study reported increased risks of myocardial infarction, stroke, invasive breast cancer, pulmonary emboli, and deep vein thrombosis in postmenopausal women during 5 years of treatment with conjugated equine estrogens (CE 0.625 mg) combined with medroxyprogesterone acetate (MPA 2.5 mg) relative to placebo. Other doses of conjugated estrogens with medroxyprogesterone, and other combinations of estrogens and progestins were not studied in the WHI and, in the absence of comparable data, these risks should be assumed to be similar. Because of these risks, estrogens with or without progestins should be prescribed at the lowest effective doses and for the shortest duration consistent with treatment goals and risks for the individual woman.

The WHI Memory Study (WHIMS), a substudy of WHI, reported increased risk of developing probable dementia in postmenopausal women 65 years of age or older during 5.2 years of treatment with daily conjugated estrogens 0.625 mg alone and during 4 years of treatment with oral conjugated estrogens 0.625 mg combined with medroxyprogesterone acetate 2.5 mg relative to placebo. It is unknown whether this finding applies to younger postmenopausal women.

In the absence of comparable data, these risks should be assumed to be similar. Because of these risks, estrogens with or without progestins should be prescribed at the lowest effective doses and for the shortest duration consistent with treatment goals and risks for the individual woman.

Indications

Estrogens are most commonly used as a component of combination contraceptives or as hormone replacement therapy in postmenopausal women. Benefits in postmenopausal women include relief of moderate to severe vasomotor symptoms and decreased risk of osteoporosis. Hormone replacement therapy also may be used in vaginal and vulvar atrophy and in hypoestrogenism caused by hypogonadism, castration, or primary ovarian failure. Less commonly, select breast or prostate cancer patients with advanced disease may receive estrogens as palliative therapy. Refer to individual agents for specific indications.

Administration and Dosage

Concomitant progestin therapy: When estrogen is prescribed for a postmenopausal woman with a uterus, also initiate progestin to reduce the risk of endometrial cancer. A woman without a uterus does not need progestin.

ESTRADIOL TRANSDERMAL SYSTEM:

Initiation of therapy –

Treatment of menopausal symptoms: Start with the 0.025 to 0.05 mg system applied to the skin once (*Climara*) or twice weekly. Adjust dose as necessary to control symptoms. Do not make dosage increases until after the first month of therapy. Use the lowest dosage necessary to control symptoms, especially in women with an intact uterus. Make attempts to taper or discontinue the drug at 3- to 6-month intervals.

Prevention of postmenopausal osteoporosis: Initiate with lowest dose as soon as possible after menopause. Adjust dosage if necessary. Discontinuation may reestablish natural rate of bone loss.

In women who are not taking oral estrogens or in women switching from another estradiol transdermal therapy, start treatment immediately. In women who are currently taking oral estrogens, start treatment 1 week after withdrawal of oral therapy or sooner if symptoms reappear in less than 1 week.

Therapeutic regimen – Therapy may be given continuously in patients who do not have an intact uterus. In patients with an intact uterus, therapy may be given on a cyclic schedule (eg, 3 weeks on followed by 1 week off).

Alora, Estraderm, Vivelle, and *Vivelle-Dot* are applied twice a week; *Climara* and *Menostar* are applied once a week.

Application of system – Place adhesive side of the system on a clean, dry area on the trunk of the body (including the buttocks and abdomen). Do not apply to breasts or to a site exposed to sunlight. Rotate application site with an interval of at least 1 week between applications to a particular site. The area should not be oily, damaged, or irritated. Avoid the waistline, because tight clothing may rub the system off. Also avoid application to areas where sitting would dislodge the system. Apply the system immediately after opening pouch and removing protective liner. Press firmly in place with the palm for approximately 10 seconds. Make sure there is good contact, especially around the edges. In the unlikely event that a system should fall off, the same system may be reapplied (except *Climara* or *Menostar*). If necessary, apply a new system. In the event that a *Climara* or *Menostar* system falls off, apply a new system for the remainder of the 7-day dosing interval. In either case, continue the original treatment schedule.

ESTRADIOL, ORAL:

Moderate to severe vasomotor symptoms, vulvar/vaginal atrophy associated with menopause – Use the lowest dose and for the shortest duration consistent with treatment goals and risks for the individual woman. Periodically reevaluate patients as clinically appropriate to determine if treatment is still necessary. Attempt to discontinue or taper medication at 3- to 6-month intervals. Initiate treatment at the lowest dose. Titrate to determine the minimal effective dose for maintenance therapy. Administer micronized estradiol cyclically (eg, 3 weeks on and 1 week off). Administer estradiol acetate once daily.

Hypoestrogenism caused by hypogonadism, castration, or primary ovarian failure – Treatment usually is initiated with a dose of 1 to 2 mg daily, adjusted as necessary to control presenting symptoms; determine the minimal effective dose for maintenance therapy by titration.

Prostatic cancer – For palliation only. Administer 1 to 2 mg 3 times daily. Judge efficacy of therapy by phosphatase determinations and symptomatic improvement.

Breast cancer – For palliation only. The usual dose is 10 mg 3 times daily for at least 3 months.

Osteoporosis prevention – Administer cyclically (eg, 23 days on and 5 days off) 0.5 mg/day as soon as possible after menopause. Adjust dosage if necessary to control concurrent menopausal symptoms.

ESTRADIOL VALERATE IN OIL: For intramuscular (IM) injection only. Inject deeply into the upper outer quadrant of the gluteal muscle.

Moderate to severe vasomotor symptoms, vulval and vaginal atrophy associated with menopause and female hypoestrogenism caused by hypogonadism, castration, or primary ovarian failure – 10 to 20 mg every 4 weeks.

Prostatic carcinoma (advanced, androgen-dependent) – 30 mg or more every 1 or 2 weeks.

CONJUGATED ESTROGENS, ORAL:

Moderate to severe vasomotor symptoms and/or moderate to severe symptoms of vulvar and vaginal atrophy associated with menopause – Start at the lowest dose. Therapy may be given continuously with no interruption, or in cyclical regimens (eg, 25 days on followed by 5 days off) as is medically appropriate on an individualized basis.

Female hypogonadism – 0.3 to 0.625 mg daily, administered cyclically (eg, 3 weeks on and 1 week off). Doses are adjusted depending on the severity of symptoms and responsiveness of the endometrium.

The dosage may be gradually titrated upward at 6- to 12-month intervals as needed to achieve appropriate bone age advancement and eventual epiphyseal closure. Chronic dosing with 0.625 mg is sufficient to induce artificial cyclic menses with sequential progestin treatment and to maintain bone mineral density after skeletal maturity is achieved.

Female castration and primary ovarian failure – 1.25 mg/day cyclically. Adjust according to severity of symptoms and patient response. For maintenance, adjust to lowest effective level.

Osteoporosis prevention – 0.625 mg/day, cyclically or continuously.

Breast cancer, metastatic (for palliation) – 10 mg 3 times/day for at least 3 months.

Prostatic carcinoma (for palliation) – 1.25 to 2.5 mg 3 times/day. Judge efficacy by phosphatase determinations and symptomatic improvement.

CONJUGATED ESTROGENS, PARENTERAL:

Abnormal uterine bleeding caused by hormonal imbalance in the absence of organic pathology – Usual dose is one 25 mg injection IV or IM. Repeat in 6 to 12 hours if necessary. Inject slowly to obviate the occurrence of flushes.

ESTERIFIED ESTROGENS:

Moderate to severe vasomotor symptoms – 1.25 mg daily, administered cyclically. If the patient has not menstruated within the last 2 months or more, cyclic administration is started arbitrarily. If the patient is menstruating, cyclic administration is started on day 5 of bleeding. For short-term use only; discontinue medication as promptly as possible.

Atrophic vaginitis and kraurosis vulvae – 0.3 to 1.25 mg or more daily. Administer cyclically. For short-term use only; discontinue medication as promptly as possible.

Female hypogonadism – Cyclically, administer 2.5 to 7.5 mg/day in divided doses for 20 days followed by a 10-day rest period. If bleeding does not occur by the end of this period, repeat the same dosage schedule. The number of courses of estrogen therapy necessary to produce bleeding varies depending on endometrial responsiveness.

If bleeding occurs before the end of the 10-day period, begin an estrogen-progestin cyclic regimen of 2.5 to 7.5 mg/day in divided doses for 20 days. During the last 5 days of estrogen therapy, give an oral progestin. If bleeding occurs before this regimen is concluded, discontinue therapy; resume on the fifth day of bleeding.

Female castration and primary ovarian failure – Give 1.25 mg/day, cyclically.

Prostatic carcinoma (inoperable, progressing) – 1.25 to 2.5 mg 3 times/day. Judge efficacy of therapy by symptomatic response and phosphatase determinations.

Breast cancer (inoperable, progressing) – 10 mg 3 times/day for at least 3 months.

ESTROPIPATE:

Moderate to severe vasomotor symptoms, vulval and vaginal atrophy associated with menopause – Give cyclically for short-term use. Choose the lowest dose and regimen that will control symptoms. Usual dosage range is 0.75 to 6 mg estropipate/day.

If a patient with vasomotor symptoms has not menstruated within the last 2 months or more, start cyclic administration arbitrarily. If the patient is menstruating, start cyclic administration on day 5 of bleeding.

Female hypogonadism – 1.5 to 9 mg estropipate (calculated as 1.25 to 7.5 mg estrone sulfate)/day for the first 3 weeks, followed by a rest period of 8 to 10 days. Repeat if bleeding does not occur by the end of the rest period. The duration of therapy necessary to produce withdrawal bleeding will vary according to the responsiveness of the endometrium. If satisfactory withdrawal bleeding does not occur, give an oral progestin in addition to estrogen during the third week of the cycle.

Female castration or primary ovarian failure – A daily dose of 1.5 to 9 mg estropipate may be given for the first 3 weeks of a theoretical cycle, followed by a rest period of 8 to 10 days.

Osteoporosis prevention – 0.75 mg/day estropipate for 25 days of a 31-day cycle per month.

SYNTHETIC CONJUGATED ESTROGENS, A:

Vasomotor symptoms (0.45, 0.625, 0.9, 1.25 mg only) – Initial doses of 0.45 mg/day are recommended with dosage adjustment based on individual patient response.

Vulvar and vaginal atrophy (0.3 mg only) – 0.3 mg/day.

SYNTHETIC CONJUGATED ESTROGENS, B:

Moderate to severe vasomotor symptoms associated with menopause – Initial dose is 0.3 mg daily. Subsequent dosage adjustment may be made based upon the individual patient response.

Vaginal dryness/vulvar and vaginal atrophy – 0.3 mg once daily.

ESTRADIOL CYPIONATE IN OIL: For IM use only.

Moderate to severe vasomotor symptoms associated with menopause – Usual dosage range is 1 to 5 mg IM, every 3 to 4 weeks. Attempt to discontinue or taper medication at 3- to 6-month intervals.

Female hypogonadism – 1.5 to 2 mg IM at monthly intervals.

MISCELLANEOUS ESTROGENS, TOPICAL:

Topical emulsion – Use the lowest effective dose and for the shortest duration consistent with treatment goals and risks for the individual women. Periodically reevaluate patients as clinically appropriate (eg, at 3-month to 6-month intervals) to determine if treatment is still necessary. For the treatment of moderate to severe vasomotor symptoms associated with menopause, the single approved dose of estradiol topical emulsion is 3.48 g/day. The lowest effective dose for this indication has not been determined.

Application:

1.) Apply in a comfortable sitting position to clean, dry skin on both legs each morning. Open each pouch individually.
2.) Allow the application areas to dry completely before covering with clothing to avoid transfer to other individuals.
3.) On completion of application, wash both hands with soap and water to remove any residual estradiol.

Gel –

Divigel: Divigel 0.1% at doses of 0.25, 0.5, and 1 g/day, is indicated for topical use in the treatment of moderate to severe vasomotor symptoms associated with menopause.

Use the lowest effective dose. Generally, women should be started at 0.25 g daily. Subsequent dosage adjustments may be made based upon the individual patient response. The dose should be periodically reassessed by the health care provider.

Application – *Divigel* should be applied once daily on the skin of either the right or left upper thigh. The application surface area should be about 5 to 7 inches. The entire contents of a unit dose packet should be applied each day. To avoid skin irritation, apply to the right or left upper thigh on alternating days. Do not apply to the face, breasts, or irritated skin, or in or around the vagina. After application, the gel should be allowed to dry before dressing. The application site should not be washed within 1 hour of applying *Divigel*. Wash hands after application.

Elestrin: Apply 1 pump per day (0.87 g/day) to the upper arm. Subsequent dose adjustment may be made based upon the patient's response.

Estrogel: Estrogel 1.25 g is the single approved dose for the treatment of moderate to severe vasomotor symptoms and/or moderate to severe symptoms of vulvar and vaginal atrophy associated with menopause. The lowest effective dose of *Estro-*

gel for these indications has not been determined. When prescribing solely for the treatment of moderate to severe symptoms of vulvar and vaginal atrophy, topical vaginal products should be considered.

Spray – Estradiol transdermal spray therapy should be initiated with 1 spray per day. Dosage adjustment should be guided by the clinical response.

Application: One, 2, or 3 sprays are applied each morning to adjacent, non-overlapping areas on the inner surface of the forearm, starting near the elbow. Sprays should be allowed to dry for approximately 2 minutes and the site should not be washed for 30 minutes. Application of estradiol transdermal spray to other skin surfaces has not been adequately studied. Estradiol transdermal spray should not be applied to skin surfaces other the forearm.

Priming: Before applying the first dose from a new applicator, the pump should be primed by spraying 3 sprays with the cover on. The container should be held upright and vertical for spraying.

Actions

Pharmacology: The primary source of estrogen in normally cycling adult women is the ovarian follicle, which secretes 70 to 500 mcg of estradiol daily. This is converted primarily to estrone, which circulates in roughly equal proportion to estradiol, and to small amounts of estriol. After menopause, most endogenous estrogen is produced by conversion of androstenedione to estrone by peripheral tissues. Thus, estrone is the most abundant circulating estrogen in postmenopausal women. Estradiol is the principal intracellular human estrogen and is substantially more potent than estrone or estriol at the receptor.

Pharmacokinetics:

Absorption/Distribution – Estrogens used in therapy are well absorbed through the skin, mucous membranes, and GI tract. When applied for a local action, absorption is usually sufficient to cause systemic effects. When conjugated for parenteral administration, the rate of absorption of oily preparations is slowed with a prolonged duration of action, such that a single IM injection of estradiol valerate or estradiol cypionate is absorbed over several weeks. Conjugated estrogens are well absorbed from the GI tract. The tablet releases conjugated estrogens slowly over several hours. The distribution of exogenous estrogens is similar to that of endogenous estrogens.

Transdermal system: In contrast to oral estradiol, the skin metabolizes estradiol via the transdermal system only to a small extent. Therefore, transdermal use produces therapeutic serum levels of estradiol with lower circulating levels of estrone and estrone conjugates, and requires smaller total doses.

Metabolism/Excretion – Metabolism and inactivation occur primarily in the liver. During cyclic passage through the liver, estrogens are degraded to less active estrogenic compounds conjugated with sulfuric and glucuronic acids.

Contraindications

Known or suspected breast cancer, except in appropriately selected patients being treated for metastatic disease; known or suspected estrogen-dependent neoplasia; undiagnosed abnormal genital bleeding; active deep vein thrombosis, pulmonary edema, or a history of these conditions; active or recent (eg, within past year) arterial thromboembolic disease (eg, stroke, MI); active thrombophlebitis or thromboembolic disorders; history of thrombophlebitis, thrombosis or thromboembolic disorders associated with previous estrogen use (except when used in treatment of breast or prostatic malignancy); known or suspected pregnancy; porphyria (estradiol vaginal tablets only); hypersensitivity to any product component.

Warnings/Precautions

Induction of malignant neoplasms: Estrogens and estrogen/progestin therapy may increase the risk of endometrial carcinoma, breast cancer, and ovarian cancer.

Gallbladder disease: There is a 2- to 3-fold increase in risk of gallbladder disease in women receiving postmenopausal estrogens.

Cardiovascular disorders: Estrogen and estrogen/progestin therapy have been associated with an increased risk of cardiovascular events (eg, MI and stroke, venous thrombosis, PE [venous thromboembolism]). Manage risk factors for cardiovascular disease appropriately.

Hepatic adenoma: Benign hepatic adenomas appear to be associated with the use of oral contraceptives (OCs).

Dementia: In the WHIMS, 4,532 generally healthy postmenopausal women 65 years of age and older were studied, of whom 35% were 70 to 74 years of age and 18% were 75 years of age or older. After an average follow-up of 4 years, 40 women being treated with 0.625 mg conjugated estrogens plus 2.5 mg medroxyprogesterone acetate (1.8%, n = 2,229) and 21 women in the placebo group (0.9%, n = 2,303) received diagnoses of probable dementia.

Familial hyperlipoproteinemia: Estrogen therapy may be associated with massive elevations of plasma triglycerides leading to pancreatitis and other complications in patients with familial defects of lipoprotein metabolism.

Hypercalcemia: Estrogens may lead to severe hypercalcemia in patients with breast cancer and bone metastases. If this occurs, discontinue the drug and take appropriate measures to reduce the serum calcium level.

Glucose tolerance: A worsening of glucose tolerance has been observed in a significant percentage of patients on estrogen-containing OCs. Carefully observe diabetic patients receiving estrogen.

Visual abnormalities: Retinal vascular thrombosis has been reported. Discontinue medication pending examination if there is sudden partial or complete loss of vision or a sudden onset of proptosis, diplopia, or migraine.

Hypothyroidism: Estrogen administration leads to increased thyroid-binding globulin (TBG) levels.

Depression: OCs appear to be associated with an increased incidence of mental depression.

Uterine leiomyomata: Preexisting uterine leiomyomata may increase in size during estrogen use.

Elevated blood pressure: In a small number of case reports, substantial increases in blood pressure have been attributed to idiosyncratic reactions to estrogens. Monitor blood pressure at regular intervals with estrogen use.

Hypercoagulability: Some studies have shown that women taking estrogen replacement therapy have hypercoagulability, primarily related to decreased antithrombin activity. This effect appears dose- and duration-dependent and is less pronounced than that associated with OC use.

History/Physical exam: Before initiating estrogens, take complete medical and family history. Pretreatment and periodic history and physical exams every 12 months should include blood pressure, breasts, abdomen, pelvic organs, and a Papanicolaou smear.

Vaginal products: Estradiol vaginal ring may not be suitable for women with narrow, short, or stenosed vaginas. Women with signs or symptoms of vaginal irritation should alert their physician.

If a vaginal infection develops during use of the estradiol vaginal ring, remove the ring and reinsert only after the infection has been appropriately treated.

Conjugated estrogens vaginal cream exposure has been reported to weaken latex condoms. Consider its potential to weaken and contribute to the failure of condoms, diaphragms, or cervical caps made of latex or rubber.

Excessive estrogenic stimulation: Certain patients may develop undesirable manifestations of excessive estrogenic stimulation (eg, abnormal or excessive uterine bleeding, mastodynia). Advise the pathologist of estrogen therapy when relevant specimens are submitted.

Fluid retention: Estrogens may cause some degree of fluid retention; conditions which might be influenced by this factor (eg, asthma, epilepsy, migraine, cardiac or renal dysfunction) require careful observation.

Calcium and phosphorus metabolism: Calcium and phosphorus metabolism is influenced by estrogens; use caution in patients with metabolic bone diseases associated with hypercalcemia or in renal function impairment.

Endometrial hyperplasia: Prolonged unopposed estrogen therapy may increase risk of endometrial hyperplasia.

Exacerbations of other conditions: Endometriosis may be exacerbated with administration of estrogen therapy. Estrogen therapy also may cause an exacerbation of asthma, diabetes mellitus, epilepsy, migraine, or porphyria; use with caution in patients with these conditions.

Benzyl alcohol: Benzyl alcohol, contained in some of these products as a preservative, has been associated with a fatal "gasping syndrome" in premature infants.

Hepatic function impairment: Patients with a history of jaundice during pregnancy have an increased risk of recurrence while on estrogen-containing OCs. If jaundice develops in any patient on estrogen, discontinue medication and investigate the cause. Estrogens may be poorly metabolized in impaired liver function; use with caution.

Pregnancy: Category X.

Lactation: Estrogens have been shown to decrease the quantity and quality of breast milk and may be excreted in breast milk. Administer only when clearly needed.

Children: Estrogen therapy has been used for the induction of puberty in adolescents with some forms of pubertal delay. Safety and efficacy in children have not otherwise been established.

Drug Interactions

Drugs that may be affected by estrogens include oral anticoagulants, tricyclic antidepressants, hydantoins, corticosteroids, and thyroid hormones.

Drugs that may affect estrogens include barbiturates, rifampin, hydantoins, topiramate, and CYP 3A4 inducers and inhibitors.

Drug/Lab test interactions: Certain endocrine and liver function tests may be affected by estrogen-containing OCs. Expect these similar changes with larger doses:

Increased sulfobromophthalein retention.

Increased prothrombin time, partial thromboplastin time, platelet aggregation time, platelet count, and factors II, VII, VIII, IX, X, XII, VII-X complex, II-VII-X complex, and β-thromboglobulin; decreased antithrombin III, antifactor Xa; increased fibrinogen, plasminogen, norepinephrine-induced platelet aggregability.

Increased TBG leading to increased circulating total thyroid hormone, as measured by PBI, T_4 by column, or T_4 by radioimmunoassay. Free T_3 resin uptake is decreased, reflecting the elevated TBG; free T_4 concentration is unaltered.

Impaired glucose tolerance; decreased pregnanediol excretion; reduced response to metyrapone test; reduced serum folate concentration.

Increased plasma high-density lipoprotein (HDL) and HDL-2 subfraction concentrations, reduced low-density lipoprotein cholesterol concentration levels, increased triglyceride levels.

Adverse Reactions

Significant adverse reactions include abdominal cramps, aggravation of porphyria, amenorrhea during and after treatment, bloating, breakthrough bleeding, breast tenderness/enlargement/secretion, change in menstrual flow, changes in libido, chloasma or melasma (may persist when drug is discontinued), cholestatic jaundice, convulsions, dermatitis, dizziness, dysmenorrhea, edema, erythema nodosum/multiforme, headache, hemorrhagic eruption, intolerance to contact lenses, mental depression, migraine, nausea, pain at injection site, premenstrual-like syndrome, postinjection flare, redness and irritation at application site with the estradiol transdermal system (17%), spotting, steepening of corneal curvature, sterile abscess, urticaria, vomiting.

MISCELLANEOUS ESTROGENS, VAGINAL

Tablets; vaginal: estradiol 25 mcg (equivalent to estradiol hemihydrate 25.8 mcg) (*Rx*)	*Vagifem* (Novo Nordisk)
Cream; vaginal: estradiol 0.1 mg/g (*Rx*)	*Estrace Vaginal* (Warner Chilcott)
conjugated estrogens 0.625 mg/g (*Rx*)	*Premarin Vaginal* (Wyeth-Ayerst)
Ring; vaginal: estradiol 2 mg[a] (*Rx*)	*Estring* (Pharmacia)
estradiol acetate 0.05 mg[b]/day and estradiol acetate 0.1 mg[c]/day (*Rx*)	*Femring* (Warner Chilcott)

[a] Releases estradiol, approximately 7.5 mcg per 24 hours, in a consistent, stable manner over 90 days. Dimensions: outer diameter, 55 mm; cross-sectional diameter, 9 mm; core diameter, 2 mm.
[b] Central core contains estradiol acetate 12.4 mg that releases 0.05 mg/day for 3 months. Dimensions: outer diameter, 56 mm; cross-sectional diameter, 7.6 mm; core diameter, 2 mm.
[c] Central core contains estradiol acetate 24.8 mg that releases 0.1 mg/day for 3 months. Dimensions: outer diameter, 56 mm; cross-sectional diameter, 7.6 mm; core diameter, 2 mm.

Warning:

Estrogens increase the risk of endometrial cancer: Close clinical surveillance of all women taking estrogens is important. Undertake adequate diagnostic measures, including endometrial sampling when indicated, to rule out malignancy in all cases of undiagnosed persistent or recurring abnormal vaginal bleeding. There is no evidence that the use of "natural" estrogens results in a different endometrial risk profile than synthetic estrogens of equivalent estrogen dose.

Cardiovascular and other risks: Do not use estrogens with or without progestins for the prevention of cardiovascular disease or dementia. The Women's Health Initiative (WHI) study reported increased risks of stroke and deep vein thrombosis in postmenopausal women (50 to 79 years of age) during 6.8 years of treatment with conjugated estrogens 0.625 mg relative to placebo. The WHI study reported increased risks of myocardial infarction (MI), stroke, invasive breast cancer, pulmonary emboli, and deep vein thrombosis in postmenopausal women (50 to 79 years of age) during 5 years of treatment with oral conjugated estrogens 0.625 mg combined with medroxyprogesterone 2.5 mg relative to placebo. The Women's Health Initiative Memory Study, a substudy of WHI, reported increased risk of developing probable dementia in postmenopausal women 65 years of age or older during 5.2 years of treatment with oral conjugated estrogens alone and during 4 years of treatment with conjugated estrogens combined with medroxyprogesterone, relative to placebo. It is unknown whether this finding applies to younger postmenopausal women. Other doses of conjugated estrogens and medroxyprogesterone acetate, and other combinations and dosage forms of estrogens and progestins, were not studied in the WHI clinical trials and, in the absence of comparable data, these risks should be assumed to be similar. Because of these risks, prescribe estrogens with or without progestins at the lowest effective doses and for the shortest duration consistent with treatment goals and risks for the individual woman.

Indications

Vulvar/Vaginal atrophy: Treatment of urogenital symptoms associated with postmenopausal atrophy of the vagina and/or the lower urinary tract.

Atrophic vaginitis: Treatment of atrophic vaginitis.

Kraurosis vulvae: For the treatment of kraurosis vulvae.

Dyspareunia (Premarin only): For the treatment of moderate to severe dyspareunia, a symptom of vulvar and vaginal atrophy caused by menopause.

Vasomotor symptoms (Femring only): Treatment of moderate to severe vasomotor symptoms associated with menopause.

Administration and Dosage

Choose the lowest dose that will control symptoms and discontinue medication as promptly as possible. Attempt to discontinue or taper medication at 3- to 6-month intervals.

Conjugated estrogens:

Atrophic vaginitis and kraurosis vulvae – Administer cyclically; 3 weeks on and 1 week off. For short-term use only. Give 0.5 to 2 g/day intravaginally, depending on the severity of the condition.

Dyspareunia (Premarin only) – 0.5 mg administered intravaginally in a twice-weekly (eg, Monday and Thursday) continuous regimen or in a cyclic regimen of 21 days of therapy followed by 7 days off of therapy.

Estradiol:

Cream – 2 to 4 g/day for 1 or 2 weeks. Gradually reduce to 50% of initial dosage. A maintenance dose of 1 g 1 to 3 times/week may be used after restoration of the vaginal mucosa has been achieved.

Ring – Press into an oval and insert as deeply as possible into the upper ⅓ of the vaginal vault. The ring is to remain in place continuously for 3 months, after which it should be removed and, if appropriate, replaced by a new ring.

If the ring is removed or falls out at any time during the 90-day treatment period, rinse the ring in lukewarm water and re-insert.

Estradiol hemihydrate: Using the supplied applicator, gently insert into the vagina as far as it can comfortably go without force.

Initial dose – 1 tablet inserted vaginally once daily for 2 weeks. Administer treatment at the same time each day.

Maintenance dose – 1 tablet inserted vaginally twice weekly.

The need to continue therapy should be assessed by the physician with the patient. Attempt to discontinue or taper medication at 3- to 6-month intervals.

Concomitant progestin therapy: When estrogen is prescribed for a postmenopausal woman with a uterus, also initiate progestin to reduce the risk of endometrial cancer. A woman without a uterus does not need progestin.

Actions

Pharmacology: The signs and symptoms of vulvovaginal epithelial atrophy (atrophic vaginitis) may be alleviated by the topical application of an estrogenic hormone.

Warnings/Precautions

Vaginal bleeding: Uterine bleeding might be provoked by excessive administration in menopausal women. Evaluation may be required to differentiate this uterine bleeding from carcinoma. Breast tenderness and vaginal discharge may result from excessive estrogenic stimulation; endometrial withdrawal bleeding may occur if use is suddenly discontinued.

Vaginal products: Estradiol vaginal ring may not be suitable for women with narrow, short, or stenosed vaginas.

If a vaginal infection develops during use of the estradiol vaginal ring, remove the ring and reinsert only after the infection has been appropriately treated.

Conjugated estrogens vaginal cream exposure has been reported to weaken latex condoms. Consider its potential to weaken and contribute to the failure of condoms, diaphragms, or cervical caps made of latex or rubber.

Pregnancy: Category X.

ESTROGENS AND PROGESTINS COMBINED

Tablets, oral: 0.3 mg conjugated estrogens/1.5 mg medroxyprogesterone acetate, 0.45 mg conjugated estrogens/1.5 mg medroxyprogesterone, 0.625 mg conjugated estrogens/2.5 mg medroxyprogesterone acetate, 0.625 mg conjugated estrogens/5 mg medroxyprogesterone acetate (*Rx*)	*Prempro* (Wyeth-Ayerst)
0.625 mg conjugated estrogens, 0.625 mg conjugated estrogens/5 mg medroxyprogesterone acetate (*Rx*)	*Premphase* (Wyeth-Ayerst)
0.5 mg drospirenone/1 mg estradiol per day (*Rx*)	*Angeliq* (Bayer)
3 mg drospirenone/0.02 mg ethinyl estradiol (*Rx*)	YAZ (Bayer)
2.5 mcg ethinyl estradiol/0.5 mg norethindrone acetate, 5 mcg ethinyl estradiol/1 mg norethindrone acetate (*Rx*)	*Femhrt* (Warner Chilcott)
0.5 mg estradiol/0.1 mg norethindrone acetate, 1 mg estradiol/0.5 mg norethindrone acetate (*Rx*)	Various, *Activella* (Novo Nordisk)
1 mg estradiol; 1 mg estradiol/0.09 mg norgestimate (*Rx*)	*Prefest* (Barr/Duramed)
Transdermal patch: 0.045 mg estradiol/0.015 mg levonorgestrel per day (*Rx*)	*ClimaraPro* (Bayer)
0.05 mg estradiol/0.14 mg norethindrone acetate per day; 0.05 mg estradiol/0.25 mg norethindrone acetate per day (*Rx*)	*CombiPatch* (Novartis)

Warning:

Do not use estrogens with or without progestins for the prevention of cardiovascular disease or dementia.

The Woman's Health Initiative (WHI) study reported increased risks of myocardial infarction, stroke, invasive breast cancer, pulmonary emboli, and deep vein thrombosis in postmenopausal women (50 to 79 years of age) during 5 years of treatment with oral conjugated equine estrogens 0.625 mg combined with medroxyprogesterone acetate 2.5 mg relative to placebo.

The WHI Memory Study (WHIMS), a sub-study of WHI, reported increased risk of developing probably dementia in postmenopausal women 65 years of age and older during 4 years of treatment with oral conjugated estrogens plus medroxyprogesterone acetate relative to placebo. It is unknown whether this finding applies to younger postmenopausal women.

Other doses of oral conjugated estrogens with medroxyprogesterone acetate, and other combinations and dosage forms of estrogens and progestins were not studied in the WHI clinical trials. In the absence of comparable data, these risks should be assumed to be similar. Because of these risks, estrogens with or without progestins should be prescribed at the lowest effective doses and for the shortest duration consistent with treatment goals and risks for the individual woman.

Indications

In women with an intact uterus for the treatment of moderate to severe vasomotor symptoms associated with menopause; treatment of vulval and vaginal atrophy (*Femhrt* and *ClimaraPro* excluded); osteoporosis prevention (*CombiPatch* and *Angeliq* excluded); treatment of hypoestrogenism caused by hypogonadism, castration, or primary ovarian failure (*CombiPatch* only).

When prescribing solely for the prevention of postmenopausal osteoporosis, consider therapy only for women at significant risk of osteoporosis; carefully consider nonestrogen medications.

Administration and Dosage

Limit the use of estrogen, alone or in combination with a progestin, to the lowest effective dose available and for the shortest duration consistent with treatment goals and risks for the individual woman. Periodically re-evaluate patients as clinically appropriate (eg, 3- to 6-month intervals) to determine if treatment is still necessary.

Patients should be started at the lowest dose.

Prempro: One 0.625 mg/2.5 mg tablet once daily; can increase to 0.625 mg/5 mg once daily.

Premphase: One 0.625 mg conjugated estrogens tablet once daily on days 1 through 14 and one 0.625 mg conjugated estrogen/5 mg medroxyprogesterone tablet once daily on days 15 through 28.

Activella and Femhrt: One tablet daily.

Angeliq: One tablet daily. Women who are already using a product containing estrogen should stop taking that product before starting *Angeliq*.

Prefest: One pink tablet daily for 3 days, followed by 1 white tablet daily for 3 days. This regimen is repeated continuously without interruption.

CombiPatch: Replace the patch system twice weekly. Advise women that monthly withdrawal bleeding often occurs.

Apply to a smooth (fold-free) clean, dry area of the skin on the lower abdomen. Do not apply to or near the breasts and avoid the waistline. The sites of application must be rotated; allow an interval of at least 1 week between applications to the same site.

Continuous combined regimen – Apply twice weekly during a 28-day cycle. Irregular bleeding may occur particularly in the first 6 months.

Continuous sequential regimen – It can be applied as a sequential regimen in combination with an estradiol-only transdermal delivery system.

ClimaraPro: Apply a new system weekly during a 28-day cycle. Women often experience withdrawal bleeding at the completion of the cycle. The first day of this bleeding would be an appropriate time to begin therapy.

Place on a smooth (fold-free), clean, dry area of the skin on the lower abdomen. Do not apply to or near the breasts. The area selected should not be oily (which can impair adherence of the system), damaged, or irritated. Avoid the waistline since tight clothing may rub the system off or modify drug delivery. The sites of application must be rotated with an interval of at least 1 week allowed between applications to the same site.

Menopause and vulval/vaginal atrophy: Re-evaluate patients at 3- to 6-month intervals to determine the need for continued treatment.

Osteoporosis: The mainstays of prevention and management of osteoporosis are estrogen and calcium; exercise and nutrition may be important adjuncts.

Monitoring: For women who have a uterus, adequate diagnostic measures, such as endometrial sampling, when indicated, should be undertaken to rule out malignancy in cases of undiagnosed persistent or recurring abnormal vaginal bleeding. Patients should be evaluated for breast abnormalities in accordance with good clinical practice.

ESTROGEN AND ANDROGEN COMBINATIONS

Tablets: 0.625 mg esterified estrogens and 1.25 mg methyltestosterone (*Rx*)	Various, *Estratest* H.S. (Solvay), *Covaryx* H.S. (Centrix)
1.25 mg esterified estrogens and 2.5 mg methyltestosterone (*Rx*)	Various, *Estratest* (Solvay), *Covaryx* (Centrix)

Warning:

Estrogens have been reported to increase the risk of endometrial carcinoma.

Close clinical surveillance of all women taking estrogens is important. In all cases of undiagnosed, persistent, or recurring abnormal vaginal bleeding, adequate diagnostic measures should be undertaken to rule out malignancy.

Do not use estrogens during pregnancy.

The use of female sex hormones, estrogens and progestogens, during early pregnancy may seriously damage the offspring.

Refer to the Warning Box in the Estrogens group monograph for more information.

Indications

Moderate to severe vasomotor symptoms: Moderate to severe vasomotor symptoms associated with menopause in patients not improved with estrogens alone.

Administration and Dosage

Oral: Give cyclically for short-term use only.

Use the lowest dose that will control symptoms and discontinue medication as promptly as possible.

Administer cyclically (eg, 3 weeks on and 1 week off). Make attempts to discontinue or taper medication at 3- to 6-month intervals.

Usual dosage range – One 1.25/2.5 mg tablet or one to two 0.625/1.25 mg tablets daily, as recommended by the physician.

Closely monitor treated patients with an intact uterus for signs of endometrial cancer and take appropriate diagnostic measures to rule out malignancy in the event of persistent or recurring abnormal vaginal bleeding.

RALOXIFENE

Tablets: 60 mg (*Rx*) *Evista* (Eli Lilly)

Warning:

Increased risk of venous thromboembolism and death from stroke: Increased risk of deep vein thrombosis and pulmonary embolism have been reported with raloxifene. Women with active venous thromboembolism (VTE) or a history of VTE should not take raloxifene.

Increased risk of death caused by stroke occurred in a trial in postmenopausal women with documented coronary heart disease or increased risk for major coronary reactions. Consider the risk-benefit balance in women at risk for stroke.

Indications

Osteoporosis, prevention, and treatment: Prevention and treatment of osteoporosis in postmenopausal women.

Reduction in the risk of invasive breast cancer in postmenopausal women with osteoporosis: Reduction in the risk of invasive breast cancer in postmenopausal women with osteoporosis.

Reduction in risk of invasive breast cancer in postmenopausal women at high risk of invasive breast cancer: Reduction in risk of invasive breast cancer in postmenopausal women at high risk of invasive breast cancer.

Administration and Dosage

The recommended dosage is 60 mg/day, which may be administered any time of day without regard to meals.

Calcium/Vitamin D supplementation: For osteoporosis treatment or prevention, supplemental calcium and/or vitamin D should be added to the diet if daily intake is inadequate.

Actions

Pharmacology: Raloxifene is a selective estrogen receptor modulator (SERM) that reduces resorption of bone and decreases overall bone turnover.

Pharmacokinetics:

Absorption – Raloxifene is absorbed rapidly after oral administration with approximately 60% of an oral dose adsorbed. However, presystemic glucuronide conjugation is extensive and absolute bioavailability is only 2%.

Distribution – The apparent volume of distribution is 2,348 L/kg and is not dose-dependent. Raloxifene and the monoglucuronide conjugates are highly bound to plasma proteins (95%).

Metabolism – Raloxifene undergoes extensive first-pass metabolism to the glucuronide conjugates. Raloxifene is not metabolized by CYP-450 pathways. Plasma elimination half-life to 27.7 hours after single dose oral dosing and 32.5 after multiple dose oral dosing.

Excretion – Raloxifene is primarily excreted in feces; less than 6% of the raloxifene dose is eliminated in urine as glucuronide conjugates and less than 0.2% is excreted unchanged in urine.

Contraindications

Women who are breast-feeding or who are or may become pregnant (see Warnings); women with active or a history of VTE, including deep vein thrombosis, pulmonary embolism, and retinal vein thrombosis; hypersensitivity to raloxifene or other constituents of the drug.

Warnings/Precautions

Venous thromboembolic events: An analysis of raloxifene-treated women showed an increased risk of venous thromboembolic events defined as DVT and pulmonary embolism. Other venous thromboembolic events could also occur. A less serious event, superficial thrombophlebitis, has been reported more frequently with raloxifene. The greatest risk for DVT and pulmonary embolism occurs during the first 4 months of treatment. Discontinue raloxifene at least 72 hours prior to and during prolonged immobilization (eg, postsurgical recovery, prolonged bed rest), and resume therapy only after the patient is fully ambulatory. Advise patients to avoid prolonged restrictions of movement during travel.

Death caused by stroke: Consider the risk-benefit balance in women at risk for stroke, such as atrial fibrillation, cigarette smoking, hypertension, prior stroke or transient ischemic attack.

Premenopausal use: There is no indication for premenopausal use of raloxifene.

Breast abnormalities: Raloxifene has not been associated with breast enlargement, breast pain, or an increased risk of breast cancer. Investigate any unexplained breast abnormality occurring during raloxifene therapy.

Cardiovascular disease: Do not use raloxifene for the primary or secondary prevention of cardiovascular disease.

Concurrent estrogen therapy: The concurrent use of raloxifene and systemic estrogen or hormone replacement therapy (ERT or HRT) has not been studied in prospective clinical trials; therefore, concomitant use is not recommended.

Hypertriglyceridemia: Limited clinical data suggest that some women with histories of marked hypertriglyceridemia (more than 5.6 mmol/L or more than 500 mg/dL) in response to treatment with oral estrogen or estrogen plus progestin may develop increased levels of triglycerides when treated with raloxifene. Monitor serum triglycerides in women with this medical history when they are taking raloxifene.

History of breast cancer: Raloxifene has not been adequately studied in women with a history of breast cancer.

Use in men: There is no indication for the use of raloxifene in men. Raloxifene has not been adequately studied in men, and its use is not recommended.

Unexplained uterine bleeding: Investigate any unexplained uterine bleeding as clinically indicated. Raloxifene- and placebo-treated groups had similar incidences of endometrial proliferation.

Breast abnormalities: Investigate any unexplained breast abnormalities occurring during raloxifene therapy. Raloxifene does not eliminate the risk of breast cancer.

Renal function impairment: Use raloxifene with caution in patients with moderate or severe renal function impairment. Safety and efficacy have not been established in patients with moderate or severe renal function impairment.

Hepatic function impairment: Use raloxifene with caution in patients with hepatic function impairment. Safety and efficacy have not been established in patients with hepatic function impairment.

Carcinogenesis: In long term carcinogenicity studies in animals there was an increased incidence of ovarian tumors, testicular interstitial cell tumors, and prostatic adenocarcinomas.

Fertility impairment: Raloxifene delayed and disrupted embryo implantation resulting in prolonged gestation and reduced litter size.

Pregnancy: Category X.

Lactation: Raloxifene should not be used by breast-feeding women.

Children: Raloxifene should not be used in children.

Monitoring: If raloxifene is given concurrently with warfarin or other coumarin derivatives, monitor prothrombin time more closely when starting or stopping therapy with raloxifene; monitor triglycerides in women with a history of hypertriglyceridemia.

Drug Interactions

Drugs that may interact with raloxifene include ampicillin and cholestyramine. Raloxifene may affect warfarin and systemic estrogens.

Highly protein-bound drugs: Use caution when raloxifene is coadministered with other highly protein-bound drugs, such as diazepam, diazoxide, and lidocaine.

Adverse Reactions

Adverse reactions occurring in at least 3% of patients include hot flashes; depression; insomnia; vertigo; rash; nausea; diarrhea; dyspepsia; vomiting; flatulence; GI disorder; vaginitis; UTI; cystitis; leukorrhea; uterine disorder; endometrial disorder; weight gain; peripheral edema; arthralgia; myalgia; leg cramps; arthritis; tendon disorder; sinusitis; rhinitis; bronchitis; pharyngitis; increased cough; infection; flu syndrome; headache; chest pain; fever.

PROGESTINS

MEDROXYPROGESTERONE	
Tablets, oral: 2.5, 5, and 10 mg (*Rx*)	Various, *Provera* (Pharmacia and Upjohn)
MEGESTROL ACETATE	
Tablets, oral: 20 and 40 mg (*Rx*)	Various, *Megace* (Bristol-Myers Oncology)
Suspension, oral: 40 mg/mL, 125 mg/mL (*Rx*)	Various, *Megace* (Bristol-Myers Oncology), *Megace ES* (Par Pharmaceutical, Inc.)
NORETHINDRONE ACETATE	
Tablets, oral: 5 mg (*Rx*)	Various, *Aygestin* (Barr)
PROGESTERONE	
Suppositories; vaginal: 25, 50, 100, 200, and 400 mg (*Rx*)	*First Progesterone* (Curtis Pharma)
PROGESTERONE (MICRONIZED)	
Capsules, oral: 100 and 200 mg (*Rx*)	*Prometrium* (Abbott)
Insert, vaginal: 100 mg (*Rx*)	*Endometrin* (Ferring Pharmaceuticals)
PROGESTERONE IN OIL	
Injection: 50 mg/mL (*Rx*)	Various
PROGESTERONE GEL	
Vaginal gel: 4% and 8% (*Rx*)	*Crinone* (Danbury Pharmacal)

Warning:

Progestins and estrogens should not be used for the prevention of cardiovascular disease.

The Women's Health Initiative (WHI) study reported increased risks of myocardial infarction (MI), stroke, invasive breast cancer, pulmonary emboli, and deep vein thrombosis in postmenopausal women (50 to 79 years of age) during 5 years of treatment with oral conjugated estrogens 0.625 mg combined with medroxyprogesterone acetate 2.5 mg relative to placebo.

The Women's Health Initiative Memory Study (WHIMS), a substudy of WHI, reported increased risk of developing probable dementia in postmenopausal women 65 years of age or older during 4 years of treatment with oral conjugated estrogens plus medroxyprogesterone acetate relative to placebo. It is unknown whether this finding applies to younger postmenopausal women.

Other doses of oral conjugated estrogens with medroxyprogesterone and other combinations and dosage forms of estrogens and progestins were not studied in the WHI clinical trials. In the absence of comparable data and product-specific studies, the relevance of the WHI findings to other products has not been established. Therefore, the risks should be assumed to be similar for all estrogen and progestin products. Because of these risks, estrogens with or without progestins should be prescribed at the lowest effective doses and for the shortest duration consistent with treatment goals and risks for the individual women.

Pregnancy: Progestins have been used beginning with the first trimester of pregnancy to prevent habitual abortion or treat threatened abortion; however, there is no adequate evidence that such use is effective. There is evidence of potential harm to the fetus when given during the first 4 months of pregnancy. Therefore, the use of such drugs during the first 4 months of pregnancy is not recommended.

The cause of abortion is generally a defective ovum, which progestational agents could not be expected to influence. In addition, progestational agents have uterine relaxant properties that may cause a delay in spontaneous abortion when given to patients with fertilized defective ova.

Indications

Norethindrone: Secondary amenorrhea; abnormal uterine bleeding caused by hormonal imbalance in the absence of organic pathology, such as submucous fibroids or uterine cancer; endometriosis.

Megestrol:

Tumors (tablets only) – Palliative treatment of advanced carcinoma of the breast or endometrium.

AIDS wasting syndrome (oral suspension only) – Treatment of anorexia, cachexia, or an unexplained, significant weight loss in patients with a diagnosis of AIDS.

Medroxyprogesterone tablets:

Endometrial hyperplasia – To reduce the incidence of endometrial hyperplasia in nonhysterectomized postmenopausal women receiving conjugated estrogens 0.625 mg.

Secondary amenorrhea/abnormal uterine bleeding – For secondary amenorrhea and for abnormal uterine bleeding due to hormonal imbalance in the absence of organic pathology, such as fibroids or uterine cancer.

Progesterone capsules and gel: Progesterone supplementation or replacement as part of an Assisted Reproductive Technology (ART) treatment for infertile women with progesterone deficiency (8% gel).

Endometrial hyperplasia (capsules) – For use in the prevention of endometrial hyperplasia in nonhysterectomized postmenopausal women who are receiving conjugated estrogens tablets.

Secondary amenorrhea – For use in secondary amenorrhea (capsules); the 4% gel is for the treatment of secondary amenorrhea, and the 8% gel is for women who have failed to respond to treatment with the 4% gel.

Progesterone in oil injection: For amenorrhea and abnormal uterine bleeding caused by hormonal imbalance in the absence of organic pathology, such as submucous fibroids or uterine cancer.

Progesterone (micronized) vaginal insert: To support embryo implantation and early pregnancy by supplementation of corpus luteal function as part of an ART treatment program for infertile women.

Administration and Dosage

MEDROXYPROGESTERONE ACETATE:

Secondary amenorrhea – 5 to 10 mg/day for 5 to 10 days. To induce an optimum secretory transformation of an endometrium that has been adequately primed with estrogen, give 10 mg daily for 10 days. Start therapy any time. Withdrawal bleeding usually occurs 3 to 7 days after therapy ends.

Abnormal uterine bleeding due to hormonal imbalance in the absence of organic pathology – 5 to 10 mg/day for 5 to 10 days, beginning on the 16th or 21st day of the menstrual cycle. To produce an optimum secretory transformation of an endometrium that has been adequately primed, give 10 mg/day for 10 days, beginning on the 16th day of the cycle. Withdrawal bleeding usually occurs 3 to 7 days after discontinuing therapy. Patients with recurrent episodes of abnormal uterine bleeding may benefit from planned menstrual cycling.

Endometrial hyperplasia – 5 or 10 mg daily for 12 to 14 consecutive days per month, beginning on day 1 or 16 of the cycle.

MEGESTROL ACETATE:

Tablets –

Breast cancer: 160 mg/day (40 mg 4 times a day).

Endometrial carcinoma: 40 to 320 mg/day in divided doses. At least 2 months of continuous treatment is considered an adequate period for determining the efficacy of megestrol acetate.

Oral suspension (40 mg/mL) – 800 mg/day (20 mL/day). Shake container well before use.

Extra strength oral suspension (125 mg/mL) – 625 mg/day (5 mL/day or 1 teaspoon daily). Shake container well before use.

NORETHINDRONE ACETATE: Norethindrone acetate differs from norethindrone only in potency; the acetate is approximately twice as potent.

Secondary amenorrhea; abnormal uterine bleeding due to hormonal imbalance in the absence of organic pathology – 2.5 to 10 mg/day for 5 to 10 days during the second half of the theoretical menstrual cycle. Withdrawal bleeding usually occurs within 3 to 7 days.

Endometriosis –

Initial dose: 5 mg/day for 2 weeks; increase in increments of 2.5 mg/day every 2 weeks up to 15 mg/day. Therapy may be held at this level for 6 to 9 months or until breakthrough bleeding demands temporary termination.

PROGESTERONE IN OIL: For IM use. The drug is irritating at the injection site.

Amenorrhea – Administer 5 to 10 mg/day for 6 to 8 consecutive days. If ovarian activity has produced a proliferative endometrium, expect withdrawal bleeding 48 to 72 hours after the last injection. Spontaneous normal cycles may follow.

Functional uterine bleeding – Administer 5 to 10 mg/day for 6 doses. Bleeding should cease within 6 days. When estrogen also is given, begin progesterone after 2 weeks of estrogen therapy. Discontinue injections when menstrual flow begins.

PROGESTERONE CAPSULES:

Prevention of endometrial hyperplasia – Give as a single daily dose in the evening, 200 mg orally for 12 days sequentially per 28-day cycle, to postmenopausal women with a uterus who are receiving daily conjugated estrogen tablets.

Secondary amenorrhea – Give as a single daily dose of 400 mg in the evening for 10 days.

PROGESTERONE GEL:

Infertility – Administer 90 mg of 8% gel vaginally once daily in women who require progesterone supplementation. In women with partial or complete ovarian failure, administer 90 mg of 8% gel vaginally twice daily. If pregnancy occurs, continue treatment until placental autonomy is achieved, no more than 10 to 12 weeks.

Secondary amenorrhea – Administer 45 mg (4% gel) vaginally every other day up to a total of 6 doses. For women who fail to respond, a trial of 8% gel every other day up to a total of 6 doses may be instituted.

PROGESTERONE VAGINAL INSERT: 100 mg administered vaginally 2 or 3 times daily starting at oocyte retrieval and continuing for up to 10 weeks total duration. Efficacy in women 35 years of age and older has not been clearly established. The appropriate dose of progesterone in this age group has not been determined.

Actions

Pharmacology: Progesterone, a principle of corpus luteum, is the primary endogenous progestational substance. Progestins (progesterone and derivatives) transform proliferative endometrium into secretory endometrium. They inhibit the secretion of pituitary gonadotropins, which in turn prevents follicular maturation and ovulation. They also inhibit spontaneous uterine contraction. Progestins may demonstrate some estrogenic, anabolic, or androgenic activity. The precise mechanism by which megestrol produces effects in anorexia and cachexia is unknown.

Pharmacokinetics: Absorption of oral tablets and parenteral oily solutions of progestins is rapid. The hormone undergoes prompt hepatic transformation.

Contraindications

Hypersensitivity to progestins; thrombophlebitis, thromboembolic disorders, cerebral hemorrhage or patients with a history of these conditions; impaired liver function or disease; carcinoma of the breast; undiagnosed vaginal bleeding; missed abortion; as a diagnostic test for pregnancy; known or suspected pregnancy; prophylactic use to avoid weight loss (megestrol).

Warnings/Precautions

Ophthalmologic effects: Discontinue medication pending examination if there is a sudden partial or complete loss of vision, or if there is sudden onset of proptosis, diplopia, or migraine. If papilledema or retinal vascular lesions are present, discontinue use.

Thrombotic disorders: Thrombotic disorders (thrombophlebitis, cerebrovascular disorders, retinal thrombosis, pulmonary embolism) occasionally occur in patients taking progestins.

HIV-infected women: Although megestrol has been used extensively in women for endometrial and breast cancers, its use in HIV-infected women has been limited. All the women in the clinical trials reported breakthrough bleeding.

Fertility impairment: Medroxyprogesterone acetate at high doses is an antifertility drug. High doses would be expected to impair fertility until the cessation of treatment.

Causes of weight loss: Institute therapy with megestrol for weight loss only after treatable causes of weight loss are sought and addressed.

Respiratory infections: Long-term treatment may increase the risk of respiratory infections.

Pretreatment physical examination: Pretreatment physical examination should include breasts and pelvic organs, as well as Papanicolaou smear.

Fluid retention: Fluid retention may occur; therefore, conditions influenced by this factor (epilepsy, migraine, asthma, or cardiac or renal function impairment) require careful observation.

Depression: Observe patients who have a history of psychic depression. Discontinue the drug if the depression recurs to a serious degree.

Glucose tolerance: A decrease in glucose tolerance has been observed in a small percentage of patients on estrogen-progestin combination drugs. Carefully observe diabetic patients receiving progestin therapy.

Menopause: The age of the patient constitutes no absolute limiting factor, although treatment with progestins may mask the onset of the climacteric.

Photosensitivity: Photosensitization (photoallergy or phototoxicity) may occur; therefore, caution patients to take protective measures (ie, sunscreens, protective clothing) against exposure to sunlight or ultraviolet light (eg, tanning beds) until tolerance is determined.

Pregnancy: Category D (progesterone injection); *Category X* (norethindrone acetate). Use is not recommended. See Warning Box.

Lactation: Detectable amounts of progestins enter the milk of mothers receiving these agents. The effect on the breast-feeding infant has not been determined.

Medroxyprogesterone does not adversely affect lactation and may increase milk production and duration of lactation if given in the puerperium.

Children: Safety and efficacy of megestrol acetate suspension in children have not been established.

Drug Interactions

Drugs that may interact with progestins include aminoglutethimide and rifampin.

Drug/Lab test interactions: Laboratory test results of hepatic function, coagulation tests (increase in prothrombin, Factors VII, VIII, IX, and X), thyroid, metyrapone test and endocrine functions, may be affected by progestins or estrogens. A decrease in glucose tolerance has been observed in a small percentage of patients on estrogen-progestin combination drugs. Pregnanediol determination may be altered by the use of progestins.

Adverse Reactions

Adverse reactions that may occur include breakthrough bleeding, spotting, change in menstrual flow, amenorrhea, changes in cervical erosion and cervical secretions; breast changes (tenderness); masculinization of the female fetus; edema; changes in weight (increase or decrease); cholestatic jaundice; rash (allergic) with and without pruritus; acne; melasma or chloasma; mental depression; alopecia; hirsutism; thromboembolic phenomena including thrombophlebitis and pulmonary embolism; sensitivity reactions ranging from pruritus and urticaria to generalized rash (medroxyprogesterone acetate).

For information concerning adverse reactions associated with combined estrogen-progestin therapy, refer to the Oral Contraceptives monograph.

Megestrol: Adverse reactions occurring in at least 3% of patients include diarrhea; impotence; rash; flatulence; hypertension; asthenia; insomnia; nausea; anemia; fever; libido decreased; hyperglycemia; headache.

CONTRACEPTIVE PRODUCTS

MONOPHASIC ORAL CONTRACEPTIVES	
Tablets: Estrogens (ethinyl estradiol, mestranol), progestins (desogestrel, drospirenone, ethynodiol diacetate, levonorgestrel, norethindrone, norethindrone acetate, norgestimate, norgestrel) (*Rx*)	*Alesse* (Wyeth-Ayerst), *Apri, Aviane* (Barr), *Balziva* (Barr),*Beyaz* (Bayer Healthcare), *Brevicon* (Watson), *Cryselle* (Barr), *Desogen* (Organon), *Femcon Fe* (Warner Chilcott), *Jolessa, Junel 21, Junel Fe, Kariva, Kelnor, Lessina* (Barr), *Levora* (Watson), *Loestrin* (Teva), *Lo/Ovral* (Wyeth Ayerst), *Low-Ogestrel, Lutera* (Watson), *Lybrel* (Wyeth), *Microgestin Fe* (Watson), *Mircette* (Duramed), *Modicon* (Ortho-McNeil), *Mononessa, Necon* (Watson), *Nordette-28* (Barr/Duramed), *Norinyl* (Watson), *Nortrel* (Barr), *Ocella* (Barr), *Ogestrel* (Watson), *Ortho-Cept, Ortho-Cyclen, Ortho-Novum* (Ortho-McNeil), *Ovcon* (Warner Chilcott), *Ovcon 35 Fe* (Warner Chilcott), *Ovral* (Wyeth-Ayerst), *Portia*, (Barr), *Quasense, Reclipsen* (Watson), *Seasonale* (Duramed), *Solia* (Prasco), *Sprintec* (Barr), *Sronyx* (Watson), *Yasmin* (Berlex), *YAZ* (Bayer), *Zenchent* (Watson), *Zovia* (Watson)
BIPHASIC ORAL CONTRACEPTIVES	
Tablets: Desogestrel, estrogen (ethinyl estradiol), progestin (norethindrone), levonorgestrel (*Rx*)	*Kariva* (Barr), *LoSeasonique* (Teva), *Mircette* (Duramed), *Necon 10/11* (Watson), *Ortho-Novum 10/11* (Ortho-McNeil), *Seasonique* (Duramed)
TRIPHASIC ORAL CONTRACEPTIVES	
Tablets: Estrogen (ethinyl estradiol), progestin (desogestrel, levonorgestrel, norethindrone, norethindrone acetate, norgestimate) (*Rx*)	*Aranelle* (Barr), *Cesia* (Prasco), *Cyclessa* (Organon), *Enpresse* (Barr), *Estrostep Fe* (Warner Chilcott), *Leena, Necon 7/7/7* (Watson), *Ortho-Novum 777, Ortho Tri-Cyclen, Ortho Tri-Cyclen Lo* (Ortho-McNeil), *Tri-Levlen* (Berlex), *TriNessa* (Watson), *Tri-Norinyl* (Watson), *Triphasil* (Wyeth-Ayerst), *Tri-Previfem* (Teva), *Tri-Sprintec* (Barr), *Trivora* (Watson), *Velivet* (Barr)
PROGESTIN-ONLY PRODUCTS	
Tablets: 0.35 mg norethindrone (*Rx*)	Various, *Camila, Errin* (Barr), *Heather* (Glenmark), *Jolivette* (Watson), *Ortho-Micronor* (Ortho-McNeil), *Nor-QD, Nora-BE* (Watson)
NORELGESTROMIN/ETHINYL ESTRADIOL TRANSDERMAL SYSTEM	
Patch: 6 mg norelgestromin, 0.75 mg ethinyl estradiol/total patch content (*Rx*)	*Ortho Evra* (Ortho-McNeil)
ETONOGESTREL/ETHINYL ESTRADIOL VAGINAL RING	
Ring: 11.7 mg etonogestrel, 2.7 mg ethinyl estradiol/sachet (*Rx*)	*NuvaRing* (Organon)
EMERGENCY CONTRACEPTIVES	
Tablets; oral: levonorgestrel 0.75 mg (*otc*)	*Next Choice*[a] (Watson), *Plan B*[b] (Duramed)
levonorgestrel 1.5 mg (*otc*)	*Plan B One-Step*[a] (Duramed)
ulipristal 30 mg (*Rx*)	*ella* (Watson Pharma)

[a] *Next Choice* and *Plan B One-Step* are approved for over-the-counter status for women ≥ 17 years of age. They are available by prescription only for women < 17 years of age.

[b] *Plan B* is approved for over-the-counter status for women ≥ 18 years of age. It is available by prescription only for women ≤ 17 years of age.

Warning:

Cigarette smoking: Cigarette smoking increases the risk of cardiovascular adverse reactions from hormonal contraceptive use. This risk increases with age and with heavy smoking (15 or more cigarettes per day) and is quite marked in women more than 35 years of age. Women who use hormonal contraceptives should not smoke.

Indications

Contraceptive: For the prevention of pregnancy. Start new patients on preparations containing estrogen 35 mcg or less.

Emergency contraceptives: For the prevention of pregnancy following unprotected intercourse or a known or suspected contraceptive failure.

Acne vulgaris (Ortho Tri-Cyclen and Estrostep only): For the treatment of moderate acne vulgaris in females 15 years of age and older who have no known contraindications to oral contraceptive therapy, desire contraception, have achieved menarche, and are unresponsive to topical antiacne medications.

Administration and Dosage

Acne: The timing of dosing with *Ortho Tri-Cyclen* or *Estrostep* for acne should follow the guidelines for use of *Ortho Tri-Cyclen* or *Estrostep* as an oral contraceptive. The dosage regimen for treatment of facial acne uses a 21-day active and a 7-day inert schedule. Take 1 active tablet daily for 21 days followed by 1 inert tablet for 7 days. After 28 tablets have been taken, a new course is started the next day.

Emergency contraceptives:

Levonorgestrel –

Next Choice and Plan B: 1 tablet should be taken within 72 hours after unprotected intercourse. The second tablet should be taken 12 hours after the first dose.

Plan B One-Step: Instruct patients to take as soon as possible within 72 hours after unprotected intercourse or a known or suspected contraceptive failure.

Administration:

Plan B – If the user vomits within 1 hour of taking either dose of medication, instruct her to contact her health care provider to discuss whether to repeat that dose.

Next Choice and Plan B One-Step – If vomiting occurs within 2 hours of taking the tablet, consider repeating the dose.

Ulipristal –

Adults: 1 tablet orally as soon as possible within 120 hours (5 days) after unprotected intercourse or a known or suspected contraceptive failure.

Children: Use before menarche is not indicated.

Administration: May be taken with or without food. If vomiting occurs within 3 hours of ulipristal intake, consider repeating the dose.

Progestin-only contraception: 1 tablet every day at the same time. Administration is continuous, with no interruption between pill packs. Every time a pill is taken late, especially if a pill is missed, pregnancy is more likely.

Missed dose – If the patient is more than 3 hours late or misses 1 or more tablets, she should take a missed pill as soon as remembered, then go back to taking progestin-only pills (POPs) at the regular time, but should use a backup method (eg, condom, spermicide) every time she has sexual intercourse for the next 48 hours.

Breast-feeding – If fully breast-feeding (not giving baby any food or formula), start POPs 6 weeks after delivery. If partially breast-feeding (giving baby some food or formula), start taking POPs by 3 weeks after delivery.

Switching pills – If switching from the combined pills to POPs, take the first POP the day after the last active combined pill is finished. Do not take any of the 7 inactive pills from the combined pill pack. Many women have irregular periods after switching to POPs; this is normal and to be expected. If switching from POPs to the combined pills, take the first active combined pill on the first day of menses, even if the POP pack is not finished. If switching to another brand of POPs, start the new brand any time. If breast-feeding, switch to another method of birth control at any time, except do not switch to the combined pills until breast-feeding is stopped or until at least 6 months after delivery.

Combined:

Sunday-start packaging – Take the first tablet on the first Sunday after menstruation begins. If menstruation begins on Sunday, take the first tablet on that day.

21-day regimen – Day 1 of the cycle is the first day of menstrual bleeding. Take 1 tablet daily for 21 days. No tablets are taken for 7 days. Whether bleeding has stopped or not, start a new course of 21 days.

28-day regimen – To eliminate the need to count the days between cycles, some products contain 7 inert or iron-containing tablets to permit continuous daily dosage during the entire 28-day cycle. Take the 7 tablets on the last 7 days of the cycle.

84-day regimen – The dosage of *Seasonale* is 1 pink (active) tablet per day for 84 consecutive days, followed by 7 days of white (inert) tablets. Withdrawal bleeding should occur during the 7 days following discontinuation of pink active tablets. During the first cycle, the patient should not place contraceptive reliance on *Seasonale* until a pink tablet has been taken daily for 7 consecutive days; the patient should use a nonhormonal backup method of birth control (such as condoms or spermicide) during those 7 days. The patient should consider the possibility of ovulation and conception prior to initiation of medication.

Biphasic and triphasic oral contraceptives – Follow instructions on the dispensers or packs. As with the monophasic oral contraceptives, 1 tablet is taken each day; however, as the color of the tablet changes, the strength of the tablet also changes (ie, the estrogen/progestin ratio varies).

Missed dose –

One tablet: Take it as soon as remembered, or take 2 tablets the next day. Alternatively, take 1 tablet, discard the other missed tablet, continue as scheduled and use another form of contraception until menses.

2 consecutive tablets: Take 2 tablets as soon as remembered with the next pill at the usual time, or take 2 tablets/day for the next 2 days, then resume the regular schedule. Use an additional form of contraception for the 7 days after pills are missed, preferably for the remainder of the cycle. If 2 active pills are missed in a row in the third week and the patient is a Sunday starter, 1 pill should be taken every day until Sunday. On Sunday, the rest of the pack should be discarded and a new pack of pills started that same day. If 2 active pills are missed in a row in the third week and the patient is a day 1 starter, the rest of the pill pack should be discarded and a new pack started that same day. Menses may not occur this month but this is expected.

Three consecutive tablets: If the patient is a Sunday starter, she should keep taking 1 pill every day until Sunday. On Sunday, the rest of the pack should be discarded and a new pack of pills started that same day. If she is a day 1 starter, the rest of the pill pack should be discarded and a new pack started that same day. Menses may not occur this month, but this is expected. If menses do not occur 2 months in a row, the health care provider should be contacted because of the possibility of pregnancy. Pregnancy may result from sexual intercourse during the 7 days after the pills are missed. Use another birth control method (eg, condoms, foam) as a back-up method for those 7 days.

Missed menstrual period: If the patient has not adhered to the prescribed dosage regimen, consider possible pregnancy after the first missed period; withhold oral contraceptives until ruling out pregnancy and use a nonhormonal method of contraception. If the patient has adhered to the prescribed regimen and misses 2 consecutive periods, rule out pregnancy before continuing the contraceptive regimen.

After several months of treatment, menstrual flow may reduce to a point of virtual absence. This reduced flow may occur as a result of medication and is not indicative of pregnancy.

Postpartum administration: Postpartum administration in non–breast-feeding mothers may begin at the first postpartum examination (4 to 6 weeks), regardless of whether spontaneous menstruation has occurred. Also, start no earlier than 4 to 6 weeks after a midtrimester pregnancy termination.

Dosage adjustments: Adverse reactions noted during the initial cycles may be transient; if they continue, dosage adjustments may be indicated. Many adverse reactions are related to the potency of the estrogen or progestin in the products. The following table summarizes these dose-related adverse reactions.

Achieving Proper Hormonal Balance in an Oral Contraceptive

Estrogen		Progestin	
Excess	Deficiency	Excess	Deficiency
Nausea, bloating Cervical mucorrhea, polyposis Melasma Hypertension Migraine headache Breast fullness or tenderness Edema	Early or midcycle breakthrough bleeding Increased spotting Hypomenorrhea	Increased appetite Weight gain Tiredness, fatigue Hypomenorrhea Acne, oily scalp[a] Hair loss, hirsutism[a] Depression Monilial vaginitis Breast regression	Late breakthrough bleeding Amenorrhea Hypermenorrhea

[a] Result of androgenic activity of progestins.

Pharmacological Effects of Progestins Used in Oral Contraceptives[a]

	Progestin	Estrogen	Androgen
Desogestrel	++++	0	+++
Levonorgestrel	++++	0	++++
Norgestrel	+++	0	+++
Ethynodiol diacetate	++	+++	+
Norgestimate	++	0	++
Norethindrone acetate	++	++	++
Norethindrone	++	++	++

[a] *Symbol Key: ++++ – pronounced effect +++ – moderate effect*
++ – low effect + – slight effect 0 – no effect

Minimize the previously listed effects by adjusting the estrogen/progestin balance or dosage. The following table categorizes products by their estrogenic, progestational, and androgenic activity. Because overall activity is influenced by the interaction of components, including androgenic and antiestrogenic activity, it is difficult to precisely classify products; placement in the table is only approximate. Differences between products within a group are probably not clinically significant.

Estimated Relative Oral Contraceptive Progestin/Estrogen/Androgen Activity

	Ingredients[a]	Brand-name examples	Progestin activity	Estrogen activity	Androgen activity
Monophasic	Levonorgestrel 0.1 mg/EE 20 mcg	*Alesse, Aviane, Lessina, Levlite*	Low	Low	Low
	Norgestimate 0.25 mg/EE 35 mcg	*Ortho-Cyclen, Sprintec*		Intermediate	
	Norethindrone 0.5 mg/EE 35 mcg	*Brevicon, Modicon, Necon 0.5/35, Nortrel 0.5/35*		High	
	Norethindrone 0.4 mg/EE 35 mcg	*Ovcon-35*			
	levonorgestrel 0.15 mg/EE 30 mcg	*Levlen, Levora, Nordette, Portia*	Intermediate	Low	Intermediate
	Norgestrel 0.3 mg/ 30 mcg EE	*Cryselle, Lo-Ovral, Low-Ogestrel*			
	Norethindrone 1 mg/mestranol 50 mcg	*Necon 1/50, Norinyl 1+50, Ortho-Novum 1/50*		Intermediate	
	Norethindrone 1 mg/EE 35 mcg	*Necon 1/35, Norinyl 1+35, Nortrel 1/35, Ortho-Novum 1/35*		High	
	Norethindrone 1 mg/EE 50 mcg	*Ovcon-50*			
	Norethindrone acetate 1 mg/ EE 20 mcg	*Loestrin 21 1/20, Loestrin Fe 1/20, Microgestin Fe 1/20*	High	Low	
	Norethindrone acetate 1.5 mg/ EE 30 mcg	*Loestrin 21 1.5/30, Loestrin Fe 1.5/30, Microgestin Fe 1.5/30*			High
	Ethynodiol diacetate 1 mg/EE 35 mcg	*Demulen 1/35, Zovia 1/35E*			Low
	Desogestrel/EE 0.15 mg to 20 mcg and EE 10 mcg	*Kariva, Mircette*			
	Desogestrel 0.15 mg/ EE 30 mcg	*Apri, Desogen, Ortho-Cept*	High	Intermediate	
	Ethynodiol diacetate 1 mg/EE 50 mcg	*Demulen 1/50, Zovia 1/50E*			
	Norgestrel 0.5 mg/ EE 50 mcg	*Ovral, Ogestrel*		High	High
	Drospirenone 3 mg/ EE 30 mcg	*Yasmin*	No data	Intermediate[b]	None[b]

Estimated Relative Oral Contraceptive Progestin/Estrogen/Androgen Activity					
	Ingredients[a]	Brand-name examples	Progestin activity	Estrogen activity	Androgen activity
Biphasic	Norethindrone/ EE 0.5 to 35/ 1 to 35 mg to mcg	*Necon 10/11, Ortho-Novum 10/11*	Intermediate	High	Low
Triphasic	Norgestimate/EE 0.18 to 25/0.215 to 25/0.25 to 25 mg to mcg	*Ortho Tri-Cyclen Lo*	Low	Low	
	Levonorgestrel/EE 0.05 to 30/0.075 to 40/0.125 to 30 mg to mcg	*Enpresse, Tri-Levlen, Triphasil, Trivora*		Intermediate	
	Norgestimate/EE 0.18 to 35/0.215 to 35/0.25 to 35 mg to mcg	*Ortho Tri-Cyclen*			
	Norethindrone/EE 0.5 to 35/1 to 35/0.5 to 35 mg to mcg	*Tri-Norinyl*		High	
	Norethindrone/EE 0.5 to 35/0.75 to 35/1 to 35 mg to mcg	*Necon 7/7/7, Ortho-Novum 7/7/7*	Intermediate		
	Norethindrone/EE 1 to 20/1 to 30/1 to 35 mg to mcg	*Estrostep Fe*	High	Low	Intermediate
	Desogestrel/EE 0.1 to 25/0.125 to 25/ 0.15 to 25 mg to mcg	*Cyclessa*			Low

[a] EE = ethinyl estradiol.

[b] Preclinical studies have shown that drospirenone has no androgenic, estrogenic, glucocorticoid, antiglucocorticoid, or antiandrogenic activity.

Patch:

Use – This system uses a 28-day (4-week) cycle. A new patch is applied each week for 3 weeks (21 days total). Week 4 is patch-free. Withdrawal bleeding is expected to begin during this time.

Apply every new patch on the same day of the week. This day is known as the "Patch Change Day."

On the day after week 4 ends, a new 4-week cycle is started by applying a new patch. Under no circumstances should there be more than a 7 day patch-free interval between dosing cycles. If there are more than 7 patch-free days, the woman may not be protected from pregnancy and back-up contraception (eg, condoms, spermicide, diaphragm) must be used for 7 days.

The patient must choose 1 option:

First day start – For first day start, apply the first patch during the first 24 hours of the menstrual period. If therapy starts after day 1 of the menstrual cycle, a nonhormonal back-up contraceptive (eg, condoms, spermicide, diaphragm) should be used concurrently for the first 7 consecutive days of the first treatment cycle.

Sunday start – For Sunday start, apply the first patch on the first Sunday after the menstrual period starts. Use back-up contraception for the first week of the first cycle. If the menstrual period begins on a Sunday, the first patch should be applied on that day and no back-up contraception is needed.

Application – Apply the patch to clean, dry, intact, healthy skin on the buttock, abdomen, upper outer arm, or upper torso in a place where it will not be rubbed by tight clothing. The patch should not be placed on skin that is red, irritated, or cut, nor should it be placed on the breasts.

To prevent interference with the adhesive properties of the patch, no topical products should be applied to the skin area where the patch is or will be placed.

Patch changes may occur at any time on the change day. Apply each new patch to a new spot on the skin to help avoid irritation, although they may be kept within the same anatomic area.

If a patch is partially or completely detached –

For less than 1 day (up to 24 hours): Try to reapply it to the same place or replace it with a new patch immediately. No back-up contraception is needed. The woman's "patch change day" will remain the same.

For more than 1 day (24 hours or more) or if the woman is not sure how long the patch has been detached: The woman may not be protected from pregnancy. Stop the current contraceptive cycle and start a new cycle immediately by applying a new patch. There is now a new "day 1" and a new "patch change day." Back-up contraception (eg, condoms, spermicide, diaphragm) must be used for the first week of the new cycle.

Do not reapply a patch if it is no longer sticky, if it has become stuck to itself or another surface, if it has other material stuck to it, or if it has previously become loose or fallen off. If a patch cannot be reapplied, a new patch should be applied immediately. Do not use supplemental adhesives or wraps to hold the patch in place.

If the woman forgets to change her patch –

At the start of any patch cycle (week 1/day 1): She may not be protected from pregnancy. Apply the first patch of the new cycle as soon as she remembers. There is now a new "patch change day" and a new "day 1." Use back-up contraception for the first week of the new cycle.

In the middle of the patch cycle (week 2/day 8 or week 3/day 15):

For 1 or 2 days (up to 48 hours) – Apply a new patch immediately. The next patch should be applied on the usual "patch change day." No back-up contraception is needed.

For more than 2 days (48 hours or more) – She may not be protected from pregnancy. Stop the current contraceptive cycle and start a new 4-week cycle immediately by putting on a new patch. There is now a new "patch change day" and a new "day 1." Use back-up contraception for 1 week.

At the end of the patch cycle (week 4/day 22): If the woman forgets to remove her patch, take it off as soon as remembered. The next cycle should be started on the usual "patch change day," which is the day after day 28. No back-up contraception is needed.

Change day adjustment – If the woman wishes to change her patch change day, complete the current cycle, removing the third patch on the correct day. During the patch-free week, select an earlier patch change day by applying a new patch on the desired day. In no case should there be more than 7 consecutive patch-free days.

Switching from an oral contraceptive – Treatment with the norelgestromin/ethinyl estradiol transdermal patch should begin on the first day of withdrawal bleeding. If there is no withdrawal bleeding within 5 days of the last active (hormone-containing) tablet, pregnancy must be ruled out. If therapy starts later than the first day of withdrawal bleeding, a nonhormonal contraceptive should be used concurrently for 7 days. If more than 7 days elapse after taking the last active oral contraceptive tablet, consider the possibility of ovulation and conception.

Use after childbirth – Women who elect not to breast-feed should start contraceptive therapy with the norelgestromin/ethinyl estradiol transdermal patch no sooner than 4 weeks after childbirth. If a woman begins using the patch postpartum and has not yet had a period, consider the possibility of ovulation and conception occurring prior to use of the patch and instruct her to use an additional method of contraception (eg, condoms, spermicide, diaphragm) for the first 7 days.

Use after abortion or miscarriage – After an abortion or miscarriage that occurs in the first trimester, the patch may be started immediately. An additional method of contraception is not needed if the patch is started immediately. If use of the patch is not started within 5 days following a first trimester abortion, the woman should follow the instructions for a woman starting the patch for the first time. In the meantime, advise her to use a nonhormonal contraceptive method. Ovulation may occur within 10 days after an abortion or miscarriage.

Do not start the patch any earlier than 4 weeks after a second trimester abortion or miscarriage. When the patch is used postpartum or postabortion, the increased risk of thromboembolic disease must be considered.

Breakthrough bleeding or spotting – In the event of breakthrough bleeding or spotting (bleeding that occurs on the days that the patch is worn), continue treatment. If breakthrough bleeding persists longer than a few cycles, consider a cause other than the patch.

In the event of no withdrawal bleeding (bleeding that should occur during the patch-free week), resume treatment on the next scheduled change day. If the patch has been used correctly, the absence of withdrawal bleeding is not necessarily an indication of pregnancy. Nevertheless, consider the possibility of pregnancy, especially if absence of withdrawal bleeding occurs in 2 consecutive cycles. Discontinue the patch if pregnancy is confirmed.

Skin irritation – If patch use results in uncomfortable irritation, the patch may be removed and a new patch may be applied to a different location until the next change day. Only 1 patch should be worn at a time.

Missed menstrual period – If the woman has not adhered to the prescribed schedule, consider the possibility of pregnancy at the time of the first missed period. Discontinue hormonal contraceptive use if pregnancy is confirmed.

If the woman has adhered to the prescribed regimen and misses 1 period, she should continue using her contraceptive patches.

If the woman has adhered to the prescribed regimen and misses 2 consecutive periods, rule out pregnancy. Discontinue use of the patch if pregnancy is confirmed.

Vaginal ring: One etonogestrel/ethinyl vaginal ring is inserted in the vagina by the patient. The ring remains in place continuously for 3 weeks. Remove for a 1-week break, during which withdrawal bleeding usually occurs. Insert a new ring 1 week after the last ring was removed on the same day of the week as it was inserted in the previous cycle. Withdrawal bleeding usually starts on day 2 to 3 after removal of the ring. To maintain contraceptive effectiveness, insert the new ring 1 week after the previous one was removed even if menstrual bleeding has not finished.

Insertion – Choose the insertion position that is most comfortable, for example standing with one leg up, squatting, or lying down. Compress the ring and insert into the vagina. The exact position of the ring inside the vagina is not critical for its function. Insert the contraceptive vaginal ring on the appropriate day and leave in place for 3 consecutive weeks.

Removal – Remove the vaginal ring by hooking the index finger under the forward rim or by grasping the rim between the index and middle finger and pulling it out. Place the used ring in the sachet (foil pouch) and discard in a waste receptacle out of the reach of children and pets. Do not flush in the toilet.

Starting the contraceptive vaginal ring – Consider the possibility of ovulation and conception prior to the first use of the contraceptive vaginal ring.

No preceding hormonal contraceptive use in the preceding cycle: Insert the contraceptive vaginal ring on the first day of the woman's cycle (ie, the first day of her menstrual bleeding). The contraceptive vaginal ring may also be started on days 2 to 5 of the woman's cycle, but in this case a barrier method, such as male condoms or spermicide, is recommended for the first 7 days of contraceptive vaginal ring use in the first cycle.

Changing from a combined hormonal contraceptive: The woman may switch from her previous combined hormonal contraceptive on any day, but at the latest on the day following the usual hormone-free interval, if she has been using her hormonal method consistently and correctly, or if it is reasonably certain that she is not pregnant.

Changing from a progestin-only method (minipill, implant, or injection) or from a progestin-releasing intrauterine system: The woman may switch on any day from the minipill. She should switch from an implant or the intrauterine system on the day of its removal, and from an injectable on the day when the next injection would be due. In all of these cases, advise the patient to use an additional method of contraception for the first 7 days after insertion of the ring.

Following complete first-trimester abortion: The patient may start using the contraceptive vaginal ring within the first 5 days following a complete first trimester abortion and does not need to use an additional method of contraception. If use is not started within 5 days following a first trimester abortion, the patient should follow the instructions for "No preceding hormonal contraceptive use in the past month." Advise the patient to use a nonhormonal contraceptive method.

Following delivery or second-trimester abortion: Initiate the use of the contraceptive vaginal ring 4 weeks postpartum in women who elect not to breast-feed. Advise women who are breast-feeding not to use the contraceptive vaginal ring but to use other forms of contraception until the child is weaned. Initiate use of the contraceptive vaginal ring 4 weeks after a second-trimester abortion. When the contraceptive vaginal ring is used postpartum or postabortion, consider the increased risk of thromboembolic disease. If the patient begins using the contraceptive vaginal ring postpartum and has not yet had a period, consider the possibility of ovulation and conception occurring prior to initiation of the contraceptive vaginal ring. Instruct the patient to use an additional method of contraception for the first 7 days.

Inadvertent removal, expulsion, or prolonged ring-free interval: If the contraceptive vaginal ring has been out during the 3-week use period, rinse with cool to lukewarm water and reinsert as soon as possible, at the latest within 3 hours. If the ring has been out of the vagina for more than 3 hours, contraceptive effectiveness may be reduced. Use an additional method of contraception until the contraceptive vaginal ring has been used continuously for 7 days.

Ring-free interval of more than 3 hours – If the ring has been out of the vagina for more than 3 hours, contraceptive effectiveness may be reduced.

During weeks 1 and 2: Reinsert the ring as soon as she remembers. A barrier method (eg, condoms, spermicides) must be used until the ring has been used continuously for 7 days.

During week 3: Discard that ring. One of the following 2 options should be chosen:

1.) Insert a new ring immediately. Inserting a new ring will start the next 3-week–use period. The woman may not experience a withdrawal bleed from her previous cycle. However, breakthrough spotting or bleeding may occur.
2.) Have a withdrawal bleeding and insert a new ring no later than 7 days (7 × 24 hours) from the time the previous ring was removed or expelled. This option should only be chosen if the ring was used continuously for the preceding 7 days.

A barrier method (eg, condoms, spermicides) must be used until the new ring has been used continuously for 7 days.

Ring-free interval of more than 1 week – Consider the possibility of pregnancy if the ring-free interval has been extended beyond 1 week. Use an additional method of contraception (eg, male condoms, spermicide) until the contraceptive vaginal ring has been used continuously for 7 days.

Consider the possibility of pregnancy if the ring-free interval has been extended beyond 1 week. Use an additional method of contraception until the contraceptive vaginal ring has been used continuously for 7 days.

Prolonged use: If the contraceptive vaginal ring has been left in place for up to 1 extra week (ie, up to 4 weeks total), remove it and insert a new ring after a 1-week ring-free interval. Rule out pregnancy if the contraceptive vaginal ring has been left in place for more than 4 weeks. Use an additional method of contraception until the contraceptive vaginal ring has been used continuously for 7 days.

In the event of a missed menstrual period: If the patient has not adhered to the prescribed regimen, consider the possibility of pregnancy at the time of the first missed period and discontinue the use of the contraceptive vaginal ring if pregnancy is confirmed.

Rule out pregnancy if the patient has adhered to the prescribed regimen and misses 2 consecutive periods.

Actions

Pharmacology: Oral contraceptives include estrogen-progestin combinations and progestin-only products.

Progestin-only – Progestin-only oral contraceptives prevent conception by suppressing ovulation in about 50% of users, thickening the cervical mucus to inhibit sperm penetration, lowering the midcycle luteinizing hormone (LH) and follicle-stimulating hormone (FSH) peaks, slowing the movement of the ovum through the fallopian tubes, and altering the endometrium.

Combination oral contraceptives – Combination oral contraceptives inhibit ovulation by suppressing the gonadotropins, FSH, and LH. Additionally, alterations in the genital tract, including cervical mucus (which inhibits sperm penetration) and the endometrium (which reduces the likelihood of implantation), may contribute to contraceptive effectiveness.

Vaginal ring – The contraceptive vaginal ring is a nonbiodegradable, flexible, transparent, colorless to almost colorless combination contraceptive vaginal ring containing etonogestrel and ethinyl estradiol. When placed in the vagina, each ring releases on average etonogestrel 0.12 mg/day and ethinyl estradiol 0.015 mg/day of over a 3-week period of use.

There are 3 types of combination oral contraceptives: monophasic, biphasic, and triphasic.

Monophasic – Fixed dosage of estrogen to progestin throughout the cycle.

Biphasic – Amount of estrogen remains the same for the first 21 days of the cycle. Decreased progestin:estrogen ratio in first half of cycle allows endometrial proliferation. Increased ratio in second half provides adequate secretory development.

Triphasic – Estrogen amount remains the same or varies throughout cycle. Progestin amount varies.

Emergency contraceptives –

Levonorgestrel: Levonorgestrel is believed to act principally by preventing ovulation or fertilization (by altering tubal transport of sperm and/or ova). In addition, it may inhibit implantation (by altering the endometrium).

Ulipristal: Ulipristal is a selective progesterone receptor modulator with antagonistic and partial agonistic effects (a progesterone agonist/antagonist) at the progesterone receptor.

Pharmacokinetics:

Estrogens – Ethinyl estradiol is rapidly absorbed, with peak concentrations attained in 1 to 2 hours. It undergoes considerable first-pass elimination. Mestranol is demethylated to ethinyl estradiol. Ethinyl estradiol is approximately 97% to 98% bound to plasma albumin. Half-life varies from 6 to 20 hours. It is excreted in bile and urine as conjugates and undergoes some enterohepatic recirculation.

Progestins – Peak concentrations of norethindrone occur 0.5 to 4 hours after oral administration; it undergoes first-pass metabolism with an overall bioavailability of approximately 65%. Levonorgestrel reaches peak concentrations between 0.5 to 2 hours, does not undergo a first-pass effect, and is completely bioavailable. Norethindrone and levonorgestrel are chiefly metabolized by reduction followed by conjugation. Desogestrel is rapidly and completely absorbed and converted into 3-keto-desogestrel, the biologically active metabolite. Relative bioavailability is approximately 84%. Maximum concentrations of the metabolite are reached at approximately 1.4 hours. Norgestimate is well absorbed; peak serum concentrations are observed within 2 hours followed by a rapid decline to levels generally below assay within 5 hours. However, a major metabolite, 17-deacetyl norgestimate, appears rapidly in serum with concentrations greatly exceeding that of the parent. Both norethynodrel and ethynodiol diacetate are converted to norethindrone. Peak serum concentrations of drospirenone are reached 1 to 3 hours after administration. Progestins are bound to albumin (79% to 95%) and to sex hormone binding globulin (except drospirenone). Terminal half-life of the progestins are as follows: Norethindrone, 5 to 14 hours; levonorgestrel, 11 to 45 hours; desogestrel (metabolite), 38 ± 20 hours; norgestimate (metabolite), 12 to 30 hours; drospirenone, 30 hours. Progestin-only administration results in lower steady-state serum progestin levels and a shorter elimination half-life than coadministration with estrogens.

Patch – Following application, norelgestromin and ethinyl estradiol rapidly appear in the serum, plateau by about 48 hours, and are maintained at steady state throughout the wear period. The metabolites of norelgestromin and ethinyl estradiol are eliminated by renal and fecal pathways.

Vaginal ring – Etonogestrel and ethinyl estradiol released by the vaginal ring are rapidly absorbed. Bioavailability of etonogestrel after vaginal administration is about 100%. Bioavailability of ethinyl estradiol after vaginal administration is about 55.6%, which is comparable to that with oral administration of ethinyl estradiol. Etonogestrel is about 66% bound to albumin in blood. Ethinyl estradiol is highly bound to albumin.

In vitro data show that both etonogestrel and ethinyl estradiol are metabolized in liver microsomes by the CYP-450 3A4 isoenzyme. Etonogestrel and ethinyl estradiol are primarily eliminated in urine, bile, and feces.

Emergency contraceptives –

Levonorgestrel: Levonorgestrel is rapidly and completely absorbed after oral administration (bioavailability about 100%). Levonorgestrel does not appear to be extensively metabolized by the liver.

Plan B – Levonorgestrel in serum is primarily protein bound. The elimination half-life of levonorgestrel following single dose administration as *Plan B* (0.75 mg) is 24.4 ± 5.3 hours. Levonorgestrel and its metabolites are primarily excreted in the urine.

Plan B One-Step and Next Choice – Levonorgestrel is about 97.5% to 99% protein-bound. About 45% of levonorgestrel and its metabolites are excreted in the urine and about 32% are excreted in feces.

Ulipristal: Maximum plasma concentrations of ulipristal and the active metabolite were reached at 0.9 and 1 hour, respectively. Ulipristal is highly bound (more than 94%) to plasma proteins. Ulipristal metabolism is predominantly mediated by CYP3A4. The terminal half-life is estimated to be 32.4 ± 6.3 hours.

Contraindications

Thrombophlebitis; thromboembolic disorders; history of deep-vein thrombophlebitis; cerebral vascular disease; myocardial infarction (MI); coronary artery disease; known or suspected breast carcinoma or estrogen-dependent neoplasia; carcinoma of endometrium; hepatic adenomas/carcinomas; undiagnosed abnormal genital bleeding; known or suspected pregnancy; cholestatic jaundice of pregnancy/jaundice with prior pill use; hypersensitivity to any component of the product; acute liver disease; uncontrolled hypertension; headaches with focal neurological symptoms; diabetes with vascular complications; major surgery with prolonged immobility.

Yasmin: Renal function impairment, hepatic function impairment, adrenal insufficiency, heavy smoking (15 or more cigarettes per day), and over 35 years of age.

Warnings/Precautions

Cigarette smoking: See Warning Box.

Smoking in combination with oral contraceptive use has been shown to contribute substantially to the incidence of MIs in women in their mid-30s or older, with smoking accounting for the majority of excess cases. Mortality rates associated with circulatory disease have been shown to increase substantially in smokers, especially in those 35 years of age and older who use oral contraceptives.

Hyperkalemia: Yasmin contains the progestin drospirenone that has antimineralocorticoid activity, including the potential for hyperkalemia in high-risk patients, comparable with a 25 mg dose of spironolactone. Do not use *Yasmin* in patients with conditions that predispose to hyperkalemia. Women receiving daily, long-term treatment for chronic conditions or diseases with medications that may increase serum potassium should have their serum potassium level checked during the first treatment cycle.

Hormone exposure via patch: The pharmacokinetic profile for norelgestromin/ethinyl estradiol patch is different from the pharmacokinetic profole for oral contraceptives in that it has a higher steady-state concentrations and lower peak concentrations. Increased estrogen exposure may increase the risk of adverse reactions, including venous thromboembolism.

Risks of oral contraceptive use: The use of oral contraceptives is associated with increased risk of thromboembolism, stroke, myocardial infarction (MI), hypertension, hepatic neoplasia, and gallbladder disease, although risk of serious morbidity or mortality is very small in healthy women without underlying risk factors.

Existing pregnancy: Ulipristal is not indicated for termination of an existing pregnancy. Exclude pregnancy before prescribing ulipristal.

Repeat use: Levonorgestrel is not recommended for routine use as a contraceptive.

Ulipristal is for occasional use as an emergency contraceptive. It should not replace a regular method of contraception. Repeated use of ulipristal within the same menstrual cycle is not recommended.

Mortality: Mortality associated with all methods of birth control is low and below that associated with childbirth, with the exception of oral contraceptive use in women 35 or older who smoke and 40 and older who do not smoke. The Fertility and Maternal Health Drugs Advisory Committee recommended that the benefits of low-dose oral contraceptive use by healthy nonsmoking women older than 40 years of age may outweigh the possible risks. Like all women, older women who take oral contraceptives should take an oral contraceptive that contains the least amount of estrogen and progestin that is compatible with a low failure rate and individual patient needs.

Thromboembolism: Be alert to the earliest symptoms of thromboembolic and thrombotic disorders. Should any of these occur or be suspected, discontinue the drug immediately.

The risk of nonfatal venous thrombosis with third-generation oral contraceptives (desogestrel, gestodene, and norgestimate) is 2 to 3 times the risk of second-generation oral contraceptives. The risk of development of deep vein thrombosis was found to be 2 to 5 times higher with low-estrogen, desogestrel-containing oral contraceptives than with second-generation monophasic and triphasic preparations.

MI – MI risk associated with oral contraceptive use is increased. This risk is primarily in smokers or women with other underlying risk factors for coronary artery disease such as hypertension, hypercholesterolemia, morbid obesity, and diabetes. The risk is very low in women younger than 30 years of age.

Long-term use – Data suggest that the increased risk of MI persists after discontinuation of long-term oral contraceptive use; the highest risk group includes women 40 to 49 years of age who used oral contraceptives for 5 years or more.

Cerebrovascular diseases – Oral contraceptives increase the risks of cerebrovascular events (thrombotic and hemorrhagic strokes). In general, the risk is greatest in hypertensive women older than 35 years of age who also smoke.

Dose-related risk – A positive association is observed between the amount of estrogen and progestin in oral contraceptives and the risk of vascular disease. A decline in serum high-density lipoprotein (HDL) has occurred with progestins and has been associated with an increased incidence of ischemic heart disease. Because estrogens increase HDL cholesterol, the net effect depends on a balance achieved between doses of estrogen and progestin and the activity of the progestin used in the contraceptives.

Age – The risk of cerebrovascular and circulatory disease in oral contraceptive users is substantially increased in women 35 years of age and older with other risk factors (eg, smoking, uncontrolled hypertension, hypercholesterolemia [low-density lipoprotein 190], obesity, diabetes).

Postsurgical thromboembolism – Risk is increased 2- to 4-fold. If possible, discontinue oral contraceptives at least 4 weeks before and 2 weeks after surgery and during and following prolonged immobilization because oral contraceptives are associated with an increased risk of thromboembolism.

Subarachnoid hemorrhage – Subarachnoid hemorrhage has been increased by oral contraceptive use.

Persistence of risk – An increased risk may persist for 6 years or more after discontinuation of oral contraceptive use for cerebrovascular disease and 9 years or more for MI in users 40 to 49 years of age who had used oral contraceptives 5 years or more. This information is based on studies that used oral contraceptives containing estrogen 50 mcg or more.

Note: The associations between oral contraceptives and cardiovascular disease are based on epidemiological studies whose conclusions have been criticized for several reasons: National trends of cardiovascular mortality are incompatible with these risk estimates; excess deaths may not be attributable entirely to smoking; the clinical diagnosis of thromboembolism is often unreliable.

Ocular lesions: Ocular lesions such as optic neuritis or retinal thrombosis have been associated with the use of hormonal contraceptives.

Risks of use immediately preceding pregnancy: Some extensive epidemiological studies have revealed no increased risk of birth defects in oral contraceptive users prior to pregnancy.

Carcinoma: While there are conflicting reports, the overall evidence in the literature suggests that use of oral contraceptives is not associated with an increase in the risk of developing breast cancer, regardless of age and parity of first use. Women with breast cancer should not use oral contraceptives because the role of female hormones in breast cancer has not been fully determined.

Studies have reported an increased risk of endometrial carcinoma associated with the prolonged use of estrogen in postmenopausal women. The risk appears to be decreased in oral contraceptive users because of the progestin component. Users appear about half as likely to develop ovarian and endometrial cancer as women who have never used oral contraceptives. The protective effect from endometrial cancer lasts up to 15 years after the pills are stopped.

Close clinical surveillance of all women taking oral contraceptives is essential; they should be reexamined at least once a year. In all cases of undiagnosed persistent or recurrent abnormal vaginal bleeding, rule out malignancy. Monitor women with a strong family history of breast cancer or who have breast nodules, fibrocystic disease of the breast, cervical dysplasia, or abnormal mammograms.

Hepatic lesions (adenomas, focal nodular hyperplasia, hepatocellular carcinoma, etc): Rarely, benign and malignant hepatic adenomas have been associated with the use of hormonal contraceptives. Severe abdominal pain, shock, or death may be due to rupture and hemorrhage of a liver tumor.

Carbohydrate metabolism: Some users of progestin-only oral contraceptives may experience slight deterioration in glucose tolerance, with increases in plasma insulin. Monitor prediabetic and diabetic women closely.

Lipid profile: Triglycerides may increase.

Elevated blood pressure: Elevated blood pressure and hypertension may occur within a few months of beginning use. The prevalence increases with the duration of use and age. Incidence of hypertension may directly correlate with increasing dosages of progestin. Discontinue use if elevated blood pressure occurs. Encourage women with a history of hypertension or hypertension-related diseases during pregnancy, or renal disease to use another method of contraception.

Headaches: Onset or exacerbation of migraine or development of headache with a new pattern which is recurrent, persistent, or severe, requires hormonal contraceptive discontinuation and evaluation.

Bleeding irregularities: Breakthrough bleeding (BTB), spotting, and amenorrhea are frequent reasons for discontinuing hormonal contraceptives. Changing to an oral contraceptive with a higher estrogen content may minimize menstrual irregularity, but consider the increased risk of thromboembolic disease. Consider short-term estrogen supplements.

Seasonale – When prescribing *Seasonale*, the convenience of fewer planned menses (4 per year instead of 13 per year) should be weighed against the inconvenience of increased intermenstrual bleeding and/or spotting.

Progestin-only products – Episodes of irregular, unpredictable spotting, and BTB within the first year are the most frequently encountered adverse reactions and are the major reasons why women discontinue hormonal contraceptive use.

Vaginal ring – Breakthrough bleeding and spotting are sometimes encountered in women using the contraceptive vaginal ring. If abnormal bleeding persists or is severe, rule out the possibility of organic pathology or pregnancy. Rule out pregnancy in the event of amenorrhea.

Emergency contraceptives –

Levonorgestrel: Menstrual bleeding patterns are often irregular among women using progestin-only oral contraceptives and in clinical studies of levonorgestrel for postcoital and emergency contraceptive use.

Ulipristal: After ulipristal intake, menses sometimes occurs earlier or later than expected by a few days.

Menopause: Treatment with hormonal contraceptives may mask the onset of the climacteric.

Lipid disorders: Closely follow women taking oral contraceptives who are being treated for hyperlipidemias.

Uterine fibroids: Preexisting uterine leiomyomata (uterine fibroids) may increase in size. However, there is no evidence of this with low-dose hormonal contraceptives.

Depression: The incidence of depression in oral contraceptive users ranges from less than 5% to 30%. Pyridoxine deficiency may be a factor in the depression. Women who become significantly depressed when using hormonal contraceptives should stop the medication and use another form of contraception.

Fluid retention: Oral contraceptives may cause fluid retention.

Body weight 90 kg or more (198 lbs):

Patch – Results of clinical trials suggest that the norelgestromin/ethinyl estradiol transdermal patch may be less effective in women with body weight 90 kg or more (198 lbs) than in women with lower body weights.

Hepatic function: Patients with a history of jaundice during pregnancy have an increased risk of recurrence of jaundice. If jaundice develops, discontinue the medication.

Contact lenses: Contact lens wearers who develop changes in vision or lens tolerance should be assessed by an ophthalmologist; consider temporary or permanent cessation of wear.

Vaginal use: The contraceptive vaginal ring may not be suitable in conditions that make the vagina more susceptible to vaginal irritation or ulceration.

The contraceptive vaginal ring may interfere with the correct placement and position of a diaphragm. A diaphragm is not recommended as a backup method with contraceptive vaginal ring use.

Expulsion – The contraceptive vaginal ring can be accidentally expelled, for example, when it has not been inserted properly, or while removing a tampon, moving the bowels, straining, or with severe constipation. If this occurs, rinse the vaginal ring with cool to lukewarm (not hot) water and reinsert promptly. If the contraceptive vaginal ring is lost, insert a new vaginal ring and continue the regimen without alteration. If the ring has been out of the vagina for more than 3 hours, contraceptive effectiveness may be reduced and an additional method of contraception (eg, male condom, spermicide) must be used until the ring has been used continuously for 7 days. Vaginal stenosis, cervical prolapse, rectoceles, and cystoceles are conditions that under some circumstances may make expulsion more likely to occur.

Serum folate levels: Serum folate levels may be depressed by therapy.

Acute intermittent porphyria: Estrogens have been reported to precipitate attacks of acute intermittent porphyria.

Vomiting/Diarrhea: Several cases of oral contraceptive failure have been reported in association with vomiting or diarrhea. If significant GI disturbance occurs, a back-up method of contraception for the remainder of the cycle is recommended.

Sexually transmitted diseases (STDs): Advise patients that hormonal contraceptives do not protect against HIV infection and other STDs.

Fertility impairment: Fertility impairment may occur in women discontinuing oral contraceptives; however, impairment diminishes with time.

Fertility following use of ulipristal – A rapid return of fertility is likely following treatment with ulipristal for emergency contraception; therefore, routine contraception should be continued or initiated as soon as possible following use of ulipristal to ensure ongoing prevention of pregnancy. Use of ulipristal may reduce the contraceptive action of regular hormonal contraceptive methods. Therefore, after use of ulipristal, a reliable barrier method of contraception should be used with subsequent acts of intercourse that occur in that same menstrual cycle.

Pregnancy: Category X. Rule out pregnancy before initiating or continuing the any hormonal contraceptives, and always consider it if withdrawal bleeding does not occur or for any patient who has missed 2 consecutive periods.

Ectopic as well as intrauterine pregnancy may occur in contraceptive failures. Consider a history of ectopic pregnancy a contraindication of using levonorgestrel emergency contraception. However, a history of ectopic pregnancy is not a contraindication of using ulipristal emergency contraception.

Pregnancy test – Do not administer contraceptives to induce withdrawal bleeding as a test for pregnancy.

Lactation: Hormonal contraceptives may interfere with lactation, decreasing both the quantity and the quality of breast milk. A small amount of oral contraceptive steroids is excreted in breast milk. A few adverse reactions on the breast-feeding infant have been reported, including jaundice and breast enlargement.

Levonorgestrel – The American Academy of Pediatrics classifies levonorgestrel as usually compatible with breast-feeding.

Ulipristal – It is not known if ulipristal is excreted in human milk. Use of ulipristal by breast-feeding women is not recommended.

Vaginal ring – Advise women who are breast-feeding not to use the contraceptive vaginal ring but to use other forms of contraception until the child is weaned.

Children: Safety and efficacy are expected to be the same for postpubertal adolescents up to 16 years of age (18 years of age for ulipristal). Use of these products before menarche is not indicated.

Elderly: This vaginal ring has not been studied in women 65 years of age and older and is not indicated in this population.

Monitoring: Pretreatment and annual exams should include blood pressure, breasts, abdomen and pelvic organs, including Papanicolaou smear. Perform preventative measures and screening, which should include total and HDL cholesterol within 5-year intervals. Advise the pathologist of oral contraceptive therapy when relevant specimens are submitted. Do not prescribe for more than 1 year without another physical exam.

Emergency contraceptives – A follow-up physical or pelvic examination is recommended if there is any doubt concerning the general health or pregnancy status of any woman after taking levonorgestrel. Evaluate patients who complain of lower abdominal pain after taking ulipristal for the possibility of ectopic pregnancy.

Drug Interactions

Drugs that may affect oral contraceptives include antibiotics, atorvastatin, barbiturates, carbamazepine, CYP3A4 inducers (barbiturates, bosentan, carbamazepine, felbamate, griseofulvin, oxcarbazepine, phenytoin, rifampin, St. John's wort, topiramate), CYP3A4 inhibitors (eg, itraconazole, ketoconazole), hydantoins, nonnucleoside reverse transcriptase inhibitors, primidone, protease inhibitors, and miconazole (vaginal ring).

Drugs that may be affected by oral contraceptives include anticoagulants, benzodiazepines, beta blockers, caffeine, corticosteroids, cyclosporine, prednisolone, theophyllines, tricyclic antidepressants, lamotrigine, and selegiline.

Drug/Lab test interactions: Estrogen-containing hormonal contraceptives may cause the following alterations in serum, plasma or blood, unless specified otherwise.

Increased – Factors I (prothrombin), VII, VIII, IX, X; fibrinogen; norepinephrine-induced platelet aggregation; thyroid binding globulin, leading to increased total thyroid hormone (as measured by protein bound iodine or T_4); corticosteroid levels;

triglycerides and phospholipids; aldosterone; amylase; gamma-glutamyltranspeptidase; iron binding capacity; sex-hormone-binding globulins are increased and result in elevated levels of total circulating sex steroids (combination); corticoids; transferrin; prolactin; renin activity; vitamin A.

Decreased – Antithrombin III; free T_3 resin uptake; response to metyrapone test; folate; glucose tolerance; albumin; cholinesterase; haptoglobin; tissue plasminogen activator; zinc; vitamin B_{12}; sex-hormone-binding globulin, thyroxine due to decrease in thyroid-binding globulin (progestin-only).

Adverse Reactions

Serious adverse reactions that may occur include thrombophlebitis and venous thrombosis with or without embolism; pulmonary embolism; coronary thrombosis; MI; cerebral thrombosis; arterial thromboembolism; cerebral hemorrhage; hypertension; gallbladder disease; hepatic adenomas or benign liver tumors; mesenteric thrombosis. Other adverse reactions that may occur include nausea and vomiting (10% to 30% of patients during the first cycle, less common with low doses, and majority resolve in 3 months); abdominal cramps; bloating; breakthrough bleeding (majority, more than 80%, resolve in 3 months); spotting; change in menstrual flow; amenorrhea during and after treatment; change in cervical erosion and cervical secretions; vaginal candidiasis; temporary infertility after discontinuation; melasma (may persist); rash (allergic); migraine; mental depression; headache; dizziness; contact lens intolerance; edema; weight change; changes in corneal curvature (steepening); neuro-ocular lesions; upper respiratory tract infection; leukorrhea; sinusitis; breast tenderness/enlargement/secretion; diminution in lactation when given immediately postpartum; cholestatic jaundice; invasive cervical cancer; prevalence of cervical chlamydia trachomatis may be increased.

Device-related: Device-related events (foreign body sensation, coital problems, device expulsion), vaginal symptoms (discomfort/vaginitis/leukorrhea), headache, emotional lability, and weight gain.

Topical administration: The most common adverse reactions reported by 9% to 22% or women using the contraceptive patch were the following, in decreasing order of significance: breast symptoms, headache, application site reaction, nausea, upper respiratory tract infection, menstrual cramps, and abdominal pain.

Levonorgestrel: Abdominal pain, breast tenderness, delay of menses (more than 7 days), diarrhea, dizziness, fatigue, headache, heavier menstrual bleeding, lighter menstrual bleeding, nausea, vomiting.

Ulipristal: Abdominal and upper abdominal pain, dizziness, dysmenorrhea, fatigue, headache.

LEVONORGESTREL INTRAUTERINE SYSTEM

Intrauterine device: 52 mg (releases approximately levonorgestrel 20 mcg/day) (*Rx*)	*Mirena* (Bayer)

> **Warning:**
> Patients should be counseled that this product does not protect against HIV infection (AIDS) and other sexually transmitted diseases.

Indications

Contraception: For intrauterine contraception for up to 5 years. Thereafter, if continued contraception is desired, the system should be replaced. The intrauterine system is recommended for women who have had at least 1 child.

Administration and Dosage

Insertion: Insert with the provided inserter into the uterine cavity within 7 days of the onset of menstruation or immediately after the first trimester abortion by carefully following the insertion instructions. It can be replaced by a new system at any time during the menstrual cycle. The system should not remain in the uterus after 5 years.

Continuing contraception after removal: If a patient with regular cycles wants to start a different birth control method, remove the system during the first 7 days of the menstrual cycle and start the new method. If a patient with irregular cycles or amenorrhea wants to start a different birth control method, or if you remove the system after the seventh day of the menstrual cycle, start the new method at least 7 days before removal.

Actions

Pharmacology: Studies of the levonorgestrel-releasing intrauterine system prototypes have suggested several mechanisms that prevent pregnancy: Thickening of cervical mucus preventing passage of sperm into the uterus; inhibition of sperm capacitation or survival; alteration of the endometrium. Low doses of levonorgestrel can be administered into the uterine cavity with the levonorgestrel-releasing intrauterine delivery system. Initially, levonorgestrel is released at a rate of 20 mcg/day. This rate decreases progressively to half that value after 5 years.

Pharmacokinetics:

Absorption/Distribution – Following insertion of levonorgestrel-releasing intrauterine system, the initial release of levonorgestrel into the uterine cavity is 20 mcg/day. A stable plasma level of levonorgestrel 150 to 200 pg/mL occurs after the first few weeks. Levonorgestrel levels after long-term use of 12, 24, and 60 months were 180 pg/mL, 192, and 159, respectively. The plasma concentrations achieved by the intrauterine system are lower than those seen with levonorgestrel contraceptive implants and with oral contraceptives.

Metabolism/Excretion – Levonorgestrel in serum is primarily bound to proteins (mainly sex hormone-binding globulin) and is extensively metabolized to a large number of inactive metabolites. The elimination half-life of levonorgestrel after daily oral doses is approximately 17 hours; both the parent drug and its metabolites are primarily excreted in the urine.

Contraindications

Pregnancy or suspicion of pregnancy; congenital or acquired uterine anomaly, including fibroids if they distort the uterine cavity; acute pelvic inflammatory disease (PID) or a history of PID, unless there has been a subsequent intrauterine pregnancy; postpartum endometritis or infected abortion in the past 3 months; known or suspected uterine or cervical neoplasia, or unresolved, abnormal Pap smear; genital bleeding of unknown etiology; untreated acute cervicitis or vaginitis, including bacterial vaginosis or other lower genital tract infections until infection is controlled; acute liver disease or liver tumor (benign or malignant); conditions associated with increased susceptibility to pelvic infections; a previously inserted intrauterine device that has not been removed; hypersensitivity to any component of this product; known or suspected carcinoma of the breast.

Warnings/Precautions

Ectopic pregnancy: Evaluate women who become pregnant while using the intrauterine system for ectopic pregnancy. Up to half of pregnancies that occur with the intrauterine system in place are ectopic.

Tell women who choose the intrauterine system about the risks of ectopic pregnancy, including the loss of fertility. Teach them to recognize and promptly report any symptoms of ectopic pregnancy to their health care provider. Women with a history of ectopic pregnancy, tubal surgery, or pelvic infection carry a higher risk of ectopic pregnancy.

Intrauterine pregnancy: If pregnancy should occur with the intrauterine system in place, the intrauterine system should be removed.

Septic abortion – In patients becoming pregnant with an IUD in place, septic abortion, with septicemia, septic shock, and death, may occur

Continuation of pregnancy – If a woman becomes pregnant with intrauterine system in place, and if the intrauterine system cannot be removed or the woman chooses not to have it removed, she should be warned that failure to remove the system increases the risk of miscarriage, sepsis, premature labor and premature delivery

Long-term effects and congenital anomalies – When pregnancy continues with the intrauterine system in place, long-term effects on the offspring are unknown. Because of the intrauterine administration of levonorgestrel and local exposure to the hormone, the possibility of teratogenicity following exposure to the intrauterine system cannot be completely excluded.

Sepsis: As of September 2006, 9 cases of group A streptococcal (GAS) sepsis out of an estimated 9.9 million levonorgestrel-releasing intrauterine system users had been reported. In some cases, severe pain occurred within hours of insertion followed by sepsis within days. Because death from GAS sepsis is more likely if treatment is delayed, it is important to be aware of these rare but serious infections.

Pelvic inflammatory disease (PID): The intrauterine system is contraindicated in the presence of known or suspected PID or in women with a history of PID, unless there has been a subsequent intrauterine pregnancy. Use of IUDs has been associated with an increased risk of PID. The highest risk of PID occurs shortly after insertion (usually within the first 20 days thereafter). PID is often associated with a sexually transmitted disease, and the intrauterine system does not protect against sexually transmitted disease. Women who have ever had PID are at increased risk for a recurrence or reinfection.

PID warning to levonorgestrel-releasing intrauterine system users – All women who choose the intrauterine system must be informed prior to insertion about the possibility of PID, and that PID can cause tubal damage leading to ectopic pregnancy or infertility, or in infrequent cases can necessitate hysterectomy, or can cause death.

Asymptomatic PID – PID may be asymptomatic but still result in tubal damage and its sequelae.

Treatment of PID – Following a diagnosis of PID, or suspected PID, bacteriologic specimens should be obtained and antibiotic therapy should be initiated promptly. Removal of the intrauterine system after initiation of antibiotic therapy is usually appropriate

Irregular bleeding and amenorrhea: The intrauterine system can alter the bleeding pattern. During the first 3 to 6 months of intrauterine system use, the number of bleeding and spotting days may be increased and bleeding patterns may be irregular. Amenorrhea develops in approximately 20% of levonorgestrel-releasing intrauterine system users by 1 year. The possibility of pregnancy should be considered if menstruation does not occur within 6 weeks of the onset of previous menstruation.

Embedment: Partial penetration or embedment of the intrauterine system in the myometrium may decrease contraceptive effectiveness and can result in difficult removal.

Perforation: An IUD may perforate the uterus or cervix, most often during insertion, although the perforation may not be detected until some time later. If perforation occurs, the IUD must be removed and surgery may be required. Adhesions, peritonitis, intestinal perforations, intestinal obstruction, abscesses and erosion of adjacent viscera have been reported with IUDs.

Expulsion: Partial or complete expulsion of the intrauterine system may occur. Symptoms of the partial or complete expulsion of any intrauterine device may include bleeding or pain. If expulsion has occurred, the intrauterine system may be replaced within 7 days of a menstrual period after pregnancy has been ruled out.

Ovarian cysts: Because the contraceptive effect of the intrauterine system is mainly due to its local effect, ovulatory cycles with follicular rupture usually occur in women of fertile age using the intrauterine system. Sometimes atresia of the follicle is delayed and the follicle may continue to grow. Enlarged follicles have been diagnosed in about 12% of the subjects using the intrauterine system

Breast cancer: Women who currently have or have had breast cancer should not use hormonal contraception because breast cancer is a hormone-sensitive tumor.

Sexually transmitted diseases: Patients should be counseled that this product does not protect against HIV infection (AIDS) and other sexually transmitted diseases

Prior to insertion: Prior to insertion, the physician, nurse, or other trained health professional must provide the patient with the patient package insert. The patient should be told that some bleeding such as irregular or prolonged bleeding and spotting, or cramps may occur during the first few weeks after insertion. If her symptoms continue or are severe, she should report them to her health care provider

Observe strict asepsis during insertion. The presence of organisms capable of establishing PID cannot be determined by appearance, and intrauterine device insertion may be associated with introduction of vaginal bacteria into the uterus. Administration of antibiotics may be considered, but the utility of this treatment is unknown.

Patient evaluation and clinical considerations: A complete medical and social history, including that of the partner, should be obtained to determine conditions that might influence the selection of an IUD for contraception. The health care provider should determine that the patient is not pregnant.

Postpartum: The intrauterine system should not be inserted until 6 weeks postpartum or until involution of the uterus is complete in order to reduce the incidence of perforation and expulsion.

Valvular/Congenital heart disease: Patients with certain types of valvular or congenital heart disease and surgically constructed systemic-pulmonary shunts are at increased risk of infective endocarditis. Use of an intrauterine system in these patients may represent a potential source of septic emboli. Patients with known congenital heart disease who may be at increased risk should be treated with appropriate antibiotics at the time of insertion and removal. Patients requiring chronic corticosteroid therapy or insulin for diabetes should be monitored with special care for infection.

Special risk patients: Patients requiring long-term corticosteroid therapy or insulin for diabetes should be monitored with special care for infection.

Use the intrauterine system with caution in patients who have a coagulopathy or are receiving anticoagulants; in patients with marked increase of blood pressure; in patients with severe arterial disease, such as stroke or myocardial infarction; and in patients with migraine, focal migraine with asymmetrical visual loss, or other symptoms indicating transient cerebral ischemia, or an exceptionally severe headache.

Coagulopathy/Anticoagulant therapy: Use with caution in patients who have a coagulopathy or are receiving anticoagulants

Vaginitis/Cervicitis: Use in patients with vaginitis or cervicitis should be postponed until proper treatment has eradicated the infection and until it has been shown that the cervicitis is not due to gonorrhea or chlamydia.

Prophylactic antibiotics: Because IUD insertion may be associated with introduction of vaginal bacteria into the uterus, strict asepsis should be observed at insertion. Administration of antibiotics may be considered, but the utility of this treatment is unknown.

Syncope/Bradycardia: Syncope, bradycardia, or other neurovascular episodes may occur during insertion or removal of the intrauterine system, especially in patients with a predisposition to these conditions or cervical stenosis.

Continuation and removal: The intrauterine system must be replaced every 5 years because contraceptive effectiveness after 5 years has not been established. User complaints of pain, odorous discharge, bleeding, fever, genital lesions or sores should be promptly responded to and prompt examination recommended. If examination during visits subsequent to insertion reveals that the length of the threads has changed from the length at time of insertion, and the system is verified as displaced, it should be removed. Because the intrauterine system may be displaced, patients should be reexamined and evaluated shortly after the first postinsertion menses, but definitely within 3 months after insertion. The intrauterine system should be removed for the following medical reasons: Menorrhagia or metrorrhagia producing anemia; acquired immune deficiency syndrome (AIDS); sexually transmitted disease; pelvic infection; endometritis; symptomatic genital actinomycosis; intractable pelvic pain; severe dyspareunia; pregnancy; endometrial or cervical malignancy; uterine or cervical perforation. Removal of the system should also be considered if any of the following conditions arise for the first time: migraine; focal migraine with asymmetrical visual loss or other symptoms indicating transient cerebral ischemia; exceptionally severe headache; jaundice; marked increase of blood pressure; severe arterial disease such as stroke or myocardial infarction (MI).

Sexually transmitted disease (STDs): Should the patient's relationship cease to be mutually monogamous, or should her partner become HIV positive, or acquire a sexually transmitted disease, she should be instructed to report this change to her clinician immediately. Removal of the system should be considered.

Pregnancy during use: In the event a pregnancy is confirmed during intrauterine system use, take the following steps: determine whether pregnancy is ectopic and take appropriate measures if it is; inform the patient of the risks of leaving the intrauterine system in place or removing it during pregnancy, and of the lack of data on long-term effects on the offspring of women who have had the system in place during conception or gestation; if possible, remove the intrauterine system after the patient has been warned of the risks of removal. If removal is difficult, counsel and offer the patient pregnancy termination; if the intrauterine system is left in place, closely follow the patient's course.

Removal of the intrauterine system: Remove the intrauterine system for the following medical reasons: menorrhagia and/or metrorrhagia producing anemia, AIDS, STDs, pelvic infection, endometritis, symptomatic genital actinomycosis, intractable pelvic pain, severe dyspareunia, pregnancy, endometrial or cervical malignancy, uterine or cervical perforation.

Also consider the removal of the intrauterine system if any of the following conditions arise for the first time: migraine or focal migraine with asymmetrical visual loss or other symptoms indicating transient cerebral ischemia, exceptionally severe headache, jaundice, marked increase of blood pressure, severe arterial disease such as stroke or myocardial infarction.

Removal may be associated with pain and/or bleeding or neurovascular episodes.

Glucose tolerance: May affect glucose tolerance, and the blood glucose concentration should be monitored in diabetic users of the intrauterine system.

Pregnancy: Category X. In the event a pregnancy is confirmed during levonorgestrel-releasing intrauterine system use, take the following steps: determine whether pregnancy is ectopic and take appropriate measures if it is; inform patient of the risks of leaving the system in place or removing it during pregnancy; if possible, the intrauterine system should be removed after the patient has been warned of the risks of removal but, if removal is difficult, the patient should be counseled and offered pregnancy termination; and, if the intrauterine system is left in place, closely follow the patient's course.

Lactation: Levonorgestrel has been identified in small quantities in the breast milk of lactating women using the intrauterine system.

Children: Safety and efficacy of the levonorgestrel-releasing intrauterine system have been established in women of reproductive age. Use of this product before menarche is not indicated.

Elderly: The intrauterine system has not been studied in women older than 65 years of age and is not currently approved for use in this population.

Drug Interactions

CYP3A4 inducers: The effectiveness of levonorgestrel is reduced by hepatic enzyme-inducing drugs, such as phenytoin, carbamazepine, phenobarbital, and rifampin.

The anticoagulant activity of warfarin may be enhanced by levonorgestrel.

Adverse Reactions

Adverse reactions reported by at least 5% of patients include abdominal pain, abnormal Pap smear, acne, back pain, breast pain, decreased libido, depression, dysmenorrhea, headache, hypertension, leukorrhea, nausea, nervousness, sinusitis, skin disorder, upper respiratory tract infection, vaginitis, and weight increase. Other reported adverse reactions occurring in less than 3% of patients include anemia, cervicitis, dyspareunia, eczema, failed insertion, hair loss, migraine, vomiting.

ETONOGESTREL

Implant: 68 mg (*Rx*)	*Implanon* (Organon)

Indications

Contraception: For the prevention of pregnancy.

Administration and Dosage

The etonogestrel implant is a long-acting (up to 3 years), reversible contraceptive method.

All health care providers performing insertions and/or removals of the etonogestrel implant must receive instruction and training and, where appropriate, supervision prior to inserting or removing the etonogestrel implant. Insert the etonogestrel implant subdermally in the inner side of the upper arm (nondominant arm) about 6 to 8 cm (2½ to 3 inches) above the elbow crease overlying the groove between the biceps and the triceps. The etonogestrel implant must be inserted by the expiration date stated on the packaging. The etonogestrel implant must be removed by the end of the third year and may be replaced by a new implant at the time of removal if continued contraceptive protection is desired.

Administration: Rule out pregnancy before inserting the etonogestrel implant.

Timing of insertion depends on the patient's recent history as follows:

No preceding hormonal contraceptive use in the past month – Counting the first day of menstruation as day 1, the etonogestrel implant must be inserted between days 1 through 5, even if the woman is still bleeding.

Switching from a combination hormonal contraceptive – The etonogestrel implant may be inserted:

- any time within 7 days after the last active (estrogen plus progestin) oral contraceptive tablet
- any time during the 7-day ring-free period of *NuvaRing* (etonogestrel/ethinyl estradiol vaginal ring)
- any time during the 7-day patch-free period of a transdermal contraceptive system

Switching from a progestin-only method – There are several types of progestin-only methods. The etonogestrel implant insertion must be performed as follows:

- any day of the month when switching from a progestin-only pill. Do not skip any days between the last pill and insertion of the etonogestrel implant.
- on the same day as contraceptive implant removal.
- on the same day as removal of a progestin-containing intrauterine device.
- on the day when the next contraceptive injection would be due.

Following a first trimester abortion: The etonogestrel implant may be inserted immediately following a complete first trimester abortion. If the etonogestrel implant is not inserted within 5 days following a first trimester abortion, follow the instructions under "No preceding hormonal contraceptive use in the past month."

Following delivery or a second trimester abortion: The etonogestrel implant may be inserted between 21 to 28 days postpartum if not exclusively breast-feeding or between 21 to 28 days following a second trimester abortion. If more than 4 weeks have elapsed, pregnancy should be excluded, and the patient should use a nonhormonal method of birth control during the first 7 days after the insertion. If the patient is exclusively breast-feeding, insert the etonogestrel implant after the fourth postpartum week.

Actions

Pharmacology: The contraceptive effect of the etonogestrel implant is achieved by several mechanisms that include suppression of ovulation, increased viscosity of the cervical mucus, and alterations in the endometrium.

Pharmacokinetics:

Absorption – After subdermal insertion of etonogestrel implant, etonogestrel is released into the circulation and is approximately 100% bioavailable.

Distribution – The apparent volume of distribution averages about 201 L. Etonogestrel is approximately 32% bound to sex hormone-binding globulin and 66% bound to albumin in blood.

Metabolism – In vitro data show that etonogestrel is metabolized in liver microsomes by the CYP-450 3A4 isoenzyme.

Excretion – The elimination half-life of etonogestrel is approximately 25 hours. Excretion of etonogestrel and its metabolites, either as free steroid or as conjugates, is mainly in urine and to a lesser extent in feces.

Special populations –

Hepatic function impairment: Etonogestrel is metabolized by the liver; therefore, use in patients with active liver disease is contraindicated.

Overweight women: The efficacy of the etonogestrel implant in overweight women has not been defined because women who weighed more than 130% of their ideal body weight were not studied.

Contraindications

Do not use the etonogestrel implant in women who have known or suspected pregnancy, current or past history of thrombosis or thromboembolic disorders, hepatic tumors (benign or malignant) or active liver disease, undiagnosed abnormal genital bleeding, known or suspected carcinoma of the breast or personal history of breast cancer, or hypersensitivity to any of the components of the etonogestrel implant.

Warnings/Precautions

Experience with etonogestrel implant:

Complications of insertion and removal – Insert the etonogestrel implant subdermally so that it is palpable after insertion. Failure to insert the etonogestrel implant properly may go unnoticed unless the implant is palpated immediately after insertion. Deep insertions may lead to difficult or impossible removals. Failure to remove the etonogestrel implant may result in infertility, ectopic pregnancy, or inability to stop a drug-related adverse reaction. Undetected failure to insert the etonogestrel implant may lead to an unintended pregnancy.

Ectopic pregnancies – Be alert to the possibility of an ectopic pregnancy among patients using the etonogestrel implant who become pregnant or complain of lower abdominal pain.

Bleeding irregularities – Patients who use the etonogestrel implant are likely to have changes in their vaginal bleeding patterns that are often unpredictable. These may include changes in bleeding frequency or duration, or amenorrhea.

Interaction with antiepileptic and other drugs – The etonogestrel implant is not recommended for women who chronically take drugs that are potent hepatic enzyme inducers because etonogestrel levels may be substantially reduced in these women.

Ovarian cysts – If follicular development occurs, atresia of the follicle is sometimes delayed, and the follicle may continue to grow beyond the size it would attain in a normal cycle. Generally, these enlarged follicles disappear spontaneously. Rarely, they can require surgery.

Thrombosis – There have been postmarketing reports of serious thromboembolic events, including cases of pulmonary emboli (some fatal) and strokes, in patients using the etonogestrel implant. Remove the etonogestrel implant in the event of a thrombosis.

Experience with combination (progestin plus estrogen) oral contraceptives:

Thromboembolic disorders and other vascular problems – Epidemiological investigations have associated the use of combination hormonal contraceptives with an increased incidence of venous thromboembolism, deep venous thrombosis, retinal vein thrombosis, and pulmonary embolism.

Cigarette smoking – Cigarette smoking increases the risk of serious cardiovascular adverse reactions from the use of combination hormonal contraceptives. This risk increases with age and with heavy smoking (15 or more cigarettes per day) and is quite marked in women older than 35 years of age who smoke. While this is believed to be an estrogen-related effect, it is not known whether a similar risk exists with progestin-only methods.

Elevated blood pressure – An increase in blood pressure has been reported in women taking combination hormonal contraceptives, and this increase is more likely with continued use and with older patients.

Carcinoma of the breast and reproductive organs – Women with breast cancer should not use hormonal contraceptives because breast cancer may be hormonally sensitive.

Hepatic neoplasia – Benign hepatic adenomas have been associated with the use of combination oral contraceptives, although the incidence of benign tumors is rare in the United States.

Gallbladder disease – Earlier studies have reported an increased lifetime relative risk of gallbladder surgery in users of combination oral contraceptives and estrogens.

Carbohydrate and lipid metabolic effects: The etonogestrel implant may induce mild insulin resistance and small changes in glucose concentrations of unknown clinical significance. Carefully observe women with diabetes or impaired glucose tolerance while using the etonogestrel implant.

Contact lenses: Contact lens wearers who develop visual changes or changes in lens tolerance should be assessed by an ophthalmologist.

Depression: Carefully observe women with a history of depression. Consider removing the etonogestrel implant in patients who become significantly depressed.

Fluid retention: Steroid contraceptives may cause some degree of fluid retention. It is unknown if the etonogestrel implant causes fluid retention.

Liver function: If jaundice develops in any patient using the etonogestrel implant, remove the etonogestrel implant.

Physical examination and follow-up: Perform a complete medical evaluation, including history and physical examination and relevant laboratory tests, prior to etonogestrel implant insertion or reinsertion.

Return to ovulation: In clinical trials, pregnancies occurred as early as during the first week after removal of the etonogestrel implant. Therefore, a patient should restart contraception immediately after removal of the etonogestrel implant if she still needs to prevent pregnancy.

Sexually transmitted diseases: This product does not protect against infection from HIV or other sexually transmitted diseases.

Weight gain: In clinical studies, mean weight gain in US etonogestrel implant users was 2.8 pounds after 1 year and 3.7 pounds after 2 years.

Fertility impairment: Fertility returned after withdrawal from treatment.

Pregnancy: The etonogestrel implant is not indicated for use during pregnancy.

Remove the etonogestrel implant if maintaining a pregnancy.

Lactation: Based on limited data, the etonogestrel implant may be used during lactation after the fourth postpartum week. Use of the etonogestrel implant before the fourth postpartum week has not been studied.

Small amounts of etonogestrel are excreted in breast milk.

Children: Safety and efficacy of the etonogestrel implant have been established in women of reproductive age. No clinical studies have been conducted in women younger than 18 years of age.

Elderly: This product has not been studied in women older than 65 years of age and is not indicated in this population.

Drug Interactions

Drugs that can affect etonogestrel include anticonvulsants, antifungals, barbiturates, hydantoins, protease inhibitors, rifamycins, and St. John's wort.

Drugs that may be affected by etonogestrel include lamotrigine and selegiline.

Adverse Reactions

Adverse reactions occurring in at least 3% of patients include abdominal pain, acne, back pain, breast pain, depression, dizziness, dysmenorrhea, emotional lability, headache, influenza-like symptoms, insertion site pain, leukorrhea, nausea, nervousness, pain, pharyngitis, sinusitis, upper respiratory tract infection, vaginal bleeding irregularities, vaginitis, and weight increase.

MEDROXYPROGESTERONE ACETATE

Injection: 104 mg (160 mg/mL) (*Rx*)	*depo-subQ provera 104* (Pfizer)
150 and 400 mg/mL (*Rx*)	Various, *Depo-Provera* (Pharmacia Corp.)

Warning:
Contraceptive injection: Patients should be counseled that this product does not protect against HIV infection (AIDS) or other sexually transmitted diseases.

Indications

Contraception (104 mg subcutaneous and 150 mg/mL IM): Medroxyprogesterone acetate contraceptive injection is indicated only for the prevention of pregnancy.

Endometrial/Renal carcinoma (400 mg/mL): Adjunctive therapy and palliative treatment of inoperable, recurrent, and metastatic endometrial or renal carcinoma.

Administration and Dosage

Shake the vial vigorously just before use to ensure that the dose being administered represents a uniform suspension.

Contraception:

Intramuscular (IM) injection – 150 mg every 3 months (13 weeks) administered by deep, IM injection in the gluteal or deltoid muscle.

To ensure the patient is not pregnant at the time of the first injection, the first injection must be given only during the first 5 days of a normal menstrual period; only within the first 5 days postpartum if not breast-feeding; and, if exclusively breast-feeding, only at the sixth postpartum week. If the time interval between injections is greater than 13 weeks, the health care provider should determine that the patient is not pregnant before administering the drug.

Subcutaneous injection – 104 mg every 3 months (12 to 14 weeks) administered subcutaneously into the anterior thigh or abdomen.

Switching from other methods of contraception – When switching from other contraceptive methods, give medroxyprogesterone in a manner than ensures continuous contraceptive coverage. For example, patients switching from combined (estrogen plus progestin) contraceptives should have their first injection within 7 days after the last day of using that method (7 days after taking the last active pill, removing the patch or ring). Similarly, contraceptive coverage will be maintained in switching from IM (150 mg) to subcutaneous (104 mg) provided the next injection is given within the prescribed dosing period for the IM (150 mg).

Endometrial/Renal carcinoma: Initially, doses of 400 to 1,000 mg IM weekly are recommended. If improvement is noted within a few weeks or months and the disease appears stabilized, it may be possible to maintain improvement with as little as 400 mg monthly. Medroxyprogesterone acetate is not recommended as primary therapy, but as adjunctive and palliative treatment in advanced inoperable cases including those with recurrent or metastatic disease.

Actions

Pharmacology: Medroxyprogesterone 150 mg/mL, when administered IM at the recommended dose to women every 3 months, inhibits the secretion of gonadotropins which, in turn, prevents follicular maturation and ovulation and results in endometrial thinning. These actions produce its contraceptive effect.

Medroxyprogesterone 400 mg/mL, administered parenterally in the recommended doses to women with adequate endogenous estrogen, transforms proliferative endometrium into secretory endometrium.

Pharmacokinetics: Following a single 150 mg IM dose, medroxyprogesterone concentrations increase for approximately 3 weeks to reach peak plasma concentrations of 1 to 7 ng/mL. The levels then decrease exponentially until they become undetectable (less than 100 pg/mL) between 120 to 200 days following injection. The apparent half-life following IM administration is approximately 50 days.

Contraindications

Known or suspected pregnancy or as a diagnostic test for pregnancy; undiagnosed vaginal bleeding; known or suspected malignancy of breast; active thrombophlebitis, or current or past history of thromboembolic disorders, or cerebral vascular disease; liver dysfunction or disease; hypersensitivity to medroxyprogesterone or any of its other ingredients.

Warnings/Precautions

Bleeding irregularities (150 mg/mL): Most women experience disruption of menstrual bleeding patterns. If abnormal bleeding persists or is severe, institute appropriate investigation to rule out the possibility of organic pathology, and institute appropriate treatment when necessary.

Bone mineral density changes: Use of medroxyprogesterone may be considered among the risk factors for development of osteoporosis. The rate of bone loss is greatest in the early years of use and then subsequently approaches the normal rate of age-related fall.

Thromboembolic disorders: Be alert to the earliest manifestations of thrombotic disorders. If any of these occur or are suspected, do not readminister the drug.

Ocular disorders: Do not readminister pending examination if there is a sudden partial or complete loss of vision or if there is a sudden onset of proptosis, diplopia, or migraine. If examination reveals papilledema or retinal vascular lesions, do not readminister.

Physical examination: The pretreatment and annual history and physical examination should include special reference to breast and pelvic organs, as well as a Papanicolaou smear.

Fluid retention: Because progestational drugs may cause some degree of fluid retention, conditions which might be influenced by this condition, such as epilepsy, migraine, asthma, cardiac or renal dysfunction, require careful observation.

150 mg/mL:

Weight changes – There is a tendency for women to gain weight while on medroxyprogesterone therapy.

Return of fertility – Medroxyprogesterone has a prolonged contraceptive effect. It is expected that 68% of women who do become pregnant may conceive within 12 months, 83% may conceive within 15 months and 93% may conceive within 18 months from the last injection.

Convulsions – There have been a few reported cases of convulsions in patients who were treated with medroxyprogesterone acetate contraceptive injection.

Carbohydrate metabolism – A decrease in glucose tolerance has been observed in some patients. Carefully observe diabetic patients during therapy.

Liver function – If jaundice develops, consider not readministering the drug.

400 mg/mL:

Vaginal bleeding – In cases of breakthrough bleeding, as in all cases of irregular bleeding per vaginum, nonfunctional causes should be borne in mind and adequate diagnostic measures undertaken.

Masking of climacteric – The age of the patient constitutes no absolute limiting factor although treatment with progestin may mask the onset of the climacteric.

Use with estrogen – Studies of the addition of a progestin product to an estrogen replacement regimen for 7 or more days of a cycle of estrogen administration have reported a lowered incidence of endometrial hyperplasia.

A decrease in glucose tolerance has been observed in a small percentage of patients on estrogen-progestin combination treatment. The mechanism of this decrease is obscure. For this reason, diabetic patients should be carefully observed while receiving such therapy.

Prolonged use – The effect of prolonged use of medroxyprogesterone acetate injection at the recommended doses on pituitary, ovarian, adrenal, hepatic, and uterine function is not known.

Multidose use – When multidose vials are used, special care to prevent contamination of the contents is essential. Although initially sterile, any multidose use of vials may lead to contamination unless strict aseptic technique is observed. There is some evidence that benzalkonium chloride is not an adequate antiseptic for sterilizing medroxyprogesterone acetate injection multi-dose vials. A povidone-iodine solution or similar product is recommended to cleanse the vial top prior to aspiration of contents.

Depression: Patients who have a history of psychic depression should be carefully observed and the drug not be readministered if the depression recurs.

Hypersensitivity reactions: Anaphylaxis and anaphylactoid reaction have been reported with the use of medroxyprogesterone acetate contraceptive injection. If an anaphylactic reaction occurs, appropriate therapy should be instituted. Serious anaphylactic reactions require emergency medical treatment.

Carcinogenesis: Long-term case-controlled surveillance of users found slight or no increased overall risk of breast cancer and no overall increased risk of ovarian, liver, or cervical cancer and a prolonged, protective effect of reducing the risk of endometrial cancer in the population of users.

Pregnancy: Category X.

Lactation: Detectable amounts of the drug have been identified in the milk of mothers receiving medroxyprogesterone. In breast-feeding mothers treated with medroxyprogesterone, milk composition, quality, and amount are not adversely affected. Infants exposed to medroxyprogesterone via breast milk have been studied for developmental and behavioral effects through puberty; no adverse effects have been noted.

Children: Safety and efficacy in children have not been established.

Drug Interactions

Drugs that may interact with medroxyprogesterone include aminoglutethimide.

Drug/Lab test interactions: The following laboratory tests may be affected by medroxyprogesterone: Plasma and urinary steroid levels are decreased; gonadotropin levels are decreased; sex-hormone binding globulin concentrations are decreased; protein bound iodine and butanol extractable protein bound iodine may increase; T_3 uptake values may decrease; coagulation test values for prothrombin (Factor II), and Factors VII, VIII, IX, and X may increase. Sulfobromophthalein and other liver function test values may be increased; the effects of medroxyprogesterone acetate on lipid metabolism are inconsistent. Both increases and decreases in total cholesterol, triglycerides, low-density lipoprotein (LDL) cholesterol, and high-density lipoprotein (HDL) cholesterol have been observed.

Adverse Reactions

Common (at least 3%) adverse reactions include menstrual irregularities; weight changes; headache; nervousness; abdominal pain; discomfort; asthenia; dizziness.

ANDROGENS

FLUOXYMESTERONE	
Tablets: 10 mg (*c-iii*)	Various, *Androxy* (Upsher-Smith)
METHYLTESTOSTERONE	
Tablets: 10 mg (*c-iii*)	Various, *Methitest* (Global)
25 mg (*c-iii*)	Various
Tablets (buccal): 10 mg (*c-iii*)	Various
Capsules: 10 mg (*c-iii*)	*Android* (Valeant), *Testred* (Valeant), *Virilon* (Star)
TESTOSTERONE ENANTHATE (IN OIL)	
Injection: 200 mg/mL (*c-iii*)	Various, *Delatestryl* (Savient)
TESTOSTERONE CYPIONATE (IN OIL)	
Injection: 100 mg/mL, 200 mg/mL (*c-iii*)	Various, *Depo-Testosterone* (Pharmacia)
TESTOSTERONE PELLETS	
Pellets: 75 mg (*c-iii*)	*Testopel* (Bartor Pharmacal)
TESTOSTERONE TRANSDERMAL SYSTEM	
Patch: 24.3 mg testosterone (*c-iii*)	*Androderm* (Watson Pharma)
12.2 mg testosterone (*c-iii*)	*Androderm* (Watson Pharma)
TESTOSTERONE GEL	
Gel: 1% testosterone (*c-iii*)	*AndroGel 1%* (Unimed Pharm), *Testim* (Auxilum Pharm)
TESTOSTERONE, BUCCAL	
Buccal system: 30 mg testosterone (*c-iii*)	*Striant* (Columbia)

Anabolic steroids are classified as a *c-iii* controlled substance under the anabolic steroids act of 1990.

Indications

Men:

Replacement therapy – Replacement therapy in hypogonadism associated with a deficiency or absence of endogenous testosterone. Appropriate adrenal cortical and thyroid hormone replacement therapy are still necessary, however, and are of primary importance.

Primary hypogonadism (congenital or acquired): Testicular failure due to cryptorchidism, bilateral torsion, orchitis, vanishing testis syndrome, or orchidectomy; Klinefelter syndrome, chemotherapy, or toxic damage from alcohol or heavy metals.

Hypogonadotropic hypogonadism (congenital or acquired): Idiopathic gonadotropin or luteinizing hormone releasing hormone deficiency or pituitary-hypothalamic injury from tumors, trauma, or radiation.

Delayed puberty: To stimulate puberty in carefully selected males with clearly delayed puberty. Brief treatment with conservative doses may be justified if these patients do not respond to psychological support.

Women:

Metastatic cancer – May be used secondarily in women with advancing inoperable metastatic (skeletal) breast cancer who are 1 to 5 years postmenopausal. Primary goals of therapy include ablation of the ovaries. This treatment has been used in premenopausal women with breast cancer who have benefited from oophorectomy and have a hormone-responsive tumor.

Administration and Dosage

FLUOXYMESTERONE:

Men –

Hypogonadism: 5 to 20 mg/day.

Delayed puberty: Carefully titrate dosage using a low dose, appropriate skeletal monitoring, and by limiting the duration of therapy to 4 to 6 months.

Women –

Inoperable breast carcinoma: 10 to 40 mg/day in divided doses. Continue for 1 month for a subjective response and 2 to 3 months for an objective response.

METHYLTESTOSTERONE:

Men –

Replacement therapy: Replacement therapy in androgen-deficient men is 10 to 50 mg of methyltestosterone daily.

Delayed puberty – Doses used in delayed puberty generally are in the lower range of that given previously, and for a limited duration, for example, 4 to 6 months.

Women –

Inoperable breast cancer: 50 to 200 mg/day orally. Follow women closely because androgen therapy occasionally appears to accelerate the disease. Shorter acting androgen preparations may be preferred rather than those with prolonged activity for treating breast carcinoma, particularly during the early stages of androgen therapy.

TESTOSTERONE, LONG-ACTING: For IM use only. Individualize dosage. In general, more than 400 mg/month is not required because of the prolonged action of the preparation.

Male hypogonadism –

Replacement therapy (eunuchism): 50 to 400 mg every 2 to 4 weeks.

Males with delayed puberty – 50 to 200 mg every 2 to 4 weeks for a limited duration.

Palliation of inoperable breast cancer in women – 200 to 400 mg every 2 to 4 weeks. Androgen therapy occasionally appears to accelerate metastatic breast carcinoma.

TESTOSTERONE TRANSDERMAL SYSTEM:

Androderm – The usual starting dose is one 5 mg system or two 2.5 mg systems applied nightly for 24 hours, providing a total dose of 5 mg/day.

Apply the adhesive side of the system to a clean, dry area of the skin on the back, abdomen, upper arms, or thighs. Avoid bony prominences, such as the shoulder and hip areas. Do NOT apply to the scrotum. Rotate the sites of application, with an interval of 7 days between applications to the same site. The area selected should not be oily, damaged, or irritated.

To ensure proper dosing, the morning serum testosterone concentration may be measured following system application the previous evening. If the serum concentration is outside the normal range, repeat sampling with assurance of proper system adhesion, as well as appropriate application time. Confirmed serum concentrations outside the normal range may require increasing the dosage regimen to 7.5 mg, or decreasing the regimen to 2.5 mg, maintaining nightly application. Because of variability in analytical values among diagnostic laboratories, this laboratory work and any later analysis for assessing the effect of therapy should be performed at the same laboratory so results can be more easily compared.

Nonvirilized patient – Dosing may be initiated with 2.5 mg system nightly.

Storage/Stability – Do not store outside the pouch provided. Damaged systems should not be used. The drug reservoir may be burst by excessive pressure or heat. Discard systems in household trash in a manner that prevents accidental application or ingestion by children, pets, or others.

TESTOSTERONE PELLETS:

Replacement therapy – The dosage guideline for testosterone pellets for replacement therapy in androgen-deficient men is 150 to 450 mg subcutaneous every 3 to 6 months.

Delayed puberty – Dosages used in delayed puberty generally are in the lower range of those listed for replacement therapy and a duration (eg, 4 to 6 months).

Determination of dose – The number of pellets to be implanted depends upon the minimal daily requirement of testosterone propionate determined by a gradual reduction of the amount administered parenterally. The usual ratio is as follows: implant two 75 mg pellets for each 25 mg of testosterone propionate required weekly. Thus, when a patient requires injections of 75 mg/week, it is usually necessary to implant 450 mg (6 pellets). With required injections of 50 mg/week, implantation of 300 mg (4 pellets) may suffice for approximately 3 months. With lower requirements by injection, correspondingly lower amounts may be implanted. It has been found that approximately ⅓ of the material is absorbed in the first month, ¼ in the second month, and ⅙ in the third month. Adequate effect of the pellets ordinarily continues for 3 to 4 months, sometimes as long as 6 months.

Dose selection – Pellet implantation is much less flexible for dosage adjustment compared with oral administration or intramuscular injection of oil solutions or aqueous suspensions. Therefore, great care should be used when estimating the amount of testosterone needed.

Discontinuation – In the face of complications in which the effects of testosterone should be discontinued, the pellets would have to be removed. In addition, there are times when the pellets may slough out. This accident is usually traceable to superficial implantation or to neglect in regard to aseptic precautions.

Implanter kit –

Sterilization: The implanter kit must be sterilized prior to use. The implanter kit may be sterilized by steam in an autoclave at 121°C (250°F) for a minimum of 15 minutes. Standard procedures for sterilizing surgical instruments should be followed.

Implantation procedure:

Implantation area – The pellets are fat-soluable and implanted subcutaneously. In most men, an area on the anterior abdominal wall is selected 1 inch medial to the anterior superior iliac spine, avoiding previous scars. An area on either buttocks may be chosen so that implantation is made beneath the external gluteus muscle.

Preparation – The skin is cleaned with an accepted antiseptic preparation and then anesthetized with 2 to 3 mL of local anaesthetic. Some health care providers use an epinephrine solution to ensure minimal capillary bleeding.

Implantation – The clinically indicated pellets are placed in a sterile tray. The *Bardani* implanter with stylet (solid tube with pointed end) in place is inserted parallel to the inguinal ligament and directed subcutaneously to the depth of the bolt (about 5 cm). When the stylet is removed, the pellets are placed in the groove of the implanter with the sterilized tissue forceps. The sterilized tray should be held beneath the implanter as the pellets are inserted, in case 1 is dropped inadvertently. A pellet that falls into the sterilized tray may be replaced, but a pellet that becomes contaminated must be discarded because it cannot be resterilized. The plunger (solid tube with blunt end) is then inserted and the pellets are eased into the fatty tissues. The implanter is removed and a dry dressing is given to the patient to apply with pressure for a few minutes. Cover the puncture site with an adhesive bandage.

TESTOSTERONE GEL: The recommended starting dose of 1% testosterone gel is 5 g (to deliver 50 mg of testosterone) applied once daily (preferably in the morning) to clean, dry, intact skin of the shoulders and upper arms or abdomen (*AndroGel* only). Upon opening the packet(s), squeeze the entire contents into the palm of the hand and immediately apply it to the application sites. Allow application sites to dry for a few minutes prior to dressing. Wash hands with soap and water after application. Cover the application sites with clothing after gel has dried.

Do not apply the gel to the genitals. Do not apply *Testim* to the abdomen.

For optimal absorption of testosterone from *AndroGel*, it appears reasonable to wait 5 to 6 hours after application prior to showering or swimming. Showering or swimming after just 1 hour should have a minimal effect on the amount absorbed if done infrequently. Do not wash the sites of application for at least 2 hours after application of *Testim*.

Measure serum testosterone levels 14 days after initiation of therapy to ensure proper dosing. If the serum testosterone concentration is below the normal range, or if the desired clinical response is not achieved, the dose may be increased from 5 to 7.5 g (*AndroGel*) or 10 g (*Testim*) and from 7.5 to 10 g (*AndroGel*), as instructed by the physician.

In order to prevent transfer to another person, instruct patients to wear clothing to cover the application sites. If direct skin-to-skin contact with another person is anticipated, the application sites must be washed thoroughly with soap and water.

In order to maintain serum testosterone levels in the normal range, instruct patients not to wash the sites of application for at least 2 hours after application.

TESTOSTERONE, BUCCAL: The recommended dosing schedule is the application of 1 buccal system (30 mg) to the gum region twice daily, morning and evening (about 12 hours apart). Testosterone buccal should be placed in a comfortable position just above the incisor tooth on either side of the mouth. With each application, testosterone should be rotated to alternate sides of the mouth.

Upon opening the packet, the rounded side surface of the buccal system should be placed against the gum and held firmly in place with a finger over the lip and against the product for 30 seconds to ensure adhesion. Testosterone buccal is designed to stay in position until removed. If the buccal system fails to properly adhere to the gum or falls off during the 12-hour dosing interval, the old buccal system should be removed and a new one applied. If the buccal system falls out of position within 4 hours before the next dose, a new buccal system should be applied and may remain in place until the time of next regularly scheduled dosing.

Take care to avoid dislodging the buccal system and check to see if testosterone buccal is in place following brushing of teeth, use of mouthwash, and consumption of food or beverages. Testosterone buccal should not be chewed or swallowed. To remove testosterone, gently slide it downwards from the gum toward the tooth to avoid scratching the gum.

Actions

Pharmacology: Testosterone, produced by the Leydig cells of the testis, is the primary natural androgen. In women, small amounts are synthesized by the ovary and adrenal cortex.

Endogenous androgens are responsible for the normal growth and development of the male sex organs and for maintenance of secondary sex characteristics. Androgens are responsible for the growth spurt of adolescence and for the termination of linear growth by fusion of the epiphyseal growth centers. During administration of exogenous androgens, endogenous testosterone release is inhibited through feedback inhibition of pituitary luteinizing hormone. Large doses of exogenous androgens may suppress spermatogenesis through feedback inhibition of pituitary follicle-stimulating hormone.

Pharmacokinetics:

Absorption –

Oral: Testosterone is metabolized by the gut and 44% is cleared by the liver in the first pass. The synthetic androgens are less extensively metabolized by the liver, have longer half-lives, and are more suitable than testosterone for oral administration.

IM: Testosterone esters in oil injected IM are absorbed slowly from the lipid phase; thus, testosterone cypionate and enanthate can be given at intervals of 2 to 4 weeks.

Topical gel: Absorption of testosterone into the blood continues for the entire 24-hour dosing interval. Serum concentrations approximate the steady-state level by the end of the first 24 hours and are at steady state by the second or third day of dosing.

When the topical gel treatment is discontinued after achieving steady state, serum testosterone levels remain in the normal range for 24 to 48 hours but return to their pretreatment levels by the fifth day after the last application.

Transdermal:

Androderm – Following application to nonscrotal skin, testosterone is continuously absorbed during the 24-hour dosing period. Daily application of 2 systems at approximately 10:00 pm results in a serum testosterone concentration profile that mimics the normal circadian variation observed in healthy young men. Maximum concentrations occur in the early morning hours with minimum concentrations in the evening.

Distribution – Testosterone in plasma is approximately 98% bound to a specific testosterone-estradiol binding globulin. There are considerable variations in the reported half-life of testosterone, ranging from 10 to 100 minutes. The half-life of testosterone cypionate IM is approximately 8 days; for oral fluoxymesterone, it is approximately 9.2 hours; and for methyltestosterone it is 2.5 to 3 hours.

Metabolism/Excretion – There are considerable variations in the reported half-life of testosterone, ranging from 10 to 100 minutes. The half-life of testosterone cypionate IM is approximately 8 days; for oral fluoxymesterone, it is approximately 9.2 hours; and for methyltestosterone it is 2.5 to 3 hours. Inactivation of testosterone occurs primarily in the liver. About 90% of a testosterone dose is excreted in the urine as conjugates of testosterone and its metabolites; about 6% of a dose is excreted in the feces.

Contraindications

Patients with serious cardiac, hepatic, or renal diseases; hypersensitivity to the drug; in men with carcinomas of the breast or prostate; pregnancy (see Warnings).

Pregnant women should avoid skin contact with *AndroGel* application sites in men. Testosterone may cause fetal harm. In the event that unwashed or unclothed skin to which *AndroGel* has been applied does come in direct contact with the skin of a pregnant woman, wash the general area of contact on the woman with soap and water as soon as possible. In vitro studies show that residual testosterone is removed from the skin surface by washing with soap and water.

Warnings/Precautions

Athletic performance: Although the anabolic steroids are generally the agents that are abused for enhancement of athletic performance, androgens have also been used for such purposes. However, these drugs are not safe and effective for this use and have a potential risk of serious adverse reactions.

Sleep apnea: The treatment of hypogonadal men with testosterone esters may potentiate sleep apnea in some patients, especially those with risk factors such as obesity or chronic lung diseases.

Product interchange: Do not use testosterone cypionate interchangeably with testosterone propionate because of differences in duration of action.

Breast cancer: Androgen therapy may cause hypercalcemia by stimulating osteolysis.

Hepatotoxicity: Prolonged use of high doses of androgens has been associated with the development of potentially life-threatening peliosis hepatis, hepatic neoplasms, and hepatocellular carcinoma. Cholestatic hepatitis and jaundice occur with fluoxymesterone and methyltestosterone at relatively low doses. Drug-induced jaundice is reversible when the medication is discontinued.

Oligospermia: Oligospermia and reduced ejaculatory volume may occur after prolonged administration or excessive dosage.

Edema: Edema, with or without congestive heart failure, may be a serious complication in patients with preexisting cardiac, renal, or hepatic disease.

Gynecomastia: Gynecomastia frequently develops and occasionally persists in patients being treated for hypogonadism.

Bone maturation: Use cautiously in healthy males with delayed puberty. Monitor bone maturation by assessing bone age of the wrist and hand every 6 months.

Virilization: Observe women for signs of virilization (deepening voice, hirsutism, acne, clitoromegaly, and menstrual irregularities). Discontinue therapy at the time of evidence of mild virilism to prevent irreversible virilization.

Hypercholesterolemia: Serum cholesterol may be altered during therapy.

Tartrazine sensitivity: Some of these products contain tartrazine, which may cause allergic-type reactions (including bronchial asthma) in susceptible individuals. Although the incidence of tartrazine sensitivity in the general population is low, it is frequently seen in patients who also have aspirin hypersensitivity. Specific products containing tartrazine are identified in the product listings.

Special risk: Patients with benign prostatic hypertrophy may develop acute urethral obstruction. Priapism or excessive sexual stimulation may develop. Oligospermia may occur after prolonged administration or excessive dosage. If any of these reactions appear, stop administration. If restarted, use a lower dosage. Avoid stimulation to the point of increasing nervous, mental, and physical activities beyond the patient's cardiovascular capacity.

Carcinogenesis: There are rare reports of hepatocellular carcinoma in patients receiving long-term therapy with androgens in high doses.

Pregnancy: Category X.

Lactation: It is not known whether androgens are excreted in breast milk.

Children: Use androgens very cautiously in children; the drugs should only be given by specialists who are aware of the adverse reactions on bone maturation. Androgens may accelerate bone maturation without producing compensatory gain in linear growth. This adverse reaction may result in compromised adult stature. The younger the child, the greater the risk of compromising final mature height.

Benzyl alcohol – Benzyl alcohol-containing products have been associated with a fatal "gasping syndrome" in premature infants. Refer to product listings.

Elderly: Elderly men, or men in general, treated with androgens may be at an increased risk of developing prostatic hypertrophy, prostatic carcinoma, and prostatic hyperplasia.

Monitoring: Frequently determine urine and serum calcium levels during the course of therapy in women with disseminated breast carcinoma. Periodically perform liver function tests, prostate specific antigen, cholesterol, and high-density lipoprotein. To ensure proper dosing, measure serum testosterone concentrations. Make periodic (every 6 months) x-ray examinations of bone age during treatment of prepubertal males to determine the rate of bone maturation and the effects of the androgen therapy on the epiphyseal centers. Check hemoglobin and hematocrit periodically for polycythemia in patients who are receiving high doses of androgens.

Drug Interactions

Androgens may affect anticoagulants, corticosteroids/ACTH, cyclosporineinsulin, oxyphenbutazone, and propranolol.

Drug/Lab test interactions:

Thyroid function tests – Decreased levels of thyroxine-binding globulin, resulting in decreased total T_4 serum levels and increased resin uptake of T_3 and T_4. Free thyroid hormone levels remain unchanged, and there is no clinical evidence of thyroid dysfunction.

Adverse Reactions

Adverse reactions occurring in 3% or more of patients include abnormal lab tests (including abnormal hemoglobin, hematocrit, triglycerides, serum lipids, potassium glucose, creatinine, bilirubin, liver function tests), acne, application site itching/erythema/discomfort, breast pain/tenderness, burning sensation, burn-like blister under system, dizziness/vertigo, gynecomastia, headache, libido decreased, other application site reactions, peripheral edema, prostate disorder, pruritus, UTI/Prostatitis.

Women – Amenorrhea and other menstrual irregularities; inhibition of gonadotropin secretion and virilization, including deepening voice and clitoral enlargement.

FINASTERIDE

Tablets: 1 mg (*Rx*)	*Propecia* (Merck)
5 mg (*Rx*)	Various, *Proscar* (Merck)

Indications

Androgenetic alopecia (Propecia only): Treatment of male pattern hair loss (vertex and anterior mid-scalp) in patients between 18 and 41 years of age.

Benign prostatic hyperplasia (BPH) (Proscar only): Treatment of symptomatic BPH in men with an enlarged prostate to improve symptoms, reduce acute urinary retention risk, and reduce the risk of the need for surgery including transurethral resection of the prostate (TURP) and prostatectomy.

Administration and Dosage

Benign prostatic hyperplasia: Recommended dose is 5 mg once/day, with or without meals.

Finasteride can be administered alone or in combination with the alpha-blocker doxazosin.

Although early improvement may be seen, at least 6 to 12 months of therapy may be necessary to assess whether a beneficial response has been achieved.

Androgenetic alopecia: 1 mg once/day, with or without meals. Daily use for at least 3 months is necessary before benefit is observed. Continued use is recommended to sustain benefit. Withdrawal of treatment leads to reversal of effect within 12 months.

Actions

Pharmacology: Finasteride is a competitive and specific inhibitor of steroid 5α-reductase, an intracellular enzyme that converts testosterone into the potent androgen 5α-dihydrotestosterone (DHT).

Pharmacokinetics: Finasteride is well absorbed after oral administration, with a mean bioavailability of approximately 64%, which is unaffected by food.

Finasteride undergoes extensive hepatic metabolism through oxidative pathways to inactive compounds that are eliminated primarily through the bile.

Approximately 90% is bound to plasma proteins. The half-life of finasteride is 4.8 to 6 hours following 1 and 5 mg/day dosing, respectively.

Contraindications

Hypersensitivity to finasteride or any component of this product; use in women or children; pregnancy or use, including handling of crushed or broken tablets, in women who may potentially be pregnant.

Warnings/Precautions

Exposure of women/risk to male fetus: Women should not handle crushed or broken finasteride tablets when they are pregnant or may become pregnant because of the possibility of finasteride absorption and the subsequent potential risk to a male fetus.

Obstructive uropathy: Because not all patients demonstrate a response to finasteride, carefully monitor patients with a large residual urinary volume or severely diminished urinary flow for obstructive uropathy. These patients may not be candidates for this therapy.

Prostate cancer evaluation/Effects on PSA: Finasteride causes a decrease in serum PSA levels in patients with BPH even in the presence of prostate cancer. Consider this reduction when evaluating PSA laboratory data; it does not suggest a beneficial effect of finasteride on prostate cancer. In controlled clinical trials, finasteride did not appear to alter the rate of prostate cancer detection.

Carefully evaluate any sustained increases in PSA levels while on finasteride, including consideration of noncompliance to therapy.

Hepatic function impairment: Use caution in those patients with liver function abnormalities since finasteride is metabolized extensively in the liver.

Pregnancy: Category X.

Lactation: Finasteride is not indicated for use in women. It is not known whether finasteride is excreted in breast milk.

Children: Finasteride is not indicated for use in children; safety and efficacy in children have not been established.

Monitoring: Monitor patients with BPH for prostate cancer (eg, digital rectal examinations) prior to initiating therapy and periodically thereafter. Monitor for obstructive uropathy in patients with large residual urinary volume and/or severely diminished urinary flow.

Drug Interactions

Drug/Lab test interactions: PSA serum levels are decreased by approximately 50% in patients with BPH treated with finasteride.

Adverse Reactions

Adverse reactions occurring in 3% or more of patients include abnormal ejaculation, asthenia, decreased libido, decreased volume of ejaculate, dizziness, impotence, postural hypotension.

DUTASTERIDE

Capsules: 0.5 mg (*Rx*)	*Avodart* (GlaxoSmithKline)

Indications

Benign prostatic hyperplasia (BPH):

Monotherapy – For the treatment of symptomatic BPH in men with an enlarged prostate to improve symptoms, reduce the risk of acute urinary retention, and reduce the risk of the need for BPH-related surgery.

Combination therapy – For the treatment of symptomatic BPH in men with an enlarged prostate in combination with the alpha-blocker tamsulosin.

Administration and Dosage

Maximum dosage is 0.5 mg taken orally once daily. Swallow the capsules whole. Dutasteride may be administered with or without food.

Monotherapy: 0.5 mg (1 capsule) taken orally once daily.

Combination therapy: 0.5 mg (1 capsule) taken once daily and tamsulosin 0.4 mg taken once daily.

Preparation for administration: Dutasteride is a hormonal agent and is also considered a teratogen. Follow safe handling procedures when preparing, administering, or dispensing dutasteride.

Dutasteride is absorbed through the skin. Dutasteride should not be handled by women who are pregnant or who may become pregnant because of the potential for absorption and the subsequent potential risk to a developing male fetus. If contact is made with a leaking capsule, the contact area should be washed immediately with soap and water.

Actions

Pharmacology: Dutasteride inhibits the conversion of testosterone to 5 alpha-dihydrotestosterone (DHT), the androgen primarily responsible for the initial development and subsequent enlargement of the prostate gland. Testosterone is converted to DHT by the enzyme 5 alpha-reductase, which exists as 2 isoforms, type 1 and type 2.

Dutasteride is a competitive and specific inhibitor of type 1 and type 2 5 alpha-reductase isoenzymes.

Effect on DHT and testosterone – The maximum effect of daily doses of dutasteride on the reduction of DHT is dose dependent and is observed within 1 to 2 weeks.

Pharmacokinetics:

Absorption – Following administration of a single 0.5 mg dose, time to peak serum concentrations (T_{max}) of dutasteride occurs within 2 to 3 hours. Absolute bioavailability in 5 healthy subjects is approximately 60% (range, 40% to 94%). When the drug is administered with food, the maximum serum concentrations were reduced by 10% to 15%.

Distribution – There is a large volume of distribution (300 to 500 L); the drug is highly bound to plasma albumin (99%) and alpha-1 acid glycoprotein (96.6%).

Metabolism/Excretion – Dutasteride is extensively metabolized in humans. Dutasteride is metabolized by the CYP3A4 isoenzyme to 2 minor mono-hydroxylated metabolites.

The terminal elimination half-life of dutasteride is approximately 5 weeks at steady state.

Special populations –

Gender: Dutasteride is contraindicated in pregnancy and women of childbearing potential and is not indicated for use in other women.

Contraindications

Pregnancy; women of childbearing potential; children, patients with previously demonstrated, clinically significant hypersensitivity (eg, serious skin reactions, angioedema) to dutasteride or other 5 alpha-reductase inhibitors.

Warnings/Precautions

Exposure of women/risk to male fetus: Women who are pregnant or may be pregnant should not handle dutasteride capsules because of the possibility of absorption of dutasteride and the potential risk of a fetal anomaly to a male fetus.

Other urological diseases: Lower urinary tract symptoms of BPH can be indicative of other urological diseases, including prostate cancer.

Prostate effects: Dutasteride reduces total serum prostate-specific antigen (PSA) concentration by approximately 40% following 3 months of treatment and by 50% following 6, 12, and 24 months of treatment. Establish a new baseline PSA concentration after 3 to 6 months of treatment, and use this new value to assess potentially cancer-related changes in PSA. To interpret an isolated PSA value in a man treated with dutasteride for 6 months or more, double the PSA value for comparison with normal values in untreated men. The free-to-total PSA ratio remains constant at month 12, even under the influence of dutasteride.

Blood donation: Men being treated with dutasteride should not donate blood until at least 6 months have passed following their last dose. The purpose of this deferred period is to prevent administration of dutasteride to a pregnant female transfusion recipient.

Reproductive effects: The clinical significance of dutasteride's effect on semen characteristics for an individual patient's fertility is not known.

Hepatic function impairment: Because dutasteride is extensively metabolized, exposure could be higher in patients with hepatic function impairment.

Pregnancy: Category X.

Lactation: It is not known whether dutasteride is excreted in human breast milk. Do not use dutasteride in breast-feeding women.

Children: Use in children is contraindicated. Safety and effectiveness in children have not been established.

Monitoring: Assess patients to rule out other urological diseases prior to treatment with dutasteride and periodically thereafter.

Carefully monitor patients with a large residual urinary volume and/or severely diminished urinary flow.

Perform digital rectal examinations, as well as other evaluations for prostate cancer, prior to initiating therapy with dutasteride and periodically thereafter.

Drug Interactions

CYP-450: Drugs that may affect dutasteride include ritonavir, ketoconazole, verapamil, diltiazem, cimetidine, troleandomycin, and ciprofloxacin.

Drug/Lab test interactions:

Effects on PSA – PSA levels generally decrease in patients treated with dutasteride as the prostate volume decreases. Establish a new baseline PSA concentration after 3 to 6 months of treatment with dutasteride.

Adverse Reactions

Adverse reaction occurring in 3% or more of patients included transient impotence and decreased libido within the first 6 months.

BENIGN PROSTATIC HYPERPLASIA (BPH) COMBINATIONS

Capsules; oral: dutasteride 0.5 mg/tamsulosin hydrochloride 0.4 mg (*Rx*)	*Jalyn* (GlaxoSmithKline)

Indications

Benign prostatic hyperplasia: For the treatment of symptomatic benign prostatic hyperplasia in men with an enlarged prostate.

Administration and Dosage

1 capsule once daily approximately 30 minutes after the same meal each day.

Dutasteride/tamsulosin should not be used in combination with strong inhibitors of CYP3A4 (eg, ketoconazole).

The capsules should be swallowed whole and not chewed or opened. Contact with the contents of the capsule may result in irritation of the oropharyngeal mucosa.

Dutasteride is absorbed through the skin. Capsules should not be handled by women who are pregnant or who may become pregnant because of the potential for absorption of dutasteride and the subsequent potential risk to a developing male fetus.

DANAZOL

Capsules: 50, 100, and 200 mg (*Rx*)	Various

Warning:

Use of danazol in pregnancy is contraindicated. A sensitive test (eg, beta subunit test if available) capable of determining early pregnancy is recommended immediately prior to start of therapy. Additionally, a nonhormonal method of contraception should be used during therapy. If a patient becomes pregnant while taking danazol, discontinue administration of the drug and apprise the patient of the potential risk to the fetus.

Thromboembolism, thrombotic and thrombophlebitic events, including sagittal sinus thrombosis and life-threatening or fatal strokes have been reported.

Experience with long-term therapy with danazol is limited. Peliosis hepatis and benign hepatic adenoma have been observed with long-term use. Peliosis hepatis and hepatic adenoma may be silent until complicated by acute, potentially life-threatening intra-abdominal hemorrhage. Therefore, alert the physician to this possibility. Attempts should be made to determine the lowest dose that will provide adequate protection (see Warnings).

Danazol has been associated with several cases of benign intracranial hypertension also known as pseudotumor cerebri. Early signs and symptoms of benign intracranial hypertension include papilledema, headache, nausea, and vomiting, and visual disturbances. Screen patients with these symptoms for papilledema and, if present, advise the patients to discontinue danazol immediately and refer them to a neurologist for further diagnosis and care.

Indications

Endometriosis: For the treatment of endometriosis amenable to hormonal management.

Fibrocystic breast disease: Danazol is usually effective in decreasing nodularity, pain, and tenderness, but it alters hormone levels; recurrence of symptoms is very common after cessation of therapy.

Hereditary angioedema: For the prevention of attacks of angioedema in males and females.

Administration and Dosage

Endometriosis: Begin therapy during menstruation or make sure the patient is not pregnant. Administer 800 mg/day in 2 divided doses to best achieve amenorrhea and rapid response to painful symptoms. Downward titration to a dose sufficient to maintain amenorrhea may be considered depending upon response. Initially, for mild cases, give 200 to 400 mg in 2 divided doses.

Fibrocystic breast disease: Begin therapy during menstruation or make sure patient is not pregnant. Dosage ranges from 100 to 400 mg/day in 2 divided doses.

Hereditary angioedema: Recommended starting dose is 200 mg 2 or 3 times/day. After a favorable initial response, determine continuing dosage by decreasing the dosage by 50% or less at intervals of at least 1 to 3 months if frequency of attacks prior to treatment dictates. If an attack occurs, increase dosage by 200 mg/day or less.

Actions

Pharmacology: A synthetic androgen derived from ethisterone, danazol suppresses the pituitary-ovarian axis by inhibiting the output of pituitary gonadotropins. Danazol depresses the output of both follicle-stimulating hormone (FSH) and luteinizing hormone (LH). Danazol acts by direct enzymatic inhibition of sex steroid synthesis and competitively inhibits binding of steroids to their cytoplasmic receptors in target tissues.

Endometriosis – In endometriosis, danazol alters the normal and ectopic endometrial tissue so that it becomes inactive and atrophic.

Hereditary angioedema – Danazol prevents attacks of the disease characterized by episodic edema of the abdominal viscera, extremities, face, and airway that may be disabling and, if the airway is involved, fatal. In addition, danazol partially or completely corrects the primary biochemical abnormality of hereditary angioedema. It increases the levels of the deficient C1 esterase inhibitor, thereby increasing the serum levels of the C4 component of the complement system.

Pharmacokinetics: Blood levels of danazol do not increase proportionately with increases in dose. When the dose is doubled, plasma levels increase only approximately 35% to 40%.

Contraindications

Undiagnosed abnormal genital bleeding; markedly impaired hepatic, renal, or cardiac function; pregnancy and lactation; patients with porphyria.

Warnings/Precautions

Thrombotic events: Thromboembolism, thrombotic and thrombophlebitic events including sagittal sinus thrombosis and life-threatening or fatal strokes have been reported.

Hepatic events: Experience with long-term therapy with danazol is limited. Peliosis hepatis and benign hepatic adenoma have been observed with long-term use (see Black Box Warning).

Intracranial hypertension: Danazol has been associated with several cases of benign intracranial hypertension (also known as pseudotumor cerebri) (see Black Box Warning).

Lipoprotein alterations: A temporary alteration of lipoproteins in the form of decreased high density lipoproteins (HDL) and possibly increased low density lipoproteins (LDL) has been reported during danazol therapy.

Carcinoma of the breast: Carcinoma of the breast should be excluded before initiating therapy for fibrocystic breast disease.

Long-term experience: Long-term experience with danazol is limited. Long-term therapy with other steroids alkylated at the 17 position has been associated with serious toxicity (cholestatic jaundice, peliosis hepatitis). Similar toxicity may develop after long-term danazol.

Androgenic effects: Androgenic effects may not be reversible even when the drug is discontinued. Watch patients closely for signs of virilization.

Fluid retention: Conditions influenced by edema require careful observation.

Hepatic dysfunction: Hepatic dysfunction has been reported; perform periodic liver function tests.

Lipoproteins: Monitor HDL and LDL periodically.

Semen: Semen should be checked for volume, viscosity, sperm count, and motility every 3 to 4 months, especially in adolescents.

Porphyria: Danazol administration has been reported to cause exacerbation of the manifestations of acute intermittent porphyria.

Pregnancy: Category X.

Lactation: Breastfeeding is contraindicated in patients taking danazol.

Children: Safety and efficacy in children has not been established.

Drug Interactions

Drugs that maybe affected by danazol are carbamazepine, cyclosporine, and warfarin.

Adverse Reactions

Significant adverse reactions include edema; vaginitis; nervousness; emotional lability; hepatic dysfunction; elevated blood pressure; pelvic pain; carpal tunnel syndrome; sleep disorders; fatigue; tremor; visual disturbances; anxiety; depression; gastroenteritis.

GLUCOCORTICOIDS

BETAMETHASONE	
Solution; oral: 0.6 mg/5 mL (*Rx*)	*Celestone* (Schering)
BETAMETHASONE SODIUM PHOSPHATE AND BETAMETHASONE ACETATE	
Injection: 3 mg acetate and 3 mg sodium phosphate/mL (*Rx*)	*Celestone Soluspan* (Prometheus)
BUDESONIDE	
Capsules; oral: 3 mg micronized budesonide (*Rx*)	*Entocort EC* (Prometheus)
CORTISONE	
Tablets; oral: 25 mg (*Rx*)	Various
DEXAMETHASONE	
Tablets; oral: 0.5, 0.75, 1, 1.5, 2, 4, and 6 mg (*Rx*)	Various, *DexPak 6 Day*, *DexPak 13 Day*, *DexPak 10 Day* (ECR)
Elixir; oral: 0.5 mg per 5 mL (*Rx*)	Various, *Baycadron* (Wockhardt)
Solution; oral: 0.5 mg per 5 mL (*Rx*)	Various
Solution (concentrate); oral: 1 mg/mL (*Rx*)	*Dexamethasone Intensol* (Roxane)
DEXAMETHASONE SODIUM PHOSPHATE	
Injection: 4 and 10 mg/mL (*Rx*)	Various
HYDROCORTISONE	
Tablets; oral: 5 mg (*Rx*)	Various, *Cortef* (Upjohn)
10 and 20 mg (*Rx*)	Various, *Cortef* (Upjohn)
HYDROCORTISONE SODIUM SUCCINATE	
Injection: 100, 250, 500, and 1,000 mg per vial (*Rx*)	*A-Hydrocort* (Hospira), *Solu-Cortef* (Pfizer)
METHYLPREDNISOLONE	
Tablets; oral: 2, 4, 8, 16, 24, and 32 mg (*Rx*)	Various, *Medrol* (Upjohn)
METHYLPREDNISOLONE SODIUM SUCCINATE	
Injection, powder for solution: 40, 125, and 500 mg and 1 g per vial (*Rx*)	Various, *A-Methapred* (Hospira), *Solu-Medrol* (Pfizer)
2 g (*Rx*)	*Solu-Medrol* (Pfizer)
METHYLPREDNISOLONE ACETATE	
Injection, suspension: 20, 40, and 80 mg/mL (*Rx*)	Various, *Depo-Medrol* (Upjohn)
PREDNISOLONE	
Tablets; oral: 5 mg (*Rx*)	Various, *Millipred* (Laser)
Syrup; oral: 15 mg per 5 mL (*Rx*)	Various, *Prelone* (Aero)
Suspension; oral: 15 mg per 5 mL (equiv. to prednisolone acetate 16.7 mg) (*Rx*)	*Flo-Pred* (Taro)
PREDNISOLONE SODIUM PHOSPHATE	
Tablets, orally disintegrating; oral: 10, 15, 30 mg (as base)	*Orapred ODT* (Sciele)
Solution; oral: 5 mg per 5 mL (*Rx*)	Various, *Pediapred* (Celltech Pharmaceuticals)
10 mg per 5 mL (*Rx*	*Millipred* (Laser)
15 mg per 5 mL (*Rx*	*Orapred* (Sciele)
20 mg per 5 mL (*Rx*	*Veripred 20* (Hawthorn)
PREDNISONE	
Tablets; oral: 1 mg (*Rx*)	Various
2.5 mg (*Rx*)	
5 mg (*Rx*)	
10 mg (*Rx*)	
20 and 50 mg (*Rx*)	
Solution; oral: 5 mg/mL, 5 mg per 5 mL (*Rx*)	
TRIAMCINOLONE HEXACETONIDE	
Injection; suspension: 5 mg/mL (*Rx*)	*Aristospan Intralesional* (Sandoz)
20 mg/mL (*Rx*)	*Aristospan Intra-articular* (Sandoz)
TRIAMCINOLONE ACETONIDE	
Injection; suspension: 10 mg/mL (*Rx*)	*Kenalog-10* (Bristol-Myers Squibb)
40 mg/mL (*Rx*)	*Kenalog-40* (Bristol-Myers Squibb)
Injection, gel suspension: 80 mg/mL	*Trivaris* (Allergan)

Indications

Allergic states: Control of severe or incapacitating allergic conditions intractable to conventional treatment in serum sickness and drug hypersensitivity reactions. Parenteral therapy is indicated for urticarial transfusion reactions and acute noninfectious laryngeal edema (epinephrine is the drug of first choice).

Collagen diseases: For exacerbation of maintenance therapy in selected cases of systemic lupus erythematosus, acute rheumatic carditis, or systemic dermatomyositis (polymyositis).

Dermatologic diseases: Pemphigus; bullous dermatitis herpetiformis; severe erythema multiforme (Stevens-Johnson syndrome); mycosis fungoides; severe psoriasis; angioedema or urticaria; exfoliative, severe seborrheic, contact, or atopic dermatitis.

Diagnostic testing: Adrenocortical hyperfunction (**dexamethasone**).

Edematous states: To induce diuresis or remission of proteinuria in the nephrotic syndrome (without uremia) of the idiopathic type or that caused by lupus erythematosus.

Endocrine disorders: Primary or secondary adrenal cortical insufficiency (**hydrocortisone** or **cortisone** is the drug of choice; synthetic analogs may be used in conjunction with mineralocorticoids; in infancy, mineralocorticoid supplementation is important); congenital adrenal hyperplasia; nonsuppurative thyroiditis; hypercalcemia associated with cancer.

Parenteral – Acute adrenal cortical insufficiency (**hydrocortisone** or **cortisone** is drug of choice); preoperatively or in serious trauma or illness with known adrenal insufficiency or when adrenal cortical reserve is doubtful; shock unresponsive to conventional therapy if adrenal cortical insufficiency exists or is suspected.

GI diseases: Ulcerative colitis; regional enteritis (Crohn disease); intractable sprue.

Hematologic disorders: Idiopathic thrombocytopenic purpura (ITP) and secondary thrombocytopenia in adults; acquired (autoimmune) hemolytic anemia; Diamond-Blackfan anemia; erythroblastopenia (red blood cell anemia); congenital (erythroid) hypoplastic anemia.

Intralesional administration: Keloids; localized hypertrophic, infiltrated, inflammatory lesions of lichen planus, psoriatic plaques, granuloma annulare, lichen simplex chronicus (neurodermatitis); discoid lupus erythematosus; necrobiosis lipoidica diabeticorum; alopecia areata. May be useful in cystic tumors of an aponeurosis or tendon (ganglia).

Neoplastic diseases: Palliative management of leukemias and lymphomas in adults; acute leukemia in childhood.

Ophthalmic: Severe acute and chronic allergic and inflammatory processes involving the eye and its adnexa.

Rheumatic disorders: Adjunctive therapy for short-term use (acute episode or exacerbation) in psoriatic arthritis; rheumatoid arthritis (RA), including juvenile RA; ankylosing spondylitis; acute and subacute bursitis; acute, nonspecific tenosynovitis; acute gouty arthritis; posttraumatic osteoarthritis; synovitis of osteoarthritis; epicondylitis.

Respiratory diseases: Acute exacerbations of chronic obstructive pulmonary disease (COPD); asthma (distinct from allergic asthma); fulminating or disseminated pulmonary tuberculosis when used concurrently with appropriate antituberculous chemotherapy; hypersensitivity pneumonitis; idiopathic eosinophilic pneumonias; idiopathic pulmonary fibrosis; *Pneumocystis carinii* pneumonia (PCP) associated with hypoxemia occurring in an HIV-positive individual who is also under treatment with appropriate anti-PCP antibiotics; and symptomatic sarcoidosis. Studies support the efficacy of systemic corticosteroids for the treatment of the following conditions: allergic bronchopulmonary aspergillosis and idiopathic bronchiolitis obliterans with organizing pneumonia; symptomatic sarcoidosis; Loeffler syndrome not manageable by other means; berylliosis; fulminating or disseminated pulmonary tuberculosis when used concurrently with appropriate antituberculous chemotherapy; aspiration pneumonitis; idiopathic eosinophilic pneumonias (**dexamethasone**).

Nervous system: Acute exacerbations of multiple sclerosis (MS); cerebral edema associated with primary or metastatic brain tumor, craniotomy, or head injury (**dexamethasone**).

Miscellaneous: Acute or chronic solid organ rejection (with or without other agents); tuberculous meningitis with subarachnoid block or impending block when accompanied by appropriate antituberculous chemotherapy; in trichinosis with neurologic or myocardial involvement.

Triamcinolone: Treatment of pulmonary emphysema where bronchospasm or bronchial edema plays a significant role, and diffuse interstitial pulmonary fibrosis (Hamman-Rich syndrome); in conjunction with diuretic agents to induce a diuresis in refractory CHF and in cirrhosis of the liver with refractory ascites; and for postoperative dental inflammatory reactions.

Administration and Dosage

The maximal activity of the adrenal cortex is between 2 and 8 am, and it is minimal between 4 pm and midnight. Exogenous corticosteroids suppress adrenocortical activity the least when given at the time of maximal activity (am). Therefore, administer glucocorticoids in the morning prior to 9 am.

Maintenance therapy: Decrease initial dosage in small amounts to the lowest dosage that maintains an adequate clinical response. If the drug is to be stopped after more than a few days of treatment, it usually should be withdrawn gradually.

Dosage adjustment: Changes in clinical status resulting from remissions or exacerbations of the disease, individual drug responsiveness, and the effect of stress (ie, surgery, infection, trauma) may require dosage adjustment.

Withdrawal of therapy: If, after long-term therapy, the drug is to be stopped, it must be withdrawn gradually. If spontaneous remission occurs in a chronic condition, discontinue treatment gradually.

Alternate-day therapy: Alternate-day therapy is a dosing regimen in which twice the usual daily dose is administered every other morning. The purpose is to provide the patient requiring long-term treatment with the beneficial effects of corticosteroids while minimizing pituitary-adrenal suppression, the Cushingoid state, withdrawal symptoms, and growth suppression in children. The benefits of alternate-day therapy are only achieved by using the intermediate-acting agents.

Intra-articular injection: Dose depends on the joint size and varies with the severity of the condition. In chronic cases, injections may be repeated at intervals of at least 1 to 5 weeks depending upon the degree of relief obtained from the initial injection. Injection must be made into the synovial space.

Miscellaneous (tendinitis, epicondylitis, ganglion): In tendinitis or tenosynovitis, inject into the tendon sheath rather than into the substance of the tendon. In epicondylitis, outline the area of greatest tenderness and infiltrate the drug into the area.

Injections for local effect in dermatologic conditions: Avoid injection of sufficient material to cause blanching, since this may be followed by a small slough. One to 4 injections are usually employed.

BETAMETHASONE:

Betamethasone, oral –

Initial dosage: 0.6 to 7.2 mg/day.

Betamethasone sodium phosphate and acetate – Betamethasone sodium phosphate provides prompt activity, while betamethasone acetate affords sustained activity.

Systemic: Not for intravenous (IV) use.

Initial dose – 0.5 to 9 mg/day. Dosage ranges are 33% to 50% of the oral dose given every 12 hours. In certain acute, life-threatening situations, dosages exceeding the usual may be justified and may be in multiples of oral dosages.

Bursitis, tenosynovitis, peritendinitis: 1 mL given intrabursally.

RA and osteoarthritis: 0.5 to 2 mL given intra-articularly.

Very large joints – 1 to 2 mL.

Large joints – 1 mL.

Medium joints – 0.5 to 1 mL.

Small joints – 0.25 to 0.5 mL.

Dermatologic conditions: 0.2 mL/cm^2 intradermally.

Maximum dose – 1 mL/week.

Foot disorders – The following doses are recommended at 3- to 7-day intervals:

Bursitis:

Under heloma durum or heloma molle – 0.25 to 0.5 mL.

Under calcaneal spur – 0.5 mL.

Over hallux rigidus or digiti quinti varus – 0.5 mL.

Tenosynovitis, periostitis of cuboid: 0.5 mL.

Acute, gouty arthritis: 0.5 to 1 mL.

BUDESONIDE:

Adults – Take 9 mg once daily in the morning for up to 8 weeks. Swallow capsules whole; do not chew or break. For recurring episodes of active Crohn disease, a repeat 8-week course of budesonide can be given. Following an 8-week course of treatment and once the patient's symptoms are controlled, 6 mg is recommended once daily for maintenance for up to 3 months. If symptom control is still maintained at 3 months, an attempt to taper to complete cessation is recommended. Continued treatment for more than 3 months has not been shown to provide substantial clinical benefit.

Patients with mild to moderately active Crohn disease have been switched from oral prednisolone to budesonide with no reported episodes of adrenal insufficiency. Prednisolone tapering should begin concomitantly with initiating budesonide treatment.

Hepatic function impairment: Monitor patients with moderate to severe liver disease for increased signs and/or symptoms of hypercorticism. Consider reducing the dose of budesonide in these patients.

CYP3A4 inhibitors: If concomitant administration with ketoconazole or any other CYP3A4 inhibitor is indicated, closely monitor patients for increased signs and/or symptoms of hypercorticism. Consider reduction in budesonide dose.

CORTISONE:

Initial dosage – 25 to 300 mg/day. In less severe diseases, lower doses may suffice.

DEXAMETHASONE:

Dexamethasone, oral –

Initial dosage: 0.75 to 9 mg/day.

Children: The range of initial doses is 0.02 to 0.3 mg/kg/day in 3 or 4 divided doses (0.6 to 9 mg/m^2 body surface area [BSA]/day).

Maintenance dosage: Decrease initial dosage in small decrements at appropriate time intervals until the lowest dosage that maintains an adequate clinical response is reached. If the drug is to be stopped after more than a few days of treatment, it usually should be withdrawn gradually.

Discontinuation of long-term therapy: If, after long-term therapy, the drug is to be stopped, it is recommended that it be withdrawn gradually, rather than abruptly.

Acute exacerbation of multiple sclerosis: Daily doses of dexamethasone 30 mg for a week followed by 4 to 12 mg every other day for one month have been shown to be effective.

Acute, self-limited allergic disorders or acute exacerbations of chronic allergic disorders: The following dosage schedule combining parenteral (dexamethasone sodium phosphate injection 4 mg/mL) and oral (0.75 mg tablets) therapy is suggested: first day, 1 or 2 mL intramuscularly (IM); second day, 4 tablets in 2 divided doses; third day, 4 tablets in 2 divided doses; fourth day, 2 tablets in 2 divided doses; fifth day, 1 tablet; sixth day, 1 tablet; seventh day, no treatment; eighth day, follow-up visit.

Palliative management of recurrent or inoperable brain tumors: 2 mg 2 or 3 times/day for maintenance therapy.

Administration of Intensol: Mix with liquid (eg, water, juices, soda-like beverages) or semi-solid food (eg, applesauce, pudding). Use the provided calibrated dropper to administer prescribed amount of *Intensol* into a liquid or semi-solid food. Stir gently for a few seconds. Consume the entire amount of liquid or food immediately; do not store for future use.

Suppression tests: For Cushing syndrome, give 1 mg at 11 pm. Draw blood for plasma cortisol determination the following day at 8 am. For greater accuracy, give

0.5 mg every 6 hours for 48 hours. Collect 24-hour urine to determine 17-hydroxycorticosteroid excretion.

Test to distinguish Cushing syndrome due to pituitary adrenocorticotropic hormone excess from Cushing syndrome due to other causes – Give 2 mg every 6 hours for 48 hours. Collect 24-hour urine to determine 17-hydroxycorticosteroid excretion.

Dexamethasone sodium phosphate –

Initial dosage: 0.5 to 9 mg daily. When the IV route is used, dosage should usually be the same as the oral dosage. However, in certain acute, life-threatening situations, dosages exceeding the usual may be justified and may be in multiples of the oral dosages.

Cerebral edema: In adults, administer an initial IV dose of 10 mg, followed by 4 mg IM every 6 hours until maximum response has been noted. Response is usually noted within 12 to 24 hours. Dosage may be reduced after 2 to 4 days and gradually discontinued over 5 to 7 days. For palliative management of patients with recurrent or inoperable brain tumors, maintenance therapy with either the injection or tablets in a dosage of 2 mg 2 or 3 times daily may be effective.

Unresponsive shock: Reported regimens range from 1 to 6 mg/kg as a single IV injection, to 40 mg initially followed by repeated IV injections every 2 to 6 hours while shock persists.

HYDROCORTISONE (Cortisol):

Hydrocortisone, oral –

Initial dosage: 20 to 240 mg/day.

Hydrocortisone sodium succinate – May be administered IV or IM. The initial dose is 100 to 500 mg, and may be repeated at 2-, 4-, or 6-hour intervals depending on patient response and clinical condition.

METHYLPREDNISOLONE:

Methylprednisolone, oral –

Initial dose: 4 to 48 mg/day; adjust until a satisfactory response is noted. Determine maintenance dose by decreasing initial dose in small decrements at appropriate intervals until reaching the lowest effective dose.

Dosepak 21 therapy: Six 4 mg tablets on day 1. Decrease by 1 tablet per day.

Methylprednisolone sodium succinate –

Initial dose: 10 to 40 mg IV, administered over 1 to several minutes. Give subsequent doses IV or IM.

Infants and children: Not less than 0.5 mg/kg/24 hours.

High-dose therapy: For high-dose therapy, give 30 mg/kg IV, infused over 10 to 20 minutes. May repeat every 4 to 6 hours, not beyond 48 to 72 hours.

Methylprednisolone acetate – Not for IV use. As a temporary substitute for oral therapy, administer the total daily dose as a single IM injection. For prolonged effect, give a single weekly dose.

Adrenogenital syndrome: A single 40 mg injection IM every 2 weeks.

RA: Weekly IM maintenance dose varies from 40 to 120 mg.

Dermatologic lesions: 40 to 120 mg IM weekly for 1 to 4 weeks. In severe dermatitis, relief may result within 8 to 12 hours of a single dose of 80 to 120 mg IM. In chronic contact dermatitis, repeated injections every 5 to 10 days may be necessary. In seborrheic dermatitis, a weekly dose of 80 mg IM may be adequate.

Asthma and allergic rhinitis: 80 to 120 mg IM.

Intra-articular and soft tissue: 4 to 80 mg.

Intralesional: 20 to 60 mg.

PREDNISOLONE:

Prednisolone, prednisolone acetate –

Initial dosage: 5 to 60 mg/day.

Multiple sclerosis: In treatment of acute exacerbations of MS, 200 mg daily for a week followed by 80 mg every other day for 1 month.

Dose/Volume Chart for Prednisolone Syrup	
Prednisolone dose (mg)	Volume of syrup
15 mg	5 mL (1 teaspoonful)
10 mg	3.33 mL (⅔ teaspoonful)
7.5 mg	2.5 mL (½ teaspoonful)
5 mg	1.66 mL (⅓ teaspoonful)

Prednisolone sodium phosphate –

Intra-articular, intralesional, or soft tissue administration: 2 to 30 mg.

Oral:

Initial dosage – 5 to 60 mg/day.

Multiple sclerosis (acute exacerbations) – 200 mg daily for a week, followed by 80 mg every other day or dexamethasone 4 to 8 mg every other day for 1 month.

Tablets, orally disintegrating – Do not break or use partial orally disintegrating tablets. Use an appropriate formulation of prednisolone if indicated dose cannot be obtained using orally disintegrating tablets. This may become important in the treatment of conditions that require tapering doses that cannot be adequately accommodated by orally disintegrating tablets, eg, tapering the dose below 10 mg.

The initial dose may vary from 10 to 60 mg (prednisolone base) per day, depending on the specific disease entity being treated.

Prednisolone orally disintegrating tablets are packaged in a blister. Patients should be instructed not to remove the tablet from the blister until just prior to dosing. The blister pack should then be peeled open, and the orally disintegrating tablet placed on the tongue, where tablets may be swallowed whole as any conventional tablet, or allowed to dissolve in the mouth, with or without the assistance of water. Orally disintegrating tablet dosage forms are friable and are not intended to be cut, split, or broken.

In children, the initial dose of prednisolone may vary depending on the specific disease entity being treated. The range of initial doses is 0.14 to 2 mg/kg/day in 3 or 4 divided doses (4 to 60 mg/m^2 bsa/day).

The standard regimen used to treat nephrotic syndrome in children is 60 mg/m^2/day given in 3 divided doses for 4 weeks, followed by 4 weeks of single dose alternate-day therapy at 40 mg/m^2/day.

The National Heart, Lung, and Blood Institute recommended dosing for systemic prednisone, prednisolone, or methylprednisolone in children whose asthma is uncontrolled by inhaled corticosteroids and long-acting bronchodilators is 1 to 2 mg/kg/day in single or divided doses. It is further recommended that short course, or burst therapy, be continued until a child achieves a peak expiratory flow rate of 80% of his or her personal best or symptoms resolve. This usually requires 3 to 10 days of treatment.

Prednisolone Equivalent Dosages to Various Glucocorticoids[a]

Drug	Prednisolone ODT 10 mg	Prednisolone oral solution 5 mg	Prednisolone oral solution 15 mg
Betamethasone	1.75 mg	0.75 mg	2.25 mg
Cortisone	50 mg	25 mg	75 mg
Dexamethasone	1.75 mg	0.75 mg	2.25 mg
Hydrocortisone	40 mg	20 mg	60 mg
Methylprednisolone	8 mg	4 mg	12 mg
Paramethasone	4 mg	2 mg	6 mg
Prednisolone	10 mg	5 mg	15 mg
Prednisone	10 mg	5 mg	15 mg
Triamcinolone	8 mg	4 mg	12 mg

[a] Dose relationships apply only to oral or intravenous (IV) administration of these compounds. When these substances or their derivatives are injected intramuscularly or into joint spaces, their relative properties may be greatly altered.

These dose relationships apply only to oral or IV administration of these compounds. When these substances or their derivatives are injected intramuscularly or into joint spaces, their relative properties may be greatly altered.

PREDNISONE: Initial dosage varies from 5 to 60 mg/day. Prednisone is inactive and must be metabolized to prednisolone. This may be impaired in patients with liver disease.

TRIAMCINOLONE:

Triamcinolone hexacetonide – Not for IV use.

Intra-articular: 2 to 20 mg average.

Intralesional or sublesional: Up to 0.5 mg per square inch of affected area.

Triamcinolone acetonide –

Systemic:

Kenalog-40 and Trivaris –

Initial dose: The suggested initial dose is 60 mg, injected deeply into the gluteal muscle. Atrophy of subcutaneous fat may occur if the injection is not properly given.

Acute exacerbations of multiple sclerosis: 160 mg daily for a week, followed by 64 mg every other day for 1 month.

Intra-articular or intrabursal administration and for injection into tendon sheaths:

Initial dose – 2.5 to 5 mg for smaller joints and 5 to 15 mg for larger joints. For adults, doses up to 10 mg for smaller areas and up to 40 mg for larger areas are usually sufficient.

Intradermal: Use only 3 or 10 mg/mL. Initial dose varies; limit to 1 mg per site.

Children –

Intra-articular:

Usual dose – May vary from 2.5 to 5 mg for smaller joints and from 5 to 15 mg for larger joints, depending on the specific disease entity being treated.

Kenalog-40 and Trivaris only:

Initial dose – May vary depending on the specific disease entity being treated. The range of initial dosages is 0.11 to 1.6 mg/kg/day in 3 or 4 divided doses (3.2 to 48 mg/m^2 body surface area per day).

Actions

Pharmacology: The naturally occurring adrenal cortical steroids have both anti-inflammatory (glucocorticoid) and salt-retaining (mineralocorticoid) properties. These compounds are used as replacement therapy in adrenocortical deficiency states and may be used for their anti-inflammatory effects.

Pharmacokinetics: **Hydrocortisone** and most of its congeners are readily absorbed from the GI tract; altered onsets and durations are usually achieved with injections of suspensions and esters. Hydrocortisone is metabolized by the liver, which is the rate-limiting step in its clearance. The metabolism and excretion of the synthetic glucocorticoids generally parallel hydrocortisone. Induction of hepatic enzymes will increase the metabolic clearance of hydrocortisone and the synthetic glucocorticoids.

Glucocorticoid Equivalencies, Potencies, and Half-Life

Glucocorticoid	Equivalent potency dose (mg)[a]	Anti-inflammatory potency[a]	Sodium-retaining potency	Half-life plasma (min)
Short-acting				
Cortisone	25	0.8	2	30
Hydrocortisone	20	1	2	80 to 118
Intermediate-acting				
Methylprednisolone	4	5	0	78 to 188
Prednisone	5	4	1	60
Prednisolone	5	4	1	115 to 212
Triamcinolone	4	5	0	200+
Long-acting				
Betamethasone	0.6 to 0.75	20 to 30	0	300+
Dexamethasone	0.75	20 to 30	0	110 to 210

[a] When converting doses, use only equivalent potency column, not anti-inflammatory potency column.

Contraindications

Systemic fungal infections; hypersensitivity to the drug; IM use in ITP; administration of live virus vaccines (eg, smallpox) in patients receiving immunosuppressive corticosteroid doses (see Warnings).

Warnings/Precautions

Infections: Corticosteroids may mask signs of infection, and new infections may appear during their use. There may be decreased resistance and inability of the host defense mechanisms to prevent dissemination of the infection. Restrict use in active tuberculosis to cases of fulminating or disseminated disease in which the corticosteroid is used for disease management with appropriate chemotherapy. Corticosteroids may exacerbate systemic fungal infections and may activate latent amebiasis.

Hepatitis: Corticosteroids may be harmful in chronic active hepatitis positive for hepatitis B surface antigen.

Ocular effects: Prolonged use may produce posterior subcapsular cataracts, glaucoma with possible damage to the optic nerves, and may enhance the establishment of secondary ocular infections caused by fungi or viruses.

Fluid and electrolyte balance: Average and large doses of **hydrocortisone** or **cortisone** can cause elevation of blood pressure, salt and water retention, and increased excretion of potassium. These effects are less likely to occur with the synthetic derivatives except when used in large doses.

Immunosuppression: During therapy, do not use live virus vaccines (eg, smallpox). Do not immunize patients who are receiving corticosteroids, especially high doses, because of possible hazards of neurological complications and a lack of antibody response. This does not apply to patients receiving corticosteroids as replacement therapy.

Adrenal suppression: Prolonged therapy of pharmacologic doses may lead to hypothalamic-pituitary-adrenal suppression. The degree of adrenal suppression varies with the dosage, relative glucocorticoid activity, biological half-life, and duration of glucocorticoid therapy within each individual. Adrenal suppression may be minimized by the use of intermediate-acting glucocorticoids (**prednisone, prednisolone, methylprednisolone**) on an alternate-day schedule.

Stress: In patients receiving or recently withdrawn from corticosteroid therapy subjected to unusual stress, increased dosage of rapidly acting corticosteroids is indicated before, during, and after stressful situations, except in patients on high-dose therapy.

Cardiovascular: Reports suggest an apparent association between corticosteroid use and left ventricular free wall rupture after a recent myocardial infarction.

Use the lowest possible dose: Make a benefit/risk decision in each individual case as to the size of the dose, duration of treatment, and the use of daily or intermittent therapy because complications of treatment are dependent on these factors.

Steroid psychosis: Steroid psychosis is characterized by a delirious or toxic psychosis with clouded sensorium. Other symptoms may include euphoria, insomnia, mood swings, personality changes, and severe depression. The onset of symptoms usually occurs within 15 to 30 days. Predisposing factors include doses greater than **prednisone** 40 mg equivalent, female predominance, and, possibly, a family history of psychiatric illness.

Multiple sclerosis: Although corticosteroids are effective in speeding the resolution of acute exacerbations of MS, they do not affect the ultimate outcome or natural history of the disease.

Repository injections: To minimize the likelihood and severity of atrophy, do not inject subcutaneously, avoid injection into the deltoid, and avoid repeated IM injections into the same site, if possible. Repository injections are not recommended as initial therapy in acute situations.

Local injections: Intra-articular injection may produce systemic and local effects. A marked increase in pain accompanied by local swelling, further restriction of joint motion, fever, and malaise is suggestive of septic arthritis. Frequent intra-articular injection may damage joint tissues.

Hypersensitivity reactions: Anaphylactoid reactions have occurred rarely with corticosteroid therapy.

Renal function impairment: Edema may occur in the presence of renal disease with a fixed or decreased glomerular filtration rate.

Special risk: Use with caution in the following situations: Nonspecific ulcerative colitis if there is a probability of impending perforation, abscess, or other pyogenic infection; diverticulitis; fresh intestinal anastomoses; hypertension; CHF; thromboembolitic tendencies; thrombophlebitis; osteoporosis; exanthema; Cushing syndrome; antibiotic-resistant infections; convulsive disorders; metastatic carcinoma; myasthenia gravis; vaccinia; varicella; diabetes mellitus; hypothyroidism, cirrhosis (enhanced effect of corticosteroids).

Pregnancy: Corticosteroids cross the placenta (**prednisone** has the poorest transport). Chronic maternal ingestion during the first trimester has shown a 1% incidence of cleft palate in humans. Hypoadrenalism has occurred.

Lactation: Corticosteroids appear in breast milk and could suppress growth, interfere with endogenous corticosteroid production, or cause other unwanted effects in the breast-feeding infant. However, large doses for short periods may not harm the infant. Alternatives to consider include waiting 3 to 4 hours after the dose before breast-feeding and using **prednisolone** rather than **prednisone**.

Children: Carefully observe growth and development of infants and children on prolonged corticosteroid therapy.

Elderly: Consider the risk/benefit factors of steroid use. Consider lower doses because of body changes caused by aging (ie, diminution of muscle mass and plasma volume).

Monitoring: Observe patients for weight increase, edema, hypertension, and excessive potassium excretion, as well as for less obvious signs of adrenocortical steroid-induced untoward effects. Monitor for a negative nitrogen balance due to protein catabolism. Evaluate blood pressure and body weight, and do routine laboratory studies, including 2-hour postprandial blood glucose and serum potassium and a chest x-ray at regular intervals during prolonged therapy. Upper GI x-rays are desirable in patients with known or suspected peptic ulcer disease or significant dyspepsia or in patients complaining of gastric distress.

Drug Interactions

Drugs that may be affected by glucocorticoids include anticholinesterases, anticoagulants, cyclosporine, digitalis glycosides, isoniazid, nondepolarizing neuromuscular blockers, potassium-depleting agents (eg, diuretics), salicylates, somatrem, and theophyllines. Drugs that may affect corticosteroids include aminoglutethimide, barbiturates, cholestyramine, oral contraceptives, ephedrine, estrogens, hydantoins, ketoconazole, macrolide antibiotics, and rifampin.

CYP3A4 inhibitors: If coadministration with a CYP3A4 inhibitor is indicated, closely monitor patients for increased signs or symptoms of hypercorticism. Consider reduction in **budesonide** dose.

Drug/Lab test interactions: Urine glucose and serum cholesterol levels may increase. Decreased serum levels of potassium, T_3, and a minimal decrease of T_4 may occur. Thyroid I^{131} uptake may be decreased. False-negative results with the nitroblue-tetrazolium test for bacterial infection. **Dexamethasone**, given for cerebral edema, may alter the results of a brain scan (decreased uptake of radioactive material).

Adverse Reactions

Adverse reactions that may occur include abdominal distension, acneiform eruptions, aggravation of preexisting psychiatric conditions, allergic dermatitis, anaphylactoid/hypersensitivity reactions, cardiac arrhythmias or electrocardiogram changes caused by potassium deficiency, convulsions, development of Cushingoid state (eg, moonface, buffalo hump, supraclavicular fat pad enlargement, central obesity), erythema, fatigue, glaucoma, glycosuria, headache, hirsutism, hyperglycemia, hypertension, hypocalcemia, hypokalemia, hypotension or shock-like reactions, impaired wound healing, increased appetite and weight gain, increased intraocular pressure, increased sweating, insomnia, malaise, menstrual irregularities, metabolic alkalosis, muscle mass loss, muscle weakness, myocardial rupture following recent myocardial infarction, nausea, neuritis/paresthesias, osteoporosis, pancreatitis, petechiae/ecchymoses, purpura, sodium and fluid retention, spontaneous fractures, steroid psychoses, suppression of growth in children, syncopal episodes, tendon rupture, thin fragile skin, thromboembolism or fat embolism, thrombophlebitis, ulcerative esophagitis, urticaria, vomiting, vertigo.

MIGLITOL

Tablets: 25, 50, and 100 mg (*Rx*) *Glyset* (Pfizer)

Indications

Type 2 diabetes: Monotherapy adjunct to diet to improve glycemic control in patients with type 2 diabetes whose hyperglycemia cannot be managed by diet alone.

Combination therapy – In combination with a sulfonylurea when diet plus either miglitol or a sulfonylurea alone do not result in adequate glycemic control. The effect of miglitol to enhance glycemic control is additive to that of sulfonylureas when used in combination, presumably because the mechanism of action is different.

Administration and Dosage

The use of miglitol must be viewed as a treatment in addition to diet and not as a substitute for diet or as a convenient mechanism for avoiding dietary restraint.

Initial dosage: The recommended starting dosage is 25 mg, given orally 3 times/day at the start (with the first bite) of each main meal. However, some patients may benefit by starting at 25 mg once daily to minimize GI adverse effects and gradually increasing the frequency of administration to 3 times/day.

Maintenance dosage: The usual maintenance dose of miglitol is 50 mg 3 times/day although some patients may benefit from increasing the dose to 100 mg 3 times/day. In order to allow adaptation to potential adverse effects, initiate miglitol therapy at a dosage of 25 mg 3 times/day, the lowest effective dosage, and then gradually titrate upward. After 4 to 8 weeks of the 25 mg 3 times/day regimen, increase the dosage to 50 mg 3 times/day for about 3 months if measured. Measure glycosylated hemoglobin level if not satisfactory, the dosage may be further increased to 100 mg 3 times/day, the maximum recommended dosage. If no further reduction in postprandial glucose or glycosylated hemoglobin levels is observed with titration to 100 mg 3 times/day, consider lowering the dose.

Maximum dosage: The maximum recommended dosage is 100 mg 3 times/day.

Combination with sulfonylureas: Because its mechanism of action is different, the effect of miglitol to enhance glycemic control is additive to that of sulfonylureas when used in combination. Miglitol given in combination with a sulfonylurea will cause a further lowering of blood glucose and may increase the risk of hypoglycemia caused by the additive effects of the 2 agents.

Actions

Pharmacology: Miglitol is an alpha-glucoside inhibitor that delays the digestion of ingested carbohydrates resulting in a smaller rise in blood glucose concentration following meals. Miglitol reduces levels of glycosylated hemoglobin in patients with type 2 (non-insulin-dependent) diabetes mellitus.

In contrast to sulfonylureas and thiazolidinediones, miglitol does not enhance insulin secretion. Miglitol has minor inhibitory activity against lactase and, at recommended doses, would not be expected to induce lactose intolerance.

Pharmacokinetics:

Absorption – Absorption of miglitol is saturable at high doses; a dose of 25 mg is completely absorbed, whereas a dose of 100 mg is only 50% to 70% absorbed. Peak concentrations are reached in 2 to 3 hours.

Distribution – The protein binding of miglitol is negligible (less than 4%). Miglitol has a volume of distribution of 0.18 L/kg, consistent with distribution primarily into the extracellular fluid.

Metabolism – No metabolites have been detected in plasma, urine, or feces, indicating a lack of either systemic or presystemic metabolism.

Excretion – Miglitol is eliminated by renal excretion as unchanged drug. Following a 25 mg dose, more than 95% of the dose is recovered in the urine within 24 hours. The elimination half-life from plasma is approximately 2 hours.

Contraindications

Diabetic ketoacidoses; inflammatory bowel disease; colonic ulceration; partial intestinal obstruction; patients predisposed to intestinal obstruction; chronic intestinal diseases associated with marked disorders of digestion or absorption or with conditions that may deteriorate as a result of increased gas formation in the intestine; hypersensitivity to the drug or any of its components.

Warnings/Precautions

GI: GI symptoms are the most common reactions to miglitol. The incidence of diarrhea and abdominal pain tend to diminish considerably with continued treatment.

Hypoglycemia: Because of its mechanism of action, miglitol, when administered alone, should not cause hypoglycemia. It may increase the hypoglycemic potential of the sulfonylurea. Use oral glucose (dextrose), whose absorption is not delayed by miglitol, instead of sucrose (cane sugar) in the treatment of mild to moderate hypoglycemia. Sucrose, whose hydrolysis to glucose and fructose is inhibited by miglitol, is unsuitable for the rapid correction of hypoglycemia. Severe hypoglycemia may require the use of either IV glucose infusion or glucagon injection.

Blood glucose control: When diabetic patients are exposed to stress such as fever, trauma, infection or surgery, a temporary loss of control of blood glucose may occur. At such times, temporary insulin therapy may be necessary.

Renal function impairment: Plasma concentrations of miglitol in renally impaired volunteers were proportionally increased relative to the degree of renal dysfunction. Long-term clinical trials in diabetic patients with significant renal dysfunction (serum creatinine more than 2 mg/dL) have not been conducted. Treatment of these patients with miglitol is not recommended.

Pregnancy: Category B.

Lactation: Although the levels of miglitol reached in breast milk are exceedingly low, do not administer miglitol to a breast-feeding woman.

Children: Safety and efficacy have not been established.

Monitoring: Monitor therapeutic response to miglitol by periodic blood glucose tests. Measurement of glycosylated hemoglobin levels is recommended for the monitoring of long-term glycemic control.

Drug Interactions

Drugs that may affect miglitol include digestive enzymes and intestinal adsorbents. Drugs that may be affected by miglitol include digoxin, glyburide, metformin, propranolol, and ranitidine.

Adverse Reactions

Adverse reactions may include skin rash (4.3%, generally transient), flatulence (41.5%), diarrhea (28.7%), and abdominal pain (11.7%).

Lab test abnormalities: Low serum iron (9.2%) usually does not persist in the majority of cases and is not associated with reductions in hemoglobin or changes in other hematologic indices.

PRAMLINTIDE ACETATE

Solution for injection: 0.6 and 1 mg/mL (*Rx*) *Symlin* (Amylin)

> **Warning:**
> Pramlintide is used with insulin and has been associated with an increased risk of insulin-induced severe hypoglycemia, particularly in patients with type 1 diabetes. When severe hypoglycemia associated with pramlintide use occurs, it is seen within 3 hours following a pramlintide injection. If severe hypoglycemia occurs while operating a motor vehicle, heavy machinery, or while engaging in other high-risk activities, serious injuries may occur. Appropriate patient selection, careful patient instruction, and insulin dose adjustments are critical elements for reducing this risk.

Indications

Pramlintide is given at mealtimes.

Type 1 diabetes mellitus: For type 1 diabetes, as an adjunct treatment in patients who use mealtime insulin therapy and who have failed to achieve desired glucose control despite optimal insulin therapy.

Type 2 diabetes mellitus: For type 2 diabetes, as an adjunct treatment in patients who use mealtime insulin therapy and who have failed to achieve desired glucose control despite optimal insulin therapy, with or without a concurrent sulfonylurea agent and/or metformin.

Administration and Dosage

Initiation of pramlintide therapy:

Patients with insulin-using type 2 diabetes – In patients with insulin-using type 2 diabetes, initiate pramlintide at a dose of 60 mcg and increase to a dose of 120 mcg as tolerated. Patients should initiate pramlintide at 60 mcg subcutaneously, immediately prior to major meals. Patients should reduce preprandial, rapid-acting, or short-acting insulin dosages, including fixed-mix insulins (eg, 70/30) by 50%.

Dosage adjustments: Increase the pramlintide dose to 120 mcg when no clinically significant nausea has occurred for 3 to 7 days. Patients should make pramlintide dose adjustments only as directed by the health care provider. If significant nausea persists at the 120 mcg dose, decrease the pramlintide dose to 60 mcg.

Patients with type 1 diabetes – In patients with type 1 diabetes, initiate pramlintide at a dose of 15 mcg and titrate at 15 mcg increments to a maintenance dose of 30 or 60 mcg as tolerated.

Patients should initiate pramlintide at a starting dose of 15 mcg subcutaneously, immediately prior to major meals. Patients should reduce preprandial, rapid-acting, or short-acting insulin dosages, including fixed-mix insulins (eg, 70/30) by 50%.

Dosage adjustments: Increase the pramlintide dose to the next increment (30, 45, or 60 mcg) when no clinically significant nausea has occurred for at least 3 days. Patients should only make pramlintide dose adjustments as directed by a health care provider. If significant nausea persists at the 45 or 60 mcg dose level, decrease the pramlintide dose to 30 mcg. If the 30 mcg dose is not tolerated, consider discontinuation of pramlintide therapy.

Optimizing therapy (type 1 and type 2 diabetic patients): After a maintenance dose of pramlintide is achieved, instruct both insulin-using patients with type 1 or type 2 diabetes to adjust insulin doses to optimize glycemic control once the target dose of pramlintide is achieved and nausea (if experienced) has subsided. Patients should only make insulin dose adjustments as directed by a health care provider.

Advise patients to contact a health care provider in the event of recurrent nausea or hypoglycemia. Patients should view an increased frequency of mild to moderate hypoglycemia as a warning sign of increased risk for severe hypoglycemia.

Administration: Administer pramlintide subcutaneously immediately prior to each major meal (250 kcal or more or containing 30 g or more of carbohydrate).

Pramlintide should be at room temperature before injection to reduce potential injection-site reactions. Administer each pramlintide dose subcutaneously into the abdomen or thigh (administration into the arm is not recommended because of variable absorption). Rotate injection sites so that the same site is not used repeatedly. The injection site selected should also be distinct from the site chosen for any concomitant insulin injection.

- Always administer pramlintide and insulin as separate injections.
- Do not mix pramlintide with any type of insulin.
- If dose is missed, wait until the next scheduled dose and administer the usual amount.

Vials – To administer pramlintide from vials, use a U-100 insulin syringe (preferably a 0.3 mL [0.3 cc] size) for optimal accuracy. If using a syringe calibrated for use with U-100 insulin, use the following chart to measure the microgram dosage in unit increments. Always use separate, new syringes and needles to give pramlintide injections.

Pramlintide Dose Conversion to Insulin Unit Equivalents

Pramlintide dosage prescribed (mcg)	Increment using a U-100 syringe (units)	Volume (cc or mL)
15	2.5	0.025
30	5	0.05
45	7.5	0.075
60	10	0.1
120	20	0.2

Pen-injectors: The pen-injector is available in 2 presentations:

- 60 pen-injector for doses of 15, 30, 45, and 60 mcg
- 120 pen-injector for doses of 60 and 120 mcg.

The patient should be advised:

- to confirm they are using the correct pen-injector that will deliver their prescribed dose
- on proper use of the pen-injector, emphasizing how and when to set up a new pen-injector
- not to transfer pramlintide from the pen-injector to a syringe. Doing so could result in a higher dose than intended because pramlintide in the pen-injector is a higher concentration than pramlintide in the pramlintide vial
- not to share the pen-injector and needles with others
- that needles are not included with the pen-injector and must be purchased separately
- which needle length and gauge should be used
- to use a new needle for each injection.

Discontinuation of therapy: Discontinue pramlintide therapy if any of the following occur:

- recurrent unexplained hypoglycemia that requires medical assistance
- persistent clinically significant nausea
- noncompliance with self-monitoring of blood glucose concentrations
- noncompliance with insulin dose adjustments
- noncompliance with scheduled health care professional contacts or recommended clinic visits.

Actions

Pharmacology: Pramlintide is a synthetic analog of human amylin, a naturally occurring neuroendocrine hormone synthesized by pancreatic beta cells that contributes to glucose control during the postprandial period.

Pharmacokinetics:

Absorption – The absolute bioavailability of a single subcutaneous dose of pramlintide is approximately 30% to 40%.

Injection of pramlintide into the arm showed higher exposure with greater variability compared with exposure after injection of pramlintide into the abdominal area or thigh.

Distribution – Pramlintide does not bind extensively to blood cells or albumin (approximately 40% of the drug is unbound in plasma).

Metabolism/Excretion – In healthy subjects, the half-life of pramlintide is approximately 48 minutes. Pramlintide is metabolized primarily by the kidneys. AUC values are relatively constant with repeat dosing, indicating no bioaccumulation.

Pharmacodynamics – In clinical studies in patients with insulin-using type 1 or type 2 diabetes, pramlintide administration resulted in a reduction in mean postprandial glucose concentrations, reduced glucose fluctuations, and reduced food intake. Pramlintide doses differ for insulin-using type 1 or type 2 patients.

Reduction in postprandial glucose concentrations: Pramlintide administered subcutaneously immediately prior to a meal reduced plasma glucose concentrations after the meal when used with regular insulin or rapid-acting insulin analogs.

Contraindications

Known hypersensitivity to pramlintide acetate or any of its components, including metacresol; diagnosis of gastroparesis; hypoglycemia.

Warnings/Precautions

Patient selection: Proper patient selection is critical to safe and effective use of pramlintide.

Before initiation of therapy, review the patient's HbA_{1c}, recent blood glucose monitoring data, history of insulin-induced hypoglycemia, current insulin regimen, and body weight. Only consider pramlintide therapy in patients with insulin-using type 1 or type 2 diabetes who fulfill the following criteria:

- have failed to achieve adequate glycemic control despite individualized insulin management;
- are receiving ongoing care under the guidance of a health care professional skilled in the use of insulin and supported by the services of diabetes educator(s).

Do not consider patients for pramlintide therapy if they meet any of the following criteria:

- poor compliance with current insulin regimen,
- poor compliance with prescribed self-blood glucose monitoring,
- have an HbA_{1c} greater than 9%,
- recurrent severe hypoglycemia requiring assistance during the past 6 months,
- presence of hypoglycemia unawareness,
- confirmed diagnosis of gastroparesis,
- require the use of drugs that stimulate GI motility,
- children.

Hypoglycemia: Pramlintide alone does not cause hypoglycemia. However, pramlintide is indicated to be coadministered with insulin therapy, and, in this setting, pramlintide increases the risk of insulin-induced severe hypoglycemia, particularly in patients with type 1 diabetes. Severe hypoglycemia associated with pramlintide occurs within the first 3 hours following a pramlintide injection.

Drugs that increase the susceptibility to hypoglycemia – The addition of any antihyperglycemic agent (eg, pramlintide) to an existing regimen of 1 or more antihyperglycemic agents (eg, insulin, sulfonylurea) or to other agents that may increase the risk of hypoglycemia may necessitate further insulin dose adjustments and particularly close monitoring of blood glucose.

Hypersensitivity reactions:

Local – Patients may experience redness, swelling, or itching at the site of injection. These minor reactions usually resolve within a few days to a few weeks. In some instances, these reactions may be related to factors other than pramlintide, such as irritants in a skin-cleansing agent or improper injection technique.

Hazardous tasks: Severe hypoglycemia associated with pramlintide occurs within the first 3 hours following a pramlintide injection. If severe hypoglycemia occurs while operating a motor vehicle, heavy machinery, or while engaging in other high-risk activities, serious injuries may occur.

Pregnancy: Category C.

Lactation: It is unknown whether pramlintide is excreted in human milk.

Children: Safety and efficacy of pramlintide in children have not been established.

Monitoring: Monitor blood glucose frequently, including pre- and post-meals and at bedtime.

Drug Interactions

Drugs that alter GI motility/absorption: Because of its effects on gastric emptying, do not consider pramlintide therapy for patients taking drugs that alter GI motility (eg, anticholinergic agents such as atropine) and agents that slow the intestinal absorption of nutrients (eg, alpha-glucosidase inhibitors). Patients using these drugs have not been studied in clinical trials.

Pramlintide delays absorption of concomitantly administered drugs: Pramlintide has the potential to delay the absorption of coadministered oral medications. When the rapid onset of an orally coadministered agent is a critical determinant of effectiveness (eg, analgesics), administer the agent at least 1 hour prior to or 2 hours after pramlintide injection.

Adverse Reactions

Adverse reactions (excluding hypoglycemia) commonly associated with pramlintide (at least 3%) when coadministered with a fixed dose of insulin in insulin-using type 2 diabetic patients and in type 1 diabetic patients are listed in the following: abdominal pain, allergic reaction, anorexia, arthralgia, coughing, dizziness, fatigue, headache, inflicted injury, nausea, pharyngitis, vomiting.

GI: Most adverse events were gastrointestinal in nature. The incidence of nausea was higher at the beginning of pramlintide treatment and decreased with time in most patients. The incidence and severity of nausea are reduced when pramlintide is gradually titrated to the recommended doses.

Severe hypoglycemia: Pramlintide alone (without the coadministration of insulin) does not cause hypoglycemia. However, pramlintide is indicated as an adjunct treatment in patients who use mealtime insulin therapy, and coadministration of pramlintide with insulin may increase the risk of insulin-induced hypoglycemia, particularly in patients with type 1 diabetes.

EXENATIDE

Injection, solution: 250 mcg/mL (*Rx*)	*Byetta* (Amylin Pharmaceuticals)

Indications

Type 2 diabetes mellitus: As adjunctive therapy to diet and exercise to improve glycemic control in adult patients with type 2 diabetes mellitus.

Administration and Dosage

Dosage: Initiate at 5 mcg per dose administered twice daily at any time within the 60-minute period before the morning and evening meals. Exenatide should not be administered after a meal. The dose of exenatide can be increased to 10 mcg twice daily after 1 month of therapy. Each dose should be administered as a subcutaneous injection in the thigh, abdomen, or upper arm.

Renal function impairment: Use caution when escalating doses of exenatide from 5 to 10 mcg in patients with moderate renal impairment (creatinine clearance [CrCl] 30 to 50 mL/min).

Actions

Pharmacology: Incretins enhance glucose-dependent insulin secretion. Exenatide is an incretin mimetic agent that mimics the enhancement of glucose-dependent insulin secretion by the pancreatic beta-cell, suppresses inappropriately elevated glucagon secretion, and slows gastric emptying.

Pharmacokinetics:

Absorption – After subcutaneous administration, exenatide reaches median peak plasma concentrations in 2.1 hours.

Distribution – The mean apparent volume of distribution of a single dose of exenatide is 28.3 L.

Metabolism/Excretion – Exenatide is predominantly eliminated by glomerular filtration. The mean terminal half-life is 2.4 hours.

Contraindications

Known hypersensitivity to this product or any of its components.

Warnings/Precautions

Insulin: Exenatide is not a substitute for insulin in insulin-requiring patients. Do not use exenatide in patients with type 1 diabetes or for the treatment of diabetic ketoacidosis.

Acute pancreatitis: Postmarketing cases of acute pancreatitis have been reported in patients treated with exenatide. Do not resume treatment with exenatide if pancreatitis is confirmed and an alternative etiology for the pancreatitis has not been identified.

Renal effects: There have been postmarketing reports of altered renal function, including increased serum creatinine, renal impairment, worsened chronic renal failure, and acute renal failure, sometimes requiring hemodialysis or kidney transplantation.

Renal function impairment: Exenatide is not recommended for use in patients with end-stage renal disease or severe renal function impairment (CrCl less than 30 mL/min). Use exenatide with caution in patients with renal transplantation.

GI disease: Exenatide has not been studied in patients with severe GI disease, including gastroparesis. Its use is commonly associated with GI adverse reactions, including nausea, vomiting, and diarrhea. The use of exenatide is not recommended in patients with severe GI disease.

Immunogenicity: Patients may develop anti-exenatide antibodies following treatment with exenatide. In most patients who develop antibodies, antibody titers diminish with time.

Hypersensitivity reactions: There have been postmarketing reports of serious hypersensitivity reactions (eg, anaphylaxis, angioedema) in patients treated with exenatide.

Fertility impairment: Administration of pramlintide 0.3, 1, or 3 mg/kg/day (8, 17, and 82 times the exposure resulting from the maximum recommended human dose based on body surface area, respectively) had no significant effects on fertility in male or female rats. The highest dose of 3 mg/kg/day resulted in dystocia in 8 of 12 female rats secondary to significant decreases in serum calcium levels.

Pregnancy: Category C.

Lactation: It is not known whether exenatide is excreted in human milk.

Children: Safety and efficacy of exenatide have not been established in children.

Monitoring: Monitor glycemic control and international normalized ratio (INR) in patients who are also taking warfarin.

Monitor patients for signs and symptoms of hypersensitivity reactions and pancreatitis.

Drug Interactions

Use exenatide with caution in patients receiving oral medications that require rapid GI absorption. For oral medications that are dependent on threshold concentrations for efficacy, such as contraceptives and antibiotics, advise patients to take those drugs at least 1 hour before exenatide. If such drugs are to be administered with food, advise patients to take them with a meal or snack when exenatide is not administered.

Drugs that may be affected by exenatide include acetaminophen, digoxin, lovastatin, oral antibiotics, oral contraceptives, other hypoglycemic agents (eg meglitinides, sulfonylureas), and warfarin.

Drug/Food interactions: Do not administer exenatide after a meal; administer exenatide 60 minutes before the 2 main meals of the day, approximately 6 hours or more apart.

Adverse Reactions

Adverse reactions occurring in at least 3% of patients include the following: asthenia, diarrhea, dizziness, dyspepsia, feeling jittery, gastroesophageal reflux disease, headache, hyperhidrosis, hypoglycemia, nausea, vomiting.

LIRAGLUTIDE

Injection, solution: 6 mg/mL (*Rx*)	*Victoza* (Novo Nordisk)

Warning:

Thyroid C-cell tumor risk: Liraglutide causes dose-dependent and treatment-duration–dependent thyroid C-cell tumors at clinically relevant exposures in both genders of rats and mice. It is unknown whether liraglutide causes thyroid C-cell tumors, including medullary thyroid carcinoma, in humans, as human relevance could not be ruled out by clinical or nonclinical studies. Liraglutide is contraindicated in patients with a personal or family history of medullary thyroid carcinoma and in patients with multiple endocrine neoplasia syndrome type 2 (MEN2). Based on the findings in rodents, monitoring with serum calcitonin or thyroid ultrasound was performed during clinical trials, but this may have increased the number of unnecessary thyroid surgeries. It is unknown whether monitoring with serum calcitonin or thyroid ultrasound will mitigate human risk of thyroid C-cell tumors. Counsel patients regarding the risk and symptoms of thyroid tumors.

Indications

Type 2 diabetes mellitus: As an adjunct to diet and exercise to improve glycemic control in adults with type 2 diabetes mellitus.

Important limitations of use: Because of the uncertain relevance of the rodent thyroid C-cell tumor findings to humans, prescribe liraglutide only to patients for whom the potential benefits are considered to outweigh the potential risk. Liraglutide is not recommended as first-line therapy for patients who have inadequate glycemic control on diet and exercise.

In clinical trials of liraglutide, there were more cases of pancreatitis with liraglutide than with comparators. Liraglutide has not been studied sufficiently in patients with a history of pancreatitis to determine whether these patients are at increased risk for pancreatitis while using liraglutide. Use with caution in patients with a history of pancreatitis.

The concurrent use of liraglutide and insulin has not been studied.

Administration and Dosage

General dosing: The 0.6 mg dose is a starting dose intended to reduce GI symptoms during initial titration and is not effective for glycemic control.

Adults:

Type 2 diabetes mellitus –

Initial dosage: 0.6 mg subcutaneously per day for 1 week.

Dosage titration: After 1 week at 0.6 mg/day subcutaneously, the dose should be increased to 1.2 mg. If the 1.2 mg dose does not result in acceptable glycemic control, the dose can be increased to 1.8 mg.

Concomitant therapy: When initiating liraglutide, consider reducing the dose of administered insulin secretagogues (such as sulfonylureas) to reduce the risk of hypoglycemia.

Administration: Liraglutide can be administered once daily at any time of day, independently of meals, and can be injected subcutaneously in the abdomen, thigh, or upper arm. The injection site and timing can be changed without dose adjustment.

Actions

Pharmacology: Liraglutide is an acylated glucagonlike peptide 1 (GLP-1) receptor agonist. Like GLP-1(7-37), liraglutide activates the GLP-1 receptor, a membrane-bound cell-surface receptor coupled to adenylyl cyclase by the stimulatory G-protein, Gs, in pancreatic beta cells. Liraglutide increases intracellular cyclic AMP (cAMP), leading to insulin release in the presence of elevated glucose concentrations. Liraglutide also decreases glucagon secretion in a glucose-dependent manner.

Pharmacokinetics:

Absorption – Following subcutaneous administration, maximum concentrations of liraglutide are achieved at 8 to 12 hours postdosing. The mean peak (C_{max}) and total (AUC) exposures of liraglutide were 35 ng/mL and 960 ng•h /mL, respectively, for a subcutaneous single dose of 0.6 mg. Absolute bioavailability of liraglutide following subcutaneous administration is approximately 55%.

Distribution – The mean apparent volume of distribution after subcutaneous administration of liraglutide 0.6 mg is approximately 13 L. Liraglutide is extensively bound to plasma protein (more than 98%).

Metabolism – Liraglutide is endogenously metabolized in a similar manner to large proteins without a specific organ as a major route of elimination.

Excretion – The mean apparent clearance following subcutaneous administration of a single dose of liraglutide is approximately 1.2 L/h with an elimination half-life of approximately 13 hours, making liraglutide suitable for once-daily administration.

Contraindications

Patients with a personal or family history of medullary thyroid carcinoma or in patients with MEN2.

Warnings/Precautions

Thyroid C-cell tumors: Liraglutide causes dose-dependent and treatment-duration–dependent thyroid C-cell tumors (adenomas and/or carcinomas) at clinically relevant exposures in both genders of rats and mice.

Pancreatitis: In clinical trials of liraglutide, there were 7 cases of pancreatitis among liraglutide-treated patients and 1 case among comparator-treated patients (2.2 vs 0.6 cases per 1,000 patient-years). After initiation of liraglutide and after dose increases, observe patients carefully for signs and symptoms of pancreatitis (including persistent severe abdominal pain sometimes radiating to the back and that may or may not be accompanied by vomiting). Use with caution in patients with a history of pancreatitis.

Macrovascular outcomes: There have been no clinical studies establishing conclusive evidence of macrovascular risk reduction with liraglutide or any other antidiabetic drug.

Insulin: Liraglutide is not a substitute for insulin. Do not use liraglutide in patients with type 1 diabetes mellitus or for the treatment of diabetic ketoacidosis because it would not be effective in these settings.

Gastroparesis: Liraglutide slows gastric emptying.

Immunogenicity: Consistent with the potentially immunogenic properties of protein and peptide pharmaceuticals, patients treated with liraglutide may develop anti-liraglutide antibodies.

Renal function impairment: There is limited experience in patients with mild, moderate, and severe renal impairment, including end-stage renal disease. No dose adjustment of liraglutide is recommended for patients with renal impairment.

Hepatic function impairment: There is limited experience in patients with mild, moderate, or severe hepatic impairment. No dose adjustment of liraglutide is recommended for patients with hepatic impairment.

Pregnancy: Category C.

Lactation: It is not known whether liraglutide is excreted in human milk. Because many drugs are excreted in human milk and because of the potential for tumorigenicity shown for liraglutide in animal studies, decide whether to discontinue breast-feeding or liraglutide.

Children: Safety and effectiveness of liraglutide have not been established in children. Liraglutide is not recommended for use in children.

Elderly: No overall differences in safety or effectiveness were observed between these patients and younger patients, but greater sensitivity of some older individuals cannot be ruled out.

Monitoring: Periodically measure blood glucose and HbA_{1c} with a goal of decreasing these levels toward the normal range.

Although routine monitoring of serum calcitonin is of uncertain value in patients treated with liraglutide, if serum calcitonin is measured and found to be elevated, refer the patient to an endocrinologist for further evaluation.

Observe patients carefully for signs and symptoms of pancreatitis, including persistent severe abdominal pain.

Drug Interactions

Oral medications: Liraglutide causes a delay of gastric emptying, and thereby has the potential to impact the absorption of administered oral medications.

Drugs that may interact with liraglutide include the following: antidiabetic agents (eg, sulfonylureas), acetaminophen, atorvastatin, digoxin, and griseofulvin.

Adverse Reactions

Liraglutide Injection vs Glimepiride Adverse Reactions (≥ 5%):

CNS – Dizziness, headache.

GI – Constipation, diarrhea, nausea, vomiting.

Respiratory – Nasopharyngitis, sinusitis, upper respiratory tract infection.

Miscellaneous – Back pain, hypertension, influenza, urinary tract infection.

SAXAGLIPTIN

Tablets; oral: 2.5 and 5 mg (*Rx*)	*Onglyza* (Bristol-Myers Squibb)

Indications

Type 2 diabetes mellitus: As an adjunct to diet and exercise to improve glycemic control in adults with type 2 diabetes mellitus.

Administration and Dosage

Adults:

Type 2 diabetes mellitus – 2.5 or 5 mg once daily.

Elderly: Take care in dose selection based on renal function.

Renal function impairment:

Moderate to severe renal impairment (creatinine clearance 50 mL/min or less) – 2.5 mg once daily.

End-stage renal disease requiring hemodialysis – 2.5 mg once daily after hemodialysis.

Strong CYP3A4/5 inhibitors: The dosage of saxagliptin is 2.5 mg once daily when coadministered with CYP3A4/5 inhibitors (eg, atazanavir, clarithromycin, indinavir, itraconazole, ketoconazole, nefazodone, nelfinavir, ritonavir, saquinavir, telithromycin).

Actions

Pharmacology: Saxagliptin is a competitive dipeptidyl peptidase-4 (DPP4) inhibitor that slows the inactivation of the incretin hormones, thereby increasing their bloodstream concentrations and reducing fasting and postprandial glucose concentrations in a glucose-dependent manner in patients with type 2 diabetes mellitus.

Pharmacokinetics:

Absorption – The median time to maximum concentration following the 5 mg once-daily dose was 2 hours for saxagliptin and 4 hours for its active metabolite.

Effect of food: Saxagliptin may be administered with or without food.

Distribution – The in vitro protein binding of saxagliptin and its active metabolite in human serum is negligible. Therefore, changes in blood protein levels in various disease states (eg, renal impairment, hepatic impairment) are not expected to alter the disposition of saxagliptin.

Metabolism – The metabolism of saxagliptin is primarily mediated by CYP3A4/5. The major metabolite of saxagliptin is also a DPP4 inhibitor, which is one-half as potent as saxagliptin.

Excretion – Saxagliptin is eliminated by both renal and hepatic pathways. Following a single oral dose of saxagliptin 5 mg to healthy subjects, the mean plasma terminal half-life for saxagliptin and its active metabolite was 2.5 and 3.1 hours, respectively.

Contraindications

None known.

Warnings/Precautions

Pregnancy: Category B.

Lactation: It is not known whether saxagliptin is secreted in human milk. Because many drugs are secreted in human milk, exercise caution when saxagliptin is administered to a breast-feeding woman.

Children: Safety and effectiveness of saxagliptin in children have not been established.

Elderly: Saxagliptin and its active metabolite are eliminated in part by the kidney. Because elderly patients are more likely to have decreased renal function, take care in dose selection in elderly patients based on renal function.

Drug Interactions

Drugs that may affect saxagliptin include aluminum hydroxide/magnesium hydroxide/simethicone, CYP3A4/5 inducers, famotidine, glyburide, metformin, moderate CYP3A4/5 inhibitors, simvastatin, and strong CYP3A4/5 inhibitors. Drugs that may be affected by saxagliptin include antidiabetic agents, diltiazem, glyburide, ketoconazole, and pioglitazone.

Adverse Reactions

Adverse reactions occurring in 3% or more of patients include headache, hypoglycemia, nasopharyngitis, peripheral edema, upper respiratory tract infection, and urinary tract infection.

SITAGLIPTIN PHOSPHATE

Tablets: 25, 50, and 100 mg (*Rx*)	*Januvia* (Merck)

Indications

Type 2 diabetes mellitus: As an adjunct to diet and exercise to improve glycemic control in patients with type 2 diabetes mellitus as monotherapy or in combination with metformin or a peroxisome proliferator–activated receptor- (PPAR) gamma agonist (eg, thiazolidinediones) when the single agent alone, with diet and exercise, does not provide adequate glycemic control.

Administration and Dosage

Dosage: 100 mg once daily as monotherapy or as combination therapy with metformin or a PPAR-gamma agonist (eg, thiazolidinediones). Sitagliptin can be taken with or without food.

Renal function impairment: For patients with mild renal function impairment (creatinine clearance [CrCl] 50 mL/min or more), no dosage adjustment for sitagliptin is required.

For patients with moderate renal function impairment (CrCl 30 mL/min or more to less than 50 mL/min), the dosage of sitagliptin is 50 mg once daily.

For patients with severe renal function impairment (CrCl less than 30 ml/min) or with end-stage renal disease (ESRD) requiring hemodialysis or peritoneal dialysis, the dosage of sitagliptin is 25 mg once daily. Sitagliptin may be administered without regard to the timing of hemodialysis.

Actions

Pharmacology: Sitagliptin is a dipeptidyl peptidase-4 inhibitor that is believed to exert its actions in patients with type 2 diabetes by slowing the inactivation of incretin hormones. Concentrations of the active intact hormones are increased by sitagliptin, thereby increasing and prolonging the action of these hormones. Incretin hormones, including glucagon-like peptide-1 and glucose-dependent insulinotropic polypeptide, are released by the intestine throughout the day, and levels are increased in response to a meal.

Pharmacokinetics:

Absorption – After oral administration of a 100 mg dose to healthy subjects, sitagliptin was rapidly absorbed, with peak plasma concentrations (median time to reach maximum concentration) occurring 1 to 4 hours postdose. Plasma area under the curve (AUC) of sitagliptin increased in a dose-proportional manner. Following a single oral 100 mg dose to healthy volunteers, mean plasma AUC of sitagliptin was 8.52 mcM•h, maximum effective plasma concentration was 950 nM, and apparent terminal half-life ($t_{1/2}$) was 12.4 hours. Plasma AUC of sitagliptin increased approximately 14% following 100 mg doses at steady state compared with the first dose. The intra- and intersubject coefficients of variation for sitagliptin AUC were small (5.8% and 15.1%). The pharmacokinetics of sitagliptin were generally similar in healthy subjects and in patients with type 2 diabetes. The absolute bioavailability of sitagliptin is approximately 87%.

Distribution – The mean volume of distribution at steady state following a single 100 mg intravenous dose of sitagliptin to healthy subjects is approximately 198 L. The fraction of sitagliptin reversibly bound to plasma proteins is low (38%).

Metabolism – Approximately 79% of sitagliptin is excreted unchanged in the urine, with metabolism being a minor pathway of elimination.

Excretion – The apparent terminal $t_{1/2}$ following a 100 mg oral dose of sitagliptin was approximately 12.4 hours and renal clearance was approximately 350 mL/min. Elimination of sitagliptin occurs primarily via renal excretion and involves active tubular secretion.

Contraindications

None known.

Warnings/Precautions

Use with medications known to cause hypoglycemia: Rates of hypoglycemia reported with sitagliptin were similar to rates in patients taking placebo. The use of sitagliptin in combination with medications known to cause hypoglycemia, such as sulfonylureas or insulin, has not been adequately studied.

Renal function impairment: A dosage adjustment is recommended in patients with moderate or severe renal function impairment and in patients with ESRD requiring hemodialysis or peritoneal dialysis. Assessment of renal function is recommended prior to initiation of sitagliptin and periodically thereafter.

Carcinogenesis: A 2-year carcinogenicity study was conducted in male and female rats given oral doses of sitagliptin 50, 150, and 500 mg/kg/day. There was an increased incidence of combined liver adenoma/carcinoma in males and females and of liver carcinoma in females at 500 mg/kg.

Fertility impairment: No adverse effect on fertility was observed at 125 mg/kg (approximately 12 times human exposure at the maximum recommended human dose of 100 mg/day based on AUC comparisons).

Pregnancy: Category B.

Lactation: Sitagliptin is secreted in the milk of lactating rats at a milk to plasma ratio of 4:1. It is not known whether sitagliptin is excreted in human milk. Because many drugs are excreted in human milk, exercise caution when sitagliptin is administered to a breast-feeding woman.

Children: Safety and efficacy of sitagliptin in children younger than 18 years of age of age have not been established.

Elderly: This drug is known to be substantially excreted by the kidneys. Because elderly patients are more likely to have decreased renal function, take care in dose selection in the elderly; it may be useful to assess renal function in these patients prior to initiating dosing and periodically thereafter.

Monitoring: Because there is a need for dosage adjustment based upon renal function, assessment of renal function is recommended prior to initiation of sitagliptin and periodically thereafter.

Drug Interactions

None known.

Adverse Reactions

The most common adverse reactions, reported in 5% or more of patients treated with sitagliptin and more commonly than in patients treated with placebo are headache, nasopharyngitis, and upper respiratory tract infection.

REPAGLINIDE

Tablets: 0.5, 1, and 2 mg (*Rx*)	*Prandin* (Novo Nordisk)

Indications

Type 2 diabetes mellitus: As an adjunct to diet and exercise to lower the blood glucose in patients with type 2 diabetes mellitus whose hyperglycemia cannot be controlled by diet and exercise alone.

Repaglinide is also indicated for combination therapy use (with metformin or thiazolidinediones) to lower blood glucose in patients whose hyperglycemia cannot be controlled by diet and exercise plus monotherapy with any of the following agents: metformin, sulfonylureas, repaglinide, or thiazolidinediones. If glucose control has not been achieved after a suitable trial of combination therapy, give consideration to discontinuing these drugs and using insulin.

Administration and Dosage

There is no fixed dosage regimen for the management of type 2 diabetes with repaglinide.

Repaglinide doses are usually taken within 15 minutes of the meal, but time may vary from immediately preceding the meal to as long as 30 minutes before the meal.

Starting dose: For patients not previously treated or whose glycosylated hemoglobin (HbA_{1c}) is less than 8%, the starting dose is 0.5 mg with each meal. For patients previously treated with blood glucose-lowering agents and whose HbA_{1c} is 8% or more, the initial dose is 1 or 2 mg before each meal.

Dose adjustment: Determine dosing adjustments by blood glucose response, usually fasting blood glucose (FPG). Double the preprandial dose up to 4 mg with each meal until satisfactory blood glucose response is achieved. At least 1 week should elapse to assess response after each dose adjustment.

Dose range: Dose range is 0.5 to 4 mg taken with meals. Repaglinide may be dosed preprandially 2, 3, or 4 times daily in response to changes in the patient's meal pattern. Maximum recommended daily dose is 16 mg.

Patient management: Monitor long-term efficacy by measurement of HbA_{1c} levels approximately every 3 months. When hypoglycemia occurs in patients taking a combination of repaglinide and a thiazolidinedione or repaglinide and metformin, reduce the dose of repaglinide.

Patients receiving other oral hypoglycemic agents: When repaglinide is used to replace therapy with other oral hypoglycemic agents, it may be started the day after the final dose is given. Observe patients carefully for hypoglycemia. When transferred from longer half-life sulfonylureas (eg, chlorpropamide), close monitoring may be indicated for up to 1 week or more.

Combination therapy: If repaglinide monotherapy does not result in adequate glycemic control, metformin or a thiazolidinedione may be added. Or, if metformin or thiazolidinedione therapy does not provide adequate control, repaglinide may be added. The starting dose and dose adjustments for combination therapy are the same as repaglinide monotherapy. Carefully adjust the dose of each drug to determine the minimal dose required.

Renal function impairment: Patients with type 2 diabetes who have severe renal function impairment should initiate repaglinide with the 0.5 mg dose; subsequently, carefully titrate patients.

Actions

Pharmacology: Repaglinide is a nonsulfonylurea hypoglycemic agent of the meglitinide class. It lowers blood glucose levels by stimulating the release of insulin. This action is dependent on functioning beta cells in the pancreatic islets. Insulin release is glucose-dependent and diminishes at low glucose concentrations.

Pharmacokinetics:

Absorption – After oral administration, repaglinide is rapidly and completely absorbed from the GI tract. Peak plasma drug levels occur within 1 hour. The mean absolute bioavailability is 56%.

Distribution – Protein binding and binding to human serum albumin was more than 98%.

Metabolism – Repaglinide is completely metabolized by oxidative biotransformation and direct conjugation with glucuronic acid after either an IV or oral dose. The majority of metabolites are an oxidated dicarboxylic acid (M2), the aromatic amine (M1), and the acyl glucuronide (M7).

Excretion – Repaglinide is rapidly eliminated from the blood stream with a half-life of about 1 hour.

Contraindications

Diabetic ketoacidosis, with or without coma (treat with insulin); type 1 diabetes; hypersensitivity to the drug or its inactive ingredients.

Warnings/Precautions

Use with insulin: Repaglinide is not indicated for use in combination with NPH-insulin.

Hypoglycemia: Hepatic function impairment may cause elevated repaglinide blood levels and may diminish gluconeogenic capacity, both of which increase the risk of serious hypoglycemia. Elderly, debilitated, or malnourished patients, and those with adrenal, pituitary, or hepatic function impairment are particularly susceptible to the hypoglycemic action of glucose-lowering drugs.

The frequency of hypoglycemia is greater in patients with type 2 diabetes who have not been previously treated with oral hypoglycemic agents or whose HbA_{1c} is less than 8%. Administer with meals to lessen the risk of hypoglycemia.

Hypoglycemia may be difficult to recognize in the elderly and in people taking beta-andrenergic-blocking drugs. Hypoglycemia is more likely to occur when caloric intake is deficient, after severe or prolonged exercise, when alcohol is ingested, or when more than 1 glucose-lowering drug is used.

Secondary failure: It may be necessary to discontinue repaglinide and administer insulin if the patient is exposed to stress (eg, fever, trauma, infection, surgery). The effectiveness of any hypoglycemic drug in lowering blood glucose to a desired level decreases in many patients over a period of time, which may be due to progression of the severity of diabetes or to diminished responsiveness to the drug. This phenomenon is known as secondary failure, to distinguish it from primary failure in which the drug is ineffective in an individual patient when the drug is first given. Adequate adjustments of dose and adherence to diet should be assessed before classifying a patient as a secondary failure.

Hepatic function impairment: Patients with liver function impairment may be exposed to higher concentrations of repaglinide and its metabolites. Use repaglinide cautiously in patients with liver function impairment. Utilize longer intervals between dose adjustments to allow full assessment of response.

Pregnancy: Category C.

Lactation: It is not known whether repaglinide is excreted in breast milk. Because the potential for hypoglycemia in breast-feeding infants may exist, a decision should be made as to whether repaglinide should be discontinued in breast-feeding mothers, or if mothers should discontinue breast-feeding.

Children: No studies have been performed in children.

Monitoring: Periodically monitor FPG and HbA_{1c} levels.

Drug Interactions

Drugs that may affect repaglinide include CYP-450 inhibitors (eg, clarithromycin, erythromycin, ketoconazole, miconazole), CYP-450 inducers (eg, barbiturates, carbamazepine, rifampin), beta blockers, calcium channel blockers, chloramphenicol, corticosteroids, coumarins, estrogens, gemfibrozil, isoniazid, itraconazole, levonorgestrel and ethinyl estradiol, MAOIs, nicotinic acid, NSAIDs, oral contraceptives, phenothiazines, phenytoin, probenecid, salicylates, simvastatin, sulfonamides, sympathomimetics, thiazides and other diuretics, and thyroid products.

Drugs that may be affected by repaglinide include levonorgestrel and ethinyl estradiol.

Drug/Food interactions: When given with food, mean C_{max} and AUC of repaglinide were decreased. Administer repaglinide before meals.

Adverse Reactions

The most common adverse reactions leading to discontinuation during trials were hyperglycemia, hypoglycemia, and related symptoms.

Adverse reactions occurring in at least 3% of patients include arthralgia, back pain, bronchitis, cardiovascular events, chest pain, constipation, diarrhea, dyspepsia, headache, hypoglycemia, nausea, paresthesia, rhinitis, sinusitis, upper respiratory tract infection, urinary tract infection, vomiting.

NATEGLINIDE

Tablets: 60 and 120 mg (*Rx*)	*Starlix* (Novartis)

Indications

Type 2 diabetes mellitus:

Monotherapy – To lower blood glucose in patients with type 2 diabetes whose hyperglycemia cannot be adequately controlled by diet and physical exercise and who have not been chronically treated with other antidiabetic agents.

Combination therapy – In patients whose hyperglycemia is inadequately controlled with metformin or after a therapeutic response to a thiazolidinedione, nateglinide may be added to, but not substituted for, metformin.

Do not switch patients whose hyperglycemia is not adequately controlled with glyburide or other insulin secretagogues to nateglinide; do not add nateglinide to their treatment regimen.

Administration and Dosage

Monotherapy and combination with metformin or a thiazolidinedione: The recommended starting and maintenance dose of nateglinide, alone or in combination with metformin, is 120 mg 3 times/day before meals.

The 60 mg dose of nateglinide, alone or in combination with metformin or a thiazolidinedione, may be used in patients who are near goal HbA_{1c} when treatment is initiated.

Take 1 to 30 minutes prior to meals.

Actions

Pharmacology: Nateglinide lowers blood glucose levels by stimulating insulin secretion from the pancreas. This action is dependent upon functioning beta-cells in the pancreatic islets.

Pharmacokinetics:

Absorption – Following oral administration immediately prior to a meal, nateglinide is rapidly absorbed with mean peak plasma drug concentrations (C_{max}) generally occurring within 1 hour (T_{max}) after dosing. Absolute bioavailability is estimated to be approximately 73%.

Distribution – Nateglinide is extensively bound (98%) to serum proteins, primarily serum albumin.

Metabolism – The major routes of metabolism are hydroxylation followed by glucuronide conjugation.

Nateglinide is predominantly metabolized by CYP-450 isoenzymes CYP2C9 (70%) and CYP3A4 (30%).

Excretion – Nateglinide and its metabolites are rapidly and completely eliminated following oral administration, with an average elimination half-life of about 1.5 hours.

Contraindications

Known hypersensitivity to the drug or its inactive ingredients; type 1 diabetes; diabetic ketoacidosis.

Warnings/Precautions

Diet/Exercise: Use of nateglinide must be viewed as a treatment in addition to diet and not as a substitute for diet or as a convenient mechanism for avoiding dietary restraint.

Hypoglycemia: Geriatric patients, malnourished patients, and those with adrenal or pituitary insufficiency are more susceptible to the glucose-lowering effect of these treatments. Hypoglycemia may be difficult to recognize in patients with autonomic neuropathy or those who use beta-blockers. Administer nateglinide before meals to reduce the risk of hypoglycemia. Patients who skip meals should also skip their scheduled dose of nateglinide to reduce the risk of hypoglycemia.

Secondary failure: Transient loss of glycemic control may occur with fever, infection, trauma, or surgery. Insulin therapy may be needed instead of nateglinide therapy at such times. Secondary failure, or reduced effectiveness of nateglinide over a period of time, may occur.

Hepatic function impairment: Use nateglinide with caution in patients with chronic liver disease. Use with caution in patients with moderate to severe liver disease because such patients have not been studied.

Pregnancy: Category C.

Lactation: It is not known whether nateglinide is excreted in human milk. Because many drugs are excreted in human milk, do not administer nateglinide to a breast-feeding woman.

Children: The safety and efficacy of nateglinide in children have not been established.

Monitoring: Periodically assess response to therapies with glucose values and HbA_{1c} levels.

Drug Interactions

Nateglinide is predominantly metabolized by the CYP-450 isozyme CYP2C9 (70%) and to a lesser extent CYP3A4 (30%). Nateglinide is a potential inhibitor of the CYP2C9 isoenzyme in vivo as indicated by its ability to inhibit the in vitro metabolism of tolbutamide. Inhibition of CYP3A4 metabolic reactions was not detected in in vitro experiments.

Drugs that may affect nateglinide include nonsteroidal anti-inflammatory agents (NSAIDs), salicylates, monoamine oxidase inhibitors, rifamycins, MAOIs, and nonselective beta-adrenergic blocking agents, thiazides, corticosteroids, thyroid products, and sympathomimetics.

Drug/Food interactions: Peak plasma levels were significantly reduced when nateglinide was administered 10 minutes prior to a liquid meal.

Adverse Reactions

Adverse reactions occurring in at least 3% of patients include arthropathy, back pain, diarrhea, dizziness, flu symptoms, upper respiratory tract infection.

ACARBOSE

Tablets: 25, 50, and 100 mg (*Rx*)	Various, *Precose* (Bayer)

Indications

Type 2 diabetes: As monotherapy as an adjunct to diet to lower blood glucose in patients with type 2 diabetes whose hyperglycemia cannot be managed on diet alone.

Acarbose also may be used with a sulfonylurea when diet plus either acarbose or a sulfonylurea do not result in adequate glycemic control.

Administration and Dosage

Dosage of acarbose must be individualized while not exceeding the maximum recommended dose of 100 mg 3 times/day for patients more than 60 kg and 50 mg 3 times/day for patients less than 60 kg.

During treatment initiation and dose titration, use 1 hour postprandial plasma glucose to determine the therapeutic response to acarbose and identify the minimum effective dose for the patient. Thereafter, measure glycosylated hemoglobin at intervals of about 3 months.

Initial dosage: The recommended starting dosage is 25 mg given 3 times/day at the start (with the first bite) of each main meal. However, some patients may benefit from more gradual dose titration to minimize GI side effects. This may be achieved by initiating treatment at 25 mg once per day and subsequently increasing the frequency of administration to achieve 25 mg three times daily.

Maintenance dosage: Adjust dosage at 4- to 8-week intervals based on 1-hour postprandial glucose levels and on tolerance. After the initial dosage of 25 mg 3 times/day, the dosage can be increased to 50 mg 3 times/day. Some patients may benefit from further increasing the dosage to 100 mg 3 times/day. The maintenance dose ranges from 50 to 100 mg 3 times/day. However, because patients with low body weight may be at increased risk for elevated serum transaminases, consider only patients with body weight more than 60 kg for dose titration above 50 mg 3 times/day. If no further reduction in postprandial glucose or glycosylated hemoglobin levels is observed with titration to 100 mg 3 times/day, consider lowering the dose. Once an effective and tolerated dosage has been established, it should be maintained.

Coadministration: Acarbose given in combination with a sulfonylurea or insulin will cause a further lowering of blood glucose and may increase the hypoglycemic potential of the sulfonylurea.

Actions

Pharmacology: Acarbose, an alpha-glucosidase inhibitor, is a complex oligosaccharide that delays the digestion of ingested carbohydrates, thereby resulting in a smaller rise in blood glucose concentration following meals. As a consequence of plasma glucose reduction, acarbose reduces levels of glycosylated hemoglobin.

Because its mechanism of action is different, the effect of acarbose to enhance glycemic control is additive to that of sulfonylureas when used in combination. In contrast to sulfonylureas, acarbose does not enhance insulin secretion.

Pharmacokinetics:

Absorption – Following oral dosing, peak plasma concentrations were attained 14 to 24 hours after dosing, while peak plasma concentrations of active drug were attained at about 1 hour.

Metabolism – Acarbose is metabolized exclusively within the GI tract, principally by intestinal bacteria, but also by digestive enzymes. A fraction of these metabolites (about 34% of the dose) was absorbed and subsequently excreted in the urine.

Excretion – The fraction of acarbose that is absorbed as intact drug is almost completely excreted by the kidneys. When acarbose was given IV, 89% of the dose was recovered in the urine as active drug within 48 hours. In contrast, less than 2% of an oral dose was recovered in the urine as active (ie, parent compound and active metabolite) drug. The plasma elimination half-life of acarbose activity is about 2 hours in healthy volunteers.

Contraindications

Hypersensitivity to the drug; diabetic ketoacidosis or cirrhosis; inflammatory bowel disease; colonic ulceration; partial intestinal obstruction or predisposition to intestinal obstruction; chronic intestinal diseases associated with marked disorders of digestion or absorption; conditions that may deteriorate as a result of increased gas formation in the intestine.

Warnings/Precautions

Diet/Physical activity: The use of acarbose must be viewed by both the physician and patient as a treatment in addition to diet, and not as a substitute for diet or as a convenient mechanism for avoiding dietary restraint.

Hypoglycemia: Because of its mechanism of action, acarbose alone should not cause hypoglycemia in the fasted or postprandial state. It may increase the hypoglycemic potential of the sulfonylurea. Use oral glucose (dextrose), whose absorption is not inhibited by acarbose, instead of sucrose (cane sugar) in the treatment of mild-to-moderate hypoglycemia. Severe hypoglycemia may require the use of either IV glucose infusion or glucagon injection.

Loss of blood glucose control: When diabetic patients are exposed to stress such as fever, trauma, infection or surgery, a temporary loss of control of blood glucose may occur. At such times, temporary insulin therapy may be necessary.

Hematocrit: Small reductions in hematocrit occurred.

Calcium/Vitamin B_6: Low serum calcium and low plasma vitamin B_6 levels were associated with acarbose therapy but were thought to be either spurious or of no clinical significance.

Renal function impairment: Patients with severe renal function impairment (creatinine clearance [CrCl] less than 25 mL/min/1.73 m^2) attained about 5 times higher peak plasma concentrations of acarbose and 6 times larger AUCs than volunteers with normal renal function. Treatment of these patients with acarbose is not recommended.

Carcinogenesis: In rats, acarbose treatment resulted in a significant increase in the incidence of renal tumors (adenomas and adenocarcinomas) and benign Leydig cell tumors. Further studies showed that the increased incidence of renal tumors found in the original studies did not occur.

Pregnancy: *Category B.*

Lactation: It is not known whether this drug is excreted in breast milk. Do not administer to a breast-feeding woman.

Children: Safety and efficacy have not been established.

Lab test abnormalities:

Elevated serum transaminase levels – Treatment-emergent elevations of serum transaminases (AST and /or ALT) above the upper limit of normal (ULN), greater than 1.8 × ULN, and greater than 3 × ULN occurred. These elevations were asymptomatic, reversible, more common in females, and, in general, were not associated with other evidence of liver dysfunction. In addition, these serum transaminase elevations appeared to be dose related.

A few cases of fulminant hepatitis with fatal outcome have been reported; the relationship to acarbose is unclear.

Monitoring: Monitor therapeutic response to acarbose by periodic blood glucose tests. Measurement of glycosylated hemoglobin levels is recommended for the monitoring of long-term glycemic control. Acarbose, particularly at doses in excess of 50 mg 3 times/day may give rise to elevations of serum transaminases and, in rare instances, hyperbilirubinemia. It is recommended that serum transaminase levels be checked every 3 months during the first year of the treatment with acarbose and periodically thereafter. If elevated transaminases are observed, a reduction in dosage or withdrawal of therapy may be indicated, particularly if the elevations persist.

Drug Interactions

Drugs that may interact with acarbose include digestive enzymes, intestinal adsorbents (eg, charcoal) and digoxin.

Certain drugs tend to produce hyperglycemia and may lead to loss of blood glucose control. These drugs include the thiazides and other diuretics, corticosteroids, phenothiazines, thyroid products, estrogens, oral contraceptives, phenytoin, nicotinic acid, sympathomimetics, calcium channel blocking drugs, and isoniazid.

Adverse Reactions

GI symptoms are the most common reaction to acarbose. In trials, the incidences of abdominal pain, diarrhea, and flatulence were 21%, 33%, and 77%, respectively, with acarbose 50 to 300 mg 3 times/day. Rarely, hypersensitive skin reactions, such as rash, may occur.

INSULIN

INSULIN INJECTION (REGULAR)	
Injection: 100 units/mL (human insulin [rDNA]) (*Rx*)	*Humulin R* (Lilly), *Novolin R* (Novo Nordisk)
ISOPHANE INSULIN SUSPENSION (NPH; insulin combined with protamine and zinc)	
Injection: 100 units/mL (human insulin [rDNA]) (*Rx*)	*Humulin N* (Lilly), *Novolin N* (Novo Nordisk)
ISOPHANE INSULIN SUSPENSION (NPH) AND INSULIN INJECTION (REGULAR)	
Injection: 100 units/mL as 70% isophane insulin and 30% insulin injection (human insulin [rDNA]) (*Rx*)	*Humulin 70/30* (Lilly), *Novolin 70/30* (Novo Nordisk)
Injection: 100 units/mL as 50% isophane insulin and 50% insulin injection (human insulin [rDNA]) (*Rx*)	*Humulin 50/50* (Lilly)
INSULIN ANALOG INJECTION	
Injection: 100 units/mL (human insulin lispro [rDNA]) (*Rx*)	*Humalog* (Lilly), *Humalog Mix 50/50* (Lilly), *Humalog Mix 75/25*[a] (Lilly)
100 units/mL (human insulin aspart [rDNA]) (*Rx*)	*NovoLog* (Novo Nordisk)
INSULIN DETEMIR	
Injection: 100 units/mL (*Rx*)	*Levemir* (Novo Nordisk)
INSULIN GLARGINE	
Injection: 100 units/mL (insulin glargine [rDNA]) (*Rx*)	*Lantus* (Aventis)
INSULIN GLULISINE	
Injection: 100 units/mL (*Rx*)	*Apidra* (Sanofi-Aventis)
INSULIN REGULAR CONCENTRATE	
Injection: 500 units/mL (*Rx*)	*Humulin R Regular U-500 (Concentrated)* (Lilly)

[a] Contains 75% insulin lispro protamine suspension and 25% insulin lispro injection (rDNA).

Indications

Type 1 diabetes mellitus (insulin-dependent).

Type 2 diabetes mellitus (non-insulin-dependent) that cannot be properly controlled by diet, exercise, and weight reduction.

In hyperkalemia, infusion of glucose and insulin produces a shift of potassium into cells and lowers serum potassium levels.

Severe ketoacidosis/diabetic coma: Insulin injection (regular insulin) may be given intravenously (IV) or intramuscularly (IM) for rapid effect in severe ketoacidosis or diabetic coma.

Highly purified (single component) and human insulins: Local insulin allergy, immunologic insulin resistance, injection-site lipodystrophy; temporary insulin use (ie, surgery, acute stress type 2 diabetes, gestational diabetes); newly diagnosed diabetic patients.

Insulin aspart: Because insulin aspart has a more rapid onset and a shorter duration of action than human regular insulin, insulin aspart normally should be used in regimens together with an intermediate or long-acting insulin. *NovoLog* may be infused subcutaneously by external insulin pumps.

Insulin detemir: Treatment of adult and children with type 1 diabetes mellitus or adult patients with type 2 diabetes mellitus who require basal (long-acting) insulin for the control of hyperglycemia.

Insulin lispro: Insulin lispro has a more rapid onset and shorter duration of action than regular human insulin. Therefore, in patients with type 1 diabetes, use in regimens that include a longer-acting insulin. However, in patients with type 2 diabetes, insulin lispro may be used without a longer-acting insulin when used in combination therapy with sulfonylureas.

Insulin glargine: Once-daily subcutaneous administration for the control of hyperglycemia.

Insulin glulisine: Insulin glulisine has a more rapid onset and shorter duration of action than regular human insulin. It normally should be used in regimens that include a longer-acting insulin or basal insulin analog. Insulin glulisine also may be infused subcutaneously by external insulin infusion pumps.

Insulin concentrated: Treatment of diabetic patients with marked insulin resistance (requirements greater than 200 units/day).

Administration and Dosage

INSULIN: Human regular insulin is best given 30 to 60 minutes before a meal. Administer maintenance doses subcutaneously.

Children and adults – 0.5 to 1 units/kg/day.

Adolescents (during growth spurt) – 0.8 to 1.2 units/kg/day.

INSULIN ASPART: Give immediately before a meal. In a meal-related treatment regimen, 50% to 70% of this requirement may be provided by insulin aspart and the remainder provided by an intermediate-acting or long-acting insulin. Patients may require more basal insulin in relation to bolus insulin and more total insulin when using insulin aspart compared with regular human insulin to prevent premeal hyperglycemia.

Because of the fast onset of action of insulin aspart, administer close to a meal (start of meal within 5 to 10 minutes after injection).

Fixed ratio insulins are typically dosed on a twice-daily basis (ie, before breakfast and supper), with each dose intended to cover 2 meals or a meal and snack.

Children –

Novolog: Novolog is approved for use in children for subcutaneous daily injections (studies included children 2 years of age and older) and for subcutaneous continuous infusion by external insulin pump (studies included children 4 years of age and older).

Insulin pump – Approximately 50% of the total dose is given as meal-related boluses and the remainder as basal infusion. Additional basal insulin injections or higher basal rates in external subcutaneous infusion pumps may be necessary. Change the insulin in the reservoir, the infusion sets, and the infusion set insertion site every 48 hours or sooner to assure the activity of insulin aspart and proper pump function.

IV administration – IV administration of insulin aspart is possible under medical supervision with close monitoring of blood glucose and potassium levels to avoid hypoglycemia and hypokalemia. For IV use, insulin aspart should be used at concentrations from 0.05 to 1 unit/mL. Insulin aspart has been shown to be stable in infusion fluids such as sodium chloride 0.9%.

Mixing of insulins – If insulin aspart is mixed with neutral protamine Hagedorn (NPH) human insulin, insulin aspart should be drawn into the syringe first. The injection should be made immediately after mixing. Mixtures should not be administered IV.

The effects of mixing insulin aspart with insulin preparations produced by other manufacturers have not been studied.

When used in external subcutaneous infusion pumps for insulin, insulin aspart should not be mixed with any other insulins or diluent.

INSULIN DETEMIR:

Dosage –

Once daily dosing: Administer with the evening meal or at bedtime.

Twice-daily dosing: Administer evening dose with the evening meal, at bedtime, or 12 hours after the morning dose.

Injection sites – Administer by subcutaneous injection in the thigh, abdominal wall, or upper arm.

Insulin-naïve patients with type 2 diabetes – 0.1 to 0.2 units/kg once daily in the evening or 10 units once or twice daily, and adjust the dose to achieve glycemic targets.

INSULIN GLARGINE: Give insulin glargine subcutaneously once daily at the same time every day. The dose may be administered at any time during the day. IV administration of the usual subcutaneous dose could result in severe hypoglycemia.

Insulin glargine must not be diluted or mixed with any other insulin or solution.

Children – Insulin glargine can be safely administered to children 6 years of age and older. Administration to children younger than 6 years of age has not been studied. The dose recommendation for changeover to insulin glargine is the same as described for adults.

Initial dosing – In a clinical study with insulin-naive patients treated with oral antidiabetic drugs, insulin glargine was started at an average dose of 10 units once daily, and adjusted to a total daily dose ranging from 2 to 100 units.

Changeover to insulin glargine – If changing from a treatment regimen with an intermediate- or long-acting insulin to a regimen with insulin glargine, the amount and timing of short-acting insulin, fast-acting insulin analog, or the dose of any oral antidiabetic drug may need to be adjusted. In clinical studies, when patients were transferred from once-daily NPH human insulin or ultralente human insulin to once-daily insulin glargine, the initial dose was usually not changed. However, when patients were transferred from twice-daily NPH to insulin glargine once daily, the initial dose was usually reduced by about 20% (compared with total daily units of NPH human insulin) and then adjusted based on patient response.

Mixing and diluting – Insulin glargine must not be diluted or mixed with any other insulin or solution.

INSULIN GLULISINE: Give within 15 minutes before a meal or within 20 minutes after starting a meal. Insulin glulisine is intended for subcutaneous administration and for use by external infusion pump or by IV administration in a clinical setting.

For IV use, insulin glulisine should be used at a concentration of insulin glulisine 0.05 to 1 unit/mL in infusion systems with the infusion fluid, sterile 0.9% sodium chloride solution, using polyvinyl chloride (PVC) infusion bags with a dedicated infusion line. The use of other bags and tubing has not been studied.

For subcutaneous administration, do not mix insulin glulisine with any other type of insulin than NPH.

INSULIN LISPRO: Insulin lispro is intended for subcutaneous administration. When used as a meal-time insulin, give insulin lispro within 15 minutes before or immediately after a meal.

Compatibility – Insulin lispro may be diluted with sterile diluent for *Humalog*, *Humulin N*, *Humulin 50/50*, *Humulin 70/30*, and *NPH Iletin* to a concentration of 1:10 (equivalent to U-10) or 1:2 (equivalent to U-50). Diluted insulin lispro may remain in patient use for 28 days when stored at 5°C (41°F) and for 14 days when stored at 30°C (86°F).

Children (Humalog only) – Safety and efficacy in children younger than 18 years of age have not been determined for *Humalog Mix*. Adjustment of basal insulin may be required. To improve accuracy of dosing in children, a diluent may be used. If the diluent is added directly to the vial, the shelf life may be reduced.

INSULIN CONCENTRATED: Administer subcutaneously. Do not inject IM or IV.

Concentrated insulin injection frequently has a duration similar to repository insulin; a single dose demonstrates activity for 24 hours.

Hypoglycemic reactions – Hypoglycemia when using this concentrated insulin can be prolonged and severe. Deep secondary hypoglycemic reactions may develop 18 to 24 hours after the original injection of concentrated insulin.

Actions

Pharmacology: Insulin and its analogs lower blood glucose levels by stimulating peripheral glucose uptake and inhibiting hepatic glucose production. Insulin, secreted by the beta cells of the pancreas, is the principal hormone required for proper glucose use in normal metabolic processes.

The bioavailability of the insulins is identical when given subcutaneously. Human insulin is the insulin of choice for patients with insulin allergy, insulin resistance, all pregnant patients with diabetes, and any patient who uses insulin intermittently.

Pharmacokinetics and Compatibility of Various Insulins

	Insulin preparations	Half-life (h)	Onset (h)	Peak (h)	Duration (h)	Compatible mixed with
Rapid-Acting	Insulin injection (regular)	–	0.5 to 1	–	8 to 12	All
	Prompt insulin zinc suspension (semilente)	–	1 to 1.5	5 to 10	12 to 16	Lente
	Lispro insulin solution	1	0.25	0.5 to 1.5	2 to 5	Ultralente, NPH
	Insulin aspart solution	1.5	0.25	1 to 3	3 to 5	[a]
	Insulin glulisine	0.7	–	0.5 to 1.5	1 to 2.5	NPH
Intermediate-Acting	Isophane insulin suspension (NPH)	–	1 to 1.5	4 to 12	24	Regular
	Insulin zinc suspension (lente)	–	1 to 2.5	7 to 15	24	Regular, semilente
Long-Acting	Insulin glargine solution	–	1.1	5[b]	24[c]	None
	Protamine zinc insulin suspension (PZI)	–	4 to 8	14 to 24	36	Regular

[a] See the following section.

[b] No pronounced peak; small amounts of insulin glargine are slowly released, resulting in a relatively constant concentration/time profile over 24 hours.

[c] Studies only conducted up to 24 hours.

Mixing of insulins – The effects of mixing insulin aspart or lispro with insulins of animal source or insulin preparations produced by other manufacturers have not been studied (see Warnings).

Do not administer mixtures IV. Inject all mixtures immediately after mixing.

Always draw clear regular insulin into the syringe first. Do not alter order of mixing insulins. Each type of insulin used must be of the same concentration (units/mL).

NPH/regular combinations of insulin are stable and are absorbed as if injected separately. Mixtures of regular insulin with lente must be mixed and injected immediately.

Manufacturer premixed formulations remain stable for 1 month at room temperature or for 3 months refrigerated. These mixtures also can be stored in prefilled plastic or glass syringes for 1 week to possibly 14 days under refrigeration. Slightly agitate to remix the insulins. Check for normal appearance.

Semilente, ultralente, and lente insulins may be mixed in any ratio. These mixtures are stable 1 month at room temperature or 3 months under refrigeration.

Insulin aspart: If insulin aspart is mixed with NPH human insulin, draw insulin aspart into the syringe first. Do not mix insulin aspart with crystalline zinc insulin preparations. When used in external subcutaneous infusion pumps for insulin, do not mix with any other insulins or diluent.

Insulin lispro: If insulin lispro is mixed with a longer-acting insulin, draw lispro into the syringe first to prevent clouding of the lispro by the longer-acting insulin.

Insulin glulisine: If insulin glulisine is mixed with NPH human insulin, draw insulin glulisine into the syringe first. Inject immediately after mixing. Do not mix insulin glulisine with insulin preparations other than NPH. When it is used in a pump, do not mix insulin glulisine with other insulins or with a diluent.

Contraindications

During episodes of hypoglycemia and in patients sensitive to any ingredient of the product.

Warnings/Precautions

Change insulins: Change insulins cautiously and under medical supervision. Changes in purity, strength, brand, type, or species source may require dosage adjustment.

Insulin resistance: Insulin resistance occurs rarely. Insulin-resistant patients require more than 200 units of insulin/day for more than 2 days in the absence of ketoacidosis or acute infection.

Hypoglycemia: Hypoglycemia may result from excessive insulin dose or may be caused by: Increased work or exercise without eating; food not being absorbed in the usual manner because of postponement or omission of a meal or in illness with vomiting, fever, or diarrhea; when insulin requirements decline.

Diabetic ketoacidosis: Diabetic ketoacidosis may result from stress, illness, or insulin omission, or may develop slowly after a long period of insulin control. Hyperglucagonemia, hyperglycemia, and ketoacidosis may result.

Symptoms of Hypoglycemia vs Ketoacidosis

Reaction	Onset	Urine glucose/ acetone	Symptoms				
			CNS	Respiration	Mouth/GI	Skin	Miscellaneous
Hypoglycemic reaction (insulin reaction)	sudden	0/0	fatigue, weakness, nervousness, confusion, headache, diplopia, convulsions, psychoses, dizziness, unconsciousness	rapid, shallow	numb, tingling, hunger, nausea	pallor, moist, shallow, or dry	normal or noncharacteristic pulse, eyeballs normal
Ketoacidosis (diabetic coma)	gradual (hours or days)	+/+	drowsiness, dim vision	air hunger	thirst, acetone breath, nausea, vomiting, abdominal pain, loss of appetite	dry, flushed	rapid pulse, soft eyeballs

Lipodystrophy:

Lipoatrophy – Lipoatrophy is the breakdown of adipose tissue at the insulin injection site causing a depression in the skin.

Lipohypertrophy – Lipohypertrophy is the result of repeated insulin injection into the same site. This condition may be avoided by rotating the injection site.

Diet: Patients must follow a prescribed diet and exercise regularly. Determine the time, number, and amount of individual doses and distribution of food among the meals of the day. Do not change this regimen unless prescribed otherwise.

Hyperthyroidism/Hypothyroidism: Hyperthyroidism may cause an increase in the renal clearance of insulin. Therefore, patients may need more insulin to control their diabetes. Hypothyroidism may delay insulin turnover, requiring less insulin to control diabetes.

Hypersensitivity reactions: May require discontinuation of insulin.

Local – Occasionally, redness, swelling, and itching at the injection site may develop. This reaction occurs if the injection is not properly made, if the skin is sensitive to the cleansing solution, or if the patient is allergic to insulin or insulin additives (eg, preservatives).

Systemic – Systemic reactions are less common and may present as a rash, shortness of breath, fast pulse, sweating, a drop in blood pressure, bronchospasm, shock, anaphylaxis, or angioedema and may be life-threatening.

Insulin aspart, insulin glulisine – Localized reactions and generalized myalgias have been reported with the use of cresol as an injectable excipient.

Renal/Hepatic function impairment: Careful glucose monitoring and dose adjustments of insulin may be necessary in these patients. Insulin requirements may be reduced in patients with renal function impairment.

Pregnancy: Category B; Category C (insulin glargine, insulin aspart, insulin glulisine).

Lactation: Breast-feeding women may require adjustments in insulin dose and diet. It is unknown whether insulin glargine, insulin aspart, or insulin glulisine are excreted in significant amounts in breast milk.

Children: Safety and efficacy in patients younger than 12 years of age have not been established.

Insulin glargine – Safety and efficacy of insulin glargine have been established in children 6 to 15 years of age with type 1 diabetes.

Humalog – *Humalog* can be used in combination with sulfonylureas in children older than 3 years of age.

Drug Interactions

Drugs That Decrease the Hypoglycemic Effect of Insulin		
Acetazolamide	Dextrothyroxine	Niacin
AIDS antivirals	Diazoxide	Nicotine
Albuterol	Diltiazem	Phenothiazines
Antipsychotic medications (atypical [eg, olanzapine, clozapine])	Diuretics	Phenytoin
	Dobutamine	Progestogens (eg, oral contraceptives)
	Epinephrine	
Asparaginase	Estrogens	Protease inhibitors
Calcitonin	Ethacrynic acid	Somatropin
Contraceptives, oral	Glucagon	Terbutaline
Corticosteroids	Isoniazid	Thiazide diuretics
Cyclophosphamide	Lithium carbonate	Thyroid hormones
Danazol	Morphine sulfate	

Drugs That Increase the Hypoglycemic Effect of Insulin		
ACE inhibitors	Disopyramide	Phenylbutazone
Alcohol	Fluoxetine	Propoxyphene
Anabolic steroids	Fibrates	Pyridoxine
Antidiabetic products, oral	Guanethidine	Salicylates
	Lithium carbonate	Somatostatin analog (eg, octreotide)
Beta-blockers[a]	MAO inhibitors	
Calcium	Mebendazole	Sulfinpyrazone
Chloroquine	Pentamidine[b]	Sulfonamides
Clofibrate	Pentoxifylline	Tetracyclines
Clonidine		

[a] Nonselective beta-blockers may delay recovery from hypoglycemic episodes and mask their signs/symptoms. Cardioselective agents may be alternatives.
[b] May sometimes be followed by hyperglycemia.

Adverse Reactions

Human insulin: Hypoglycemia and hypokalemia are among the potential clinical adverse reactions associated with the use of all insulins. Other adverse reactions commonly associated with human insulin therapy include the following:

Dermatologic – Injection-site reaction, lipodystrophy, pruritus, rash.

Lab test abnormalities – Hypoglycemia, hypokalemia.

Miscellaneous – Allergic reactions; sodium retention and edema may occur, particularly if previously poor metabolic control is improved by intensified insulin therapy; antibody production.

SULFONYLUREAS

CHLORPROPAMIDE	
Tablets: 100 and 250 mg (*Rx*)	Various
GLIMEPIRIDE	
Tablets: 1, 2, and 4 mg (*Rx*)	Various, *Amaryl* (Aventis)
GLIPIZIDE	
Tablets: 5 and 10 mg (*Rx*)	Various, *Glucotrol* (Pfizer)
Tablets, extended-release: 2.5, 5, and 10 mg (*Rx*)	Various, *Glucotrol XL* (Pfizer)
GLYBURIDE	
Tablets: 1.25, 2.5, and 5 mg (*Rx*)	Various, *DiaBeta* (Hoechst Marion Roussel)
Tablets, micronized: 1.5, 3, 4.5, and 6 mg (*Rx*)	Various, *Glynase PresTab* (Pharmacia & Upjohn)
TOLAZAMIDE	
Tablets: 100, 250, and 500 mg (*Rx*)	Various
TOLBUTAMIDE	
Tablets: 500 mg (*Rx*)	Various

Indications

As an adjunct to diet and exercise to lower the blood glucose in patients with type 2 (non-insulin-dependent) diabetes mellitus whose hyperglycemia cannot be controlled by diet and exercise alone.

Glimepiride:

Combination with insulin – Glimepiride is also indicated for use in combination with insulin to lower blood glucose in patients whose hyperglycemia cannot be controlled by diet and exercise in conjunction with an oral hypoglycemic agent. Combined use of glimepiride and insulin may increase the potential for hypoglycemia.

Combination metformin therapy – Glimepiride may be used concomitantly with metformin when diet, exercise, and glimepiride or metformin alone do not result in adequate glycemic control.

Glyburide:

Combination with metformin – Glyburide also may be used concomitantly with metformin when diet and glyburide or diet and metformin alone do not result in adequate glycemic control (see Metformin monograph).

Administration and Dosage

Short-term administration: Short-term administration of sulfonylureas may be sufficient during periods of transient loss of control in patients usually well controlled on diet.

Transfer from other hypoglycemic agents:

Sulfonylureas – When transferring patients from one oral hypoglycemic agent to another, no transitional period and no initial or priming dose is necessary. However, when transferring patients from chlorpropamide, exercise particular care during the first 2 weeks because the prolonged retention of chlorpropamide in the body and subsequent overlapping drug effects may provoke hypoglycemia.

Insulin – During insulin withdrawal period, test blood for glucose and urine for ketones 3 times/day and report results to physician daily.

Insulin Requirement When Instituting Sulfonylurea Therapy	
Insulin dose	Insulin requirement
< 20 units	Start directly on oral agent and discontinue insulin abruptly.
20 to 40 units	Initiate oral therapy with concurrent 25% to 50% reduction in insulin dose. Further reduce insulin as response is observed. With glyburide, insulin may be discontinued immediately.
> 40 units	Initiate oral therapy with concurrent 20% to 50% reduction in insulin dose. Further reduce insulin as response is observed.

Elderly patients: Elderly patients may be particularly sensitive to these agents; therefore, start with a lower initial dose before breakfast, and check blood and urine glucose during the first 24 hours of therapy.

Acute complications: During the course of intercurrent complications (eg, ketoacidosis, severe trauma, major surgery, infections, severe diarrhea, nausea, vomiting), supportive therapy with insulin may be necessary.

Combination insulin therapy: Concurrent administration of insulin and an oral sulfonylurea (generally glipizide or glyburide) has been used with some success in type 2 diabetic patients who are difficult to control with diet and sulfonylurea therapy alone.

CHLORPROPAMIDE:

Initial dose – 250 mg/day in the mild to moderately severe, middle-aged, stable diabetic patient; use 100 to 125 mg/day in older, debilitated, or malnourished patients, and patients with impaired renal/hepatic function.

Maintenance therapy – No more than 100 to 250 mg/day. Severe diabetics may require 500 mg/day. Avoid doses greater than 750 mg/day.

Patients on insulin –

Transferal of Type 2 Diabetes Patients on Insulin to Chlorpropamide Monotherapy

Insulin dose	Initial chlorpropamide dose	Insulin withdrawal
≤ 40	250 mg/day	Not necessary; may be discontinued abruptly.
> 40	250 mg/day	Reduce insulin dose by 50%; further reduce as response is observed. Consider hospitalization during the transition period.

GLIMEPIRIDE:

Initial dose – 1 to 2 mg once daily, given with breakfast or the first main meal. Patients sensitive to hypoglycemic drugs should begin at 1 mg once daily; titrate carefully.

Maximum starting dose is 2 mg or less.

Maintenance dose – 1 to 4 mg once daily. The maximum recommended dose is 8 mg once daily. After a dose of 2 mg is reached, increase dose at increments of no more than 2 mg at 1 to 2 week intervals based on the patient's blood glucose response. Monitor long-term efficacy by measurement of HbA_{1c} levels, for example, every 3 to 6 months.

Combination metformin therapy – If patients do not respond adequately to the maximal dose of glimepiride monotherapy, addition of metformin may be considered.

Combination insulin therapy – The recommended dose is 8 mg once daily with the first main meal with low-dose insulin.

Patients on other oral antidiabetic agents – When transferring patients to glimepiride, no transition period is necessary. No exact dosage relationship exists between glimepiride and the other oral hypoglycemic agents.

GLIPIZIDE:

Immediate release –

Initial dose: 5 mg, given approximately 30 minutes before breakfast to achieve the greatest reduction in postprandial hyperglycemia. Elderly patients or those with liver disease may be started on 2.5 mg of the immediate-release formulation.

Adjust dosage in 2.5 to 5 mg increments, as determined by blood glucose response. Several days should elapse between titration steps. If response to a single dose is not satisfactory, dividing that dose may prove effective. The maximum recommended once daily dose is 15 mg. The maximum recommended total daily dose is 40 mg.

Maintenance dose: Some patients may be controlled on a once-a-day regimen, while others show better response with divided dosing. Divide total daily doses greater than 15 mg and give before meals of adequate caloric content. Total daily doses greater than 30 mg have been safely given on a twice daily basis to long-term patients.

Extended release –

Initial dose: 5 mg/day, given with breakfast. The recommended dose for elderly patients is also 5 mg/day. HbA_{1c} level measured at 3-month intervals is the preferred means of monitoring response to therapy. Measure HbA_{1c} as extended release therapy is initiated at the 5 mg dose and repeated approximately 3 months later.

If the first test result suggests that glycemic control over the preceding 3 months was inadequate, the dose may be increased to 10 mg. Make subsequent dosage adjustments at 3-month intervals. If no improvement is seen after 3 months of therapy with a higher dose, resume the previous dose. Base decisions that use fasting blood glucose to adjust therapy on at least 2 similar consecutive values obtained at least 7 days after the previous dose adjustment.

Maintenance dose: Most patients will be controlled with 5 or 10 mg taken once daily. However, some patients may require up to the maximum recommended daily dose of 20 mg. While the glycemic control of selected patients may improve with doses that exceed 10 mg, clinical studies conducted to date have not demonstrated an additional group average reduction of HbA_{1c} beyond what was achieved with the 10 mg dose.

Immediate vs extended release: Patients receiving immediate-release glipizide may be switched safely to the extended-release tablets once a day at the nearest equivalent total daily dose. Patients receiving immediate-release tablets also may be titrated to the appropriate dose of the extended-release tablets starting with 5 mg once daily.

Combination therapy: When used in combination with other oral blood glucose-lowering agents, add the second agent at the lowest recommended dose and observe patients carefully.

Patients on other oral antidiabetic agents – No transition period is necessary when transferring patients to the extended-release tablets. Observe patients carefully (1 to 2 weeks) when being transferred from longer half-life sulfonylureas (ie, chlorpropamide) to the extended release tablets due to potential overlapping of drug effect.

Patients on insulin –

Transferal of Type 2 Diabetes Patients on Insulin to Glipizide Monotherapy

Insulin dose	Initial glipizide dose	Insulin withdrawal
< 20	5 mg/day	Not necessary; may be discontinued abruptly.
> 20	5 mg/day	Reduce insulin dose by 50%; further reduce as response is observed. Consider hospitalization during the transition period.

GLYBURIDE (Glibenclamide):

Nonmicronized (DiaBeta) –

Initial dose: 2.5 to 5 mg/day, administered with breakfast or the first main meal. For patients who may be more sensitive to hypoglycemic drugs, start at 1.25 mg/day.

Maintenance dose: 1.25 to 20 mg/day. Give as a single dose or in divided doses. Increase in increments of 2.5 mg or less at weekly intervals based on the patient's blood glucose response. Daily doses greater than 20 mg are not recommended.

Micronized (Glynase) –

Initial dose: 1.5 to 3 mg/day, administered with breakfast or the first main meal. For patients who may be more sensitive to hypoglycemic drugs, start at 0.75 mg/day.

Maintenance dose: 0.75 to 12 mg/day. Give as a single dose or in divided doses; some patients, particularly those receiving more than 6 mg/day, may have a more satisfactory response with twice-daily dosing. Increase in increments of no more than 1.5 mg at weekly intervals based on the patient's blood glucose response. Daily doses greater than 12 mg are not recommended.

Concomitant metformin: Add glyburide gradually to the dosing regimen of patients who have not responded to the maximum dose of metformin monotherapy after 4 weeks. (Refer to the Metformin monograph.) The desired control of blood glucose may be obtained by adjusting the dose of each drug. With concomitant therapy, the risk of hypoglycemia associated with sulfonylurea therapy continues and may be increased.

Patients on other oral antidiabetic agents: Transfer patients from other oral antidiabetic regimens to glyburide conservatively. When transferring patients from oral hypoglycemic agents other than chlorpropamide, no transition period and no initial priming dose is necessary. When transferring patients from chlorpropamide, exercise care during the first 2 weeks because the prolonged retention of chlorpropamide in the body and subsequent overlapping drug effects may provoke hypoglycemia.

Patients on insulin:

Transferal of Type 2 Diabetes Patients on Insulin to Glyburide Monotherapy		
Insulin dose	Initial glyburide dose	Insulin withdrawal
< 20	1.5-3 mg/day micronized, 2.5-5 mg/day nonmicronized	Not necessary; may be discontinued abruptly.
20 to 40	3 mg/day micronized, 5 mg/day nonmicronized	Not necessary; may be discontinued abruptly.
> 40	3 mg/day micronized, 5 mg/day nonmicronized	Reduce insulin dose by 50%; further reduce as response is observed. Consider hospitalization during the transition period.

TOLAZAMIDE:

Initial dose – 100 to 250 mg/day with breakfast or the first main meal. If fasting blood sugar (FBS) is less than 200 mg/dL, use 100 mg/day, or 250 mg/day if FBS is greater than 200 mg/dL. If patients are malnourished, underweight, elderly or not eating properly, use 100 mg once a day. Adjust dose to response. If greater than 500 mg/day is required, give in divided doses twice daily. Doses greater than 1 g/day are not likely to improve control.

Maintenance dose – The usual maintenance dose is 100 to 1,000 mg/day with the average maintenance dose being 250 to 500 mg/day. Following initiation of therapy, dosage adjustment is made in increments of 100 to 250 mg at weekly intervals based on the patient's blood glucose response.

Patients on other oral antidiabetic agents – Transfer patients from other oral antidiabetes regimens to tolazamide conservatively. When transferring patients from oral hypoglycemic agents other than chlorpropamide to tolazamide, no transition period or initial priming dose is necessary. Consider 250 mg chlorpropamide to provide approximately the same degree of blood control as 250 mg tolazamide. Observe the patient carefully for hypoglycemia during the transition period from chlorpropamide to tolazamide (1 or 2 weeks) due to the prolonged retention of chlorpropamide in the body and the possibility of a subsequent overlapping drug effect. If patient is receiving less than 1 g/day tolbutamide, begin at 100 mg/day of tolazamide. If patient is receiving 1 g/day or more, initiate 250 mg/day tolazamide as a single dose.

Patients on insulin –

Transferal of Type 2 Diabetes Patients on Insulin to Tolazamide Monotherapy		
Insulin dose	Initial tolazamide dose	Insulin withdrawal
< 20	100 mg/day	Not necessary; may be discontinued abruptly.
20 to 40	250 mg/day	Not necessary; may be discontinued abruptly
> 40	250 mg/day	Reduce insulin by 50%; further reduce as response is observed. Consider hospitalization during the transition period.

TOLBUTAMIDE:

Initial dose – 1 to 2 g/day (range, 0.25 to 3 g). A maintenance dose greater than 2 g/day is seldom required. Daily doses greater than 3 g are not recommended. Total dose may be taken in the morning, but divided doses may allow increased GI tolerance.

Patients on other oral antidiabetic agents – Transfer patients from other oral antidiabetes regimens to tolbutamide conservatively. When transferring patients from oral hypoglycemic agents other than chlorpropamide to tolbutamide, no transition period and no initial or priming doses are necessary. However, when transferring patients from chlorpropamide, exercise particular care during the first 2 weeks because of the prolonged retention of chlorpropamide in the body and the possibility that subsequent overlapping drug effects might provoke hypoglycemia.

Patients on insulin –

Transferal of Type 2 Diabetes Patients on Insulin to Tolbutamide Monotherapy		
Insulin dose	Initial tolbutamide dose	Insulin withdrawal
< 20	1 to 2 g/day	Not necessary; may be discontinued abruptly.
20 to 40	1 to 2 g/day	Reduce insulin dose by 30% to 50%; further reduce as response is observed.
> 40	1 to 2 g/day	Reduce insulin dose by 20%; further reduce as response is observed. Consider hospitalization during the transition period.

Occasionally, conversion to tolbutamide in the hospital may be advisable in candidates who require more than 40 units of insulin daily. During this conversion period when insulin and tolbutamide are being used, hypoglycemia rarely may occur. During insulin withdrawal, have patients test urine for glucose and acetone at least 3 times/day and report results to their physician. The appearance of persistent acetonuria with glycosuria indicates that the patient is a type 1 diabetes patient who requires insulin therapy.

Actions

Pharmacology: The sulfonylurea hypoglycemic agents appear to lower blood glucose by stimulating insulin release from beta cells in the pancreatic islets possibly due to increased intracellular cAMP. These agents are only effective in patients with some capacity for endogenous insulin production. They may improve the binding between insulin and insulin receptors or increase the number of insulin receptors.

General clinical characteristics that favor successful sulfonylurea monotherapy following insulin withdrawal include the following:

- Onset of diabetes at 35 years of age or older
- Obese or normal body weight
- Duration of diabetes less than 10 years
- Absence of ketoacidosis
- Fasting serum glucose 200 mg/dL or less
- Postprandial blood glucose values less than 250 mg/dL
- Insulin requirement less than 40 units/day
- Absence of renal or hepatic dysfunction

Pharmacokinetics: All sulfonylureas are strongly bound to plasma proteins, primarily albumin.

Major Pharmacokinetic Parameters of the Sulfonylureas							
Sulfonylureas	Approximate equivalent doses (mg)	Doses/day	Serum t½ (h)	Onset (h)	Duration (h)	Renal excretion (%)	Active metabolites
First generation							
Chlorpropamide	250 to 375	1	36	1	24 to 60	100	Yes
Tolazamide	250 to 375	1 to 2	7	4 to 6	12 to 24	100	Yes
Tolbutamide	1,000 to 1,500	2 to 3	4.5 to 6.5	1	6 to 12	100	No
Second generation							
Glipizide	10	1 to 2	2 to 4	1 to 3	10 to 24	80 to 85	No
Glyburide Nonmicronized	5	1 to 2	10	2 to 4	16 to 24	50	Yes[a]
Micronized	3	1 to 2	≈ 4	1	12 to 24	50	Yes[a]
Glimepiride	NA[b]	1	≈ 9	2 to 3	24	60	Yes

[a] Weakly active.
[b] Not applicable.

Contraindications

Hypersensitivity to sulfonylureas; diabetes complicated by ketoacidosis, with or without coma; sole therapy of type 1 (insulin-dependent) diabetes mellitus; diabetes when complicated by pregnancy.

Warnings/Precautions

The administration of oral hypoglycemic drugs: The administration of oral hypoglycemic drugs has been associated with increased cardiovascular mortality as compared with treatment with diet alone or diet plus insulin.

Patients treated for 5 to 8 years with diet plus tolbutamide (1.5 g/day) had a rate of cardiovascular mortality approximately 2.5 times that of patients treated with diet alone. A significant increase in total mortality was not observed.

Bioavailability: Micronized glyburide 3 mg tablets provide serum concentrations that are *not* bioequivalent to those from the conventional formulation (nonmicronized) 5 mg tablets.

Hypoglycemia: All sulfonylureas may produce severe hypoglycemia. Proper patient selection, dosage and instructions are important to avoid hypoglycemic episodes.

Asymptomatic patients: Controlling blood glucose in type 2 diabetes with sulfonylureas has not been definitely established to be effective in preventing the long-term cardiovascular or neural complications of diabetes.

Loss of blood glucose control: When a patient stabilized on any diabetic regimen is exposed to stress such as fever, trauma, infection, or surgery, a loss of control may occur. At such times, it may be necessary to discontinue the drug and give insulin.

Disulfiram-like syndrome: A sulfonylurea-induced facial flushing or breathlessness reaction may occur when some sulfonylureas are administered with alcohol.

Syndrome of inappropriate secretion of antidiuretic hormone (SIADH): Water retention and dilutional hyponatremia have occurred after administration of sulfonylureas to type 2 diabetes patients, especially those with CHF or hepatic cirrhosis.

Renal/Hepatic function impairment: Hepatic function impairment may result in inadequate release of glucose in response to hypoglycemia. Renal function impairment may cause decreased elimination of sulfonylureas leading to accumulation producing hypoglycemia.

Pregnancy: *Category* C; *Category* B (glyburide).

Lactation: Chlorpropamide and tolbutamide are excreted in breast milk. It is not known if other sulfonylureas are excreted in breast milk.

Children: Safety and efficacy in children have not been established.

Elderly: In elderly, debilitated, or malnourished patients, and patients with impaired renal or hepatic function, the initial and maintenance dosing should be conservative to avoid hypoglycemic reactions.

Monitoring:

Treatment Goals for Type 2 Diabetes Mellitus

Patient population	Average preprandial glucose (mg/dL)	HbA_{1c}[a] (%)
ADA general recommendations[b]	80 to 120	< 7
Healthy, relatively young	80 to 120	< 8
Elderly and patients with serious medical conditions	100 to 140	< 9

[a] Glycosylated hemoglobin.
[b] American Diabetes Association 1999 Clinical Practice Recommendations.

During the transitional period, test the urine for glucose and acetone at least 3 times/day and have the results reviewed by a physician frequently. Measurement of glycosylated hemoglobin also is useful. It is important that patients be taught to correctly and frequently self-monitor blood glucose.

Drug Interactions

Drugs that may affect sulfonylureas include androgens, anticoagulants, azole antifungals, barbiturates, beta blockers, calcium channel blockers, charcoal, chloramphenicol, cholestyramine, ciprofloxacin, clofibrate, corticosteroids, diazoxide, estrogens, ethanol, fluconazole, gemfibrozil, histamine H_2 antagonists, hydantoins, isoniazid, magnesium salts, methyldopa, MAO inhibitors, nicotinic acid, oral contraceptives, phenothiazines, probenecid, rifampin, salicylates, sulfinpyrazone, sulfonamides, sympathomimetics, thiazide diuretics, thyroid agents, tricyclic antidepressants, urinary acidifiers, and urinary alkalinizers. Drugs that may be affected by sulfonylureas include digitalis glycosides.

Drug/Lab test interactions: A metabolite of tolbutamide in the urine may give a false-positive reaction for albumin if measured by the acidification-after-boiling test, which causes the metabolite to precipitate. There is no interference with the sulfosalicylic acid test.

Drug/Food interactions: Absorption of glipizide is delayed by approximately 40 minutes when taken with food; the drug is more effective when given approximately 30 minutes before a meal. The other sulfonylureas may be taken with food.

Adverse Reactions

GI disturbances (eg, nausea, epigastric fullness, heartburn) are the most common reactions. Other adverse reactions may include hypoglycemia, disulfiram-like reactions; allergic skin reactions; eczema; pruritus; erythema; urticaria; photosensitivity reactions; leukopenia; thrombocytopenia; aplastic anemia; agranulocytosis; hemolytic anemia; pancytopenia; weakness; paresthesia; tinnitus; fatigue; dizziness; vertigo; malaise; elevated liver function tests.

METFORMIN HYDROCHLORIDE

Tablets, oral: 500, 850, and 1,000 mg (*Rx*)	Various, *Glucophage* (Bristol-Myers Squibb)
Tablets, extended-release, oral: 500 mg (*Rx*)	Various, *Fortamet* (First Horizon), *Glucophage XR* (Bristol-Myers Squibb), *Glumetza* (Depomed)
750 mg (*Rx*)	*Glucophage XR* (Bristol-Myers Squibb)
1,000 mg (*Rx*)	*Fortamet* (First Horizon), *Glumetza* (Depomed)
Solution, oral: 500 mg/5 mL (*Rx*)	*Riomet* (Ranbaxy)

Warning:

Lactic acidosis: Lactic acidosis is a rare, but serious, metabolic complication that can occur because of metformin accumulation during treatment; when it occurs, it is fatal in approximately 50% of cases. Lactic acidosis also may occur in association with a number of pathophysiologic conditions, including diabetes mellitus, and whenever there is significant tissue hypoperfusion and hypoxemia. Lactic acidosis is characterized by elevated blood lactate levels (more than 5 mmol/L), decreased blood pH, electrolyte disturbances with an increased anion gap, and an increased lactate/pyruvate ratio. When metformin is implicated as the cause of lactic acidosis, metformin plasma levels of 5 mcg/mL or more are generally found.

continued on next page

Warning: (cont.)

The reported incidence of lactic acidosis in patients receiving metformin is very low (approximately 0.03 cases/1,000 patient-years, with approximately 0.015 fatal cases/1,000 patient-years). In more than 20,000 patient-years exposure to metformin in clinical trials, there were no reports of lactic acidosis. Reported cases have occurred primarily in diabetic patients with significant renal function impairment, including intrinsic renal disease and renal hypoperfusion, often in the setting of multiple concomitant medical/surgical problems and multiple concomitant medications. Patients with congestive heart failure (CHF) requiring pharmacologic management, in particular those with unstable or acute CHF who are at risk of hypoperfusion and hypoxemia, are at increased risk of lactic acidosis. The risk of lactic acidosis increases with the degree of renal function impairment and the patient's age. Therefore, the risk of lactic acidosis may be significantly decreased by regular monitoring of renal function in patients taking metformin and by use of the minimum effective dose. In particular, treatment of the elderly should be accompanied by careful monitoring of renal function. Do not initiate metformin treatment in patients 80 years of age and older unless measurement of creatinine clearance (CrCl) demonstrates that renal function is not reduced, because these patients are more susceptible to developing lactic acidosis. In addition, promptly withhold metformin in the presence of any condition associated with hypoxemia, dehydration, or sepsis. Because impaired hepatic function may significantly limit the ability to clear lactate, generally avoid using metformin in patients with clinical or laboratory evidence of hepatic disease. Caution patients against excessive alcohol intake (acute or chronic) because alcohol potentiates the effects of metformin on lactate metabolism. In addition, temporarily discontinue metformin prior to any intravascular radiocontrast study and for any surgical procedure.

The onset of lactic acidosis often is subtle and accompanied only by nonspecific symptoms such as malaise, myalgias, respiratory distress, increasing somnolence, and nonspecific abdominal distress. There may be associated hypothermia, hypotension, and resistant bradyarrhythmias with more marked acidosis. The patient and the patient's health care provider must be aware of the possible importance of such symptoms. Instruct the patient to notify the health care provider immediately if these symptoms occur. Withdraw metformin until the situation is clarified. Serum electrolytes, ketones, blood glucose, and, if indicated, blood pH, lactate levels, and blood metformin levels may be useful. Once a patient is stabilized on any dose of metformin, GI symptoms, which are common during initiation of therapy, are unlikely to be drug related. Later occurrence of GI symptoms could be caused by lactic acidosis or other serious disease.

Levels of fasting venous plasma lactate above the upper limit of normal but less than 5 mmol/L in patients taking metformin do not necessarily indicate impending lactic acidosis and may be explained by other mechanisms, such as poorly controlled diabetes or obesity, vigorous physical activity, or technical problems in sample handling.

Suspect lactic acidosis in any diabetic patient with metabolic acidosis lacking evidence of ketoacidosis (ketonuria and ketonemia).

Lactic acidosis is a medical emergency that must be treated in a hospital setting. In a patient with lactic acidosis who is taking metformin, immediately discontinue the drug and promptly institute general supportive measures. Because metformin is dialyzable (with a clearance of up to 170 mL/min under good hemodynamic conditions), prompt hemodialysis is recommended to correct the acidosis and remove the accumulated metformin. Such management often results in prompt reversal of symptoms and recovery.

Indications

Type 2 diabetes: As monotherapy, as an adjunct to diet and exercise to improve glycemic control in patients with type 2 diabetes. Metformin immediate-release (IR) tablets and oral solution are indicated in patients 10 years of age and older. Metformin extended-release (ER) tablets are indicated in patients 17 years of age and older (18 years of age and older for *Glumetza*).

Metformin may be used concomitantly with a sulfonylurea or insulin to improve glycemic control in adults 17 years of age and older (18 years of age and older for *Glumetza*).

Administration and Dosage

Individualize dosage on the basis of efficacy and tolerance, while not exceeding the maximum recommended daily dose of metformin IR 2,550 mg in adults and 2,000 mg in children (10 to 16 years of age); the maximum recommended daily dose of metformin ER in adults is 2,000 mg (2,500 mg with *Fortamet*). Give metformin IR in divided doses with meals and give metformin ER once daily with the evening meal. Start at a low dose, with gradual dose escalation, to reduce GI adverse reactions.

Short-term administration may be sufficient during periods of transient loss of control in patients usually well controlled on diet alone.

Metformin ER must be swallowed whole and never crushed or chewed. Occasionally, the inactive ingredients will be eliminated in the feces as a soft, hydrated mass, while the 1,000 mg ER tablets will leave an insoluble shell.

Adults:

Metformin IR tablets and solution – The usual starting dose is 500 mg twice/day or 850 mg once/day, given with meals. Make dosage increases in increments of 500 mg weekly or 850 mg every 2 weeks, up to a total of 2,000 mg/day, given in divided doses. Patients also can be titrated from 500 mg twice/day to 850 mg twice/day after 2 weeks. Metformin IR may be given to a maximum daily dose of 2,550 mg/day. Doses above 2,000 mg may be better tolerated given 3 times/day with meals.

Metformin ER – The usual starting dose is 500 mg once/day (or 1,000 mg once/day with *Glumetza* and *Fortamet*) with the evening meal. Make dosage increases in increments of 500 mg weekly, up to a maximum of 2,000 mg once/day (or 2,500 mg once/day with *Fortamet*) with the evening meal. If glycemic control is not achieved on 2,000 mg once/day, consider a trial of 1,000 mg twice/day. If higher doses of metformin are required, use metformin IR tablets at total daily doses up to 2,550 mg administered in divided daily doses.

Conversion from metformin IR to ER – Patients receiving metformin IR may be safely switched to metformin ER once daily at the same total daily dose, up to 2,000 mg once/day (2,500 mg for *Fortamet*). Closely monitor glycemic control and make dosage adjustments accordingly.

Children: The usual starting dose of metformin IR is 500 mg twice a day, given with meals. Make dosage increases in increments of 500 mg/week up to a maximum of 2,000 mg/day given in divided doses.

The safety and efficacy of metformin ER tablets have not been established.

Transfer from other antidiabetic therapy: When transferring patients from standard oral hypoglycemic agents other than chlorpropamide to metformin, generally no transition period is necessary. When transferring patients from chlorpropamide, exercise care during the first 2 weeks because of the prolonged retention of chlorpropamide leading to overlapping drug effects and possible hypoglycemia.

Concomitant metformin and sulfonylurea therapy in adults: If patients have not responded to 4 weeks of the maximum dose of metformin monotherapy, consider gradual addition of an oral sulfonylurea while continuing metformin at the maximum dose.

If patients have not satisfactorily responded to 1 to 3 months of concomitant therapy with the maximum doses of metformin and an oral sulfonylurea, consider institution of insulin therapy and discontinuation of these oral agents.

Concomitant metformin IR or ER and insulin therapy in adults: Continue the current insulin dose. Initiate metformin IR or ER therapy at 500 mg once/day in patients on insulin therapy. For patients not responding adequately, increase the dose of metformin IR or ER by 500 mg after approximately 1 week and by 500 mg every week thereafter until adequate glycemic control is achieved. It is recommended that the insulin dose be decreased 10% to 25% when fasting plasma glucose (FPG) concentrations decrease to less than 120 mg/dL in patients receiving concomitant insulin and metformin IR or ER.

Special patient populations: Initial and maintenance dosing should be conservative in patients with advanced age because of the potential for decreased renal function. Base any dosage adjustment on a careful assessment of renal function. Generally, do not titrate elderly, debilitated, or malnourished patients to the maximum dose. Do not initiate metformin IR and ER treatment in patients 80 years of age and older unless measurement of CrCl demonstrates that renal function is not reduced.

Actions

Pharmacology: Metformin decreases hepatic glucose production, decreases intestinal absorption of glucose, and improves insulin sensitivity (increases peripheral glucose uptake and utilization). Metformin does not produce hypoglycemia and does not cause hyperinsulinemia. With metformin therapy, insulin secretion remains unchanged while fasting insulin levels and day-long plasma insulin response may actually decrease.

Pharmacokinetics:

Absorption/Distribution – The absolute bioavailability of metformin IR 500 mg given under fasting conditions is approximately 50% to 60%. Food decreases the extent and slightly delays the absorption of metformin.

Metformin is negligibly bound to plasma proteins; steady-state plasma concentrations are reached within 24 to 48 hours.

The extent of metformin absorption from metformin ER at 2,000 mg once-daily dose is similar to the same total daily dose administered as metformin IR 1,000 mg twice daily.

Metabolism/Excretion – Metformin is excreted unchanged in the urine and does not undergo hepatic metabolism or biliary excretion. Tubular secretion is the major route of elimination. The elimination half-life is approximately 17.6 hours.

Contraindications

Renal disease or renal function impairment (eg, as suggested by serum creatinine levels greater than or equal to 1.5 mg/dL [males], greater than or equal to 1.4 mg/dL [females], or abnormal CrCl) that may also result from conditions such as cardiovascular collapse (shock), acute myocardial infarction (MI), and septicemia; CHF requiring pharmacologic treatment; hypersensitivity to metformin; acute or chronic metabolic acidosis, including diabetic ketoacidosis, with or without coma. Treat diabetic ketoacidosis with insulin.

Metformin should be temporarily discontinued in patients undergoing radiologic studies involving intravascular administration of iodinated contrast materials because use of such products may result in acute alteration of renal function.

Warnings/Precautions

Lactic acidosis: Lactic acidosis is a rare, but serious, metabolic complication that can occur because of metformin accumulation during treatment; when it occurs, it is fatal in approximately 50% of cases (see Warning Box).

Hypoxic states: Cardiovascular collapse (shock), acute CHF, acute MI, and other conditions characterized by hypoxemia have been associated with lactic acidosis and may cause prerenal azotemia. If such events occur, discontinue metformin.

Surgical procedures: Temporarily suspend metformin for surgical procedures (unless minor and not associated with restricted intake of food and fluids). Do not restart until the patient's oral intake has resumed and renal function is normal.

Vitamin B_{12} levels: A decrease of previously normal serum vitamin B_{12} levels has been observed in patients receiving metformin.

Hypoglycemia: Hypoglycemia does not occur in patients receiving metformin alone under usual circumstances, but could occur with deficient caloric intake, strenuous exercise not compensated by caloric supplementation, or during concomitant use with other glucose-lowering agents (such as sulfonylureas) or ethanol.

Loss of blood glucose control: When a patient stabilized on any diabetic regimen is exposed to stress such as fever, trauma, infection, or surgery, a temporary loss of glycemic control may occur. At such times, it may be necessary to withhold metformin and temporarily administer insulin. Metformin may be reinstituted after the acute episode is resolved.

Should secondary failure occur with metformin or sulfonylurea monotherapy, combined therapy with metformin and sulfonylurea may result in a response. Should secondary failure occur with combined therapy, it may be necessary to consider therapeutic alternatives, including initiation of insulin therapy.

Iodinated contrast materials: Radiologic studies involving the use of intravascular iodinated contrast materials (ie, IV urogram, IV cholangiography, angiography, and CT scans with intravascular contrast materials) can lead to acute alteration of renal function and have been associated with lactic acidosis in patients receiving metformin. Therefore, in patients in whom any such study is planned, temporarily discontinue metformin at the time of or prior to the procedure, and withhold for 48 hours subsequent to the procedure; reinstitute only after renal function has been reevaluated and found to be normal.

Renal function impairment: Metformin is contraindicated in patients with renal disease or renal function impairment that also may result from conditions such as CV collapse (shock), acute MI, and septicemia.

Hepatic function impairment: Because hepatic function impairment has been associated with cases of lactic acidosis, avoid metformin in patients with clinical or laboratory evidence of hepatic disease.

Pregnancy: Category B.

Lactation: Decide whether to discontinue breast-feeding or to discontinue the drug, taking into account the importance of the drug to the mother.

Children: Safety and efficacy of metformin IR for the treatment of type 2 diabetes have been established in children 10 to 16 years of age who demonstrated a similar response in glycemic control to that seen in adults. A maximum daily dose of 2,000 mg is recommended.

Safety and efficacy of metformin ER in children have not been established.

Elderly: Do not initiate metformin therapy in patients 80 years of age and older unless measurements of CrCl demonstrates that renal function is not reduced. Use metformin with caution as age increases. Generally, do not titrate elderly patients to the maximum dose of metformin.

Monitoring: Before initiation of therapy and at least annually thereafter, assess renal function. In patients at risk of renal function impairment, assess renal function more frequently and discontinue the drug if renal function impairment is present.

Promptly evaluate patients previously well controlled on metformin who develop laboratory abnormalities or clinical illness for evidence of ketoacidosis or lactic acidosis. If acidosis of either form occurs, stop metformin immediately and initiate other appropriate corrective measures.

Monitor response to all diabetic therapies by periodic measurements of FPG and HbA_{1c} levels. Thereafter, monitor both glucose and HbA_{1c}.

Perform initial and periodic monitoring of hematologic parameters and renal function at least on an annual basis.

Drug Interactions

Drugs that may affect metformin include alcohol, cationic drugs, cimetidine, furosemide, iodinated contrast material, and nifedipine.

Drugs that may be affected by metformin include glyburide and furosemide.

Certain drugs tend to produce hyperglycemia and may lead to loss of glycemic control. These drugs include thiazide and other diuretics, corticosteroids, phenothiazines, thyroid products, estrogens, oral contraceptives, phenytoin, nicotinic acid, sympathomimetics, calcium channel blocking drugs, and isoniazid.

Food decreases the extent and slightly delays the absorption of metformin, as shown by an approximately 40% lower mean C_{max}, a 25% lower AUC, and a 35-minute prolongation of T_{max} following administration of a single metformin 850 mg tablet with food.

Adverse Reactions

Adverse reactions occurring in at least 3% of patients include the following:

Metformin IR – Abdominal discomfort, asthenia, diarrhea, flatulence, headache, ingestion, nausea, vomiting.

Metformin ER – Adverse reactions occurring in more than 5% of patients include headache, diarrhea, dyspepsia, nausea, rhinitis, accidental injury, infection, and hypoglycemia.

Adverse reaction occurring in 1% to 5% of patients include hypertension, asthenia, dizziness, hypoesthesia, sinus headache, tremor, contusion, abdominal distension, abdominal pain, dyspepsia, flatulence, gastroenteritis viral, loose stools, toothache, upper abdominal pain, vomiting, muscle cramp, muscle strain, myalgia, pain in limb, nasal congestion, seasonal allergy, ear pain, chest pain, fungal infection, tonsillitis, tooth abscess.

THIAZOLIDINEDIONES

ROSIGLITAZONE MALEATE	
Tablets; oral: 2, 4, and 8 mg (*Rx*)	*Avandia* (GlaxoSmithKline)
PIOGLITAZONE HYDROCHLORIDE	
Tablets; oral: 15, 30, and 45 mg (*Rx*)	*Actos* (Takeda Pharmaceuticals America)

Warning:

Congestive heart failure (CHF): Thiazolidinediones cause or exacerbate CHF in some patients. After initiation of a thiazolidinedione and after dose increases, observe patients carefully for signs and symptoms of heart failure (including excessive, rapid weight gain, dyspnea, and/or edema). If these signs and symptoms develop, manage the heart failure according to the current standards of care. Furthermore, discontinuation or dose reduction of the thiazolidinedione must be considered.

Thiazolidinediones are not recommended in patients with symptomatic heart failure. Initiation of thiazolidinediones in patients with New York Heart Association class III or IV heart failure is contraindicated.

Indications

Pioglitazone:

Type 2 diabetes – Monotherapy as an adjunct to diet and exercise to improve glycemic control.

In combination with metformin, insulin, a sulfonylurea, or metformin and a sulfonylurea when diet, exercise, and a single agent do not result in adequate glycemic control.

Rosiglitazone:

Type 2 diabetes – Monotherapy as an adjunct to diet and exercise in patients with type 2 diabetes mellitus.

Also for use in combination with a sulfonylurea, metformin, or metformin and a sulfonylurea when diet, exercise, and a single agent do not result in adequate glycemic control.

Administration and Dosage

PIOGLITAZONE: Take without regard to meals.

Monotherapy – Initiate at 15 or 30 mg once daily. For patients who respond inadequately, the dose can be increased in increments up to 45 mg once daily.

Combination therapy –

Sulfonylureas: Initiate pioglitazone in combination with a sulfonylurea at 15 or 30 mg once daily. Decrease the dose of the sulfonylurea if patients report hypoglycemia.

Metformin: Initiate pioglitazone in combination with metformin at 15 or 30 mg once daily.

Insulin: Initiate pioglitazone in combination with insulin at 15 or 30 mg once daily. Continue the current insulin dose upon initiation of pioglitazone therapy. Decrease the insulin dose by 10% to 25% if the patient reports hypoglycemia or if plasma glucose concentrations decrease to less than 100 mg/dL.

Maximum recommended dose – Do not exceed more than 45 mg once daily of pioglitazone.

ROSIGLITAZONE MALEATE:

Monotherapy – The usual starting dose is 4 mg, administered as a single dose once daily or in divided doses twice daily.

Combination therapy – When rosiglitazone is added to existing therapy, the current dose of sulfonylurea, insulin, or metformin can be continued upon initiation of rosiglitazone therapy.

Metformin: The usual starting dose of rosiglitazone in combination with metformin is 4 mg as a single dose once daily or in divided doses twice daily.

Insulin: Continue the insulin dose upon initiation of rosiglitazone therapy. Dose rosiglitazone at 4 mg daily.

Sulfonylureas: When used in combination with sulfonylurea, the recommended dose of rosiglitazone is 4 mg as a single dose once daily or in divided doses twice daily. If patients report hypoglycemia, decrease the dose of sulfonylurea.

Sulfonylurea plus metformin: The usual starting dose of rosiglitazone in combination with a sulfonylurea plus metformin is 4 mg administered as either a single dose once daily or divided doses twice daily. If patients report hypoglycemia, the dose of the sulfonylurea should be decreased.

Maximum recommended dose: The dose of rosiglitazone should not exceed 8 mg/day as a single dose or divided twice daily. Doses of rosiglitazone higher than 4 mg/day in combination with insulin are not currently indicated.

Actions

Pharmacology: **Rosiglitazone** and **pioglitazone**, members of the thiazolidinediones class of antidiabetic agents, improve glycemic control by improving insulin sensitivity. Studies indicate that they improve sensitivity to insulin in muscle and adipose tissue and inhibit hepatic gluconeogenesis.

Pharmacokinetics:

Pharmacokinetics of Thiazolidinediones

Parameters	Pioglitazone	Rosiglitazone
Absorption		
Bioavailability	—	99%
T_{max} [a]	2 h[b]	1 h
Food effect	Delay in T_{max} (3 to 4 h)	Delay in T_{max} (1.75 h);
Distribution		
Volume of distribution	≈ 0.63 L/kg[c]	17.6 L
Protein binding	> 99%	≈ 99.8%
Metabolism		
Mechanism	Hydroxylation, oxidation, CYP2C8, CYP3A4, CYP 1A1	N-demethylation, hydroxylation, conjugation CYP2C8, CYP2C9 (minor)

Pharmacokinetics of Thiazolidinediones		
Parameters	Pioglitazone	Rosiglitazone
Excretion		
Site	Urine (15% to 30%), feces	Urine (64%), feces (23%)
Elimination half-life	3 to 7 h	3 to 4 h

[a] T_{max} = time to maximum plasma concentration.
[b] In the fasting state.
[c] Following single oral doses.

Contraindications

Initiation in patients with established NYHA class III or IV heart failure; hypersensitivity or allergy to **pioglitazone** or **rosiglitazone** or any of their components.

Warnings/Precautions

Cardiac effects: Thiazolidinediones can cause fluid retention, which may exacerbate or lead to heart failure.

Rosiglitazone is not recommended in patients with symptomatic heart failure. Initiation of rosiglitazone is not recommended for patients experiencing an acute coronary event. Initiate **pioglitazone** at the lowest approved dose if it is prescribed for patients with systolic heart failure (NYHA class II).

Edema: Use **pioglitazone** and **rosiglitazone** with caution in patients with edema.

Use with caution in patients at risk for heart failure and monitor patients at risk for heart failure for signs and symptoms of heart failure.

Fractures: An increased incidence of bone fractures was noted in women taking thiazolidinediones.

Hematologic: **Rosiglitazone** and **pioglitazone** may cause decreases in hemoglobin and hematocrit.

Hepatotoxicity: Check liver enzymes prior to the initiation of therapy. Do not initiate therapy in patients with increased baseline liver enzyme levels (ALT more than 2.5 times the upper limit of normal [ULN]). If at any time ALT levels increase to more than 3 times the ULN, recheck liver enzyme levels as soon as possible. If ALT levels remain more than 3 times the ULN, discontinue therapy.

If any patient develops symptoms suggesting hepatic dysfunction, check liver enzymes. If jaundice is observed, discontinue therapy.

Hypoglycemia: Patients receiving **pioglitazone** or **rosiglitazone** in combination with insulin or oral hypoglycemics (eg, sulfonylureas) may be at risk for hypoglycemia.

Macular edema: Macular edema has been reported in postmarketing experience.

Ovulation: In premenopausal anovulatory patients with insulin resistance, thiazolidinedione treatment may result in resumption of ovulation. These patients may be at risk for pregnancy.

Type 1 diabetes: **Pioglitazone** and **rosiglitazone** are active only in the presence of insulin. Therefore, do not use in type 1 diabetes patients or for the treatment of diabetic ketoacidosis.

Weight gain: Dose-related weight gain was seen with **rosiglitazone** and **pioglitazone** alone and combination with other hypoglycemic agents.

Pregnancy: Category C.

Lactation: Do not administer to breast-feeding women.

Children: Safety and efficacy have not been established in patients under 18 years of age.

Monitoring: Perform periodic fasting blood glucose and HbA_{1c} measurements to monitor therapeutic response. Liver enzyme monitoring is recommended prior to initiation of therapy in all patients and periodically thereafter.

After initiation or with dose increase, carefully monitor patients for adverse reactions related to fluid retention, weight gain, or signs and symptoms of CHF exacerbation.

Drug Interactions

Drugs that may affect **pioglitazone** include atorvastatin, CYP2C8 inhibitors (eg, gemfibrozil, ketoconazole, trimethoprim), gatifloxacin, gemfibrozil, insulin, and ketoconazole. Drugs that may be affected by **pioglitazone** include atorvastatin, glyburide, hormonal contraceptives (eg, ethinyl estradiol), insulin, midazolam, nevirapine, nifedipine, and nitrates (eg, nitroglycerin).

Adverse Reactions

Pioglitazone – Adverse reactions that occurred in at least 3% of patients included the following: aggravated diabetes mellitus, edema, headache, myalgia, pharyngitis, sinusitis, tooth disorder, upper respiratory tract infection.

Rosiglitazone – Adverse reactions that occurred in at least 3% of patients included the following: back pain, edema, fatigue, headache, hyperglycemia, injury, sinusitis, upper respiratory tract infection.

Lab test abnormalities:

Pioglitazone – Decreased alkaline phosphatase, AST, gamma-glutamyl transferase, hematocrit, hemoglobin, triglycerides; increased ALT, creatinine phosphokinase, high-density lipoprotein (HDL).

Rosiglitazone – decreased free fatty acids, hematocrit, hemoglobin, white blood cells; increased ALT, bilirubin, HDL, low-density lipoprotein, total cholesterol.

ANTIDIABETIC COMBINATION PRODUCTS

GLYBURIDE/METFORMIN HYDROCHLORIDE	
Tablets; oral: Glyburide 1.25 mg/metformin 250 mg, glyburide 2.5 mg/metformin 500 mg, and glyburide 5 mg/metformin 500 mg (*Rx*)	Various, *Glucovance* (Bristol-Myers Squibb)
GLIPIZIDE/METFORMIN HYDROCHLORIDE	
Tablets; oral: Glipizide 2.5 mg/metformin 250 mg, glipizide 2.5 mg/metformin 500 mg, and glipizide 5 mg/metformin 500 mg (*Rx*)	Various, *Metaglip* (Bristol-Myers Squibb)
PIOGLITAZONE HYDROCHLORIDE/GLIMEPIRIDE	
Tablets; oral: Pioglitazone 30 mg/glimepiride 2 mg and pioglitazone 30 mg/glimepiride 4 mg (*Rx*)	*Duetact* (Takeda Pharmaceuticals America)
PIOGLITAZONE HYDROCHLORIDE/METFORMIN HYDROCHLORIDE	
Tablets; oral: Pioglitazone 15 mg/metformin 500 mg and pioglitazone 15 mg/metformin 850 mg (*Rx*)	*ActoPlus Met* (Takeda)
Tablets, extended-release; oral: Pioglitazone 15 mg/metformin 1,000 mg XR and pioglitazone 30 mg/metformin 1,000 mg XR (*Rx*)	*ActoPlus Met XR* (Takeda)
REPAGLINIDE/METFORMIN HYDROCHLORIDE	
Tablets; oral: Repaglinide 1 mg/metformin 500 mg and repaglinide 2 mg/metformin 500 mg (*Rx*)	*PrandiMet* (Novo Nordisk)
ROSIGLITAZONE/GLIMEPIRIDE	
Tablets; oral: Rosiglitazone 4 mg/glimepiride 1 mg, rosiglitazone 4 mg/glimepiride 2 mg, rosiglitazone 4 mg/glimepiride 4 mg, rosiglitazone 8 mg/glimepiride 2 mg, rosiglitazone 8 mg/glimepiride 4 mg (*Rx*)	*Avandaryl* (GlaxoSmithKline)
ROSIGLITAZONE/METFORMIN HYDROCHLORIDE	
Tablets; oral: Rosiglitazone 2 mg/metformin 500 mg, rosiglitazone 2 mg/metformin 1,000 mg, rosiglitazone 4 mg/metformin 500 mg, and rosiglitazone 4 mg/metformin 1,000 mg (*Rx*)	*Avandamet* (GlaxoSmithKline)
SAXAGLIPTIN/METFORMIN	
Tablets, extended-release; oral: Saxagliptin 5 mg/metformin 500 mg, saxagliptin 5 mg/metformin 1,000 mg, saxagliptin 2.5 mg/metformin 1,000 mg (*Rx*)	*Kombiglyze XR* (Bristol-Myers Squibb)
SITAGLIPTIN/METFORMIN HYDROCHLORIDE	
Tablets; oral: Sitagliptin 50 mg/metformin 500 mg, sitagliptin 50 mg/metformin 1,000 mg (*Rx*)	*Janumet* (Merck)

Warning:

Congestive heart failure: Thiazolidinediones cause or exacerbate congestive heart failure (CHF) in some patients. After initiation of thiazolidinediones, and after dose increases, observe patients carefully for signs and symptoms of heart failure (including excessive, rapid weight gain, dyspnea, and/or edema). If these signs and symptoms develop, the heart failure should be managed according to the current standards of care. Furthermore, discontinuation or dose reduction of thiazolidinediones must be considered.

Thiazolidinediones are not recommended in patients with symptomatic heart failure. Initiation of thiazolidinediones in patients with established New York Heart Association (NYHA) class III or IV heart failure is contraindicated.

continued on next page

Warning: (cont.)

Lactic acidosis: Lactic acidosis is a rare but serious complication that can occur because of **metformin** accumulation during treatment with **metformin** combinations; when it occurs, it is fatal in approximately 50% of cases. Lactic acidosis may also occur in association with a number of pathophysiologic conditions, including diabetes mellitus, and whenever there is a significant tissue hypoperfusion and hypoxemia. Lactic acidosis is characterized by elevated blood lactate levels (greater than 5 mmol/L), decreased blood pH, electrolyte disturbances with an increased anion gap, and an increased lactate/pyruvate ratio. When **metformin** is implicated as the cause of lactic acidosis, **metformin** plasma levels greater than 5 mcg/mL are generally found.

The reported incidence of lactic acidosis in patients receiving **metformin** is very low (approximately 0.03 cases per 1,000 patient years, with approximately 0.015 fatal cases per 1,000 patient years). In more than 20,000 patient years' exposure to metformin in clinical trials, there were no reports of lactic acidosis. Reported cases have occurred primarily in diabetic patients with significant renal function impairment, including intrinsic renal disease and renal hypoperfusion, often in the setting of multiple concomitant medical/surgical problems and multiple concomitant medications. Patients with CHF requiring pharmacologic management, in particular those with unstable or acute CHF who are at risk of hypoperfusion and hypoxemia, are at increased risk of lactic acidosis. The risk of lactic acidosis increases with the degree of renal function impairment and the patient's age. Therefore, the risk of lactic acidosis may be significantly decreased by regular monitoring of renal function in patients taking **metformin** combinations. In particular, accompany treatment of elderly patients with careful monitoring of renal function. Do not initiate treatment with **metformin** combinations in patients 80 years of age and older unless measurement of creatinine clearance (CrCl) demonstrates that renal function is not reduced, because these patients are more susceptible to developing lactic acidosis. In addition, promptly withhold **metformin** combinations in the presence of any condition associated with hypoxemia, dehydration, or sepsis. Because hepatic function impairment may significantly limit the ability to clear lactate, generally avoid **metformin** combinations in patients with clinical or laboratory evidence of hepatic disease. Caution patients against excessive alcohol intake, either acute or chronic, when taking **metformin** combinations because alcohol potentiates the effects of **metformin** on lactate metabolism. In addition, temporarily discontinue **metformin** combination therapy prior to any intravascular radio contrast study and for any surgical procedure.

The onset is often subtle, accompanied only by nonspecific symptoms, such as malaise, myalgias, respiratory distress, increasing somnolence, and nonspecific abdominal distress. There may be associated hypothermia, hypotension, and resistant bradyarrhythmias with more marked acidosis. The patient and the patient's health care provider must be aware of the possible importance of such symptoms and instruct patients to immediately notify their health care provider if symptoms occur. Withdraw **metformin** combinations until the situation is clarified. Serum electrolytes, ketones, blood glucose, and, if indicated, blood pH, lactate levels, and even blood **metformin** levels may be useful. Once a patient is stabilized on any dose level of metformin combination, GI symptoms, which are common during initiation of therapy, are unlikely to be drug related. Later occurrence of GI symptoms could be caused by lactic acidosis or other serious disease.

Levels of fasting venous plasma lactate above the upper limit of normal (ULN) but less than 5 nmol/L in patients taking **metformin** combinations do not necessarily indicate impending lactic acidosis and may be explainable by other mechanisms, such as poorly controlled diabetes or obesity, vigorous physical activity, or technical problems in sample handling.

continued on next page

Warning: (cont.)

Suspect lactic acidosis in any diabetic patient with metabolic acidosis lacking evidence of ketoacidosis (eg, ketonemia, ketonuria).

Lactic acidosis is a medical emergency that must be treated in a hospital setting. Immediately discontinue **metformin** combination therapy in a patient with lactic acidosis and promptly institute general supportive measures. Because **metformin** is dialyzable (with a clearance of up to 170 mL/min under good hemodynamic conditions), prompt hemodialysis is recommended to correct the acidosis and remove the accumulated metformin. Such management often results in prompt reversal of symptoms and recovery.

Indications

Glyburide/Metformin and glipizide/metformin combinations:

Type 2 diabetes – Initial and second-line therapy.

Pioglitazone/Glimepiride combination:

Type 2 diabetes – As an adjunct to diet and exercise to improve glycemic control in patients with type 2 diabetes mellitus who are already treated with a thiazolidinedione and a sulfonylurea or who have inadequate glycemic control on a thiazolidinedione alone or sulfonylurea alone.

Pioglitazone/Metformin combination:

Type 2 diabetes – In patients who are already being treated with a combination of **pioglitazone** and **metformin** or whose diabetes is not adequately controlled with **metformin** or **pioglitazone** alone.

Repaglinide/Metformin combination:

Type 2 diabetes – As an adjunct to diet and exercise to improve glycemic control in adults with type 2 diabetes mellitus who are already treated with a meglitinide and metformin or who have inadequate glycemic control on a meglitinide alone or metformin alone.

Rosiglitazone/Glimepiride combination:

Type 2 diabetes – As an adjunct to diet and exercise to improve glycemic control in patients with type 2 diabetes mellitus when treatment with dual **rosiglitazone** and **glimepiride** therapy is appropriate.

Rosiglitazone/Metformin combination:

Type 2 diabetes – As an adjunct to diet and exercise to improve glycemic control in adults with type 2 diabetes mellitus when treatment with both **rosiglitazone** and **metformin** is appropriate.

Saxagliptin/Metformin combination:

Type 2 diabetes mellitus – As an adjunct to diet and exercise to improve glycemic control in adults with type 2 diabetes mellitus when treatment with both **saxagliptin** and **metformin** is appropriate.

Sitagliptin/Metformin combination:

Type 2 diabetes – As an adjunct to diet and exercise to improve glycemic control in adults with type 2 diabetes mellitus who are not adequately controlled on **metformin** or **sitagliptin** alone or in patients already being treated with the combination of **sitagliptin** and **metformin**.

Administration and Dosage

Specific patient populations: **Metformin** combination products are not recommended for use during pregnancy or in children. Initial and maintenance dosing should be conservative in patients with advanced age. Do not titrate elderly, debilitated, or malnourished patients to the maximum dose to avoid the risk of hypoglycemia.

GLYBURIDE/METFORMIN and GLIPIZIDE/METFORMIN: See Warning Box at the beginning of the monograph.

Initial therapy –

Starting dose:

Glyburide/Metformin – Glyburide 1.25 mg/metformin 250 mg once or twice daily with meals. Increase dosage in increments of glyburide 1.25 mg/metformin

250 mg/day every 2 weeks. As initial therapy in patients with baseline HbA_{1C} of more than 9% or a fasting plasma glucose (FPG) of more than 200 mg/dL, a starting dosage of glyburide 1.25 mg/metformin 250 mg twice daily with the morning and evening meals may be used.

Glipizide/Metformin – Glipizide 2.5 mg/metformin 250 mg once a day with a meal. For patients whose FPG is 280 to 320 mg/dL, consider a starting dose of glipizide 2.5 mg/metformin 500 mg twice daily. Increase dosage by 1 tablet per day every 2 weeks up to a maximum of glipizide 10 mg/metformin 1,000 mg or glipizide 10 mg/metformin 2,000 mg per day given in divided doses.

Previously treated patients (second-line therapy) –

Starting dose:

Glyburide/Metformin – Glyburide 2.5 mg/metformin 500 mg or glyburide 5 mg/metformin 500 mg twice daily with meals.

Titrate the daily dose by no more than glyburide 5 mg/metformin 500 mg up to a maximum dose of glyburide 20 mg/metformin 2,000 mg/day. The starting dose should not exceed the daily dose of **glyburide** and **metformin** already being taken.

Glipizide/Metformin – Glipizide 2.5 mg/metformin 500 mg or glipizide 5 mg/metformin 500 mg twice daily with the morning and evening meals. The starting dose should not exceed the daily doses of **glipizide** or **metformin** already being taken. Titrate the daily dose by no more than glipizide 5 mg/metformin 500 mg up to a maximum dose of glipizide 20 mg/metformin 2,000 mg per day.

Addition of thiazolidinediones to glyburide/metformin therapy – Initiate thiazolidinediones at its recommended starting dose. In patients who develop hypoglycemia when receiving **glyburide/metformin** and a thiazolidinedione, consider reducing the dose of the glyburide component of **glyburide/metformin**.

PIOGLITAZONE/GLIMEPIRIDE:

Maximum dose – Pioglitazone 45 mg/glimepiride 8 mg per day.

Dosage – Administer once daily with the first main meal.

Patients currently on glimepiride monotherapy: Initiate at pioglitazone 30 mg/glimepiride 2 mg or pioglitazone 30 mg/glimepiride 4 mg tablet strengths once daily.

Patients currently on pioglitazone monotherapy: Initiate at pioglitazone 30 mg/glimepiride 2 mg once daily.

Patients switching from combination therapy of pioglitazone plus glimepiride as separate tablets: Pioglitazone 30 mg/glimepiride 2 mg or pioglitazone 30 mg/glimepiride 4 mg tablet strengths based on the dose of **pioglitazone** and **glimepiride** already being taken.

Patients currently on a different sulfonylurea monotherapy or switching from combination therapy of pioglitazone plus a different sulfonylurea: Start dosage at pioglitazone 30 mg/glimepiride 2 mg once daily.

Hepatic function impairment – Therapy with **pioglitazone/glimepiride** should not be initiated if the patient exhibits clinical evidence of active liver disease or increased serum transaminase levels (ALT greater than 2.5 times the ULN) at start of therapy. Liver enzyme monitoring is recommended in all patients prior to initiation of therapy and periodically thereafter.

Special risk patients – In elderly, debilitated, or malnourished patients or in patients with renal or hepatic function impairment, the initial dosing, dose increments, and maintenance dosage of **pioglitazone/glimepiride** should be conservative to avoid hypoglycemic reactions. Start these patients at glimepiride 1 mg prior to prescribing **pioglitazone/glimepiride**.

Pioglitazone/glimepiride is not recommended for use in children or during pregnancy or lactation.

Congestive heart failure – The lowest approved dose of **pioglitazone/glimepiride** therapy should be prescribed to patients with type 2 diabetes and systolic dysfunction only after titration from **pioglitazone** 15 to 30 mg of has been safely tolerated. If subsequent dose adjustment is necessary, patients should be carefully monitored for weight gain, edema, or signs and symptoms of CHF exacerbation.

PIOGLITAZONE/METFORMIN: See Warning Box at the beginning of the monograph.

Maximum dose –

Immediate-release: Pioglitazone 45 mg/metformin 2,550 mg per day.

Extended-release: Pioglitazone 45 mg/metformin extended-release (ER) 2,000 mg per day.

Initial dose – Selecting the starting dose of pioglitazone/metformin should be based on the patient's current regimen of pioglitazone and/or metformin.

Immediate-release: Pioglitazone 15 mg/metformin 500 mg or pioglitazone 15 mg/metformin 850 mg once or twice daily with food.

Extended-release: Pioglitazone 15 mg/metformin ER 1,000 mg or pioglitazone 30 mg/metformin ER 1,000 mg once daily with the evening meal.

Special populations – **Pioglitazone/metformin** is not recommended for use in children or pregnancy.

Renal function impairment: Monitoring of renal function is necessary to aid in prevention of metformin-associated lactic acidosis, particularly in elderly patients. Pioglitazone/metformin should only be used in patients with normal renal function.

Hepatic function impairment: Therapy with **pioglitazone/metformin** should not be initiated if the patient exhibits clinical evidence of active liver disease or increased serum transaminase levels (ALT greater than 2.5 times the ULN) at start of therapy. Liver enzyme monitoring is recommended in all patients prior to initiation of therapy with **pioglitazone/metformin** and periodically thereafter.

Elderly: Any dosage adjustment should be based on a careful assessment of renal function. Generally, elderly, debilitated, and malnourished patients should not be titrated to the maximum dose of pioglitazone/metformin.

Administration – Pioglitazone/metformin should be given in divided daily doses with meals to reduce the GI adverse reactions associated with metformin.

Pioglitazone/metformin ER must be swallowed whole and not chewed, cut, or crushed. Inform patients that the inactive ingredients may occasionally be eliminated in the feces as a soft mass that may resemble the original tablet.

REPAGLINIDE/METFORMIN:

Recommended dosing – Administer 2 to 3 times a day up to a maximum daily dose of repaglinide 10 mg/metformin 2,500 mg. No more than repaglinide 4 mg/metformin 1,000 mg should be taken per meal.

Patients inadequately controlled with metformin monotherapy – The recommended starting dose of repaglinide/metformin is repaglinide 1 mg/metformin 500 mg administered twice daily with meals, with gradual dose escalation.

Patients inadequately controlled with meglitinide monotherapy – The recommended starting dose of the metformin component of repaglinide/metformin should be metformin 500 mg twice a day, with gradual dose escalation.

Patients currently using repaglinide and metformin concomitantly – Repaglinide/metformin can be initiated at the dose of repaglinide and metformin similar to (but not exceeding) the patient's current doses.

Maximum dose – Repaglinide 10 mg/metformin 2,500 mg per day; or repaglinide 4 mg/metformin 1,000 mg per meal.

Administration – Repaglinide/metformin doses should be taken within 15 minutes prior to the meal, but can vary from immediately preceding the meal up to 30 minutes before the meal. Patients who skip a meal should be instructed to skip the repaglinide/metformin dose for that meal.

ROSIGLITAZONE/GLIMEPIRIDE:

Dosage – Rosiglitazone 4 mg/glimepiride 1 mg administered once daily with the first meal of the day. For patients already treated with a sulfonylurea or thiazolidinedione, consider a starting dose of rosiglitazone 4 mg/glimepiride 2 mg.

When switching from combination therapy of **rosiglitazone** plus **glimepiride** as separate tablets, the usual starting dose of **rosiglitazone/glimepiride** is the dose of **rosiglitazone** and **glimepiride** already being taken.

Dose titration –

Previously treated with thiazolidinedione monotherapy: For patients previously treated with thiazolidinedione monotherapy and switched to **rosiglitazone/glimepiride**, dose titration of the **glimepiride** component of **rosiglitazone/glimepiride** is recommended if patients are not adequately controlled after 1 to 2 weeks.

Increases in glimepiride component: The **glimepiride** component may be increased in no more than 2 mg increments. After an increase in the **glimepiride** component, dose titration of **rosiglitazone/glimepiride** is recommended if patients are not adequately controlled after 1 to 2 weeks.

Previously treated with sulfonylurea monotherapy: For patients previously treated with sulfonylurea monotherapy and switched to **rosiglitazone/glimepiride**, it may take 2 weeks to see a reduction in blood glucose and 2 to 3 months to see the full effect of the **rosiglitazone** component. Therefore, dose titration of the **rosiglitazone** component of **rosiglitazone/glimepiride** is recommended if patients are not adequately controlled after 8 to 12 weeks.

Maximum dose – The maximum recommended daily dose is **rosiglitazone** 8 mg/**glimepiride** 4 mg.

ROSIGLITAZONE/METFORMIN: See Warning Box at the beginning of the monograph.

Initial therapy – Rosiglitazone 2 mg/metformin 500 mg administered once or twice daily. For patients with glycosylated hemoglobin (HBA_{1c}) more than 11% or a FPG more than 270 mg/dL, a starting dosage of rosiglitazone 2 mg/metformin 500 mg twice daily may be considered. The dose of **rosiglitazone/metformin** may be increased in increments of rosiglitazone 2 mg/metformin 500 mg per day to a maximum of rosiglitazone 8 mg/metformin 2,000 mg per day given in divided doses if patients are not adequately controlled after 4 weeks.

Patients inadequately controlled with rosiglitazone or metformin monotherapy – After an increase in **metformin** dosage, dose titration is recommended if patients are not adequately controlled after 1 to 2 weeks. After an increase in **rosiglitazone** dosage, dose titration is recommended if patients are not adequately controlled after 8 to 12 weeks.

Patients inadequately controlled on metformin monotherapy – **rosiglitazone** 4 mg plus the dose of **metformin** already being taken (see the following table).

Patients inadequately controlled on rosiglitazone monotherapy – **Metformin** 1,000 mg plus the dose of **rosiglitazone** already being taken (see the following table).

Rosiglitazone/Metformin Starting Dose

	Usual *Avandamet* starting dose	
Prior therapy (total daily dose)	Tablet strength	Number of tablets
Metformin hydrochloride[a]		
1,000 mg/day	2 mg/ 500 mg	1 tablet twice daily
2,000 mg/day	2 mg/ 1,000 mg	1 tablet twice daily
Rosiglitazone		
4 mg/day	2 mg/ 500 mg	1 tablet twice daily
8 mg/day	4 mg/ 500 mg	1 tablet twice daily

[a] For patients on doses of **metformin hydrochloride** between 1,000 and 2,000 mg/day, initiation of **rosiglitazone/metformin** requires individualization of therapy.

When switching from combination therapy of rosiglitazone plus metformin as separate tablets – Starting dose is the dose of **rosiglitazone** and **metformin** already being taken.

If additional glycemic control is needed – The daily dose may be increased by increments of **rosiglitazone** 4 mg and/or **metformin** 500 mg, up to the maximum recommended total daily dose of rosiglitazone 8 mg/metformin 2,000 mg.

Elderly – Elderly patients should not be titrated to the maximum dose of rosiglitazone/metformin. Carefully titrate rosiglitazone/metformin to establish the minimum dose for adequate glycemic effect. Monitor renal function regularly in elderly patients, particularly those 80 years of age and older, and, generally, do not titrate rosiglitazone/metformin to the maximum dose of the metformin component (ie, 2,000 mg).

Renal function impairment – Any dosage adjustment should be based on a careful assessment of renal function. Patients with serum creatinine levels above the ULN for their age should not receive rosiglitazone/metformin.

Debilitated/malnourished patients – Generally, debilitated and malnourished patients should not be titrated to the maximum dose of rosiglitazone/metformin.

Hepatic function impairment – Do not initiate therapy if the patient exhibits clinical evidence of active liver disease or increased serum transaminase levels (ALT more than 2.5 times ULN at start of therapy). Liver enzyme monitoring is recommended in all patients prior to initiation of therapy with **rosiglitazone/metformin** and periodically thereafter.

Administration – Rosiglitazone/metformin is generally given in divided doses with meals.

SAXAGLIPTIN/METFORMIN:

General dosing considerations – The dosage should be individualized on the basis of the patient's current regimen, effectiveness, and tolerability. Saxagliptin/metformin ER should generally be administered once daily with the evening meal, with gradual dose titration to reduce the GI adverse effects associated with metformin.

Adults – The recommended starting dosage of saxagliptin/metformin ER in patients who need saxagliptin 5 mg and who are not currently treated with metformin is saxagliptin 5 mg/metformin ER 500 mg once daily with gradual dose escalation to reduce the GI adverse effects due to metformin.

In patients treated with metformin, the dose of saxagliptin/metformin ER should provide metformin at the dose already being taken or the nearest therapeutically appropriate dose. Following a switch from metformin immediate release to metformin ER, glycemic control should be closely monitored and dosage adjustments made accordingly.

Patients who need saxagliptin 2.5 mg in combination with metformin ER may be treated with saxagliptin 2.5 mg/metformin ER 1,000 mg. Patients who need saxagliptin 2.5 mg who are either metformin naíve or who require a dose of metformin higher than 1,000 mg should use the individual components.

The maximum daily recommended dose is 5 mg for saxagliptin and 2,000 mg for metformin ER.

Strong CYP3A4/5 inhibitors: The maximum recommended dosage of saxagliptin is 2.5 mg once daily when coadministered with strong cytochrome P450 3A4/5 (CYP3A4/5) inhibitors (eg, ketoconazole, atazanavir, clarithromycin, indinavir, itraconazole, nefazodone, nelfinavir, ritonavir, saquinavir, telithromycin). For these patients, limit the dosage of the combination to saxagliptin 2.5 mg/metformin ER 1,000 mg once daily.

Administration – Saxagliptin/metformin ER must be swallowed whole and never crushed, cut, or chewed. Occasionally, the inactive ingredients of saxagliptin/metformin ER will be eliminated in the feces as a soft, hydrated mass that may resemble the original tablet.

SITAGLIPTIN/METFORMIN:

Dosing recommendations – The starting dose of **sitagliptin/metformin** should be based on the patient's current regimen. **Sitagliptin/metformin** should be given twice daily with meals.

Do not exceed the maximum recommended daily dose of **sitagliptin** 100 mg and **metformin** 2,000 mg.

Patients inadequately controlled on metformin monotherapy – The usual starting dose of **sitagliptin/metformin** should be equal to 100 mg total daily dose (50 mg twice daily) of **sitagliptin** plus the dose of **metformin** already being taken. For patients taking **metformin** 850 mg twice daily, the recommended starting dosage of **sitagliptin/metformin** is **sitagliptin** 50 mg/**metformin** 1,000 mg twice daily.

Patients inadequately controlled on sitagliptin monotherapy – The usual starting dosage of **sitagliptin/metformin** is **sitagliptin** 50 mg/**metformin** 500 mg twice daily. Patients may be titrated up to **sitagliptin** 50 mg/**metformin** 1,000 mg twice daily. Patients taking **sitagliptin** monotherapy dose-adjusted for renal function impairment should not be switched to **sitagliptin/metformin**.

Patients switching from sitagliptin coadministered with metformin – **Sitagliptin/metformin** may be initiated at the dose of **sitagliptin** and **metformin** already being taken.

THYROID HORMONES

LEVOTHYROXINE SODIUM	
Tablets: 0.025, 0.05, 0.075, 0.088, 0.1, 0.112, 0.125, 0.137, 0.15, 0.175, 0.2, and 0.3 mg (*Rx*)	Various, *Levothroid* (Forest), *Levoxyl* (Jones Pharma), *Synthroid* (Abbott), *Thyro-Tabs* (Lloyd), *Unithroid* (Lannett)
Powder for injection, lyophilized: 200 and 500 mcg (*Rx*)	Various
LIOTHYRONINE SODIUM	
Tablets: 5, 25, and 50 mcg (*Rx*)	Various, *Cytomel* (Monarch)
Injection: 10 mcg/mL (*Rx*)	Various, *Triostat* (JHP Pharmaceutical)
LIOTRIX (64.8 mg = 1 grain)	
Tablets: ¼, ½, 1, 2, and 3 grains (T_4:T_3 content in a 4:1 ratio, mcg-for-mcg basis) (*Rx*)	*Thyrolar* (Forest)
THYROID DESICCATED (64.8 mg = 1 grain)[a]	
Tablets: 15 and 30 mg (*Rx*)	*Armour Thyroid* (Forest)
16.25 mg (*Rx*)	*Nature-Throid* (RLC Labs)
32.4 mg (*Rx*)	*Nature-Throid*, *Westhroid* (Western Research Labs)
32.5 mg (*Rx*)	Various
60 mg (*Rx*)	*Armour Thyroid* (Forest)
64.8 mg (*Rx*)	*Nature-Throid*, *Westhroid* (Western Research Labs)
65 mg (*Rx*)	Various
90 and 120 mg (*Rx*)	*Armour Thyroid* (Forest)
129.6 mg (*Rx*)	*Nature-Throid*, *Westhroid* (Western Research Labs)
130 mg (*Rx*)	Various
180 mg (*Rx*)	*Armour Thyroid* (Forest)
194.4 mg (*Rx*)	*Nature-Throid*, *Westhroid* (Western Research Labs)
195 mg (*Rx*)	Various
240 and 300 mg (*Rx*)	*Armour Thyroid* (Forest)
Capsules: 7.5, 15, 30, 60, 90, 120, 150, 180, and 240 mg (*Rx*)	*Bio-Throid* (Bio-Tech)

[a] Porcine derived.

Warning:

Drugs with thyroid hormone activity, alone or with other therapeutic agents, have been used for the treatment of obesity. In euthyroid patients, doses within the range of daily hormonal requirements are ineffective for weight reduction. Larger doses may produce serious or even life-threatening manifestations of toxicity, particularly when given in association with sympathomimetic amines such as those used for their anorectic effects.

Indications

Hypothyroidism: As replacement or supplemental therapy in hypothyroidism of any etiology, except transient hypothyroidism during the recovery phase of subacute thyroiditis.

Pituitary TSH suppressants: In the treatment or prevention of various types of euthyroid goiters, including thyroid nodules, subacute, or chronic lymphocytic thyroiditis (Hashimoto), multinodular goiter, and in the management of thyroid cancer (except liothyronine).

Diagnostic use (except levothyroxine): Diagnostic use in suppression tests to differentiate suspected hyperthyroidism from euthyroidism.

Myxedema coma/precoma (injection only): For the treatment of myxedema coma/precoma.

Administration and Dosage

Synthetic derivatives include levothyroxine (T_4), liothyronine (T_3), and liotrix (a 4 to 1 mixture of T_4 and T_3).

Generally, institute thyroid therapy at relatively low doses and slowly increase in small increments until the desired response is obtained. Administer thyroid as a single daily dose, preferably before breakfast.

Treatment of choice: Treatment of choice for hypothyroidism is T_4 because of its consistent potency and prolonged half-life.

Thyroid cancer: Exogenous thyroid hormone may produce regression of metastases from follicular and papillary carcinoma of the thyroid and is used as ancillary therapy of these conditions with radioactive iodine. Larger doses than those used for replacement therapy are required.

Laboratory tests: Laboratory tests useful in the diagnosis and evaluation of thyroid function are listed in the following table, indicating the alterations noted in various thyroid disorders.

Laboratory Tests for Diagnosis and Evaluation of Thyroid Function

↕ ↑ = Increased ↓ = Decreased N = Normal X = Contraindicated	Pregnancy	Primary hypothyroidism	Secondary hypothyroidism	Hyperthyroidism	T_3 thyrotoxicosis	Normal values
Free T_4 (unbound)	N	↓	↓	↑	N	12 to 32 pmol/L
Total T_4	↑	↓	↓	↑	N	55 to 160 nmol/L
T_3	↑	↓	↓	↑	↑	0.6 to 3.1 nmol/L
RAIU[a]	X	↓	-	↑	–	5% to 30%
Free thyroxine index (FT_4I)	N	↓	↓	↑	-	6.5 to 12.5[b] 1.3 to 3.9[c]
TSH[a]	N	↑	N/↓	↓	↓	0.4 to 4.2 milliunits/L

[a] RAIU = radioactive iodine uptake; TSH = thyroid-stimulating hormone
[b] T_4 uptake method
[c] $TT_4 \times RT_3U$ method

Dosage equivalents of thyroid products: In changing from one thyroid product to another, the following dosage equivalents may be used. However, each patient may still require dosage adjustments because these equivalents are only estimates.

LEVOTHYROXINE SODIUM (T_4; L-thyroxine): Take levothyroxine in the morning on an empty stomach, at least 30 minutes before any food is eaten. Take levothyroxine at least 4 hours apart from drugs that are known to interfere with its absorption.

Hypothyroidism in adults and children in whom growth and puberty are complete – The average full replacement dose of levothyroxine is approximately 1.7 mcg/kg/day (eg, 100 to 125 mcg/day for a 70 kg adult). Older patients may require less than 1 mcg/kg/day.

For most patients older than 50 years of age or for patients younger than 50 years of age with underlying cardiac disease, an initial starting dose of 25 to 50 mcg/day of levothyroxine is recommended, with gradual increments in dose at 6- to 8-week intervals, as needed. The recommended starting dose of levothyroxine sodium in elderly patients with cardiac disease is 12.5 to 25 mcg/day, with gradual dose increments at 4- to 6-week intervals.

Dosage adjustment: The levothyroxine dose generally is adjusted in 12.5 to 25 mcg increments until the patient with primary hypothyroidism is clinically euthyroid and the serum TSH has normalized.

Severe hypothyroidism – In patients with severe hypothyroidism, the recommended initial levothyroxine dose is 12.5 to 25 mcg/day with increases of 25 mcg/day every 2 to 4 weeks.

IV or IM: IV or IM injection can be substituted for the oral dosage form when oral ingestion is precluded for long periods of time. The initial parenteral dosage should be approximately one-half of the previously established oral dosage. A daily maintenance dose of 50 to 100 mcg parenterally should suffice to maintain the euthyroid state once established. Close observation of the patient, with individual adjustment of the dosage as needed, is recommended.

Subclinical hypothyroidism – If this condition is treated, a lower levothyroxine dose (eg, 1 mcg/kg/day) than that used for full replacement may be adequate to normalize the serum TSH level.

Myxedema coma – Oral thyroid hormone drug products are not recommended to treat this condition; administer thyroid hormone products formulated for IV.

In myxedema coma or stupor, without concomitant severe heart disease, 200 to 500 mcg of levothyroxine for injection may be administered IV as a solution containing 100 mcg/mL. Do not add to other IV fluids. Although the patient may show evidence of increased responsivity within 6 to 8 hours, full therapeutic effect may not be evident until the following day. An additional 100 to 300 mcg or more may be given on the second day if evidence of significant and progressive improvements has not occurred. Maintain continued daily administration of lesser amounts parenterally until the patient is fully capable of accepting a daily oral dose.

TSH suppression in well-differentiated thyroid cancer and thyroid nodules – The target level for TSH suppression in these conditions has not been established in controlled studies. In addition, the efficacy of TSH suppression for benign nodular disease is controversial. Therefore, individualize the dose of levothyroxine used for TSH suppression based on the specific disease and the patient being treated.

In the treatment of well-differentiated (papillary and follicular) thyroid cancer, levothyroxine is used as an adjunct to surgery and radioiodine therapy. Generally, TSH is suppressed to less than 0.1 milliunits/L, and this usually requires a levothyroxine dose of greater than 2 mcg/kg/day. However, in patients with high-risk tumors, the target level for TSH suppression may be less than 0.01 milliunits/L.

In the treatment of benign nodules and nontoxic multinodular goiter, TSH generally is suppressed to a higher target (eg, 0.1 to 0.5 or 1 milliunits/L).

Special populations – Exercise caution when administering levothyroxine to patients with underlying cardiovascular disease, to the elderly, and to those with concomitant adrenal insufficiency.

Children – Follow the recommendations in the following table. In infants with congenital or acquired hypothyroidism, institute therapy with full doses as soon as diagnosis is made.

Levothyroxine tablets may be given to infants and children who cannot swallow intact tablets. Crush the proper dose tablet and suspend in a small amount (5 to 10 mL) of water. The suspension can be given by spoon or dropper. Do not store the suspension for any period of time. Do not use foods that decrease absorption of levothyroxine, such as soybean infant formula, for administering levothyroxine sodium tablets.

Infants and children: Levothyroxine therapy usually is initiated at full replacement doses, with the recommended dose per body weight decreasing with age (see table). However, in children with chronic or severe hypothyroidism, an initial 25 mcg/day dose of levothyroxine is recommended with increments of 25 mcg every 2 to 4 weeks until the desired effect is achieved.

Hyperactivity in an older child can be minimized if the starting dose is one-fourth of the recommended full replacement dose and the dose is then increased on a weekly basis by an amount equal to one-fourth of the full-recommended replacement dose until the full recommended replacement dose is reached.

Newborns: The recommended starting dose is 10 to 15 mcg/kg/day. Consider a lower starting dose (eg, 25 mcg/day) in infants at risk for cardiac failure; the dose should be increased in 4 to 6 weeks as needed. In infants with very low (less than 5 mcg/dL) or undetectable serum T_4 concentrations, the recommended initial starting dose is 50 mcg/day of levothyroxine.

Recommended Pediatric Dosage for Congenital Hypothyroidism	
Age	Daily dose per kg (mcg)[a]
0 to 3 mo	10 to 15
3 to 6 mo	8 to 10
6 to 12 mo	6 to 8
1 to 5 y	5 to 6
6 to 12 y	4 to 5
> 12 y (growth/puberty incomplete)	2 to 3
> 12 y (growth/puberty complete)	1.7

[a] The dose should be adjusted based on clinical response and laboratory parameters.

LIOTHYRONINE SODIUM (T_3):

Mild hypothyroidism – Starting dose is 25 mcg/day. Daily dosage may be increased by up to 25 mcg every 1 or 2 weeks. Usual maintenance dose is 25 to 75 mcg/day.

Congenital hypothyroidism – Starting dose is 5 mcg/day, with a 5 mcg increment every 3 to 4 days until the desired response is achieved. Infants a few months old may require only 20 mcg/day for maintenance. At 1 year of age, 50 mcg/day may be required. Above 3 years, full adult dosage may be necessary.

Simple (nontoxic) goiter – Starting dose is 5 mcg/day. Dosage may be increased every 1 to 2 weeks by 5 or 10 mcg every 1 to 2 weeks. When 25 mcg/day is reached, dosage may be increased every 1 to 2 weeks by 12.5 or 25 mcg. Usual maintenance dosage is 75 mcg/day.

Thyroid suppression therapy – 75 to 100 mcg/day for 7 days; radioactive iodine uptake is determined before and after administration of the hormone.

Myxedema – Starting dose is 5 mcg/day. This may be increased by 5 to 10 mcg/day every 1 to 2 weeks. When 25 mcg/day is reached, dosage may be increased by 5 or 25 mcg every 1 or 2 weeks. Usual maintenance dose is 50 to 100 mcg/day.

Myxedema coma/precoma (injection only) – For IV use only; do not give IM or subcutaneously. Give doses at least 4 hours, and not more than 12 hours, apart. Giving at least 65 mcg/day initially is associated with lower mortality.

An initial IV dose ranging from 25 to 50 mcg is recommended in the emergency treatment of myxedema complications in adults. In patients with known or suspected cardiovascular disease, an initial dose of 10 to 20 mcg is suggested.

A single dose of liothyronine administered IV produces a detectable metabolic response in as little as 2 to 4 hours and a maximum therapeutic response within 2 days.

Switching to oral therapy: Resume oral therapy as soon as the clinical situation has been stabilized and the patient is able to take oral medication. If oral levothyroxine is used, keep in mind that there is a delay of several days in the onset of action; discontinue IV therapy gradually.

Elderly or children – Start therapy with 5 mcg/day; increase only by 5 mcg increments at the recommended intervals.

Exchange therapy – When switching a patient to liothyronine from thyroid levothyroxine or thyroglobulin, discontinue the other medication, initiate liothyronine at a low dosage, and increase gradually according to the patient's response. Liothyronine has a rapid onset of action and that residual effects of the other thyroid preparation may persist for the first several weeks of therapy.

LIOTRIX:

Hypothyroidism –

Initial dosage: Usual starting dose is 1 tablet of *Thyrolar ½* with increments of 1 tablet of *Thyrolar ¼* every 2 to 3 weeks. A lower starting dose, 1 tablet/day *Thyrolar ¼* is recommended in patients with long-standing myxedema, particularly if cardiovascular impairment is suspected

Maintenance dosage: Most patients require 1 tablet *Thyrolar 1* to 1 tablet *Thyrolar 2* per day; failure to respond to 1 tablet *Thyrolar 3* suggests lack of compliance or malabsorption.

Dosage readjustment – Readjust dosage within the first 4 weeks of therapy after proper clinical and laboratory evaluations including serum levels of T_4 bound and free, and TSH.

Thyroid cancer: Larger amounts of thyroid hormone than those used for replacement therapy are required.

Diagnostic agent – For adults, the usual suppressive dose of T_4 is 1.56 mcg/kg of body weight per day given for 7 to 10 days. These doses usually yield normal serum T_4 and T_3 levels and lack of response to TSH.

Children – In infants with congenital hypothyroidism, institute therapy with full doses as soon as diagnosis is made.

Recommended Pediatric Dosage for Congenital Hypothyroidism

Age	Dose per day in mcg		
	T_3/T_4	to	T_3/T_4
0 to 6 mo	3.1/12.5	to	6.25/25
6 to 12 mo	6.25/25	to	9.35/37.5
1 to 5 y	9.35/37.5	to	12.5/50
6 to 12 y	12.5/50	to	18.75/75
Over 12 y			> 18.75/75

THYROID DESICCATED:

Hypothyroidism –

Initial dosage: Usual starting dose is 30 mg, with increments of 15 mg every 2 to 3 weeks. Use 15 mg/day in patients with long-standing myxedema, particularly if cardiovascular impairment is suspected.

Maintenance dosage: 60 to 120 mg/day; failure to respond to 180 mg doses suggests lack of compliance or malabsorption.

Thyroid cancer – Larger amounts of thyroid hormone than those used for replacement therapy are required.

Diagnostic agent – For adults, the usual suppressive dose of T_4 is 1.56 mcg/kg of body weight per day given for 7 to 10 days.

Children – In infants with congenital hypothyroidism, institute therapy with full doses as soon as diagnosis is made.

Recommended Pediatric Dosage for Congenital Hypothyroidism

Age	Dose per day (mg)	Daily dose per kg (mg)
0 to 6 mo	7.5 to 30	2.4 to 6
6 to 12 mo	30 to 45	3.6 to 4.8
1 to 5 y	45 to 60	3 to 3.6
6 to 12 y	60 to 90	2.4 to 3
> 12 y	> 90	1.2 to 1.8

Special populations – Initiate therapy in low doses (15 to 30 mg) in patients with angina pectoris or the elderly, in whom there is a greater likelihood of occult cardiac disease.

Actions

Pharmacology: Thyroid hormones enhance oxygen consumption by most tissues of the body and increase the basal metabolic rate and metabolism of carbohydrates, lipids, and proteins in the body.

Pharmacokinetics:

Absorption – Absorption of orally administered T_4 varies from 40% to 80%. T_4 absorption is increased by fasting and decreased in malabsorption syndromes and by certain foods, such as soybean infant formula. Dietary fiber decreases bioavailability of T_4. Absorption also may decrease with age. The hormones in natural preparations are absorbed in a manner similar to the synthetic hormones.

Excretion – Thyroid hormones are primarily eliminated by the kidneys.

Various Pharmacokinetic Parameters of Thyroid Hormones				
Hormone	Ratio in thyroglobulin	Biologic potency	Half-life (days)	Protein binding (%)[a]
Levothyroxine (T_4)	10 to 20	1	6 to 7[b]	99+
Liothyronine (T_3)	1	4	≤ 2.5	99+

[a] Includes TBG, TBPA, and TBA.
[b] 3 to 4 days in hyperthyroidism, 9 to 10 days in hypothyroidism.

Contraindications

Diagnosed but uncorrected adrenal cortical insufficiency; untreated thyrotoxicosis; hypersensitivity to active or extraneous constituents.

Levothyroxine is contraindicated in patients with untreated subclinical (suppressed serum TSH level with normal T_3 and T_4 levels) and in patients with acute MI.

Concomitant use of *Triostat* and artificial rewarming of patients is contraindicated.

Warnings/Precautions

Obesity: In euthyroid patients, hormonal replacement doses are ineffective for weight reduction. Larger doses may produce serious or even life-threatening toxicity, particularly when given with sympathomimetic amines such as anorexiants.

Infertility: Thyroid hormone therapy is unjustified for the treatment of male or female infertility unless the condition is accompanied by hypothyroidism.

Cardiovascular disease: Use caution in suspected cardiovascular disease, particularly the coronary arteries, is suspect. This includes patients with angina or the elderly, in whom there is a greater likelihood of occult cardiac disease. Initiate therapy with low doses.

Endocrine disorders: Thyroid hormone therapy in patients with concomitant diabetes mellitus or insipidus or adrenal insufficiency (Addison disease) exacerbates the intensity of their symptoms.

Autoimmune polyglandular syndrome – Chronic autoimmune thyroiditis may occur in association with other autoimmune disorders. Treat patients with concomitant adrenal insufficiency with replacement glucocorticoids prior to initiation of treatment. Failure to do so may precipitate an acute adrenal crisis when thyroid hormone therapy is initiated. Patients with diabetes mellitus may require upward adjustments of their antidiabetic therapeutic regimens.

Nontoxic diffuse goiter or nodular thyroid disease: Use caution when administering levothyroxine to patients with nontoxic diffuse goiter or nodular thyroid disease in order to prevent precipitation of thyrotoxicosis. If the serum TSH is already suppressed, do not administer levothyroxine.

Severe and prolonged hypothyroidism: In severe and prolonged hypothyroidism, supplemental adrenocortical steroids may be necessary.

Morphologic hypogonadism and nephrosis: Rule out morphologic hypogonadism and nephrosis prior to initiating therapy.

Myxedema: Start dosage at a very low level and increase gradually. Myxedema coma therapy requires simultaneous administration of glucocorticoids.

Hyperthyroid effects: In rare instances, the administration of thyroid hormone may precipitate a hyperthyroid state or may aggravate existing hyperthyroidism.

Decreased bone density: In women, long-term levothyroxine therapy has been associated with increased bone resorption, thereby decreasing bone mineral density, especially in postmenopausal women on greater than replacement doses or in women who are receiving suppressive doses of levothyroxine.

Pregnancy: Category A.

Lactation: Minimal amounts of thyroid hormones are excreted in breast milk. Thyroid is not associated with serious adverse reactions.

Children:

Congenital hypothyroidism – The incidence of congenital hypothyroidism is relatively high (1:4000). Routine determinations of serum T_4 and/or TSH are strongly advised in neonates.

Monitoring: Treatment of patients with thyroid hormones requires the periodic assessment of thyroid status by means of appropriate laboratory tests. The TSH suppression test can be used to test the effectiveness of any thyroid preparation.

The frequency of TSH monitoring during levothyroxine dose titration is generally recommended at 6- to 8-week intervals until normalization. For patients who have recently initiated levothyroxine therapy and whose serum TSH has normalized or in patients who have had their dosage or brand of levothyroxine changed, measure the serum TSH concentration after 8 to 12 weeks.

Drug Interactions

Drugs that may affect thyroid hormones include amiodarone, glucocorticoids, PTU, aluminum and magnesium containing antacids, bile acid sequestrants, calcium carbonate, iron salts, sodium polystyrene sulfonate, simethicone, sucralfate, beta blockers, carbamazepine, hydantoins, phenobarbital, rifamycins, estrogens, oral contraceptives, furosemide, heparin, hydantoins, NSAIDs, salicylates, SSRIs, tri- and tetra-cyclic antidepressants, and sympathomimetics. Drugs that may be affected by thyroid hormones include beta-blockers, tri- and tetra-cyclic antidepressants, anticoagulants, antidiabetic agents: biguanides, meglitinides, sulfonylureas, thiazolidinediones, and insulin, digitalis glycosides, growth hormones, ketamine, radiographic agents, sympathomimetics and theophylline.

Drug/Lab test interactions: Consider changes in TBG concentration when interpreting T_4 and T_3 values. In such cases, measure the unbound (free) hormone and/or free T_4 index (FT_4I). Pregnancy, infectious hepatitis, estrogens, estrogen-containing oral contraceptives, and acute intermittent porphyria increase TBG concentrations. Decreases in TBG concentrations are observed in nephrosis, severe hypoproteinemia, severe liver disease, and acromegaly, and after androgen or corticosteroid therapy. Familial hyper- or hypothyroxine binding globulinemias have been described.

Medicinal or dietary iodine interferes with all in vivo tests of radioiodine uptake, producing low uptakes that may not reflect a true decrease in hormone synthesis.

Cytokines: Interferon-α and interleukin-2 – Therapy with interferon-α has been associated with the development of antithyroid microsomal antibodies in 20% of patients and some have transient hypothyroidism, hyperthyroidism, or both. Patients who have antithyroid antibodies before treatment are at higher risk of thyroid dysfunction during treatment. Interleukin-2 has been associated with transient painless thyroiditis in 20% of patients.

Drugs that may reduce TSTH secretion include dopamine and dopamine agonists, glucocorticoids, and octreotide. Drugs that may decrease thyroid hormone secretion include aminoglutethimide, amiodarone, iodine, lithium, methimazole, PTU, sulfonamides, and tolbutamide. Drugs that may increase thyroid hormone secretion may include amiodarone, and iodide. Drugs that may alter serum TBG concentrations include estrogen-containing contraceptives, oral estrogens, heroin and methadone, 5-fluorouracil, mitotane, and tamoxifen. Drugs that are associated with thyroid hormone and/or TSH level alterations by various mechanisms include chloral hydrate, diazepam, ethionamide, lovastatin, metoclopramide, 6-mercaptopurine, nitroprusside, para-aminosalicylate sodium, perphenazine, excessive topical use of resorcinol and thiazide diuretics.

Drug/Food interactions: Fasting increases the absorption of T_4 from the GI tract.

Adverse Reactions

Adverse reactions other than those indicating hyperthyroidism caused by therapeutic overdosage, initially or during the maintenance period, are rare. Symptoms of overdosage include the following: Palpitations; tachycardia; arrhythmias; angina; cardiac arrest; increased pulse and blood pressure; CHF; MI; tremors; headache; nervousness; insomnia; hyperactivity; anxiety, irritability; emotional lability; diarrhea; vomiting; abdominal cramps; hypersensitivity reactions to inactive ingredients; weight loss; fatigue; increased appetite; menstrual irregularities; excessive sweating; heat intolerance; fever; muscle weakness; dyspnea; hair loss; flushing; decreased bone mineral density; impaired fertility; increase in liver function tests.

Children – Pseudotumor cerebri; slipped capital femoral epiphysis; craniosynostosis; premature closure of the epiphyses.

Liothyronine injection only – Hypotension; phlebitis; twitching.

ANTITHYROID AGENTS

METHIMAZOLE	
Tablets; oral: 5 and 10 mg (*Rx*)	Various, *Northyx* (Centrix), *Tapazole* (Monarch)
15 and 20 mg (*Rx*)	*Northyx* (Centrix)
PROPYLTHIOURACIL	
Tablets; oral: 50 mg (*Rx*)	Various

Warning:

Propylthiouracil:

Hepatotoxicity – Severe liver injury and acute liver failure, in some cases fatal, have been reported in patients treated with propylthiouracil. These reports of hepatic reactions include cases requiring liver transplantation in adults and children. Reserve propylthiouracil for patients who cannot tolerate methimazole and in whom radioactive iodine therapy or surgery are not appropriate treatments for the management of hyperthyroidism.

Pregnancy – Because of the risk of fetal abnormalities associated with methimazole, propylthiouracil may be the treatment of choice when an antithyroid drug is indicated during or just prior to the first trimester of pregnancy.

Indications

Hyperthyroidism: Long-term therapy may lead to disease remission. Also used to ameliorate hyperthyroidism in preparation for subtotal thyroidectomy or radioactive iodine therapy.

Propylthiouracil is also used when thyroidectomy is contraindicated or not advisable.

Administration and Dosage

METHIMAZOLE: Usually given in 3 equal doses at approximately 8 hour intervals.

Adults –

Initial: 15 mg daily for mild hyperthyroidism, 30 to 40 mg/day for moderately severe hyperthyroidism and 60 mg/day for severe hyperthyroidism.

Maintenance: 5 to 15 mg/day.

Children –

Initial: 0.4 mg/kg/day.

Maintenance: Approximately ½ the initial dose.

PROPYLTHIOURACIL: Usually given in 3 equal doses at approximately 8 hour intervals.

Adults –

Initial: 300 mg/day. In patients with severe hyperthyroidism, very large goiters, or both, the initial dosage is usually 400 mg/day; an occasional patient will require 600 to 900 mg/day initially.

Maintenance: Usually, 100 to 150 mg/day.

Children –

6 years of age and older: Initial dose is 50 mg/day.

Maintenance: Determined by patient response.

Off-label dosing for children:

Younger than 6 years of age –

Initial: 5 to 7 mg/kg/day in divided every 8 hours.

Maintenance: ⅓ to ⅔ the initial dose divided every 8 to 12 hours when the patient is euthyroid.

Neonates – 5 to 10 mg/kg/day divided every 8 hours.

Actions

Pharmacology: Propylthiouracil and methimazole inhibit the synthesis of thyroid hormones and, thus, are effective in the treatment of hyperthyroidism. They do not inactivate existing thyroxine (T_4) and triiodothyronine (T_3) nor do they interfere with the effectiveness of exogenous thyroid hormones. Propylthiouracil partially inhibits the peripheral conversion of T_4 to T_3.

Pharmacokinetics:

Various Pharmacokinetic Parameters of Antithyroid Agents						
Antithyroid agent	Bioavailability (%)	Protein binding (%)	Transplacental passage	Breast milk levels (M:P)[a]	Half-life (h)	Excreted in urine (%)
Methimazole	80 to 95	0	High	High (1)	6 to 13	< 10
Propylthiouracil	80 to 95	75 to 80	Low	Low (0.1)	1 to 2	< 35

[a] Approximate milk:plasma ratio.

Contraindications

Hypersensitivity to antithyroid drugs; lactation.

Warnings/Precautions

Agranulocytosis: Agranulocytosis is potentially the most serious side effect of therapy. Leukopenia, thrombocytopenia and aplastic anemia (pancytopenia) may also occur.

Hemorrhagic effects: Because propylthiouracil may cause hypoprothrombinemia and bleeding, monitor prothrombin time during therapy, especially before surgical procedures.

Pregnancy: Category D. These agents, used judiciously, are effective drugs in hyperthyroidism complicated by pregnancy. Because they readily cross the placenta and can induce goiter and even cretinism in the developing fetus, it is important that a sufficient, but not excessive, dose be given. If an antithyroid agent is needed, propylthiouracil is preferred because it is less likely than methimazole to cross the placenta and induce fetal/neonatal complications.

Lactation: Postpartum patients receiving antithyroid preparations should not nurse their babies. However, if necessary, the preferred drug is propylthiouracil.

Children: In several case reports, propylthiouracil hepatotoxicity has occurred in children.

Monitoring: Monitor thyroid function tests periodically during therapy.

Drug Interactions

Drugs that may interact with antithyroid agents include anticoagulants.

Adverse Reactions

Agranulocytosis is the most serious effect.

BISPHOSPHONATES

ALENDRONATE SODIUM	
Tablets; oral: 5, 10, 35, 40, and 70 mg (as base) (*Rx*)	Various, *Fosamax* (Merck)
Solution; oral: 70 mg (as base) (*Rx*)	*Fosamax* (Merck)
ETIDRONATE DISODIUM (ORAL)	
Tablets; oral: 200 and 400 mg (*Rx*)	Various, *Didronel* (Procter & Gamble)
IBANDRONATE SODIUM	
Tablets; oral: 150 mg (as base) (*Rx*)	*Boniva* (Genentech)
Injection: 1 mg/mL (as base) (*Rx*)	
PAMIDRONATE DISODIUM	
Injection, lyophilized powder for solution: 30 and 90 mg (*Rx*)	Various, *Aredia* (Novartis)
Injection: 3, 6, and 9 mg/mL (*Rx*)	Various
RISEDRONATE SODIUM	
Tablets; oral: 5, 30, 35, and 150 mg (*Rx*)	*Actonel* (Procter & Gamble Pharmaceuticals)
Tablets, delayed release; oral: 35 mg	*Atelvia* (Warner Chilcott)
TILUDRONATE SODIUM	
Tablets; oral: 240 mg (equiv. to 200 mg tiludronic acid) (*Rx*)	*Skelid* (Sanofi-Aventis)
ZOLEDRONIC ACID	
Injection, solution; concentrate: 4 mg per 5 mL (*Rx*)	*Zometa* (Novartis)
Injection, solution: 5 mg per 100 mL (*Rx*)	*Reclast* (Novartis)
BISPHOSPHONATE COMBINATIONS	
Tablets; oral: 70 mg alendronate/70 mcg vitamin D_3[a] and 70 mg alendronate/140 mcg vitamin D_3[b] (*Rx*)	*Fosamax D* (Merck)
35 mg risedronate/1,250 mg calcium carbonate[c] (*Rx*)	*Actonel with Calcium* (Procter & Gamble)

[a] Equivalent to 2,800 units of vitamin D.
[b] Equivalent to 5,600 units of vitamin D.
[c] Equivalent to 500 mg elemental calcium.

Indications

Osteoporosis:

In postmenopausal women (alendronate, risedronate [delayed release treatment only], ibandronate oral, ibandronate IV [treatment only], alendronate/cholecalciferol, zoledronic acid [Reclast, treatment only]) – For the treatment and prevention of osteoporosis in postmenopausal women.

Glucocorticoid-induced (alendronate, risedronate, zoledronic acid [Reclast, only]) – Treatment and prevention of glucocorticoid-induced osteoporosis in men and women who are either initiating or continuing systemic glucocorticoid treatment for chronic diseases in a daily dosage equivalent to prednisone 7.5 mg or more and who have low bone mineral density.

In men (alendronate, alendronate/cholecalciferol, risedronate, zoledronic acid [Reclast, only]) – As treatment to increase bone mass in men with osteoporosis.

Paget disease of bone: For treatment of Paget disease of bone where alkaline phosphatase is at least 2 times the upper limit of normal, or those who are symptomatic or at risk for future complications from their disease (**alendronate, risedronate, tiludronate, zoledronic acid** [*Reclast*]); treatment of symptomatic Paget disease (**etidronate**); treatment of moderate to severe Paget disease (**pamidronate**).

Heterotopic ossification (etidronate): Prevention and treatment of heterotopic ossification following total hip replacement or caused by spinal injury.

Hypercalcemia of malignancy: For the treatment of hypercalcemia of malignancy (**zoledronic acid** [*Zometa*]); for the treatment of moderate or severe hypercalcemia associated with malignancy, with or without bone metastases (**pamidronate** patients with epidermoid or nonepidermoid tumors respond to pamidronate).

Breast cancer/Multiple myeloma (pamidronate): For the treatment of osteolytic bone metastases of breast cancer and osteolytic lesions of multiple myeloma.

Multiple myeloma and bone metastases of solid tumors (zoledronic acid [Zometa]): For the treatment of multiple myeloma and bone metastases from solid tumors.

Administration and Dosage

ALENDRONATE AND ALENDRONATE/CHOLECALCIFEROL: Alendronate and alendronate/cholecalciferol must be taken at least 30 minutes before the first food, beverage, or medication of the day with plain water only. Swallow alendronate only upon arising for the day. Take with a full glass of water and avoid lying down for at least 30 minutes and until after the first food of the day. Do not take alendronate at bedtime or before arising for the day. To facilitate gastric emptying, follow the oral solution with at least 60 mL (¼ cup) of water.

Osteoporosis in postmenopausal women –

Treatment: 70 mg tablet once weekly or one 10 mg tablet once daily, or 1 bottle of 70 mg oral solution once weekly.

Prevention: 35 mg tablet once weekly or one 5 mg tablet once daily.

Osteoporosis in men – 10 mg once daily, one 70 mg tablet, or 1 bottle of 70 mg oral solution once weekly, or one alendronate 70 mg/cholecalciferol 2,800 units tablet once weekly.

Glucocorticoid-induced osteoporosis – 5 mg once daily. For postmenopausal women not receiving estrogen, the recommended dose is 10 mg once daily.

Paget disease of bone – 40 mg once a day for 6 months.

Retreatment: Retreatment with alendronate may be considered, following a 6-month posttreatment evaluation period, in patients who have relapsed based on increases in serum alkaline phosphatase. Retreatment also may be considered in those who failed to normalize their serum alkaline phosphatase.

Calcium/Vitamin D supplementation – The recommended intake of vitamin D is 400 to 800 units daily. Alendronate/cholecalciferol is intended to provide 7 days' worth of vitamin D 400 units daily in a single, once-weekly dose.

ETIDRONATE DISODIUM (ORAL): Administer as a single dose. If GI discomfort occurs, divide the dose. To maximize absorption, avoid the following within 2 hours of dosing:

1.) Food, especially items high in calcium, such as milk or milk products.
2.) Vitamins with mineral supplements or antacids high in metals (eg, calcium, iron, magnesium, aluminum).

Paget disease –

Initial treatment: 5 to 10 mg/kg/day (not to exceed 6 months) or 11 to 20 mg/kg/day (not to exceed 3 months). Reserve doses higher than 10 mg/kg/day for use when lower doses are ineffective, when there is an overriding requirement for suppression of increased bone turnover, or when prompt reduction of elevated cardiac output is required. Doses higher than 20 mg/kg/day are not recommended.

Retreatment: Initiate only after an etidronate-free period of at least 90 days and when there is evidence of active disease process.

Heterotopic ossification –

Caused by spinal cord injury: 20 mg/kg/day for 2 weeks, followed by 10 mg/kg/day for 10 weeks; total treatment period is 12 weeks. Institute as soon as feasible following the injury, preferably prior to evidence of heterotopic ossification.

Total hip replacement: 20 mg/kg/day for 1 month before and for 3 months after surgery; total treatment period is 4 months.

IBANDRONATE SODIUM:

Oral –

Prevention or treatment of postmenopausal osteoporosis: One 2.5 mg tablet taken once daily. Alternatively, one 150 mg tablet taken once monthly on the same date each month.

Administration: To maximize absorption and clinical benefit, patients should take ibandronate at least 60 minutes before the first food or drink (other than water) of the day or before taking any oral medication or supplementation, including calcium, antacids, or vitamins.

Swallow whole with a full glass of plain water (180 to 240 mL; 6 to 8 oz) while the patient is standing or sitting in an upright position. Patients should not lie down for 60 minutes after taking ibandronate.

Missed monthly dose: If the once-monthly dose is missed and the patient's next scheduled ibandronate day is more than 7 days away, instruct the patient to take 1 ibandronate 150 mg tablet in the morning following the date that it is remembered. The patient then should return to the original schedule.

The patient must not take two 150 mg tablets within the same week. If the patient's next scheduled ibandronate day is only 1 to 7 days away, the patient must wait until his next scheduled ibandronate day to take the tablet.

Injection – Ibandronate injection must only be administered intravenously (IV). Do not administer ibandronate injection intra-arterially or paravenously.

Patients must receive supplemental calcium and vitamin D.

Treatment of postmenopausal osteoporosis: 3 mg every 3 months administered over 15 to 30 seconds.

Missed doses: If the dose is missed, administer the injection as soon as it can be rescheduled. Do not administer more frequently than once every 3 months.

Renal function impairment – Ibandronate is not recommended for use in patients with severe renal function impairment, patients with serum creatinine more than 200 mcmol/L (2.3 mg/dL), or creatinine clearance (CrCl, measured or estimated) less than 30 mL/min.

Admixture incompatibilities – Ibandronate injection must not be mixed with calcium-containing solutions or other IV administered drugs.

PAMIDRONATE DISODIUM:

Hypercalcemia of malignancy –

Moderate hypercalcemia: (corrected serum calcium of about 12 to 23.5 mg/dL) 60 to 90 mg given as a *single-dose* IV infusion over at least 2 to 24 hours. Longer infusions (eg, more than 2 hours) may reduce the risk for renal toxicity.

Severe hypercalcemia: (corrected serum calcium higher than 13.5 mg/dL) 90 mg given by initial *single-dose*, IV infusion over 2 to 24 hours. Longer infusions (eg, more than 2 hours) may reduce the risk for renal toxicity.

Retreatment: Retreatment may be carried out if serum calcium does not return to normal or remain normal after initial treatment. Allow a minimum of 7 days to elapse before retreatment. Retreatment is identical to initial therapy.

Paget disease – 30 mg daily, given as a 4 hour infusion on 3 consecutive days for a total dose of 90 mg.

Retreatment: When clinically indicated, retreat at the dose of initial therapy.

Osteolytic bone metastases of breast cancer – 90 mg administered over a 2-hour infusion every 3 to 4 weeks.

Osteolytic bone lesions of multiple myeloma – 90 mg given as a 4-hour infusion on a monthly basis. Patients with marked Bence-Jones proteinuria and dehydration should receive adequate hydration prior to pamidronate infusion.

Admixture incompatibility – Do not mix with calcium-containing infusion solutions, such as Ringer's solution. Give in a single IV solution and line separate from all other drugs.

RISEDRONATE:

Immediate release – Take once daily at least 30 minutes before the first food or drink of the day other than water.

Take while in an upright position with a full glass (6 to 8 ounces; 180 to 240 mL) of plain water and avoid lying down for 30 minutes to minimize the possibility of GI adverse reactions.

Instruct patients that if they miss a dose of risedronate 35 mg once weekly, they should take 1 tablet on the morning after they remember and return to taking 1 tablet once weekly, as originally scheduled on their chosen day.

If both tablets of risedronate 75 mg on 2 consecutive days per month are missed and the next month's scheduled doses are more than 7 days away, take 1 risedronate 75 mg tablet on the morning after the day it is remembered and then the other tablet on the next consecutive morning. If only 1 risedronate 75 mg tablet is missed, take the missed tablet on the morning after the day it is remembered. Instruct patients to then return to taking their risedronate 75 mg dose on 2 consecutive days per month, as originally scheduled.

If 1 or both tablets of risedronate 75 mg on 2 consecutive days per month are missed and the next month's scheduled doses are within 7 days, instruct patients to wait until their next month's scheduled doses and then continue taking risedronate 75 mg on 2 consecutive days per month.

If the dose of risedronate 150 mg once a month is missed and the next month's scheduled dose is more than 7 days away, instruct the patient to take the missed tablet on the morning after the day it is remembered. Instruct patients to then return to taking their risedronate 150 mg once a month. If the dose of risedronate 150 mg once a month is missed and the next month's scheduled dose is within 7 days, instruct patients to wait until their next month's scheduled dose.

Delayed release – Delayed-release risedronate should be taken in the morning immediately following breakfast.

Delayed-release risedronate should be swallowed whole while in an upright position and with at least 4 oz of plain water. Tablets should not be chewed, cut, or crushed. Patients should not lie down for 30 minutes after taking the medication.

Paget disease (immediate release only) – 30 mg once daily for 2 months.

Treatment/Prevention of postmenopausal osteoporosis – 5 mg daily, 35 mg once per week, or 75 mg taken on 2 consecutive days for a total of 2 tablets per month. Alternatively, one 150 mg tablet taken orally once a month may be considered.

Calcium/Vitamin D supplementation: Patients should receive supplemental calcium and vitamin D if dietary intake is inadequate. Calcium supplements and calcium-, aluminum-, and magnesium-containing medications may interfere with the absorption of risedronate and should be taken at a different time of the day.

Men with osteoporosis (immediate release only) – One 35 mg tablet orally taken once a week.

Osteoporosis in postmenopausal women (treatment) –

Delayed release: 35 mg once per week.

Treatment/Prevention of glucocorticoid-induced osteoporosis (immediate release only) – 5 mg orally taken daily.

Renal function impairment – Risedronate is not recommended for use in patients with severe renal function impairment (CrCl less than 30 mL/min).

TILUDRONATE: Administer a single 400 mg/day oral dose, taken with 6 to 8 ounces of plain water only for a period of 3 months. Do not take within 2 hours of food. Take calcium or mineral supplements at least 2 hours before or after tiludronate.

Retreatment – Following therapy, allow an interval of 3 months to assess response.

ZOLEDRONIC ACID:

Zometa –

Hypercalcemia of malignancy:

Dose – The maximum recommended dose in hypercalcemia of malignancy (albumin-corrected serum calcium at least 12 mg/dL [3 mmol/L]) is 4 mg given as a single dose IV infusion over not less than 15 minutes.

Retreatment – Retreatment with 4 mg may be considered if serum calcium does not return to normal or remain normal after initial treatment. It is recommended that a minimum of 7 days elapse before retreatment.

Multiple myeloma and metastatic bone lesions from solid tumors: 4 mg infused over 15 minutes every 3 or 4 weeks.

Calcium/Vitamin D supplementation – Administer patients an oral calcium supplement of 500 mg and a multiple vitamin containing vitamin D 400 units daily.

Renal function impairment:

Recommended Zoledronic Acid Dose for Patients with Mild to Moderate Renal Function Impairment

Baseline CrCl (mL/min)	Recommended dose[a]
> 60	4 mg
50 to 60	3.5 mg
40 to 49	3.3 mg
30 to 39	3 mg

[a] Doses calculated assuming target area under the curve of 0.66 (mg•h/L) (CrCl = 75 mL/min).

In the clinical studies, treatment was resumed only when the creatinine returned to within 10% of the baseline value. Reinitiate zoledronic acid at the same dose as that prior to treatment interruption.

Reclast –

Osteoporosis in men and postmenopausal women; glucocorticoid-induced osteoporosis:

Dose – 5 mg infusion once a year given IV over no less than 15 minutes.

Calcium/Vitamin D supplementation – An average of calcium 1,200 mg and vitamin D 800 to 1,000 units daily is recommended for osteoporosis in men and in postmenopausal women.

Paget disease of bone:

Dose – 5 mg infusion over no less than 15 minutes at a constant infusion rate. Administer as a single IV solution through a separate vented infusion line.

Retreatment – After a single treatment with zoledronic acid in Paget disease, an extended remission period is observed. Retreatment with zoledronic acid may be considered in patients who have relapsed, based on increases in serum alkaline phosphatase, or in those patients who failed to achieve normalization of their serum alkaline phosphatase, or in those patients with symptoms, as dictated by medical practice.

Calcium/Vitamin D supplementation – To reduce the risk of hypocalcemia, all patients should receive elemental calcium 1,500 mg daily in divided doses (750 mg 2 times a day or 500 mg 3 times a day) and vitamin D 800 units daily, particularly in the 2 weeks following zoledronic acid administration.

Administration – Administration of acetaminophen following zoledronic acid may reduce the incidence of acute-phase reactions symptoms.

Renal function impairment – The recommended dose in patients with CrCl 35 mL/min or more is zoledronic acid (*Reclast* only) 5 mg infused over no less than 15 minutes at a constant infusion rate. No adjustments are necessary in patients on *Zometa*.

Admixture incompatibilities: Zoledronic acid solution for infusion must not be allowed to come in contact with any calcium or other divalent cation-containing solutions.

Actions

Pharmacology: Bisphosphonates act primarily on bone. Their major pharmacologic action is the inhibition of normal and abnormal bone resorption. There is no evidence that the bisphosphonates are metabolized.

Pharmacokinetics:

Alendronate – Mean steady-state volume of distribution (exclusive of bone) is 28 L or more. Protein binding in plasma is about 78%.

Etidronate – The plasma half-life of etidronate is 1 to 6 hours. Within 24 hours, about half the absorbed dose is excreted in urine. The remainder is chemically adsorbed to bone and is slowly eliminated.

Pamidronate – Pamidronate is exclusively eliminated by renal excretion. The mean half-life is approximately 28 hours.

Risedronate – The mean steady-state volume of distribution is 6.3 L/kg; plasma protein binding is about 24%. Mean oral bioavailability is 0.63% and is decreased when administered with food.

Tiludronate – Bioavailability is reduced by food. Tiludronic acid is approximately 90% bound to human serum protein. The mean plasma elimination half-life was approximately 150 hours.

Contraindications

Hypersensitivity to bisphosphonates or any component of the products; hypocalcemia (**alendronate, risedronate**); abnormalities of the esophagus that delay esophageal emptying, such as stricture or achalasia (**alendronate**); inability to stand or sit upright for at least 30 minutes (**alendronate, risedronate**); clinically overt osteomalacia (**etidronate**).

Warnings/Precautions

GI irritation/disorders: Bisphosphonates cause local irritation of the upper GI mucosa. Alert health care providers to any signs or symptoms signaling a possible esophageal reaction, and instruct patients to discontinue bisphosphonates and seek medical attention if they develop dysphagia, odynophagia, retrosternal pain, or new or worsening heartburn.

Use caution when bisphosphonates are given to patients with active upper GI problems (such as dysphagia, esophageal diseases, gastritis, duodenitis, or ulcers). **Etidronate** therapy has been withheld from patients with enterocolitis because diarrhea is seen in some patients, particularly at higher doses.

Osteoporosis (alendronate): Consider causes other than estrogen deficiency and aging; consider glucocorticoid use.

Paget disease (etidronate): Response may be slow and may continue for months after treatment discontinuation. Do not increase dosage prematurely or initiate retreatment until after at least a 90-day, drug-free interval.

Asthma (zoledronic acid): While not observed in clinical trials with zoledronic acid, administration of other bisphosphonates has been associated with bronchoconstriction in aspirin-sensitive asthmatic patients.

Hypercalcemia: Carefully monitor standard hypercalcemia-related metabolic parameters, such as serum levels of calcium, phosphate, and magnesium, as well as serum creatinine. Do not use loop diuretics until the patient is adequately rehydrated; use with caution in combination with zoledronic acid in order to avoid hypocalcemia. Use **zoledronic acid** with caution with other nephrotoxic drugs.

Concomitant use with estrogen/hormone replacement therapy (alendronate): Two clinical studies have shown that the degree of suppression of bone turnover (as assessed by mineralizing surface) was significantly greater with the combination than with either component alone.

Nutrition: Patients should maintain adequate nutrition, particularly an adequate intake of calcium and vitamin D.

Osteoid: **Etidronate** suppresses bone turnover and may retard mineralization of osteoid laid down during the bone accretion process. In patients with fractures, especially of long bones, it may be advisable to delay or interrupt treatment until callus is evident.

Fracture: In Paget patients, treatment regimens of **etidronate** exceeding the recommended daily maximum dose of 20 mg/kg or continuous administration for periods greater than 6 months may be associated with an increased risk of fracture.

Hypocalcemia: Hypocalcemia has occurred with **pamidronate** therapy. Rare cases of symptomatic hypocalcemia (including tetany) occurred during pamidronate treatment. If hypocalcemia occurs, consider short-term calcium therapy.

Hypocalcemia must be corrected before therapy initiation with **alendronate** and **risedronate**. Also effectively treat other disturbances of mineral metabolism (eg, vitamin D deficiency).

Renal function impairment:

Alendronate – No dosage adjustment is necessary in mild to moderate renal function impairment (CrCl 35 to 60 mL/min). Alendronate use is not recommended in more severe renal function impairment (CrCl less than 35 mL/min).

Alendronate/Cholecalciferol – Not recommended for patients with severe renal function impairment (CrCl less than 35 mL/min) because of lack of experience.

Pamidronate – Bisphosphonates, including pamidronate, have been associated with renal toxicity manifested as deterioration of renal function and potential renal failure.

In patients receiving pamidronate for bone metastases who show evidence of deterioration in renal function, withhold treatment until renal function returns to baseline. In a clinical study, pamidronate treatment was resumed only when the creatinine returned to within 10% of the baseline value.

Ibandronate – Ibandronate is not recommended for use in patients with severe renal function impairment (CrCl less than 30 mL/min).

Risedronate – Risedronate is not recommended for patients with severe renal function impairment (CrCl less than 30 mL/min). No dosage adjustment is needed when CrCl is greater than 30 mL/min.

Tiludronate – Tiludronate is not recommended for patients with severe renal failure (CrCl less than 30 mL/min).

Zoledronic acid – Single doses of zoledronic acid should not exceed 4 mg (*Zometa*) and the duration of infusion should be no less than 15 minutes. Zoledronic acid treatment is not recommended in patients with bone metastases with severe renal function impairment.

Pregnancy: *Category D* (zoledronic acid); *Category C* (alendronate, oral and IV etidronate, pamidronate, risedronate, and tiludronate).

Lactation: It is not known whether these drugs are excreted in breast milk. Because **zoledronic acid** binds to bone long-term, do not administer to a breast-feeding woman.

Children: Safety and efficacy for use in children have not been established. Children have been treated with **etidronate** at doses recommended for adults to prevent heterotopic ossifications or soft tissue calcifications.

Monitoring: Carefully monitor standard hypercalcemia-related metabolic parameters, such as serum levels of calcium, phosphate, magnesium, and potassium following **pamidronate** and **zoledronic acid** initiation. Also, closely monitor electrolytes, creatinine, as well as complete blood cell count, and differential and hematocrit/hemoglobin. Carefully monitor patients who have preexisting anemia, leukopenia, or thrombocytopenia in the first 2 weeks following treatment.

Drug Interactions

Drugs that may interact with **alendronate** include aspirin and ranitidine. Drugs that may interact with **tiludronate** include aspirin and indomethacin. Calcium supplements and antacids may interact with **alendronate**, **etidronate**, **risedronate**, or **tiludronate**. Warfarin may interact with etidronate. Drugs that may interact with **zoledronic acid** include aminoglycosides and loop diuretics.

Drug/Food interactions: Bioavailability of **alendronate** was decreased when given 0.5 or 1 hour before breakfast versus 2 hours before, and bioavailability was negligible when alendronate was given with or 2 hours after breakfast. Concomitant coffee or orange juice reduced bioavailability by 60%. Take alendronate in the morning at least 30 minutes before the first meal, beverage, or medication.

Absorption of **etidronate** may be reduced by foods. Take on an empty stomach 2 hours before a meal.

Bioavailability of **tiludronate** was reduced when administered with, or 2 hours after, breakfast compared with administration after an overnight fast and 4 hours before a standard breakfast.

Mean oral bioavailability of **risedronate** is decreased when given with food. Take at least 30 minutes before the first food or drink of the day other than water.

Adverse Reactions

Adverse reactions occurring in at least 3% of patients include the following:

Alendronate: Abdominal pain, bone/skeletal pain, constipation, diarrhea, dyspepsia, nausea.

Etidronate: Abnormal hepatic function, constipation, convulsions, dyspnea, fever, fluid overload, hypomagnesemia, hypophosphatemia, nausea, stomatitis, taste perversion.

Pamidronate:

In patients receiving 90 mg for osteolytic bone metastases and osteolytic lesions – Abdominal pain, anemia, anorexia, anxiety, arthralgia, asthenia, bone/skeletal pain, constipation, coughing, diarrhea, dyspepsia, dyspnea, fatigue, fever, granulocytopenia, headache, hypocalcemia, hypokalemia, hypomagnesemia, hypophosphatemia, insomnia, metastases, myalgia, nausea, pain, pleural effusion, serum creatinine abnormal, sinusitis, thrombocytopenia, upper respiratory infection, urinary tract infection, vomiting.

In patients receiving 90 mg over 24 hours (HCM) – Anemia, atrial fibrillation, anorexia, constipation, fatigue, fever, GI hemorrhage, hypertension, hypocalcemia, hypokalemia, hypomagnesemia, hypophosphatemia, hypothyroidism, infusion site reaction, moniliasis, nausea, rales/rhinitis, somnolence, syncope, tachycardia.

In patients receiving 60 mg over 4 hours (HCM) – Anorexia, constipation, dyspepsia, fever, hypokalemia, hypomagnesemia, leukopenia, nausea, psychosis, uremia, vomiting.

In patients receiving 60 mg over 24 hours (HCM) – Fever, hypokalemia, hypomagnesemia, hypophosphatemia, infusion site reaction, upper respiratory infection.

Risedronate (including all treatment regimens): Abdominal pain, accidental injury, amblyopia, anxiety, arthralgia, arthritis, asthenia, back pain, belching, bone disorder/fracture, bone/skeletal pain, bronchitis, bursitis, cataract, chest pain, colitis, conjunctivitis, constipation, coughing, cystitis, depression, diarrhea, dizziness, dry eye, dyspepsia, dyspnea, ecchymosis, edema/peripheral edema, flatulence, gastroenteritis, headache, hypertension, influenza-like symptoms, infection, insomnia, joint disorder, leg/muscle cramps, myalgia, myasthenia, nausea, neck pain, neoplasm, neuralgia, overdose, pain, pharyngitis, pneumonia, pruritus, rales/rhinitis, rash, sinusitis, tendon disorder, tinnitus, urinary tract infection, vertigo.

Tiludronate: Accidental injury, back pain, diarrhea, dizziness, dyspepsia, headache, influenza-like symptoms, nausea, pain, paresthesia, rales/rhinitis, sinusitis, upper respiratory infection, and vomiting.

Zoledronic acid: Abdominal pain, agitation, alopecia, anemia, anorexia, anxiety, arthralgia, asthenia, back pain, bone/skeletal pain, cancer progression, confusion, constipation, coughing, decreased appetite, decreased weight, dehydration, depression, dermatitis, diarrhea, dizziness, dyspnea, edema/peripheral edema, fatigue, fever, headache, hypesthesia, hypokalemia, hypomagnesemia, hypophosphatemia, hypotension, insomnia, moniliasis, myalgia, nausea, neoplasm, neutropenia, paresthesia, rigors, upper respiratory infection, vomiting, urinary tract infection.

ANTIDOTES

Various Detoxification Agents and Their Uses

Drug (trade name)	Toxic/Overdosed substance
Dimercaprol (*BAL In Oil*)	Arsenic, gold, mercury, lead
Deferoxamine mesylate (*Desferal*)	Iron
Deferasirox (*Exjade*)	Iron
Dexrazoxane (*Zinecard*)	Doxorubicin-induced cardiomyopathy
Digoxin immune fab (*Digibind, Digifab*)	Digoxin, digitoxin
Edetate calcium disodium (*Calcium Disodium Versenate*)	Lead
Flumazenil (*Romazicon*)	Benzodiazepines
Fomepizole (*Antizol*)	Ethylene glycol, methanol
Mesna (*Mesnex*)	Ifosfamide-induced hemorrhagic cystitis
Methylene blue (Various)	Nitrites
Narcotic antagonists Naloxone (*Narcan*) Naltrexone (*ReVia*)	Opioids
Physostigmine salicylate	Anticholinergics (including tricyclic antidepressants)
Pralidoxime Cl (*Protopam Cl*)	Organophosphates Anticholinesterases
Sodium thiosulfate (Various)	Cyanide Cisplatin-induced nephrotoxicity Cisplatin extravasation
Sodium nitrite (Various)	Cyanide
Succimer (*Chemet*)	Lead
Trientene (*Syprine*)	Copper
Other agents used additionally as antidotes:	
Acetylcysteine (*Mucomyst, Mucosil*)	Acetaminophen
Amyl nitrite, Na Nitrite, Na Thiosulfate (*Cyanide antidote kit*)	Cyanide
Anticholinesterases Pyridostigmine Br Neostigmine Br (*Prostigmin*) Edrophonium Cl (*Enlon, Reversol*)	Nondepolarizing muscle relaxants
Atropine (Various)	Cholinergic agents: Organophosphates, carbamates, pilocarpine, physostigmine, or choline esters.
Glucagon	Insulin-induced hypoglycemia, beta-blockers
Hydroxocobalamin (Various)	Cyanide poisoning
Leucovorin calcium (*Wellcovorin*)	Folic acid antagonists (eg, methotrexate)
Protamine sulfate (Various)	Heparin
Pyridoxine	Isoniazid
Vitamin K_1 (Various)	Oral anticoagulants

Various Detoxification Agents and Their Uses	
Drug (trade name)	Toxic/Overdosed substance
Nonspecific therapy of overdoses include the following:	
Activated charcoal (Various)	Nonspecific, supportive therapies of overdoses. See also General Management of Acute Overdosage.
Cathartics	
Osmotic diuretics	
Polyethylene glycol electrolyte solution (*GoLYTELY*)	
Syrup of ipecac (Various)	
Urinary acidifiers	
Urinary alkalinizers	

TRIENTINE HYDROCHLORIDE

Capsules: 250 mg (*Rx*) *Syprine* (Merck)

Indications

Wilson disease: Treatment of patients with Wilson disease who are intolerant of penicillamine.

Administration and Dosage

Take on an empty stomach at least 1 hour before or 2 hours after meals and at least 1 hour apart from any other drug, food, or milk. Swallow the capsules whole and do not open or chew.

Adults: Initially, 750 to 1250 mg/day in divided doses 2, 3, or 4 times/day. May increase to a maximum of 2,000 mg/day.

Children 12 years of age and under: Initially, 500 to 750 mg/day in divided doses 2, 3, or 4 times/day. May increase to a maximum of 1,500 mg/day.

Increase the daily dose only when the clinical response is not adequate or the concentration of free serum copper is persistently above 20 mcg/dL. Determine optimal long-term maintenance dosage at 6- to 12-month intervals.

Actions

Pharmacology: Wilson disease (hepatolenticular degeneration) is an inherited metabolic defect resulting in excess copper accumulation, possibly because the liver lacks the mechanism to excrete free copper into the bile. Hepatocytes store excess copper, but when their capacity is exceeded, copper is released into the blood and is taken up into extrahepatic sites. Treat this condition with a low copper diet and chelating agents that bind copper to facilitate its excretion from the body. Trientine is a chelating compound for removal of excess copper from the body.

Warnings/Precautions

Not indicated for the following: Not indicated for cystinuria; rheumatoid arthritis; biliary cirrhosis.

Patient supervision: Patients should remain under regular medical supervision throughout the period of drug administration.

Iron deficiency anemia: Closely monitor patients (especially women) for evidence of iron deficiency anemia.

Hypersensitivity: There are no reports of hypersensitivity in patients given trientine for Wilson disease. However, there have been reports of asthma, bronchitis, and dermatitis occurring after prolonged environmental exposure in workers who use trientine as a hardener of epoxy resins. Observe patients closely for signs of possible hypersensitivity.

Pregnancy: Category C.

Lactation: It is not known whether this drug is excreted in breast milk. Exercise caution when administering to a breast-feeding woman.

Children: Safety and efficacy for use in children have not been established. Trientine has been used clinically in children as young as 6 years of age with no reported adverse effects.

Elderly: In general, dose selection should be cautious, usually starting at the low end of the dosing range, reflecting the greater frequency of decreased hepatic, renal, or cardiac function, and of concomitant disease or other drug therapy.

Monitoring: The most reliable index for monitoring treatment is the determination of free copper in the serum, which equals the difference between quantitatively determined total copper and ceruloplasmin-copper. Adequately treated patients will usually have less than 10 mcg free copper/dL of serum.

Therapy may be monitored with a 24-hour urinary copper analysis periodically (ie, every 6 to 12 months). Urine must be collected in copper-free glassware. Because a low copper diet should keep copper absorption down to less than 1 mg/day, the patient probably will be in the desired state of negative copper balance if 0.5 to 1 mg of copper is present in a 24-hour collection of urine.

Drug Interactions

Mineral supplements: In general, do not give mineral supplements; they may block the absorption of trientine. However, iron deficiency may develop, especially in children and menstruating or pregnant women, or as a result of the low copper diet recommended for Wilson disease. If necessary, iron may be given in short courses, but because iron and trientine each inhibit absorption of the other, allow 2 hours to elapse between administration of trientine and iron.

SUCCIMER (DMSA)

Capsules: 100 mg (*Rx*) — *Chemet* (Sanofi-Synthelabo)

Indications

Lead poisoning: Treatment of lead poisoning in children with blood lead levels above 45 mcg/dL. Not indicated for prophylaxis of lead poisoning in a lead-containing environment; always accompany succimer use with identification and removal of the source of lead exposure.

Administration and Dosage

Start dosage at 10 mg/kg or 350 mg/m^2 every 8 hours for 5 days; initiation of therapy at higher doses is not recommended (see table). Reduce frequency of administration to 10 mg/kg or 350 mg/m^2 every 12 hours (two-thirds of initial daily dosage) for an additional 2 weeks of therapy. A course of treatment lasts 19 days. Repeated courses may be necessary if indicated by weekly monitoring of blood lead concentration. A minimum of 2 weeks between courses is recommended unless blood lead levels indicate the need for more prompt treatment.

Succimer Pediatric Dosing Chart

Weight			
lbs	kg	Dose (mg)[a]	Number of capsules[a]
18 to 35	8 to 15	100	1
36 to 55	16 to 23	200	2
56 to 75	24 to 34	300	3
76 to 100	35 to 44	400	4
> 100	> 45	500	5

[a] To be administered every 8 hours for 5 days, followed by dosing every 12 hours for 14 days.

In young children who cannot swallow capsules, succimer can be administered by separating the capsule and sprinkling the medicated beads on a small amount of soft food or putting them in a spoon and following with a fruit drink.

Identification of the lead source in the child's environment and its abatement are critical to successful therapy. Chelation therapy is not a substitute for preventing further exposure to lead and should not be used to permit continued exposure to lead.

Patients who have received calcium EDTA with or without dimercaprol may use succimer for subsequent treatment after an interval of 4 weeks. Data on the concomitant use of succimer with calcium EDTA with or without dimercaprol are not available, and such use is not recommended.

Adequately hydrate all patients undergoing treatment.

Actions

Pharmacology: Succimer is an orally active, heavy metal chelating agent; it forms water soluble chelates and, consequently, increases the urinary excretion of lead.

Pharmacokinetics: In a study in healthy adult volunteers, after a single dose of 16, 32, or 48 mg/kg, absorption was rapid but variable, with peak blood levels between 1 and 2 hours. Approximately 49% of the dose was excreted: 39% in the feces, 9% in the urine, and 1% as carbon dioxide from the lungs. Because fecal excretion probably represented nonabsorbed drug, most of the absorbed drug was excreted by the kidneys. The apparent elimination half-life was about 2 days.

Contraindications

History of allergy to the drug.

Warnings/Precautions

Lead exposure: Not a substitute for effective abatement of lead exposure.

Neutropenia: Mild to moderate neutropenia has been observed in some patients receiving succimer. While a causal relationship to succimer has not been definitely established, neutropenia has been reported with other drugs in the same chemical class. Obtain a complete blood count with white blood cell differential and direct platelet counts prior to and weekly during treatment. Withhold or discontinue therapy if the absolute neutrophil count (ANC) is below 1,200/mcL and follow the patient closely to document recovery of the ANC to above 1,500/mcL or to the patient's baseline neutrophil count. There is limited experience with reexposure in patients who have developed neutropenia. Therefore, rechallenge such patients only if the benefit of succimer therapy clearly outweighs the potential risk of another episode of neutropenia and then only with careful patient monitoring.

Infection – Instruct patients treated with succimer to report promptly any signs of infection. If infection is suspected, immediately conduct the above laboratory tests.

Rebound blood lead levels: After therapy, monitor patients for rebound of blood lead levels by measuring the levels at least once weekly until stable.

Renal function: Adequately hydrate all patients undergoing treatment. Exercise caution in using succimer therapy in patients with compromised renal function. Limited data suggest that succimer is dialyzable but that the lead chelates are not.

Hepatic function: Transient mild elevations of serum transaminases have been observed in 6% to 10% of patients during the course of therapy. Monitor serum transaminases before the start of therapy and at least weekly during therapy. Closely monitor patients with a history of liver disease. No data are available regarding the metabolism of succimer in patients with liver disease.

Repeated courses: Clinical experience is limited. The safety of uninterrupted dosing longer than 3 weeks has not been established and is not recommended.

Allergic reactions: The possibility of allergic or other mucocutaneous reactions must be borne in mind upon readministration (and during initial courses). Monitor patients requiring repeated courses during each treatment course.

Pregnancy: Category C.

Lactation: It is not known whether this drug is excreted in breast milk. Discourage mothers requiring therapy from breast-feeding their infants.

Children: Safety and efficacy in children younger than 12 months of age have not been established.

Drug Interactions

Chelation therapy (eg, EDTA): Coadministration of succimer with other chelation therapy is not recommended.

Drug/Lab test interactions: Succimer may interfere with serum and urinary laboratory tests.

Adverse Reactions

The most common reactions were GI symptoms or increases in serum transaminases (10%) and rashes (4%). Mild to moderate neutropenia has occurred in some patients receiving succimer. The following table presents adverse reactions reported with the administration of succimer for the treatment of lead and other heavy metal intoxication.

Succimer Adverse Reactions (%)[a]

Body system/adverse reaction	Children (n = 191)	Adults (n = 134)
GI:		
Nausea; vomiting; diarrhea; appetite loss; hemorrhoidal symptoms; loose stools; metallic taste in mouth	12%	20.9%
Body as a whole:		
Back, stomach, head, rib, flank pain; abdominal cramps; chills; fever; flu-like symptoms; heavy head/tired; head cold; headache; moniliasis	5.2%	15.7%
Metabolic:		
Elevated AST, ALT, alkaline phosphatase, serum cholesterol	4.2%	10.4%
CNS:		
Drowsiness; dizziness; sensorimotor neuropathy; sleepiness; paresthesia	1%	12.7%
Dermatologic:		
Papular rash; herpetic rash; rash; mucocutaneous eruptions; pruritus	2.6%	11.2%
Special senses:		
Cloudy film in eye; ears plugged; otitis media; watery eyes	1%	3.7%
Respiratory:		
Sore throat; rhinorrhea; nasal congestion; cough	3.7%	0.7%
GU:		
Decreased urination; voiding difficulty; proteinuria increased	0%	3.7%
Other:		
Arrhythmia	0%	1.8%
Mild to moderate neutropenia; increased platelet count; intermittent eosinophilia	0.5%	1.5%
Kneecap pain; leg pains	0%	3%

[a] Incidence regardless of attribution or dosage.

METHYLNALTREXONE BROMIDE

Injection, solution: 12 mg per 0.6 mL (*Rx*) — *Relistor* (Wyeth)

Indications

Opioid-induced constipation: For the treatment of opioid-induced constipation in patients with advanced illness who are receiving palliative care when response to laxative therapy has not been sufficient. Use beyond 4 months has not been studied.

Administration and Dosage

8 mg for patients weighing 38 to less than 62 kg (84 to less than 136 lbs) or 12 mg for patients weighing 62 to 114 kg (136 to 251 lbs). The usual schedule is 1 dose every other day, as needed, but no more frequently than 1 dose in a 24-hour period. Patients whose weight falls outside of these ranges should be dosed at 0.15 mg/kg.

Renal function impairment: In patients with severe renal function impairment (creatinine clearance [CrCl] less than 30 mL/min), dose reduction of methylnaltrexone by one-half is recommended.

Administration: Methylnaltrexone is administered as a subcutaneous injection only and should be injected in the upper arm, abdomen, or thigh.

Actions

Pharmacology: Methylnaltrexone functions as a peripherally acting muopioid receptor antagonist in tissues such as the GI tract, thereby decreasing the constipating effects of opioids without impacting opioid-mediated analgesic effects on the CNS.

Pharmacokinetics:

Absorption – Following subcutaneous administration, methylnaltrexone is absorbed rapidly, with peak concentrations achieved at approximately 0.5 hours.

Distribution – The fraction of methylnaltrexone bound to human plasma proteins is 11% to 15.3%.

Excretion – Methylnaltrexone is eliminated primarily as unchanged drug. The terminal half-life is approximately 8 hours.

Contraindications

In patients with known or suspected mechanical GI obstruction.

Warnings/Precautions

Severe or persistent diarrhea: If severe or persistent diarrhea occurs during treatment, advise patients to discontinue therapy.

Peritoneal catheters: Use of methylnaltrexone has not been studied in patients with peritoneal catheters.

Renal function impairment: Dose reduction to one-half is recommended in patients with severe renal function impairment (CrCl less than 30 mL/min).

Pregnancy: Category B.

Lactation: It is not known whether this drug is excreted in human milk. Because many drugs are excreted in human milk, exercise caution when methylnaltrexone is administered to a breast-feeding woman.

Children: Safety and effectiveness have not been established in children.

Drug Interactions

None known.

Adverse Reactions

Adverse reactions occurring in ≥ 5% of patients include abdominal pain, diarrhea, dizziness, flatulence, and nausea.

NALOXONE HYDROCHLORIDE

Injection: 0.4 and 1 mg/mL (*Rx*)	Various, *Narcan* (DuPont Pharm)

Indications

For the complete or partial reversal of narcotic depression, including respiratory depression, induced by opioids including natural and synthetic narcotics, propoxyphene, methadone, nalbuphine, butorphanol, and pentazocine. Also indicated for the diagnosis of suspected acute opioid overdosage.

Administration and Dosage

Give IV, IM, or subcutaneously. The most rapid onset of action is achieved with IV use, which is recommended in emergency situations.

Adults:

Narcotic overdose (known or suspected) – Initial dose is 0.4 to 2 mg IV; may repeat IV at 2- to 3-minute intervals. If no response is observed after 10 mg has been administered, question the diagnosis of narcotic-induced or partial narcotic-induced toxicity.

Postoperative narcotic depression (partial reversal) – Smaller doses are usually sufficient. Titrate dose according to the patient's response.

Initial dose: Inject in increments of 0.1 to 0.2 mg IV at 2- to 3-minute intervals to the desired degree of reversal.

Repeat doses: Repeat doses may be required within 1- or 2-hour intervals depending on the amount, type (ie, short- or long-acting) and time interval since last administration of narcotic. Supplemental IM doses have produced a longer lasting effect.

Children:

Narcotic overdose (known or suspected) – Initial dose is 0.01 mg/kg IV; give a subsequent dose of 0.1 mg/kg if needed. If an IV route is not available, may be given IM or subcutaneously in divided doses.

Postoperative narcotic depression – Follow the recommendations and cautions under adult administration guidelines. For initial reversal of respiratory depression, inject in increments of 0.005 to 0.01 mg IV at 2- to 3-minute intervals to desired degree of reversal.

Neonates:

Narcotic-induced depression – Initial dose is 0.01 mg/kg IV, IM, or subcutaneously; may be repeated in accordance with adult administration guidelines.

Actions

Pharmacology: The mechanism of action is not fully understood; evidence suggests that it antagonizes the opioid effects by competing for the same receptor sites.

Pharmacokinetics:

Distribution – After parenteral use, naloxone is rapidly distributed in the body. It is metabolized in the liver, primarily by glucuronide conjugation.

Excretion – Naloxone is excreted in the urine. The serum half-life in adults ranged from 30 to 81 minutes; in neonates, 3.1 ± 0.5 hours.

Onset, peak, and duration – Onset of action of IV naloxone is generally apparent within 2 minutes; it is only slightly less rapid when given subcutaneously or IM. Duration of action of 1 to 4 hours depends upon dose and route. IM use produces a more prolonged effect than IV use.

Contraindications

Hypersensitivity to these agents.

Warnings/Precautions

Drug dependence: Administer cautiously to people who are known or suspected to be physically dependent on opioids, including newborns of mothers with narcotic dependence. Reversal of narcotic effect will precipitate acute abstinence syndrome.

Repeat administration: The patient who has satisfactorily responded should be kept under continued surveillance. Administer repeated doses as necessary, because the duration of action of some narcotics may exceed that of the narcotic antagonist.

Respiratory depression: Not effective against respiratory depression due to nonopioid drugs.

Other supportive therapy: Maintain a free airway and provide artificial ventilation, cardiac massage, and vasopressor agents; employ when necessary to counteract acute narcotic overdosage.

Cardiovascular effects: Several instances of hypotension, hypertension, pulmonary edema, and ventricular tachycardia and fibrillation have been reported in postoperative patients.

Pregnancy: Category B.

Lactation: It is not known whether the drug is excreted in breast milk.

Adverse Reactions

Abrupt reversal of narcotic depression may result in nausea, vomiting, sweating, tachycardia, increased blood pressure, and tremulousness.

In postoperative patients, excessive dosage may result in excitement and significant reversal of analgesia, hypotension, hypertension, pulmonary edema, and ventricular tachycardia and fibrillation.

NALTREXONE HYDROCHLORIDE

Tablets: 50 mg (*Rx*)	Various, *ReVia* (Barr)
Suspension for injection, extended-release: 380 mg per vial (*Rx*)	*Vivitrol* (Alkermes, Inc.)

Warning:

Hepatotoxicity: Naltrexone has the capacity to cause hepatocellular injury when given in excessive doses.

Naltrexone is contraindicated in acute hepatitis or liver failure. Carefully consider its use in patients with active liver disease in light of its hepatotoxic effects.

The margin of separation between the apparently safe dose of naltrexone and the dose causing hepatic injury appears to be only 5-fold or less. Naltrexone does not appear to be a hepatotoxin at the recommended doses.

Warn patients of the risk of hepatic injury and advise them to stop the use of naltrexone and seek medical attention if they experience symptoms of acute hepatitis.

Indications

Narcotic addiction: Blockade of the effects of exogenously administered opioids.

Alcoholism: Treatment of alcohol dependence.

Administration and Dosage

If there is any question of occult opioid dependence, perform a naloxone challenge test. Do not attempt treatment until naloxone challenge is negative.

Alcoholism: A dose of 50 mg once daily is recommended for most patients.

Narcotic dependence: Initiate treatment using the following guidelines:

1.) Do not attempt treatment until the patient has remained opioid-free for 7 to 10 days.
2.) Administer a naloxone challenge test (see below). If signs of opioid withdrawal are still observed following challenge, do not treat with naltrexone. The naloxone challenge can be repeated in 24 hours.
3.) Initiate treatment carefully, with an initial dose of 25 mg of naltrexone. If no withdrawal signs occur, start the patient on 50 mg/day thereafter.

Naloxone challenge test: The naloxone challenge test may be administered by either intravenous (IV) or subcutaneous routes.

IV: Inject naloxone 0.2 mg.

Observe for 30 seconds for signs or symptoms of withdrawal. If no evidence of withdrawal is observed, inject 0.6 mg of naloxone. Observe for an additional 20 minutes.

Subcutaneous: Administer naloxone 0.8 mg.

Observe for 20 minutes for signs or symptoms of withdrawal.

Interpretation of the challenge: Monitor vital signs and observe the patient for signs and symptoms of opioid withdrawal. If signs or symptoms of withdrawal appear, the test is positive and no additional naloxone should be administered.

Warning: If the test is positive, do not initiate naltrexone therapy. Repeat the challenge in 24 hours. If the test is negative, naltrexone therapy may be started if no other contraindications are present.

Injection: 380 mg delivered intramuscularly (IM) every 4 weeks or once a month. The injection should be administered by a health care provider as an IM gluteal injection, alternating buttocks, using the carton components provided. Naltrexone must not be administered IV.

If patients miss doses, they should be instructed to receive the next dose as soon as possible. Pretreatment with oral naltrexone is not required before using naltrexone injection.

Reinitiation of treatment in patients previously discontinued – There are no data to specifically address reinitiation of treatment.

Switching from oral naltrexone for alcohol dependence – There are no systematically collected data that specifically address the switch from oral naltrexone to naltrexone injection.

Preparation for administration – Naltrexone must be suspended only in the diluent supplied in the carton and must be administered with the needle supplied in the carton. All components (ie, the microspheres, diluent, preparation needle, and an administration needle with safety device) are required for administration. A spare administration needle is provided in case of clogging. Do not substitute any other components for the components of the carton.

Maintenance treatment: Once the patient has been started on naltrexone, 50 mg every 24 hours will produce adequate clinical blockade of the actions of parenterally administered opioids. A flexible dosing regimen may be employed. Thus, patients may receive 50 mg every weekday with a 100 mg dose on Saturday, 100 mg every other day, or 150 mg every third day.

Actions

Pharmacology: Naltrexone is a pure opioid antagonist. It markedly attenuates or completely blocks, reversibly, the subjective effects of IV administered opioids.

Pharmacokinetics:

Absorption – Although well-absorbed orally, naltrexone is subject to significant first-pass metabolism with oral bioavailability estimates ranging from 5% to 40%. Following oral administration, naltrexone undergoes rapid and nearly complete absorption with approximately 96% of the dose absorbed from the GI tract. Peak plasma levels of both naltrexone and 6-β-naltrexol occur within 1 hour of dosing.

Injection: Naltrexone is an extended-release, microsphere formulation of naltrexone designed to be administered by IM gluteal injection every 4 weeks or once a month. After IM injection, the naltrexone plasma concentration time profile is characterized by a transient initial peak, which occurs approximately 2 hours after injection, followed by a second peak observed approximately 2 to 3 days later. Beginning approximately 14 days after dosing, concentrations slowly decline, with measurable levels for greater than 1 month.

Maximum plasma concentration and area under the curve for naltrexone and 6β-naltrexol (the major metabolite) following naltrexone administration are dose proportional. Compared with daily oral dosing with naltrexone 50 mg over 28 days, total naltrexone exposure is 3- to 4-fold higher following administration of a single dose of naltrexone 380 mg. Steady state is reached at the end of the dosing interval following the first injection. There is minimal accumulation (less than 15%) of naltrexone or 6β-naltrexol upon repeat administration of naltrexone.

Distribution – The volume of distribution for naltrexone after IV administration is estimated to be 1,350 L. In vitro, naltrexone is 21% bound to plasma proteins.

Significantly less 6β-naltrexol is generated following IM administration of naltrexone than with administration of oral naltrexone because of a reduction in first-pass hepatic metabolism.

Metabolism/Excretion – The major metabolite of naltrexone is 6-β-naltrexol. The activity of naltrexone is believed to be due to both parent and the 6-β-naltrexol metabolite. The mean elimination half-life values for naltrexone and 6-β-naltrexol are 4 and 13 hours, respectively.

Renal elimination is primarily by glomerular filtration. Parent drug and metabolites are excreted primarily by the kidney; however, urinary excretion of unchanged naltrexone accounts for less than 2% of an oral dose, and fecal excretion is a minor elimination pathway. The urinary excretion of unchanged and conjugated 6-β-naltrexone accounts for 43% of an oral dose. Naltrexone and its metabolites may undergo enterohepatic recycling.

Contraindications

Patients receiving opioid analgesics; opioid-dependent patients; patients in acute opioid withdrawal; failed naloxone challenge; positive urine screen for opioids; history of sensitivity to naltrexone; acute hepatitis or liver failure.

Warnings/Precautions

Eosinophilic pneumonia: If a person receiving naltrexone develops progressive dyspnea and hypoxemia, consider diagnosis of eosinophilic pneumonia. Consider the possibility of eosinophilic pneumonia in patients who do not respond to antibiotics.

Hepatotoxicity: Naltrexone has the capacity to cause direct hepatocellular injury when given in excessive doses. It is contraindicated in acute hepatitis or liver failure, and its use in patients with active liver disease must be carefully considered in light of its hepatotoxic effects.

Warn patients of the risk of hepatic injury and advise them to stop naltrexone and seek medical attention if they experience symptoms of acute hepatitis.

Although no cases of hepatic failure have ever been reported, consider this as a possible risk of treatment.

Abstinence precipitation/syndrome: Unintended precipitation of abstinence or exacerbation of a preexisting subclinical abstinence syndrome may occur; therefore, patients should remain opioid-free for a minimum of 7 to 10 days before starting naltrexone.

Severe opioid withdrawal syndromes: Severe opioid withdrawal syndromes precipitated by accidental naltrexone ingestion have occurred in opioid-dependent individuals. Withdrawal symptoms usually appear within 5 minutes or less of ingestion and may last up to 48 hours.

Surmountable blockade: While naltrexone is a potent antagonist with a prolonged pharmacologic effect (24 to 72 hours), the blockade produced by naltrexone is surmountable. This poses a potential risk to individuals who attempt to overcome the blockade by self-administering large amounts of opioids. Any attempt by a patient to overcome the antagonism by taking opioids is very dangerous and may lead to fatal overdose.

Use with narcotics: Patients taking naltrexone may not benefit from opioid-containing medicines. Use a nonopioid-containing alternative, if available.

Ultra-rapid opioid withdrawal: Safe use of naltrexone in rapid opiate detoxification programs has not been established.

Injection-site reactions: Naltrexone injections may be followed by pain, tenderness, induration, or pruritus.

Suicide: The risk of suicide is increased in patients with substance abuse with or without concomitant depression. This risk is not abated by treatment with naltrexone.

Renal function impairment: Naltrexone and its primary metabolite are excreted primarily in the urine, and caution is recommended in administering the drug to patients with renal function impairment.

Pregnancy: Category C.

Lactation: It is not known if naltrexone is excreted in breast milk.

Children: Safety for use in children younger than 18 years of age has not been established.

Monitoring: A high index of suspicion for drug-related hepatic injury is critical if the occurrence of liver damage induced by naltrexone is to be detected at the earliest possible time.

Drug Interactions

Drugs that may be affected by naltrexone include opioid-containing products and thioridazine.

Adverse Reactions

Adverse reactions associated with treatment of alcoholism include nausea, headache, dizziness, nervousness, fatigue, insomnia, and vomiting.

Reactions associated with treatment of narcotic addiction include difficulty sleeping, anxiety, nervousness, headache, low energy, irritability, increased energy, dizziness, abdominal cramps/pain, nausea, vomiting, loss of appetite, diarrhea, constipation, joint/muscle pain, delayed ejaculation, decreased potency, skin rash, chills, and increased thirst.

FLUMAZENIL

Injection: 0.1 mg/mL (*Rx*) — *Romazicon* (Hoffman-La Roche)

Indications

Reversal of benzodiazepine sedation: For the complete or partial reversal of the sedative effects of benzodiazepines in cases where general anesthesia has been induced or maintained with benzodiazepines, where sedation has been produced with benzodiazepines for diagnostic and therapeutic procedures, and for the management of benzodiazepine overdose.

Administration and Dosage

For IV use only. To minimize the likelihood of pain at the injection site, administer flumazenil through a freely running IV infusion into a large vein.

Individualization of dosage: In high-risk patients, it is important to administer the smallest amount of flumazenil that is effective. The 1-minute wait between individual doses in the dose-titration recommended for general clinical populations may be too short for high-risk patients because it takes 6 to 10 minutes for any single dose of flumazenil to reach full effects. Slow the rate of administration of flumazenil administered to high-risk patients.

Reversal of conscious sedation or in general anesthesia: The recommended initial dose is 0.2 mg (2 mL) administered IV over 15 seconds. If the desired level of consciousness is not obtained after waiting an additional 45 seconds, a further dose of 0.2 mg (2 mL) can be injected and repeated at 60 second intervals where necessary (up to a maximum of 4 additional times) to a maximum total dose of 1 mg (10 mL). Individualize the dose based on the patient's response, with most patients responding to doses of 0.6 to 1 mg.

In the event of resedation, repeated doses may be administered at 20-minute intervals as needed. For repeat treatment, administer no more than 1 mg (given as 0.2 mg/min) at any one time, and give no more than 3 mg in any 1 hour.

Suspected benzodiazepine overdose: The recommended initial dose is 0.2 mg (2 mL) administered IV over 30 seconds. If the desired level of consciousness is not obtained after waiting 30 seconds, a further dose of 0.3 mg (3 mL) can be administered over another 30 seconds. Further doses of 0.5 mg (5 mL) can be administered over 30 seconds at 1-minute intervals up to a cumulative dose of 3 mg.

Most patients with benzodiazepine overdose will respond to a cumulative dose of 1 to 3 mg, and doses beyond 3 mg do not reliably produce additional effects.

If a patient has not responded 5 minutes after receiving a cumulative dose of 5 mg, the major cause of sedation is likely not to be due to benzodiazepines, and additional flumazenil is likely to have no effect.

In the event of resedation, repeated doses may be given at 20-minute intervals if needed. For repeat treatment, give no more than 1 mg (given as 0.5 mg/min) at any one time and give no more than 3 mg in any 1 hour.

Actions

Pharmacology: Flumazenil antagonizes the actions of benzodiazepines on the CNS and competitively inhibits the activity at the benzodiazepine recognition site on the GABA/benzodiazepine receptor complex.

The duration and degree of reversal of benzodiazepine effects are related to the dose and plasma concentrations of flumazenil. The onset of reversal is usually evident within 1 to 2 minutes after the injection is completed. Within 3 minutes, 80% response will be reached, with the peak effect occurring at 6 to 10 minutes.

Pharmacokinetics: After IV administration, flumazenil has an initial distribution half-life of 7 to 15 minutes and a terminal half-life of 41 to 79 minutes. Peak concentrations of flumazenil are proportional to dose, with an apparent initial volume of distribution of 0.5 L/kg. After redistribution the apparent volume of distribution ranges from 0.77 to 1.6 L/kg. Protein binding is approximately 50%.

Flumazenil is a highly extracted drug. Clearance of flumazenil occurs primarily by hepatic metabolism and is dependent on hepatic blood flow. In healthy volunteers, total clearance ranges from 0.7 to 1.3 L/h/kg, with less than 1% of the administered dose eliminated unchanged in urine. Elimination of drug is essentially complete within 72 hours, with 90% to 95% appearing in urine and 5% to 10% in feces.

Contraindications

Hypersensitivity to flumazenil or to benzodiazepines; benzodiazepine use for control of a potentially life-threatening condition; in patients who are showing signs of serious cyclic antidepressant overdose.

Warnings/Precautions

Seizures: The use of flumazenil has been associated with the occurrence of seizures. These are most frequent in patients who have been on benzodiazepines for long-term sedation or in overdose cases where patients are showing signs of serious cyclic antidepressant overdose. Individualize the dosage of flumazenil and be prepared to manage seizures.

Seizure risk: The reversal of benzodiazepine effects may be associated with the onset of seizures in certain high-risk populations.

Most convulsions associated with flumazenil administration require treatment and have been successfully managed with benzodiazepines, phenytoin, or barbiturates.

Hypoventilation: Monitor patients who have received flumazenil for the reversal of benzodiazepine effects (after conscious sedation or general anesthesia) for resedation, respiratory depression or other residual benzodiazepine effects for an appropriate period (120 minutes or less) based on the dose and duration of effect of the benzodiazepine employed, because flumazenil has not been established as an effective treatment for hypoventilation due to benzodiazepine administration.

Flumazenil may not fully reverse postoperative airway problems or ventilatory insufficiency induced by benzodiazepines. In addition, even if flumazenil is initially effective, such problems may recur because the effects of flumazenil wear off before the effects of many benzodiazepines.

Return of sedation: Resedation is least likely in cases where flumazenil is administered to reverse a low dose of a short-acting benzodiazepine. It is most likely in cases where a large single or cumulative dose of a benzodiazepine has been given in the course of a long procedure along with neuromuscular blocking agents and multiple anesthetic agents.

Intensive Care Unit (ICU): Use with caution in the ICU because of the increased risk of unrecognized benzodiazepine dependence in such settings.

Overdose situations: Flumazenil is intended as an adjunct to, not as a substitute for, proper management of airway, assisted breathing, circulatory access and support, internal decontamination by lavage and charcoal, and adequate clinical evaluation.

Head injury: Use with caution in patients with head injury as flumazenil may be capable of precipitating convulsions or altering cerebral blood flow in patients receiving benzodiazepines.

Neuromuscular blocking agents: Do not use flumazenil until the effects of neuromuscular blockade have been fully reversed.

Psychiatric patients: Flumazenil may provoke panic attacks in patients with a history of panic disorder.

Drug- and alcohol-dependent patients: Use with caution in patients with alcoholism and other drug dependencies due to the increased frequency of benzodiazepine tolerance and dependence observed in these patient populations.

Tolerance to benzodiazepines: Flumazenil may cause benzodiazepine withdrawal symptoms in individuals who have been taking benzodiazepines long enough to have some degree of tolerance. Slower titration rates of 0.1 mg/min and lower total doses may help reduce the frequency of emergent confusion and agitation.

Physical dependence on benzodiazepines: Flumazenil is known to precipitate withdrawal seizures in patients who are physically dependent on benzodiazepines, even if such dependence was established in a relatively few days of high-dose sedation in ICU environments. The risk of either seizures or resedation in such cases is high and patients have experienced seizures before regaining consciousness. Use flumazenil in such settings with extreme caution, because use of flumazenil in this situation has not been studied and no information as to dose and rate of titration is available.

Pain on injection: To minimize the likelihood of pain or inflammation at the injection site, administer flumazenil through a freely flowing IV infusion into a large vein. Local irritation may occur following extravasation into perivascular tissues.

Respiratory disease: Appropriate ventilatory support is the primary treatment of patients with serious lung disease who experience serious respiratory depression due to benzodiazepines rather than the administration of flumazenil.

Ambulatory patients: Effects may wear off before a long-acting benzodiazepine is completely cleared from the body.

Mixed drug overdosage: Particular caution is necessary when using flumazenil in cases of mixed drug overdosage; toxic effects of other drugs taken in overdose (especially cyclic antidepressants) may emerge with reversal of the benzodiazepine effect by flumazenil.

Hepatic function impairment: Mean total clearance is decreased to 40% to 60% of normal in patients with moderate liver dysfunction and to 25% of normal in patients with severe liver dysfunction compared with age-matched healthy subjects. This results in a prolongation of the half-life from 0.8 hours in healthy subjects to 1.3 hours in patients with moderate hepatic function impairment and 2.4 hours in severely impaired patients.

Pregnancy: Category C.

Labor and delivery – The use of flumazenil to reverse the effects of benzodiazepines used during labor and delivery is not recommended because the effects of the drug in the newborn are unknown.

Lactation: It is not known whether flumazenil is excreted in breast milk.

Children: Flumazenil is not recommended for use in children.

Monitoring: Monitor patients for resedation, respiratory depression, or other persistent or recurrent agonist effects for an adequate period of time after administration of flumazenil.

Drug Interactions

Drug/Food interactions: Ingestion of food during an IV infusion of flumazenil results in a 50% increase in flumazenil clearance, most likely due to the increased hepatic blood flow that accompanies a meal.

Adverse Reactions

Adverse reactions may include death, convulsions, headache, injection site pain, increased sweating, fatigue, cutaneous vasodilation, nausea, vomiting, dizziness, agitation, dry mouth, tremors, palpitations, insomnia, dyspnea, hyperventilation, emotional lability, abnormal/blurred vision, and paresthesia.

Chapter 4

CARDIOVASCULAR AGENTS

CARDIAC GLYCOSIDES

DIGOXIN	
Tablets: 0.125 and 0.25 mg (*Rx*)	Various, *Lanoxin* (GlaxoSmithKline)
Elixir, pediatric: 0.05 mg/mL (*Rx*)	Various
Injection: 0.25 mg/mL (*Rx*)	Various, *Lanoxin* (GlaxoSmithKline)
Injection, pediatric: 0.1 mg/mL (*Rx*)	Various, *Lanoxin* (GlaxoSmithKline)

Indications

Congestive heart failure (CHF) all degrees: Increased cardiac output results in diuresis and general amelioration of disturbances characteristic of right heart failure (venous congestion, edema) and left heart failure (dyspnea, orthopnea, cardiac asthma).

Atrial flutter: Digitalis slows the heart; normal sinus rhythm may appear. Often, flutter is converted to atrial fibrillation with a slow ventricular rate.

Administration and Dosage

Recommended dosages of digoxin may require considerable modification because of individual sensitivity of the patient to the drug, the presence of associated conditions, or the use of concurrent medications. In selecting a dose of digoxin, the following factors must be considered:

1.) The body weight of the patient. Calculate doses based upon lean (ie, ideal) body weight.
2.) The patient's renal function, preferably evaluated on the basis of estimated creatinine clearance (Ccr).
3.) The patient's age. Infants and children require different doses of digoxin than adults.
4.) Concomitant disease states, concurrent medications, or other factors likely to alter the pharmacokinetic or pharmacodynamic profile of digoxin.

Serum digoxin concentrations: About 66% of adults considered adequately digitalized (without evidence of toxicity) have serum digoxin concentrations ranging from 0.8 to 2 ng/mL. Consequently, interpret the serum concentration of digoxin in the overall clinical context, and do not use an isolated measurement as the basis for increasing or decreasing the dose of the drug.

To allow adequate time for equilibration of digoxin between serum and tissue, perform sampling of serum concentrations just before the next scheduled dose of the drug. If this is not possible, perform sampling at least 6 to 8 hours after the last dose, regardless of the route of administration or the formulation used.

Heart failure:

Adults – Digitalization may be accomplished by either of 2 general approaches that vary in dosage and frequency of administration but reach the same endpoint in terms of total amount of digoxin accumulated in the body.

1.) If rapid digitalization is considered medically appropriate, it may be achieved by administering a loading dose based upon projected peak digoxin body stores. Calculate maintenance dose as a percentage of the loading dose.
2.) Obtain more gradual digitalization beginning an appropriate maintenance dose, thus allowing digoxin body stores to accumulate slowly. Steady-state serum digoxin concentration will be achieved in approximately 5 half-lives of the drug for the individual patient. Depending upon the patient's renal function, this will take between 1 and 3 weeks.

Atrial fibrillation: Peak digoxin body stores larger than the 8 to 12 mcg/kg required for most patients with heart failure and normal sinus rhythm have been used for control of ventricular rate in patients with atrial fibrillation. Titrate doses of digoxin used for the treatment of chronic atrial fibrillation to the minimum dose that achieves the desired ventricular rate control without causing undesirable side effects. Data are not available to establish the appropriate resting or exercise target rates that should be achieved.

Renal function impairment: In children with renal disease, digoxin must be carefully titrated based upon clinical response.

Rapid digitalization with a loading dose: Peak digoxin body stores of 8 to 12 mcg/kg should provide therapeutic effect with minimum risk of toxicity in most patients with heart failure and normal sinus rhythm. Because of altered digoxin distribution and elimination, projected peak body stores for patients with renal insufficiency should be conservative (ie, 6 to 10 mcg/kg; see Precautions).

Administer the loading dose in several portions, with roughly half the total given as the first dose. Additional fractions of this planned total dose may be given at 6- to 8-hour intervals, with careful assessment of clinical response before each additional dose.

If the patient's clinical response necessitates a change from the calculated loading dose of digoxin, then base calculation of the maintenance dose upon the amount actually given.

Digoxin injection is frequently used to achieve rapid digitalization, with conversion to digoxin tablets or capsules for maintenance therapy. If patients are switched from IV to oral digoxin formulations, make allowances for differences in bioavailability when calculating maintenance dosages (see Pharmacology).

Tablets – A single initial dose of 500 to 750 mcg (0.5 to 0.75 mg) of digoxin tablets usually produces a detectable effect in 0.5 to 2 hours that becomes maximal in 2 to 6 hours. Additional doses of 125 to 375 mcg (0.125 to 0.375 mg) may be given cautiously at 6- to 8-hour intervals until clinical evidence of an adequate effect is noted. The usual amount of digoxin tablets that a 70 kg patient requires to achieve 8 to 12 mcg/kg peak body stores is 750 to 1250 mcg (0.75 to 1.25 mg).

Injection – A single initial IV dose of 400 to 600 mcg (0.4 to 0.6 mg) of injection usually produces a detectable effect in 5 to 30 minutes that becomes maximal in 1 to 4 hours. Additional doses of 100 to 300 mcg (0.1 to 0.3 mg) may be given cautiously at 6- to 8-hour intervals until clinical evidence of an adequate effect is noted. The usual amount of injection that a 70 kg patient requires to achieve 8 to 12 mcg/kg peak body stores is 600 to 1000 mcg (0.6 to 1 mg).

Dosage adjustment when changing preparations: The difference in bioavailability between digoxin injection or capsules and pediatric elixir or tablets must be considered when changing patients from 1 dosage form to another.

The absolute bioavailability of the capsule formulation is greater than that of the standard tablets and near that of the IV dosage form. As a result, the doses recommended for the capsules are the same as those for injection. Adjustments in dosage will seldom be necessary when converting a patient from the IV formulation to capsules.

Doses of 100 mcg (0.1 mg) and 200 mcg (0.2 mg) of digoxin capsules are approximately equivalent to 125 mcg (0.125 mg) and 250 mcg (0.25 mg) doses of tablets and pediatric elixir, respectively.

Maintenance dosing: The doses of digoxin used in controlled trials in patients with heart failure have ranged from 125 to 500 mcg (0.125 to 0.5 mg) once daily. In these studies, the digoxin dose has been generally titrated according to the patient's age, lean body weight, and renal function. Therapy is generally initiated at a dose of 250 mcg (0.25 mg) once daily in patients younger than 70 years of age with good renal function, at a dose of 125 mcg (0.125 mg) once daily in patients older than 70 years of age or with impaired renal function, and at a dose of 62.5 mcg (0.0625 mg) in patients with marked renal impairment. Doses may be increased every 2 weeks according to clinical response.

In a subset of approximately 1,800 patients enrolled in a trial (wherein dosing was based on an algorithm similar to that in the table below) the mean (± SD) serum digoxin concentrations at 1 month and 12 months were approximately 1.01 ng/mL and approximately 0.97 ng/mL, respectively.

Base the maintenance dose upon the percentage of the peak body stores lost each day through elimination. The following formula has had wide clinical use:

Tablets:

Maintenance dosing –

Usual Digoxin Tablet Daily Maintenance Dose Requirements (mcg) for Estimated Peak Body Stores of 10 mcg/kg							
Corrected Ccr (mL/min/70 kg)[a]	Lean Body Weight (kg/lbs)						Number of days before steady-state achieved[b]
	50/110	60/132	70/154	80/176	90/198	100/220	
0	62.5	125	125	125	187.5	187.5	22
10	125	125	125	187.5	187.5	187.5	19
20	125	125	187.5	187.5	187.5	250	16
30	125	187.5	187.5	187.5	250	250	14
40	125	187.5	187.5	250	250	250	13
50	187.5	187.5	250	250	250	250	12
60	187.5	187.5	250	250	250	375	11
70	187.5	250	250	250	250	375	10
80	187.5	250	250	250	375	375	9
90	187.5	250	250	250	375	500	8
100	250	250	250	375	375	500	7

[a] Ccr is corrected to 70 kg body weight or 1.73 m^2 body surface area. For adults, if only serum creatinine concentrations (Scr) are available, a Ccr (corrected to 70 kg body weight) may be estimated in men as (140 − Age)/Scr. For women, multiply this result by 0.85. Note: This equation cannot be used for estimating Ccr in infants or children.

[b] If no loading dose is administered.

Infants and children – In general, divided daily dosing is recommended for infants and young children younger than 10 years of age. In the newborn period, renal clearance of digoxin is diminished and observe suitable dosage adjustments. This is especially pronounced in the premature infant. Beyond the immediate newborn period, children generally require proportionally larger doses than adults on the basis of body weight or body surface area. Children older than 10 years of age require adult dosages in proportion to their body weight. Some researchers have suggested that infants and young children tolerate slightly higher serum concentrations than do adults.

Daily maintenance doses for each age group are given in the table below and should provide therapeutic effects with minimum risk of toxicity in most patients with heart failure and normal sinus rhythm. These recommendations assume the presence of normal renal function:

Daily Digoxin Maintenance Doses in Children with Normal Renal Function	
Age	Daily maintenance dose (mcg/kg)
2 to 5 years	10 to 15
5 to 10 years	7 to 10
> 10 years	3 to 5

Pediatric elixir:

Usual digitalizing and maintenance dosing –

Usual Digitalizing and Maintenance Dosages for Pediatric Elixir in Children with Normal Renal Function Based on Lean Body Weight		
Age	Oral digitalizing[a] dose (mcg/kg)	Daily maintenance dose[b] (mcg/kg)
Premature	20 to 30	20% to 30% of oral digitalizing dose[c]
Full-term	25 to 35	25% to 35% of oral digitalizing dose[c]
1 to 24 months	35 to 60	
2 to 5 years	30 to 40	
5 to 10 years	20 to 35	
> 10 years	10 to 15	

[a] IV digitalizing doses are 80% of oral digitalizing doses.
[b] Divided daily dosing is recommended for children younger than 10 years of age.
[c] Projected or actual digitalizing dose providing clinical response.

Gradual digitalization with a maintenance dose – More gradual digitalization also can be accomplished by beginning an appropriate maintenance dose. The range of percentages provided in the above table can be used in calculating this dose for patients with normal renal function.

Injection: Slow infusion of injection is preferable to bolus administration. Rapid infusion of digitalis glycosides has been shown to cause systemic and coronary arteriolar constriction, which may be clinically undesirable. Caution is thus advised and injection probably should be administered over a period of 5 minutes or more. Mixing injection with other drugs in the same container or simultaneous administration in the same intravenous line is not recommended.

Parenteral administration of digoxin should be used only when the need for rapid digitalization is urgent or when the drug cannot be taken orally. IM injection can lead to severe pain at the injection site, thus IV administration is preferred. If the drug must be administered by the IM route, inject it deep into the muscle followed by massage. Do not inject more than 500 mcg (2 mL) into a single site.

If tuberculin syringes are used to measure very small doses, one must be aware of the problem of inadvertent overadministration of digoxin. Do not flush the syringe with the parenteral solution after its contents are expelled into an indwelling vascular catheter.

Admixture compatibility – Digoxin injection can be administered undiluted or diluted with a 4-fold or greater volume of sterile water for injection, 0.9% sodium chloride injection, or 5% dextrose injection. The use of less than 4-fold volume of diluent could lead to precipitation of the digoxin. Immediate use of the diluted product is recommended.

Maintenance dose –

Usual Daily Maintenance Dose Requirements (mcg) of Digoxin Injection for Estimated Peak Body Stores of 10 mcg/kg[a]							
	Lean body weight (kg/lb)						
Corrected Ccr (mL/min/70 kg)[b]	50/110	60/132	70/154	80/176	90/198	100/220	Number of days before steady-state achieved[c]
0	75	75	100	100	125	150	22
10	75	100	100	125	150	150	19
20	100	100	125	150	150	175	16
30	10	125	150	150	175	200	14
40	100	125	150	175	200	225	13
50	125	150	175	200	225	250	12
60	125	150	175	200	225	250	11

Usual Daily Maintenance Dose Requirements (mcg) of Digoxin Injection for Estimated Peak Body Stores of 10 mcg/kg[a]							
	Lean body weight (kg/lb)						
Corrected Ccr (mL/min/70 kg)[b]	50/110	60/132	70/154	80/176	90/198	100/220	Number of days before steady-state achieved[c]
70	150	175	200	225	250	275	10
80	150	175	200	250	275	300	9
90	150	200	225	250	300	325	8
100	175	200	250	275	300	350	7

[a] Daily maintenance doses have been rounded to the nearest 25 mcg increment.
[b] Ccr is corrected to 70 kg body weight or 1.73 m^2 body surface area. For adults, if only serum creatinine concentrations (Scr) are available, a Ccr (corrected to 70 kg body weight) may be estimated in men as (140 – Age)/Scr. For women, this result should be multiplied by 0.85. Note: This equation cannot be used for estimating Ccr in infants or children.
[c] If no loading dose is administered.

Pediatric injection:

Digitalizing and maintenance dosages –

Usual Digitalizing and Maintenance Dosages for Digoxin Pediatric Injection in Children with Normal Renal Function Based on Lean Body Weight		
Age	IV digitalizing[a] dose (mcg/kg)	Daily IV maintenance dose[b] (mcg/kg)
Premature	15 to 25	20% to 30% of the IV digitalizing dose[c]
Full-term	20 to 30	25% to 35% of the IV digitalizing dose[c]
1 to 24 months	30 to 50	
2 to 5 years	25 to 35	
5 to 10 years	15 to 30	
≥ 10 years	8 to 12	

[a] IV digitalizing doses are 80% of oral digitalizing doses.
[b] Divided daily dosing is recommended for children younger than 10 years of age.
[c] Projected or actual digitalizing dose providing clinical response.

Gradual digitalization with a maintenance dose – More gradual digitalization also can be accomplished by beginning an appropriate maintenance dose. The range of percentages provided in the table above can be used in calculating this dose for patients with normal renal function.

Actions

Pharmacology: Digoxin inhibits sodium-potassium ATPase, leading to an increase in the intracellular concentration of sodium and thus, (by stimulation of sodium-calcium exchange) an increase in the intracellular concentration of calcium. The pharmacologic consequences of these direct and indirect effects are the following: An increase in the force and velocity of myocardial systolic contraction (positive inotropic action); a decrease in the degree of activation of the sympathetic nervous system and renin-angiotensin system (neurohormonal deactivating effect); and slowing of the heart rate and decreased conduction velocity through the AV node (vagomimetic effect).

Hemodynamic effects – Digoxin produces hemodynamic improvement in patients with heart failure. Short- and long-term therapy with the drug increases cardiac output and lowers pulmonary artery pressure, pulmonary capillary wedge pressure, and systemic vascular resistance.

Pharmacokinetics:

Absorption – Following oral administration, peak serum concentrations of digoxin occur at 1 to 3 hours. Absorption of digoxin from the tablets has been demonstrated to be 60% to 80% complete compared with an identical IV dose of digoxin (absolute bioavailability) or capsules (relative bioavailability).

Distribution – Digoxin has a large apparent volume of distribution. Digoxin crosses the blood-brain barrier and the placenta. Approximately 25% of digoxin in the plasma is bound to protein. Serum digoxin concentrations correlate best with lean (ie, ideal) body weight, not total body weight.

Metabolism – Only a small percentage (16%) of a dose of digoxin is metabolized.

Excretion – Elimination of digoxin follows first-order kinetics. Following IV administration to healthy volunteers, 50% to 70% of a digoxin dose is excreted unchanged in the urine. Digoxin is not effectively removed from the body by dialysis, exchange transfusion, or during cardiopulmonary bypass because most of the drug is bound to tissue and does not circulate in the blood.

Contraindications

Ventricular fibrillation; hypersensitivity to digoxin or other digitalis preparations.

Warnings/Precautions

Sinus node disease and AV block: The drug may cause severe sinus bradycardia or sinoatrial block in patients with preexisting sinus node disease and may cause advanced or complete heart block in patients with preexisting incomplete AV block. Consider inserting a pacemaker before treatment with digoxin.

Accessory AV pathway (Wolff-Parkinson-White syndrome): After IV digoxin therapy, some patients with paroxysmal atrial fibrillation or flutter and a coexisting accessory AV pathway have developed increased antegrade conduction across the accessory pathway bypassing the AV node, leading to a very rapid ventricular response or ventricular fibrillation. Unless conduction down the accessory pathway has been blocked (either pharmacologically or by surgery), do not use digoxin in such patients.

Use in patients with preserved left ventricular systolic function: Patients with certain disorders involving heart failure associated with preserved left ventricular ejection fraction may be particularly susceptible to toxicity of the drug.

Electrolyte disorders: In patients with hypokalemia or hypomagnesemia, toxicity may occur despite serum digoxin concentrations less than 2 ng/mL, because potassium or magnesium depletion sensitizes the myocardium to digoxin. Therefore, it is desirable to maintain normal serum potassium and magnesium concentrations in patients being treated with digoxin.

Hypercalcemia from any cause predisposes the patient to digitalis toxicity. Calcium, particularly when administered rapidly by the IV route, may produce serious arrhythmias in digitalized patients. On the other hand, hypocalcemia can nullify the effects of digoxin in humans; thus, digoxin may be ineffective until serum calcium is restored to normal.

Thyroid disorders and hypermetabolic states: Hypothyroidism may reduce the requirements for digoxin. Heart failure or atrial arrhythmias resulting from hypermetabolic or hyperdynamic states (eg, hyperthyroidism, hypoxia, arteriovenous shunt) are best treated by addressing the underlying condition. Atrial arrhythmias associated with hypermetabolic states are particularly resistant to digoxin treatment. Care must be taken to avoid toxicity if digoxin is used.

Acute MI: Use digoxin with caution in patients with acute MI. The use of inotropic drugs in some patients in this setting may result in undesirable increases in myocardial oxygen demand and ischemia.

Electrical cardioversion: It may be desirable to reduce the dose of digoxin for 1 to 2 days prior to electrical cardioversion of atrial fibrillation to avoid the induction of ventricular arrhythmias, but physicians must consider the consequences of increasing the ventricular response if digoxin is withdrawn. If digitalis toxicity is suspected, delay elective cardioversion. If it is not prudent to delay cardioversion, select the lowest possible energy level to avoid provoking ventricular arrhythmias.

Renal function impairment: Digoxin is primarily excreted by the kidneys; therefore, patients with impaired renal function require smaller than usual maintenance doses of digoxin (see Administration and Dosage).

Pregnancy: Category C.

Lactation: Exercise caution when digoxin is administered to a breast-feeding woman.

Children: Newborn infants display considerable variability in tolerance. Premature and immature infants are particularly sensitive; reduce dosage and individualize digitalization according to infant's degree of maturity.

Lab test abnormalities: Periodically assess serum electrolytes and renal function (serum creatinine concentrations); the frequency of assessments will depend on the clinical setting.

Drug Interactions

Increased digoxin serum levels: The following agents may increase digoxin serum levels, possibly increasing its therapeutic and toxic effects: Alprazolam, amiodarone, anticholinergics, benzodiazepines, bepridil, captopril, cyclosporine, diltiazem, diphenoxylate, erythromycin, esmolol, felodipine, flecainide, hydroxychloroquine, ibuprofen, indomethacin, itraconazole, nifedipine, omeprazole, propafenone, propantheline, quinidine, quinine, tetracycline, tolbutamide, and verapamil.

Decreased GI absorption of digitalis glycosides: May be caused by the following agents, possibly decreasing the serum levels and therapeutic effects: Aminoglutethimide, aminoglycosides (oral), aminosalicylic acid, antacids (aluminum or magnesium salts), antihistamines, antineoplastics, barbiturates, cholestyramine, colestipol, hydantoins, hypoglycemic agents (oral), kaolin/pectin, metoclopramide, neomycin, penicillamine, rifampin, sucralfate, and sulfasalazine.

Other drugs that may interact with cardiac glycosides include the following: Albuterol, amphotericin B, beta-blockers, calcium, disopyramide, loop diuretics, nondepolarizing muscle relaxants, potassium-sparing diuretics, succinylcholine, sympathomimetics, thiazide diuretics, thioamines, and thyroid hormones.

Drug/Lab test interactions: The use of therapeutic doses of digoxin may cause prolongation of the PR interval and depression of the ST segment on the electrocardiogram. Digoxin may produce false positive ST-T changes on the electrocardiogram during exercise testing.

Drug/Food interactions: When digoxin tablets are taken after meals, the rate of absorption is slowed but total amount absorbed is usually unchanged. However, when taken with meals high in bran fiber, the amount absorbed may be reduced.

Adverse Reactions

Digoxin adverse reactions are dose-dependent and occur at doses higher than those needed to achieve a therapeutic effect. Cardiac adverse reactions accounted for approximately 50%, GI disturbances for approximately 25%, and CNS and other toxicity for approximately 25% of these adverse reactions. However, available evidence suggests that the incidence and severity of digoxin toxicity has decreased substantially in recent years.

Adverse reactions occurring in at least 3% of patients include the following: Headache, dizziness, mental disturbances, nausea, diarrhea, and death.

NITRATES

AMYL NITRITE	
Inhalant: 0.3 mL (*Rx*)	Various
ISOSORBIDE DINITRATE (ORAL)	
Tablets: 5, 10, 20, 30, and 40 mg (*Rx*)	Various, *Isordil Titradose* (Wyeth-Ayerst)
Tablets, extended-release: 40 mg (*Rx*)	Various, *Isochron* (Forest)
Tablets, sublingual; oral: 2.5 and 5 mg (*Rx*)	Various
Capsules, sustained-release: 40 mg (*Rx*)	Various, *Isordil Tembids* (Wyeth-Ayerst), *Dilatrate-SR* (Schwarz Pharma)
ISOSORBIDE DINITRATE (SUBLINGUAL)	
Tablets, sublingual: 2.5 and 5 mg (*Rx*)	Various, *Isordil* (Wyeth-Ayerst)
ISOSORBIDE MONONITRATE (ORAL)	
Tablets: 10 and 20 mg (*Rx*)	*Monoket* (Schwarz Pharma), *ISMO* (Reddy Pharmaceuticals)
Tablets, extended-release: 30, 60, and 120 mg (*Rx*)	*Imdur* (Key)
NITROGLYCERIN (IV)	
Injection: 5 mg/mL (*Rx*)	Various, *Tridil* (Faulding)
Injection solution: 100, 200, and 400 mcg/mL in 5% dextrose (*Rx*)	Various
NITROGLYCERIN (SUBLINGUAL)	
Tablets, sublingual: 0.3, 0.4, and 0.6 mg (*Rx*)	Various, *Nitrostat* (Parke-Davis), *NitroTab* (Able)
NITROGLYCERIN (LINGUAL)	
Aerosol spray, lingual: 0.4 mg/metered spray (*Rx*)	*NitroMist* (Par)
NITROGLYCERIN (EXTENDED-RELEASE)	
Capsules, extended-release: 2.5, 6.5, and 9 mg (*Rx*)	Various, *Nitro-Time* (Time-Cap Labs)
NITROGLYCERIN (TOPICAL)	
Ointment: 2% (*Rx*)	Various, *Nitro-Bid* (Savage)
NITROGLYCERIN TRANSDERMAL SYSTEMS	
Patch: 0.1, 0.2, 0.3, 0.4, 0.6, and 0.8 mg/h (*Rx*)	Various, *Nitro-Dur* (Key)
NITROGLYCERIN (TRANSLINGUAL)	
Spray: 0.4 mg/dose (*Rx*)	*Nitrolingual* (Sciele Pharma)

Indications

Acute angina (nitroglycerin sublingual or translingual spray; isosorbide dinitrate sublingual; amyl nitrite): For relief of acute anginal episodes; prophylaxis prior to events likely to provoke an attack.

Angina prophylaxis (nitroglycerin topical, transdermal, translingual spray, oral sustained release; isosorbide dinitrate; isosorbide mononitrate): Prophylaxis and long-term management of recurrent angina.

Nitroglycerin IV: Control of blood pressure in perioperative hypertension associated with surgical procedures, especially cardiovascular procedures, such as endotracheal intubation, anesthesia, skin incision, sternotomy, cardiac bypass, and in the immediate postsurgical period.

CHF associated with acute MI; treatment of angina pectoris unresponsive to organic nitrates or β-blockers; production of controlled hypotension during surgical procedures.

Administration and Dosage

AMYL NITRITE: Usual adult dose is 0.3 mL by inhalation, as required.

Crush the capsule and wave under the nose; 2 to 6 inhalations from one capsule are usually sufficient to produce the desired effect. May repeat in 3 to 5 minutes.

ISOSORBIDE DINITRATE, ORAL:

Tablets – Initial dose is 5 to 20 mg; maintenance dose is 10 to 40 mg 2 to 3 times daily.

Extended-release/Sustained-release – The initial dose is 40 mg; maintenance controlled release dose is 40 to 80 mg every 8 to 12 hours. Do not crush or chew these preparations.

Tolerance – Tolerance to these agents may develop. Consider administering the short-acting preparations 2 or 3 times/day (last dose no later than 7 pm) and the sustained release preparations once daily or twice daily at 8 am and 2 pm.

ISOSORBIDE DINITRATE, SUBLINGUAL:

Angina pectoris – Usual starting dose is 2.5 to 5 mg for sublingual tablets. Titrate upward until angina is relieved or side effects limit the dose.

Acute prophylaxis – A patient anticipating activity likely to cause angina should take 1 sublingual tablet (2.5 to 5 mg) approximately 15 minutes before the activity is expected to begin.

ISOSORBIDE MONONITRATE:

Tablets – 20 mg twice/day, with the 2 doses given 7 hours apart. A starting dose of 5 mg might be appropriate for people of particularly small stature, but should be increased to no more than 10 mg by the second or third day of therapy. Suggested regimen is to give first dose on awakening and second dose 7 hours later.

Tablets, extended-release – Initially, 30 or 60 mg once daily. After several days, the dosage may be increased to 120 mg once daily. Rarely 240 mg may be required. Suggested regimen is to give in the morning on arising. Do not crush or chew extended release tablets, and swallow them with a half glassful of liquid.

NITROGLYCERIN, IV:

Dosage requirements – The usual starting adult dose in clinical studies using polyvinyl chloride (PVC) administration sets was 25 mcg/min. When using a nonabsorbing infusion set, the initial dosage should be 5 mcg/min delivered through an infusion pump capable of exact and constant delivery of the drug. Initial titration should be in 5 mcg/min increments, with increases every 3 to 5 minutes until some response is noted. If no response occurs at 20 mcg/min, increments of 10 and even 20 mcg/min can be used. Once a partial blood pressure response is observed, reduce the dose and lengthen the interval between increments.

NITROGLYCERIN, SUBLINGUAL: Dissolve 1 tablet under tongue or in buccal pouch (between cheek and gum) at first sign of an acute anginal attack. Repeat approximately every 5 minutes until relief is obtained. Take no more than 3 tablets in 15 minutes. May be used prophylactically 5 to 10 minutes prior to activities which might precipitate an acute attack.

AEROSOL SPRAY:

Dosage – At the onset of attack, spray 1 or 2 metered doses onto or under the tongue. A spray may be repeated approximately every 5 minutes as needed. No more than 3 metered doses are recommended within a 15-minute period. If chest pain persists, prompt medical attention is recommended. May be used prophylactically 5 to 10 minutes prior to engaging in activities that might precipitate an acute attack.

Administration – During application the patient should rest, ideally in the sitting position. Do not shake container. The container should be held vertically with the valve head uppermost and the spray orifice as close to the mouth as possible. The dose should preferably be sprayed onto the tongue by pressing the button firmly and the mouth should be closed immediately after each dose. Do not inhale spray. The medication should not be expectorated or the mouth rinsed for 5 to 10 minutes following administration. Instruct patients to familiarize themselves with the position of the spray orifice, which can be identified by the finger rest on top of the valve, in order to facilitate oriehuntation for administration at night.

Priming – Each metered spray of nitroglycerin lingual spray delivers 48 mg of solution containing nitroglycerin 400 mcg after an initial priming of 1 spray. It will remain adequately primed for 6 weeks. If the product is not used within 6 weeks it can be adequately reprimed with 1 spray. There are 60 or 200 metered sprays per bottle. However, the total number of available doses is dependent on the number of sprays per use (1 or 2 sprays) and the frequency of repriming.

NITROGLYCERIN, EXTENDED-RELEASE: The usual starting dose is 2.5 to 6.5 mg, 3 or 4 times/day. The dose may be increased 2 to 4 times/day over a period of days or weeks. Doses as high as 26 mg given 4 times/day have been reported effective.

Give the smallest effective dose 2 to 4 times/day.

Capsules must be swallowed; not for chewing or sublingual use.

NITROGLYCERIN, TOPICAL:

Usual therapeutic dose – Apply 2 daily ½ inch (7.5 mg) doses, 1 applied on rising in the morning and 1 applied 6 hours later. The dose can be doubled and even doubled again in patients tolerating this dose but failing to respond to it.

One inch (25 mm) of ointment contains approximately 15 mg nitroglycerin.

NITROGLYCERIN TRANSDERMAL SYSTEMS: Patient instructions for application are provided with products.

Apply once daily to a skin site free of hair and not subject to excessive movement. Do not apply to distal parts of extremities. Avoid areas with cuts/irritations.

Starting dose – 0.2 to 0.4 mg/h. Doses between 0.4 and 0.8 mg/h have shown continued effectiveness for 10 to 12 hours/day for at least 1 month of intermittent administration. Although the minimum nitrate-free interval has not been defined, data show that a nitrate-free interval of 10 to 12 hours is sufficient. Thus, an appropriate dosing schedule would include a daily "patch-on" period of 12 to 14 hours and a "patch-off" period of 10 to 12 hours. Tolerance is a major factor limiting efficacy when the system is used continuously for more than 12 hours each day.

NITROGLYCERIN, TRANSLINGUAL: At the onset of attack, spray 1 or 2 metered doses onto or under the tongue. No more than 3 metered doses are recommended within 15 minutes. May use prophylactically 5 to 10 minutes prior to activities which might precipitate an acute attack. Do not inhale spray.

Actions

Pharmacology: The principal pharmacological action of nitrates is relaxation of the vascular smooth muscle and consequent dilation of peripheral arteries and especially the veins. Dilation of the veins promotes peripheral pooling of blood and decreases venous return to the heart, thereby reducing left ventricular end-diastolic pressure and pulmonary capillary wedge pressure (preload). Arteriolar relaxation reduces systemic vascular resistance, systolic arterial pressure, and mean arterial pressure (afterload). Dilation of the coronary arteries also occurs. The relative importance of preload reduction, afterload reduction, and coronary dilation remains undefined.

Pharmacokinetics:

Doseform, Onset, and Duration of Available Nitrates

Nitrates	Dosage form	Onset (minutes)	Duration
Amyl nitrate	Inhalant	0.5	3 to 5 min
Nitroglycerin	IV	1 to 2	3 to 5 min
	Sublingual	1 to 3	30 to 60 min
	Translingual spray	2	30 to 60 min
	Transmucosal tablet	1 to 2	3 to 5 hours[a]
	Oral, sustained release	20 to 45	3 to 8 hours
	Topical ointment	30 to 60	2 to 12 hours[b]
	Transdermal	30 to 60	up to 24 hours[c]
Isosorbide dinitrate	Sublingual	2 to 5	1 to 3 hours
	Oral	20 to 40	4 to 6 hours
	Oral, sustained release	up to 4 hours	6 to 8 hours
Isosorbide mononitrate	Oral	30 to 60	nd[d]

[a] A significant antianginal effect can persist for 5 hours if the tablet has not completely dissolved.
[b] Depends on total amount used per unit of surface area.
[c] Tolerance may develop after 12 hours.
[d] nd = No data.

Contraindications

Amyl nitrite: Patients with glaucoma, recent head trauma, cerebral hemorrhage, and pregnancy.

Isosorbide dinitrate: Allergic reactions to isosorbide dinitrate or any of its ingredients.

Isosorbide mononitrate: Hypersensitivity or idiosyncratic reactions to other nitrates or nitrites.

Nitroglycerin: Allergic reactions to organic nitrates.

Patients who are using certain drugs for erectile dysfunction (eg, sildenafil citrate), because these drugs have been shown to potentiate the hypotensive effects of organic nitrates (sublingual tablets, lingual spray, transdermal).

Allergy to the adhesives used in the transdermal patches (transdermal).

Patients with early MI, severe anemia, increased intracranial pressure, known hypersensitivity to nitroglycerin (sublingual tablets).

Patients with pericardial tamponade, restrictive cardiomyopathy, constrictive pericarditis, solutions containing dextrose in patients with known allergy to corn or corn products (IV).

Warnings/Precautions

MI: In acute MI, use nitrates only under close clinical observation and with hemodynamic monitoring. In general, do not use a long-acting form because its effects are difficult to terminate rapidly if excessive hypotension or tachycardia develop.

Arcing: A cardioverter/defibrillator should not be discharged through a paddle electrode that overlies a transdermal nitroglycerin system.

Postural hypotension: Postural hypotension may occur, even with small doses.

Polyvinyl chloride (PVC) tubing: Because of the problem of nitroglycerin absorption by PVC tubing, use nitroglycerin IV with the least absorptive infusion tubing (ie, non-PVC tubing) available.

IV filters: Some in-line IV filters also absorb nitroglycerin; avoid these filters.

Hemolysis/Pseudoagglutination: Do not administer solutions containing dextrose without electrolytes through the same administration set as blood because this may result in pseudoagglutination or hemolysis.

Electrolyte concentrations: The IV administration of solutions may cause fluid overloading, resulting in dilution of serum electrolyte concentrations, overhydration, and congested states of pulmonary edema.

Flammability: Amyl nitrite is very flammable. Do not use where it would become ignited.

Angina: Nitrate therapy may aggravate angina caused by hypertrophic cardiomyopathy.

Tolerance: Use only the smallest dose required for effective relief of the acute anginal attack. Excessive use of sublingual nitroglycerin may lead to the development of tolerance.

Severe hypotension: Severe hypotension, particularly with upright posture, may occur with small doses of nitrates.

Withdrawal: Chest pain, acute MI, and even sudden death have occurred during temporary withdrawal of nitrates from industrial workers who have had long-term exposure to unknown doses of organic nitrates, demonstrating the existence of true physical dependence.

Nitrate-free interval: Several clinical trials of nitroglycerin in patients with angina pectoris have evaluated regimens that incorporated a 10- to 12-hour nitrate-free interval.

Fluid load: Lower concentrations of nitroglycerin IV and nitroglycerin in dextrose injection increase the potential precision of dosing, but these concentrations increase the total fluid volume that must be delivered to patients. Total fluid load may be a dominant consideration in patients with compromised function of the heart, liver, and/or kidneys.

Nitroglycerin infusions: Administer nitroglycerin IV and nitroglycerin in dextrose infusions only via an infusion pump that can maintain a constant infusion rate.

Diabetes mellitus: Use solutions containing dextrose with caution in patients with known subclinical or overt diabetes mellitus.

Discontinuation: Discontinue sublingual nitroglycerin if blurring of vision or drying of the mouth occurs. Excessive dosages of nitroglycerin may produce severe headaches.

Drug abuse and dependence: Volatile nitrites, including amyl nitrite, are abused for sexual stimulation, with headache as a common side effect.

Pregnancy: *Category* C (nitroglycerin, isosorbide dinitrate, isosorbide mononitrate [ie, *ISMO*], amyl nitrite); *Category B* (isosorbide mononitrate ER [ie, *Imdur*], isosorbide mononitrate [ie, *Monoket*]).

Lactation: It is not know whether nitrates are excreted in breast milk.

Children: Safety and efficacy for use in children have not been established.

Elderly: Clinical experience for organic nitrates reported in the literature identified a potential for severe hypotension and increased sensitivity to nitrates in the elderly. Nitrate therapy may aggravate the angina caused by hypertrophic cardiomyopathy, particularly in the elderly.

Use caution in dose selection for an elderly patient, usually starting at the low end of the dosing range, reflecting the greater frequency of decreased hepatic, renal, or cardiac function, and of concomitant disease or other drug therapy.

Drug Interactions

Drugs that may interact with nitrates include alcohol, alteplase, aspirin, beta-blockers, calcium channel blockers, dihydroergotamine, heparin, nondepolarizing muscle relaxants, phenothiazines, phosphodiesterase inhibitors (eg, sildenafil, tadalafil, vardenafil), and vasodilators.

Drug/Lab test interactions: Nitrates may interfere with the *Zlatkis-Zak* color reaction causing a false report of decreased serum cholesterol.

Drug/Food interactions: Concomitant food intake may decrease the rate (increase in T_{max}) but not the extent (AUC) of absorption of isosorbide mononitrate.

Adverse Reactions

Amyl nitrite: Mild transitory headache, dizziness, and flushing of the face. The following adverse reactions may occur in susceptible patients: cold sweat, hypotension, involuntary passing of urine and feces, nausea, pallor, restlessness, syncope, tachycardia, vomiting, weakness.

Isosorbide mononitrate tablets:

Cardiovascular – Cardiovascular disorder, chest pain.

CNS – Dizziness, emotional lability, fatigue, headache.

Dermatologic – Pruritus, rash.

GI – Abdominal pain, diarrhea, nausea, vomiting.

Respiratory – Increased cough, upper respiratory tract infection.

Miscellaneous – Allergic reaction, flushing, pain.

Isosorbide mononitrate ER tablets:

Cardiovascular – Angina pectoris aggravated, arrhythmia, arrhythmia atrial, atrial fibrillation, bradycardia, bundle branch block, cardiac failure, extrasystole, heart murmur, heart sound abnormal, hypertension, hypotension, MI, palpitation, Q-wave abnormality, tachycardia, ventricular tachycardia (5% or less).

CNS – Dizziness, headache.

Dermatologic – Acne, hair texture abnormal, increased sweating, pruritus, rash, skin nodule.

GI – Abdominal pain, constipation, diarrhea, dry mouth, dyspepsia, flatulence, gastric ulcer, gastritis, glossitis, hemorrhagic gastric ulcer, hemorrhoids, loose stools, melena, nausea, vomiting.

GU – Atrophic vaginitis, breast pain, impotence, polyuria, renal calculus, urinary tract infection.

Hematologic – Hypochromic anemia, purpura, thrombocytopenia.

Hepatic – ALT increase, AST increase.

Metabolic/Nutritional – Edema, hyperuricemia, hypokalemia.

Musculoskeletal – Arthralgia, frozen shoulder, muscle weakness, musculoskeletal pain, myalgia, myositis, tendon disorder, torticollis.

Respiratory – Bronchitis, bronchospasm, coughing, dyspnea, increased sputum, nasal congestion, pharyngitis, pneumonia, pulmonary infiltration, rales, rhinitis, sinusitis.

Special senses – Conjunctivitis, earache, photophobia, tinnitus, tympanic membrane perforation, vision abnormal.

Miscellaneous – Asthenia, back pain, bacterial infection, chest pain, fever, flu-like symptoms, flushing, hot flushes, intermittent claudication, leg ulcer, malaise, moniliasis, ptosis, rigors, varicose vein, viral infection.

Nitroglycerin lingual spray: Headache, hypotension.

More than 2% – Dizziness, headache, paresthesia.

Nitroglycerin sublingual: Dizziness, headache, palpitation, vertigo, weakness.

Nitroglycerin ointment, transdermal, IV, ER capsules, and isosorbide dinitrate: Headache.

The most frequent adverse reactions with transdermal nitroglycerin were as follows: headache (63%); light-headedness (6%); hypotension and/or syncope (4%); increased angina (2%).

ANTIARRHYTHMIC AGENTS

Optimal therapy of cardiac arrhythmias requires documentation, accurate diagnosis, and modification of precipitating causes, and if indicated, proper selection and use of antiarrhythmic drugs. These drugs are classified according to their effects on the action potential of cardiac cells and their presumed mechanism of action.

Class I: Local anesthetics or membrane-stabilizing agents that depress phase 0.

IA *(quinidine, procainamide, disopyramide)* – Depress phase 0 and prolong the action potential duration.

IB *(tocainide, lidocaine, phenytoin, mexiletine)* – Depress phase 0 slightly and may shorten the action potential duration. Although arrhythmia is not a labeled indication for phenytoin, it is commonly used in treatment of digitalis-induced arrhythmias.

IC *(flecainide, encainide, propafenone)* – Marked depression of phase 0. Slight effect on repolarization. Profound slowing of conduction. Encainide was voluntarily withdrawn from the market, but is still available on a limited basis.

Moricizine – Moricizine is a Class I agent that shares some of the characteristics of the Class IA, B, and C agents.

Class II *(propranolol, esmolol, acebutolol):* Depress phase 4 depolarization.

Class III *(bretylium, amiodarone):* Produce a prolongation of phase 3 (repolarization).

Class IV *(verapamil):* Depress phase 4 depolarization and lengthen phases 1 and 2 of repolarization.

Sotalol: Sotalol has both Class II (beta blocking) and III properties; Class III effects are seen at doses greater than 160 mg.

Digitalis glycosides (digoxin): Digitalis glycosides (digoxin) cause a decrease in maximal diastolic potential and action potential duration and increase the slope of phase 4 depolarization.

Adenosine: Adenosine slows conduction time through the AV node and can interrupt the reentry pathways through the AV node.

Serum drug levels: Some antiarrhythmic drugs (eg, quinidine) can produce toxic effects that can be easily confused with the symptoms for which the drug has been prescribed. Drug serum levels are important in evaluating toxic or subtherapeutic dosage regimens of most of the antiarrhythmic drugs.

Proarrhythmic effects: Antiarrhythmic agents may cause new or worsened arrhythmias. It is essential that each patient be evaluated electrocardiographically and clinically prior to and during therapy to determine whether the response to the drug supports continued treatment.

Antiarrhythmic Electrophysiology/Electrocardiogram Effects

Anti-arrhythmic		Electrophysiology[a]										ECG changes[a]				
		Automaticity		Conduction velocity			Refractory period									
Group	Drug	SA node	Ectopic pacemaker	Atrium	AV node	His-Purkinje	Atrium	AV node	His-Purkinje	Ventricle	Accessory pathways[b]	Heart rate	PR interval	QRS complex	QT_c interval	JT interval
I	Moricizine[c]	0	↓	0	↓	↓	±	0	0	0-↑	↑	0-↑	↑	↑	0	↓
	Quinidine	±	↓	↓	±	↓	↑↑	0-↑[d]	↑↑	↑	↑	±	±	↑	↑	↑
	Procainamide	±	↓	↓	±	↓	↑	0-↑[d]	↑↑	↑	↑↑	±	±	↑	↑	↑
	Disopyramide	±	↓	↓	±	↓	↑↑	0-↑[d]	↑↑	↑	↑	±	±	↑	↑	↑
	Lidocaine	0	↓	—	0	0	0	±	±	±	↑-↓	0	0	0	0-↓	0
	Phenytoin	↓-0	↓	—	0	0	0	±	±	±	—	±	0-↓	0	↓	0
	Tocainide	0-↓	↓	0	0	0	↓	↓	±	↓	↑	0	0	0	0-↓	0
	Mexiletine	↓	↓	0	0	0	0	±	↑	↑	↑	—	0	0	0	0
	Flecainide	↓	↓	↓↓	↓	↓↓	0	0	↑	↑	↑↑	0	↑[e]	↑↑[e]	0-↑[e]	0
	Propafenone	0	↓	0	↓	↓	0	↑	↑	↑	↑	0	↑[e]	↑	0-↑[e]	0
II	Propranolol	↓	↓	±	↓	0-↓	±	↑	0	0	0-↑	↓	0-↑	0	0-↓	0
	Esmolol	↓	↓	±	↓	0-	±	↑	0	0	0-↑	↓	0-↑	0	0-↓	0
	Acebutolol	↓	↓	±	↓	0	±	↑	0	0	0-↑	↓	0-↑	0	0-↓	0
III	Bretylium	↑	↑	0	0	0-↑	0	↓-0-↑[g]	↑	0-↑	±	0	0	0	0	↑
	Amiodarone	↓	↓	↓	↓	↓	↑	↑	↑	↑	↑	↓	↑	↑	↑↑	↑↑
	Sotalol[h]	↓	↓	0	↓	0	↑↑	↑	↑↑	↑↑	↑	↓	↑	0	↑↑	↑↑
IV	Verapamil	↓	↓	0	↓	0	0	↑	0	0	0	↓	↑	0	0	0
—	Digoxin	0-↓	↑	±	↓	0-↓	±	↑	0	↓	↓-↑	↓	↑	0	↓	↓
—	Adenosine	↓	↓	0	↓	0	0	↑	0	0	0	↑	↑	0	0	—

[a] These values assume therapeutic levels.
[b] Accessory pathways occur in Wolff-Parkinson-White syndrome (preexcitation phenomena) and possibly other abnormal conditions.
[c] Does not belong to any of the 3 subclasses (A, B or C), but does have some properties of each.
[d] Retrograde AV node RP↑; antegrade RP not affected.
[e] Dose-related increases.
[f] Withdrawn from the market; however, available on a limited basis.
[g] Due to a complex balance of direct and indirect autonomic effects.
[h] Has both Class II (beta-blocking) and III properties; Class III effects are seen at doses greater than 160 mg.

Antiarrhythmic Pharmacokinetics

Group	Drug	Onset (h) (oral)[a]	Duration (h)	Half-life (h)	Protein binding (%)	Excreted unchanged (%)	Therapeutic serum level (mcg/mL)	Toxic serum levels (mcg/mL)
I A	Moricizine	2	10-24	1.5-3.5[b]	95	< 1	Not applicable	—
	Quinidine	0.5	6-8	6-7	80-90	10-50	2-6	> 8
	Procainamide	0.5	3+	2.5-4.7	14-23	40-70	4-8	> 16
	Disopyramide	0.5	6-7	4-10	20-60[c]	40-60	2-8	> 9
B	Lidocaine	—	0.25[d]	1-2	40-80	< 3	1.5-6	> 7
	Phenytoin	0.5-1	24+	22-36[e]	87-93	< 5	10-20	> 20
	Tocainide	—	—	11-15	10-20	28-55	4-10	> 10
	Mexiletine	—	—	10-12	50-60	10	0.5-2	> 2
C	Flecainide	—	—	12-27	40	30	0.2-1	> 1
	Propafenone	—	—	2-10[j]	97	< 1	0.06-1	—
II	Propranolol	0.5	3-5	2-3	90-95	< 1	0.05-0.1	—
	Esmolol	< 5 min	very short	0.15	55	< 2	—	—
	Acebutolol	—	24-30	3-4	26	15-20	—	—
III	Bretylium	—	6-8	5-10	0-8	> 80	0.5-1.5	—
	Amiodarone	1-3 wk[k]	weeks to months	26-107 days	96	negli-gible	0.5-2.5	> 2.5
	Sotalol	—	—	12	0	100	—	—
IV	Verapamil	0.5	6	3-7	90	3-4	0.08-0.3	—
—	Digoxin	0.5-2	24+	30-40	20-25	60	0.5-2 ng/mL	> 2.5 ng/mL
—	Adenosine	(34 sec IV)	1-2 min	< 10 sec	—	0 (enters body pool)	Not applicable	—

[a] Within 1 to 5 minutes with IV use.
[b] Half-life may be prolonged in patients after multiple dosing.
[c] Protein binding is concentration-dependent.
[d] Very short after discontinuation of IV infusion.
[e] Half-life increases with increasing dosage.
[f] Withdrawn from the market; however, available on a limited basis.
[g] Half-life 6 to 11 hours in less than 10% of patients (poor metabolizers).
[h] More than 50% in poor metabolizers.
[i] MODE (3-methoxy-O-demethyl encainide) and ODE (O-demethyl encainide), metabolites more active than encainide on a per mg basis.
[j] Half-life 10 to 32 hours in less than 10% of patients (slow metabolizers).
[k] Onset of action may occur in 2 to 3 days.

DRONEDARONE

Tablets; oral: 400 mg (*Rx*)	*Multaq* (Sanofi-Aventis)

Warning:

Dronedarone is contraindicated in patients with New York Heart Association (NYHA) class IV heart failure or NYHA class II to III heart failure with a recent decompensation requiring hospitalization or referral to a specialized heart failure clinic.

In a placebo-controlled study in patients with severe heart failure requiring recent hospitalization or referral to a specialized heart failure clinic for worsening symptoms (the ANDROMEDA study), patients given dronedarone had a greater than 2-fold increase in mortality. Do not give such patients dronedarone.

Indications

Paroxysmal or persistent atrial fibrillation or paroxysmal or persistent atrial flutter: To reduce the risk of cardiovascular hospitalization in patients with paroxysmal or persistent atrial fibrillation or paroxysmal or persistent atrial flutter, with a recent episode of atrial fibrillation/atrial flutter and associated cardiovascular risk factors (ie, older than 70 years of age, hypertension, diabetes, prior cerebrovascular accident, left atrial diameter 50 mm or more or left ventricular ejection fraction [LVEF] less than 40%), who are in sinus rhythm or who will be cardioverted.

Administration and Dosage

Treatment with class I or III antiarrhythmics (eg, amiodarone, flecainide, propafenone, quinidine, disopyramide, dofetilide, sotalol) or drugs that are strong inhibitors of CYP3A4 (eg, ketoconazole) must be stopped before taking dronedarone.

Adults: 400 mg orally twice daily with morning and evening meals.

Actions

Pharmacology: Dronedarone has antiarrhythmic properties belonging to all 4 Vaughan-Williams classes, but the contribution of each of these activities to the clinical effect is unknown.

Pharmacokinetics:

Absorption – After oral administration, peak plasma concentrations of dronedarone and the main active metabolite are reached within 3 to 6 hours; steady state is reached within 4 to 8 days of treatment.

Effect of food: The bioavailability of dronedarone is increased by meals. It increases to approximately 15% when dronedarone is administered with a high-fat meal.

Distribution – The plasma protein binding of dronedarone is greater than 98%.

Metabolism – Dronedarone is extensively metabolized, mainly by CYP3A.

Excretion – Approximately 6% of the labeled dose was excreted in urine and 84% was excreted in feces. The elimination half-life of dronedarone ranges from 13 to 19 hours.

Contraindications

NYHA class IV heart failure or NYHA class II to III heart failure with a recent decompensation requiring hospitalization or referral to a specialized heart failure clinic; second- or third-degree atrioventricular (AV) block or sick sinus syndrome (except when used in conjunction with a functioning pacemaker); bradycardia less than 50 bpm; concomitant use of strong CYP3A inhibitors, such as ketoconazole, itraconazole, voriconazole, cyclosporine, telithromycin, clarithromycin, nefazodone, and ritonavir; concomitant use of drugs or herbal products that prolong the QT interval and might increase the risk of torsades de pointes, such as phenothiazine antipsychotics, tricyclic antidepressants, certain oral macrolide antibiotics, and class I and III antiarrhythmics; QTc Bazett interval 500 ms or more or PR interval more than 280 ms; severe hepatic impairment; pregnancy; breast-feeding mothers.

Warnings/Precautions

Heart failure: Advise patients to consult a health care provider if they develop signs or symptoms of heart failure, such as weight gain, dependent edema, or increasing shortness of breath. If heart failure develops or worsens, consider the suspension or discontinuation of dronedarone.

Concomitant use with potassium-depleting diuretics: Potassium levels should be within the normal range prior to administration of dronedarone and maintained in the normal range during administration of dronedarone.

QT interval prolongation: Dronedarone induces a moderate (average of about 10 ms, but much greater effects have been observed) QTc (Bazett) prolongation. If the QTc Bazett interval is 500 ms or more, stop dronedarone.

Renal effects: Serum creatinine levels increase by about 0.1 mg/dL following treatment initiation. The elevation has a rapid onset, reaches a plateau after 7 days, and is reversible after discontinuation. Use this increased value as the patient's new baseline.

Women of childbearing potential: Premenopausal women who have not undergone a hysterectomy or oophorectomy must use effective contraception while using dronedarone. Dronedarone caused fetal harm in animal studies at doses equivalent to recommended human doses.

Hepatic function impairment: Dronedarone is contraindicated in severe hepatic impairment.

Pregnancy: Category X.

Lactation: Dronedarone is contraindicated in breast-feeding women.

Children: Safety and efficacy in children younger than 18 years of age have not been established.

Drug Interactions

Drugs that may affect dronedarone include beta-blockers, calcium channel blockers, class I and III antiarrhythmics, CYP3A4 inducers, CYP3A4 inhibitors, phenothiazine antipsychotics, tricyclic antidepressants, and P-glycoprotein substrates.

Drugs that may be affected by dronedarone include beta-blockers, calcium channel blockers, tricyclic antidepressants, CYP2D6 and 3A substrates, P-glycoprotein substrates, simvastatin, warfarin.

Drug/Food interactions: Instruct patients to avoid grapefruit beverages while taking dronedarone.

Adverse Reactions

Adverse reactions occurring in 3% or more of patients include abdominal pain, diarrhea, nausea, asthenic conditions, bradycardia, serum creatinine increased at least 10% five days after treatment initiation, skin and subcutaneous tissue reactions (eg, generalized, macular, maculopapular, and erythematous rash; pruritus; eczema; dermatitis; allergic dermatitis), QTc Bazett prolonged (longer than 450 ms in men, longer than 470 ms in women).

QUINIDINE

QUINIDINE SULFATE	
Tablets: 200 and 300 mg (*Rx*)	Various, *Quinora* (Key Pharm)
Tablets, sustained-release: 300 mg (*Rx*)	Various
QUINIDINE GLUCONATE	
Tablets, sustained-release: 324 mg (*Rx*)	Various
Injection: 80 mg/mL (*Rx*)	Various

Indications

Oral: Premature atrial, AV junctional and ventricular contractions; paroxysmal atrial (supraventricular) tachycardia; paroxysmal AV junctional rhythm; atrial flutter; paroxysmal and chronic atrial fibrillation; established atrial fibrillation when therapy is appropriate; paroxysmal ventricular tachycardia not associated with complete heart block; maintenance therapy after electrical conversion of atrial fibrillation or flutter.

Parenteral: When oral therapy is not feasible or when rapid therapeutic effect is required.

Quinidine gluconate – Life-threatening *Plasmodium falciparum* malaria.

Administration and Dosage

Test dose: Administer a single 200 mg tablet of quinidine sulfate or 200 mg IM quinidine gluconate to determine whether the patient has an idiosyncratic reaction.

Adjust the dosage to maintain plasma concentration between 2 to 6 mcg/mL.

Oral:

Premature atrial and ventricular contractions – 200 to 300 mg 3 or 4 times/day.

Paroxysmal supraventricular tachycardias – 400 to 600 mg every 2 or 3 hours until the paroxysm is terminated.

Atrial flutter – Administer quinidine after digitalization. Individualize dosage.

Conversion of atrial fibrillation – 200 mg every 2 or 3 hours for 5 to 8 doses, with subsequent daily increases until sinus rhythm is restored or toxic effects occur. Do not exceed a total daily dose of 3 to 4 g in any regimen.

Maintenance therapy – 200 to 300 mg 3 or 4 times/day. Other patients may require larger doses or more frequent administration than the usually recommended schedule.

Sustained-release forms – 300 to 600 mg every 8 or 12 hours.

Parenteral:

IM – In the treatment of acute tachycardia, the initial dose is 600 mg quinidine gluconate. Subsequently, 400 mg quinidine gluconate can be repeated as often as every 2 hours.

IV – In approximately 50% of patients who respond successfully to quinidine, the arrhythmia can be terminated by 330 mg quinidine gluconate or less (or its equivalent in other salts); as much as 500 to 750 mg may be required. Inject slowly.

QUINIDINE GLUCONATE – *P. falciparum malaria* – The following 2 regimens are effective empirically. As soon as practical, institute standard oral antiplasmodial therapy.

1.) Loading: 15 mg/kg in 250 mL normal saline infused over 4 hours followed by; Maintenance: beginning 24 hours after the beginning of the loading dose, 7.5 mg/kg infused over 4 hours, every 8 hours for 7 days or until oral therapy can be instituted.
2.) Loading: 10 mg/kg in 250 mL normal saline infused over 1 to 2 hours, followed immediately by; Maintenance: 0.02 mg/kg/min for up to 72 hours or until parasitemia decreases to less than 1% or oral therapy can be instituted.

Children:

Oral (quinidine sulfate) – 30 mg/kg/day or 900 mg/m^2/day in 5 divided doses.

IV (quinidine gluconate) – 2 to 10 mg/kg/dose every 3 to 6 hours as needed; however, this route is not recommended.

Actions

Pharmacology: Quinidine, a class IA antiarrhythmic, depresses myocardial excitability, conduction velocity and contractility.

Pharmacokinetics:

Absorption/Distribution –

Anhydrous Quinidine Alkaloid Content in Various Salts

Quinidine salts	Quinidine content		Time to peak plasma levels (hours)
	Active drug	Absorbed	
Quinidine sulfate	83%	73%	1 to 3[a]
Quinidine gluconate	62%	70%	3-5

[a] 3 to 5 hours for sustained release form.

Quinidine is rapidly absorbed from the GI tract. Maximum effects of quinidine gluconate occur 30 to 90 minutes after IM administration; onset is more rapid after IV administration. Activity persists for at least 6 to 8 hours. The average therapeutic serum levels are reported to be 2 to 7 mcg/mL. Toxic reactions may occur at levels from 5 to 8 mcg/mL or more. Quinidine is 80% to 90% bound to plasma proteins; the unbound fraction may be significantly increased in patients with hepatic insufficiency.

Metabolism/Excretion – From 60% to 80% of a dose is metabolized via the liver into several metabolites. Quinidine is excreted unchanged (10% to 50%) in the urine within 24 hours. The elimination half-life ranges from 4 to 10 hours in healthy patients, with a mean of 6 to 7 hours. Urinary acidification facilitates quinidine elimination, and alkalinization retards it. In patients with cirrhosis, the elimination half-life may be prolonged and the volume of distribution increased.

Contraindications

Hypersensitivity or idiosyncrasy to quinidine or other cinchona derivatives manifested by thrombocytopenia, skin eruption or febrile reactions; myasthenia gravis; history of thrombocytopenic purpura associated with quinidine administration; digitalis intoxication manifested by arrhythmias or AV conduction disorders; complete heart block; left bundle branch block or other severe intraventricular conduction defects exhibiting marked QRS widening or bizarre complexes; complete AV block with an AV nodal or idioventricular pacemaker; aberrant ectopic impulses and abnormal rhythms due to escape mechanisms; history of drug-induced torsade de pointes; history of long QT syndrome.

Warnings/Precautions

Hepatotoxicity: Hepatotoxicity (including granulomatous hepatitis) due to quinidine hypersensitivity has occurred.

Atrial flutter or fibrillation: Reversion to sinus rhythm may be preceded by a progressive reduction in degree of AV block to a 1:1 ratio, which results in an extremely rapid ventricular rate. Prior to use in atrial flutter, pretreat with digitalis preparation.

Cardiotoxicity: Cardiotoxicity (eg, increased PR and QT intervals, 50% widening of QRS complex, ventricular tachyarrhythmias, frequent ventricular ectopic beats, or tachycardia) dictates immediate discontinuation of quinidine; closely monitor the ECG.

Large oral doses may reduce the arterial pressure by means of peripheral vasodilation. Serious hypotension is more likely with parenteral use.

Use quinidine with extreme caution in incomplete AV block, because complete block and asystole may result. The drug may cause unpredictable dysrhythmias in digitalized patients. Use cautiously in patients with partial bundle branch block, severe CHF, and hypotensive states due to the depressant effects of quinidine on myocardial contractility and arterial pressure.

Parenteral therapy: The dangers of parenteral use of quinidine are increased in the presence of AV block or absence of atrial activity. Administration is more hazardous in patients with extensive myocardial damage. Use of quinidine in digitalis-induced cardiac arrhythmia is extremely dangerous because the cardiac glycoside may already have caused serious impairment of intracardiac conduction system. Too rapid IV administration of as little as 200 mg may precipitate a fall of 40 to 50 mm Hg in arterial pressure.

Syncope: Syncope occasionally occurs in patients on long-term quinidine therapy, usually resulting from ventricular tachycardia or fibrillation.

Renal, hepatic, or cardiac insufficiency: Use with caution in renal, cardiac, or hepatic insufficiency because of potential toxicity.

Potassium balance: The effect of quinidine is enhanced by potassium and reduced if hypokalemia is present. The risk of drug-induced torsade de pointes is increased by concomitant hypokalemia.

Hypersensitivity reactions: Asthma, muscle weakness, and infection with fever prior to quinidine administration may mask hypersensitivity reactions to the drug.

Pregnancy: Category C.

Lactation: Quinidine is excreted into breast milk with a milk:serum ratio of approximately 0.71. The American Academy of Pediatrics considers quinidine to be compatible with breast-feeding.

Children: Safety and efficacy have not been established.

Monitoring: Perform periodic blood counts and liver and kidney function tests. Discontinue use if blood dyscrasias or signs of hepatic or renal disorders occur. Frequently measure arterial blood pressure during IV use.

Drug Interactions

Drugs that may affect quinidine include amiodarone, antacids, barbiturates, cholinergic drugs, cimetidine, disopyramide, hydantoins, nifedipine, rifampin, sucralfate, urinary alkalinizers and verapamil. Drugs that may be affected by quinidine include anticholinergics, anticoagulants, beta-blockers, cardiac glycosides, disopyramide, nondepolarizing neuromuscular blockers, procainamide, propafenone, succinylcholine, and tricyclic antidepressants.

Drug/Lab test interactions: Triamterene and quinidine have similar fluorescence spectra; thus, triamterene will interfere with the fluorescent measurement of quinidine serum levels.

Adverse Reactions

Adverse reactions may include nausea, vomiting, abdominal pain, diarrhea, anorexia; cinchonism (ringing in the ears, hearing loss, headache, nausea, dizziness, vertigo, light-headedness, disturbed vision); headache; fever; vertigo; apprehension; excitement; confusion; delirium; dementia; depression; acute hemolytic anemia; hypoprothrombinemia; thrombocytopenic purpura; agranulocytosis; thrombocytopenia; leukocytosis; mydriasis; blurred vision; disturbed color perception; reduced vision field; night blindness, photophobia; rash; urticaria; cutaneous flushing with intense pruritus; photosensitivity; eczema; psoriasis; abnormalities of pigmentation; arthralgia; myalgia; disturbed hearing; lupus erythematosus; hepatitis; cardiac asystole; ventricular ectopy; idioventricular rhythms; paradoxical tachycardia; arterial embolism; hypotension; ventricular extrasystoles; complete AV block; ventricular flutter.

PROCAINAMIDE

Tablets: 375 and 500 mg (*Rx*)	*Pronestyl* (Apothecon)
Tablets, sustained-release: 250, 500, and 1,000 mg (*Rx*)	Various
Capsules: 250 and 375 mg (*Rx*)	Various
Injection: 100 and 500 mg/mL (*Rx*)	Various

Warning:

The prolonged administration often leads to the development of a positive antinuclear antibody (ANA) test, with or without symptoms of a lupus erythematosus-like syndrome. If a positive ANA titer develops, assess the benefit/risk ratio related to continued procainamide therapy.

Mortality: In the National Heart, Lung, and Blood Institute's Cardiac Arrhythmia Suppression Trial (CAST), a long-term, multicentered, randomized, double-blind study in patients with asymptomatic nonlife-threatening ventricular arrhythmias who had an MI more than 6 days but less than 2 years previously, an excessive mortality or nonfatal cardiac arrest rate was seen in patients treated with encainide or flecainide (7.7%) compared with that seen in patients assigned to matched placebo-treated groups (3%). The averaged duration of treatment with encainide or flecainide in this study was 10 months.

The applicability of these results to other populations (eg, those without recent MIs) is uncertain. Considering the known proarrhythmic properties of procainamide and the lack of evidence of improved survival for any antiarrhythmic drug in patients without life-threatening arrhythmias, the use of procainamide and other antiarrhythmic agents should be reserved for patients with life-threatening ventricular arrhythmias.

Blood dyscrasias: Agranulocytosis, bone marrow depression, neutropenia, hypoplastic anemia, and thrombocytopenia in patients receiving procainamide have been reported at a rate of approximately 0.5%. Most of these patients received procainamide within the recommended dosage range. Fatalities have occurred (with approximately 20% to 25% mortality in reported cases of agranulocytosis). Because most of these events have been noted during the first 12 weeks of therapy, it is recommended that complete blood counts (CBC), including white cell, differential, and platelet counts be performed at weekly intervals for the first 3 months of therapy, and periodically thereafter. Perform CBC promptly if the patient develops any signs of infection (eg, fever, chills, sore throat, stomatitis), bruising, or bleeding. If any of these hematologic disorders are identified, discontinue therapy. Blood counts usually return to normal within 1 month of discontinuation. Use caution in patients with preexisting marrow failure or cytopenia of any type.

Indications

Treatment of documented ventricular arrhythmias, such as sustained ventricular tachycardia, that are judged to be life-threatening. Because of the proarrhythmic effects, use with lesser arrhythmias is generally not recommended.

Because procainamide has the potential to produce serious hematologic disorders (0.5%), particularly leukopenia or agranulocytosis (sometimes fatal), reserve its use for patients in whom the benefits of treatment clearly outweigh the risks.

Avoid treatment of patients with asymptomatic ventricular premature depolarizations.

Unlabeled uses:

Atrial fibrillation/flutter – Procainamide has been used to convert atrial fibrillation/flutter to sinus rhythm.

For the treatment of hemodynamically stable ventricular tachycardia in children, procainamide (loading dose of 15 mg/kg IV infused over 30 to 60 minutes) may be considered as an alternative agent to amiodarone.

Administration and Dosage

Oral: Oral dosage forms are preferable for less urgent arrhythmias as well as for long-term maintenance after initial parenteral therapy. Individualize dosage based on clinical assessment of the degree of underlying myocardial disease, the patient's age and renal function.

As a general guide, for younger adult patients with normal renal function, an initial total daily oral dose of 50 mg/kg or less may be used, given in divided doses every 3 hours, to maintain therapeutic blood levels. For older patients, especially those older than 50 years of age, or for patients with renal, hepatic, or cardiac insufficiency, lesser amounts or longer intervals may produce adequate blood levels and decrease the probability of occurrence of dose-related adverse reactions. Administer the total daily dose in divided doses at 3-, 4-, or 6-hour intervals and adjust according to the patient's response.

Guidelines to Provide up to 50 mg/kg/day Procainamide

Weight		Dose every 3 hours (standard formulation)	Dose every 6 hours (standard formulation and sustained release)	Dose every 12 hours (*Procanbid* sustained release tablets only)
lb	kg			
88-110	40-50	250 mg	500 mg	1 g
132-154	60-70	375 mg	750 mg	1.5 g
176-198	80-90	500 mg	1 g	2 g
> 220	> 100	625 mg	1.25 g	2.5 g

Sustained-release products are not recommended for initial therapy. Total dosage (50 mg/kg/day) may be given in divided doses every 6 hours.

Parenteral: Useful for arrhythmias that require immediate suppression and for maintenance of arrhythmia control. IV therapy allows most rapid control of serious arrhythmias, including those following MI; use in circumstances where close observation and monitoring of the patient are possible, such as in hospital or emergency facilities. IM administration is less apt to produce temporary high plasma levels but therapeutic plasma levels are not obtained as rapidly as with IV administration.

IM administration – IM administration may be used as an alternative to the oral route for patients with less threatening arrhythmias but who are nauseated or vomiting, who are ordered to receive nothing by mouth preoperatively, or who may have malabsorptive problems. An initial daily dose of 50 mg/kg may be estimated. Divide this amount into fractional doses of ⅛ to ¼ to be injected IM every 3 to 6 hours until oral therapy is possible. If more than 3 injections are given, assess patient factors such as age and renal function, clinical response and, if available, blood levels of procainamide and NAPA in adjusting further doses for that individual. For treatment of arrhythmias associated with anesthesia or surgery, the suggested dose is 100 to 500 mg by IM injection.

IV –

Dilutions and Rates for IV Infusions of Procainamide

Infusion	Final concentration	Infusion volume[a]	Procainamide to be added	Infusion rate
Initial loading infusion	20 mg/mL	50 mL	1,000 mg	1 mL/min (for up to 25 to 30 min)
Maintenance infusion[b]	2 mg/mL	500 mL	1,000 mg	1 to 3 mL/min
	or			
	4 mg/mL	250 mL	1,000 mg	0.5 to 1.5 mL/min

[a] All infusions should be made up to final volume with 5% dextrose injection, USP.

[b] The maintenance infusion rates are calculated to deliver 2 to 6 mg/min depending on body weight, renal elimination rate and steady-state plasma level needed to maintain control of the arrhythmia. The 4 mg/mL maintenance concentration may be preferred if total infused volume must be limited.

Cautiously administer the IV injection to avoid a possible hypotensive response. Initial arrhythmia control, under blood pressure and ECG monitoring, may usually be accomplished safely within 30 minutes by either of the 2 methods that follow:

1) Slowly direct injection into a vein or into tubing of an established infusion line at a rate not to exceed 50 mg/min. It is advisable to dilute the 500 mg/mL concentrations prior to IV injection to facilitate control of dosage rate. Doses of 100 mg may be administered every 5 minutes at this rate until the arrhythmia is suppressed or until 500 mg has been administered, after which it is advisable to wait 10 minutes or longer to allow for more distribution into tissues before resuming.

2) Alternatively, a loading infusion containing 20 mg/mL (1 g diluted to 50 mL with 5% dextrose injection, USP) may be administered at a constant rate of 1 mL/min for 25 to 30 minutes to deliver 500 to 600 mg. Some effects may be seen after infusion of the first 100 or 200 mg; it is unusual to require more than 600 mg to achieve satisfactory antiarrhythmic effects.

The maximum advisable dosage to be given either by repeated bolus injections or such loading infusion is 1 g.

To maintain therapeutic levels, a more dilute IV infusion at a concentration of 2 mg/mL is convenient (1 g in 500 mL 5% dextrose injection), and may be administered at 1 to 3 mL/min. If daily total fluid intake must be limited, a 4 mg/mL concentration (1 g in 250 mL of 5% dextrose injection) administered at 0.5 to 1.5 mL/min will deliver an equivalent 2 to 6 mg/min. Assess the amount needed in a given patient to maintain the therapeutic level principally from the clinical response. Adjust based on close observation. A maintenance infusion rate of 50 mcg/kg/min to a person with a normal renal procainamide elimination half-life of 3 hours should produce a plasma level of about 6.5 mcg/mL.

Terminate IV therapy if persistent conduction disturbances or hypotension develop. As soon as the patient's basic cardiac rhythm appears to be stabilized, oral antiarrhythmic maintenance therapy is preferable (if indicated and possible). A period of approximately 3 to 4 hours (one half-life for renal elimination, ordinarily) should elapse after the last IV dose before administering the first dose of oral procainamide.

Children: The following doses have been suggested.

Oral – 15 to 50 mg/kg/day divided every 3 to 6 hours; maximum 4 g/day.

IM – 20 to 30 mg/kg/day.

IV – Loading dose: 3 to 6 mg/kg/dose over 5 minutes. Maintenance: 20 to 80 mcg/kg/min continuous infusion. Maximum 100 mg/dose or 2 g/day.

Actions

Pharmacology: Procainamide, a class IA antiarrhythmic, increases the effective refractory period of the atria, and to a lesser extent the bundle of His-Purkinje system and ventricles of the heart.

Electrophysiology – The ECG may show slight sinus tachycardia and widened QRS complexes and, less regularly, prolonged QT and PR intervals, as well as some decrease in QRS and T-wave amplitude.

Pharmacokinetics:

Absorption/Distribution – Oral procainamide is resistant to digestive hydrolysis, and the drug is well absorbed from the entire small intestinal surface, but individual patients vary in their completeness of absorption. Following oral use, plasma levels peak at approximately 45 to 120 minutes. Following IM injection, plasma levels peak in 15 to 60 minutes. IV use can produce therapeutic plasma levels within minutes. About 15% to 20% is reversibly bound to plasma proteins. The apparent volume of distribution eventually reaches approximately 2 L/kg with a half-life of approximately 5 minutes.

Metabolism/Excretion – A significant fraction of the circulating procainamide may be metabolized in hepatocytes to N-acetylprocainamide (NAPA), ranging from 16% to 33% of an administered dose. NAPA also has significant antiarrhythmic activity and somewhat slower renal clearance than procainamide. The elimination half-life of procainamide is 3 to 4 hours in patients with normal renal function, but reduced creatinine clearance (Ccr) and advancing age each prolong the elimination half-life. Half-life and renal clearance are also reduced in infants. Thirty percent to 60% of the drug is excreted as unchanged procainamide, and 6% to 52% as the NAPA derivative. Both procainamide and NAPA are eliminated by active tubular secretion as well as by glomerular filtration.

Contraindications

Complete heart block; idiosyncratic hypersensitivity; lupus erythematosus; torsades de pointes.

Warnings/Precautions

Blood dyscrasias: Agranulocytosis, bone marrow depression, neutropenia, hypoplastic anemia and thrombocytopenia in patients receiving procainamide have been reported at a rate of approximately 0.5%. Fatalities have occurred (with approximately 20% to 25% mortality in reported cases of agranulocytosis). Perform complete blood counts including white cell, differential, and platelet counts at weekly intervals for the first 3 months of therapy, and periodically thereafter. Perform complete blood counts promptly if the patient develops any signs of infection (eg, fever, chills, sore throat, stomatitis), bruising, or bleeding. If any of these hematologic disorders are identified, discontinue therapy. Blood counts usually return to normal within 1 month of discontinuation. Use caution in patients with preexisting marrow failure or cytopenia of any type.

Mortality: Considering the known proarrhythmic properties of procainamide and the lack of evidence of improved survival for any antiarrhythmic drug in patients without life-threatening arrhythmias, reserve the use of procainamide and other antiarrhythmic agents for patients with life-threatening ventricular arrhythmias.

Complete heart block: Do not administer to patients with complete heart block because of its effects in suppressing nodal or ventricular pacemakers and the hazard of asystole. If significant slowing of ventricular rate occurs during treatment without evidence of AV conduction appearing, stop procainamide. In cases of second-degree AV block or various types of hemiblock, avoid or discontinue procainamide because of the possibility of increased severity of block, unless the ventricular rate is controlled by an electrical pacemaker.

Torsades de pointes: Procainamide may aggravate this special type of ventricular extrasystole or tachycardia instead of suppressing it.

Lupus erythematosus: If the lupus erythematosus-like syndrome develops in a patient with recurrent life-threatening arrhythmias not controlled by other agents, corticosteroid suppressive therapy may be used concomitantly with procainamide. Because the procainamide-induced lupoid syndrome rarely includes the dangerous pathologic renal changes, therapy may not necessarily have to be stopped unless the symptoms of serositis and the possibility of further lupoid effects are of greater risk than the benefit of procainamide in controlling arrhythmias. Patients with rapid acetylation capability are less likely to develop the lupoid syndrome after prolonged therapy.

Digitalis intoxication: Exercise caution in the use of procainamide in arrhythmias associated with digitalis intoxication. Procainamide can suppress digitalis-induced arrhythmias; however, if there is concomitant marked disturbance of AV conduction, additional depression of conduction and ventricular asystole or fibrillation may result. Consider use of procainamide only if discontinuation of digitalis, and therapy with potassium, lidocaine, or phenytoin are ineffective.

First-degree heart block: Exercise caution if the patient exhibits or develops first-degree heart block while taking procainamide; dosage reduction is advised. If the block persists despite dosage reduction, evaluate the continuation of procainamide on the basis of current benefit vs risk of increased heart block.

Predigitalization for atrial flutter or fibrillation: Cardiovert or digitalize patients with atrial flutter or fibrillation prior to procainamide administration to avoid enhancement of AV conduction, which may result in ventricular rate acceleration beyond tolerable limits. Adequate digitalization reduces the possibility of sudden increase in ventricular rate.

CHF: Use with caution in patients with CHF and in those with acute ischemic heart disease or cardiomyopathy because even slight depression of myocardial contractility may further reduce cardiac output of the damaged heart.

Concurrent antiarrhythmic agents: Concurrent antiarrhythmic agents may produce enhanced prolongation of conduction or depression of contractility and hypotension, especially in patients with cardiac decompensation. Reserve concurrent use of procainamide with other Class IA antiarrhythmic agents (eg, quinidine, disopyramide) for patients with serious arrhythmias unresponsive to a single drug and use only if close observation is possible.

Myasthenia gravis: Procainamide administration in myasthenia gravis patients may be hazardous without optimal adjustment of anticholinesterase medications and other precautions. Immediately after initiation of therapy, closely observe patients for muscular weakness if myasthenia gravis is a possibility.

Renal insufficiency: Renal insufficiency may lead to accumulation of high plasma levels from conventional oral doses of procainamide, with effects similar to those of overdosage unless dosage is adjusted for the individual patient.

Embolization: In conversion of atrial fibrillation to normal sinus rhythm by any means, dislodgment of mural thrombi may lead to embolization.

Hypersensitivity reactions: In patients sensitive to procaine or other ester-type local anesthetics, cross-sensitivity to procainamide is unlikely; however, consider the possibility. Do not use procainamide if it produces acute allergic dermatitis, asthma or anaphylactic symptoms.

Sulfite sensitivity: Some of these products contain sulfites that may cause allergic-type reactions including anaphylactic symptoms and life-threatening or less severe asthmatic episodes. Sulfite sensitivity is seen more frequently in asthmatic or atopic nonasthmatic persons.

Pregnancy: *Category C.*

Lactation: Both procainamide and NAPA are excreted in breast milk and absorbed by the breast-feeding infant. Discontinue breast-feeding or the drug, taking into account the importance of the drug to the mother.

Children: Safety and efficacy have not been established. However, see Administration and Dosage.

Monitoring: After achieving and maintaining therapeutic plasma concentrations and satisfactory ECG and clinical responses, continue frequent periodic monitoring of vital signs and ECG. If evidence of QRS widening of more than 25% or marked prolongation of the QT interval occurs, concern for overdosage is appropriate; reduction in dosage is advisable if a 50% increase occurs. Elevated serum creatinine or urea nitrogen, reduced Ccr or history of renal insufficiency, as well as use in older patients (older than 50 years of age), provide grounds to anticipate that less than the usual dosage and longer time intervals between doses may suffice. If facilities are available for measurement of plasma procainamide and NAPA levels or acetylation capability, individual dose adjustment for optimal therapeutic levels may be easier, but close observation of clinical effectiveness is the most important criterion.

Drug Interactions

Drugs that may affect procainamide include amiodarone, anticholinergics, antiarrhythmics, beta-blockers, ethanol, histamine H_2 antagonists, propranolol, quinidine, quinolones, thioridazine, trimethoprim, and ziprasidone. Drugs that may be affected by procainamide include neuromuscular blockers (succinylcholine). Tests that depend on fluorescence measurement may also be affected.

Adverse Reactions

Significant adverse reactions include a lupus erythematosus-like syndrome of arthralgia, pleural or abdominal pain, and sometimes arthritis, pleural effusion, pericarditis, fever, chills, myalgia, and possibly related hematologic or skin lesions (after prolonged administration); neutropenia; thrombocytopenia; agranulocytosis (after repeated use; deaths have occurred); anorexia; nausea; vomiting; abdominal pain; bitter taste; diarrhea.

DISOPYRAMIDE

Capsules: 100 and 150 mg (*Rx*)	Various, *Norpace* (Searle)
Capsules, extended-release: 100 and 150 mg (*Rx*)	Various, *Norpace CR* (Searle)

Warning:

In the National Heart, Lung, and Blood Institute's Cardiac Arrhythmia Suppression Trial (CAST), a long-term, multicenter, randomized, double-blind study in patients with asymptomatic non-life-threatening ventricular arrhythmias who had an MI more than 6 days but less than 2 years previously, an excessive mortality or nonfatal cardiac arrest rate (7.7%) was seen in patients treated with encainide or flecainide compared with that seen in patients assigned to carefully matched placebo-treated groups (3%). The average duration of treatment with encainide or flecainide in this study was 10 months.

The applicability of the CAST results to other populations (eg, those without recent MI) is uncertain. Considering the known proarrhythmic properties of disopyramide and the lack of evidence of improved survival for any antiarrhythmic drug in patients without life-threatening arrhythmias, the use of disopyramide as well as other antiarrhythmic agents should be reserved for patients with life-threatening ventricular arrhythmias.

Indications

Treatment of documented ventricular arrhythmias (eg, sustained ventricular tachycardia) considered to be life-threatening.

Administration and Dosage

Individualize dosage. Initiate treatment in the hospital.

Adults: 400 to 800 mg/day. The recommended dosage for most adults is 600 mg/day. For patients less than 50 kg (110 pounds), give 400 mg/day. Divide the total daily dose and administer every 6 hours in the immediate release form or every 12 hours in the controlled-release form.

In the event of increased anticholinergic side effects, plasma levels of disopyramide should be monitored and the dose of the drug adjusted accordingly. A reduction of the dose by one third, from the recommended 600 mg/day to 400 mg/day, would be reasonable, without changing the dosing interval.

Children: Divide daily dosage and administer equal doses every 6 hours or at intervals according to patient needs. Closely monitor plasma levels and therapeutic response. Hospitalize patients during initial treatment and start dose titration at the lower end of the ranges provided below:

Suggested Total Daily Disopyramide Dosage in Children[a]

Age (years)	Disopyramide (mg/kg/day)
< 1	10 to 30
1 to 4	10 to 20
4 to 12	10 to 15
12 to 18	6 to 15

[a] Prepare a 1 to 10 mg/mL suspension by adding contents of the immediate release capsule to cherry syrup, NF. The resulting suspension, when refrigerated, is stable for 1 month; shake thoroughly before measuring dose. Dispense in an amber glass bottle. Do not use the controlled-release form to prepare the solution.

Initial loading dose: For rapid control of ventricular arrhythmia, give an initial loading dose of 300 mg immediate release (200 mg for patients less than 50 kg [110 lbs]). Therapeutic effects are attained in 30 minutes to 3 hours. If there is no response or no evidence of toxicity within 6 hours of the loading dose, 200 mg every 6 hours may be administered instead of the usual 150 mg. If there is no response within 48 hours, discontinue the drug or carefully monitor subsequent doses of 250 or 300 mg every 6 hours.

Do not use the controlled-release form initially if rapid plasma levels are desired.

Severe refractory ventricular tachycardia: A limited number of patients have tolerated up to 1600 mg/day (400 mg every 6 hours), resulting in plasma levels up to 9 mcg/mL. Hospitalize patients for close evaluation and continuous monitoring.

Cardiomyopathy or possible cardiac decompensation: Do not administer a loading dose, and limit the initial dosage to 100 mg immediate release every 6 to 8 hours. Make subsequent dosage adjustments gradually.

Renal/Hepatic function impairment: For patients with moderate renal insufficiency (Ccr greater than 40 mL/min) or hepatic insufficiency, the recommended dosage is 400 mg/day given in divided doses (either 100 mg every 6 hours for immediate release or 200 mg every 12 hours for controlled release).

In severe renal insufficiency (Ccr up to 40 mL/min), the recommended dosage is 100 mg of the immediate release form given at the intervals shown in the table below, with or without an initial loading dose of 150 mg.

Disopyramide Dosage in Renal Impairment

Creatinine clearance (mL/min)	Loading dose (mg)	Dose (mg)	Dosage interval (h)
30-40	150	100	8
15-30	150	100	12
< 15	150	100	24

Transfer to disopyramide: Use the regular maintenance schedule, without a loading dose, 6 to 12 hours after the last dose of quinidine or 3 to 6 hours after the last dose of procainamide. Where withdrawal of quinidine or procainamide is likely to produce life-threatening arrhythmias, consider hospitalization.

When transferring from immediate to controlled release, start maintenance schedule of controlled release 6 hours after the last dose of immediate release.

Actions

Pharmacology:

Mechanism of action – Disopyramide is a class IA antiarrhythmic agent that decreases the rate of diastolic depolarization (phase 4), decreases the upstroke velocity (phase 0), increases the action potential duration of normal cardiac cells, and prolongs the refractory period (phases 2 and 3). It also decreases the disparity in refractoriness between infarcted and adjacent normally perfused myocardium and does not affect alpha- or beta-adrenergic receptors.

Pharmacokinetics:

Absorption/Distribution – Following oral administration of immediate-release disopyramide, the drug is rapidly and almost completely (approximately 90%) absorbed. Peak plasma levels usually occur within 2 hours. Therapeutic plasma levels of disopyramide are 2 to 4 mcg/mL. Protein binding is concentration-dependent and varies from 50% to 65%; it is difficult to predict the concentration of the free drug when total drug is measured.

Metabolism/Excretion – About 50% is excreted in the urine as the unchanged drug and 30% as metabolites (20% mono-N-dealkyldisopyramide [MND]). The plasma concentration of MND is approximately one-tenth that of disopyramide. The mean plasma half-life is 6.7 hours (range, 4 to 10 hours). In impaired renal function, half-life values ranged from 8 to 18 hours. Therefore, decrease the dose in renal failure to avoid drug accumulation.

Immediate-release vs controlled-release – Following multiple doses, steady-state plasma levels of between 2 and 4 mcg/mL were attained following either 150 mg every 6 hours (immediate release) or 300 mg every 12 hours (controlled release).

Contraindications

Cardiogenic shock; preexisting second- or third-degree AV block (if no pacemaker is present); congenital QT prolongation; sick sinus syndrome; hypersensitivity to disopyramide.

Warnings/Precautions

Proarrhythmic effects: Because of the proarrhythmic effects, use with lesser arrhythmias is generally not recommended.

Asymptomatic ventricular premature contractions: Avoid treatment of patients with this condition.

Survival: Antiarrhythmic drugs have not been shown to enhance survival in patients with ventricular arrhythmias.

Negative inotropic properties:

Heart failure/hypotension – May cause or aggravate CHF or produce severe hypotension, especially in patients with depressed systolic function. Do not use in patients with uncompensated or marginally compensated CHF or hypotension unless secondary to cardiac arrhythmia. Treat patients with a history of heart failure with careful attention to the maintenance of cardiac function, including optimal digitalization. If hypotension occurs or CHF worsens, discontinue use; restart at a lower dosage after adequate cardiac compensation has been established.

Do not give a loading dose to patients with myocarditis or other cardiomyopathy; closely monitor initial dosage and subsequent adjustments.

QRS widening – QRS widening (greater than 25%), although unusual, may occur; discontinue use in such cases.

QT_c prolongation – QT_c prolongation and worsening of the arrhythmia, including ventricular tachycardia and fibrillation, may occur. Patients who have QT prolongation in response to quinidine may be at particular risk. Disopyramide has been associated with torsade de pointes. If QT prolongation greater than 25% is observed and if ectopy continues, monitor closely and consider discontinuing the drug.

Atrial tachyarrhythmias: Digitalize patients with atrial flutter or fibrillation prior to administration to ensure that enhancement of AV conduction does not increase ventricular rate beyond acceptable limits.

Conduction abnormalities: Use caution in patients with sick sinus syndrome, Wolff-Parkinson-White syndrome or bundle branch block.

Heart block: If first-degree heart block develops, reduce dosage. If the block persists, drug continuation must depend upon the benefit compared with the risk of higher degrees of heart block. Development of second- or third-degree AV block or unifascicular, bifascicular, or trifascicular block requires discontinuation of therapy, unless ventricular rate is controlled by a ventricular pacemaker.

Concomitant antiarrhythmic therapy: Reserve concomitant use of disopyramide with other class IA antiarrhythmics or propranolol for life-threatening arrhythmias unresponsive to a single agent. Such use may produce serious negative inotropic effects or may excessively prolong conduction, particularly with cardiac decompensation.

Hypoglycemia: Hypoglycemia has been reported in rare instances. Monitor blood glucose levels in patients with CHF, chronic malnutrition, hepatic disease, and in those taking drugs which could compromise normal glucoregulatory mechanisms in the absence of food.

Anticholinergic activity: Do not use in patients with urinary retention, glaucoma, or myasthenia gravis unless adequate overriding measures are taken. Males with benign prostatic hypertrophy are at particular risk of having urinary retention. In patients with a family history of glaucoma, measure intraocular pressure before initiating therapy.

Potassium imbalance: Disopyramide may be ineffective in *hypo*kalemia and its toxic effects may be enhanced in *hyper*kalemia. Correct any potassium deficit before instituting therapy.

Renal function impairment: Reduce dosage in impaired renal function. Carefully monitor ECG for signs of overdosage. The controlled-release form is not recommended for patients with severe renal insufficiency (Ccr up to 40 mL/min).

Hepatic function impairment: Impairment increases plasma half-life; reduce dosage in such patients. Carefully monitor the ECG. Patients with cardiac dysfunction have a higher potential for hepatic impairment.

Pregnancy: Category C.

Lactation: Disopyramide has been detected in breast milk.

Drug Interactions

Drugs that may affect disopyramide include antiarrhythmics, beta blockers, cisapride, clarithromycin, erythromycin, fluoroquinolones, hydantoins, quinidine, thioridazine, rifampin, verapamil, and ziprasidone. Drugs that may be affected by disopyramide include quinidine, anticoagulants, and digoxin.

Adverse Reactions

The most serious adverse reactions are hypotension and CHF. The most common reactions are anticholinergic and are dose-dependent. These may be transitory, but may be persistent or severe. Urinary retention is the most serious anticholinergic effect. Adverse reactions occurring in 3% or more of patients include urinary retention, frequency and urgency; dizziness; fatigue; headache; nausea; pain; bloating; gas; dry mouth; urinary hesitancy; constipation; blurred vision; dry nose; eyes and throat; muscle weakness; malaise; aches/pain.

LIDOCAINE HYDROCHLORIDE

Injection: (for IM administration) 300 mg/3 mL automatic injection device (*Rx*)	*LidoPen Auto-Injector* (Survival Technology)
(for direct IV administration) 1% (10 mg/mL), 2% (20 mg/mL) (*Rx*)	Various, *Xylocaine Hydrochloride IV for Cardiac Arrhythmias* (Astra)
(for IV admixtures) 10% (100 mg/mL) (*Rx*)	Various
(for IV admixtures) 4% (40 mg/mL), 20% (200 mg/mL) (*Rx*)	Various, *Xylocaine Hydrochloride IV for Cardiac Arrhythmias* (Astra)
(for IV infusion) 0.2% (2 mg/mL), 0.4% (4 mg/mL), 0.8% (8 mg/mL) (*Rx*)	Various

Indications

IV: Acute management of ventricular arrhythmias occurring during cardiac manipulation, such as cardiac surgery or in relation to acute myocardial infarction (MI).

IM: Single doses are justified in the following exceptional circumstances: When ECG equipment is not available to verify the diagnosis but the potential benefits outweigh the possible risks; when facilities for IV administration are not readily available; by the patient in the prehospital phase of suspected acute MI, directed by qualified medical personnel viewing the transmitted ECG.

Unlabeled uses: In pediatric patients with cardiac arrest, less than 10% develop ventricular fibrillation, and others develop ventricular tachycardia; the hemodynamically compromised child may develop ventricular couplets or frequent premature ventricular beats. In these cases, administer 1 mg/kg lidocaine by the IV, intraosseous, or endotracheal route. A second 1 mg/kg dose may be given in 10 to 15 minutes. Start a lidocaine infusion if the second dose is required; a third bolus may be needed in 10 to 15 minutes to maintain therapeutic levels.

Administration and Dosage

IM: 300 mg. The deltoid muscle is preferred. Avoid intravascular injection. Use only the 10% solution for IM injection.

The *LidoPen Auto-Injector* unit is for self-administration into deltoid muscle or anterolateral aspect of thigh. Patient instructions are provided with product.

Replacement therapy – As soon as possible, change patient to IV lidocaine or to an oral antiarrhythmic preparation for maintenance therapy. However, if necessary, an additional IM injection may be administered after 60 to 90 minutes.

IV: Use only lidocaine injection without preservatives, clearly labeled for IV use. Monitor ECG constantly to avoid potential overdosage and toxicity.

IV bolus – IV bolus is used to establish rapid therapeutic blood levels. Continuous IV infusion is necessary to maintain antiarrhythmic effects. The usual dose is 50 to 100 mg, given at a rate of 25 to 50 mg/min. If the initial injection does not produce the desired clinical response, give a second bolus dose after 5 minutes. Give no more than 200 to 300 mg/hour.

Reduce loading (bolus) doses – Reduce loading (bolus) doses in patients with congestive heart failure (CHF) or reduced cardiac output and in the elderly. However, some investigators recommend the usual loading dose be administered and only the maintenance dosage be reduced.

IV continuous infusion – IV continuous infusion is used to maintain therapeutic plasma levels following loading doses in patients in whom arrhythmias tend to recur and who cannot receive oral antiarrhythmic drugs. Administer at a rate of 1 to 4 mg/min (20 to 50 mcg/kg/min). Reduce maintenance doses in patients with heart failure or liver disease, or who are also receiving other drugs known to decrease clearance of lidocaine or decrease liver blood flow and in patients older than 70 years of age. Reassess the rate of infusion as soon as the cardiac rhythm stabilizes or at the earliest signs of toxicity. Change patients to oral antiarrhythmic agents for maintenance therapy as soon as possible. It is rarely necessary to continue IV infusions for prolonged periods. Use a precision volume control IV set for continuous IV infusion.

Children – The American Heart Association's Standards and Guidelines recommend a bolus dose of 1 mg/kg, followed by an infusion of 30 mcg/kg/min. The following dosage has also been suggested:

Loading dose – Loading dose, 1 mg/kg/dose given IV or intratracheally every 5 to 10 min to desired effect, maximum total dose 5 mg/kg; Maintenance: 20 to 50 mcg/kg/min.

Actions

Pharmacology: Therapeutic concentrations of lidocaine attenuate phase 4 diastolic depolarization, decrease automaticity and cause a decrease or no change in excitability and membrane responsiveness. Action potential duration and effective refractory period (ERP) of Purkinje fibers and ventricular muscle are decreased, while the ratio of ERP to action potential duration is increased. Lidocaine raises ventricular fibrillation threshold. AV nodal conduction time is unchanged or shortened. Lidocaine increases the electrical stimulation threshold of the ventricle during diastole.

Pharmacokinetics:

Absorption/Distribution – Lidocaine is ineffective orally; it is most commonly administered IV with an immediate onset (within minutes) and brief duration (10 to 20 minutes) of action following a bolus dose. Continuous IV infusion of lidocaine (1 to 4 mg/min) is necessary to maintain antiarrhythmic effects. Following IM administration, therapeutic serum levels are achieved in 5 to 15 minutes and may persist for up to 2 hours. Higher and more rapid serum levels are achieved by injection into the deltoid muscle. Therapeutic serum levels are 1.5 to 6 mcg/mL; serum levels greater than 6 to 10 mcg/mL are usually toxic. Lidocaine is approximately 50% protein bound (concentration-dependent).

Metabolism/Excretion – Extensive biotransformation in the liver (approximately 90%) results in at least 2 active metabolites, monoethylglycinexylidide and glycinexylidide. Lidocaine exhibits a biphasic half-life. The distribution phase is approximately 10 minutes. The elimination half-life is 1.5 to 2 hours; half-life may be 3 hours or more following infusions of more than 24 hours. Any condition that alters liver function, including changes in liver blood flow, which could result from severe CHF or shock, may alter lidocaine kinetics. Less than 10% of the parent drug is excreted unchanged in the urine. Renal elimination plays an important role in the elimination of the metabolites.

Contraindications

Hypersensitivity to amide local anesthetics; Stokes-Adams syndrome; Wolff-Parkinson-White syndrome; severe degrees of sinoatrial, atrioventricular (AV), or intraventricular block in the absence of an artificial pacemaker.

Warnings/Precautions

Survival: Prophylactic single dose lidocaine administered in a monitored environment does not appear to affect mortality in the earliest phase of acute MI, and may harm some patients who are later shown not to have suffered an acute MI.

Constant ECG monitoring: Constant ECG monitoring is essential for proper administration. Have emergency resuscitative equipment and drugs immediately available.

IV use: Signs of excessive depression of cardiac conductivity should be followed by dosage reduction and, if necessary, prompt cessation of IV infusion.

IM use: May increase creatine phosphokinase levels. Use of the enzyme determination without isoenzyme separation, as a diagnostic test for acute MI, may be compromised.

Cardiac effects: Use with caution and in lower doses in patients with CHF, reduced cardiac output, digitalis toxicity accompanied by AV block and in the elderly.

In sinus bradycardia or incomplete heart block, lidocaine administration for the elimination of ventricular ectopy without prior acceleration in heart rate (eg, by atropine, isoproterenol or electric pacing) may promote more frequent and serious ventricular arrhythmias or complete heart block. Use with caution in patients with hypovolemia and shock, and all forms of heart block.

Acceleration of ventricular rate – Acceleration of ventricular rate may occur when administered to patients with atrial flutter or fibrillation.

Malignant hyperthermia: Amide local anesthetic administration has been associated with acute onset of fulminant hypermetabolism of skeletal muscle known as malignant hyperthermic crisis. Recognition of early unexplained signs of tachycardia, tachypnea, labile blood pressure, and metabolic acidosis may precede temperature elevation. Successful outcome depends on early diagnosis, prompt discontinuance of the triggering agent and institution of treatment, including oxygen, supportive measures, and IV dantrolene sodium.

Hypersensitivity reactions: Hypersensitivity reactions may occur. Refer to Management of Acute Hypersensitivity Reactions.

Renal/Hepatic function impairment: Use caution with repeated or prolonged use in liver or renal disease; possible toxic accumulation may occur.

Pregnancy: Category B.

Lactation: Exercise caution when administering to a breast-feeding woman.

Children: Safety and efficacy have not been established; reduce dosage. The IM auto-injector device is not recommended in children less than 50 kg.

Drug Interactions

Drugs that may affect lidocaine include beta-blockers, cimetidine, procainamide, tocainide, and succinylcholine.

Adverse Reactions

Significant drug interactions include light-headedness; nervousness; drowsiness; dizziness; apprehension; confusion; mood changes; hallucinations; tremors; convulsions; unconsciousness; hypotension; bradycardia; cardiovascular collapse, which may lead to cardiac arrest; febrile response; soreness/infection at the injection site; venous thrombosis or phlebitis extending from the site of injection; extravasation; vomiting; respiratory depression/arrest.

PROPAFENONE HYDROCHLORIDE

Tablets: 150, 225, and 300 mg (*Rx*)	*Rythmol* (Various, eg Reliant)
Capsules, extended-release: 225, 325, and 425 mg (*Rx*)	*Rythmol SR* (Reliant)

Warning:

In the National Heart, Lung, and Blood Institute's Cardiac Arrhythmia Suppression Trial (CAST), a long-term, multicenter, randomized, double-blind study in patients with asymptomatic non-life-threatening ventricular arrhythmias who had an MI more than 6 days but less than 2 years previously, an increased rate of death or reversed cardiac arrest rate (7.7%) was seen in patients treated with encainide or flecainide (Class 1C antiarrhythmics) compared with that seen in patients assigned to placebo (3%). The average duration of treatment with encainide or flecainide in this study was 10 months.

The applicability of the CAST results to other populations (eg, those without recent MI) or other antiarrhythmic drugs is uncertain, but at present, it is prudent to consider any 1C antiarrhythmic to have a significant risk in patients with structural heart disease. Given the lack of any evidence that these drugs improve survival, antiarrhythmic agents should generally be avoided in patients with nonlife-threatening ventricular arrhythmias, even if the patients are experiencing unpleasant, but not life-threatening symptoms or signs.

Indications

Treatment of documented life-threatening ventricular arrhythmias, such as sustained ventricular tachycardia.

Atrial fibrillation/flutter:

Immediate-release (IR) – To prolong the time to recurrence of paroxysmal atrial fibrillation/flutter associated with disabling symptoms in patients without structural heart disease.

Extended-release (ER) – To prolong the time to recurrence of symptomatic atrial fibrillation in patients with structural heart disease.

Because of the proarrhythmic effects of propafenone, reserve its use for patients in whom the benefits of treatment outweigh the risks. The use of propafenone is not recommended in patients with less severe ventricular arrhythmias, even if the patients are symptomatic.

Administration and Dosage

IR: Individually titrate on the basis of response and tolerance. Initiate with 150 mg every 8 hours (450 mg/day). Dosage may be increased at a minimum of 3 to 4 day intervals to 225 mg every 8 hours (675 mg/day) and, if necessary, to 300 mg every 8 hours (900 mg/day). The safety and efficacy of dosages exceeding 900 mg/day have not been established. In those patients in whom significant widening of the QRS complex or second- or third-degree AV block occurs, consider dose reduction.

As with other antiarrhythmics, in the elderly or patients with marked previous myocardial damage, increase dose more gradually during initial treatment phase.

SR: Individually titrate on the basis of response and tolerance. Therapy should be initiated with 225 mg given every 12 hours. Dosage may be increased at a minimum of 5-day intervals to 325 mg given every 12 hours. If additional therapeutic effect is needed, the dose may be increased to 425 mg given every 12 hours.

The SR capsules can be taken with or without food. Do not crush or further divide the contents of the capsule.

Actions

Pharmacology: Propafenone is a Class IC antiarrhythmic with local anesthetic effects and direct stabilizing action on myocardial membranes.

Pharmacokinetics:

Absorption/Distribution – Propafenone is nearly completely absorbed after oral administration with peak plasma levels occurring approximately 3.5 hours after administration. It exhibits extensive first-pass metabolism resulting in a dose-dependent and dosage-form-dependent absolute bioavailability. Propafenone follows a nonlinear pharmacokinetic disposition presumably due to saturation of first-pass hepatic metabolism as the liver is exposed to higher concentrations of propafenone and shows a very high degree of interindividual variability.

Metabolism/Excretion – There are 2 genetically determined patterns of propafenone metabolism. In more than 90% of patients, the drug is rapidly and extensively metabolized with an elimination half-life of 2 to 10 hours. These patients metabolize propafenone into two active metabolites: 5-hydroxypropafenone and N-depropylpropafenone. They both are usually present in concentrations less than 20% of propafenone. The saturable hydroxylation pathway is responsible for the nonlinear pharmacokinetic disposition.

Contraindications

Uncontrolled CHF; cardiogenic shock; sinoatrial, AV and intraventricular disorders of impulse generation or conduction (eg, sick sinus node syndrome, AV block) in the absence of an artificial pacemaker; bradycardia; marked hypotension; bronchospastic disorders; manifest electrolyte imbalance; hypersensitivity to the drug.

Warnings/Precautions

Mortality: An excessive mortality or nonfatal cardiac arrest rate was seen in patients treated with encainide or flecainide compared with that seen in patients assigned to carefully matched placebo-treated groups.

Proarrhythmic effects: Propafenone may cause new or worsened arrhythmias. Such proarrhythmic effects range from an increase in frequency of PVCs to the development of more severe ventricular tachycardia, ventricular fibrillation or torsade de pointes, which may lead to fatal consequences. It is essential that each patient be evaluated electrocardiographically and clinically prior to, and during therapy to determine whether response to propafenone supports continued use.

Non-life-threatening arrhythmias: Use of propafenone is not recommended in patients with less severe ventricular arrhythmias, even if the patients are symptomatic.

Survival: There is no evidence from controlled trials that the use of propafenone favorably affects survival or the incidence of sudden death.

Nonallergic bronchospasm (eg, chronic bronchitis, emphysema): In general, these patients should not receive propafenone or other agents with beta-adrenergic blocking activity.

CHF: New or worsened CHF has occurred in 3.7% of patients.

As propafenone exerts both beta blockade and a (dose-related) negative inotropic effect on cardiac muscle, fully compensate patients with CHF before receiving propafenone. If CHF worsens, discontinue propafenone unless CHF is due to the cardiac arrhythmia and, if indicated, restart at a lower dosage only after adequate cardiac compensation has been established.

Conduction disturbances: Propafenone causes first-degree AV block. Average PR interval prolongation and increases in QRS duration are closely correlated with dosage increases and concomitant increases in propafenone plasma concentrations. Development of second- or third-degree AV block requires a reduction in dosage or discontinuation of propafenone. Bundle branch block and intraventricular conduction delay have occurred. Bradycardia has also occurred. Patients with sick sinus node syndrome should not be treated with propafenone.

Effects on pacemaker threshold: Pacing and sensing thresholds of artificial pacemakers may be altered. Monitor and program pacemakers accordingly during therapy.

Hematologic disturbances: Agranulocytosis with fever and sepsis has occurred. Unexplained fever or decrease in white cell count, particularly during the first 3 months of therapy, warrants consideration of possible agranulocytosis/granulocytopenia.

Elevated ANA titers: Positive ANA titers have occurred. They have been reversible upon cessation of treatment and may disappear even with continued therapy. Carefully evaluate patients who develop an abnormal ANA test and, if persistent or worsening elevation of ANA titers is detected, consider discontinuing therapy.

Renal/Hepatic changes: Renal changes have been observed in the rat following 6 months of oral administration of propafenone at doses of 180 and 360 mg/kg/day (2 to 4 times the maximum recommended human dose). Both inflammatory and noninflammatory changes in the renal tubules with accompanying interstitial nephritis were observed.

Neuromuscular dysfunction: Exacerbation of myasthenia gravis has been reported during propafenone therapy.

Renal function impairment: A considerable percentage of propafenone metabolites are excreted in the urine. Administer cautiously in impaired renal function.

Hepatic function impairment: Propafenone is highly metabolized by the liver; administer cautiously to patients with impaired hepatic function. The clearance of propafenone is reduced and the elimination half-life increased in patients with significant hepatic dysfunction. The dose of propafenone should be approximately 20% to 30% of the dose given to patients with normal hepatic function.

Pregnancy: Category C.

Lactation: Propafenone is excreted in breast milk. Decide whether to discontinue breastfeeding or to discontinue the drug, taking into account the importance of the drug to the mother.

Children: The safety and efficacy in children have not been established.

Elderly: Because of the possible increased risk of impaired hepatic or renal function in this age group, use with caution. The effective dose may be lower in these patients.

Drug Interactions

Drugs that inhibit CYP2D6, CYP1A2, and CYP3A4 might lead to increased plasma levels of propafenone. Drugs that may affect propafenone include local anesthetics, cimetidine, quinidine, cisapride, rifampin, ritonavir, and SSRIs. Drugs that may be affected by propafenone include anticoagulants, beta blockers, cisapride, cyclosporine, desipramine, digoxin, mexiletine, and theophylline.

Adverse Reactions

Adverse reactions occurring in at least 3% of patients include angina; first-degree AV block; CHF; intraventricular conduction delay; palpitations; proarrhythmia; ventricular tachycardia; dizziness; fatigue; headache; constipation; dyspepsia; nausea/vomiting; unusual taste; blurred vision; dyspnea. About 20% of patients discontinued treatment due to adverse reactions.

MEXILETINE HYDROCHLORIDE

Capsules: 150, 200, and 250 mg (*Rx*) Various, *Mexitil* (Boehringer Ingelheim)

Warning:

Mortality: In the National Heart, Lung and Blood Institute's Cardiac Arrhythmia Suppression Trial (CAST), a long-term, multicentered, randomized, double-blind study in patients with asymptomatic non-life-threatening ventricular arrhythmias who had an MI more than 6 days but less than 2 years previously, an excessive mortality or nonfatal cardiac arrest rate was seen in patients treated with encainide or flecainide (7.7%) compared with that seen in patients assigned to matched placebo-treated groups (3%). The average duration of treatment with encainide or flecainide in this study was 10 months.

The applicability of these results to other populations (eg, those without recent MI) is uncertain. Considering the known proarrhythmic properties of mexiletine and the lack of evidence of improved survival for any antiarrhythmic drug in patients without life-threatening arrhythmias, the use of mexiletine as well as other antiarrhythmic agents should be reserved for patients with life-threatening ventricular arrhythmia.

Indications

Treatment of documented, life-threatening ventricular arrhythmias, such as sustained ventricular tachycardia. Because of the proarrhythmic effects of mexiletine, use with lesser arrhythmias is generally not recommended.

Administration and Dosage

Individualize dosage. Administer with food or antacids.

Perform clinical and ECG evaluation as needed to determine whether the desired antiarrhythmic effect has been obtained and to guide titration and dose adjustment.

Initial dose: 200 mg every 8 hours when rapid control of arrhythmia is not essential, with a minimum of 2 to 3 days between adjustments. Adjust dose in 50 or 100 mg increments.

Control can be achieved in most patients with 200 to 300 mg given every 8 hours. If satisfactory response is not achieved at 300 mg every 8 hours, and the patient tolerates mexiletine well, try 400 mg every 8 hours. The severity of CNS side effects increases with total daily dose; do not exceed 1,200 mg/day.

Renal/hepatic function impairment: In general, patients with renal failure will require the usual doses of mexiletine. Patients with severe liver disease, however, may require lower doses and must be monitored closely. Similarly, marked right-sided CHF can reduce hepatic metabolism and reduce the dose needed.

Loading dose: When rapid control of ventricular arrhythmia is essential, administer an initial loading dose of 400 mg, followed by a 200 mg dose in 8 hours. Onset of therapeutic effect is usually observed within 30 minutes to 2 hours.

Twice-daily dosage: If adequate suppression is achieved on a dose of 300 mg or less every 8 hours, the same total daily dose may be given in divided doses every 12 hours with monitoring. The dose may be adjusted to a maximum of 450 mg every 12 hours.

Transferring to mexiletine: When transferring from other Class I oral antiarrhythmics to mexiletine, based on theoretical considerations, initiate with a 200 mg dose, and titrate to response as described above, 6 to 12 hours after the last dose of quinidine sulfate, 3 to 6 hours after the last dose of procainamide, 6 to 12 hours after the last disopyramide dose or 8 to 12 hours after the last tocainide dose.

Hospitalize patients in whom withdrawal of the previous antiarrhythmic agent is likely to produce life-threatening arrhythmias.

When transferring from lidocaine to mexiletine, stop the lidocaine infusion when the first oral dose of mexiletine is administered. Maintain the IV line until suppression of the arrhythmia appears satisfactory. Consider the similarity of adverse effects of lidocaine and mexiletine and the additive potential.

Actions

Pharmacology:

Mechanism – Structurally like lidocaine, mexiletine inhibits the inward sodium current, thus reducing the rate of rise of the action potential, Phase 0. Mexiletine decreases the effective refractory period (ERP) in Purkinje fibers. The decrease in ERP is of lesser magnitude than the decrease in action potential duration (APD), with a resulting increase in ERP/APD ratio.

Hemodynamic effects – Small decreases in cardiac output and increases in systemic vascular resistance have occurred, with no significant negative inotropic effect. Blood pressure and pulse rate remain essentially unchanged. Mild depression of myocardial function has been observed following IV mexiletine (dosage form not available in the US) in patients with cardiac disease.

Electrophysiology – Mexiletine is a local anesthetic and a Class IB antiarrhythmic compound with electrophysiologic properties similar to lidocaine.

Pharmacokinetics:

Absorption/Distribution – Mexiletine is well absorbed (approximately 90%) from the GI tract. The absorption rate is reduced in clinical situations (such as acute MI) in which gastric emptying time is increased.

Peak blood levels are reached in 2 to 3 hours. The therapeutic range is approximately 0.5 to 2 mcg/mL. An increase in the frequency of CNS adverse effects has been observed when plasma levels exceed 2 mcg/mL. It is 50% to 60% bound to plasma protein with a volume of distribution of 5 to 7 L/kg.

Metabolism/Excretion – Mexiletine is metabolized in the liver primarily by CYP2D6, although it is a substrate for CYP1A2. The most active minor metabolite is N-methylmexiletine, which is less than 20% as potent as mexiletine. Urinary excretion of N-methylmexiletine is less than 0.5%.

In healthy subjects, the elimination half-life is 10 to 12 hours. Hepatic impairment prolongs it to a mean of 25 hours. Little change in half-life occurs with reduced renal function. In eight patients with creatinine clearance less than 10 mL/min, the mean plasma elimination half-life was 15.7 hours; in seven patients with creatinine clearance between 11 and 40 mL/min, the mean half-life was 13.4 hours.

Contraindications

Cardiogenic shock; preexisting second- or third-degree AV block (if no pacemaker).

Warnings/Precautions

Proarrhythmia: Mexiletine can worsen arrhythmias; it is uncommon in patients with less serious arrhythmias (frequent premature beats or nonsustained ventricular tachycardia) but is of greater concern in patients with life-threatening arrhythmias, such as sustained ventricular tachycardia.

Survival: Antiarrhythmic drugs have not been shown to enhance survival in patients with ventricular arrhythmias.

Initial therapy: As with other antiarrhythmics, initiate therapy in the hospital.

Mortality: Considering the known proarrhythmic properties of mexiletine and the lack of evidence of improved survival for any antiarrhythmic drug in patients without life-threatening arrhythmias, the use of mexiletine should be reserved for patients with life-threatening ventricular arrhythmia.

Cardiovascular effects: If a ventricular pacemaker is operative, patients with second- or third-degree heart block may be treated with mexiletine if continuously monitored. Exercise caution in such patients or in patients with preexisting sinus node dysfunction or intraventricular conduction abnormalities.

Use with caution in patients with hypotension and severe CHF.

AST elevation and liver injury: Elevations of AST more than 3 times the upper limit of normal occurred in about 1% of both mexiletine-treated and control patients.

Rare instances of severe liver injury, including hepatic necrosis, have been reported. Carefully evaluate patients in whom an abnormal liver test has occurred, or who have signs or symptoms suggesting liver dysfunction.

Hematologic effects: Marked leukopenia (neutrophils less than 1,000/mm^3) or agranulocytosis were seen in 0.06%; milder depressions of leukocytes were seen in 0.08% and thrombocytopenia was observed in 0.16%. Many of these patients were seriously ill and were receiving concomitant medications with known hematologic adverse effects. Rechallenge with mexiletine in several cases was negative. If significant hematologic changes are observed, carefully evaluate the patient and, if warranted, discontinue mexiletine. Blood counts usually return to normal within 1 month of discontinuation.

CNS effects: Convulsions occurred in about 2 of 1,000 patients. Convulsions occurred in patients with and without a history of seizures. Use with caution in patients with a known seizure disorder.

Urinary pH: Avoid concurrent drugs or diets which may markedly alter urinary pH. Minor fluctuations in urinary pH associated with normal diet do not affect mexiletine excretion.

Hepatic function impairment: Since mexiletine is metabolized in the liver, and hepatic impairment prolongs the elimination half-life, carefully monitor patients with liver disease. Observe caution in patients with hepatic dysfunction secondary to CHF.

Abnormal liver function tests have been reported, some in the first few weeks of therapy with mexiletine. Most have occurred along with CHF or ischemia; their relationship to mexiletine has not been established.

Pregnancy: Category C.

Lactation: Mexiletine appears in breast milk in concentrations similar to those in plasma. If mexiletine is essential, consider alternative infant feeding.

Children: Safety and efficacy in children have not been established.

Drug Interactions

Drugs that may affect mexiletine include aluminum-magnesium hydroxide, atropine, narcotics, cimetidine, fluvoxamine, hydantoins, metoclopramide, propafenone, rifampin, urinary acidifiers, and urinary alkalinizers.

Drugs that may be affected by mexiletine include cimetidine, caffeine, and theophylline.

CYP450 system: Because mexiletine is a substrate for CYP2D6 and CYP1A2, inhibition or induction of either of these enzymes would be expected to alter mexiletine concentrations.

Adverse Reactions

The most frequent adverse reactions were upper GI distress, tremor, lightheadedness, and coordination difficulties. These reactions were generally not serious, dose-related, and reversible if the dosage was reduced, if the drug was taken with food or antacids or if it was discontinued.

Other adverse events occurring in at least 3% of patients include palpitations, chest pain, nervousness, changes in sleep habits, headache, blurred vision/visual disturbances, paresthesias/numbness, weakness, fatigue, diarrhea, constipation, rash, nonspecific edema, dyspnea/respiratory.

Postmarketing: There have been isolated, spontaneous reports of pulmonary changes including pulmonary infiltration and pulmonary fibrosis during mexiletine therapy with or without other drugs or diseases that are known to produce pulmonary toxicity.

FLECAINIDE ACETATE

Tablets: 50, 100, and 150 mg (*Rx*) *Tambocor* (Graceway Pharmaceuticals)

Warning:

Mortality: Flecainide was included in the National Heart Lung and Blood Institute's Cardiac Arrhythmia Suppression Trial (CAST), a long-term, multicenter, randomized, double-blind study in patients with asymptomatic non-life-threatening ventricular arrhythmias who had an MI more than 6 days but less than 2 years previously. An excessive mortality or nonfatal cardiac arrest rate was seen in patients treated with flecainide compared with that seen in patients assigned to a carefully matched placebo-treated group. This rate was 5.1% for flecainide and 2.3% for the matched placebo. The average duration of treatment with flecainide in this study was 10 months.

The applicability of the CAST results to other populations (eg, those without recent MI) is uncertain, but at present, it is prudent to consider the risks of Class IC agents (including flecainide), coupled with the lack of any evidence of improved survival, generally unacceptable in patients without life-threatening ventricular arrhythmias, even if the patients are experiencing unpleasant, but not life-threatening, symptoms or signs.

Ventricular proarrhythmic effects in patients with atrial fibrillation/flutter: A review of the world literature revealed reports of 568 patients treated with oral flecainide for paroxysmal atrial fibrillation/flutter (PAF). Ventricular tachycardia was experienced in 0.4% of these patients. Of 19 patients in the literature with chronic atrial fibrillation (CAF), 10.5% experienced ventricular tachycardia (VT) or ventricular fibrillation (VF). Flecainide is not recommended for use in patients with CAF. Case reports of ventricular proarrhythmic effects in patients treated with flecainide for atrial fibrillation/flutter have included increased premature ventricular contractions (PVCs), VT, VF, and death.

As with other Class I agents, patients treated with flecainide for atrial flutter have been reported with 1:1 atrioventricular conduction due to slowing the atrial rate. A paradoxical increase in the ventricular rate also may occur in patients with atrial fibrillation who receive flecainide. Concomitant negative chronotropic therapy such as digoxin or beta-blockers may lower the risk of this complication.

Indications

Atrial fibrillation: For the prevention of paroxysmal atrial fibrillation/flutter (PAF) associated with disabling symptoms and paroxysmal supraventricular tachycardias (PSVT), including atrioventricular nodal reentrant tachycardia, atrioventricular reentrant tachycardia, and other supraventricular tachycardias of unspecified mechanism associated with disabling symptoms in patients without structural heart disease.

Ventricular arrhythmias: Prevention of documented life-threatening ventricular arrhythmias, such as sustained ventricular tachycardia.

Not recommended in patients with less severe ventricular arrhythmias even if the patients are symptomatic. Because of proarrhythmic effects of flecainide, reserve use for patients in whom benefits outweigh risks.

Administration and Dosage

For patients with sustained ventricular tachycardia, initiate therapy in the hospital and monitor rhythm.

Do not increase dosage more frequently than once every 4 days, because optimal effect may not be achieved during the first 2 to 3 days of therapy.

An occasional patient not adequately controlled by (or intolerant of) a dose given at 12-hour intervals may be dosed at 8-hour intervals.

Once the arrhythmia is controlled, it may be possible to reduce the dose, as necessary, to minimize side effects or effects on conduction.

PSVT and PAF: The recommended starting dose is 50 mg every 12 hours. Doses may be increased in increments of 50 mg twice daily every 4 days until efficacy is achieved. For PAF patients, a substantial increase in efficacy without a substantial increase in discontinuation for adverse experiences may be achieved by increasing the flecainide dose from 50 to 100 mg twice/day. The maximum recommended dose for patients with paroxysmal supraventricular arrhythmias is 300 mg/day.

Sustained ventricular tachycardia:

Initial dose – 100 mg every 12 hours. Increase in 50 mg increments twice daily every 4 days until effective. Most patients do not require more than 150 mg every 12 hours (300 mg/day). Maximum dose is 400 mg/day.

Use of higher initial doses and more rapid dosage adjustments have resulted in an increased incidence of proarrhythmic events and CHF, particularly during the first few days of dosing. A loading dose is not recommended.

CHF or MI – Use cautiously in patients with a history of CHF or myocardial dysfunction (see Warnings).

Renal function impairment: In severe renal impairment (Ccr 35 mL/min/1.73 m^2 or less), the initial dosage is 100 mg once daily (or 50 mg twice/day). Frequent plasma level monitoring is required to guide dosage adjustments. In patients with less severe renal disease, initial dosage is 100 mg every 12 hours. Increase dosage cautiously at intervals greater than 4 days, observing the patient closely for signs of adverse cardiac effects or other toxicity. It may take more than 4 days before a new steady-state plasma level is reached following a dosage change. Monitor plasma levels to guide dosage adjustments.

Transfer to flecainide: Theoretically, when transferring patients from another antiarrhythmic to flecainide, allow at least 2 to 4 plasma half-lives to elapse for the drug being discontinued before starting flecainide at the usual dosage. Consider hospitalization of patients in whom withdrawal of a previous antiarrhythmic is likely to produce life-threatening arrhythmias.

Administration with amiodarone: When flecainide is given in the presence of amiodarone, reduce the usual flecainide dose by 50% and monitor the patient closely for adverse effects. Plasma level monitoring is strongly recommended to guide dosage with such combination therapy.

Plasma level monitoring: The majority of patients treated successfully had trough plasma levels between 0.2 and 1 mcg/mL. The probability of adverse experiences, especially cardiac, may increase with higher trough plasma levels, especially levels greater than 1 mcg/mL. Monitor trough plasma levels periodically, especially in patients with severe or moderate chronic renal failure or severe hepatic disease and CHF, as drug elimination may be slower.

Actions

Pharmacology: Flecainide has local anesthetic activity and belongs to the membrane stabilizing (Class I) group of antiarrhythmic agents; it has electrophysiologic effects characteristic of the IC class of antiarrhythmics.

Pharmacokinetics:

Absorption/Distribution – Oral absorption is nearly complete. Peak plasma levels are attained at approximately 3 hours. The plasma half-life ranges from 12 to 27 hours after multiple oral doses. Steady-state levels are approached in 3 to 5 days; once at steady-state, no accumulation occurs during chronic therapy. Plasma levels are approximately proportional to dose. In patients with congestive heart failure (CHF; NYHA class III), the rate of flecainide elimination from plasma is moderately slower than for healthy subjects. Plasma protein binding is about 40% and is independent of plasma drug level over the range of 0.015 to about 3.4 mcg/mL.

Metabolism/Excretion – About 30% of a single oral dose (range, 10% to 50%) is excreted in urine unchanged. The two major urinary metabolites are meta-O-dealkylated flecainide (active, but about as potent) and the meta-O-dealkylated lactam (inactive). These two metabolites (primarily conjugated) account for most of the remaining portion of the dose. With increasing renal impairment, the extent of unchanged drug in urine is reduced and the half-life is prolonged. Hemodialysis removes only about 1% of an oral dose as unchanged flecainide.

Contraindications

Preexisting second- or third-degree AV block, right bundle branch block when associated with a left hemiblock (bifascicular block), unless a pacemaker is present to sustain the cardiac rhythm if complete heart block occurs; recent myocardial infarction (MI); presence of cardiogenic shock; hypersensitivity to the drug.

Warnings/Precautions

Mortality: An excessive mortality or nonfatal cardiac arrest rate was seen in patients treated with flecainide compared with that seen in a carefully matched placebo-treated group.

Ventricular proarrhythmic effects in patients with atrial fibrillation/flutter: Flecainide is not recommended for use in patients with chronic atrial fibrillation. Case reports of ventricular proarrhythmic effects in patients treated with flecainide for atrial fibrillation/flutter have included increased premature ventricular contractions (PVCs), ventricular tachycardia (VT), ventricular fibrillation (VF), and death.

Non-life-threatening ventricular arrhythmias: It is prudent to consider the risks of Class IC agents, coupled with the lack of any evidence of improved survival, generally unacceptable in patients whose ventricular arrhythmias are not life-threatening, even if the patients are experiencing unpleasant but not life-threatening symptoms or signs.

Proarrhythmic effects: Flecainide can cause new or worsened arrhythmias. Such proarrhythmic effects range from an increase in frequency of PVCs to the development of more severe ventricular tachycardia.

Sick sinus syndrome: Use only with extreme caution; the drug may cause sinus bradycardia, sinus pause, or sinus arrest. The frequency probably increases with higher trough plasma levels.

Heart failure: Flecainide has a negative inotropic effect and may cause or worsen CHF, particularly in patients with cardiomyopathy, preexisting severe heart failure (NYHA functional class III or IV), or low ejection fractions (less than 30%). The initial dosage should be no more than 100 mg twice/day; monitor patients carefully. Give close attention to maintenance of cardiac function, including optimal digitalis, diuretic or other therapy. Where CHF has developed or worsened during treatment, the time of onset has ranged from a few hours to several months after starting therapy. Some patients who develop reduced myocardial function while on flecainide can continue with adjustment of digitalis or diuretics; others may require dosage reduction or discontinuation of flecainide. When feasible, monitor plasma flecainide levels. Keep trough plasma levels less than 1 mcg/mL.

Cardiac conduction: Flecainide slows cardiac conduction in most patients to produce dose-related increases in PR, QRS, and QT intervals. The degree of lengthening of PR and QRS intervals does not predict either efficacy or the development of cardiac adverse effects. Patients may develop new first-degree AV heart block. Use caution and consider dose reductions. The JT interval (QT minus QRS) only widens approximately 4% on the average. Rare cases of torsade de pointes-type arrhythmias have occurred.

If second-or third-degree AV block, or right bundle branch block associated with a left hemiblock occurs, discontinue therapy unless a ventricular pacemaker is in place to ensure an adequate ventricular rate.

Electrolyte disturbance: Hypokalemia or hyperkalemia may alter the effects of Class I antiarrhythmic drugs. Correct preexisting hypokalemia or hyperkalemia before administration.

Effects on pacemaker thresholds: Flecainide increases endocardial pacing thresholds and may suppress ventricular escape rhythms. These effects are reversible. Use with caution in patients with permanent pacemakers or temporary pacing electrodes. Do not administer to patients with existing poor thresholds or nonprogrammable pacemakers unless suitable pacing rescue is available.

Urinary pH: Flecainide elimination is altered by urinary pH; alkalinization decreases, and acidification increases flecainide renal excretion.

Hepatic function impairment: Because flecainide elimination from plasma can be markedly slower in patients with significant hepatic impairment, do not use in such patients unless the potential benefits outweigh the risks. If used, make dosage increases very cautiously when plasma levels have plateaued (after more than 4 days).

Pregnancy: Category C.

Lactation: Flecainide is excreted in breast milk; determine whether to discontinue breast-feeding or discontinue the drug, taking into account the importance of the drug to the mother.

Children: Safety and efficacy for use in children younger than 18 years of age have not been established.

Based on several studies flecainide appears to be beneficial in treating supraventricular and ventricular arrhythmias in children. Elimination half-life is shorter and volume of distribution is smaller.

Elderly: Patients up to 80 years of age and above have been safely treated with usual doses.

Drug Interactions

Drugs that may affect flecainide include amiodarone, cimetidine, cisapride, disopyramide, propranolol, ritonavir, urinary acidifiers/alkalinizers, and verapamil. Smoking may also have an effect. Drugs that may be affected by flecainide include cisapride, propranolol, and digoxin.

Adverse Reactions

Adverse interactions occurring in at least 3% of patients include dizziness; dyspnea; headache; nausea; fatigue; palpitation; chest pain; asthenia; tremor; constipation; edema; abdominal pain; visual disturbances.

In post-MI patients with asymptomatic PVCs and nonsustained ventricular tachycardia, flecainide therapy was associated with a 5.1% rate of death and nonfatal cardiac arrest, compared with a 2.3% rate in a matched placebo group.

AMIODARONE HYDROCHLORIDE

Tablets: 100, 200, and 400 mg (*Rx*)	Various, *Cordarone* (Wyeth-Ayerst), *Pacerone* (Upsher Smith)
Injection: 50 mg/mL (*Rx*)	Various, *Cordarone* (Wyeth-Ayerst)

Warning:

Oral:

Life-threatening arrhythmias – Amiodarone is intended for use only in patients with the indicated life-threatening arrhythmias because its use is accompanied by substantial toxicity.

Potentially fatal toxicities – Amiodarone has several potentially fatal toxicities, the most important of which is pulmonary toxicity (hypersensitivity pneumonitis or interstitial/alveolar pneumonitis). Pulmonary toxicity has been fatal approximately 10% of the time. Liver injury is common with amiodarone, but is usually mild and evidenced only by abnormal liver enzymes. However, overt liver disease can occur and has been fatal in a few cases. Like other antiarrhythmics, amiodarone can exacerbate the arrhythmia (ie, by making the arrhythmia less well tolerated or more difficult to reverse).

High-risk patients – Even in patients at high risk of arrhythmic death, in whom the toxicity of amiodarone is an acceptable risk, amiodarone poses major management problems that could be life-threatening in a population at risk of sudden death; every effort should be made to utilize alternative agents first.

Patients with the indicated arrhythmias must be hospitalized while the loading dose of amiodarone is given, and a response generally requires at least 1 week, usually 2 or more. Because absorption and elimination are variable, maintenance-dose selection is difficult, and it is not unusual to require dosage decrease or discontinuation of treatment. The time at which a previously controlled life-threatening arrhythmia will recur after discontinuation or dose adjustment is unpredictable, ranging from weeks to months. The patient is obviously at great risk during this time and may need prolonged hospitalization. Attempts to substitute other antiarrhythmic agents when amiodarone must be stopped will be made difficult by the gradually, but unpredictably, changing amiodarone body burden. A similar problem exists when amiodarone is not effective; it still poses the risk of an interaction with whatever subsequent treatment is tried.

Indications

Ventricular arrhythmias:

Oral – Only for treatment of the following documented life-threatening recurrent ventricular arrhythmias that do not respond to documented adequate doses of other antiarrhythmics or when alternative agents are not tolerated:

1.) Recurrent ventricular fibrillation (VF).

2.) Recurrent hemodynamically unstable ventricular tachycardia (VT).

Parenteral – Initiation of treatment and prophylaxis of frequently recurring VF and hemodynamically unstable VT in patients refractory to other therapy. It can also be used to treat patients with VT/VF for whom oral amiodarone is indicated, but who are unable to take oral medication.

During or after treatment with IV amiodarone, patients may be transferred to oral amiodarone therapy. Use IV amiodarone for acute treatment until the patient's ventricular arrhythmias are stabilized. Most patients require this therapy for 48 to 96 hours, but IV amiodarone may be given safely for longer periods if needed.

Administration and Dosage

Oral: In order to ensure that an antiarrhythmic effect will be observed without waiting several months, loading doses are required. Individual patient titration is suggested. Because of the food effect on absorption, amiodarone should be administered consistently with regard to meals.

Life-threatening ventricular arrhythmias (VF or hemodynamically unstable VT) – Administer the loading dose in a hospital. Loading doses of 800 to 1,600 mg/day are required for 1 to 3 weeks (occasionally longer) until initial therapeutic response occurs. Administer in divided doses with meals for total daily doses of at least 1,000 mg, or when GI intolerance occurs. If side effects become excessive, reduce the dose. Elimination of recurrence of VF and tachycardia usually occurs within 1 to 3 weeks, along with reduction in complex and total ventricular ectopic beats.

Dose titration/adjustment – When starting amiodarone therapy, attempt to gradually discontinue prior antiarrhythmic drugs. When adequate arrhythmia control is achieved, or if side effects become prominent, reduce dose to 600 to 800 mg/day for 1 month and then to the maintenance dose, usually 400 mg/day. Some patients may require larger maintenance doses, up to 600 mg/day, and some can be controlled on lower doses. Amiodarone may be administered as a single daily dose, or in patients with severe GI intolerance, as twice daily dosing.

Parenteral: The recommended starting dose of amiodarone injection is about 1,000 mg over the first 24 hours of therapy, delivered by the following infusion regimen:

Amiodarone IV Dose Recommendations During the First 24 Hours	
Loading infusions	
First rapid	150 mg over the *first* 10 min (15 mg/min). Add 3 mL amiodarone IV (150 mg) to 100 mL D5W (concentration, 1.5 mg/mL). Infuse 100 mL/10 min.
Followed by slow	360 mg over the *next* 6 hours (1 mg/min). Add 18 mL amiodarone IV (900 mg) to 500 mL D5W (concentration, 1.8 mg/mL).
Maintenance infusion	540 mg over the *remaining* 18 hours (0.5 mg/min). Decrease the rate of the slow loading infusion to 0.5 mg/min.

After the first 24 hours, continue the maintenance infusion rate of 0.5 mg/min (720 mg/24 hours) utilizing a concentration of 1 to 6 mg/mL (amiodarone injection concentrations greater than 2 mg/mL should be administered via a central venous catheter). Use an in-line filter during administration. In the event of breakthrough episodes of VF or hemodynamically unstable VT, 150 mg supplemental infusions of amiodarone IV mixed in 100 mL D5W may be given. Administer such infusions over 10 minutes to minimize the potential for hypotension.

Amiodarone injection concentrations greater than 2 mg/mL should be administered via a central venous catheter. Use an in-line filter during administration.

Amiodarone IV infusions exceeding 2 hours must be administered in glass or polyolefin bottles containing D5W.

Amiodarone adsorbs to polyvinyl chloride (PVC) tubing, and the clinical trial dose administration schedule was designed to account for this adsorption; therefore its use is recommended.

Admixture incompatibility – Amiodarone IV in D5W, in a concentration of 4 mg/mL, forms a precipitate and is incompatible with the following drugs: Aminophylline, cefamandole, cefazolin, mezlocillin, heparin (no amiodarone concentration stated), and sodium bicarbonate (amiodarone concentration of 3 mg/mL).

IV to oral transition:

Recommendations for Oral Amiodarone Dosage After IV Infusion	
Duration of amiodarone IV infusions[a]	Initial daily dose of oral amiodarone
< 1 week	800 to 1,600 mg
1 to 3 weeks	600 to 800 mg
> 3 weeks[b]	400 mg

[a] Assuming a 720 mg/day infusion (0.5 mg/min).
[b] Amiodarone IV is not intended for maintenance treatment.

Actions

Pharmacology: Amiodarone possesses electrophysiologic characteristics of all 4 Vaughan Williams Classes but has predominantly Class III antiarrhythmic effects. The antiarrhythmic effect may be due to at least 2 major properties: Prolongation of the myocardial cell-action potential duration and refractory period, and noncompetitive α- and β-adrenergic inhibition.

Pharmacokinetics:

Absorption – Following oral administration, amiodarone is slowly and variably absorbed; bioavailability is approximately 50%. Maximum plasma concentrations are attained 3 to 7 hours after a single dose. The onset of action may occur in 2 to 3 days, but more commonly takes 1 to 3 weeks, even with loading doses.

Peak concentrations after 10-minute infusions of 150 mg in patients with VF or hemodynamically unstable VT range between 7 and 26 mg/L. Due to rapid distribution, serum concentrations decline to 10% of peak values within 30 to 45 minutes after the end of the infusion.

Distribution – Amiodarone has a very large but variable volume of distribution, averaging about 60 L/kg. The drug is highly protein bound (approximately 96%).

Metabolism – Amiodarone is metabolized principally by CYP3A4. Because grapefruit juice is known to inhibit CYP3A4-mediated metabolism of oral amiodarone, grapefruit juice should not be taken during treatment with oral amiodarone.

Excretion – Following discontinuation of chronic oral therapy, amiodarone has a biphasic elimination with an initial one-half reduction of plasma levels after 2.5 to 107 days. A much slower terminal plasma elimination phase shows a half-life of the parent compound of approximately 53 days. For the metabolite, mean plasma elimination half-life was approximately 61 days. Antiarrhythmic effects persist for weeks or months after the drug is discontinued.

The main route of elimination is via hepatic excretion into bile; some enterohepatic recirculation may occur. The drug has a very low plasma clearance with negligible renal excretion. Neither amiodarone nor its metabolite is dialyzable.

Contraindications

Hypersensitivity to the drug or any of its components, including iodine.

Oral: Severe sinus-node dysfunction, causing marked sinus bradycardia; second- and third-degree AV block; when episodes of bradycardia have caused syncope (except when used in conjunction with a pacemaker).

Parenteral: Marked sinus bradycardia; second- and third-degree AV block unless a functioning pacemaker is available; cardiogenic shock.

Warnings/Precautions

Potentially fatal toxicities: See Warning Box for more information.

Life-threatening arrhythmias: See Warning Box for more information.

Ophthalmologic effects:

Oral – Optic neuropathy or neuritis may occur at any time following initiation of therapy, in some cases, visual impairment has progressed to permanent blindness. Corneal microdeposits appear in virtually all adults treated with amiodarone. They give rise to symptoms such as visual halos or blurred vision in as many as 10% of patients. Corneal microdeposits are reversible upon reduction of dose or drug discontinuation. Asymptomatic microdeposits are not a reason to reduce dose or stop treatment.

Pulmonary toxicity:

Oral – Amiodarone may cause a clinical syndrome of cough and progressive dyspnea accompanied by functional, radiographic, gallium scan, and pathological data consistent with pulmonary toxicity. The frequency varies from 2% to 17%; fatalities occur in about 10% of cases. However, in patients with life-threatening arrhythmias, discontinuation of amiodarone therapy due to suspected drug-induced pulmonary toxicity should be undertaken with caution, as the most common cause of death in these patients is sudden cardiac death.

Any new respiratory symptom suggests pulmonary toxicity, therefore repeat and evaluate the history, physical exam, chest x-ray, gallium scan, and pulmonary function tests (with diffusion capacity). In some cases, rechallenge at a lower dose has not resulted in return of interstitial/alveolar pneumonitis.

Hypersensitivity pneumonitis: Hypersensitivity pneumonitis usually appears earlier in the course of therapy, and rechallenging these patients results in a more rapid recurrence of greater severity.

Interstitial/alveolar pneumonitis: Interstitial/alveolar pneumonitis is characterized by findings of diffuse alveolar damage, interstitial pneumonitis or fibrosis in lung biopsy specimens. A diagnosis of amiodarone-induced interstitial/alveolar pneumonitis should lead to dose reduction or to withdrawal of amiodarone to establish reversibility. With these measures, a reduction in symptoms of amiodarone-induced pulmonary toxicity was usually noted within the first week.

Pulmonary fibrosis –

IV: Only 1 of more than 1,000 patients treated with amiodarone IV in clinical studies developed pulmonary fibrosis.

Cardiac effects:

Oral –

Proarrhythmias: Amiodarone can cause serious exacerbation of the presenting arrhythmia, a risk that may be enhanced by concomitant antiarrhythmics. In addition, amiodarone has caused symptomatic bradycardia, heart block, or sinus arrest with suppression of escape foci. Treat bradycardia by slowing the infusion rate or discontinuing amiodarone IV. In some patients, inserting a pacemaker is required. Cardiac conduction abnormalities are infrequent and reversible on discontinuation.

IV –

Hypotension: Hypotension is the most common adverse effect seen with amiodarone IV. Clinically significant hypotension during infusions was seen most often in the first several hours of treatment and appeared to be related to the rate of infusion. Treat hypotension initially by slowing the infusion; additional standard therapy may be needed.

Bradycardia and AV block: Drug-related bradycardia in clinical trials for life-threatening VT/VF; it was not dose-related. Treat bradycardia by slowing the infusion rate or discontinuing amiodarone injection. Inserting a pacemaker is required.

Proarrhythmia: Amiodarone injection may cause a worsening of existing arrhythmias or precipitate a new arrhythmia. Proarrhythmia, primarily torsades de pointes, has been associated with prolongation of the QTc interval to 500 ms or greater.

Hepatic effects:

Oral – Elevated hepatic enzyme levels (AST and ALT) are frequent, and in most cases are asymptomatic. If the increase exceeds 3 times normal, or doubles in a patient with an elevated baseline, consider discontinuation or dosage reduction.

Parenteral – Elevations of blood hepatic enzyme values, ALT, AST, and GGT, are seen commonly in patients with immediately life-threatening VT/VF.

In patients with life-threatening arrhythmias, weigh the potential risk of hepatic injury against the potential benefit of therapy. Monitor carefully for evidence of progressive hepatic injury. Give consideration to reducing the rate of administration or withdrawing amiodarone IV in such cases.

CNS effects: Chronic administration of oral amiodarone in rare instances may lead to the development of peripheral neuropathy that may resolve when amiodarone is discontinued, but this resolution has been slow and incomplete.

Thyroid abnormalities: Amiodarone inhibits peripheral conversion of thyroxine (T_4) to triiodothyronine (T_3), prompting increased T_4 levels, increased levels of inactive reverse T_3 and decreased levels of T_3. It is also a potential source of large amounts of inorganic iodine. It can cause hypothyroidism or hyperthyroidism. High plasma iodide levels, altered thyroid function, and abnormal thyroid function tests may persist for several weeks or even months following amiodarone withdrawal.

Hypothyroidism – Hypothyroidism is best managed by amiodarone dose reduction and thyroid hormone supplement.

Hyperthyroidism – Hyperthyroidism usually poses a greater hazard to the patient than hypothyroidism because of the possibility of arrhythmia breakthrough or aggravation. If any new signs of arrhythmia appear, consider the possibility of hyperthyroidism. Aggressive medical treatment is indicated, including, dose reduction or withdrawal of amiodarone.

Surgery:

IV and oral – Close perioperative monitoring is recommended in patients undergoing general anesthesia who are on amiodarone therapy as they may be more sensitive to the myocardial depressant and conduction effects of halogenated inhalational anesthetics.

Hypotension postbypass –

Oral: Rare occasions of hypotension upon discontinuation of cardiopulmonary bypass during open-heart surgery in patients receiving amiodarone have been reported.

Pulmonary toxicity: There have been postmarketing reports of acute-onset (days to weeks) pulmonary injury in patients treated with amiodarone IV. Findings have included pulmonary infiltrates on X-ray, bronchospasm, wheezing, fever, dyspnea, cough, hemoptysis, and hypoxia.

Adult respiratory distress syndrome (ARDS): ARDS has been reported in clinical studies and in patients who have undergone either cardiac or noncardiac surgery.

Electrolyte disturbances: Correct potassium or magnesium deficiency before therapy begins as these disorders can exaggerate the degree of QTc prolongation and increase the potential for torsades de pointes.

Benzyl alcohol (IV): Benzyl alcohol, contained in some of these products as a preservative, has been associated with a fatal "gasping syndrome" in premature infants.

Photosensitivity: Amiodarone has induced photosensitization in about 10% of patients. During long-term treatment, a blue-gray discoloration of the exposed skin may occur; some protection may be afforded by sun barrier creams or protective clothing.

Pregnancy: *Category D.*

Lactation: Amiodarone is excreted in breast milk. When amiodarone therapy is indicated, advise the mother to discontinue breast-feeding.

Children: Safety and efficacy for use in children have not been established. Amiodarone is not recommended in children.

Elderly: In general, dose selection for an elderly patient should be cautious, usually starting at the low end of the dosing range, reflecting the greater frequency of decreased hepatic, renal, or cardiac function, and of concomitant disease or other drug therapy.

Monitoring: Perform baseline chest x-rays and pulmonary function tests, including diffusion capacity before therapy initiation. Repeat a history, physical exam, and chest x-ray every 3 to 6 months.

Monitor thyroid function at baseline and periodically during therapy, particularly in the elderly and in any patient with a history of thyroid nodules, goiter, or other thyroid dysfunction.

Perform regular ophthalmic examination, including fundoscopy and slit-lamp examination, during administration of amiodarone.

Monitor liver enzymes on a regular basis.

Closely monitor FiO_2 and the determinants of oxygen delivery to the tissues (eg, SaO_2, PaO_2) in patients on amiodarone.

Drug Interactions

Drugs that may affect amiodarone include azole antifungal agents, cholestyramine, cimetidine, fluoroquinolones, hydantoins, macrolide antibiotics, protease inhibitors, rifamycins, and St. John's wort.

Drugs that may be affected by amiodarone include anticoagulants, beta-blockers, calcium channel blockers, cisapride, cyclosporine, dextromethorphan, digoxin, disopyramide, fentanyl, flecainide, HMG-CoA reductase inhibitors, hydantoins, lidocaine, methotrexate, procainamide, quinidine, theophylline, thioridazine, vardenafil, ziprasidone.

Drug/Lab test interactions: Amiodarone alters the results of thyroid function tests, causing an increase in serum T_4 and serum reverse T_3 levels and a decline in serum T_3 levels. Despite these biochemical changes, most patients remain clinically euthyroid.

Drug/Food interactions: Grapefruit juice inhibits metabolism of oral amiodarone in the intestinal mucosa, resulting in increased amiodarone AUC and C_{max}. Consider this information when changing from intravenous amiodarone to oral amiodarone. Because of the food effect on absorption, amiodarone should be administered consistently with regard to meals.

Adverse Reactions

Oral – Adverse reactions occurring in 3% or more of patients include the following: abnormal gait/ataxia, abnormal liver function tests, anorexia, congestive heart failure, constipation, dizziness, exacerbation of arrythmias, fibrosis, lack of coordination, malaise and fatigue, nausea, paresthesia, peripheral neuropathy, poor coordination and gait, photosensitivity, pulmonary inflammation, solar dermatitis, tremor and involuntary movements, visual disturbances, vomiting.

Parenteral – The most important treatment-emergent adverse effects were hypotension, asystole/cardiac arrest/electromechanical dissociation (EMD), cardiogenic shock, CHF, bradycardia, liver function test abnormalities, VT, and AV block. The most common adverse effects leading to discontinuation of IV therapy were hypotension, asystole/cardiac arrest/EMD, VT, and cardiogenic shock. Adverse reactions occurring in at least 3% of patients include nausea.

CALCIUM CHANNEL BLOCKING AGENTS

AMLODIPINE	
Tablets; oral: 2.5, 5, and 10 mg (*Rx*)	Various, *Norvasc* (Pfizer), *Amvaz* (Reddy)
CLEVIDIPINE BUTYRATE	
Injection, solution: 0.5 mg/mL (*Rx*)	*Cleviprex* (The Medicines Co)
DILTIAZEM HYDROCHLORIDE	
Tablets; oral: 30, 60, 90, and 120 mg (*Rx*)	Various, *Cardizem* (Biovail)
Tablets, extended-release; oral: 120, 180, 240, 300, 360, 420 mg (*Rx*)	*Cardizem LA* (Abbott)
Capsules, extended-release; oral: 60 and 90 mg (*Rx*)	Various
120, 180, and 240 mg (*Rx*)	Various, *Cardizem CD* (Biovail), *CartiaXT* (Andrx), *Diltia XT* (Andrx), *Dilt-CD* (Apotex), *Tiazac* (Forest), *Taztia XT* (Andrx)
300 mg (*Rx*)	Various, *Cardizem CD* (Biovail), *CartiaXT* (Andrx), *Dilt-CD* (Apotex), *Tiazac* (Forest), *Taztia XT* (Andrx)
360 mg (*Rx*)	Various, *Cardizem CD* (Biovail), *Tiazac* (Forest), *Taztia XT* (Andrx)
420 mg (*Rx*)	Various, *Tiazac* (Forest)
Injection, solution: 5 mg/mL (*Rx*)	Various
Injection, powder for solution: 25 mg (*Rx*)	*Cardizem* (Bioavail)
FELODIPINE	
Tablets, extended-release; oral: 2.5, 5, and 10 mg (*Rx*)	Various
ISRADIPINE	
Tablets, controlled-release; oral: 5 and 10 mg (*Rx*)	*DynaCirc CR* (Reliant)
Capsules; oral: 2.5 and 5 mg (*Rx*)	Various
NICARDIPINE HYDROCHLORIDE	
Capsules; oral: 20 and 30 mg (*Rx*)	Various
Capsules, sustained-release; oral: 30, 45, and 60 mg (*Rx*)	*Cardene SR* (EKR Therapeutics)
Injection, solution: 0.1 and 0.2 mg/mL (*Rx*)	*Cardene I.V.* (EKR Therapeutics)
2.5 mg/mL (*Rx*)	
NIFEDIPINE	
Tablets, extended-release; oral: 30, 60, and 90 mg (*Rx*)	Various, *Adalat CC* (Schering), *Afeditab CR* (Watson), *Nifediac CC*, *Nifedical XL* (Teva), *Procardia XL* (Pfizer)
Capsules; oral: 10 and 20 mg (*Rx*)	Various, *Procardia* (Pfizer)
NIMODIPINE	
Capsules, liquid-filled; oral: 30 mg (*Rx*)	Various
NISOLDIPINE	
Tablets, extended-release; oral: 8.5, 17, 20, 25.5, 30, 34, and 40 mg (*Rx*)	Various, *Sular* (Sciele Pharma)
VERAPAMIL HYDROCHLORIDE	
Tablets; oral: 40, 80, and 120 mg (*Rx*)	Various
Tablets, extended-release; oral: 120 mg (*Rx*)	Various, *Calan SR* (Pfizer), *Isoptin SR* (FSC)
180 and 240 mg (*Rx*)	Various, *Calan SR*, *Covera-HS* (Pfizer), *Isoptin SR* (FSC)
Capsules, extended-release; oral: 120, 180, 240, and 360 mg (*Rx*)	Various, *Verelan* (Schwarz Pharma)
100, 200, and 300 mg (*Rx*)	Various, *Verelan PM* (Schwarz Pharma)
Injection: 2.5 mg/mL (*Rx*)	Various

Warning:

Nimodipine: Do not administer nimodipine intravenously (IV) or by other parenteral routes. Deaths and serious, life-threatening adverse reactions have occurred when the contents of nimodipine capsules have been injected parenterally.

Indications

Calcium Channel Blocking Agents – Summary of Indications[a]

Indications	Amlodipine	Clevidipine	Diltiazem	Diltiazem SR	Diltiazem ER	Diltiazem IV	Felodipine	Isradipine	Nicardipine	Nicardipine SR	Nicardipine IV	Nifedipine	Nifedipine ER	Nimodipine	Nisoldipine	Verapamil	Verapamil SR	Verapamil ER	Verapamil IV
Angina pectoris																			
Vasospastic	✓		✓		✓							✓	✓[b]			✓		✓[c]	
Chronic stable	✓		✓		✓				✓			✓	✓[b]			✓		✓[c]	
Unstable																✓		✓[c]	
Hypertension	✓	✓		✓	✓		✓	✓	✓	✓	✓		✓		✓	✓	✓	✓	
Subarachnoid hemorrhage														✓					
Atrial fibrillation/ flutter						✓													✓
Paroxysmal supraventricular tachycardia						✓										✓[d]			✓

[a] For more detailed information, see the information following and individual drug monographs.
[b] Except *Adalat* CC.
[c] *Covera-HS* only.
[d] For prophylaxis of repetitive paroxysmal supraventricular tachycardia.

Administration and Dosage

Swallow extended-release tablets and sustained-release capsule forms whole; do not bite, open, chew, crush, or divide.

AMLODIPINE: May be taken without regard to meals.

Hypertension – Usual dose is 5 mg once daily. Maximum dose is 10 mg once daily. Small, fragile, or elderly patients or patients with hepatic function impairment may be started on 2.5 mg once daily; or when adding amlodipine to other antihypertensive therapy. In general, titrate over 7 to 14 days; proceed more rapidly if clinically warranted.

Angina (chronic stable or vasospastic) – 5 to 10 mg, using the lower dose for elderly patients and patients with hepatic function impairment. Most patients require 10 mg.

CLEVIDIPINE:

Monitoring – Monitor blood pressure and heart rate continually during infusion, and then until vital signs are stable.

Rebound hypertension: Patients who receive prolonged clevidipine infusions and are not transitioned to other antihypertensive therapies should be monitored for the possibility of rebound hypertension for at least 8 hours after the infusion is stopped.

Initial dosage – Initiate the IV infusion at 1 to 2 mg/h.

Dosage titration – The dose may be doubled at short (90-second) intervals initially. As the blood pressure approaches the goal, the increase in doses should be less than doubling and the time between dose adjustments should be lengthened to every 5 to 10 minutes. An approximately 1 to 2 mg/h increase will generally produce an additional 2 to 4 mm Hg decrease in systolic pressure.

Maintenance dosage – The desired therapeutic response for most patients occurs at doses of 4 to 6 mg/h. Patients with severe hypertension may require doses of up to 32 mg/h.

Duration of therapy – There is little experience with infusion durations beyond 72 hours at any dose.

Hepatic/Renal function impairment – An initial infusion rate of 1 to 2 mg/h is appropriate in these patients.

Administration – Clevidipine is intended for IV use.

Admixture compatibility –

Incompatibility: Clevidipine should not be administered in the same line as other medications.

Compatibility: Clevidipine should not be diluted, but it can be administered with the following:

- water for injection
- sodium chloride 0.9% injection
- dextrose 5% injection
- dextrose 5% in sodium chloride 0.9% injection
- dextrose 5% in Ringer's lactate injection
- Ringer's lactate injection
- 10% amino acid.

DILTIAZEM HYDROCHLORIDE:

Oral –

Tablets, immediate-release: Start with 30 mg 4 times/day before meals and at bedtime; gradually increase dosage to 180 to 360 mg (given in divided doses 3 or 4 times/day) at 1- to 2-day intervals until optimum response is obtained. The average optimum dosage range appears to be 180 to 360 mg/day.

Tablets, extended-release: Intended for once daily administration. Switch to once daily extended-release diltiazem tablets at the nearest equivalent total daily dose.

Swallow tablets whole; do not crush or chew. Take tablets at about the same time once every day, either in the morning or at bedtime.

Hypertension – Starting dose is 180 to 240 mg once daily. Maximum effect usually is observed by 14 days of therapy. Maximum dose is 540 mg daily.

Angina – Initial dose of 180 mg may be increased at intervals of 7 to 14 days if adequate response is not obtained. Doses above 360 mg appear not to confer any additional benefit.

Extended-release capsules:

Hypertension – Start with 60 to 120 mg twice daily or 180 to 240 mg once daily. Optimum dosage range is 240 to 360 mg/day. Individual patients may respond to higher doses of up to 480 mg once daily.

Angina – Start with 120 or 180 mg once daily. Individual patients may respond to higher doses of up to 480 mg once daily. Titrate dose change over 7 to 14 days.

Cardizem CD and Cartia XT –

Hypertension: 180 to 240 mg once daily. Maximum effect is usually achieved by 14 days of therapy. Usual range is 240 to 360 mg once daily; experience with doses more than 360 mg is limited.

Angina: Start with 120 or 180 mg once daily. Some patients may respond to higher doses of up to 480 mg once daily. Titration may be carried out over a 7- to 14-day period.

Dilacor XR and Diltia XT –

Hypertension: 180 to 240 mg once daily. Patients, particularly those 60 years of age or older, may respond to a lower dose of 120 mg. Usual range is 180 to 480 mg once daily. Do not exceed 540 mg once daily.

Angina: Start with 120 mg once daily, which may be titrated to doses of up to 480 mg once daily. When necessary, titrate over a 7- to 14-day period.

Administration in the morning on an empty stomach is recommended.

Tiazac –

Hypertension: Usual starting doses are 120 to 240 mg once daily. Maximum effect is usually observed by 14 days of therapy. The usual dosage range is 120 to 540 mg once daily.

Angina: Start with a dose of 120 to 180 mg once daily. Patients may respond to higher doses of up to 540 mg once daily. Titration should be carried out over 7 to 14 days.

Parenteral –

Direct IV single injections (bolus): The initial dose is 0.25 mg/kg as a bolus administered over 2 minutes (20 mg is the dose for the average patient). If response is inadequate, a second dose may be administered after 15 minutes. The second bolus dose should be 0.35 mg/kg administered over 2 minutes (25 mg is the dose for the average patient). Individualize subsequent IV bolus doses. Dose patients with low body weights on a mg/kg basis. Some patients may respond to an initial dose of 0.15 mg/kg, although duration of action may be shorter.

Continuous IV infusion: Immediately following bolus administration of 20 mg (0.25 mg/kg) or 25 mg (0.35 mg/kg) and reduction of heart rate, begin an IV infusion. The recommended initial infusion rate is 10 mg/h. The infusion rate may be increased in 5 mg/h increments up to 15 mg/h as needed, if further reduction in heart rate is required. The infusion may be maintained for up to 24 hours.

Concomitant therapy: Concomitant therapy with β-blockers or digitalis is usually well tolerated, but the effects of coadministration cannot be predicted, especially in patients with left ventricular dysfunction or cardiac conduction abnormalities.

Use caution in titrating dosages for patients with renal or hepatic function impairment, since dosage requirements are not available.

FELODIPINE: The recommended starting dose is 5 mg once daily. The dosage can be decreased to 2.5 mg or increased to 10 mg once daily. Adjustments should occur at intervals of not less than 2 weeks. The recommended dosage range is 2.5 to 10 mg once daily.

ISRADIPINE:

Capsules – Recommended initial dose is 2.5 mg twice daily. Response usually occurs within 2 to 3 hours; maximal response may require 2 to 4 weeks. If a satisfactory response does not occur, the dose may be adjusted in increments of 5 mg/day at 2 to 4 week intervals up to a maximum of 20 mg/day.

Tablets, controlled-release – Recommended initial dose is 5 mg once daily. Response usually occurs within 2 hours with the peak response occurring 8 to 10 hours post-dose. If necessary, the dose may be adjusted in increments of 5 mg at 2- to 4-week intervals up to a maximum dose of 20 mg/day.

Swallow controlled-release tablets whole; do not bite or divide.

NICARDIPINE HYDROCHLORIDE:

Oral –

Angina (immediate-release only): Usual initial dose is 20 mg 3 times/day (range, 20 to 40 mg 3 times/day). Allow at least 3 days before increasing dose.

Hypertension (immediate-release only): Initial dose is 20 mg 3 times/day (range, 20 to 40 mg 3 times/day). The maximum BP-lowering effect occurs approximately 1 to 2 hours after dosing.

Hypertension (sustained-release): Initial dose is 30 mg twice daily. Effective doses range from 30 to 60 mg twice daily.

Renal function impairment: Titrate dose beginning with 20 mg 3 times/day (immediate-release) or 30 mg twice/day (sustained-release).

Hepatic function impairment: Starting dose is 20 mg twice/day (immediate-release) with individual titration.

Parenteral –

Hypertension:

Initial dosage –

Premixed injection (0.1 mg/mL): 50 mL/h (5 mg/h).

Premixed injection (0.2 mg/mL): 25 mL/h (5 mg/h).

Vials: 50 mL/h (5 mg/h).

Dosage titration –

Premixed injection (0.1 mg/mL): If desired blood pressure reduction is not achieved at initial dosage, the infusion rate may be increased by 25 mL/h (2.5 mg/h) every 15 minutes, until desired blood pressure reduction is achieved. For a more rapid blood pressure reduction, initiate therapy at 50 mL/h (5 mg/h). If desired blood pressure reduction is not achieved at this dose, the infusion rate may be increased by 25 mL/h (2.5 mg/h) every 5 minutes until desired blood pressure is achieved. Following achievement of the blood pressure goal, the infusion rate should be decreased to 30 mL/h (3 mg/h).

Premixed injection (0.2 mg/mL): If desired blood pressure reduction is not achieved at initial dosage, the infusion rate may be increased by 12.5 mL/h (2.5 mg/h) every 15 minutes until desired blood pressure reduction is achieved. For a more rapid blood pressure reduction, initiate therapy at 25 mL/h (5 mg/h). If desired blood pressure reduction is not achieved at this dose, the infusion rate may be increased by 12.5 mL/h (2.5 mg/h) every 5 minutes until desired blood pressure is achieved. Following achievement of the blood pressure goal, the infusion rate should be decreased to 15 mL/h (3 mg/h).

Vials: If desired blood pressure reduction is not achieved at initial dosage, the infusion rate may be increased by 25 mL/h (2.5 mg/h) every 15 minutes until desired blood pressure reduction is achieved. For more rapid blood pressure reduction, titrate every 5 minutes.

Maintenance dosage – Adjust the rate of infusion as needed to maintain desired response.

Discontinuation – When treating acute hypertensive episodes in patients with chronic hypertension, discontinuation of infusion is followed by a 50% offset of action in 30 ± 7 minutes, but plasma levels of drug and gradually decreasing antihypertensive effects exist for approximately 50 hours.

Hypotension or tachycardia – If there is concern of impending hypotension or tachycardia, discontinue the infusion. When blood pressure has stabilized, infusion may be restarted at low doses (eg, 30 to 50 mL/h) and adjusted to maintain desired blood pressure.

Premixed injection (0.1 mg/mL): 30 to 50 mL/h (3 to 5 mg/h).

Premixed injection (0.2 mg/mL): 15 to 25 mL/h (3 to 5 mg/h).

Vials: 30 to 50 mL/h (3 to 5 mg/h).

Impaired cardiac, hepatic, or renal function – Caution is advised when titrating nicardipine IV in patients with congestive heart failure or impaired hepatic or renal function.

Administration – Nicardipine injection is administered by slow continuous infusion. The infusion site should be changed every 12 hours if administered via peripheral vein.

Premixed injection: Do not use plastic container in series connections. Such use could result in air embolism because of residual air being drawn from the primary container before the administration of the fluid from the secondary container is complete.

Oral to injection therapy:

Equivalent Nicardipine Doses: Oral vs IV Infusion	
Oral dose	Equivalent IV infusion rate
20 mg every 8 h	0.5 mg/h
30 mg every 8 h	1.2 mg/h
40 mg every 8 h	2.2 mg/h

Injection to oral therapy: If treatment includes transfer to an oral antihypertensive other than nicardipine, generally initiate therapy upon discontinuation of the infusion. If oral nicardipine is to be used, administer the first dose of a 3-times-daily regimen 1 hour prior to discontinuation of the infusion.

Elderly – Dose selection for an elderly patient should be cautious, usually starting at the low end of the dosing range, reflecting the greater frequency of decreased hepatic, renal, or cardiac function, and of concomitant disease or drug therapy.

NIFEDIPINE:

Initial dosage (capsule) – 10 mg 3 times/day; swallow whole. Usual range is 10 to 20 mg 3 times/day. Some patients, especially those with coronary artery spasm, respond to 20 to 30 mg 3 or 4 times/day. More than 180 mg/day is not recommended.

Titrate throughout 7 to 14 days to assess response.

Sustained-release –

Procardia XL/Nifedical XL: 30 or 60 mg once daily. Titrate over a 7- to 14-day period. Titration may proceed more rapidly if the patient is frequently assessed. Titration to doses more than 120 mg is not recommended.

Angina patients maintained on the capsule formulation may be switched to the sustained release tablet at the nearest equivalent total daily dose. Experience with doses more than 90 mg in angina is limited.

Adalat CC: Administer once daily on an empty stomach. In general, titrate over a 7- to 14-day period starting with 30 mg once daily. Usual maintenance dose is 30 to 60 mg once daily. Titration to doses more than 90 mg daily is not recommended.

Concomitant drug therapy – Concomitant drug therapy with β-blockers may be beneficial in chronic stable angina.

NIMODIPINE: Commence therapy within 96 hours of the subarachnoid hemorrhage (SAH), using 60 mg every 4 hours for 21 consecutive days.

If the capsule cannot be swallowed (eg, time of surgery, unconscious patient), make a hole in both ends of the capsule with an 18 gauge needle and extract the contents into a syringe. Empty the contents into the patient's in situ nasogastric tube and wash down the tube with 30 mg normal saline.

NISOLDIPINE:

Dosage –

Initial dosage: The dosage of nisoldipine must be adjusted to each patient's needs. Therapy usually should be initiated with 17 mg orally once daily, then increased by 8.5 mg per week or longer intervals to attain adequate control of blood pressure.

Maintenance dosage: Usual maintenance dosage is 17 to 34 mg once daily. Blood pressure response increases over the 8.5 to 34 mg daily dose range, but adverse reaction rates also increase.

Maximum dosage: Dosages beyond 34 mg once daily are not recommended.

Concomitant drug therapy – Nisoldipine has been used safely with diuretics, angiotensin-converting enzyme (ACE) inhibitors, and beta-blocking agents.

Elderly/Hepatic function impairment – Patients older than 65 years of age or patients with hepatic function impairment are expected to develop higher plasma concentrations of nisoldipine. Their blood pressure should be monitored closely during any dosage adjustment. A starting dose not exceeding 8.5 mg daily is recommended in these patient groups.

Administration – Nisoldipine tablets should be administered orally once daily. Nisoldipine should be taken on an empty stomach (1 hour before or 2 hours after a meal). Administration with a high-fat meal can lead to excessive peak drug concentration and should be avoided. Grapefruit products should be avoided before and after dosing. Nisoldipine is an extended-release dosage form and tablets should be swallowed whole, not bitten, divided, or crushed.

VERAPAMIL HYDROCHLORIDE: Avoid verapamil in patients with severe left ventricular dysfunction (eg, ejection fractions less than 30%) or moderate to severe symptoms of cardiac failure and in patients with any degree of ventricular dysfunction if they are receiving a beta-adrenergic blocker.

Do not exceed 480 mg/day; safety and efficacy are not established.

Lower initial doses may be warranted in patients who may have an increased response to verapamil (eg, elderly people, those of small stature, those with hepatic function impairment). Base upward titration on therapeutic efficacy and safety evaluated approximately 24 hours after dosing. The antihypertensive effects of verapamil are evident within the first week of therapy.

Immediate-release –

Angina: Usual initial dose is 80 to 120 mg 3 times/day; 40 mg 3 times/day may be warranted if patients have increased response to verapamil (eg, decreased hepatic function, elderly). Base upward titration of safety and efficacy evaluated about 8 hours after dosing. Increase dosage daily (eg, unstable angina) or weekly until optimum clinical response is obtained.

Arrhythmias: Dosage range in digitalized patients with chronic atrial fibrillation is 240 to 320 mg/day in divided doses 3 or 4 times/day. Dosage range for prophylaxis of paroxysmal supraventricular tachycardia (PSVT) (non-digitalized patients) is 240 to 480 mg/day in divided doses 3 or 4 times/day. In general, maximum effects will be apparent during the first 48 hours of therapy.

Hypertension: The usual initial monotherapy dose is 80 mg 3 times/day (240 mg/day). Daily dosages of 360 and 480 mg have been used, but there is no evidence that dosages more than 360 mg provide added effect.

Extended-release – Swallow whole; do not chew, break, or crush the tablets.

Capsules: The usual daily dose is 240 mg once daily in the morning.

Tablets: Initiate therapy with 180 mg given in the morning.

Covera-HS tablets: Initiate therapy with 180 mg/day at bedtime. Dose range is between 180 and 540 mg per day given at bedtime.

Verelan PM: Usual daily dose is 200 mg/day at bedtime.

Sustained-release – When switching from the immediate-release formulation, total daily dose (in mg) may remain the same.

Calan SR and Isoptin SR: Initiate therapy with 180 mg given in the morning with food.

Sustained-release characteristics are not altered when the tablet is divided in half.

Verelan: Usual daily dose is 240 mg once daily in the morning.

Pellet-filled capsules: Do not chew or crush the contents of the capsule. Pellet-filled capsules also may be administered by carefully opening the capsule and sprinkling the pellets on a spoonful of applesauce. Swallow the applesauce immediately without chewing and follow with a glass of cool water to ensure complete swallowing of the pellets. Use any pellet/applesauce mixture immediately and do not store for future use. Subdividing the contents of the capsule is not recommended.

Parenteral (supraventricular tachyarrhythmias or atrial flutter or fibrillation) –

Adults:

Initial dose – 5 to 10 mg (0.075 to 0.15 mg/kg body weight) given as an IV bolus over at least 2 minutes.

Repeat dose – 10 mg (0.15 mg/kg body weight) 30 minutes after the first dose if the initial response is not adequate. An optimal interval for subsequent IV doses has not been determined and should be individualized for each patient.

Elderly patients – Administer the dose over at least 3 minutes to minimize the risk of untoward drug effects.

Children:

Initial dose –

0 to 1 year of age: Administer 0.1 to 0.2 mg/kg body weight (usual single-dose range, 0.75 to 2 mg) as an IV bolus over at least 2 minutes under continuous electrocardiogram (ECG) monitoring.

1 to 15 years of age: Administer 0.1 to 0.3 mg/kg body weight (usual single-dose range, 2 to 5 mg) as an IV bolus over at least 2 minutes. Do not exceed 5 mg.

Repeat dose – Repeat initial dose 30 minutes after the first dose if the initial response is not adequate (under continuous ECG monitoring). An optimal interval for subsequent IV doses has not been determined and should be individualized for each patient. Do not exceed a single dose of 10 mg in patients 1 to 15 years of age.

Administration: For IV use only. Give verapamil injection as a slow IV injection over at least a 2-minute time period under continuous ECG and blood pressure monitoring.

Use only if solution is clear and vial seal is intact. Discard any unused amount of the solution immediately following withdrawal of any portion of contents.

Admixture incompatibilities: For stability reasons, this product is not recommended for dilution with sodium lactate injection in polyvinyl chloride bags. Verapamil is physically compatible and chemically stable for at least 24 hours at 25°C (77°F) protected from light in most common large-volume parenteral solutions.

Avoid admixing verapamil injection with albumin, amphotericin B, hydralazine, and trimethoprim with sulfamethoxazole. Verapamil injection will precipitate in any solution with a pH above 6.

Actions

Pharmacology: The calcium channel blockers share the ability to inhibit movement of calcium ions across the cell membrane. The effects on the cardiovascular system include depression of mechanical contraction of myocardial and smooth muscle and depression of both impulse formation (automaticity) and conduction velocity. Calcium channel blockers are classified by structure as follows: Diphenylalkylamines – verapamil; benzothiazepines – diltiazem; dihydropyridines – amlodipine, felodipine, isradipine, nicardipine, nifedipine, nimodipine, nisoldipine.

Pharmacokinetics:

Calcium Channel Blocking Agents: Pharmacokinetics[a]

	Parameters	Amlodipine	Diltiazem	Felodipine	Isradipine	Nicardipine	Nifedipine	Nimodipine	Nisoldipine	Verapamil
Pharmacokinetics	Extent of absorption (oral) (%)	nd	nd	≈ 100	90 to 95	≈ 100	100	nd	nd	> 90
	Absolute bioavailability (oral) (%)	64 to 90	40	≈ 20	15 to 24	≈ 35	45 to 75 (IR) 84 to 89 (ER)	≈ 13	≈ 5	20 to 35 (IR)
	Volume of distribution	nd	≈ 305 L (IV)	10 L/kg	3 L/kg	8.3 L/kg (IV)	nd	nd	nd	nd
	T_{max} (h)	6 to 12	2 to 4 (IR) 10 to 14 (ER) 6 to 11 (SR)	2.5 to 5	1.5 (IR) 7 to 18 (CR)	0.5 to 2 (IR) 1 to 4 (SR)	0.5 (IR) 6 (ER)	1	6 to 12	1 to 2 (IR) ≈ 11 (ER) ≈ 7 to 9 (SR)
	Protein binding (%)	93	70 to 80	> 99	95	> 95	92 to 98	> 95	> 99	≈ 90
	Metabolism	Hepatic	Hepatic	Hepatic	Hepatic	Hepatic	Hepatic	Hepatic	Hepatic	Hepatic
	Major metabolites	90% converted to inactive	Desacetyl-diltiazem[c]	6 inactive	Mono acids and cyclic lactone[d]	nd	Inactive	Numerous, inactive	5 major urinary metabolites	Norverapamil[e]
	Half-life, elimination (h)	30 to 50	3 to 4.5 (IR) 4 to 9.5 (ER) 5 to 7 (SR) ≈ 3.4 (IV)	11 to 16	8	2 to 4	≈ 2 (IR) ≈ 7 (ER)	≈ 8 to 9[h]	7 to 12	2.8 to 7.4[i] 4.5 to 12[j] ≈ 12 (SR) 2 to 5 (IV)
	Clearance, systemic	nd	≈ 65 L/h (IV)	≈ 0.8 L/min	1.4 L/min	0.4 L/h•kg (IV)	nd	nd	nd	nd
	Excreted unchanged in urine (%)	10	2 to 4	±	0	< 1	< 0.1	< 1	trace	3 to 4
	Excreted in urine (%)	nd	nd	70	60 to 65	60 (oral) 49 (IV)	60 to 80	nd	60 to 80	≈ 70
	Excreted in feces (%)	nd	nd	10	25 to 30	35 (oral) 43 (IV)	15	nd	nd	≥ 16

Calcium Channel Blocking Agents: Pharmacokinetics[a]										
	Parameters	Amlodipine	Diltiazem	Felodipine	Isradipine	Nicardipine	Nifedipine	Nimodipine	Nisoldipine	Verapamil
ECG Changes	Heart rate	±	0-↓	↑↑	↑	↑↑	0-↑		±	±
	QRS complex	0	nd	0	0	0	nd		0	nd
	PR interval	0	↑	0	0	0	nd		0	↑
	QT interval	0	nd	0	↑	↑	nd		0	nd
Hemodynamics	Myocardial contractility	0-↓	0-↓	0-↓	↓	0-↓	0-↓	na	0-↓	↓↓
	Cardiac output/index	↑	0-↑	nd	↑	↑↑	↑		nd	±
	Peripheral vascular resistance	↓↓	↓↓[k]	↓↓[k]	↓↓	↓↓↓	↓↓↓		↓↓[k]	↓↓

[a] ↑↑↑ or ↓↓↓ = pronounced effect; ↑↑ or ↓↓ = moderate effect; ↑ or ↓ = slight effect; ± = negligible amount or effect; nd = no data; na = not applicable.
[b] Activity of metabolites is unknown.
[c] 25% to 50% as potent a coronary vasodilator as diltiazem; plasma levels are 10% to 20% of the parent drug.
[d] Of 6 metabolites identified, accounting for more than 75%.
[e] Major metabolite; cardiovascular activity is approximately 20% that of verapamil.
[f] Following cessation of multiple dosing.
[g] During a given dosing interval.
[h] Earlier elimination rates are much more rapid, equivalent to a half-life of 1 to 2 hours.
[i] After single doses.
[j] After repetitive doses.
[k] Dose-related.

Contraindications

Hypersensitivity to the drug; hypersensitivity to dihydropyridine calcium channel blockers (**nisoldipine**); sick sinus syndrome or second- or third-degree AV block except with a functioning pacemaker, hypotension less than 90 mm Hg systolic (**diltiazem** and **verapamil**).

Diltiazem: Acute MI and pulmonary congestion.

Injectable –

- Sick sinus syndrome except in the presence of a functioning ventricular pacemaker.
- Second- or third-degree AV block except in the presence of a functioning ventricular pacemaker.
- Severe hypotension or cardiogenic shock.
- Hypersensitivity to the drug.
- Do not be administer IV diltiazem and IV beta-blockers together or in close proximity (within a few hours).
- Atrial fibrillation or atrial flutter associated with an accessory bypass tract such as in Wolff-Parkinson-White syndrome or short PR syndrome.
- Initial use of injectable forms of diltiazem should be, if possible, in a setting where monitoring and resuscitation capabilities, including DC cardioversion/defibrillation, are present. Once familiarity of the patient's response is established, use in an office setting may be acceptable.
- Ventricular tachycardia.
- In newborns, because of the presence of benzyl alcohol (*Cardizem Lyo-Ject Syringe* only).

Verapamil: Severe left ventricular dysfunction; cardiogenic shock and severe congestive heart failure (CHF), unless secondary to a supraventricular tachycardia amenable to verapamil therapy and in patients with atrial flutter or atrial fibrillation and an accessory bypass tract.

Verapamil IV – Do not administer concomitantly with IV β-adrenergic blocking agents (within a few hours), because both may depress myocardial contractility and AV conduction; ventricular tachycardia (VT), because use in patients with wide-complex VT (QRS 0.12 seconds or more) can result in marked hemodynamic deterioration and ventricular fibrillation; atrial fibrillation or atrial flutter associated with an accessory bypass tract.

Nicardipine: Advanced aortic stenosis.

Warnings/Precautions

Hypotension: Hypotension, usually modest and well tolerated, may occasionally occur during initial therapy or with dosage increases, and may be more likely in patients taking concomitant β-blockers.

CHF: CHF has developed rarely, usually in patients receiving a β-blocker, after beginning **nifedipine**.

Oral verapamil may precipitate heart failure. Control patients with milder ventricular dysfunction with digitalis or diuretics before verapamil, if possible.

Use **diltiazem**, **nicardipine**, **isradipine**, **felodipine**, and **amlodipine** with caution in CHF patients.

Cardiac conduction: **IV verapamil** slows AV nodal conduction and SA nodes; it rarely produces second- or third-degree AV block, bradycardia, and in extreme cases, asystole. This is more likely to occur in patients with sick sinus syndrome.

Oral verapamil – Oral verapamil may lead to first-degree AV block and transient bradycardia, sometimes accompanied by nodal escape rhythms.

IV diltiazem – If second- or third-degree AV block occurs in sinus rhythm, discontinue and institute appropriate supportive measures.

Premature ventricular contractions (PVCs): During conversion or marked reduction in ventricular rate, benign complexes of unusual appearance (sometimes resembling PVCs) may occur after **IV verapamil**.

Hypertrophic cardiomyopathy: Serious adverse effects were seen in 120 patients with hypertrophic cardiomyopathy (especially with pulmonary artery wedge pressure more than 20 mm Hg and left ventricular outflow obstruction) who received oral **verapamil** at doses up to 720 mg/day. Sinus bradycardia occurred in 11%, second-degree AV block in 4%, and sinus arrest in 2%.

Withdrawal syndrome: Abrupt withdrawal of calcium channel blockers may be associated with an exacerbation of angina. Gradually taper the dose.

β-blocker withdrawal: Patients recently withdrawn from β-blockers may develop a withdrawal syndrome with increased angina, probably related to increased sensitivity to catecholamines. Initiation of **nifedipine** will not prevent this occurrence and might exacerbate it by provoking reflex catecholamine release. Taper β-blockers rather than stopping them abruptly before beginning nifedipine.

Gradually reduce beta-blocker dose over 8 to 10 days with nicardipine administration.

Hepatic function impairment: The pharmacokinetics, bioavailability, and patient response to **verapamil** and **nifedipine** may be significantly affected by hepatic cirrhosis.

Because **amlodipine**, **diltiazem**, **nicardipine**, **felodipine**, and **nimodipine** are extensively metabolized by the liver, use with caution in patients with hepatic function impairment or reduced hepatic blood flow.

Renal function impairment: The pharmacokinetics of **diltiazem** and **verapamil** in patients with renal function impairment are similar to the pharmacokinetic profile of patients with normal renal function. However, caution is still advised. **Nifedipine**'s plasma concentration is slightly increased in patients with renal function impairment. **Nicardipine**'s mean plasma concentrations, AUC, and maximum concentration were about 2-fold higher in patients with mild renal function impairment.

Increased angina: Occasional patients have increased frequency, duration, or severity of angina on starting **nifedipine** or **nicardipine**, or at the time of dosage increases.

Duchenne muscular dystrophy: **Verapamil** may decrease neuromuscular transmission in patients with Duchenne muscular dystrophy and prolong recovery from the neuromuscular blocking agent vecuronium. Decrease in verapamil dosage may be necessary.

Acute hepatic injury: In rare instances, symptoms consistent with acute hepatic injury, as well as significant elevations in enzymes such as alkaline phosphatase, CPK, LDH, AST, and ALT, have occurred with **diltiazem** and **nifedipine**.

Elevations of transaminases with and without concomitant elevations in alkaline phosphatase and bilirubin have occurred with **verapamil**.

Isolated cases of elevated LDH, alkaline phosphatase, and ALT levels have occurred rarely with **nimodipine**.

Clinically significant transaminase elevations have occurred in approximately 1% of patients receiving these agents; however, no patient became clinically symptomatic or jaundiced, and values returned to normal when the drug was stopped.

Edema: Edema, mild to moderate, typically associated with arterial vasodilation and not due to left ventricular dysfunction, occurs in 10% to 30% of patients receiving **nifedipine**. It occurs primarily in the lower extremities and usually responds to diuretics. In patients with CHF, differentiate this peripheral edema from the effects of decreasing left ventricular function.

Peripheral edema, generally mild and not associated with generalized fluid retention, may occur with **felodipine** within 2 to 3 weeks of therapy initiation. The incidence is both age- and dose-dependent, with frequency ranging from 10% in patients less than 50 years of age taking 5 mg/day to 30% in patients more than 60 years of age taking 20 mg/day.

Pregnancy: Category C.

Lactation: Discontinue breast-feeding while taking **amlodipine**, **diltiazem**, **nicardipine**, **verapamil**, or **nimodipine**. If using **felodipine**, **isradipine**, **nifedipine**, or **nisoldipine**, decide whether to discontinue breast-feeding or discontinue the drug, taking into account the importance of the drug to the mother.

Children: Safety and efficacy of oral **verapamil**, **diltiazem**, **felodipine**, **amlodipine**, **nicardipine**, **nifedipine**, **nisoldipine**, and **isradipine** have not been established. Use of *Procardia* in the pediatric population is not recommended.

Controlled studies of **IV verapamil** have not been conducted in children, but uncontrolled experience indicates that results of treatment are similar to those in adults. Patients younger than 6 months of age may not respond to IV verapamil; this resistance may be related to a developmental difference of AV node responsiveness.

Elderly: **Verapamil**, **nifedipine**, and **felodipine** may cause a greater hypotensive effect than that seen in younger patients, probably due to age-related changes in drug disposition.

Drug Interactions

Drugs that may affect calcium blockers include amiodarone, antineoplastics, azole antifungals, barbiturates, beta blockers, calcium salts, carbamazepine, , cisapride, cyclosporine, erythromycin, H_2 antagonists, hydantoins, melatonin, nafcillin, oxcarbazepine, quinupristine/dalfopristin, moricizine, quinidine, rifampin, ritonavir, sparfloxacin, St. John's wort, valproic acid.

Drugs that may be affected by calcium blockers include anesthetics, antiarrhythmic agents, antineoplastics, benzodiazepines, buspirone, carbamazepine, digoxin, dofetilide, ethanol, HMG-CoA reductase inhibitors, imipramine, lithium, lovastatin, methylprednisolone, moricizine, nondepolarizing muscle relaxants, prazosin, quinidine, sirolimus, tacrolimus, theophyllines, and vincristine.

Diltiazem and **verapamil** inhibit other CYP3A4 substrates, whereas the dihydropyridines do not.

Drug/Food interactions: **Nifedipine**, **amlodipine**, and **verapamil** may be administered without regard to meals.

Bioavailability of **felodipine** is not affected by food, but increased more than 2-fold when taken with doubly concentrated grapefruit juice versus water or orange juice.

Avoid high-fat meals and grapefruit juice with **nisoldipine**.

Adverse Reactions

Generally not serious; rarely requires discontinuation or dosage adjustment.

Calcium Channel Blocker Adverse Reactions (%)[a]

	Adverse reactions	Amlodipine	Diltiazem oral (IV)[b]	Felodipine	Isradipine[b]	Nicardipine oral (IV)[b]	Nifedipine[b]	Nimodipine	Nisoldipine	Verapamil oral (IV)[b]
Cardiovascular	Angina increased					5.6[c]	≤ 1			
	AV block (1°, 2°, or 3°)		≤ 7.6 (< 1)			(†)			≤ 1	0.8 to 1.7
	Bradycardia	≤ 1	≤ 6 (< 1)				< 1	≤ 1		1.4 (1.2)
	Edema	1.8 to 14.6[d]	≤ 6 (< 1)		3.5 to 35.9[c]	0.6 to 1	10 to 30[c]	≤ 1.2[c]		1.7 to 3
	ECG abnormalities		≤ 4.1			0.6 (1.4)		≤ 1.4		2
	Hypotension	≤ 1	< 2	0.5 to 1.5	≤ 1	† (5.6)	< 1	≤ 8.1[c]	≤ 1	0.7 to 2.5
	Hypotension, symptomatic		(3.2)							(1.5)
	Palpitations	0.7 to 4.5[c]	≤ 2	0.4 to 2.5	1 to 5.1[c]	2.8 to 4.1	≤ 7	< 1	3	≤ 1
	Peripheral edema		2 to 15 (4.3)	2 to 17.4		(†)	7 to 29[c]		7 to 29[c]	3.7
	Tachycardia	≤ 1	< 2	0.5 to 1.5	≤ 3.4	0.8 to 3.4 (3.5)	≤ 1	≤ 1.4		
	Vasodilation		≤ 3			4.7 to 5.5 (0.7)			4	
CNS	Asthenia	1 to 2	≤ 4 (< 1)	2.2 to 3.9		0.9 to 5.8 (0.7)	≤ 4			2
	Dizziness/ Lightheadedness	≤ 3.4[c]	≤ 10 (< 1)	2.7 to 3.7	3.4 to 8	1.6 to 6.9 (1.4)	4 to 27	< 1	3 to 10[c]	3 to 4.7 (1.2)
	Drowsiness				≤ 1					
	Fatigue/ Lethargy	4.5[c]			≤ 8.5[c]		4 to 5.9			1.7 to 4.5
	Headache	7.3	≤ 12 (< 1)	10.6 to 14.7	10.3 to 22	6.2 to 8.2	10 to 23	≤ 4.1[c]	22	2.2 to 12.1 (1.2)
	Nervousness	≤ 1	≤ 2	0.5 to 1.5	≤ 1	0.6	≤ 7		≤ 1	
	Tremor	≤ 1	< 2			0.6	≤ 8		≤ 1	
	Weakness				≤ 1.2		10 to 12			

Calcium Channel Blocker Adverse Reactions (%)[a]

	Adverse reactions	Amlodipine	Diltiazem oral (IV)[b]	Felodipine	Isradipine[b]	Nicardipine oral (IV)[b]	Nifedipine[b]	Nimodipine	Nisoldipine	Verapamil oral (IV)[b]
GI	Abdominal discomfort	1.6	1	0.5 to 1.5	≤ 5.1	(0.7)	< 3			(0.6)
	Anorexia	≤ 1	< 2						≤ 1	
	Constipation	≤ 1	≤ 3.6 (< 1)	0.3 to 1.5	≤ 3.8	0.6	≤ 3.3			3.9 to 11.7
	Diarrhea	≤ 1	≤ 2	0.5 to 1.5	≤ 3.4		< 3	≤ 4.2	≤ 1	≤ 2.4
	Dry mouth	≤ 1	< 2 (< 1)	0.5 to 1.5	≤ 1	0.4 to 1.4	< 3		≤ 1	≤ 1
	Dyspepsia	1 to 2	≤ 6	0.5 to 3.9		0.8 to 1.5 (†)	< 3		≤ 1	2.5 to 2.7
	GI distress									≤ 1
	Nausea	2.9[c]	≤ 2.2 (< 1)	1 to 1.7	1 to 5.1	1.9 to 2.2 (4.9)	2 to 11	0.6 to 1.4	2	1.7 to 2.7 (0.9)
	Vomiting	≤ 0.1	≤ 2 (< 1)	0.5 to 1.5	≤ 1.3	0.4 to 0.6 (4.9)	≤ 1	< 1		
Respiratory	Cough	≤ 0.1		0.8 to 1.7	≤ 1		≤ 6			
	Dyspnea	1 to 2	≤ 6 (< 1)	0.5 to 1.5	≤ 3.4	0.6 (0.7)	≤ 6	≤ 1.2	≤ 1	1.4
	Nasal congestion		< 2				≤ 6			
	Pharyngitis		1.4 to 6	0.5 to 1.5			< 1		≤ 5	3
	Rhinitis	≤ 0.1	≤ 9.6			†			≤ 1	2.7
	Upper respiratory infection			0.7 to 3.9			≤ 1			5.4
	Wheezing						6	< 1		
Miscellaneous	Flu-like illness/ syndrome/ symptoms		≤ 2.3	0.5 to 1.5					≤ 1	3.7
	Flushing	0.7 to 4.5[d]	≤ 3 (1.7)	3.9 to 6.9	1.2 to 5.1[c]	5.6 to 9.7	≤ 25	≤ 2.1		0.6 to 0.8
	Injection site reactions		(3.9)			(1.4)				
	Infection		≤ 6			†				12.1
	Muscle cramps	1 to 2	< 2	0.5 to 1.5			≤ 8	≤ 1.4		≤ 1
	Pain	≤ 1	≤ 6			0.6	< 3			
	Sore throat					†	6			
	Tinnitus	≤ 1	< 2			† (†)	≤ 1		≤ 1	≤ 1
	Urinary frequency	≤ 1		0.5 to 1.5	1.3 to 3.4	≤ 0.6 (†)	≤ 3		≤ 1	≤ 1

[a] Data are pooled from separate studies and are not necessarily comparable.
[b] Includes data for SR/ER form.
[c] Dose-related.
[d] Dose-related and higher in females.
[f] †Occurs, no incidence reported.

VASOPRESSORS USED IN SHOCK

Vasopressors: Sympathomimetic agents are used in shock to treat hypoperfusion in normovolemic patients and in patients unresponsive to whole blood or plasma volume expanders. These agents increase myocardial contractility, constrict capacitance vessels, and dilate resistance vessels. In cardiogenic shock or advanced shock from other causes associated with a low cardiac output, they may be combined with vasodilators (eg, nitroprusside, nitroglycerin) to maintain blood pressure while the vasodilator improves myocardial performance. Nitroprusside is used to reduce preload and afterload and improve cardiac output. Nitroglycerin directly relaxes the venous vasculature and decreases preload.

Pharmacology: Sympathomimetic agents produce α-adrenergic stimulation (vasoconstriction), β_1-adrenergic stimulation (increase myocardial contractility, heart rate, automaticity, and AV conduction), and β_2-adrenergic activity (peripheral vasodilation). Dopamine also causes vasodilation of the renal and mesenteric, cerebral, and coronary beds by dopaminergic receptor activation.

Monitoring: Monitoring shock patients and their response to drugs requires special vigilance. Monitor heart rate, blood pressure, and ECG continuously. Record urine output and fluid intake frequently. Due to rapid and life-threatening changes that can occur in the hemodynamically unstable patient, optimal drug selection, dose titration, and management is probably best achieved with the use of invasive hemodynamic monitoring.

Administration: Administration only should be via the IV route using a large-bore, free flowing IV in the antecubital vein, or a central vein due to unpredictable absorption. Small IVs in the extremities are both unreliable and unsafe for vasopressor administration. Frequent monitoring of the IV sites for extravasation injury is essential when vasopressor agents are being used.

Prolonged, high-dose therapy: Prolonged, high-dose therapy can produce cyanosis and tissue necrosis of distal extremities. The principle of using the lowest dose that produces an adequate response for the shortest period of time is very important when using these agents.

Plasma volume depletion: Prolonged use of vasopressors may result in plasma volume depletion; correct this by appropriate fluid and electrolyte replacement therapy. If plasma volumes are not corrected, hypotension may recur when these drugs are discontinued.

Acidosis: Acidosis lessens the response to vasopressors; therefore, correct acidosis if it exists or develops during the course of vasopressor therapy.

Avoid continuous IV therapy: Acute tolerance develops during continuous IV administration. High concentration/low volume (250 mL) vasopressor solutions administered with the aid of an infusion control device allows for maximum dosing flexibility because fluids and drugs can be regulated independently and the development of tolerance is minimized.

Effects of Vasopressors Used in Shock

+++ pronounced effect
++ *moderate effect*
+ *slight effect*
0 *no effect*
↑ *increase*
↓ *decrease*

		Sites of action: Heart		Sites of action: Blood vessels		Hemodynamic response			
		Contractility (Inotropic)	SA Node Rate (Chronotropic)	Vasoconstriction	Vasodilatation	Renal Perfusion	Cardiac Output	Total Peripheral Resistance	Blood Pressure
		β_1	β_1	α	β_2				
Inotropic	Isoproterenol	+++	+++	0	+++	↑[a] or ↓[b]	↑	↓	↑[c]↓[d]
	Dobutamine	+++	0 to +[e]	0 to +[e]	+	0	↑	↓	↑
	Dopamine	+++	+ to ++[e]	+ to +++[e]	0 to +[f]	↑[e]	↓	↓[e] or ↑	0 to ↑
Mixed	Epinephrine	+++	+++	+++[e]	++[e]	↓	↑	↓	↑[c]↓[d]
	Norepinephrine	++	++[g]	+++	0	↓	0 or ↓	↑	↑
	Ephedrine	++	++	+	0 to +	↓	↑	↑ or ↓	↑
	Mephentermine	+	+	+	++	↑ or ↓	↑	0 to ↑	↑
Pressors	Metaraminol	+	+	++	0	↓	↓	↑	↑
	Methoxamine	0	0[g]	+++	0	↓	0 or ↓	↑	↑
	Phenylephrine	0	0[g]	+++	0	↓	↓	↑	↑

[a] Cardiogenic or septicemic shock.
[b] Normotensive patient.
[c] Systolic effect.
[d] Diastolic effect.
[e] Effects are dose dependent.
[f] Dilates renal and splanchnic beds via dopaminergic effect at doses less than 10 mcg/kg/min.
[g] Decreased heart rate may result from reflex mechanisms.

Common Dilutions and Infusion Rates for Selected Drugs Used in Shock

Drug	Usual Dilution for IV Infusion	Infusion Rate
Isoproterenol	2 mg (10 mL) in 500 mL D5W (4 mcg/mL) or 1 mg (5 mL) in 250 mL D5W	5 mcg/min
Dobutamine	250 mg in 250 to 500 mL NS or D5W (500 to 1000 mcg/mL)	2.5 to 15 mcg/kg/min
Dopamine	200 to 800 mg in 250 to 500 mL NS or D5W (400 to 3200 mcg/mL)	Low dose – 2.5 to 10 mcg/kg/min High dose – 20 to 50 mcg/kg/min
Norepinephrine	4 mg in 250 mL of D5W (16 mcg/mL)	Initial: 8 to 12 mcg/min Maintenance: 2 to 4 mcg/min

VASODILATOR COMBINATIONS

Tablets: 20 mg isosorbide dinitrate/37.5 mg hydralazine hydrochloride (*Rx*)	*BiDil* (NitroMed)

Indications

Heart failure: For the treatment of heart failure as an adjunct to standard therapy in self-identified black patients to improve survival, to prolong time to hospitalization for heart failure, and to improve patient-reported functional status.

Administration and Dosage

One tablet 3 times daily; may be titrated to a maximum tolerated dose not to exceed 2 tablets 3 times daily.

BETA-ADRENERGIC BLOCKING AGENTS

ACEBUTOLOL HYDROCHLORIDE	
Capsules; oral: 200 and 400 mg (*Rx*)	Various, *Sectral* (Reddy Pharmaceuticals)
ATENOLOL	
Tablets; oral: 25, 50, and 100 mg (*Rx*)	Various, *Tenormin* (AstraZeneca)
BETAXOLOL HYDROCHLORIDE	
Tablets; oral: 10 and 20 mg (*Rx*)	*Kerlone* (Sanofi)
BISOPROLOL FUMARATE	
Tablets; oral: 5 and 10 mg (*Rx*)	Various, *Zebeta* (Lederle)
CARTEOLOL HYDROCHLORIDE	
Tablets; oral: 2.5 and 5 mg (*Rx*)	*Cartrol* (Abbott)
ESMOLOL HYDROCHLORIDE	
Injection: 10, 20, or 250 mg/mL (*Rx*)	*Brevibloc*, *Brevibloc Double Strength* (Baxter)
METOPROLOL	
Tablets; oral: 25 mg (*Rx*)	Various
50 and 100 mg (*Rx*)	Various, *Lopressor* (Novartis)
Tablets, extended-release; oral: 25, 50, 100, and 200 mg (*Rx*)	Various, *Toprol XL* (AstraZeneca)
Injection: 1 mg/mL (*Rx*)	Various, *Lopressor* (Novartis)
NADOLOL	
Tablets; oral: 20, 40, 80, 120, and 160 mg (*Rx*)	Various, *Corgard* (Monarch)
NEBIVOLOL	
Tablets; oral: 2.5, 5, and 10 mg (*Rx*)	*Bystolic* (Forest Laboratories)
PENBUTOLOL SULFATE	
Tablets; oral: 20 mg (*Rx*)	*Levatol* (Schwarz Pharma)
PINDOLOL	
Tablets; oral: 5 and 10 mg (*Rx*)	Various, *Visken* (Novartis)
PROPRANOLOL	
Tablets; oral: 10, 20, 40, 60, and 80 mg (*Rx*)	Various
Capsules, extended-release; oral: 60, 80, 120, and 160 mg (*Rx*)	Various, *Inderal LA* (Wyeth-Ayerst), *InnoPran XL* (GlaxoSmithKline)
Solution; oral: 4 and 8 mg/mL (*Rx*)	Various
Injection: 1 mg/mL (*Rx*)	Various, *Inderal* (Wyeth-Ayerst)
SOTALOL HYDROCHLORIDE	
Tablets; oral: 80, 120, 160, and 240 mg (*Rx*)	Various, *Betapace* (Bayer)
80, 120, 160 mg (*Rx*)	*Betapace* AF (Bayer)
Injection, solution, concentrate: 15 mg/mL (*Rx*)	Various
TIMOLOL MALEATE	
Tablets; oral: 5, 10, and 20 mg (*Rx*)	Various, *Blocadren* (Merck)

Warning:

Atenolol, metoprolol, nadolol, propranolol, timolol: There have been reports of exacerbation of angina and, in some cases, myocardial infarction and ventricular arrythmias, following abrupt discontinuation of beta-adrenergic blocking agents therapy. Therefore, when discontinuance of beta-adrenergic blocking agents is planned, gradually reduce the dosage over at least a few weeks, and caution the patient against interruption or cessation of therapy without a health care provider's advice. If beta-adrenergic blocking agents therapy is interrupted and exacerbation of angina occurs or acute coronary insufficiency develops, it is usually advisable to promptly reinstitute beta-adrenergic blocking agents therapy and take other measures appropriate for the management of angina pectoris. Because coronary artery disease may be unrecognized, it may be prudent to follow the above advice in patients who are given beta-adrenergic blocking agents for other indications.

Sotalol: To minimize the risk of induced arrhythmia, place patients initiated or reinitiated on sotalol or sotalol AF for a minimum of 3 days (on their maintenance dose) in a facility that can provide cardiac resuscitation, continuous electrocardiographic monitoring, and calculations of creatinine clearance (CrCl). For detailed instructions regarding dose selection and special cautions for people with renal impairment, see Administration and Dosage.

Do not substitute sotalol for sotalol AF because of significant differences in labeling (eg, patient package insert, dosing administration, safety administration).

Indications

Beta-Adrenergic Blocking Agents – Summary of Indications

Indications ✓= labeled	Acebutolol	Atenolol	Betaxolol	Bisoprolol	Carteolol	Esmolol	Metoprolol	Nadolol	Nebivolol	Penbutolol	Pindolol	Propranolol	Sotalol	Timolol
Hypertension	✓	✓	✓	✓	✓		✓	✓	✓	✓	✓	✓		✓
Angina pectoris		✓					✓	✓				✓[a]		
Cardiac arrhythmias														
Supraventricular arrhythmias/ tachycardias						✓						✓[b]		
Sinus tachycardia						✓								
Intraoperative and postoperative tachycardia and hypertension						✓								
Ventricular arrhythmias/ tachycardias												✓	✓[c]	
Premature ventricular contractions	✓											✓		
Digitalis-induced tachyarrhythmias												✓		
Resistant tachyarrhythmias (during anesthesia)												✓		
Maintenance of normal sinus rhythm													✓	
MI		✓					✓					✓[b]		✓
CHF (stable)[d]							✓[e]							
Pheochromocytoma												✓[b]		
Migraine prophylaxis												✓[a]		✓
Hypertrophic subaortic stenosis												✓[a]		
Essential tremors												✓[b]		

[a] Except *InnoPram XL*.
[b] Except extended-release.
[c] Not *Betapace AF*.
[d] CHF = congestive heart failure; see Precautions or Warnings.
[e] *Toprol-XL* 25 mg only.

Administration and Dosage

ACEBUTOLOL HYDROCHLORIDE:

Hypertension –

Initial dose: 400 mg in uncomplicated mild to moderate hypertension. May be given as a single daily dose, but 200 mg twice/day may be required for adequate control. Optimal response usually occurs with 400 to 800 mg/day (range, 200 to 1,200 mg/day given twice daily).

Ventricular arrhythmia –

Initial dose: 400 mg (200 mg twice/day). Increase dosage gradually until optimal response is obtained, usually 600 to 1,200 mg/day.

Elderly – Because bioavailability increases approximately 2-fold, older patients may require lower maintenance doses. Avoid doses greater than 800 mg/day.

Renal/Hepatic function impairment – Reduce the daily dose by 50% when CrCl is less than 50 mL/min. Reduce by 75% when it is less than 25 mL/min. Use cautiously in patients with impaired hepatic function.

ATENOLOL:

Hypertension –

Initial dosage: 50 mg once daily, used alone or in combination with other antihypertensive agents. If an optimal response is not achieved, increase to 100 mg/day. Dosage greater than 100 mg/day is unlikely to produce any further benefit.

Angina pectoris –

Initial dosage: 50 mg/day. If an optimal response is not achieved within 1 week, increase to 100 mg/day. Some patients may require 200 mg/day for optimal effect.

With once-daily dosing, 24-hour control is achieved by giving doses larger than necessary to achieve an immediate maximum effect. The maximum early effect on exercise tolerance occurs with doses of 50 to 100 mg, but the effect at 24 hours is attenuated, averaging approximately 50% to 75% of that with once-daily doses of 200 mg.

Acute myocardial infarction –

Oral: In patients who tolerate the full 10 mg intravenous (IV) dose, initiate 50 mg tablets 10 minutes after the last IV dose followed by another 50 mg dose 12 hours later. Thereafter, administer 100 mg once daily or 50 mg twice/day for 6 to 9 days longer or until discharge from the hospital.

If there is any question concerning the use of IV atenolol, eliminate the IV administration and use the tablets at a dosage of 100 mg once daily or 50 mg twice/day for 7 days or longer.

Renal function impairment –

Atenolol Dosage Adjustments in Severe Renal Impairment

CrCl (mL/min/1.73 m^2)	Elimination half-life (h)	Maximum dosage
15 to 35	16 to 27	50 mg/day
< 15	> 27	50 mg every other day

Hemodialysis – Give 25 or 50 mg after each dialysis.

BETAXOLOL HYDROCHLORIDE:

Initial dose – 10 mg once daily, alone or added to diuretic therapy. If the desired response is not achieved the dose can be doubled. Increasing the dose to more than 20 mg has not produced a statistically significant additional hypertensive effect; however, the 40 mg dose is well tolerated.

Elderly – Consider reducing the starting dose to 5 mg.

Renal function impairment – In patients with renal impairment, clearance of betaxolol declines with decreasing renal function.

In patients with severe renal impairment and those undergoing dialysis, the initial dose is 5 mg once daily. If the desired response is not achieved, dosage may be increased by 5 mg/day increments every 2 weeks to a maximum dose of 20 mg/day.

BISOPROLOL FUMARATE: May be given without regard to meals.

Initial dose – 5 mg once daily. In some patients, 2.5 mg may be appropriate. If the antihypertensive effect of 5 mg is inadequate, the dose may be increased to 10 mg and then, if necessary, to 20 mg once daily.

Renal/Hepatic function impairment – In patients with renal dysfunction (CrCl less than 40 mL/min) or hepatic impairment (hepatitis or cirrhosis), use an initial daily dose of 2.5 mg.

CARTEOLOL HYDROCHLORIDE:

Initial dose – 2.5 mg as a single daily dose, either alone or with a diuretic. If adequate response is not achieved, gradually increase to 5 and 10 mg as single daily doses. Doses greater than 10 mg/day are unlikely to produce further benefit and may decrease response.

Maintenance – 2.5 to 5 mg once daily.

Renal function impairment –

Carteolol Dosage in Renal Impairment

CrCl (mL/min/1.73 m^2)	Dosage interval (h)
> 60	24
20 to 60	48
< 20	72

ESMOLOL HYDROCHLORIDE:

Supraventricular tachycardia – 50 to 200 mcg/kg/min; average dose is 100 mcg/kg/min, although dosages as low as 25 mcg/kg/min have been adequate. Dosages as high as 300 mcg/kg/min provide little added effect and an increased rate of adverse effects and are not recommended.

Dosage in Supraventricular Tachycardia

	Loading dose (over 1 minute)		Maintenance dose (over 4 minutes)	
Time (minutes)	mcg/kg/min	mg/kg/min	mcg/kg/min	mg/kg/min
0 to 1	500	0.5		
1 to 5			50	0.05
5 to 6	500	0.5		
6 to 10			100	0.1
10 to 11	500	0.5		
11 to 15			150	0.15
15 to 16	—	—		
16 to 20			200[a]	0.2[a]
> 20 (24 hours)			Maintenance dose titrated to heart rate or other clinical end point	

[a] As the desired heart rate or end point is approached, the loading infusion may be omitted and the maintenance infusion titrated to 300 mcg/kg/min (0.3 mg/kg/min) or downward as appropriate. Maintenance dosages more than 200 mcg/kg/min (0.2 mg/kg/min) have not been shown to have significantly increased benefits. The interval between titration steps may be increased.

If adequate therapeutic effect is not observed within 5 minutes, repeat loading dose and follow with maintenance infusion increased to 100 mcg/kg/min. Continue titration procedure, repeating loading infusion, increasing maintenance infusion by increments of 50 mcg/kg/min (for 4 minutes). As the desired heart rate or a safety end point (eg, lowered blood pressure) is approached, omit loading infusion and titrate the maintenance dosage up or down to end point. Also, if desired, increase interval between titration steps from 5 to 10 minutes.

This specific dosage regimen has not been intraoperatively studied. Because of the time required for titration, it may not be optimal for intraoperative use.

The safety of dosages greater than 300 mcg/kg/min has not been studied.

In the event of an adverse reaction, reduce dosage or discontinue the drug. If a local infusion-site reaction develops, use an alternative site. Avoid butterfly needles.

Transfer to alternative agents – After achieving adequate heart rate control and stable clinical status, transition to alternative antiarrhythmic agents may be accomplished.

Reduce the dosage of esmolol as follows: 30 minutes after the first dose of the alternative agent, reduce esmolol infusion rate by 50%. Following the second dose of the alternative agent, monitor patient's response and, if satisfactory control is maintained for the first hour, discontinue esmolol infusion.

Intraoperative and postoperative tachycardia and hypertension –

Immediate control: For intraoperative treatment of tachycardia and hypertension, give an 80 mg (approximately 1 mg/kg) bolus dose over 30 seconds followed by a 150 mcg/kg/min infusion, if necessary. Adjust the infusion rate as required up to 300 mcg/kg/min to maintain desired heart rate or blood pressure.

Gradual control: For postoperative tachycardia and hypertension, the dosing schedule is the same as that used in supraventricular tachycardia.

Withdrawal effects – The use of esmolol infusions for up to 24 hours has been well documented. Limited data indicate that esmolol is well tolerated for up to 48 hours.

Preparation of solution –

250 mg/mL ampule: Aseptically prepare a 10 mg/mL infusion by adding two 2,500 mg ampules to a 500 mL container or one 2,500 mg ampule to a 250 mL container of one of the IV fluids listed in Compatibility/Stability. This yields a final concentration of 10 mg/mL. The diluted solution is stable for 24 hours or more at room temperature. Esmolol has been well tolerated when administered via a central vein.

The 250 mg/mL strength is concentrated and is not for direct IV injection; dilute prior to infusion. Do not mix with sodium bicarbonate. Do not mix with other drugs prior to dilution in a suitable IV fluid.

10 mg/mL: This dosage form is prediluted to provide a ready to use 10 mg/mL concentration. It may be used to administer an esmolol loading dose infusion by hand-held syringe while the maintenance infusion is being prepared.

Compatibility/Stability – Esmolol, at a final concentration of 10 mg/mL, is compatible with the following solutions and is stable for 24 hours or more at controlled room temperature or under refrigeration: 5% dextrose injection; 5% dextrose in Lactated Ringer's injection; 5% dextrose in Ringer's injection; 5% dextrose and 0.9% or 0.45% sodium chloride injection; Lactated Ringer's injection; potassium chloride (40 mEq/L) in 5% dextrose injection; 0.9% or 0.45% sodium chloride injection.

Esmolol is *not* compatible with 5% sodium bicarbonate injection.

METOPROLOL:

Tablets (immediate-release) and injection –

Hypertension:

Initial dosage – 100 mg/day in single or divided doses, used alone or added to a diuretic taken with or immediately after meals. The dosage may be increased at weekly (or longer) intervals until optimum blood pressure reduction is achieved.

Maintenance dosage – 100 to 450 mg/day. Dosages greater than 450 mg/day have not been studied. While once daily dosing is effective and can maintain a reduction in blood pressure throughout the day, lower doses (especially 100 mg) may not maintain a full effect at the end of the 24-hour period; larger or more frequent daily doses may be required.

Angina pectoris:

Initial dosage – 100 mg/day in 2 divided doses. Dosage may be gradually increased at weekly intervals until optimum clinical response is obtained or a pronounced slowing of heart rate occurs. Effective dosage range is 100 to 400 mg/day. Dosages above 400 mg/day have not been studied.

Myocardial infarction:

Early treatment – During the early phase of definite or suspected acute myocardial infarction, initiate treatment as soon as possible. Administer 3 IV bolus injections of 5 mg each at approximately 2-minute intervals.

In patients who tolerate the full IV dose (15 mg), give 50 mg orally every 6 hours 15 minutes after the last IV dose and continue for 48 hours. Thereafter, administer a maintenance dosage of 100 mg twice daily.

In patients who do not tolerate the full IV dose, start with 25 or 50 mg orally every 6 hours (depending on the degree of intolerance) 15 minutes after the last IV dose or as soon as the clinical condition allows.

Late treatment – Patients with contraindications to early treatment, patients who do not tolerate the full early treatment, and patients in whom therapy is delayed for any other reason should be started at 100 mg orally twice daily as soon as their clinical condition allows. Continue for 3 months or more.

Extended-release tablets, – The extended-release tablets are for once daily administration. When switching from metoprolol immediate-release tablets to extended-release, use the same daily dose.

Hypertension: The usual initial dosage is 50 to 100 mg/day in a single dose whether used alone or added to a diuretic. The dosage may be increased at weekly (or longer) intervals until optimum blood pressure reduction is achieved. Dosages greater than 400 mg/day have not been studied.

Angina pectoris: The usual initial dosage is 100 mg/day in a single dose. The dosage may be gradually increased at weekly intervals until optimum clinical response has been obtained or there is a pronounced slowing of the heart rate. Dosages greater than 400 mg/day have not been studied.

Congestive heart failure: Prior to initiation of therapy, stabilize the dosing of diuretics, angiotensin-converting inhibitors, and digitalis (if used). The recommended starting dose is 25 mg once daily for 2 weeks in patients with New York Heart Association class II heart failure and 12.5 mg once daily in patients with more severe heart failure. Double the dose every 2 weeks to the highest dosage level tolerated by the patient or up to 200 mg. If transient worsening of heart failure occurs, it may be treated with increased dose of diuretics, and it may be necessary to lower the dose of metoprolol or temporarily discontinue it. The dose should not be increased until symptoms of worsening heart failure have been stabilized; initial difficulty with titration should not preclude later attempts to introduce metoprolol. If patients with heart failure experience symptomatic bradycardia, reduce the dose.

NADOLOL:

Angina pectoris –

Initial dose: 40 mg/day. Gradually increase dosage in 40 to 80 mg increments at 3- to 7-day intervals until optimum clinical response is obtained or there is pronounced slowing of the heart rate.

Maintenance dosage: Usual dosage is 40 to 80 mg once daily. Up to 160 to 240 mg once daily may be needed. The safety and efficacy of dosages exceeding 240 mg/day have not been established.

Hypertension –

Initial dose: 40 mg once daily, alone or in addition to diuretic therapy. Gradually increase dosage in 40 to 80 mg increments until optimum blood pressure reduction is achieved.

Maintenance dose: Usual dose is 40 to 80 mg once daily. Up to 240 to 320 mg once daily may be needed.

Renal function impairment –

Nadolol Dosage Adjustments in Renal Failure

CrCl (mL/min/1.73^2)	Dosage interval (h)
> 50	24
31 to 50	24 to 36
10 to 30	24 to 48
< 10	40 to 60

NEBIVOLOL HYDROCHLORIDE: For most patients, 5 mg once daily with or without food as monotherapy or in combination with other agents. For patients requiring further reduction in blood pressure, the dose can be increased at 2-week intervals, up to 40 mg.

Renal function impairment – In patients with severe renal function impairment (CrCl less than 30 mL/min), the recommended initial dosage is 2.5 mg once daily; upward titration should be performed cautiously if needed.

Hepatic function impairment – In patients with moderate hepatic function impairment, the recommended initial dosage is 2.5 mg once daily; upward titration should be performed cautiously if needed. Nebivolol has not been studied in patients with severe hepatic function impairment and, therefore, is not recommended in that population.

PENBUTOLOL SULFATE: Usual starting and maintenance dose is 20 mg once daily. Doses of 40 to 80 mg have been well tolerated but have not shown greater antihypertensive effect. A dose of 10 mg also lowers blood pressure, but the full effect is not seen for 4 to 6 weeks.

PINDOLOL: 5 mg twice daily, alone or with other antihypertensive agents. Response usually occurs within the first week of treatment. Maximal response may take as long as or occasionally longer than 2 weeks. If a satisfactory reduction in blood pressure does not occur within 3 to 4 weeks, adjust dose in increments of 10 mg/day at 2- to 4-week intervals to a maximum of 60 mg/day.

PROPRANOLOL HYDROCHLORIDE:

Propranolol Dosage Based on Indication[a]

Indication	Initial dosage	Usual range	Maximum daily dosage
Arrhythmias		10 to 30 mg 3 to 4 times a day (given before meals and at bedtime)	
Hypertension	40 mg twice a day or 80 mg once daily (ER)	120 to 240 mg/day (given 2 to 3 times a day) or 80 to 160 mg once daily (ER)	640 mg
Angina	80 mg once daily (ER)	80 to 320 mg 2, 3, or 4 times a day or 160 mg once daily (ER)	320 mg
Atrial fibrillation		10 to 30 mg 3 or 4 times daily before meals and at bedtime	
MI	40 mg 3 times daily	180 to 240 mg/day (given 2 or 3 times a day)	240 mg
IHSS[b]		20 to 40 mg 3 to 4 times a day (given before meals and at bedtime) or 80 to 160 mg once daily (ER)	
Pheochromocytoma		Preoperatively: 60 mg/day × 3 days preoperatively (in divided doses) Management of inoperable brain tumor: 30 mg/day in divided doses, concomitantly with an alpha-adrenergic blocking agent	
Inoperable tumor		30 mg/day (in divided doses)	
Migraine	80 mg/day once daily (ER) or in divided doses	160 to 240 mg once daily (ER) or in divided doses	
Essential tremor	40 mg twice a day	120 mg/day	320 mg

[a] ER = extended release.
[b] IHSS = idiopathic hypertrophic subaortic stenosis.

Extended-release capsules – The extended-release capsule should be administered once daily. Administer *InnoPran XL* at bedtime (approximately 10 PM) consistently either on an empty stomach or with food. The starting dose is 80 mg, and titration may be needed to a dose of 120 mg or higher. Doses of *InnoPran XL* more than 120 mg had no additional effects on blood pressure. The time needed for full antihypertensive response is usually achieved within 2 to 3 weeks.

Parenteral –

Usual dose: 1 to 3 mg. Do not exceed 1 mg/min. If necessary, give a second dose after 2 minutes. Thereafter, do not give additional drug in under 4 hours. Transfer to oral therapy as soon as possible.

Pediatrics – IV use is not recommended.

Oral dosage for treating hypertension requires titration, beginning with a 1 mg/kg/day dosage regimen (eg, 0.5 mg/kg twice daily). May be increased at 3- to 5-day intervals to a maximum of 16 mg/kg/day.

The usual pediatric dosage range is 2 to 4 mg/kg/day in 2 equally divided doses (eg, 1 to 2 mg/kg twice daily). Dosage calculated by weight generally produces plasma levels in a therapeutic range similar to that in adults. Do not use dosages of more than 16 mg/kg/day.

SOTALOL HYDROCHLORIDE:

Oral –

Betapace: The recommended initial dose is 80 mg twice daily. This dose may be increased if necessary to 240 or 320 mg/day (120 to 160 mg twice a day). A therapeutic response is usually obtained at a total daily dose of 160 to 320 mg/day given in 2 or 3 divided doses. Some patients with life-threatening refractory ventricular arrhythmias may require doses as high as 480 to 640 mg/day.

Adjust dosage gradually, allowing 3 days between dosing increments to attain steady-state plasma concentrations and allow monitoring of QT intervals.

Renal function impairment –

Sotalol Dosing Interval in Renal Impairment

CrCl (mL/min)	Dosing interval (hours)[a]
≥ 60	12
30 to 59	24
10 to 29	36 to 48
< 10	Individualize dosage

[a] The initial dose of 80 mg and subsequent doses should be administered at these intervals. See following paragraph for dosage escalations.

Dose escalations in renal impairment should be done after administration of at least 5 to 6 doses at appropriate intervals.

Exercise extreme caution in the use of sotalol in patients with renal failure undergoing hemodialysis. The half-life of sotalol is prolonged (up to 69 hours) in anuric patients. However, sotalol can be partly removed by dialysis, with subsequent partial rebound in concentrations when dialysis is completed. Safety (heart rate, QT interval) and efficacy (arrhythmia control) must be closely monitored.

Betapace AF: Therapy with *Betapace* AF must be initiated (and if necessary, titrated) in a setting that provides continuous electrocardiogram (ECG) monitoring and in the presence of personnel trained in the management of serious ventricular arrhythmias. Continue to monitor patients in this way for a minimum of 3 days on the maintenance dose. In addition, do not discharge patients within 12 hours of electrical or pharmacological conversion to normal sinus rhythm.

The baseline QT interval must be 450 msec or less in order for a patient to be started on *Betapace* AF therapy. During initiation and titration, monitor the QT interval 2 to 4 hours after each dose. If the QT interval prolongs to 500 msec or more, the dose must be reduced or the drug discontinued.

Modify the dosing interval according to the following table.

***Betapace AF* Dosing Interval in Renal Impairment**

CrCl (mL/min)	Dosing interval (hours)
> 60	12
40 to 60	24
< 40	Contraindicated

The recommended initial dose of *Betapace* AF is 80 mg and is initiated as shown in the dosing algorithm described in the following information. The 80 mg dose can be titrated upward to 120 mg during initial hospitalization or after discharge on 80 mg in the event of recurrence by rehospitalization and repetition of the same steps used during the initiation of therapy.

Anticoagulate patients with atrial fibrillation according to usual medical practice. Correct hypokalemia before initiation of *Betapace* AF therapy.

Patients to be discharged on *Betapace* AF therapy from an inpatient setting should have an adequate supply of *Betapace* AF to allow uninterrupted therapy until the patient can fill a *Betapace* AF prescription.

Initiation of therapy –

1.) Electrocardiographic assessment: If the baseline QT is greater than 450 msec, *Betapace* AF is contraindicated.
2.) Starting dose: The starting dose is 80 mg twice daily if the CrCl is greater than 60 mL/min and 80 mg once daily if the CrCl is 40 to 60 mL/min. If the CrCl is less than 40 mL/min, *Betapace* AF is contraindicated.
3.) Begin continuous ECG monitoring with QT interval measurements 2 to 4 hours after each dose.
4.) If the 80 mg dose level is tolerated and the QT interval remains less than 500 msec after at least 3 days (after 5 or 6 doses if patient is receiving once daily dosing), the patient can be discharged. Alternatively, during hospitalization, the dose can be increased to 120 mg twice daily and the patient followed for 3 days on this dose (followed for 5 or 6 doses if the patient is receiving once daily doses).

Upward titration of dose – If the 80 mg dose level (given once or twice daily) does not reduce the frequency of relapses of atrial fibrillation/atrial flutter (AFIB/AFL) and is tolerated without excessive QT interval prolongation (ie, 520 msec or more), the dose level may be increased to 120 mg (once or twice daily). As proarrhythmic events can occur with each upward dosage adjustment, steps 2 through 5 should be followed when increasing the dose level. If the 120 mg dose does not reduce the frequency of early relapse of AFIB/AFL and is tolerated without excessive QT interval prolongation (520 msec or more), an increase to 160 mg (once or twice daily) can be considered. Steps 2 through 5 should be used again to introduce such an increase.

Maintenance of Betapace AF therapy – Regularly re-evaluate renal function and QT if medically warranted. If QT is at least 520 msec, reduce the dose of *Betapace* AF therapy and carefully monitor patients until QT returns to less than 520 msec. If the QT interval is 520 msec or more while on the lowest maintenance dose level (80 mg), discontinue the drug. If renal function deteriorates, reduce the daily dose in half by administering the drug once daily as described in Initiation of Therapy, step 3.

Special considerations – The maximum recommended dose in patients with a calculated CrCl greater than 60 mL/min is 160 mg twice/day.

A patient who misses a dose should not double the next dose. The next dose should be taken at the usual time.

Transfer to sotalol from other antiarrhythmic therapy – Before starting sotalol, generally withdraw previous antiarrhythmic therapy under careful monitoring for a minimum of 2 to 3 plasma half-lives if the patient's clinical condition permits. Treatment has been initiated in some patients receiving IV lidocaine without ill effect. After discontinuation of amiodarone, do not initiate sotalol until the QT interval is normalized.

Transfer to Betapace AF from Betapace – Patients with a history of symptomatic AFIB/AFL who are currently receiving *Betapace* for the maintenance of normal sinus rhythm should be transferred to *Betapace* AF because of the significant differences in labeling (ie, patient package insert for *Betapace* AF, dosing, administration, safety information).

Injection – Start sotalol therapy only if the baseline QT interval is less than 450 ms. During initiation and titration, monitor the QT interval after the completion of each infusion. If the QT interval prolongs to 500 ms or greater, reduce the dose, decrease the infusion rate, or discontinue the drug.

Administer sotalol twice daily in patients with a CrCl greater than 60 mL/min or once daily in patients with a CrCl between 40 and 60 mL/min. Sotalol is not recommended in patients with a CrCl less than 40 mL/min. The recommended initial IV dose of sotalol is 75 mg (once or twice daily) and is initiated as shown in the dosing algorithm that follows. The 75 mg dose can be titrated upward to 112.5 or 150 mg after at least 3 days.

Conversion from oral to IV:

Conversion From Oral to IV Sotalol	
Oral dose once or twice daily	IV dose once or twice daily administered over 5 hours
80 mg	75 mg (5 mL sotalol injection)
120 mg	112.5 mg (7.5 mL sotalol injection)
160 mg	150 mg (10 mL sotalol injection)

Initiation of IV sotalol therapy: The starting dose of IV sotalol is 75 mg infused over 5 hours once or twice daily based on the CrCl. Monitor ECG for excessive increase in QTc.

Dosage titration: If the 75 mg dose of IV sotalol does not reduce the frequency of relapses of symptomatic AFIB/AFL and is tolerated without excessive (to greater than 500 ms) QTc prolongation, increase the dose to 112.5 mg infused over 5 hours once or twice daily depending upon the CrCl. Continue to monitor QTc during dose escalations.

Dose for ventricular arrhythmias: The recommended initial dose of IV sotalol is 75 mg infused over 5 hours once or twice daily based on the CrCl. The dosage may be increased in increments of 75 mg/day every 3 days. The usual therapeutic effect is observed with oral dosages of 80 to 160 mg once or twice a day (corresponding to sotalol 75 to 150 mg IV). Oral dosages as high as 240 to 320 mg once or twice a day (corresponding to sotalol 225 to 300 mg IV) have been utilized in patients with refractory life-threatening arrhythmias.

Children: IV sotalol has not been studied in children.

TIMOLOL MALEATE:

Hypertension –

Initial dosage: 10 mg twice/day used alone or added to a diuretic.

Maintenance dosage: 20 to 40 mg/day. Titrate, depending on blood pressure and heart rate. Increases to a maximum of 60 mg/day divided into 2 doses may be necessary. There should be an interval of at least 7 days between dosage increases.

Myocardial infarction (long-term prophylactic use in patients who have survived the acute phase of myocardial infarction) – 10 mg twice/day.

Migraine – Initial dosage is 10 mg twice/day. During maintenance therapy, the 20 mg/day dosage may be given as a single dose. Total daily dosage may be increased to a maximum of 30 mg in divided doses or decreased to 10 mg once daily, depending on clinical response and tolerability. Discontinue if a satisfactory response is not obtained after 6 to 8 weeks of the maximum daily dosage.

Actions

Pharmacology:

Pharmacologic/Pharmacokinetic Properties of Beta-Adrenergic Blocking Agents

0 – none + – low ++ – moderate +++ – high Drug	Adrenergic-receptor blocking activity	Membrane stabilizing activity	Intrinsic sympathomimetic activity	Lipid solubility	Extent of absorption (%)	Absolute oral bioavailability (%)	Half-life (h)	Protein binding (%)	Metabolism/ Excretion
Acebutolol	β_1[a]	+[b]	+	Low	90	20 to 60	3 to 4	26	Hepatic; renal excretion 30% to 40%; nonrenal excretion 50% to 60% (bile; intestinal wall)
Atenolol	β_1[a]	0	0	Low	50	50 to 60	6 to 7	6 to 16	≈ 50% excreted unchanged in feces
Betaxolol	β_1[a]	+	0	Low	≈ 100	89	14 to 22	≈ 50	Hepatic; > 80% recovered in urine, 15% unchanged
Bisoprolol	β_1[a]	0	0	Low	≥ 90	80	9 to 12	≈ 30	≈ 50% excreted unchanged in urine, remainder as inactive metabolites; < 2% excreted in feces.
Esmolol	β_1[a]	0	0	Low	na[c]	na[c]	0.15	55	Rapid metabolism by esterases in cytosol of red blood cells
Metoprolol	β_1[a]	0[b]	0	Moderate	≈ 100	40 to 50	3 to 7	12	Hepatic; renal excretion, < 5% unchanged
Metoprolol, long-acting						77[d]			
Carteolol	β_1 β_2	0	++	Low	85	85	6	23 to 30	50% to 70% excreted unchanged in urine
Nadolol	β_1 β_2	0	0	Low	30	30 to 50	20 to 24	30	Urine, unchanged
Penbutolol	β_1 β_2	0	+	High	≈ 100	≈ 100	≈ 5	80 to 98	Hepatic (conjugation, oxidation); renal excretion of metabolites (17% as conjugate)
Pindolol	β_1 β_2	0	+++	Low	> 95	≈ 100	3 to 4[e]	40	Urinary excretion of metabolites (60% to 65%) and unchanged drug (35% to 40%)
Propranolol	β_1 β_2	++	0	High	< 90	30	3 to 5	90	Hepatic; < 1% excreted unchanged in urine
Propranolol, long-acting						9 to 18	8 to 11		
Sotalol	β_1 β_2	0	0	Low	nd[f]	90 to 100	12	0	Not metabolized; excreted unchanged in urine
Timolol	β_1 β_2	0	0	Low to moderate	90	75	4	< 10	Hepatic; urinary excretion of metabolites and unchanged drug

[a] Inhibits β_2 receptors (bronchial and vascular) at higher doses.
[b] Detectable only at doses much greater than required for beta blockade.
[c] Not applicable (available IV only).
[d] Average bioavailability; not absolute.
[e] In elderly hypertensive patients with normal renal function, half-life variable: 7 to 15 hours.
[f] No data.

Contraindications

Sinus bradycardia; greater than first degree heart block; cardiogenic shock; CHF, unless secondary to a tachyarrhythmia treatable with beta-blockers; overt cardiac failure; hypersensitivity to beta-blocking agents.

Acebutolol, carteolol: Persistently severe bradycardia.

Carteolol, nadolol, penbutolol, pindolol, propranolol, sotalol, and timolol: Bronchial asthma or bronchospasm, including severe chronic obstructive pulmonary disease.

Metoprolol: Treatment of MI in patients with a heart rate less than 45 beats/min; significant heart block greater than first degree (PR interval 0.24 seconds or more); systolic blood pressure less than 100 mm Hg; moderate to severe cardiac failure.

Sotalol: Congenital or acquired long QT syndromes.

Warnings/Precautions

Proarrhythmia: Like other antiarrhythmic agents, **sotalol** can provoke new or worsened ventricular arrhythmias in some patients, including sustained ventricular tachycardia or ventricular fibrillation, with potentially fatal consequences.

Cardiac failure: Sympathetic stimulation is a vital component supporting circulatory function in CHF, and beta-blockade carries the potential hazard of further depressing myocardial contractility and precipitating more severe failure.

Wolff-Parkinson-White syndrome: In several cases, the tachycardia was replaced by a severe bradycardia, requiring a demand pacemaker after **propranolol** administration with as little as 5 mg.

Abrupt withdrawal: The occurrence of a beta-blocker withdrawal syndrome is controversial. However, hypersensitivity to catecholamines has been observed in patients withdrawn from beta-blocker therapy. Exacerbation of angina, myocardial infarction, ventricular arrhythmias, and death have occurred after abrupt discontinuation of therapy. Reduce dosage gradually over 1 to 2 weeks and carefully monitor the patient.

Because coronary artery disease may be unrecognized, do not discontinue therapy abruptly, even in patients treated only for hypertension, as abrupt withdrawal may result in transient symptoms.

Peripheral vascular disease: Treatment with beta-antagonists reduces cardiac output and can precipitate or aggravate the symptoms of arterial insufficiency in patients with peripheral or mesenteric vascular disease.

Nonallergic bronchospasm (eg, chronic bronchitis, emphysema): In general, do not administer beta-blockers to patients with bronchospastic diseases. Administer **nadolol, timolol, penbutolol, propranolol, sotalol**, and **pindolol** with caution, because they may block bronchodilation produced by endogenous or exogenous catecholamine stimulation of $beta_2$ receptors.

Because of their relative $beta_1$ selectivity, low doses of **metoprolol, acebutolol, bisoprolol**, and **atenolol** may be used with caution in patients with bronchospastic disease who do not respond to, or cannot tolerate, other antihypertensive treatment.

Bradycardia: **Metoprolol** produces a decrease in sinus heart rate in most patients; this decrease is greatest among patients with high initial heart rates and least among patients with low initial heart rates.

Pheochromocytoma: It is hazardous to use **propranolol** or **atenolol** unless alpha-adrenergic blocking drugs are already in use, because this would predispose to serious blood pressure elevation.

Sinus bradycardia: Sinus bradycardia (heart rate less than 50 beats/min) occurred in 13% of patients receiving **sotalol** in clinical trials and led to discontinuation in about 3%. Bradycardia itself increases risk of torsade de pointes.

Electrolyte disturbances: Do not use **sotalol** in patients with hypokalemia or hypomagnesemia prior to correction of imbalance.

Hypotension: If hypotension (systolic blood pressure up to 90 mm Hg) occurs, discontinue drug and carefully assess the patient's hemodynamic status and extent of myocardial damage.

Anaphylaxis: Anaphylaxis has occurred and may include symptoms such as profound hypotension, bradycardia with or without AV nodal block, severe sustained bronchospasm, hives, and angioedema. Deaths have occurred.

Anesthesia and major surgery: Necessity, or desirability, of withdrawing beta-blockers prior to major surgery is controversial. Beta-blockade impairs the heart's ability to respond to beta-adrenergically mediated reflex stimuli. While this might help prevent arrhythmic response, risk of excessive myocardial depression during general anesthesia may be enhanced, and difficulty restarting and maintaining heart beat has occurred. If beta-blockers are withdrawn, allow 48 hours between the last dose and anesthesia. Others may recommend withdrawal of beta-blockers well before surgery takes place.

Atrioventricular block: **Metoprolol** slows atrioventricular conduction and may produce significant first (PR interval, 0.26 seconds or more), second; or third-degree heart block. Acute myocardial infarction also produces heart block.

Sick sinus syndrome: Use **sotalol** only with extreme caution in patients with sick sinus syndrome associated with symptomatic arrhythmias, because it may cause sinus bradycardia, sinus pauses, or sinus arrest.

Concomitant use of calcium channel blockers (atenolol): Bradycardia and heart block can occur and the left ventricular end diastolic pressure can rise when beta-blockers are administered with verapamil or diltiazem. Patients with preexisting conduction abnormalities or left ventricular dysfunction are particularly susceptible.

Recent acute myocardial infarction (sotalol): Sotalol can be used safely and effectively in the long-term treatment of life-threatening ventricular arrhythmias following a myocardial infarction. However, experience in the use of sotalol to treat cardiac arrhythmias in the early phase of recovery from acute myocardial infarction is limited and, at least at high initial doses, is not reassuring. In the first 2 weeks after the myocardial infarction, caution is advised and careful dose titration is especially important, particularly in patients with markedly impaired ventricular function.

Intraoperative and postoperative tachycardia and hypertension: Do not use esmolol as the treatment for hypertension in patients in whom the increased blood pressure is primarily caused by the vasoconstriction associated with hypothermia.

Diabetes/Hypoglycemia: Beta-adrenergic blockade may blunt premonitory signs and symptoms (eg, tachycardia, blood pressure changes) of acute hypoglycemia. Nonselective beta-blockers may potentiate insulin-induced hypoglycemia.

Thyrotoxicosis: Beta-adrenergic blockers may mask clinical signs (eg, tachycardia) of developing or continuing hyperthyroidism. Abrupt withdrawal may exacerbate symptoms of hyperthyroidism, including thyroid storm.

In contrast, propranolol may be beneficial in reducing the symptoms of thyrotoxicosis.

Serum lipid concentrations: Beta-blockers may alter serum lipids, including an increase in the concentration of total triglycerides, total cholesterol, and low-density lipoprotein and very low-density lipoprotein cholesterol, and a decrease in the concentration of high-density lipoprotein cholesterol.

Muscle weakness: Beta-blockade has potentiated muscle weakness consistent with certain myasthenic symptoms (eg, diplopia, ptosis, generalized weakness).

Renal/Hepatic function impairment: Use with caution.

Pregnancy: *Category D* (**atenolol**).

Category C (**betaxolol, bisoprolol, carteolol, esmolol, metoprolol, nadolol, penbutolol, propranolol, timolol**).

Category B (**acebutolol, pindolol, sotalol**).

Lactation: In general, instruct mothers receiving these drugs to not breast-feed.

Children: Safety and efficacy for use in children have not been established.

IV administration of **propranolol** is not recommended in children; however, oral propranolol has been used.

Drug Interactions

Drugs that may affect beta blockers include aluminum salts, barbiturates, calcium blockers, calcium salts, cholestyramine, cimetidine, colestipol, diphenhydramine, flecainide, haloperidol, hydralazine, hydroxychloroquine, loop diuretics, monoamine oxidase inhibitors, nonsteroidal anti-inflammatory drugs, oral contraceptives, penicillins (ampicillin), phenothiazines, propafenone, quinidine, quinolones (ciprofloxacin), rifampin, salicylates, selective serotonin reuptake inhibitors, sulfinpyrazone, thioamines, and thyroid hormones.

Drugs that may be affected by beta blockers include anticoagulants, benzodiazepines, clonidine, disopyramide, epinephrine, ergot alkaloids, flecainide, gabapentin, haloperidol, hydralazine, lidocaine, nondepolarizing muscle relaxants, phenothiazines, prazosin, sulfonylureas, and theophylline.

Drug/Lab test interactions: These agents may produce hypoglycemia and interfere with glucose or insulin tolerance tests. **Propranolol** and **betaxolol** may interfere with the glaucoma screening test because of a reduction in intraocular pressure.

Drug/Food interactions: Food enhances the bioavailability of **metoprolol** and **propranolol**; this effect is not noted with **nadolol**, **bisoprolol**, or **pindolol**. The rate of **carteolol** and **penbutolol** absorption is slowed by the presence of food; however, extent of absorption is not appreciably affected. **Sotalol** absorption is reduced approximately 20% by a standard meal.

Adverse Reactions

Most adverse effects are mild and transient and rarely require withdrawal of therapy.

Cardiovascular: Abnormal ECG, bradycardia, chest pain, CHF, edema, first-, second-, and third-degree heart block, flushing, hypertension, hypotension, pallor, palpitations, peripheral ischemia, peripheral vascular insufficiency, presyncope and syncope, pulmonary edema, shortness of breath, supraventricular tachycardia, tachycardia, torsade de pointes and other serious new ventricular arrhythmias, vasodilation, worsening of angina and arterial insufficiency.

CNS: Acute mental changes in the elderly; anxiety; change in behavior; diminished concentration/memory; dizziness; hallucinations; headache; incoordination; increase in signs and symptoms of myasthenia gravis; insomnia; lethargy; mental depression; mood change; nervousness; paresthesias; peripheral neuropathy; restlessness; sedation; sleep disturbances; somnolence; tiredness/fatigue; vertigo.

It has been suggested that the more lipophilic the beta-blocker, the higher the CNS penetration and subsequent incidence of adverse CNS effects.

Dermatologic: Acne; alopecia; dry skin; eczema; erythematous rash; flushing; increased pigmentation; pruritus; psoriasis; purpura; rash; skin irritation; sweating/hyperhidrosis.

Endocrine: Hyperglycemia; hypoglycemia; unstable diabetes.

GI: Abdominal discomfort/pain, anorexia, appetite disorder, bloating, constipation, diarrhea, dry mouth, dyspepsia, flatulence, gastric/epigastric pain, gastritis, heartburn, nausea, taste distortion, vomiting.

GU: Dysuria, impotence or decreased libido, nocturia, sexual dysfunction, urinary retention or frequency.

Hematologic: Agranulocytosis, bleeding, eosinophilia, hyperlipidemia, leukopenia, nonthrombocytopenic or thrombocytopenic purpura, thrombocytopenia.

Hypersensitivity: Anaphylaxis, angioedema, erythematous rash, fever combined with aching and sore throat, laryngospasm, pharyngitis, photosensitivity reaction, respiratory distress.

Musculoskeletal: Arthralgia, arthritis, back/neck pain, extremity pain, joint pain, localized pain, muscle cramps/pain, myalgia, twitching/tremor.

Ophthalmic: Abnormal lacrimation, blurred vision, conjunctivitis, dry/burning eyes, eye irritation/discomfort, ocular pain/pressure.

Respiratory: Asthma, bronchial obstruction, bronchospasm, cough, dyspnea, laryngospasm with respiratory distress, nasal stuffiness, pharyngitis, rhinitis, sinusitis, wheezing.

Miscellaneous: Asthenia, death, earache, facial swelling, fever, malaise, Raynaud's phenomenon, speech disorder, weight gain, weight loss.

Lab test abnormalities: **Propranolol** may elevate blood urea levels in patients with severe heart disease. **Propranolol** and **metoprolol** may cause elevated serum transaminase, alkaline phosphatase, and lactate dehydrogenase.

Minor persistent elevations in AST and ALT have occurred in 7% of patients treated with **pindolol**. Elevations of AST and ALT of 1 to 2 times normal have occurred with **bisoprolol** (3.9% to 6.2%).

LABETALOL HYDROCHLORIDE

Tablets: 100, 200, and 300 mg (*Rx*) — Various, *Trandate* (Faro Pharmaceuticals)
Injection: 5 mg/mL (*Rx*)

Indications

Oral: Hypertension, alone or with other agents, especially thiazide and loop diuretics.

Parenteral: For control of blood pressure in severe hypertension.

Administration and Dosage

Oral:

Initial dose – 100 mg twice/day, alone or added to a diuretic. After 2 or 3 days, using standing BP as an indicator, titrate dosage in increments of 100 mg twice/day, every 2 or 3 days.

Maintenance dose – 200 to 400 mg twice/day. Patients with severe hypertension may require 1.2 to 2.4 g/day. Should side effects (principally nausea or dizziness) occur with twice daily dosing, the same total daily dose given 3 times/day may improve tolerability. Titration increments should not exceed 200 mg twice/day.

Parenteral:

Repeated IV injection – Initially, 20 mg (0.25 mg/kg for an 80 kg patient) slowly over 2 minutes. Additional injections of 40 or 80 mg can be given at 10 minute intervals until a desired supine BP is achieved or a total of 300 mg has been injected. The maximum effect usually occurs within 5 minutes of each injection.

Slow continuous infusion – Give at a rate of 3 mL/min (2 mg/min). Continue infusion until satisfactory response is obtained; then discontinue infusion and start oral labetalol. Effective IV dose range is 50 to 200 mg, up to 300 mg.

Transfer to oral dosing (hospitalized patients): Begin oral dosing when supine diastolic BP begins to rise. Recommended initial dose is 200 mg, then 200 or 400 mg, 6 to 12 hours later, depending on BP response. Thereafter, proceed as follows:

Inpatient Titration Instructions

IV regimen	Oral daily dose[a]
200 mg twice a day	400 mg
400 mg twice a day	800 mg
800 mg twice a day	1600 mg
1200 mg twice a day	2400 mg

[a] Total daily dose may be given in 3 divided doses.

Actions

Pharmacology: Labetalol combines both selective, competitive postsynaptic α_1-adrenergic blocking, and nonselective, competitive β-adrenergic blocking activity. The α- and β-blocking actions decrease BP. Standing BP is lowered more than supine.

Pharmacokinetics:

Absorption/Distribution – Oral labetalol is completely absorbed; peak plasma levels occur in 1 to 2 hours. Steady-state plasma levels during repetitive dosing are reached by about the third day. Due to an extensive first-pass effect, absolute bioavailability is 25%. Protein binding is approximately 50%.

Metabolism/Excretion – Metabolism is mainly through conjugation to glucuronide metabolites, which are excreted in urine and in feces (via bile). Elimination half-life is 5.5 to 8 hours. About 55% to 60% of a dose appears in urine as conjugates or unchanged drug in the first 24 hours.

Onset/Peak/Duration –

Oral: The peak effects of single oral doses occur within 2 to 4 hours and lasts 8 to 12 hours. The maximum, steady-state BP response upon oral, twice-a-day dosing occurs within 24 to 72 hours.

IV: The maximum effect of each IV injection of labetalol at each dose level occurs within 5 minutes. Following discontinuation of IV therapy, BP approaches pretreatment baseline values in 16 to 18 hours.

Contraindications

Bronchial asthma; overt cardiac failure; greater than first-degree heart block; cardiogenic shock; severe bradycardia.

Warnings/Precautions

Cardiac failure: Avoid use in overt CHF; may be used with caution in patients with a history of heart failure who are well compensated. CHF has been observed in patients receiving labetalol.

Patients without history of cardiac failure (latent cardiac insufficiency): Continued depression of myocardium with β-blockers can lead to cardiac failure.

Withdrawal: Hypersensitivity to catecholamines has been seen in patients withdrawn from β-blockers. When discontinuing chronic labetalol, particularly in ischemic heart disease, gradually reduce dosage over 1 to 2 weeks and carefully monitor.

Nonallergic bronchospasm (eg, chronic bronchitis, emphysema): Patients with bronchospastic disease should, in general, not receive β-blockers.

Diabetes mellitus and hypoglycemia: β-blockade may prevent the appearance of premonitory signs and symptoms of acute hypoglycemia. β-blockade also reduces insulin release; it may be necessary to adjust antidiabetic drug dose.

Major surgery: Withdrawing β-blockers prior to major surgery is controversial. Protracted severe hypotension and difficulty restarting or maintaining heartbeat have been reported with beta blockers.

Rapid decreases of BP: Observe caution when reducing severely elevated BP. Achieve desired BP lowering over as long a time as possible.

Hypotension: Symptomatic postural hypotension is most likely to occur 2 to 4 hours after a dose, especially following a large initial dose or upon large changes in dose. It is likely to occur if patients are tilted or allowed to assume the upright position 3 hours or less of receiving labetalol injection.

Hepatic function impairment: Drug metabolism may be diminished.

Jaundice or hepatic dysfunction – Jaundice or hepatic dysfunction has rarely been associated with labetalol.

Pregnancy: Category C.

Lactation: Small amounts are excreted in breast milk.

Children: Safety and efficacy for use in children have not been established.

Elderly: Bioavailability is increased in elderly patients.

Drug Interactions

Drugs that may interact with labetalol include beta-adrenergic agonists, cimetidine, glutethimide, halothane, and nitroglycerin.

Drug/Lab test interactions: A labetalol metabolite may falsely increase urinary catecholamine levels when measured by a nonspecific trihydroxyindole reaction.

Drug/Food interactions: Food may increase bioavailability of the drug.

Adverse Reactions

Significant adverse reactions include fatigue; headache; drowsiness; paresthesias; difficulty in micturition; diarrhea; reversible increases in serum transaminases; dyspnea; bronchospasm; asthenia; muscle cramps; nausea; vomiting; fever with aching and sore throat; toxic myopathy; rashes; systemic lupus erythematosus; vision abnormality; hypoesthesia; ventricular arrhythmias; intensification of AV block; mental depression; scalp tingling.

CARVEDILOL

Tablets: 3.125, 6.25, 12.5, and 25 mg (*Rx*)	Various, *Coreg* (GlaxoSmithKline)
Capsules, extended-release[a]: 10, 20, 40, and 80 mg (as phosphate) (*Rx*)	*Coreg CR* (GlaxoSmithKline)

[a] Contains immediate- and controlled-release microparticles.

Indications

Essential hypertension: Management of essential hypertension. It can be used alone or in combination with other antihypertensive agents, especially thiazide-type diuretics.

Congestive heart failure (CHF): For the treatment of mild to severe heart failure of ischemic or cardiomyopathic origin, usually in addition to diuretics, angiotensin-converting enzyme (ACE) inhibitors, and digitalis, to increase survival, and to reduce the risk of hospitalization.

Left ventricular dysfunction (LVD) following myocardial infarction (MI): To reduce cardiovascular mortality in clinically stable patients who have survived the acute phase of an MI and have a left ventricular ejection fraction of 40% or less (with or without symptomatic heart failure).

Administration and Dosage

Immediate-release (IR) tablets:

Hypertension – 6.25 mg twice daily. If this dose is tolerated, maintain the dose for 7 to 14 days, and then increase to 12.5 mg twice daily, if needed, based on trough blood pressure. Maintain this dose for 7 to 14 days and then be adjust upward to 25 mg twice/day if tolerated and needed. The full antihypertensive effect of carvedilol is seen within 7 to 14 days. Total daily dose should not exceed 50 mg. Carvedilol should be taken with food.

CHF – 3.125 mg twice daily for 2 weeks. If this dose is tolerated, increased to 6.25, 12.5, and 25 mg twice daily over successive intervals of at least 2 weeks. A maximum dose of 50 mg twice daily has been administered to patients weighing over 85 kg (187 lbs) with mild to moderate heart failure.

Reduce the dose of carvedilol if patients experience bradycardia (heart rate less than 55 beats/minute).

LVD following MI – 6.25 mg twice daily and increased after 3 to 10 days, based on tolerability to 12.5 mg twice daily, then again to the target dose of 25 mg twice daily. A lower starting dose may be used (3.125 mg twice daily) and/or the rate of up-titration may be slowed if clinically indicated. Maintain patients on lower doses if higher doses are not tolerated.

Discontinuation – Because carvedilol has β-blocking activity, do not discontinue abruptly. Severe exacerbation of angina and the occurrence of MI and ventricular arrhythmias have been reported. Instead, discontinue over 1 or 2 weeks.

Extended-release (ER) tablets:

Switching from IR to ER carvedilol – Patients controlled with carvedilol IR tablets alone or in combination with other medications may be switched to carvedilol ER capsules based on the total daily doses shown in the following table.

Carvedilol Dosing Conversion

Daily dosage of carvedilol IR tablets	Daily dosage of carvedilol ER capsules
6.25 mg (3.125 mg twice daily)	10 mg once daily
12.5 mg (6.25 mg twice daily)	20 mg once daily
25 mg (12.5 mg twice daily)	40 mg once daily
50 mg (25 mg twice daily)	80 mg once daily

Administration – Carvedilol should be taken once daily in the morning with food. Carvedilol should be swallowed as a whole capsule. Carvedilol and/or its contents should not be crushed, chewed, or taken in divided doses.

The administration of carvedilol with alcohol (including prescription and over-the-counter medications that contain ethanol) should be separated by at least 2 hours.

Alternative administration: The capsules may be carefully opened and the beads sprinkled over a spoonful of applesauce. The applesauce should not be warm because it could affect the modified-release properties of this formulation. The mixture of drug and applesauce should be consumed immediately in its entirety. The drug and applesauce mixture should not be stored for future use. Absorption of the beads sprinkled on other foods has not been tested.

Heart failure – 10 mg once daily for 2 weeks. Patients who tolerate a dosage of 10 mg once daily may have their dose increased to 20, 40, and 80 mg over successive intervals of at least 2 weeks. Patients should be maintained on lower doses if higher doses are not tolerated.

Left ventricular dysfunction following MI – It is recommended that carvedilol be started at 20 mg once daily and increased after 3 to 10 days, based on tolerability, to 40 mg once daily, then again to the target dosage of 80 mg once daily. Patients should be maintained on lower doses if higher doses are not tolerated.

Hypertension – 20 mg once daily. If this dosage is tolerated, the dosage should be maintained for 7 to 14 days, and then increased to 40 mg once daily if needed. This dosage should also be maintained for 7 to 14 days and then can be adjusted upward to 80 mg once daily if tolerated and needed. It is anticipated that the full antihypertensive effect of carvedilol would be seen within 7 to 14 days, as had been demonstrated with carvedilol IR. Total daily dose should not exceed 80 mg.

Addition of a diuretic to carvedilol or carvedilol to a diuretic can be expected to produce additive effects and exaggerate the orthostatic component of carvedilol action.

Actions

Pharmacology: Carvedilol, an antihypertensive agent, is a racemic mixture in which nonselective β-adrenoreceptor blocking activity is present in the S(−) enantiomer and α-adrenergic blocking activity is present in both R(+) and S(−) enantiomers at equal potency. Carvedilol has no intrinsic sympathomimetic activity.

Carvedilol (1) reduces cardiac output, (2) reduces exercise- or isoproterenol-induced tachycardia, and (3) reduces reflex orthostatic tachycardia. Significant β-blocking effect is usually seen within 1 hour of drug administration.

Carvedilol also (1) attenuates the pressor effects of phenylephrine, (2) causes vasodilation, and (3) reduces peripheral vascular resistance. These effects contribute to the reduction of blood pressure and usually are seen within 30 minutes of drug administration.

Pharmacokinetics:

Absorption/Distribution – Carvedilol is rapidly and extensively absorbed following oral administration of carvedilol IR tablets, with absolute bioavailability of approximately 25% to 35% due to a significant degree of first-pass metabolism. Carvedilol ER capsules have approximately 85% of the bioavailability of carvedilol IR tablets. Following oral administration, the apparent mean terminal elimination half-life generally ranges from 7 to 10 hours. Plasma concentrations achieved are proportional to the oral dose administered.

Carvedilol is more than 98% bound to plasma proteins (primarily albumin). It has a steady-state volume of distribution of approximately 115 L, indicating substantial distribution into extravascular tissues. Plasma clearance ranges from 500 to 700 mL/min.

Metabolism/Excretion – Carvedilol is extensively metabolized. Following oral administration in healthy volunteers, carvedilol accounted for only about 7% of the total in plasma as measured by area under the curve. Less than 2% of the dose was excreted unchanged in the urine. The metabolites of carvedilol are excreted primarily via the bile into the feces.

Contraindications

Bronchial asthma (2 cases of death from status asthmaticus have been reported in patients receiving single doses of carvedilol) or related bronchospastic conditions, second- or third-degree atrioventricular (AV) block, sick sinus syndrome or severe bradycardia (unless a permanent pacemaker is in place), cardiogenic shock or decompensated heart failure requiring the use of IV inotropic therapy (such patients should first be weaned from IV therapy before initiating carvedilol), clinically manifest hepatic function impairment, hypersensitivity to any component of the drug.

Warnings/Precautions

Cessation of therapy: Because carvedilol has β-blocking activity, do not discontinue abruptly. Severe exacerbation of angina and the occurrence of MI and ventricular arrhythmias have been reported. Instead, discontinue over 1 or 2 weeks.

Bronchial asthma: Two cases of death from status asthmaticus have occurred in patients receiving single doses of carvedilol.

Bronchospasm, nonallergic (eg, chronic bronchitis, emphysema): In general, do not give β-blockers to patients with bronchospastic disease. However, carvedilol may be used with caution in patients who do not respond to, or cannot tolerate, other antihypertensive agents. If carvedilol is used, it is prudent to use the smallest effective dose so that inhibition of endogenous or exogenous β-agonists is minimized.

Worsening cardiac failure: Worsening cardiac failure or fluid retention may occur during up-titration of carvedilol. If such symptoms occur, increase diuretics and do not advance the carvedilol dose until clinical stability resumes. Occasionally, it is necessary to lower the carvedilol dose or temporarily discontinue it. Such episodes do not preclude subsequent successful titration of carvedilol.

Peripheral vascular disease: β-blockers can precipitate or aggravate symptoms of arterial insufficiency in patients with peripheral vascular disease. Exercise caution.

Hypotension and postural hypotension: Hypotension and postural hypotension occurred in 9.7% and syncope in 3.4% of CHF patients receiving carvedilol, compared with 3.6% and 2.5% of placebo patients, respectively. The risk for these events was highest during the first 30 days of dosing.

Anesthesia and major surgery: If carvedilol treatment is to be continued perioperatively, take particular care with anesthetic agents, which depress myocardial function.

Diabetes and hypoglycemia: β-blockers may mask some of the manifestations of hypoglycemia, particularly tachycardia. Nonselective β-blockers may potentiate insulin-induced hypoglycemia and delay recovery of serum glucose levels. Caution patients subject to spontaneous hypoglycemia, or diabetic patients receiving insulin or oral hypoglycemic agents, about these possibilities and use carvedilol with caution.

Effects on glycemic control in patients with type 2 diabetes: In CHF patients with diabetes, carvedilol therapy may lead to worsening hyperglycemia, which responds to intensification of hypoglycemic therapy. It is recommended that blood glucose be monitored when carvedilol dosing is initiated, adjusted, or discontinued.

Thyrotoxicosis: β-adrenergic blockade may mask clinical signs of hyperthyroidism, such as tachycardia. Abrupt withdrawal of β-blockade may be followed by an exacerbation of the symptoms of hyperthyroidism or may precipitate thyroid storm.

Pheochromocytoma: In patients with pheochromocytoma, an α-blocking agent should be initiated prior to use of any β-blocking agent. Although carvedilol has both α- and β-blocking pharmacologic activities, there has been no experience with its use in this condition. Therefore, use caution in administering carvedilol.

Prinzmetal variant angina: Agents with nonselective β-blocking activity may provoke chest pain in patients with Prinzmetal variant angina. Although the α-blocking activity of carvedilol may prevent such symptoms, take caution with patients suspected of having Prinzmetal variant angina.

Cardiovascular effects: Because carvedilol has β-blocking activity, it should not be discontinued abruptly, particularly in patients with ischemic heart disease. Instead, discontinue over 1 to 2 weeks.

In clinical trials, carvedilol caused bradycardia in about 2% of patients. If pulse rate drops below 55 beats/min, reduce the dosage.

Hypersensitivity reactions: While taking β-blockers, patients with a history of severe anaphylactic reaction to a variety of allergens may be more reactive to repeated challenge, either accidental, diagnostic, or therapeutic. Such patients may be unresponsive to the usual doses of epinephrine used to treat allergic reaction.

Renal/Hepatic function impairment: Rarely, use of carvedilol in patients with CHF has resulted in deterioration of renal function. Patients at risk appear to be those with low blood pressure (systolic BP less than 100 mm Hg), ischemic heart disease, and diffuse vascular disease or underlying renal insufficiency. Renal function returned to baseline when carvedilol was stopped. Discontinue the drug or reduce dosage if worsening of renal function occurs.

Use of carvedilol in patients with clinically manifest hepatic function impairment is not recommended. Mild hepatocellular injury, confirmed by rechallenge, has occurred rarely with carvedilol therapy.

Photosensitivity: Photosensitivity may occur; therefore, caution patients to take protective measures (eg, sunscreens, protective clothing) against exposure to ultraviolet light or sunlight until tolerance is determined.

Pregnancy: Category C.

Lactation: It is not known whether this drug is excreted in breast milk.

Children: Safety and efficacy in patients younger than 18 years of age have not been established.

Elderly: Plasma levels of carvedilol average about 50% higher in the elderly compared with young subjects. With the exception of dizziness (8.8% in the elderly vs 6% in younger patients), there were no events for which the incidence in the elderly exceeded that in the younger population by more than 2%.

Monitoring: Regular monitoring of blood glucose is recommended in patients taking insulin or oral hypoglycemics. Monitor renal function during up-titration, discontinuation, or dosage reduction in patients at risk for renal function deterioration. Monitor for worsening of heart failure or fluid retention.

Drug Interactions

Drugs that may affect carvedilol include cimetidine, CYP-4502D6 inhibitors (eg, propafenone, quinidine), rifampin, selective serotonin reuptake inhibitors (eg, fluoxetine, paroxetine), hydroxychloroquine, and diphenhydramine. Additionally, alcohol, catecholamine depleting agents, clonidine, and salicylates may affect carvedilol ER.

Drugs that may be affected by carvedilol include antidiabetic agents, calcium blockers, clonidine, cyclosporine, disopyramide, catecholamine depleting agents (eg, reserpine), and digoxin.

Drug/Food interactions: When taken with food, rate of absorption is slowed but extent of bioavailability is not affected. Taking with food minimizes the risk of orthostatic hypotension.

Adverse Reactions

CHF patients – Reactions occurring in 3% or more of patients include abdominal pain, abnormal vision, angina pectoris, arthralgia, asthenia, bradycardia, BUN increase, chest pain, diarrhea, digoxin level increased, dizziness, fatigue, fever, generalized and dependent edema, headache, hypercholesterolemia, hyperglycemia, hypotension, increased cough, nausea, nonprotein nitrogen increase, rales, syncope, upper respiratory tract infection, vomiting, weight increase.

Hypertensive patients – Adverse reactions occurring in 3% or more of patients include dizziness.

ANTIHYPERTENSIVES

Agents used in hypertension therapy are listed in the following tables:

Pharmacological Effects of Antihypertensive Agents

↑ = increase ⇧ = slight increases 0 = no change ⇩ = slight decrease ↓ = decrease	Onset (min)	Peak effect[a] (h)	Duration of action[b] (h)	Plasma volume	Plasma renin activity	RBF GFR[c]	Peripheral resistance	Cardiac output	Heart rate	LVH	Total cholesterol	HDL	LDL	Triglycerides
Antiadrenergic Agents – Centrally Acting														
Methyldopa	120	2-6	12-24	↑	⇩/0	⇩/0	↓	⇩/0	⇩/0	↓	0	0	0	0
Clonidine	30-60	2-5	12-24	↑	⇩	⇩/0	↓	⇩/0	↓	↓	0	0	0	0
Guanabenz	60	2-4	6-12	0	↓	0	↓	0	↓	↓	0	0	0	0
Guanfacine		1-4	24	⇩/0	↓		↓	0	⇩	↓	0	0	0	0
Antiadrenergic Agents – Peripherally Acting														
Reserpine	days	6-12	6-24	↑	⇩/0	⇩/0	↑	0/↓	↑					
Guanethidine		6-8	24-48	↑	⇩/0	⇩/0	↓	0/↓	↑					
Guanadrel	30-120	4-6	9-14	↑		0	↑	0	↓					
Doxazosin		2-3								↓	↓	↑	0/↓	↓
Prazosin	120-130	1-3	6-12	0/⇧	⇩/0	0	↓	0/⇧	0/⇧	↓	↓	↑	0/↑	↓
Terazosin	15	1-2	12-24	0	0	0	↑	⇧	⇧	↓	↓	↑	0/↓	↓
Antiadrenergic Agents – Beta-Adrenergic Blockers														
Acebutolol		3-8	24-30				⇩	↓	↓	0/↓	0/↑	↓	↑	0/↑
Atenolol		2-4	24 +	⇩/0	↓	↓/0	0	↓	↓	↓	0/↑	↓	↑	0/↑
Betaxolol								↓	↓		0/↑	↓	↑	0/↑
Bisoprolol								↓	↓		0			0
Carteolol		1-3	24 +					↓	↓		0			0
Metoprolol		1.5	13-19	⇩/0	↓	⇩/0	0/↓	↓	↓	↓	0/↑	↓	↑	0/↑
Nadolol		3-4	17-24	⇩/0	↓	0	0	↓	↓	↓	0/↑	↓	↑	0/↑
Penbutolol		1.5-3	20 +		↓	⇩	0	↓	↓		0	0/↑	0	↑/↓
Pindolol		1	24 +		0	0	↓	⇩	↓	0/↓	0	0/↑	0	↑/↓
Propranolol		2-4	8-12	⇩/0	↓	↓	⇩/0	↓	↓	↓	0	0/↑	0	↑/↓
Timolol		1-3	12	⇩/0	↓		0	↓	↓	↓	0	0/↑	0	↑/↓
Antiadrenergic Agents – Alpha/Beta-Adrenergic Blocker														
Labetalol		2-4	8-12	↑	↓	0/↑	↓	0	↓	↓				
Carvedilol	30						↓	↓	↓					
Angiotensin Converting Enzyme (ACE) Inhibitors														
Benazepril	60	0.5-1	24		↑	RBF ↑ GFR 0	↓	0/↑	0	↓	0	0	0	0
Captopril	15-30	0.5-1.5	6-12	⇧	↑	RBF ↑ GFR 0	↓	0/↑	0	↓	0	0	0	0
Enalapril	60	4-6	24	0/⇧	↑	RBF ↑ GFR 0	↓	↑	0	↓	0	0	0	0
Enalaprilat	15	3-4	≈ 6		↑	RBF ↑ GFR 0	↓	↑	0	↓	0	0	0	0
Fosinopril	60	≈ 3	24		↑	RBF ↑ GFR 0	↓	0/↑	0	↓	0	0	0	0
Lisinopril	60	≈ 7	24		↑	RBF ↑ GFR 0	↓	0	0	↓	0	0	0	0
Quinapril	60	1	24		↑	RBF ↑ GFR 0	↓	0/↑	0	↓	0	0	0	0
Ramipril	60-120	1	24		↑	RBF ↑ GFR 0	↓	0/↑	0	↓	0	0	0	0

Pharmacological Effects of Antihypertensive Agents

↑ = increase ⇧ = slight increases 0 = no change ⇩ = slight decrease ↓ = decrease	Onset (min)	Peak effect[a] (h)	Duration of action[b] (h)	Plasma volume	Plasma renin activity	RBF GFR[c]	Peripheral resistance	Cardiac output	Heart rate	LVH	Total cholesterol	HDL	LDL	Triglycerides
Calcium Channel Blocking Agents														
Amlodipine	gradual	6-12	> 24	0	0	↑	↓↓↓	0	0	↓	0	0	0	0
Diltiazem SR	30-60	6-11					↓	0-↑	↓-0	↓	0	0	0	0
Felodipine	120-300	2.5-5					↓↓↓	↑	↑	↓	0	0	0	0
Isradipine	120	1.5					↓↓↓	↑	↑/↓	↓	0	0	0	0
Nicardipine	20	0.5-2			⇧/↑	⇧	↓	↑	↑	↓	0	0/⇧	0	0
Nifedipine SR	20	6					↓↓↓	↑↑	↑	↓	0	0	0	0
Verapamil	30	1-2.2			0/⇧	0	↓	↑/↓	↑/↓	↓	0	0/⇧	0	0
Diuretics														
Thiazides & deriv.	60-120	4-12	6-72	↓	↑	↓	↓	↓	0	0/↓	↑	0	↑	↑
Loop diuretics	within 60	1-2	4-8	↓	↑	↓	↓	↓	0	0/↓	↑	0	↑	↑
Amiloride	120	6-10	24	↓	↑	0	↓	↓	0					
Spironolactone	24-48 h	48-72	48-72	↓	↑	0	↓	0	0					
Triamterene	2-4 h	6-8	12-16											
Vasodilators														
Hydralazine	45	0.5-2	6-8	↑	↑	↑	↓	↑	↑	↑				
Minoxidil	30	2-3	24-72	↑	↑	0	↓	↑	↑	↑				
Agents For Hypertensive Emergencies/Urgencies														
Phentolamine	immed.		5-10 min	⇧	↑	↑	↓	0/↑	↑					
Phenoxy-benzamine	gradual	2-3	24 +	⇧	↑	↑	↓	↑	↓					
Metyrosine		6 +	2-3 days				↓		↓					
Agents For Pheochromocytoma														
Nitroprusside	0.5-1		3-5 min	↑	↑	0	↓	⇩	⇧		NA[d]			
Diazoxide	1-2	5 min	< 12	↑	↑	↑	↓	↑	↑					
Trimethaphan camsylate	1-2		10-15 min	↑	↓	0	↓	↓	↓					
Nitroglycerin (IV)	immed.		tran-sient	0	0		↓	↑	↑					
Captopril[e]				⇧	↑	RBF ↑ GFR 0	↓	0/↑	0					
Enalaprilat[e]					↑	RBF ↑ GFR 0	↓	↑	0					
Hydralazine[e]	10-20		3-6											
Labetalol[e]	5-10		3-6	↑	↓	0/↑	↓	0	↓					
Nicardipine[e]	1-5		3-6		⇧/↑	⇧	↓	↑	↑					
Nifedipine[e]							↓↓↓	↑↑	↑					
Phentolamine[e]	1-2		3-10 min											
Miscellaneous Agents														
Mecamylamine	30-120		6-12+	↑	↓	↓	↓	↓	↑					
Pargyline		4-21 days	3 weeks			↓	↓	0	0					
Tolazoline							↓							

[a] Peak clinical effect following a single oral dose, except where indicated.
[b] Duration of action is frequently dose-dependent.
[c] Renal blood flow and glomerular filtration rate.
[d] NA = Not applicable.
[e] Unlabeled use.

Stepped-Care Antihypertensive Regimen: The Fifth-Report of the Joint National Committee on Detection, Evaluation, and Treatment of High Blood Pressure. *Arch Intern Med* 1993;153:154-83.

Experience in treating essential hypertension (systolic blood pressure [BP] 140 mm Hg or greater and/or diastolic BP 90 mm Hg or greater) demonstrates the benefits of pharmacotherapy. Reducing BP decreases cardiovascular mortality and morbidity in patients with hypertension. Antihypertensive therapy protects against stroke, left ventricular hypertrophy, CHF, and progression to more severe hypertension. In addition to drug therapy, life-style modifications of adjunctive value include weight reduction, sodium and alcohol restriction, smoking cessation, regular exercise, and a diet low in saturated fat.

Hypertension Categories

Range (mm Hg)		
Systolic	Diastolic	Category[a]
< 130	< 85	Normal BP
130-139	85-89	High normal BP
140-159	90-99	Stage 1 (mild) hypertension
160-179	100-109	Stage 2 (moderate) hypertension
180-209	110-119	Stage 3 (severe) hypertension
≥ 210	≥ 120	Stage 4 (very severe) hypertension

[a] When systolic and diastolic BP fall into different categories, select the higher category to classify the patient's BP (eg, classify 165/95 mm Hg as Stage 2, 170/115 mm Hg as Stage 3). Isolated systolic hypertension is systolic BP 140 mm Hg or greater and diastolic BP less than 90 mm Hg (stage appropriately).

For purposes of risk classification and management, specify presence or absence of target-organ disease and additional risk factors in addition to classifying hypertension stages. For example, classify a diabetic patient with Stage 3 hypertension and left ventricular hypertrophy as "Stage 3 hypertension with target-organ disease (left ventricular hypertrophy) and with one additional risk factor (diabetes)."

The *stepped-care approach* begins with life-style modifications. If BP remains at least 140/90 mm Hg for 3 to 6 months, start antihypertensive therapy, especially in patients with target-organ disease or other risk factors for cardiovascular disease. Initiate therapy with one agent, increase the dosage gradually, then add or substitute agents with gradual increases in doses until the therapeutic goal is achieved, side effects become intolerable or maximum dosages are reached. Try life-style modifications first.

Stepped-Care Approach

I. Life-style modifications	Weight reduction Moderation of alcohol intake Regular physical activity	Reduction of sodium intake Smoking cessation
II. Inadequate response	Continue life-style modifications Initial pharmacological selection[a] 1) Diuretics or beta blockers[b] 2) ACE inhibitors, calcium blockers, $alpha_1$ blockers, alpha-beta blocker[c]	
III. Inadequate response	1) Increase drug dose, or; 2) Substitute another drug, or; 3) Add a second agent from a different class.[d]	
IV. Inadequate response	Add a second or third agent or diuretic if not already prescribed.[d]	

[a] Initial drug therapy is monotherapy for Stage 1 and Stage 2 hypertension.

[b] Preferred because a reduction in morbidity and mortality has been demonstrated.

[c] Equally effective in reducing BP; however, these have not been tested in long-term controlled trials to demonstrate reduction of morbidity and mortality. Reserve for special indications or when preferred agents are unacceptable or ineffective.

[d] Supplemental antihypertensive agents, which include centrally acting $alpha_2$-agonists (clonidine, guanabenz, guanfacine, methyldopa), peripheral-acting adrenergic antagonists (guanadrel, guanethidine, rauwolfia alkaloids) and direct vasodilators (hydralazine, minoxidil), are not routinely well suited for initial monotherapy.

Diuretics – Generally initiate therapy with a thiazide or other oral diuretic. Thiazide-type diuretics are drugs of choice; hydrochlorothiazide or chlorthalidone are generally preferred. Reserve loop diuretics for selected patients. This therapy alone may control many cases of mild hypertension. Consider treating diuretic-induced hypokalemia (less than 3.5 mEq/L) with potassium supplementation or by adding a potassium-sparing diuretic to therapy.

Beta-adrenergic blocking agents – Beta-adrenergic blocking agents also may be used as initial drug monotherapy. Beta blockers are effective in older patients, but less effective in black people. Beta-adrenergic blocking agents decrease cardiac output without effects on vascular resistance. In addition, they inhibit renin release.

Calcium channel blockers, ACE inhibitors, labetalol, and alpha$_1$ blockers – Calcium channel blockers, ACE inhibitors, labetalol, and alpha$_1$ blockers may be used as initial monotherapy, although they are not routinely preferred over diuretics and beta-blockers. Black people tend to respond better to calcium blockers than ACE inhibitors; labetalol may be more effective in black people than other beta-blockers.

Antiadrenergic agents – Antiadrenergic agents (central and peripheral adrenergic inhibitors) are considered supplemental agents and are used when the initial drug therapy fails to achieve the desired effect. Diuretics are usually continued to provide synergistic effects and to prevent secondary fluid accumulation that may occur with use of antiadrenergic agents alone. Combination therapy also may minimize untoward reactions, which are more common at the higher doses necessary when a single drug is used alone.

Decreased adrenergic tone results in reduced cardiac output or decreased peripheral vascular resistance. Methyldopa, guanabenz, guanfacine, and clonidine act mainly in the CNS. Although reserpine has been used for years, other agents are preferred. Guanadrel is a peripheral antiadrenergic similar to guanethidine.

Vasodilators: Vasodilators also are considered supplemental agents and are not suited for initial monotherapy. A 3 drug regimen should include agents acting by different mechanisms. Hydralazine and minoxidil have direct vasodilating actions. In order to prevent reflex tachycardia caused by decreased peripheral resistance, these agents are most effective when used with a diuretic and a β-blocker. Minoxidil's undesirable side effects limit its use to severely hypertensive patients who do not respond to minimum doses of a diuretic and 2 other agents.

Antihypertensive drug withdrawal syndrome – Antihypertensive drug withdrawal syndrome may occur after discontinuation of antihypertensives.

To circumvent problems, encourage patient compliance, avoid excessive doses, avoid combining sympatholytics and β-blockers, and maintain antihypertensive medication in surgical patients. When discontinuing medication, taper the dose slowly, one drug at a time; use special caution in patients with coronary artery or cerebrovascular disease.

Treatment generally includes reinstitution of therapy, bed rest/sedation and, perhaps, therapy similar to treatment of malignant hypertension.

Step-down therapy – Attempt to decrease the dosage or the number of antihypertensive agents in patients; have them maintain life-style modifications. It may be possible to accomplish this in a deliberate, slow, progressive manner if the patient has been effectively controlled for 1 year and at least 4 visits.

METHYLDOPA AND METHYLDOPATE HYDROCHLORIDE

Tablets: 250 and 500 mg methyldopa (*Rx*)	Various
Injection: 50 mg methyldopate hydrochloride/mL (*Rx*)	

Indications

Hypertension.

Methyldopate hydrochloride may be used to initiate treatment of acute hypertensive crises; however, due to its slow onset of action, other agents may be preferred for rapid reduction of blood pressure.

Administration and Dosage

Oral:

Adults –

Initial therapy: 250 mg, 2 or 3 times/day in the first 48 hours. Adjust dosage at intervals of not less than 2 days until adequate response is achieved. To minimize sedation, increase dosage in the evening. By adjustment of dosage, morning hypotension may be prevented without sacrificing control of afternoon blood pressure.

Maintenance therapy: 500 mg to 3 g daily in 2 to 4 doses. Methyldopa is usually administered in 2 divided doses; some patients may be controlled with a single daily dose given at bedtime.

Concomitant drug therapy: When methyldopa is given with antihypertensives other than thiazides, limit the initial dosage to 500 mg/day in divided doses; when added to a thiazide, the dosage of thiazide need not be changed.

Children – Individualize dosage. Initial oral dosage is based on 10 mg/kg/day in 2 to 4 doses. The maximum daily dosage is 65 mg/kg or 3 g, whichever is less.

IV: Add dose to 100 mL 5% dextrose or give in 5% dextrose in water in a concentration of 10 mg/mL. Administer over 30 to 60 minutes. When control has been obtained, substitute oral therapy starting with the same parenteral dosage schedule.

Adults – 250 to 500 mg every 6 hours as required (maximum 1 g every 6 hours).

Children – 20 to 40 mg/kg/day in divided doses every 6 hours. The maximum daily dosage is 65 mg/kg or 3 g, whichever is less.

Tolerance: Tolerance may occur, usually between the second and third month of therapy. Adding a diuretic or increasing the dosage of methyldopa frequently restores blood pressure control. A thiazide is recommended if therapy was not started with a thiazide or if effective control of blood pressure cannot be maintained on 2 g methyldopa daily.

Discontinuation: Methyldopa has a relatively short duration of action; therefore, withdrawal is followed by return of hypertension, usually within 48 hours. This is not complicated by an overshoot of blood pressure above pretreatment levels.

Impaired renal function: Methyldopa is largely excreted by the kidneys; patients with impaired renal function may respond to smaller doses.

Actions

Pharmacology: The proposed mechanism of action of methyldopa is probably due to the drug's metabolism to alpha-methyl norepinephrine, which lowers arterial pressure by the stimulation of central inhibitory α-adrenergic receptors, false neurotransmission or reduction of plasma renin activity.

Pharmacokinetics:

Absorption/Distribution – Following oral administration, methyldopa is variably absorbed. The mean bioavailability is approximately 50%. Methyldopa crosses the blood-brain barrier and is converted in the CNS to active alpha-methylnoradrenaline. Methyldopa crosses the placental barrier and appears in cord blood and breast milk. A decrease in BP occurs within 4 to 6 hours following IV or oral administration and lasts 10 to 16 hours or 12 to 24 hours, respectively.

Metabolism/Excretion – Methyldopa is extensively metabolized. Approximately 17% of a dose of methyldopate hydrochloride appears in plasma as free methyldopa. The average T_{max} is 2 hours. The total volume of distribution is about 0.6 L/kg. Approximately 70% (oral) and approximately 49% (IV) of the drug that is absorbed is excreted in the urine as methyldopa and its mono-O-sulfate conjugate. Methyldopa is less than 20% bound to plasma proteins. The drug is removed by dialysis.

Contraindications

Active hepatic disease, such as acute hepatitis or active cirrhosis; if previous methyldopa therapy has been associated with liver disorders; coadministration with MAOIs; hypersensitivity to any component of these formulations, including sulfites.

Warnings/Precautions

Positive Coombs' test/Hemolytic anemia: With prolonged therapy, 10% to 20% of patients develop a positive direct Coombs' test, usually between 6 and 12 months of therapy.

This is associated rarely with hemolytic anemia, which could lead to potentially fatal complications and is difficult to predict. Perform baseline and periodic blood counts to detect hemolytic anemia. If Coombs'-positive hemolytic anemia occurs, discontinue methyldopa; anemia usually remits promptly.

Blood transfusions: Should the need for transfusion arise in a patient receiving methyldopa, perform both a direct and indirect Coombs' test.

Edema/Weight gain: Some patients taking methyldopa experience clinical edema or weight gain, which may be controlled by use of a diuretic. Do not continue methyldopa if edema progresses or signs of heart failure appear.

Hepatotoxicity: Fever has occasionally occurred within the first 3 weeks of therapy, sometimes associated with eosinophilia or abnormalities in 1 liver function test or more. Jaundice with or without fever may occur, usually within the first 2 to 3 months of therapy. Incidence of elevated serum transaminase levels and impaired hepatic function ranges from 1% to 27%.

Perform periodic determinations of hepatic function, particularly during the first 6 to 12 weeks of therapy or when an unexplained fever occurs.

Hematologic disorders: Rarely, a reversible reduction of the white blood cell (WBC) count with a primary effect on granulocytes has been seen.

Paradoxical pressor response: Paradoxical pressor response has been reported with IV methyldopa.

Involuntary choreoathetotic movements: Involuntary choreoathetotic movements have been observed rarely in patients with severe bilateral cerebrovascular disease. Should these occur, discontinue methyldopa therapy.

Sedation: Usually transient, sedation may occur during initial therapy or whenever the dose is increased.

Urine discoloration: Rarely, when urine is exposed to air, it may darken because of breakdown of methyldopa or its metabolites.

Sulfite sensitivity: These products contain sulfites that may cause allergic-type reactions in certain susceptible people. Sulfite sensitivity is seen more frequently in asthmatic or atopic nonasthmatic people.

Renal function impairment: The active metabolites of methyldopa accumulate in uremia. Use with caution in renal failure. Prolonged hypotension has been reported.

Hypertension has recurred occasionally after dialysis in patients given methyldopa because the drug is removed by this procedure.

Hepatic function impairment: Use with caution in patients with previous liver disease or dysfunction.

Pregnancy: *Category B* (oral); *Category C* (IV).

Lactation: Methyldopa is excreted in breast milk.

Elderly: Syncope in older patients may be related to an increased sensitivity and advanced arteriosclerotic vascular disease. May be avoided by lower doses.

Monitoring: Blood count, Coombs' tests, and liver function tests are recommended before initiating therapy and at periodic intervals. Perform periodic determinations of hepatic function, particularly during the first 6 to 12 weeks of therapy or when an unexplained fever occurs.

Drug Interactions

Drugs that may affect methyldopa include levodopa, nonselective beta-blockers (eg, propranolol), and ferrous sulfate or gluconate.

Drugs that may be affected by methyldopa include haloperidol, levodopa, lithium, sympathomimetics, MAOIs, anesthetics, and phenothiazines.

Drug/Lab test interactions: Methyldopa may interfere with tests for: Urinary uric acid by phosphotungstate method; serum creatinine by alkaline picrate method; AST by colorimetric methods. Because methyldopa causes fluorescence in urine samples at the same wavelengths as catecholamines, falsely high levels of urinary catecholamines may occur and will interfere with the diagnosis of pheochromocytoma.

Adverse Reactions

Possible adverse reactions include fever; lupus-like syndrome; rise in BUN; myalgia; septic shock-like syndrome; headache; asthenia; weakness; dizziness; symptoms of cerebrovascular insufficiency; paresthesias; parkinsonism; Bell's palsy; decreased mental acuity; involuntary choreoathetotic movements; psychic disturbances; verbal memory impairment; bradycardia; prolonged carotid sinus hypersensitivity; aggravation of angina pectoris; pericarditis; myocarditis; orthostatic hypotension; edema/weight gain (usually relieved by a diuretic; discontinue methyldopa if edema progresses or signs of heart failure appear); nausea; vomiting; constipation; diarrhea; colitis; sore or "black" tongue; pancreatitis; liver disorders; positive Coombs' test, bone marrow depression; leukopenia; granulocytopenia; thrombocytopenia; positive tests for antinuclear antibody, LE cells and rheumatoid factor; rash; toxic epidermal necrolysis; gynecomastia; lactation; amenorrhea.

CLONIDINE HYDROCHLORIDE

Tablets: 0.1 mg, 0.2 mg, and 0.3 mg (*Rx*)	Various, *Catapres* (Boehringer-Ingelheim)
Transdermal system: 2.5 mg (release rate 0.1 mg/24 h) (*Rx*)	*Catapres-TTS-1* (Boehringer-Ingelheim)
5 mg (release rate 0.2 mg/24 h) (*Rx*)	*Catapres-TTS-2* (Boehringer-Ingelheim)
7.5 mg (release rate 0.2 mg/24 h) (*Rx*)	*Catapres-TTS-3* (Boehringer-Ingelheim)
Tablets, modified-release; oral: 0.1 mg (*Rx*)	*Jenloga* (UPM)

Indications

Hypertension.

Unlabeled uses: Clonidine has been evaluated for use in the following conditions:

Clonidine Unlabeled Uses

Use	Dosage[a]
Alcohol withdrawal	0.3 to 0.6 mg every 6 hours
Constitutional growth delay in children	0.0375 to 0.15 mg/m^2/day
Diabetic diarrhea	0.15 to 1.2 mg/day or 0.3 mg/24-hour patch (1 to 2 patches/week)
Gilles de la Tourette syndrome	0.15 to 0.2 mg/day
Hypertensive "urgencies" (diastolic > 120 mm Hg)	Initially 0.1 to 0.2 mg, followed by 0.05 to 0.1 mg every hour to a maximum of 0.8 mg
Menopausal flushing	0.1 to 0.4 mg/day or 0.1 mg/24-hour patch
Methadone/opiate detoxification	15 to 16 mcg/kg/day
Pheochromocytoma diagnosis (overnight clonidine suppression test)	0.3 mg
Postherpetic neuralgia	0.2 mg/day
Reduction of allergen-induced inflammatory reactions in patients with extrinsic asthma	0.15 mg for 3 days
Smoking cessation facilitation	0.15 to 0.4 mg/day or 0.2 mg/24-hour patch
Ulcerative colitis	0.3 mg 3 times a day

[a] Dosage given as oral unless otherwise specified.

Administration and Dosage

Oral: Individualize dosage.

Initial dose – 0.1 mg twice daily (immediate release) or 0.1 mg at bedtime (modified release). The elderly may benefit from a lower initial dose.

Maintenance dose – Increments of 0.1 or 0.2 mg/day may be made until desired response is achieved; most common range is 0.2 to 0.6 mg/day given in divided doses. The maximum dose is 2.4 mg/day. Minimize sedative effects by slowly increasing the daily dosage and giving the majority of the daily dose at bedtime.

Children – 0.2 to 0.6 mg/day in divided doses. The maximum dose is 2.4 mg/day. The initial dose is 0.1 mg tablet twice daily (morning and bedtime). Increments of 0.1 mg/day may be made at weekly intervals if necessary until the desired response is achieved.

Unlabeled route of administration – Sublingual clonidine, using a dosage of 0.2 to 0.4 mg/day, may be effective in hypertensive patients unable to take oral medication. The onset occurs within 30 to 60 minutes and blood pressure appears to be maintained on a twice daily regimen.

Renal Impairment – Adjust dosage according to degree of renal impairment and carefully monitor patients. Because only a minimal amount of clonidine is removed during hemodialysis, there is no need to give supplemental clonidine following dialysis.

Transdermal: Apply to a hairless area of intact skin on upper arm or torso, once every 7 days. Use a different skin site from the previous application. If the system loosens during the 7-day wearing, apply the adhesive overlay directly over the system to ensure good adhesion.

For initial therapy, start with the 0.1 mg system. If, after 1 or 2 weeks, desired blood pressure reduction is not achieved, add another 0.1 mg system or use a larger system. Dosage greater than two 0.3 mg systems usually does not improve efficacy. Note that the antihypertensive effect of the system may not commence until 2 to 3 days after application. Therefore, when substituting the transdermal system in patients on prior antihypertensive therapy, a gradual reduction of prior drug dosage is advised. Previous antihypertensive treatment may have to be continued, particularly in patients with severe hypertension.

Actions

Pharmacology: Initially, clonidine stimulates peripheral α-adrenergic receptors producing transient vasoconstriction. Stimulation of alpha-adrenergic in the brain stem results in reduced sympathetic outflow from the CNS and a decrease in peripheral resistance, renal vascular resistance, heart rate, and blood pressure.

Pharmacokinetics:

Immediate release – Blood pressure declines within 30 to 60 minutes after an oral dose. The peak plasma level occurs in approximately 3 to 5 hours with a plasma half-life of 12 to 16 hours. About 50% of the absorbed dose is metabolized in the liver. In patients with impaired renal function, half-life increases to 30 to 40 hours. Clonidine and its metabolites are excreted mainly in the urine. About 40% to 60% of the absorbed dose is recovered in the urine as unchanged drug in 24 hours.

Modified release – Following oral administration of modified-release clonidine, peak clonidine levels are reached in 4 to 7 hours. The absorption of clonidine from modified-release clonidine is not affected by food. The plasma half-life of modified-release clonidine averages 13 hours.

Transdermal system – The system, a 0.2 mm thick film with 4 layers, contains a drug reservoir of clonidine, released at an approximately constant rate for 7 days.

Therapeutic plasma levels, achieved 2 to 3 days after initial application, are lower than during oral therapy with equipotent doses. When system is removed, therapeutic plasma clonidine levels persist for approximately 8 hours and then decline slowly over several days; blood pressure returns gradually to pretreatment levels. Elimination half-life is approximately 19 hours.

Contraindications

Hypersensitivity to clonidine or any component of adhesive layer of transdermal system.

Warnings/Precautions

Use with caution in patients with severe coronary insufficiency, recent MI, cerebrovascular disease, or chronic renal failure.

Tolerance: Tolerance may develop, necessitating a reevaluation of therapy.

Rebound hypertension: Do not discontinue therapy without consulting a physician. Discontinue therapy by reducing the dose gradually over 2 to 4 days to avoid a rapid rise in blood pressure.

If an excessive rise in blood pressure occurs, it can be reversed by resumption of therapy or by IV phentolamine, phenoxybenzamine, or prazosin. Direct vasodilators and captopril also have been used. If therapy is to be discontinued in patients receiving β-blockers and clonidine concurrently, discontinue β-blockers several days before the gradual withdrawal of clonidine.

Rebound hypertension also has occurred following discontinuation of the transdermal patch.

Ophthalmologic effects: Perform periodic eye examinations, because retinal degeneration has been noted in animal studies.

Perioperative use: Continue administration of clonidine to within 4 hours of surgery and resume as soon as possible thereafter. Carefully monitor blood pressure and institute appropriate measures to control it. If transdermal therapy is started during the perioperative period, note that therapeutic plasma levels are not achieved until 2 to 3 days after initial application.

Sensitization to transdermal clonidine: In patients who develop an allergic reaction to transdermal clonidine, oral clonidine hydrochloride substitution may elicit a similar reaction.

Pregnancy: Category C.

Lactation: Clonidine is excreted in breast milk.

Children: Safety and efficacy for use in children have not been established.

Drug Interactions

Drugs that may interact with clonidine include beta-adrenergic blocking agents and tricyclic antidepressants.

Adverse Reactions

Oral:

Immediate release – Adverse reactions may include dry mouth; drowsiness; dizziness; sedation; constipation; anorexia; malaise; nausea and vomiting; parotid pain; mild transient abnormalities in liver function tests; gynecomastia; CHF; orthostatic symptoms; palpitations, tachycardia and bradycardia; Raynaud's phenomenon; ECG abnormalities; conduction disturbances, arrhythmias, sinus bradycardia; dreams or nightmares; insomnia; hallucinations; delirium; nervousness; anxiety; depression; headache; rash, angioneurotic edema, hives, urticaria; hair thinning and alopecia; pruritus; impotence; decreased sexual activity; difficulty in micturition; weakness; muscle or joint pain; increased sensitivity to alcohol; dryness, itching or burning of the eyes; dryness of the nasal mucosa; pallor; fever; weakly positive Coombs' test.

Modified release – The incidence of adverse reactions progressively increased with increasing doses and was notably less in the 0.2 mg/day treatment group compared with the 0.4 and 0.6 mg/day treatment groups. The majority of adverse reactions were mild. No inferences regarding differences in adverse reactions between modified-release clonidine and other clonidine formulations is warranted.

Transdermal system: Adverse reactions may include dry mouth, drowsiness (the most frequent systemic reactions); constipation; nausea; change in taste; fatigue; headache; sedation; insomnia; nervousness; dizziness; impotence/sexual dysfunction; transient localized skin reactions; hyperpigmentation; edema; excoriation; burning; papules; throbbing; generalized macular rash.

ALPHA-1-ADRENERGIC BLOCKERS

ALFUZOSIN HYDROCHLORIDE	
Tablets, extended-release; oral: 10 mg (*Rx*)	*Uroxatral* (Sanofi-Synthelabo)
DOXAZOSIN MESYLATE	
Tablets; oral: 1, 2, 4, and 8 mg (as base) (*Rx*)	Various, *Cardura* (Pfizer)
Tablets, extended-release; oral: 4 and 8 mg (as base) (*Rx*)	*Cardura XL* (Pfizer)
PRAZOSIN	
Capsules; oral: 1, 2, and 5 mg (as base) (*Rx*)	Various, *Minipress* (Pfizer)
SILODOSIN	
Capsules; oral: 4 and 8 mg (*Rx*)	*Rapaflo* (Watson Pharma)
TAMSULOSIN HYDROCHLORIDE	
Capsules; oral: 0.4 mg (*Rx*)	*Flomax* (Abbott)
TERAZOSIN	
Tablets; oral: 1, 2, 5, and 10 mg (as base) (*Rx*)	Various
Capsules; oral: 1, 2, 5, and 10 mg (as base) (*Rx*)	Various, *Hytrin* (Abbott)

Indications

Hypertension (**doxazosin** *[except extended-release]*, **prazosin**, **terazosin**)*:* For the treatment of hypertension, alone or in combination with other antihypertensive agents.

Alfuzosin, doxazosin, silodosin, tamsulosin, and terazosin: Treatment of symptomatic benign prostatic hyperplasia (BPH).

Administration and Dosage

ALFUZOSIN:

Benign prostatic hyperplasia – Alfuzosin extended-release 10 mg/day tablet taken immediately after the same meal each day. Do not chew or crush tablets.

DOXAZOSIN MESYLATE:

Benign prostatic hyperplasia – Initial dosage is 1 mg given once daily in the morning or evening.

Maintenance: Dosage may then be increased to 2 mg and thereafter to 4 and 8 mg once daily, the maximum recommended dose for BPH. The recommended titration interval is 1 to 2 weeks. Evaluate blood pressure routinely.

Extended-release tablet: Administer the initial dose, 4 mg once daily, with breakfast. The dose may be increased to 8 mg, the maximum recommended dose, at 3 to 4 week intervals. If administration is discontinued for several days, restart using the 4 mg once daily dose. Tablets should be swallowed whole and must not be chewed, divided, cut, or crushed.

If switching from immediate to extended release, initiate with the lowest dose (4 mg once daily). Prior to starting therapy with extended-release tablets, the final evening dose of immediate-release tablets should not be taken.

Hypertension –

Initial dosage: 1 mg once daily. Postural effects are most likely to occur between 2 and 6 hours after a dose.

Maintenance dose: Depending on the standing blood pressure response, dosage may be increased to 2 mg and, if necessary, to 4, 8, and 16 mg to achieve the desired reduction in blood pressure. Increases in dose beyond 4 mg increase the likelihood of excessive postural effects.

PRAZOSIN:

Hypertension –

Initial dose: 1 mg 2 or 3 times daily. When increasing dosages, give the new dose increment at bedtime to reduce syncopal episodes.

Maintenance dose: 6 to 15 mg/day in divided doses. Doses higher than 20 mg usually do not increase efficacy; however, a few patients may benefit from up to 40 mg/day.

Children – A dose of 0.5 to 7 mg 3 times a day has been suggested.

Concomitant therapy – When adding a diuretic or other antihypertensive agent, reduce dosage to 1 or 2 mg 3 times a day and then retitrate.

SILODOSIN:

Benign prostatic hyperplasia – 8 mg orally once daily with a meal.

Renal function impairment – Silodosin is contraindicated in patients with severe renal impairment (creatinine clearance [CrCl] less than 30 mL/min). In patients with moderate renal impairment (CrCl 30 to 50 mL/min), the dosage should be reduced to 4 mg once daily taken with a meal. No dosage adjustment is needed in patients with mild renal impairment (CrCl 50 to 80 mL/min).

Hepatic function impairment – No dosage adjustment is needed in patients with mild or moderate hepatic impairment.

TAMSULOSIN:

Benign prostatic hyperplasia – 0.4 mg once daily, administered approximately 30 minutes following the same meal each day. Do not crush, chew, or open capsules.

For those patients who fail to respond to the 0.4 mg dose after 2 to 4 weeks of dosing, the dose can be increased to 0.8 mg once daily. If administration is discontinued or interrupted for several days, start therapy again with the 0.4 mg once-daily dose.

TERAZOSIN:

Hypertension –

Initial dose: 1 mg at bedtime for all patients. Do not exceed this dose.

Subsequent doses: Slowly increase the dose to achieve the desired blood pressure response. The recommended dose range is 1 to 5 mg daily; however, some patients may benefit from doses as high as 20 mg/day. If response is substantially diminished at 24 hours, consider an increased dose or a twice-daily regimen.

Benign prostatic hyperplasia –

Initial dose: 1 mg at bedtime is the starting dose for all patients; do not exceed as an initial dose.

Subsequent doses: Increase the dose in a stepwise fashion to 2, 5, or 10 mg daily to achieve desired improvement of symptoms or flow rates. Doses of 10 mg once daily are generally required for clinical response; therefore, treatment with 10 mg for a minimum of 4 to 6 weeks may be required.

Concomitant therapy – Observe caution when terazosin is administered concomitantly with other antihypertensive agents (eg, calcium antagonists) to avoid the possibility of significant hypotension. When adding a diuretic or other antihypertensive agent, dosage reduction and retitration may be necessary.

Actions

Pharmacology: **Alfuzosin** and **silodosin** exhibit selectivity for alpha-1-adrenergic receptors in the lower urinary tract. **Alfuzosin** and **silodosin** are not intended for use as antihypertensive drugs.

Doxazosin, **prazosin**, and **terazosin** selectively block alpha-1-adrenergic receptors. Blockade of the alpha-1-adrenergic receptor decreases urethral resistance and may relieve the obstruction and improve urine flow and BPH symptoms.

Tamsulosin selectively inhibits the alpha-1A-adrenergic receptor. Approximately 70% of the alpha-1-adrenergic receptors in the human prostate are of the alpha-1A subtype. Tamsulosin is not intended for use as an antihypertensive drug.

Terazosin decreases blood pressure gradually within 15 minutes following oral administration. Terazosin treatment in normotensive men with BPH did not result in a clinically significant blood pressure-lowering effect.

Pharmacokinetics: **Prazosin** is extensively metabolized. The metabolites of prazosin are active. Duration of antihypertensive effect is 10 hours.

Terazosin undergoes minimal hepatic first-pass metabolism; nearly all of the circulating dose is in the form of parent drug.

Alfuzosin, doxazosin, and **tamsulosin** are extensively metabolized in the liver.

Pharmacokinetics of Alpha-1-Adrenergic Blockers						
Parameters	Alfuzosin	Doxazosin	Prazosin	Silodosin	Tamsulosin	Terazosin
Oral bioavailability	49% (fed state)	≈ 65%	nd	32%	> 90% (fasting state)	nd
Peak plasma level, time	8 h (fed state)	≈ 2 to 3 h	≈ 3 h	≈ 2.6 h	4 to 5 h (fasting state) 6 to 7 h (fed state)	≈ 1 h
Protein binding	82% to 90%	≈ 98%	High	97%	94% to 99%	90% to 94%
Metabolism	Extensively metabolized by the liver, mainly by oxidation, O-demethylation, and N-dealkylation.	First-pass metabolism; extensively metabolized by the liver, mainly by O-demethylation or hydroxylation	Extensively metabolized, primarily by demethylation and conjugation	Extensive metabolism through glucuronidation, alcohol, and aldehyde dehydrogenase, and CYP3A4 pathways.	CYP450	nd
Half-life	10 h	≈ 22 h	2 to 3 h	≈ 13.3 h	9 to 15 h	≈ 12 h
Excretion	Feces: 69% urine: 24%	Feces: ≈ 63% urine: ≈ 9%	Bile and feces	Feces: 54.9% urine: 33.5%	Feces: 21% urine: 76%	Feces: ≈ 60% urine: ≈ 40%

[a] nd = no data

Contraindications

Hypersensitivity to quinazolines (eg, **doxazosin**, **prazosin**, **tamsulosin**, **terazosin**).

Alfuzosin: Moderate or severe hepatic insufficiency; coadministration with potent CYP3A4 inhibitors (eg, ketoconazole, itraconazole, ritonavir)

Silodosin: Severe renal impairment; coadministration with potent CYP3A4 inhibitors (eg, ketoconazole, clarithromycin, itraconazole, ritonavir)

Warnings/Precautions

"First-dose" effect: **Prazosin**, **terazosin**, **doxazosin**, **silodosin**, **alfuzosin**, and **tamsulosin**, like other alpha-adrenergic blocking agents, can cause marked hypotension (especially postural hypotension) and syncope with sudden loss of consciousness with the first few doses. Anticipate a similar effect if therapy is interrupted for more than a few doses, if dosage is increased rapidly, or if another antihypertensive drug is introduced.

The "first-dose" phenomenon may be minimized by limiting the initial dose to 1 mg of terazosin or prazosin (given at bedtime) or doxazosin.

Weight gain: There was a tendency for patients to gain weight during **terazosin** therapy.

Cholesterol: During controlled clinical studies, **terazosin** and **doxazosin** were associated with small decreases in low-density lipoprotein and cholesterol.

Prostatic carcinoma: Examine patients prior to starting therapy with **terazosin** to rule out the presence of carcinoma of the prostate.

Coronary insufficiency: Discontinue **alfuzosin** if symptoms of angina pectoris appear or worsen.

Hemodilution: Small but statistically significant decreases in hematocrit, hemoglobin, white blood cells, total protein, and albumin were observed in controlled clinical trials with **terazosin**. These laboratory findings suggest the possibility of hemodilution.

Leukopenia/Neutropenia: In hypertensive patients receiving **doxazosin**, mean white blood cell counts (WBC) and neutrophil counts were decreased by 2.4% and 1%, respectively, compared with placebo, a phenomenon seen with other alpha-blocking drugs. In patients with BPH, the incidence of clinically significant WBC abnormalities was 0.4%. No patients became symptomatic as a result of the low counts. WBCs and neutrophil counts returned to normal after drug discontinuation.

Intraoperative floppy iris syndrome: Intraoperative floppy iris syndrome has been observed during cataract surgery in some patients on alpha-1 blockers or previously treated with alpha-1 blockers.

Cardiotoxicity: An increased incidence of myocardial necrosis or fibrosis occurred in rats and mice following 6 to 18 months of **doxazosin** 40 to 80 mg/kg/day. There is no evidence that similar lesions occur in humans.

Patients with congenital or acquired QT prolongation: The QT effect of **alfuzosin** 40 mg did not appear as large as that of the active control moxifloxacin. Consider this observation in clinical decisions to prescribe **alfuzosin** for patients with a known history of QT prolongation or patients who are taking medications known to prolong QT.

Priapism: Rarely, alpha-$_1$ antagonists have been associated with priapism.

Renal function impairment: Exercise caution when **alfuzosin** is administered in patients with severe renal insufficiency. Reduce **silodosin** dose in patients with moderate renal impairment; exercise caution and monitor for adverse reactions.

Hepatic function impairment: Administer **doxazosin**, **silodosin**, and **alfuzosin** with caution to patients with evidence of impaired hepatic function or to patients receiving drugs known to influence hepatic metabolism.

Pregnancy: *Category* C (**prazosin, terazosin, doxazosin**); *Category* B (**silodosin, alfuzosin, tamsulosin**).

Lactation: Safety has not been established.

Children: Safety and efficacy for use in children have not been established.

Drug Interactions

Drugs that may affect alpha-1-adrenergic blockers include alcohol, beta blockers, cimetidine, CYP 3A4 inhibitors, indomethacin, phosphodiesterase type 5 inhibitors, P-gp inhibitors, and verapamil.

Drugs that may be affected by alpha-1-adrenergic blockers include beta blockers, clonidine, and phosphodiesterase type 5 inhibitors.

Drug/Lab test interactions: False-positive results may occur in screening tests for pheochromocytoma in patients who are being treated with **prazosin**.

Adverse Reactions

Alpha-1 adrenergic blocker adverse reactions occurring in 3% or more of patients when used for the treatment of hypertension:

Doxazosin – Asthenia, dizziness, edema, fatigue/malaise, headache, nausea, rhinitis, somnolence.

Prazosin – Asthenia, blurred vision/amblyopia, conjunctivitis/reddened sclera/eye pain, constipation, depression, diarrhea, dizziness, drowsiness, dry mouth, dyspnea, edema, epistaxis, headache, lack of energy, nasal congestion, nausea, nervousness, palpitations, postural hypotension/hypertension, rash, syncope, urinary frequency, vertigo, weakness.

Terazosin – Asthenia, dizziness, dyspnea, headache, nasal congestion, nausea, palpitations, peripheral edema, shoulder/neck/back/extremity pain, somnolence.

Alpha-1 adrenergic blocker adverse reactions occurring in 3% or more of patients when used for the treatment of BPH:

Alfuzosin – Dizziness.

Doxazosin – Dizziness, fatigue, headache, somnolence.

Silodosin – Abnormal ejaculation, dizziness.

Tamsulosin – Abnormal ejaculation, asthenia, chest pain, diarrhea, dizziness, headache, increased cough, infection, nausea, pharyngitis/rhinitis, shoulder/neck/back/extremity pain, sinusitis, somnolence.

Terazosin – Asthenia, dizziness, headache, postural hypotension/hypertension, somnolence.

HYDRALAZINE HYDROCHLORIDE

Tablets: 10, 25, 50, and 100 mg (*Rx*)	Various, *Apresoline* (Ciba)
Injection: 20 mg/mL (*Rx*)	

Indications

Oral: Essential hypertension, alone or in combination with other agents.

Parenteral: Severe essential hypertension when the drug cannot be given orally or when the need to lower blood pressure is urgent.

Unlabeled uses: Hydralazine in doses up to 800 mg 3 times/day has been effective in reducing afterload in the treatment of congestive heart failure (CHF), severe aortic insufficiency, and after valve replacement.

Administration and Dosage

Bioavailability of hydralazine tablets is enhanced by the concurrent ingestion of food.

Initiate therapy: Initiate therapy in gradually increasing dosages; individualize dosage. Start with 10 mg 4 times daily for the first 2 to 4 days, increase to 25 mg 4 times daily for the balance of the first week.

Second and subsequent weeks: Increase dosage to 50 mg 4 times daily.

Maintenance: Adjust dosage to lowest effective level. Twice daily dosage may be adequate. In a few resistant patients, up to 300 mg/day may be required for a significant antihypertensive effect. In such cases, consider a lower dosage of hydralazine combined with a thiazide or reserpine or a beta-blocker. However, when combining therapy, individual titration is essential to ensure the lowest possible therapeutic dose of each drug.

Children –

Initial: 0.75 mg/kg/day in 4 divided doses. Dosage may be increased gradually over the next 3 to 4 weeks to a maximum of 7.5 mg/kg or 200 mg daily.

Parenteral: Therapy in the hospitalized patient may be initiated IV or IM. Use parenterally only when the drug cannot be given orally. Usual dose is 20 to 40 mg, repeated as necessary. Certain patients (especially those with marked renal damage) may require a lower dose. Check blood pressure frequently; it may begin to fall within a few minutes after injection; average maximal decrease occurs in 10 to 80 minutes. Where there is a previously existing increased intracranial pressure, lowering the blood pressure may increase cerebral ischemia. Most patients can transfer to the oral form in 24 to 48 hours.

Children – 0.1 to 0.2 mg/kg/dose every 4 to 6 hours as needed.

Eclampsia – A dose of 5 to 10 mg every 20 minutes as an IV bolus has been recommended. If there is no effect after 20 mg, try another agent.

Stability: Use hydralazine injection as quickly as possible after drawing through a needle into a syringe. Hydralazine changes color after contact with a metal filter.

Actions

Pharmacology: Hydralazine exerts a peripheral vasodilating effect through a direct relaxation of vascular smooth muscle.

Pharmacokinetics: Hydralazine is rapidly absorbed after oral use. Half-life is 3 to 7 hours. Protein binding is 87%, and bioavailability is 30% to 50%. Plasma levels vary widely among individuals. Peak plasma concentrations occur 1 to 2 hours after ingestion; duration of action is 6 to 12 hours. Hypotensive effects are seen 10 to 20 minutes after parenteral use and last 2 to 4 hours. Slow acetylators generally have higher plasma levels of hydralazine and require lower doses to maintain control of blood pressure. Hydralazine undergoes extensive hepatic metabolism; it is excreted in the urine as active drug (12% to 14%) and metabolites.

Contraindications

Hypersensitivity to hydralazine; coronary artery disease; mitral valvular rheumatic heart disease.

Warnings/Precautions

Lupus erythematosus: Hydralazine may produce a clinical picture simulating systemic lupus erythematosus including glomerulonephritis. Symptoms usually regress when the drug is discontinued, but residual effects have been detected years later. Long-term treatment with steroids may be necessary.

Perform complete blood counts and antinuclear antibody (ANA) titer determinations before and during prolonged therapy, even in the asymptomatic patient. These studies also are indicated if the patient develops arthralgia, fever, chest pain, continued malaise, or other unexplained signs or symptoms. If the ANA titer reaction is positive, carefully weigh benefits to be derived from hydralazine.

Cardiovascular: The "hyperdynamic" circulation caused by hydralazine may accentuate specific cardiovascular inadequacies. It may reduce the pressor responses to epinephrine. Postural hypotension may result from hydralazine. Use with caution in patients with cerebral vascular accidents.

Coronary artery disease – Myocardial stimulation produced by hydralazine can cause anginal attacks and ECG changes of myocardial ischemia. The drug has been implicated in the production of MI. Use with caution in patients with suspected coronary artery disease.

Pulmonary hypertension – Use hydralazine with caution in patients with pulmonary hypertension. Severe hypotension may result. Monitor carefully.

Lipids – Hydralazine may cause some decrease in total cholesterol.

Peripheral neuritis: Peripheral neuritis evidenced by paresthesias, numbness, and tingling, has been observed. Add pyridoxine to the regimen if symptoms develop.

Hematologic effects: Blood dyscrasias consisting of reduction in hemoglobin and red cell count, leukopenia, agranulocytosis, and purpura have been reported. If such abnormalities develop, discontinue therapy. Periodic blood counts are advised.

Tartrazine sensitivity: Some of these products contain tartrazine, which may cause allergic-type reactions in susceptible individuals. Tartrazine sensitivity is frequently seen in patients who also have aspirin hypersensitivity.

Renal function impairment: In hypertensive patients with normal kidneys who are treated with hydralazine, there is evidence of increased renal blood flow and a maintenance of glomerular filtration rate. Renal function may improve where control values were below normal prior to administration. Use with caution in patients with advanced renal damage.

Pregnancy: Category C.

Lactation: Hydralazine is excreted in breast milk.

Children: Safety and efficacy for use in children have not been established.

Drug Interactions

Drugs that may interact with hydralazine include beta blockers (eg, metoprolol, propranolol) and indomethacin.

Drug/Food interactions: Taking with food results in higher plasma hydralazine levels.

Adverse Reactions

Possible adverse reactions include headache; anorexia; nausea; vomiting; diarrhea; palpitations; tachycardia; angina pectoris; toxic reactions (particularly the LE cell syndrome); lacrimation; conjunctivitis; dizziness; tremors; psychotic reactions; rash; urticaria; pruritus; fever; chills; arthralgia; eosinophilia; constipation; paralytic ileus; lymphadenopathy; splenomegaly; nasal congestion; flushing; edema; muscle cramps; hypotension; paradoxical pressor response; dyspnea; urination difficulty; adverse reactions with hydralazine are usually reversible when dosage is reduced. However, it may be necessary to discontinue the drug.

MINOXIDIL

Tablets: 2.5 and 10 mg (*Rx*)	Various

Warning:

Minoxidil may produce serious adverse effects. It can cause pericardial effusion, occasionally progressing to tamponade; it can exacerbate angina pectoris. Reserve for hypertensive patients who do not respond adequately to maximum therapeutic doses of a diuretic and 2 other antihypertensive agents.

In experimental animals, minoxidil caused several kinds of myocardial lesions and other adverse cardiac effects (see Warnings).

Administer under close supervision, usually concomitantly with a beta-adrenergic blocking agent, to prevent tachycardia and increased myocardial workload. Usually, it must be given with a diuretic, frequently one acting in the ascending limb of the loop of Henle, to prevent serious fluid accumulation. When first administering minoxidil, hospitalize and monitor patients with malignant hypertension and those already receiving guanethidine to avoid too rapid or large orthostatic decreases in blood pressure.

Indications

Severe hypertension: Severe hypertension that is symptomatic or associated with target organ damage, and is not manageable with maximum therapeutic doses of a diuretic plus two other antihypertensives.

Topical minoxidil is used for the treatment of male pattern baldness (alopecia androgenetica) of the vertex of the scalp. Use of the tablets, in any formulation, to promote hair growth is not an approved use.

Administration and Dosage

Adults and children (12 years of age or older): Initial dosage is 5 mg/day as a single dose. Daily dosage can be increased to 10, 20, then 40 mg in single or divided doses if required. Effective range is usually 10 to 40 mg/day. Maximum dosage is 100 mg/day.

Children: Initial dosage is 0.2 mg/kg/day as a single dose. Dose may be increased in 50% to 100% increments until optimum BP control is achieved. Effective range is usually 0.25 to 1 mg/kg/day. Maximum dosage is 50 mg/day.

Dose frequency: If supine diastolic pressure has been reduced less than 30 mm Hg, administer the drug only once a day; if reduced more than 30 mm Hg, divide the daily dosage into 2 equal parts.

Dosage adjustment intervals: Dosage adjustment intervals, which must be carefully titrated, should be 3 or more days because the full response to a given dose is not obtained until then.

Concomitant drug therapy:

Diuretics – Use minoxidil with a diuretic in patients relying on renal function for maintaining salt and water balance. Diuretics have been used at the following dosages when starting minoxidil therapy: hydrochlorothiazide (50 mg twice daily) or other thiazides at equally effective doses; chlorthalidone (50 to 100 mg/day); furosemide (40 mg twice daily). If excessive salt and water retention results in a weight gain of more than 2.3 kg (5 lb), change diuretic therapy to furosemide. In furosemide-treated patients, increase dosage in accordance with their needs.

Beta-blockers/Other sympathetic nervous system suppressants – When beginning therapy, the β-blocker dosage should be equal to 80 to 160 mg/day propranolol in divided doses. If β-blockers are contraindicated, use methyldopa 250 to 750 mg twice daily; give for at least 24 hours before starting minoxidil due to delay in onset. Clonidine may also be used to prevent tachycardia induced by minoxidil; usual dosage is 0.1 to 0.2 mg twice daily.

Actions

Pharmacology: Minoxidil is a direct-acting peripheral vasodilator. Minoxidil elicits a reduction of peripheral arteriolar resistance. The exact mechanism of action on the vascular smooth muscle is unknown.

Pharmacokinetics:

Absorption/Distribution – Minoxidil is at least 90% absorbed from the GI tract. Plasma levels of the parent drug reach a maximum within the first hour and decline rapidly thereafter. Minoxidil is not protein bound; it concentrates in arteriolar smooth muscle.

Onset/Duration: The extent and time course of BP reduction by minoxidil do not correspond closely to its plasma concentration. When minoxidil is administered chronically, once or twice a day, the time required to achieve maximum effect on BP is inversely related to the size of the dose. Thus, maximum effect is achieved on 10 mg/day within 7 days, on 20 mg/day within 5 days and on 40 mg/day within 3 days.

Metabolism/Excretion – 90% is metabolized, predominantly by conjugation with glucuronic acid. Average plasma half-life is 4.2 hours.

Contraindications

Hypersensitivity to any component of the product; pheochromocytoma (because the drug may stimulate secretion of catecholamines from the tumor through its antihypertensive action); acute MI; dissecting aortic aneurysm.

Warnings/Precautions

Mild hypertension: Because of the potential for serious adverse effects, use in milder degrees of hypertension is not recommended.

Cardiac lesions: Autopsies did not reveal right atrial or other hemorrhage pathology of the kind seen in animals.

ECG changes: Rarely, a large negative amplitude of the T wave may encroach upon the ST segment, but the ST segment is not independently altered. These changes usually disappear with continuance of treatment and revert to the pretreatment state if therapy is discontinued.

Fluid and electrolyte balance: Monitor fluid and electrolyte balance and body weight. Give with a diuretic to prevent fluid retention and possible CHF; a loop diuretic is usually required. If used without a diuretic, retention of several hundred mEq salt and corresponding volumes of water can occur in a few days, leading to increased plasma and interstitial fluid volume and local or generalized edema.

Refractory fluid retention rarely may require discontinuation of minoxidil. Under close medical supervision, it may be possible to resolve refractory salt retention by discontinuing the drug for 1 or 2 days, and then resuming treatment in conjunction with vigorous diuretic therapy.

Tachycardia/Angina: Minoxidil increases heart rate; this can be prevented by coadministration of a β-adrenergic blocking drug or other sympathetic nervous system suppressants. In addition, angina may worsen or appear for the first time during treatment, probably because of the increased oxygen demands associated with increased heart rate and cardiac output. This can usually be prevented by sympathetic blockade.

Pericardial effusion: Pericardial effusion, occasionally with tamponade, has occurred in approximately 3% of treated patients not on dialysis, especially those with inadequate or compromised renal function. Many cases were associated with connective tissue disease, the uremic syndrome, CHF or fluid retention, but were instances in which these potential causes of effusion were not present. Observe patients closely for signs of pericardial disorder. Perform echocardiographic studies if suspicion arises. More vigorous diuretic therapy, dialysis, pericardiocentesis, or surgery may be required. If the effusion persists, consider drug withdrawal.

Hazard of rapid control of BP: In patients with very severe BP elevation, too rapid control of BP can precipitate syncope, cerebrovascular accidents, MI and ischemia of special sense organs with resulting decrease or loss of vision or hearing. Patients with compromised circulation or cryoglobulinemia also may suffer ischemic episodes of affected organs. Although such events have not been unequivocally associated with minoxidil use, experience is limited.

Hospitalize any patient with malignant hypertension during initial treatment to ensure that blood pressure is not falling more rapidly than intended.

Hemodilution: Hematocrit, hemoglobin, and erythrocyte count usually fall about 7% initially and then recover to pretreatment levels.

Myocardial infarction: Minoxidil has not been used in patients who have had an MI within the preceding month. A reduction in arterial pressure with the drug might further limit blood flow to the myocardium, although this might be compensated by decreased oxygen demand because of lower BP.

Hypertrichosis: Elongation, thickening, and enhanced pigmentation of fine body hair develops within 3 to 6 weeks after starting therapy in approximately 80% of patients. It is usually first noticed on the temples, between the eyebrows, between the hairline and the eyebrows, or in the sideburn area of the upper lateral cheek, later extending to the back, arms, legs, and scalp. After discontinuation, 1 to 6 months may be required for restoration to pretreatment appearance. No endocrine abnormalities have been found to explain the abnormal hair growth; thus, it is hypertrichosis without virilism.

Hypersensitivity reactions: Manifested as a skin rash, hypersensitivity reactions occur in fewer than 1% of patients and rare reports of bullous eruptions and Stevens-Johnson syndrome.

Renal function impairment: Renal failure or dialysis patients may require smaller doses; closely supervise to prevent cardiac failure or exacerbation of renal failure.

Carcinogenesis: Dietary administration of minoxidil to mice for up to 2 years was associated with an increased incidence of malignant lymphomas in females at all dose levels (10, 25, and 63 mg/kg/day) and an increased incidence of hepatic nodules in males (63 mg/kg/day).

Fertility impairment: There was a dose-dependent reduction in conception rate.

Pregnancy: Category C.

Lactation: Minoxidil is excreted in breast milk; do not breast-feed while taking minoxidil.

Children: Use in children is limited, particularly in infants. The recommendations under Administration and Dosage are only a rough guide; careful titration is essential.

Lab test abnormalities: Repeat tests that are abnormal at initiation of minoxidil therapy to ascertain whether improvement or deterioration is occurring under therapy. Initially, perform such tests frequently, at 1 to 3 month intervals, and as stabilization occurs, at 6 to 12 month intervals.

Monitoring: Monitor initially and periodically thereafter body weight, blood pressure, fluid, and electrolyte balance; signs and symptoms of pericardial effusion; ECG changes; CBC; alkaline phosphatase; renal function tests.

Drug Interactions

Drugs that may interact with minoxidil include guanethidine.

Adverse Reactions

Adverse reactions may include Stevens-Johnson syndrome; pericardial effusion; T-wave changes; rebound hypertension (following gradual withdrawal in children); decreased initial hematocrit, hemoglobin and erythrocyte counts; nausea; vomiting; temporary edema; alkaline phosphatase/serum creatinine/BUN increase, hypertrichosis.

ACE INHIBITORS

BENAZEPRIL HYDROCHLORIDE	
Tablets: 5, 10, 20, and 40 mg (*Rx*)	Various, *Lotensin* (Novartis)
CAPTOPRIL	
Tablets: 12.5, 25, 50, and 100 mg (*Rx*)	Various, *Capoten* (Par)
ENALAPRIL	
Tablets: 2.5, 5, 10, and 20 mg (*Rx*)	Various, *Vasotec* (Merck)
Injection: 1.25 mg enalaprilat/mL (*Rx*)	*Vasotec I.V.* (Merck)
FOSINOPRIL SODIUM	
Tablets: 10, 20, and 40 mg (*Rx*)	*Monopril* (Bristol-Myers Squibb)
LISINOPRIL	
Tablets: 2.5, 5, 10, 20, 30, and 40 mg (*Rx*)	Various, *Prinivil* (Merck), *Zestril* (Zeneca)
MOEXIPRIL HYDROCHLORIDE	
Tablets: 7.5 and 15 mg (*Rx*)	Various, *Univasc* (Schwarz Pharma)
PERINDOPRIL ERBUMINE	
Tablets: 2, 4, and 8 mg (*Rx*)	Various, *Aceon* (Solvay Pharm.)
QUINAPRIL HYDROCHLORIDE	
Tablets: 5, 10, 20, and 40 mg (*Rx*)	Various, *Accupril* (Parke-Davis)
RAMIPRIL	
Capsules: 1.25, 2.5, 5, and 10 mg (*Rx*)	Various, *Altace* (Monarch)
TRANDOLAPRIL	
Tablets: 1, 2, and 4 mg (*Rx*)	*Mavik* (Knoll)

Warning:

Pregnancy: When used in pregnancy during the second and third trimesters, angiotensin-converting enzyme (ACE) inhibitors can cause injury and even death to the developing fetus. When pregnancy is detected, discontinue the ACE inhibitor as soon as possible.

Indications

Hypertension: The ACE inhibitors are effective alone and in combination with other antihypertensive agents, especially thiazide-type diuretics. Blood pressure (BP)-lowering effects of ACE inhibitors and thiazides are approximately additive.

Heart failure: Some ACE inhibitors are effective in the management of congestive heart failure (CHF), usually as adjunctive therapy and in patients who demonstrate clinical signs of CHF or have evidence of left ventricular systolic dysfunction within the first few days after an acute myocardial infarction (MI).

MI (lisinopril): Treatment of hemodynamically stable patients within 24 hours of acute MI, to improve survival. Patients should receive, as appropriate, the standard recommended treatments such as thrombolytics, aspirin and beta-blockers.

Left ventricular dysfunction (LVD): Various ACE inhibitors have demonstrated improved survival and decreased rates of development of overt heart failure in patients with varying degrees of LVD (from modest, asymptomatic to severe with CHF).

Diabetic nephropathy (captopril): Treatment of diabetic nephropathy (proteinuria greater than 500 mg/day) in patients with type 1 insulin-dependent diabetes mellitus and retinopathy.

Heart failure post-MI/left-ventricular dysfunction post-MI (trandolapril, ramipril): For stable patients who have evidence of left-ventricular systolic dysfunction or who are symptomatic from CHF within the first few days after sustaining acute MI.

Essential hypertension (perindopril): For the treatment of patients with essential hypertension. It may be used alone or given with other classes of antihypertensives, especially thiazide diuretics.

Stable coronary artery disease (CAD) (perindopril): Perindopril is indicated in patients with stable CAD to reduce the risk of cardiovascular mortality or nonfatal myocardial infarction (MI). Perindopril can be used with conventional treatment for management of CAD, such as antiplatelet, antihypertensive, or lipid-lowering therapy.

Reduction in risk of MI, stroke, and death from cardiovascular causes (ramipril): In patients 55 years of age or older at high risk of developing a major cardiovascular event because of a history of coronary artery disease, stroke, peripheral vascular disease, or diabetes that is accompanied by at least 1 other cardiovascular risk factor (eg, hypertension, elevated total cholesterol levels, low high-density lipoprotein levels, cigarette smoking, documented microalbuminuria).

Administration and Dosage

BENAZEPRIL HYDROCHLORIDE:

Initial dose – 10 mg once daily for patients not receiving a diuretic.

Maintenance dosage – 20 to 40 mg/day as a single dose or 2 divided doses. Total daily doses above 80 mg have not been evaluated. If blood pressure is not controlled with benazepril alone, add a diuretic.

Renal function impairment – 5 mg once daily in patients with creatinine clearance (CrCl) of less than 30 mL/min/1.73 m^2 (serum creatinine greater than 3 mg/dL). Dosage may be titrated upward until BP is controlled or to a maximum of 40 mg/day.

Children 6 years of age and older – 0.2 mg/kg once per day as monotherapy. Doses above 0.6 mg/kg (or in excess of 40 mg daily) have not been studied in children.

CAPTOPRIL: Administer 1 hour before meals.

Hypertension –

Initial: 25 mg 2 or 3 times/day. If satisfactory BP reduction is not achieved after 1 or 2 weeks, increase to 50 mg 2 or 3 times/day. If BP is not controlled after 1 or 2 weeks at this dose, add a modest dose of a thiazide diuretic.

If further BP reduction is required, increase to 100 mg captopril 2 or 3 times/day and then, if necessary, to 150 mg 2 or 3 times/day (while continuing diuretic). Do not exceed daily dose of 450 mg.

Accelerated or malignant hypertension: Promptly initiate captopril at 25 mg 2 or 3 times daily under close supervision. Increase dose every 24 hours or less until a satisfactory response is obtained or the maximum dose is reached.

Heart failure – Usual initial dosage is 25 mg 3 times daily. After 50 mg 3 times daily is reached, delay further dosage increases, where possible, for at least 2 weeks to determine if a satisfactory response occurs. Do not exceed a daily dose of 450 mg.

LVD after MI – Initiate as early as 3 days following an MI. After a single 6.25 mg dose, initiate at 12.5 mg 3 times daily, then increase to 25 mg 3 times daily to a target of 50 mg 3 times daily over the next several weeks as tolerated.

Diabetic nephropathy – Recommended dose for long-term use is 25 mg 3 times daily.

Renal function impairment – Reduce initial dosage and use smaller increments for titration, (1- to 2-week intervals). After the desired therapeutic effect is achieved, slowly back-titrate to the minimal effective dose.

ENALAPRIL:

Oral –

Hypertension:

Patients taking diuretics – Discontinue the diuretic, if possible, for 2 to 3 days before beginning therapy to reduce the likelihood of hypotension. If the diuretic cannot be discontinued, use an initial dose of 2.5 mg under medical supervision for at least 2 hours and until BP has stabilized for at least an additional hour.

Patients not taking diuretics – Initial dose is 5 mg once a day. The usual dosage range is 10 to 40 mg/day as a single dose or in 2 divided doses.

Renal function impairment – Titrate the dosage upward until BP is controlled or until a maximum dose of 40 mg/day. Use initial dose of 5 mg/day in normal and mild renal function impairment, in moderate to severe renal function impairment, and in dialysis patients on dialysis days.

Heart failure: Recommended starting dose is 2.5 mg twice daily. The usual range is 2.5 to 20 mg/day given in 2 divided doses. The maximum daily dose is 40 mg.

Renal function impairment or hyponatremia –

Serum sodium less than 130 mEq/L or with serum creatinine greater than 1.6 mg/dL: Initiate at 2.5 mg/day. Increase to 2.5 mg twice daily, then 5 mg twice daily and higher as needed, usually at intervals of 4 days or more. The maximum daily dose is 40 mg.

Asymptomatic left ventricular dysfunction: 2.5 mg twice daily, titrated as tolerated to the targeted daily dose of 20 mg in divided doses.

Parenteral (enalaprilat) – For intravenous (IV) administration only.

Hypertension: 1.25 mg every 6 hours IV over 5 minutes.

The dose for patients being converted to IV from oral therapy is 1.25 mg every 6 hours. For conversion from IV to oral therapy, the recommended initial dose of tablets is 5 mg/day for patients with CrCl greater than 30 mL/min and 2.5 mg/day for patients with CrCl 30 mL/min or less.

Patients taking diuretics: Starting dose for hypertension is 0.625 mg IV over 5 minutes. If there is inadequate clinical response after 1 hour, repeat the 0.625 dose.

For conversion from IV to oral therapy, the recommended initial dose of enalapril maleate tablets for patients who have responded to 0.625 mg enalaprilat every 6 hours is 2.5 mg once a day with subsequent dosage adjustment as needed.

Renal function impairment: Administer 1.25 mg every 6 hours for patients with CrCl greater than 30 mL/min. For CrCl 30 mL/min or less, initial dose is 0.625 mg. If there is inadequate clinical response after 1 hour, the 0.625 mg dose may be repeated. For dialysis patients, initial dose is 0.625 mg or less administered over 5 minutes or more.

For conversion from IV to oral therapy, the recommended initial dose is 5 mg once a day for patients with CrCl greater than 30 mL/min and 2.5 mg once daily for patients with CrCl 30 mL/min or less.

FOSINOPRIL SODIUM:

Initial dose – 10 mg once daily.

Maintenance dosage – Usual range is 20 to 40 mg/day but some patients appear to have a further response to 80 mg. If trough response is inadequate, consider dividing the daily dose.

LISINOPRIL:

Hypertension –

Initial therapy: 10 mg once/day. The usual dosage range is 20 to 40 mg/day as a single daily dose.

Diuretic-treated patients: Discontinue the diuretic, if possible, for 2 to 3 days before beginning therapy to reduce the likelihood of hypotension. If the diuretic cannot be discontinued, use an initial dose of 5 mg under medical supervision for at least 2 hours and until BP has stabilized for at least an additional hour.

Renal function impairment: For hypertension, titrate dosage upward until BP is controlled or to a maximum of 40 mg daily.

Lisinopril Dosage in Renal Function Impairment

Renal status	CrCl (mL/min)	Initial dose (mg/day)
Normal function to mild impairment	> 30	10
Moderate to severe impairment	≥ 10 to ≤ 30	5
Dialysis patients	< 10	2.5[a]

[a] Adjust dosage or dosing interval depending on the BP response.

Heart failure –

Initial dose: 5 mg once daily with diuretics and digitalis. Usual effective dosage range is 5 to 20 mg/day as a single dose. In patients with hyponatremia, initiate dose at 2.5 mg once daily. If used with diuretics, initial dose is 5 mg/day.

Renal function impairment or hyponatremia: In patients with heart failure who have hyponatremia (serum sodium less than 130 mEq/L) or moderate to severe renal function impairment (CrCl 30 mL/min or less or serum creatinine greater than 3 mg/dL), therapy with lisinopril should be initiated at a dose of 2.5 mg once a day under close medical supervision.

Acute MI – In hemodynamically stable patients within 24 hours of the onset of symptoms of acute MI, the first dose is 5 mg, followed by 5 mg after 24 hours, 10 mg after 48 hours and then 10 mg once daily. Continue dosing for 6 weeks. Patients with a low systolic BP (120 mm Hg or less) when treatment is started or during the first 3 days after the infarct should be given a lower 2.5 mg dose. If hypotension occurs (systolic BP 100 mm Hg or less), a daily maintenance dose of 5 mg may be given with temporary reductions to 2.5 mg if needed. If prolonged hypotension occurs (systolic BP less than 90 mm Hg for more than 1 hour), withdraw lisinopril.

Elderly – Make dosage adjustments with particular caution.

Children (6 years of age and older) – The usual recommended starting dosage is 0.07 mg/kg once daily (up to 5 mg total). Dosage should be adjusted according to blood pressure response. Doses above 0.61 mg/kg (or in excess of 40 mg) have not been studied in children.

Lisinopril is not recommended in children younger than 6 years of age or in children with a glomerular filtration rate less than 30 mL/min per 1.73 min^2.

MOEXIPRIL HYDROCHLORIDE:

Initial dose – In patients not receiving diuretics, 7.5 mg 1 hour prior to meals once daily. If control is not adequate, increase the dose or divide the dosing.

Maintenance dose – 7.5 to 30 mg daily in 1 or 2 divided doses 1 hour before meals.

Concomitant diuretics – Discontinue diuretic 2 to 3 days prior to beginning moexipril, if possible. If blood pressure is not controlled, resume diuretic therapy. If diuretic cannot be discontinued, use an initial dose of moexipril 3.75 mg.

Renal function impairment – Cautiously use 3.75 mg once daily in patients with CrCl of 40 mL/min/1.73 m^2 or less. Dosage may be titrated to a maximum of 15 mg/day.

PERINDOPRIL:

In uncomplicated hypertensive patients – Initial dose is 4 mg once a day. Maximum of 16 mg/day. May be administered in 2 divided doses.

Stable CAD – Initial dose of 4 mg once daily for 2 weeks, and then increased to a maintenance dosage of 8 mg once daily. In elderly patients, perindopril should be given as a 2 mg dose once daily in the first week, followed by 4 mg once daily in the second week, and 8 mg once daily for maintenance dosage, if tolerated.

Use in elderly patients – The recommended initial dosage is 4 mg daily in 1 or 2 divided doses.

Use in concomitant diuretics – If BP is not adequately controlled with perindopril alone, a diuretic may be added. In patients currently being treated with a diuretic, symptomatic hypotension occasionally can occur following the initial dose of perindopril. To reduce likelihood of such reaction, the diuretic should, if possible, be discontinued 2 to 3 days prior to beginning perindopril therapy. Then, if BP is not controlled with perindopril alone, resume the diuretic.

If the diuretic cannot be discontinued, use an initial dose of 2 to 4 mg daily in 1 or 2 divided doses with careful medical supervision for several hours and until BP has stabilized. Titrate the dosage as described above.

Use in patients with impaired renal function – In patients with CrCl less than 30 mL/min, safety and efficacy have not been established. For patients CrCl more than 30 mL/min, the initial dosage should be 2 mg/day, and dosage should not exceed 8 mg/day.

QUINAPRIL HYDROCHLORIDE:

Hypertension –

Initial dose: 10 or 20 mg once daily for patients not on diuretics. Dosage should be adjusted according to blood pressure response measured at peak (2 to 6 hours after dosing) and trough (predosing). Dosage adjustments should be made at intervals of at least 2 weeks.

Elderly (65 years of age or older): 10 mg once daily.

Renal function impairment: Initial dose is 10 mg with CrCl greater than 60 mL/min, 5 mg with CrCl 30 to 60 mL/min and 2.5 mg with CrCl 10 to 30 mL/min.

Concomitant diuretics: If blood pressure is not adequately controlled with quinapril monotherapy, a diuretic may be added. In patients who are currently being treated with a diuretic, symptomatic hypotension occasionally can occur following the initial dose of quinapril. To reduce the likelihood of hypotension, the diuretic should, if possible, be discontinued 2 to 3 days prior to beginning therapy with quinapril. Then, if blood pressure is not controlled with quinapril alone, diuretic therapy should be resumed.

If the diuretic cannot be discontinued, an initial dose of 5 mg quinapril should be used with careful medical supervision for several hours and until blood pressure has stabilized.

The dosage should subsequently be titrated (as previously above) to the optimal response.

CHF – 5 mg twice/day. Titrate patients at weekly intervals until an effective dose, usually 20 to 40 mg/day given in 2 equally divided doses, is reached.

Dose adjustments in patients with heart failure and renal impairment or hyponatremia: Initial dose is 5 mg in patients with a creatinine clearance greater than 30 mL/min and 2.5 mg in patients with a creatinine clearance of 10 to 30 mL/min. If the initial dose is well tolerated, quinapril may be administered the following day as a twice-daily regimen. The dose may be increased at weekly intervals based on clinical and hemodynamic response.

RAMIPRIL:

Reduction in risk of MI, stroke, and death from cardiovascular causes –

Initial dose: 2.5 mg once daily for 1 week, 5 mg once daily for the next 3 weeks, and then increase to maintenance dose.

Maintenance dosage: 10 mg once daily. If the patient is hypertensive or recently post-MI, give as a divided dose.

Renal function impairment: In patients with CrCl of less than 40 mL/min/1.73 m^2 (serum creatinine greater than 2.5 mg/dL) 25% of the normal dose should be expected to induce full therapeutic levels of ramiprilat.

Hypertension –

Initial dose: 2.5 mg once daily in patients not receiving a diuretic.

Maintenance dosage: 2.5 to 20 mg/day as a single dose or in two equally divided doses. If BP is not controlled, a diuretic can be added.

Renal function impairment: 1.25 mg once daily in patients with CrCl of less than 40 mL/min/1.73 m^2 (serum creatinine greater than 2.5 mg/dL). Dosage may be titrated upward until BP is controlled or to a maximum of 5 mg/day.

Heart failure post-MI – Starting dose is 2.5 mg twice daily. A patient who becomes hypotensive at this dose may be switched to 1.25 mg twice daily, all patients should then be titrated toward a target dose of 5 mg twice daily, with dosage increases being approximately 3 weeks apart. Reduce the dose of any concomitant diuretic.

Renal function impairment: 1.25 mg once daily in patients with CrCl of less than 40 mL/min/1.73 m^2 (serum creatinine greater than 2.5 mg/dL). Dosage may be increased to 1.25 mg twice daily up to a maximum dose of 2.5 mg twice daily.

Alternative route of administration – Ramipril capsules are usually swallowed whole. However, the capsules may be opened and the contents sprinkled on a small amount of applesauce or mixed in apple juice or water.

TRANDOLAPRIL:

Hypertension –

Initial dose: 1 mg/day (2 mg in black patients). Make dosage adjustments at intervals of 1 week or more.

Maintenance – Patients inadequately treated with once daily dosing at 4 mg may be treated with twice-daily dosing.

Concomitant diuretic – In patients being treated with a diuretic, symptomatic hypotension can occasionally occur following the initial dose of trandolapril. To reduce the likelihood of hypotension, if possible, discontinue the diuretic 2 to 3 days prior to beginning therapy with trandolapril. If BP is not controlled with trandolapril alone, resume diuretic therapy. If the diuretic cannot be discontinued, give an initial dose of trandolapril 0.5 mg with careful medical supervision for several hours until BP has stabilized. Titrate dosage as previously described to the optimal response.

Heart failure post-MI or LVD post-MI –

Initial dose: 1 mg/day

Target dose: 4 mg/day.

Renal/Hepatic function impairment – For patients with a CrCl less than 30 mL/min or with hepatic cirrhosis, the recommended starting dose is 0.5 mg/day.

Actions

Pharmacology: The ACE inhibitors appear to act primarily through suppression of the renin-angiotensin-aldosterone system.

These agents prevent the conversion of angiotensin I to angiotensin II by inhibiting ACE. ACE inhibitors may also inhibit local angiotensin II at vascular and renal sites and attenuate the release of catecholamines from adrenergic nerve endings.

Some ACE inhibitors have demonstrated a beneficial effect on the severity of heart failure and an improvement in maximal exercise tolerance in patients with heart failure. In these patients, ACE inhibitors significantly decrease peripheral (systemic vascular) resistance, BP (afterload), pulmonary capillary wedge pressure (preload), pulmonary vascular resistance and heart size and increase cardiac output and exercise tolerance time.

Pharmacokinetics:

Pharmacokinetics of the Active Moieties of ACE Inhibitors

ACE inhibitor	Onset/ Duration (h)	Protein binding	Effect of food on absorption	Active metabolite	Half-life: Normal renal function	Half-life: Impaired renal function	Elimination (24 h): Total	Elimination (24 h): Unchanged
Benazepril	1/24	≈ 96.7% (≈ 95.3%)[a]	slightly reduced	benazeprilat	10-11 h[a]	prolonged	11% to 12% bile[a]	trace
Captopril	nd[b]/ dose-related	≈ 25% to 30%	reduced		< 2 h	prolonged	> 95% urine	40% to 50% in urine
Enalapril	1/24	nd[b]	none	enalaprilat	1.3 h (11 h)[a]	nd[b]	94% urine and feces	54% in urine (40%)[a]
Enalaprilat	0.25/≈6	na[c]	na[d]		11 h	prolonged	nd[b]	> 90% in urine
Fosinopril	1/24	≈ 99.4%	slightly reduced	fosinoprilat	≈ 12 h[a]	prolonged negligible clinical effect	50% urine, 50% feces	negligible
Lisinopril	1/24	na[c]	none	-	12 h	prolonged	nd[b]	100% in urine
Moexipril	1.5/24	≈ 50%	markedly reduced	moexiprilat	2 to 9 h[a]	prolonged	13% urine, 53% feces	1% in urine, 1% in feces
Quinapril	1/24	≈ 97%	reduced	quinaprilat	2 h[a]	prolonged	≈60% urine, ≈37% feces	trace
Ramipril	1-2/24	≈ 73% (≈ 56%)[a]	slightly reduced	ramiprilat	13 to 17 h[a]	prolonged	≈ 60% urine, ≈ 40% feces	< 2%
Trandolapril	4/24	≈ 80%	reduced	trandolaprilat	≈ 5 h (≈ 10 h)[a]	prolonged	33% urine, 56% feces	nd[b]

[a] Of active metabolite.
[b] nd – No data.
[c] na – Not applicable.
[d] na – Not applicable; available IV only.

Contraindications

Hypersensitivity to these products.

Warnings/Precautions

Neutropenia/Agranulocytosis: Neutropenia (less than 1,000/mm^3) with myeloid hypoplasia resulted from **captopril** use. About half of the neutropenic patients developed systemic or oral cavity infections or other features of agranulocytosis. Neutropenia/agranulocytosis has occurred rarely with **enalapril** or **lisinopril** and in 1 patient on **quinapril**. Data are insufficient to show that **moexipril, ramipril, quinapril, benazepril, trandolapril,** or **fosinopril** do not cause agranulocytosis at similar rates. Periodically monitor white blood cell counts.

Angioedema: Angioedema has occurred. It may occur at any time during treatment, especially following the first dose of **enalapril** (0.2%), **captopril, lisinopril, trandolapril** (0.13%), **benazepril** (approximately 0.5%), **quinapril**(0.1%), or **moexipril** (less than 0.5%). Angioedema associated with laryngeal edema may be fatal. Black patients receiving ACE inhibitor monotherapy have been reported to have a higher incidence of angioedema compared with non-blacks.

Proteinuria: Total urinary proteins more than 1 g/day were seen in 0.7% of **captopril** patients. Nephrotic syndrome occurred in approximately 20% of these cases.

Hypotension:

First-dose effect – ACE inhibitors may cause a profound fall in BP following the first dose.

Heart failure – In heart failure, where the BP was either normal or low, transient decreases in mean BP greater than 20% occurred in approximately 50% of the patients.

Hyperkalemia: Elevated serum potassium (at least 0.5 mEq/L greater than the upper limit of normal) was observed in 0.4% of hypertensive patients given **trandolapril**, approximately 1% of hypertensive patients given **benazepril, enalapril, ramipril**, or **moexipril**; approximately 2% of patients receiving **quinapril** or **lisinopril**, approximately 2.6% of hypertensive patients given **fosinopril**, and approximately 4.8% of CHF patients given lisinopril. Hyperkalemia also occurred with **captopril**.

Valvular stenosis: Theoretically, patients with aortic stenosis might be at risk of decreased coronary perfusion when treated with vasodilators, because they do not develop as much afterload reduction as others.

Surgery/Anesthesia: In patients undergoing major surgery or during anesthesia with agents that produce hypotension, ACE inhibitors will block angiotensin II formation secondary to compensatory renin release.

Cough: Chronic cough has occurred with the use of all ACE inhibitors. Characteristically, the cough is nonproductive, persistent and resolves within 1 to 4 days after therapy discontinuation.

The incidence of cough, although still reported as 0.5% to 3% by some manufacturers, appears to range from 5% to 25% and has been reported to be as high as 39%, resulting in discontinuation rates as high as 15%.

Renal function impairment: Some hypertensive patients with renal disease, particularly those with severe renal artery stenosis, have developed increases in serum urea nitrogen and serum creatinine after reduction of BP.

In patients with severe CHF whose renal function may depend on the activity of the renin-angiotensin-aldosterone system, treatment with ACE inhibitors may be associated with oliguria or progressive azotemia and, rarely, with acute renal failure or death.

Impaired renal function decreases **lisinopril** elimination. The elimination half-life of quinaprilat increases as CrCl decreases. Dosage adjustment may be necessary for **quinapril, benazepril, ramipril,** and **lisinopril**. Impaired renal function decreases total clearance of fosinoprilat and approximately doubles the area under the curve.

Hepatic function impairment: Patients with impaired liver function could develop markedly elevated plasma levels of unchanged **fosinopril** or **ramipril**. In patients with alcoholic or biliary cirrhosis, the rate, but not extent of fosinopril hydrolysis was reduced. Quinaprilat concentrations are reduced in alcoholic cirrhosis.

Pregnancy: *Category* C (first trimester); *Category D* (second and third trimesters).

Lactation: Several ACE inhibitors have been detected in breast milk. Do not administer **trandolapril** or **ramipril** to breast-feeding mothers. It is not known whether **lisinopril**, **moexipril**, or **ramipril** is excreted in breast milk. Discontinue breastfeeding or the drug.

Children: Safety and efficacy have not been established. Use **captopril** in children only when other measures for controlling BP have not been effective.

Elderly: Elderly patients may have higher blood levels and area under the curve of **lisinopril**, **ramiprilat**, **quinaprilat**, and **moexiprilat**. This may relate to decreased renal function rather than to age itself.

Drug Interactions

Drugs that may affect ACE inhibitors may include antacids, capsaicin, indomethacin, phenothiazines, probenecid, and rifampin. Drugs that may be affected by ACE inhibitors include allopurinol, digoxin, lithium, potassium preparations/potassium-sparing diuretics, and tetracycline.

Drug/Lab test interactions: Captopril may cause a false-positive test for urine acetone.

Fosinopril may cause a false low measurement of serum digoxin levels with the *Digi-Tab RIA Kit for Digoxin* other kits such as the *Coat-A-Count RIA Kit*, may be used.

Drug/Food interactions: Food significantly reduces the bioavailability of **captopril** by 30% to 40%. Administer captopril 1 hour before meals. The rate and extent of **quinapril** absorption are diminished moderately (25% to 30%) when administered during a high-fat meal. The rate, but not extent, of **ramipril** and **fosinopril** absorption is reduced by food. Food does not reduce the GI absorption of **benazepril**, **enalapril**, and **lisinopril**.

Adverse Reactions

Adverse reactions may include chest pain, cough, diarrhea, dizziness, dysgeusia, dyspepsia, fatigue, headache, hypotension, myalgia, rash, and syncope.

ANGIOTENSIN II RECEPTOR ANTAGONISTS

CANDESARTAN CILEXETIL	
Tablets; oral: 4, 8, 16, and 32 mg (*Rx*)	*Atacand* (AstraZeneca)
EPROSARTAN MESYLATE	
Tablets; oral: 600 mg (*Rx*)	*Teveten* (KOS Pharmaceuticals)
IRBESARTAN	
Tablets; oral: 75, 150, and 300 mg (*Rx*)	*Avapro* (Bristol-Myers Squibb/Sanofi-Synthelabo)
LOSARTAN POTASSIUM	
Tablets; oral: 25, 50, and 100 mg (*Rx*)	*Cozaar* (Merck)
OLMESARTAN MEDOXOMIL	
Tablets; oral: 5, 20, and 40 mg (*Rx*)	*Benicar* (Daiichi Sankyo)
TELMISARTAN	
Tablets; oral: 20, 40, and 80 mg (*Rx*)	*Micardis* (Boehringer Ingelheim)
VALSARTAN	
Capsules; oral: 40, 80, 160, and 320 mg (*Rx*)	*Diovan* (Novartis)

Warning:

Pregnancy: When used in pregnancy (especially during the second and third trimesters), drugs that act directly on the renin-angiotensin system can cause injury and even death to the developing fetus. When pregnancy is detected, discontinue angiotensin II receptor antagonists as soon as possible.

Indications

Hypertension: Treatment of hypertension alone or in combination with other antihypertensive agents.

Nephropathy in type 2 diabetes (irbesartan, losartan): Treatment of diabetic nephropathy with an elevated serum creatinine and proteinuria in patients with type 2 diabetes and a history of hypertension.

Heart failure (candesartan, valsartan): Treatment of heart failure (New York Heart Association class II to IV).

Hypertensive patients with left ventricular hypertrophy (losartan): Used to reduce the risk of stroke in patients with hypertension and left ventricular hypertrophy, but there is evidence that this benefit does not apply to black patients.

Postmyocardial infarction (valsartan): In clinically stable patients with left ventricular failure or left ventricular dysfunction following myocardial infarction (MI), valsartan is indicated to reduce cardiovascular mortality.

Cardiovascular risk reduction (telmisartan): For reduction of the risk of MI, stroke, or death from cardiovascular causes in patients 55 years of age and older at high risk of developing major cardiovascular events who are unable to take angiotensin-converting enzyme (ACE) inhibitors.

Administration and Dosage

CANDESARTAN:

Hypertension – Administer with or without food. The usual starting dose is 16 mg once daily when used as monotherapy in patients who are not volume-depleted. Candesartan can be administered once or twice daily with total daily doses ranging from 8 to 32 mg.

For patients with possible intravascular volume depletion, consider administering a lower dose.

Heart failure – Initial dosage is 4 mg once daily. The target dosage is 32 mg once daily, which is achieved by doubling the dose at approximately 2-week intervals, as tolerated.

EPROSARTAN:

Hypertension – The usual starting dosage is 600 mg once daily when used as monotherapy in patients who are not volume-depleted. Eprosartan can also be administered once or twice daily with total daily doses ranging from 400 to 800 mg.

Elderly and hepatic/renal function impairment – No initial dosing adjustment is generally necessary in patients with moderate and severe renal function impairment, with maximum dose not exceeding 600 mg/day.

IRBESARTAN:

Hypertension – The initial dosage is 150 mg once daily with or without food. Patients may be titrated to 300 mg once daily.

Patients not adequately treated by the maximum dose of 300 mg once daily are unlikely to derive additional benefit from a higher dose or twice-daily dosing.

Nephropathy in type 2 diabetes – The recommended target maintenance dose is 300 mg once daily.

Children younger than 6 years of age – Safety and efficacy have not been established.

Children 6 to 12 years of age – Initial dose is 75 mg once daily. Titrate patients requiring further reduction in blood pressure to 150 mg once daily.

Adolescents 13 to 16 years of age – Initial dose is 150 mg once daily. Titrate patients requiring further reduction in blood pressure to 300 mg once daily. Higher doses are not recommended.

Volume- and salt-depleted patients – A lower initial dose of 75 mg is recommended.

LOSARTAN POTASSIUM:

Hypertension – The usual starting dose is 50 mg once daily with 25 mg used in patients with possible depletion of intravascular volume or a history of hepatic function impairment. Administer with or without food once or twice daily with total daily doses ranging from 25 to 100 mg.

Pediatric hypertensive patients 6 years of age and older – The usual starting dosage is 0.7 mg/kg once daily (up to 50 mg total) administered as a tablet or suspension. Doses above 1.4 mg/kg (or in excess of 100 mg) daily have not been studied in children.

Losartan is not recommended in children younger than 6 years of age or in children with a glomerular filtration rate less than 30 mL/min per 1.73 m^2.

Hypertensive patients with left ventricular hypertrophy – The usual starting dose is 50 mg once daily. Add hydrochlorothiazide 12.5 mg/day and/or increase the dose of losartan to 100 mg once daily followed by an increase in hydrochlorothiazide to 25 mg once daily based on blood pressure response.

Nephropathy in type 2 diabetes – The usual starting dose is 50 mg once daily. Increase the dose to 100 mg once daily based on blood pressure response.

OLMESARTAN:

Hypertension – The usual starting dose is 20 mg once daily with or without food when used as monotherapy in patients who are not volume-contracted. For patients requiring further reduction in blood pressure after 2 weeks of therapy, the dose may be increased to 40 mg. Doses above 40 mg do not appear to have greater effect. Twice-daily dosing offers no advantage over the same total dose given once daily.

For patients with possible depletion of intravascular volume, consider using a lower starting dose.

Children 6 to 16 years of age –

Children weighing 20 to less than 35 kg (44 to less than 77 lb):

Maximum dose – 20 mg once daily.

Initial dosage – 10 mg once daily.

Dosage adjustment – After 2 weeks of therapy, the dosage of olmesartan may be increased to a maximum of 20 mg once daily.

Children weighing 35 kg (77lb) or more:

Maximum dose – 40 mg once daily.

Initial dosage – 20 mg once daily.

Dosage adjustment – After 2 weeks of therapy, the dosage of olmesartan may be increased to a maximum of 40 mg once daily.

TELMISARTAN:

Cardiovascular risk reduction – 80 mg once a day.

Hypertension – The usual starting dose is 40 mg/day. Usual dosage range is 20 to 80 mg. May be administered with or without food.

Special risk patients: Patients on dialysis may develop orthostatic hypotension; monitor blood pressure closely. Initiate treatment under close medical supervision for patients with biliary obstructive disorders or hepatic function impairment.

VALSARTAN:

Hypertension – The recommended starting dose is 80 or 160 mg once daily, with or without food, when used as monotherapy in patients who are not volume-depleted. A usual dose range is 80 to 320 mg once daily. The full antihypertensive effect usually is seen in 2 to 4 weeks.

If additional antihypertensive effect is required, increase dose to 160 or 320 mg or add a diuretic.

Children: For children who can swallow tablets, the usual recommended starting dosage is 1.3 mg/kg once daily (up to 40 mg total). The dosage should be adjusted according to blood pressure response. Dosages higher than 2.7 mg/kg (up to 160 mg) once daily have not been studied in children 6 to 16 years of age.

For children who cannot swallow tablets, or children for whom the calculated dosage (mg/kg) does not correspond to the available tablet strengths of valsartan, the use of a suspension is recommended. When the suspension is replaced by a tablet, the dose of valsartan may have to be increased. The exposure to valsartan with the suspension is 1.6 times more than with the tablet.

Heart failure – The recommended starting dose is 40 mg twice daily. Titrate 80 and 160 mg twice daily to the highest dose, as tolerated. Consider reducing the dose of concomitant diuretics.

Postmyocardial infarction – May be initiated as early as 12 hours after an MI. The recommended starting dosage is 20 mg twice daily. Dosage may be increased within 7 days to 40 mg twice daily, with subsequent titrations to a target dosage of 160 mg twice daily, as tolerated. If symptomatic hypotension or renal function impairment occur, consider a dosage reduction.

Hepatic/Renal function impairment – Exercise care when dosing patients with severe hepatic or renal function impairment.

Actions

Pharmacology: Angiotensin II receptor antagonists block the vasoconstrictor and aldosterone-secreting effects of angiotensin II by selectively blocking the binding of angiotensin II to the AT_1 receptor found in many tissues.

Angiotensin II receptor antagonists do not inhibit angiotensin-converting enzymes (ACE) (kininase II, the enzyme that converts angiotensin I to angiotensin II and degrades bradykinin), nor do they bind to or block other hormone receptors or ion channels known to be important in cardiovascular regulation.

Pharmacokinetics:

Angiotensin II Receptor Antagonists Pharmacokinetics

Parameters	Candesartan	Eprosartan	Irbesartan	Losartan (metabolite)[a]	Olmesartan	Telmisartan	Valsartan
Bioavailability	≈ 15%	≈ 13%	60% to 80%	≈ 33%	≈ 26%	42%/58% (40 mg/ 160 mg)	≈ 25%
Food effect (AUC/C_{max})	no effect	↓< 25%	no effect	↓10%/↓14%	no effect	↓6%/↓20% (40 mg AUC/ 160 mg AUC)	↓40%/↓50%
Plasma bound	> 99%	≈ 98%	90%	98.7% (99.8%)	99%	> 99.5%	95%
T_{max}	3 to 4 h	1 to 2 h	1.5 to 2 h	1 h (3 to 4 h)	1 to 2 h	0.5 to 1 h	2 to 4 h
Metabolism	O-deethylation	glucuronidation	CYP2C9	CYP2C9; CYP3A4	none	conjugation	unknown
Terminal half-life	≈ 9 h	5 to 9 h	11 to 15 h	≈ 2 h (6 to 9 h)	≈ 13 h	≈ 24 h	≈ 6 h[b]

[a] Active.
[b] IV dosing.

Contraindications

Hypersensitivity to any component of these products.

Warnings/Precautions

Hypotension/Volume- or salt-depleted patients: In patients who are intravascularly volume-depleted (eg, those treated with diuretics), symptomatic hypotension may occur. Correct these conditions prior to administration.

Race: **Losartan** was effective in reducing blood pressure regardless of race, although the effect was somewhat less in black patients (usually a low-renin population). In healthy black subjects, **irbesartan** AUC values were approximately 25% greater than in white subjects.

Cough: In trials where **valsartan** was compared with an ACE inhibitor with or without placebo, the incidence of dry cough was significantly greater in the ACE inhibitor group (7.9%) than in the groups who received valsartan (2.6%) or placebo (1.5%). In patients who had dry cough when previously receiving ACE inhibitors, the incidences of cough in patients who received angiotensin II receptor antagonists, hydrochlorothiazide, or lisinopril were about 22.5%, about 18%, and 69%, respectively.

There was no significant difference in the incidence of cough between **losartan**, **olmesartan**, **eprosartan**, or **telmisartan** and placebo. **Irbesartan** use was not associated with an increased incidence of dry cough, as is typically associated with ACE inhibitor use.

Potassium supplements: Tell patients receiving **losartan** not to use potassium supplements or salt substitutes containing potassium without consulting the prescribing health care provider.

Lab test abnormalities:

Liver function tests – Occasional elevations of liver enzymes or serum bilirubin have occurred.

Creatinine/Blood urea nitrogen (BUN) – Minor increases in BUN or serum creatinine were observed with **candesartan**, **losartan**, **valsartan**, **irbesartan**, and **eprosartan**.

Hemoglobin and hematocrit – Small decreases in hemoglobin and hematocrit occurred in patients treated with angiotensin II receptor antagonists but were rarely of clinical importance. Decreases of more than 20% in hemoglobin and hematocrit were observed in 0.4% and 0.8%, respectively, of **valsartan** patients, versus 0.1% and 0.1% with placebo.

Serum potassium – Increases in serum potassium were observed in some patients treated with angiotensin II receptor antagonists but was rarely of clinical importance.

Renal function impairment: In patients whose renal function may depend on the activity of the renin-angiotensin-aldosterone system (eg, patients with severe CHF), treatment with ACE inhibitors and angiotensin receptor antagonists has been associated with oliguria or progressive azotemia and with acute renal failure or death (rarely). No dosage adjustment is necessary for patients with renal function impairment unless they are volume-depleted. Angiotensin II receptor antagonists are not dialyzable.

Hepatic function impairment:

Losartan – Compared with healthy subjects, the total plasma clearance in patients with hepatic function impairment was about 50% lower and the oral bioavailability was about 2 times higher. A lower starting dose is recommended.

Valsartan – On average, patients with mild to moderate long-term liver disease have twice the exposure to valsartan of healthy volunteers. In general, no dosage adjustment is needed in patients with mild to moderate liver disease. However, exercise care in this patient population.

Olmesartan – Increases in $AUC_{0-\infty}$ and C_{max} were observed in patients with moderate hepatic function impairment compared with those in matched controls, with an increase in AUC of about 60%.

Telmisartan – As the majority of telmisartan is eliminated by biliary excretion, patients with biliary obstructive disorders or hepatic function impairment can be expected to have reduced clearance. Use telmisartan with caution in these patients.

Pregnancy: *Category* C (first trimester); *Category D* (second and third trimesters).

Lactation: It is not known if angiotensin II receptor antagonists are excreted in human breast milk.

Children: Safety and efficacy have not been established in children younger than 6 years of age.

Elderly: No dosage adjustment is necessary when initiating angiotensin II receptor antagonists in the elderly.

Drug Interactions

Drugs that may interact with **losartan** include cimetidine, phenobarbital, fluconazole, indomethacin, and rifamycins.

Drugs that may interact with **telmisartan** include digoxin and warfarin.

In vitro studies show significant inhibition of the formation of oxidized **irbesartan** metabolites with the known cytochrome CYP2C9 substrates/inhibitors, tolbutamide, and nifedipine. However, clinical consequences were negligible.

CYP-450: In vitro studies show significant inhibition of the formation of the active metabolite of **losartan** by inhibitors of CYP-450 3A4 (eg, ketoconazole, troleandomycin) or P-450 2C9 (sulfaphenazole). The consequences of concomitant use of losartan and these inhibitors have not been examined.

Potassium: Concomitant use of potassium-sparing diuretics, potassium supplements, or salt substitutes containing potassium and angiotensin II receptor antagonists may lead to increases in serum potassium.

Adverse Reactions

Adverse reactions occurring in at least 3% of patients include cough, diarrhea, dizziness, fatigue, pain, pharyngitis, rhinitis, sinusitis, upper respiratory tract infection, and viral infection.

ALISKIREN

Tablets: 150 and 300 mg (*Rx*)	*Tekturna* (Novartis)

Warning:

Use in pregnancy: When used in pregnancy during the second and third trimesters, drugs that act directly on the renin-angiotensin system can cause injury and even death to the developing fetus. When pregnancy is detected, discontinue aliskiren as soon as possible.

Indications

Hypertension: For the treatment of hypertension. It may be used alone or in combination with other antihypertensive agents.

Administration and Dosage

Patients should establish a routine pattern for taking aliskiren with regard to meals. High-fat meals decrease absorption substantially.

The usual recommended starting dosage of aliskiren is 150 mg once daily. In patients whose blood pressure is not adequately controlled, the daily dose may be increased to 300 mg.

The antihypertensive effect of a given dose is substantially attained (85% to 90%) by 2 weeks.

Aliskiren may be coadministered with other antihypertensive agents. Most exposure to date is with diuretics and an angiotensin receptor blocker (valsartan).

Actions

Pharmacology: Aliskiren is a direct renin inhibitor, decreasing plasma renin activity and inhibiting the conversion of angiotensin to Ang I. Whether aliskiren affects other renin-angiotensin-aldosterone system components is not known.

Pharmacokinetics:

Absorption/Distribution – Aliskiren is a poorly absorbed drug with an approximate accumulation half-life of 24 hours. Steady-state blood levels are reached in about 7 to 8 days. Following oral administration, peak plasma concentrations of aliskiren are reached within 1 to 3 hours. When taken with a high-fat meal, mean area under the curve (AUC) and maximum drug concentration (C_{max}) of aliskiren are decreased 71% and 85%, respectively.

Metabolism/Excretion – About one-fourth of the absorbed dose appears in the urine as parent drug. How much of the absorbed dose is metabolized is unknown. Based on the in vitro studies, the major enzyme responsible for aliskiren metabolism appears to be CYP3A4.

Contraindications

None known.

Warnings/Precautions

Head and neck angioedema: Angioedema of the face, extremities, lips, tongue, glottis, and/or larynx has been reported in patients treated with aliskiren. This may occur at any time during treatment. Promptly discontinue aliskiren and provide appropriate therapy and monitoring until complete and sustained resolution of signs and symptoms has occurred.

Hypotension: An excessive fall in blood pressure was rarely seen (0.1%) in patients with uncomplicated hypertension treated with aliskiren alone. Hypotension also was infrequent (less than 1%) during combination therapy with other antihypertensive agents. In patients with an activated renin-angiotensin system, such as volume- or salt-depleted patients, symptomatic hypotension could occur after initiation of treatment with aliskiren. Correct this condition prior to administration of aliskiren or start the treatment under close medical supervision.

Hyperkalemia: Increases in serum potassium more than 5.5 mEq/L were infrequent with aliskiren alone. However, when used in combination with an ACE inhibitor in a diabetic population, increases in serum potassium were more frequent. Routine monitoring of electrolytes and renal function is indicated in this population.

Renal function impairment: Patients with greater than moderate renal function impairment, a history of dialysis, nephrotic syndrome, or renovascular hypertension were excluded from clinical trials of aliskiren in hypertension. Exercise caution in these patients.

Pregnancy: *Category* C (first trimester); *Category D* (second and third trimesters).

Fetal/Neonatal morbidity and mortality – Drugs that act directly on the renin-angiotensin system can cause fetal and neonatal morbidity and death when administered to pregnant women.

Lactation: It is not known whether aliskiren is excreted in human breast milk.

Children: Safety and efficacy in children have not been established.

Monitoring: Aliskiren, when used in combination with an ACE inhibitor in a diabetic population, caused increases in serum potassium. Routine monitoring of electrolytes and renal function is indicated in this population.

Drug Interactions

Drugs that may interact with aliskiren include irbesartan, potent P-glycoprotein inhibitors (eg, atorvastatin, cyclosporine, ketoconazole), thiazide diuretics, ACE inhibitor drugs that increase potassium levels, potassium-sparing diuretics, potassium supplements, salt, substitues containing potassium, and furosemide.

Adverse Reactions

Adverse reactions occurring in at least 1% of patients include back pain, cough, diarrhea, dizziness, fatigue, headache, rash, nasopharyngitis, and upper respiratory infection.

Lab test abnormalities:

Creatine kinase – Increases in creatine kinase were recorded in about 1% of aliskiren monotherapy patients versus 0.5% of placebo patients.

Hemoglobin and hematocrit – Small decreases in hemoglobin and hematocrit were observed.

BUN, creatinine – Minor increases in BUN or serum creatinine were observed in less than 7% of patients with essential hypertension treated with aliskiren alone versus 6% on placebo.

EPLERENONE

Tablets: 25 and 50 mg (*Rx*)	*Inspra* (Searle)

Indications

Congestive heart failure (CHF) post-myocardial infarction (MI): To improve survival of stable patients with left ventricular systolic dysfunction (ejection fraction 40% or less) and clinical evidence of CHF after an acute MI.

Hypertension: Treatment of hypertension alone or in combination with other antihypertensive agents.

Administration and Dosage

The recommended starting dose is 50 mg administered once daily. The full therapeutic effect is apparent within 4 weeks. For patients with an inadequate response to 50 mg once daily, increase the dosage to 50 mg twice daily. Higher dosages are not recommended.

CHF post-MI: 50 mg once daily. Initiate treatment at 25 mg once daily and titrate to the target dose of 50 mg once daily, preferably within 4 weeks as tolerated by the patient.

Eplerenone Dose Adjustment in CHF		
Serum potassium (mEq/L)	Action	Dose adjustment
< 5	Increase	25 mg every other day to 25 mg every day 25 mg every day to 50 mg every day
5 to 5.4	Maintain	No adjustment
5.5 to 5.9	Decrease	50 mg every day to 25 mg every day 25 mg every day to 25 mg every other day 25 mg every other day to withhold
≥ 6	Withhold	—

Eplerenone can be restarted at a dose of 25 mg every other day when serum potassium levels have fallen below 5.5 mEq/L. Measure serum potassium before initiating eplerenone therapy, within the first week, and at 1 month after the start of treatment or dose adjustment. Periodically assess serum potassium thereafter. Factors such as patient characteristics and serum potassium levels may indicate that additional monitoring is appropriate.

For patients receiving weak CYP3A4 inhibitors (eg, erythromycin, saquinavir, verapamil, fluconazole), reduce the starting dose to 25 mg once daily.

Actions

Pharmacology: Eplerenone blocks the binding of aldosterone, a component of the renin-angiotensin-aldosterone system (RAAS).

Pharmacokinetics:

Absorption – Mean peak plasma concentrations are reached approximately 1.5 hours following oral administration. Steady state is reached within 2 days. Absorption is not affected by food.

Distribution – The plasma protein binding of eplerenone is about 50%. The apparent volume of distribution at steady state ranged from 43 to 90 L. Eplerenone does not preferentially bind to red blood cells.

Metabolism – Eplerenone is primarily metabolized via CYP3A4. Inhibitors of CYP3A4 increase blood levels of eplerenone.

Excretion – The elimination half-life of eplerenone is approximately 4 to 6 hours. The apparent plasma clearance is approximately 10 L/h.

Special populations –

Age and race: At steady state, elderly subjects had increases in C_{max} (22%) and AUC (45%) compared with younger subjects. At steady state, C_{max} was 19% lower and AUC was 26% lower in blacks.

Contraindications

All patients with the following conditions: Serum potassium greater than 5.5 mEq/L at initiation; Ccr 30 mL/min or less; concomitant use with the following potent CYP3A4 inhibitors: Ketoconazole, itraconazole, nefazodone, troleandomycin, clarithromycin, ritonavir, and nelfinavir.

Also contraindicated for the treatment of hypertension in patients with the following conditions: Type 2 diabetes with microalbuminuria; serum creatinine greater than 2 mg/dL in males or greater than 1.8 mg/dL in females; Ccr less than 50 mL/min; concomitant use of potassium supplements or potassium-sparing diuretics (amiloride, spironolactone, or triamterene).

Warnings/Precautions

Hyperkalemia: The principal risk of eplerenone is hyperkalemia. Hyperkalemia can cause serious, sometimes fatal arrhythmias. This risk can be minimized by patient selection, avoidance of certain concomitant treatments, dose reduction of eplerenone, and monitoring. The rates of hyperkalemia increase with declining renal function. Treat patients with CHF post-MI who have serum creatinine levels greater than 2 mg/dL (males) or greater than 1.8 mg/dL (females), patients who have Ccr 50 mL/min or less, and diabetic patients with CHF post-MI, including those with proteinuria, with caution.

Renal function impairment: No correlation was observed between plasma clearance of eplerenone and creatinine clearance. Eplerenone is not removed by hemodialysis.

Hepatic function impairment: In 16 subjects with mild to moderate hepatic impairment who received 400 mg of eplerenone, no elevations of serum potassium above 5.5 mEq/L were observed. The mean increase in serum potassium was 0.12 mEq/L in patients with hepatic impairment and 0.13 mEq/L in normal controls. The use of eplerenone in patients with severe hepatic impairment has not been evaluated.

Pregnancy: *Category B.*

Lactation: The concentration of eplerenone in human breast milk after oral administration is unknown.

Children: Safety and efficacy have not been established in pediatric patients.

Drug Interactions

Drugs that may affect eplerenone include ACE inhibitors, angiotensin II antagonists, CYP3A4 inhibitors, NSAIDs, and St. John's wort. Drugs that may be affected by eplerenone include lithium.

Adverse Reactions

Adverse reactions occurring in at least 3% of patients include hyperkalemia and dizziness, increased creatinine (more than 0.5 mg/dL).

ANTIHYPERLIPIDEMIC AGENTS

Lowering cholesterol levels can arrest or reverse atherosclerosis in all vascular beds and can significantly decrease the morbidity and mortality associated with atherosclerosis. Each 10% reduction in cholesterol levels is associated with an approximately 20% to 30% reduction in the incidence of coronary heart disease. Hyperlipidemia, particularly elevated serum cholesterol and low density lipoprotein (LDL) levels, is a risk factor in the development of atherosclerotic cardiovascular disease.

Treatment of hyperlipidemia is based on the assumption that lowering serum lipids decreases morbidity and mortality of atherosclerotic cardiovascular disease.

The cornerstone of treatment in primary hyperlipidemia is diet restriction and weight reduction. Limit or eliminate alcohol intake. Use drug therapy in conjunction with diet, and after maximal efforts to control serum lipids by diet alone prove unsatisfactory, when tolerance to or compliance with diet is poor or when hyperlipidemia is severe and risk of complications is high. Treat contributory diseases such as hypothyroidism or diabetes mellitus.

Positive risk factors for CHD (other than high LDL) include: Age (men 45 years of age or older; women 55 years of age or older or women who go through premature menopause without estrogen replacement therapy); family history of premature CHD; smoking; hypertension (greater than 140/90 mm Hg); low HDL cholesterol (less than 35 mg/dL); obesity (more than 30% overweight); and diabetes mellitus. Physical inactivity is not listed but should also be considered.

Negative risk factors include: High HDL cholesterol (60 mg/dL or more); subtract one risk factor if the patient's HDL is at this level.

All Americans (except children younger than 2 years of age) should adopt a diet that reduces total dietary fat, decreases intake of saturated fat, increases intake of polyunsaturated fat, and reduces daily cholesterol intake to no more than 250 to 300 mg.

The following treatments guidelines are provided by the National Cholesterol Education Program Expert Panel on Detection, Evaluation and Treatment of High Blood Cholesterol in Adults 20 years of age and older.

Classification of Total and HDL Cholesterol Levels

Level (mg/dL)	Classification
< 200 (5.2 mmol/L)	desirable
200 to 239 (5.2 to 6.2 mmol/L)	borderline-high
≥ 240 (6.2 mmol/L)	high
HDL < 35 (0.9 mmol/L)	low

1.) Total blood cholesterol less than 200 mg/dL: HDL 35 mg/dL or more, repeat total cholesterol and HDL measurements within 5 years or with physical exam; provide education on general population eating pattern, physical activity, and risk factor education. HDL less than 35 mg/dL, do lipoprotein analysis; base further action on LDL levels.

2.) Total blood cholesterol 200 to 239 mg/dL: HDL 35 mg/dL or more and less than 2 risk factors, provide information on dietary modification, physical activity, and risk factor reduction; reevaluate in 1 to 2 years, repeat total and HDL cholesterol measurements, and reinforce nutrition and physical activity education. HDL less than 35 mg/dL or at least 2 risk factors, analyze lipoprotein; base further action on LDL levels.

3.) Total blood cholesterol 240 mg/dL or more: Analyze lipoprotein; base further action on LDL levels.

Classification of LDL- Cholesterol Levels

Level (mg/dL)	Classification
< 130 (3.4 mmol/L)	desirable
130 to 159 (3.4 to 4.1 mmol/L)	borderline-high
≥ 160 (4.1 mmol/L)	high

4.) LDL 160 mg/dL or more without CHD and with less than 2 risk factors: Dietary treatment.
5.) LDL 130 mg/dL or more without CHD and with at least 2 risk factors: Dietary treatment.
6.) LDL 190 mg/dL or more without CHD and with less than 2 other risk factors, or LDL 160 mg/dL or more without CHD and with at least 2 other risk factors: Drug treatment.

Elevations and treatment associated with each type of hyperlipidemia follow:

Hyperlipidemias and Their Treatment[a]

	Hyperlipidemia type					
	I	IIa	IIb	III	IV	V
Lipids						
Cholesterol	N-⇧	↑	↑	N-↑	N-⇧	N-↑
Triglycerides	↑	N	↑	N-↑	↑	↑
Lipoproteins						
Chylomicrons	↑	N	N	N	N	↑
VLDL (pre-β)	N-⇧	N-↓	↑	N-⇧	↑	↑
ILDL (broad-β)[b]				↑		
LDL (β)	↓	↑	↑	↑	N-⇩	↓
HDL (α)	↓	N	N	N	N-⇩	↓
Treatment	Diet	Diet Bile acid sequestrants Dextrothyroxine Nicotinic acid Probucol HMG-CoA reductase inhibitors	Diet Bile acid sequestrants[c] Clofibrate[d] Gemfibrozil[e] Nicotinic acid HMG-CoA reductase inhibitors	Diet Clofibrate Gemfibrozil Nicotinic acid	Diet Clofibrate Gemfibrozil Nicotinic acid Fenofibrate	Diet Clofibrate Gemfibrozil Nicotinic acid Fenofibrate

[a] N = normal ↑ = increase ↓ = decrease ⇧ = slight increase ⇩ = slight decrease
[b] An abnormal lipoprotein.
[c] Particularly useful if hypercholesterolemia predominates.
[d] With high serum triglyceride levels and moderately elevated cholesterol.
[e] In patients with inadequate response to weight loss, bile acid sequestrants, and nicotinic acid.

Antihyperlipidemic Drug Effects[a]

	Lipids		Lipoproteins		
Drug	Cholesterol	Triglycerides	VLDL (pre-β)	LDL (β)	HDL
Atorvastatin	↓	↓	↓	↓	↑
Cerivastatin	↓	↓	↓	↓	↑
Cholestyramine	↓	→↑	→↑	↓	→↑
Clofibrate[b]	↓	↓	↓	→↓	→↑
Colestipol	↓	→↑	↑	↓	→↑
Dextrothyroxine[b]	↓	→	→	↓	→
Fenofibrate	↓	↓	↓	↑	↑
Fluvastatin	↓	↓	↓	↓	↑
Gemfibrozil	↓	↓	↓	→↓	↑
Lovastatin	↓	↓	↓	↓	↑
Nicotinic Acid	↓	↓	↓	↓	↑
Pravastatin	↓	↓	↓	↓	↑
Simvastatin	↓	↓	↓	↓	↑

[a] ↓ = decrease ↑ = increase → = unchanged.
[b] These agents are no longer commonly used as antihyperlipidemics.

BILE ACID SEQUESTRANTS

CHOLESTYRAMINE	
Powder for suspension; oral: anhydrous cholestyramine resin 4 g per 9 g powder (*Rx*)	Various, *Questran* (Par)
anhydrous cholestyramine resin 4 g per 5.7 g powder (*Rx*)	*Cholestyramine Light* (Eon, Novopharm)
anhydrous cholestyramine resin 4 g per 5.5 g powder (*Rx*)	*Prevalite* (Upsher Smith)
anhydrous cholestyramine resin 4 g per 6.4 g powder (*Rx*)	*Questran Light* (Par)
COLESEVELAM HYDROCHLORIDE	
Tablets; oral: 625 mg (*Rx*)	*Welchol* (Daiichi Pharm)
Powder for suspension; oral: 1.875 and 3.75 g (*Rx*)	
COLESTIPOL HYDROCHLORIDE	
Tablets; oral: 1 g (*Rx*)	Various, *Colestid* (Pharmacia)
Granules for suspension; oral: colestipol hydrochloride 5 g/dose, colestipol hydrochloride 5 g per 7.5 g powder (*Rx*)	

Indications

Hyperlipoproteinemia: Adjunctive therapy for the reduction of elevated serum cholesterol in patients with primary hypercholesterolemia (elevated LDL) who do not respond adequately to diet.

Biliary obstruction (cholestyramine only): Relief of pruritus associated with partial biliary obstruction.

Type 2 diabetes mellitus (colesevelam only): As an adjunct to diet and exercise to improve glycemic control in adults with type 2 diabetes mellitus.

Administration and Dosage

Although generally given 3 to 4 times daily, there appears to be no advantage to dosing more frequently than twice daily.

CHOLESTYRAMINE:

Adults – 4 g 1 to 2 times daily.

Children – 240 mg/kg/day of anhydrous cholestyramine resin in 2 to 3 divided doses, normally not to exceed 8 g/day with dosage titration based on response and tolerance.

Maintenance dose – 8 to 16 g/day divided into 2 doses. Use gradual increases in dose with periodic assessment of lipid/lipoprotein levels at intervals of at least 4 weeks. Maximum recommended daily dose is 24 g.

Suggested time of administration is at mealtime but may be modified to avoid interference with absorption of other medications. Although the recommended dosing schedule is twice daily, it may be given in 1 to 6 doses per day.

Preparation – Mix the contents of 1 powder packet or 1 level scoopful with 60 to 180 mL (2 to 6 fl oz) water or noncarbonated beverage. Do not take in dry form. Always mix with water or other fluids, highly fluid soups, or pulpy fruits, such as applesauce or crushed pineapple.

Constipation – In patients with preexisting constipation, the starting dosage should be 1 packet or 1 scoop once daily for 5 to 7 days, increasing to twice daily with monitoring of constipation and of serum lipoproteins, at least twice, 4 to 6 weeks apart.

COLESEVELAM: Advise patients to take colesevelam with liquid and a meal. To avoid esophageal distress, colesevelam for oral suspension should not be taken in its dry form.

Adults –

Primary hyperlipidemia: 6 tablets once daily or 3 tablets twice daily whether used as monotherapy or in combination with a statin or 3.75 g powder once daily or 1.875 g powder twice daily.

Concomitant therapy – Colesevelam can be dosed at the same time as a statin, or the 2 drugs can be dosed apart.

Type 2 diabetes mellitus: 6 tablets once daily or 3 tablets twice daily or 3.75 g powder once daily or 1.875 g powder twice daily.

Children (10 to 17 years of age) –

Primary hypercholesterolemia: 3.75 g powder once daily or 1.875 g powder twice daily taken with meals.

Because of the tablet size, colesevelam tablets are not recommended for use in children.

COLESTIPOL HYDROCHLORIDE:

Granules –

Adults: 5 to 30 g colestipol per day given once or in divided doses. The starting dose should be 5 g once or twice daily with a daily increment of 5 g at 1- or 2-month intervals.

Preparation: Mix in liquids, soups, cereals, or pulpy fruits. Do not take dry. Add the prescribed amount to a glassful (at least 90 mL) of liquid; stir until completely mixed. Colestipol will not dissolve. May also mix with carbonated beverages slowly stirred in a large glass. Rinse glass with a small amount of additional beverage to ensure that all the medication is taken.

Tablets – 2 to 16 g/day given once or in divided doses. The starting dose should be 2 g once or twice daily. Dosage increases of 2 g, once or twice daily, should occur at 1 or 2 month intervals.

Swallow tablets whole; do not cut, chew, or crush.

Constipation –

Tablets: 2 g once or twice daily.

Oral suspension: 1 packet or 1 scoop once daily for 5 to 7 days, increasing to twice daily with monitoring of constipation and of serum lipoproteins, at least twice, 4 to 6 weeks apart.

Actions

Pharmacology: Bile acid sequestering resins bind bile acids in the intestine to form an insoluble complex, which is excreted in the feces. This results in a partial removal of bile acids from the enterohepatic circulation, preventing their absorption.

The fall in LDL concentration is apparent in 4 to 7 days. The decline in serum cholesterol is usually evident by 1 month. When the resins are discontinued, serum cholesterol usually returns to baseline within 1 month. Cholesterol may rise even with continued use; determine serum levels periodically.

Contraindications

Hypersensitivity to bile acid sequestering resins or any components of the products; complete biliary obstruction (cholestyramine only); bowel obstruction (colesevelam only).

Warnings/Precautions

Powder: To avoid accidental inhalation or esophageal distress, do not take powder or granules dry. Mix with fluids.

Phenylketonurics: Some products may contain phenylalanine.

Calcified material: Calcified material has been observed in the biliary tree and the gall bladder; however, this may be due to liver disease and not drug-related.

Malabsorption: Because they sequester bile acids, these resins may interfere with normal fat absorption and digestion and may prevent absorption of fat-soluble vitamins such as A, D, E, and K.

Chronic use of resins may be associated with increased bleeding tendency due to hypoprothrombinemia associated with vitamin K deficiency.

Reduced folate: Reduction of serum or red cell folate has been reported over long-term administration of cholestyramine. Consider supplementation with folic acid.

Hyperchloremic acidosis: Prolonged use may cause hyperchloremic acidosis, especially in younger and smaller patients where relative dosage may be higher.

Constipation: These agents may produce or severely worsen preexisting constipation. Fecal impaction may occur and hemorrhoids may be aggravated.

Monitoring: Determine serum cholesterol levels at baseline, then frequently during the first few months of therapy and periodically thereafter. Periodically measure serum triglyceride levels to detect significant changes.

Diet: Before instituting therapy, vigorously attempt to control serum cholesterol with an appropriate dietary regimen and weight reduction.

Thyroid function: While there have been no reports of hypothyroidism induced in individuals with normal thyroid function, the theoretical possibility exists, particularly in patients with limited thyroid reserve.

Contributing diseases: Prior to initiating therapy, investigate and treat diseases contributing to increased blood cholesterol (eg, alcoholism, diabetes mellitus, dysproteinemias, hypothyroidism, nephrotic syndrome, obstructive liver disease, other drug therapy).

GI: The safety and efficacy of colesevelam in patients with dysphagia, swallowing disorders, severe GI motility disorders, or major GI tract surgery have not been established. Use with caution.

Pregnancy: *Category* B (colesevelam). *Category* C (cholestyramine and colestipol). These agents are not absorbed systemically, and are not expected to cause fetal harm when administered during pregnancy in recommended doses.

Lactation: Exercise caution when administering to a breast-feeding woman. The possible lack of proper vitamin absorption may have an effect on breast-feeding infants.

Children:

Cholestyramine – Dosage schedules have not been established.

Colestipol and colesevelam – Safety and efficacy have not been established.

Drug Interactions

Cholestyramine and colestipol resins may delay or reduce the absorption of concomitant oral medication by binding the drugs in the gut. Take other drugs at least 1 hour before or 4 to 6 hours after these agents.

Drugs that may be affected by bile acid sequestrants include anticoagulants; corticosteroids; digitalis glycosides; doxepin; estrogens/progestins; furosemide; gemfibrozil; glipizide; HMG-CoA reductase inhibitors; hydrocortisone; imipramine; mycophenolate; NSAIDs; penicillin G; phenobarbital; phosphate supplements; propranolol; tetracyclines; thiazide diuretics; thyroid hormones; ursodiol; valproic acid; verapamil, sustained-release; vitamins A, D, E, and K.

Adverse Reactions

Cholestyramine/Colestipol:

GI –

Most common: Constipation; infection; flatulence.

Less frequent: Abdominal pain/distention/cramping; GI bleeding; belching; bloating; nausea; vomiting; diarrhea; loose stools; indigestion; dyspepsia; heartburn; anorexia; steatorrhea; rhinitis; pharyngitis.

Miscellaneous – Transient and modest elevations of AST, ALT, and alkaline phosphatase (colestipol); liver function abnormalities (cholestyramine); pain, flu syndrome, accidental injury, asthenia (colesevelam); headache (including migraine and sinus); anxiety; vertigo; dizziness; light-headedness; insomnia; fatigue; tinnitus; syncope; drowsiness; urticaria; dermatitis; asthma; wheezing; rash; backache; muscle/joint pains; hematuria; dysuria; burnt odor to urine; diuresis; uveitis; anorexia; weight loss/gain; increased libido; swollen glands; edema; weakness; shortness of breath; swelling of hands/feet.

Colesevelam: Abdominal pain; accidental injury; asthenia; back pain; constipation; diarrhea; dyspepsia; flatulence; flu syndrome; headache; infection; nausea; pain; pharyngitis; rhinitis.

HMG-CoA REDUCTASE INHIBITORS

ATORVASTATIN CALCIUM	
Tablets; oral: 10, 20, 40, and 80 mg (as base) (*Rx*)	*Lipitor* (Pfizer)
FLUVASTATIN	
Capsules; oral: 20 and 40 mg (as base) (*Rx*)	*Lescol* (Novartis)
Tablets, extended-release; oral: 80 mg (as base) (*Rx*)	*Lescol XL* (Novartis)
LOVASTATIN	
Tablets; oral: 10, 20, and 40 mg (*Rx*)	Various, *Mevacor* (Merck)
Tablets, extended-release; oral: 10, 20, 40, and 60 mg (*Rx*)	*Altoprev* (Sciele)
PITAVASTATIN	
Tablets; oral: 1, 2, and 4 mg (*Rx*)	*Livalo* (Kowa)
PRAVASTATIN SODIUM	
Tablets; oral: 10, 20, 40, and 80 mg (*Rx*)	Various, *Pravachol* (Bristol-Myers Squibb)
ROSUVASTATIN CALCIUM	
Tablets; oral: 5, 10, 20, and 40 mg (as base) (*Rx*)	*Crestor* (AstraZeneca)
SIMVASTATIN	
Tablets; oral: 5, 10, 20, 40, and 80 mg (*Rx*)	Various, *Zocor* (Merck)
Tablets, disintegrating; oral: 10, 20, 40, and 80 mg (*Rx*)	Various

Indications

Antihyperlipidemics:

HMG-CoA Reductase Inhibitors – Summary of Indications[a]

Indication	Atorvastatin	Fluvastatin	Lovastatin	Pitavastatin	Pravastatin	Rosuvastatin	Simvastatin
Food and Drug Administration–approved indications							
Primary prevention of CV disease in patients with multiple risk factors for CHD, diabetes, peripheral vascular disease, history of stroke, or other cerebrovascular disease to:							
Reduce angina risk	✓		✓				
Reduce MI risk	✓				✓		✓
Reduce stroke risk	✓						✓
Reduce risk for revascularization procedures	✓		✓		✓		✓
Reduce risk of CV mortality					✓		✓
Secondary prevention of CV events in patients with clinically evident CHD to:							
Reduce risk of MI	✓				✓		✓
Reduce risk of stroke	✓				✓		✓
Reduce risk for revascularization procedures	✓	✓			✓		✓
Reduce risk of hospitalization for CHF	✓						
Reduce angina risk	✓						
Slow progression of coronary atherosclerosis		✓	✓		✓	✓	
Reduce risk of total mortality by reducing coronary death					✓		✓

HMG-CoA Reductase Inhibitors – Summary of Indications[a]

Indication	Atorvastatin	Fluvastatin	Lovastatin	Pitavastatin	Pravastatin	Rosuvastatin	Simvastatin
Hypercholesterolemia							
Primary hypercholesterolemia (heterozygous familial and nonfamilial)	✓	✓	✓	✓	✓	✓	✓
Adolescents with heterozygous familial hypercholesterolemia	✓	✓	✓		✓		✓
Homozygous familial hypercholesterolemia	✓					✓	✓
Mixed dyslipidemia (Fredrickson types IIa and IIb)	✓	✓	✓	✓	✓	✓	✓
Hypertriglyceridemia (Fredrickson type IV)	✓				✓	✓	✓
Primary dysbetalipoproteinemia (Fredrickson type III)	✓				✓	✓	✓

[a] HMG-CoA = 3-hydroxy-3-methylglutaryl coenzyme A; CV = cardiovascular; CHD = coronary heart disease; MI = myocardial infarction; CHF = congestive heart failure.
[a] Includes heterozygous familial and nonfamilial hypercholesterolemia.
[b] Immediate-release only.
[c] Includes Fredrickson types IIa and IIb.
[d] Includes Fredrickson type IV.
[e] Includes Fredrickson type III.
[f] Children 10 to 16 years of age.
[g] Adolescents 10 to 17 years of age.
[h] Extended-release only.

Administration and Dosage

ATORVASTATIN CALCIUM:

Hypercholesterolemia (heterozygous familial and nonfamilial), mixed dyslipidemia (Fredrickson type IIa and IIb), and prevention of cardiovascular disease – 10 to 20 mg once/day. Patients who require a more than 45% reduction in LDL-C may be started at 40 mg once/day. Dosage range is 10 to 80 mg once/day, at any time of the day, with or without food. After initiation and/or upon dose titration, analyze lipid levels within 2 to 4 weeks and adjust dosing accordingly.

Heterozygous familial hypercholesterolemia in children 10 to 17 years of age – 10 mg/day; the maximum dose is 20 mg/day. Make adjustments at intervals of 4 weeks or more.

Homozygous familial hypercholesterolemia – 10 to 80 mg/day.

Concomitant lipid-lowering therapy – Atorvastatin may be used in combination with a bile acid–binding resin for additive effect. Generally, avoid the combination of HMG-CoA reductase inhibitors and fibrates.

FLUVASTATIN: For patients requiring LDL-C reduction to a goal of 25% or more, the starting dose is either 40 mg, 80 mg as a single extended-release dose, or 80 mg in divided doses of the 40 mg capsule given twice daily. For patients requiring LDL-C reduction to a goal of less than 25%, a starting dose of 20 mg may be used. The recommended dosing range is 20 to 80 mg/day.

Children – The starting dose is 20 mg. Dose adjustments, up to a maximum daily dose of 40 mg twice daily or 80 mg extended-release once daily, should be made at 6-week intervals.

Concomitant lipid-lowering therapy – When administering a bile acid resin and fluvastatin, administer fluvastatin at bedtime, at least 2 hours following the resin.

LOVASTATIN: Give immediate-release tablets once/day with meals and give extended-release tablets once/day in the evening at bedtime.

Adults –

Immediate-release: 20 mg once/day with the evening meal. Dosage range is 10 to 80 mg/day in a single dose or 2 divided doses. Start patients requiring reductions in LDL-C of 20% or more on 20 mg/day. Give a starting dose of 10 mg for patients requiring smaller reductions. Adjust at intervals of 4 weeks or more. Maximum dose is 80 mg/day.

Extended-release: 20, 40, or 60 mg once/day given in the evening at bedtime. The dosing range is 10 to 60 mg/day in single doses. Consider a starting dose of 10 mg for patients requiring smaller reductions. Adjust at intervals of 4 weeks or more. Swallow whole; do not chew or crush.

Adolescents 10 to 17 years of age with heterozygous familial hypercholesterolemia (immediate-release only) – The dosing range is 10 to 40 mg/day; the maximum recommended dose is 40 mg/day. Start patients requiring reductions in LDL-C of 20% or more on 20 mg/day. Consider a starting dose of 10 mg for patients requiring smaller reductions. Adjust at intervals of 4 weeks or more.

Concomitant lipid-lowering therapy – Generally, avoid use of lovastatin with fibrates or niacin. If lovastatin is used in combination with gemfibrozil, other fibrates, or lipid-lowering doses (1 g/day or more) of niacin, the dose of lovastatin should not exceed 20 mg/day.

Concomitant cyclosporine – 10 mg/day in patients taking cyclosporine. Maximum dose is 20 mg/day.

Concomitant amiodarone or verapamil (immediate-release only) – In patients taking amiodarone or verapamil concomitantly with lovastatin, the dose should not exceed 40 mg/day.

Renal function impairment – In patients with severe renal function impairment (creatine clearance [CrCl] less than 30 mL/min), carefully consider dosage increases more than 20 mg/day.

PITAVASTATIN:

Adults –

Primary hyperlipidemia and mixed dyslipidemia: Maximum dose is 4 mg once daily; the recommended starting dose is 2 mg. The dosage range is 1 to 4 mg orally once daily at any time of the day with or without food.

After initiation or upon titration of pitavastatin, lipid levels should be analyzed after 4 weeks and the dosage adjusted accordingly.

Renal function impairment – Patients with moderate renal impairment (glomerular filtration rate [GFR] 30 to less than 60 mL/min/1.73 m^2) and end-stage renal disease receiving hemodialysis should receive a starting dose of pitavastatin 1 mg once daily and a maximum dose of 2 mg once daily. Pitavastatin should not be used in patients with severe renal impairment (GFR less than 30 mL/min/1.73 m^2) not yet on hemodialysis.

Concomitant medications –

Erythromycin: 1 mg once daily should not be exceeded in patients taking erythromycin.

Rifampin: 2 mg once daily should not be exceeded in patients taking rifampin.

PRAVASTATIN SODIUM: Pravastatin can be administered as a single dose at any time of the day, with or without food.

Adults – 40 mg once/day. If a daily dose of 40 mg does not achieve desired cholesterol levels, 80 mg once/day is recommended.

Children –

Children 8 to 13 years of age (inclusive): 20 mg once daily. Doses greater than 20 mg have not been studied in this patient population.

Adolescents 14 to 18 years of age: 40 mg once daily. Doses greater than 40 mg have not been studied in this patient population.

Concomitant immunosuppressants – In patients taking immunosuppressive drugs, begin therapy with 10 mg once/day at bedtime and titrate to higher doses with caution. Most patients treated with this combination received a maximum dose of 20 mg/day.

Concomitant lipid-lowering therapy – When administering a bile acid–binding resin (eg, cholestyramine, colestipol) and pravastatin, give pravastatin either 1 hour or more before or at least 4 hours following the resin. Generally, avoid the combined use of pravastatin and fibrates.

Renal/Hepatic function impairment – Use a starting dose of 10 mg/day in significant renal or hepatic function impairment.

ROSUVASTATIN CALCIUM:

Hypercholesterolemia (heterozygous familial and nonfamilial), mixed dyslipidemia, hypertriglyceridemia, primary dysbetalipoproteinemia (type III hyperlipoproteinemia), and atherosclerosis – The dosage range is 5 to 40 mg once daily. The starting dosage is 10 to 20 mg once daily. After initiation or upon dose titration, analyze lipid levels within 2 to 4 weeks.

Homozygous familial hypercholesterolemia – 20 mg once daily. The maximum daily dose is 40 mg.

Concomitant cyclosporine – Limit therapy to 5 mg once daily.

Concomitant lopinavir/ritonavir or atazanavir/ritonavir therapy – Limit therapy to 10 mg once daily.

Concomitant lipid-lowering therapy – If used in combination with gemfibrozil, limit the dose to 10 mg once daily.

Administration – Administer as a single dose at any time of the day, with or without food.

Asian patients – Initiate therapy with 5 mg once daily should be considered for Asian patients.

Renal function impairment – For patients with severe renal function impairment (CrCl less than 30 mL/min/1.73 m^2) not on hemodialysis, start dosing at 5 mg once daily. Do not exceed 10 mg once daily.

Hepatic function impairment – Use caution in patients who consume substantial quantities of alcohol or have a history of liver disease. Active liver disease or unexplained persistent transaminase elevations are contraindications to the use of rosuvastatin.

SIMVASTATIN: Dosage range is 5 to 80 mg/day. Adjust dose at intervals of 4 weeks or more.

Homozygous familial hypercholesterolemia – 40 mg/day in the evening or 80 mg/day in 3 divided doses of two 20 mg doses and 1 evening dose of 40 mg.

Prevention of coronary events – 20 to 40 mg once a day in the evening. For patients at high risk, starting dosage is 40 mg/day.

Adolescents 10 to 17 years of age with heterozygous familial hypercholesterolemia – 10 mg once a day in the evening. Dosing range is 10 to 40 mg/day; maximum dose is 40 mg/day. Adjust at intervals of 4 weeks or more.

Concomitant cyclosporine – In patients taking cyclosporine concomitantly, begin therapy with 5 mg/day; do not exceed 10 mg/day. Simvastatin orally-disintegrating tablets are not available in the 5 mg dosage strength. Other simvastatin 5 mg tablets should be used if a 5 mg dose is needed.

Concomitant amiodarone or verapamil – In patients taking amiodarone or verapamil concomitantly, the dose should not exceed 20 mg/day.

Concomitant lipid-lowering therapy – Simvastatin is effective alone or when used concomitantly with bile-acid sequestrants. If simvastatin is used in combination with gemfibrozil, the dose of simvastatin should not exceed 10 mg/day.

Renal function impairment – Exercise caution when simvastatin is administered to patients with severe renal function impairment. Initiate therapy in these patients with 5 mg/day.

Administration –

Orally disintegrating tablets: Place the orally disintegrating tablet on the tongue where it will dissolve and then be swallowed with saliva. If necessary, follow with water.

Actions

Pharmacology: These agents specifically competitively inhibit 3-hydroxy-3-methylglutaryl-coenzyme A (HMG-CoA) reductase, the enzyme that catalyzes the early rate-limiting step in cholesterol biosynthesis, conversion of HMG-CoA to mevalonate. This conversion is an early rate-limiting step in cholesterol biosynthesis.

The rank order for statins, based on LDL-C–lowering potencies, is as follows: **rosuvastatin > atorvastatin > simvastatin > pravastatin = lovastatin > fluvastatin.**

Pharmacokinetics:

HMG-CoA Reductase Inhibitor Pharmacokinetics[a]

	Atorvastatin	Fluvastatin	Lovastatin	Pitavastatin	Pravastatin	Rosuvastatin	Simvastatin
Bioavailability	≈ 14%; first-pass metabolism (CYP3A4)	24%; saturable first-pass metabolism (CYP2C9); mean relative bioavailability is ≈ 29% for ER compared with IR	< 5%; extensive first-pass metabolism (CYP3A4); bioavailability for ER was 190% compared with IR	51%	34% absorbed; absolute bioavailability 17%; extensive first-pass metabolism	≈ 20%	< 5%; extensive first-pass metabolism (CYP3A4)
Effect of food	Decreased rate and extent of absorption 25% and 9%, respectively; not clinically significant	Decreased rate, but not extent, of absorption (IR); Delayed T_{max} (6 h) and increased bioavailability by ≈ 50% (ER)	Decreased bioavailability (ER)	Decreased rate by 43%, but does not significantly reduce extent	Decreased bioavailability; not clinically significant	Decreased rate 20%, but not extent of absorption	
Protein binding	≥ 98%	98%	> 95%	> 99%	≈ 50%	88%	≈ 95%
Half-life	14 h[b]	< 3 h (IR); ≈ 9 (ER)	3 to 4 h (IR)	12 h	77 h[c]	≈ 19 h	
Metabolic enzymes	Extensive CYP3A4	Extensive CYP2C9, CYP3A4	Extensive CYP3A4	Marginal CYP2C9	Extensive sulfation	Minor CYP2C9	Extensive CYP3A4
Excretion	Biliary; < 2% (urine)	≈ 5% (urine); ≈ 90% (feces)	10% (urine); 83% (feces)	15% (urine); 79% (feces)	≈ 20% (urine); 70% (feces)	90% (feces)	13% (urine); 60% (feces)
Effects of renal/hepatic impairment	Plasma levels not affected by renal disease; markedly increased with chronic alcoholic liver disease; C_{max} and AUC are 4-fold greater and 16-fold greater in patients with Child-Pugh score A disease and Child-Pugh score B disease, respectively.	Potential drug accumulation with hepatic insufficiency.	Increased plasma concentration with severe renal disease.	Plasma concentrations are increased in mild to moderate hepatic impairment; rate and extent of absorption are increased 60% and 79%, respectively, in patients with moderate renal impairment.	Potential drug accumulation with renal or hepatic insufficiency; mean AUC varied 18-fold in cirrhotic patients, and peak values varied 47-fold.	Increased plasma concentrations with severe renal impairment and hepatic disease.	Higher systemic exposure may occur in hepatic and severe renal insufficiency.

[a] IR = immediate-release; C_{max} = maximal drug concentration; T_{max} = time to maximal drug concentration; AUC = area under the curve.

[b] For unmetabolized **atorvastatin** only. The half-life of inhibitory activity for HMG-CoA reductase is 20 to 30 hours because of the contribution of active metabolites.

[c] Parent plus metabolites.

Contraindications

Hypersensitivity to any component of these products; active liver disease or unexplained persistent elevated hepatic transaminases; pregnancy, lactation; coadministration with cyclosporine (**pitavastatin** only).

Warnings/Precautions

Liver dysfunction: Use with caution in patients who consume substantial quantities of alcohol or who have a history of liver disease or have signs suggestive of liver disease.

Skeletal muscle effects: Cases of rhabdomyolysis with acute renal failure secondary to myoglobinuria have been reported with statins, and rare fatalities have occurred. Myopathy (ie, muscle pain, tenderness, or weakness with creatine phosphokinase [CPK] values above 10 times the upper limit of normal [ULN]) and uncomplicated myalgia have also been reported.

Endocrine effects: Statins interfere with cholesterol synthesis and lower circulating cholesterol levels and, as such, might theoretically blunt adrenal or gonadal steroid hormone production. Small declines in total testosterone with no commensurate elevation in luteinizing hormone have been noted with the use of **fluvastatin. Pravastatin** showed inconsistent results with regard to possible effects on basal steroid hormone levels; **atorvastatin, lovastatin, rosuvastatin**, and **simvastatin** did not reduce basal plasma cortisol concentration, basal plasma testosterone concentration, or impair adrenal reserve.

Homozygous familial hypercholesterolemia: HMG-CoA reductase inhibitors are less effective in patients with the rare homozygous familial hypercholesterolemia, possibly because they have no functional LDL receptors.

Ophthalmic effects: There was a high prevalence of baseline lenticular opacities in the patient population included in the early clinical trials with **lovastatin.**

Hypersensitivity reactions: An apparent hypersensitivity syndrome has occurred. Refer to Management of Acute Hypersensitivity Reactions.

Renal function impairment: Closely monitor patients with renal function impairment.

Hepatic function impairment: Marked persistent increases (greater than 3 times ULN) in serum transaminases occurred in patients treated with all agents ranging in frequency from less than 1% to 2.7%.

Pregnancy: Category X.

Lactation: **Atorvastatin** and **rosuvastatin** are excreted in the milk of rats and is likely to be excreted in breast milk. It is not known whether **lovastatin, pitavastatin,** and **simvastatin** are excreted in breast milk. A small amount of **pravastatin** is excreted in breast milk. **Fluvastatin** is present in breast milk in a 2:1 ratio (milk:plasma). Because of the potential for serious adverse reactions in breast-feeding infants, caution women taking these drugs not to breast-feed their infants.

Children: Safety and efficacy have not been established for **atorvastatin, simvastatin,** and **lovastatin** immediate-release in prepubertal patients and patients younger than 10 years of age. Safety and efficacy have not been established in patients younger than 8 years of age for **pravastatin**. Safety and efficacy of **lovastatin** ER, **pitavastatin**, and **rosuvastatin** have not been established in children.

Elderly: Elderly patients are at higher risk of myopathy; use HMG-CoA reductase inhibitors with caution in elderly patients.

Monitoring:

HMG-CoA Reductase Inhibitors – Recommended Monitoring							
	Atorvastatin	Fluvastatin	Lovastatin	Pitavastatin	Pravastatin	Rosuvastatin	Simvastatin
Efficacy							
Lipids	2 to 4 weeks after initiation or dosage titration	4 weeks after initiation and periodically thereafter	Periodically	4 weeks after initiation or dosage titration	4 weeks after initiation or dosage titration	2 to 4 weeks after initiation or dosage titration	4 weeks after initiation and periodically thereafter

HMG-CoA Reductase Inhibitors – Recommended Monitoring							
	Atorvastatin	Fluvastatin	Lovastatin	Pitavastatin	Pravastatin	Rosuvastatin	Simvastatin
Toxicity							
Liver function tests	Before initiation, at 12 weeks after initiation and any dose increase, and semiannually thereafter	Before initiation and at 12 weeks after initiation and any dose increase	Before initiation in patients with a history of liver disease, or when clinically indicated; in all patients prior to use of 40 mg/day dosage; and when clinically indicated	Before initiation, at 12 weeks following the initiation of therapy and any elevation of dose, and periodically (eg, semiannually) thereafter	Before initiation and when clinically indicated	Before initiation, at 12 weeks after initiation and any dose increase, and semiannually thereafter	Before initiation and when clinically indicated; for dosages of 80 mg/day, patients should receive an additional test prior to titration, 3 months after titration, and semiannually for the first year

For **lovastatin**, perform liver function tests (LFTs) before initiating therapy, at 6 and 12 weeks after initiation of therapy or after dose elevation, and periodically thereafter (at approximately 6-month intervals). For **rosuvastatin**, **fluvastatin**, and **atorvastatin**, it is recommended that LFTs be performed prior to and at 12 weeks following both the initiation of therapy and any elevation in dose and periodically (eg, semiannually) thereafter. For **pravastatin** and **simvastatin**, perform LFTs prior to the initiation of therapy, prior to elevation of dose, and when otherwise clinically indicated. For patients titrated to the 80 mg dose of simvastatin, perform LFTs prior to titration, 3 months after titration to the 80 mg dose, and periodically thereafter (eg, semiannually) for the first year of treatment. Pay special attention to patients who develop elevated serum transaminase levels. If transaminase levels progress, particularly if they rise to 3 times the ULN and are persistent, discontinue the drug.

Because HMG-CoA reductase inhibitors may increase CPK and transaminase levels, consider this in the differential diagnosis of chest pain in patients treated with these agents.

Closely monitor patients with renal impairment receiving pravastatin or simvastatin.

Drug Interactions

Drugs that may affect HMG-CoA reductase inhibitors include amiodarone, antacids, azole antifungals, bile acid sequestrants, bosentan, carbamazapine, cilostazole, cisapride, colchicine, cyclosporine, danazol, diltiazem, fibric acid derivatives, glyburide, histamine H_2 antagonists (eg, cimetidine, ranitidine), hydantoins, imatinib, isradipine, macrolides (eg, clarithromycin, erythromycin), nefazodone, niacin, nicotinic acid, NNRTIs, omeprazole, propranolol, protease inhibitors, quinine, rifamycins, St. John's wort, telithromycin, and verapamil.

Drugs that may be affected by HMG-CoA reductase inhibitors include benzodiazepines, cisapride, clopidogrel, colchicine, hormonal contraceptives, diclofenac, digoxin, fibric acid derivatives, glyburide, niacin, verapamil, and warfarin.

Atorvastatin, **lovastatin**, and **simvastatin** are primarily metabolized by CYP3A4; they may interact with CYP3A4 inhibitors.

Fluvastatin is primarily metabolized by CYP2C9; it may interact with CYP2C9 inhibitors.

Drug/Food interactions: Under fasting conditions, **lovastatin** (immediate-release) levels are approximately two-thirds of those found when given immediately after meals; **lovastatin** (immediate-release) should be taken with meals. When **lovastatin** (ER) was given after a meal, plasma concentrations were approximately 0.5 to 0.6 times those found when **lovastatin** (ER) was administered in a fasting state.

Fibers such as oat bran and pectin may decrease GI absorption of HMG-CoA reductase inhibitors. If coadministration cannot be avoided, separate the administration times by as much as possible.

Grapefruit juice – Coadministration with large quantities of grapefruit juice (at least 1 quart daily) may result in increased plasma levels of **lovastatin, simvastatin**, or **atorvastatin**, increasing the risk of myopathy. Avoid concurrent use.

Adverse Reactions

HMG-CoA Reductase Inhibitor Adverse Reactions[a]							
Adverse reaction	Atorvastatin	Fluvastatin[b]	Lovastatin[b]	Pitavastatin	Pravastatin[c]	Rosuvastatin	Simvastatin
Cardiovascular							
Angina pectoris	< 2%	—	—	—	3.1%	—	—
Atrial fibrillation	—	—	—	—	—	—	5.7%
CNS							
Asthenia	≤ 3.8%	—	1.2% to 3%	—	PM[d]	2.7%	✔[d]
Dizziness	≥ 2%	✔	0.5% to 2%	—	1% to 2.2%	4%	PM[d]
Headache	2.5% to 16.7%	4.7% to 8.9%	2.1% to 7%	✔	1.7% to 1.9%	5.5% to 6.4%	7.4%
Insomnia	≥ 2%	0.8% to 2.7%	0.5% to 1%	—	< 1%	—	4%
Vertigo	—	✔	✔	—	< 1%	—	4.5%
Dermatologic							
Eczema	< 2%	—	—	—	—	—	4.5%
Rash	1.1% to 3.9%	—	0.8% to 1.3%	—	1.3% to 2.1%	✔[d]	✔[d]
GI							
Abdominal pain/cramps	≤ 3.8%	3.7% to 4.9%	2% to 2.5%	—	2% to 2.4%	2.4%	7.3%
Acid regurgitation	—	—	0.5% to 1%	—	—	—	—
Constipation	≤ 2.5%	—	2% to 3.5%	3.6%	1.2% to 2.4%	2.4%	6.6%
Diarrhea	≤ 5.3%	3.3% to 4.9%	2.2% to 3%	2.6%	2%	—	✔[d]
Dysgeusia	< 2%	—	0.8%	—	—	—	—
Dyspepsia	1.3% to 2.8%	3.5% to 7.9%	1% to 1.6%	—	3.5%	—	✔[d]
Flatulence	1.1% to 2.8%	1.4% to 2.6%	3.7% to 4.5%	—	1.2% to 2.7%	—	✔[d]
Gastroenteritis/ Gastritis	< 2%	—	—	—	—	≥ 2%	4.9%
Musculoskeletal							
Arthralgia	≤ 5.1%	✔	0.5% to 5%	✔	PM[d]	10.1%	PM[d]
Arthropathy	—	3.2%	—	—	—	—	—
Back pain	≤ 3.8%	—	5%	3.9%	—	—	—
Muscle cramps/pain	—	✔	0.6% to 1.1%	—	2% to 6%	12.7%	PM[d]
Myalgia	≤ 5.6%	3.8% to 5%	1.8% to 3%	3.1%	0.6% to 1.4%	2.8%	3.7%
Myopathy	✔[d]	✔[d]	✔[d]	—	PM[d]	✔[d]	0.02% to 0.53%
Respiratory							
Bronchitis	≥ 2%	1.8% to 2.6%	—	—	—	—	6.6%
Sinusitis	≤ 6.4%	2.6% to 3.5%	4% to 6%	—	—	—	2.3%

HMG-CoA Reductase Inhibitor Adverse Reactions[a]							
Adverse reaction	Atorvastatin	Fluvastatin[b]	Lovastatin[b]	Pitavastatin	Pravastatin[c]	Rosuvastatin	Simvastatin
Miscellaneous							
Accidental trauma	≤ 4.2%	4.2% to 5.1%	4% to 6%	—	—	—	—
ALT > 3 × ULN	0.2% to 2.3%	0.2% to 4.9%	1.9%	—	≤ 1.2%	2.2%	≈1%
Diabetes mellitus	—	—	—	—	—	—	4.2%
Fatigue	PM[d]	1.6% to 2.7%	—	—	1.9% to 3.4%	—	—
Flu syndrome	≤ 3.2%	5.1% to 7.1%	5%	—	—	—	—
Infection	2.8% to 10.3%	—	11% to 16%	—	—	—	—
Pain	—	—	3% to 5%	—	1.4%	≥ 2%	—
Urinary tract infection	≥ 2%	1.6% to 2.7%	2% to 3%	—	—	—	3.2%

[a] All reactions. Data are pooled from separate studies and are not necessarily comparable.
[b] Immediate-release and ER combined.
[c] Includes short-term and long-term studies.
[d] ✔ = reported, no evidence given; PM = postmarketing

GEMFIBROZIL

Tablets; oral: 600 mg (*Rx*) — Various, *Lopid* (Parke-Davis)

Indications

Hypertriglyceridemia: Hypertriglyceridemia in adults (types IV and V hyperlipidemia) who present a risk of pancreatitis and do not respond to diet. Consider therapy for those with triglyceride elevations between 1,000 and 2,000 mg/dL and who have a history of pancreatitis or recurrent abdominal pain typical of pancreatitis.

Reducing coronary heart disease risk: Consider gemfibrozil therapy in those type IIb patients who have low high-density lipoprotein (HDL) cholesterol levels in addition to elevated low-density lipoprotein (LDL) cholesterol and triglycerides and who have not responded to weight loss, dietary therapy, exercise, and other pharmacologic agents.

Gemfibrozil is not useful for the hypertriglyceridemia of type I hyperlipidemia.

Administration and Dosage

Adults: 1,200 mg daily in 2 divided doses 30 minutes before the morning and evening meals.

Actions

Pharmacology: Gemfibrozil is a lipid-regulating agent that decreases serum triglycerides and very low density lipoprotein (VLDL) cholesterol and increases HDL cholesterol. While modest decreases in total and LDL cholesterol may be observed with gemfibrozil therapy, treatment of patients with elevated triglycerides caused by type IV hyperlipoproteinemia often results in a rise in LDL-cholesterol. Gemfibrozil usually raises HDL cholesterol significantly in type IIb patients with elevations of both serum LDL cholesterol and triglycerides.

Pharmacokinetics:

Absorption/Distribution – Gemfibrozil is well absorbed from the GI tract. Peak plasma levels occur in 1 to 2 hours. Gemfibrozil is highly bound to plasma proteins.

Metabolism/Excretion – Gemfibrozil mainly undergoes oxidation to form a hydroxymethyl and a carboxyl metabolite. Approximately 70% is excreted in the urine, mostly as the glucuronide conjugate.

Contraindications

Hepatic or severe renal dysfunction, including primary biliary cirrhosis; preexisting gallbladder disease; hypersensitivity to gemfibrozil; concurrent use with repaglinide.

Warnings/Precautions

Gallstones: If cholelithiasis is suspected, perform gallbladder studies. Discontinue therapy if gallstones are found.

Concomitant anticoagulants: Exercise caution when anticoagulants are given in conjunction with gemfibrozil. Reduce the dosage of the anticoagulant.

Skeletal muscle effects: Concomitant therapy with gemfibrozil and an HMG-CoA reductase inhibitor is associated with an increased risk of skeletal muscle toxicity manifested as rhabdomyolysis, markedly elevated creatine kinase levels and myoglobinuria, leading in a high proportion of cases to acute renal failure and death. Because of an observed marked increased risk of myopathy and rhabdomyolysis, the specific combination of gemfibrozil and cerivastatin is absolutely contraindicated. If myositis is suspected or diagnosed, gemfibrozil therapy should be withdrawn.

Monitoring therapy: Perform adequate pretreatment laboratory studies. Obtain periodic determinations of serum lipids during administration. Withdraw the drug after 3 months if response is inadequate.

Hematologic – Mild hemoglobin, hematocrit, and white blood cell decreases have been observed. Perform periodic blood counts during the first 12 months of administration.

Liver function – Abnormal elevations of AST, ALT, LDH, bilirubin, and alkaline phosphatase have occurred and are usually reversible on drug discontinuation. Perform periodic liver function studies and terminate therapy if abnormalities persist.

Blood glucose – Gemfibrozil has a moderate hyperglycemic effect; carefully monitor blood glucose levels during therapy.

Renal function impairment: There have been reports of worsening renal insufficiency on the addition of gemfibrozil therapy in individuals with baseline plasma creatinine greater than 2 mg/dL. In such patients, consider the use of alternative therapy against the risks and benefits of a lower dose of gemfibrozil.

Pregnancy: Category C.

Lactation: Decide whether to discontinue breast-feeding or the drug, taking into account the importance of the drug to the mother.

Children: Safety and efficacy in children have not been established.

Drug Interactions

Drugs that may affect gemfibrozil include colestipol. Drugs that may be affected by gemfibrozil include oral anticoagulants, bexarotene, cyclosporine, HMG-CoA reductase inhibitors, loperamide, montelukast, repaglinide, sulfonylureas, thiazolidinediones, and tiagabine.

Adverse Reactions

Adverse reactions occurring in at least 3% of patients include abdominal pain, diarrhea, dyspepsia, fatigue, and GI reactions.

FENOFIBRATE

Tablets; oral: 48 and 145 mg (*Rx*)	*Tricor* (Abbott)
50 mg (*Rx*)	*Triglide* (Sciele)
54 mg (*Rx*)	Various, *Lofibra* (Gate)
107 mg (*Rx*)	Various
160 mg (*Rx*)	Various, *Lofibra* (Gate), *Triglide* (Sciele)
Capsules; oral: 43 and 130 mg (micronized fenofibrate) (*Rx*)	*Antara* (Reliant)
50 and 150 mg (*Rx*)	*Lipofen* (Proethic)
67, 134, and 200 mg (micronized fenofibrate) (*Rx*)	Various, *Lofibra* (Gate)
Capsules, delayed release; oral: 45 and 135 mg (*Rx*)	*Trilipix* (Abbott)

Indications

Hypercholesterolemia: Adjunctive therapy to diet for the reduction of low-density lipoprotein-cholesterol (LDL-C), total-C, triglycerides, and apolipoprotein B (apo B) and to increase high-density lipoprotein-cholesterol (HDL-C) in adult patients with primary hypercholesterolemia or mixed dyslipidemia (Fredrickson types IIa and IIb).

Hypertriglyceridemia: Adjunctive therapy to diet for treatment of adults with hypertriglyceridemia (Fredrickson types IV and V hyperlipidemia).

Combination therapy with statins for mixed dyslipidemia (fenofibric acid): As an adjunct to diet in combination with a statin to reduce triglycerides and increase HDL-C in patients with mixed dyslipidemia and coronary heart disease (CHD) or a CHD risk equivalent who are on optimal statin therapy.

CHD risk equivalents comprise:

- other clinical forms of atherosclerotic disease (eg, abdominal aortic aneurysm, peripheral arterial disease, symptomatic carotid artery disease),
- diabetes,
- multiple risk factors that confer a 10-year risk for CHD greater than 20%.

Administration and Dosage

Give *Lofibra* capsules and tablets and *Lipofen* capsules with meals, optimizing the bioavailability of the medication. The other fenofibrate formulations (*Antara, Tricor, Triglide, Trilipix*) can be given without regard to meals.

Adjust dosage if necessary following repeat lipid determinations at 4- to 8-week intervals. Consider reducing the dose of fenofibrate if lipid levels fall significantly below the targeted range. Withdraw therapy in patients who do not have an adequate response after 2 months of treatment with the maximum recommended dose.

Fenofibrate Dosing Recommendations

Dosing regimen	*Antara*	*Lipofen*[a]	*Lofibra* tablets[a]	*Lofibra* capsules[a]	*Tricor*	*Triglide*	*Trilipix*
Primary hypercholesterolemia or mixed hyperlipidemia	Initial dose: 130 mg/day	Initial dose: 150 mg/day	Initial dose: 160 mg/day	Initial dose: 200 mg/day	Initial dose: 145 mg/day	Initial dose: 160 mg/day	Initial dose: 135 mg/day
Hypertriglyceridemia	Initial dose: 43 to 130 mg/day	Initial dose: 50 to 150 mg/day	Initial dose: 54 to 160 mg/day	Initial dose: 67 to 200 mg/day	Initial dose: 48 to 145 mg/day	Initial dose: 50 to 160 mg/day	Initial dose: 45 to 135 mg/day
	Max dose: 130 mg/day	Max dose: 150 mg/day	Max dose: 160 mg/day	Max dose: 200 mg/day	Max dose: 145 mg/day	Max dose: 160 mg/day	Max dose: 135 mg/day
Renal function impairment	Initial dose: 43 mg/day	Initial dose: 50 mg/day	Initial dose: 54 mg/day	Initial dose: 67 mg/day	Initial dose: 48 mg/day	Initial dose: 50 mg/day	Initial dose: 45 mg/day
Elderly	Initial dose: 43 mg/day	Initial dose: 50 mg/day	Initial dose: 54 mg/day	Initial dose: 67 mg/day	Initial dose: 48 mg/day	Initial dose: 50 mg/day	Base on renal function
Combination therapy with statin for mixed dyslipidemia							Initial dose: 135 mg/day

[a] Taken with meals.

Actions

Pharmacology: Fenofibrate increases lipolysis and elimination of triglyceride-rich particles from plasma by activating lipoprotein lipase and reducing production of apoprotein C III (an inhibitor of lipoprotein lipase activity). The resulting fall in triglycerides produces an alteration in the size and composition of LDL.

Pharmacokinetics:

Absorption/Distribution – Fenofibrate is well absorbed from the GI tract. Peak plasma levels of fenofibric acid occur within 3 to 8 hours after administration and steady-state plasma levels are achieved within 5 to 7 days of dosing. Serum protein binding is approximately 99%.

Metabolism – Fenofibrate is rapidly hydrolyzed by esterases to the active metabolite, fenofibric acid. Fenofibric acid is primarily conjugated with glucuronic acid.

Excretion – Fenofibrate is eliminated with a half-life of 16 to 23 hours. It is mainly excreted in urine in the form of metabolites, primarily fenofibric acid; approximately 60% of the dose appears in urine and 25% in feces.

Contraindications

Hepatic or severe renal dysfunction, including primary biliary cirrhosis, and patients with unexplained persistent liver function abnormality; preexisting gallbladder disease; hypersensitivity to fenofibrate.

Warnings/Precautions

Cholelithiasis: Fenofibrate, like clofibrate and gemfibrozil, may increase cholesterol excretion into the bile, leading to cholelithiasis. If cholelithiasis is suspected, gallbladder studies are indicated. Discontinue therapy if gallstones are found.

Initial therapy: Ascertain that lipid levels are consistently abnormal before instituting fenofibrate therapy. Control serum lipids with appropriate diet, exercise, weight loss in obese patients, and control of any medical problems (eg, diabetes mellitus, hypothyroidism) that are contributing to the lipid abnormalities. If possible, discontinue or change medications known to exacerbate hypertriglyceridemia (eg, beta-blockers, estrogens, thiazides) prior to triglyceride-lowering drug therapy.

Hematologic changes: Mild to moderate hemoglobin, hematocrit, and white blood cell decreases have been observed following initiation of fenofibrate therapy. However, these levels stabilize during long-term administration.

Pancreatitis: This may represent a failure of efficacy in patients with severe hypertriglyceridemia, a direct drug effect, or a secondary phenomenon mediated through biliary tract stone or sludge formation and obstruction of the common bile duct.

Skeletal muscle effects: The use of fibrates alone may occasionally be associated with myopathy. Treatment has been associated on rare occasions with rhabdomyolysis, usually in patients with renal function impairment. Consider myopathy in any patient with diffuse myalgias, muscle tenderness or weakness, or marked elevations of creatine phosphokinase (CPK) levels.

Hypersensitivity reactions: Acute hypersensitivity reactions have occurred.

Renal function impairment: Minimize the dosage in patients who have creatinine clearance less than 50 mL/min.

Hepatic function impairment: Fenofibrate is associated with increases in serum transaminases (AST or ALT). Increases to more than 3 times the upper limit of normal (ULN) occurred.

Pregnancy: Category C.

Lactation: Do not use fenofibrate in breast-feeding mothers.

Children: Safety and efficacy in children have not been established.

Elderly: Fenofibric acid is known to be substantially excreted by the kidney, and the risk of adverse reactions may be greater in patients with renal function impairment. Because elderly patients are more likely to have decreased renal function, take care in dose selection.

Monitoring: Obtain periodic determination of serum lipids during initial therapy to establish the lowest effective dose. Withdraw therapy in patients who do not have an adequate response after 2 months of treatment with the maximum recommended dose. Perform liver function tests regularly. Perform regular periodic monitoring of liver function and discontinue therapy if enzyme levels persist above 3 times the ULN.

Drug Interactions

Drugs that may interact with fenofibrate include oral anticoagulants, bile acid sequestrants, cyclosporine, and HMG-CoA reductase inhibitors.

Drug/Food interactions: The absorption of micronized fenofibrate is increased when administered with food.

Adverse Reactions

Adverse reactions occurring in at least 3% of patients include abdominal pain, abnormal liver function tests, ALT and AST increased, back pain, headache, increased CPK, and respiratory disorder.

EZETIMIBE

Tablets: 10 mg (*Rx*)	*Zetia* (Merck/Schering-Plough)

Indications

Primary hypercholesterolemia:

Monotherapy – As adjunctive therapy to diet for the reduction of elevated total cholesterol (total-C), low density lipoprotein cholesterol (LDL-C), and apolipoprotein B (Apo B) in patients with primary (heterozygous familial and nonfamilial) hypercholesterolemia.

Combination therapy with HMG-CoA reductase inhibitors – In combination with an HMG-CoA reductase inhibitor as adjunctive therapy to diet for the reduction of elevated total-C, LDL-C, and Apo B in patients with primary (heterozygous familial and nonfamilial) hypercholesterolemia.

Homozygous familial hypercholesterolemia (HoFH): With atorvastatin or simvastatin for the reduction of elevated total-C and LDL-C levels in patients with HoFH as an adjunct to other lipid-lowering treatments (eg, LDL apheresis) or if such treatments are unavailable.

Homozygous sitosterolemia: As adjunctive therapy to diet for the reduction of elevated sitosterol and campesterol levels in patients with homozygous familial sitosterolemia.

Mixed hyperlipidemia:

Combination therapy with fenofibrate – In combination with fenofibrate as adjunctive therapy to diet for the reduction of total-C, LDL-C, apo B, and non–high-density lipoprotein cholesterol (non–HDL-C) in patients with mixed hyperlipidemia.

Administration and Dosage

Dose: The recommended dose of ezetimibe is 10 mg once daily administered with or without food.

Coadministration with HMG-CoA reductase inhibitors or fenofibrate: For convenience, the daily dose of ezetimibe may be taken at the same time as the HMG-CoA reductase inhibitor or fenofibrate.

Coadministration with bile acid sequestrants: Dosing of ezetimibe should occur at least 2 hours before or at least 4 hours after administration of a bile acid sequestrant.

Actions

Pharmacology: Ezetimibe inhibits the absorption of cholesterol, leading to a decrease in the delivery of intestinal cholesterol to the liver. This causes a reduction of hepatic cholesterol stores and an increase in clearance of cholesterol from the blood.

Pharmacokinetics:

Absorption – After oral administration, ezetimibe is absorbed and extensively conjugated to a pharmacologically active phenolic glucuronide (ezetimibe-glucuronide). Mean ezetimibe peak plasma concentrations were attained within 4 to 12 hours.

Distribution – Ezetimibe and ezetimibe-glucuronide are highly bound (greater than 90%) to human plasma proteins.

Metabolism/Excretion – Ezetimibe is primarily metabolized in the small intestine and liver via glucuronide conjugation with subsequent biliary and renal excretion. Ezetimibe is slowly eliminated from plasma with a half-life of approximately 22 hours.

Special populations –

Gender: Plasma concentrations for total ezetimibe were slightly higher (less than 20%) in women than in men.

Contraindications

Hypersensitivity to any component of the medication.

The combination of ezetimibe with an HMG-CoA reductase inhibitor is contraindicated in patients with active liver disease or unexplained persistent elevations in serum transaminases.

All HMG-CoA reductase inhibitors are contraindicated in pregnant and breast-feeding women. When ezetimibe is administered with an HMG-CoA reductase inhibitor in a woman of childbearing potential, refer to the pregnancy category and product labeling for the HMG-CoA reductase inhibitor.

Warnings/Precautions

Hyperlipidemia, secondary causes: Prior to initiating therapy with ezetimibe, exclude or, if appropriate, treat secondary causes for dyslipidemia. Perform a lipid profile to measure total-C, LDL-C, HDL-C, and TG.

Liver enzymes: When ezetimibe is coadministered with an HMG-CoA reductase inhibitor, perform liver function tests at initiation of therapy.

Skeletal muscle effects: In clinical trials, there was no excess of myopathy or rhabdomyolysis associated with ezetimibe compared with the relevant control arm (placebo or HMG-CoA reductase inhibitor alone). However, myopathy and rhabdomyolysis are known adverse reactions to HMG-CoA reductase inhibitors and other lipid-lowering drugs.

Hepatic function impairment: Because of the unknown effects of the increased exposure to ezetimibe in patients with moderate or severe hepatic insufficiency, ezetimibe is not recommended in these patients.

Pregnancy: Category C.

Lactation: It is not known whether ezetimibe is excreted in human breast milk.

Children: Treatment with ezetimibe in children (younger than 10 years of age) is not recommended.

Monitoring: Obtain a lipid panel before therapy and periodically thereafter. At the time of hospitalization for an acute coronary event, take lipid measures on admission or within 24 hours.

Drug Interactions

Drugs that may interact with ezetimibe include antacids, cholestyramine, fibric acid derivatives, and cyclosporine.

Drug/Food interactions: Ezetimibe may be administered with or without food.

Adverse Reactions

Adverse reactions occurring in at least 3% of patients include diarrhea, abdominal pain, back pain, arthralgia, sinusitis. In combination with HMG-CoA reductase inhibitors reactions included headache, myalgia, pharyngitis, URI, chest pain.

ANTIHYPERLIPIDEMIC COMBINATIONS

EZETIMIBE/SIMVASTATIN	
Tablets; oral: ezetimibe 10 mg/simvastatin 10 mg, ezetimibe 10 mg/simvastatin 20 mg, ezetimibe 10 mg/simvastatin 40 mg, ezetimibe 10 mg/simvastatin 80 mg (*Rx*)	*Vytorin* (Merck/Schering-Plough)
NIACIN (EXTENDED-RELEASE)/LOVASTATIN	
Tablets; oral: niacin 500 mg/lovastatin 20 mg, niacin 1,000 mg/lovastatin 20 mg, and niacin 1,000 mg/lovastatin 40 mg (*Rx*)	*Advicor* (Abbott)
NIACIN/SIMVASTATIN	
Tablets, extended-release; oral: niacin extended-release 500 mg/simvastatin 20 mg, niacin extended-release 750 mg/simvastatin 20 mg, niacin extended-release 1,000 mg/simvastatin 20 mg (*Rx*)	*Simcor* (Abbott)

Indications

Homozygous familial hypercholesterolemia (ezetimibe/simvastatin): For reducing elevated total cholesterol (total-C) and low-density lipoprotein cholesterol (LDL-C) in patients with homozygous familial hypercholesterolemia, as an adjunct to other lipid-lowering treatments (eg, LDL apheresis) or if such treatments are unavailable.

Hypercholesterolemia (**niacin/simvastatin**)*:* For the reduction of total cholesterol, LDL-C, apolipoprotein B (apo B), non–high-density liproprotein cholesterol (HDL-C), or triglycerides, or to increase HDL-C in patients with primary hypercholesterolemia and mixed dyslipidemia (Fredrickson type IIa and IIb) when treatment with simvastatin monotherapy or niacin extended-release monotherapy is considered inadequate.

Hypertriglyceridemia (niacin/simvastatin): For the reduction of triglycerides in patients with hypertriglyceridemia (Fredrickson type IV hyperlipidemia) when treatment with simvastatin monotherapy or niacin extended-release monotherapy is considered inadequate.

Primary hypercholesterolemia (ezetimibe/simvastatin): Adjunctive therapy to diet for reducing elevated total-C, LDL-C, Apo B, triglyceride, and non-HDL-C, and increasing HDL-C in patients with primary (heterozygous familial and nonfamilial) hypercholesterolemia or mixed hyperlipidemia.

Primary hypercholesterolemia/mixed dyslipidemia (niacin extended release/lovastatin): For the treatment of primary hypercholesterolemia (heterozygous familial and nonfamilial) and mixed dyslipidemia (Fredrickson Types IIa and IIb) in the following: Patients treated with lovastatin who require further triglyceride lowering or HDL raising who may benefit from having niacin added to their regimen; patients treated with niacin who require further LDL lowering who may benefit from having lovastatin added to their regimen.

Administration and Dosage

EZETIMIBE/SIMVASTATIN: The patient should be placed on a standard cholesterol-lowering diet before receiving ezetimibe/simvastatin and should continue on this diet during treatment. Individualize the dosage according to the baseline LDL-C level, the recommended goal of therapy, and the patient's response. Take ezetimibe/simvastatin as a single daily dose in the evening, with or without food.

Primary hypercholesterolemia – The recommended usual starting dose is ezetimibe 10 mg/simvastatin 20 mg daily. Initiation of therapy with ezetimibe 10 mg/simvastatin 10 mg daily may be considered for patients requiring less aggressive LDL-C reductions. Patients who require a larger reduction in LDL-C (more than 55%) may be started at ezetimibe 10 mg/simvastatin 40 mg daily. After initiation or titration of ezetimibe/simvastatin, lipid levels may be analyzed after 2 or more weeks and dosage adjusted, if needed.

Homozygous familial hypercholesterolemia – The recommended dosage for patients with homozygous familial hypercholesterolemia is ezetimibe 10 mg/simvastatin 40 mg daily or ezetimibe 10 mg/simvastatin 80 mg daily in the evening. Use ezetimibe/

simvastatin as an adjunct to other lipid-lowering treatments (eg, LDL apheresis) in these patients or if such treatments are unavailable.

Hepatic function impairment – Use is not recommended in patients with moderate or severe hepatic insufficiency.

Renal function impairment – For patients with severe renal insufficiency, do not start ezetimibe/simvastatin unless the patient has already tolerated treatment with simvastatin at a dose of 5 mg or higher. Exercise caution when ezetimibe/simvastatin is administered to these patients, and monitor them closely.

Chinese patients taking lipid-modifying doses (niacin 1 g/day or more) of niacin-containing products – Because of an increased risk for myopathy, caution should be used when treating Chinese patients with ezetimibe/simvastatin coadministered with lipid-modifying doses (niacin 1 g/day or more) of niacin-containing products. Because the risk for myopathy is dose-related, Chinese patients should not receive ezetimibe 10 mg/simvastatin 80 mg coadministered with lipid-modifying doses of niacin-containing products.

Concomitant bile acid sequestrants – Give ezetimibe/simvastatin either 2 hours or more before or 4 hours or more after administration of a bile acid sequestrant.

Concomitant cyclosporine or danazol – Exercise caution when initiating ezetimibe/simvastatin in the setting of cyclosporine. In patients taking cyclosporine or danazol, do not start ezetimibe/simvastatin unless the patient has already tolerated treatment with simvastatin at a dose of 5 mg or higher. Do not exceed ezetimibe 10 mg/simvastatin 10 mg daily.

Concomitant amiodarone or verapamil – In patients taking amiodarone or verapamil concomitantly with ezetimibe/simvastatin, do not exceed ezetimibe 10 mg/simvastatin 20 mg daily.

Concomitant lipid-lowering therapy – The safety and efficacy of ezetimibe administered with fibrates have not been established. Therefore, the combination of ezetimibe/simvastatin and fibrates should be avoided.

NIACIN EXTENDED RELEASE/LOVASTATIN: The usual recommended starting dose for extended-release niacin tablets is 500 mg at bedtime. Niacin extended-release tablets must be titrated and the dose should not be increased by more than 500 mg every 4 weeks up to a maximum dose of 2,000 mg/day, to reduce the incidence and severity of side effects. Patients already receiving a stable dose of niacin extended-release tablets may be switched directly to a niacin-equivalent dose of niacin extended-release/lovastatin tablets.

The usual recommended starting dose of lovastatin is 20 mg once/day. Make dose adjustments at intervals of 4 weeks or more. Patients already receiving a stable dose of lovastatin may receive concomitant dosage titration with niacin extended-release tablets, and switch to niacin extended-release/lovastatin tablets once a stable dose of niacin extended-release tablets has been reached.

Take niacin extended-release/lovastatin tablets at bedtime, with a low-fat snack, and individualize dose according to patient response.

Take whole; do not break, chew, or crush before swallowing. Do not increase the dose by more than 500 mg/day (based on the niacin extended release component) every 4 weeks. The lowest dose of niacin extended-release/lovastatin tablets is 500mg/20 mg. Doses greater than 2,000/40 mg/day are not recommended. If therapy is discontinued for an extended period (greater than 7 days), begin reinstitution of therapy with the lowest dose.

NIACIN/SIMVASTATIN: Niacin extended-release/simvastatin tablets should be taken whole and not broken, crushed, or chewed before swallowing. They should be taken as a single daily dose at bedtime, with a low-fat snack.

Starting dose – Patients not taking niacin extended-release and patients taking niacin products other than niacin extended-release should start niacin extended-release/simvastatin at a single 500 mg/20 mg tablet daily at bedtime.

Dose modification – The dose of niacin extended-release should not be increased by more than 500 mg daily every 4 weeks (see the following table).

Recommended Niacin Extended-Release Initial Titration Schedule	
Week(s)	Daily dose of niacin extended-release
1 to 4	500 mg
5 to 8	1,000 mg
[a]	1,500 mg
[a]	2,000 mg

[a] After week 8, titrate to patient response and tolerance. If response to 1,000 mg daily is inadequate, increase dose to 1,500 mg daily; may subsequently increase dose to 2,000 mg daily. Daily dose should not be increased more than 500 mg in a 4-week period, and doses higher than 2,000 mg daily are not recommended.

Maintenance dose – The recommended maintenance dose for niacin extended-release/simvastatin is 1,000 mg/20 mg to 2,000 mg/40 mg (two 1,000 mg/20 mg tablets) once daily depending on patient tolerability and lipid levels.

Maximum dose – The efficacy and safety of doses of niacin extended-release/simvastatin more than 2,000 mg/40 mg daily are not recommended.

Interruption of therapy – If niacin extended-release/simvastatin therapy is discontinued for an extended period of time (more than 7 days), retitration as tolerated is recommended.

Interchangeability – Niacin extended-release/simvastatin should only be substituted for equivalent doses of niacin extended-release (*Niaspan*).

Pretreatment – Flushing may be reduced in frequency or severity by pretreatment with aspirin or other nonsteroidal anti-inflammatory drugs (approximately 30 minutes prior to niacin extended-release/simvastatin dose).

AMLODIPINE BESYLATE/ATORVASTATIN CALCIUM

Tablets; oral: amlodipine besylate 2.5 mg/atorvastatin calcium 10 (as base), amlodipine besylate 2.5 mg/atorvastatin calcium 20 (as base), amlodipine besylate 2.5 mg/atorvastatin calcium 40 (as base), amlodipine besylate 5 mg/atorvastatin calcium 10 mg (as base), amlodipine besylate 5 mg/atorvastatin calcium 20 mg (as base), amlodipine besylate 5 mg/atorvastatin calcium 40 mg (as base), amlodipine besylate 5 mg/atorvastatin calcium 80 mg (as base), amlodipine besylate 10 mg/atorvastatin calcium 10 mg (as base), amlodipine besylate 10 mg/atorvastatin calcium 20 mg (as base), amlodipine besylate 10 mg/atorvastatin calcium 40 mg (as base), amlodipine besylate 10 mg/atorvastatin calcium 80 mg (as base) (*Rx*)	*Caduet* (Pfizer)

See individual drug monographs for more information.

Indications

Indicated in patients for whom treatment with both amlodipine and atorvastatin is appropriate.

Amlodipine: For the treatment of hypertension, chronic stable angina, and confirmed or suspected vasospastic angina (Prinzmetal or Variant angina).

Atorvastatin: As an adjunct to diet to reduce elevated total-cholesterol (C), LDL-C, apo B, and triglyceride levels and to increase HDL-C in patients with primary hypercholesterolemia (heterozygous familial and nonfamilial) and mixed dyslipidemia (Fredrickson types IIa and IIb); as an adjunct to diet for the treatment of patients with elevated serum triglyceride levels (Fredrickson type IV); for the treatment of patients with primary dysbetalipoproteinemia (Fredrickson type III); to reduce total-C and LDL-C in patients with homozygous familial hypercholesterolemia as an adjunct to other lipid-lowering treatments (eg, LDL apheresis) or if such treatments are unavailable; to reduce total-C, LDL-C, and apo B levels in boys and postmenarchal girls (10 to 17 years of age with heterozygous familial hypercholesterolemia).

Administration and Dosage

Individualize dosage. Lipid-altering agents should be used in addition to a diet restricted in saturated fat and cholesterol, only when the response to diet and other nonpharmacological measures has been inadequate.

Amlodipine/Atorvastatin may be substituted for its individually titrated components. Patients may be given the equivalent dose of amlodipine/atorvastatin or a dose of amlodipine/atorvastatin with increased amounts of amlodipine, atorvastatin, or both for additional antianginal effects, blood pressure lowering, or lipid-lowering effect.

As initial therapy for one indication and continuation of treatment of the other, the recommended starting dose of amlodipine/atorvastatin should be selected based on the continuation of the component being used and the recommended starting dose of the added monotherapy. The maximum dose of the amlodipine component is 10 mg once daily. The maximum dose of the atorvastatin component is 80 mg/day.

Concomitant therapy: Atorvastatin may be used in combination with a bile acid-binding resin for additive effect. The combination of HMG-CoA reductase inhibitors and fibrates generally should be avoided.

RANOLAZINE

Tablets, extended-release: 500 and 1,000 mg (*Rx*)	*Ranexa* (CV Therapeutics)

Indications

Chronic angina: For the treatment of chronic angina.

Administration and Dosage

Adults: Initiate at 500 mg twice daily and increase to 1,000 mg twice daily as needed. The maximum recommended daily dose of ranolazine is 1,000 mg twice daily.

Ranolazine may be taken with or without meals. Ranolazine should be swallowed whole and not crushed, broken, or chewed.

Actions

Pharmacology: Ranolazine has antianginal and anti-ischemic effects that do not depend upon reductions in heart rate or blood pressure. The mechanism of action of ranolazine is unknown.

Pharmacokinetics:

Absorption/Distribution – Steady state is generally achieved within 3 days of twice daily dosing. Peak plasma concentrations of ranolazine are reached between 2 and 5 hours. The bioavailability of ranolazine is 76%.

Metabolism/Excretion – The apparent terminal half-life of ranolazine is 7 hours. Ranolazine is metabolized rapidly and extensively in the liver and intestine; less than 5% is excreted unchanged in urine and feces; it is metabolized mainly by CYP3A and to a lesser extent by CYP2D6.

Contraindications

Patients taking strong inhibitors of CYP3A, patients taking inducers of CYP3A, and those with clinically significant hepatic impairment.

Warnings/Precautions

QT prolongation: Ranolazine has been shown to prolong the QTc interval in a dose-related manner.

Avoid ranolazine use in patients with known QT prolongation (eg, congenital long QT syndrome, uncorrected hypokalemia), patients with known history of ventricular tachycardia, and patients receiving drugs that prolong the QTc interval, such as class Ia (eg, quinidine) and class III (eg, dofetilide, sotalol) antiarrhythmics and antipsychotics (eg, thioridazine, ziprasidone).

Tumor promotion: A published study reported that ranolazine promoted tumor formation and progression to malignancy when given to mice at a dosage of 30 mg/kg twice daily.

Use in patients with diabetes mellitus: Ranolazine produces small reductions in hemoglobin A_{1c} (HbA_{1c}) in patients with diabetes. Do not consider ranolazine a treatment for diabetes.

Renal function impairment: In patients with varying degrees of renal impairment, ranolazine plasma levels increased up to 50%. The pharmacokinetics of ranolazine have not been assessed in patients on dialysis.

Hepatic function impairment: Because the QTc-prolonging effect is increased approximately 3-fold in patients with hepatic dysfunction, ranolazine is contraindicated in patients with mild, moderate, or severe liver disease.

Pregnancy: Category C.

Lactation: It is not known whether ranolazine is excreted in human milk. Decide whether to discontinue breast-feeding or ranolazine, taking into account the importance of the drug to the mother.

Children: Safety and efficacy in children have not been established.

Elderly: Use caution when selecting dose for an elderly patient, usually starting at the low end of the dosing range, reflecting the greater frequency of decreased cardiac, hepatic, or renal function, and of concomitant disease or other drug therapy.

Monitoring: Regularly monitor blood pressure after initiation of ranolazine in patients with severe renal function impairment. Obtain baseline and follow-up ECGs to evaluate effects on QT interval. Monitor HbA_{1c} regularly.

Drug Interactions

Drugs that may affect ranolazine include aprepitant, carbamazepine, clarithromycin, cyclosporine, diltiazem, itraconazole, ketoconazole, macrolides, nefazodone, paroxetine, phenobarbital, phenytoin, drugs that prolong the QT interval, protease inhibitors, rifamycins, St. John's wort, and verapamil.

Drugs that may be affected by ranolazine include digoxin and simvastatin.

Drug/Food interactions:

Grapefruit – Concomitant use may increase ranolazine plasma levels and QTc prolongation. Avoid coadministration.

Adverse Reactions

The most commonly observed adverse reactions occurring in patients receiving ranolazine include dizziness, headache, constipation, nausea, and syncope.

Chapter 5

RENAL & GENITOURINARY AGENTS

ALPROSTADIL (Prostaglandin E_1; PGE_1)

Injection, aqueous: 10, 20, and 40 mcg/mL (*Rx*)	*Caverject* (Pharmacia & Upjohn)
Powder for injection, lyophilized: 5, 10, 20, and 40 mcg/mL (after reconstitution) (*Rx*)	
Powder for injection, lyophilized: 10 mcg per 0.5 mL, 20 mcg per 0.5 mL (after reconstitution) (*Rx*)	*Caverject Impulse* (Pharmacia & Upjohn)
5, 10, 20, and 40 mcg/mL (after reconstitution) (*Rx*)	*Edex* (Schwarz Pharma)
Pellet: 125, 250, 500, or 1000 mcg (*Rx*)	*Muse* (Vivus)

Indications

Erectile dysfunction: Treatment of erectile dysfunction caused by neurogenic, vasculogenic, psychogenic, or mixed etiology.

Intracavernosal alprostadil may be a useful adjunct to other diagnostic tests in the diagnosis of erectile dysfunction (*Caverject* only).

Administration and Dosage

Intercavernosal: The first alprostadil injections must be done at the physician's office by medically trained personnel. The injection site is usually along the dorsolateral aspect of the proximal third of the penis. Avoid visible veins. Alternate the side of the penis that is injected and the site of injection.

The dose of alprostadil that is selected for self-injection treatment should provide the patient with an erection that is satisfactory for sexual intercourse and that is maintained for no longer than 1 hour. If the duration of erection is more than 1 hour, reduce the dose.

Initial titration – The patient must stay in the physician's office until complete detumescence occurs. If there is no response, then the next higher dose may be given within 1 hour. If there is a response, then wait at least 1 day before the next dose is given.

Erectile dysfunction of vasculogenic, psychogenic, or mixed etiology – Do not give more than 2 doses within a 24-hour period during initial titration. If there is no response to the initial 2.5 mcg dose, the second dose may be increased to 7.5 mcg within 1 hour. If additional titration is required, doses in increments of 5 to 10 mcg may be given at least 24 hours apart.

Erectile dysfunction of pure neurogenic etiology (spinal cord injury) – Initiate dosage titration at 1.25 mcg. The dose may be increased by 1.25 mcg to a dose of 2.5 mcg within 1 hour. Do not give more than 2 doses within a 24-hour period during initial titration. If additional titration is required, a dose of 5 mcg may be given during the next 24 hours. Doses in increments of 5 mcg may be given at least 24 hours apart until the dose that produces an erection suitable for intercourse and does not exceed a duration of 1 hour is reached.

Adjunct to the diagnosis of erectile dysfunction (Caverject only) – Patients are monitored for the occurrence of an erection after an intracavernosal injection of alprostadil. Use a single dose of alprostadil that induces a rigid erection.

Maintenance therapy – The first injections of alprostadil must be done at the physician's office by medically trained personnel. The recommended frequency of injection is 3 times/week or less, with at least 24 hours between each dose.

Intraurethral: Administer as needed to achieve an erection. The onset of effect is within 5 to 10 minutes after administration. The duration of effect is approximately 30 to 60 minutes. A medical professional should instruct each patient on proper technique for administering alprostadil prior to self-administration. The maximum frequency of use is no more than 2 systems per 24-hour period.

Initiation of therapy – Titrate dose under the supervision of a physician to test a patient's response to alprostadil, to demonstrate proper administration technique and to monitor for evidence of hypotension. Individually titrate patients to the lowest dose that is sufficient for sexual intercourse. If necessary, increase the dose (or decrease) on separate occasions in a stepwise manner until the patient achieves an erection that is sufficient for sexual intercourse.

Actions

Pharmacology: Alprostadil induces erection by relaxation of trabecular smooth muscle and by dilation of cavernosal arteries.

Pharmacokinetics:

Absorption – For treatment of erectile dysfunction, alprostadil is administered by injection into the corpora cavernosa or inserted intraurethrally.

Intracavernosal: Following intracavernosal injection of 20 mcg, mean peripheral plasma concentrations at 30 to 60 minutes after injection (89 to 102 pcg/mL, respectively) were not significantly greater than baseline levels of endogenous alprostadil (96 pcg/mL).

Intraurethral: The transurethral absorption of alprostadil is rapid, with approximately 80% of an administered dose absorbed within 10 minutes. The mean time to the maximum plasma PGE_1 concentration after a 1000 mcg intraurethral dose is approximately 16 minutes.

Distribution –

Intracavernosal: Alprostadil is bound in plasma primarily to albumin (81% bound).

Intraurethral: The half-life is short, varying between 30 seconds and 10 minutes.

Metabolism – Following IV administration, 80% of circulating alprostadil is metabolized in one pass through the lungs, primarily by beta- and omega-oxidation. The near-complete pulmonary first-pass metabolism of PGE_1 is the primary factor influencing the systemic pharmacokinetics of alprostadil and is a reason that peripheral venous plasma levels of PGE_1 are low or undetectable (less than 2 pg/mL) following alprostadil administration. The enzyme catalyzing this process has been isolated from many tissues in the lower GU tract including the urethra, prostate, and corpus cavernosum.

Excretion – The metabolites of alprostadil are excreted primarily by the kidney, with almost 90% of an administered IV dose excreted in urine within 24 hours post-dose. The remainder of the dose is excreted in the feces.

Contraindications

Hypersensitivity to the drug; conditions that might predispose patients to priapism (eg, sickle cell anemia or trait, multiple myeloma, leukemia); patients with anatomical deformation of the penis; patients with penile implants (intracavernosal); use in women, children, or newborns; use in men for whom sexual activity is inadvisable or contraindicated; for sexual intercourse with a pregnant woman unless the couple uses a condom barrier.

Intraurethral: Urethral stricture; balanitis; severe hypospadias; patients with acute or chronic urethritis; thrombocythemia; polycythemia.

Warnings/Precautions

Priapism: Prolonged erection (lasting more than 4 to 6 or fewer hours) and priapism (erection lasting more than 6 hours) have occurred in patients using alprostadil. To minimize the chances of prolonged erection or priapism, titrate slowly to the lowest effective dose.

Penile fibrosis: Regular follow-up of patients, with careful examination of the penis, is strongly recommended to detect signs of penile fibrosis.

Penile pain: Penile pain after intracavernosal administration was reported. In the majority of the cases, penile pain was rated mild or moderate in intensity.

Hematoma/Ecchymosis: In most cases, hematoma/ecchymosis was judged to be a complication of a faulty injection technique.

Hemodynamic changes: Hemodynamic changes, manifested as decreases in blood pressure and increases in pulse rate, principally at doses more than 20 mcg, were observed during clinical studies, and appeared to be dose-dependent.

Erectile dysfunction: Diagnose and treat underlying treatable medical causes of erectile dysfunction prior to initiation of therapy.

Pulmonary disease: The pulmonary extraction of alprostadil following intravascular administration was reduced by 15% in patients with acute respiratory distress syndrome (ARDS).

Pregnancy: *Category* C. Do not use for sexual intercourse with a pregnant woman unless the couple uses a condom barrier.

Children: *Caverject* is not indicated for use in newborns or children. However, alprostadil (*Prostin VR Pediatric*) is used in newborns to maintain the patency of the ductus arteriosus in neonates with congenital heart defects.

Drug Interactions

Drugs that may interact with alprostadil include anticoagulants and vasoactive agents.

Adverse Reactions

Adverse reactions occurring in at least 3% of patients receiving alprostadil by intracavernosal administration include bleeding, ecchymosis, hematoma, penile angulation, penis disorder, penile fibrosis, penile pain, and prolonged erection.

Adverse reactions in at least 3% of patients receiving alprostadil by intraurethral administration include accidental injury, dizziness, flu syndrome, headache, hypotension, pain, penile pain, testicular pain, urethral bleeding/spotting, urethral burning, urethral pain, and URI.

The most common drug-related adverse event reported by female partners during clinical studies was vaginal burning/itching (5.8%).

PHOSPHODIESTERASE TYPE 5 INHIBITORS

SILDENAFIL CITRATE	
Tablets; oral: 20 mg (*Rx*)	*Revatio* (Pfizer)
25, 50, and 100 mg (*Rx*)	*Viagra* (Pfizer)
Injection, solution: 10 mg per 12.5 mL (*Rx*)	*Revatio* (Pfizer)
TADALAFIL	
Tablets; oral: 2.5, 5, 10, and 20 mg (*Rx*)	*Cialis* (Eli Lilly)
20 mg (*Rx*)	*Adcirca* (Eli Lilly)
VARDENAFIL HYDROCHLORIDE	
Tablets; oral: 2.5, 5, 10, and 20 mg (*Rx*)	*Levitra* (Schering-Plough)
Tablets, disintegrating oral: 10 mg	*Staxyn* (Schering-Plough)

Indications

Erectile dysfunction (except Revatio): Treatment of erectile dysfunction.

Pulmonary arterial hypertension (Revatio and Adcirca): For the treatment of pulmonary arterial hypertension (World Health Organization [WHO] Group I) to improve exercise ability.

Administration and Dosage

SILDENAFIL:

Erectile dysfunction – 50 mg taken as needed approximately 1 hour before sexual activity. However, sildenafil may be taken anywhere from 4 hours to 30 minutes before sexual activity. The dose may be increased to a maximum recommended dose of 100 mg or decreased to 25 mg. The maximum recommended dosing frequency is once per day.

Pulmonary arterial hypertension – 20 mg orally 3 times daily, taken approximately 4 to 6 hours apart, with or without food. Treatment with doses higher than 20 mg 3 times daily is not recommended.

Injection: 10 mg (corresponding to 12.5 mL) administered as an IV bolus injection 3 times a day. Do not adjust for body weight. The 10 mg injection has a similar effect to the 20 mg oral dose.

Renal function impairment – Consider an initial sildenafil dose of 25 mg in patients with severe renal impairment.

Hepatic function impairment – Consider an initial sildenafil dose of 25 mg in patients with hepatic cirrhosis.

Dosage adjustment – Consider a starting dose of 25 mg in the following patients: Older than 65 years of age, hepatic impairment, severe renal impairment, and concomitant use of potent CYP-450 3A4 inhibitors (eg, erythromycin, ketoconazole, itraconazole, saquinavir).

Concomitant use with protease inhibitors: Do not exceed a maximum single dose of sildenafil 25 mg within a 48-hour period (eg, ritonavir).

Concomitant use with nitrates: Administration in patients who use nitric oxide donors or nitrates in any form is contraindicated.

Concomitant use with alpha-blockers: Do not take 50 or 100 mg doses of sildenafil within 4 hours of alpha-blocker administration. A 25 mg dose of sildenafil may be taken at any time.

TADALAFIL: Tadalafil may be taken without regard to food.

Erectile dysfunction –

As needed use: 10 mg taken prior to anticipated sexual activity. The dose may be increased to 20 mg or decreased to 5 mg. The maximum recommended dosing frequency is once daily in most patients.

Tadalafil was shown to improve erectile function for up to 36 hours following dosing.

Once daily use: The recommended starting dose of tadalafil for once daily use is 2.5 mg, taken at approximately the same time every day, without regard to timing of sexual activity. The tadalafil dose for once daily use may be increased to 5 mg.

Concomitant therapy:

Alpha-blockers – Patients should be stable on alpha-blocker therapy prior to initiating tadalafil treatment; initiate at the lowest recommended dose.

CYP3A4 inhibitors – The once-daily dose should not exceed 2.5 mg.

Nitrates – Concomitant use is contraindicated. In a life-threatening situation, at least 48 hours should elapse after the last dose of tadalafil before nitrate administration is considered.

Maximum dosage: 20 mg for as needed use; 5 mg for once daily use.

Pulmonary arterial hypertension (Adcirca) – 40 mg (two 20 mg tablets) once daily. Dividing the dose over the course of the day is not recommended.

Renal function impairment –

Cialis: For patients with moderate (CrCl 31 to 50 mL/min) renal insufficiency, a starting dose of 5 mg not more than once daily is recommended, and the maximum dose is 10 mg not more than once every 48 hours. For patients with severe (CrCl less than 30 mL/min and on hemodialysis) renal insufficiency on hemodialysis, the maximum recommended dose is 5 mg once every 72 hours.

Once daily use: For patients with severe renal insufficiency (CrCl less than 30 mL/min and on hemodialysis), once daily use is not recommended.

Pulmonary arterial hypertension:

Mild to moderate renal insufficiency (CrCl 31 to 80 mL/min) – Start dosing at 20 mg once daily. Increase to 40 mg once daily based on individual tolerability.

Severe renal insufficiency (CrCl less than 30 mL/min and on hemodialysis) – Avoid use because of increased tadalafil exposure (area under the curve [AUC]), limited clinical experience, and the lack of ability to influence clearance by dialysis.

Hepatic function impairment –

As-needed use: In severe hepatic impairment (Child-Pugh class C), the use of tadalafil is not recommended.

Once-daily use:

Mild or moderate hepatic insufficiency (Child-Pugh class A or B) – Caution is advised.

Cialis: In mild or moderate hepatic impairment (Child-Pugh class A or B), do not exceed 10 mg once daily.

Adcirca: Because of limited clinical experience in patients with mild or moderate hepatic impairment (Child-Pugh class A or B), consider a starting dosage of 20 mg/day.

Concomitant medications with Adcirca – In patients receiving ritonavir, start tadalafil at 20 mg once daily. Increase to 40 mg once daily based on individual tolerability.

Avoid the use of tadalafil during the initiation of ritonavir. Stop tadalafil at least 24 hours prior to starting ritonavir. After at least 1 week, resume tadalafil 20 mg once daily. Increase to 40 mg once daily based on individual tolerability.

VARDENAFIL HYDROCHLORIDE: 10 mg taken orally approximately 60 minutes before sexual activity. The dose may be increased to a maximum recommended dose of 20 mg or decreased to 5 mg. Vardenafil can be taken with or without food.

Maximum dose –

Film-coated tablets: 20 mg/dose once daily.

Orally disintegrating tablets: 10 mg/day according to the prescribing information.

Dosage adjustment –

Film-coated tablets: The dose may be increased to a maximum recommended dose of 20 mg or decreased to 5 mg based on efficacy and adverse reactions.

Elderly – Consider a starting dose of 5 mg in patients 65 years of age and older.

Hepatic function impairment –

Film-coated tablets: A starting dose of 5 mg is recommended in patients with moderate hepatic impairment (Child-Pugh B). The maximum dose should not exceed 10 mg.

Orally disintegrating tablets: Do not use in patients with moderate (Child-Pugh B) or severe (Child-Pugh C) hepatic impairment.

Concomitant medications – The dosage of vardenafil may require adjustment in patients receiving certain CYP3A4 inhibitors. For ritonavir, do not exceed a single dose of vardenafil 2.5 mg in a 72-hour period. For indinavir, ketoconazole 400 mg/day, and itraconazole 400 mg/day, do not exceed a single dose of vardenafil 2.5 mg in a 24-hour period. For ketoconazole 200 mg/day, itraconazole 200 mg/day, and erythromycin, do not exceed a single dose of vardenafil 5 mg in a 24-hour period.

Alpha-blockers – For alpha-blockers, caution is advised when phosphodiesterase type 5 inhibitors are used concomitantly with alpha-blockers because of the potential for an additive effect on blood pressure. Initiate concomitant treatment only if the patient is stable on alpha-blocker therapy. In those patients who are stable on alpha-blocker therapy, initiate vardenafil therapy at a dose of 5 mg (2.5 mg when used concomitantly with certain CYP3A4 inhibitors).

Orally disintegrating tablets – In those patients who are stable on alpha-blocker therapy, phosphodiesterase type 5 (PDE5) inhibitors should be initiated at the lowest recommended starting dose. In patients taking alpha-blockers, do not initiate vardenafil therapy. Lower doses of vardenafil film-coated tablets should be used as initial therapy in these patients. Patients taking alpha-blockers who have previously used vardenafil film-coated tablets may change to orally disintegrated tablets at the advice of their health care provider.

Concomitant therapy with CYP3A4 inhibitors –

Orally disintegrating tablets: Do not use with potent or moderate CYP3A4 inhibitors, such as ketoconazole, itraconazole, ritonavir, indinavir, saquinavir, atazanavir, clarithromycin, and erythromycin.

Concomitant therapy with nitrates: Concomitant use with nitrates in any form is contraindicated.

Administration –

Orally disintegrating tablets: Should be placed on the tongue where it will disintegrate. Should be taken without liquid, immediately upon removal from the blister.

Actions

Pharmacology: **Sildenafil**, **tadalafil**, and **vardenafil** are selective inhibitors of phosphodiesterase type 5.

Pharmacokinetics:

Absorption/Distribution –

Phosphodiesterase Type 5 Inhibitors Pharmacokinetics

Parameters	Sildenafil	Tadalafil	Vardenafil
Bioavailability	Approximately 40%	Not determined	Approximately 15%
T_{max}	0.5 to 2 h (median, 1 h)[a]	0.5 to 6 h (median, 2 h)[b]	0.5 to 2 h (median, 1 h)[c]
Onset of action	Approximately 30 min	Approximately 30 min	Approximately 20 min[d]
Maximum effect	no data	no data	45 to 90 min[d]
Duration of action	≥ 4 h	36 h	< 5 h
Protein binding[e]	Approximately 96%	94%	Approximately 95%
Metabolism	CYP3A4 (major) CYP2C9 (minor)	CYP3A4	CYP3A4 (major) CYP3A5, CYP2C isoforms (minor)
Terminal half-life	Approximately 4 h	17.5 h	4 to 5 h

[a] Oral dosing in the fasted state.
[b] Single oral dose.
[c] Single oral dose of 20 mg; fasted state.
[d] Based on animal studies.
[e] For parent drug and major circulating metabolite.

Metabolism/Excretion – **Sildenafil**, **tadalafil**, and **vardenafil** are cleared predominantly by the CYP3A4 (major route), 3A5 (major route; vardenafil), and CYP2C9 (minor route) hepatic isoenzymes.

Contraindications

Hypersensitivity to any component of the tablet; administration with nitrates (either regularly and/or intermittently) and nitric oxide donors (because of the potentiation of hypotension).

Warnings/Precautions

Priapism: Prolonged erections more than 4 hours and priapism (painful erections more than 6 hours in duration) have been infrequently reported. In the event of an erection that persists more than 4 hours, advise the patient to seek immediate medical assistance.

Cardiovascular effects: Treatments for erectile dysfunction, including these agents, generally should not be used in men for whom sexual activity is inadvisable because of their underlying cardiovascular status.

Patients with the following underlying conditions can be particularly sensitive to the actions of vasodilators, including **sildenafil**, **tadalafil**, and **vardenafil**: Those with left ventricular outflow obstruction (eg, aortic stenosis, idiopathic hypertrophic subaortic stenosis) and those with severely impaired autonomic control of blood pressure.

Erectile dysfunction: Undertake thorough medical history and physical examination to diagnose erectile dysfunction, determine potential underlying causes, and identify appropriate treatment.

The safety and efficacy of combinations of **sildenafil** or **vardenafil** with other treatments for erectile dysfunction have not been studied. Therefore, the use of such combinations is not recommended.

Deformation of penis: Use agents for the treatment of erectile dysfunction with caution in patients with anatomical deformation of the penis or in patients who have conditions that may predispose them to priapism.

Bleeding disorders: **Sildenafil**, **tadalafil**, and **vardenafil** have no effect on bleeding time when taken alone or with aspirin.

Visual disturbances: Single oral doses of phosphodiesterase inhibitors have demonstrated transient, dose-related impairment of color discrimination (blue/green), with peak effects near the time of peak plasma levels. The findings were most evident 1 hour after administration and diminishing but still present 6 hours after administration.

Retinitis pigmentosa: There is no safety information on the administration of **sildenafil** or **vardenafil** to patients with known hereditary degenerative retinal disorders, including retinitis pigmentosa. Therefore, administer with caution to these patients.

Renal function impairment: In volunteers with severe renal impairment (CrCl 30 mL/min or less), **sildenafil** clearance was reduced. There is no clinical data on the safety or efficacy of **vardenafil** in patients with end-stage renal disease requiring dialysis.

Limit **tadalafil** to 5 mg not more than once every 72 hours in patients with severe renal insufficiency or end-stage renal disease. The starting dose in patients with a moderate degree of renal insufficiency should be 5 mg not more than once daily, and the maximum dose should be limited to 10 mg not more than once in every 48 hours. No dose adjustment is required in patients with mild renal insufficiency.

In patients with moderate (CrCl 30 to 50 mL/min) to severe (CrCl less than 30 mL/min) renal impairment, the AUC of vardenafil was 20% to 30% higher. No dosage adjustment for vardenafil is required.

Hepatic function impairment: In volunteers with hepatic cirrhosis, **sildenafil** clearance was reduced. Consider an initial sildenafil dose of 25 mg in these patients. In patients with mild or moderate hepatic impairment, do not exceed a 10 mg dose of **tadalafil**. Because of insufficient information in patients with severe hepatic impairment, use in these patients is not recommended. In volunteers with mild and moderate hepatic impairment (Child-Pugh A), the C_{max} and AUC following a 10 mg **vardenafil** dose were increased. Consequently, a starting dose of 5 mg is recommended for patients with moderate hepatic impairment, and the maximum dose should not exceed 10 mg. Vardenafil is not recommended in patients with severe (Child-Pugh C) hepatic impairment.

Pregnancy: Category B.

Lactation: These agents are not indicated for use in women.

Children: These agents are not indicated for use in newborns and children.

Elderly: Consider an initial **sildenafil** dose of 25 mg in these patients. Consider a lower starting dose of **vardenafil** (5 mg) in patients 65 years of age and older.

Drug Interactions

CYP-450 system: Phosphodiesterase type 5 inhibitors are metabolized principally by the CYP-450 isoforms 3A4 (major route), 3A5 (major route; **vardenafil**), and 2C9 (minor route; **sildenafil**, vardenafil). Therefore, inhibitors of these isoenzymes may increase phosphodiesterase type 5 inhibitor concentrations, and inducers of these isoenzymes may decrease phosphodiesterase type 5 inhibitor concentrations. See the Administration and Dosage sections of the individual monographs for dosing recommendations.

Drugs that affect phosphodiesterase type 5 inhibitors include the following: alcohol, alpha-blockers, amlodipine, angiotensin II receptor blockers, antacids, azole antifungals, beta-blockers, bosentan, cimetidine, diuretics, enalapril, macrolides, metoprolol, nifedipine, nitrates, protease inhibitors, rifampin, tacrolimus.

Drugs that may be affected by phosphodiesterase type 5 inhibitors include: alpha-blockers, amlodipine, angiotensin II receptor blockers, anticoagulants, bosentan, enalapril, metoprolol, nifedipine, nitrates, protease inhibitors.

Drug/Food interactions: When taken with a high-fat meal, the rate of **sildenafil** absorption is reduced, with a mean delay in T_{max} of 60 minutes and a mean reduction in C_{max} of 29%. High-fat meals caused a reduction in C_{max} of **vardenafil** by 18% to 50%.

Adverse Reactions

Adverse reactions occurring in 3% or more of patients receiving these agents during clinical trials included abnormal vision (mild and transient, predominantly color tinge to vision but also increased sensitivity to light or blurred vision), accidental injury, back pain, diarrhea, dyspepsia, flushing, flu syndrome, headache, limb pain, myalgia, nasal congestion, rhinitis, sinusitis, urinary tract infection.

PENICILLAMINE

Capsules: 250 mg (*Rx*)	*Cuprimine* (Valeant Pharmaceuticals)
Tablets: 250 mg (*Rx*)	*Depen Titratabs* (Meda Pharmaceuticals)

Indications

Rheumatoid arthritis.

Wilson's disease (hepatolenticular degeneration).

Cystinuria.

Administration and Dosage

Give penicillamine on an empty stomach at least 1 hour before meals or 2 hours after meals and at least 1 hour apart from any other drug, food, or milk.

Wilson's disease: Initial dosage is 1 g/day for children or adults. This may be increased, as indicated by the urinary copper analyses, but it is seldom necessary to exceed 2 g/day. In patients who cannot tolerate 1 g/day initially, initiating dosage with 250 mg/day and increasing gradually allows closer control of the drug. Give on an empty stomach in 4 divided doses, 30 minutes to 1 hour before meals and at bedtime (2 hours or more after the evening meal).

Cystinuria:

Adult dosage – 2 g/day (range, 1 to 4 g/day) in 4 divided doses.

Pediatric dosage – 30 mg/kg/day in 4 divided doses. If 4 equal doses are not feasible, give the larger portion at bedtime. Initiating dosage with 250 mg/day, and increasing gradually, allows closer control of the drug and may reduce the incidence of adverse reactions.

Patients should drink about a pint of fluid at bedtime and another pint once during the night when urine is more concentrated and more acid than during the day. The greater the fluid intake, the lower the dosage of penicillamine required.

Rheumatoid arthritis: Administer on an empty stomach at least 1 hour before meals and at least 1 hour apart from any other drug, food, or milk.

Initial therapy: A single daily dose of 125 or 250 mg. Thereafter, increase dose at 1- to 3-month intervals by 125 or 250 mg/day as patient response and tolerance indicate. If satisfactory remission is achieved, continue the dose. If there is no improvement and if there are no signs of potentially serious toxicity after 2 to 3 months with doses of 500 to 750 mg/day, continue increases of 250 mg/day at 2- to 3-month intervals until satisfactory remission occurs or toxicity develops. If there is no discernible improvement after 3 to 4 months of treatment with 1 to 1.5 g/day, assume the patient will not respond and discontinue the drug.

Maintenance therapy: Many patients respond to less than or equal to 500 to 750 mg/day. In patients who respond but who evidence incomplete disease suppression after the first 6 to 9 months of treatment, increase daily dosage by 125 or 250 mg/day at 3-month intervals. Dosage more than 1 g/day is unusual, but 1.5 g/day or less has been required.

Dosage frequency: Dosages 500 mg/day or less can be given as a single daily dose. Administer dosages greater than 500 mg/day in divided doses.

Actions

Pharmacology:

Rheumatoid arthritis – The mechanism of action of penicillamine in rheumatoid arthritis is unknown. The onset of therapeutic response may not be seen for 2 or 3 months in those patients who respond.

Wilson's disease – Penicillamine is a chelating agent that removes excess copper in patients with Wilson's disease. Noticeable improvement may not occur for 1 to 3 months.

Poisoning – Penicillamine also forms soluble complexes with iron, mercury, lead, and arsenic, which are readily excreted by the kidneys. The drug may be used to treat poisoning by these metals.

Cystinuria – Penicillamine reduces excess cystine excretion in cystinuria. Penicillamine with conventional therapy decreases crystalluria and stone formation and may decrease the size of or dissolve existing stones. This is done, at least in part, by disulfide interchange between penicillamine and cystine, resulting in a substance more soluble than cystine and readily excreted.

Pharmacokinetics: It is well absorbed from the GI tract after oral administration (40% to 70%); peak plasma levels occur in 1 to 3 hours. Most (80%) of the plasma penicillamine is protein bound, primarily to albumin. Penicillamine is rapidly excreted in the urine; 50% is excreted in the feces. Metabolites may be detected in the urine for up to 3 months after stopping the drug. Half-life ranges are 1.7 to 3.2 hours.

Contraindications

History of penicillamine-related aplastic anemia or agranulocytosis; rheumatoid arthritis patients with a history or other evidence of renal insufficiency; pregnancy; breastfeeding.

Warnings/Precautions

Fatalities: Penicillamine has been associated with fatalities due to aplastic anemia, agranulocytosis, thrombocytopenia, Goodpasture's syndrome, and myasthenia gravis.

Hematologic: Leukopenia (2%) and thrombocytopenia (4%) have occurred. A reduction in WBC below 3,500, neutrophils less than 2,000/mm^3, or monocytes greater than 500/mm^3 mandate permanent withdrawal of therapy.

Hepatotoxicity: Penicillamine has been associated with a mild elevation of hepatic enzymes that usually returns to normal even with continuation of the drug.

Autoimmune syndromes: Autoimmune syndromes that may be caused by penicillamine include polymyositis, diffuse alveolitis and dermatomyositis, Goodpasture's syndrome, myasthenic syndrome, pemphigus, and obliterative bronchiolitis.

Pemphigoid-type: Pemphigoid-type reactions characterized by bullous lesions have required discontinuation of penicillamine and treatment with corticosteroids.

Lupus erythematosus: Certain patients will develop a positive antinuclear antibody (ANA) test and some may show a lupus erythematosus-like syndrome similar to other drug-induced lupus, but it is not associated with hypocomplementemia and may be present without nephropathy. A positive ANA test does not mandate drug discontinuance; however, a lupus erythematosus-like syndrome may develop later.

Sensitivity reactions: Once instituted for Wilson's disease or cystinuria, continue treatment with penicillamine on a daily basis. Interruptions for even a few days have been followed by sensitivity reactions after reinstitution of therapy.

Drug fever: Drug fever may appear in some patients, usually in the second to third week of therapy; it is sometimes accompanied by a macular cutaneous eruption.

Dermatologic: Skin rashes are the most frequent (44% to 50%) adverse reactions. Early rash occurs during the first few months of treatment and is more common.

A late rash: A late rash is less commonly seen, usually after 6 months or more of treatment, and requires drug discontinuation. It usually appears on the trunk, is accompanied by intense pruritus, and is usually unresponsive to topical corticosteroids.

Pemphigoid rash: Pemphigoid rash, the most serious dermatologic reaction occurs most often after 6 to 9 months of penicillamine.

Oral ulcerations: Oral ulcerations may develop that may have the appearance of aphthous stomatitis. Although rare, cheilosis, glossitis, and gingivostomatitis have been reported.

Hypogeusia: Hypogeusia occurs in 25% to 33% of patients, except for a lesser incidence in Wilson's disease (4%).

Dietary supplementation: Because of their dietary restriction, give patients with Wilson's disease, cystinuria, and rheumatoid arthritis whose nutrition is impaired 25 mg/day of pyridoxine during therapy, because penicillamine increases the requirement for this vitamin.

Iron deficiency may develop, especially in children and in menstruating women. This may be caused by diet. If necessary, give iron in short courses. A period of

2 hours should elapse between administration of penicillamine and iron, because orally administered iron reduces the effects of penicillamine.

Effects of penicillamine on collagen and elastin: Effects of penicillamine on collagen and elastin make it advisable to consider a reduction in dosage to 250 mg/day when surgery is contemplated.

Penicillamine may cause increased skin friability at sites subject to pressure or trauma, such as shoulders, elbows, knees, toes, and buttocks.

Hypersensitivity reactions: Allergic reactions occur in approximately 33% of patients. They are more common at the start of treatment, and occur as generalized rashes or drug fever. Discontinue treatment and reinstitute at a low dosage such as 250 mg/day, with gradual increases. Administering prednisolone 20 mg/day for the first few weeks of penicillamine therapy reduces the severity of these reactions. Antihistamines may control pruritus.

Renal function impairment: Proteinuria and hematuria may develop and may be a warning sign of membranous glomerulopathy, which can progress to a nephrotic syndrome.

Pregnancy: Category D.

Lactation: Safety has not been established.

Children: The efficacy of penicillamine in juvenile rheumatoid arthritis has not been established.

Monitoring: When indicated, monitor drug toxicity or efficacy through urinalysis. In rheumatoid arthritis patients, discontinue the drug if unexplained gross hematuria or persistent microscopic hematuria develops. Perform liver function tests and an annual x–ray for renal stones.

Monitor white and differential blood cell count, hemoglobin determination, and direct platelet count every 2 weeks for the first 6 months of penicillamine therapy and monthly thereafter.

Drug Interactions

Drugs that may affect penicillamine include gold therapy, antimalarial or cytotoxic drugs, iron salts, antacids, and food.

Drugs that may be affected by penicillamine include digoxin.

Adverse Reactions

Penicillamine has a high incidence (greater than 50%) of untoward reactions, some of which are potentially fatal.

Adverse reactions that may occur in 3% or more of patients include anorexia; epigastric pain; nausea; vomiting; diarrhea; blunting/diminution/total loss of taste; taste perversion; thrombocytopenia; generalized pruritus; early and late rashes; proteinuria.

FLAVOXATE

Tablets: 100 mg (*Rx*)	*Urispas* (ALZA)

Indications

For the symptomatic relief of dysuria, urgency, nocturia, suprapubic pain, frequency, and incontinence as may occur in cystitis, prostatitis, urethritis, urethrocystitis/urethrotrigonitis.

Not indicated for definitive treatment but is compatible with drugs used to treat urinary tract infections.

Administration and Dosage

Adults and children older than 12 years of age: 100 or 200 mg 3 or 4 times/day. Reduce the dose when symptoms improve.

Actions

Pharmacology: Counteracts smooth muscle spasm of the urinary tract and exerts its effect directly on the muscle.

Contraindications

Pyloric or duodenal obstruction; obstructive intestinal lesions or ileus; achalasia; GI hemorrhage; obstructive uropathies of the lower urinary tract.

Warnings/Precautions

Glaucoma: Give cautiously in patients with suspected glaucoma.

Pregnancy: Category B.

Lactation: It is not known whether this drug is excreted in breast milk. Use caution when flavoxate is administered to a nursing woman.

Children: Safety and efficacy in children younger than 12 years of age have not been established.

Adverse Reactions

Nausea; vomiting; dry mouth; nervousness; vertigo; headache; drowsiness; mental confusion (especially in the elderly patient); hyperpyrexia; blurred vision; increased ocular tension; disturbance in eye accommodation; urticaria and other dermatoses; dysuria; tachycardia; palpitations; eosinophilia; leukopenia.

OXYBUTYNIN CHLORIDE

Tablets: 5 mg (*Rx*)	Various
Tablets, extended-release: 5, 10, 15 mg (*Rx*)	Various, *Ditropan XL* (Ortho-McNeil)
Syrup: 5 mg/5 mL (*Rx*)	Various
Transdermal system: 36 mg delivering 3.9 mg oxybutynin per day. (*Rx*)	*Oxytrol* (Watson)
Gel, topical: 10%. (*Rx*)	*Gelnique* (Watson)

Indications

Bladder instability/Overactive bladder: For the relief of symptoms of bladder instability/treatment of overactive bladder associated with voiding in patients with uninhibited and reflex neurogenic bladder (eg, urgency, frequency, urinary leakage, urge incontinence, dysuria).

Administration and Dosage

Oxybutynin immediate-release tablets:

Adults – 5 mg (tablets or syrup) 2 or 3 times/day. Maximum dose is 5 mg 4 times/day.

Children (older than 5 years of age) – 5 mg (tablets or syrup) 2 times/day. Maximum dose is 5 mg 3 times/day.

Oxybutynin ER tablets: 5 mg once daily. Dosage may be adjusted in 5 mg increments to achieve a balance of efficacy and tolerability (up to a maximum of 30 mg/day). Dosage adjustments may proceed at approximately weekly intervals.

The ER tablets may be administered with or without food and must be swallowed whole with the aid of liquids, and not be chewed, divided, or crushed.

Transdermal system: Apply system to dry, intact skin on the abdomen, hip, or buttock. Select a new application site with each new system to avoid reapplication to the same site within 7 days.

The dose is one 3.9 mg/day system applied twice weekly (every 3 to 4 days).

Topical: Apply 1 g (1 sachet) once daily to dry, intact skin on the abdomen, upper arms/shoulders, or thighs.

Application sites should be rotated. Oxybutynin gel should not be applied to the same site on consecutive days. Oxybutynin gel is for topical application only and should not be ingested. Apply immediately after the sachets are opened and contents expelled.

Actions

Pharmacology: Oxybutynin exerts direct antispasmodic effect on smooth muscle and inhibits the muscarinic action of acetylcholine on smooth muscle.

In patients with conditions characterized by involuntary bladder contractions, oxybutynin increases vesical capacity, diminishes frequency of uninhibited contractions of the detrusor muscle, and delays initial desire to void. Oxybutynin thus decreases urgency and the frequency of incontinent episodes and voluntary urination.

Oxybutynin is well tolerated in patients administered the drug from 30 days to 2 years.

Pharmacokinetics:

ER tablets – Following the first dose of oxybutynin ER tablets, oxybutynin plasma concentrations rise for 4 to 6 hours; thereafter, steady concentrations are maintained for up to 24 hours, minimizing fluctuations between peak and trough concentrations associated with oxybutynin.

Steady-state oxybutynin plasma concentrations are achieved by day 3 of repeated oxybutynin ER dosing, with no observed drug accumulation or change in oxybutynin and desethyloxybutynin pharmacokinetic parameters.

Transdermal system – Following application of the first 3.9 mg/day transdermal system, oxybutynin plasma concentration increases for approximately 24 to 48 hours, reaching average maximum concentrations of 3 to 4 ng/mL. Thereafter, steady concentrations are maintained for up to 96 hours. Absorption of oxybutynin is bioequivalent when oxybutynin transdermal system is applied to the abdomen, buttocks, or hip.

Topical – Oxybutynin is transported across intact skin and into the systemic circulation by passive diffusion across the stratum corneum. Steady-state concentrations are achieved within 7 days of continuous dosing. Absorption of oxybutynin is similar when oxybutynin gel is applied to the abdomen, upper arm/shoulders, or thighs.

Contraindications

Urinary retention, gastric retention, or uncontrolled narrow-angle glaucoma and in patients who are at risk for these conditions; known hypersensitivity to oxybutynin or other components of these product.

Warnings/Precautions

Heat prostration: When administered in the presence of high environmental temperature, heat prostration (fever and heat stroke) may occur because of decreased sweating.

Diarrhea: Diarrhea may be an early symptom of incomplete intestinal obstruction, especially in patients with ileostomy or colostomy; discontinue treatment.

Flammable gel: Oxybutynin is an alcohol-based gel and is therefore flammable. Instruct patients to avoid open fire or smoking until gel has dried.

GI disorders: Doses administered to patients with ulcerative colitis may suppress GI motility and produce paralytic ileus and precipitate or aggravate toxic megacolon.

Administer ER tablets with caution to patients with GI obstructive disorders because of the risk of gastric retention.

The ER tablets and transdermal system, like other anticholinergic drugs, may decrease GI motility and should be used with caution in patients with conditions such as ulcerative colitis, intestinal atony, and myasthenia gravis.

Use the ER tablets and transdermal system with caution in patients who have gastroesophageal reflux or who are concurrently taking drugs (such as bisphosphonates) that can cause or exacerbate esophagitis.

As with other nondeformable material, use caution when administering the ER tablets to patients with preexisting severe GI narrowing (pathologic or iatrogenic). There have been rare reports of obstructive symptoms in patients with known strictures in association with the ingestion of other drugs in nondeformable controlled-release formulations.

Skin transference: Transfer of oxybutynin to another person can occur when vigorous skin-to-skin contact is made with the application site. Cover the application site with clothing after the gel has dried if direct skin-to-skin contact at the application site is anticipated.

Urinary retention: Administer ER tablets with caution to patients with clinically significant bladder outflow obstruction because of the risk of urinary retention.

Use with caution: Use with caution in the elderly and patients with autonomic neuropathy and hepatic or renal disease.

Cardiac and other effects: Symptoms of hyperthyroidism, coronary heart disease, CHF, cardiac arrhythmias, tachycardia, hypertension, hiatal hernia, and prostatic hypertrophy may be aggravated.

Renal/Hepatic function impairment: Use ER tablets with caution in patients with hepatic or renal impairment.

Hazardous tasks: Patients should use caution while driving or performing other tasks requiring alertness, coordination, or physical dexterity.

Pregnancy: Category B.

Lactation: It is not known whether this drug is excreted in breast milk. Exercise caution when administering to a nursing woman.

Children: Safety and efficacy in children (younger than 5 years of age for immediate-release tablets) have not been established.

Drug Interactions

Drugs that interact with oxybutynin include atenolol, digoxin, haloperidol, phenothiazines, amantadine, and anticholinergic agents.

Adverse Reactions

Adverse reactions occurring in 3% or more of patients – Palpitations; vasodilation; dizziness; insomnia; rash; constipation; dry mouth; nausea; urinary hesitance and retention.

Immediate-release tablets: Tachycardia; drowsiness; hallucinations; restlessness; decreased sweating; decreased GI motility; amblyopia; cycloplegia; decreased lacrimation; mydriasis; asthenia; impotence; suppression of lactation.

Extended-release tablets: Somnolence; headache; diarrhea; dyspepsia; blurred vision; dry eyes; asthenia; pain; rhinitis; urinary tract infection; hypertension; nervousness; confusion; dry skin; flatulence; gastroesophageal reflux; increased post-void residual volume; cystitis; upper respiratory tract infection; cough; sinusitis; bronchitis; dry nasal and sinus mucous membranes; pharyngitis; abdominal pain; accidental injury; back pain; flu syndrome; arthritis.

Topical: Dry mouth; upper respiratory tract infection; application-site reactions; urinary tract infection.

TOLTERODINE TARTRATE

Tablets: 1 and 2 mg (*Rx*)	*Detrol* (Pharmacia)
Capsules, extended-release: 2 and 4 mg (*Rx*)	*Detrol LA* (Pharmacia)

Indications

Overactive bladder: Treatment of patients with an overactive bladder with symptoms of urinary frequency, urgency, or urge incontinence.

Administration and Dosage

Immediate-release: The initial recommended dose is 2 mg twice/day. The dose may be lowered to 1 mg twice/day based on individual response and tolerability. For patients with significantly reduced hepatic function or who are currently taking drugs that are inhibitors of cytochrome P450 3A4, the recommended dose is 1 mg twice/day.

Extended-release (ER): The recommended dose is 4 mg once daily taken with liquids and swallowed whole. The dose may be lowered to 2 mg/day based on individual response and tolerability; however, limited efficacy data is available for the 2 mg capsules.

For patients with significantly reduced hepatic or renal function or who are currently taking drugs that are potent inhibitors of CYP3A4, the recommended dose of the ER capsules is 2 mg/day.

Actions

Pharmacology: Tolterodine is a competitive muscarinic receptor antagonist for overactive bladder. Urinary bladder contraction and salivation are mediated via cholinergic muscarinic receptors.

After oral administration, tolterodine is metabolized in the liver, resulting in the formation of the 5-hydroxymethyl derivative, a major active metabolite. The 5-hydroxymethyl metabolite, which exhibits antimuscarinic activity similar to that of tolterodine, contributes significantly to the therapeutic effect.

Tolterodine has a pronounced effect on bladder function in healthy volunteers. The main effects following a 6.4 mg single dose of tolterodine were an increase in residual urine, reflecting an incomplete emptying of the bladder, and a decrease in detrusor pressure.

Pharmacokinetics:

Absorption – Tolterodine is rapidly absorbed; 77% or more is absorbed, but absolute bioavailability is highly variable (10% to 74%). Maximum steady-state serum concentrations (C_{max}) typically occur within 1 to 2 hours. The pharmacokinetics of tolterodine are dose-proportional over the range of 1 to 4 mg.

Distribution – Tolterodine is highly bound to plasma proteins, primarily α_1-acid glycoprotein. The 5-hydroxymethyl metabolite is not extensively protein bound, with unbound fraction concentrations averaging approximately 36%.

Metabolism – Tolterodine undergoes extensive and variable first-pass hepatic metabolism following oral dosing. The primary metabolic route involves the oxidation of the 5-methyl group mediated by the cytochrome P450 2D6 leading to the formation of an active 5-hydroxymethyl metabolite. Further metabolism leads to formation of the 5-carboxylic acid and N-dealkylated 5-carboxylic acid metabolites, which account for approximately 51% and approximately 29% of the metabolites recovered in the urine, respectively.

Variability in metabolism: A subset (approximately 7%) of the population is devoid of CYP2D6, the enzyme responsible for the formation of the 5-hydroxymethyl metabolite of tolterodine. The identified pathway of metabolism for these individuals ("poor metabolizers") is by dealkylation via cytochrome P450 3A4 (CYP3A4) to *N*-dealkylated tolterodine. The remainder of the population is referred to as "extensive metabolizers." Pharmacokinetic studies revealed that tolterodine is metabolized at a slower rate in poor metabolizers than in extensive metabolizers; this results in significantly higher serum concentrations of tolterodine and in negligible concentrations of the 5-hydroxymethyl metabolite.

Excretion – Following a 5 mg oral dose in healthy volunteers, 77% was recovered in urine and 17% was recovered in feces. Less than 1% (less than 2.5% in poor metabolizers) of the dose was recovered as intact tolterodine, and 5% to 14% (less than 1% in poor metabolizers) was recovered as the active 5-hydroxymethyl metabolite.

Special populations –

Renal insufficiency: Exposure levels of other metabolites of tolterodine were significantly higher (10- to 30-fold) in renally impaired patients.

Hepatic function impairment: The elimination half-life of tolterodine was longer in cirrhotic patients (mean, 8.7 hours) than in healthy, young, and elderly volunteers (mean, 2 to 4 hours). The clearance of oral tolterodine was substantially lower in cirrhotic patients (approximately 1.1 L/h/kg) than in the healthy volunteers (approximately 5.7 L/h/kg).

Contraindications

Urinary retention; gastric retention; uncontrolled narrow-angle glaucoma; hypersensitivity to the drug or its ingredients.

Warnings/Precautions

Urinary/Gastric retention: Administer with caution to patients with clinically significant bladder outflow obstruction because of the risk of urinary retention and to patients with GI obstructive disorders, such as pyloric stenosis, because of the risk of gastric retention.

Controlled narrow-angle glaucoma: Use with caution in patients being treated for narrow-angle glaucoma.

Renal/Hepatic function impairment: Patients with significantly reduced hepatic function should not receive doses greater than 1 mg twice/day (greater than 2 mg/day for ER capsules). Treat patients with renal impairment with caution.

Pregnancy: Category C.

Lactation: It is not known whether tolterodine is excreted in human breast milk; therefore, discontinue administration during nursing.

Children: Safety and efficacy have not been established.

Drug Interactions

Fluoxetine: Fluoxetine is a potent inhibitor of cytochrome P450 2D6 activity. No dose adjustment is required when tolterodine and fluoxetine are coadministered.

Cytochrome P450:

3A4 inhibitors – Patients receiving cytochrome P450 3A4 inhibitors, such as macrolide antibiotics (erythromycin and clarithromycin), antifungal agents (ketoconazole, itraconazole, and miconazole), or cyclosporine or vinblastine should not receive doses of tolterodine greater than 1 mg twice/day (greater than 2 mg/day for ER capsules).

2D6 – Tolterodine is not expected to influence the pharmacokinetics of drugs that are metabolized by cytochrome P450 2D6, such as flecainide, vinblastine, carbamazepine, and tricyclic antidepressants.

Drug/Food interactions: Food intake increases the bioavailability of tolterodine (average increase 53%). This change is not expected to be a safety concern and adjustment of dose is not needed.

Adverse Reactions

Adverse reactions occurring in 3% or more of patients include the following: Dry mouth, headache, dizziness, somnolence, abdominal pain, constipation, dyspepsia, xerophthalmia (extended- and immediate-release); diarrhea, fatigue, flu-like syndrome (immediate-release).

TROSPIUM CHLORIDE

Tablets; oral: 20 mg (*Rx*)	*Sanctura* (Odyssey, Indevus)
Capsules, extended-release; oral: 60 mg (*Rx*)	*Sanctura XR* (Allergan)

Indications

Overactive bladder: For the treatment of overactive bladder with symptoms of urge urinary incontinence, urgency, and urinary frequency.

Administration and Dosage

Immediate-release tablets: 20 mg twice daily. Dose at least 1 hour before meals or give on an empty stomach.

Extended-release capsules: One 60 mg capsule daily in the morning. Trospium extended-release should be dosed with water on an empty stomach, at least 1 hour before a meal.

Renal function impairment:

Immediate-release tablets – For patients with severe renal impairment (creatinine clearance [CrCl] less than 30 mL/min), the recommended dose is 20 mg once daily at bedtime.

Extended-release capsules – Not recommended for use in patients with severe renal function impairment (CrCl less than 30 mL/min).

Elderly: In elderly patients 75 years of age and older, dose may be titrated down to 20 mg once daily based upon tolerability.

Actions

Pharmacology: Trospium is an antispasmodic, antimuscarinic agent. Trospium antagonizes the effect of acetylcholine on muscarinic receptors in cholinergically innervated organs. Its parasympatholytic action reduces the tonus of smooth muscle in the bladder.

Pharmacokinetics:

Absorption – After oral administration, less than 10% of the dose is absorbed. Mean absolute bioavailability of a 20 mg dose is 9.6% (range, 4% to 16.1%). Peak plasma concentrations (C_{max}) occur between 5 and 6 hours postdose.

Distribution – Protein binding ranged from 50% to 85%. The apparent volume of distribution for a 20 mg oral dose is 395 (± 140) L.

Metabolism – Of the 10% of the dose absorbed, metabolites account for approximately 40% of the excreted dose following oral administration. The major metabolic pathway is hypothesized as ester hydrolysis with subsequent conjugation. CYP-450 is not expected to contribute significantly to the elimination of trospium.

Excretion – The plasma half-life for trospium following oral administration is approximately 20 hours. After administration of oral trospium, the majority of the dose (85.2%) was recovered in feces and a smaller amount (5.8%) was recovered in urine; 60% of the radioactivity excreted in urine was unchanged trospium.

Contraindications

Patients with urinary retention, gastric retention, or uncontrolled narrow-angle glaucoma and patients at risk for these conditions; hypersensitivity to the drug or its ingredients.

Warnings/Precautions

Decreased GI motility: Administer trospium with caution to patients with GI obstructive disorders because of the risk of gastric retention. Use with caution in patients with conditions such as ulcerative colitis, intestinal atony, and myasthenia gravis.

Narrow-angle glaucoma: In patients being treated for narrow-angle glaucoma, only use trospium if the potential benefits outweigh the risks and, in that circumstance, only with careful monitoring.

Risk of urinary retention: Administer trospium with caution to patients with clinically significant bladder outflow obstruction because of the risk of urinary retention.

Renal function impairment: Dose modification is recommended in patients with severe renal insufficiency (CrCl less than 30 mL/min). In such patients, administer trospium as 20 mg once daily at bedtime.

Hepatic function impairment: Use caution when administering trospium in patients with moderate or severe hepatic dysfunction.

Pregnancy: *Category* C.

Lactation: It is not known whether this drug is excreted in human milk. Exercise caution when administering trospium to a breast-feeding mother. Use during lactation only if the potential benefit justifies the potential risk to the newborn.

Children: Safety and efficacy in children have not been established.

Elderly: In 2 studies, the incidence of commonly reported anticholinergic adverse reactions in patients treated with trospium (including dry mouth, constipation, dyspepsia, UTI, and urinary retention) was higher in patients 75 years of age and older compared with younger patients. This effect may be related to an enhanced sensitivity to anticholinergic agents in this patient population. Therefore, based upon tolerability, the dose frequency of trospium may be reduced to 20 mg once daily in patients 75 years of age and older.

Drug Interactions

Drugs that may affect trospium include other anticholinergic agents; drugs eliminated by active tubular secretion.

Drugs that may be affected by trospium include those eliminated by active tubular secretion (eg, digoxin, metformin, morphine, pancuronium, procainamide, tenofovir, and vancomycin).

Drug/Food interactions: It is recommended that trospium be taken at least 1 hour prior to meals or on an empty stomach.

Adverse Reactions

Adverse reactions occurring in 3% or more of patients included dry mouth, constipation, and headache.

DARIFENACIN HYDROBROMIDE

Tablets, extended-release: 7.5 and 15 mg (*Rx*) — *Enablex* (Novartis)

Indications

Overactive bladder: For the treatment of overactive bladder with symptoms of urge urinary incontinence, urgency, and frequency.

Administration and Dosage

Take tablets once daily with liquid, and with or without food. Swallow whole; do not chew, divide, or crush.

Recommended dose: 7.5 mg once daily. The dose may be increased to 15 mg once daily, as early as 2 weeks after starting therapy.

Hepatic function impairment – For patients with moderate hepatic impairment, do not exceed a daily dose of darifenacin 7.5 mg. Darifenacin is not recommended for use in patients with severe hepatic impairment.

Coadministration with CYP450 inhibitors – When coadministered with potent CYP3A4 inhibitors (eg, ketoconazole, itraconazole, ritonavir, nelfinavir, clarithromycin, nefazodone), do not exceed a daily dose of darifenacin 7.5 mg.

Actions

Pharmacology: Darifenacin is a competitive muscarinic receptor antagonist.

Pharmacokinetics:

Absorption – The oral bioavailability at steady-state is estimated to be 15% and 19% for 7.5 and 15 mg tablets, respectively.

Peak plasma concentrations are reached approximately 7 hours after multiple dosing, and steady-state plasma concentrations are achieved by the sixth day of dosing.

Distribution – Darifenacin is approximately 98% bound to plasma proteins.

Metabolism – Darifenacin is extensively metabolized by the liver by cytochrome P-450 enzymes CYP2D6 and CYP3A4.

Excretion – Following administration of an oral dose approximately 60% was recovered in the urine and 40% in the feces. The elimination half-life of darifenacin following chronic dosing is approximately 13 to 19 h.

Contraindications

In patients with urinary retention, gastric retention, or uncontrolled narrow-angle glaucoma and in patients who are at risk for these conditions; known hypersensitivity to the drug or its ingredients.

Warnings/Precautions

Narrow-angle glaucoma: Use with caution in patients being treated for narrow-angle glaucoma and only when the potential benefits outweigh the risks.

Decreased GI motility: Administer with caution to patients with GI obstructive disorders; use with caution in patients with conditions such as severe constipation, ulcerative colitis, and myasthenia gravis.

Risk of urinary retention: Administer with caution to patients with clinically significant bladder outflow obstruction because of the risk of urinary retention.

Pregnancy: Category C.

Lactation: It is not known whether darifenacin is excreted into human milk. Use caution before administering to a breastfeeding woman.

Children: The safety and efficacy have not been established.

Drug Interactions

Drugs that may interact with darifenacin include moderate and potent CYP3A4 inhibitors, anticholinergic drugs, CYP2D6 substrates, and digoxin.

Adverse Reactions

Adverse reactions occurring in 3% or more of patients include abdominal pain, accidental injury, constipation, dry mouth, dyspepsia, flu syndrome, headache, nausea, urinary tract infection.

SOLIFENACIN SUCCINATE

Tablets: 5 and 10 mg (*Rx*)	*Vesicare* (Astellas)

Indications

Overactive bladder: For the treatment of overactive bladder with symptoms of urge urinary incontinence, urgency, and urinary frequency.

Administration and Dosage

The recommended dose is 5 mg once daily. If 5 mg is well tolerated, the dose may be increased to 10 mg once daily.

Take with liquids and swallow whole. Administer with or without food.

Renal function impairment: For patients with severe renal impairment (CrCl less than 30 mL/min), a daily dose greater than 5 mg is not recommended.

Hepatic function impairment: For patients with moderate hepatic impairment (Child-Pugh B), a daily dose greater than 5 mg is not recommended. Use in patients with severe hepatic impairment (Child Pugh C) is not recommended.

Dose adjustment with CYP3A4 inhibitors: When administered with therapeutic doses of ketoconazole or other potent CYP3A4 inhibitors, a daily dose greater than 5 mg is not recommended.

Actions

Pharmacology: Solifenacin is a competitive muscarinic receptor antagonist. Muscarinic receptors plays a role in contractions of urinary bladder smooth muscle and stimulation of salivary secretion.

Pharmacokinetics:

Absorption – After oral administration, peak plasma levels are reached within 3 to 8 hours. The absolute bioavailability of solifenacin is approximately 90%, and plasma concentrations are proportional to the dose administered.

Distribution – Solifenacin is approximately 98% bound to human plasma proteins, principally to α_1-acid glycoprotein.

Metabolism – Solifenacin is extensively metabolized in the liver. The primary pathway for elimination is by way of CYP3A4.

Excretion – Following administration, 69.2% was recovered in the urine and 22.5% in the feces. The elimination half-life of solifenacin following chronic dosing is approximately 45 to 68 hours.

Contraindications

In patients with urinary retention, gastric retention, uncontrolled narrow-angle glaucoma, and in patients who have demonstrated hypersensitivity to the drug substance or other components of the product.

Warnings/Precautions

Bladder outflow obstruction: Administer solifenacin with caution to patients with clinically significant bladder outflow obstruction because of the risk of urinary retention.

GI obstructive disorders and decreased GI motility: Use solifenacin with caution in patients with decreased GI motility.

Controlled narrow-angle glaucoma: Use solifenacin with caution in patients being treated for narrow-angle glaucoma. Solifenacin is contraindicated in patients with uncontrolled narrow-angle glaucoma.

Patients with congenital or acquired QT prolongation: In a study of the effect of solifenacin on the QT interval, the QT prolonging effect appeared less with solifenacin 10 mg than with 30 mg (3 times the maximum recommended dose), and the effect of solifenacin 30 mg did not appear as large as that of the positive control moxifloxacin at its therapeutic dose. Consider this observation when prescribing solifenacin for patients with a known history of QT prolongation or patients who are taking medications known to prolong the QT interval.

Renal function impairment: Doses greater than 5 mg are not recommended in patients with severe renal impairment (CrCl less than 30 mL/min).

Hepatic function impairment: Doses greater than 5 mg are not recommended in patients with moderate hepatic impairment (Child-Pugh B). Solifenacin is not recommended for patients with severe hepatic impairment (Child-Pugh C).

Pregnancy: Category C.

Lactation: It is not known whether solifenacin is excreted in human milk. Because many drugs are excreted in human milk, do not administer solifenacin during breastfeeding.

Children: The safety and efficacy of solifenacin in pediatric patients have not been established.

Drug Interactions

P450 system: In vitro drug metabolism studies have shown that solifenacin is a substrate of CYP3A4. Inducers or inhibitors of CYP3A4 may alter solifenacin pharmacokinetics.

Ketoconazole: It is recommended not to exceed a 5 mg daily dose of solifenacin when administered with therapeutic doses of ketoconazole or other potent CYP3A4 inhibitors.

Adverse Reactions

The most common adverse reactions reported in patients were dry mouth and constipation.

Adverse reactions occurring in 3% or more of patients include blurred vision, constipation, dry mouth, dyspepsia, nausea, urinary tract infection.

FESOTERODINE

Tablets, extended-release: 4 mg, 8 mg (*Rx*) *Toviaz* (Pfizer)

Indications

Overactive bladder: For the treatment of overactive bladder with symptoms of urge urinary incontinence, urgency, and frequency.

Administration and Dosage

Adults:

Usual dosage – 8 mg once daily.

Initial dosage – 4 mg once daily.

Concomitant therapy – The daily dose should not exceed 4 mg in patients taking potent CYP3A4 inhibitors (eg, clarithromycin, itraconazole, ketoconazole).

Renal function impairment: Doses of more than 4 mg are not recommended in patients with severe renal insufficiency.

Administration: Fesoterodine tablets should be taken with liquid and swallowed whole; do not chew, divide, or crush the tablets. May be administered with or without food.

Actions

Pharmacology: Fesoterodine is a competitive muscarinic receptor antagonist. Muscarinic receptors play a role in contractions of urinary bladder smooth muscle and stimulation of salivary secretion.

Pharmacokinetics:

Absorption/Distribution – After oral administration, fesoterodine is well absorbed. Bioavailability of the active metabolite is 52%. Maximum plasma levels are reached after approximately 5 hours.

Plasma protein binding of the active metabolite is approximately 50%, and is primarily bound to albumin and alpha-1 acid glycoprotein.

Metabolism/Excretion – Fesoterodine is rapidly and extensively hydrolyzed to its active metabolite via 2 major pathways involving CYP2D6 and CYP3A4.

The apparent half-life following oral administration is approximately 7 hours.

Contraindications

Urinary retention; gastric retention; uncontrolled narrow-angle glaucoma; known hypersensitivity to the drug or its ingredients.

Warnings/Precautions

Bladder outlet obstruction: Administer fesoterodine with caution to patients with clinically significant bladder outlet obstruction because of the risk of urinary retention.

GI motility: Use fesoterodine, like other antimuscarinic drugs, with caution in patients with decreased GI motility, such as those with severe constipation.

Controlled narrow-angle glaucoma: Use fesoterodine with caution in patients being treated for narrow-angle glaucoma.

Myasthenia gravis: Use fesoterodine with caution in patients with myasthenia gravis, a disease characterized by decreased cholinergic activity at the neuromuscular junction.

Renal function impairment: Doses of fesoterodine of more than 4 mg are not recommended in patients with severe renal insufficiency.

Hepatic function impairment: There are no dosing adjustments for patients with mild or moderate hepatic function impairment. Fesoterodine is not recommended for use in patients with severe hepatic function impairment.

Pregnancy: Category C.

Lactation: It is not known whether fesoterodine is excreted in human milk. Do not administer during breast-feeding unless the potential benefit outweighs the potential risk to the neonate.

Children: The safety and effectiveness of fesoterodine in children have not been established.

Elderly: The incidence of antimuscarinic adverse reactions, including constipation, dizziness (at 8 mg only), dry mouth, dyspepsia, increase in residual urine, and urinary tract infection, was higher in patients 75 years of age and older as compared with younger patients.

Drug Interactions

Drugs that may interact with fesoterodine include CYP3A4 inducers (eg, rifampin), CYP3A4 inhibitors (eg, clarithromycin, erythromycin, itraconazole, ketoconazole), and anticholinergic agents.

Adverse Reactions

Adverse reactions occurring in at least 3% of patients treated with fesoterodine include constipation, dry eyes, dry mouth, and urinary tract infection.

THIAZIDES AND RELATED DIURETICS

CHLOROTHIAZIDE	
Tablets; oral: 250 and 500 mg (*Rx*)	Various
Suspension; oral: 250 mg per 5 mL (*Rx*)	*Diuril* (Salix)
Injection, lyophilized powder for solution: 500 mg (as sodium) (*Rx*)	*Diuril* (Ovation)
CHLORTHALIDONE	
Tablets; oral: 15, 25, 50, and 100 mg (*Rx*)	Various, *Thalitone* (Monarch)
HYDROCHLOROTHIAZIDE	
Tablets; oral: 12.5 and 100 mg (*Rx*)	Various
25 mg (*Rx*)	Various, *HydroDIURIL* (Merck), *Hydro-Par* (Parmed)
50 mg (*Rx*)	Various, *Ezide* (Econo Med), *Hydro-Par* (Parmed)
Capsules; oral: 12.5 mg (*Rx*)	Various, *Microzide* (Watson)
INDAPAMIDE	
Tablets; oral: 1.25 and 2.5 mg (*Rx*)	Various
METHYCLOTHIAZIDE	
Tablets; oral: 2.5 and 5 mg (*Rx*)	Various, *Enduron* (Abbott)
METOLAZONE	
Tablets; oral: 2.5, 5 and 10 mg (*Rx*)	Various, *Zaroxolyn* (UCB Pharma)

Indications

Edema: Adjunctive therapy in edema associated with congestive heart failure (CHF), hepatic cirrhosis, and corticosteroid and estrogen therapy. Useful in edema due to renal dysfunction (eg, nephrotic syndrome, acute glomerulonephritis, chronic renal failure).

Indapamide – Indapamide alone is indicated for edema associated with CHF.

Hypertension: As the sole therapeutic agent or to enhance other antihypertensive drugs in more severe forms of hypertension.

Administration and Dosage

CHLOROTHIAZIDE: Reserve IV route for patients unable to take oral medication or for emergency situations.

Adults –

Edema: 0.5 to 1 g (10 to 20 mL) once or twice/day, orally or IV. Many patients with edema respond to intermittent therapy (ie, administration on alternate days or 3 to 5 days each week).

Hypertension (oral forms only): The starting dosage is 0.5 or 1 g (10 to 20 mL) a day as a single or divided dose. Rarely, some patients may require up to 2 g (40 mL) a day in divided doses.

Infants and children –

Oral: 10 to 20 mg/kg (5 to 10 mg/lb) per day in single or 2 divided doses, not to exceed 375 mg/day (2.5 to 7.5 mL or ½ to 1½ teaspoonfuls of the oral suspension daily) in infants 2 years of age and younger or 1 g/day in children 2 to 12 years of age. In infants younger than 6 months of age, doses of up to 30 mg/kg (15 mg/pound) per day in 2 divided doses may be required.

IV use: IV use is not generally recommended.

CHLORTHALIDONE: Give as a single dose with food in the morning. Maintenance doses may be lower than initial doses.

Edema – Initiate therapy with 50 to 100 mg daily, or 100 mg on alternate days. Some patients may require 150 or 200 mg at these intervals. However, dosages above this level do not usually create a greater response.

Hypertension – Initiate therapy with a single dose of 25 mg/day. If response is insufficient after a suitable trial, increase to 50 mg. For additional control, increase dosage to 100 mg once daily, or add a second antihypertensive.

Note: Doses greater than 25 mg/day are likely to potentiate potassium excretion but provide no further benefit in sodium excretion or blood pressure reduction.

HYDROCHLOROTHIAZIDE:

Capsules –

Hypertension: 1 capsule given once daily whether given alone or in combination with other antihypertensives. Total daily doses greater than 50 mg are not recommended.

Tablets –

Adults:

Edema – The usual adult dosage is 25 to 100 mg daily as a single or divided dose. Many patients with edema respond to intermittent therapy, ie, administration on alternate days or on 3 to 5 days each week.

Hypertension – The usual initial dose in adults is 25 mg daily given as a single dose. The dose may be increased to 50 mg daily, given as a single or 2 divided doses. Doses above 50 mg are often associated with marked reductions in serum potassium (see Precautions).

Patients usually do not require doses in excess of 50 mg of hydrochlorothiazide daily when used concomitantly with other antihypertensive agents.

Infants and children:

For diuresis and for control of hypertension – The usual pediatric dosage is 0.5 to 1 mg per pound (1 to 2 mg/kg) per day in single or 2 divided doses, not to exceed 37.5 mg/day in infants up to 2 years of age or 100 mg/day in children 2 to 12 years of age. In infants less than 6 months of age, doses up to 1.5 mg per pound (3 mg/kg) per day in 2 divided doses may be required (see Warnings, Children).

INDAPAMIDE:

Edema of congestive heart failure –

Adults: 2.5 mg as a single daily dose in the morning. If response is not satisfactory after 1 week, increase to 5 mg once daily.

Hypertension –

Adults: 1.25 mg as a single daily dose taken in the morning. If the response to 1.25 mg is not satisfactory after 4 weeks, increase the daily dose to 2.5 mg taken once daily. If the response to 2.5 mg is not satisfactory after 4 weeks, the daily dose may be increased to 5 mg taken once daily, but consider adding another antihypertensive.

METHYCLOTHIAZIDE:

Edema –

Adults: 2.5 to 10 mg once daily. Maximum effective single dose is 10 mg.

Hypertension –

Adults: 2.5 to 5 mg once daily. If blood pressure control is not satisfactory after 8 to 12 weeks with 5 mg once daily, add another antihypertensive.

METOLAZONE: Individualize dosage.

Zaroxolyn –

Mild to moderate essential hypertension: 2.5 to 5 mg once daily.

Edema of renal disease/cardiac failure: 5 to 20 mg once daily.

Mykrox –

Mild to moderate hypertension: 0.5 mg as a single daily dose taken in the morning. If response is inadequate, increase the dose to 1 mg daily. Do not increase dosage if blood pressure is not controlled with 1 mg. Rather, add another antihypertensive agent with a different mechanism of action.

Actions

Pharmacology: Thiazide diuretics increase the urinary excretion of sodium and chloride in approximately equivalent amounts. They inhibit reabsorption of sodium and chloride in the cortical thick ascending limb of the loop of Henle and the early distal tubules. Other common actions include: Increased potassium and bicarbonate excretion, decreased calcium excretion and uric acid retention. At maximal therapeutic dosages all thiazides are approximately equal in diuretic efficacy.

The antihypertensive action requires several days to produce effects. Administration for less than or equal to 2 to 4 weeks is usually required for optimal therapeutic effect. The duration of the antihypertensive effect of the thiazides is sufficiently long to adequately control blood pressure with a single daily dose.

Pharmacokinetics:

Pharmacokinetics of Thiazides and Related Diuretics						
Diuretic	Onset (hours)	Peak (hours)	Duration (hours)	Equivalent dose (mg)	Percent absorbed	Half-life (hours)
Chlorothiazide	2[b]	4[b]	16 to 12	500	10 to 21[c]	0.75 to 2
Chlorthalidone	2 to 3	2 to 6	24 to 72	50	64[c]	40
Hydrochlorothiazide	2	4 to 6	16 to 12	50	65 to 75	5.6 to 14.8
Indapamide	1 to 2	≤ 2	up to 36	2.5	93	≈ 14
Methyclothiazide	2	6	24	5	nd[a]	nd[a]
Metolazone	1	2	12 to 24	5	65	nd[a]

[a] nd = No data.
[b] Following IV use, onset of action is 15 minutes; peak occurs in 30 minutes.
[c] Bioavailability may be dose-dependent.

Contraindications

Anuria; renal decompensation; hypersensitivity to thiazides or related diuretics or sulfonamide-derived drugs; hepatic coma or precoma (**metolazone**).

Warnings/Precautions

Parenteral use: Use IV **chlorothiazide** only when patients are unable to take oral medication or in an emergency. In infants and children, IV use is not recommended.

Lupus erythematosus: Lupus erythematosus exacerbation or activation has occurred.

Fluid/Electrolyte balance: Perform initial and periodic determinations of serum electrolytes, BUN, uric acid and glucose. Observe patients for clinical signs of fluid or electrolyte imbalance (eg, hyponatremia, hypochloremic alkalosis, hypokalemia, changes in serum and urinary calcium).

Hypokalemia – Hypokalemia may develop during concomitant corticosteroids, ACTH, and especially with brisk diuresis, with severe liver disease or cirrhosis, vomiting or diarrhea, or after prolonged therapy.

Hyponatremia/Hypochloremia – A chloride deficit is generally mild and usually does not require specific treatment, except in extraordinary circumstances (as in liver or renal disease). Thiazide-induced hyponatremia has been associated with death and neurologic damage in elderly patients.

Hypomagnesemia – Thiazide diuretics have been shown to increase urinary excretion of magnesium, resulting in hypomagnesemia.

Hypercalcemia – Calcium excretion may be decreased by thiazide diuretics.

Hyperuricemia – Hyperuricemia may occur or acute gout may be precipitated in certain patients receiving thiazides, even in those patients without a history of gouty attacks.

Glucose tolerance – Hyperglycemia may occur with thiazide diuretics.

Lipids: Thiazides may cause increased concentrations of total serum cholesterol, total triglycerides and LDL (but not HDL) in some patients, although these appear to return to pretreatment levels with long-term therapy.

Hypersensitivity reactions: Hypersensitivity reactions may occur in patients with or without a history of allergy or bronchial asthma; cross-sensitivity with sulfonamides may also occur. Refer to Management of Acute Hypersensitivity Reactions.

Renal function impairment: Use with caution in severe renal disease because these agents may precipitate azotemia. Cumulative effects of the drug may develop in patients with impaired renal function. Monitor renal function periodically. **Metolazone** is the only thiazide-like diuretic that may produce diuresis in patients with GFR less than 20 mL/min. Indapamide may also be useful in patients with impaired renal function.

Photosensitivity: Photosensitization may occur.

Pregnancy: *Category B* (chlorothiazide, chlorthalidone, hydrochlorothiazide, indapamide, metolazone); *Category C* (methyclothiazide). Routine use during normal pregnancy is inappropriate.

Lactation: Thiazides may appear in breast milk. Discontinue nursing or the drug.

Children: Chlorthalidone, hydrochlorothiazide, methyclothiazide, metolazone – Safety and efficacy have not been established. Metolazone is not recommended for use in children. In infants and children, IV use of chlorothiazide has been limited and is generally not recommended.

Drug Interactions

Drugs that may be affected by thiazides include the following: Allopurinol; anesthetics; anticoagulants; antigout agents; antineoplastics; calcium salts; diazoxide; digitalis glycosides; insulin; lithium; loop diuretics; methyldopa; nondepolarizing muscle relaxants; sulfonylureas; vitamin D. Drugs that may affect thiazides include: Amphotericin B; anticholinergics; bile acid sequestrants; corticosteroids; methenamines; NSAIDs.

Drug/Lab test interactions: Thiazides may decrease serum PBI levels without signs of thyroid disturbance. Thiazides also may cause diagnostic interference of serum electrolyte, blood, and urine glucose levels (usually only in patients with a predisposition to glucose intolerance), serum bilirubin levels, and serum uric acid levels. In uremic patients, serum magnesium levels may be increased.

Adverse Reactions

Adverse Reactions of Thiazides and Related Diuretics

Adverse reaction	Chlorothiazide	Chlorthalidone	Hydrochlorothiazide	Indapamide	Methyclothiazide	Metolazone
Cardiovascular						
Orthostatic hypotension	✓		✓	< 5%	✓	< 2%[a]
Palpitations				< 5%		< 2%[b]
CNS						
Dizziness/Lightheadedness	✓	✓	✓	≥ 5%	✓	10%[b]
Vertigo	✓	✓	✓	< 5%	✓	✓[c]
Headache	✓	✓	✓	≥ 5%	✓	9%[b]
Paresthesias	✓	✓	✓		✓	✓[c]
Xanthopsia	✓	✓	✓		✓	
Weakness	✓	✓	✓	≥ 5%	✓	< 2%[d]
Restlessness/Insomnia	✓	✓	✓	< 5%	✓	✓[c]
Drowsiness				< 5%		✓[c]
Fatigue/Lethargy/Malaise/Lassitude				≥ 5%		4%[b]
Anxiety				≥ 5%		< 2%[c]
Depression				< 5%		< 2%[b]
Nervousness				≥ 5%		< 2%[c]
Blurred vision (may be transient)	✓		✓	< 5%		✓[c]
GI						
Anorexia	✓	✓	✓	< 5%	✓	✓[c]
Gastric irritation/epigastric distress	✓	✓	✓	< 5%	✓	
Nausea	✓	✓	✓	< 5%	✓	< 2%[b]
Vomiting	✓	✓	✓	< 5%	✓	< 2%[d]
Abdominal pain/cramping/bloating	✓	✓	✓	< 5%	✓	< 2%[b]
Diarrhea	✓	✓	✓	< 5%	✓	< 2%[b]
Constipation	✓	✓	✓	< 5%	✓	< 2%[b]
Jaundice (intrahepatic/cholestatic)	✓	✓	✓		✓	✓[c]
Pancreatitis	✓	✓	✓		✓	✓[c]
Dry mouth				< 5%		< 2%[a]

Adverse Reactions of Thiazides and Related Diuretics

Adverse reaction	Chlorothiazide	Chlorthalidone	Hydrochlorothiazide	Indapamide	Methyclothiazide	Metolazone
GU						
Nocturia				<5%		<2%[a]
Impotence/Reduced libido	✓	✓	✓	<5%	✓	<2%[b]
Hematologic						
Leukopenia	✓	✓	✓		✓	✓[c]
Thrombocytopenia	✓	✓	✓		✓	
Agranulocytosis	✓	✓	✓		✓	✓[c]
Aplastic/Hypoplastic anemia	✓	✓	✓		✓	✓[c]
Dermatologic						
Purpura	✓	✓	✓		✓	✓[c]
Photosensitivity/ Photosensitivity dermatitis	✓	✓	✓		✓	✓[c]
Rash	✓	✓	✓	<5%	✓	<2%[b]
Urticaria	✓	✓	✓			✓[c]
Necrotizing angiitis, vasculitis, cutaneous vasculitis	✓	✓	✓	<5%	✓	✓[b]
Pruritus				<5%		<2%[a]
Metabolic						
Hyperglycemia	✓	✓	✓	<5%	✓	✓[c]
Glycosuria	✓	✓	✓	<5%	✓	✓[c]
Hyperuricemia	✓	✓	✓	<5%	✓	
Miscellaneous						
Muscle cramp/spasm	✓	✓	✓	≥5%	✓	6%[b]

[a] Percentage of occurrence refers to rapidly acting doseform; however this adverse reaction also occurred with the slow acting doseform.
[b] IV doseform.
[c] Possibly with life-threatening anaphylactic shock.
[d] Slow acting doseform only.

LOOP DIURETICS

BUMETANIDE	
Tablets: 0.5, 1, and 2 mg (*Rx*)	Various
Injection: 0.25 mg/mL (*Rx*)	
ETHACRYNIC ACID	
Tablets: 25 mg (as ethacrynic acid) (*Rx*)	*Edecrin* (Aton Pharma)
Powder for Injection: 50 mg (as ethacrynate sodium) per vial (*Rx*)	*Edecrin Sodium* (Aton Pharma)
FUROSEMIDE	
Tablets: 20, 40, and 80 mg (*Rx*)	Various, *Lasix* (Hoechst-Roussel)
Oral Solution: 10 mg/mL (*Rx*)	
Injection: 10 mg/mL (*Rx*)	

Warning:
These agents are potent diuretics; excess amounts can lead to a profound diuresis with water and electrolyte depletion.

Indications

Edema: Edema associated with CHF, hepatic cirrhosis, and renal disease, including the nephrotic syndrome. Particularly useful when greater diuretic potential is desired.

Parenteral administration is indicated when a rapid onset of diuresis is desired (eg, acute pulmonary edema), when GI absorption is impaired or when oral use is not practical for any reason. As soon as it is practical, replace with oral therapy.

Hypertension (furosemide, oral): Alone or in combination with other antihypertensive drugs.

Ethacrynic acid:

Ascites – Short-term management of ascites due to malignancy, idiopathic edema, and lymphedema.

Congenital heart disease, nephrotic syndrome – Short-term management of hospitalized pediatric patients, other than infants.

Pulmonary edema, acute – Adjunctive therapy.

Administration and Dosage

BUMETANIDE:

Oral – 0.5 to 2 mg/day, given as a single dose. If diuretic response is not adequate, give a second or third dose at 4- to 5-hour intervals, up to a maximum daily dose of 10 mg. An intermittent dose schedule, given on alternate days or for 3 to 4 days with rest periods of 1 to 2 days in between, is the safest and most effective method for the continued control of edema. In patients with hepatic failure, keep the dose to a minimum, and if necessary, increase the dose carefully.

Parenteral – Initially, 0.5 to 1 mg IV or IM. Administer IV over a period of 1 to 2 minutes. If the initial response is insufficient, give a second or third dose at intervals of 2 to 3 hours; do not exceed a daily dosage of 10 mg. End parenteral treatment and start oral treatment as soon as possible.

Renal function impairment – In patients with severe chronic renal insufficiency, a continuous infusion of bumetanide (12 mg over 12 hours) may be more effective and less toxic than intermittent bolus therapy.

ETHACRYNIC ACID:

Oral –

Initial therapy: Give minimally effective dose (usually, 50 to 200 mg/day) on a continuous or intermittent dosage schedule to produce gradual weight loss of 2.2 to 4.4 kg/day (1 to 2 lb/day). Adjust dose in 25 to 50 mg increments. Higher doses, up to 200 mg twice daily, achieved gradually, are most often required in patients with severe, refractory edema.

Children: Initial dose is 25 mg. Make careful increments of 25 mg to achieve maintenance. Dosage for infants has not been established.

Maintenance therapy: Administer intermittently after an effective diuresis is obtained using an alternate daily schedule or more prolonged periods of diuretic therapy interspersed with rest periods.

Parenteral – Do not give subcutaneously or IM because of local pain and irritation. The usual IV dose for the average adult is 50 mg, or 0.5 to 1 mg/kg. Give slowly through the tubing of a running infusion or by direct IV injection over several minutes. Usually, only 1 dose is necessary; occasionally, a second dose may be required; use a new injection site to avoid thrombophlebitis. A single IV dose, not exceeding 100 mg, has been used. Insufficient pediatric experience precludes recommendation for this age group.

FUROSEMIDE:

Oral –

Edema: 20 to 80 mg/day as a single dose. Depending on response, administer a second dose 6 to 8 hours later. If response is not satisfactory, increase by increments of 20 or 40 mg, no sooner than 6 to 8 hours after previous dose, until desired diuresis occurs. This dose should then be given once or twice daily (eg, at 8 am and 2 pm). Dosage may be titrated up to 600 mg/day in patients with severe edema.

Mobilization of edema may be most efficiently and safely accomplished with an intermittent dosage schedule; the drug is given 2 to 4 consecutive days each week. With doses greater than 80 mg/day, clinical and laboratory observations are advisable.

Hypertension: 40 mg twice a day; adjust according to response. If the patient does not respond, add other antihypertensive agents. Reduce dosage of other agents by at least 50% as soon as furosemide is added to prevent excessive drop in blood pressure.

Infants and children: 2 mg/kg. If diuresis is unsatisfactory, increase by 1 or 2 mg/kg, no sooner than 6 to 8 hours after previous dose. Doses greater than 6 mg/kg are not recommended. For maintenance therapy, adjust dose to the minimum effective level. A dose range of 0.5 to 2 mg/kg twice daily has also been recommended.

CHF and chronic renal failure: It has been suggested that doses as high as 2 to 2.5 g/day or more are well tolerated and effective in these patients.

Parenteral –

Edema: Initial dose: 20 to 40 mg IM or IV. Give the IV injection slowly (1 to 2 minutes). If needed, another dose may be given in the same manner 2 hours later. The dose may be raised by 20 mg and given no sooner than 2 hours after previous dose, until desired diuretic effect is obtained. This dose should then be given once or twice daily. Administer high-dose parenteral therapy as a controlled infusion at a rate 4 mg/min or less.

Acute pulmonary edema: The usual initial dose is 40 mg IV (over 1 to 2 minutes). If response is not satisfactory within 1 hour, increase to 80 mg IV (over 1 to 2 minutes).

Infants and children: 1 mg/kg IV or IM given slowly under close supervision. If diuretic response after the initial dose is not satisfactory, increase the dosage by 1 mg/kg, no sooner than 2 hours after previous dose, until desired effect is obtained. Doses greater than 6 mg/kg are not recommended.

CHF and chronic renal failure: It has been suggested that doses as high as 2 to 2.5 g/day or more are well tolerated and effective in these patients. For IV bolus injections, the maximum should not exceed 1 g/day given over 30 minutes.

Actions

Pharmacology: Furosemide and ethacrynic acid inhibit primarily reabsorption of sodium and chloride, not only in proximal and distal tubules, but also the loop of Henle. In contrast, bumetanide is more chloruretic than natriuretic and may have an additional action in the proximal tubule; it does not appear to act on the distal tubule.

Pharmacokinetics: These agents are metabolized and excreted primarily through the urine. Protein binding of these agents exceeds 90%. Furosemide is metabolized approximately 30% to 40%, and its urinary excretion is 60% to 70%. Oral administration of bumetanide revealed that 81% was excreted in urine, 45% of it as unchanged drug.

Pharmacokinetic Parameters of the Loop Diuretics								
Diuretic	Bioavailability (%)	Half-life (min)	Onset of action (min)	Peak (min)	Duration (h)	Dosage (mg)	Relative potency	Doses/ day
Bumetanide								
Oral	72-96	60-90[d]	30-60	60-120	4-6	0.5-2	≈ 40	1
IV			within minutes	15-30	0.5-1	0.5-1	≈ 40	1-3
Ethacrynic acid								
Oral	≈100	60	≤ 30	120	6-8	50-100	0.6-0.8	1-2
IV			≤ 5	15-30	2	50	0.6-0.8	1-2
Furosemide								
Oral	60-64[a]	≈ 120[e]	≤ 60	60-120[b]	6-8	20-80	1	1-2
IV or IM			≤ 5[c]	30	2	20-40	1	

[a] Decreased in uremia and nephrosis.
[b] Decreased in CHF.
[c] Somewhat delayed after IM administration.
[d] Prolonged in renal disease.
[e] Prolonged in renal failure, uremia, and in neonates.

Contraindications

Anuria; hypersensitivity to these compounds or to sulfonylureas; infants (ethacrynic acid); patients with hepatic coma or in states of severe electrolyte depletion until the condition is improved or corrected (bumetanide).

Warnings/Precautions

Dehydration: Excessive diuresis may result in dehydration and reduction in blood volume with circulatory collapse and the possibility of vascular thrombosis and embolism, particularly in elderly patients.

Hepatic cirrhosis and ascites: In these patients, sudden alterations of electrolyte balance may precipitate hepatic encephalopathy and coma. Do not institute therapy until the basic condition is improved.

Ototoxicity: Tinnitus, reversible and irreversible hearing impairment, deafness, and vertigo with a sense of fullness in the ears have been reported. Deafness is usually reversible and of short duration (1 to 24 hours); however, irreversible hearing impairment has occurred. Usually, ototoxicity is associated with rapid injection, with severe renal impairment, with doses several times the usual dose, and with concurrent use with other ototoxic drugs.

Systemic lupus erythematosus: Systemic lupus erythematosus may be exacerbated or activated.

Thrombocytopenia: Because there have been rare spontaneous reports of thrombocytopenia with **bumetanide**, observe regularly for possible occurrence.

Monitoring: Observe for blood dyscrasias, liver or kidney damage, or idiosyncratic reactions. Perform frequent serum electrolyte, calcium, glucose, uric acid, CO_2, creatinine, and BUN determinations during the first few months of therapy and periodically thereafter.

Cardiovascular effects: Too vigorous a diuresis, as evidenced by rapid and excessive weight loss, may induce an acute hypotensive episode. In elderly cardiac patients, avoid rapid contraction of plasma volume and the resultant hemoconcentration to prevent thromboembolic episodes, such as cerebral vascular thromboses and pulmonary emboli.

Electrolyte imbalance: Electrolyte imbalance may occur, especially in patients receiving high doses with restricted salt intake. Perform periodic determinations of serum electrolytes.

Hypokalemia: Hypokalemia prevention requires particular attention to the following: Patients receiving digitalis and diuretics for CHF, hepatic cirrhosis, and ascites; in aldosterone excess with normal renal function; potassium-losing nephropathy; certain diarrheal states; or where hypokalemia is an added risk to the patient (eg, history of ventricular arrhythmias).

Hypomagnesemia: Loop diuretics increase the urinary excretion of magnesium.

Hypocalcemia: Serum calcium levels may be lowered (rare cases of tetany have occurred).

Hyperuricemia: Asymptomatic hyperuricemia can occur, and rarely, gout may be precipitated.

Glucose: Increases in blood glucose and alterations in glucose tolerance tests (fasting and 2 hour postprandial sugar) have been observed.

Lipids: Increases in LDL and total cholesterol and triglycerides with minor decreases in HDL cholesterol may occur.

Hypersensitivity reactions: Patients with known sulfonamide sensitivity may show allergic reactions to **furosemide** or **bumetanide**. Bumetanide use following instances of allergic reactions to furosemide suggests a lack of cross-sensitivity. Refer to Management of Acute Hypersensitivity Reactions.

Renal function impairment: If increasing azotemia, oliguria, or reversible increases in BUN or creatinine occur during treatment of severe progressive renal disease, discontinue therapy.

Photosensitivity: Photosensitization (photoallergy or phototoxicity) may occur.

Pregnancy: Category B (ethacrynic acid); *Category* C (furosemide, bumetanide). Since furosemide may increase the incidence of patent ductus arteriosus in preterm infants with respiratory-distress syndrome, use caution when administering before delivery.

Lactation: **Furosemide** appears in breast milk.

Children: Safety and efficacy for use of **bumetanide** in children younger than 18 years of age, and **ethacrynic acid** in infants (oral) and children (IV) have not been established.

Furosemide – Furosemide stimulates renal synthesis of prostaglandin E_2 and may increase the incidence of patent ductus arteriosus when given in the first few weeks of life, to premature infants with respiratory-distress syndrome.

Drug Interactions

Loop diuretics may affect the following drugs: Aminoglycosides; anticoagulants; chloral hydrate; digitalis glycosides; lithium; nondepolarizing neuromuscular blockers; propranolol; sulfonylureas; theophyllines. Loop diuretics may be affected by the following drugs: Charcoal; cisplatin; clofibrate; hydantoins; NSAIDs; probenecid; salicylates; thiazide diuretics.

Drug/Food interactions: The bioavailability of **furosemide** is decreased and its degree of diuresis reduced when administered with food.

Adverse Reactions

Adverse reactions associated with loop diuretics include nausea; vomiting; diarrhea; gastric irritation; headache; fatigue; dizziness; thrombocytopenia; rash; orthostatic hypotension; hyperuricemia; hyperglycemia; electrolyte imbalance (decreased chloride, potassium and sodium); dehydration.

Bumetanide: Adverse reactions may include impaired hearing, ear discomfort, dry mouth, pain, renal failure, weakness, arthritic pain, muscle cramps, ECG changes, chest pain, hives, pruritus, itching, sweating, hyperventilation.

Ethacrynic acid: Adverse reactions may include anorexia, pain, GI bleeding, severe neutropenia, agranulocytosis, fever, chills, confusion, fatigue, malaise, sense of fullness in the ears, blurred vision, tinnitus, hearing loss (irreversible), rash.

Furosemide: Adverse reactions may include anorexia, cramping, constipation, blurred vision, hearing loss, restlessness, fever, anemia, purpura, thrombocytopenia, agranulocytosis, photosensitivity, urticaria, pruritus, thrombophlebitis, muscle spasm, weakness.

POTASSIUM-SPARING DIURETICS

Actions

Pharmacology: In the kidney, potassium is filtered at the glomerulus and then absorbed parallel to sodium throughout the proximal tubule and thick ascending limb of the loop of Henle, so that only minor amounts reach the distal convoluted tubule. As a result, potassium appearing in urine is secreted at the distal tubule and collecting duct. The potassium-sparing diuretics interfere with sodium reabsorption at the distal tubule, thus decreasing potassium secretion. They exert a weak diuretic and antihypertensive effect when used alone. Their major use is to enhance the action and counteract the kaliuretic effect of thiazide and loop diuretics.

Spironolactone – Spironolactone, a competitive inhibitor of aldosterone, binds to aldosterone receptors of the distal tubule and prevents the formation of a protein important in sodium transport. It is effective in primary and secondary hyperaldosteronism. Spironolactone is effective in lowering systolic and diastolic blood pressure in primary hyperaldosteronism and essential hypertension, although aldosterone secretion may be normal in benign essential hypertension.

Amiloride and triamterene – **Amiloride** and **triamterene** not only inhibit sodium reabsorption induced by aldosterone, but they also inhibit basal sodium reabsorption. They are not aldosterone antagonists, but act directly on the renal distal tubule, cortical collecting tubule and collecting duct. They induce a reversal of polarity of the transtubular electrical-potential difference and inhibit active transport of sodium and potassium. Amiloride may inhibit sodium, potassium-ATPase.

Potassium-Sparing Diuretics: Pharmacological and Pharmacokinetic Properties

Parameters	Amiloride	Spironolactone	Triamterene
Pharmacology			
Tubular site of action	Proximal = distal	Distal	Distal
Mechanism of action	Na^+, K^+–ATPase inhibition; Na^+/H^+ exchange mechanism inhibition (proximal tubule)	Aldosterone antagonism	Membrane effect
Action:			
Onset (hours)	2	24 to 48	2 to 4
Peak (hours)	6 to 10	48 to 72	6 to 8
Duration (hours)	24	48 to 72	12 to 16
Pharmacokinetics			
Bioavailability	15% to 25%	> 90%	30% to 70%
Protein binding	23%	≥ 98%[a]	50% to 67%
Half-life (hours)	6 to 9	20[b]	3
Active metabolites	none	canrenone	hydroxytriamterene sulfate
Peak plasma levels (hours)	3 to 4	canrenone: 2 to 4	3
Excreted unchanged in urine	≈ 50%[c]	†[d]	≈ 21%
Dosage			
Daily dose (mg)	5 to 20	25 to 400	200 to 300

[a] Canrenone > 98%.
[b] 10 to 35 hours for canrenone.
[c] 40% excreted in stool within 72 hours.
[d] Metabolites primarily excreted in urine, but also in bile.

AMILORIDE HYDROCHLORIDE

Tablets: 5 mg (*Rx*)	*Midamor* (Merck)

Indications

Adjunctive treatment with thiazide or loop diuretics in CHF or hypertension to: Help restore normal serum potassium in patients who develop hypokalemia on the kaliuretic diuretic; prevent hypokalemia in patients who would be at particular risk if hypokalemia were to develop (eg, digitalized patients or patients with significant cardiac arrhythmias).

Unlabeled uses: Amiloride (10 to 20 mg/day) may be useful in reducing lithium-induced polyuria without increasing lithium levels as is seen with thiazide diuretics.

Administration and Dosage

Administer with food.

Concomitant therapy: Add amiloride 5 mg/day to the usual antihypertensive or diuretic dosage of a kaliuretic diuretic. Increase dosage to 10 mg/day, if necessary; doses greater than 10 mg are usually not needed. If persistent hypokalemia is documented with 10 mg, increase the dose to 15 mg, then 20 mg, with careful titration of the dose and careful monitoring of electrolytes.

In patients with CHF, potassium loss may decrease after an initial diuresis; reevaluate the need or dosage for amiloride. Maintenance therapy may be intermittent.

Single drug therapy: The starting dose is 5 mg/day. Increase to 10 mg/day, if necessary; doses greater than 10 mg are usually not needed. If persistent hypokalemia is documented with 10 mg, increase the dose to 15 mg, then 20 mg, with careful monitoring of electrolytes.

Contraindications

Hypersensitivity to amiloride; serum potassium greater than 5.5 mEq/L; antikaliuretic therapy or potassium supplementation; renal function impairment patients receiving spironolactone or triamterene.

Warnings/Precautions

Hyperkalemia: Amiloride may cause hyperkalemia (serum potassium greater than 5.5 mEq/L) that, if uncorrected, is potentially fatal. Monitor serum potassium carefully. Symptoms of hyperkalemia include paresthesias, muscular weakness, fatigue, flaccid paralysis of the extremities, bradycardia, shock, and ECG abnormalities.

Diabetes mellitus: Avoid use of amiloride in diabetic patients. If it is used, monitor serum electrolytes and renal function frequently. Discontinue use 3 days or more before glucose tolerance testing.

Metabolic or respiratory acidosis: Cautiously institute amiloride in severely ill patients in whom respiratory or metabolic acidosis may occur, such as patients with cardiopulmonary disease or poorly controlled diabetes. Monitor acid-base balance frequently. Shifts in acid-base balance alter the ratio of extracellular/intracellular potassium; the development of acidosis may be associated with rapid increases in serum potassium.

Electrolyte imbalance and BUN increases: Hyponatremia and hypochloremia may occur when amiloride is used with other diuretics. Increases in BUN levels usually accompany vigorous fluid elimination, especially when diuretic therapy is used in seriously ill patients, such as those who have hepatic cirrhosis with ascites and metabolic alkalosis, or those with resistant edema.

Renal function impairment: Anuria, acute or chronic renal insufficiency and evidence of diabetic nephropathy are contraindications because potassium retention is accentuated and may result in the rapid development of hyperkalemia. Do not give to patients with evidence of renal impairment (BUN greater than 30 mg/dL or serum creatinine greater than 1.5 mg/dL) or diabetes mellitus without continuous monitoring of serum electrolytes, creatinine, and BUN levels.

Hepatic function impairment: In patients with preexisting severe liver disease, hepatic encephalopathy (manifested by tremors, confusion, and coma, and increased jaundice) may occur. Because amiloride is not metabolized by the liver, drug accumulation is not anticipated in patients with hepatic dysfunction, but accumulation can occur if hepatorenal syndrome develops.

Pregnancy: Category B.

Lactation: It is not known whether amiloride is excreted in breast milk.

Children: Safety and efficacy for use in children have not been established.

Drug Interactions

Drugs that may interact include digoxin, potassium preparations, ACE inhibitors, and NSAIDs.

Adverse Reactions

Possible adverse reactions include headache, nausea, anorexia, diarrhea, vomiting.

SPIRONOLACTONE

Tablets: 25, 50, and 100 mg (*Rx*)	Various, *Aldactone* (Searle)

Indications

Primary hyperaldosteronism: Diagnosis of primary hyperaldosteronism.

Short-term preoperative treatment of patients with primary hyperaldosteronism.

Long-term maintenance therapy for patients with discrete aldosterone-producing adrenal adenomas who are poor operative risks, or who decline surgery.

Long-term maintenance therapy for patients with bilateral micronodular or macronodular adrenal hyperplasia (idiopathic hyperaldosteronism).

Edematous conditions when other therapies are inappropriate or inadequate:

CHF – Management of edema and sodium retention; also indicated with digitalis.

Cirrhosis of the liver accompanied by edema or ascites – For maintenance therapy in conjunction with bed rest and the restriction of fluid and sodium.

Nephrotic syndrome – For nephrotic patients when treatment of the underlying disease, restriction of fluid and sodium intake, and the use of other diuretics do not provide an adequate response.

Essential hypertension: Usually in combination with other drugs.

Hypokalemia: Hypokalemia and the prophylaxis of hypokalemia in patients taking digitalis.

Severe heart failure (NYHA class III to IV): To increase survival and to reduce the need for hospitalization for heart failure when used in addition to standard therapy.

Unlabeled uses: Spironolactone has been used in combination with an oral contraceptive for treatment of polycystic ovary syndrome (PCOS) hirsutism due to its antiandrogenic properties.

Administration and Dosage

Spironolactone may be administered in single or divided doses.

Diagnosis of primary hyperaldosteronism: As initial diagnostic measure to provide presumptive evidence of primary hyperaldosteronism in patients on normal diets, as follows:

Long test – 400 mg/day for 3 to 4 weeks. Correction of hypokalemia and hypertension provides presumptive evidence for diagnosis of primary hyperaldosteronism.

Short test – 400 mg/day for 4 days. If serum potassium increases but decreases when spironolactone is discontinued, consider a presumptive diagnosis of primary hyperaldosteronism.

Maintenance therapy for hyperaldosteronism: 100 to 400 mg/day in preparation for surgery. For patients unsuitable for surgery, employ the drug for long-term maintenance therapy at lowest possible dose.

Edema:

Adults (CHF, hepatic cirrhosis, nephrotic syndrome) – Initially, 100 mg/day (range, 25 to 200 mg/day). When given as the sole diuretic agent, continue for ≥ 5 days at the initial dosage level, then adjust to the optimal level. If after 5 days an adequate diuretic response has not occurred, add a second diuretic, which acts more proximally in the renal tubule. Because of the additive effect of spironolactone with such diuretics, an enhanced diuresis usually begins on the first day of combined treatment; combined therapy is indicated when more rapid diuresis is desired. Spironolactone dosage should remain unchanged when other diuretic therapy is added.

Children – 3.3 mg/kg/day (1.5 mg/lb/day) administered in single or divided doses.

Essential hypertension:

Adults – Initially, 50 to 100 mg/day in single or divided doses. May also be combined with diuretics, which act more proximally, and with other antihypertensive agents. Continue treatment for 2 weeks or more because the maximal response may not occur sooner. Individualize dosage.

Children – A dose of 1 to 2 mg/kg twice/day has been recommended.

Hypokalemia: 25 to 100 mg/day. Useful in treating diuretic-induced hypokalemia when oral potassium supplements or other potassium-sparing regimens are considered inappropriate.

Severe heart failure:

Initial dosage – 25 mg once daily if the patient's serum potassium is 5 mEq/L or less and the patient's serum creatinine is 2.5 mg/dL or less.

Dosage adjustment – Patients who can tolerate 25 mg once daily may have their dosage increased to 50 mg once daily as clinically indicated. Patients who do not tolerate the 25 mg once-daily dose may have their dosage reduced to 25 mg every other day.

Unlabeled uses:

Adults –

Hirsutism in women: Used as monotherapy or in combination therapy at dosages ranging from 50 to 200 mg daily in 1 to 2 divided doses.

Children –

Diagnosis of primary aldosteronism: 125 to 375 mg/m^2/day orally divided 2 to 4 times daily.

Diuretic:

Older than 29 days of age – 1 to 3.3 mg/kg/day orally divided once to 4 times daily.

29 days of age and younger – 1 to 3 mg/kg/day orally divided once to twice daily.

Contraindications

Anuria; acute renal insufficiency; significant impairment of renal function; hyperkalemia; patients receiving amiloride or triamterene.

Warnings/Precautions

Hyperkalemia: Carefully evaluate patients for possible fluid and electrolyte balance disturbances. Hyperkalemia may occur with impaired renal function or excessive potassium intake and can cause cardiac irregularities that may be fatal. Ordinarily, do not give potassium supplements with spironolactone.

Hyponatremia: Hyponatremia may be caused or aggravated by spironolactone, especially in combination with other diuretics. Symptoms include dry mouth, thirst, lethargy, drowsiness.

Gynecomastia: Gynecomastia may develop and appears to be related to dosage and duration of therapy. It is normally reversible when therapy is discontinued.

Reversible hyperchloremic metabolic acidosis: Reversible hyperchloremic metabolic acidosis, usually in association with hyperkalemia, occurs in some patients with decompensated hepatic cirrhosis, even in the presence of normal renal function.

Renal function impairment: Use of spironolactone may cause a transient elevation of BUN, especially in patients with preexisting renal impairment. The drug may cause mild acidosis.

Carcinogenesis: Spironolactone was a tumorigen in chronic toxicity studies in rats.

Pregnancy: Spironolactone or its metabolites may cross the placental barrier.

Lactation: Canrenone, a metabolite of spironolactone, appears in breast milk. The labeling suggests that an alternative method of infant feeding be instituted when using spironolactone; however, the American Academy of Pediatrics considers the drug to be compatible with breast-feeding.

Drug Interactions

Drugs that may affect spironolactone include ACE inhibitors, salicylates, and food. Drugs that may be affected by spironolactone include anticoagulants, digitalis glycosides, mitotane, digoxin, and potassium preparations.

Adverse Reactions

Adverse reactions are usually reversible upon discontinuation of the drug.

Possible adverse reactions include cramping; diarrhea; gastric bleeding; ulceration; gastritis; vomiting; drowsiness; lethargy; headache; mental confusion; ataxia; irregular menses; carcinoma of the breast.

TRIAMTERENE

Capsules: 50 and 100 mg (*Rx*)	*Dyrenium* (Wellspring Pharmaceuticals)

Indications

Edema: Edema associated with CHF, hepatic cirrhosis, and the nephrotic syndrome; steroid-induced edema, idiopathic edema, and edema due to secondary hyperaldosteronism.

May be used alone or with other diuretics, either for additive diuretic effect or antikaliuretic (potassium-sparing) effect. It promotes increased diuresis in patients resistant or only partially responsive to other diuretics because of secondary hyperaldosteronism.

Administration and Dosage

Individualize dosage.

When used alone, the usual starting dose is 100 mg twice/daily after meals. When combined with other diuretics or antihypertensives, decrease the total daily dosage of each agent initially, and then adjust to the patient's needs. Do not exceed 300 mg/day.

Contraindications

Patients receiving spironolactone or amiloride; anuria; severe hepatic disease; hyperkalemia; hypersensitivity to triamterene; severe or progressive kidney disease or dysfunction, with the possible exception of nephrosis; preexisting elevated serum potassium (impaired renal function, azotemia) or patients who develop hyperkalemia while on triamterene.

Warnings/Precautions

Hyperkalemia: Abnormal elevation of serum potassium levels (5.5 mEq/L or more) can occur. Hyperkalemia is more likely to occur in patients with renal impairment and diabetes (even without evidence of renal impairment), and in the elderly or severely ill. Because uncorrected hyperkalemia may be fatal, serum potassium levels must be monitored at frequent intervals, especially when dosages are changed or with any illness that may influence renal function.

When triamterene is added to other diuretic therapy, or when patients are switched to triamterene from other diuretics, discontinue potassium supplementation.

Electrolyte imbalance: In CHF, renal disease, or cirrhosis, electrolyte imbalance may be aggravated or caused by diuretics. The use of full doses of a diuretic when salt intake is restricted can result in a low salt syndrome.

Renal stones: Triamterene has been found in renal stones with other usual calculus components. Use cautiously in patients with histories of stone formation.

Hematologic effects: Triamterene is a weak folic acid antagonist. Because cirrhotics with splenomegaly may have marked variations in hematological status, it may contribute to the appearance of megaloblastosis in cases where folic acid stores have been depleted. Perform periodic blood studies in these patients.

Metabolic acidosis: Triamterene may cause decreasing alkali reserve with a possibility of metabolic acidosis.

Diabetes mellitus: Triamterene may raise blood glucose levels for adult-onset diabetes; dosage adjustments of hypoglycemic agents may be necessary. Concurrent use with chlorpropamide may increase the risk of severe hyponatremia.

Hypersensitivity reactions: Monitor patients regularly for blood dyscrasias, liver damage, or other idiosyncratic reactions.

Renal function impairment: Perform periodic BUN and serum potassium determinations to check kidney function, especially in patients with suspected or confirmed renal insufficiency and in elderly or diabetic patients; diabetic patients with nephropathy are especially prone to develop hyperkalemia.

Hepatic function impairment: Triamterene is extensively metabolized in the liver. The overall diuretic response may not be affected.

Photosensitivity: Photosensitization is likely to occur; avoid prolonged exposure to sunlight.

Pregnancy: Category B.

Lactation: If the drug is essential, the patient should stop nursing.

Children: Safety and efficacy have not been established.

Drug Interactions

Drugs that may affect triamterene include ACE inhibitors, cimetidine, and indomethacin. Drugs that may be affected by triamterene include amantadine and potassium preparations. Triamterene will interfere with the fluorescent measurement of quinidine serum levels.

Adverse Reactions

Diarrhea; nausea; vomiting; jaundice; liver enzyme abnormalities. Azotemia; elevated BUN/creatinine; increased serum uric acid levels (in patients predisposed to gouty arthritis); thrombocytopenia; megaloblastic anemia; weakness; dizziness; hypokalemia; headache; dry mouth; anaphylaxis.

CARBONIC ANHYDRASE INHIBITORS

ACETAZOLAMIDE	
Tablets; oral: 125 and 250 mg (*Rx*)	Various
Capsules, extended-release; oral: 500 mg (*Rx*)	Various, *Diamox Sequels* (Barr)
Powder for injection, lyophilized: 500 mg (*Rx*)	Various
METHAZOLAMIDE	
Tablets; oral: 25 and 50 mg (*Rx*)	Various

Warning:

Fatalities have occurred, although rarely, because of severe reactions to sulfonamides, including Stevens-Johnson syndrome, toxic epidermal necrolysis, fulminant hepatic necrosis, agranulocytosis, aplastic anemia, and other blood dyscrasias. Sensitizations may recur when a sulfonamide is readministered irrespective of the route of administration. If signs of hypersensitivity or other serious reactions occur, discontinue use of this drug.

Caution is advised for patients receiving concomitant high-dose aspirin and acetazolamide because anorexia, tachypnea, lethargy, coma, and death have been reported.

Indications

Glaucoma: For adjunctive treatment of open-angle glaucoma and secondary glaucoma; preoperatively in acute angle-closure glaucoma when delay of surgery is desired to lower intraocular pressure (IOP).

Acetazolamide:

Acute mountain sickness – For the prevention or amelioration of symptoms associated with acute mountain sickness in climbers attempting rapid ascent and in those who are susceptible to acute mountain sickness despite gradual ascent.

Edema – For adjunctive treatment of edema due to CHF, drug-induced edema, and centrencephalic epilepsy (petit mal, unlocalized seizures).

Administration and Dosage

ACETAZOLAMIDE:

Adults –

Acute congestive (closed-angle) glaucoma, chronic simple (open-angle) glaucoma, secondary glaucoma:

Extended-release capsules – 500 mg 2 times a day.

It may be necessary to adjust the dose, but it has usually been found that a dose in excess of 1 g does not produce an increased effect. The dosage should be adjusted with careful individual attention both to symptomatology and intraocular tension. In all cases, continuous supervision by a health care provider is advisable.

Conversion: In those unusual instances in which adequate control is not obtained by the twice-a-day administration of acetazolamide extended-release capsules, the desired control may be established by means of tablets or parenteral. Use tablets or parenteral in accordance with the more frequent dosage schedules recommended for these dosage forms, such as 250 mg every 4 hours, or an initial dose of 500 mg followed by 250 or 125 mg every 4 hours, depending on the case in question.

Tablets – 250 mg every 4 hours, although some cases have responded to 250 mg twice daily on short-term therapy. In some acute cases, it may be more satisfactory to administer an initial dose of 500 mg followed by 125 or 250 mg every 4 hours depending on the individual case.

Concomitant therapy: A complementary effect has been noted when used in conjunction with miotics or mydriatics as the case demanded.

Acute mountain sickness: 500 to 1,000 mg daily in divided doses using tablets or extended-release capsules, as appropriate. In circumstances of rapid ascent, such as in rescue or military operations, the higher dose level of 1,000 mg is recommended. It is preferable to initiate dosing 24 to 48 hours before ascent.

Continue for 48 hours while at high altitude, or longer as necessary to control symptoms.

Congestive heart failure:

Tablets – 250 to 375 mg once daily in the morning (5 mg/kg).

Failures in therapy may be because of overdosage or too frequent dosage.

If, after an initial response, the patient fails to continue to lose edema fluid, do not increase the dose but allow for kidney recovery by skipping medication for a day. Acetazolamide yields best diuretic results when given on alternate days, or for 2 days alternating with a day of rest.

The use of acetazolamide does not eliminate the need for other therapy such as digitalis, bed rest, and salt restriction.

Drug-induced edema:

Tablets – 250 to 375 mg once a day for 1 or 2 days, alternating with a day of rest.

Seizures:

Tablets – 8 to 30 mg/kg in divided doses. Although some patients respond to a low dose, the optimum range appears to be from 375 to 1,000 mg daily. However, some investigators feel that daily doses in excess of 1 g do not produce any better results than a 1 g dose.

When acetazolamide is given in combination with other anticonvulsants, it is suggested that the starting dosage should be 250 mg once daily in addition to the existing medications. This can be increased to levels as previously indicated.

Children (12 years of age and older) –

Acute mountain sickness:

Extended-release capsules – 500 to 1,000 mg daily, in divided doses as appropriate. In circumstances of rapid ascent, such as in rescue or military operations, the higher dose level of 1,000 mg is recommended. It is preferable to initiate dosing 24 to 48 hours before ascent.

Continue for 48 hours while at high altitude, or longer as necessary to control symptoms.

Glaucoma: 500 mg 2 times a day.

It may be necessary to adjust the dose, but it has usually been found that a dose in excess of 1 g does not produce an increased effect. The dosage should be adjusted with careful individual attention both to symptomatology and intraocular tension. In all cases, continuous supervision by a health care provider is advisable.

Administration –

Extended-release capsules: Usually 1 capsule is administered in the morning and 1 capsule in the evening.

METHAZOLAMIDE:

Glaucoma – 50 to 100 mg 2 or 3 times/day. May be used with miotic and osmotic agents.

Actions

Pharmacology: These agents are nonbacteriostatic sulfonamides that inhibit the enzyme carbonic anhydrase. This action reduces the rate of aqueous humor formation, resulting in decreased IOP.

Pharmacokinetics:

Pharmacokinetics of Carbonic Anhydrase Inhibitors

Carbonic anhydrase inhibitor	IOP Lowering Effects			Relative inhibitor potency
	Onset (h)	Peak effect (h)	Duration (h)	
Acetazolamide				
Tablets	1 to 1.5	1 to 4	8 to 12	1
Sustained release capsules	2	3 to 6	18 to 24	
Injection (IV)	2 min	15 min	4 to 5	
Methazolamide	2 to 4	6 to 8	10 to 18	†[a]

[a] † Quantitative data not available; reported to be more active than acetazolamide.

Contraindications

Hypersensitivity to these agents; depressed sodium or potassium serum levels; marked kidney and liver disease or dysfunction; suprarenal gland failure; hyperchloremic acidosis; adrenocortical insufficiency; severe pulmonary obstruction with inability to increase alveolar ventilation since acidosis may be increased (dichlorphenamide); cirrhosis (acetazolamide, methazolamide); long-term use in chronic noncongestive angle-closure glaucoma.

Warnings/Precautions

Dose increases: Increasing the dose of **acetazolamide** does not increase diuresis and may increase drowsiness or paresthesia; it often results in decreased diuresis. However, very large doses have been given with other diuretics to promote diuresis in complete refractory failure.

Pulmonary conditions: These drugs may precipitate or aggravate acidosis. Use with caution in patients with pulmonary obstruction or emphysema when alveolar ventilation may be impaired.

Cross-sensitivity: Cross-sensitivity between antibacterial sulfonamides and sulfonamide derivative diuretics, including acetazolamide and various thiazides, has been reported.

Hepatic function impairment: Use of **methazolamide** in this condition could precipitate hepatic coma.

Pregnancy: Category C.

Lactation: Safety has not been established.

Children: Safety and efficacy for use in children have not been established.

Monitoring: Monitor for hematologic reactions common to sulfonamides. Obtain baseline CBC and platelet counts before therapy and at regular intervals during therapy.

Hypokalemia – Hypokalemia may develop when severe cirrhosis is present, during concomitant use of steroids or ACTH, and with interference with adequate oral electrolyte intake.

Drug Interactions

Drugs that may interact with carbonic anhydrase inhibitors include cyclosporine, primidone, salicylates, and diflunisal.

Adverse Reactions

Sulfonamide-type adverse reactions may occur.

CNS: Convulsions; weakness; malaise; fatigue; nervousness; drowsiness; depression; dizziness; disorientation; confusion; ataxia; tremor; tinnitus; headache.

Dermatologic: Urticaria; pruritus; skin eruptions; rash (including erythema multiforme, Stevens-Johnson syndrome, toxic epidermal necrolysis); photosensitivity.

GI: Melena; anorexia; nausea; vomiting; constipation; taste alteration; diarrhea.

Hematologic: Bone marrow depression; thrombocytopenia; thrombocytopenic purpura; hemolytic anemia; leukopenia; pancytopenia; agranulocytosis.

Renal: Hematuria; glycosuria; urinary frequency.

Miscellaneous: Weight loss; fever; decreased/absent libido; impotence; electrolyte imbalance; hepatic insufficiency.

Chapter 6

RESPIRATORY AGENTS

SYMPATHOMIMETICS

ALBUTEROL	
Tablets: 2 and 4 mg (as sulfate) (*Rx*)	Various
Tablets, extended release: 4 and 8 mg (as sulfate) (*Rx*)	Various, *VoSpire ER* (Dava)
Syrup: 2 mg (as sulfate) per 5 mL (*Rx*)	Various
Aerosol: Delivers 90 mcg (as sulfate)/actuation (*Rx*)	Various, *ProAir HFA* (Teva), *Proventil HFA* (Key), *Ventolin HFA* (GlaxoSmithKline)
Solution for inhalation: 0.083% (2.5 mg per 3 mL) and 0.5% (5 mg/mL) (as sulfate) (*Rx*)	Various, *Proventil* (Schering)
0.021% (0.63 mg per 3 mL) and 0.042% (1.25 mg per 3 mL) (as sulfate) (*Rx*)	Various, *AccuNeb* (Dey)
ARFORMOTEROL TARTRATE	
Solution for inhalation: 15 mcg (equivalent to arformoterol tartrate 22 mcg) (*Rx*)	*Brovana* (Sepracor)
EPHEDRINE SULFATE	
Capsules: 25 mg (*otc*)	Various
Injection: 50 mg/mL (*Rx*)	
EPINEPHRINE	
Aerosol: 0.22 mg epinephrine/spray (*otc*)	Various, *Primatene Mist* (Wyeth)
Solution, inhalation: 2.25% racepinephrine hydrochloride (1.125% epinephrine base) (*otc*)	*S2* (Nephron)
Solution, intranasal: 1:1,000 (1 mg/mL) as hydrochloride (*Rx*)	*Adrenalin Chloride Solution* (JHP Pharmaceuticals)
Injection: 1:10,000 (0.1 mg/mL) (*Rx*)	Various
1:2,000 (0.15 mg per 0.3 mL) (*Rx*)	*EpiPen Jr* (Dey)
1:1,000 (0.15 mg per 0.15 mL) (*Rx*)	*Twinject* (Sciele)
1:1,000 (0.3 mg per 0.3 mL) (*Rx*)	Various, *EpiPen* (Dey)
1:1,000 (1 mg/mL) (*Rx*)	Various
FORMOTEROL FUMARATE	
Solution for inhalation: 20 mcg per 2 mL (*Rx*)	*Perforomist* (Dey)
Inhalation powder in capsules: 12 mcg (*Rx*)	*Foradil Aerolizer* (Schering)
ISOPROTERENOL HYDROCHLORIDE	
Injection: (1:5,000 solution) 0.2 mg/mL (*Rx*)	Various
LEVALBUTEROL	
Solution for inhalation: 0.31 mg per 3 mL (as hydrochloride), 0.63 mg per 3 mL (as hydrochloride), 1.25 mg per 3 mL (as hydrochloride) (*Rx*)	*Xopenex* (Sepracor)
Solution for inhalation, concentrate: 1.25 mg per 0.5 mL (*Rx*)	Various
Aerosol: Delivers 45 mcg/actuation (as tartrate) (*Rx*)	*Xopenex HFA* (Sepracor)
METAPROTERENOL SULFATE	
Tablets: 10 and 20 mg (*Rx*)	Various
Syrup: 10 mg per 5 mL (*Rx*)	
PIRBUTEROL ACETATE	
Aerosol: Delivers 0.2 mg (as acetate)/actuation (*Rx*)	*Maxair Autohaler* (Graceway Pharmaceuticals)
SALMETEROL XINAFOATE	
Powder for inhalation: 50 mcg (as base) (*Rx*)	*Serevent Diskus* (GlaxoSmithKline)
TERBUTALINE SULFATE	
Tablets: 2.5 and 5 mg (*Rx*)	Various
Injection: 1 mg/mL (*Rx*)	

Warning:

Asthma-related death: Long-acting beta-2 agonists may increase the risk of asthma-related death. Data from a large placebo-controlled US study that compared the safety of salmeterol or placebo added to usual asthma therapy showed an increase in asthma-related deaths in patients receiving salmeterol. This finding is considered a class effect of long-acting beta-2 agonists. All long-acting beta-2 agonists are contraindicated in patients with asthma without the use of a long-term asthma control medication. Currently available data are inadequate to determine whether current use of inhaled corticosteroids or other long-term asthma control drugs mitigates the increased risk of asthma related-death from long-acting beta-2 adrenergic agonists.

Because of this risk, use of formoterol for the treatment of asthma without a concomitant long-term asthma control medication, such as an inhaled corticosteroid, is contraindicated. Use formoterol only as additional therapy for patients with asthma who are currently taking but are inadequately controlled on a long-term asthma control medication, such as an inhaled corticosteroid. Once asthma control is achieved and maintained, assess the patient at regular intervals and step down therapy (eg, discontinue long-acting beta-2 agonist) if possible without loss of asthma control and maintain the patient on a long-term asthma control medication, such as an inhaled corticosteroid. Do not use long-acting beta-2 agonists for patients whose asthma is adequately controlled on low- or medium-dose inhaled corticosteroids.

Children and adolescents: Available data from controlled clinical trials suggest that long-acting beta-2 agonists increase the risk of asthma-related hospitalization in children and adolescents. For children and adolescents with asthma who require addition of a long-acting beta-2 agonist to an inhaled corticosteroid, a fixed-dose combination product containing both an inhaled corticosteroid and a long-acting beta-2 agonist should ordinarily be used to ensure adherence with both drugs. In cases where use of a separate long-term asthma control medication (eg, inhaled corticosteroid) and a long-acting beta-2 agonist is clinically indicated, appropriate steps must be taken to ensure adherence with both treatment components. If adherence cannot be ensured, a fixed-dose combination product containing both an inhaled corticosteroid and a long-acting beta-2 agonist is recommended.

Indications

Sympathomimetics: According to the National Asthma Education and Prevention Program's Expert Panel Report II, long-acting beta-2 -agonists (eg, **salmeterol**) are used concomitantly with anti-inflammatory medications for long-term control of symptoms, especially nocturnal symptoms. They also prevent exercise-induced bronchospasm (EIB). Short-acting beta-2 agonists (eg, **albuterol**, **pirbuterol**) are the therapy of choice for relief of acute symptoms and prevention of EIB.

Albuterol: Relief and prevention of bronchospasm in patients with reversible obstructive airway disease; prevention of EIB.

Arformoterol:

Chronic obstructive pulmonary disease (COPD) – For the long-term, twice-daily (morning and evening) maintenance treatment of bronchoconstriction in patients with COPD, including chronic bronchitis and emphysema. Arformoterol is for use by nebulization only.

Ephedrine sulfate:

Asthma – Ephedrine sulfate injection is indicated in the treatment of allergic disorders, such as bronchial asthma. Oral ephedrine is indicated for temporary relief of shortness of breath, tightness of chest, and wheezing caused by bronchial asthma. Eases breathing for asthma patients by reducing spasms of bronchial muscles.

Epinephrine:

Inhalation – For temporary relief of shortness of breath, tightness of chest, and wheezing caused by bronchial asthma.

Injection – To relieve respiratory distress due to bronchospasm, to provide rapid relief of hypersensitivity reactions to drugs and other allergens, and to prolong the action of anesthetics used in local and regional anesthesia.

As a hemostatic agent in treating mucosal congestion of hay fever, rhinitis, and acute sinusitis and in syncope because of complete heart block or carotid sinus hypersensitivity; for symptomatic relief of serum sickness, urticaria, or angioneurotic edema; for resuscitation in cardiac arrest following anesthetic accidents; in simple (open-angle) glaucoma; for relaxation of uterine musculature and to inhibit uterine contractions.

Treatment and prophylaxis of cardiac arrest in the absence of ventricular fibrillation and attacks of transitory atrioventricular (AV) heart block with syncopal seizures (Stokes-Adams syndrome), and to stimulate the heart in syncope due to complete heart block or carotid sinus sensitivity and is used for resuscitation in cardiac arrest following anesthetic accidents.

Formoterol fumarate:

Asthma/Bronchospasm (inhalation powder only) – For the treatment of asthma and in the prevention of bronchospasm only as concomitant therapy with a long-term asthma control medication in adults and children 5 years of age and older with reversible obstructive airways disease, including patients with symptoms of nocturnal asthma.

EIB (inhalation powder only) – For the acute prevention of EIB in adults and children 5 years of age and older when administered on an occasional, as-needed basis.

COPD – For long-term, twice daily (morning and evening) administration in the maintenance of bronchoconstriction in patients with COPD, including chronic bronchitis and emphysema.

Formoterol inhalation solution is not indicated to treat acute deteriorations of COPD.

Isoproterenol:

Injection – Management of bronchospasm during anesthesia.

Isoproterenol and phenylephrine bitartrate: Treatment of bronchospasm associated with acute and chronic asthma; reversible bronchospasm that may be associated with emphysema or chronic bronchitis.

Levalbuterol: For the treatment or prevention of bronchospasm in patients with reversible obstructive airway disease.

Metaproterenol: For bronchial asthma and reversible bronchospasm.

Pirbuterol: Prevention and reversal of bronchospasm in patients 12 years of age and older with reversible bronchospasm, including asthma. Use with or without concurrent theophylline or steroid therapy.

Salmeterol:

Asthma/Bronchospasm – Treatment of asthma and in the prevention of bronchospasm in patients 4 years of age and older with reversible obstructive airway disease, including patients with symptoms of nocturnal asthma.

EIB – Prevention of EIB in patients 4 years of age and older.

COPD – Maintenance treatment of bronchospasm associated with COPD (including emphysema and chronic bronchitis).

Terbutaline: Prevention and reversal of bronchospasm in patients 12 years of age and older with asthma.

Administration and Dosage

ALBUTEROL:

Inhalation aerosol –

Adults and children 4 years of age and older (12 years of age and older for Proventil): 2 inhalations every 4 to 6 hours. In some patients, 1 inhalation every 4 hours may be sufficient. More frequent administration or a larger number of inhalations is not recommended.

Maintenance therapy (Proventil only): For maintenance therapy or to prevent exacerbation of bronchospasm, 2 inhalations 4 times/day should be sufficient.

Prevention of EIB:

Adults and children 4 years of age and older (12 years of age and older for Proventil) – 2 inhalations 15 minutes prior to exercise.

Inhalation solution –

Adults and children 12 years of age and older: 2.5 mg 3 to 4 times/day by nebulization. Dilute 0.5 mL of the 0.5% solution with 2.5 mL sterile normal saline. Deliver over approximately 5 to 15 minutes.

Children 2 to 12 years of age (15 kg or more): 2.5 mg (1 unit dose vial) 3 to 4 times/day by nebulization. Children weighing less than 15 kg who require less than 2.5 mg/dose (ie, less than a full unit dose vial) should use the 0.5% inhalation solution. Deliver over approximately 5 to 15 minutes.

AccuNeb: The usual starting dosage for patients 2 to 12 years of age is 1.25 or 0.63 mg administered 3 or 4 times/day, as needed, by nebulization. More frequent administration is not recommended. Deliver over 5 to 15 minutes. *AccuNeb* has not been studied in the setting of acute attacks of bronchospasm.

Tablets –

Adults and children 12 years of age and older: Usual starting dosage is 2 or 4 mg 3 or 4 times/day. Do not exceed a total daily dose of 32 mg. Use doses greater than 4 mg 4 times/day only when the patient fails to respond. If a favorable response does not occur, cautiously increase stepwise, up to a maximum of 8 mg 4 times/day, as tolerated.

Children 6 to 12 years of age: Usual starting dosage is 2 mg 3 to 4 times/day. For those who fail to respond to the initial starting dosage, cautiously increase stepwise, but do not exceed 24 mg/day in divided doses.

Elderly patients and those sensitive to beta-adrenergic stimulants: Start with 2 mg 3 or 4 times/day. If adequate bronchodilation is not obtained, increase dosage gradually to as much as 8 mg 3 or 4 times/day.

Tablets, extended release –

Adults and children older than 12 years of age: Usual recommended dose is 8 mg every 12 hours; in some patients, 4 mg every 12 hours may be sufficient. In unusual circumstances (eg, low adult body weight), initial doses may be 4 mg every 12 hours and progress to 8 mg every 12 hours according to response. The dose may be cautiously increased stepwise under health care provider supervision to a maximum of 32 mg/day in divided doses (eg, every 12 hours) if symptoms are not controlled.

Children 6 to 12 years of age: Usual recommended dose is 4 mg every 12 hours. The dose may be cautiously increased stepwise under health care provider supervision to a maximum of 24 mg/day in divided doses (eg, every 12 hours) if symptoms are not controlled.

Switching to extended-release tablets: Patients maintained on regular-release albuterol tablets or syrup can be switched to extended-release tablets. A 4 mg extended-release tablet every 12 hours is equivalent to a regular 2 mg tablet every 6 hours. Multiples of this regimen up to the maximum recommended dose also apply.

Syrup –

Adults and children older than 12 years of age: Usual dose is 2 or 4 mg 3 or 4 times/day. Give doses greater than 4 mg 4 times/day only when patient fails to respond. If a favorable response does not occur, cautiously increase, but do not exceed 8 mg 4 times/day.

Children 6 to 12 years of age: Usual starting dose is 2 mg 3 or 4 times/day. If patient does not respond to 2 mg 4 times/day, cautiously increase stepwise. Do not exceed 24 mg/day in divided doses.

Children 2 to 6 years of age: Initiate at 0.1 mg/kg 3 times/day. Do not exceed 2 mg 3 times/day. If the patient does not respond to the initial dose, increase stepwise to 0.2 mg/kg 3 times/day. Do not exceed 4 mg 3 times/day.

Elderly patients and those sensitive to beta-adrenergic stimulation: Restrict initial dose to 2 mg 3 or 4 times/day. Individualize dosage thereafter.

ARFORMOTEROL: 15 mcg administered twice a day (morning and evening) by nebulization.

Maximum dose is 30 mcg/day.

Concomitant therapy – Discontinue use of inhaled, short-acting beta-2 agonists on a regular basis (eg, 4 times a day) and use them only for symptomatic relief of acute respiratory symptoms.

EPHEDRINE SULFATE:

Adults and children 12 years of age and older – Oral dosage is 12.5 to 25 mg every 4 hours, not to exceed 150 mg in 24 hours.

Adults – The usual parenteral dose is 25 to 50 mg administered subcutaneously or intramuscularly (IM), or 5 to 25 mg administered slowly intravenously (IV) repeated every 5 to 10 minutes, if necessary.

Children –

Capsules: For use in children younger than 12 years of age, consult a health care provider.

Injection: The usual subcutaneous, IV, or IM dose is 0.5 to 0.75 mg/kg or 16.7 to 25 mg/m^2 every 4 to 6 hours.

EPINEPHRINE:

Inhalation –

Adults and children 4 years of age and older:

Rx – Treatment should be started at the first symptoms. One to 3 inhalations not more often than every 3 hours.

OTC – Start with 1 inhalation, then wait at least 1 minute. If not relieved, use once more. Do not use again for at least 3 hours. Each inhalation delivers epinephrine 0.22 mg.

Intranasal –

Adults and children 6 years of age and older: Apply locally as drops or spray or with a sterile swab, as required. See product labeling for dilution instructions.

Injection –

Anaphylaxis:

1:1,000 (1 mg/mL) – 0.2 to 1 mg (mL) subcutaneously or intramuscularly (IM). Start with a small dose and increase if required. Repeat every 10 to 15 minutes as needed.

1:10,000 (0.1 mg/mL) – 0.1 to 0.25 mg (1 to 2.5 mL) administered slowly IV. May repeat every 5 to 15 minutes as needed.

Asthma:

1:1,000 (1 mg/mL) – 0.2 to 1 mg (mL) subcutaneously. Start with a small dose and increase if required. May also be given IM, but the subcutaneous route is preferred.

1:10,000 (0.1 mg/mL) – 0.1 to 0.25 mg (1 to 2.5 mL) injected slowly IV.

Cardiac stimulation:

1:1,000 (1 mg/mL) solution – The effect of IV administration of 1:10,000 (0.1 mg/mL) may only last a few minutes, so the IV dose may be followed with 0.3 mg (0.3 mL) of 1:1,000 (1 mg/mL) solution administered subcutaneously.

1:10,000 (0.1 mg/mL) – 0.1 to 1 mg (1 to 10 mL) of 1:10,000 (0.1 mg/mL) solution, repeated every 5 minutes, if necessary. Epinephrine is administered by IV injection and/or, in cardiac arrest, by intracardiac injection.

Intraspinal use – Usual dose is 0.2 to 0.4 mL (0.2 to 0.4 mg) of 1:1,000 (1 mg/mL) solution added to anesthetic spinal fluid mixture. Epinephrine 1:100,000 (0.01 mg/mL) to 1:20,000 (0.05 mg/mL) is the usual concentration employed for use with local anesthetics.

Ophthalmologic use – For producing conjunctival decongestion, controlling hemorrhage, producing mydriasis, and reducing intraocular pressure, use a concentration of 1:10,000 (0.1 mg/mL) to 1:1,000 (1 mg/mL).

FORMOTEROL: Administer formoterol capsules only by the oral inhalation route and only using the *Aerolizer Inhaler*. Do not ingest formoterol (ie, swallowed) orally. Always store capsules in the blister, and only remove immediately before use.

Inhalation solution – Patients should not take the inhalation solution by mouth. It should be administered by the orally inhaled route via a standard jet nebulizer connected to an air compressor.

Inhalation powder – Administer only by the oral inhalation route and only using the inhaler supplied. Patients must not exhale into the device. The inhaler should not be used with any other capsules.

Asthma/Bronchospasm – For adults and children 5 years of age and older, the usual dosage is the inhalation of the contents of one 12 mcg formoterol capsule every 12 hours using the inhaler supplied. The patient must not exhale into the device. The total daily dose of formoterol should not exceed 1 capsule twice daily (24 mcg total daily dose). If symptoms arise between doses, take an inhaled short-acting beta-2 -agonist for immediate relief.

Prevention of EIB – For adults and adolescents 12 years of age and older, the usual dosage is the inhalation of the contents of one 12 mcg formoterol capsule at least 15 minutes before exercise administered on an occasional as-needed basis. Additional doses should not be used for 12 hours after the administration of this drug.

COPD –

Formoterol inhalation powder: The usual dosage is the inhalation of the contents of one 12 mcg capsule every 12 hours using the inhaler supplied. A total daily dose of more than 24 mcg is not recommended.

Formoterol inhalation solution: The recommended dose of formoterol inhalation solution is one 20 mcg unit-dose vial administered twice daily (morning and evening) by nebulization. A total daily dose of more than 40 mcg is not recommended.

ISOPROTERENOL:

Injection – For the management of bronchospasm during anesthesia, dilute 1 mL (0.2 mg) of a 1:5,000 solution to 10 mL with sodium chloride injection or 5% dextrose injection. Administer an initial dose of 0.01 to 0.02 mg (0.5 to 1 mL of diluted solution) IV; repeat when necessary; or use a 1:50,000 undiluted solution and administer an initial dose of 0.01 to 0.02 mg (0.5 to 1 mL).

LEVALBUTEROL:

Xopenex –

Children 6 to 11 years of age: 0.31 mg administered 3 times/day by nebulization. Do not exceed routine dosing of 0.63 mg 3 times/day.

Adults and children 12 years of age and older: 0.63 mg administered 3 times/day, every 6 to 8 hours, by nebulization. Patients 12 years of age and older with more severe asthma or patients who do not respond adequately to a dose of levalbuterol 0.63 mg may benefit from a dosage of 1.25 mg 3 times/day.

Administration: Dilute the concentrated solution (1.25 mg per 0.5 mL) with sterile normal saline before administration by nebulization.

Drug compatibility, efficacy, and safety when mixed with other drugs in a nebulizer have not been established.

Xopenex HFA –

Adults and children 4 years of age and older: 2 inhalations (90 mcg) repeated every 4 to 6 hours; in some patients, 1 inhalation every 4 hours may be sufficient. More frequent administrations or a larger number of inhalations is not routinely recommended. Prime the inhaler before using for the first time and in cases where the inhaler has not been used for more than 3 days by releasing 4 test sprays into the air, away from the face.

Cleaning: To maintain proper use of this product, the actuator must be washed and dried thoroughly at least once a week.

METAPROTERENOL:

Syrup –

Adults: 10 mL (20 mg) 3 or 4 times a day.

Children 9 years of age and older or weight over 60 lbs: 10 mL (20 mg) 3 or 4 times a day.

Children 6 to 9 years of age or weight under 60 lbs: 5 mL (10 mg) 3 or 4 times a day.

Children younger than 6 years of age: Daily doses of approximately 1.3 to 2.6 mg/kg have been well tolerated.

Tablets –

Adults: The usual dose is 20 mg 3 to 4 times daily.

Children:

Aged 6 to 9 years or weight under 60 lbs – 10 mg 3 or 4 times a day.

Older than 9 years or weight over 60 lbs – 20 mg 3 or 4 times a day.

Younger than 6 years of age – Metaproterenol tablets are not recommended for use in children under 6 years at this time.

PIRBUTEROL:

Adults and children 12 years of age and older – 2 inhalations (0.4 mg) repeated every 4 to 6 hours. One inhalation (0.2 mg) may be sufficient for some patients.

Do not exceed a total daily dose of 12 inhalations.

SALMETEROL:

Asthma/Bronchospasm – For asthma/bronchospasm in adults and children 4 years of age and older, use 1 inhalation/disk twice daily (12 hours apart).

Prevention of EIB – 1 inhalation at least 30 minutes before exercise protects patients against EIB. Do not use additional doses of salmeterol for 12 hours after administration of this drug. In patients who are receiving salmeterol twice daily (morning and evening), do not use additional salmeterol for prevention of EIB.

COPD – 1 powder inhalation (50 mcg) twice daily (morning and evening, approximately 12 hours apart).

TERBUTALINE:

Oral –

Adults and children older than 15 years of age: 5 mg, given at 6-hour intervals, 3 times/day during waking hours. If adverse reactions are pronounced, the dose may be reduced to 2.5 mg 3 times/day. Do not exceed 15 mg in 24 hours.

Children 12 to 15 years of age: 2.5 mg 3 times/day. Do not exceed 7.5 mg in 24 hours. Not recommended for children younger than 12 years of age.

Parenteral – Usual dose is 0.25 mg subcutaneously into the lateral deltoid area. If significant improvement does not occur in 15 to 30 minutes, administer a second 0.25 mg dose. Do not exceed a total dose of 0.5 mg in 4 hours. If a patient fails to respond to a second 0.25 mg dose within 15 to 30 minutes, consider other therapeutic measures.

Actions

Pharmacology: These agents are used to produce bronchodilation. They relieve reversible bronchospasm by relaxing the smooth muscles of the bronchioles.

Sympathomimetic Bronchodilators: Pharmacologic Effects and Pharmacokinetic Properties

Sympathomimetic	Adrenergic receptor activity	Beta-2 potency[a]	Route	Onset (min)	Duration (h)
Albuterol[b]	beta-1 < beta-2	2	by mouth	within 30	4 to 8
			inhalation[c]	within 5	3 to 6
Ephedrine	alpha beta-1 beta-2	—	by mouth	15 to 60	3 to 5
			subcutaneous	> 20	≤ 1
			IM	10 to 20	≤ 1
			IV	immediate	—
Epinephrine	alpha beta-1 beta-2	—	subcutaneous	5 to 10	4 to 6
			IM	—	1 to 4
			inhalation[c]	1 to 5	1 to 3
Isoproterenol	beta-1 beta-2	1	IV	immediate	< 1
			inhalation[c]	2 to 5	1 to 3
Metaproterenol[b]	beta-1 < beta-2	15	by mouth	≈ 30	4
Pirbuterol[b]	beta-1 < beta-2	5	inhalation	within 5	5
Salmeterol[b]	beta-1 < beta-2	0.5	inhalation	within 20	12

Sympathomimetic Bronchodilators: Pharmacologic Effects and Pharmacokinetic Properties					
Sympathomimetic	Adrenergic receptor activity	Beta-2 potency[a]	Route	Onset (min)	Duration (h)
Terbutaline[b]	beta-1 < beta-2	4	by mouth	30	4 to 8
			subcutaneous	5 to 15	1.5 to 4
			inhalation	5 to 30	3 to 6

[a] Relative molar potency: 1 = most potent.
[b] These agents all have minor beta-1 activity.
[c] May be administered via aerosol or bulb nebulizer or IPPB administration.

Contraindications

Hypersensitivity to any component (allergic reactions are rare); cardiac arrhythmias associated with tachycardia (**metaproterenol**); angina, preexisting cardiac arrhythmias associated with tachycardia, known hypersensitivity to sympathomimetic amines, and ventricular arrhythmias requiring inotropic therapy, tachycardia, or heart block caused by digitalis intoxication (**isoproterenol**); patients with organic brain damage, local anesthesia of certain areas (eg, fingers, toes) because of the risk of tissue sloughing, labor, cardiac dilatation, coronary insufficiency, cerebral arteriosclerosis, organic heart disease (**epinephrine**); in those cases where vasopressors may be contraindicated; narrow-angle glaucoma, nonanaphylactic shock during general anesthesia with halogenated hydrocarbons or cyclopropane (**epinephrine, ephedrine**).

Warnings/Precautions

Extravasation: Tissue necrosis may develop if extravasation occurs. Accidental injection into the digits, hands, or feet may result in loss of blood flow to the affected area and should be avoided.

Cardiovascular effects: Use with caution in patients with cardiovascular disorders including coronary insufficiency, ischemic heart disease, history of stroke, coronary artery disease, cardiac arrhythmias, congestive heart failure, and hypertension.

Beta-adrenergic agonists can produce significant cardiovascular effects measured by pulse rate, blood pressure, symptoms, or electrocardiogram changes (eg, flattening of T-waves, prolongation of the QTc interval, and ST-segment depression).

Isoproterenol doses sufficient to increase the heart rate more than 130 bpm may increase the likelihood of inducing ventricular arrhythmias.

Ephedrine may cause hypertension resulting in intracranial hemorrhage. It may induce anginal pain in patients with coronary insufficiency or ischemic heart disease.

Large doses of inhaled or oral **salmeterol** (12 to 20 times the recommended dose) have been associated with clinically significant prolongation of the QTc interval, which has the potential for producing ventricular arrhythmias.

Use with short-acting beta-2 agonists: When patients begin treatment with **salmeterol, arformoterol**, or **formoterol**, advise those who have been taking short-acting, inhaled beta-2 agonists on a daily basis to discontinue their regular daily dosing regimen, and clearly instruct them to use short-acting, inhaled beta-2 agonists only for symptomatic relief.

Paradoxical bronchospasm: Occasionally patients have developed severe paradoxical airway resistance with repeated, excessive use of inhalation preparations. Discontinue the drug immediately and institute alternative therapy.

Usual dose response: Advise patients to contact a health care provider if they do not respond to their usual dose of a sympathomimetic amine.

Further therapy with **isoproterenol** aerosol alone is inadvisable when 3 to 5 treatments within 6 to 12 hours produce minimal or no relief.

Do not continue to use epinephrine, and seek medical assistance immediately if symptoms are not relieved within 20 minutes or become worse.

CNS effects: Sympathomimetics may produce CNS stimulation.

Long-term use: Prolonged use of **ephedrine** may produce a syndrome resembling an anxiety state; many patients develop nervousness; a sedative may be needed.

Acute symptoms: If the patient's short-acting, inhaled beta$_2$-agonist becomes less effective (eg, the patient needs more inhalations than usual), medical evaluation must be obtained immediately. Do not use long-acting beta-2 agonists for COPD symptoms.

Excessive use of inhalants: Deaths have been reported; the exact cause is unknown, but cardiac arrest following an unexpected severe acute asthmatic crisis and subsequent hypoxia is suspected.

Morbidity/Mortality: Long-acting beta-2 agonists may increase the risk of asthma-related death. Data from a large, placebo-controlled study compared the safety of **salmeterol** or placebo added to usual asthma therapy and showed and increase in asthma-related deaths in patients receiving **salmeterol**. This finding may apply to other long-acting beta-2 agonists.

Overdosage or inadvertent IV injection: Overdosage or inadvertent IV injection of conventional subcutaneous epinephrine doses may cause extremely elevated arterial pressure, which may result in cerebrovascular hemorrhage, particularly in elderly patients; severe peripheral constriction and cardiac stimulation resulting in pulmonary arterial hypertension and potentially fatal pulmonary edema; and ventricular hyperirritability, which may result in death from ventricular fibrillation.

Tolerance: Tolerance may occur with prolonged use of sympathomimetic agents, but temporary cessation of the drug restores its original effectiveness.

Benzyl alcohol: Benzyl alcohol, contained in some of these products as a preservative, has been associated with a fatal "gasping syndrome" in premature infants.

Parkinson disease: Epinephrine may temporarily increase rigidity and tremor.

Combined therapy: Concomitant use with other sympathomimetic agents is not recommended, as it may lead to deleterious cardiovascular effects. This does not preclude the judicious use of an adrenergic stimulant aerosol bronchodilator in patients receiving tablets. Do not give on a routine basis. If regular coadministration is required, consider alternative therapy.

Do not use 2 or more beta-adrenergic aerosol bronchodilators simultaneously because of the potential of additive effects.

Patients must be warned not to stop or reduce corticosteroid therapy without medical advice, even if they feel better when they are being treated with beta-2-agonists. These agents are not to be used as a substitute for oral or inhaled corticosteroids.

Hypersensitivity reactions: Hypersensitivity reactions can occur after administration of **albuterol, levalbuterol, metaproterenol, terbutaline, ephedrine, salmeterol, arformoterol, formoterol**, and possibly other bronchodilators.

Special risk: Administer with caution to patients with diabetes mellitus, hyperthyroidism, prostatic hypertrophy (**ephedrine**) or history of seizures; elderly; psychoneurotic individuals, patients with long-standing bronchial asthma and emphysema who have developed degenerative heart disease (**epinephrine**).

In patients with status asthmaticus and abnormal blood gas tensions, improvement in vital capacity and blood gas tensions may not accompany apparent relief of bronchospasm following **isoproterenol**.

Diabetes – Large doses of IV **albuterol** and IV **terbutaline** may aggravate preexisting diabetes mellitus and ketoacidosis. Relevance to the use of oral or inhaled albuterol and oral terbutaline is unknown. Diabetic patients receiving any of these agents may require an increase in dosage of insulin or oral hypoglycemic agents.

Drug abuse and dependence: Prolonged abuse of **ephedrine** can lead to symptoms of paranoid schizophrenia. Patients exhibit such signs as tachycardia, poor nutrition and hygiene, fever, cold sweat, and dilated pupils. Some measure of tolerance develops, but addiction does not occur.

Pregnancy: *Category B* (**terbutaline**). *Category C* (**albuterol, levalbuterol, arformoterol, formoterol, ephedrine, epinephrine, isoproterenol, metaproterenol, salmeterol, pirbuterol**).

Labor and delivery – Use of beta-2 active sympathomimetics inhibits uterine contractions. Other reactions include increased heart rate, transient hyperglycemia, hypokalemia, cardiac arrhythmias, pulmonary edema, cerebral and myocardial ischemia, and increased fetal heart rate and hypoglycemia in the neonate. Although these effects are unlikely with aerosol use, consider the potential for untoward effects.

Do not use parenteral **ephedrine** in obstetrics when maternal blood pressure exceeds 130/80.

Lactation: **Terbutaline, ephedrine,** and **epinephrine** are excreted in breast milk. It is not known whether other agents are excreted in breast milk.

Children:

Inhalation – Safety and efficacy for use of **pirbuterol** and **salmeterol** in children 12 years of age and younger have not been established. For **levalbuterol**, safety and efficacy in children younger than 6 years of age (inhalation solution) and 4 years of age (inhalation aerosol) have not been established. Safety and efficacy of **arformoterol** in children have not been established. Safety and efficacy of **formoterol** inhalation powder in children younger than 5 years of age have not been established; **formoterol** inhalation solution is not indicated for use in children. **Albuterol** aerosol in children younger than 4 years of age and **albuterol** solution for inhalation in children younger than 2 years of age have not been established.

Injection – Parenteral **terbutaline** is not recommended for use in children younger than 12 years of age. Administer **epinephrine** with caution to infants and children. Syncope has occurred following administration to asthmatic children.

Oral – **Terbutaline** is not recommended for use in children younger than 12 years of age. Safety and efficacy of **albuterol** have not been established for children younger than 2 years (syrup), 6 years (tablets), and 6 years (tablets, extended release) of age.

Elderly: Lower doses may be required due to increased sympathomimetic sensitivity.

Lab test abnormalities:

Hypokalemia – Decreases in serum potassium levels have occurred, possibly through intracellular shunting, which can produce adverse cardiovascular effects. The decrease is usually transient, not requiring supplementation.

Monitoring: Monitor patients for significant cardiovascular effects, such as pulse rate, blood pressure, and/or ECG changes (eg, flattening of T waves, prolongation of the QTc interval, ST-segment depression).

Drug Interactions

Drugs that may affect sympathomimetics include alpha-adrenergic blockers (eg, phentolamine), antihistamines, beta-blockers (eg, propranolol), cardiac glycosides (eg, digoxin), COMT inhibitors (ie, entacapone, tolcapone), diuretics, ergot alkaloids, furazolidone, general anesthetics (eg, cyclopropane, halothane), guanethidine, levothyroxine, linezolid, methyldopa, MAOIs, nitrites, oxytocic drugs (eg, ergonovine), phenothiazines (eg, chlorpromazine), rauwolfia alkaloids (ie, reserpine), steroids, TCAs (eg, amitriptyline, imipramine), xanthine derivatives (eg, aminophylline, theophylline).

Drugs that may be affected by sympathomimetics include cardiac glycosides (eg, digoxin), diuretics (eg, loop diuretics, thiazide diuretics), ergot alkaloids, guanethidine, MAOIs, xanthine derivatives (eg, aminophylline, theophylline), and bromocriptine.

Adverse Reactions

Sympathomimetic Bronchodilator Adverse Reactions (≥ 3%)[a]

	Adverse reaction	Albuterol	Arformoterol	Ephedrine	Epinephrine	Formoterol	Isoproterenol	Levalbuterol	Metaproterenol	Pirbuterol	Salmeterol	Terbutaline
Cardiovascular	Palpitations	< 1-10		✓[b]	7.8-30	✓[b]	< 5-22		0.3-4	1.3-1.7	1-3	≤ 23
	Tachycardia	1-10		✓	≤ 2.6	✓	2-12	2-12	< 17	1.2-1.3	1-3	1.3-3
	Blood pressure changes/hypertension	1-5			✓	✓	2-5	< 2	0.3			< 1
	Chest tightness/pain/ discomfort, angina	< 3	7		≤ 2.6	1.9–3.2	✓	< 2	0.2	< 1.3		1.3-1.5
	PVCs, arrhythmias, skipped beats			✓	✓	✓	< 1-3			< 1		≈ 4
CNS	Tremor	< 1-24.2	< 2		16-18	1.9	< 15	6.8	1-33	1.3-6	4	< 5-38
	Dizziness/vertigo	< 1-7		✓	3.3-7.8	1.6-2.4	1.5-5	1.4-2.7	1-4	0.6-1.2	≥ 3	1.3-10
	Shakiness/ nervousness/ tension	1-20		✓	8.5-31	✓	< 15	2.8-9.6	2.6-14	4.5-7	1-3	< 5-31
	Drowsiness	< 1			8.2-14		< 5		0.7			< 5-11.7
	Hyperactivity/ Hyperkinesia, excitement	1-20					✓			< 1		
	Headache	2-22		✓	3.3-10	✓	1.5-10	7.6-11.9	≤ 4	1.3-2	28	7.8-10
	Insomnia	1-11		✓	✓	1.5–2.4	1.5	< 2	1.8	< 1		✓
GI	Nausea/Vomiting	2-15		✓	1-11.5	2.4-4.9	< 15	< 10.5	< 14	≤ 1.7	1-3	1.3-10
	Heartburn/GI distress/ disorder	≤ 5					≤ 5-10	1.4-2.7	≤ 4		1-3	< 10
	Dry mouth	< 3				1.2-3.3		< 2	0.4	< 1.3		
	Diarrhea	1	6			4.9		≤ 6	0.7	< 1.3	1-3	
Respiratory	Cough	< 1-5					1-5	1.4-4.1	≤ 4	1.2	7	
	Dyspnea	1.5	4		≤ 2	2.1	≤ 1.5					≤2
	Bronchospasm	1-15.4					≤ 18					
	Throat dryness/ irritation, pharyngitis	≤ 6				3.5	3.1	3-10.4	≤ 4	< 1	≥ 3	✓

[a] Data pooled for all routes of administration, all age groups, from separate studies, and are not necessarily comparable.
[b] ✓ = Reported; no incidence given.

Adverse reactions are generally transient, and no cumulative effects have been reported. It is usually not necessary to discontinue treatment; however, in selected cases, temporarily reduce the dosage.

Albuterol:

Respiratory – Bronchitis (1.5% to 4%); epistaxis (1% to 3%).

Miscellaneous – Increased appetite, stomachache (3%); muscle cramps (1% to 3%).

Isoproterenol:

Respiratory – Bronchitis (5%).

Formoterol:

Respiratory – Upper respiratory tract infection (7.4%); serious asthma exacerbations (some fatal) (up to 6.4%); bronchitis (4.6%); nasopharyngitis (3.3%).

Miscellaneous – Viral infection (17.2%); back pain (4.2%).

Levalbuterol:

Dermatologic – Rash (0% to 7.5%); urticaria (0% to 3%).

Respiratory – Asthma (9% to 9.4%); rhinitis (2.7% to 11.1%); sinusitis (1.4% to 4.2%).

Miscellaneous – Viral infection (6.9% to 12.3%); fever (3% to 9.1%); flu syndrome (1.4% to 4.2%); accidental injury (0% to 9.2%); asthenia (3%); pain (1.4% to 4%).

Metaproterenol:

Metabolic – GI distress (3%).

Salmeterol:

Musculoskeletal – Joint/back pain, muscle cramp/contractions, myalgia/myositis, muscular soreness (1% to 3%).

Respiratory – Nasopharyngitis, upper respiratory tract infection (14%); nasal cavity/sinus disease (6%); lower respiratory tract infection, sinus headache (4%); allergic rhinitis (3% or more); laryngitis, rhinitis, tracheitis/bronchitis (1% to 3%).

Miscellaneous – Giddiness, influenza (3% or more); dental pain, dysmenorrhea, malaise/fatigue, rash/skin eruption, urticaria, viral gastroenteritis (1% to 3%).

XANTHINE DERIVATIVES

AMINOPHYLLINE	
Tablets; oral: 100 mg (equiv. to 79 mg theophylline), 200 mg (equiv. to 158 mg theophylline) (*Rx*)	Various
Injection: 25 mg (equiv. to 19.75 mg theophylline) per mL (*Rx*). For IV use.	Various
DYPHYLLINE	
Tablets; oral: 200 or 400 mg (*Rx*)	Various
Elixir; oral: 100 mg per 15 mL (33.3 or mg per 5 mL) (*Rx*)	*Dylix* (Lunsco)
THEOPHYLLINE	
Tablets, extended-release (12-hour); oral: 100, 200, 300, and 450 mg (*Rx*)	Various, *Theochron* (Caraco Pharmaceutical)
Tablets, extended-release (24 hours): 400 and 600 mg (*Rx*)	Various
Capsules, extended-release (12-hour); oral: 125 and 200 mg (*Rx*)	Various
Capsules, extended-release (24-hour); oral: 100, 200, 300, and 400 mg (*Rx*)	*Theo-24*[a] (Actient Pharmaceuticals)
Elixir; oral: 80 mg per 15 mL (*Rx*)	*Elixophyllin* (Caraco Pharmaceutical)
Injection; solution: 0.8, 1.6, 2, 3.2, and 4 mg/mL(*Rx*)	Various

[a] Patients receiving once daily doses ≥ 13 mg/kg or ≥ 900 mg (whichever is less) should avoid eating a high-fat–content morning meal or should take medication at least 1 hour before eating. If patient cannot comply with this regimen, place on alternative therapy.

Indications

Symptomatic relief or prevention of bronchial asthma and reversible bronchospasm associated with chronic bronchitis and emphysema.

Administration and Dosage

AMINOPHYLLINE:

Individual dosage – Effective use of theophylline occurs when the theophylline concentration is maintained from 10 to 20 mcg/mL.

Although the 20 mcg/mL level remains appropriate as a critical value (above which toxicity is more likely to occur) for safety purposes, additional data indicate that serum theophylline concentrations required to produce maximum physiologic benefit may fluctuate with the degree of bronchospasm.

Calculate dosage on the basis of lean (ideal) body weight where mg/kg doses are presented.

Dosage guidelines –

Note: Status asthmaticus should be considered a medical emergency. Optimal therapy for such patients frequently requires parenterally administered additional medication and close monitoring, preferably in an intensive care setting.

Theophylline Oral Dosing Initiation and Titration in Children (1 to 15 Years of Age) and Adults (16 to 60 Years of Age)[a]		
Titration step	Children < 45 kg	Children > 45 kg and adults
Starting dosage	12 to 14 (15.2 to 17.7[b]) mg/kg/day up to a maximum of 300 (380[b]) mg/day divided every 4 to 6 h	300 (380[b]) divided every 6 to 8 h
After 3 days, if tolerated, increase dosage to:	16 (20.3[b]) mg/kg/day up to a maximum of 400 (507[b]) mg/day divided every 4 to 6 h	400 (507[b]) mg/day divided every 6 to 8 h
After 3 more days, if tolerated, increase dosage to:	20 (25.3[b]) mg/kg/day up to a maximum of 600 (760[b]) mg/day divided every 4 to 6 h	600 (760[b]) mg/day divided every 6 to 8 h

[a] Patients with more rapid metabolism, clinically identified by higher than average dose requirements, should receive a smaller dose more frequently to prevent breakthrough symptoms resulting from low trough concentrations before the next dose. A reliably absorbed slow-release formulation will decrease fluctuations and permit longer dosing intervals.
[b] Aminophylline equivalent.

Patients with risk factors for impaired clearance, elderly patients (older than 60 years of age), and those in whom it is not feasible to monitor theophylline concentrations – In children 1 to 15 years of age, the final theophylline dose should not exceed 16 mg/kg/day (equivalent to aminophylline 20.3 mg), up to a maximum of 400 mg/day (equivalent to aminophylline 507 mg) in the presence of risk factors for reduced theophylline clearance or if it is not feasible to monitor serum theophylline concentrations. In adolescents 16 years of age and adults, including elderly patients, the final theophylline dose should not exceed 400 mg/day (equivalent to aminophylline 507 mg) in the presence of risk factors for reduced theophylline clearance or if it is not feasible to monitor serum theophylline concentrations.

Loading dose for acute bronchodilation – A single dose of theophylline 5 mg/kg in a patient who has not received any theophylline in the previous 24 hours will produce an average peak serum theophylline concentration of 10 mcg/mL (range, 5 to 15 mcg/mL). If dosing with theophylline is to be continued beyond the loading dose, the previous guidelines should be used and serum theophylline concentration monitored at 24-hour intervals to adjust final dosage.

Dosage adjustment –

Dosage Adjustment Based on Serum Theophylline Concentration	
Peak serum concentration	Dosage adjustment
< 9.9 mcg/mL	If symptoms are not controlled and current dosage is tolerated, increase dose about 25%. Recheck serum concentration after 3 days for further dosage adjustment.
10 to 14.9 mcg/mL	If symptoms are controlled and current dosage is tolerated, maintain dose and recheck serum concentration at 6- to 12-month intervals.[a] If symptoms are not controlled and current dosage is tolerated, consider adding additional medication(s) to treatment regimen.
15 to 19.9 mcg/mL	Consider a 10% decrease in dose to provide greater margin of safety even if current dosage is tolerated.[a]
20 to 24.9 mcg/mL	Decrease dose by 25%, even if no adverse reactions are present. Recheck serum concentration after 3 days to guide further dosage adjustment.

Dosage Adjustment Based on Serum Theophylline Concentration	
Peak serum concentration	Dosage adjustment
25 to 30 mcg/mL	Skip next dose and decrease subsequent doses at least 25%, even if no adverse reactions are present. Recheck serum concentration after 3 days to guide further dosage adjustment. If symptomatic, consider whether overdose treatment is indicated.
> 30 mcg/mL	Treat overdose as indicated. If theophylline is subsequently resumed, decrease dose by at least 50% and recheck serum concentration after 3 days to guide further dosage adjustment.

[a] Dose reduction and/or serum theophylline concentration measurement is indicated whenever adverse reactions are present, physiologic abnormalities that can reduce theophylline clearance occur (eg, sustained fever), or a drug that interacts with theophylline is added or discontinued.

Aminophylline injection –

Dosage: In a patient who has received no theophylline in the previous 24 hours, a loading dose of theophylline 4.6 mg/kg IV (5.7 mg/kg as aminophylline), calculated on the basis of ideal body weight and administered over 30 minutes, on average, will produce a maximum postdistribution serum concentration of 10 mcg/mL, with a range of 6 to 16 mcg/mL. When a loading dose becomes necessary in the patient who has already received theophylline, estimation of the serum concentration based upon the history is unreliable, and an immediate serum level determination is indicated.

A loading dose should not be given before obtaining a serum theophylline concentration if the patient has received any theophylline in the previous 24 hours.

A serum concentration obtained 30 minutes after an IV loading dose, when distribution is complete, can be used to assess the need for and size of subsequent loading doses, if clinically indicated, and for guidance of continuing therapy. Once a serum concentration of 10 to 15 mcg/mL has been achieved with the use of a loading dose(s), a constant IV infusion is started.

The following table contains initial theophylline infusion rates following an appropriate loading dose recommended for patients in various age groups and clinical circumstances.

Initial Theophylline Infusion Rates Following an Appropriate Loading Dose		
Patient population	Age	Theophylline infusion rate (mg/kg/h)[a], [b]
Neonates	≤ 24 days (postnatal)	1 mg/kg every 12 h[c]
	> 24 days (postnatal)	1.5 mg/kg every 12 h[c]
Infants	6 to 52 wk	mg/kg/h = 0.008 × age in wk + 0.21
Young children	1 to 9 y	0.8
Older children	9 to 12 y	0.7
Adolescents (cigarette or marijuana smokers)	12 to 16 y	0.7
Adolescents (nonsmokers)	12 to 16 y	0.5[d]
Adults (otherwise healthy nonsmokers)	16 to 60 y	0.4[d]
Elderly patients	> 60 y	0.3[e]

Initial Theophylline Infusion Rates Following an Appropriate Loading Dose		
Patient population	Age	Theophylline infusion rate (mg/kg/h)[a], [b]
Cardiac decompensation, cor pulmonale, hepatic function impairment, sepsis with multiorgan failure, or shock		0.2[e]

[a] To achieve a target concentration of 10 mcg/mL, aminophylline = theophylline divided by 0.8. Use ideal body weight for obese patients.
[b] Lower initial dosage may be required for patients receiving other drugs that decrease theophylline clearance (eg, cimetidine).
[c] To achieve a target concentration of 7.5 mcg/mL for neonatal apnea.
[d] Not to exceed 900 mg/day, unless serum levels indicate the need for a larger dose.
[e] Not to exceed 400 mg/day, unless serum levels indicate the need for a larger dose.

Final Dosage Adjustment Based on Serum Theophylline Concentration	
Peak serum concentration	Dosage adjustment
< 9.9 mcg/mL	If symptoms are not controlled and current dosage is tolerated, increase infusion rate by approximately 25%. Recheck serum concentration after 12 hours in children and 24 hours in adults for further dosage adjustments.
10 to 14.9 mcg/mL	If symptoms are controlled and current dosage is tolerated, maintain infusion rate and recheck serum concentration at 24-hour intervals.[a] If symptoms are not controlled and current dosage is tolerated, consider adding additional medication(s) to treatment regimen.
15 to 19.9 mcg/mL	Consider 10% decrease in infusion rate to provide greater margin of safety, even if current dosage is tolerated.[a]
20 to 24.9 mcg/mL	Decrease infusion rate by 25%, even if no adverse reactions are present. Recheck serum concentration after 12 hours in children and 24 hours in adults to guide further dosage adjustment.
25 to 30 mcg/mL	Stop infusion for 12 hours in children and 24 hours in adults and decrease subsequent infusion rate at least 25%, even if no adverse reactions are present. Recheck serum concentration after 12 hours in children and 24 hours in adults to guide further dosage adjustment. If symptomatic, stop infusion and consider whether overdose treatment is indicated.
> 30 mcg/mL	Stop the infusion and treat overdose as indicated. If theophylline is subsequently resumed, decrease infusion rate by at least 50% and recheck serum concentration after 12 hours in children and 24 hours in adults to guide further dosage adjustment.

[a] Dose reduction and/or serum theophylline concentration measurement is indicated whenever adverse reactions are present, physiologic abnormalities that can reduce theophylline clearance occur (eg, sustained fever), or a drug that interacts with theophylline is added or discontinued.

Special populations – In patients with cor pulmonale, cardiac decompensation, or hepatic function impairment, or in those taking drugs that markedly reduce theophylline clearance (eg, cimetidine), the initial theophylline infusion rate should not exceed 17 mg/h (21 mg/h as aminophylline), unless serum concentrations can be monitored at 24-hour intervals. In these patients, 5 days may be required before steady state is reached.

DYPHYLLINE: Dyphylline is a derivative of theophylline; it is not a theophylline salt and is not metabolized to theophylline in vivo. Although dyphylline is 70% theophylline by molecular weight ratio, the amount of dyphylline equivalent to a given amount of theophylline is not known. Specific dyphylline serum levels may be used to monitor therapy; serum theophylline levels will not measure dyphylline. The minimal effective therapeutic concentration is 12 mcg/mL.

Tablets –

Adults: Up to 15 mg/kg every 6 hours.

Elixir –

Adults: 30 to 60 mL (2 to 4 tablespoons) every 6 hours.

Renal function impairment – Appropriate dosage adjustments should be made in patients with renal function impairment.

Children – Safety and efficacy have not been established.

THEOPHYLLINE: Individualize dosage. Base dosage adjustments on clinical response and improvement in pulmonary function. Monitor serum levels to maintain levels in the therapeutic range of 10 to 20 mcg/mL.

Calculate dosages on the basis of lean body weight. Dosages should be equivalent based on anhydrous theophylline content.

Individualize frequency of dosing – With immediate-release products, dosing every 6 hours is generally required, especially in children; intervals 8 hours or less may be satisfactory in adults. When converting from an immediate-release to a sustained-release product, the total daily dose should remain the same, and only the dosing interval adjusted.

Infants younger than 1 year of age (Elixophyllin) –

Theophylline Dosing Initiation and Titration in Infants < 1 Year of Age[a]

Age	Initial dosage	Final dosage
Premature neonates		Adjusted to maintain a peak steady-state serum theophylline concentration of 5 to 10 mcg/mL in neonates and 10 to 15 mcg/mL in older infants. Because the time required to reach steady state is a function of theophylline half-life, up to 5 days may be required to achieve steady state in a premature neonate, while only 2 to 3 days may be required in an infant 6 months of age without other risk factors for impaired clearance in the absence of a loading dose. If a serum theophylline concentration is obtained before steady state is achieved, the maintenance dose should not be increased, even if the serum theophylline concentration is less than 10 mcg/mL.
< 24 days postnatal	1 mg/kg every 12 hours	
≥ 24 days postnatal	1.5 mg/kg every 12 hours	
Full term infants and infants ≤ 52 weeks of age		
Up to 26 weeks of age	Divide dose[a] into 3 equal amounts administered at 8-hour intervals	
26 weeks of age and older	Divide dose[a] into 4 equal amounts administered at 6-hour intervals	

[a] Total daily dose (mg) = ([0.2 × age in weeks] + 5) × (kg body weight)

Children less than 45 kg without risk factors for impaired clearance –

Theophylline Dosing Initiation and Titration for Children < 45 kg Without Risk Factors for Impaired Clearance

Titration step	Children (1 to 15 years of age)	Children (1 to 15 years of age)	Children (6 to 15 years of age)	Children (12 to 15 years of age)
	Elixophyllin	Theophylline extended-release capsules	Theophylline extended-release tablets, *Theochron*	*Theo-24, Uniphyl*
Starting dosage	12 to 14 mg/kg/day, up to a maximum of 300 mg/day divided every 4 to 6 hours[a]	12 to 14 mg/kg/day, up to a maximum of 300 mg/day divided every 8 to 12 hours[a]	12 to 14 mg/kg/day, up to a maximum of 300 mg/day divided every 12 hours[a]	12 to 14 mg/kg/day, up to a maximum of 300 mg/day given once every 24 hours[a]

Theophylline Dosing Initiation and Titration for Children < 45 kg Without Risk Factors for Impaired Clearance				
	Children (1 to 15 years of age)	Children (1 to 15 years of age)	Children (6 to 15 years of age)	Children (12 to 15 years of age)
Titration step	*Elixophyllin*	Theophylline extended-release capsules	Theophylline extended-release tablets, *Theochron*	*Theo-24, Uniphyl*
After 3 days, if tolerated, increase dose to:	16 mg/kg/day, up to a maximum of 400 mg/day divided every 4 to 6 hours[a]	16 mg/kg/day, up to a maximum of 400 mg/day divided every 8 to 12 hours[a]	16 mg/kg/day, up to a maximum of 400 mg/day divided every 12 hours[a]	16 mg/kg/day, up to a maximum of 400 mg/day given once every 24 hours[a]
After 3 more days, if tolerated and needed, increase dose to:	20 mg/kg/day, up to a maximum of 600 mg/day divided every 4 to 6 hours[a]	20 mg/kg/day, up to a maximum of 600 mg/day divided every 8 to 12 hours[a]	20 mg/kg/day, up to a maximum of 600 mg/day divided every 12 hours[a]	20 mg/kg/day, up to a maximum of 600 mg/day given once every 24 hours[a]

[a] Patients with more rapid metabolism, clinically identified by higher-than-average dose requirements, should receive a smaller dose more frequently to prevent breakthrough symptoms resulting from low trough concentrations before the next dose. A reliably-absorbed, slow-release formulation will decrease fluctuations and permit longer dosing intervals.

Children 45 kg or more and adults without risk factors for impaired clearance –

Theophylline Dosing Initiation and Titration for Children > 45 kg and Adults Without Risk Factors for Impaired Clearance				
Titration step	*Elixophyllin*	Theophylline extended-release capsules	Theophylline extended-release tablets, *Theochron*	*Theo-24, Uniphyl*
Starting dosage	300 mg/day divided every 6 to 8 hours[b]	300 mg/day divided every 8 to 12 hours[b]	300 mg/day divided every 12 hours[b]	300 to 400 mg/day[a] given once every 24 hours[b]
After 3 days, if tolerated, increase dose to:	400 mg/day divided every 6 to 8 hours[b]	400 mg/day divided every 8 to 12 hours[b]	400 mg/day divided every 12 hours[b]	400 to 600 mg/day[a] given once every 24 hours[b]
After 3 more days, if tolerated and needed, increase dose to:	600 mg/day divided every 6 to 8 hours[b]	600 mg/day divided every 8 to 12 hours[b]	600 mg/day divided every 12 hours[b]	As with all theophylline products, doses greater than 600 mg should be titrated according to blood level.

[a] If caffeine-like adverse reactions occur, consideration should be given to a lower dose and titrating the dose more slowly.

[b] Patients with more rapid metabolism, clinically identified by higher-than-average dose requirements, should receive a smaller dose more frequently to prevent breakthrough symptoms resulting from low trough concentrations before the next dose. A reliably-absorbed, slow-release formulation will decrease fluctuations and permit longer dosing intervals.

Patients with risk factors for impaired clearance, elderly patients older than 60 years of age, and patients not feasible to monitor serum theophylline concentrations –

Theophylline Dosing in Patients With Risk Factors for Impaired Clearance, Patients ≥ 60 Years of Age, and Patients Not Feasible to Monitor Serum Theophylline Concentrations	
Patients with risk factor	Theophylline dose
Theo-24, Uniphyl	
Children 12 to 15 years of age	Final theophylline dose should not exceed 16 mg/kg/day, up to a maximum of 400 mg/day
Adolescents 16 years of age and older and adults, including elderly patients	Final theophylline dose should not exceed 400 mg/day

Theophylline Dosing in Patients With Risk Factors for Impaired Clearance, Patients ≥ 60 Years of Age, and Patients Not Feasible to Monitor Serum Theophylline Concentrations	
Patients with risk factor	Theophylline dose
Elixophyllin, theophylline extended-release capsules	
Children 1 to 15 years of age	Final theophylline dose should not exceed 16 mg/kg/day, up to a maximum of 400 mg/day
Adolescents 16 years of age and older and adults, including elderly patients	Final theophylline dose should not exceed 400 mg/day
Theophylline extended-release tablets, *Theochron*	
Children 6 to 15 years of age	Final theophylline dose should not exceed 16 mg/kg/day, up to a maximum of 400 mg/day
Adolescents 16 years of age and older and adults, including elderly patients	Final theophylline dose should not exceed 400 mg/day

Dosage adjustment guided by serum theophylline concentrations –

Dosage Adjustment Guided by Serum Theophylline Concentrations	
Theophylline concentration	Theophylline dosage adjustment
< 9.9 mcg/mL	If symptoms are not controlled and current dosage is tolerated, increase dose about 25%. Recheck serum concentration after 3 days for further dosage adjustment.
10 to 14.9 mcg/mL	If symptoms are controlled and current dosage is tolerated, maintain dose and recheck serum concentration at 6- to 12-month intervals.[a] If symptoms are not controlled and current dosage is tolerated, consider adding additional medication(s) to treatment regimen.
15 to 19.9 mcg/mL	Consider 10% decrease in dose to provide greater margin of safety, even if current dosage is tolerated.[a]
20 to 24.9 mcg/mL	Decrease dose by 25%, even if no adverse reactions are present. Recheck serum concentration after 3 days to guide further dosage adjustment.
25 to 30 mcg/mL	Skip next dose and decrease subsequent doses at least 25%, even if no adverse reactions are present. Recheck serum concentration after 3 days to guide further dosage adjustment. If symptomatic, consider whether overdose treatment is indicated.
> 30 mcg/mL	Treat overdose as indicated. If theophylline is subsequently resumed, decrease dose by at least 50% and recheck serum concentration after 3 days to guide further dosage adjustment.

[a] Dose reduction and/or serum theophylline concentration measurement is indicated whenever adverse reactions are present, physiologic abnormalities that can reduce theophylline clearance occur (eg, sustained fever), or a drug that interacts with theophylline is added or discontinued.

Once-daily dosing – Once-daily dosing should be considered only after the patient has been gradually and satisfactorily treated to therapeutic levels with every-12-hours dosing. Once-daily dosing should be based on the dosing guidelines in the previous tables and should be initiated at the end of the last every-12-hour dosing interval. If symptoms recur or signs of toxicity appear during the once-daily dosing interval, dosing on the every-12-hours basis should be reinstituted.

Loading dose for acute bronchodilation – A single 5 mg/kg dose of theophylline in a patient who has not received any theophylline in the previous 24 hours will produce an average peak serum theophylline concentration of 10 mcg/mL (range, 5 to 15 mcg/mL). If dosing with theophylline is to be continued beyond the loading dose, follow the guidelines in the previous tables and monitor serum theophylline concentrations at 24-hour intervals to adjust final dosage.

Theophylline injection – In a patient who has received no theophylline in the previous 24 hours, a loading dose of theophylline 4.6 mg/kg IV, calculated on the basis of ideal body weight and administered over 30 minutes, on average, will produce a maximum postdistribution serum concentration of 10 mcg/mL, with a range of 6 to 16 mcg/mL. When a loading dose becomes necessary in the patient who has already received theophylline, estimation of the serum concentration based upon the history is unreliable and an immediate serum level determination is indicated.

A serum concentration obtained 30 minutes after an IV loading dose, when distribution is complete, can be used to assess the need for and size of subsequent loading doses, if clinically indicated, and for guidance of continuing therapy. Once a serum concentration of 10 to 15 mcg/mL has been achieved with the use of a loading dose(s), a constant IV infusion is started.

Initial Theophylline Infusion Rates Following an Appropriate Loading Dose

Patient population	Age	Theophylline infusion rate (mg/kg/h)[a,b]
Neonates	Postnatal age ≤ 24 days	1 mg/kg every 12 h[c]
	Postnatal age > 24 days	1.5 mg/kg every 12 h[c]
Infants	6 to 52 weeks	mg/kg/h = (0.008) (age in weeks) + 0.21
Young children	1 to 9 years	0.8
Older children	9 to 12 years	0.7
Adolescents (cigarette or marijuana smokers)	12 to 16 years	0.7
Adolescents (nonsmokers)	12 to 16 years	0.5[d]
Adults (otherwise healthy nonsmokers)	16 to 60 years	0.4[d]
Elderly	> 60 years	0.3[e]
Cardiac decompensation, cor pulmonale, liver function impairment, sepsis with multiorgan failure, or shock		0.2[e]

[a] To achieve a target concentration of 10 mcg/mL, use ideal body weight for obese patients.
[b] Lower initial dosage may be required for patients receiving other drugs that decrease theophylline clearance (eg, cimetidine).
[c] To achieve a target concentration of 7.5 mcg/mL for neonatal apnea.
[d] Not to exceed 900 mg/day, unless serum levels indicate the need for a larger dose.
[e] Not to exceed 400 mg/day, unless serum levels indicate the need for a larger dose.

Dosage adjustment based on serum theophylline concentration: The following table contains recommendations for final theophylline dosage adjustment based on serum theophylline concentrations.

Theophylline Final Dosage Adjustment Guided by Serum Concentration	
Peak serum concentration	Dosage adjustment
< 9.9 mcg/mL	If symptoms are not controlled and current dosage is tolerated, increase infusion rate about 25%. Recheck serum concentration after 12 hours in children and 24 hours in adults for further dosage adjustment.
10 to 14.9 mcg/mL	If symptoms are controlled and current dosage is tolerated, maintain infusion rate and recheck serum concentration at 24-hour intervals.[a] If symptoms are not controlled and current dosage is tolerated, consider adding additional medication(s) to treatment regimen.
15 to 19.9 mcg/mL	Consider a 10% decrease in infusion rate to provide greater margin of safety, even if current dosage is tolerated.[a]
20 to 24.9 mcg/mL	Decrease infusion rate by 25%, even if no adverse reactions are present. Recheck serum concentration after 12 hours in children and 24 hours in adults to guide further dosage adjustment.
25 to 30 mcg/mL	Stop infusion for 12 hours in children and 24 hours in adults and decrease subsequent infusion rate at least 25%, even if no adverse reactions are present. Recheck serum concentration after 12 hours in children and 24 hours in adults to guide further dosage adjustment. If symptomatic, stop infusion and consider whether overdose treatment is indicated.
> 30 mcg/mL	Stop the infusion and treat overdose as indicated (see recommendations for chronic overdosage). If theophylline is subsequently resumed, decrease infusion rate by at least 50% and recheck serum concentration after 12 hours in children and 24 hours in adults to guide further dosage adjustment.

[a] Dose reduction and/or serum theophylline concentration measurement is indicated whenever adverse reactions are present, physiologic abnormalities that can reduce theophylline clearance occur (eg, sustained fever), or a drug that interacts with theophylline is added or discontinued.

Actions

Pharmacology: The methylxanthines (theophylline, its soluble salts and derivatives) directly relax the smooth muscle of the bronchi and pulmonary blood vessels, stimulate the CNS, induce diuresis, increase gastric acid secretion, reduce lower esophageal sphincter pressure, and inhibit uterine contractions. Theophylline is also a central respiratory stimulant. Aminophylline has a potent effect on diaphragmatic contractility in healthy people and may then be capable of reducing fatigability, thereby improving contractility in patients with chronic obstructive airways disease.

Pharmacokinetics:

Absorption – Theophylline is well absorbed from oral liquids and uncoated plain tablets; maximal plasma concentrations are reached in 2 hours. Rectal absorption from suppositories is slow and erratic; the oral route is generally preferred. Enteric-coated tablets and some sustained-release dosage forms may be unreliably absorbed.

Distribution – Average volume of distribution is 0.45 L/kg (range, 0.3 to 0.7 L/kg). Theophylline does not distribute into fatty tissue. Approximately 40% is bound to plasma protein. Therapeutic serum levels generally range from 10 to 20 mcg/mL.

Metabolism/Excretion – Xanthines are biotransformed in the liver (85% to 90%) to 1, 3-dimethyluric acid, 3-methylxanthine and 1-methyluric acid; 3-methylxanthine accumulates in concentrations approximately 25% of those of theophylline.

Excretion is by the kidneys; less than 15% of the drug is excreted unchanged. Elimination kinetics vary greatly. Plasma elimination half-life averages about 3 to

15 hours in adult nonsmokers, 4 to 5 hours in adult smokers (1 to 2 packs per day), 1 to 9 hours in children, and 20 to 30 hours for premature neonates. In neonates, theophylline is metabolized partially to caffeine. The premature neonate excretes approximately 50% unchanged theophylline and may accumulate the caffeine metabolite. A prolonged half-life may occur in congestive heart failure, liver dysfunction, alcoholism, respiratory infections, and patients receiving certain other drugs (see Drug Interactions).

Equivalent dose –

Theophylline Content and Equivalent Dose of Various Theophylline Salts

Theophylline salts	Theophylline (%)	Equivalent dose (mg)
Theophylline anhydrous	100	100
Theophylline monohydrate	91	110
Aminophylline anhydrous	86	116
Aminophylline dihydrate	79	127
Oxtriphylline	64	156

Dyphylline – Dyphylline, a chemical derivative of theophylline, is not a theophylline salt as are the other agents. It is about one-tenth as potent as theophylline. Following oral administration, dyphylline is 68% to 82% bioavailable. Peak plasma concentrations are reached within 1 hour, and its half-life is 2 hours. The minimal effective therapeutic concentration is 12 mcg/mL. It is not metabolized to theophylline, and 83% ± 5% is excreted unchanged in the urine.

Contraindications

Hypersensitivity to any xanthine; peptic ulcer; underlying seizure disorders (unless receiving appropriate anticonvulsant medication).

Aminophylline: Hypersensitivity to ethylenediamine.

Aminophylline rectal suppositories: Irritation or infection of rectum or lower colon.

Warnings/Precautions

Status asthmaticus: Status asthmaticus is a medical emergency and is not rapidly responsive to usual doses of conventional bronchodilators. Oral theophylline products alone are not appropriate for status asthmaticus.

Toxicity: Excessive doses may cause severe toxicity; monitor serum levels to ensure maximum benefit with minimum risk.

Serious adverse effects such as ventricular arrhythmias, convulsions, or even death may appear as the first sign of toxicity without previous warning. Less serious signs of toxicity (eg, nausea, restlessness) may occur frequently when initiating therapy but are usually transient; when such signs are persistent during maintenance therapy, they are often associated with serum concentrations greater than 20 mcg/mL. Serious toxicity is not reliably preceded by less severe adverse effects.

Cardiac effects: Theophylline may cause dysrhythmias or worsen pre-existing arrhythmias.

Use with caution: Cardiac disease; hypoxemia; hepatic disease; hypertension; congestive heart failure; alcoholism; elderly (particularly men); and neonates.

GI effects: Use cautiously in peptic ulcer. Local irritation may occur; centrally mediated GI effects may occur with serum levels are greater than 20 mcg/mL. Reduced lower esophageal pressure may cause reflux, aspiration, and worsening of airway obstruction.

Pregnancy: Category C.

Lactation: Theophylline distributes readily into breast milk.

Children: Sufficient numbers of infants younger than 1 year of age have not been studied in clinical trials to support use in this age group; however, there is evidence that the use of dosage recommendations for older infants and young children may result in the development of toxic serum levels.

Drug Interactions

Agents that may decrease theophylline levels include aminoglutethimide, barbiturates, carbamazepine, charcoal, hydantoins, isoniazid, ketoconazole, loop diuretics, rifampin, smoking (cigarettes and marijuana), sulfinpyrazone, sympathomimetics (beta-agonists), and thioamines.

Agents that may increase theophylline levels include allopurinol, beta blockers (nonselective), calcium channel blockers, carbamazepine, cimetidine, corticosteroids, disulfiram, ephedrine, influenza virus vaccine, interferon, isoniazid, loop diuretics, macrolides, mexiletine, oral contraceptives, quinolones, thiabendazole, and thyroid hormones.

The following agents may be affected by theophylline: benzodiazepines, beta-agonists, halothane, ketamine, lithium, nondepolarizing muscle relaxants, propofol, ranitidine, and tetracyclines. Probenecid may increase the effects of dyphylline.

Drug/Food interactions: Theophylline elimination is increased (half-life shortened) by a low carbohydrate, high protein diet and charcoal broiled beef (because of a high polycyclic carbon content). Conversely, elimination is decreased (prolonged half-life) by a high carbohydrate, low protein diet. Food may alter the bioavailability and absorption pattern of certain sustained-release preparations. Some sustained-release preparations may be subject to rapid release of their contents when taken with food, resulting in toxicity. It appears that consistent administration in the fasting state allows predictability of effects.

Adverse Reactions

Adverse reactions/toxicity are uncommon at serum theophylline levels less than 20 mcg/mL.

Levels greater than 20 mcg/mL – Diarrhea, headache, insomnia, irritability, nausea, and vomiting.

Levels greater than 35 mcg/mL – Brain damage, cardiac arrhythmias, death, hyperglycemia, hypotension, seizures, tachycardia (greater than 10 mcg/mL in premature newborns).

Other – Alopecia, fever, flushing, hyperglycemia, inappropriate antidiuretic hormone syndrome, and rash. Ethylenediamine in aminophylline can cause sensitivity reactions, including exfoliative dermatitis and urticaria.

Cardiovascular: Circulatory failure, extrasystoles, hypotension, life-threatening ventricular arrhythmias, palpitations, tachycardia.

CNS: Convulsions, headache, insomnia, irritability; muscle twitching, reflex hyperexcitability, and restlessness.

GI: Diarrhea, epigastric pain, hematemesis, nausea, rectal irritation or bleeding (aminophylline suppositories), vomiting. Therapeutic doses of theophylline may induce gastroesophageal reflux during sleep or while recumbent, increasing the potential for aspiration, which can aggravate bronchospasm.

Renal: Potentiation of diuresis, proteinuria.

Respiratory: Respiratory arrest, tachypnea.

CORTICOSTEROIDS

BECLOMETHASONE	
Aerosol: 40 and 80 mcg/actuation (*Rx*)	QVAR (IVAX)
BUDESONIDE	
Powder: 90 mcg (each actuation delivers ≈ 80 mcg) per metered dose and 180 mcg (each actuation delivers ≈ 160 mcg) per metered dose (*Rx*)	*Pulmicort Flexhaler* (AstraZeneca)
Inhalation suspension: 0.25 mg per 2 mL, 0.5 mg per 2 mL (*Rx*)	Various, *Pulmicort Respules* (AstraZeneca)
1 mg per 2 mL (*Rx*)	*Pulmicort Respules* (AstraZeneca)
CICLESONIDE	
Solution; inhalation: 80 and 160 mcg/actuation (*Rx*)	*Alvesco* (Sepracor)
FLUNISOLIDE	
Aerosol: Each actuation delivers ≈ 250 mcg (*Rx*)	*AeroBid* (Forest), *AeroBid-M* (Forest)
Each actuation delivers ≈ 80 mcg flunisolide hemihydrate (78 mcg flunisolide) (*Rx*)	*AeroSpan* (Forest)
FLUTICASONE	
Aerosol: 44, 110, and 220 mcg/actuation (*Rx*)	*Flovent HFA* (GlaxoSmithKline)
Powder for inhalation: 50, 100, and 250 mcg/actuation (*Rx*)	*Flovent Diskus* (GlaxoSmithKline)
MOMETASONE	
Powder for inhalation: 110 mcg (delivers mometasone furoate 100 mcg)/actuation (*Rx*)	*Asmanex Twisthaler* (Schering)
220 mcg (delivers mometasone furoate 200 mcg)/actuation (*Rx*)	*Asmanex Twisthaler* (Schering)
TRIAMCINOLONE	
Aerosol; inhalation: 75 mcg per actuation (*Rx*)	*Azmacort* (KOS)

Warning:

Particular care is needed in patients who are transferred from systemically active corticosteroids to inhaled corticosteroids because deaths because of adrenal insufficiency have occurred in patients with asthma during and after transfer from systemic corticosteroids to aerosol corticosteroids. After withdrawal from systemic corticosteroids, a number of months are required for recovery of hypothalamic-pituitary-adrenal (HPA) function. Patients who have been previously maintained on 20 mg/day or more of prednisone (or its equivalent) may be most susceptible, particularly when their systemic corticosteroids have been almost completely withdrawn. During this period of HPA suppression, patients may exhibit signs and symptoms of adrenal insufficiency when exposed to trauma, surgery, or infection (particularly gastroenteritis) or other conditions associated with severe electrolyte loss. Although inhaled corticosteroids may provide control of asthmatic symptoms during these episodes, in recommended doses they supply less than normal physiological amounts of glucocorticoid systemically and do not provide the mineralocorticoid activity that is necessary for coping with these emergencies. During periods of stress or a severe asthmatic attack, instruct patients who have been withdrawn from systemic corticosteroids to resume systemic corticosteroids (in large doses) immediately and to contact their health care provider for further instruction. Also instruct these patients to carry a warning card indicating that they may need supplementary systemic corticosteroids during periods of stress or a severe asthma attack.

Indications

Asthma, chronic: Maintenance and prophylactic treatment of asthma; includes patients who require systemic corticosteroids and those who may benefit from systemic dose reduction/elimination; for the maintenance treatment of asthma and as a prophylactic therapy in children (12 months to 8 years of age [**budesonide respules**], 12 years of age and older [**ciclesonide**], 6 years of age and older [**flunisolide hemihydrate**], 4 years of age and older [**mometasone** and **fluticasone**]).

Administration and Dosage

Estimated Comparative Daily Dosages for Inhaled Corticosteroids (Adults)[a]			
Drug	Low dose	Medium dose	High dose
Beclomethasone dipropionate 42 mcg/puff 84 mcg/puff	168 to 504 mcg 4 to 12 puffs 2 to 6 puffs	504 to 840 mcg 12 to 20 puffs 6 to 10 puffs	> 840 mcg > 20 puffs > 10 puffs
Flunisolide 250 mcg/puff	500 to 1,000 mcg 2 to 4 puffs	1,000 to 2,000 mcg 4 to 8 puffs	> 2,000 mcg > 8 puffs
Fluticasone MDI:[b] 44, 110, 220 mcg/puff	88 to 264 mcg 2 to 6 puffs (44 mcg) or 2 puffs (110 mcg)	264 to 660 mcg 2 to 6 puffs (110 mcg)	> 660 mcg > 6 puffs (110 mcg) or > 3 puffs (220 mcg)
Triamcinolone acetonide 75 mcg/puff	450 to 600 mcg 6 to 8 puffs	600 mcg 8 puffs	> 900 to 1,200 mcg > 12 to 16 puffs

[a] *Guidelines for the Diagnosis and Management of Asthma.* Expert Panel Report 2. National Institutes of Health. National Heart, Lung, and Blood Institute. February 1997. http://www.lungusa.org/asthma/astnhlbi.html.
[b] MDI = Metered dose inhaler.

Estimated Comparative Daily Dosages for Inhaled Corticosteroids (Children)[a]			
Drug	Low dose	Medium dose	High dose
Beclomethasone dipropionate (6 to 12 years of age) 42 mcg/puff 84 mcg/puff	84 to 336 mcg 2 to 8 puffs 1 to 4 puffs	336 to 672 mcg 8 to 16 puffs 4 to 8 puffs	> 672 mcg > 16 puffs > 8 puffs
Flunisolide (6 to 15 years of age) 250 mcg/puff	500 to 750 mcg 2 to 3 puffs	1,000 to 1,250 mcg 4 to 5 puffs	> 1,250 mcg > 5 puffs
Fluticasone (≥ 12 years of age) MDI:[b] 44, 110 mcg/puff	88 to 176 mcg 2 to 4 puffs (44 mcg)	176 to 440 mcg 4 to 10 puffs (44 mcg) or 2 to 4 puffs (110 mcg)	> 440 mcg > 4 puffs (110 mcg)
Triamcinolone acetonide (6 to 12 years of age) 75 mcg/puff	225 to 600 mcg 3 to 8 puffs	300 to 600 mcg 4 to 8 puffs	> 900 mcg > 12 puffs

[a] *Guidelines for the Diagnosis and Management of Asthma.* Expert Panel Report 2. National Institutes of Health. National Heart, Lung, and Blood Institute. February 1997. http://www.lungusa.org/asthma/astnhlbi.html.
[b] MDI = Metered dose inhaler.

Patients receiving concomitant systemic steroids: Slowly wean patients from systemic corticosteroids after transferring to steroid inhalers. Monitor lung function (FEV_1 or AM PEFR), beta-agonist use, and asthma symptoms during withdrawal of oral corticosteroids. Transfer to steroid inhalant and subsequent management may be more difficult because of slow HPA function recovery that may last up to 12 months.

Stabilize the patient's asthma before treatment is started. Initially, use aerosol concurrently with usual maintenance dose of systemic steroid. After approximately 1 week, start gradual withdrawal of the systemic steroid by reducing the daily or alternate daily dose. Make the next reduction after 1 to 2 weeks, depending on response. Generally, these decrements should not exceed 25% of the prednisone dose or its equivalent. A slow rate of withdrawal cannot be overemphasized.

BECLOMETHASONE: Test aerosol by spraying 2 times into the air before first use and when the product has not been used for over 10 days. Rinse mouth after inhalation.

The safety and efficacy in children younger than 5 years of age have not been established.

Expect improvement in asthma symptoms within the first or second week of starting treatment, but do not expect maximum benefit until 3 to 4 weeks of therapy. For patients who do not respond adequately to the starting dose after 3 to 4 weeks of therapy, higher doses may provide additional asthma control.

Recommended Doses in Patients ≥ 5 Years of Age		
Previous therapy	Recommended starting dose	Highest recommended dose
Adults and adolescents		
Bronchodilators alone	40 to 80 mcg twice daily	320 mcg twice daily
Inhaled corticosteroids	40 to 160 mcg twice daily	320 mcg twice daily
Children 5 to 11 years of age		
Bronchodilators alone	40 mcg twice daily	80 mcg twice daily
Inhaled corticosteroids	40 mcg twice daily	80 mcg twice daily

Patients not receiving systemic corticosteroids – Follow the doses recommended previously. Improvement in pulmonary function is usually apparent within 1 to 4 weeks after the start of therapy. Once the desired effect is achieved, consider tapering to the lowest effective dose.

Concomitant systemic corticosteroid therapy – See Administration in the group monograph.

BUDESONIDE:

Budesonide Recommended Starting Dose and Highest Recommended Dose		
Previous therapy	Recommended starting dose[a]	Highest recommended dose
Turbuhaler		
Adults		
Bronchodilators alone	200 to 400 mcg twice/day	400 mcg twice/day
Inhaled corticosteroids[b]	200 to 400 mcg twice/day	800 mcg twice/day
Oral corticosteroids	400 to 800 mcg twice/day	800 mcg twice/day
Children ≥ 6 years of age[c]		
Bronchodilators alone	200 mcg twice/day	400 mcg twice/day
Inhaled corticosteroids[b]	200 mcg twice/day	400 mcg twice/day
Oral corticosteroids	The highest recommended dose in children is 400 mcg twice/day.	
Respules		
Children 12 months to 8 years of age		
Bronchodilators alone	0.5 mg total daily dose administered once or twice daily in divided doses	0.5 mg total daily dose
Inhaled corticosteroids	0.5 mg total daily dose administered once or twice daily in divided doses	1 mg total daily dose
Oral corticosteroids	1 mg total daily dose administered as 0.5 mg twice/day or 1 mg once daily	1 mg total daily dose

[a] 200 mcg released with each actuation delivers approximately 160 mcg to the patient (*Turbuhaler*).
[b] In patients with mild to moderate asthma who are well controlled on inhaled corticosteroids, dosing budesonide 200 or 400 mcg once daily may be considered. Administer budesonide once daily in the morning or evening.
[c] Insufficient information is available to warrant use in children younger than 6 years of age.

Budesonide Flexhaler – A definitive comparative therapeutic ratio between budesonide *Flexhaler* and budesonide *Turbuhaler* has not been established. For patients who have been on budesonide *Turbuhaler* the dose of budesonide *Flexhaler* may not be predicted by the dose of that product. The clinical response of budesonide *Flexhaler* compared with budesonide *Turbuhaler* tends to be lower. Dose appropriately any patient who is switched from budesonide *Turbuhaler* to budesonide *Flexhaler*, taking into account the dosing recommendations and titrating the dose as dictated by the clinical response.

Budesonide *Flexhaler* Recommended Dosages		
	Recommended starting dose	Highest recommended dose
Adults	360 mcg twice daily[a]	720 mcg twice daily
Children	180 mcg twice daily[b]	360 mcg twice daily

[a] In some patients, a starting dose of 180 mcg twice daily may be adequate.
[b] In some patients, a starting dose of 360 mcg twice daily may be appropriate.

Dose titration: As with any inhaled corticosteroid, select the dosage that would be appropriate based upon the patient's disease severity and titrate the dosage downward over time to the lowest level that maintains proper asthma control. In adult patients who are well controlled, a dosage of 180 mcg twice daily may be considered. If the 180 mcg twice daily dose does not provide adequate control, increase the dose.

Budesonide respules – Administer by the inhaled route via jet nebulizer connected to an air compressor in asthmatic patients 12 months to 8 years of age. Improvement in asthma control can occur within 2 to 8 days of initiation of treatment, although maximum benefit may not be achieved for 4 to 6 weeks. Downward-titrate to the lowest effective dose once asthma stability is achieved. In symptomatic children not responding to nonsteroidal therapy and in patients who require maintenance therapy of their asthma, a starting dose of 0.25 mg once daily may also be considered.

If once-daily treatment does not provide adequate control of asthma symptoms, increase the total daily dose or administer as a divided dose.

Ultrasonic nebulizers are not suitable for the administration of budesonide respules and are not recommended. The effects of mixing budesonide respules with other nebulizable medications has not been assessed; administer separately in the nebulizer.

Patients maintained on chronic oral corticosteroids – Initially use concurrently with the patient's usual maintenance dose of systemic corticosteroid. Initiate at 1 mg/day.

CICLESONIDE:

Adults –

Patients who receive bronchodilators alone: The maximum dose is 160 mcg twice daily. The initial dose is 80 mcg twice daily. For patients who do not respond adequately to the starting dose after 4 weeks of therapy, higher doses may provide additional asthma control. After asthma stability has been achieved, titrate to the lowest effective dosage.

Patients who receive inhaled corticosteroids: The maximum dose is 320 mcg twice daily. The initial dose is 80 mcg twice daily. For patients who do not respond adequately to the starting dose after 4 weeks of therapy, higher doses may provide additional asthma control. After asthma stability has been achieved, titrate to the lowest effective dosage.

Patients who receive oral corticosteroids: The maximum dose is 320 mcg twice daily. The initial dose is 320 mcg twice daily. After asthma stability has been achieved, it is desirable to titrate to the lowest effective dosage. Prednisone should be reduced gradually, no sooner than 2.5 mg/day on a weekly basis, beginning after 1 week or more of therapy with ciclesonide.

FLUNISOLIDE:

Adults – Two inhalations (500 mcg) twice daily, morning and evening (total daily dose 1,000 mcg). Do not exceed 4 inhalations twice daily (2,000 mcg).

Children 6 to 15 years of age – Two inhalations twice daily, morning and evening (total daily dose 1,000 mcg). Higher doses have not been studied. Safety and efficacy for use in children younger than 6 years of age have not been established. With chronic use, monitor children for growth as well as for effects on the HPA axis.

Patients not receiving systemic steroids – In responsive patients, pulmonary function usually improves within 1 to 4 weeks.

FLUNISOLIDE HEMIHYDRATE: The onset and degree of symptom relief with orally inhaled corticosteroids is usually apparent within 2 to 4 weeks after the start of treatment. For patients who do not respond adequately to the starting dose after 3 to 4 weeks of therapy, higher doses may provide additional asthma control.

Adults – The recommended starting dose is 160 mcg twice daily. Do not exceed a maximum dose of 320 mcg twice daily.

Children 6 to 11 years of age – The recommended starting dose is 80 mcg twice daily. Do not exceed a maximum dose of 160 mcg twice daily.

FLUTICASONE: Advise patients to rinse mouth after inhalation.

Administer Fluticasone by the orally inhaled route only in patients 4 years of age and older. Individual patients will experience a variable time to onset and degree of symptom relief. Maximum benefit may not be achieved for 1 to 2 weeks or longer after starting treatment.

After asthma stability has been achieved, titrate to the lowest effective dose to reduce side effect possibility. For patients not responding adequately to the starting dose after 2 weeks, higher doses may provide additional asthma control.

Adults –

Recommended Adult Dosages for Fluticasone Aerosol

Previous therapy	Recommended starting dosage	Highest recommended dosage
Bronchodilators alone	88 mcg twice daily	440 mcg twice daily
Inhaled corticosteroids	88 to 220 mcg twice daily[a]	440 mcg twice daily
Oral corticosteroids[b]	440 mcg twice daily	880 mcg twice daily

[a] For patients currently receiving inhaled corticosteroid therapy, starting doses > 88 mcg twice daily may be considered for patients with poorer asthma control or those who have previously required doses of inhaled corticosteroids that are in the higher range for that specific agent.

[b] See Concomitant Therapy With Oral Corticosteroids.

Recommended Adult Dosages for Fluticasone *Diskus*[a]

Previous therapy	Recommended starting dosage	Highest recommended dosage
Bronchodilators alone	100 mcg twice daily	500 mcg twice daily
Inhaled corticosteroids	100 to 250 mcg twice daily	500 mcg twice daily
Oral corticosteroids	500 to 1,000 mcg twice daily	1,000 mcg twice daily

[a] Starting dosages > 100 mcg twice daily for adults may be considered for patients with poorer asthma control or those who have previously required doses of inhaled corticosteroids that are in the higher range for that specific agent.

Children –

Recommended Pediatric Dosages for Fluticasone Aerosol

Previous therapy	Recommended starting dosage	Highest recommended dosage
≥ 12 years of age		
Bronchodilators alone	88 mcg twice daily	440 mcg twice daily
Inhaled corticosteroids	88 to 220 mcg twice daily[a]	440 mcg twice daily
Oral corticosteroids	440 mcg twice daily	880 mcg twice daily
4 to 11 years of age[b]		
–	88 mcg twice daily	88 mcg twice daily

[a] For patients currently receiving inhaled corticosteroid therapy, starting doses > 88 mcg twice daily may be considered for patients with poorer asthma control or those who have previously required doses of inhaled corticosteroids that are in the higher range for that specific agent.

[b] Recommended pediatric dosage is 88 mcg twice daily regardless of prior therapy.

Recommended Pediatric Dosages for Fluticasone *Diskus*[a]		
Previous therapy	Recommended starting dosage	Highest recommended dosage
≥ 12 years of age		
Bronchodilators alone	100 mcg twice daily	500 mcg twice daily
Inhaled corticosteroids	100 to 250 mcg twice daily	500 mcg twice daily
Oral corticosteroids[b]	500 to 1,000 mcg twice daily[c]	1,000 mcg twice daily
4 to 11 years of age[d]		
Bronchodilators alone	50 mcg twice daily	100 mcg twice daily
Inhaled corticosteroids	50 mcg twice daily	100 mcg twice daily

[a] Starting dosages > 100 mcg twice daily for children ≥ 12 years of age and > 50 mcg twice daily for children 4 to 11 years of age may be considered for patients with poorer asthma control or those who have previously required doses of inhaled corticosteroids that are in the higher range for that specific agent.
[b] See Concomitant Therapy With Oral Corticosteroids.
[c] The choice of starting dosage should be made on the basis of individual patient assessment. A controlled clinical study of 111 oral corticosteroid–dependent patients with asthma showed few significant differences between the 2 doses of fluticasone *Diskus* on safety and efficacy end points. However, inability to decrease the dose of oral corticosteroids further during corticosteroid reduction may be indicative of the need to increase the dose of fluticasone *Diskus* up to the maximum of 1,000 mcg twice daily.
[d] Because individual responses may vary, children previously maintained on other inhaled corticosteroids may require dosage adjustments upon transfer to fluticasone *Diskus*.

Priming – Fluticasone aerosol should be primed before using for the first time by releasing 4 test sprays into the air away from the face, shaking well before each spray. In cases where the inhaler has not been used for more than 7 days or when it has been dropped, prime the inhaler again by shaking well and releasing 1 test spray into the air away from the face.

Concomitant systemic corticosteroid therapy – For patients currently receiving chronic oral corticosteroids, reduce prednisone no faster than 2.5 to 5 mg/day on a weekly basis, beginning after at least 1 week of aerosol therapy. Monitor patients for signs of asthma instability, including serial objective measures of airflow, and for signs of adrenal insufficiency. Decrease fluticasone dosage to the lowest effective dose once prednisone reduction is complete.

MOMETASONE: For patients 12 years of age and older who do not respond adequately to the starting dose after 2 weeks of therapy, higher doses may provide additional asthma control.

The recommended starting doses and highest recommended daily dose for mometasone treatment in patients 4 years of age and older based on prior asthma therapy are provided in the following table.

Mometasone Recommended Dosages		
Previous therapy	Recommended starting dosage	Highest recommended daily dose
Patients ≥ 12 years of age who received bronchodilators alone	220 mcg once daily in the evening[a]	440 mcg[b]
Patients ≥ 12 years of age who received inhaled corticosteroids	220 mcg once daily in the evening[a]	440 mcg[b]
Patients ≥ 12 years of age who received oral corticosteroids[c]	440 mcg twice daily	880 mcg
Children 4 to 11 years of age[d]	110 mcg once daily in the evening[a]	110 mcg[a]

[a] When administered once daily, mometasone should only be taken in the evening.
[b] The 440 mcg daily dose may be administered in divided doses of 220 mcg twice daily or as 440 mcg once daily.
[c] For patients currently receiving chronic oral corticosteroid therapy, reduce prednisone no faster than 2.5 mg/day on a weekly basis, beginning after at least 1 week of mometasone therapy. Carefully monitor patients for signs of asthma instability, including serial objective measures of airflow, and for signs of adrenal insufficiency. Once prednisone reduction is complete, reduce the dosage of mometasone to the lowest effective dosage.
[d] Recommended pediatric dose is 110 mcg once daily in the evening regardless of prior therapy.

TRIAMCINOLONE:

Adults – The usual dosage is 2 inhalations (150 mg) 3 to 4 times/day or 4 inhalations (300 mcg) twice daily. Do not exceed a maximum daily intake of 16 inhalations (1,200 mcg). Higher initial doses (12 to 16 inhalations/day) may be considered in patients with more severe asthma.

Children 6 to 12 years of age – The usual dosage is 1 or 2 inhalations (75 to 150 mcg) 3 to 4 times/day or 2 to 4 inhalations (150 to 300 mcg) twice daily. Do not exceed a maximum daily intake of 12 inhalations (900 mcg). Clinical data are insufficient with respect to use in children younger than 6 years of age.

Patients not receiving systemic steroids – Follow previous directions. In responsive patients, an improvement in pulmonary function is usually apparent within 1 to 2 weeks, but maximum benefit may not be achieved for 2 weeks or more.

Administration – Shake well before use. Rinsing the mouth after inhalation is advised.

Patients maintained on systemic corticosteroids – Clinical studies have shown that triamcinolone may be effective in the management of patients with asthma dependent or maintained on systemic corticosteroids and may permit replacement or significant reduction in the dosage of systemic corticosteroids.

The patient's asthma should be reasonably stable before treatment with triamcinolone is started. Initially, triamcinolone should be used concurrently with the patient's usual maintenance dose of a systemic corticosteroid. After approximately 1 week, gradual withdrawal of the systemic corticosteroid is started by reducing the daily or alternate daily dose. Reductions may be made after an interval of 1 or 2 weeks, depending on the response of the patient. A slow rate of withdrawal is strongly recommended. Generally, these decrements should not exceed prednisone 2.5 mg or its equivalent. During withdrawal, some patients may experience symptoms of systemic corticosteroid withdrawal (eg, joint and/or muscular pain, lassitude, depression) despite maintenance or even improvement in pulmonary function. Such patients should be encouraged to continue with the inhaler but should be monitored for objective signs of adrenal insufficiency. If evidence of adrenal insufficiency occurs, the systemic corticosteroid doses should be increased temporarily; thereafter, withdrawal should continue more slowly. Inhaled corticosteroids should be used with caution when used chronically in patients receiving prednisone regimens, either daily or on alternate days.

During periods of stress or a severe asthma attack, transfer patients may require supplementary treatment with systemic corticosteroids.

Actions

Pharmacology: These agents are synthetic adrenocortical steroids with basic glucocorticoid actions and effects. Glucocorticoids may decrease number and activity of inflammatory cells, enhance effect of beta-adrenergic drugs on cyclic adenosine monophosphate production, inhibit bronchoconstrictor mechanisms, or produce direct smooth muscle relaxation. Inhaler use provides effective local steroid activity with minimal systemic effect.

Pharmacokinetics:

Pharmacokinetics of Inhaled Corticosteroids

Parameters	Corticosteroids				
	Beclomethasone	Budesonide	Flunisolide	Fluticasone	Triamcinolone
Absorption					
Systemic bioavailability from lungs	≈ 20%	25%	40%	20%	21.5%
Distribution					
Protein binding	87%	85% to 90%	NA	91%	≈ 68%

Pharmacokinetics of Inhaled Corticosteroids

Parameters	Corticosteroids				
	Beclomethasone	Budesonide	Flunisolide	Fluticasone	Triamcinolone
Metabolism					
Site	Liver (CYP3A)	Liver (CYP3A)	Liver	Liver (CYP3A4)	Mostly from liver, less extensively from the kidneys
Excretion					
Site	Feces, urine (< 10%)	Urine (≈ 60%), feces	Renal (50%), feces (40%)	Feces, urine (< 0.02%)	Urine (≈ 40%), feces (≈ 60%)
$T_{½}$	2.8 h	2.8 h	≈ 1.8 h	3.1 h	1.5 h

Contraindications

Relief of acute bronchospasm; primary treatment of status asthmaticus or other acute episodes of asthma when intensive measures are required; hypersensitivity to any ingredient; systemic fungal infections; persistently positive sputum cultures for *Candida albicans*.

Vanceril: Relief of asthma that can be controlled by bronchodilators and other nonsteroid medications; in patients who require systemic corticosteroid treatment infrequently; treatment of nonasthmatic bronchitis.

Warnings/Precautions

Infections: Localized fungal infections with *C. albicans* or *Aspergillus niger* have occurred in the mouth, pharynx, and occasionally in the larynx. Use inhaled corticosteroids with caution, if at all, in patients with active or quiescent tuberculous infection of the respiratory tract; untreated systemic fungal, bacterial, parasitic, or viral infection; or ocular herpes simplex.

Acute asthma: These products are not bronchodilators and are not for rapid relief of bronchospasm.

Bronchospasm: Bronchospasm may occur with an immediate increase in wheezing following dosing; treat immediately with a fast-acting inhaled bronchodilator.

Combination with prednisone: Combination therapy of inhaled corticosteroids with systemic corticosteroids may increase the risk of HPA suppression compared with a therapeutic dose of either one alone. Use inhaled corticosteroids with caution in patients already receiving prednisone.

Replacement therapy: Transfer from systemic steroid therapy may unmask allergic conditions previously suppressed. During withdrawal from oral steroids, some patients may experience withdrawal symptoms despite maintenance or improvement of respiratory function.

Steroid withdrawal: During withdrawal from oral steroids, some patients may experience symptoms of systemically active steroid withdrawal (eg, joint or muscular pain, lassitude, depression), despite maintenance or even improvement of respiratory function. Although steroid withdrawal effects are usually transient and not severe, severe and even fatal exacerbation of asthma can occur if the previous daily oral corticosteroid requirement had significantly exceeded 10 mg/day of prednisone or equivalent.

HPA suppression: Inhaled corticosteroids may permit control of asthmatic symptoms with less HPA suppression. Because these agents are absorbed and can be systemically active, the beneficial effects in minimizing or preventing HPA dysfunction may be expected only when recommended dosages are not exceeded. Take particular care in observing patients postoperatively or during periods of stress for evidence of a decrease in adrenal function.

Flunisolide – Because of the possibility of higher systemic absorption, monitor patients using **flunisolide** for any evidence of systemic corticosteroid effect. If such changes occur, discontinue slowly, consistent with accepted procedures for discontinuing oral corticosteroids. When **flunisolide** is used chronically at 2 mg/day, monitor patients periodically for effects on the HPA axis.

Glaucoma: Rare instances of glaucoma, increased intraocular pressure, and cataracts have been reported following the inhaled administration of corticosteroids.

Pulmonary infiltrates: Pulmonary infiltrates with eosinophilia may occur with **beclomethasone** or **flunisolide**.

Reduction in growth velocity: Closely follow the growth of adolescents taking corticosteroids, and weigh the benefits of corticosteroid therapy and asthma control against the possibility of growth suppression.

Pregnancy: *Category* C; *Category* B (**budesonide** only).

Lactation: Glucocorticoids are excreted in breast milk. It is not known whether inhaled corticosteroids are excreted in breast milk, but it is likely.

Children: Insufficient information is available to warrant use in children younger than 6 years of age or younger than 12 years of age with **fluticasone** and **beclomethasone**. Monitor growth in children and adolescents because there is evidence that oral corticosteroids may suppress growth in a dose-related fashion, particularly in higher doses for extended periods.

Drug Interactions

Ketoconazole: A potent inhibitor of CYP-450 3A4 may increase plasma levels of **budesonide** and **fluticasone** during concomitant dosing. The clinical significance is unknown. Use caution.

Adverse Reactions

Local: Coughing, dry mouth, facial edema, flu syndrome, hoarseness/dysphonia, rash, throat irritation, wheezing.

Systemic: Suppression of HPA function has occurred. Deaths caused by adrenal insufficiency have occurred during and after transfer from systemic to aerosol corticosteroids.

Beclomethasone: Adverse reactions occurring in 3% or more of patients include coughing, dysmenorrhea, dyspepsia, headache, nasal congestion, pharyngitis, rhinitis, sinusitis, upper respiratory tract infection, viral infections.

Budesonide: Adverse reactions occurring in 3% or more of patients include back pain, conjunctivitis, coughing, ear infection, epistaxis, fever, flu syndrome, headache, otitis media, pain, pharyngitis, rhinitis, sinusitis, upper respiratory tract infection, viral infections, voice alteration.

Flunisolide: Adverse reactions occurring in 3% or more of patients include abdominal pain, anorexia, chest congestion, chest pain, cold symptoms, coughing, diarrhea, dizziness, ear infection, edema, eczema, fever, general flu, headache, heartburn, hoarseness, irritability, itching/pruritus, loss of smell or taste, menstrual disturbance, nasal and sinus congestion, nausea, nervousness, oral candidiasis, palpitations, rash, rhinitis, runny nose, shakiness, sinus drainage/infection, sinusitis, sneezing, sore throat, sputum, unpleasant taste, upper respiratory tract infection, upset stomach, vomiting, wheezing.

Fluticasone: Adverse reactions occurring in 3% or more of patients include allergic rhinitis, diarrhea, dysphonia, fever, headache, influenza, menstrual disturbance, nasal congestion, nasal discharge, oral candidiasis, pharyngitis, rhinitis, sinusitis, upper respiratory tract infection.

Triamcinolone: Adverse reactions occurring in 3% or more of patients include back pain, flu syndrome, headache, pharyngitis, sinusitis.

ACETYLCYSTEINE (N-Acetylcysteine)

Solution: 10% and 20% (*Rx*)	Various

Indications

Mucolytic: Adjuvant therapy for abnormal, viscid, or inspissated mucus secretions in chronic bronchopulmonary disease (chronic emphysema, emphysema with bronchitis, chronic asthmatic bronchitis, tuberculosis, bronchiectasis, primary amyloidosis of lung); acute bronchopulmonary disease (pneumonia, bronchitis, tracheobronchitis); pulmonary complications of cystic fibrosis; tracheostomy care; pulmonary complications associated with surgery; use during anesthesia; posttraumatic chest conditions; atelectasis due to mucus obstruction; diagnostic bronchial studies (bronchograms, bronchospirometry, bronchial wedge catheterization).

Antidote: To prevent or lessen hepatic injury that may occur following ingestion of a potentially hepatotoxic quantity of acetaminophen.

Administration and Dosage

Nebulization (face mask, mouth piece, tracheostomy): 1 to 10 mL of the 20% solution or 2 to 20 mL of the 10% solution every 2 to 6 hours; the dose for most patients is 3 to 5 mL of the 20% solution or 6 to 10 mL of the 10% solution 3 to 4 times/day.

Nebulization (tent, croupette): Very large volumes are required, occasionally up to 300 mL during a treatment period. The dose is the volume of solution that will maintain a very heavy mist in the tent or croupette for the desired period. Administration for intermittent or continuous prolonged periods, including overnight, may be desirable.

Instillation:

Direct – 1 to 2 mL of a 10% to 20% solution as often as every hour.

Tracheostomy – 1 to 2 mL of a 10% to 20% solution every 1 to 4 hours by instillation into the tracheostomy.

May be introduced directly into a particular segment of the bronchopulmonary tree by inserting (under local anesthesia and direct vision) a plastic catheter into the trachea. Instill 2 to 5 mL of the 20% solution by a syringe connected to the catheter.

Percutaneous intratracheal catheter – 1 to 2 mL of the 20% solution or 2 to 4 mL of the 10% solution every 1 to 4 hours by a syringe attached to the catheter.

Diagnostic bronchograms: 2 or 3 administrations of 1 to 2 mL of the 20% solution or 2 to 4 mL of the 10% solution by nebulization or by instillation intratracheally, prior to the procedure.

Equipment compatibility: Certain materials in nebulization equipment react with acetylcysteine, especially certain metals (notably iron and copper) and rubber. Where materials may come into contact with acetylcysteine solution, use parts made of the following materials: Glass, plastic, aluminum, anodized aluminum, chromed metal, tantalum, sterling silver, or stainless steel. Silver may become tarnished after exposure, but this is not harmful to the drug action or to the patient.

Admixture incompatibility: Tetracycline, chlortetracycline, oxytetracycline, erythromycin lactobionate, amphotericin B, and sodium ampicillin are incompatible when mixed in the same solution with acetylcysteine. Administer from separate solutions. Iodized oil, chymotrypsin, trypsin, and hydrogen peroxide are also incompatible.

Actions

Pharmacology: The mucolytic action of acetylcysteine is related to the sulfhydryl group in the molecule, which acts directly to split disulfide linkages between mucoprotein molecular complexes, resulting in depolymerization and a decrease in mucus viscosity. The mucolytic activity of acetylcysteine increases with increasing pH.

Acetylcysteine also reduces the extent of liver injury following acetaminophen overdose. It is thought that acetylcysteine protects the liver by maintaining or restoring glutathione levels, or by acting as an alternate substrate for conjugation with, and thus, detoxification of, the reactive metabolite of acetaminophen.

Pharmacokinetics: Following a 200 to 400 mg oral dose, peak plasma concentrations of 0.35 to 4 mg/L are achieved within 1 to 2 hours. Protein binding is approximately

50% 4 hours postdose. Volume of distribution is 0.33 to 0.47 L/kg. The terminal half-life of reduced acetylcysteine is 6.25 hours. Approximately 70% of total body clearance is nonrenal.

Contraindications

Hypersensitivity to acetylcysteine. As an antidote, there are no contraindications.

Warnings/Precautions

Bronchial secretions: An increased volume of liquefied bronchial secretions may occur; when cough is inadequate, maintain an open airway by mechanical suction if necessary. When there is a large mechanical block due to a foreign body or local accumulation, clear the airway by endotracheal aspiration, with or without bronchoscopy.

Asthmatics: Carefully observe asthmatics under treatment with acetylcysteine. If bronchospasm progresses, discontinue medication immediately.

Antidotal use:

Allergic effects – Generalized urticaria has been observed rarely. If this or other allergic symptoms appear, discontinue treatment unless it is deemed essential and the allergic symptoms can be otherwise controlled.

Hepatic effects – If encephalopathy due to hepatic failure occurs, discontinue treatment to avoid further administration of nitrogenous substances.

Vomiting – Vomiting, occasionally severe and persistent, occurs as a symptom of acute acetaminophen overdose. Treatment with oral acetylcysteine may aggravate vomiting. Evaluate patients at risk of gastric hemorrhage concerning the risk of upper GI hemorrhage vs the risk of developing hepatic toxicity. Diluting acetylcysteine minimizes its propensity to aggravate vomiting.

Disagreeable odor: Administration may initially produce a slight disagreeable odor which soon disappears.

Face mask use: A face mask may cause stickiness on the face after nebulization; remove with water.

Solution color: Solution color may change in the opened bottle, but does not significantly impair the drug's safety or efficacy.

Continued nebulization: Continued nebulization of acetylcysteine with a dry gas results in concentration of drug in the nebulizer due to evaporation. Extreme concentration may impede nebulization and drug delivery. Dilute with Sterile Water for Injection as concentration occurs.

Pregnancy: *Category B.*

Lactation: It is not known whether this drug is excreted in breast milk.

Adverse Reactions

Adverse reactions may include stomatitis; nausea; vomiting; fever; rhinorrhea; drowsiness; clamminess; chest tightness; bronchoconstriction; bronchospasm; irritation to the tracheal and bronchial tracts.

Antidotal use – Large doses of oral acetylcysteine may result in nausea, vomiting, and other GI symptoms. Rash (with or without mild fever), pruritus, angioedema, bronchospasm, tachycardia, hypotension, and hypertension have occurred.

IPRATROPIUM BROMIDE

Aerosol: Each actuation delivers 17 mcg (*Rx*)	*Atrovent HFA* (Boehringer Ingelheim)
Solution for Inhalation: 0.02% (500 mcg/vial) (*Rx*)	Various
Nasal spray: 0.03% (21 mcg/spray) and 0.06% (42 mcg/spray) (*Rx*)	Various, *Atrovent* (Boehringer Ingelheim)

Indications

Bronchospasm (solution and aerosol): Used alone or in combination with other bronchodilators (especially beta-adrenergics) as a bronchodilator for maintenance treatment of bronchospasm associated with chronic obstructive pulmonary disease (COPD), including chronic bronchitis and emphysema.

Rhinorrhea:

Perennial rhinitis (0.03% nasal spray) – Symptomatic relief of rhinorrhea associated with allergic and nonallergic perennial rhinitis in patients 6 years of age or older.

Common cold (0.06% nasal spray) – Symptomatic relief of rhinorrhea associated with the common cold or seasonal allergic rhinitis in patients 5 years of age or older.

Administration and Dosage

Aerosol: The usual dose is 2 inhalations (36 mcg) 4 times/day. Patients may take additional inhalations as required; however, do not exceed 12 inhalations in 24 hours.

Solution: The usual dose is 500 mcg (1 unit dose vial) administered 3 to 4 times/day by oral nebulization, with doses 6 to 8 hours apart. The solution can be mixed in the nebulizer with albuterol if used within 1 hour.

Nasal spray:

0.03% (patients 6 years of age or older) – The usual dose is 2 sprays (42 mcg) per nostril 2 or 3 times/day (total dose, 168 to 252 mcg/day). Optimum dosage varies.

0.06% (patients 5 years of age or older) –

For symptomatic relief or rhinorrhea associated with the common cold: Recommended dose is 2 sprays (84 mcg) per nostril 3 or 4 times/day (total dose, 504 to 672 mcg/day). Optimum dosage varies.

Children 5 to 11 years of age – Recommended dose is 2 sprays (84 mcg) per nostril 3 times/day (total dose, 504 mcg/day).

The safety and efficacy of use for more than 4 days in patients with the common cold have not been established.

For symptomatic relief of rhinorrhea associated with seasonal allergic rhinitis: The recommended dose of ipratropium bromide 0.06% nasal spray is 2 sprays (84 mcg) per nostril 4 times daily (total dose 672 mcg/day) in adults and children 5 years of age and older.

The safety and efficacy of the use of ipratropium bromide 0.06% nasal spray beyond 3 weeks in patients with seasonal allergic rhinitis have not been established.

Actions

Pharmacology: Ipratropium for oral inhalation is an anticholinergic (parasympatholytic) agent that appears to inhibit vagally mediated reflexes by antagonizing the action of acetylcholine. The bronchodilation following inhalation is primarily a local, site-specific effect, not a systemic one.

Ipratropium bromide (nasal) has antisecretory properties and, when applied locally, inhibits secretions from the serous and seromucous glands lining the nasal mucosa.

Pharmacokinetics:

Absorption – Ipratropium bromide is poorly absorbed into the systemic circulation following oral administration. Much of an inhaled dose is swallowed (inhalation).

Distribution – Ipratropium is minimally bound (0% to 9%).

Metabolism/Excretion – Ipratropium is partially metabolized to inactive products. The half-life of elimination is about 2 hours after inhalation, nasal, or IV administration.

Contraindications

Hypersensitivity to ipratropium, atropine, or its derivatives.

Warnings/Precautions

Acute bronchospasm: Ipratropium HFA inhalation aerosol is not indicated for the initial treatment of acute episodes of bronchospasm where rescue therapy is required for rapid response.

Special risk patients: Use with caution in patients with narrow-angle glaucoma, prostatic hypertrophy, or bladder neck obstruction.

Hypersensitivity reactions: Immediate hypersensitivity reactions may occur after administration of ipratropium as demonstrated by rare cases of urticaria, angioedema, rash, bronchospasm, anaphylaxis, and oropharyngeal edema.

Special risk: Ipratropium bromide nasal spray should be used with caution in patients with narrow-angle glaucoma, prostatic hypertrophy, or bladder neck obstruction.

Pregnancy: Category B.

Lactation: It is not known whether this drug is excreted in breast milk.

Children:

HFA aerosol – Safety and efficacy in children have not been established.

Solution – Safety and efficacy in children younger than 12 years of age have not been established.

Drug Interactions

Ipratropium has been used concomitantly with other drugs, including beta-adrenergic bronchodilators, sympathomimetic bronchodilators, methylxanthines, steroids, commonly used in the treatment of chronic obstructive pulmonary disease, without adverse drug reactions.

Anticholinergic agents: There is some potential for an additive interaction with concomitantly used anticholinergic medications.

Solution incompatibility: Advise patients that ipratropium inhalation solution can be mixed in the nebulizer with albuterol or metaproterenol if used within 1 hour.

Adverse Reactions

Adverse reactions from **inhalational products** may include back or chest pain, bronchitis, cough, changes to COPD exacerbation, dizziness, dry mouth, dyspepsia, dyspnea, epistaxis, GI distress, headache, influenza-like symptoms, nausea, nervousness, pharyngitis, rhinitis, sinusitis, upper respiratory tract infection, urinary tract infection.

Adverse reactions from **nasal spray** may include dry mouth/throat, epistaxis, headache, nasal dryness, other nasal symptoms, pharyngitis, taste perversion, and upper respiratory tract infection.

TIOTROPIUM BROMIDE

Capsule, powder for administration; inhalation: 18 mcg (as base) (*Rx*)	*Spiriva* (Boehringer Ingelheim)

Indications

Chronic obstructive pulmonary disease: For the long-term, once-daily, maintenance treatment of bronchospasm associated with chronic obstructive pulmonary disease (COPD), including chronic bronchitis and emphysema; to reduce exacerbations in COPD patients.

Administration and Dosage

Dose: Two inhalations of the contents of 1 capsule, once daily, with the *HandiHaler* inhalation device.

Administration: Tiotropium capsules are for inhalation only; do not swallow.

For administration, a capsule is placed into the center chamber of the *HandiHaler* device. The capsule is pierced by pressing and releasing the green piercing button on the side of the *HandiHaler* device. The medication is dispersed into the air stream when the patient inhales through the mouth piece.

Actions

Pharmacology: Tiotropium is a long-acting, antimuscarinic agent, which is often referred to as an anticholinergic. In the airways, it exhibits pharmacological effects through inhibition of M_3-receptors at the smooth muscle, leading to bronchodilation. The bronchodilation following inhalation of tiotropium is predominantly a site-specific effect.

Pharmacokinetics:

Absorption – The majority of a delivered dose is deposited in the GI tract and, to a lesser extent, in the lung, the intended organ. The absolute bioavailability of

19.5% suggests that the fraction reaching the lung is highly bioavailable. Maximum tiotropium plasma concentrations were observed 5 minutes after inhalation.

Distribution – Tiotropium shows a volume of distribution of 32 L/kg, indicating that the drug binds extensively to tissues. The drug is bound 72% to plasma proteins. At steady state, peak plasma levels in COPD patients were 17 to 19 pg/mL when measured 5 minutes after an 18 mcg dry powder inhalation dose and decreased rapidly in a multicompartmental manner. Steady-state trough plasma concentrations were 3 to 4 pg/mL.

Metabolism – The extent of biotransformation appears to be small. In vitro experiments with human liver microsomes and human hepatocytes suggest that a fraction of the administered dose (74% of an intravenous dose is excreted unchanged in the urine, leaving 25% for metabolism) is metabolized by cytochrome P450-dependent oxidation and subsequent glutathione conjugation to a variety of phase 2 metabolites. This enzymatic pathway can be inhibited by CYP450 2D6 and 3A4 inhibitors (eg, quinidine, ketoconazole, and gestodene).

Excretion – The terminal elimination half-life is between 5 and 6 days following inhalation. After dry powder inhalation, urinary excretion is 14% of the dose, the remainder being mainly nonabsorbed drug in the gut, which is eliminated via the feces. The renal clearance of tiotropium exceeds the creatinine clearance (CrCl), indicating active secretion into the urine. After chronic, once-daily inhalation by patients with COPD, pharmacokinetic steady state was reached after 2 to 3 weeks with no accumulation thereafter.

Contraindications

Hypersensitivity to ipratropium or tiotropium.

Warnings/Precautions

Acute bronchospasm: Tiotropium is intended as a once-daily maintenance treatment for COPD and is not indicated for the initial treatment of acute episodes of bronchospasm (ie, rescue therapy).

Narrow-angle glaucoma: Use tiotropium with caution in patients with narrow-angle glaucoma.

Urinary retention: Use tiotropium with caution in patients with urinary retention.

Hypersensitivity reactions: Immediate hypersensitivity reactions, including angioedema, may occur after administration of tiotropium. If such a reaction occurs, stop therapy at once and consider alternative treatment.

Renal function impairment: As a predominantly renally-excreted drug, closely monitor patients with moderate to severe renal impairment (CrCl 50 mL/min or less) treated with tiotropium for anticholinergic adverse reactions.

Pregnancy: Category C.

Lactation: It is not known whether tiotropium is excreted in human milk. Exercise caution if administering to a breast-feeding woman.

Children: Safety and efficacy have not been established.

Elderly: Advanced age was associated with a decrease of tiotropium renal clearance, which may be explained by decreased renal function. In the placebo-controlled studies, a higher frequency of dry mouth, constipation, and urinary tract infections was observed with increasing age in the tiotropium group.

Drug Interactions

Anticholinergic agents: The coadministration of tiotropium with other anticholinergic-containing drugs (eg, ipratropium) has not been studied and, therefore, is not recommended.

Adverse Reactions

Adverse reactions occurring in 3% or more of patients include abdominal pain, accidents, chest pain (nonspecific), constipation, dry mouth, dyspepsia, edema (dependent), epistaxis, infection, moniliasis, myalgia, pharyngitis, rash, rhinitis, sinusitis, upper respiratory tract infection, urinary tract infection, vomiting.

IPRATROPIUM BROMIDE AND ALBUTEROL SULFATE

Aerosol: Each actuation delivers 18 mcg ipratropium bromide and 103 mcg albuterol sulfate (*Rx*)	*Combivent* (Boehringer Ingelheim)
Inhalation solution: 0.5 mg ipratropium bromide and 3 mg albuterol sulfate (equiv. to 2.5 mg albuterol base) (*Rx*)	Various, *DuoNeb* (Dey)

Indications

Bronchospasm: Use in patients with chronic obstructive pulmonary disease (COPD) on a regular aerosol bronchodilator who continue to have evidence of bronchospasm and require a second bronchodilator.

Administration and Dosage

Combivent: Shake well before using.

The recommended dose is 2 inhalations 4 times/day. Patients may take additional inhalations as required; however, advise the patient not to exceed 12 in 24 hours. It is recommended to "test spray" 3 times before using the first time and in cases where the aerosol has not be used for more than 24 hours.

DuoNeb: The recommended dose is one 3 mL vial administered 4 times/day via nebulization with up to 2 additional 3 mL doses allowed per day, if needed. Administer via jet nebulizer connected to an air compressor with an adequate air flow, equipped with mouthpiece or suitable face mask.

The use of these agents can be continued as medically indicated to control recurring bouts of bronchospasm. If a previously effective regimen fails to provide the usual relief, medical advice should be sought immediately, as this is often a sign of worsening COPD, which would require reassessment of therapy.

CROMOLYN SODIUM (Disodium Cromoglycate)

Solution for inhalation: 20 mg per 2 mL (*Rx*)	Various
Nasal Solution: 40 mg/mL. Each actuation delivers 5.2 mg (*otc*)	Various, *Nasalcrom* (Pharmacia)
Oral concentrate: 100 mg per 5 mL (*Rx*)	*Gastrocrom* (Celltech)

Indications

Bronchial asthma (inhalation solution, aerosol): As prophylactic management of bronchial asthma. Cromolyn is given on a regular, daily basis in patients with frequent symptomatology requiring a continuous medication regimen.

Prevention of bronchospasm (inhalation solution, aerosol): To prevent acute bronchospasm induced by exercise, toluene diisocyanate, environmental pollutants, and known antigens.

Allergic rhinitis (nasal solution): To prevent and treat allergic rhinitis caused by airborne pollens from trees, grasses, or ragweed, and by mold, animals, and dust. To prevent and relieve the following nasal symptoms: Runny/itchy nose, sneezing, and allergic stuffy nose.

Mastocytosis (oral): Improves diarrhea, flushing, headaches, vomiting, urticaria, abdominal pain, nausea and itching in some patients.

Unlabeled uses: Cromolyn has been used as an alternative therapy in refractory forms of chronic urticaria/angioedema. Oral cromolyn has been used for the treatment of food allergies and mucosal and serosal eosinophilic gastroenteritis.

Administration and Dosage

Nebulizer solution:

Adults and children 2 or more years of age –

Asthma: 1 vial by nebulization 4 times/day at regular intervals. The effectiveness of therapy depends upon administration at regular intervals.

Prevention of acute bronchospasm: 1 vial administered by nebulization shortly before exposure to the precipitating factor.

Administration – For oral inhalation use only. Not for injection. Cromolyn should be used in a power-driven nebulizer with an adequate airflow rate equipped with a suitable face mask or mouthpiece. Cromolyn inhalation solution is poorly absorbed when swallowed and is not effective by this route of administration.

Admixture compatibility – Drug stability and safety of cromolyn sodium inhalation solution when mixed with other drugs in a nebulizer have not been established.

Nasal solution:

Adults and children 2 years of age and older – One spray in each nostril 3 to 4 times/day at regular intervals every 4 to 6 hours. Maximum effects may not be seen for 1 to 2 weeks. Clear the nasal passages before administering the spray and inhale through the nose during administration.

Oral:

Adults (13 or more years of age) – 200 mg (2 ampules) 4 times/day, 30 minutes before meals and at bedtime.

Children 2 to 12 years of age – 100 mg (1 ampule) 4 times/day 30 minutes before meals and bedtime.

If satisfactory control of symptoms is not achieved within 2 to 3 weeks, the dosage may be increased but should not exceed 40 mg/kg/day.

The effect of therapy is dependent upon its administration at regular intervals as directed. Not for inhalation or injection.

Maintenance – Once a therapeutic response has been achieved the dose may be reduced to the minimum required to maintain the patient with a lower degree of symptomatology. To prevent relapses, maintain the dosage.

Concomitant corticosteroid treatment: Continue concomitant corticosteroid treatment and bronchodilators following the introduction of cromolyn. If the patient improves, attempt to decrease corticosteroid dosage. Even if the steroid-dependent patient fails to improve following cromolyn use, attempt gradual tapering of steroid dosage while maintaining close patient supervision. Consider reinstituting steroid therapy for a patient subjected to significant stress while being treated or within 1 year (occasionally up to 2 years) after steroid treatment has been terminated, in case of adrenocortical insufficiency. When the inhalation of cromolyn is impaired, a temporary increase in the amount of steroids or other agents may be required.

Cautiously withdraw cromolyn in cases where its use has permitted a reduction in the maintenance dose of steroids as there may be a sudden reappearance of asthma that will require immediate therapy and possible reintroduction of corticosteroids.

Nonsteroidal agents: Add cromolyn (inhalation solution and aerosol) to the patient's existing treatment regimen (eg, bronchodilators). Concomitant medications may be decreased gradually when a clinical response to cromolyn is evident (approximately 2 to 4 weeks) and asthma is under good control. Titrate the frequency of cromolyn administration downward to the lowest effective level if concomitant medications are discontinued or required on no more than an as-needed basis. The usual decrease is from 4 to 3 ampules/vials per day for the nebulizer solution, or from 2 metered inhalations 4 times/day to 3 times/day to twice daily for the inhalation aerosol. Gradually reduce dosage to avoid asthma exacerbations. Clinical deterioration in these patients whose dosage has been decreased to less than 4 ampules/vials or 4 inhalations per day may require an increase in cromolyn dosage and the introduction of, or increase in, symptomatic medications.

Actions

Pharmacology: Cromolyn is an anti-inflammatory agent. It has no intrinsic bronchodilator, antihistaminic, anticholinergic, vasoconstrictor, or glucocorticoid activity. The drug inhibits the release of mediators, histamine, and SRS-A (the slow-reacting substance of anaphylaxis, a leukotriene) from the mast cell. Cromolyn acts locally on the lung to which it is directly applied.

Pharmacokinetics: After inhalation, approximately 8% is absorbed from the lung and is rapidly excreted unchanged in bile and urine. The remainder is either exhaled, or deposited in the oropharynx, swallowed and excreted via the alimentary tract.

Cromolyn is poorly absorbed from the GI tract. No more than 1% of an administered dose is absorbed after oral administration, the remainder excreted in the feces.

Contraindications

Hypersensitivity to cromolyn or to any ingredient contained in these products.

Warnings/Precautions

Acute asthma: Cromolyn has no role in the treatment of acute asthma, especially status asthmaticus; it is a prophylactic drug with no benefit for acute situations.

Respiratory effects: Occasionally, patients experience cough or bronchospasm following inhalation.

Dosing reduction/discontinuation: Asthma may recur if drug is reduced below recommended dosage or discontinued.

Hypersensitivity reactions: Severe anaphylactic reactions may occur rarely.

Renal/Hepatic function impairment: Decrease the dose or discontinue the drug in these patients.

Pregnancy: *Category* B.

Lactation: Safety for use in the nursing mother has not been established.

Children:

Aerosol – Safety and efficacy in children younger than 2 years of age are not established.

Nebulizer solution – Safety and efficacy in children younger than 2 years of age not established.

Nasal solution – Safety and efficacy in children younger than 2 years of age are not established.

Oral – In term infants up to 6 months of age, data suggest the dose not exceed 20 mg/kg/day. Reserve use in children younger than 2 years of age for patients with severe disease in which potential benefits clearly outweigh risks.

Adverse Reactions

The most frequently reported adverse reactions attributed to cromolyn sodium (on the basis of recurrence following readministration) involve the respiratory tract and include bronchospasm (sometimes severe, associated with a precipitous fall in pulmonary function [FEV_1]), cough, laryngeal edema (rare), nasal congestion (sometimes severe), pharyngeal irritation, and wheezing.

Adverse reactions associated with **aerosol** may include throat irritation or dryness, bad taste, cough, wheeze, and nausea.

Reactions from the **nebulizer solution** may include cough, nasal congestion, wheezing, sneezing, nasal itching, epistaxis, nose burning, serum sickness, and stomach ache.

Adverse events associated with the **nasal solution** may include sneezing, nasal stinging, and nasal irritation.

Adverse reactions from oral concentrate may include headache and diarrhea.

NASAL DECONGESTANTS

NAPHAZOLINE HYDROCHLORIDE	
Solution: 0.05% (*otc*)	*Privine* (Insight)
OXYMETAZOLINE HYDROCHLORIDE	
Solution: 0.05% (*otc*)	Various, *Afrin 12-Hour, Afrin Severe Congestion, Afrin No-Drip 12-Hour, Afrin No-Drip 12-Hour Extra Moisturizing, Afrin Extra Moisturizing 12 Hour Relief, Afrin Sinus 12 Hour Relief, Duration* (Schering-Plough Healthcare), *Genasal* (Goldline), *Nasal Decongestant, Maximum Strength* (Taro), *Nasal Relief* (Rugby), *Twice-A-Day 12-Hour Nasal* (Major), *Neo-Synephrine 12-Hour Extra Moisturizing* (Bayer), *Dristan 12-Hr Nasal* (Wyeth), *Duramist Plus 12-Hr Decongestant* (Pfeiffer), *Nōstrilla 12-Hour* (Heritage), *Nōstrilla Complete Congestion Relief 12-Hour, Nōstrilla Conditioning Double-Moisture* (Insight), *Vicks Sinex 12-Hour Long-Acting, Vicks Sinex 12-Hour Ultra Fine Mist for Sinus Relief* (Proctor & Gamble)
PHENYLEPHRINE HYDROCHLORIDE	
Tablets: 10 mg (*otc*)	*Sudafed PE* (Pfizer), *Sudogest PE* (Major)
Oral liquid: 7.5 mg per 5 mL (*otc*)	*Lusonal* (WraSer)
Solution, concentrate: 2.5 mg per mL (*otc*)	*Little Colds Decongestant Drops for Infants & Children* (Vetco)
Solution: 2.5 mg per 5 mL (*otc*)	*Pediacare Children's Decongestant* (Pfizer)
Nasal solution: 0.125% (*otc*)	*Little Noses Gentle Formula, Infants & Children* (Vetco)
0.25% (*otc*)	*Neo-Synephrine Mild Strength* (Bayer Corp.), *Rhinall* (Scherer)
0.5% (*otc*)	*Neo-Synephrine Regular Strength* (Bayer Corp.), *Vicks Sinex Ultra Fine Mist* (Proctor & Gamble)
1% (*otc*)	Various, *4-Way Fast Acting* (Novartis Consumer), *Neo-Synephrine Extra Strength* (Bayer Corp.)
PSEUDOEPHEDRINE HYDROCHLORIDE	
Tablets: 30 mg (*otc*)	Various, *Congest Aid* (Zee Medical), *Genaphed* (Goldline), *Sudafed* (McNeil), *Simply Stuffy* (McNeil Consumer)
60 mg (*otc*)	Various
Tablets, extended-release: 120 mg (*otc*)	Various, *Sudafed 12-Hour* (McNeil), *Maximum Strength 12-Hour Non-Drowsy Extentabs* (Whitehall-Robins)
Tablets, controlled-release: 240 mg (*otc*)	*Sudafed 24-Hour* (McNeil)
Liquid: 15 mg per 5 mL (*otc*)	Various, *Sudafed Children's* (McNeil)
30 mg per 5 mL (*otc*)	Various, *Silfedrine, Children's* (Silarx), *Unifed* (Altaire)
Syrup: 30 mg per 5 mL (*otc*)	*SudoGest Children's Congestion* (Harvard Drug)
Drops: 7.5 mg per 0.8 mL (*otc*)	Various, *Kid Kare* (Rugby)
Gel: 15 mg per 5 mL (*Rx*)	*ElixSure Congestion* (Taro)
TETRAHYDROZOLINE HYDROCHLORIDE	
Solution: 0.05% (*Rx*)	*Tyzine Pediatric* (Kenwood)
0.1% (*Rx*)	*Tyzine* (Kenwood)
XYLOMETAZOLINE HYDROCHLORIDE	
Solution: 0.05% (*otc*)	*Otrivin Pediatric Nasal* (Novartis Consumer)
0.1% (*otc*)	*Otrivin, 4-Way Nasal Decongestant Moisturizing Relief* (Novartis Consumer)
NASAL DECONGESTANT COMBINATIONS	
Solution: 0.5% phenylephrine hydrochloride and 0.2% pheniramine maleate (*otc*)	*Dristan Fast Acting Formula* (Whitehall-Robins)
NASAL DECONGESTANT INHALERS	
Inhaler: 250 mg propylhexedrine (*otc*)	*Benzedrex* (B.F. Ascher)
50 mg l-desoxyephedrine (*otc*)	*Vicks Vapor Inhaler* (Proctor & Gamble Consumer)

NASAL PRODUCTS

Solution: Sodium chloride (*otc*)	Various, *Pretz Moisturizing*, *Pretz Irrigation* (Parnell), *Afrin Saline* (Schering-Plough Healthcare), *Simply Saline* (Blairex)
0.4% Sodium chloride (*otc*)	*SalineX* (Muro)
0.65% Sodium chloride (*otc*)	*Ayr Saline* (B.F. Ascher), *Breathe Free* (Thompson Medical), *HuMist Moisturizing Mist* (Scherer), *NaSal* (Bayer Corp.), *Nasal Moist* (Blairex), *Ocean* (Fleming and Co.), *Mycinaire Saline Mist* (Pfeiffer)
15% polyethylene glycol per 5% propylene glycol, 15% polyethylene glycol per 20% propylene glycol (*otc*)	*Rhinaris Lubricating Mist* (Pharmascience)
Zinc acetate, zinc gluconate (*otc*)	*Nasal•Ease with Zinc*, *Nasal•Ease with Zinc Gluconate* (Health Care Products)

Indications

Oral: For temporary relief of nasal congestion due to the common cold, hay fever, or other upper respiratory allergies, and nasal congestion associated with sinusitis; to promote nasal or sinus drainage.

Topical: Symptomatic relief of nasal and nasopharyngeal mucosal congestion due to the common cold, sinusitis, hay fever, or other upper respiratory allergies.

Administration and Dosage

Recommended Dosage Guidelines for Oral and Topical Nasal Decongestants (Dosage Maximum per 24 h)[a]

Drug and route	Adults ≥ 12 years of age	Children 6 to < 12 years of age	Children 2 to < 6 years of age
Naphazoline			
Topical			
Sprays	0.05%: 1 or 2 sprays in each nostril no more than q 6 h (4 doses per 24 h)	not recommended	not recommended
Drops	0.05%: 1 or 2 drops in each nostril no more than q 6 h (4 doses per 24 h)	not recommended	not recommended
Oxymetazoline hydrochloride			
Topical			
Sprays	0.05%: 2 or 3 sprays in each nostril q 10 to 12 h (2 doses per 24 h)	same as adults	not recommended
Phenylephrine hydrochloride			
Oral	10-20 mg q 4 h (120 mg per 24 h)	10 mg q 4 h (60 mg per 24 h)	0.25% drops: 1 mL q 4 h (6 doses per 24 h); (15 mg per 24 h)
Topical			
Sprays	0.25%, 0.5%, 1%: 2 to 3 sprays in each nostril no more than q 4 h (6 doses per 24 h)	0.25%: 2 to 3 sprays in each nostril no more than q 4 h (6 doses per 24 h)	not recommended
Drops	0.25%, 0.5%, 1%: 2 to 3 drops in each nostril no more than q 4 h (6 doses per 24 h)		0.125%: 2 to 3 drops in each nostril no more than q 4 h (6 doses per 24 h)
Pseudoephedrine hydrochloride			
Oral	60 mg q 4 to 6 h (240 mg per 24 h)	30 mg q 4 to 6 h (120 mg per 24 h)	15 mg q 4 to 6 h (60 mg per 24 h)
Oral SR, CR	120 mg SR q 12 h or 240 mg CR q 24 h (240 mg per 24 h)	not recommended	not recommended
Tetrahydrozoline hydrochloride			
Topical			
Sprays	0.1%: 3 to 4 sprays in each nostril prn, no more than q 3 h (8 doses per 24 h)	same as adults	not recommended
Drops	0.1%: 2 to 4 drops in each nostril prn, no more than q 3 h (8 doses per 24 h)	same as adults	0.05%: 2 to 3 drops in each nostril prn no more than q 3 h (8 doses per 24 h)

Recommended Dosage Guidelines for Oral and Topical Nasal Decongestants (Dosage Maximum per 24 h)[a]			
Drug and route	Adults ≥ 12 years of age	Children 6 to < 12 years of age	Children 2 to < 6 years of age
Xylometazoline hydrochloride			
Topical			
Sprays	0.1%: 1 to 3 sprays in each nostril q 8 to 10 h (3 doses per 24 h)	0.05%: 1 spray in each nostril q 8 to 10 h (3 doses per 24 h)	same dose for 2 to 12 years of age
Drops	0.1%: 2 to 3 drops in each nostril q 8 to 10 h (3 doses per 24 h)	0.05%: 2 to 3 drops in each nostril q 8 to 10 h (3 doses per 24 h)	same dose for 2 to 12 years of age

[a] Refer to manufacturer's directions. SR = sustained release; CR = controlled release; ER = extended release

Actions

Pharmacology: Decongestants act on the adrenergic receptors in the nasal mucosa by affecting the blood vessels' sympathetic tone and provoking vasoconstriction.

Decongestants improve nasal ventilation by shrinking swollen nasal mucosa. Constriction in the mucous membranes results in their shrinkage; this promotes drainage, thus improving ventilation and the stuffy feeling.

Oral agents are not as effective as topical products, especially on an immediate basis, but generally have a longer duration of action, cause less local irritation and are not associated with rebound congestion (rhinitis medicamentosa).

Contraindications

Monoamine oxidase inhibitor (MAOI) therapy; hypersensitivity.

Oral:

Sustained-release pseudoephedrine – Children younger than 12 years of age.

Oral:

Sustained release pseudoephedrine and naphazoline – Children younger than 12 years of age.

Topical:

Tetrahydrozoline – 0.1% solution in children younger than 6 years of age; 0.05% solution in infants younger than 2 years of age.

Warnings/Precautions

Hypertension: Hypertensive patients should use these products only with medical advice, as they may experience a change in blood pressure because of the added vasoconstriction. Studies suggest pseudoephedrine is the drug of choice. Sustained-action preparations may affect the cardiovascular system to a lesser degree.

Excessive use: Do not exceed recommended dosage. If nervousness, dizziness, or sleeplessness occur, discontinue use and have the patient consult a physician. Do not take topical products for more than 3 days or oral products for more than 7 days. If symptoms do not improve or are accompanied by a fever, the patient should consult a physician.

Rebound congestion (rhinitis medicamentosa): May occur following topical application after the vasoconstriction subsides. Patients may increase the amount of drug and frequency of use, producing toxicity and perpetuating the rebound congestion.

Treatment – A simple but uncomfortable solution is to completely withdraw the topical medication. A more acceptable method is to gradually withdraw therapy by initially discontinuing the medication in one nostril, followed by total withdrawal. Substituting an oral decongestant for a topical one may also be useful.

Acute use: Use topical decongestants only in acute states and not longer than 3 to 5 days. Use sparingly (especially the imidazolines) in all patients, particularly infants, children, and patients with cardiovascular disease.

Stinging sensation: Some individuals may experience a mild, transient stinging sensation after topical application.

Sulfite sensitivity: Some of the nasal decongestant products contain sulfites that may cause allergic-type reactions including anaphylactic symptoms and life-threatening or less severe asthmatic episodes in certain susceptible people. Products containing sulfites are identified in the product listings.

Special risk: Administer with caution to patients with thyroid disease, diabetes mellitus, cardiovascular disease, coronary artery disease, hypertension, peripheral vascular disease, heart disease, ischemic heart disease, increased intraocular pressure, or prostatic hypertrophy.

Oral – Rarely, some tablets may cause bowel obstruction or blockage, usually in people with severe narrowing of the bowel, esophagus, stomach, or intestine. If a patient has had obstruction or narrowing of the bowel, have him or her consult a physician before taking oral tablet products. Advise patients to contact their physician if they experience persistent abdominal pain or vomiting.

Pregnancy: Category C.

Lactation:

Oral preparations – Consult a physician before using.

Topical – It is not known if these agents are excreted in breast milk.

Children: Use in children is product specific.

Elderly: Patients 60 years of age and older are more likely to experience adverse reactions to sympathomimetics. Overdosage may cause hallucinations, convulsions, CNS depression, and death.

Drug Interactions

Most interactions listed apply to sympathomimetics when used as vasopressors; however, consider the interaction when using the nasal decongestants.

Drugs that may affect nasal decongestants include beta blockers, furazolidone, guanethidine, methyldopa, MAO inhibitors, rauwolfia alkaloids, tricyclic antidepressants, urinary acidifiers, and urinary alkalinizers.

Drugs that may be affected by nasal decongestants include guanethidine.

Adverse Reactions

Arrhythmias; palpitations; tachycardia; transient hypertension; bradycardia; headache; lightheadedness; dizziness; drowsiness; tremor; insomnia; nervousness; restlessness; giddiness; psychological disturbances; prolonged psychosis; weakness; nausea; gastric irritation; hypersensitivity reactions such as rash, urticaria, leukopenia, agranulocytosis, and thrombocytopenia; orofacial dystonia; sweating; blepharospasm; urinary retention may occur in patients with prostatic hypertrophy.

Topical use – Burning; stinging; sneezing; dryness; local irritation; rebound congestion.

INTRANASAL STEROIDS

BECLOMETHASONE DIPROPIONATE	
Spray: 42 mcg/actuation (*Rx*)	*Beconase AQ* (GlaxoSmithKline)
BUDESONIDE	
Spray: 32 mcg/actuation (*Rx*)	*Rhinocort Aqua* (AstraZeneca)
CICLESONIDE	
Spray: 50 mcg/actuation (*Rx*)	*Omnaris* (Nycomed US Inc.)
FLUNISOLIDE	
Solution: 0.025% (25 mcg/actuation) (*Rx*)	*Flunisolide* (Bausch & Lomb)
FLUTICASONE PROPIONATE	
Spray: 50 mcg/actuation (*Rx*)	Various, *Flonase* (GlaxoSmithKline)
Spray, suspension; intranasal: 27.5 mcg/spray (as furoate) (*Rx*)	*Veramyst* (GlaxoSmithKline)
MOMETASONE FUROATE MONOHYDRATE	
Spray: 50 mcg/actuation (*Rx*)	*Nasonex* (Schering)

Indications

Intranasal Steroids Indications[a]

Condition	Beclomethasone	Budesonide	Ciclesonide	Flunisolide	Fluticasone	Mometasone
Nasal polyps	✓					✓
Nonallergic (vasomotor) rhinitis	✓				✓	
Perennial allergic rhinitis	✓	✓	✓	✓	✓	✓
Seasonal allergic rhinitis	✓	✓	✓	✓	✓	✓[b]
Recurrent chronic sinusitis[c]		X			X	X

[a] ✓ = approved use; X = unlabeled use.
[b] Treatment and prophylaxis.
[c] As adjunctive therapy with an antibiotic and/or decongestant.

Administration and Dosage

Improvement in symptoms usually becomes apparent within a few days. However, relief may not occur in some patients for as long as 2 weeks. Do not continue beyond 3 weeks in absence of significant symptomatic improvement.

BECLOMETHASONE DIPROPIONATE:

Adults and children 12 years of age and older – 1 or 2 nasal inhalations (42 to 84 mcg) in each nostril twice daily (total dose, 168 to 336 mcg/day).

Children 6 to 11 years of age – 1 nasal inhalation in each nostril twice daily (168 mcg). Patients not adequately responding or those with more severe symptoms may use 2 sprays in each nostril twice daily (336 mcg/day).

Maximum dosage – 2 sprays in each nostril twice daily (336 mcg/day).

Maintenance dose – Once adequate control is achieved, decrease the dosage to 1 spray in each nostril twice daily.

BUDESONIDE:

Adults and children 6 years of age and older – 1 spray in each nostril once daily (64 mcg/day). Some patients who do not achieve symptom control at the recommended starting dose may benefit from an increased dose.

Maximum dose –

Adults 12 years of age and older: 4 sprays in each nostril once daily (256 mcg/day).

Children 6 to 11 years of age: 2 sprays in each nostril once daily (128 mcg/day).

Maintenance dose – After the desired clinical effect is obtained, reduce the maintenance dose to the smallest amount necessary to control symptoms.

CICLESONIDE:

Perennial allergic rhinitis –

Adults and adolescents 12 years of age and older: 200 mcg/day, administered as 2 sprays (50 mcg/spray) in each nostril once daily.

Seasonal allergic rhinitis –

Adults and children 6 years of age and older: 200 mcg/day, administered as 2 sprays (50 mcg/spray) in each nostril once daily.

Maximum dose – The maximum total daily dose should not exceed 2 sprays in each nostril (200 mcg/day).

FLUNISOLIDE:

Adults – 2 sprays (50 mcg) in each nostril 2 times/day (total dose 200 mcg/day). May increase to 2 sprays in each nostril 3 times/day (total dose 300 mcg/day). Maximum daily dose is 8 sprays in each nostril (400 mcg/day).

Children (6 to 14 years of age) – Starting dose is 1 spray (25 mcg) in each nostril 3 times/day or 2 sprays (50 mcg) in each nostril 2 times/day (total dose 150 to 200 mcg/day). Maximum daily dose is 4 sprays in each nostril (200 mcg/day).

Maintenance dose – After desired clinical effect is obtained, reduce maintenance dose to smallest amount necessary to control symptoms. Some patients with perennial rhinitis may be maintained on 1 spray in each nostril per day.

FLUTICASONE FUROATE:

Adults – 110 mcg once daily administered as 2 sprays (27.5 mcg/spray) in each nostril. When symptoms have been controlled, reduce the dosage to 55 mcg (1 spray in each nostril) once daily.

Children 2 to 11 years of age – 55 mcg once daily administered as 1 spray (27.5 mcg/spray) in each nostril. Children not adequately responding to 55 mcg may use 110 mcg (2 sprays in each nostril) once daily. Once symptoms have been controlled, the dosage may be decreased to 55 mcg once daily.

FLUTICASONE PROPIONATE:

Adults – 2 sprays (50 mcg each) per nostril once daily (total daily dose, 200 mcg). The same dosage divided into 100 mcg given twice daily is also effective. Dosage may be reduced to 100 mcg (1 spray per nostril) once daily for maintenance therapy. Maximum total daily dosage should not exceed 200 mcg/day.

Some patients 12 years of age and older with seasonal allergic rhinitis may find as-needed use of fluticasone propionate nasal spray (not to exceed 200 mcg daily) effective for symptom control. Greater symptom control may be achieved with scheduled regular use.

Adolescents 4 years of age and older – 100 mcg (1 spray per nostril per day). Patients not adequately responding to 100 mcg may use 200 mcg (2 sprays/nostril). Depending on response, dosage may be decreased to 100 mcg daily. Total daily dosage should not exceed 200 mcg/day.

Children younger than 4 years of age – Use not recommended.

MOMETASONE FUROATE MONOHYDRATE:

Allergic rhinitis –

Adults and children 12 years of age and older: 2 sprays (50 mcg) in each nostril once daily (total daily dose, 200 mcg).

In patients with a known seasonal allergen, prophylaxis with mometasone (200 mcg/day) is recommended 2 to 4 weeks prior to the anticipated start of the pollen season.

Children 2 to 11 years of age: 1 spray (50 mcg) in each nostril once daily (total daily dose, 100 mcg).

Nasal polyps –

Adults 18 years of age and older: 2 sprays (50 mcg each) in each nostril twice daily (total daily dose of 400 mcg); 2 sprays (50 mcg each) in each nostril once daily (total daily dose of 200 mcg) is also effective.

Actions

Pharmacology: These drugs have potent glucocorticoid and weak mineralocorticoid activity. The mechanisms responsible for the anti-inflammatory action of corticosteroids on the nasal mucosa are unknown. These agents, when administered topically, exert direct local anti-inflammatory effects with minimal systemic effects.

Pharmacokinetics: The amount of an intranasal dose that reaches systemic circulation is generally low, and metabolism is rapid.

Contraindications

Untreated localized infections involving the nasal mucosa (flunisolide); hypersensitivity to the drug or any component of the product.

Warnings/Precautions

Effect on growth: Intranasal corticosteroids may cause a reduction in growth velocity when administered to children.

Excessive doses/sensitivity: If recommended doses of intranasal corticosteroids are exceeded or if individuals are particularly sensitive or predisposed by virtue of recent systemic steroid therapy, symptoms of hypercorticism may occur, including, very rarely, menstrual irregularities, acneiform lesions, and cushingoid features.

Infections: Localized infections of the nose and pharynx with *Candida albicans* have developed only rarely.

Use with caution in patients with active or quiescent tuberculosis infections of the respiratory tract, or in untreated fungal, bacterial, or systemic viral infections, or ocular herpes simplex.

Individuals receiving immunosuppressant agents are more susceptible to infections than healthy individuals. Avoid exposure to chicken pox or measles.

Long-term treatment: Examine patients periodically over several months or longer for possible changes in the nasal mucosa.

Nasal septum perforation: Rare instances of nasal septum perforation have been reported following the intranasal application of corticosteroids.

Nasopharyngeal irritation: If persistent nasopharyngeal irritation occurs, it may be an indication to stop therapy.

Ophthalmic effects: Rare instances of cataracts, glaucoma, and increased intraocular pressure have been reported following intranasal application of corticosteroids.

Respiratory effects: Rare instances of wheezing have been reported following intranasal application of corticosteroids.

Special senses: Temporary or permanent loss of the sense of smell and taste has been reported with flunisolide use.

Systemic corticosteroids: The combined administration of alternate-day systemic prednisone with these products may increase the likelihood of hypothalamic-pituitary-adrenal (HPA) suppression.

Systemic effects: Although systemic absorption is low when used in recommended dosage, HPA suppression and other systemic effects may occur, especially with excessive doses.

Vasoconstrictors: In the presence of excessive nasal mucosa secretion or edema of the nasal mucosa, the drug may fail to reach the site of intended action. In such cases, use a nasal vasoconstrictor during the first 2 to 3 days of therapy.

Wound healing: Because of the inhibitory effect of corticosteroids on wound healing in patients who have experienced recent nasal septal ulcers, recurrent epistaxis, nasal surgery, or trauma, use nasal steroids with caution until healing has occurred.

Hypersensitivity reactions: Rare cases of immediate and delayed hypersensitivity reactions, including angioedema, urticaria, rash, and bronchospasm, have occurred.

Hepatic function impairment: Reduced liver function may affect the elimination of corticosteroids. The systemic availability of oral **budesonide** was doubled by compromised liver function.

Pregnancy: Category C.

Carefully observe infants born of mothers who have received substantial doses of corticosteroids during pregnancy for signs of adrenal insufficiency.

Lactation: It is not known whether these drugs are excreted in breast milk. Because other corticosteroids are excreted in human milk, use caution when administering to breast-feeding women.

Children:

Beclomethasone, budesonide, flunisolide, triamcinolone – Safety and efficacy for use in children younger than 6 years of age have not been established.

Ciclesonide – Safety and effectiveness for seasonal and perennial allergic rhinitis in children 12 years of age and older have been established.

Fluticasone – Safety and efficacy for use in children younger than 4 years of age have not been established.

Mometasone – Safety and efficacy for use in children younger than 2 years of age have not been established.

Drug Interactions

Drugs that may affect intranasal steroids include cimetidine, inhibitors of CYP3A4 (eg, ketoconazole, itraconazole, clarithromycin, erythromycin, cimetidine, ritonavir).

Adverse Reactions

Adverse reactions associated with intranasal steroids include abdominal pain, aches and pains, aftertaste, arthralgia, asthma symptoms, bronchitis, burning, chest pain, conjunctivitis, cough, diarrhea, dryness, dysmenorrhea, dyspepsia, earache, epistaxis, fever, flu-like symptoms, headache, lightheadedness, loss of taste/smell, mild nasopharyngeal irritation, myalgia, nasal irritation, nasopharyngitis, nausea, otitis media, pharyngitis, pharyngolaryngeal pain, rhinitis, rhinorrhea, sinusitis, sneezing, stinging, throat discomfort, upper respiratory tract infection, viral infection, vomiting, watery eyes, wheezing.

ANTIHISTAMINES

AZELASTINE HYDROCHLORIDE	
Spray, solution; intranasal: 137 and 205.5 mcg/spray (*Rx*)	*Astelin* (Medpointe)
BROMPHENIRAMINE	
Tablets, chewable; oral: 12 mg (*Rx*)	Various, *BrōveX CT* (Athlon)
Tablets, extended release; oral: 6 mg (as maleate and tannate) (*Rx*)	*LoHist 12 Hour* (Larken)
Capsules, extended release; oral: 12 mg (as maleate) (*Rx*)	*Lodrane 24* (ECR Pharmaceuticals)
Liquid; oral: 2 mg per 5 mL (*Rx*)	*VaZol* (WraSer)
Suspension; oral: 4 mg per 5 mL, 8 mg per 5 mL, 10 mg per 5 mL, 12 mg per 5 mL (*Rx*)	Various, *BrōveX* (Athlon), *Lodrane XR* (ECR Pharmaceuticals), *J-Tan* (Jaymec Pharmaceuticals), *P-tex* (Poly Pharmaceuticals)
CARBINOXAMINE MALEATE	
Tablets; oral: 4 mg (*Rx*)	Various, *Palgic* (Pamlab)
Tablets, timed release; oral: 8 mg (*Rx*)	*Histex CT* (Teamm Pharm)
Capsules, extended release; oral: 10 mg (*Rx*)	*Histex I/E*[a] (Teamm Pharm)
Liquid; oral: 1.67 mg per 5 mL (*Rx*)	*Pediatex* (Zyber Pharmaceuticals)
4 mg per 5 mL (*Rx*)	Various, *Histex Pd* (Teamm Pharm), *Palgic* (Pamlab)
Suspension; oral: 3.2 mg per 5 mL (*Rx*)	*Pediatex 12* (Zyber)
CETIRIZINE HYDROCHLORIDE	
Tablets; oral: 5 mg (*otc*)	Various
10 mg (*otc*)	Various, *Zyrtec Hives Relief*, *Zyrtec Allergy* (McNeil Consumer)
Tablets, chewable; oral: 5 and 10 mg (*otc*)	*Zyrtec Children's Allergy* (McNeil Consumer)
Syrup; oral: 1 mg per mL (*otc*)	Various, *Zyrtec Children's Hive Relief*, *Zyrtec Children's Allergy* (McNeil Consumer)
CHLORPHENIRAMINE	
Tablets; oral: 4 mg (as maleate) (*otc*)	Various, *Aller-Chlor* (Rugby), *Allergy* (Major), *Allergy Relief* (Zee Medical)
Tablets, chewable; oral: 2 mg (as maleate) (*otc*)	*Chlo-Amine* (Hollister-Stier)
Tablets, extended release; oral: 8 mg (as maleate) (*otc*)	*Chlor-Trimeton Allergy 8 Hour* (Schering-Plough Healthcare)
12 mg (as maleate) (*otc*)	*Chlor-Trimeton Allergy 12 Hour* (Schering-Plough Healthcare)
16 mg (as maleate) (*otc*)	*Efidac 24*[b] (Hogil)
Caplet; oral: 8 mg (as tannate) (*Rx*)	*ED-CHLOR-TAN* (Edwards Pharmaceuticals)
Capsules, extended release; oral: 12 mg (as maleate) (*Rx*)	*QDALL AR*[c] (Atley)
Capsules, sustained release; oral: 8 and 12 mg (as maleate) (*Rx*)	Various
Syrup; oral: 2 mg per 5 mL (*otc*)	*Aller-Chlor* (Rugby)
Suspension; oral: 4 mg (as maleate) per 5 mL (*Rx*)	*Pediox-S* (Atley)
CLEMASTINE FUMARATE	
Tablets; oral: 1.34 mg as fumarate (equiv. to clemastine 1 mg) (*otc*)	Various, *Dayhist-1* (Major), *Tavist Allergy* (Novartis Consumer Health)
2.68 mg (equiv. to clemastine 2 mg) (*Rx*)	Various
Syrup; oral: 0.67 mg (equiv. to clemastine 0.5 mg) per 5 mL (*Rx*)	Various
CYPROHEPTADINE HYDROCHLORIDE	
Tablets; oral: 4 mg (*Rx*)	Various
Syrup; oral: 2 mg per 5 mL (*Rx*)	Various
DESLORATADINE	
Tablets; oral: 5 mg (*Rx*)	*Clarinex* (Schering)
Tablets, rapidly disintegrating; oral: 2.5 and 5 mg (*Rx*)	*Clarinex RediTabs* (Schering)
Syrup; oral: 2.5 mg per 5 mL (*Rx*)	*Clarinex* (Schering)
DEXCHLORPHENIRAMINE MALEATE	
Tablets, extended release; oral: 4 and 6 mg (*Rx*)	Various
Syrup; oral: 2 mg per 5 mL (*Rx*)	(Morton Grove)

DIPHENHYDRAMINE	
Tablets; oral: 25 mg (as hydrochloride) (*otc*)	Various, *Banophen* (Major), *Benadryl Allergy Ultratabs* (Pfizer), *Diphenhist Captabs* (Rugby), *Dormin* (Randob), *Miles Nervine* (Miles), *Nytol* (Block), *Simply Sleep* (McNeil), *Sleep-eze 3* (Whitehall), *Sleepwell 2-nite* (Rugby), *Sominex* (SmithKline Beecham)
50 mg (as hydrochloride) (*otc*)	*AllerMax Maximum Strength Caplets* (Pfeiffer), *Compoz Nighttime Sleep Aid* (Medtech), *40 Winks* (Roberts Med), *Maximum Strength Nytol* (Block), *Midol PM* (Sterling Health), *Snooze Fast* (BDI), *Sominex* (SmithKline-Beecham), *Twilite* (Pfeiffer)
Tablets, chewable; oral: 12.5 mg (as hydrochloride) (*otc*)	*Benadryl Allergy* (Pfizer)
25 mg (as tannate) (*Rx*)	*Dytan* (Hawthorn)
Tablets, disintegrating; oral: 12.5 mg (equiv. to 19 mg citrate) (*otc*)	*Children's Benadryl Allergy Fastmelt* (Pfizer)
Capsules; oral: 25 mg (as hydrochloride) (*otc/Rx*)	Various, *Banophen* (Major), *Benadryl Allergy Kapseals* (Pfizer), *Benadryl Dye-Free Allergy Liqui-Gels* (Pfizer), *Compoz Gel Caps* (Medtech) *Dormin* (Randob) *Diphenhist* (Rugby), *Genahist* (Goldline)
50 mg (as hydrochloride) (*otc/Rx*)	Various *Maximum Strength Sleepinal* (Thompson), *Maximum Strength Unisom SleepGels* (Pfizer)
Strips, disintegrating; oral: 12.5 mg (as hydrochloride) (*otc*)	*Triaminic Children's Allergy* (Novartis Consumer Health), *Triaminic Cough & Runny Nose* (Novartis Consumer Health)
25 mg (as hydrochloride) (*otc*)	*Benadryl Allergy Quick Dissolve Strips* (Pfizer), *Triaminic MultiSymptom* (Novartis Consumer Health)
Liquid; oral: 12.5 mg per 5 mL (*otc*)	*AllerMax* (Pfeiffer), *Altaryl Children's Allergy* (Altaire), *Benadryl Children's Allergy* (Pfizer), *Benadryl Children's Dye-Free Allergy* (Pfizer), *Diphen AF* (Morton Grove), *Genahist* (Goldline), *Q-dryl* (Qualitest Pharmaceuticals), *Scot-Tussin Allergy Relief Formula Clear* (Scot-Tussin)
Solution; oral: 12.5 mg per 5 mL (as hydrochloride) (*otc*)	*Diphenhist* (Rugby), *PediaCare Children's Nighttime Cough* (Pfizer)
Elixir; oral: 12.5 mg per 5 mL (as hydrochloride) (*otc*)	*Banophen Allergy* (Major), *Siladryl* (Silarx)
Syrup; oral: 12.5 mg per 5 mL (*Rx*)	Various, *Silphen Cough* (Silarx), *Tusstat* (Century)
Suspension; oral: 25 mg per 5 mL (as tannate) (*Rx*)	*Dytan* (Hawthorn)
Injection: 50 mg/mL (as hydrochloride) (*Rx*)	Various, *Benadryl* (Parke-Davis)
FEXOFENADINE HYDROCHLORIDE	
Tablets; oral: 30 mg (*Rx*)	Various
60 and 180 mg (*Rx*)	Various, *Allegra* (Sanofi-Aventis)
Tablets, disintegrating; oral: 30 mg (*Rx*)	*Allegra ODT* (Sanofi-Aventis)
Suspension; oral: 6 mg/mL (*Rx*)	*Allegra* (Sanofi-Aventis)
HYDROXYZINE	
Tablets; oral (as hydrochloride): 10, 25, and 50 mg (*Rx*)	Various
Capsules; oral (as pamoate): 25, 50, and 100 mg (*Rx*)	Various, *Vistaril* (Pfizer)
Syrup; oral (as hydrochloride): 10 mg per 5 mL (*Rx*)	Various
Injection (as hydrochloride): 25 and 50 mg/mL (*Rx*)	Various
LEVOCETIRIZINE	
Tablets; oral: 5 mg (*Rx*)	*Xyzal* (UCB)
Solution; oral: 2.5 mg per 5 mL (*Rx*)	*Xyzal* (UCB)
LORATADINE	
Tablets; oral: 10 mg (*otc*)	Various, *Claritin 24-hour Allergy*, *Claritin Hives Relief* (Schering), *Clear-Atadine* (Major)
Tablets, chewable; oral: 5 mg (*otc*)	*Claritin Children's Allergy* (Schering-Plough Healthcare)
Tablets, disintegrating; oral: 5 mg (*otc*)	*Claritin RediTabs* (Schering-Plough)

10 mg (*otc*)	*Alavert* (Wyeth Consumer), *Claritin RediTabs* (Schering-Plough Healthcare), *Triaminic Allerchews* (Novartis), *Dimetapp Children's ND Non-Drowsy Allergy* (Wyeth), *Non-Drowsy Allergy Relief* (Major), *Clear-Atadine Children's* (Major)
Syrup; oral: 5 mg per 5 mL (*otc*)	Various, *Claritin* (Schering), *Claritin Children's Allergy* (Schering), *Clear-Atadine Children's* (Major), *Dimetapp Children's ND Non-Drowsy Allergy* (Wyeth), *Alavert Children's* (Wyeth), *Non-Drowsy Allergy Relief for Kids* (Major)
OLOPATADINE HYDROCHLORIDE	
Spray, solution; intranasal: 0.6% (*Rx*)	*Patanase* (Alcon Labs)
PROMETHAZINE HYDROCHLORIDE	
Tablets; oral: 12.5, 25, and 50 mg (*Rx*)	Various, *Phenergan* (Wyeth Labs)
Syrup; oral: 6.25 mg per 5 mL (*Rx*)	Various
Suppositories: 12.5 and 25 mg (*Rx*)	Various, *Phenadoz* (Paddock), *Phenergan* (Wyeth Labs)
50 mg (*Rx*)	Various
Injection; solution: 25 and 50 mg/mL (*Rx*)	Various, *Phenergan* (Wyeth Labs)
TRIPROLIDINE HYDROCHLORIDE	
Liquid; oral: 1.25 mg per 5 mL (*Rx*)	Various, *Zymine* (Vindex Pharmaceuticals)
Suspension; oral: 2.5 mg per 5 mL (*Rx*)	*Zymine XR* (Vindex)

[a] 2 mg immediate-release and 8 mg extended-release.
[b] 4 mg immediate-release and 12 mg controlled-release.
[c] 2 mg immediate-release and 10 mg sustained-release.

Warning:

Promethazine: Do not use promethazine in children younger than 2 years of age because of the potential for fatal respiratory depression.

Postmarketing cases of respiratory depression, including fatalities, have been reported with the use of promethazine in children younger than 2 years of age. A wide range of weight-based doses of promethazine have resulted in respiratory depression in these patients.

Exercise caution when administering promethazine to children 2 years of age and older. It is recommended that the lowest effective dose of promethazine be used in children 2 years of age and older and that coadministration of other drugs with respiratory-depressant effects be avoided.

Indications

Oral: Relief of symptoms associated with the following: perennial and seasonal allergic rhinitis; vasomotor rhinitis; allergic conjunctivitis (eg, caused by inhalant allergens or food); temporary relief of sneezing, itchy or watery eyes, itchy nose or throat, and runny nose caused by hay fever (allergic rhinitis) or other respiratory allergies and the common cold; allergic and nonallergic pruritic symptoms; mild, uncomplicated, allergic skin manifestations of urticaria and angioedema; uncomplicated skin manifestations of chronic idiopathic urticaria; amelioration of allergic reactions to blood or plasma; dermatographism; adjunctive therapy in anaphylactic reactions; lacrimation.

Parenteral: When oral therapy is not possible or contraindicated.

Brompheniramine: VaZol also is indicated for the temporary relief of runny nose and sneezing caused by the common cold; treatment of allergic and nonallergic pruritic symptoms; temporary relief of mild, uncomplicated urticaria and angioedema; amelioration of allergic reactions to blood or plasma; adjunctive therapy in anaphylactic reactions.

Cetirizine, desloratadine, fexofenadine, levocetirizine: Also indicated for chronic idiopathic urticaria.

Cyproheptadine: Hypersensitivity reactions: perennial and seasonal allergic rhinitis; vasomotor rhinitis; allergic conjunctivitis caused by inhalant allergens and foods; mild, uncomplicated allergic skin manifestations of urticaria and angioedema;

amelioration of allergic reactions to blood or plasma; cold urticaria; dermatographism; adjunctive anaphylactic therapy.

Diphenhydramine: Also indicated for active treatment of motion sickness (injection only); for parkinsonism in the elderly intolerant of more potent agents, for mild cases in other age groups, and in combination with centrally-acting anticholinergics; as a cough suppressant (oral liquids); insomnia (oral only).

Hydroxyzine: Symptomatic relief of anxiety and tension associated with psychoneurosis and as an adjunct in organic disease states in which anxiety is manifest.

Management of pruritus caused by allergic conditions such as chronic urticaria, atopic and contact dermatoses and in histamine-mediated pruritus.

As a sedative when used as premedication and following general anesthesia.

Intramuscular only – For the acutely disturbed or hysterical patient; the acute or chronic alcoholic with anxiety withdrawal symptoms or delirium tremens; allay anxiety; adjunctive therapy in asthma.

Antiemetic (parenteral only): In controlling nausea and vomiting (excluding nausea and vomiting of pregnancy). As pre- and postoperative and pre- and postpartum adjunctive medication to control emesis.

Analgesia, adjunctive therapy (parenteral only): As pre- and postoperative and pre- and postpartum adjunctive medication to permit reduction in narcotic dosage.

Olopatadine (intranasal): For the relief of the symptoms of seasonal allergic rhinitis in patients 6 years of age and older.

Promethazine: Promethazine is also indicated for preoperative, postoperative, or obstetric sedation; prevention and control of nausea and vomiting associated with certain types of anesthesia and surgery; an adjunct to analgesics for control of postoperative pain; sedation and relief of apprehension, and to produce light sleep; antiemetic effect in postoperative patients; active and prophylactic treatment of motion sickness (oral and rectal only).

Administration and Dosage

AZELASTINE: Before initial use, prime the delivery system with 4 sprays or until a fine mist appears. When at least 3 days have elapsed since last use, re-prime the pump with 2 sprays or until a fine mist appears.

Seasonal allergic rhinitis –

Adults and children 12 years of age and older: 1 or 2 sprays per nostril twice daily. The Astepro 205.5 mcg/spray solution can also be administered as 2 sprays per nostril once daily.

Children 5 to 11 years of age (Astelin): 1 spray per nostril twice daily.

Perennial allergic rhinitis (Astepro 205.5 mcg/spray) –

Adults and children 12 years of age and older: 2 sprays per nostril twice daily.

Vasomotor rhinitis (Astelin) –

Adults and children 12 years of age and older: 2 sprays per nostril twice daily.

BROMPHENIRAMINE TANNATE:

Extended-release tablets – Take with food, water, or milk to minimize gastric irritation. Swallow whole; do not crush tablets.

Adults and children older than 12 years of age: 1 or 2 tablets (6 to 12 mg) every 12 hours.

Children 6 to 12 years of age: 1 tablet (6 mg) every 12 hours.

Tablets, chewable –

Adults and children 12 years of age and older: 1 or 2 tablets (12 to 24 mg) every 12 hours, up to 4 tablets (48 mg) in 24 hours.

Children 6 to younger than 12 years of age: ½ to 1 tablet (6 to 12 mg) every 12 hours, up to 2 tablets (24 mg) in 24 hours.

Children 2 to younger than 6 years of age: ½ tablet (6 mg) every 12 hours, up to 1 tablet (12 mg) in 24 hours.

Extended-release capsules – Take with food, water, or milk to minimize gastric irritation. Swallow whole; do not crush capsules.

Adults and children 12 years of age and older: 1 or 2 capsules (12 to 24 mg) once daily.

Children 6 to younger than 12 years of age: 1 capsule (12 mg) once daily.

Oral suspension – Shake well before use.

Adults and children 12 years of age and older: 5 to 10 mL (12 to 24 mg) every 12 hours, up to 20 mL (48 mg) in 24 hours.

Children 6 to younger than 12 years of age: 5 mL (12 mg) every 12 hours, up to 10 mL (24 mg) in 24 hours.

Children 2 to younger than 6 years of age: 2.5 mL (6 mg) every 12 hours, up to 5 mL (12 mg) in 24 hours.

Children 12 months to 2 years of age: 1.25 mL (3 mg) every 12 hours, up to 2.5 mL (6 mg) in 24 hours.

Oral liquid –

Adults and children older than 12 years of age: 10 mL (4 mg) 4 times daily.

Children 6 to 12 years of age: 5 mL (2 mg) 4 times daily.

Children 2 to 6 years of age: 2.5 mL (1 mg) 4 times daily

Children younger than 2 years of age: Titrate dosage individually based on 0.5 mg/kg/day in equally divided doses, 4 times daily.

Lodrane XR –

Adults and children older than 12 years of age: 5 mL every 12 hours, not to exceed 2 doses in 24 hours.

Children 6 to 12 years of age: 2.5 mL every 12 hours, not to exceed 2 doses in 24 hours.

Children 2 to 6 years of age: 1.25 mL every 12 hours, not to exceed 2 doses in 24 hours.

Children younger than 2 years of age: As recommended by a health care provider.

CARBINOXAMINE MALEATE:

Tablets –

Histex CT: Histex CT tablets are not recommended for children younger than 6 years of age. Tablets may be broken in half for ease of administration, but should not be crushed or chewed.

Adults and children 12 years of age and older – 1 tablet (8 mg) twice daily (every 12 hours).

Children 6 to 12 years of age – ½ tablet twice daily (every 12 hours).

Palgic:

Adults – 1 or 2 tablets (4 to 8 mg) 3 to 4 times daily.

Children 6 years of age and older – 1 to 1½ tablets (4 to 6 mg) 3 or 4 times daily.

Children 3 to 6 years of age – ½ to 1 tablet (2 to 4 mg) 3 or 4 times daily.

Children 1 to 3 years of age – ½ tablet (2 mg) 3 or 4 times daily.

Capsules –

Adults and children 12 years of age and older: 1 capsule every 12 hours, up to 2 a day.

Liquids –

Histex Pd:

Adults and children 6 years of age and older – 5 mL 4 times per day.

Children –

18 months to 6 years of age: 2.5 mL 4 times per day.

9 to 18 months of age: 1.25 to 2.5 mL 4 times per day.

Palgic:

Adults – 5 or 10 mL 3 to 4 times per day.

Children –

Older than 6 years of age: 5 to 7.5 mL 3 or 4 times per day.

3 to 6 years of age: 2.5 to 5 mL 3 or 4 times per day.

1 to 3 years of age: 2.5 mL 3 or 4 times per day.

Pediatex:

Adults and children 6 years of age and older – 10 mL 4 times per day.

Children –

18 months to 6 years of age: 5 mL 4 times per day.

9 to 18 months of age: 3.75 to 5 mL 4 times per day.

6 to 9 months of age: 3.75 mL 4 times per day.

3 to 6 months of age: 2.5 mL 4 times per day.

1 to 3 months of age: 1.25 mL 4 times per day.

Oral suspension –

Adults and children 12 years of age and older: 2 to 4 teaspoonsful every 12 hours.

Children 6 to 12 years of age: 1 to 2 teaspoonsful every 12 hours.

Children 2 to 6 years of age: ½ to 1 teaspoonful every 12 hours.

CETIRIZINE HYDROCHLORIDE: May be given with or without food.

Adults and children 12 years of age and older – 5 or 10 mg once daily depending on symptom severity.

Children –

6 to 11 years of age: 5 or 10 mg once daily depending on symptom severity.

2 to younger than 6 years of age: 2.5 mg once daily of the oral solution. May increase to a maximum dose of 5 mg/day as 5 mg once daily or as 2.5 mg given every 12 hours.

Elderly (77 years of age and older) – 5 mg once daily as recommended.

Renal/Hepatic function impairment – In patients 12 years of age and older with decreased renal function (creatinine clearance [CrCl] 11 to 31 mL/min), hemodialysis patients (CrCl less than 7 mL/min), and in hepatically impaired patients, 5 mg once daily is recommended.

CHLORPHENIRAMINE MALEATE: Individualize dosage.

Tablets or syrup –

Adults and children 12 years of age and older: 4 mg every 4 to 6 hours. Do not exceed 24 mg in 24 hours.

Children 6 to 12 years of age: 2 mg (break 4 mg tablets in half) every 4 to 6 hours. Do not exceed 12 mg in 24 hours.

Children younger than 6 years of age: Consult a health care provider.

Tablets, extended-release –

Adults and children 12 years of age and older: 8 mg every 8 to 12 hours or 12 mg every 12 hours. Do not exceed 24 mg in 24 hours.

Efidac 24:

Adults and children 12 years of age and older – 16 mg with liquid every 24 hours. Do not exceed 16 mg in 24 hours. Swallow each tablet whole; do not divide, crush, chew, or dissolve.

Capsules, extended-release –

Adults and children 12 years of age and older: 12 mg once daily, not to exceed 24 mg in 24 hours.

Capsules, sustained-release –

Adults and children 12 years of age and older: 8 or 12 mg every 12 hours, up to 16 to 24 mg/day.

Children 6 to 12 years of age: 8 mg at bedtime or during the day as indicated.

Caplets –

Adults and children 12 years of age and older: 8 mg every 12 hours, up to 16 to 24 mg/day.

Children 6 to 12 years of age: Consult a health care provider.

Oral suspension –

Adults and children 12 years of age and older: 5 to 10 mL every 12 hours, up to 20 mL/day.

Children 6 to younger than 12 years of age: 2.5 to 5 mL every 12 hours, up to 10 mL/day.

Children 2 to younger than 6 years of age: 1.25 mL every 12 hours, up to 5 mL/day.

Younger than 2 years of age: As directed by a health care provider.

CLEMASTINE FUMARATE:

Allergic rhinitis –

Adults: 1.34 mg every 12 hours or twice daily. Do not exceed 8.04 mg for the syrup or 2.68 mg for the tablets in 24 hours.

Children 6 to 12 years of age (syrup only): 0.67 mg twice daily. Single doses of up to 2.25 mg have been well tolerated. Do not exceed 4.02 mg/day.

Urticaria/Angioedema –

Adults: 2.68 mg twice daily, not to exceed 8.04 mg/day.

Children 6 to 12 years of age (syrup only): 1.34 mg twice daily, not to exceed 4.02 mg/day.

CYPROHEPTADINE HYDROCHLORIDE:

Adults – 4 to 20 mg/day. Initiate therapy with 4 mg 3 times/day. Most patients require 12 to 16 mg/day and occasionally as much as 32 mg/day. Do not exceed 0.5 mg/kg/day.

Children – Calculate total daily dosage as approximately 0.25 mg/kg or 8 mg/m^2.

7 to 14 years of age: 4 mg 2 or 3 times/day. Do not exceed 16 mg/day.

2 to 6 years of age: 2 mg 2 or 3 times/day. Do not exceed 12 mg/day.

DESLORATADINE:

Adults and children 12 years of age and older – 5 mg once daily. In patients with liver or renal impairment, a starting dose of 5 mg every other day is recommended.

Place rapidly disintegrating tablets on the tongue immediately after opening the blister. Administer with or without water.

Children 6 to 11 years of age – 2.5 mg once daily.

Children 12 months to 5 years of age – 1.25 mg once daily.

Children 6 to 11 months of age – 1 mg once daily.

Renal/Hepatic function impairment – In adults, a starting dose of one 5 mg tablet every other day is recommended.

DEXCHLORPHENIRAMINE MALEATE:

Adults 12 years of age and older – 4 to 6 mg at bedtime, or every 8 to 10 hours.

Children 6 to 12 years of age – 4 mg/day, preferably at bedtime.

DIPHENHYDRAMINE HYDROCHLORIDE: Individualize dosage.

Hypersensitivity reactions, type I/Antiparkinsonism/Motion sickness –

Oral:

Adults – 25 to 50 mg, every 4 to 6 hours, not to exceed 300 mg/day.

Children 6 to younger than 12 years of age – 12.5 to 25 mg, every 4 to 6 hours, not to exceed 150 mg/day.

Children 2 to younger than 6 years of age – For diphenhydramine tannate oral suspension, 12.5 to 25 mg every 12 hours.

Parenteral: Administer intravenously (IV) or deeply intramuscularly (IM).

Adults – 10 to 50 mg administered IV at a rate generally not exceeding 25 mg/min, or deep IM; 100 mg if required. Maximum daily dosage is 400 mg.

Children – 5 mg/kg/day or 150 mg/m^2/day in 4 divided doses. Maximum daily dosage is 300 mg. Administer IV at a rate generally not exceeding 25 mg/min, or deep IM.

Insomnia (12 years of age and older) – 38 to 76 mg of diphenhydramine citrate before bedtime.

Antitussive (syrup only) –

Adults: 25 mg every 4 hours, not to exceed 150 mg in 24 hours.

Children:

6 to 12 years of age – 12.5 mg every 4 hours, not to exceed 75 mg in 24 hours.

2 to 6 years of age – 6.25 mg every 4 hours, not to exceed 25 mg in 24 hours.

FEXOFENADINE:

Fexofenadine Dosing Guidelines

	Seasonal allergic rhinitis	Chronic idiopathic urticaria
Tablets		
Adults and children 12 years of age and older	60 mg twice daily or 180 mg once daily	60 mg twice daily or 180 mg once daily
Children 6 to 11 years of age	30 mg twice daily	30 mg twice daily
ODT[a]		
Children 6 to 11 years of age	30 mg twice daily	30 mg twice daily

Fexofenadine Dosing Guidelines		
	Seasonal allergic rhinitis	Chronic idiopathic urticaria
Suspension		
Children 2 to 11 years of age	30 mg (5 mL) twice daily	30 mg (5 mL) twice daily
Children 6 months to younger than 2 years of age	NA	15 mg (2.5 mL) twice daily

[a] ODT = orally disintegrating tablet.

Fexofenadine Starting Doses in Patients With Renal Function Impairment		
	Seasonal allergic rhinitis	Chronic idiopathic urticaria
Tablets		
Adults and children 12 years of age and older	60 mg once daily	60 mg once daily
Children 6 to 11 years of age	30 mg once daily	30 mg once daily
ODT		
Children 6 to 11 years of age	30 mg once daily	30 mg once daily
Suspension		
Children 2 to 11 years of age	30 mg (5 mL) once daily	30 mg (5 mL) once daily
Children 6 months to younger than 2 years of age	NA	15 mg (2.5 mL) once daily

Administration –

Tablets: Take with water.

ODT: Fexofenadine ODT is designed to disintegrate on the tongue, followed by swallowing with or without water, and should be taken on an empty stomach. Fexofenadine ODT is not intended to be chewed. Fexofenadine ODT should not be removed from the original blister package until time of administration.

Suspension: Shake oral suspension well before each use.

HYDROXYZINE: Administer by deep IM only; may be given without further dilution. Avoid IV, subcutaneous, or intra-arterial administration. Do not administer IM injections into the lower and mid-third of the upper arm.

Anxiety – The efficacy of hydroxyzine as an antianxiety agent for long-term use (longer than 4 months) has not been assessed; periodically reevaluate its usefulness.

Oral:

Adults – 50 to 100 mg 4 times a day.

Children (older than 6 years of age) – 50 to 100 mg/day in divided doses.

Children (younger than 6 years of age) – 50 mg/day in divided doses.

Pruritus –

Oral:

Adults – 25 mg 3 or 4 times/day.

Children –

6 years of age: 50 to 100 mg/day in divided doses.

Younger than 6 years of age: 50 mg/day in divided doses.

Sedation (oral only) –

Adults: 50 to 100 mg. Hydroxyzine may potentiate concomitant narcotics and barbiturates; reduce dosages accordingly. Atropine and other belladonna alkaloids may be given as appropriate.

Children: 0.6 mg/kg.

Antiemetic/Analgesia, adjunctive therapy (parenteral only) –

Adults: 25 to 100 mg IM. Reduce dosage of concomitant CNS depressants and narcotics by as much as 50%.

Children: 1.1 mg/kg (0.5 mg/lb) IM. Reduce dosage of concomitant CNS depressants and narcotics by as much as 50%.

LEVOCETIRIZINE: Levocetirizine can be taken without regard to food consumption.

Adults and children 12 years of age and older – The recommended dosage of levocetirizine is 5 mg (1 tablet or 10 mL of oral solution) once daily in the evening. Some patients may be adequately controlled by 2.5 mg (half of a tablet or 5 mL of oral solution) once daily in the evening.

Children 6 to 11 years of age – The recommended dosage of levocetirizine is 2.5 mg (half of a tablet or 5 mL of oral solution) once daily in the evening. The 2.5 mg dose should not be exceeded because the systemic exposure with 5 mg is approximately twice that of adults.

Children 6 months to 5 years of age – 1.25 mg (2.5 mL oral solution) once daily in the evening. The 1.25 mg once daily dose should not be exceeded based on comparable exposure to adults receiving 5 mg.

Renal function impairment – In adults and children 12 years of age and older with the following:

Mild renal function impairment (CrCl 50 to 80 mL/min): A dosage of 2.5 mg once daily is recommended.

Moderate renal function impairment (CrCl 30 to 50 mL/min): A dosage of 2.5 mg once every other day is recommended.

Severe renal function impairment (CrCl 10 to 30 mL/min): A dosage of 2.5 mg twice weekly (administered once every 3 to 4 days) is recommended.

End-stage renal disease (CrCl less than 10 mL/min) and hemodialysis: These patients should not receive levocetirizine.

Hepatic function impairment – No dose adjustment is needed in patients with hepatic function impairment alone. In patients with both hepatic and renal function impairment, adjustment of the dose is recommended.

LORATADINE:

Adults and children 6 years of age and older – 10 mg once daily.

Children 2 to 5 years of age – 5 mg (5 mL) syrup once daily.

Hepatic/Renal function impairment (glomerular filtration rate less than 30 mL/min) –

Adults and children 6 years of age and older: 10 mg every other day as starting dose.

Children 2 to 5 years of age: 5 mg every other day as starting dose.

Rapidly disintegrating tablets – Place tablets on the tongue. Administer with or without water. Use within 6 months of opening laminated foil pouch and immediately upon opening individual tablet blister.

OLOPATADINE: Olopatadine nasal spray should be primed before the initial use and when the spray has not been used for more than 7 days. Before the initial use, prime olopatadine nasal spray by releasing 5 sprays, or until a fine mist appears. When the nasal spray has not been used for more than 7 days, re-prime by releasing 2 sprays. The correct amount of medication cannot be assured before the initial priming and after 240 sprays have been used, even though the bottle is not completely empty.

Adults and children 12 years of age and older – 2 sprays per nostril twice daily.

6 to 11 years of age – 1 spray per nostril twice daily.

PROMETHAZINE HYDROCHLORIDE: The preferred parenteral route of administration is deep IM injection; properly administered IV doses are well tolerated, but this method is associated with increased hazard. IV administration should not exceed 25 mg/mL at a rate no more than 25 mg/min. Avoid subcutaneous and intra-arterial injection. Use is contraindicated in patients younger than 2 years of age.

Hypersensitivity reactions, Type I –

Adults and children older than 2 years of age: Usual dose is 25 mg at bedtime; 12.5 mg before meals and at bedtime may be given, if necessary. Single 25 mg doses at bedtime or 6.25 to 12.5 mg taken 3 times daily will usually suffice. Doses of 25 mg will control minor transfusion reactions of an allergic nature.

Parenteral:

Adults – 25 mg; may repeat dose within 2 hours if needed.

Children 2 years of age and older – Dose should not exceed half the adult dose.

Sedation –

Oral/Rectal: If used for preoperative sedation, administer the night before surgery to relieve apprehension and produce quiet sleep.

Adults – 25 to 50 mg at bedtime.

Children older than 2 years of age – 12.5 to 25 mg at bedtime.

Parenteral:

Adults – 25 to 50 mg at bedtime for nighttime sedation. Doses of 50 mg provide sedation and relieve apprehension during early stages of labor. When labor is definitely established, 25 to 75 mg may be given IM or IV with an appropriately reduced dose of any desired narcotic. If necessary, promethazine injection with a reduced dose of analgesic may be repeated once or twice at 4-hour intervals. Do not exceed 100 mg per 24 hours for patients in labor.

Children 2 to 12 years of age – Do not exceed half the adult dose.

Antiemetic –

Oral/Rectal:

Adults – Usual dose is 25 mg; doses of 12.5 to 25 mg may be repeated every 4 to 6 hours as needed.

Children more than 2 years of age – Usual dose is 25 mg or 0.5 mg/lb; doses of 12.5 to 25 mg may be repeated every 4 to 6 hours as needed.

Antiemetics are not recommended for treatment of uncomplicated vomiting in children; limit use to prolonged vomiting of known etiology.

Parenteral:

Adults – Usual dose is 12.5 to 25 mg, may repeat every 4 hours as needed. If used postoperatively, reduce doses of concomitant analgesics or barbiturates accordingly.

Children 2 to 12 years of age – Do not exceed half the adult dose. Do not use when etiology of vomiting is unknown.

Motion sickness (oral and rectal only) –

Adults: Usual dose is 25 mg twice/day; take first dose 30 to 60 minutes before anticipated travel; repeat 8 to 12 hours later if needed. On successive travel days, take 25 mg upon rising and again before the evening meal.

Children older than 2 years of age: 12.5 to 25 mg twice/day.

Pre- and postoperative use –

Oral/Rectal:

Adults – For preoperative use, 50 mg administered with an appropriately reduced dose of narcotic or barbiturate and the required amount of a belladonna alkaloid. For postoperative use, 25 to 50 mg doses in adults.

Children older than 2 years of age – For preoperative use, 0.5 mg/lb in combination with an appropriately reduced dose of narcotic or barbiturate and the appropriate dose of an atropine-like drug. For postoperative use, 12.5 to 25 mg in children.

Parenteral:

Adults – 25 to 50 mg in combination with appropriately reduced doses of analgesics, hypnotics, and atropine-like drugs as appropriate.

Children 2 to 12 years of age – 0.5 mg/lb in combination with an appropriately reduced dose of narcotic or barbiturate and the appropriate dose of an atropine-like drug.

Use in children – Contraindicated in children younger than 2 years of age because of the potential for fatal respiratory depression. The extrapyramidal symptoms that can occur secondary to promethazine administration may be confused with the CNS signs of undiagnosed primary disease (eg, encephalopathy, Reye syndrome). Avoid use in children whose signs and symptoms may suggest Reye syndrome or other hepatic diseases.

TRIPROLIDINE HYDROCHLORIDE:

Adults and children (12 years of age and older) – 10 mL every 4 to 6 hours, not to exceed 40 mL in 24 hours.

Children –

6 to 12 years of age: 5 mL every 4 to 6 hours, not to exceed 20 mL in 24 hours.

4 to 6 years of age: 3.75 mL every 4 to 6 hours, not to exceed 15 mL in 24 hours.

2 to 4 years of age: 2.5 mL every 4 to 6 hours, not to exceed 10 mL in 24 hours.

4 months to 2 years of age: 1.25 mL every 4 to 6 hours, not to exceed 5 mL in 24 hours.

TRIPROLIDINE TANNATE:

Dosage –

Adults and children 12 years of age and older: 10 mL every 12 hours.

Children 6 to younger than 12 years of age: 5 mL every 12 hours.

Children 2 to younger than 6 years of age: 2.5 mL every 12 hours.

Actions

Pharmacology:

Antihistamines: Dosage and Effects

Antihistamine	Sedative effects	Antihistaminic activity	Anticholinergic activity	Antiemetic effects
First-Generation (nonselective)				
Alkylamines				
Brompheniramine	+[a]	+++[a]	++	—
Chlorpheniramine	+	++[a]	++	—
Dexchlorpheniramine	+	+++	++	—
Pheniramine	++	—	—	—
Triprolidine	+	—	—	—
Ethanolamines				
Carbinoxamine	+++	—	+++	—
Clemastine	++	+ to ++	+++	++ to +++
Diphenhydramine	+++	+ to ++	+++	++ to +++
Phenothiazines				
Promethazine	+++	+++	+++	++++[a]
Piperazines				
Hydroxyzine	+++	++ to +++	++	+++
Piperidines				
Azatadine	++	++	++	—
Cyproheptadine	+	++	++	—
Second-Generation (peripherally selective)				
Phthalazinone				
Azelastine[b]	±	++ to +++	±	—
Piperazine				
Cetirizine	+	++ to +++	±	—
Piperidines				
Desloratadine	±	—	±	—
Fexofenadine	±	—	±	—
Loratadine	±	++ to +++	±	—

[a] ++++ = very high, +++ = high, ++ = moderate, + = low, ± = low to none.

[b] Some effects may be enhanced or reduced as a result of administration via the nasal route.

Antihistamines are reversible, competitive H_1 receptor antagonists that reduce or prevent most of the physiologic effects that histamine normally induces at the H_1 receptor site. First-generation antihistamines bind nonselectively to central and peripheral H_1 receptors and can result in CNS stimulation or depression. Second-generation antihistamines are selective for peripheral H_1 receptors and, as a group, are less sedating. First-generation agents with strong anticholinergic properties bind to central muscarinic receptors and produce antiemetic effects.

Pharmacokinetics:

First-generation agents – Pharmacokinetics of first-generation agents have not been extensively studied. These agents are generally well absorbed following oral administration, have an onset of action within 15 to 30 minutes, are maximal within 1 to 2 hours, and have a duration of approximately 4 to 6 hours, although some are longer acting. Most are metabolized by the liver. Antihistamine metabolites and small amounts of unchanged drug are excreted in urine.

Second-generation agents – Intranasal administration of **azelastine** yields peak levels in 2 to 3 hours, with an elimination half-life of 22 hours. Metabolism by the P-450 system results in steady-state peak levels of a major active metabolite (desmethyl-azelastine), which are 20% to 50% of **azelastine** levels. The elimination half-life of the metabolite is predicted to be 54 hours. The major route of excretion is via feces.

Pharmacokinetics of Peripherally Selective H_1 Antagonists (Oral)

	Onset of action	T_{max}[a] (h)	Elimination t½ (h)	Protein binding (%)
Cetirizine	rapid	1	8.3	93
Fexofenadine	rapid	2.6	14.4	60 to 70
Loratadine	rapid	1.3 to 2.5[b]	8.4 to 28[c]	97 (75)[c]

[a] T_{max} = time to maximum plasma concentration.
[b] All active constituents (parent drug and active metabolites)
[c] Active metabolite

Olopatadine – Olopatadine was absorbed with individual maximum plasma concentration (C_{max}) observed between 30 minutes and 1 hour after twice-daily intranasal administration in healthy subjects. The average absolute bioavailability of intranasal olopatadine is 57%. Olopatadine was bound predominately to human serum albumin. Olopatadine is not extensively metabolized. The plasma elimination half-life of olopatadine is 8 to 12 hours.

Contraindications

First-generation antihistamines: Hypersensitivity to specific or structurally-related antihistamines; newborns or premature infants; breast-feeding mothers; monoamine oxidase (MAO) therapy; pregnancy (**hydroxyzine**); angle-closure glaucoma, stenosing peptic ulcer, symptomatic prostatic hypertrophy, bladder neck obstruction, pyloroduodenal obstruction, elderly, debilitated patients (**cyproheptadine**). Hydroxyzine injection is for IM use only. Do not inject subcutaneously, IV, or intra-arterially.

Second-generation antihistamines: Hypersensitivity to specific or structurally-related antihistamines. **Desloratadine** is contraindicated in those who are hypersensitive to **loratadine**. **Cetirizine** is contraindicated in those who are hypersensitive to **hydroxyzine**.

Warnings/Precautions

Neuroleptic malignant syndrome: A potentially fatal symptom complex sometimes referred to as neuroleptic malignant syndrome (NMS) has been reported in association with **promethazine** alone or in combination with antipsychotic drugs. Clinical manifestations of NMS are hyperpyrexia, muscle rigidity, altered mental status, and evidence of autonomic instability (eg, irregular pulse or blood pressure, tachycardia, diaphoresis, cardiac dysrhythmias).

CNS depression: Antihistamines may impair the mental and/or physical abilities required for the performance of potentially hazardous tasks, such as driving a vehicle or operating machinery. The impairment may be amplified by concomitant use of other CNS depressants, such as alcohol, sedatives/hypnotics (including barbiturates), narcotics, narcotic analgesics, general anesthetics, tricyclic antidepressants, and tranquilizers. Therefore, either eliminate such agents or give in reduced dosage in the presence of certain antihistamines with strong CNS depressant effects.

When given concomitantly with **promethazine**, reduce the dose of barbiturates by at least one half, and reduce the dose of the narcotics by one quarter to one half. Individualize dosage. Excessive amounts of promethazine relative to a narcotic may lead to restlessness and motor hyperactivity in the patient with pain.

Special risk patients: Use antihistamines with caution in patients with narrow-angle glaucoma, stenosing peptic ulcer, pyloroduodenal obstruction, symptomatic prostatic hypertrophy, bladder neck obstruction, bronchial asthma, increased intraocular pressure, hyperthyroidism, cardiovascular disease, and hypertension.

Respiratory depression: Avoid sedatives and CNS depressants in patients with compromised respiratory function (eg, chronic obstructive pulmonary disease, sleep apnea).

Respiratory disease: In general, antihistamines are not recommended to treat lower respiratory tract symptoms, because their anticholinergic effects may cause thickening of secretions and impair expectoration. However, several reports indicate antihistamines can be safely used in asthmatic patients with severe perennial allergic rhinitis.

Seizure threshold: **Promethazine** may lower the seizure threshold; consider this when giving to people with known seizure disorders or when giving in combination with narcotics or local anesthetics that also may affect seizure threshold.

Hematologic: Use **promethazine** with caution in bone marrow depression. Leukopenia and agranulocytosis have been reported, usually when used with other toxic agents.

Anticholinergic effects: Antihistamines have varying degrees of atropine-like actions; use with caution in patients with a predisposition to urinary retention, history of bronchial asthma, increased intraocular pressure, hyperthyroidism, cardiovascular disease, or hypertension.

Olopatadine:

Epistaxis and nasal ulceration – In placebo (vehicle)-controlled clinical trials of 2 weeks' to 6 months' duration, epistaxis and nasal ulcerations were reported.

Nasal septal perforation – Nasal septal perforations were reported in 1 patient treated with the investigational formulation of olopatadine and 2 patients treated with the vehicle. In a 6-month trial with olopatadine, which does not contain povidone, there were no reports of nasal septal perforation. Before starting olopatadine, conduct a nasal examination to ensure that patients are free of nasal disease other than allergic rhinitis. Perform nasal examinations periodically for signs of adverse reactions on the nasal mucosa, and consider stopping olopatadine if patients develop nasal ulcerations.

Phenothiazines: Use phenothiazines with caution in patients with cardiovascular disease, liver dysfunction, or ulcer disease. Promethazine has been associated with cholestatic jaundice.

Use cautiously in people with acute or chronic respiratory impairment, particularly children, because phenothiazines may suppress the cough reflex. If hypotension occurs, epinephrine is not recommended because phenothiazines may reverse its usual pressor effect and cause a paradoxical further lowering of blood pressure. Because these drugs have an antiemetic action, they may obscure signs of intestinal obstruction, brain tumor, or overdosage of toxic drugs.

Phenothiazines elevate prolactin levels.

Phenylketonurics: Inform phenylketonuric patients that some of these products contain phenylalanine.

Tartrazine sensitivity: Some of these products contain tartrazine (FD & C yellow #5), which may cause allergic-type reactions (including bronchial asthma) in susceptible individuals. Although the incidence of sensitivity is low, it is frequently seen in patients who also have aspirin hypersensitivity. Specific products containing tartrazine are identified in the product listings.

Hypersensitivity reactions: Hypersensitivity reactions may occur, and any of the usual manifestations of drug allergy may develop.

Renal/Hepatic function impairment: Use a lower initial dose of **loratadine, desloratadine,** and **cetirizine** in patients with renal or hepatic impairment.

Hazardous tasks: May cause drowsiness and reduce mental alertness; patients should not drive or perform tasks requiring alertness, coordination, or physical dexterity.

Photosensitivity: Photosensitization may occur.

Pregnancy: Category B – **azatadine, cetirizine, chlorpheniramine, clemastine, cyproheptadine, dexchlorpheniramine, diphenhydramine, loratadine.**

Category C – **azelastine, brompheniramine, carbinoxamine, desloratadine, fexofenadine, hydroxyzine, olopatadine, phenyltoloxamine, promethazine, triprolidine.**

Lactation: Antihistamine therapy is contraindicated in breast-feeding mothers.

Children: Antihistamines may diminish mental alertness; conversely, they may occasionally produce excitation, particularly in the young child.

Promethazine is not recommended in children younger than 2 years of age. Exercise caution when administering promethazine to children because of the potential for fatal respiratory depression. Limit antiemetics to prolonged vomiting of known etiology. Avoid use in children whose signs and symptoms may suggest Reye syndrome or other hepatic diseases. In children with dehydration, there is an increased susceptibility to dystonias with the use of promethazine.

Elderly: Antihistamines are more likely to cause dizziness, excessive sedation, syncope, toxic confusional states, and hypotension in elderly patients. Dosage reduction may be required. Phenothiazine side effects (extrapyramidal signs, especially parkinsonism, akathisia, and persistent dyskinesia) are more prone to develop in the elderly.

Drug Interactions

Drugs that may affect antihistamines include aluminum/magnesium-containing acids, cimetidine, erythromycin, ketoconazole, MAO inhibitors, and rifamycins (eg, rifampin). Drugs that may be affected by antihistamines include alcohol and CNS depressants, beta-blockers, MAO inhibitors, metyrapone, nefazodone, selective serotonin reuptake inhibitors, and venlafaxine.

See the Antipsychotic Agents monograph for drug interactions that relate to **promethazine.**

Drug/Lab test interactions: Diagnostic pregnancy tests based on hCG may result in false-negative or false-positive interpretations in patients on promethazine. Increased blood glucose has occurred in **promethazine** patients.

Phenothiazines may increase serum cholesterol, spinal fluid protein, and urinary urobilinogen levels; decrease protein bound iodine; yield false-positive urine bilirubin tests; and interfere with urinary ketone and steroid determinations.

Discontinue antihistamines approximately 4 days prior to skin testing procedures; these drugs may prevent or diminish otherwise positive reactions to dermal reactivity indicators.

Drug/Food interactions: Food increased the area under the curve (AUC) of **loratadine** by approximately 40% and the metabolite by approximately 15%; absorption was delayed by 1 hour. Although not expected to be clinically important, take on an empty stomach.

Certain fruit juices (ie, apple, orange, grapefruit) administered with **fexofenadine** significantly reduced the AUC and C_{max} of fexofenadine. Therefore, fexofenadine's clinical effect may be decreased. It would be prudent for patients to take fexofenadine with a liquid other than these juices.

Adverse Reactions

Adverse reactions may include the following: acute labyrinthitis; agranulocytosis; anaphylactic shock; anemias; anorexia; aplastic anemia; asthma; blurred vision; bradycardia; cardiac arrest; catatonic-like states; chest tightness; chills; confusion; constipation; convulsions; dermatitis; diarrhea; diplopia; disorientation; disturbed coordination; disturbing dreams/nightmares; dizziness; drowsiness (often transient); drug rash; dry mouth, nose, and throat; dysuria; early menses; ECG changes, including blunting of T-waves and prolongation of the QT interval; elevated spinal fluid proteins; elevation of plasma cholesterol levels; epigastric distress, especially ethylenediamines; erythema; euphoria; excessive perspiration; excitation; extrasystoles; faintness; fatigue; grand mal seizures; glycosuria; gynecomastia; hallucinations; headache; hemolytic anemia; high or prolonged glucose tolerance curves; hypertension; hypoplastic anemia; hypotension; hysteria; increased appetite and weight gain; increases and decreases in blood pressure; induced lactation; inhibition of ejaculation; insomnia; lassitude; leukopenia; lupus erythematosus-like syndrome; nasal stuffiness; nausea; neuritis; obstructive jaundice (usually reversible upon discontinuation); oculogyric crisis; palpitations; pancytopenia; paresthesias; peripheral, angioneurotic, and laryngeal edema; pharyngitis; photosensitivity; postural hypotension; pseudoschizophrenia; reflex tachycardia; respiratory depression; restlessness; sedation; sore throat; stomatitis; tachycardia; thickening of bronchial secretions; thrombocytopenia; thrombocytopenic purpura; tingling, heaviness, and weakness of the hands; tinnitus; tissue necrosis following subcutaneous administration of IV **promethazine**; tongue protrusion (usually in association with IV administration or excessive dosage); torticollis; tremor; urinary frequency; urinary retention; urticaria; venous thrombosis at injection site (IV **promethazine**); vertigo; vomiting; weakness; wheezing.

Extrapyramidal reactions may occur with high doses; these reactions usually respond to dose reduction.

Nasal spray: Asthma; bitter taste; conjunctivitis; cough; dysesthesia; epistaxis; eye abnormality; eye pain; glossitis; headache, increased ALT; nasal burning; nasal ulcerations; paroxysmal sneezing; pharyngitis; rhinitis; sinusitis; somnolence; taste loss; temporomandibular dislocation; ulcerative and aphthous stomatitis; watery eyes.

These antihistamines infrequently cause typical phenothiazine adverse effects. See the Antipsychotic Agents monograph for a complete discussion.

DEXTROMETHORPHAN HBr

Gelcaps: 15 mg (*otc*)	*Robitussin CoughGels* (Wyeth)
30 mg (*otc*)	*DexAlone* (DexGen)
Lozenges: 5 mg (*otc*)	*Hold DM* (B.F. Ascher), *Scot-Tussin DM Cough Chasers* (Scot-Tussin)
7.5 mg (*otc*)	*Trocal* (Textilease)
10 mg (*otc*)	*Sucrets DM Cough Suppressant* (Insight Pharmaceuticals), *Sucrets DM Cough Formula* (Insight Pharmaceuticals)
Strips, orally disintegrating: 7.5 mg (*otc*)	*Triaminic Thin Strips Long Acting Cough* (Novartis Consumer Health)
15 mg (*otc*)	*Theraflu Thin Strips Long Acting Cough* (Novartis Consumer Health)
Liquid: 5 mg per 5 mL (*otc*)	*Simply Cough* (McNeil-PCP)
10 mg per 15 mL (3.33 mg per 5 mL) (*otc*)	*Creo-Terpin* (Lee)
10 mg per 5 mL (*otc*)	*Vicks 44 Cough Relief* (Proctor and Gamble)
12.5 mg per 5 mL (*otc*)	*Buckley's Cough Mixture* (Novartis Consumer Health)
15 mg per 5 mL (*otc*)	*Robitussin Maximum Strength Cough* (Whitehall-Robins)
Syrup: 5 mg per 5 mL (*otc*)	*Creomulsion for Children* (Summit)
7.5 mg per 5 mL (*otc*)	*Robitussin Pediatric Cough* (Whitehall-Robins), *ElixSure Children's Cough* (Taro Consumer), *Triaminic Long Acting Cough* (Novartis Consumer Health)
10 mg per 5 mL (*otc*)	*Silphen DM* (Silarx)
20 mg per 15 mL (*otc*)	*Creomulsion Adult Formula* (Summit)
Oral solution: 7.5 mg per 5 mL (*otc*)	*Children's PediaCare Long-Acting Cough* (Pfizer)
Oral suspension: 30 mg dextromethorphan tannate per 5 mL (*Rx*)	*AeroTuss 12* (AeroPharm)
Oral suspension, extended-release: Dextromethorphan polistirex equivalent to 30 mg dextromethorphan HBr per 5 mL (*otc*)	*Delsym* (Celltech)
Drops: 3.75 mg per 0.8 mL (*otc*)	*PediaCare Infants' Long-Acting Cough* (Pfizer Consumer Health)
7.5 mg/mL (*otc*)	*Little Colds Cough Formula* (Vetco)
Freezer pops: 7.5 mg per 25 mL (per pop) (*otc*)	*PediaCare Infants' Long-Acting Cough* (Pfizer Consumer Health)

Indications

Temporarily relieves cough caused by minor throat and bronchial irritation as may occur with the common cold or inhaled irritants.

Administration and Dosage

Gelcaps:

Adults and children 12 years of age and older – 30 mg every 6 to 8 hours. Do not exceed 120 mg in 24 hours. Do not use in children less than 12 years of age.

Lozenges:

Adults and children 12 years of age and older – 5 to 15 mg every 1 to 4 hours up to 120 mg/day.

Children 6 to younger than 12 years of age – 5 to 10 mg every 1 to 4 hours up to 60 mg/day. Do not give to children under 6 years of age unless directed by a physician.

Liquid and syrup:

Adults and children 12 years of age and older – 10 to 20 mg every 4 hours or 30 mg every 6 to 8 hours up to 120 mg/day.

Children –

6 to younger than 12 years of age: 15 mg every 6 to 8 hours up to 60 mg/day.

2 to younger than 6 years of age: 7.5 mg every 6 to 8 hours up to 30 mg/day.

Extended-release suspension:

Adults and children 12 years of age and older – 60 mg every 12 hours up to 120 mg/day.

Children –

6 to younger than 12 years of age: 30 mg every 12 hours up to 60 mg/day.

2 to younger than 6 years of age: 15 mg every 12 hours up to 30 mg/day.

Strips: Allow the strip to dissolve on the tongue.

Adults and children 12 years of age and older – 30 mg every 6 to 8 hours, up to 120 mg/day.

Children 6 to younger than 12 years of age – 15 mg every 6 to 8 hours, up to 60 mg/day.

Oral solution: If needed, repeat dose every 6 to 8 hours. Do not exceed 4 doses in 24 hours.

Children 6 to younger than 12 years of age – 10 mL every 6 to 8 hours.

Children 2 to younger than 6 years of age – 5 mL every 6 to 8 hours.

Children younger than 2 years of age – Consult a doctor.

Freezer pops:

Children 6 to younger than 12 years of age – Two freezer pops (50 mL as liquid). If needed, repeat dose every 6 to 8 hour; do not exceed 4 doses in 24 hours.

Children 2 to younger than 6 years of age – One freezer pop (25 mL as liquid). If needed, repeat dose every 6 to 8 hour; do not exceed 4 doses in 24 hours.

Drops:

Children 2 to 3 years of age – One dropperful (2 dropperfuls *PediaCare*) for a total of 7.5 mg. If needed, repeat every 6 to 8 hours, up to 30 mg/day.

Actions

Pharmacology: Dextromethorphan is the d-isomer of the codeine analog of levorphanol. Its cough suppressant action is due to a central action on the cough center in the medulla. Dextromethorphan 15 to 30 mg equals 8 to 15 mg codeine as an antitussive.

Pharmacokinetics: Dextromethorphan is rapidly absorbed from the GI tract. It undergoes metabolism in the liver and is then excreted in the urine as unchanged drug and demethylated metabolites.

Contraindications

Hypersensitivity to any component.

Warnings/Precautions

Use: For persistent or chronic cough or cough accompanied by excessive secretions, consult a doctor before use.

Anecdotal reports of abuse of dextromethorphan-containing cough/cold products has increased, especially among teenagers.

Pregnancy: Category C.

Lactation: It is not known if dextromethorphan is excreted in breast milk.

Drug Interactions

Drugs that may interact with dextromethorphan include MAO inhibitors, quinidine, and sibutramine.

Adverse Reactions

Adverse reactions may include dizziness, drowsiness, and GI disturbances.

BENZONATATE

Capsules: 100 and 200 mg (*Rx*)	Various, *Tessalon Perles* (Forest)

Indications

Symptomatic relief of cough.

Administration and Dosage

Adults and children (older than 10 years of age): 100 to 200 mg 3 times/day, up to 600 mg/day.

Actions

Pharmacology: Benzonatate anesthetizes stretch receptors in respiratory passages, lungs, and pleura, dampening their activity, and reducing the cough reflex. It has no inhibitory effect on the respiratory center in recommended dosage. Onset of action is 15 to 20 minutes; effects last 3 to 8 hours.

Contraindications

Hypersensitivity to benzonatate or related compounds (eg, tetracaine).

Warnings/Precautions

Behavior changes: Isolated instances of bizarre behavior, including mental confusion and visual hallucinations, have been reported in patients taking benzonatate in combination with other prescribed drugs.

CNS effects: Benzonatate has been associated with adverse CNS effects possibly related to a prior sensitivity to similar agents or interaction with concomitant medication.

Local anesthesia: Release of benzonatate in the mouth can produce a temporary local anesthesia of the oral mucosa. Swallow the capsules without chewing.

Hypersensitivity reactions: Severe hypersensitivity reactions (eg, bronchospasm, laryngospasm, cardiovascular collapse) have been reported that may be related to local anesthesia from sucking or chewing the capsule instead of swallowing it. Severe reactions have required intervention with vasopressor agents and supportive measures.

Pregnancy: Category C.

Lactation: It is not known whether this drug is excreted in breast milk.

Adverse Reactions

Sedation; headache; dizziness; mental confusion; visual hallucinations; constipation; nausea; GI upset; pruritus; skin eruptions; nasal congestion; sensation of burning in the eyes; a vague "chilly" sensation; chest numbness; hypersensitivity.

DEXTROMETHORPHAN HBr and BENZOCAINE

Lozenges: 5 mg dextromethorphan and 2 mg benzocaine (*otc*)	*Cough X* (B.F. Ascher)
7.5 mg dextromethorphan and 5 mg benzocaine (*otc*)	*Cēpacol Ultra Sore Throat Plus Cough* (Combe)
10 mg dextromethorphan HBr and 15 mg benzocaine (*otc*)	*Tetra-Formula* (Reese Pharm.)

Indications

Temporarily suppresses cough caused by minor throat and bronchial irritants that may occur with the common cold. Also for the temporary relief of occasional minor irritation and sore throat.

Administration and Dosage

Do not use for more than 2 days for sore throat or for more than 7 days for cough unless directed by a doctor. Do not use for persistent or chronic cough such as occurs with smoking, asthma, emphysema, or if cough is accompanied by excessive phlegm unless directed by a doctor. Allow lozenge to dissolve slowly in the mouth.

Cough-X:

Adults and children 6 years of age and older – One lozenge every 2 hours as needed, not to exceed 12 lozenges in 24 hours or as directed by a physician.

Children 2 to 6 years of age – One lozenge every 4 hours not to exceed 6 lozenges in 24 hours, or as directed by a physician.

In children, take care to prevent choking on lozenge.

Tetra-Formula:

Adults and children 6 years of age and older – Dissolve 1 lozenge slowly in the mouth; do not chew. May be repeated every 4 hours or as directed by a physician.

Children under 6 years of age – Consult a physician.

ZAFIRLUKAST

Tablets: 10 and 20 mg (*Rx*)	*Accolate* (AstraZeneca)

Indications

Asthma: Prophylaxis and chronic treatment of asthma in adults and children 5 years of age and older.

Administration and Dosage

Because food reduces bioavailability of zafirlukast, take at least 1 hour before or 2 hours after meals.

Adults and children 12 years of age and older: The recommended dose of zafirlukast is 20 mg twice daily.

Children 5 to 11 years of age: The recommended dose of zafirlukast is 10 mg twice daily.

Actions

Pharmacology: Zafirlukast is a selective and competitive leukotreine receptor antagonist of leukotreine D_4 and E_4, components of slow-reacting substance of anaphylaxis. Leukotriene production and receptor occupation have been correlated with airway edema, smooth muscle constriction, and altered cellular activity associated with the inflammatory process, which contribute to the signs and symptoms of asthma.

Pharmacokinetics: Oral zafirlukast is rapidly absorbed. Peak plasma concentrations are achieved 3 hours after dosing. The mean terminal elimination half-life is approximately 10 hours. Zafirlukast is more than 99% bound to plasma proteins, predominantly albumin.

Zafirlukast is extensively metabolized. Urinary excretion accounts for approximately 10% of the dose, and the remainder is excreted in the feces. Liver microsomes that hydroxylate metabolites of zafirlukast are formed through the cytochrome P450 2C9 (CYP2C9) enzyme pathway.

Additional studies show that zafirlukast inhibits the CYP3A4 and CYP2C9 isoenzymes.

Contraindications

Hypersensitivity to zafirlukast or any of its inactive ingredients.

Warnings/Precautions

Acute asthma attacks: Zafirlukast is not indicated for use in the reversal of bronchospasm in acute asthma attacks, including status asthmaticus. Continue zafirlukast during acute exacerbations of asthma.

Hepatic effects: Cases of life-threatening hepatic failure have been reported. Cases of liver injury without other attributable cause have been reported from postmarketing adverse reaction surveillance of patients who have received the recommended dosage of zafirlukast (40 mg/day). In most, but not all, postmarketing reports, the patient's symptoms abated and the liver enzymes returned to normal or near normal after stopping zafirlukast. In rare cases, patients have either presented with fulminant hepatitis or progressed to hepatic failure, liver transplantation, and death.

Eosinophilia: In rare cases, patients taking zafirlukast may present with systemic eosinophilia, sometimes presenting with clinical features of vasculitis consistent with Churg-Strauss syndrome, a condition that is often treated with systemic steroid therapy. These events usually, but not always, have been associated with the reduction of oral steroid therapy. Be alert to eosinophilia, vasculitic rash, worsening pulmonary symptoms, cardiac complications, or neuropathy presenting in their patients.

Hepatic function impairment: The clearance of zafirlukast is reduced in patients with hepatic impairment.

Pregnancy: Category B.

Lactation: Zafirlukast is excreted in breast milk.

Children: The safety and effectiveness of zafirlukast in patients younger than 5 years of age have not been established.

Elderly: The clearance of zafirlukast is reduced in elderly patients (65 years of age and older), such that maximal plasma clearance and area under the curve are approximately twice those of younger adults.

Drug Interactions

Due to zafirlukast's inhibition of cytochrome P450 2C9 and 3A4 isoenzymes, use caution with coadministration of drugs known to be metabolized by these isoenzymes.

Drugs that may affect zafirlukast include aspirin, erythromycin, and theophylline.

Drugs that may be affected by zafirlukast include warfarin.

Drug/Food interactions: The bioavailability of zafirlukast may be decreased when taken with food. Take zafirlukast at least 1 hour before or 2 hours after meals.

Adverse Reactions

Adverse reactions occurring in 3% or more of patients include headache, infection, and nausea.

MONTELUKAST SODIUM

Tablets; oral: 10 mg (as base) (*Rx*)	*Singulair* (Merck)
Tablets, chewable; oral: 4 and 5 mg (as base) (*Rx*)	
Granules; oral: 4 mg/packet (*Rx*)	

Indications

Asthma: Prophylaxis and chronic treatment of asthma in adults and pediatric patients 12 months of age and older.

Allergic rhinitis: For the relief of symptoms of allergic rhinitis (seasonal allergic rhinitis in adults and children 2 years of age and older), and perennial allergic rhinitis in adults and children 6 months of age and older.

Exercise-induced bronchoconstriction (EIB): For the prevention of EIB in patients 15 years of age and older.

Administration and Dosage

Adults and adolescents 15 years of age and older: One 10 mg tablet daily.

Children 6 to 14 years of age: One 5 mg chewable tablet daily.

Children 2 to 5 years of age: One 4 mg chewable tablet daily or 1 packet of 4 mg oral granules daily.

Children 6 to 23 months of age: One packet of 4 mg granules daily.

Administration:

Asthma (12 months of age and older) – Montelukast should be taken once daily in the evening.

Asthma/Allergic rhinitis (12 months of age and older) – Patients with both asthma and allergic rhinitis should take only 1 tablet daily in the evening.

EIB: A single dose of montelukast should be taken at least 2 hours before exercise. An additional dose should not be taken within 24 hours of a previous dose. Patients already taking 1 tablet daily for another indication (including chronic asthma) should not take an additional dose to prevent EIB. All patients should have a short-acting beta-agonist available for rescue.

Daily administration of montelukast for the chronic treatment of asthma has not been established to prevent acute episodes of EIB.

Administration of oral granules: Montelukast 4 mg oral granules can be administered directly in the mouth or dissolved in 1 teaspoonful (5 mL) of cold or room temperature baby formula or breast milk, or mixed with a spoonful of cold or room temperature soft foods; based on stability studies, use only applesauce, carrots, rice, or ice cream. Do not open the packet until ready to use. After opening the packet, the full dose (with or without mixing with food) must be administered within 15 minutes. If mixed with baby formula, breast milk, or food, the oral granules must not be stored for future use. Discard any unused portion. Montelukast oral granules are not intended to be dissolved in liquid for administration. However, liquids may be taken subsequent to administration. The granules can be administered without regard to the time of meals.

Actions

Pharmacology: Montelukast is a selective and orally active leukotriene receptor antagonist that inhibits the cysteinyl leukotrine ($CysLT_1$) receptor.

Leukotrienes are products of arachidonic acid metabolism and are released from mast cells and eosinophils. Leukotrienes and leukotriene receptor occupation have been correlated with airway edema, smooth muscle contraction, and altered cellular activity associated with the inflammatory process, which contribute to the signs and symptoms of asthma.

Pharmacokinetics: Montelukast is rapidly absorbed following oral administration. With the 10 mg film-coated tablet, the mean peak plasma concentration (C_{max}) is achieved in 3 to 4 hours (T_{max}). For the 5 mg chewable tablet, the mean C_{max} is achieved in 2 to 2.5 hours. For the 4 mg chewable tablet, the mean C_{max} is achieved 2 hours after administration. The mean oral bioavailability is 64%. Montelukast is more than 99% bound to plasma proteins and is extensively metabolized by the CYP-450 3A4 and 2C9 pathways. The steady-state volume of distribution of montelukast averages 8 to 11 L. The plasma clearance of montelukast averages 45 mL/min in healthy adults. Montelukast and its metabolites are excreted almost exclusively via the bile.

The mean plasma half-life ranged from 2.7 to 5.5 hours in healthy young adults.

Contraindications

Hypersensitivity to any component of this product.

Warnings/Precautions

Acute asthma attacks/exercise-induced bronchoconstriction: Montelukast is not indicated for use in acute asthma attacks, including status asthmaticus. Advise patients to have appropriate rescue medication available. Montelukast therapy can be continued during acute exacerbations of asthma. Patients who have exacerbations of asthma after exercise should have a short-acting inhaled beta-agonist available for rescue.

Concurrent corticosteroids: While the dose of inhaled corticosteroid may be reduced gradually under medical supervision, montelukast should not be abruptly substituted for inhaled or oral corticosteroids.

Eosinophilia: Physicians should be alert to eosinophilia, vasculitic rash, worsening pulmonary symptoms, cardiac complications, or neuropathy in their patients. In rare cases, patients on therapy with montelukast may present with systemic eosinophilia. These events usually, but not always, have been associated with the reduction of oral corticosteroid therapy.

Aspirin sensitivity: Patients with known aspirin sensitivity should continue avoidance of aspirin and nonsteroidal anti-inflammatory agents while taking montelukast.

Phenylketonurics: Inform phenylketonuric patients that the 4 and 5 mg chewable tablets contain phenylalanine.

Pregnancy: *Category B.*

Merck maintains a registry to monitor the pregnancy outcomes of pregnant women exposed to montelukast. Health care providers are encouraged to report any prenatal exposure to montelukast by calling the Pregnancy Registry at (800) 986-8999.

Lactation: It is not known if montelukast is excreted in human breast milk.

Children: The safety and efficacy in children younger than 12 months of age with asthma and younger than 6 months of age with perennial allergic rhinitis have not been established.

Elderly: No overall differences in safety or efficacy were observed between these subjects and younger subjects, but greater sensitivity of some older individuals cannot be ruled out.

Drug Interactions

Drugs that may interact with montelukast include phenobarbital, prednisone, and rifampin.

Adverse Reactions

Asthma: Adverse reactions occurring in more than 3% of patients include headache and influenza. In children 6 to 14 years of age, the following reactions occurred with a frequency of at least 2%: dyspepsia, diarrhea, fever, influenza, laryngitis, pharyngitis, nausea, otitis, sinusitis, viral infections. In children 2 to 5 years of age, the following reactions occurred with a frequency of at least 2%: abdominal pain, conjunctivitis, cough, dermatitis, diarrhea, ear pain, eczema, fever, gastroenteritis, headache, influenza, otitis, pneumonia, rash, rhinorrhea, sinusitis, urticaria, and varicella. In children 6 to 23 months of age, the following reactions occurred with a frequency of at least 2%: upper respiratory infection, wheezing, otitis media, pharyngitis, tonsillitis, cough, rhinitis.

Allergic rhinitis: In children 2 to 14 years of age, the following reactions occurred with a frequency of at least 2%: headache, otitis media, pharyngitis, upper respiratory tract infection.

ZILEUTON

Tablets, extended-release, oral: 600 mg (Rx)	*Zyflo CR* (Critical Therapeutics)

Indications

Asthma: The prophylaxis and chronic treatment of asthma in adults and children 12 years of age or older.

Administration and Dosage

Extended-release: Two 600 mg extended-release tablets twice daily within 1 hour of morning and evening meals for a total daily dose of 2,400 mg. Tablets should not be chewed, cut, or crushed. If a dose is missed, the patient should take the next dose at the scheduled time and not double the dose.

Actions

Pharmacology: Zileuton is a specific inhibitor of 5-lipoxygenase and thus inhibits leukotriene formation.

Zileuton inhibits leukotriene-dependent smooth muscle contractions. Pretreatment with zileuton attenuated bronchoconstriction caused by cold air challenge in patients with asthma.

Pharmacokinetics:

Absorption – Zileuton is rapidly absorbed upon oral administration with a mean time to peak plasma concentration (T_{max}) of 1.7 hours and a mean peak level (C_{max}) of 4.98 mcg/mL. Plasma concentrations of zileuton are proportional to dose.

Distribution – The apparent volume of distribution of zileuton is approximately 1.2 L/kg. Zileuton is 93% bound to plasma proteins, primarily to albumin, with minor binding to alpha-acid glycoprotein.

Metabolism – Several zileuton metabolites have been identified in plasma and urine. Liver microsomes have shown that zileuton and its N-dehydroxylated metabolite can be oxidatively metabolized by the CYP-450 isoenzymes 1A2, 2C9, and 3A4 (CYP1A2, CYP2C9, and CYP3A4).

Excretion – Elimination of zileuton is predominantly via metabolism with a mean terminal half-life of 2.5 hours. Zileuton activity is primarily because of the parent drug. Orally administered zileuton is well absorbed into the systemic circulation with 94.5% and 2.2% of the dose recovered in urine and feces, respectively.

Contraindications

Active liver disease or transaminase elevations 3 times or more the upper limit of normal (ULN), hypersensitivity to zileuton or any of its inactive ingredients.

Warnings/Precautions

Hepatotoxicity: Elevations of 1 or more liver function tests may occur during zileuton therapy. These laboratory abnormalities may progress, remain unchanged or resolve with continued therapy.

Acute asthma attacks: Zileuton is not indicated for use in the reversal of bronchospasm in acute asthma attacks, including status asthmaticus.

Hepatic function impairment: Use with caution in patients who consume substantial quantities of alcohol or have a history of liver disease.

Pregnancy: Category C.

Lactation: Zileuton and its metabolites are excreted in rat milk. It is not known if zileuton is excreted in breast milk.

Children: The safety and effectiveness of zileuton in children younger than 12 years of age have not been established. Zileuton ER is not appropriate for children younger than 12 years of age.

Elderly: Clinical studies with zileuton immediate-release suggests that women 65 years of age and older appear to be at increased risk of ALT elevations.

Monitoring: Evaluate hepatic transaminases at initiation of and during therapy with zileuton. Monitor serum ALT before treatment begins, once a month for the first 3 months, every 2 to 3 months for the remainder of the first year and periodically thereafter for patients receiving long-term zileuton therapy. If symptoms of liver dysfunction develop or transaminase elevations more than 5 times the ULN occur, discontinue therapy and follow transaminase levels until normal.

Drug Interactions

Liver microsomes have shown that zileuton and its N-dehydroxylated metabolite can be oxidatively metabolized by the CYP-450 isoenzymes 1A2, 2C9, and 3A4. Use caution when prescribing a medication that inhibits any of these enzymes.

Drugs that may be affected by zileuton include pimozide, propranolol, terfenadine, theophylline, and warfarin.

Drugs that may affect zileuton include CYP3A4 agents (eg, calcium channel blockers, cisapride, cyclosporine, ketoconazole).

Adverse Reactions

Adverse reactions occurring in 3% or more of patients taking zileuton immediate-release include headache, pain, abdominal pain, asthenia, accidental injury, dyspepsia, nausea, myalgia.

Adverse reactions occurring in 5% or more of patients taking zileuton extended-release include nausea, pharyngolaryngeal pain, sinusitis, headache, upper respiratory tract infection, myalgia, diarrhea.

RESPIRATORY INHALANT COMBINATIONS

FLUTICASONE PROPIONATE/SALMETEROL	
Powder; inhalation: 100 mcg fluticasone propionate per 50 mcg salmeterol, 250 mcg fluticasone propionate per 50 mcg salmeterol, 500 mcg fluticasone propionate per 50 mcg salmeterol (*Rx*)	*Advair Diskus* (GlaxoSmithKline)
Aerosol, spray; inhalation: 45 mcg fluticasone propionate per 21 mcg salmeterol, 115 mcg fluticasone propionate per 21 mcg salmeterol, 230 mcg fluticasone propionate per 21 mcg salmeterol (*Rx*)	*Advair HFA* (GlaxoSmithKline)
BUDESONIDE/FORMOTEROL	
Aerosol; inhalation: 80 mcg budesonide and 4.5 mcg formoterol/actuation, 160 mcg budesonide and 4.5 mcg formoterol/actuation (*Rx*)	*Symbicort* (AstraZeneca)
MOMETASONE FUROATE/FORMOTEROL FUMARATE	
Aerosol; inhalation: mometasone furoate 100 mcg/formoterol fumarate 5 mcg per actuation (*Rx*) mometasone furoate 200 mcg/formoterol fumarate 5 mcg per actuation	*Dulera* (Schering)

Warning:

Long-acting beta-2 adrenergic agonists (LABAs) such as formoterol, one of the active ingredients in budesonide/formoterol, increase the risk of asthma-related death. Data from a large placebo-controlled US study that compared the safety of another LABA (salmeterol) or placebo added to usual asthma therapy showed an increase in asthma-related deaths in patients receiving salmeterol. This finding with salmeterol is considered a class effect of the LABAs, including formoterol. Currently available data are inadequate to determine whether concurrent use of inhaled corticosteroids or other long-term asthma control drugs mitigates the increased risk of asthma-related death from LABAs. Available data from controlled clinical trials suggest that LABAs increase the risk of asthma-related hospitalization in pediatric and adolescent patients. Therefore, when treating patients with asthma, only use budesonide/formoterol for patients not adequately controlled on a long-term asthma control medication, such as an inhaled corticosteroid, or for patients whose disease severity clearly warrants initiation of treatment with both an inhaled corticosteroid and a LABA. Once asthma control is achieved and maintained, assess the patient at regular intervals and step down therapy (eg, discontinue budesonide/formoterol) if possible without loss of asthma control, and maintain the patient on a long-term asthma control medication such as an inhaled corticosteroid. Do not use budesonide/formoterol for patients whose asthma is adequately controlled on low- or medium-dose inhaled corticosteroids.

continued on next page

Warning: (cont.)

Asthma-related death: Long-acting $beta_2$-adrenergic agonists (LABAs), such as formoterol, one of the active ingredients in mometasone/formoterol, increase the risk of asthma-related death. Data from a large placebo-controlled US study that compared the safety of another LABA (salmeterol) with placebo added to usual asthma therapy showed an increase in asthma-related deaths in patients receiving salmeterol. This finding with salmeterol is considered a class effect of the LABAs, including formoterol. Currently available data are inadequate to determine whether concurrent use of inhaled corticosteroids or other long-term asthma control drugs mitigates the increased risk of asthma-related death from LABAs. Available data from controlled clinical trials suggest that LABAs increase the risk of asthma-related hospitalization in pediatric and adolescent patients. Therefore, when treating patients with asthma, use mometasone/formoterol only in patients not adequately controlled on a long-term asthma control medication, such as an inhaled corticosteroid, or in patients whose disease severity clearly warrants initiation of treatment with both an inhaled corticosteroid and a LABA. Once asthma control is achieved and maintained, assess the patient at regular intervals, step down therapy (eg, discontinue mometasone/formoterol) if possible without loss of asthma control, and maintain the patient on a long-term asthma control medication such as an inhaled corticosteroid. Do not use mometasone/formoterol for patients whose asthma is adequately controlled on low- or medium-dose inhaled corticosteroids.

Indications

Asthma, chronic:

Fluticasone/salmeterol Diskus – For the long-term, twice-daily maintenance treatment of asthma in patients 4 years of age and older.

Fluticasone/salmeterol hydrofluoroalkane (HFA) – For the long-term, twice-daily maintenance treatment of asthma in patients 12 years of age and older.

Budesonide/formoterol – For the long-term maintenance treatment of asthma in patients 12 years of age and older.

Chronic obstructive pulmonary disease: For the twice-daily maintenance treatment of airflow obstruction in patients with chronic obstructive pulmonary disease (COPD), including chronic bronchitis and emphysema. Budesonide 160 mcg/formoterol 4.5 mcg is the only approved dosage for the treatment of airflow obstruction in COPD.

Chronic obstructive pulmonary disease associated with chronic bronchitis:

Fluticasone/salmeterol Diskus – For the twice-daily maintenance treatment of airflow obstruction in patients with COPD, including chronic bronchitis and/or emphysema. Fluticasone 250 mcg/salmeterol 50 mcg *Diskus* is also indicated to reduce exacerbations of COPD in patients with a history of exacerbations. Fluticasone/salmeterol 250 mcg per 50 mcg twice daily is the only approved dosage for the treatment of COPD associated with chronic bronchitis. Higher doses, including fluticasone/salmeterol 500 mcg per 50 mcg, are not recommended.

Mometasone furoate/formoterol fumarate: For the treatment of asthma in patients 12 years of age and older. Mometasone/formoterol is not indicated for the relief of acute bronchospasm.

Administration and Dosage

Fluticasone/salmeterol:

Adults –

Asthma, chronic:

Usual dosage –

Diskus: 1 inhalation twice daily.

The recommended starting dosage is based on the patient's asthma severity.

HFA:

Patients not currently on inhaled corticosteroids – 2 inhalations twice daily. The recommended starting dosage is based on the patient's current asthma therapy.

Patients not adequately controlled on an inhaled corticosteroid – The following table provides the recommended starting dose for patients currently on and not adequately controlled by an inhaled corticosteroid.

Maximum dose –

Diskus: 1 inhalation of 500 mcg/50 mcg twice daily.

HFA: 2 inhalations of 230 mcg/21 mcg twice daily.

Dosage adjustment – For patients who do not respond adequately to the starting dose after 1 to 2 weeks of therapy with budesonide 80 mcg/formoterol 4.5 mcg, replacement with budesonide 160 mcg/formoterol 4.5 mcg may provide additional asthma control.

Children –

Asthma, chronic:

Usual dosage –

12 years of age and older (HFA): See Adults for dosing in children 12 years of age and older.

12 years of age and older (Diskus): See Adults for dosing in children 12 years of age and older

4 to 11 years of age: 1 inhalation of fluticasone 100 mcg/salmeterol 50 mcg twice daily (morning and evening, approximately 12 hours apart).

Diskus – Advise patients to rinse mouth after inhalation without swallowing.

Chronic obstructive pulmonary disease associated with chronic bronchitis –

Fluticasone/salmeterol Diskus: 1 inhalation (250 mcg per 50 mcg) twice/day. Higher doses are not recommended because no additional improvement in lung function was observed in clinical trials and higher doses of corticosteroids increase the risk of systemic effects.

Budesonide/formoterol:

Asthma –

Adults and children 12 years of age and older: 2 inhalations twice daily in the morning and in the evening.

Dosage increase: For patients who do not respond adequately to the starting dose after 1 to 2 weeks of therapy with budesonide 80 mcg/formoterol 4.5 mcg, increasing to budesonide 160 mcg/formoterol 4.5 mcg may provide additional asthma control.

Chronic obstructive pulmonary disease – Budesonide 160 mcg/formoterol 4.5 mcg, 2 inhalations twice daily.

If shortness of breath occurs in the period between doses, an inhaled short-acting beta-2 agonist should be taken for immediate relief.

Administration – Rinsing the mouth after every dose is advised.

Prime before using for the first time by releasing 2 test sprays into the air away from the face; shaking well for 5 seconds before each spray. If the inhaler has not been used for more than 7 days or if it has been dropped, prime the inhaler again by shaking well before each spray and releasing 2 test sprays into the air away from the face.

Discard the inhaler when the labeled number of inhalations have been used or within 3 months of removal from the foil pouch. Never immerse the canister into water to determine the amount remaining in the canister ("float test").

Maximum dosage – The maximum daily recommended dosage is budesonide 640 mcg/formoterol 18 mcg (given as 2 inhalations of budesonide 160 mcg/formoterol 4.5 mcg twice daily). Do not use more than twice daily or use more than 2 inhalations twice daily.

Onset of relief – Improvement in asthma control following inhaled administration of budesonide/formoterol can occur within 15 minutes of beginning treatment, although maximum benefit may not be achieved for 2 weeks or longer after beginning treatment.

Mometasone furoate/formoterol fumarate:

Administration – After each dose, the patient should be advised to rinse his/her mouth with water without swallowing.

Mometasone/formoterol should be primed before using for the first time by releasing 4 test sprays into the air, away from the face, shaking well before each spray. In cases in which the inhaler has not been used for more than 5 days, prime the inhaler again by releasing 4 test sprays into the air, away from the face, shaking well before each spray.

Recommended Dosages for Mometasone/Formoterol

Previous therapy	Recommended dosage	Maximum recommended daily dose
Inhaled medium-dose corticosteroids	Mometasone 100 mcg/ formoterol 5 mcg, 2 inhalations twice daily	Mometasone 400 mcg/ formoterol 20 mcg
Inhaled high-dose corticosteroids	Mometasone 200 mcg/ formoterol 5 mcg, 2 inhalations twice daily	Mometasone 800 mcg/ formoterol 20 mcg

If symptoms arise between doses, an inhaled short-acting beta$_2$-adrenergic agonist should be taken for immediate relief.

The maximum benefit may not be achieved for 1 week or longer after beginning treatment. For patients 12 years of age and older who do not respond adequately after 2 weeks of therapy, a higher strength may provide additional asthma control.

Chapter 7

CENTRAL NERVOUS SYSTEM AGENTS

MODAFINIL

Tablets, oral: 100 mg, 200 mg (*c-iv*) | *Provigil* (Cephalon)

Indications

Sleep disorder: To improve wakefulness in patients with excessive sleepiness associated with narcolepsy, obstructive sleep apnea /hypopnea syndrome(OSA/HS), and shift work sleep disorder.

In OSA/HS, as an adjunct to standard treatment(s) for the underlying obstruction. If continuous positive airway pressure is the treatment of choice for a patient, make a maximal effort to treat with continuous positive airway pressure for an adequate period of time prior to initiating modafinil. If modafinil is used adjunctively with continuous positive airway pressure, the encouragement of and periodic assessment of continuous positive airway pressure compliance is necessary.

Administration and Dosage

Narcolepsy/OSA/HS (16 years of age and older): 200 mg as a single dose in the morning.

Shift work sleep disorder (16 years of age and older): 200 mg approximately 1 hour prior to the start of the work shift.

Maximum dose: Doses of up to 400 mg/day have been well tolerated, but there is no evidence that this dose confers additional benefit beyond the 200 mg dose.

Hepatic function impairment: In patients with severe hepatic function impairment, reduce the dose to one-half of that recommended for patients with healthy hepatic function.

Actions

Pharmacology: Modafinil has wake-promoting actions like sympathomimetic agents, although the pharmacologic profile is not identical to that of sympathomimetic amines. In vitro, modafinil binds to the dopamine transporter and inhibits dopamine reuptake.

Pharmacokinetics:

Absorption/Distribution – Apparent steady states of total modafinil is reached after 2 to 4 days of dosing.

Absorption of modafinil is rapid, with peak plasma concentrations occurring at 2 to 4 hours.

Metabolism/Excretion – Modafinil is well distributed in body tissue, with an apparent volume of distribution (approximately 0.9 L/kg) that is larger than the volume of total body water (0.6 L/kg). Modafinil is moderately bound to plasma protein (approximately 60%, mainly to albumin).

The effective elimination half-life of modafinil after multiple doses is about 15 hours. The major route of elimination (approximately 90%) is metabolism, primarily by the liver, with subsequent renal elimination of the metabolites.

Contraindications

Known hypersensitivity to modafinil, armodafinil, or its inactive ingredients.

Warnings/Precautions

Dermatologic effects: Serious rash requiring hospitalization and discontinuation of treatment has been reported.

Rare cases of serious or life-threatening rash, including Stevens-Johnson syndrome, toxic epidermal necrolysis (TEN), and drug rash with eosinophilia and systemic symptoms have been reported.

Persistent sleepiness: Advise patients with abnormal levels of sleepiness that their level of wakefulness may not return to normal.

Psychiatric effects: There have been reports of psychiatric adverse experiences. Postmarketing adverse reactions have included, mania, delusions, hallucinations, and suicidal ideation.

Diagnosis of sleep disorders: Use modafinil only in patients who have had complete evaluations of their excessive sleepiness and in whom a diagnosis of narcolepsy, OSA/HS, and/or shift work sleep disorder has been made with ICSD or DSM-IV diagnostic criteria

Continuous positive airway pressure use in patients with OSA/hypopnea syndrome: If continuous positive airway pressure use is the treatment of choice for a patient, make a maximal effort to treat with continuous positive airway pressure for an adequate period of time prior to initiating modafinil. If modafinil is used adjunctively with continuous positive airway pressure, the encouragement of and periodic assessment of continuous positive airway pressure compliance is necessary.

Cardiovascular effects: It is recommended that modafinil not be used in patients with histories of left ventricular hypertrophy or in patients with mitral valve prolapse who have experienced the mitral valve prolapse syndrome when previously receiving CNS stimulants.

Hypersensitivity reactions:

Angioedema/Anaphylactoid reactions – Angioedema has been reported in postmarketing experience with modafinil. Advise patients to discontinue therapy and immediately report to their health care provider any signs or symptoms suggesting angioedema or anaphylaxis.

Multiorgan hypersensitivity reactions – Multiorgan hypersensitivity reactions, including at least one fatality in postmarketing experience, have occurred in close temporal association to the initiation of modafinil.

Hepatic function impairment: In patients with severe hepatic function impairment, with or without cirrhosis, administer modafinil at a reduced dose.

Drug abuse and dependence: Modafinil is listed in Schedule IV of the Controlled Substances Act.

Hazardous tasks: Caution patients about operating an automobile or other hazardous machinery until they are reasonably certain that modafinil therapy will not adversely affect their abilities to engage in such activities.

Pregnancy: *Category* C.

Lactation: It is not known whether modafinil or its metabolites are excreted in human milk.

Children: Modafinil is not approved for use in children for any indication.

Elderly: In elderly patients, elimination of modafinil and its metabolites may be reduced as a consequence of aging. Therefore, consider using lower doses in this population.

Monitoring: Monitor prothrombin time/international normalized ratio more frequently with warfarin coadministration. Increased monitoring of blood pressure may be appropriate in patients on modafinil.

Drug Interactions

Drugs that may be affected by modafinil include clozapine; hormonal contraceptives; estrogens; cyclosporine; CYP2C9/2C19 (eg, diazepam, propranolol, phenytoin, SSRIs, certain tricyclic antidepressants [eg, clomipramine, desipramine]); CYP1A2, CYP2B6, and CYP3A4 substrates, and triazolam.

Drugs that may affect modafinil include CYP3A4 inducers (eg, carbamazepine, phenobarbital, rifampin), CYP3A4 inhibitors (eg, itraconazole, ketoconazole), MAOIs (eg, phenelzine), methylphenidates, and dextroamphetamine.

Adverse Reactions

Adverse reactions occurring in at least 3% of patients treated with modafinil include anorexia, anxiety, back pain, chest pain, diarrhea, dizziness, dry mouth, dyspepsia, flu syndrome, headache, hypertension, insomnia, nausea, nervousness, pharyngitis, and rhinitis.

AMPHETAMINES

DEXTROAMPHETAMINE SULFATE	
Tablets; oral: 5 and 10 mg (*c-ii*)	Various, *Dextrostat* (Shire Richwood)
Capsules, extended-release; oral: 5, 10, and 15 mg (*c-ii*)	Various, *Dexedrine Spansules* (GlaxoSmithKline)
LISDEXAMFETAMINE	
Capsules; oral: 20, 30, 40, 50, 60, and 70 mg (*c-ii*)	*Vyvanse* (Shire US)
METHAMPHETAMINE HYDROCHLORIDE (Desoxyephedrine Hydrochloride)	
Tablets; oral: 5 mg (*c-ii*)	Various, *Desoxyn* (Ovation Pharm)
AMPHETAMINE MIXTURES	
Tablets; oral: 5, 7.5, 10, 12.5, 15, 20, and 30 mg mixed salts of a single entity amphetamine product (*c-ii*)	Various, *Adderall* (Shire Richwood)
Capsules; oral: 5, 10, 15, 20, 25, and 30 mg mixed salts of a single entity amphetamine product (*c-ii*)	*Adderall XR* (Shire)

Warning:

Drug dependence: Amphetamines have a high potential for abuse. Use in weight reduction programs only when alternative therapy has been ineffective. Administration for prolonged periods may lead to drug dependence and must be avoided. Pay particular attention to the possibility of subjects obtaining amphetamines for nontherapeutic use or distribution to others. Prescribe or dispense sparingly. Misuse of amphetamine may cause sudden death and serious cardiovascular adverse reactions.

Indications

Narcolepsy (amphetamine mixtures, dextroamphetamine): To improve wakefulness in patients with excessive daytime sleepiness associated with narcolepsy.

Attention deficit disorder with hyperactivity: Indicated as an integral part of a total treatment program that includes other remedial measures (eg, psychological, educational, social) for a stabilizing effect in children 3 to 16 years of age with a behavioral syndrome characterized by moderate to severe distractibility, short attention span, hyperactivity, emotional lability, and impulsivity. Do not diagnose this syndrome with finality when these symptoms are only of comparatively recent origin. Nonlocalizing (soft) neurological signs, learning disability, and abnormal electroencephalogram (EEG) may be present and a diagnosis of CNS dysfunction may be warranted.

Exogenous obesity (methamphetamine only): As a short-term adjunct in a regimen of weight reduction based on caloric restriction for patients refractory to alternative therapy (eg, repeated diets, group programs, other drugs). Weigh the limited usefulness against the possible risks inherent in use.

Administration and Dosage

Administer at the lowest effective dosage and adjust individually. Avoid late evening doses, particularly with the long-acting form, because of the resulting insomnia.

Attention deficit disorder: When treating attention deficit disorder (ADD) in children, occasionally interrupt drug administration to determine if there is a recurrence of behavioral symptoms sufficient to require continued therapy.

DEXTROAMPHETAMINE SULFATE:

Narcolepsy – 5 to 60 mg/day in divided doses. Initial dosage is 10 mg daily.

Children (6 to 12 years of age): Initial dose is 5 mg/day; increase in increments of 5 mg at weekly intervals until optimal response is obtained (maximum, 60 mg/day).

Adults (12 years of age and older): Start with 10 mg/day; raise in increments of 10 mg/day at weekly intervals. If adverse reactions appear (eg, insomnia, anorexia), reduce dose. Long-acting forms may be used for once-daily dosage. With tablets, give first dose on awakening; give additional doses at intervals of 4 to 6 hours.

Attention deficit hyperactivity disorder –

Adults: 5 mg once or twice daily; increase in increments of 5 mg at weekly intervals.

Not recommended for children younger than 3 years of age.

Children (3 to 5 years of age): 2.5 mg/day; increase in increments of 2.5 mg/day at weekly intervals until optimal response is obtained.

Children (6 years of age and older): 5 mg once or twice daily; increase in increments of 5 mg/day at weekly intervals until optimal response is obtained. Dosage rarely will exceed 40 mg/day.

Long-acting forms may be used for once-daily dosage. With tablets, give first dose on awakening; additional doses may be given at intervals of 4 to 6 hours.

LISDEXAMFETAMINE:

Attention deficit hyperactivity disorder –

Children 6 to 12 years of age: The recommended dose is 30 mg once daily in the morning, adjusted in increments of 10 or 20 mg/day and at approximately weekly intervals.

The maximum recommended dose in children is 70 mg/day.

When possible, drug administration should be interrupted occasionally to determine if there is a recurrence of behavioral symptoms sufficient to require continued therapy.

Lisdexamfetamine has not been studied in children younger than 6 or older than 12 years of age.

Lisdexamfetamine may be taken with or without food.

METHAMPHETAMINE HYDROCHLORIDE:

Attention deficit disorder with hyperactivity –

Adults and children 6 years of age and older: Initially, 5 mg once or twice/day; increase in increments of 5 mg/day at weekly intervals until an optimum response is achieved. Usual effective dose is 20 to 25 mg/day.

Total daily dose may be given in 2 divided doses. Where possible, interrupt drug administration to determine if there is a recurrence of behavioral symptoms sufficient to require continued therapy.

Obesity –

Adults and children 12 years of age and older: 5 mg 30 minutes before each meal.

Treatment duration should not exceed a few weeks. Do not use in children younger than 12 years of age.

AMPHETAMINE MIXTURES:

Tablets –

Attention deficit disorder with hyperactivity:

Adults and children 6 years of age and older – Maximum dose is 40 mg/day. Start with 5 mg once or twice daily. Daily dosage may be raised in increments of 5 mg at weekly intervals. Only in rare cases will it be necessary to exceed a total of 40 mg/day.

3 to 5 years of age – 2.5 mg daily. Daily dosage may be raised in increments of 2.5 mg at weekly intervals until optimal response is obtained.

Younger than 3 years of age – Not recommended for children younger than 3 years of age.

Narcolepsy:

Adults and children 12 years of age and older – Usual dosage is 5 to 60 mg/day in divided doses, depending on individual patient response. Start with 10 mg daily.

Daily dosage may be raised in increments of 10 mg at weekly intervals. If bothersome adverse reactions appear, dosage should be reduced.

6 to 12 years of age – Narcolepsy seldom occurs in children younger than 12 years of age; however, when it does, dextroamphetamine sulfate may be used.

Initial dosage is 5 mg daily. Daily dose may be raised in increments of 5 mg at weekly intervals until optimal response is obtained.

Extended-release capsule –

Attention deficit disorder with hyperactivity:

Adults and children 6 years of age and older – Maximum dosage is 30 mg/day. Doses more than 30 mg/day of amphetamine extended-release have not been studied.

Initial dose is 10 mg once daily in the morning if starting treatment for the first time or switching from another medication. Daily dosage may be raised in increments of 10 mg at weekly intervals.

Based on bioequivalence data, patients taking divided doses of immediate-release amphetamine may be switched to amphetamine extended-release at the same total daily dose taken once daily. Titrate at weekly intervals to appropriate efficacy and tolerability as indicated.

Younger than 6 years of age – Amphetamine extended-release has not been studied in children younger than 6 years of age.

Duration of therapy – Where possible, drug administration should be interrupted occasionally to determine if there is a recurrence of behavioral symptoms sufficient to require continued therapy.

Administration –

Tablets: Give first dose on awakening; give additional doses (1 or 2) at intervals of 4 to 6 hours.

Extended-release capsule: Given upon awakening.

Actions

Pharmacology: Amphetamines are sympathomimetic amines with CNS stimulant activity. CNS effects are mediated by release of norepinephrine from central noradrenergic neurons. Peripheral activities include elevation of systolic and diastolic blood pressures and weak bronchodilator and respiratory stimulant action.

Pharmacokinetics:

Dextroamphetamine – Following administration of 15 mg, maximum plasma dextroamphetamine concentrations were reached in approximately 3 hours (tablets) and 8 hours (extended-release capsules). The average plasma half-life was similar, approximately 12 hours.

Lisdexamfetamine – Lisdexamfetamine is rapidly absorbed from the GI tract. The time to reach maximum concentration (T_{max}) is approximately 3.5 hours following single-dose oral administration. The T_{max} of lisdexamfetamine was approximately 1 hour.

Food prolongs T_{max} by approximately 1 hour.

Approximately 96% of the oral dose radioactivity was recovered in the urine and only 0.3% recovered in the feces over a period of 120 hours. The plasma elimination half-life of lisdexamfetamine typically averaged less than 1 hour in studies of lisdexamfetamine in volunteers.

Methamphetamine – Methamphetamine is rapidly absorbed from the GI tract. The primary site of metabolism is in the liver. The biological half-life is in the range of 4 to 5 hours. Excretion occurs in the urine and is dependent on urine pH. Alkaline urine increases the drug half-life.

Amphetamine mixture – Peak plasma concentrations occur in about 3 hours (*Adderall*) and 7 hours (*Adderall XR*). Elimination half-life is 10 to 13 hours in adults and 9 to 11 hours in children. Extended-release amphetamine mixture capsules demonstrate linear pharmacokinetics. There is no unexpected accumulation at steady state. Food does not affect the extent of absorption of extended-release amphetamine mixture capsules but prolongs T_{max} by 2.5 hours.

Special populations:

Children – Children eliminated amphetamine faster than adults.

Contraindications

Advanced arteriosclerosis; symptomatic cardiovascular disease; moderate to severe hypertension; hyperthyroidism; hypersensitivity or idiosyncrasy to the sympathomimetic amines; glaucoma; agitated states; history of drug abuse; during or within 14 days following administration of monoamine oxidase inhibitors (MAOIs) (hypertensive crises may result).

Warnings/Precautions

Cardiovascular effects:

Sudden death and preexisting structural cardiac abnormalities or other serious heart problems –

Children and adolescents: Sudden death has been reported in association with CNS stimulant treatment at usual doses in children and adolescents with structural cardiac abnormalities or other serious heart problems.

Adults: Sudden death, stroke, and myocardial infarction have been reported in adults taking stimulant drugs at usual doses for attention deficit disorder with hyperactivity (ADHD).

Assessing cardiovascular status: Perform a careful history (including assessment for a family history of sudden death or ventricular arrhythmia) and physical exam to assess for the presence of cardiac disease in children, adolescents, or adults who are being considered for treatment with stimulant medications.

CNS effects:

Preexisting psychosis – Administration of stimulants may exacerbate symptoms of behavior disturbance and thought disorder in patients with preexisting psychotic disorder.

Bipolar illness – Take particular care in using stimulants to treat patients with ADHD with comorbid bipolar disorder because of concern for possible induction of mixed/manic episodes in such patients.

Emergence of new psychotic or manic symptoms – Treatment-emergent psychotic or manic symptoms (eg, delusional thinking, hallucinations, mania) in children and adolescents without a history of psychotic illness or mania can be caused by stimulants at usual doses.

Aggression – Aggressive behavior or hostility is often observed in children and adolescents with ADHD and has been reported in clinical trials and postmarketing experience of some medications indicated for the treatment of ADHD.

Tolerance: When tolerance to the anorectic effect develops, do not exceed the recommended dose in an attempt to increase the effect; rather, discontinue the drug.

Drug dependence: Amphetamines have been extensively abused. Tolerance, extreme psychological dependence, and severe social disability have occurred. Patients may increase the dosage to many times that recommended. Abrupt cessation following prolonged high dosage results in extreme fatigue, mental depression, and changes on the sleep EEG.

Manifestations of chronic intoxication – Severe dermatoses, marked insomnia, irritability, hyperactivity, and personality changes have occurred. Disorganization of thoughts, poor concentration, visual hallucinations, and compulsive behavior often occur. The most severe manifestation of chronic intoxication is psychosis, often clinically indistinguishable from paranoid schizophrenia. This is rare with oral amphetamines.

Growth inhibition: Decrements in the predicted growth (ie, weight gain, height) rate have been reported with the long-term use of stimulants in children.

Hypertension: Use cautiously, even in mild hypertension.

Prescribe or dispense: Prescribe or dispense the least amount feasible at one time to minimize the possibility of overdosage.

Potentially hazardous tasks: Amphetamines may impair the ability of the patient to engage in potentially hazardous activities such as operating machinery or vehicles; caution the patient accordingly.

Tics: Amphetamines have been reported to exacerbate motor and phonic tics and Tourette syndrome.

Attention deficit disorder: Drug treatment is not indicated in all cases.

Seizures: Stimulants may lower the convulsive threshold.

Fatigue: Do not use **methamphetamine** to combat fatigue or replace rest in healthy people.

Visual disturbance: Difficulties with accommodation and blurring of vision have been reported with stimulant treatment.

Tartrazine sensitivity: Some of these products contain tartrazine, which may cause allergic-type reactions (including bronchial asthma) in susceptible individuals.

Pregnancy: Category C.

Lactation: Amphetamines are excreted in breast milk.

Children: Safety and efficacy have not been established for the use of amphetamines as anorectic agents in children younger than 12 years of age.

Extended-release amphetamine mixture capsules are indicated for children 6 years of age and older. Effects in children 3 to 5 years of age have not been studied.

Drug Interactions

Drugs that may affect amphetamines include furazolidone, haloperidol, lithium, MAOIs, methenamine, phenothiazines, SSRIs, tricyclic antidepressants, urinary acidifiers, and urinary alkalinizers. Drugs that may be affected by amphetamines include adrenergic blockers, antihistamines, antihypertensive agents, ethosuximide, guanethidine, meperidine, norepinephrine, phenobarbital, phenothiazines, phenytoin, SSRIs, tricyclic antidepressants, and veratrum alkaloids.

Insulin requirements in diabetes mellitus may be altered in association with the use of **methamphetamine** and the concomitant dietary regimen.

Drug/Lab test interactions: Plasma **corticosteroid** levels may be increased. **Urinary steroid** determinations may be altered by amphetamines.

Adverse Reactions

Adverse reactions may include arrhythmias (at larger doses), changes in libido, constipation, diarrhea, dizziness, dry mouth, dyskinesia, dysphoria, elevation of blood pressure, euphoria, headache, impotence, insomnia, overstimulation, palpitations, reflex decrease in heart rate, restlessness, tachycardia, tremor, unpleasant taste, urticaria.

ANOREXIANTS

BENZPHETAMINE HYDROCHLORIDE	
Tablets: 50 mg (*c-iii*)	Various, *Didrex* (Pharmacia)
DIETHYLPROPION HYDROCHLORIDE	
Tablets: 25 mg (*c-iv*)	Various
Tablets, controlled-release: 75 mg (*c-iv*)	
PHENDIMETRAZINE TARTRATE	
Tablets: 35 mg (*c-iii*)	Various, *Bontril PDM* (Valeant)
Capsules, extended-release: 105 mg (*c-iii*)	Various, *Prelu-2* (Roxane), *Melfiat-105 Unicelles* (Numark), *Bontril Slow-Release* (Amerin)
PHENTERMINE HYDROCHLORIDE	
Tablets: 8 and 37.5 mg (*c-iv*)	Various, *Zantryl* (Ion), *Adipex-P* (Gate)
Capsules: 15, 18.75, 30, and 37.5 mg (*c-iv*)	Various, *Adipex-P* (Gate), *Ionamin* (Celltech), *Pro-Fast HS* (American Pharm.), *Pro-Fast SR* (American Pharm.)
SIBUTRAMINE	
Capsules: 5, 10, and 15 mg (*c-iv*)	*Meridia* (Knoll)

Indications

Exogenous obesity: As a short-term (a few weeks) adjunct in a regimen of weight reduction based on caloric restriction. Measure the limited usefulness of these agents against their inherent risks.

Sibutramine:

Obesity treatment – Management of obesity, including weight loss and maintenance of weight loss, in conjunction with a reduced calorie diet.

Administration and Dosage

Intermittent or interrupted courses of therapy may be useful in the treatment of obesity. A 3- to 6-week course of therapy followed by a discontinuation period of half the original treatment length has been suggested.

BENZPHETAMINE HYDROCHLORIDE:

Adults and children 12 years of age and older – Initiate dosage with 25 to 50 mg once per day; increase according to response. Dosage ranges from 25 to 50 mg 1 to 3 times per day.

DIETHYLPROPION HYDROCHLORIDE:

Tablets – 25 mg 3 times per day 1 hour before meals and in mid-evening if needed to overcome night hunger.

Controlled-release tablets – 75 mg once per day in mid-morning.

PHENDIMETRAZINE TARTRATE:

Tablets and capsules – 35 mg 2 or 3 times per day 1 hour before meals.

Extended-release capsules – 105 mg once per day in the morning 30 to 60 minutes before breakfast.

PHENTERMINE HYDROCHLORIDE: Take 8 mg 3 times per day 30 minutes before meals, or 15 to 37.5 mg as a single daily dose before breakfast or 10 to 14 hours before retiring.

Take *Pro-Fast HS* and *Pro-Fast SR* capsules approximately 2 hours after breakfast for appetite control. Take *Adipex-P* capsules and tablets before breakfast or 1 to 2 hours after breakfast; the tablet dosage may be adjusted to the patient's need (ie, ½ tablet [18.75 mg] daily or 18.75 mg 2 times per day may be adequate).

Swallow *Ionamin* capsules whole.

Avoid late-evening medication because of the possibility of resulting insomnia.

SIBUTRAMINE: The recommended starting dose is 10 mg administered once per day with or without food. If there is inadequate weight loss, the dose may be titrated after 4 weeks to a total of 15 mg once per day. Reserve the 5 mg dose for patients who do not tolerate the 10 mg dose. Take into account blood pressure and heart rate changes when making decisions regarding dose titration.

Doses more than 15 mg/day are not recommended. In most of the clinical trials, sibutramine was given in the morning.

The safety and efficacy of sibutramine when taken for more than 2 years have not been determined at this time.

Actions

Pharmacology: Adrenergic agents (eg, **diethylpropion, benzphetamine, phendimetrazine, phentermine**) act by modulating central norepinephrine and dopamine receptors through the promotion of catecholamine release. Aside from phentermine, other adrenergic agents are infrequently used, perhaps because of the lack of long-term, well-controlled data or the fear of their potential abuse. Older adrenergic weight-loss drugs (eg, amphetamine, methamphetamine, phenmetrazine), which strongly engage in dopamine pathways, are no longer recommended because of the risk of their abuse.

Pharmacokinetics:

Absorption – **Diethylpropion** is rapidly absorbed from the GI tract after oral administration and is extensively metabolized through a complex pathway of biotransformation involving N-dealkylation and reduction. Many of these metabolites are biologically active and may participate in the therapeutic action of diethylpropion.

Sibutramine is rapidly absorbed from the GI tract (time to maximal plasma concentration, 1.2 hours) following oral administration.

Metabolism – Sibutramine is metabolized in the liver principally by the cytochrome P450 ($3A_4$) isoenzyme.

Excretion – Most of the drug and metabolites are excreted via the kidneys.

Contraindications

Advanced arteriosclerosis; symptomatic cardiovascular disease; moderate to severe hypertension; hyperthyroidism; known hypersensitivity or idiosyncrasy to sympathomimetic amines; glaucoma; agitated states; history of drug abuse; during or up to 14 days following the administration of monoamine oxidase (MAO) inhibitors (hypertensive crises may result); coadministration with other CNS stimulants; pregnancy (benzphetamine hydrochloride); patients with anorexia nervosa; patients taking other centrally-acting, appetite-suppressant drugs (sibutramine).

Warnings/Precautions

Blood pressure and pulse: Sibutramine substantially increases blood pressure in some patients.

Concurrent monoamine oxidase inhibitors: Do not use sibutramine concomitantly with MAO inhibitors. There should be at least a 2-week interval after starting or stopping MAO inhibitors before starting treatment with sibutramine.

Serotonin syndrome (sibutramine): The rare but serious constellation of symptoms also has been reported with the concomitant use of selective serotonin reuptake inhibitors (SSRIs) and agents for migraine therapy (eg, sumatriptan, dihydroergotamine), certain opioids (eg, dextromethorphan, meperidine, pentazocine, fentanyl), lithium, or tryptophan. Because sibutramine inhibits serotonin reuptake, do not administer with other serotonergic agents.

Concomitant cardiovascular disease: Do not use sibutramine in patients with a history of coronary artery disease, congestive heart failure, arrhythmias, or stroke.

Glaucoma: Because sibutramine can cause mydriasis, use with caution in patients with narrow-angle glaucoma.

Tolerance: Tolerance to the anorectic effects may develop within a few weeks. If tolerance to the anorectic effect develops, do not exceed the recommended dose in an attempt to increase the effect; rather, discontinue the drug.

Other drugs: These agents should not be used in combination with other anorectic agents, including prescribed drugs (eg, SSRIs [eg, fluoxetine, sertraline, fluvoxamine, paroxetine]), *otc* preparations, and herbal products. When using CNS-active agents, consider the possibility of adverse interactions with alcohol.

Primary pulmonary hypertension: Primary pulmonary hypertension (PPH), a rare, frequently fatal disease of the lungs, has been reported to occur in patients receiving certain anorectic agents. The initial symptom of PPH is usually dyspnea. Other initial symptoms include the following: angina pectoris, syncope, or lower extremity edema. Advise patients to report immediately any deterioration in exercise tolerance. Discontinue treatment in patients who develop new, unexplained symptoms of dyspnea, angina pectoris, syncope, or lower extremity edema.

Valvular heart disease: Serious regurgitant cardiac valvular disease, primarily affecting the mitral, aortic, or tricuspid valves, has been reported in otherwise healthy people who had taken certain anorectic agents in combination for weight loss. The etiology of these valvulopathies has not been established, and their course in individuals after the drugs are stopped is not known.

Psychological disturbances: Psychological disturbances occurred in patients who received an anorectic agent together with a restrictive diet.

Cardiovascular disease: Use with caution and monitor blood pressure in patients with mild hypertension. Not recommended for patients with symptomatic cardiovascular disease, including arrhythmias.

Convulsions: Convulsions may increase in some epileptics receiving **diethylpropion**.

Seizures: Use **sibutramine** cautiously in patients with a history of seizures; discontinue in any patient who develops seizures.

Diabetes: Insulin requirements in diabetes mellitus may be altered in association with the use of anorexigenic drugs and the concomitant dietary restrictions.

Primary pulmonary hypertension (sibutramine): Certain centrally-acting weight loss agents that cause release of serotonin from nerve terminals have been associated with PPH.

Drug abuse and dependence: These drugs are chemically and pharmacologically related to the amphetamines and have abuse potential. Intense psychological or physical dependence and severe social dysfunction may be associated with long-term therapy or abuse. If this occurs, gradually reduce the dosage to avoid withdrawal symptoms.

Hazardous tasks: May produce dizziness, extreme fatigue, and depression after abrupt cessation of prolonged high dosage therapy; instruct patients to observe caution while driving or performing other tasks requiring alertness.

Pregnancy: *Category* X (**benzphetamine hydrochloride**); *Category* C (sibutramine, phentermine, phendimetrazine); *Category* B (diethylpropion).

Lactation: Safety for use in the breast-feeding mother has not been established.

Children: Not recommended for use in children younger than 12 years of age. The safety and efficacy of sibutramine in children younger than 16 years of age have not been established.

Drug Interactions

Drugs that may affect anorexiants include MAO inhibitors, furazolidone, and SSRIs. Drugs that may be affected by anorexiants include guanethidine and tricyclic antidepressants. Drugs that may affect **sibutramine** include alcohol, cimetidine, erythromycin, ketoconazole, and other CYP3A inhibitors. Sibutramine may affect agents that may raise blood pressure or heart rate, CNS-active drugs, MAO inhibitors, SSRIs, ergot alkaloids, lithium, certain opioids, $5HT_1$ receptor antagonists, and tryptophan.

Adverse Reactions

Adverse reactions may include the following: abdominal discomfort, agitation, agranulocytosis, anorexia, anxiety, arrhythmias, arthralgia, asthenia, back pain, bone marrow depression, blurred vision, burning sensation, change in libido, chest pain, chills, clamminess, confusion, constipation, cough increase, depression, diarrhea, dizziness, drowsiness, dry mouth, dysarthria, dyskinesia, dysmenorrhea, dyspepsia, dysphoria, dysuria, ecchymosis, elevated mood, erythema, euphoria, eye irritation, fainting, fever, flushing, flu syndrome, gynecomastia, hair loss, headache, hypertension or hypotension, impotence, incoordination, increased appetite, injury accident, insomnia, leukopenia, malaise, menstrual upset, muscle pain, myalgia, mydriasis, nausea, nervousness, overstimulation, palpitations, pharyngitis, polyuria, rash, restlessness, rhinitis, sinusitis, stomach pain, sweating excessive, tachycardia, tension, tremor, unpleasant taste, urinary frequency, urticaria, vomiting, weakness or fatigue.

OPIOID ANALGESICS

ALFENTANIL HYDROCHLORIDE	
Injection; solution: 500 mcg (as base)/mL (*c-ii*)	Various
CODEINE	
Tablets; oral: 15, 30, and 60 mg (as sulfate) (*c-ii*)	Various
Injection; solution: 15 and 30 mg/mL (as phosphate) (*c-ii*)	Various
FENTANYL CITRATE	
Tablets; buccal: 100, 200, 400, 600, and 800 mcg (*c-ii*)	*Fentora* (Cephalon)
Lozenge on a stick: 200, 400, 600, 800, 1,200, and 1,600 mcg (as base) (*c-ii*)	Various, *Actiq* (Cephalon)
Injection; solution: 50 mcg (as base)/mL (*c-ii*)	Various
FENTANYL TRANSDERMAL SYSTEM	
Patch; transdermal: 12.5, 25, 50, 75, and 100 mcg/h (*c-ii*)	Various, *Duragesic-12*, *Duragesic-25*[a], *Duragesic-50*[a], *Duragesic-75*[a], *Duragesic-100*[a] (Janssen)
FENTANYL BUCCAL FILM	
Film, soluble: 200, 400, 600, 800, and 1,200 mcg/film (*c-ii*)	*Onsolis* (Meda)
HYDROMORPHONE HYDROCHLORIDE	
Tablets; oral: 2, 4, and 8 mg (*c-ii*)	Various, *Dilaudid* (Abbott)
Tablets, extended-release; oral: 8, 12, 16 mg (*c-ii*)	*Exalgo* (Alza)
Liquid; oral: 1 mg per 1 mL (*c-ii*)	Various, *Dilaudid* (Abbott)
Suppositories; rectal: 3 mg (*c-ii*)	Various, *Dilaudid* (Abbott)
Injection; solution: 1, 2, and 4 mg/mL (*c-ii*)	Various, *Dilaudid* (Abbott)
Injection, solution, concentrate: 10 mg/mL (*c-ii*)	Various, *Dilaudid-HP* (Abbott)
Injection, lyophilized powder for solution, concentrate: 250 mg (10 mg/mL after reconstitution) (*c-ii*)	*Dilaudid-HP* (Abbott)
LEVORPHANOL TARTRATE	
Tablets; oral: 2 mg (*c-ii*)	Various
Injection; solution: 2 mg/mL (*c-ii*)	*Levo-Dromoran* (Valeant)
MEPERIDINE HYDROCHLORIDE	
Tablets; oral: 50 and 100 mg (*c-ii*)	Various, *Demerol* (Sanofi-Synthelabo)
Syrup; oral: 50 mg per 5 mL (*c-ii*)	Various, *Demerol* (Sanofi-Synthelabo)
Injection; solution: 25, 50, 75, and 100 mg/mL (*c-ii*)	Various, *Demerol* (Abbott)
METHADONE HYDROCHLORIDE	
Tablets; oral: 5 and 10 mg (*c-ii*)	Various, *Dolophine* (Roxane), *Methadose* (Mallinckrodt)
Tablets, dispersible; oral: 40 mg (*c-ii*)	Various[b], *Methadose*[b] (Mallinckrodt), *Diskets* (Cebert)
Solution; oral: 5 mg per 5 mL and 10 mg per 5 mL (*c-ii*)	*Methadone Hydrochloride* (Roxane)
Solution, concentrate; oral: 10 mg/mL (*c-ii*)	*Methadone Hydrochloride Intensol* (Roxane), *Methadose*[b] (Mallinckrodt)
Injection; solution: 10 mg/mL (*c-ii*)	*Methadone Hydrochloride* (AAI Pharma)
MORPHINE SULFATE	
Tablets; oral: 15 and 30 mg (*c-ii*)	Various
Tablets, controlled-release; oral: 15, 30, 60 mg; and 100 mg[a] (*c-ii*)	Various, *MS Contin* (Purdue Frederick), *Oramorph SR* (aaiPharma)
200 mg[a] (*c-ii*)	Various, *MS Contin* (Purdue Frederick)
Tablets, extended-release; oral: 15, 30, 60, 100 mg; and 200 mg[a] (*c-ii*)	Various
Injection; soluble tablets: 10, 15, and 30 mg (*c-ii*)	*Morphine Sulfate* (Ranbaxy)
Capsules, extended-release pellets; oral: 30 mg; 45, 60, 75, 90, and 120 mg[a] (*c-ii*)	*Avinza* (King)
Capsules, extended-release pellets; oral: 10, 20, 30, 50, 60, 80 mg; 100[a] and 200 mg[a] (*c-ii*)	*Kadian* (Alpharma)
Solution; oral: 10 mg per 5 mL, 20 mg per 5 mL (*c-ii*)	*Morphine Sulfate* (Roxane), *MSIR* (Purdue Frederick)
Solution, concentrate; oral: 20 mg/mL (*c-ii*)	Various, *MSIR* (Purdue Frederick), *Roxanol*, *Roxanol T* (aaiPharma)
100 mg per 5 mL (*c-ii*)	*Roxanol 100* (aaiPharma)
Suppositories; rectal: 5, 10, 20, and 30 mg (*c-ii*)	Various, *RMS* (Upsher-Smith)
Injection; solution: 0.5, 1, 2, 4, 5, 8, 10, 15 mg/mL (*c-ii*)	Various, *Astramorph PF* (APP Pharmaceuticals), *Duramorph* (Baxter), *Infumorph 200* (ESI Lederle)

Injection, extended-release liposomal: 10 mg/mL (*c-ii*)	*DepoDur* (Endo)
Injection; solution: 25[c] and 50 mg/mL[c] (*c-ii*)	Various, *Infumorph 500* (Baxter)
OPIUM	
Liquid; oral: anhydrous morphine equiv. to 10 mg per mL (*c-ii*)	*Opium Tincture, Deodorized* (Ranbaxy)
anhydrous morphine equiv. to 2 mg per 5 mL (*c-iii*)	*Paregoric* (Various)
OXYCODONE HYDROCHLORIDE	
Tablets; oral: 5, 10, 15, 20, and 30 mg (*c-ii*)	Various, *M-oxy* (Mallinckrodt), *Roxicodone* (aaiPharma)
Tablets, controlled-release; oral: 10, 15, 20, 30, 40, and 60 mg; and 80 mg[a] (*c-ii*)	Various, *OxyContin* (Purdue Pharma LP)
Capsules; oral: 5 mg (*c-ii*)	*Oxycodone Hydrochloride* (Ethex), *OxyIR* (Purdue Pharma)
Solution; oral: 5 mg per 5 mL (*c-ii*)	Various, *Roxicodone* (aaiPharma)
Solution, concentrate; oral: 20 mg/mL (*c-ii*)	Various, *OxyFAST* (Purdue Pharma LP), *Roxicodone Intensol* (aaiPharma)
OXYMORPHONE HYDROCHLORIDE	
Tablets; oral: 5 and 10 mg (*c-ii*)	Various, *Opana* (Endo)
Tablets, extended-release; oral: 5, 7.5, 10, 15, 20, 30, and 40 mg (*c-ii*)	*Opana ER* (Endo)
Injection, solution: 1 mg/mL (*c-ii*)	*Opana* (Endo)
REMIFENTANIL HYDROCHLORIDE	
Injection; powder for solution: 1, 2, and 5 mg (as base) (*c-ii*)	*Ultiva* (Abbott)
SUFENTANIL CITRATE	
Injection; solution: 50 mcg (as base)/mL (*c-ii*)	Various, *Sufenta* (Taylor)
TRAMADOL HYDROCHLORIDE	
Tablets; oral: 50 mg (*Rx*)	Various, *Ultram* (Janssen)
Tablets, extended-release; oral: 100, 200, and 300 mg (*Rx*)	Various, *Ryzolt* (Purdue Pharma), *Ultram ER* (Ortho-McNeil)
TAPENTADOL	
Tablets; oral: 50, 75, and 100 mg (*Rx*)	*Nucynta* (PriCara)

[a] For use in opioid-tolerant patients only.
[b] For detoxification and maintenance only.
[c] For IV use after dilution. Not for direct injection.

Warning:

Fentanyl: Fentanyl is an opioid agonist and a schedule II controlled substance with an abuse liability similar to other opioid analgesics. Fentanyl can be abused in a manner similar to other opioid agonists, legal or illicit. This should be considered when prescribing or dispensing fentanyl in situations in which the health care provider or pharmacist is concerned about in increased risk of misuse, abuse, or diversion. Schedule II opioid substances, which include morphine, oxycodone, hydromorphone, oxymorphone, and methadone, have the highest potential for abuse and risk of fatal overdose due to respiratory depression.

Serious adverse events, including deaths, in patients treated with oral transmucosal fentanyl products have been reported. Deaths occurred as a result of improper patient selection (eg, use in opioid nontolerant patients) and/or improper dosing. The substitution of fentanyl buccal soluble film for any other fentanyl product may result in fatal overdose.

The fentanyl lozenge, buccal tablet, and buccal soluble film are indicated only for the management of breakthrough cancer pain in patients with cancer already receiving and tolerant to opioid therapy for their underlying persistent cancer pain. Patients considered opioid-tolerant are those who are taking oral morphine 60 mg/day or more, transdermal fentanyl 25 mcg/h, oxycodone 30 mg/day, oral hydromorphone 8 mg/day, or an equianalgesic dose of another opioid for a week or longer.

continued on next page

Warning: (cont.)

Because life-threatening respiratory depression could occur at any dose in patients not on long-term opiates, it is contraindicated in the management of acute or postoperative pain, including headache/migraine, dental pain, or use in the emergency room. This product is not indicated for use in opioid-nontolerant patients, including those using opioids intermittently, on an as-needed basis. Deaths have occurred in opioid-nontolerant patients treated with other fentanyl products.

Instruct patients and their caregivers that this drug contains a medicine in an amount that can be fatal to a child, in individuals for whom it is not prescribed, and in those who are not opioid tolerant. Keep all units out of the reach of children, and discard opened units properly.

This medicine should be used only in the care of cancer patients and only by health care providers who are knowledgeable of and skilled in the use of schedule II opioids to treat cancer pain.

Tablet – Because of the higher bioavailability of fentanyl in the buccal tablet, when converting patients from other oral fentanyl products (including the fentanyl lozenge) to the buccal tablet, do not substitute the buccal tablet on a mcg per mcg basis. Adjust dosage as appropriate.

Buccal soluble film – When prescribing, do not convert patients on a mcg per mcg basis from any other oral transmucosal fentanyl product to fentanyl buccal soluble film. Patients beginning treatment with fentanyl buccal soluble film must begin with titration from the 200 mcg dose.

When dispensing, do not substitute an fentanyl buccal soluble film prescription for any other fentanyl product. Substantial differences exist in the pharmacokinetic profile of fentanyl buccal soluble film compared with other fentanyl products that result in clinically important differences in the extent of absorption of fentanyl. As a result of these differences, the substitution of fentanyl buccal soluble film for any other fentanyl product may result in fatal overdose.

Special care must be used when dosing fentanyl buccal soluble film. If the breakthrough pain episode is not relieved, patients should wait at least 2 hours before taking another dose.

The concomitant use of fentanyl buccal soluble film with CYP3A4 inhibitors may result in an increase in fentanyl plasma concentrations and may cause potentially fatal respiratory depression.

Because of the risk for misuse, abuse, and overdose, fentanyl buccal soluble film is available only through a restricted distribution program, called the FOCUS Program. Under the FOCUS Program, only prescribers, pharmacies, and patients registered with the program are able to prescribe, dispense, and receive fentanyl buccal soluble film. To enroll in the FOCUS Program, call 1-877-466-7654 or visit http://www.OnsolisFocus.com

Hydromorphone:

Exalgo – Hydromorphone is an opioid agonist and a schedule II controlled substance with an abuse liability similar to other opioid analgesics.

Hydromorphone is an extended-release (ER) formulation of hydromorphone hydrochloride indicated for the management of moderate to severe pain in opioid-tolerant patients when a continuous around-the-clock opioid analgesic is needed for an extended period of time. Hydromorphone ER is for use in opioid-tolerant patients only. Fatal respiratory depression could occur in patients who are not opioid tolerant. Accidental consumption of hydromorphone ER, especially in children, can result in a fatal overdose of hydromorphone. Hydromorphone ER is not indicated for the management of acute or postoperative pain. Hydromorphone ER is not intended for use as an as-needed analgesic.

continued on next page

Warning: (cont.)

High potency (HP) injection – HP injection is a highly concentrated solution of hydromorphone intended for use in opioid-tolerant patients. Do not confuse HP injection with standard parenteral formulations of injection or other opioids. Overdose and death could result.

Methadone: Deaths have been reported during initiation of methadone treatment for opioid dependence. In some cases, drug interactions with other drugs, both licit and illicit, have been suspected. However, in other cases, deaths appear to have occurred because of the respiratory or cardiac effects of methadone and too-rapid titration without appreciation for the accumulation of methadone over time. It is critical to understand the pharmacokinetics of methadone and to exercise vigilance during treatment initiation and dose titration. Patients must also be strongly cautioned against self-medicating with CNS depressants during initiation of methadone treatment.

Respiratory depression is the chief hazard associated with methadone administration. Methadone's peak respiratory depressant effects typically occur later and persist longer than its peak analgesic effects, particularly in the early dosing period. These characteristics can contribute to the cases of iatrogenic overdose, particularly during treatment initiation and dose titration.

Cases of QT interval prolongation and serious arrhythmia (torsades de pointes) have been observed during treatment with methadone. Most cases involve patients being treated for pain with large, multiple daily doses of methadone, although cases have been reported in patients receiving doses commonly used for maintenance treatment of an opioid addiction.

Conditions for the distribution and use of methadone products for the treatment of an opioid addiction – Methadone products, when used for the treatment of an opioid addiction in detoxification or maintenance programs, shall be dispensed only by opioid treatment programs (and agencies, practitioners, or institutions by formal agreement with the program sponsor) certified by the Substance Abuse and Mental Health Services Administration and approved by the designated state authority. Certified treatment programs shall dispense and use methadone in oral form only and according to the treatment requirements stipulated in the Federal Opioid Treatment Standards (42 CFR 8.12). See the following information for important regulatory exceptions to the general requirement for certification to provide opioid agonist treatment.

Failure to abide by the requirement in these regulations may result in criminal prosecution, seizure of the drug supply, revocation of the program approval, and injunction precluding operation of the program.

Regulatory exceptions to the general requirement for certification to provide opioid agonist treatment include the following:

- During inpatient care, when the patient was admitted for any condition other than concurrent opioid addiction (pursuant to 21 CFR 1306.07[c]), to facilitate the treatment of the primary admitting diagnosis.
- During an emergency period of no longer than 3 days while definitive care for the addiction is being sought in an appropriately licensed facility (pursuant to 21 CFR 1306.07[b]).

Morphine:

Avinza – *Avinza* capsules are a modified-release formulation of morphine sulfate indicated for once-daily administration for the relief of moderate to severe pain requiring continuous, around-the-clock opioid therapy for an extended period of time. *Avinza* capsules are to be swallowed whole or the contents of the capsules sprinkled on applesauce. The capsule beads are not to be chewed, crushed, or dissolved due to the risk of rapid release and absorption of a potentially fatal dose of morphine.

continued on next page

Warning: (cont.)

Kadian – Morphine, an opioid agonist and a Schedule II controlled substance, has an abuse liability similar to other opioid analgesics. Morphine can be abused in a manner similar to other opioid agonists, legal or illicit. Consider this when prescribing or dispensing *Kadian* in situations in which the health care provider or pharmacist is concerned about an increased risk of misuse, abuse, or diversion.

Kadian capsules are an extended release oral formulation of morphine indicated for the management of moderate to severe pain requiring a continuous, around-the-clock opioid analgesic for an extended period of time.

Kadian capsules are not for use as an as-needed analgesic. *Kadian* 100 and 200 mg capsules are for use in opioid-tolerant patients only. Ingestion of these capsules or of the pellets within the capsules may cause fatal respiratory depression when administered to patients not already tolerant to high doses of opioids. *Kadian* capsules are to be swallowed whole or the contents of the capsule sprinkled on applesauce. The pellets in the capsules are not to be chewed, crushed, or dissolved because of the risk of rapid release and absorption of a potentially fatal dose of morphine.

Astromorph PF, Duramorph, Infumorph – Because of the risk of severe adverse effects when the epidural or intrathecal route of administration is employed, patients must be observed in a fully equipped and staffed environment for at least 24 hours after the initial dose.

Infumorph – Infumorph is not recommended for single-dose intravenous (IV), intramuscular (IM), or subcutaneous administration because of the very large amount of morphine in the ampul and the associated risk of overdosage.

Oxycodone: Controlled-release (CR) oxycodone is an opioid agonist and a schedule II controlled substance with an abuse liability similar to morphine.

Oxycodone can be abused in a manner similar to other opioid agonists, legal or illicit. Consider this when prescribing or dispensing oxycodone CR tablets in situations where there is concern about an increased risk of misuse, abuse, or diversion.

Oxycodone CR tablets are indicated for the management of moderate to severe pain when a continuous, around-the-clock analgesic is needed for an extended period of time.

Oxycodone CR tablets are not intended for use as an as-needed analgesic.

Oxycodone 80 and 160 mg CR tablets are for use in opioid-tolerant patients only. These tablet strengths may cause fatal respiratory depression when administered to patients not previously exposed to opioids.

Oxycodone CR tablets are to be swallowed whole and are not to be broken, chewed, or crushed. Taking broken, chewed, or crushed oxycodone CR tablets leads to rapid release and absorption of a potentially fatal dose of oxycodone.

Oxymorphone extended-release (ER): Oxymorphone ER is a morphine-like opioid agonist and a Schedule II controlled substance with an abuse liability similar to other opioid analgesics. Oxymorphone can be abused in a manner similar to other opioid agonists, legal or illicit. Consider this when prescribing or dispensing oxymorphone ER in situations in which the health care provider or pharmacist is concerned about an increased risk of misuse, abuse, or diversion.

Oxymorphone ER oral formulation is indicated for the management of moderate to severe pain when a continuous, around-the-clock opioid analgesic is needed for an extended period of time. Oxymorphone ER is not intended for use on an as-needed basis.

continued on next page

> **Warning: (cont.)**
> Oxymorphone ER tablets are to be swallowed whole and not broken, chewed, dissolved, or crushed. Taking broken, chewed, dissolved, or crushed oxymorphone ER tablets leads to rapid release and absorption of a potentially fatal dose of oxymorphone.
> Patients must not consume alcoholic beverages or prescription or nonprescription medications containing alcohol while on oxymorphone ER therapy. The coingestion of alcohol with oxymorphone ER may result in increased plasma levels and a potentially fatal overdose of oxymorphone.

Indications

Alfentanil hydrochloride: As an analgesic adjunct in the maintenance of anesthesia with barbiturate/nitrous oxide/oxygen.

As an analgesic administered by continuous infusion with nitrous oxide/oxygen in the maintenance of general anesthesia.

As a primary anesthetic for induction of anesthesia in general surgery when endotracheal intubation and mechanical ventilation are required.

Analgesic component for monitored anesthesia care (MAC).

Codeine: Relief of mild to moderate pain and in combination with other respiratory agents for the treatment of cough.

Fentanyl injection:

Pain – For analgesic action of short duration during anesthesia (premedication, induction, maintenance) and in the immediate postoperative period (recovery room) as needed.

For use as a narcotic analgesic supplement in general or regional anesthesia.

For administration with a neuroleptic such as droperidol as an anesthetic premedication, for induction of anesthesia and as an adjunct in maintenance of general and regional anesthesia.

For use as an anesthetic agent with oxygen in selected high-risk patients (open heart surgery or certain complicated neurological or orthopedic procedures.

Fentanyl citrate transmucosal system, fentanyl buccal film:

Breakthrough cancer pain – For the management of breakthrough cancer pain in patients who are already receiving and are tolerant to opioid therapy.

Fentanyl transdermal system:

Pain – Management of persistent moderate to severe chronic pain in patients requiring continuous opioid analgesia for pain.

Only use in patients who are already receiving opioid therapy, who have demonstrated opioid tolerance, and who require a total daily dose at least equivalent to fentanyl transdermal system 25 mcg/h.

Hydromorphone hydrochloride: Relief of moderate to severe pain such as that caused by surgery, cancer, trauma (soft tissue and bone), biliary colic, MI, burns, and renal colic.

Extended release tablets indicated for the management of moderate to severe pain in opioid-tolerant patients requiring continuous, around-the-clock opioid analgesia for an extended period of time. Patients considered opioid tolerant are those who are taking at least oral morphine 60 mg per day, transdermal fentanyl 25 mcg/h, oral oxycodone 30 mg/day, oral hydromorphone 8 mg/day, oral oxymorphone 25 mg/day, or an equianalgesic dose of another opioid, for a week or longer.

Levorphanol tartrate:

Pain – Management of moderate to severe pain where an opioid analgesic is appropriate.

Pain/Preoperative medication (Levo-Dromoran only) – As a preoperative medication where an opioid analgesic is appropriate.

Meperidine hydrochloride:

Oral and parenteral – Relief of moderate to severe pain.

Parenteral – For preoperative medication, support of anesthesia and obstetrical analgesia.

Methadone hydrochloride:

Detoxification – For detoxification treatment of opioid addiction (heroin or other morphine-like drugs).

For maintenance treatment of opioid addiction, in conjunction with appropriate social and medical services.

Note: Outpatient maintenance and detoxification treatment may be provided only by Opioid Treatment Programs (OTPs) certified by the Federal Substance Abuse and Mental Health Services Administration (SAMHSA) and registered by the Drug Enforcement Agency (DEA). This does not preclude the maintenance treatment of a patient with concurrent opioid addiction who is hospitalized for conditions other than opioid addiction and who requires temporary maintenance during the critical period of his/her stay, or if a patient whose enrollment has been verified in a program that has been certified for maintenance treatment with methadone.

Pain (except oral concentrate and tablets for suspension) – For the treatment of moderate to severe pain not responsive to nonnarcotic analgesics.

Morphine sulfate:

Oral –

Immediate-release tablets/solution: Relief of moderate to severe pain.

Controlled/Extended/Sustained-release tablets/capsules: Relief of moderate to severe pain in those who require continuous, around-the-clock opioid therapy for an extended period of time.

Parenteral –

IV: Relief of severe pain; pain of MI; used preoperatively to sedate the patient and allay apprehension, facilitate anesthesia induction, and reduce anesthetic dosage; control postoperative pain; relieve anxiety and reduce left ventricular work by reducing preload pressure; treatment of dyspnea associated with acute left ventricular failure and pulmonary edema; produce anesthesia for open-heart surgery.

Subcutaneous/IM: Relief of severe pain; relieve preoperative apprehension; preoperative sedation; control postoperative pain; supplement to anesthesia; analgesia during labor; acute pulmonary edema; allay anxiety.

Epidural/Intrathecal: Management of pain not responsive to nonnarcotic analgesics. For treatment of intractable chronic pain (*Infumorph* only).

ER epidural: Indicated for single-dose administration by the epidural route, at the lumbar level, for the treatment of pain following major surgery. *DepoDur* is administered prior to surgery or after clamping the umbilical cord during cesarean section.

Rectal – Severe acute and chronic pain.

Opium:

Diarrhea – For treatment of diarrhea. Do not be used in diarrhea caused by poisoning until the toxic material is eliminated from the GI tract.

Oxycodone hydrochloride:

Oral solution and concentrate solution – Relief of moderate to severe pain.

Immediate-release tablets – Management of moderate to severe pain where use of an opioid analgesic is appropriate.

Controlled-release tablets – Management of moderate to severe pain when a continuous, around-the-clock analgesic is needed for an extended period of time.

Oxymorphone hydrochloride:

Oxymorphone IR – For the relief of moderate to severe acute pain when the use of an opioid is appropriate.

Oxymorphone ER – For the relief of moderate to severe pain in patients requiring continuous, around-the-clock opioid treatment for an extended period of time; not intended for use as an as-needed analgesic.

Oxymorphone injection – For relief of anxiety in patients with dyspnea associated with pulmonary edema secondary to acute left ventricular dysfunction and moderate to severe pain; as preoperative medication, support of anesthesia, and obstetrical analgesia.

Remifentanil hydrochloride:

General anesthesia – An analgesic agent for use during the induction and maintenance of general anesthesia for inpatient and outpatient procedures and for continuation as an analgesic into the immediate postoperative period.

Monitored anesthesia care – As an analgesic component of monitored anesthesia care.

Sufentanil citrate:

Analgesia – Analgesic adjunct for the maintenance of balanced general anesthesia in patients who are intubated and ventilated.

Anesthetic – As a primary anesthetic agent for the induction and maintenance of anesthesia with 100% oxygen in patients undergoing major surgical procedures. In patients who are intubated and ventilated, such as cardiovascular surgery or neurosurgical procedures in the sitting position, to provide favorable myocardial and cerebral oxygen balance or when extended postoperative ventilation is anticipated.

Epidural analgesic – For epidural administration as an analgesic combined with low-dose bupivacaine, usually 12.5 mg per administration, during labor and vaginal delivery.

Tapentadol:

Acute pain – For the relief of moderate to severe acute pain in patients 18 years of age and older.

Tramadol:

IR – Management of moderate to moderately severe pain in adults.

ER – Management of moderate to moderately severe chronic pain in adults who require around-the-clock treatment of pain for an extended period of time.

Administration and Dosage

The most important factor to be considered in determining the appropriate dose is the extent of pre-existing opioid tolerance. Reduce initial doses in elderly or debilitated patients.

The following equianalgesic dosing table is based on parenteral **morphine** 10 mg. Dosage adjustments may be needed if the elimination half-life of the new opioid differs from the current opioid (see Pharmacokinetics).

Approximate Equianalgesic Dosing of Opioid Analgesics in Adults[a,b]

	Equianalgesic dose		
Opioid	Oral	Parenteral (IM, subcutaneous, IV)	Rectal
Codeine	200 mg	120 to 130 mg	NA[c]
Fentanyl[d]	NA	0.1 mg	NA
Hydrocodone	30 mg	NA	NA
Hydromorphone	7.5 mg	1.5 mg	3 mg
Levorphanol	4 mg	2 mg	NA
Meperidine	300 mg	75 mg	NA
Methadone	10 to 20 mg	5 to 10 mg	NA
Morphine	60 mg single dose, 30 mg repeated doses	10 mg	ND[e]
Oxycodone	20 to 30 mg	NA	NA
Oxymorphone	NA	1 mg	10 mg

[a] Table is to be used for estimation only. Data are compiled from multiple references and may be based on single-dose studies.

[b] Caution: Recommended doses do not apply for adult patients with body weight less than 50 kg. Recommended doses do not apply to patients with renal or hepatic insufficiency or other conditions affecting drug metabolism and kinetics. Starting doses should be lower for elderly patients.

[c] NA = Not available commercially for this route of administration.

[d] Refer to Fentanyl Transdermal monograph for dosing conversion.

[e] ND = No data.

ALFENTANIL HYDROCHLORIDE:

Children younger than 12 years of age – Use is not recommended.

General anesthesia –

Alfentanil Dosage Range for Use During General Anesthesia

Clinical status	Induction[a] (initial dose)	Maintenance (increments/Infusion)	Total dose
Spontaneously breathing/ Assisted ventilation	8 to 20 mcg/kg	3 to 5 mcg/kg every 5 to 20 minor 0.5 to 1 mcg/kg/min	8 to 40 mcg/kg
Assisted or controlled ventilation			
Incremental injection (to attenuate response to laryngoscopy and intubation)	20 to 50 mcg/kg	5 to 15 mcg/kg every 5 to 20 min	≤ 75 mcg/kg
Continuous infusion[b] (to provide attenuation of response to intubation and incision)	50 to 75 mcg/kg	0.5 to 3 mcg/kg/min. Average infusion rate 1 to 1.5 mcg/kg/min	dependent on duration of procedure
Anesthetic induction (give slowly [over 3 min]).[c]Reduce concentration of inhalation agents by 30% to 50% for initial hour)	130 to 245 mcg/kg	0.5 to 1.5 mcg/kg/min or general anesthetic	dependent on duration of procedure
MAC[d] (for sedated and responsive spontaneously breathing patients)	3 to 8 mcg/kg	3 to 5 mcg/kg every 5 to 20 minor 0.25 to 1 mcg/kg/min	3 to 40 mcg/kg

[a] Administer induction doses of alfentanil slowly (over 3 minutes). Administration may produce loss of vascular tone and hypotension. Consider fluid replacement prior to induction.

[b] 0.5 to 3 mcg/kg/min with nitrous oxide/oxygen in general surgery. Following anesthetic induction dose, reduce infusion rate requirements by 30% to 50% for the first hour of maintenance.Vital sign changes that indicate response to surgical stress or lightening of anesthesia may be controlled by increasing rate to a max of 4 mcg/kg/min or administering bolus doses of 7 mcg/kg. If changes are not controlled after 3 bolus doses given over 5 minutes, use a barbiturate, vasodilator, and/or inhalation agent. Always adjust infusion rates downward in the absence of these signs until there is some response to surgical stimulation.Rather than an increase in infusion rate, administer 7 mcg/kg bolus doses of alfentanil or a potent inhalation agent in response to signs of lightening of anesthesia within the last 15 minutes of surgery. Discontinue infusion at least 10 to 15 minutes prior to the end of surgery.

[c] At these doses, expect truncal rigidity and use a muscle relaxant.

[d] During administration of alfentanil for MAC, infusions may be continued to the end of the procedure.

CODEINE:

Analgesic –

Adults: 15 to 60 mg orally every 4 to 6 hours; 30 mg subcutaneously or IM every 4 hours as needed. Usual dose is 15 to 60 mg.

Children: 500 mcg/kg or 15 mg/m^2 subcutaneously or IM every 4 hours as necessary.

Admixture incompatibility – Codeine is incompatible with soluble barbiturates.

FENTANYL:

Premedication – 50 to 100 mcg IM, 30 to 60 minutes prior to surgery.

Adjunct to general anesthesia –

Total low dose: 2 mcg/kg in small doses for minor, painful surgical procedures and postoperative pain relief.

Maintenance low dose: 2 mcg/kg. Additional doses are needed infrequently in minor procedures.

Total moderate dose: 2 to 20 mcg/kg. Respiratory depression necessitates artificial ventilation and careful observation of postoperative ventilation.

Maintenance moderate dose: 2 to 20 mcg/kg. Use 25 to 100 mcg IV or IM when movement and/or changes in vital signs indicate surgical stress or lightening of analgesia.

Total high dose: 20 to 50 mcg/kg for "stress free" anesthesia. Use during open heart surgery and complicated neurosurgical and orthopedic procedures where surgery is prolonged and the stress response is detrimental.

Maintenance high dose: 20 to 50 mcg/kg, ranging from 25 mcg to half the initial loading dose. Administer when vital signs indicate surgical stress and lightening of analgesia.

Adjunct to regional anesthesia – 50 to 100 mcg IM or slowly IV over 1 to 2 minutes as required.

Postoperatively (recovery room) – 50 to 100 mcg IM for the control of pain, tachypnea, and emergence delirium; repeat dose in 1 to 2 hours as needed.

Children (2 to 12 years of age) – For induction and maintenance, a reduced dose as low as 2 to 3 mcg/kg is recommended.

Elderly/Debilitated patients – Reduce initial dose in elderly and debilitated patients and patients with renal or hepatic dysfunction.

General anesthetic – 50 to 100 mcg/kg with oxygen and a muscle relaxant when attenuation of the responses to surgical stress is especially important. Up to 150 mcg/kg may be necessary.

FENTANYL CITRATE:

Fentanyl lozenge (oral transmucosal) –

Warning: See Warning Box at the beginning of the monograph.

Use has not been established with opioid-tolerant children younger than 16 years of age. Keep out of the reach of children.

Instruct the patient to suck, not chew, the lozenge. If chewed and swallowed, might result in lower peak concentrations and lower bioavailability.

Instruct the patient to consume the lozenge over a 15-minute period. Longer or shorter consumption times may produce less efficacy than reported in clinical trials. If signs of excessive opioid effects appear before the unit is consumed, remove the drug matrix from the patient's mouth immediately and decrease future doses.

Dose titration: Initial dose to treat episodes of breakthrough cancer pain should be 200 mcg. Prescribe patients an initial titration supply of six 200 mg units, thus limiting the number of units in the home during titration. Advise patients to use all units before increasing to a higher dose.

From this initial dose, patients should be closely followed and the dosage level changed until the patient reaches a dose that provides adequate analgesia using a single oral transmucosal fentanyl dosage unit per breakthrough cancer pain episode.

Redosing within a single episode during titration – Redosing may start 15 minutes after the previous unit has been completed (30 minutes after the start of the previous unit). Do not give more than 2 units for each individual breakthrough cancer pain episode.

Increasing the dose – If treatment of several consecutive breakthrough cancer pain episodes requires more than 1 fentanyl lozenge per episode, consider an increase in dose to the next higher available strength. At each new dose during titration, prescribe 6 units of the titration dose. Evaluate each new dose used in the titration period over several episodes of breakthrough cancer pain (generally 1 to 2 days) to determine whether it provides adequate efficacy with acceptable adverse reactions. The incidence of adverse reactions is likely to be greater during this initial titration period compared with later, after the effective dose is determined.

Daily limit – Instruct patients to limit consumption to 4 units/day or less. If consumption increases to more than 4 units/day, reevaluate the dose.

Discontinuation – Recommend a gradual downward titration for discontinuation because it is not known at what dose level the opioid may be discontinued without producing the signs and symptoms of abrupt withdrawal.

Dosage adjustment: Experience in a long-term study of the fentanyl lozenge in the treatment of breakthrough cancer pain suggests that dosage adjustment of both the fentanyl lozenge and the maintenance (around-the-clock) opioid analgesic may be required in some patients to continue to provide adequate relief of breakthrough cancer pain.

Fentanyl buccal tablet –

Starting dose: 100 mcg.

For patients switching from oral transmucosal fentanyl to the buccal tablet, initiate the buccal tablet dose as shown in the following table.

Fentanyl Dosing Conversion Recommendations	
Current oral transmucosal fentanyl dose	Initial fentanyl buccal tablet dose
200 mcg	100 mcg
400 mcg	100 mcg
600 mcg	200 mcg
800 mcg	200 mcg
1,200 mcg	400 mcg
1,600 mcg	400 mcg

Redosing patients within a single episode: Dosing may be repeated once during a single episode of breakthrough pain if pain is not adequately relieved by 1 fentanyl buccal tablet dose. Redosing may occur 30 minutes after the start of the administration of the fentanyl buccal tablet, and the same dosage strength should be used.

Increasing the dose: Titration should be initiated using multiples of the fentanyl 100 mcg buccal tablet. Patients needing to titrate above 100 mcg can be instructed to use two 100 mcg tablets (1 on each side of the mouth in the buccal cavity). If this dose is not successful in controlling the breakthrough pain episode, the patient may be instructed to place two 100 mcg tablets on each side of the mouth in the buccal cavity (total of four 100 mcg tablets).

To reduce the risk of overdose during titration, patients should have only one strength fentanyl buccal tablet available at any one time. Patients should be strongly encouraged to use all of their fentanyl buccal tablets of 1 strength prior to being prescribed the next strength. If this is not practical, unused fentanyl buccal tablets should be disposed of safely.

Hepatic/Renal function impairment: Caution should be exercised for patients with hepatic and/or renal function impairment, and the lowest possible dose should be used in these patients.

Current CYP3A4 inhibitor use: Particular caution should be exercised for patients receiving CYP3A4 inhibitors, and the lowest possible dose should be used in these patients.

Opening the blister package: Patients should be instructed not to open the blister until ready to administer. Patients should NOT attempt to push the tablet through the blister, as this may cause damage to the tablet.

Tablet administration: Patients should not attempt to split the tablet.

The fentanyl buccal tablet should not be sucked, chewed, or swallowed.

The fentanyl buccal tablet should be left between the cheek and gum until it has disintegrated, which usually takes approximately 14 to 25 minutes.

After 30 minutes, if remnants from the fentanyl buccal tablet remain, they may be swallowed with a glass of water.

Fentanyl buccal soluble film – Only prescribers enrolled in the FOCUS Program may prescribe fentanyl buccal soluble film.

All patients must begin treatment using 1 fentanyl 200 mcg buccal soluble film. Do not switch patients on a mcg per mcg basis from any other oral transmucosal fentanyl product to fentanyl buccal soluble film.

Titrate using multiples of 200 mcg fentanyl buccal soluble film, increasing the dose by 200 mcg in each subsequent episode. Do not use more than 4 of the fentanyl 200 mcg buccal soluble films simultaneously. When multiple fentanyl 200 mcg buccal soluble films are used, they should not be placed on top of each other and may be placed on both sides of the mouth.

Doses above fentanyl 1,200 mcg buccal soluble film should not be used.

Single doses should be separated by at least 2 hours. Fentanyl buccal soluble film should only be used once per breakthrough cancer pain episode; fentanyl buccal soluble film should not be redosed within an episode.

Once a successful dose has been found, each episode is treated with a single film. Fentanyl buccal soluble film should be limited to 4 or fewer doses per day.

FENTANYL TRANSDERMAL SYSTEM:

Warning – See Warning Box at the beginning of the monograph.

Application – Each system may be worn continuously for 72 hours.

Dose selection – Maintain each patient at the lowest dose providing acceptable pain control. Unless the patient has pre-existing opioid tolerance, use the lowest dose, 12.5 mcg/h, as the initial dose.

Upward titration may be done no more frequently than 3 days after the initial dose; thereafter, it may be done no more frequently than every 6 days. For delivery rates in excess of 100 mcg/h, multiple systems may be used.

Initial Fentanyl Transdermal Dose Based on Daily Morphine Equivalence Dose[a]

Oral 24 hour morphine (mg/day)	Fentanyl transdermal (mcg/h)
60-134[b]	25
135-224	50
225-314	75
315-404	100
405-494	125
495-584	150
585-674	175
675-764	200
765-854	225
855-944	250
945-1034	275
1035-1124	300

[a] Do not use this table to convert from fentanyl transdermal system to other therapies because this conversion to fentanyl is conservative. Use of this table for conversion to other analgesic therapies can overestimate the dose of the new agent. Overdosage of the new analgesic agent is possible.

[b] Pediatric patients initiating therapy on a fentanyl transdermal system 25 mcg/h should be opioid-tolerant and receiving oral morphine equivalents 60 mg/day or more.

Fentanyl Dose Conversion Guidelines[a]

Current analgesic	Daily dose (mg/day)			
Oral morphine	60 to 134	135 to 224	225 to 314	315 to 404
IM/IV[b] morphine	10 to 22	23 to 37	38 to 52	53 to 67
Oral oxycodone	30 to 67	67.5 to 112	112.5 to 157	157.5 to 202
IM/IV oxycodone	15 to 33	33.1 to 56	56.1 to 78	78.1 to 101
Oral codeine	150 to 447	448 to 747	748 to 1,047	1,048 to 1,347
Oral hydromorphone	8 to 17	17.1 to 28	28.1 to 39	39.1 to 51
IV hydromorphone	1.5 to 3.4	3.5 to 5.6	5.7 to 7.9	8 to 10
IM meperidine	75 to 165	166 to 278	279 to 390	391 to 503
Oral methadone	20 to 44	45 to 74	75 to 104	105 to 134
IM methadone	10 to 22	23 to 37	38 to 52	53 to 67
Recommended fentanyl transdermal system dose				
Fentanyl transdermal system	25 mcg/h	50 mcg/h	75 mcg/h	100 mcg/h

[a] This table should not be used to convert fentanyl transdermal system to other therapies because this conversion to fentanyl transdermal system is conservative. Use of this table for conversion to other analgesic therapies can overestimate the dose of the new agent. Overdosage of the new analgesic agent is possible.

[b] IM = intramuscular; IV = intravenous.

The majority of patients are adequately maintained with transdermal fentanyl administered every 72 hours. A small number of patients may require systems to be applied every 48 hours.

During the initial application, patients should use short-acting analgesics for the first 24 hours as needed until analgesic efficacy with the transdermal system is attained. Thereafter, some patients still may require periodic supplemental doses of other short-acting analgesics for breakthrough pain.

Dose titration – Base appropriate dosage increments on the daily dose of supplementary opioids, using the ratio of 45 mg/24 h of oral morphine to a 12.5 mcg/h increase in transdermal fentanyl dose.

Discontinuation – Upon system removal, it takes 17 hours or more for the fentanyl serum concentration to fall by 50% after system removal. Titrate the dose of the new analgesic based on the patient's report of pain until adequate analgesia has been attained. For patients requiring discontinuation of opioids, a gradual downward titration is recommended because it is not known at what dose level the opioid may be discontinued without producing the signs and symptoms of abrupt withdrawal.

HYDROMORPHONE HYDROCHLORIDE:

Warnings – See Warning Box at the beginning of the monograph.

Oral (immediate release) –

Tablet: 2 to 4 mg every 4 to 6 hours as needed; 4 mg or more every 4 to 6 hours for more severe pain.

Liquid: 2.5 to 10 mg every 3 to 6 hours.

Oral (extended release) – The dose range of hydromorphone ER studied in clinical trials is 8 to 64 mg. The tablets are to be administered every 24 hours with or without food. Discontinue all other ER opioids when beginning hydromorphone ER therapy. As hydromorphone ER is only for use in opioid-tolerant patients, do not begin any patient on hydromorphone ER as the first opioid.

It is critical to initiate the dosing regimen individually for each patient. Overestimating the hydromorphone ER dose when converting patients from another opioid medication can result in fatal overdose with the first dose.

In the selection of the initial dose of hydromorphone, give attention to the following:

- the daily dose, potency, and specific characteristics of the opioid the patients has been taking previously;
- the reliability of the relative potency estimate used to calculate the equivalent hydromorphone dose needed;
- the patient's degree of opioid tolerance;
- the age, general condition, and medical status of the patient;
- concurrent nonopioid analgesics and other medications, such as those with CNS activity;
- the type and severity of the patient's pain;
- the balance between pain control and adverse reactions;
- risk factors for abuse, addiction, or diversion, including a history of abuse, addiction, or diversion.

Patients receiving oral immediate-release hydromorphone may be converted to hydromorphone ER by administering a starting dose equivalent to the patient's total daily oral hydromorphone ER dose, taken once daily. The dose of hydromorphone ER can be titrated every 3 to 4 days until adequate pain relief with tolerable adverse reactions has been achieved.

For conversion from other opioids to hydromorphone ER, refer to published relative potency information, keeping in mind that conversion ratios are only approximate. In general, start hydromorphone ER therapy by administering 50% of the calculated total daily dose of hydromorphone ER (see conversion ratio table) every 24 hours. The initial dose of hydromorphone ER can be titrated until adequate pain relief with tolerable adverse reactions has been achieved. The opioid conversion provides approximate equivalent doses, which may be used as a guideline for conversion.

Conversion Ratios to Hydromorphone ER[a,b]		
Previous opioid	Approximate equivalent oral dose	Oral conversion ratio[c]
Hydromorphone	12 mg	1
Codeine	200 mg	0.06

Conversion Ratios to Hydromorphone ER[a,b]		
Previous opioid	Approximate equivalent oral dose	Oral conversion ratio[c]
Hydrocodone	30 mg	0.4
Methadone[d]	20 mg	0.6
Morphine	60 mg	0.2
Oxycodone	30 mg	0.4
Oxymorphone	20 mg	0.6

[a] Select opioid, sum the total daily dose, and then multiply the dose by the conversion ratio to calculate the approximate oral hydromorphone equivalent.
[b] The conversion ratios and approximate equivalent doses in this conversion table are only to be used for the conversion from current opioid therapy to hydromorphone ER.
[c] Ratio for conversion of oral opioid dose to approximate hydromorphone equivalent dose.
[d] It is extremely important to monitor all patients closely when converting from methadone to other opioid agonists. The ratio between methadone and other opioid agonists may vary widely as a function of previous dose exposure. Methadone has a long half-life and tends to accumulate in the plasma.

Eighteen hours following the removal of the transdermal fentanyl patch, hydromorphone ER treatment can be initiated. For each fentanyl transdermal 25 mcg/h dose the equianalgesic dose of hydromorphone is 12 mg every 24 hours. An appropriate starting dose of hydromorphone ER is 50% of the calculated total daily dose every 24 hours.

Parenteral – The starting dosage is 1 to 2 mg subcutaneously or IM every 4 to 6 hours as needed. May be given by slow IV injection over at least 2 to 3 minutes.

HP: Only give the HP strength (10 mg/mL) to patients tolerant of other narcotics. If HP hydromorphone is substituted for a different opioid analgesic, use the following equivalency table as a guide.

Approximate Equianalgesic Doses[a] (IM or Subcutaneous Administration)		
Drug	Dose (mg)	Duration compared with morphine
Butorphanol	1.5 to 2.5	Same
Heroin	4 to 5	Slightly shorter
Hydromorphone	1.3	Slightly shorter
Levorphanol	2.3	Same
Meperidine	80	Shorter
Methadone	10	Same
Morphine	10	Same
Nalbuphine	12	Same
Oxymorphone	1.1	Slightly shorter
Pentazocine	60	Shorter

[a] Equianalgesic to IM morphine 10 mg in terms of the area under the analgesic time effect curve.

Rectal – 3 mg every 6 to 8 hours.

Children – Safety and efficacy have not been established.

LEVORPHANOL TARTRATE:

IV – The usual recommended starting dose for IV administration is up to 1 mg given in divided doses by slow injection. This may be repeated in 3 to 6 hours as needed. Total daily doses of more than 4 to 8 mg IV in 24 hours are not recommended as starting doses in nonopioid tolerant patients.

IM or subcutaneous – The usual recommended starting dose for IM or subcutaneous administration is 1 to 2 mg. This may be repeated in 6 to 8 hours as needed. Total daily doses of more then 3 to 8 mg IM in 24 hours are not recommended as starting doses in nonopioid-tolerant patients.

Oral – Recommended starting dose is 2 mg. Repeat in 6 to 8 hours (*Levo-Dromoran*) or 3 to 6 hours (Levorphanol Tartrate) as needed.

Levo-Dromoran: If necessary, increase the dose to up to 3 mg every 6 to 8 hours. Higher doses may be appropriate in opioid-tolerant patients.

Levorphanol Tartrate: The effective daily dosage range is 8 to 16 mg in 24 hours in the nontolerant patient. Total oral daily doses of more than 16 mg in 24 hours are generally not recommended as starting doses in non-opioid-tolerant patients.

Chronic pain – Levorphanol is 4 to 8 times as potent as morphine and has a longer half-life. When converting a patient from morphine to levorphanol, begin the total daily dose of oral levorphanol at approximately 1/15 to 1/12 of the total daily dose of oral morphine that such patients had previously required.

Premedication (Levo-Dromoran) – Two mg levorphanol is approximately equivalent to 10 to 15 mg of morphine or 100 mg of meperidine.

MEPERIDINE HYDROCHLORIDE:

Relief of pain – While subcutaneous administration is suitable for occasional use, IM administration is preferred for repeated doses. If IV administration is required, decrease dosage and inject very slowly, preferably using a diluted solution. Meperidine is less effective when administered orally than when given parenterally. Reduce proportionately (usually by 25% to 50%) when administering concomitantly with phenothiazines and other tranquilizers.

Adults: 50 to 150 mg IM, subcutaneously, or orally every 3 to 4 hours, as necessary.

Children: 1.1 to 1.75 mg/kg (0.5 to 0.8 mg/lb) IM, subcutaneously, or orally up to adult dose, every 3 or 4 hours, as necessary.

Preoperative medication –

Adults: 50 to 100 mg IM or subcutaneously, 30 to 90 minutes before beginning anesthesia.

Children: 1.1 to 2.2 mg/kg (0.5 to 1 mg/lb) IM or subcutaneously, up to adult dose, 30 to 90 minutes before beginning anesthesia.

Support of anesthesia – Meperidine may be administered in repeated doses diluted to 10 mg/mL by slow IV injection, or by continuous IV infusion of solution diluted to 1 mg/mL.

Obstetrical analgesia – When pains become regular, administer 50 to 100 mg IM or subcutaneously; repeat at 1- to 3-hour intervals.

METHADONE HYDROCHLORIDE:

Warning – See Warning Box at the beginning of the monograph.

Detoxification –

Induction/Initial dosing: A single dose of methadone 20 to 30 mg will often be sufficient to suppress withdrawal symptoms. The initial dose should not exceed 30 mg.

Dosage adjustment: If same-day dosing adjustments are to be made, the patient should be asked to wait 2 to 4 hours for further evaluation, when peak levels have been reached. An additional 5 to 10 mg of methadone may be provided if withdrawal symptoms have not been suppressed or if symptoms reappear. The total daily dose of methadone on the first day of treatment should not ordinarily exceed 40 mg.

Short-term: For patients preferring a brief course of stabilization followed by a period of medically supervised withdrawal, it is generally recommended that the patient be titrated to a total daily dose of approximately 40 mg in divided doses to achieve an adequate stabilizing level. Stabilization can be continued for 2 to 3 days, after which the dose of methadone should be gradually decreased.

Maintenance treatment: Patients in maintenance treatment should be titrated to a dose at which opioid symptoms are prevented for 24 hours and the patient is tolerant to the sedative effects of methadone. Most commonly, clinical stability is achieved at doses between 80 and 120 mg/day.

Withdrawal maintenance treatment: It is generally suggested that dose reductions should be less than 10% of the established tolerance or maintenance doses, and that 10- to 14-day intervals should elapse between dose reductions.

Pain (except oral concentrate and dispersible tablets for suspension) –

Initiation of therapy (opioid-nontolerant patients) (oral): 2.5 to 10 mg every 8 to 12 hours, slowly titrated to effect.

Conversion from parenteral to oral methadone: Initially use a 1:2 dose ratio.

Switching from other chronic opioids: Switching a patient from another chronically administered opioid to methadone requires caution because of the uncertainty of dose conversion ratios and incomplete cross-tolerance. Deaths have occurred in opioid-tolerant patients during conversion to methadone.

Conversion ratios in many commonly used equianalgesic dosing tables do not apply in the setting of repeated methadone testing.

The following conversion scheme is derived from various consensus guidelines for converting chronic pain patients to methadone from morphine.

Oral Morphine to Oral Methadone Conversion for Chronic Administration	
Total daily baseline oral morphine dose	Estimated daily oral methadone requirement as percent of total daily morphine dose
< 100 mg	20% to 30%
100 to 300 mg	10% to 20%
300 to 600 mg	8% to 12%
600 to 1,000 mg	5% to 10%
> 1,000 mg	< 5%

The total daily methadone dose derived from the previous table may then be divided to reflect the intended dosing schedule (eg, for administration every 8 hours, divide the total daily dose by 3).

Dosage adjustment during pregnancy: Methadone clearance may be increased during pregnancy. During pregnancy, a woman's methadone dose may need to be increased or her dosing interval decreased. Methadone should be used in pregnancy only if the potential benefit justifies the potential risks to the fetus.

Administration –

Dispersible tablets and oral solution: Methadone dispersible tablets have been formulated with insoluble excipients to deter the use of this drug by injection. Dissolve each tablet in approximately 1 oz of liquid (other than grapefruit juice) and swallow. Do not swallow the tablets whole or chew tablets.

Diskets – Diskets are intended for dispersion in a liquid immediately prior to oral administration of the prescribed dose. The tablets should not be chewed or swallowed before dispersing in liquid. The tablets are cross-scored, allowing for flexible dosing adjustment. Each tablet may be broken or cut in half to yield two 20 mg doses, or in quarters to yield four 10 mg doses.

Prior to administration, the desired dose should be dispersed in approximately 120 mL (4 oz) of water, orange juice, *Tang*, citrus flavors of *Kool-Aid*, or other acidic fruit beverage prior to taking. Methadone is very soluble in water, but there are some insoluble excipients that will not entirely dissolve. If residue remains in the cup after initial administration, a small amount of liquid should be added and the resulting mixture administered to the patient.

Because *Diskets* can be administered only in 10 mg increments, they may not be the appropriate product for initial dosing or gradual dose reduction in many patients.

MORPHINE SULFATE:

Warnings – See Warning Box at the beginning of the monograph.

Oral –

IR: 5 to 30 mg every 4 hours.

Controlled/Extended/Sustained-release (CR/ER/SR): Swallow whole; do not break, chew, or crush. See below for SR capsule administration.

Initial therapy – There has been no evaluation of CR/ER/SR morphine as an initial opioid analgesic in the management of pain. It is ordinarily advisable to begin treatment using an immediate-release morphine formulation.

Reserve MS *Contin* 200 mg strength for patients who have already been titrated to a stable analgesic regimen using lower strengths of MS *Contin* or other opioids.

As the initial opioid for patients who do not have a proven tolerance to opioids, treat patient with *Avinza* initially at a dose of 30 mg once daily (at 24-hour intervals). Adjust the dose of *Avinza* in increments not greater than 30 mg every 4 days. If breakthrough pain occurs, *Avinza* may be supplemented with a small dose (5% to 15% of the total daily dose of morphine) of a short-acting analgesic.

If *Kadian* is chosen, start with 20 mg in those who do not have a proven tolerance to opioids. Increase up to 20 mg every other day.

Individualization of dosage –

Kadian: Administer one half of the estimated total daily oral morphine dose every 12 hours (twice a day) or administer the total daily oral morphine dose every 24 hours (once a day). To avoid accumulation, the dosing interval should not be reduced below 12 hours. The dose should be titrated no more frequently than every other day to allow the patient to stabilize before escalating the dose. if breakthrough pain occurs, the dose may be supplemented with a small dose (less than 20% of the total daily dose) of a short-acting analgesic. Patients who are excessively sedated after a once-daily dose or who regularly experience inadequate analgesia before the next dose should be switched to a twice daily dosing. Patients who do not have a proven tolerance to opioids should be started only on the 20 mg strength and usually should be increased at a rate not greater than 20 mg every other day.

Most patients will rapidly develop some degree of tolerance, requiring dosage adjustment until they have achieved their individual best balance between baseline analgesia and opioid adverse reactions such as confusion, sedation, and constipation. No guidance can be given as to the recommended maximal dose, especially in patients with chronic pain of malignancy. In such cases, the total dose of *Kadian* should be advanced until the desired therapeutic end point is reached or clinically significant opioid-related adverse reactions intervene.

Conversion from conventional IR oral morphine to CR/ER/SR oral morphine –

SR: Administer one-half the patient's total daily oral morphine dose as *Kadian* every 12 hours or by administering the total daily oral morphine dose as *Kadian* every 24 hours. The first dose of *Kadian* may be taken with the last dose of any IR opioid medication because of the long delay until the peak effect after administration of *Kadian*.

ER (tablets and capsules):

Tablets – Convert to morphine ER in either of 2 ways:

1.) by administering one-half the patient's 24-hour requirement as morphine ER on an every 12-hour schedule; or,
2.) by administering one-third the patient's daily requirement as morphine ER on an every 8-hour schedule.

The 15 mg ER tablet should be used for initial conversion for patient's total daily requirement is expected to be less than 60 mg. Morphine ER tablets of 30 mg strength are recommended for patients with a daily morphine requirement of 60 to 120 mg.

Capsules – Patients receiving other oral morphine formulations may be converted to *Avinza* or *Kadian* by administering the patient's total daily oral morphine dose as *Avinza* or *Kadian* once daily or by administering one half of the patient's total daily oral morphine dose as *Kadian* every 12 hours. Supplemental pain medication may be required until the response to the patient's daily *Avinza* dosage has stabilized (up to 4 days).

CR: The patient may convert in 1 of 2 ways:

1.) by administering one-half the patients 24-hour requirement as MS *Contin* or *Oramorph SR* on an every 12-hour schedule; or
2.) by administering one-third the patient's daily requirement as MS *Contin* on an every 8-hour schedule.

The 15 mg tablet of MS *Contin* should be used for initial conversion for patients whose total daily requirement is expected to be less than 60 mg. The 30 mg tablet strength is recommended for patients with a daily morphine requirement of 60 to 120 mg. The 30 mg tablet strength of *Oramorph SR* for initial conversion is recommended for patients with a daily morphine requirement of 120 mg or less.

Conversion from parenteral morphine or other opioids (parenteral or oral) to CR/ER/SR doseforms – Initial dosing regimens should be conservative. In patients whose daily morphine requirements are expected to be 120 mg/day or less, the 30 mg tablet strength is recommended for the initial titration period. Convert to the 60 or 100 mg tablet strength once a stable dose regimen is reached.

Conversion from CR/ER/SR oral morphine to parenteral opioids – To estimate the required 24-hour dose of morphine for IM use, one could employ a conversion of 1 mg morphine IM for every 6 mg of morphine as controlled-release tablet. Of course, the IM 24-hour dose would have to be divided by 6 and administered every 4 hours. This approach is recommended because it is least likely to cause overdose.

Avinza/Kadian: When converting from *Avinza* or *Kadian* to parenteral opioids, it is best to calculate an equivalent parenteral dose and then initiate treatment at half of this calculated value.

Conversion of ER (Avinza) or SR (Kadian) to other CR oral morphine formulations – *Kadian* is not bioequivalent to other CR morphine preparations. For a given dose, the same total amount of morphine is available from *Avinza* as from oral morphine solution or CR morphine tablets. Conversion from *Kadian* or *Avinza* to the same total daily dose of another CR morphine formulation may lead to either excessive sedation at peak or inadequate analgesia at trough, close observation and appropriate dosage adjustments are recommended.

Dosage reductions/adjustments –

IR: During the first 2 to 3 days of effective pain relief, the patient may sleep for many hours. This can be misinterpreted as the effect of excessive analgesic dosing rather than the first sign of relief in a pain-exhausted patient. The dose, therefore, should be maintained for at least 3 days before reduction, if respiratory activity and other vital signs are adequate. Following successful relief of severe pain, periodic attempts to reduce the narcotic dose should be made.

CR/ER/SR: If signs of excessive opioid effects are observed early in a dosing interval, the next dose should be reduced. If this adjustment leads to inadequate analgesia (ie, breakthrough pain occurs late in the dosing interval) the dosing interval may be shortened. Alternatively, a supplemental dose of a short-acting analgesic may be given. It is recommended that the dosing interval never be extended beyond 12 hours, because the administration of a very large dose may lead to acute overdosage.

Discontinuation of therapy – When the patient no longer requires therapy, doses should be tapered gradually to prevent signs and symptoms of withdrawal in the physically dependent patient.

Administration –

CR/ER/SR tablets/capsules: Swallow whole; do not break, chew, crush, or dissolve because of the risk of acute overdose.

Avinza – Capsules may be opened and the entire bead contents sprinkled on a small amount of applesauce immediately prior to ingestion. Swallow mixture without chewing or crushing beads, rinse mouth and swallow to ensure all beads have been ingested. Consume entire portion and do not divide applesauce into separate doses. Absorption of the beads sprinkled on other foods has not been tested.

Kadian – Capsules may be opened and the entire contents sprinkled on a small amount of applesauce immediately prior to ingestion.

Open the capsule and sprinkle the entire contents over approximately 10 mL of water and flush through a prewetted 16 French gastrostomy tube fitted. Flush with water. Do not administer pellets through a nasogastric tube.

May be given once or twice daily.

Concentrate oral solution: Administer with caution since the solution is a highly concentrated solution of morphine. Error in dosage or confusion between milligrams of morphine and milliliters of solution may cause significant overdosage. Dosing instructions should be clearly prescribed in milligrams of morphine and milliliters of solution. Verify correct dose and volume before administration to patient.

Subcutaneously/IM – Prepare soluble tablets in sterile water and filter through a 0.22 micron membrane filter.

Adults: 10 mg (range, 5 to 20 mg) per 70 kg every 4 hours as needed.

Children: 0.1 to 0.2 mg/kg every 4 hours as needed. Do not exceed 15 mg/dose.

Soluble tablets: Prepare soluble tablets in sterile water and filter through a 0.22 micron membrane filter.

For preanesthetic medication –

Adults: 10 mg per 70 kg of body weight (range, 5 to 20 mg).

Children (1 year of age and older): 0.1 mg per kg (maximum dose 10 mg).

For analgesia –

Adults: 10 mg per 70 kg of body weight (range, 5 to 20 mg).

Children: 0.1 to 0.2 mg/kg (maximum dose 15 mg).

IV –

Adults: 2 to 10 mg per 70 kg of body weight. A strength of 2.5 to 15 mg of morphine may be diluted in 4 to 5 mL of Water for Injection. Administer slowly over 4 to 5 minutes. Rapid IV use increases the incidence of adverse reactions (see Warnings). Do not administer IV unless a narcotic antagonist is immediately available.

For relief of pain and as preanesthetic: 10 mg every 4 hours. The usual individual dose range is 5 to 15 mg. The usual daily dose range is 12 to 120 mg.

Usual pediatric dose (analgesic): 50 to 100 mcg IV (0.05 to 0.1 mg) per kg of body weight, administered very slowly. Not to exceed 10 mg per dose.

Severe chronic pain associated with terminal cancer: A loading dose of 15 mg or more of morphine sulfate may be administered by IV push to alleviate pain.

The infusion dosage range is 0.8 to 80 mg/h, though doses up to 144 mg/h have been used. Thus, for the 1 mg/mL solution, the infusion may be run from 0.8 to 80 mg/h.

Open-heart surgery: Administer large doses (0.5 to 3 mg/kg) of morphine IV as the sole anesthetic or with a suitable anesthetic agent.

MI pain: 8 to 15 mg administered parenterally. For very severe pain, additional smaller doses may be given every 3 to 4 hours as needed.

Rectal – 10 to 30 mg every 4 hours as needed or as directed by physician.

Epidural –

Adults: Initial injection of 5 mg in the lumbar region may provide satisfactory pain relief for up to 24 hours. If adequate pain relief is not achieved within 1 hour, carefully administer incremental doses of 1 to 2 mg. Give no more than 10 mg/24 hours.

For continuous infusion, an initial dose of 2 to 4 mg/24 hours is recommended. Further doses of 1 to 2 mg may be given if pain relief is not achieved initially.

Aged or debilitated patients: Administer with extreme caution. Doses less than 5 mg may provide satisfactory pain relief for up to 24 hours.

Infumorph: The recommended initial epidural dose in patients who are not tolerant to opioids range from 3.5 to 7.5 mg/day. The usual starting dose for continuous epidural infusion, based upon limited data in patients who have some degree of opioid tolerance, is 4.5 to 10 mg/day. The dose requirements may increase significantly during treatment, frequently to 20 to 30 mg/day.

ER epidural – Patient monitoring should be continued for at least 48 hours after dosing, as delayed respiratory depression may occur.

Major orthopedic surgery: 15 mg.

Lower abdominal or pelvic surgery: 10 to 15 mg (20 mg dose of *DepoDur*).

Cesarean section: 10 mg. *DepoDur* should not be administered to women for vaginal labor and delivery.

Administration: *DepoDur* is not intended for intrathecal, IV, or IM administration. Administration of *DepoDur* into the thoracic epidural space or higher has not been evaluated and therefore is not recommended. *DepoDur* may be administered via needle or catheter at the lumbar level. *DepoDur* may be administered undiluted or may be diluted up to 5 mL total volume with preservative-free 0.9% normal saline. Do not use an in-line filter during administration of *DepoDur*.

Elderly: *DepoDur* should be administered to elderly patients (older than 65 years of age) after careful evaluation of their underlying medical condition and consideration of the risks associated with *DepoDur*. Vigilant perioperative monitoring should be exercised for elderly patients. The dose for elderly or debilitated patients should be at the low end of the dosing range.

Intrathecal –

Adult: A single injection of 0.2 to 1 mg may provide satisfactory pain relief for up to 24 hours. (Caution: This is only 0.4 to 2 mL of the 0.5 mg/mL potency or 0.2 to 1 mL of the 1 mg/mL potency.) Do not inject intrathecally 2 mL of the 0.5 mg/mL potency or 1 mL of the 1 mg/mL potency. Use in lumbar area only. Repeated intrathecal injections are not recommended. A constant IV infusion of 0.6 mg/h naloxone for 24 hours after intrathecal injection may reduce incidence of potential side effects.

Infumorph: Filter through a 5 micron or less microfilter before injecting into the microinfusion device. If dilution is required, 0.9% NaCl injection is recommended. The recommended initial lumbar intrathecal dose range in patients with no tolerance to opioids is 0.2 to 1 mg/day. The published range of doses for individuals who have some degree of opioid tolerance varies from 1 to 10 mg/day. Limited experience with continuous intrathecal infusion of morphine has shown that the daily doses have to be increased over time.

Aged or debilitated: Use extreme caution. Lower dose is usually satisfactory.

Repeat dosage: Consider alternative administration routes because experience with repeated doses by this route is limited.

OPIUM:

Caution – Opium tincture contains 25 times more morphine than paregoric. Do not confuse opium tincture with paregoric; this may lead to an overdose of morphine.

Opium tincture –

Adults: 0.6 mL 4 times/day.

Paregoric –

Adults: 5 to 10 mL 1 to 4 times/day.

Children: 0.25 to 0.5 mL/kg 1 to 4 times/day.

OXYCODONE HYDROCHLORIDE:

Warning – See Warning Box at the beginning of the monograph.

IR tablets, oral solution, immediate-release capsules –

Adults: 10 to 30 mg every 4 hours (5 mg every 6 hours for *OxyIR*, oxycodone IR capsules) as needed. More severe pain may require 30 mg or more every 4 hours.

Children: Not recommended for use in children.

Patients not currently on opioid therapy (opioid naïve): 5 to 15 mg every 4 to 6 hours as needed for pain. Patients with chronic pain should have their dosage given on an around-the-clock basis to prevent the reoccurrence of pain rather than treating the pain after it has occurred.

Severe chronic pain: Administer on a regularly scheduled basis, every 4 to 6 hours, at the lowest dosage level that will achieve adequate analgesia.

Cessation of therapy: When a patient no longer requires therapy for the treatment of pain, gradually discontinue treatment over time to prevent the development of an opioid abstinence syndrome (narcotic withdrawal). In general, therapy can be decreased by 25% to 50% per day with careful monitoring for signs and symptoms of withdrawal. If the patient develops these signs or symptoms, raise the dose to the previous level and titrate down more slowly.

Oral concentrate solutions – *Roxicodone Intensol, OxyFAST*, and *ETH-Oxydose* 20 mg/mL solution are highly concentrated solutions. Fill dropper to the level of the prescribed dose (1 mL = 20 mg; 0.75 mL = 15 mg; 0.5 mL = 10 mg; 0.25 mL = 5 mg). Add dose to approximately 30 mL (1 fluid oz) or more of juice or other liquid. May also be added to applesauce, pudding, or other semi-solid foods. The drug-food mixture should be used immediately and not stored for future use.

CR tablets – Swallow tablets whole; do not break, chew, or crush. *OxyContin* is not indicated for rectal administration.

One 160 mg tablet is comparable to two 80 mg tablets when taken on an empty stomach. However, with a high-fat meal there is a 25% greater peak plasma concentration following one 160 mg tablet. Use dietary caution when patients are initially titrated to 160 mg tablets.

CR tablets are intended for the management of moderate to severe pain when a continuous, around-the-clock analgesic is needed for an extended period of time. The CR nature of the formulation allows it to be effectively administered every 12 hours. While symmetric (same AM and PM), around-the-clock, every-12-hour dosing is appropriate for the majority of patients, some patients may benefit from asymmetric (different dose given in AM than in PM) dosing, tailored to their pain pattern. It is usually appropriate to treat a patient with only 1 opioid for around-the-clock therapy.

Patients not already taking opioids (opioid naïve): 10 mg every 12 hours. If a nonopioid analgesic (eg, aspirin, acetaminophen, NSAID) is being provided, it may be continued.

Patients currently on opioid therapy:

1.) Using standard conversion ratio estimates (see table below), multiply the mg per day of the previous opioids by the appropriate multiplication factors to obtain the equivalent total daily dose of oral oxycodone.
2.) Divide this 24-hour oxycodone dose in half to obtain the twice-daily (every 12 hours) dose of CR tablets.
3.) Round down to a dose that is appropriate for the tablet strengths available.
4.) Discontinue all other around-the-clock opioid drugs when CR tablet therapy is initiated.

Multiplication Factors for Converting the Daily Dose of Prior Opioids to the Daily Dose of Oral Oxycodone[a]

mg/day prior opioid × factor = mg/day oral oxycodone

Drug	Oral prior opioid	Parenteral prior opioid
Oxycodone	1	—
Codeine	0.15	—
Fentanyl transdermal therapeutic system	see below	see below
Hydrocodone	0.9	—
Hydromorphone	4	20
Levorphanol	7.5	15
Meperidine	0.1	0.4
Methadone	1.5	3
Morphine	0.5	3

[a] To be used only for conversion to oral oxycodone. For patients receiving high-dose parenteral opioids, a more conservative conversion is warranted. For example, for high-dose parenteral morphine, use 1.5 instead of 3 as a multiplication factor.

In all cases, supplemental analgesia should be made available in the form of IR oral oxycodone or another suitable short-acting analgesic.

Conversion from transdermal fentanyl to CR tablets: Eighteen hours following the removal of the transdermal fentanyl patch, treatment with CR tablets can be initiated. Although there has been no systematic assessment of such conversion, a conservative oxycodone dose, approximately 10 mg every 12 hours of CR tablets, should be initially substituted for each fentanyl transdermal patch 25 mcg/h. Closely follow the patient for early titration as there is very limited clinical experience with this conversion.

Dosage individualization: Titrate patients to adequate effect (generally mild or no pain with the regular use of no more than 2 doses of supplemental analgesia per 24 hours). Because steady-state plasma concentrations are approximated within 24 to 36 hours, dosage adjustment may be carried out every 1 to 2 days. It is most appropriate to increase the every-12-hour dose, not the dosing frequency. There is no clinical information on dosing intervals shorter than every 12 hours. As a guideline, except for the increase from 10 to 20 mg every 12 hours, the total daily oxycodone dose usually can be increased by 25% to 50% of the current dose at each increase.

CR tablets, 80 and 160 mg, are for use only in opioid-tolerant patients requiring daily oxycodone equivalent dosages of at least 160 mg for the 80 mg tablet and at least 320 mg for the 160 mg tablet.

Therapy cessation: When the patient no longer requires therapy with the CR tablets, taper doses gradually over several days to prevent signs and symptoms of withdrawal in the physically dependent patient.

Conversion from CR tablets to parenteral opioids: To avoid overdose, follow conservative dose conversion ratios. For patients receiving high-dose parenteral opioids, a more conservative conversion is warranted.

OXYMORPHONE HYDROCHLORIDE: Oxymorphone should be administered on an empty stomach at least 1 hour prior to or 2 hours after eating.

Oxymorphone ER tablets are to be swallowed whole and not broken, chewed, dissolved, or crushed. Taking broken, chewed, dissolved, or crushed oxymorphone ER tablets leads to rapid release and absorption of a potentially fatal dose of oxymorphone.

Initiation of therapy with oxymorphone IR tablets –

Opioid-naive patients: Patients who have not been receiving opioid analgesics should be started on oxymorphone IR in a dosing range of 10 to 20 mg every 4 to 6 hours, depending on the initial pain intensity. Patients may be started with oxymorphone IR 5 mg.

Conversion from parenteral oxymorphone to oxymorphone IR: Convert by administering 10 times the total daily parenteral oxymorphone dose as oxymorphone IR tablets, in 4 or 6 equally divided doses (eg, IV dose × 10/4). For example, approximately 10 mg of oxymorphone IR every 4 to 6 hours may be required to provide pain relief equivalent to a total daily dose of oxymorphone 4 mg IM.

Conversion from other oral opioids to oxymorphone IR: In general, it is safest to start the oxymorphone IR therapy by administering half of the calculated total daily dose of oxymorphone IR in 4 to 6 equally divided doses every 4 to 6 hours.

Initiation of therapy with oxymorphone ER –

Opioid-naive patients: 5 mg every 12 hours. Individually titrate dose at increments of 5 to 10 mg every 12 hours every 3 to 7 days.

Opioid-experienced patients:

Asymmetric dosing – While symmetric (same dose AM and PM), around-the-clock, every-12-hours dosing is appropriate for the majority of patients, some patients may benefit from asymmetric (different dose given in AM than in PM) dosing tailored to their pain pattern.

Conversion from oxymorphone IR to ER – Administer half of the patient's total daily oral oxymorphone IR dose as ER every 12 hours.

Conversion from parenteral oxymorphone to ER – Convert by administering 10 times the total daily parenteral oxymorphone dose as ER in 2 equally divided doses (eg, IV dose × 10/2). For example, approximately 20 mg of ER every 12 hours may be required to provide pain relief equivalent to a total daily dose of parenteral oxymorphone 4 mg.

Conversion from other oral opioids to oxymorphone ER – In general it is safest to start oxymorphone therapy by administering half of the calculated total daily dose of ER (see the following table) in 2 divided doses every 12 hours.

Conversion Ratios to Oxymorphone ER		
Opioid	Approximate equivalent dose (oral)	Oral conversion ratio[a]
Oxymorphone	10 mg	1
Hydrocodone	20 mg	0.5
Oxycodone	20 mg	0.5
Methadone	20 mg	0.5
Morphine	30 mg	0.333

[a] Ratio for conversion of oral opioid dose to approximate oxymorphone equivalent dose. Select opioid and multiply the dose by the conversion ratio to calculate the approximate oral oxymorphone equivalent.

- Sum the total daily dose for the opioid and multiply by the conversion ratio to calculate the oxymorphone total daily dose.
- For patients on a regimen of mixed opioids, calculate the approximate oral oxymorphone dose for each opioid and sum the totals to estimate the total daily oxymorphone dose.
- The dose of oxymorphone ER can be gradually adjusted, preferably at increments of 10 mg every 12 hours every 3 to 7 days, until adequate pain relief and acceptable adverse reactions have been achieved.

Oxymorphone injection –

Initiation of therapy:

IV – Initially, 0.5 mg. In nondebilitated patients, the dose can be cautiously increased until satisfactory pain relief is obtained.

Subcutaneous or IM – Initially, 1 to 1.5 mg every 4 to 6 hours as needed. For analgesia during labor, give 0.5 to 1 mg IM.

Conversion from oral to injection: Given an absolute oral bioavailability of approximately 10%, administering one-tenth the patient's total daily oral oxymorphone dose as oxymorphone injection in 4 or 6 equally divided doses (eg, total daily oral dose/[10 × 4]). For example, approximately oxymorphone 1 mg IM every 6 hours (4 mg IM total dose) may be required to provide pain relief equivalent to a total daily dose of oxymorphone 40 mg orally.

REMIFENTANIL HYDROCHLORIDE: For IV use only.

Administer continuous infusions of remifentanil only by an infusion device. The injection site should be close to the venous cannula.

General anesthesia – Remifentanil is not recommended as the sole agent in general anesthesia because loss of consciousness cannot be assured and because of a high incidence of apnea, muscle rigidity, and tachycardia. Remifentanil is synergistic with other anesthetics and doses of thiopental, propofol, isoflurane, and midazolam have been reduced by up to 75% with the coadministration of remifentanil.

Remifentanil Dosing Guidelines - General Anesthesia and Continuing as an Analgesic into the Postoperative Care Unit or Intensive Care Setting			
Phase	Continuous IV infusion (mcg/kg/min)	Infusion dose range (mcg/kg/min)	Supplemental IV bolus dose (mcg/kg)
Induction of anesthesia (through intubation)	0.5 to 1[a]	NA[b]	NA[b]
Maintenance of anesthesia with:			
Nitrous oxide (66%)	0.4	0.1 - 2	1
Isoflurane (0.4 to 1.5 MAC[c])	0.25	0.05 - 2	1
Propofol (100 to 200 mcg/kg/min)	0.25	0.05 - 2	1
Continuation as an analgesic into the immediate postoperative period	0.1	0.025 - 0.2	not recommended

[a] An initial dose of 1 mcg/kg may be administered over 30 to 60 seconds.
[b] No data available.
[c] MAC = monitored anesthesia care.

Children (1 year of age and older) – The table below summarizes the recommended doses in pediatric patients, predominantly American Society of Anesthesiologists (ASA) physical status I, II, or III. In pediatric patients, remifentanil was administered with nitrous oxide or nitrous oxide in combination with halothane, sevoflurane, or isoflurane.

Dosing Guidelines in Pediatric Patients — Maintenance of Anesthesia

Phase	Continuous IV infusion[a] (mcg/kg/min)	Infusion dose range (mcg/kg/min)	Supplemental IV bolus dose (mcg/kg)
Maintenance of anesthesia with:			
Halothane (0.3 to 1.5 MAC)	0.25	0.05 to 1.3	1
Sevoflurane (0.3 to 1.5 MAC)	0.25	0.05 to 1.3	1
Isoflurane (0.4 to 1.5 MAC)	0.25	0.05 to 1.3	1

[a] An initial dose of 1 mcg/kg may be administered over 30 to 60 seconds.

Induction of anesthesia – Administer at an infusion rate of 0.5 to 1 mcg/kg/min with a hypnotic or volatile agent for the induction of anesthesia. If endotracheal intubation is to occur less than 8 minutes after the start of infusion of remifentanil, then an initial dose of 1 mcg/kg may be administered over 30 to 60 seconds.

Maintenance of anesthesia – After endotracheal intubation, decrease the infusion rate of remifentanil in accordance with the dosing guidelines in the table above. Because of the rapid onset and short duration of action of remifentanil, the rate of administration during anesthesia can be titrated upward in 25% to 100% increments or downward in 25% to 50% decrements every 2 to 5 minutes to attain the desired level of μ-opioid effect. In response to light anesthesia or transient episodes of intense surgical stress, supplemental bolus doses of 1 mcg/kg may be administered every 2 to 5 minutes. At infusion rates more than 1 mcg/kg/min, consider increases in the concomitant anesthetic agents to increase the depth of anesthesia.

Continuation as an analgesic into the immediate postoperative period – Remifentanil infusions may be continued into the immediate postoperative period for select patients for whom later transition to longer-acting analgesics may be desired. The use of bolus injections of remifentanil to treat pain during the postoperative period is not recommended. When used as an IV analgesic in the immediate postoperative period, administer remifentanil initially by continuous infusion at a rate of 0.1 mcg/kg/min. The infusion rate may be adjusted every 5 minutes in 0.025 mcg/kg/min increments to balance the patient's level of analgesia and respiratory rate. Infusion rates more than 0.2 mcg/kg/min are associated with respiratory depression (respiratory rate less than 8 breaths/min).

Guidelines for discontinuation – Upon discontinuation of remifentanil, clear the IV tubing to prevent inadvertent administration at a later time.

Analgesic component of MAC (adults only) – It is strongly recommended that supplemental oxygen be supplied whenever remifentanil is administered.

Remifentanil Dosing Guidelines for Adults - Monitored Anesthesia Care

Method	Timing	Remifentanil alone	Remifentanil + midazolam 2 mg
Single IV dose	Given 90 seconds before local anesthetic	1 mcg/kg over 30 to 60 seconds	0.5 mcg/kg over 30 to 60 seconds
Continuous IV infusion	Beginning 5 minutes before local anesthetic	0.1 mcg/kg/min	0.05 mcg/kg/min
	After local anesthetic	0.05 mcg/kg/min (range: 0.025 to 0.2 mcg/kg/min)	0.025 mcg/kg/min (range: 0.025 to 0.2 mcg/kg/min)

Single dose: A single IV dose of 0.5 to 1 mcg/kg over 30 to 60 seconds may be given 90 seconds before the placement of the local or regional anesthetic block.

Continuous infusion: When used alone as an IV analgesic component of MAC, administer initially by continuous infusion at a rate of 0.1 mcg/kg/min beginning 5 minutes before placement of the local or regional anesthetic block.

Because of the risk for hypoventilation, decrease the infusion rate of remifentanil to 0.05 mcg/kg/min following placement of the block. Thereafter, rate adjustments of 0.025 mcg/kg/min at 5-minute intervals may be used to balance the patient's level of analgesia and respiratory rate. Rates greater than 0.2 mcg/kg/min are generally associated with respiratory depression (respiratory rates less than 8 breaths/min).

Bolus doses of remifentanil administered simultaneously with a continuous infusion of remifentanil to spontaneously breathing patients are not recommended.

Coronary artery bypass surgery – The table below summarizes the recommended doses for induction, maintenance, and continuation as an analgesic into the intensive care unit (ICU) in adult patients, predominantly ASA physical status III or IV. To avoid hypotension during the induction phase, it is important to consider the concomitant medication regimens used.

Dosing Recommendations — Coronary Artery Bypass Surgery

Phase	Continuous IV infusion (mcg/kg/min)	Infusion dose range (mcg/kg/min)	Supplemental IV bolus dose (mcg/kg)
Induction of anesthesia (through intubation)	1	—	—
Maintenance of anesthesia	1	0.125 to 4	0.5 to 1
Continuation as an analgesic into ICU	1	0.05 to 1	—

Individualization of dosage –

Elderly: Decrease the starting doses of remifentanil by 50% in elderly patients (older than 65 years of age). Cautiously titrate to effect.

Obesity: Base the starting dose of remifentanil on ideal body weight (IBW) in obese patients (more than 30% over their IBW).

SUFENTANIL CITRATE:

Adult Dosage Range Chart — Analgesic Component to General Anesthesia (Total Dosage Requirements of 1 mcg/kg/h or Less are Recommended)

Total dosage	Maintenance dosage
Analgesic dosages	
Incremental or infusion: 1 to 2 mcg/kg (expected duration of anesthesia is 1 to 2 hours). Approximately ≥ 75% of total sufentanil dosage may be administered prior to intubation by either slow injection or infusion titrated to individual patient response.	*Incremental:* 10 to 25 mcg (0.2 to 0.5 mL) may be administered in increments as needed when movement and/or changes in vital signs indicate surgical stress or lightening of analgesia. *Infusion:* Sufentanil may be administered as an intermittent or continuous infusion as needed in response to signs of lightening of analgesia. In absence of signs of lightening of analgesia, always adjust infusion rates downward until there is some response to surgical stimulation. Individualize supplemental dosages. Adjust maintenance infusion rates based upon the induction dose of sufentanil so that the total dose does not exceed 1 mcg/kg/h of expected surgical time. Individualize dosage and adjust to remaining operative time anticipated.

Adult Dosage Range Chart — Analgesic Component to General Anesthesia (Total Dosage Requirements of 1 mcg/kg/h or Less are Recommended)	
Total dosage	Maintenance dosage
Incremental or infusion: 2 to 8 mcg/kg (expected duration of anesthesia is 2 to 8 hours). Approximately ≤ 75% of the total calculated sufentanil dosage may be administered by slow injection or infusion prior to intubation, titrated to individual patient response.	*Incremental:* 10 to 25 mcg (0.2 to 0.5 mL) may be administered in increments as needed when movement and/or changes in vital signs indicate surgical stress or lightening of analgesia. Individualize supplemental dosages. *Infusion:* Sufentanil may be administered as an intermittent or continuous infusion as needed in response to signs of lightening of analgesia. In absence of signs of lightening of analgesia, always adjust infusion rates downward until there is some response to surgical stimulation. Adjust maintenance infusion rates based upon the induction dose of sufentanil so that the total dose does not exceed 1 mcg/kg/h of expected surgical time. Individualize dosage and adjust to remaining operative time anticipated.
Anesthetic dosages	
Incremental or infusion: 8 to 30 mcg/kg (anesthetic doses). At this anesthetic dosage range, sufentanil is generally administered as a slow injection, as an infusion, or as an injection followed by an infusion.	*Incremental:* Depending on the initial dose, maintenance doses of 0.5 to 10 mcg/kg may be administered by slow injection in anticipation of surgical stress, such as incision, sternotomy, or cardiopulmonary bypass. *Infusion:* Sufentanil may be administered by continuous or intermittent infusion as needed in response to signs of lightening of anesthesia. In the absence of lightening of anesthesia, infusion rates should always be adjusted downward until there is some response to surgical stimulation. Base the maintenance infusion rate for sufentanil upon the induction dose so that the total dose for the procedure does not exceed 30 mcg/kg.

Epidural use in labor and delivery – 10 to 15 mcg administered with bupivacaine 0.125% 10 mL with or without epinephrine. Mix sufentanil and bupivacaine together before administration. Doses can be repeated twice (for a total of 3 doses) at not less than 1-hour intervals until delivery.

Administer sufentanil by slow injection. Closely monitor respiration following each administration of an epidural injection of sufentanil.

Children (younger than 12 years of age) – For induction and maintenance of anesthesia in children undergoing cardiovascular surgery, a dose of 10 to 25 mcg/kg administered with 100% oxygen is recommended. Supplemental doses of up to 25 to 50 mcg are recommended for maintenance.

Elderly/Debilitated patients – Dosage should be reduced.

Concomitant medication – If benzodiazepines, barbiturates, inhalation agents, other opioids, or CNS depressants are used concomitantly, the dose of sufentanil and/or these agents should be reduced.

Obesity – In obese patients (more then 20% above ideal body weight), the dosage of sufentanil should be determined on the basis of lean body weight.

TAPENTADOL:

Acute pain – 50 to 100 mg every 4 to 6 hours with or without food. On the first day of dosing, the second dose may be administered as soon as 1 hour after the first dose if adequate pain relief is not attained with the first dose.

Maximum dose: 700 mg on the first day of therapy, 600 mg on subsequent days.

Discontinuation of therapy: Withdrawal symptoms may occur if tapentadol is discontinued abruptly. These symptoms may include anxiety, sweating, insomnia, rigors, pain, nausea, tremors, diarrhea, upper respiratory tract symptoms, piloerection, and, rarely, hallucinations. Withdrawal symptoms may be reduced by tapering tapentadol.

Children – Not recommended for use in children younger than 18 years of age.

Elderly – Consider starting elderly patients with the lower range of recommended doses because elderly patients are more likely to have impaired renal or hepatic function.

Severe renal function impairment – The use in this population is not recommended.

Hepatic function impairment – For moderate hepatic function impairment, initiate treatment at 50 mg with the interval between doses of no less than every 8 hours, with the maximum dose being 3 doses in 24 hours. Use is not recommended in patients with severe hepatic function impairment.

TRAMADOL:

IR – Can be administered without regard to meals.

Adults (17 years of age and older): For moderate to moderately severe chronic pain not requiring rapid onset of analgesic effect, administer 25 mg/day in the morning and titrate in 25 mg increments as separate doses every 3 days to reach 100 mg/day (25 mg 4 times/day). Thereafter, increase the dose by 50 mg as tolerated every 3 days to reach 200 mg/day (50 mg 4 times/day). After titration, administer 50 to 100 mg every 4 to 6 hours as needed for pain relief. Do not exceed 400 mg/day.

For patients requiring rapid onset of analgesic relief and for whom the benefits outweigh the risk of discontinuation due to adverse effects associated with higher initial doses, administer 50 to 100 mg every 4 to 6 hours as needed, not to exceed 400 mg/day.

ER – ER tablets must be swallowed whole, and must not be chewed, crushed, or split.

Adults (18 years of age and older):

Patients not currently on tramadol immediate-release products – Initiate at a dosage of 100 mg once daily and titrate as necessary by 100 mg increments every 5 days to relieve pain. ER tablets should not be administered at a dosage exceeding 300 mg/day.

Patients currently on tramadol immediate-release products – For patients maintained on tramadol immediate-release products, calculate the 24-hour tramadol immediate-release dose and initiate a total daily dose of tramadol ER rounded down to the next lowest 100 mg increment. The dose may subsequently be individualized according to patient need. Because of limitations in flexibility of dose selection with tramadol ER, some patients maintained on tramadol immediate-release products may not be able to convert to tramadol ER. Tramadol ER should not be administered at a dose exceeding 300 mg per day.

Elderly – Start at the low end of the dosing range. Do not exceed 300 mg/day in patients 75 years of age and older.

Renal function impairment –

Immediate-release: In patients with a creatinine clearance less than 30 mL/min, increase the dosing interval to 12 hours, with a maximum daily dose of 200 mg. Dialysis patients can receive their regular dose on the day of dialysis.

ER: ER tablets should not be used in patients with CrCl less than 30 mL/min

Hepatic function impairment –

Immediate-release: The recommended dose for patients with cirrhosis is 50 mg every 12 hours.

ER: ER tablets should not be used in patients with severe hepatic function impairment (Child-Pugh class C).

Actions

Pharmacology:

Opioid Analgesics Comparative Pharmacology[a]							
Drug	Analgesic	Antitussive	Constipation	Respiratory depression	Sedation	Emesis	Physical dependence
Phenanthrenes							
Codeine	+[b]	+++	+	+	+	+	+
Hydrocodone	++	+++	nd[c]	nd	nd	nd	++
Hydromorphone	++	++	+	++	+	+	++
Levorphanol	++	++	nd	++	++	+	++
Morphine	++	++	++	++	++	++	++
Oxycodone	++	+++	++	++	++	++	++
Oxymorphone	++	+	+++	+++	nd	+++	+++
Phenylpiperidines							
Fentanyl	++	nd	nd	+	nd	+	nd
Meperidine	++	nd	+	++	+	nd	++
Diphenylheptanes							
Methadone	++	++	+	++	+	+	+

[a] Table adapted from Catalano RB. The medical approach to management of pain caused by cancer. *Semin Oncol.* 1975;2:379-392.

[b] + = degree of activity from the least (+) to the greatest (+++).

[c] nd – No data available.

Pharmacokinetics: Pharmacokinetic profiles are summarized in the following table, using morphine as the standard. Data based on IM administration unless otherwise noted.

Opioid Analgesic Pharmacokinetics

Drug	Onset of effect	Peak effect	Duration of effect	Elimination t½	Protein binding (%)	Metabolism pathway	Active metabolites	Major excretion pathway
Alfentanil	immediate	1.5 to 2 min	< 10 min	1.5 to 1.85 h	92%	liver	—	urine
Codeine	Oral: 10 to 30 min, IV: 15 min	0.5 to 1 h	Oral: 4 to 6 h, IV: 5 h	2.5 to 3 h	—	liver	Morphine	urine
Fentanyl injection	IV: immediate, IM: 7 to 8 min	—	IV: 0.5 to 1 h, IM: 1 to 2 h	3.65 h	Alters with increasing ionization	liver	—	urine
Fentanyl transdermal	—	24 to 72 h	72 h	≈ 17 h	Decreases with increasing ionization	liver: CYP3A4	—	urine
Fentanyl transmucosal	—	—	—	7 h	80% to 85%	liver: CYP3A4	—	urine
Hydromorphone	IM/Subcutaneous: 15 min, Oral: 30 min	0.5 to 1 h	IR: 4 to 5 h, ER: 24 h, IM/Subcutaneous: 4 to 5 h	IR: 2.3 h, ER: 18.6 h, IM/Subcutaneous: 2.6 h	8% to 20%	liver: glucuronidation	—	urine
Levorphanol	IM: 15 to 30 min	Oral: 1 h	—	IV: 11 to 16 h	40%	—	—	—
Meperidine	—	—	2 to 4 h	3 to 6 (parent), < 20 h (normeperidine)	60% to 80%	liver	normeperidine	—
Methadone	Parenteral: 10 to 20 min, Oral: 30 to 60 min	—	4 h	8 to 59 h	85% to 90%	liver: primarily CYP3A4 and to lesser extent CYP2D6	—	urine and fecal
Morphine sulfate	IM/Subcutaneous: 10 to 30 min	Epidural: 10 to 15 min, Oral: 1 h	Subcutaneous/IM: 4 to 5 h	1.5 to 2 h	20% to 35%	liver: glucuronidation	morphine-6-glucuronide	urine
Oxycodone	within 60 min	—	IR: 3 to 4 h, CR[a]: 12 h	IR: 3.2 h, CR: 4.5 h	45%	liver: somewhat involves CYP2D6	noroxycodone and oxymorphone	urine
Oxymorphone	Parenteral: 5 to 10 min	—	Parenteral: 3 to 6 h	1.3 h	—	liver	—	urine
Remifentanil	rapid	—	—	10 to 20 min	70%	hydrolysis by esterases	—	urine
Tramadol	—	—	2 h (tramadol), 3 h (M1, active metabolite)	6.3 h (tramadol), 7.4 h (M1, active metabolite)	20%	liver: CYP2D6 and CYP3A4	O-desmethyl-tramadol (M1) via CYP2D6	urine

[a] CR = controlled-release

Contraindications

Hypersensitivity to the drug or known intolerance to other opioids or any components of the products.

Fentanyl:

Transmucosal – Management of acute or postoperative pain; opioid nontolerant patients.

Transdermal – Nonopioid-tolerant patients; management of acute pain or in patients who require opioid analgesia for a short period of time; management of postoperative pain, including use after outpatient day surgeries; management of mild or intermittent pain (eg, use on an as-needed basis); respiratory depression; acute or severe bronchial asthma; paralytic ileus; doses exceeding 25 mcg/h at initiation of opioid therapy.

Hydromorphone:

Oral/Suppositories – Use on as-needed basis; respiratory depression; acute or severe bronchial asthma; paralytic ileus; obstetrical analgesia (8 mg tablets, oral solution, and suppositories only); intracranial lesion associated with increased intracranial pressure (2 and 4 mg tablets only).

Injection – Patients not already receiving large amounts of parenteral narcotics (HP injection only); respiratory depression; status asthmaticus; obstetrical analgesia (hydromorphone injection).

Meperidine: In patients taking monoamine oxidase inhibitors (MAOIs) or in those who have received such agents within 14 days.

Methadone:

Injection – Respiratory depression; acute bronchial asthma; hypercarbia.

Morphine:

IR concentrated oral solution and tablets/suppositories – Respiratory insufficiency or depression; severe CNS depression; attack of bronchial asthma; heart failure secondary to chronic lung disease; cardiac arrhythmias; increased intracranial or CSF pressure; head injuries; brain tumor; acute alcoholism; delirium tremens; convulsive disorders; after biliary tract surgery; suspected surgical abdomen; surgical anastomosis; concomitantly with MAOIs or within 14 days of such treatment; paralytic ileus.

Injection – Heart failure secondary to chronic lung disease; cardiac arrhythmias; brain tumor; acute alcoholism; delirium tremens; idiosyncrasy to the drug; increased intracranial or CSF pressure; head injuries; acute bronchial asthma; upper airway obstruction. Because of its stimulating effect on the spinal cord, morphine should not be used in convulsive states (eg, status epilepticus, tetanus, strychnine poisoning); concomitantly with MAOIs or in those who have received such agents within 14 days.

Epidural/Intrathecal – Presence of infection at the injection microinfusion site; concomitant anticoagulant therapy; uncontrolled bleeding diathesis; parenterally administered corticosteroids within a 2-week period, other concomitant drug therapy or medical condition that would contraindicate the technique of epidural or intrathecal analgesia; acute bronchial asthma; upper airway obstruction.

Soluble tablets for injection – Convulsive states such as those occurring in status epilepticus, tetanus, and strychnine poisoning.

DepoDur – Respiratory depression; acute or severe bronchial asthma; upper airway obstruction; paralytic ileus; head injury; increased intracranial pressure; circulatory shock.

Sustained-release (SR)/ER/CR – Respiratory depression; acute or severe bronchial asthma; paralytic ileus.

Opium: Diarrhea caused by poisoning until the toxic material is eliminated from the GI tract; use in children (opium tincture only); convulsive states such as those occurring in status epilepticus, tetanus, and strychnine poisoning (*Paregoric* only).

Oxycodone:

CR/IR tablets (15 and 30 mg)/IR capsules (5 mg)/ER/Concentrated solution – Significant respiratory depression; acute or severe bronchial asthma; hypercarbia; paralytic ileus.

Oxymorphone: Hypersensitivity to morphine analogs; acute asthma attack; severe respiratory depression or upper airway obstruction; paralytic ileus; pulmonary edema secondary to a chemical respiratory irritant.

Remifentanil: For epidural or intrathecal administration; hypersensitivity to fentanyl analogs.

Tramadol: Acute intoxication with alcohol, hypnotics, narcotics, centrally acting analgesics, opioids, or psychotropic drugs.

Warnings/Precautions

Respiratory depression: Narcotics may be expected to produce serious or potentially fatal respiratory depression if given in an excessive dose, too frequently, or in full dosage to compromised or vulnerable patients because the doses required to produce analgesia in the general clinical population may cause serious respiratory depression in vulnerable patients.

Respiratory depression caused by opioid analgesics can be reversed by opioid antagonists, such as naloxone. Because the duration of respiratory depression may last longer than the duration of the opioid antagonist action, maintain appropriate surveillance.

Excessive doses: These products given in excessive doses, either alone or in combination with other CNS depressants (including alcohol), are a major cause of drug-related deaths.

Head injury and increased intracranial pressure: Narcotics may obscure the clinical course of patients with head injuries. The respiratory depressant effects and the capacity to elevate cerebrospinal fluid pressure may be markedly exaggerated in the presence of head injury, brain tumor, other intracranial lesions or a preexisting elevated intracranial pressure.

QT prolongation: Administer **methadone** with particular caution to patients already at risk for development of prolonged QT interval

Seizures: Seizures may be aggravated or may occur in individuals with or without a history of convulsive disorders if dosage is substantially increased above recommended levels because of tolerance. Observe patients with known seizure disorders closely for **hydromorphone**-, **meperidine**-, **morphine**-, or **tramadol**-induced seizure activity.

Parenteral therapy: Give by very slow IV injection, preferably as a diluted solution. The patient should be lying down. Rapid IV injection increases the incidence of adverse reactions. Use caution when injecting subcutaneously or IM in chilled areas or in patients with hypotension or shock because impaired perfusion may prevent complete absorption.

Limit epidural or intrathecal administration of **morphine** to the lumbar area.

Hydrochlorides of opium alkaloids – Do not administer IV.

Epidural/Intrathecal administration: Limit epidural or intrathecal administration of preservative-free **morphine** to the lumbar area. Intrathecal use has been associated with a higher incidence of respiratory depression than epidural use.

Asthma and other respiratory conditions: The use of bisulfites is contraindicated in asthmatic patients. Bisulfites and **morphine** may potentiate each other, preventing use by causing severe adverse reactions. Use with extreme caution in patients having an acute asthmatic attack, bronchial asthma, chronic obstructive pulmonary disease or cor pulmonale, a substantially decreased respiratory reserve, and preexisting respiratory depression, hypoxia, or hypercapnia. Even usual therapeutic doses of narcotics may decrease respiratory drive while simultaneously increasing airway resistance to the point of apnea. Reserve use for those whose conditions require endotracheal intubation and respiratory support or control of ventilation. In these patients, consider alternative nonopioid analgesics, and employ only under careful medical supervision at the lowest effective dose.

Hypotensive effect: Narcotic analgesics may cause severe hypotension in individuals whose ability to maintain blood pressure has been compromised by a depleted blood volume, or coadministration of drugs such as phenothiazines or general anesthetics.

Renal toxicity: *Avinza* doses over 1,600 mg/day contain a quantity of fumaric acid that has not been demonstrated to be safe, which may result in serious renal toxicity.

Acute abdominal conditions: Narcotics may obscure diagnosis or clinical course. Do not give SR **morphine** to patients with GI obstruction, particularly paralytic ileus, as there is a risk of the product remaining in the stomach for an extended period and the subsequent release of a bolus of morphine when normal gut motility is restored.

Skeletal muscle rigidity: **Alfentanil** and **fentanyl** may cause skeletal muscle rigidity, particularly of the truncal muscles. The incidence and severity of muscle rigidity is usually dose-related. Alfentanil and fentanyl may produce muscular rigidity that involves all skeletal muscles, including those of the neck and extremities.

Fever/External heat: Serum **fentanyl** concentrations may increase by approximately one third for patients with a body temperature of 40°C (104°F) because of temperature-dependent increases in fentanyl release from the transdermal system and increased skin permeability.

Supraventricular tachycardias: Use **meperidine** with caution in atrial flutter and other supraventricular tachycardias; vagolytic action may increase the ventricular response rate.

Cardiovascular effects: Limit use of **levorphanol** in acute MI or in cardiac patients with myocardial dysfunction or coronary insufficiency because the effects of levorphanol on the heart are unknown.

Administer opioids with caution to patients in circulatory shock, because vasodilation produced by the drug may further reduce cardiac output and blood pressure.

Pancreatitis/Biliary tract disease: Use opioids with caution in patients with biliary tract disease, including acute pancreatitis and in those about to undergo surgery of the biliary tract.

Urinary system disorders: Initiation of neuraxial opiate analgesia is frequently associated with disturbances of micturition, especially in males with prostatic enlargement.

Cough reflex: Exercise caution when using narcotic analgesics postoperatively and in patients with pulmonary disease because cough reflex is suppressed.

Intraoperative awareness: Intraoperative awareness has been reported in patients younger than 55 years of age when **remifentanil** has been administered with propofol infusion rates of 75 mcg/kg/min or less.

Tolerance: Some patients develop tolerance to the narcotic analgesic. This may occur after days or months of continuous therapy. The dose generally needs to be increased to obtain adequate analgesia.

Cross-tolerance – Cross-tolerance is not complete. Switching to another narcotic agonist, starting with half the predicted equianalgesic dose, may circumvent the cross-tolerance.

Renal/Hepatic function impairment: Renal and hepatic dysfunction may cause a prolonged duration and cumulative effect; smaller doses may be necessary.

Meperidine – In patients with renal dysfunction, normeperidine (an active metabolite of meperidine) may accumulate, resulting in increased CNS adverse reactions.

Special risk: Exercise caution in elderly and debilitated patients and in those suffering from conditions accompanied by hypoxia or hypercapnia when even moderate therapeutic doses may dangerously decrease pulmonary ventilation. Also exercise caution in patients sensitive to CNS depressants, including those with cardiovascular disease; myxedema; convulsive disorders; increased ocular pressure; acute alcoholism; delirium tremens; cerebral arteriosclerosis; ulcerative colitis; fever; decreased respiratory reserve (eg, emphysema, severe obesity); hypothyroidism; kyphoscoliosis; Addison's disease; prostatic hypertrophy; urethral stricture; CNS depression; coma; gallbladder disease; recent GI or GU tract surgery; toxic psychosis.

In obese patients (more than 20% above ideal body weight), determine the **alfentanil** and **remifentanil** dosage on the basis of ideal body weight.

Use **fentanyl transmucosal** with caution in patients with diabetes because it contains approximately 2 g of sugar per unit.

In patients with pheochromocytoma, **meperidine** has been reported to provoke hypertension.

Bradycardia – **Fentanyl, remifentanil**, and **alfentanil** may produce bradycardia, which may be treated with ephedrine or anticholinergic drugs, such as atropine or glycopyrrolate. Use caution when administering to patients with bradyarrhythmias.

Drug abuse and dependence: Psychological dependence, physical dependence, and tolerance may develop upon repeated administration of opioids; therefore, prescribe and administer opioids with caution.

Use opioids with caution in patients with alcoholism or other drug dependencies because of the increased frequency of opioid tolerance, dependence, and the risk of addiction observed in these patient populations. Abuse of opioids in combination with other CNS depressants can result in serious risk to the patient.

Abuse of ER dose forms by crushing, chewing, snorting, or injecting the dissolved product will result in the immediate release of the entire daily dose of the opioid and pose a significant risk to the abuser that could result in overdose and death.

Acute abstinence syndrome (withdrawal) – In chronic pain patients in whom opioid analgesics are abruptly discontinued, anticipate a severe abstinence syndrome.

Hazardous tasks: May produce drowsiness or dizziness; observe caution while driving or performing other tasks requiring alertness or physical dexterity.

Pregnancy: *Category C, Category B,* (**oxycodone**).

Labor – Narcotics cross the placental barrier and can produce depression of respiration and psycho-physiologic effects in the neonate.

Lactation: Most of these agents appear in breast milk, but effects on the infant may not be significant. Some recommend waiting 4 to 6 hours after use before nursing.

Children: Safety and efficacy of **fentanyl** (transdermal and injection) in children younger than 2 years of age are not established. Fentanyl transmucosal and **tramadol** use has not been established in children younger than 16 years of age. Hypotension has occurred in neonates with respiratory distress syndrome on **alfentanil** 20 mcg/kg.

Do not use **oxycodone** in children. Safe dosage of **codeine** has not been established for children younger than 3 years of age. Safety and efficacy have been established with **remifentanil** from birth to 12 years of age in maintenance of general anesthesia.

Safety and efficacy not established in children for **hydromorphone, levorphanol, methadone, morphine, opium, oxymorphone**.

Monitoring: Because of the possibility of delayed respiratory depression, continue monitoring patients well after surgery. Monitor vital signs routinely.

Drug Interactions

Drug/Drug interactions: Drugs that may affect narcotic analgesics include acyclovir, amiodarone, anticholinergics, azole antifungals, barbiturate anesthetics, benzodiazepines, beta blockers, calcium channel blockers, carbamazepine, cigarette smoking, cimetidine, CNS depressants, CYP2D6 inhibitors, CYP3A4 inducers, CYP3A4 inhibitors, droperidol, erythromycin, ethanol, hydantoins, lidocaine, MAOIs, neostigmine, nitrous oxide, nonnucleoside reverse transcriptase inhibitors, nucleoside reverse transcriptase inhibitors, phenothiazines, propofol, protease inhibitors, quinidine, reserpine, rifamycins, sibutramine, SSRIs, tricyclic antidepressants, and urinary acidifiers. Charcoal and cigarette smoking may also affect narcotic analgesics.

Drugs that may be affected by narcotic analgesics include barbiturate anesthetics, beta blockers, carbamazepine, desipramine, digoxin, diuretics, lidocaine, MAOIs, nucleoside reverse transcriptase inhibitors, sibutramine, skeletal muscle relaxants, SSRIs, and warfarin.

Drug/Lab test interactions: Determinations of plasma amylase or lipase levels may be unreliable for 24 hours after narcotic administration.

Adverse Reactions

Major hazards: Respiratory depression; apnea; circulatory depression; respiratory arrest; coma; shock; cardiac arrest; hypoventilation. Most cases of serious or fatal adverse events involving **levorphanol** reported to the manufacturer or the FDA have involved either the administration of large initial doses or too frequent doses of the drug to non-opioid-tolerant patients, or the simultaneous administration of levorphanol with other drugs affecting respiration. Reduce the initial levorphanol dose by approximately more than 50% when it is given to patients along with another drug affecting respiration.

Most frequent: Anxiety; apnea; asthenia; bradycardia; confusion; constipation; diarrhea; dizziness; headache; hypertension; hypotension; lightheadedness; nausea; nervousness; respiratory depression; sedation; skeletal muscle rigidity; sweating; vasodilation; vomiting. Symptoms are more prominent in ambulatory patients and in those without severe pain. Use lower doses in these patients. Some reactions may be alleviated if the ambulatory patient lies down.

NARCOTIC AGONIST-ANTAGONIST ANALGESICS

There are 2 types of narcotic agonist-antagonists: 1) Drugs which are antagonists at the μ receptor and are agonists at other receptors (ie, pentazocine), 2) partial agonists (ie, buprenorphine) that have limited agonist activity at the μ receptor. The narcotic agonist-antagonist analgesics are potent analgesic agents with a lower abuse potential than pure narcotic agonists. Because of their narcotic antagonist activity, these agents may precipitate withdrawal symptoms in those with opiate dependence.

Narcotic Agonist-Antagonist Pharmacokinetics

Agonist/Antagonist		Onset (min)	Peak (min)	Duration (h)	t½ (h)	Equivalent dose[a] (mg)	Relative antagonist activity
Buprenorphine	IM	15	60	6	2.2-3.5	0.3	equipotent with naloxone
	IV[b]						
Butorphanol	IM	< 10	30-60	3-4	2.5-4	2-3	30× pentazocine or 1/40 naloxone
Dezocine	IM	≤ 30	30-150	2-4[c]	nd	10	greater than pentazocine
	IV	≤ 15			2.4[d]		
Nalbuphine	IM	< 15[e]	60	3-6	5	10	10× pentazocine
	IV	12-30[b]	30				
Pentazocine	IM	15-20[b]	15-601	3	2.2-3.5	30	weak
	IV	12-30[b]	nd[f]				
	oral	15-30[b]	60-180				

[a] Parenteral dose equivalent to 10 mg morphine.
[b] Time to onset and peak effect shorter.
[c] Dose related.
[d] For 10 or 20 mg dose; 1.7 h for 5 mg dose.
[e] Also for subcutaneous administration.
[f] nd – no data

PENTAZOCINE

Injection: 30 mg (as lactate) per mL (*c-iv*) — *Talwin* (Hospira)

Indications

Moderate to severe pain: For the relief of moderate to severe pain.

Preoperative or preanesthetic/supplement to surgical anesthesia: For preoperative or preanesthetic medication; supplement to surgical anesthesia.

Administration and Dosage

Adults: 30 mg IM, subcutaneously or IV; may repeat every 3 to 4 hours. Doses in excess of 30 mg IV or 60 mg IM or subcutaneously are not recommended. Do not exceed a total daily dosage of 360 mg.

Use subcutaneously only when necessary; severe tissue damage is possible at injection sites. When frequent injections are needed, administer IM, constantly rotating injection sites.

Patients in labor: A single 30 mg IM dose is most common. A 20 mg IV dose, given 2 or 3 times at 2- to 3-hour intervals, has resulted in adequate pain relief when contractions become regular.

Children (younger than 12 years of age): Clinical experience is limited; use is not recommended.

Admixture incompatibility: Do not mix pentazocine in the same syringe with soluble barbiturates because precipitation will occur.

Actions

Pharmacology: Pentazocine, a potent analgesic, weakly antagonizes the effects of morphine, meperidine, and other opiates at the μ-opioid receptor.

Pharmacokinetics: Pentazocine is well absorbed from the GI tract and from subcutaneous and IM sites. Oral bioavailability is less than 20%; concentrations in plasma coincide closely with onset, intensity and duration of analgesia. It is excreted via the kidney, less than 5% unchanged.

Contraindications

Hypersensitivity to pentazocine.

Warnings/Precautions

Tissue damage: Severe sclerosis of skin, subcutaneous tissues, and underlying muscle has occurred at injection sites following multiple doses of pentazocine lactate.

Head injury and increased intracranial pressure: Pentazocine can produce effects that may obscure the clinical course of head injury patients. Use with extreme caution and only if essential.

MI: Exercise caution in the IV use of pentazocine for patients with acute MI accompanied by hypertension or left ventricular failure. Use the oral form with caution in MI patients who have nausea or vomiting.

Acute CNS manifestations: Patients receiving therapeutic doses have experienced hallucinations (usually visual), disorientation, and confusion that have cleared spontaneously.

Seizures have occurred with the use of pentazocine.

Respiratory conditions: Use caution and low dosage in patients with respiratory depression, severely limited respiratory reserve, severe bronchial asthma, obstructive respiratory conditions, and cyanosis.

Biliary tract pressure elevation: Biliary tract pressure elevation generally occurs for varying periods following narcotic use. However, some evidence suggests pentazocine causes little or no elevation in biliary tract pressures.

Patients receiving narcotics: Pentazocine is a mild narcotic antagonist. Some patients previously given narcotics, including methadone for the daily treatment of narcotic dependence, have experienced withdrawal symptoms after receiving pentazocine.

Renal/Hepatic function impairment: The drug is metabolized in liver and excreted by the kidney; administer with caution to patients with such impairment. Extensive liver disease predisposes to greater side effects and may be the result of decreased drug metabolism.

Drug abuse and dependence: Special care should be exercised in prescribing pentazocine for emotionally unstable patients and for those with a history of drug misuse. Such patients should be closely supervised when more than 4 or 5 days of therapy is contemplated. Extended use of parenteral pentazocine lactate may lead to physical or psychological dependence in some patients. When pentazocine lactate is abruptly discontinued, withdrawal symptoms such as abdominal cramps, elevated temperature, rhinorrhea, restlessness, anxiety, and lacrimation may occur. In the rare patient in whom more than minor difficulty has been encountered, reinstitution of parenteral pentazocine lactate with gradual withdrawal has ameliorated the patient's symptoms. Substituting methadone or other narcotics for pentazocine lactate in the treatment of the pentazocine abstinence syndrome should be avoided. There have been rare reports of possible abstinence syndromes in newborns after prolonged use of pentazocine lactate during pregnancy.

Hazardous tasks: May produce sedation, dizziness, and occasional euphoria; observe caution while driving or performing other tasks requiring alertness, coordination, or physical dexterity.

Pregnancy: Category C.

Labor – Use with caution in women delivering premature infants.

Lactation: Safety for use in the nursing mother has not been established.

Children: Safety and efficacy in children younger than 12 years of age have not been established.

Drug Interactions

Drugs that may interact with pentazocine include alcohol and barbiturate anesthetics.

Adverse Reactions

Significant adverse reactions include nausea; dizziness or lightheadedness; drowsiness; vomiting; euphoria; constipation; cramps; abdominal distress; anorexia; diarrhea; dry mouth; taste alteration; sedation; headache; weakness or faintness; depression; disturbed dreams; insomnia; syncope; hallucinations; tremor; irritability; excitement; tinnitus; disorientation; confusion; blurred vision; focusing difficulty; nystagmus; diplopia; miosis; edema of the face; sweating; anaphylactic reaction; rash; urticaria; soft tissue induration; nodules; cutaneous depression; ulceration (sloughing); severe sclerosis of the skin and subcutaneous tissues; diaphoresis; stinging on injection; flushed skin; dermatitis; pruritus; toxic epidermal necrolysis; decrease in blood pressure; tachycardia; circulatory depression; shock; hypertension; respiratory depression; dyspnea; transient apnea in newborns whose mothers received parenteral pentazocine during labor; depression of white blood cells (especially granulocytes); urinary retention; paresthesia; chills; neuromuscular and psychiatric muscle tremors; alterations in rate or strength of uterine contractions during labor (parenteral form).

PENTAZOCINE COMBINATIONS

Tablets; oral: pentazocine 25 mg (as hydrochloride) and acetaminophen 650 mg (*c-iv*)	Various
pentazocine 50 mg (as hydrochloride) and naloxone hydrochloride 0.5 mg (*c-iv*)	

Administration and Dosage

Adults:

Pentazocine and naloxone – 50 mg every 3 or 4 hours, increased to 100 mg if necessary, up to a maximum of 600 mg/day.

Pentazocine and acetaminophen – 1 tablet every 4 hours, up to 6 tablets/day.

Children: Not recommended for children younger than 12 years of age.

NALBUPHINE HYDROCHLORIDE

Injection: 10 and 20 mg/mL (*Rx*)	Various, *Nubain* (Endo)

Indications

Relief of moderate to severe pain.

For preoperative analgesia, as a supplement to balanced analgesia, to surgical and post-surgical anesthesia and for obstetrical analgesia during labor and delivery.

Administration and Dosage

Pain:

Adults – Usual dose is 10 mg/70 kg administered subcutaneously, IM, or IV every 3 to 6 hours as necessary. Individualize dosage. In nontolerant individuals, the recommended single maximum dose is 20 mg, with a maximum total daily dose of 160 mg.

Supplement to anesthesia:

Induction doses – 0.3 to 3 mg/kg IV administered over a 10 to 15 minute period.

Maintenance dose – 0.25 to 0.5 mg/kg in a single IV administration.

Patients dependent on narcotics: Patients dependent on narcotics may experience withdrawal symptoms upon the administration of nalbuphine. If unduly troublesome, control by slow IV administration of small increments of morphine until relief occurs. If the previous analgesic was morphine, meperidine, codeine or another narcotic with similar duration of activity, administer 25% the anticipated nalbuphine dose initially. Observe for signs of withdrawal. If untoward symptoms do not occur, progressively increase doses at appropriate intervals until analgesia is obtained.

Actions

Pharmacology: Nalbuphine is a potent analgesic with narcotic agonist and antagonist actions. Its analgesic potency is essentially equivalent to that of morphine on a milligram basis.

Pharmacokinetics: Onset of action occurs within 2 to 3 minutes after IV administration, and in less than 15 minutes following subcutaneous or IM injection. Nalbuphine is metabolized in the liver; plasma half-life is 5 hours. The duration of analgesic activity ranges from 3 to 6 hours. Approximately 7% is excreted unchanged in the urine.

Contraindications

Hypersensitivity to nalbuphine.

Warnings/Precautions

Administration: Nalbuphine should be given as a supplement to general anesthesia only by persons specifically trained in the use of IV anesthetics and management of the respiratory effects of potent opioids.

Head injury and increased intracranial pressure: The possible respiratory depressant effects and the potential of potent analgesics to elevate cerebrospinal fluid pressure may be markedly exaggerated in the presence of head injury, intracranial lesions, or a preexisting increase in intracranial pressure.

Respiratory depression: At the usual adult dose of 10 mg/70 kg, nalbuphine causes respiratory depression approximately equal to that produced by equal doses of morphine. However, nalbuphine exhibits a ceiling effect; increases in dosage beyond 30 mg produce no further respiratory depression. Respiratory depression induced by nalbuphine can be reversed by naloxone. Administer nalbuphine with caution at low doses to patients with impaired respiration (eg, from other medication, uremia, bronchial asthma, severe infection, cyanosis, or respiratory obstructions).

MI: Use with caution in patients with MI who have nausea or vomiting.

Biliary tract surgery: Use with caution in patients about to undergo biliary tract surgery because it may cause spasm of the sphincter of Oddi.

Cardiovascular effects: During evaluation of nalbuphine in anesthesia, a higher incidence of bradycardia has been reported in patients who did not receive atropine preoperatively.

Renal/Hepatic function impairment: Because nalbuphine is metabolized in the liver and excreted by the kidneys, use nalbuphine with caution in patients with renal or liver dysfunction and administer in reduced amounts.

Drug abuse and dependence: Observe caution in prescribing nalbuphine to emotionally unstable patients or to individuals with a history of opioid abuse. Closely supervise such patients when long-term therapy is contemplated.

Abrupt discontinuation after prolonged use has been followed by symptoms of narcotic withdrawal.

Hazardous tasks: May produce drowsiness. Observe caution while driving or performing other tasks requiring alertness, coordination or physical dexterity.

Pregnancy: Category B. (Category D in prolonged use or in high doses at term). Safe use in pregnancy has not been established.

Labor and delivery – May produce fetal bradycardia, respiratory depression, apnea, cyanosis, and hypotonia in the neonate. Maternal administration of naloxone during labor has normalized these effects in some cases. Use with caution in women delivering premature infants.

Lactation: Exercise caution when nalbuphine is administered to a nursing woman.

Children: Not recommended in patients younger than 18 years of age.

Drug Interactions

Drugs that may interact with nalbuphine hydrochloride include barbiturate anesthetics, cimetidine, CNS depressants.

Adverse Reactions

Adverse reactions occurring in 3% or more of patients include sedation; sweaty/clammy feeling; nausea; vomiting; dizziness; vertigo; dry mouth; headache.

BUPRENORPHINE HYDROCHLORIDE

BUPRENORPHINE HYDROCHLORIDE	
Tablets, sublingual: 2 and 8 mg (as base) (*c-iii*)	*Subutex* (Reckitt Benckiser)
Injection: 0.324 mg (equiv. to 0.3 mg buprenorphine) per mL (*c-iii*)	Various, *Buprenex* (Reckitt Benckiser)
BUPRENORPHINE HYDROCHLORIDE COMBINATIONS	
Tablets, sublingual: 2 mg buprenorphine base/0.5 mg naloxone, 8 mg buprenorphine base/2 mg naloxone (*c-iii*)	*Suboxone* (Reckitt Benckiser)

Indications

Tablets, sublingual: Treatment of opioid dependence.

Injection: Relief of moderate to severe pain.

Buprenorphine/Naloxone combination: Treatment of opioid dependence.

Administration and Dosage

Tablets: Administer sublingually as a single daily dose in the range of 12 to 16 mg/day. When taken sublingually, buprenorphine and buprenorphine/naloxone have similar clinical effects and are interchangeable. Buprenorphine tablets contain no naloxone and are preferred for use during induction.

Administration – Place tablets under the tongue until they are dissolved. The patient should continue to hold the tablets under the tongue until they dissolve; swallowing the tablets reduces the bioavailability of the drug.

Induction – To avoid precipitating withdrawal, undertake induction with buprenorphine when objective and clear signs of withdrawal are evident.

Patients taking heroin or other short-acting opioids: At treatment initiation, administer the dose of buprenorphine at least 4 hours after the patient last used opioids or, preferably, when early signs of withdrawal appear.

Patients taking methadone or other long-acting opioids: Withdrawal appears more likely in patients maintained on higher doses of methadone (more than 30 mg) and when the first buprenorphine dose is administered shortly after the last methadone dose.

Maintenance – Buprenorphine/Naloxone is the preferred medication for maintenance treatment because of the presence of naloxone in the formulation.

Reducing dosage and stopping treatment – Make the decision to discontinue therapy with buprenorphine or buprenorphine/naloxone after a period of maintenance or brief stabilization as part of a comprehensive treatment plan. Gradual and abrupt discontinuation have been used but there is not a best method of tapering the dose at the end of treatment.

Injection:

Patients 13 years of age and older – 0.3 mg IM or slow IV, every 6 hours, as needed. Repeat once (up to 0.3 mg) if required, 30 to 60 minutes after initial dosage, giving consideration to previous dose pharmacokinetics; use thereafter only as needed. In high-risk patients (eg, elderly, debilitated, presence of respiratory disease) or in patients where other CNS depressants are present, such as in the immediate postoperative period, reduce dose by about 50%. Exercise extra caution with the IV route of administration, particularly with the initial dose.

Occasionally, it may be necessary to give up to 0.6 mg. Data are insufficient to recommend single IM doses more than 0.6 mg for long-term use.

Children – Buprenorphine has been used in children 2 to 12 years of age at doses between 2 and 6 mcg/kg of body weight given every 4 to 6 hours. There is insufficient experience to recommend a dose in infants below 2 years of age, single doses greater than 6 mcg/kg of body weight, or the use of a repeat or second dose at 30 to 60 minutes (such as is used in adults).

Actions

Pharmacology: Buprenorphine is a semisynthetic centrally acting opioid analgesic derived from thebaine; a 0.3 mg dose is approximately equivalent to 10 mg morphine in analgesic effects. Buprenorphine exerts its analgesic effect via high affinity binding of CNS opiate receptors.

Its narcotic antagonist activity is approximately equipotent to naloxone.

Cardiovascular – Buprenorphine may cause a decrease or, rarely, an increase in pulse rate and blood pressure in some patients.

Respiratory effects – A therapeutic dose of 0.3 mg buprenorphine can decrease respiratory rate similarly to an equianalgesic dose of morphine (10 mg).

Pharmacokinetics: Onset of analgesic effect occurs 15 minutes after IM injection, peaks in about 1 hour, and persists up to 6 hours. When given IV, the time to onset and peak is shortened.

Buprenorphine is metabolized by the liver mediated by cytochrome P450 3A4, and its clearance is related to hepatic blood flow. Plasma protein binding is about 96%. The mean elimination half-life from plasma is 37 hours.

Contraindications

Hypersensitivity to buprenorphine.

Warnings/Precautions

Narcotic-dependent patients: Because of the narcotic antagonist activity of buprenorphine, use in physically dependent individuals may result in withdrawal effects. Buprenorphine, a partial agonist, has opioid properties that may lead to psychic dependence because of a euphoric component of the drug. The drug may not be substituted in acutely dependent narcotic addicts because of its antagonist component.

Respiratory effects: There have been occasional reports of clinically significant respiratory depression associated with buprenorphine.

Head injury/increased intracranial pressure: Buprenorphine may elevate cerebrospinal fluid (CSF) pressure; use with caution in head injury, intracranial lesions, and other states where CSF pressure may be increased. Buprenorphine can produce miosis and changes in consciousness levels that may interfere with patient evaluation.

Hepatitis: Cases of cytolytic hepatitis and hepatitis with jaundice have been observed in the addict population receiving buprenorphine both in clinical trials and in postmarketing adverse event reports.

Allergic reactions: Cases of acute and chronic hypersensitivity to buprenorphine have been reported in clinical trials and in the postmarketing experience. The most common signs and symptoms include rash, hives, and pruritus. Cases of bronchospasm, angioneurotic edema, and anaphylactic shock have been reported.

Use with caution in the following: Elderly or debilitated; severe impairment of hepatic, pulmonary or renal function; myxedema or hypothyroidism; adrenal cortical insufficiency; CNS depression or coma; toxic psychoses; prostatic hypertrophy or urethral stricture; acute alcoholism; delirium tremens; or kyphoscoliosis. Naloxone may not be effective in reversing respiratory depression.

Biliary tract dysfunction: Buprenorphine increases intracholedochal pressure to a similar degree as other opiates; administer with caution.

Acute abdominal conditions: As with other μ-opioid receptor agonists, the administration of buprenorphine or buprenorphine/naloxone may obscure the diagnosis or clinical course of patients with acute abdominal conditions.

Hepatic function impairment: Buprenorphine is metabolized by the liver; the activity may be altered in those individuals with impaired hepatic function.

Hazardous tasks: May cause dizziness or drowsiness; observe caution while driving or performing other tasks requiring alertness.

Pregnancy: Category C.

Labor and delivery – Safety and efficacy have not been established.

Lactation: It is not known whether buprenorphine is excreted in breast milk.

Children: Safety and efficacy for use in children have not been established.

Drug Interactions

Drugs that may interact with buprenorphine hydrochloride include barbiturate anesthetics, benzodiazepines, CNS depressants, CYP3A4 inducers and inhibitors, and MAOIs.

Adverse Reactions

Adverse reactions occurring in at least 3% of patients include sedation, dizziness/vertigo, headache, hypotension, nausea/vomiting, hypoventilation, miosis, sweating.

ACETAMINOPHEN (N-Acetyl-P-Aminophenol, APAP)

ACETAMINOPHEN	
Tablets; oral: 325 mg (*otc*)	Various, *Aminofen* (Dover), *Apap* (Medique), *Cetafen* (Hart Health & Safety), *Genapap* (Ivax), *Mapap Regular Strength*, (Major), *Masophen* (Mason), *Pain and Fever* (Rugby), *Pain Reliever* (Magno-Humphries), *Q-Pap* (Qualitest), *Tylenol Regular Strength*, (McNeil Consumer), *Valorin* (Otis Clapp)
500 mg (*otc*)	Various, *Aminofen Max Extra Strength* (Dover), *Anacin Aspirin Free* (Insight), *Apap* (Medique), *Cetafen Extra* (Hart Health & Safety), *Mapap* (Major), *Masophen*, *Non-Aspirin Extra Strength* (Mason), *Pain and Fever* (Rugby), *Pain Relief Extra Strength* (Basic), *Pain Reliever Extra Strength* (Magno-Humphries), *Q-Pap Extra Strength* (Qualitest), *Tylenol Extra Strength EZ Tabs*, *Tylenol Extra Strength* (McNeil Consumer), *UN-Aspirin Extra Strength* (Zee Medical), *Valorin* (Otis Clapp)
Tablets, chewable; oral: 80 mg (*otc*)	Various, *Genapap Children's* (Ivax), *Mapap Children's* (Major), *Pain and Fever Children's* (Rugby)
160 mg (*otc*)	*Mapap Junior Strength* (Major)
500 mg (*otc*)	*Tylenol Extra Strength Go Tabs* (McNeil Consumer)
Tablets, extended-release; oral: 650 mg (*otc*)	*Mapap Arthritis Pain* (Major), *Tylenol Arthritis Pain*, *Tylenol 8 Hour* (McNeil-Consumer)
Tablets, disintegrating; oral: 80 mg (*otc*)	*Quick Melts Children's Non-Aspirin* (Marlex)
160 mg (*otc*)	*Quick Melts Jr. Strength Non-Aspirin* (Marlex)
Tablets, chewable/dispersible; oral: 80 mg (*otc*)	*Tylenol Children's Meltaways* (McNeil Consumer)
160 mg (*otc*)	*Tylenol Jr. Meltaways* (McNeil Consumer)
Tablets, rapid release, oral: 500 mg (*otc*)	*Genapap Extra Strength Gelcaps* (Ivax), *Mapap Gelcaps* (Major), *Tylenol Extra Strength Rapid Release Gels* (McNeil Consumer)
Capsules; oral: 500 mg (*otc*)	Various, *Mapap* (Major), *Masophen Extra Strength* (Mason)
Liquid; oral: 160 mg per 5 mL (*otc*)	Various, *Q-Pap Children's* (Qualitest), *Silapap Children's* (Silarx)
166.6 mg per 5 mL (*otc*)	Various, *Tylenol Extra Strength*, *Tylenol Sore Throat Daytime* (McNeil Consumer)
500 mg per 5 mL (*otc*)	*Apap 500* (Cypress)
Elixir; oral: 160 mg per 5 mL (*otc*)	*Apra Children's* (Altaire), *Mapap Children's* (Major), *Q-Pap Children's* (Qualitest), *Silapap Children's* (Silarx)
Solution; oral: 160 mg per 5 mL (*otc*)	Various, *Ed-Apap Children's* (Edwards), *ElixSure Children's Fever Reducer/Pain Reliever* (Alterna), *Pain and Fever Relief Children's* (Rugby)
Solution, concentrate; oral 80 mg/mL (*otc*)	*Little Fevers* (Little Remedies)
100 mg/mL (*otc*)	*Apap Infants' Drops* (Various), *Infantaire Drops* (Altaire), *Mapap Infant Drops* (Major), *Pain and Fever Relief Children's Drops* (Rugby), *Q-Pap Infants Drops* (Qualitest), *Silapap Infants* (Silarx), *Triaminic Infants' Fever Reducer/Pain Reliever* (Novartis), *Tylenol Infants' Drops* (McNeil Consumer)
Suspension; oral: 160 mg per 5 mL (*otc*)	*Nortemp Children's* (Ballay), *Q-Pap Children's* (Qualitest), *Tylenol Children's*, *Tylenol with Flavor Creator Children's* (McNeil Consumer)
Suppositories; rectal: 80 mg (*otc*)	*FeverAll Infants* (Actavis)
120, 325, and 650 mg (*otc*)	Various, *Acephen* (G & W Labs), *FeverAll*, *FeverAll Children*, *FeverAll Junior Strength* (Actavis)
Injection, solution: 10 mg/mL (*Rx*)	*Ofirmev* (Cadence Pharmaceuticals)
ACETAMINOPHEN, BUFFERED	
Effervescent granules: 325 mg w/2.781 g sodium bicarbonate & 2.224 g citric acid/dose measure (*otc*)	*Bromo Seltzer* (Warner-Lambert)

Indications

Oral:

Adults and children at least 12 years of age – For the temporary reduction of fever and temporary relief of minor aches and pains caused by backache, the common cold, headache, menstrual cramps, minor arthritis pain, muscular aches, and toothache.

Children – Children 2 to 11 years of age: For the temporary reduction of fever and temporary relief of minor aches and pains caused by the common cold, flu, headache, sore throat, and toothache.

Injection: For the reduction of fever; for the management of mild to moderate pain and the management of moderate to severe pain with adjunctive opioid analgesics.

Administration and Dosage

Oral: If possible, use the patient's weight to determine the dose; otherwise, use age. For children, a dosage of 10 mg/kg also has been used.

General Acetaminophen Dosing

Age	Weight (lb)	Weight (kg)	Dose and frequency	Maximum daily amount
Adults and children > 12 years of age			325 to 650 mg every 4 to 6 h (immediate release) or 1,300 mg every 8 h (extended release)	4 g in 24 h
12 years	≥ 96	≥ 43.6	640 mg every 4 to 6 h	5 doses per day (3.2 g in 24 h)
11 years	72 to 95	32.7 to 42.3	480 mg every 4 to 6 h	5 doses per day (2.4 g)
9 to 10 years	60 to 71	27.3 to 32.3	400 mg every 4 to 6 h	5 doses per day (2 g in 24 h)
6 to 8 years	48 to 59	21.8 to 26.8	320 mg every 4 to 6 h	5 doses per day (1.6 g in 24 h)
4 to 5 years	36 to 47	16.4 to 21.4	240 mg every 4 h	5 doses per day (1.2 g in 24 h)
2 to 3 years	24 to 35	10.9 to 15.9	160 mg every 4 h	5 doses per day (800 mg in 24 h)
1 to 2 years[a]	18 to 23	8.2 to 10.5	120 mg every 4 h	5 doses per day (600 mg in 24 h)
4 to 11 months[a]	12 to 17	5.5 to 7.7	80 mg every 4 h	5 doses per day (400 mg in 24 h)
0 to 3 months[a]	6 to 11	2.7 to 5	40 mg every 4 h	5 doses per day (200 mg in 24 h)

[a] Unlabeled dosing.

Children's Acetaminophen Dosing by Formulation

Age	Weight (lb)	Weight (kg)	Dose given every 4 h up to 5 times per day	Acetaminophen formulation: Jr. strength chewable and disintegrating tablets (160 mg)	Children's chewable and disintegrating tablets (80 mg)	Children's liquid, solution, and suspension (160 mg per 5 mL)	Infants' concentrated drops (80 mg per 0.8 mL)
12 years	≥ 96	≥ 43.6	640 mg	4 tablets	—	—	—
11 years	72 to 95	32.7 to 42.3	480 mg	3 tablets	6 tablets	15 mL (3 tsp)	—
9 to 10 years	60 to 71	27.3 to 32.3	400 mg	2.5 tablets	5 tablets	12.5 mL (2.5 tsp)	—

Children's Acetaminophen Dosing by Formulation

Age	Weight lb	Weight kg	Dose given every 4 h up to 5 times per day	Acetaminophen formulation: Jr. strength chewable and disintegrating tablets (160 mg)	Children's chewable and disintegrating tablets (80 mg)	Children's liquid, solution, and suspension (160 mg per 5 mL)	Infants' concentrated drops (80 mg per 0.8 mL)
6 to 8 years	48 to 59	21.8 to 26.8	320 mg	2 tablets	4 tablets	10 mL (2 tsp)	—
4 to 5 years	36 to 47	16.4 to 21.4	240 mg	—	3 tablets	7.5 mL (1.5 tsp)	—
2 to 3 years	24 to 35	10.9 to 15.9	160 mg	—	2 tablets	5 mL (1 tsp)	1.6 mL (2 droppersful)
1 to 2 years[a]	18 to 23	8.2 to 10.5	120 mg	—	—	3.75 mL (¾ tsp)	1.2 mL (1.5 droppersful)
4 to 11 months[a]	12 to 17	5.5 to 7.7	80 mg	—	—	2.5 mL (½ tsp)	0.8 mL (1 dropperful)
0 to 3 months[a]	6 to 11	2.7 to 5	40 mg	—	—	—	0.4 mL (½ dropperful)

[a] Unlabeled dosing.

Administration –

Chewable tablets: Chew tablets before swallowing.

Chewable/Dispersible tablets: Dissolve in the mouth or chew before swallowing.

Elixirs, suspensions, and concentrated infants' drops: Shake well before using.

Extended-release tablets: Swallow whole; do not crush, chew, or dissolve.

Orally disintegrating tablets: Put tablet on the tongue and allow tablet to dissolve. Do not chew or swallow the tablet whole.

Injection:

Fever/Pain –

13 years of age and older:

Weighing 50 kg or more – 1,000 mg every 6 hours or 650 mg every 4 hours IV up to a maximum of 1,000 mg as a single dose and 4,000 mg/day.

Weighing less than 50 kg – 15 mg/kg every 6 hours or 12.5 mg/kg every 4 hours IV up to a maximum of 15 mg/kg (up to 750 mg) as a single dose and 75 mg/kg (up to 3,750 mg) per day.

2 to 12 years of age: 15 mg/kg every 6 hours or 12.5 mg/kg every 4 hours IV up to a maximum of 15 mg/kg as a single dose and 75 mg/kg per day.

Renal function impairment – Longer dosing intervals and a reduced total daily dose may be warranted in patients with severe renal impairment (creatinine clearance [CrCl] 30 mL/min or less).

Hepatic function impairment – Use with caution in patients with hepatic impairment or active liver disease; a reduced total daily dose may be warranted. Contraindicated in patients with severe hepatic impairment or severe active liver disease.

Administration – Administer IV over 15 minutes. Acetaminophen may be administered without further dilution.

Actions

Pharmacology: Acetaminophen is the active metabolite of phenacetin and has antipyretic and analgesic activities. In peripheral tissues, acetaminophen is a weak COX-1 and COX-2 inhibitor. Acetaminophen appears to be equivalent to aspirin as an analgesic and antipyretic agent. However, acetaminophen lacks anti-inflammatory properties, does not affect uric acid levels, and does not inhibit platelet function.

Pharmacokinetics:

Absorption/Distribution – Absorption of acetaminophen is rapid and peak plasma levels are reached in 30 to 60 minutes. Acetaminophen is distributed throughout most body fluids and is slightly bound to plasma proteins.

Metabolism/Excretion – Average elimination half-life is 2 to 3 hours; half-life is slightly prolonged in neonates (2.2 to 5 hours) and in cirrhotics.

Contraindications

Hypersensitivity to acetaminophen or any components in the products ; severe hepatic impairment or severe active liver disease (IV).

Warnings/Precautions

Alcohol warning: Patients who consume 3 or more alcoholic drinks every day should ask their health care provider whether they should take acetaminophen or other pain relievers/fever reducers. Caution chronic alcoholics to limit acetaminophen intake to 2 g or less per day.

Hepatic effects: Acetaminophen may cause liver damage (see Adverse Reactions and Overdosage).

Sore throat: If sore throat is severe, persists for more than 2 days, is accompanied by fever, headache, nausea, rash, or vomiting, tell patients to consult a health care provider promptly.

Usage: Patients should not use oral acetaminophen with any other product containing acetaminophen.

Advise patients to stop use and ask a health care provider if pain gets worse or lasts for more than 5 days (children) or more than 10 days (adults), fever gets worse or lasts for more than 3 days, redness or swelling is present, or new symptoms occur. These could be signs of a serious condition.

Hepatic function impairment: Use with caution in patients with any type of liver disease.

Pregnancy: *Category* B (oral); *Categoy* C (injection).

Lactation: Acetaminophen is excreted in breast milk in low concentrations with reported milk:plasma ratios of 0.91 to 1.42 at 1 and 12 hours, respectively. No adverse reactions in breast-feeding infants were reported, except for a single case of maculopapular rash on a breast-feeding infant. Acetaminophen is compatible with breast-feeding, according to the American Academy of Pediatrics.

Children: For children younger than 2 years of age (or less than 24 pounds), instruct patients to consult their health care provider.

The effectiveness of acetaminophen injection for the treatment of acute pain and fever has not been studied in children younger than 2 years of age.

Drug Interactions

Drugs that may affect APAP include activated charcoal, barbiturates, ethanol, hydantoins, and sulfinpyrazone.

Drugs that may be affected by acetaminophen include lamotrigine and warfarin.

Adverse Reactions

Used as directed, acetaminophen rarely causes severe toxicity or side effects.

Injection: Headache, insomnia, nausea, pyrexia, vomiting.

SALICYLATES

ASPIRIN	
Tablets, chewable: 81 mg (*otc*)	*Bayer Children's Aspirin* (Bayer), *St. Joseph Adult Chewable Aspirin* (Schering-Plough)
Tablets: 81 mg (*otc*)	*Bayer Heart Advantage* (Bayer)
325 mg (*otc*)	Various, *Genuine Bayer Aspirin* (Bayer), *Empirin* (GlaxoWellcome), *Norwich Regular Strength* (Lee)
500 mg (*otc*)	Various, *Arthritis Foundation Pain Reliever* (McNeil-CPC), *Maximum Bayer Aspirin* (Bayer), *Norwich Extra-Strength* (Lee)
Tablets, enteric-coated: 81 mg (*otc*)	*Aspir Low* (Major), *Ecotrin* (GlaxoSmithKline Consumer Healthcare), *Halfprin 81* (Kramer), *Heartline* (BDI)
162 mg (*otc*)	½ *Halfprin* (Kramer)
325 mg (*otc*)	Various, *Ecotrin* (GlaxoSmithKline)
500 mg (*otc*)	*Ecotrin Maximum Strength* (SmithKline Beecham), *Extra Strength Bayer Enteric 500 Aspirin* (Bayer)
650 mg (*otc*)	Various
Tablets, extended-release: 650 mg (*otc*)	*Extended Release Bayer 8-Hour* (Bayer)
Tablets, controlled-release: 800 mg (*Rx*)	*ZORprin* (PAR)
Tablets, delayed-release: 81 mg (*otc*)	*Bayer Low Adult Strength* (Bayer)
Suppositories: 120, 200, 300, and 600 mg (*otc*)	Various
ASPIRIN (Acetylsalicylic Acid; ASA), BUFFERED	
Tablets: 325 mg with calcium carbonate, magnesium oxide, and magnesium carbonate (*otc*)	*Tri-Buffered Bufferin* (Bristol-Myers Squibb), *Bufferin* (Novartis)
325 mg with buffers (*otc*)	Various, *Bayer Buffered Aspirin* (Bayer)
500 mg with calcium carbonate, magnesium carbonate, and magnesium oxide (*otc*)	*Extra Strength Bayer Plus* (Bayer), *Bufferin Extra Strength* (Bristol-Myers)
500 mg with 237 mg calcium carbonate, 33 mg magnesium hydroxide, 33 mg aluminum hydroxide (*otc*)	*Ascriptin Maximum Strength* (Novartis)
500 mg with 100 mg magnesium hydroxide and 27 mg aluminum hydroxide (*otc*)	*Arthritis Pain Formula* (Whitehall)
Tablets, coated: 325 mg with calcium carbonate, magnesium carbonate, and magnesium oxide (*otc*)	*Adprin-B* (Pfeiffer)
325 mg with 50 mg magnesium hydroxide, 50 mg aluminum hydroxide, and calcium carbonate (*otc*)	*Ascriptin* (Novartis)
Tablets, effervescent: 325 mg with 1.9 g sodium bicarbonate and 1 g citric acid per dry tablet, 567 mg sodium/tablet (*otc*)	*Alka-Seltzer with Aspirin* (Bayer)
325 mg with 1.7 g sodium bicarbonate and 1.2 g citric acid per dry tablet, 506 mg sodium/tablet (*otc*)	*Alka-Seltzer with Aspirin (Flavored)* (Bayer)
500 mg with 1.9 g sodium bicarbonate and 1 g citric acid (*otc*)	*Alka-Seltzer Extra Strength with Aspirin* (Bayer)
CHOLINE SALICYLATE	
Liquid: 870 mg/5 mL (*otc*)	*Arthropan* (Purdue Frederick)
MAGNESIUM SALICYLATE	
Tablets: 325, 467, 500, 545, 580, and 600 mg (*otc*)	*Original Doan's* (Novartis Consumer Health), *Backache Maximum Strength Relief* (B-M Squibb), *Extra Strength Doan's* (Novartis Consumer Health), *Magan* (Adria), *Bayer Select Maximum Strength Backache* (Sterling Health), *Mobidin* (Ascher)
SALSALATE (Salicylsalicyclic Acid)	
Capsules: 500 mg (*Rx*)	*Amigesic* (Amide), *Disalcid* (3M)
Tablets: 500 mg (*Rx*)	Various, *Disalcid* (3M), *Salflex* (Carnrick), *Salsitab* (Upsher-Smith)
750 mg (*Rx*)	Various, *Disalcid* (3M), *Salsitab* (Upsher-Smith), *Salflex* (Carnrick), *Marthritic* (Marnel)
SODIUM SALICYLATE	
Tablets, enteric-coated: 325 mg and 650 mg (*otc*)	Various

SALICYLATE COMBINATIONS

Tablets: 500 mg salicylate (as 293 mg choline salicylate and 362 mg Mg salicylate), 750 mg salicylate (as 440 mg choline salicylate and 544 mg Mg salicylate), 1,000 mg salicylate (as 587 mg choline salicylate, 725 mg Mg salicylate) (*Rx*)	*Choline Magnesium Trisalicylate* (Sidmak), *Tricosal* (Invamed)

Warning:

Children and teenagers should not use salicylates for chickenpox or flu symptoms before a doctor is consulted about Reye's syndrome, a rare but serious illness.

Indications

Mild to moderate pain; fever; various inflammatory conditions such as rheumatic fever, rheumatoid arthritis and osteoarthritis.

Aspirin: Aspirin, for reducing the risk of recurrent transient ischemic attacks (TIAs) or stroke in men who have had transient ischemia of the brain because of fibrin platelet emboli. It has not been effective in women and is of no benefit for completed strokes.

To reduce the risk of death or nonfatal myocardial infarction (MI) in patients with previous infarction or unstable angina pectoris.

Administration and Dosage

ASPIRIN (Acetylsalicylic Acid; ASA):

Minor aches and pains – 325 to 650 mg every 4 hours as needed. Some extra strength (500 mg) products suggest 500 mg every 3 hours or 1,000 mg every 6 hours.

Arthritis, other rheumatic conditions (eg, osteoarthritis) – 3.2 to 6 g/day in divided doses.

Juvenile rheumatoid arthritis: 60 to 110 mg/kg/day in divided doses (every 6 to 8 hours). When starting at lower doses (eg, 60 mg/kg/day), may increase by 20 mg/kg/day after 5 to 7 days, followed by 10 mg/kg/day after another 5 to 7 days.

Maintain a serum salicylate level of 150 to 300 mcg/mL.

Acute rheumatic fever –

Adults: 5 to 8 g/day, initially.

Children: 100 mg/kg/day for 2 weeks, then decreased to 75 mg/kg/day for 4 to 6 weeks.

Therapeutic salicylate level: Therapeutic salicylate levels 150 to 300 mcg/mL.

Transient ischemic attacks in men – 1300 mg/day in divided doses (650 mg 2 times/day, or 325 mg 4 times/day). One study indicated that a dose of 300 mg/day is as effective as the larger dose and may be associated with fewer side effects.

MI prophylaxis – 300 or 325 mg/day. This use applies to solid oral doseforms (buffered and plain) and to buffered aspirin in solution.

Children –

Analgesic/antipyretic dosage: 10 to 15 mg/kg/dose every 4 hours (see table), up to 60 to 80 mg/kg/day.

Recommended Aspirin Dosage in Children

Age (years)	Weight lbs	Weight kg	Dosage (mg every 4 hours)	No. of 81 mg tablets (every 4 hours)	No. of 325 mg tablets (every 4 hours)
2-3	24-35	10.6-15.9	162	2	½
4-5	36-47	16-21.4	243	3	
6-8	48-59	21.5-26.8	324	4	1
9-10	60-71	26.9-32.3	405	5	
11	72-95	32.4-43.2	486	6	1½
12-14	≥ 96	≥ 43.3	648	8	2

Kawasaki disease (mucocutaneous lymph node syndrome): For acute febrile period, 80 to 180 mg/kg/day; very high doses may be needed to achieve therapeutic levels. After the fever resolves, dosage may be adjusted to 10 mg/kg/day.

ASPIRIN, BUFFERED: The addition of small amounts of antacids may decrease GI irritation and increase the dissolution and absorption rates of these products. Dosing is the same as with unbuffered aspirin.

CHOLINE SALICYLATE: Has fever GI side effects than aspirin.

Adults and children (older than 12 years of age) – 870 mg every 3 to 4 hours; maximum 6 times/day. Rheumatoid arthritis patients may start with 5 to 10 mL, up to 4 times/day.

MAGNESIUM SALICYLATE: A sodium free salicylate derivative that may have a low incidence of GI upset. The product labeling and dosage are expressed as magnesium salicylate anhydrous. The possibility of magnesium toxicity exists in people with renal insufficiency.

Usual dose is 650 mg every 4 hours or 1090 mg, 3 times a day. May increase to 3.6 to 4.8 g/day in 3 or 4 divided doses.

Safety and efficacy for use in children have not been established.

SALSALATE (Salicylsalicylic Acid): After absorption, the drug is partially hydrolyzed into two molecules of salicylic acid. Insoluble in gastric secretions, it is not absorbed until it reaches the small intestine.

Usual adult dose is 3,000 mg/day given in divided doses.

SODIUM SALICYLATE: Less effective than an equal dose of aspirin in reducing pain or fever. Patients hypersensitive to aspirin may be able to tolerate sodium salicylate. Each gram contains 6.25 mEq sodium.

Usual dose – 325 to 650 mg every 4 hours.

Actions

Pharmacology: Salicylates have analgesic, antipyretic, anti-inflammatory, and antirheumatic effects. Salicylates lower elevated body temperature through vasodilation of peripheral vessels, thus enhancing dissipation of excess heat. The anti-inflammatory and analgesic activity may be mediated through inhibition of the prostaglandin synthetase enzyme complex.

Aspirin – Aspirin differs from the other agents in this group in that it more potently inhibits prostaglandin synthesis, has greater anti-inflammatory effects and irreversibly inhibits platelet aggregation.

Irreversible inhibition of platelet aggregation (aspirin) – Single analgesic aspirin doses prolong bleeding time. Aspirin (no other salicylates) inhibits platelet aggregation for the life of the platelet (7 to 10 days).

Low doses of aspirin inhibit platelet aggregation and may be more effective than higher doses. Larger doses inhibit cyclooxygenase in arterial walls, interfering with prostacyclin production, a potent vasodilator and inhibitor of platelet aggregation.

Pharmacokinetics:

Absorption/Distribution – Salicylates are rapidly and completely absorbed after oral use. Bioavailability is dependent on the dosage form, presence of food, gastric emptying time, gastric pH, presence of antacids or buffering agents and particle size. Bioavailability of some enteric coated products may be erratic. Absorption from rectal suppositories is slower, resulting in lower salicylate levels. Protein binding of salicylates is concentration-dependent.

Metabolism/Excretion – Salicylic acid is eliminated by renal excretion.

Contraindications

Hypersensitivity to salicylates or nonsteroidal anti-inflammatory drugs (NSAIDs). Use extreme caution in patients with history of adverse reactions to salicylates. Cross-sensitivity may exist between aspirin and other NSAIDs that inhibit prostaglandin synthesis, and aspirin, and tartrazine. Aspirin cross-sensitivity does not appear to occur with sodium salicylate, salicylamide, or choline salicylate. Aspirin hypersensitivity is more prevalent in those with asthma, nasal polyposis, chronic urticaria.

In hemophilia, bleeding ulcers and hemorrhagic states.

Magnesium salicylate: Magnesium salicylate in advanced chronic renal insufficiency because of Mg^{++} retention.

Warnings/Precautions

Otic effects: Discontinue use if dizziness, ringing in ears (tinnitus), or impaired hearing occurs. Tinnitus probably represents blood salicylic acid levels reaching or exceeding the upper limit of the therapeutic range.

Use in surgical patients: Avoid aspirin, if possible, for 1 week prior to surgery because of the possibility of postoperative bleeding.

Renal effects: Use with caution in chronic renal insufficiency; aspirin may cause a transient decrease in renal function, and may aggravate chronic kidney diseases (rare).

In patients with renal impairment, take precautions when administering **magnesium salicylate**.

GI effects: Use caution in those intolerant to salicylate because of GI irritation, and in gastric ulcers, peptic ulcer, mild diabetes, gout, erosive gastritis, or bleeding tendencies. **Salsalate** and **choline salicylate** may cause less GI irritation than aspirin.

Although fecal blood loss is less with enteric coated aspirin than with uncoated, give enteric coated aspirin with caution to patients with GI distress, ulcer, or bleeding problems.

Hematologic effects: Aspirin interferes with hemostasis. Avoid use if patients have severe anemia, history of blood coagulation defects, or take anticoagulants.

Long-term therapy: To avoid potentially toxic concentrations, warn patients on long-term therapy not to take other salicylates (nonprescription analgesics, etc).

Salicylism: Salicylism may require dosage adjustment.

Controlled-release aspirin: Controlled-release aspirin, because of its relatively long onset of action, is not recommended for antipyresis or short-term analgesia. Not recommended in children older than 12 years of age; contraindicated in all children with fever accompanied by dehydration.

Hypersensitivity reactions: Aspirin intolerance, manifested by acute bronchospasm, generalized urticaria/angioedema, severe rhinitis, or shock occurs in 4% to 19% of asthmatics. Symptoms occur within 3 hours after ingestion. Have epinephrine 1:1,000 immediately available.

Foods – Foods may contribute to a reaction. Some foods with 6 mg/100 g salicylate include curry powder, paprika, licorice, Benedictine liqueur, prunes, raisins, tea, and gherkins. A typical American diet contains 10 to 200 mg/day salicylate.

Hepatic function impairment: Use caution in liver damage, preexisting hypoprothrombinemia, and vitamin K deficiency.

Pregnancy: Category D (aspirin); *Category C* (salsalate, magnesium salicylate). Avoid use during pregnancy, especially in third trimester.

Lactation: Salicylates are excreted in breast milk in low concentrations.

Children: Safety and efficacy of **magnesium salicylate** or **salsalate** have not been established. Administration of **aspirin** to children (including teenagers) with acute febrile illness has been associated with the development of Reye's syndrome. Dehydrated febrile children appear more prone to salicylate intoxication.

Drug Interactions

Drugs that may affect aspirin include activated charcoal, ammonium chloride, ascorbic acid or methionine, antacids and urinary alkalinizers, carbonic anhydrase inhibitors, corticosteroids, and nizatidine. Drugs that may be affected by aspirin include alcohol, ACE inhibitors, anticoagulants (oral), beta-adrenergic blockers, heparin, loop diuretics, methotrexate, nitroglycerin, NSAIDs, probenecid and sulfinpyrazone, spironolactone, sulfonylureas and exogenous insulin, and valproic acid.

Drug/Lab test interactions: Salicylates compete with thyroid hormone for binding sites on thyroid binding pre-albumin and possibly thyroid binding globulin resulting in increases in **protein bound iodine**. Salicylates probably do not interfere with T_3 resin uptake.

Serum uric acid – Serum uric acid levels are elevated by salicylate levels less than 10 mg/dL and decreased by levels more than 10 mg/dL.

Salicylates in moderate to large (anti-inflammatory) doses cause false-negative readings for **urine glucose** by the glucose oxidase method and false-positive readings by the copper reduction method.

Salicylates in the urine interfere with **5-HIAA** determinations by fluorescent methods, but not by the nitrosonaphthol colorimetric method.

Salicylates in the urine interact with **urinary ketone** determinations by the ferric chloride (Gerhardt) method producing a reddish color.

Large doses may decrease urinary excretion of **phenolsulfonphthalein**.

Salicylates in the urine result in falsely elevated **vanillylmandelic acid (VMA)** with most tests, but falsely decrease VMA determinations by the Pisano method.

Adverse Reactions

Adverse reactions include the following: Hives; rashes; angioedema; nausea, dyspepsia (5% to 25%); heartburn; epigastric discomfort; anorexia; massive GI bleeding; occult blood loss; potentiation of peptic ulcer; persistent iron deficiency anemia; prolongation of bleeding time; leukopenia; thrombocytopenia; purpura; decreased plasma iron concentration; shortened erythrocyte survival time; fever; thirst; dimness of vision.

Miscellaneous:

Mild "salicylism" – Mild "salicylism" may occur after repeated use of large doses and consists of dizziness, tinnitus, difficulty hearing, nausea, vomiting, diarrhea, mental confusion, CNS depression, headache, sweating, hyperventilation, and lassitude. Salicylate serum concentrations correlate with pharmacological actions and adverse effects observed.

DIFLUNISAL

Tablets, oral: 250 mg and 500 mg (*Rx*)	Various (eg, Teva)

Warning:

Cardiovascular (CV) risk: Nonsteroidal anti-inflammatory drugs (NSAIDs) may cause an increased risk of serious CV thrombotic reactions, myocardial infarction (MI), and stroke, which can be fatal. This risk may increase with duration of use. Patients with CV disease or risk factors for CV disease may be at greater risk.

Diflunisal is contraindicated for the treatment of perioperative pain in the setting of coronary artery bypass graft (CABG) surgery.

GI risk: NSAIDs cause an increased risk of serious GI adverse reactions, including bleeding, ulceration, and perforation of the stomach or intestines, which can be fatal. These reactions can occur at any time during use and without warning symptoms. Elderly patients are at greater risk for serious GI reactions.

Indications

Acute or long-term symptomatic treatment of mild to moderate pain, rheumatoid arthritis, and osteoarthritis.

Administration and Dosage

Mild to moderate pain: 1,000 mg followed by 500 mg every 12 hours. Following the initial dose, some patients may require 500 mg every 8 hours.

A lower dosage may be appropriate depending on pain severity, patient response, weight, or advanced age; for example, 500 mg initially, followed by 250 mg every 8 to 12 hours.

Osteoarthritis/Rheumatoid arthritis: 250 to 1,000 mg/day in 2 divided doses. Doses more than 1,500 mg/day are not recommended.

Administration: Tablets should be swallowed whole, not crushed or chewed.

Actions

Pharmacology: Diflunisal, a salicylic acid derivative, is a nonsteroidal, peripherally acting, nonnarcotic analgesic with anti-inflammatory and antipyretic properties. Chemically, it differs from aspirin and is not metabolized to salicylic acid. Diflunisal is a prostaglandin synthetase inhibitor.

Pharmacokinetics: Diflunisal is rapidly and completely absorbed following oral administration; peak plasma concentrations occur between 2 to 3 hours, producing significant analgesia within 1 hour and maximum analgesia within 2 to 3 hours. An initial loading dose shortens the time to reach steady-state levels.

In contrast with salicylic acid, which has a plasma half-life or 2.5 hours, the plasma half-life of diflunisal is 3 to 4 times longer (8 to 12 hours).

The drug is excreted in the urine. Little or no diflunisal is excreted in the feces.

Contraindications

Hypersensitivity to diflunisal.

Treatment of perioperative pain in the setting of CABG surgery; patients who have experienced asthma, urticaria, or allergic-type reactions after taking aspirin or other NSAIDs.

Warnings/Precautions

CV effects:

CV thrombotic events – Trials of NSAIDs have shown an increased risk of serious CV thrombotic events, MI, and stroke, which can be fatal.

Hypertension – NSAIDs, including diflunisal, can lead to onset of new hypertension or worsening of preexisting hypertension. Patients taking thiazides or loop diuretics may have impaired response to these therapies when taking NSAIDs.

Fluid retention/edema – Use diflunisal with caution in patients with fluid retention or heart failure.

GI effects: NSAIDs, including diflunisal, can cause serious GI adverse reactions, including inflammation, bleeding, ulceration, and perforation of the stomach, small intestine, or large intestine, which can be fatal.

Skin reactions: NSAIDs, including diflunisal, can cause serious skin adverse reactions such as exfoliative dermatitis, Stevens-Johnson syndrome, and toxic epidermal necrolysis, which can be fatal. These serious reactions may occur without warning. Inform patients about the signs and symptoms of serious skin manifestations and discontinue use of the drug at the first appearance of skin rash or any other sign of hypersensitivity.

Corticosteroid use: Diflunisal cannot be expected to substitute for corticosteroids or to treat corticosteroid insufficiency.

Fever/Inflammation: The pharmacologic activity of diflunisal in reducing fever and inflammation may diminish the utility of these diagnostic signs in detecting complications of presumed noninfectious, painful conditions.

Ophthalmologic effects: Ophthalmologic effects have been reported with these agents.

Hematologic effects:

Anemia – Anemia is sometimes seen in patients receiving NSAIDs, including diflunisal. This may be caused by fluid retention, occult or gross GI blood loss, or an incompletely described effect upon erythropoiesis.

Platelet aggregation – NSAIDs inhibit platelet aggregation and have been shown to prolong bleeding time in some patients.

Preexisting asthma: Because cross-reactivity, including bronchospasm, between aspirin and other NSAIDs has been reported in such aspirin-sensitive patients, do not administer diflunisal to patients with this form of aspirin sensitivity and use caution in patients with preexisting asthma.

Reye syndrome: Acetylsalicylic acid has been associated with Reye syndrome. Because diflunisal is a derivative of salicylic acid, the possibility of its association with Reye syndrome cannot be excluded.

Hypersensitivity reactions: As with other NSAIDs, anaphylactic/anaphylactoid reactions may occur in patients without known prior exposure to diflunisal. Do not give diflunisal to patients with the aspirin triad. This symptom complex typically occurs in asthmatic patients who experience rhinitis with or without nasal polyps, or who exhibit severe, potentially fatal bronchospasm after taking aspirin or other NSAIDs.

Renal function impairment: Long-term administration of NSAIDs has resulted in renal papillary necrosis and other renal injury. Renal toxicity has also been seen in patients in who renal prostaglandins have a role in renal perfusion. Treatment with diflunisal is not recommended in patients with advanced renal disease. Close monitoring of the patient's renal function is advisable.

Hepatic function impairment: Borderline elevations of one or more liver tests may occur in up to 15% of patients taking NSAIDs, including diflunisal. These abnormalities may progress, may remain unchanged, or may be transient with continued therapy.

Pregnancy: Category C.

Nonteratogenic – Avoid use during pregnancy (particularly late pregnancy) because of the known effects of NSAIDs on the fetal CV system.

Lactation: Diflunisal is excreted in breast milk. Because of the potential for adverse reactions in breast-feeding infants, discontinue either breast-feeding or the drug.

Children: Use in children younger than 12 years of age is not recommended.

Elderly: Elderly patients seem to tolerate ulceration or bleeding less well than other individuals, and many spontaneous reports of fatal GI reactions are in this population.

The risk of toxic reactions to this drug may be greater in patients with renal function impairment. Because elderly patients are more likely to have decreased renal function, take care in dose selection.

Monitoring: Monitor for signs and symptoms of GI bleeding. Periodically perform a complete blood cell count and check the chemistry profile of patients on long-term treatment. Carefully monitor patients with coagulation disorders or patients receiving anticoagulants. If signs or symptoms consistent with liver or renal disease develop, systemic manifestations occur, or if abnormal liver tests persist or worsen, discontinue diflunisal. Closely monitor blood pressure during the initiation of NSAID treatment and throughout therapy.

Drug Interactions

Drugs that may be affected by diflunisal include acetaminophen; ACE inhibitors; angiotensin II antagonists; anticoagulants, oral; cyclosporine; diuretics; indomethacin; lithium; methotrexate; naproxen; NSAIDs; and sulindac.

Drugs that may affect diflunisal include antacids, aspirin, and probenecid.

Adverse Reactions

Adverse reactions that occur in 3% or more include nausea, dyspepsia, GI pain, diarrhea, vomiting, headache, rash, fatigue/tiredness, tinnitus.

DICLOFENAC SODIUM AND MISOPROSTOL

Tablets: 50 mg diclofenac sodium/200 mcg misoprostol and 75 mg diclofenac sodium/200 mcg misoprostol (*Rx*)	*Arthrotec* (Searle)

Warning:

Pregnancy: This product contains diclofenac and misoprostol. The administration of misoprostol to women who are pregnant can cause abortion, premature birth, or birth defects.

Uterine rupture has been reported when misoprostol was administered to pregnant women to induce labor or abortion beyond the eighth week of pregnancy. This drug should not be taken by pregnant women.

Patients must be advised of the abortifacient property and warned not to give the drug to others. Do not use in women of childbearing potential unless the patient requires nonsteroidal anti-inflammatory drug (NSAID) therapy and is at high risk of developing gastric or duodenal ulceration or of developing complications from gastric or duodenal ulcers associated with the use of the NSAID. In such patients, this drug may be prescribed if the patient:

- had a negative serum pregnancy test within 2 weeks prior to beginning therapy;
- is capable of complying with effective contraceptive measures;
- has received both oral and written warnings of the hazards of misoprostol, the risk of possible contraception failure, and the danger to other women of childbearing potential should the drug be taken by mistake;
- will begin using this product only on the second or third day of the next normal menstrual period.

Cardiovascular risk:

- NSAIDs may cause an increased risk of serious cardiovascular thrombotic reactions, myocardial infarction, and stroke, which can be fatal. This risk may increase with duration of use. Patients with cardiovascular disease or risk factors for cardiovascular disease may be at greater risk.
- Diclofenac/misoprostol is contraindicated for treatment of perioperative pain in the setting of coronary artery bypass graft (CABG) surgery.

GI risk:

- NSAIDs cause an increased risk of serious GI adverse reactions, including bleeding, ulceration, and perforation of the stomach or intestines, which can be fatal. These reactions can occur at any time during use and without warning symptoms. Elderly patients are at greater risk for serious GI reactions.

Indications

Arthritis: Treatment of the signs and symptoms of osteoarthritis or rheumatoid arthritis in patients at high risk of developing NSAID-induced gastric and duodenal ulcers and their complications.

Administration and Dosage

Swallow tablets whole; do not chew, crush, or dissolve. Tablets may be taken with meals to minimize GI effects.

Do not exceed a total misoprostol dose of 800 mcg/day, and do not administer more than 200 mcg of misoprostol at any one time.

Osteoarthritis: The recommended dose is diclofenac 50 mg/misoprostol 200 mcg 3 times/day. For patients who experience intolerance, diclofenac 50 mg/misoprostol 200 mcg or diclofenac 75 mg/misoprostol 200 mcg twice/day can be used but are less effective in preventing ulcers.

Rheumatoid arthritis: Recommended dose is diclofenac 50 mg/misoprostol 200 mcg 3 or 4 times/day. For patients who experience intolerance, diclofenac 50 mg/misoprostol 200 mcg or diclofenac 75 mg/misoprostol 200 mcg twice/day can be used but are less effective in preventing ulcers.

Special dosing considerations: For gastric ulcer prevention, misoprostol 200 mcg 3 and 4 times/day is therapeutically equivalent but more protective than the twice-daily regimen. For duodenal ulcer prevention, 4 times/day is more protective than the 2 or 3 times/day regimens. However, the 4 times/day regimen is less well tolerated because of usually self-limited diarrhea related to the misoprostol dose.

The total dose of misoprostol should not exceed 800 mcg/day. Do not administer more than misoprostol 200 mcg at any one time. Doses of diclofenac higher than 150 mg/day in osteoarthritis or higher than 225 mg/day in rheumatoid arthritis are not recommended.

Actions

Pharmacology: This product is a combination containing diclofenac sodium, an NSAID with analgesic properties, and misoprostol, a GI mucosal protective prostaglandin E_1 analog.

Pharmacokinetics: The pharmacokinetics following oral administration of a single dose or multiple doses of diclofenac/misoprostol to healthy subjects under fasted conditions are similar to the pharmacokinetics of the 2 individual components. Food decreases the multiple-dose bioavailability profile of both formulations.

Contraindications

Hypersensitivity to diclofenac or to misoprostol or other prostaglandins. Do not give to patients who have experienced asthma, urticaria, or other allergic-type reactions after taking aspirin or other NSAIDs; pregnancy; severe, rarely fatal anaphylactic-like reactions to diclofenac have been reported. For the treatment of perioperative pain in the setting of CABG surgery.

Warnings/Precautions

Cardiovascular effects:

Cardiovascular thrombotic events – Patients with known cardiovascular disease or risk factors for cardiovascular disease may be at greater risk for serious cardiovascular thrombotic events. To minimize the potential risk for an adverse cardiovascular event in patients treated with an NSAID, use the lowest effective dose for the shortest duration possible.

Hypertension – NSAIDs, including diclofenac/misoprostol, can lead to onset of new hypertension or worsening of preexisting hypertension, either of which may contribute to the increased incidence of cardiovascular events. Patients taking thiazides or loop diuretics may have impaired response to these therapies when taking NSAIDs.

Congestive heart failure and edema – Fluid retention and edema have been observed in some patients taking NSAIDs. Use diclofenac/misoprostol with caution in patients with fluid retention or heart failure.

GI effects:

Risk of ulceration, bleeding, and perforation – NSAIDs, including diclofenac/misoprostol, can cause serious GI adverse reactions, including inflammation, bleeding, ulceration, and perforation of the stomach, small intestine, or large intestine, which can be fatal.

Renal effects: Long-term administration of NSAIDs has resulted in renal papillary necrosis and other renal injury. Renal toxicity has also been seen in patients in whom renal prostaglandins have a compensatory role in the maintenance of renal perfusion.

Hepatic effects: Elevations of 1 or more liver tests may occur during therapy with diclofenac/misoprostol. Monitor transaminases within 4 to 8 weeks after initiating treatment with diclofenac.

Corticosteroid use: Diclofenac/misoprostol cannot be expected to substitute for corticosteroids or to treat corticosteroid insufficiency. Patients on prolonged corticosteroid therapy should have their therapy tapered slowly if a decision is made to discontinue corticosteroids.

Fever and/or inflammation: The pharmacologic activity of diclofenac/misoprostol in reducing fever and inflammation may diminish the utility of these diagnostic signs in detecting complications of presumed noninfectious, painful conditions.

Hematological effects: Patients on long-term treatment with NSAIDs should have their hemoglobin or hematocrit checked if they exhibit any signs or symptoms of anemia.

Preexisting asthma: Do not administer diclofenac/misoprostol to patients with aspirin-sensitive asthma. Use this drug with caution in patients with preexisting asthma.

Aseptic meningitis: As with other NSAIDs, aseptic meningitis with fever and coma has been observed on rare occasions in patients on diclofenac therapy. If signs or symptoms of meningitis develop in a patient on diclofenac, consider the possibility that it may be related to diclofenac.

Porphyria: Avoid the use of diclofenac/misoprostol in patients with hepatic porphyria.

Platelet aggregation: Diclofenac impairs platelet aggregation but does not affect bleeding time, plasma thrombin clotting time, plasma fibrinogen, or factors V and VII to XII.

Hypersensitivity reactions:

Anaphylactoid reactions – As with other NSAIDs, anaphylactoid reactions may occur in patients without known prior exposure to diclofenac/misoprostol. Do not give diclofenac/misoprostol to patients with the aspirin triad.

Skin reactions – NSAIDs, including diclofenac/misoprostol, can cause serious skin adverse reactions such as exfoliative dermatitis, Stevens-Johnson syndrome, and toxic epidermal necrolysis.

Renal function impairment: Treatment with diclofenac/misoprostol is not recommended in patients with advanced renal disease.

Pregnancy: *Category* X. Contraindicated in pregnancy.

Lactation: Diclofenac sodium is found in the milk of breast-feeding mothers. Because of the potential for serious adverse reactions in breast-feeding infants, this product is not recommended for breast-feeding mothers.

Children: Safety and efficacy in children have not been established.

Elderly: Because elderly patients are more likely to have decreased renal function, take care in dosage selection; it may be useful to monitor renal function.

Monitoring: Monitor for signs of symptoms of GI bleeding. Patients should have their complete blood cell counts and a chemistry profile checked periodically. Monitor blood pressure during the initiation of treatment and throughout therapy. Monitor for fluid retention and edema. Measure hepatic transaminases periodically in patients receiving long-term therapy and for 4 to 8 weeks after initiating therapy.

Carefully monitor patients who may be adversely affected by alterations in platelet function, such as those with coagulation disorders or patients receiving anticoagulants.

Drug Interactions

Drugs that may affect diclofenac/misoprostol include antacids, aspirin, azole antifungals, bile acid sequestrants, bisphosphonates, cyclosporine, SSRIs, and sucralfate. Drugs that may be affected by diclofenac/misoprostol include ACE inhibitors, aminoglycosides, anticoagulants, cyclosporine, digoxin, heparins, lithium, loop diuretics, methotrexate, oral hypoglycemic agents, potassium-sparing diuretics, thiazide diuretics.

Adverse Reactions

Adverse reactions reported in at least 3% of patients include the following: abdominal pain, diarrhea, dyspepsia, flatulence, nausea.

NAPROXEN AND LANSOPRAZOLE

Tablets and Capsules, delayed release: naproxen 500 mg/ lansoprazole 15 mg (*Rx*)	*Prevacid NapraPAC 500* (TAP Pharmaceuticals)

Indications

Nonsteroidal anti-inflammatory drug (NSAID)-associated gastric ulcers: For reducing the risk of NSAID-associated gastric ulcers in patients with a history of documented gastric ulcer who require the use of an NSAID for treatment of the signs and symptoms of rheumatoid arthritis, osteoarthritis, and ankylosing spondylitis.

Administration and Dosage

Each daily dose consists of one 15 mg lansoprazole capsule and 2 of either 375 or 500 mg naproxen tablets. Take the lansoprazole capsule and 1 of the naproxen tablets before eating in the morning with a glass of water. Take the second naproxen tablet in the evening with a glass of water. The maximum daily naproxen dose of naproxen/lansoprazole is 1,000 mg.

Swallow lansoprazole delayed-release capsules whole. Do not chew or crush.

Dosage adjustment: For naproxen/lansoprazole, no adjustment of the 15 mg lansoprazole component is necessary in patients with renal insufficiency or for the elderly. However, consider dose adjustment for the naproxen component for patients with renal insufficiency, liver disease, or the elderly.

NAPROXEN AND ESOMEPRAZOLE

Tablets, delayed-release; oral: Naproxen 375 mg/ esomeprazole 20 mg, naproxen 500 mg/esomeprazole 20 mg (*Rx*)	*Vimovo* (AstraZeneca)

Warning:

Cardiovascular risk: Naproxen, a component of naproxen/esomeprazole, may cause an increased risk of serious cardiovascular thrombotic events, myocardial infarction, and stroke, which can be fatal. This risk may increase with duration of use. Patients with cardiovascular disease or risk factors for cardiovascular disease may be at a greater risk.

Naproxen/esomeprazole is contraindicated for the treatment of perioperative pain in the setting of coronary artery bypass graft surgery.

GI risk: Nonsteroidal anti-inflammatory drugs (NSAIDs), including naproxen, a component of naproxen/esomeprazole, cause an increased risk of serious GI adverse events, including bleeding, ulceration, and perforation of the stomach or intestines, which can be fatal. These events can occur at any time during use and without warning symptoms. Elderly patients are at a greater risk for serious GI events.

Indications

Ankylosing spondylitis/osteoarthritis/rheumatoid arthritis: For the relief of signs and symptoms of osteoarthritis, rheumatoid arthritis, and ankylosing spondylitis and to decrease the risk of developing gastric ulcers in patients at risk of developing NSAID-associated gastric ulcers.

Naproxen/esomeprazole is not recommended for initial treatment of acute pain because the absorption of naproxen is delayed compared with absorption from other naproxen-containing products.

Administration and Dosage

Usual dosage is 1 tablet twice daily.

Elderly: Although total plasma concentration of naproxen is unchanged, the unbound plasma fraction of naproxen is increased in elderly patients. Use caution when high doses are required, and dosage adjustment may be required in elderly patients.

Renal function impairment: Naproxen-containing products are not recommended for use in patients with moderate to severe or severe renal impairment (creatinine clearance less than 30 mL/min).

Hepatic function impairment: Monitor patients with mild to moderate hepatic impairment closely, and consider a possible dose reduction based on the naproxen component of naproxen/esomeprazole.

Naproxen/esomeprazole is not recommended in patients with severe hepatic impairment because esomeprazole doses should not exceed 20 mg daily in these patients.

Administration: The tablets are to be swallowed whole with liquid. Do not split, chew, crush, or dissolve the tablet.

Naproxen/esomeprazole is to be taken at least 30 minutes before meals.

NONSTEROIDAL ANTI-INFLAMMATORY AGENTS

CELECOXIB	
Capsules; oral: 50, 100, 200, and 400 mg (*Rx*)	*Celebrex* (Pfizer)
DICLOFENAC	
Tablets; oral: 50 mg (as potassium) (*Rx*)	Various, *Cataflam* (Novartis)
Tablets, delayed-release; oral: 25, 50, and 75 mg (as sodium) (*Rx*)	Various, *Voltaren* (Novartis)
Tablets, extended-release; oral: 100 mg (as sodium) (*Rx*)	Various, *Voltaren-XR* (Novartis)
Capsules; oral: 25 mg (as potassium) (*Rx*)	*Zipsor* (Xanodyne)
Powder for solution; oral: 50 mg (as potassium) (*Rx*)	*Cambia* (Mipharm)
ETODOLAC	
Capsules; oral: 200 and 300 mg (*Rx*)	Various
Tablets; oral: 400 and 500 mg (*Rx*)	
Tablets, extended-release; oral: 400, 500, and 600 mg (*Rx*)	
FENOPROFEN CALCIUM	
Capsules; oral: 200, 300, and 400 mg (*Rx*)	Various, *Nalfon* (Pedinol)
Tablets; oral: 600 mg (*Rx*)	Various
FLURBIPROFEN	
Tablets; oral: 50 and 100 mg (*Rx*)	Various
IBUPROFEN	
Tablets; oral: 100 mg (*otc*)	*Junior Strength Motrin* (McNeil)
200 mg (*otc*)	Various, *Advil* (Whitehall-Robins), *Ibutab* (Zee Medical), *Midol Maximum Strength Cramp Formula* (Bayer), *Motrin IB* (McNeil), *Motrin Migraine Pain* (McNeil Consumer)
400, 600, and 800 mg (*Rx*)	Various
Tablets, chewable; oral: 50 and 100 mg (*otc*)	*Children's Motrin*, *Jr. Strength Motrin* (McNeil)
Capsules; oral: 200 mg (*otc*)	*Advil Liqui-Gels*, *Advil Migraine* (Whitehall-Robins)
Suspension; oral: 100 mg per 5 mL (*otc*)	Various, *Children's Advil* (Wyeth-Ayerst), *Children's Motrin* (McNeil-CPC), *PediaCare Fever* (Pharmacia & Upjohn)
Drops; oral: 40 mg/mL (*otc*)	Various, *Advil Pediatric Drops* (Whitehall-Robins), *Infants' Motrin* (McNeil), *PediaCare Fever* (Pharmacia & Upjohn)
Injection, solution, concentrate: 100 mg/mL	*Caldolor* (Cumberland Pharmaceuticals)
INDOMETHACIN	
Capsules; oral: 25 and 50 mg (*Rx*)	Various
Capsules, sustained-release; oral: 75 mg (*Rx*)	Various
Suspension; oral: 25 mg per 5 mL (*Rx*)	*Indocin* (Merck)
Suppositories; rectal: 50 mg (*Rx*)	Various, *Indocin* (Merck)
KETOPROFEN	
Capsules; oral: 50 and 75 mg (*Rx*)	Various
Capsules, extended-release; oral: 100, 150, and 200 mg (*Rx*)	
KETOROLAC TROMETHAMINE	
Tablets; oral: 10 mg (*Rx*)	Various
Injection; oral: 15 and 30 mg/mL (*Rx*)	
MECLOFENAMATE SODIUM	
Capsules; oral: 50 and 100 mg (as sodium) (*Rx*)	Various
MEFENAMIC ACID	
Capsules; oral: 250 mg (*Rx*)	Various, *Ponstel* (Sciele Pharma)

MELOXICAM	
Tablets; oral: 7.5 and 15 mg (*Rx*)	Various, *Mobic* (Boehringer Ingelheim/Abbott)
Suspension; oral: 7.5 mg per 5 mL (*Rx*)	
NABUMETONE	
Tablets; oral: 500 and 750 mg (*Rx*)	Various
NAPROXEN	
Tablets; oral: 200 mg (220 mg naproxen sodium) (*otc*)	Various, *Aleve* (Bayer), *Midol Extended Relief* (Bayer)
250 mg (275 mg naproxen sodium) and 500 mg (550 mg naproxen sodium) (*Rx*)	Various, *Anaprox* (Roche)
250, 375, and 500 mg (*Rx*)	Various, *Naprosyn* (Roche)
Tablets, delayed-release; oral: 375 and 500 mg (*Rx*)	Various, *EC-Naprosyn* (Roche)
Tablets, controlled-release; oral: 375 mg (412.5 mg naproxen sodium) and 500 mg (550 mg naproxen sodium) (*Rx*)	*Naprelan* (Victory)
Suspension; oral: 125 mg per 5 mL (*Rx*)	Various, *Naprosyn* (Roche)
OXAPROZIN	
Tablets; oral: 600 mg (*Rx*)	Various, *Daypro* (Searle)
600 mg (as 678 mg oxaprozin potassium) (*Rx*)	*Daypro ALTA* (Pharmacia)
PIROXICAM	
Capsules; oral: 10 and 20 mg (*Rx*)	Various, *Feldene* (Pfizer)
SULINDAC	
Tablets; oral: 150 and 200 mg (*Rx*)	Various, *Clinoril* (Merck)
TOLMETIN SODIUM	
Tablets; oral: 200 and 600 mg (as sodium) (*Rx*)	Various
Capsules; oral: 400 mg (as sodium) (*Rx*)	

Warning:

Cardiovascular (CV) risk: Nonsteroidal anti-inflammatory drugs (NSAIDs) may cause an increased risk of serious CV thrombotic events, myocardial infarction (MI), and stroke, which can be fatal. This risk may increase with duration of use. Patients with CV disease or risk factors for CV disease may be at higher risk.

Celecoxib, diclofenac, fenoprofen, flurbiprofen, ibuprofen, indomethacin, mefenamic acid, meloxicam, nabumetone, naproxen (except for controlled-release tablets), oxaprozin, piroxicam, sulindac, and tolmetin are contraindicated for the treatment of perioperative pain in the setting of coronary artery bypass graft (CABG) surgery.

GI risk: NSAIDs, including celecoxib, cause an increased risk of serious GI adverse reactions, including bleeding, ulceration, and perforation of the stomach or intestines, which can be fatal. These reactions can occur at any time during use and without warning symptoms. Elderly patients are at higher risk for serious GI events.

Cardiovascular (CV) risk: Nonsteroidal anti-inflammatory drugs (NSAIDs) may cause an increased risk of serious CV thrombotic events, myocardial infarction (MI), and stroke, which can be fatal. This risk may increase with duration of use. Patients with CV disease or risk factors for CV disease may be at higher risk.

Celecoxib, diclofenac, fenoprofen, flurbiprofen, ibuprofen, indomethacin, mefenamic acid, meloxicam, nabumetone, naproxen (except for controlled-release tablets), oxaprozin, piroxicam, sulindac, and tolmetin are contraindicated for the treatment of perioperative pain in the setting of coronary artery bypass graft (CABG) surgery.

continued on next page

Warning: (cont.)

GI risk: NSAIDs, including celecoxib, cause an increased risk of serious GI adverse reactions, including bleeding, ulceration, and perforation of the stomach or intestines, which can be fatal. These reactions can occur at any time during use and without warning symptoms. Elderly patients are at higher risk for serious GI events.

Ketorolac: Ketorolac tromethamine is indicated for the short-term (up to 5 days in adults) management of moderately severe short-term pain that requires analgesia at the opioid level. It is not indicated for minor or long-term painful conditions. Increasing the dose of ketorolac tromethamine beyond the label recommendations will not provide better efficacy but will result in increasing the risk of developing serious adverse reactions.

GI effects – Ketorolac tromethamine is contraindicated in patients with active peptic ulcer disease, in patients with recent GI bleeding or perforation, and in patients with a history of peptic ulcer disease or GI bleeding.

Renal effects – Ketorolac tromethamine is contraindicated in patients with advanced renal function impairment or in patients at risk for renal failure due to volume depletion.

Risk of bleeding – Ketorolac tromethamine inhibits platelet function and is contraindicated in patients with suspected or confirmed cerebrovascular bleeding, hemorrhagic diathesis, incomplete hemostasis, and in those at high risk of bleeding.

Ketorolac tromethamine is contraindicated as prophylactic analgesic before any major surgery and is contraindicated intraoperatively when hemostasis is critical because of the increased risk of bleeding.

Hypersensitivity – Ketorolac tromethamine is contraindicated in patients with previously demonstrated hypersensitivity to ketorolac tromethamine or allergic manifestations to aspirin or other NSAIDs.

Labor, delivery, and breast-feeding – Ketorolac tromethamine is contraindicated in labor and delivery because, through its prostaglandin synthesis inhibitory effect, it may adversely affect fetal circulation and inhibit uterine contractions.

The use of ketorolac tromethamine is contraindicated in breast-feeding mothers because of the potential adverse reactions of prostaglandin-inhibiting drugs on neonates.

Concomitant use with NSAIDs – Ketorolac tromethamine is contraindicated in patients currently receiving aspirin or NSAIDs because of the cumulative risks of inducing serious NSAID-related adverse reactions.

Dosage and administration – Oral ketorolac tromethamine is indicated only as continuation therapy to intravenous (IV)/intramuscular (IM) ketorolac tromethamine, and the combined duration of use of IV/IM ketorolac tromethamine and oral ketorolac tromethamine is not to exceed 5 days.

Indications

NSAIDs: Summary of Indications																						
Indications	Celecoxib	Diclofenac potassium	Diclofenac sodium/ Diclofenac sodium XR	Etodolac	Fenoprofen	Flurbiprofen	Ibuprofen	Ibuprofen injection	Indomethacin	Indomethacin SR	Ketoprofen	Ketoprofen SR	Ketorolac	Meclofenamate	Mefenamic acid	Meloxicam	Nabumetone	Naproxen	Oxaprozin	Piroxicam	Sulindac	Tolmetin
Rheumatoid arthritis (RA)	✔	✔	✔	✔	✔	✔	✔		✔	✔	✔	✔		✔			✔	✔	✔	✔	✔	✔
Osteoarthritis (OA)	✔	✔	✔	✔	✔	✔	✔		✔	✔	✔	✔		✔		✔	✔	✔	✔	✔	✔	✔
Ankylosing spondylitis (AS)		✔	✔[a]						✔	✔								✔			✔	
Mild to moderate pain		✔		✔	✔		✔							✔	✔[b]							
Pain	✔			✔				✔[g]			✔		✔[c]					✔				
Primary dysmenorrhea	✔	✔					✔				✔			✔	✔			✔				
Juvenile RA	✔			✔														✔				✔
Tendinitis									✔	✔								✔			✔	
Bursitis									✔	✔								✔			✔	
Short-term painful shoulder									✔	✔											✔	
Short-term gout									✔									✔			✔	
Fever							✔[d]	✔														
Familial adenomatous polyposis (FAP)	✔																					
Migraine																						
Closure of persistent patent ductus arteriosus									✔[e]													
Short-term attacks with or without aura		✔[f]																				

[a] Sodium only, not sodium XR.
[b] Therapy not to exceed 1 week.
[c] Therapy not to exceed 5 days.
[d] In children only.
[e] IV formulation only.
[f] Diclofenac oral solution is not indicated for the prophylactic therapy of migraine. The safety and effectiveness of diclofenac oral solution have not been established for cluster headache, which is present in an older, predominantly male population.
[g] IV formulation. For the management of mild to moderate pain and the management of moderate to severe pain as an adjunct to opioid analgesics in adults.

RA (except **ketorolac, mefenamic acid**) *and* OA (*except* **ketorolac** *and* **mefenamic acid**): Relief of signs and symptoms; treatment of short-term flares and exacerbation; long-term management.

Concomitant therapy – Concomitant therapy with other second-line drugs (eg, gold salts) demonstrates additional therapeutic benefit.

Use with salicylates is not recommended. The use of aspirin with NSAIDs may cause a decrease in blood levels of the nonaspirin drug.

Short-term gouty arthritis: **Indomethacin** (except ER formulation).

Mild to moderate pain (**diclofenac potassium, etodolac, fenoprofen, ibuprofen, ketoprofen, ketorolac, meclofenamate, mefenamic acid, naproxen, naproxen sodium**): Postextraction dental pain, postsurgical episiotomy pain, and soft tissue athletic injuries.

Idiopathic heavy menstrual blood loss: **Meclofenamate sodium.**

FAP (**celecoxib**): To reduce the number of adenomatous colorectal polyps in FAP as an adjunct to usual care (eg, endoscopic surveillance, surgery).

Administration and Dosage

CELECOXIB: See Warning Box at the beginning of the NSAIDs group monograph.

AS – 200 mg daily, single (once daily) or divided (twice daily) doses. If no effect is observed after 6 weeks, a trial of 400 mg daily may be worthwhile.

FAP – 400 mg twice daily with food.

OA – 200 mg/day administered as a single dose or as 100 mg twice a day.

RA – 100 to 200 mg twice a day.

Juvenile RA –

2 years of age and older and 10 to 25 kg: 50 mg capsule twice daily.

More than 25 kg: 100 mg capsule twice daily.

Method of administration: For patients who have difficulty swallowing capsules, the contents can be added to applesauce. The entire capsule contents are carefully emptied onto a level teaspoon of cool or room temperature applesauce and ingested immediately with water. The sprinkled capsule contents on applesauce are stable for up to 6 hours under refrigerated conditions (2° to 8°C [35° to 45°F]).

Short-term pain and primary dysmenorrhea – 400 mg initially, followed by an additional 200 mg dose if needed on the first day. On subsequent days, the recommended dosage is 200 mg twice daily as needed.

Renal function impairment – Not recommended in patients with severe renal function impairment.

Hepatic function impairment – In patients with moderate hepatic impairment (Child-Pugh class B), the daily dose should be reduced by approximately 50%. The use of celecoxib is not recommended in patients with severe hepatic impairment.

DICLOFENAC: See Warning Box at the beginning of the NSAIDs group monograph.

OA –

Delayed-release and as potassium: 100 to 150 mg/day in divided doses (50 mg twice/day or 3 times/day [diclofenac sodium or potassium] or 75 mg twice/day [diclofenac sodium]). Dosages greater than 200 mg/day have not been studied.

Extended-release: 100 mg/day.

RA –

Delayed-release and as potassium: 150 to 200 mg/day in divided doses (50 mg 3 or 4 times/day [diclofenac sodium or potassium] or 75 mg twice/day [diclofenac sodium]). Dosages greater than 225 mg/day of diclofenac potassium.

Extended-release: 100 mg/day. In the rare patient where diclofenac 100 mg/day extended-release tablets are unsatisfactory, the dose may be increased to 100 mg twice daily if the benefits outweigh the clinical risks of increased adverse reactions.

AS –

Immediate-release: 50 mg twice daily (range, 100 to 125 mg/day).

Delayed-release: 100 to 125 mg/day as 25 mg 4 times/day, with an extra 25 mg dose at bedtime if necessary.

Analgesia and primary dysmenorrhea (diclofenac potassium only) – 50 mg 3 times/day; 25 mg 4 times daily (oral capsules only). In some patients, an initial dose of 100 mg followed by 50 mg doses will provide better relief. After the first day, when the maximum recommended dose may be 200 mg, the total daily dose generally should not exceed 150 mg.

Migraine –

Oral solution: Administer 1 packet (50 mg) for the short-term treatment of migraine.

Interchangeability – Different formulations of oral diclofenac are not bioequivalent even if the milligram strength is the same.

Powder for oral solution – Advise patients to empty the contents of 1 packet into a cup containing 1 to 2 ounces (30 to 60 mL) of water, mix well, and drink immediately. Do not use liquids other than water. Administration of diclofenac oral solution with food may cause a reduction in effectiveness compared with administration on an empty stomach.

ETODOLAC:

Capsules and tablets –

Analgesia: For short-term pain, up to 1,000 mg, given as 200 to 400 mg every 6 to 8 hours.

OA and RA: 300 mg 2 times a day or 3 times a day, 400 mg 2 times a day, or 500 mg 2 times a day.

Extended-release tablets –

Juvenile RA	
Body weight range (kg)	Dose
20 to 30 kg	400 mg tablet × 1
31 to 45 kg	600 mg tablet × 1
46 to 60 kg	400 mg tablet × 2
> 60 kg	500 mg tablet × 2

RA and OA: 400 to 1,000 mg, given once daily, up to a maximum dose of 1,200 mg/day.

FENOPROFEN: See Warning Box at the beginning of the NSAIDs group monograph. Do not exceed 3.2 g/day. If GI upset occurs, take with meals or milk.

RA and OA – 400 to 600 mg 3 or 4 times/day.

Analgesia – 200 mg every 4 to 6 hours, as needed.

FLURBIPROFEN: See Warning Box at the beginning of the NSAIDs group monograph.

RA and OA – Initial total daily dose is 200 to 300 mg; administer in divided doses 2, 3, or 4 times/day. The largest recommended single dose is 100 mg. Doses greater than 300 mg/day are not recommended.

IBUPROFEN: See Warning Box at the beginning of the NSAIDs group monograph.

OTC –

Adults:

Capsules – Administer 2 capsules with a glass of water.

Gelcaps and tablets – Administer 1 gelcap or tablet every 4 to 6 hours while symptoms persist. If pain or fever does not respond, 2 gelcaps or tablets may be used, not to exceed 6 gelcaps or tablets in 24 hours, unless directed by a health care provider.

Children:

Chewable tablets, junior strength chewable tablets – If needed, repeat dose every 6 to 8 hours. It is not recommended to take more than 4 times a day.

50 mg chewable tablets:

Children weighing less than 36 pounds or younger than 4 years of age, consult a health care provider.

Children 36 to 47 pounds or 4 to 5 years of age: 3 tablets (150 mg).

Children 48 to 59 pounds or 6 to 8 years of age: 4 tablets (200 mg).

Children 60 to 71 pounds or 9 to 10 years of age: 5 tablets (250 mg).

Children 72 to 95 pounds or 11 years of age: 6 tablets (300 mg).

Junior strength 100 mg chewable tablets:

Children weighing less than 48 pounds and younger than 6 years of age: consult a health care provider.

Children 48 to 59 pounds or 6 to 8 years of age: 2 tablets (200 mg).

Children 60 to 71 pounds or 9 to 10 years of age: 2.5 tablets (250 mg).

Children 72 to 95 pounds or 11 years of age: 3 tablets (300 mg).

Oral suspension – 7.5 mg/kg of body weight.

Children weighing less than 24 pounds or younger than 2 years of age, consult a health care provider.

Children 24 to 35 pounds or 2 to 3 years of age: 1 teaspoonful (100 mg).

Children 36 to 47 pounds or 4 to 5 years of age: 1.5 teaspoonfuls (150 mg).

Children 48 to 59 pounds or 6 to 8 years of age: 2 teaspoonfuls (200 mg).

Children 60 to 71 pounds or 9 to 10 years of age: 2.5 teaspoonfuls (250 mg).

Children 72 to 95 pounds or 11 years of age: 3 teaspoonfuls (300 mg).

Oral suspension and oral drops – Shake well before using.

Oral drops:

Children weighing less than 24 pounds or younger than 6 months of age: consult a health care provider.

Children 12 to 17 pounds or 6 to 11 months of age: 1.25 mL (50 mg).

Children 18 to 23 pounds or 12 to 23 months of age: 1.875 mL (75 mg).

Rx – Do not exceed a 3,200 mg total daily dose. If GI complaints occur, administer ibuprofen tablets with meals or milk.

RA and OA, including flareups of long-term disease:

Suggested dosage – 1,200 mg to 3,200 mg daily (300 mg 4 times daily; 400, 600, or 800 mg 3 or 4 times daily).

Mild to moderate pain – 400 mg every 4 to 6 hours as necessary for relief of pain.

Dysmenorrhea – Beginning with the earliest onset of pain, give ibuprofen in a dose of 400 mg every 4 hours as necessary for the relief of pain.

Injection –

Fever:

Usual dosage – 400 mg IV followed by 400 mg IV every 4 to 6 hours or 100 to 200 mg IV every 4 hours as necessary.

Maximum dose – 3,200 mg/day.

Pain:

Usual dosage – 400 to 800 mg IV every 6 hours as necessary.

Maximum dose – 3,200 mg/day.

INDOMETHACIN: See Warning Box at the beginning of the NSAIDs group monograph.

Always give indomethacin capsules, oral suspension, and ER capsules with food, immediately after meals, or with antacids to reduce gastric irritation.

Moderate to severe RA (including short-term flares of long-term disease), moderate to severe AS, and moderate to severe OA – 25 mg 2 or 3 times/day. If well tolerated, increase the daily dose by 25 or 50 mg at weekly intervals until a satisfactory response is obtained or until a daily dose of 150 to 200 mg is reached.

In patients who have persistent night pain or morning stiffness, giving a large dose, up to a maximum of 100 mg of the total daily dose at bedtime, either orally or by rectal suppositories, may help to relieve pain. The total daily dose should not exceed 200 mg.

In short-term flares of long-term RA, it may be necessary to increase the dosage by 25 or, if required, by 50 mg/day.

Short-term painful shoulder (bursitis or tendinitis) – 75 to 150 mg/day in 3 or 4 divided doses. Discontinue the drug after inflammation has been controlled for several days. Usual course of therapy is 7 to 14 days.

Short-term gouty arthritis – 50 mg 3 times/day until pain is tolerable, then rapidly reduce to complete cessation of the drug. Relief of pain usually has been reported within 2 to 4 hours. Tenderness and heat usually subside in 24 to 36 hours, and swelling gradually disappears in 3 to 5 days. Do not use sustained-release form.

Sustained-release form – Do not crush. The 75 mg sustained-release capsule can be taken once/day as an alternative to the 25 mg capsule 3 times/day. However, there will be significant differences between the 2 dosing regimens in indomethacin blood levels, especially after 12 hours. One 75 mg sustained-release capsule twice/day can be substituted for the 50 mg capsule 3 times/day. Do not use sustained-release form in short-term gouty arthritis.

Children – Efficacy in children 14 years of age and younger has not been established. When using in children 2 years of age and older, closely monitor liver function. Suggested starting dose is 2 mg/kg/day in divided doses. Do not exceed 4 mg/kg/day or 150 to 200 mg/day, whichever is less.

KETOPROFEN: Take with antacids, food, or milk to minimize adverse GI reactions.

RA and OA – Do not exceed 300 mg/day for regular-release formulation or 200 mg/day for extended-release capsules.

Daily dose: 150 to 300 mg divided into 3 or 4 doses.

Starting dose: 75 mg 3 times/day or 50 mg 4 times/day. Reduce initial dose to one-half to one-third in elderly or debilitated patients or those with renal function impairment.

Mild to moderate pain, primary dysmenorrhea – 25 to 50 mg every 6 to 8 hours as needed. Give smaller dosages initially to smaller patients, the elderly, and those with renal or liver disease. Doses above 50 mg may be given, but doses above 75 mg do not display added therapeutic effects. Do not exceed 300 mg/day.

KETOROLAC TROMETHAMINE: See Warning Box at the beginning of the NSAIDs group monograph.

The combined duration of IV/IM and oral ketorolac is not to exceed 5 days. Oral use is only indicated as continuation therapy to IV/IM.

IV/IM – When administering IV/IM, the IV bolus must be given over no less than 15 seconds. Give IM administration slowly and deeply into the muscle.

Single-dose treatment:

Younger than 65 years of age – One 60 mg dose (IM); one 30 mg dose (IV).

65 years of age and older, renal function impairment, or weight less than 50 kg (110 lbs) – One 30 mg dose (IM); one 15 mg dose (IV).

Multiple-dose treatment:

Younger than 65 years of age – The recommended dose is 30 mg every 6 hours. The maximum daily dose should not exceed 120 mg.

65 years of age and older, renal function impairment, or weight less than 50 kg (110 lbs) – The recommended dose is 15 mg every 6 hours. The maximum daily dose should not exceed 60 mg.

Oral – Indicated only as continuation therapy to ketorolac IV/IM.

Transition from IV/IM to oral:

Younger than 65 years of age – 20 mg as a first oral dose for patients who received 60 mg IM single dose, 30 mg single IV dose, or 30 mg multiple dose IV/IM followed by 10 mg every 4 to 6 hours, not to exceed 40 mg in 24 hours.

65 years of age and older, renal function impairment, or weight less than 50 kg (110 lbs) – 10 mg as a first oral dose for patients who received a 30 mg IM single dose, 15 mg IV single dose, or 15 mg multiple dose IV/IM followed by 10 mg every 4 to 6 hours, not to exceed 40 mg in 24 hours.

MECLOFENAMATE SODIUM:

Mild to moderate pain – 50 mg every 4 to 6 hours; 100 mg may be required for optimal pain relief. Do not exceed daily dosage of 400 mg.

Excessive menstrual blood loss and primary dysmenorrhea – 100 mg 3 times/day for up to 6 days, starting at the onset of menstrual flow.

RA and OA –

Usual dosage: 200 to 400 mg/day in 3 or 4 equal doses.

Initial dosage: Initiate at lower dosage; increase as needed. Do not exceed 400 mg/day.

Children – Safety and efficacy in children younger than 14 years of age are not established.

MEFENAMIC ACID: See Warning Box at the beginning of the NSAIDs group monograph.

Short-term pain –

Adults (14 years of age and older): 500 mg, then 250 mg every 6 hours, as needed, usually not to exceed 1 week. Give with food.

Primary dysmenorrhea – 500 mg, then 250 mg every 6 hours. Start with the onset of bleeding and associated symptoms. Should not be necessary for longer than 2 to 3 days.

Children – Safety and efficacy in children younger than 14 years of age have not been established.

MELOXICAM: See Warning Box at the beginning of the NSAIDs group monograph.

Meloxicam may be taken without regard to meals.

Arthritis – Use the lowest dosage. The recommended starting and maintenance dose is 7.5 mg once/day. Some patients may receive additional benefit by increasing the dose to 15 mg once/day. The maximum recommended dose is 15 mg/day.

Meloxicam oral suspension may be substituted for meloxicam tablets. Shake suspension well before using.

Pauciarticular/polyarticular course juvenile RA – The recommended oral dose of meloxicam is 0.125 mg/kg once daily, up to a maximum of 7.5 mg.

Oral Suspension Juvenile RA Dosing Based on Weight		
	0.125 mg/kg	
Weight	Dose (1.5 mg/mL)	Delivered dose
12 kg (26 lbs)	1 mL	1.5 mg
24 kg (54 lbs)	2 mL	3 mg
36 kg (80 lbs)	3 mL	4.5 mg
48 kg (106 lbs)	4 mL	6 mg
≥ 60 kg (132 lbs)	5 mL	7.5 mg

NABUMETONE: See Warning Box at the beginning of the NSAIDs group monograph.

Recommended starting dose is 1,000 mg as a single dose with or without food. May be given either once or twice/day. Dosages greater than 2,000 mg/day have not been studied.

Renal function impairment – The maximum starting dosage of nabumetone in patients with moderate or severe renal function impairment should not exceed 750 or 500 mg, respectively, once daily. Following careful monitoring, daily doses may be increased to a maximum of 1,500 and 1,000 mg, respectively.

NAPROXEN: See Warning Box at the beginning of the NSAIDs group monograph.

Rx – Do not exceed 1.25 g/day naproxen (1.375 g/day naproxen sodium).

RA, OA, AS, pain, dysmenorrhea, short-term tendinitis, and bursitis:

Naproxen – 250 to 500 mg twice/day. May increase to 1.5 g/day for limited periods.

Delayed-release naproxen – 375 to 500 mg twice/day. Do not break, crush, or chew tablets.

Controlled-release naproxen – 750 mg or 1,500 mg once/day. Do not exceed 1,000 mg/day.

Naproxen sodium – 275 to 550 mg twice/day. May increase to 1.65 g for limited periods.

Juvenile arthritis:

Naproxen only (not naproxen sodium) – Total daily dose is approximately 10 mg/kg in 2 divided doses.

Suspension: Use the following as a guide:

Naproxen Suspension: Children's Dose	
Child's weight	Dose
13 kg (29 lb)	2.5 mL (0.5 tsp) twice a day
25 kg (55 lb)	5 mL (1 tsp) twice a day
38 kg (84 lb)	7.5 mL (1.5 tsp) twice a day

Short-term gout:

Naproxen – 750 mg, followed by 250 mg every 8 hours until attack subsides.

Naproxen sodium – 825 mg, then 275 mg every 8 hours until attack subsides.

Controlled-release naproxen – 1,000 to 1,500 mg once/day on the first day, followed by 1,000 mg once/day until the attack has subsided.

Mild to moderate pain, primary dysmenorrhea, short-term tendinitis, and bursitis:

Naproxen – 500 mg, followed by 250 mg every 6 to 8 hours. Do not exceed a 1.25 g total daily dose. Total daily dose should not exceed 1,000 mg.

Naproxen sodium – 550 mg, followed by 275 mg every 6 to 8 hours. Do not exceed a 1.375 g total daily dose.

Controlled-release naproxen – 1,000 mg once daily; 1,500 mg/day may be used for a limited period.

Children: Safety and efficacy in children younger than 2 years of age have not been established.

OTC –

Adults: 200 mg with a full glass of liquid every 8 to 12 hours while symptoms persist. An initial dose of 400 mg followed by 200 mg 12 hours later may give better relief. Do not exceed 600 mg in 24 hours unless otherwise directed.

Elderly (older than 65 years of age): Do not take more than 200 mg every 12 hours.

Children: Do not give to children younger than 12 years of age except under the advice and supervision of a health care provider.

OXAPROZIN: See Warning Box at the beginning of the NSAIDs group monograph.

RA – 1,200 mg once/day.

OA – 1,200 mg once/day. For patients of low body weight or with milder disease, an initial dosage of 600 mg once/day may be appropriate.

Maximum dose – 1,800 mg/day (or 26 mg/kg, whichever is lower) in divided doses.

PIROXICAM: See Warning Box at the beginning of the NSAIDs group monograph.

Initiate and maintain at a single daily dose of 20 mg. May divide daily dose. Do not assess effect of therapy for 2 weeks.

Children – Use in children has not been established.

SULINDAC: See Warning Box at the beginning of the NSAIDs group monograph.

Administer twice/day with food. The usual maximum dosage is 400 mg/day. Dosages above 400 mg/day are not recommended.

OA, RA, and AS – Initial dosage is 150 mg twice a day.

Short-term painful shoulder (short-term subacromial bursitis/supraspinatus tendinitis) and short-term gouty arthritis – 200 mg twice/day. After satisfactory response, reduce dosage accordingly.

Children – Safety and efficacy have not been established.

TOLMETIN SODIUM: See Warning Box at the beginning of the NSAIDs group monograph.

Adults –

RA and OA: Initially, 400 mg 3 times/day; preferably, include dose on arising and at bedtime. Doses more than 1,800 mg/day are not recommended.

Children (2 years of age and older) – Initially, 20 mg/kg/day in 3 or 4 divided doses. When control is achieved, usual dosage ranges from 15 to 30 mg/kg/day. Doses more than 30 mg/kg/day are not recommended.

Actions

Pharmacology: NSAIDs have analgesic, antipyretic, and anti-inflammatory activities. The major mechanism is believed to be inhibition of cyclooxygenase (COX) activity and prostaglandin synthesis.

Two COX isoenzymes have been identified: COX-1 and COX-2. Inhibition of COX-1 activity is considered a major contributor to NSAID GI toxicity. The function of the COX-2 isoenzyme is induced during pain and inflammatory stimuli.

Many NSAIDs inhibit COX-1 and COX-2. Most NSAIDs are mainly COX-1 selective (eg, **aspirin**, **indomethacin**, **ketoprofen**, **piroxicam**, **sulindac**). Others are considered slightly selective for COX-1 (eg, **ibuprofen**, **naproxen**, **diclofenac**) and others may be considered slightly selective for COX-2 (eg, **etodolac**, **nabumetone**). The mechanism of action of **celecoxib** is primarily selective inhibition of COX-2.

Pharmacokinetics:

Pharmacokinetic Parameters/Maximum Dosage Recommendations of NSAIDs

NSAID	Bioavailability (%)	Half-life (hours)	Peak (hours)	Protein binding (%)
Acetic acids				
Diclofenac	50 to 60	2	2	> 99
Indomethacin	98	4.5	2	90
Sulindac	90	7.8	2 to 4	> 93
Tolmetin	NS[a]	2 to 7	0.5 to 1	NS[a]
COX-2 inhibitors				
Celecoxib	NS[a]	11	3	97
Fenamates				
Meclofenamate	≈ 100	1.3	0.5 to 2	> 99
Mefenamic acid	NS[a]	2	2 to 4	> 90
Naphthylalkanones				
Nambumetone	> 80	22.5	9 to 12	> 99
Oxicams				
Piroxicam	NS[a]	50	3 to 5	98.5
Meloxicam	89	15 to 20	4 to 5	99.4
Propionic acids				
Fenoprofen	NS[a]	3	2	99
Flurbiprofen	NS[a]	5.7	≈ 1.5	> 99
Ibuprofen	> 80	1.8 to 2	1 to 2	99
Ketoprofen	90	2.1	0.5 to 2	> 99
Ketoprofen ER	90	5.4	6 to 7	> 99
Naproxen	95	12 to 17	2 to 4	> 99
Oxaprozin	95	42 to 50	3 to 5	> 99
Pyranocarboxylic acid				
Etodolac	≥ 80	7.3	≈ 1.5	> 99
Pyrrolizine carboxylic acid				
Ketorolac	100	5 to 6	2 to 3	99

[a] NS = Not studied.

Contraindications

NSAID hypersensitivity: Because of potential cross-sensitivity to other NSAIDs, do not give these agents to patients in whom aspirin or other NSAIDs have induced symptoms of asthma, rhinitis, urticaria, nasal polyps, angioedema, bronchospasm, and other symptoms of allergic or anaphylactoid reactions.

Fenoprofen or mefenamic acid: Pre-existing renal disease.

Mefenamic acid: Active ulceration or long-term inflammation of the upper or lower GI tract.

Celecoxib: Hypersensitivity to sulfonamides.

Ketorolac: Active peptic ulcer disease; recent GI bleeding or perforation; history of peptic ulcer disease or GI bleeding; advanced renal function impairment or patients at risk for renal failure because of volume depletion; labor and delivery; breast-feeding mothers; previously demonstrated hypersensitivity to ketorolac tromethamine; as prophylactic analgesic before any major surgery; intraoperatively when hemostasis is critical because of the increased risk of bleeding; suspected or confirmed cerebrovascular bleeding, hemorrhagic diathesis, incomplete hemostasis, and those at high risk of bleeding; patients currently receiving aspirin or NSAIDs because of the cumulative risks of inducing serious NSAID-related adverse reactions; for neuraxial (epidural or intrathecal) administration; concomitant use with probenecid. Severe, rarely fatal anaphylactic-like and asthmatic reactions have been reported in such patients receiving NSAIDs.

Warnings/Precautions

Ketorolac tromethamine: See Warning Box at the beginning of the monograph.

GI effects: Serious GI toxicity, such as bleeding, ulceration, and perforation, can occur at any time, with or without warning symptoms, in patients treated with NSAID therapy long term. Higher doses of **meloxicam** (eg, 30 mg/day) were associated with increased risk of serious GI effects; do not exceed daily doses of 15 mg.

If diarrhea occurs with **mefenamic acid** or diarrhea, GI irritation, and abdominal pain occur with **meclofenamate**, reduce dosage or temporarily discontinue use. Some patients may be unable to tolerate further therapy with these agents.

CNS effects: **Indomethacin** may aggravate depression or other psychiatric disturbances, epilepsy, and parkinsonism. Some of these agents may also cause headaches (highest incidence with **fenoprofen**, **indomethacin**, **ketorolac**, and **celecoxib**).

Steroid dosage: If reduced or eliminated during therapy, reduce slowly and observe patient closely for evidence of adverse reactions, including adrenal insufficiency and exacerbation of symptoms.

Porphyria: Avoid the use of NSAIDs in patients with hepatic porphyria.

Platelet aggregation: NSAIDs can inhibit platelet aggregation; the effect is quantitatively less and of shorter duration than that seen with aspirin. These agents prolong bleeding time in healthy subjects.

Preexisting asthma: Because cross-reactivity, including bronchospasm, between aspirin and other NSAIDs has been reported in such aspirin-sensitive patients, do not administer NSAIDs to patients with this form of aspirin sensitivity, and use the drug with caution in patients with preexisting asthma.

Hematologic effects: Decreased hemoglobin or hematocrit levels rarely have required discontinuation.

Aseptic meningitis: Aseptic meningitis with fever and coma has been observed on rare occasions in patients on NSAIDs therapy, although it is probably more likely to occur in patients with systemic lupus erythematosus.

CV effects: May cause fluid retention and peripheral edema. Use caution in compromised cardiac function, hypertension, in patients on long-term diuretic therapy, or other conditions predisposing to fluid retention. Agents may be associated with significant deterioration of circulatory hemodynamics in severe heart failure and hyponatremia.

Ophthalmologic effects: Effects include blurred or diminished vision, scotomata, changes in color vision, corneal deposits, and retinal disturbances, including maculas.

Infection: NSAIDs may mask the usual signs of infection.

Renal effects: Short-term renal insufficiency, interstitial nephritis with hematuria, nephrotic syndrome, proteinuria, hyperkalemia, hyponatremia, renal papillary necrosis, and other renal medullary changes may occur.

Hepatic effects: Borderline liver function test elevations may occur in about 15% of patients and may progress, remain essentially unchanged, or become transient with continued therapy.

Pancreatitis: Pancreatitis has occurred in patients receiving **sulindac**.

Auditory effects: Perform periodic auditory function tests during long-term **fenoprofen** therapy in patients with impaired hearing.

Heavy menstrual blood loss evaluation: Prior to prescribing **meclofenamate** for heavy blood flow and primary dysmenorrhea, make a thorough risk/benefit assessment.

Dermatologic effects: Promptly discontinue **mefenamic acid** if rash occurs. A combination of dermatologic and allergic signs and symptoms suggestive of serum sickness occasionally have occurred in conjunction with the use of **piroxicam**.

Concomitant therapy: Do not use **naproxen sodium** and **naproxen** concomitantly; both drugs circulate as naproxen anion.

Do not use **diclofenac** immediate-release, delayed-release, or extended-release tablets concomitantly with other diclofenac-containing products because they also circulate in plasma as diclofenac anion.

Hypersensitivity reactions: A potentially fatal apparent hypersensitivity syndrome has occurred with **sulindac**.

Anaphylactoid reactions have occurred in patients without known exposure to NSAIDs, but they typically occur in asthmatic patients who experience rhinitis with or without nasal polyps, or who exhibit severe, potentially fatal bronchospasm after taking aspirin or other NSAIDs.

Renal function impairment: NSAID metabolites are eliminated primarily by kidneys; use with caution in those with renal function impairment. In cases of advanced kidney disease, treatment with **piroxicam** and **meloxicam** is not recommended. Reduce dosage to avoid excessive accumulation.

Use **sulindac** with caution in patients with a history of renal lithiasis and keep patients well hydrated while receiving the drug.

Hepatic function impairment: Dose reduction may be needed with **naproxen**. Use caution in patients with hepatic function impairment or a history of liver disease.

Photosensitivity: Photosensitivity may occur.

Pregnancy: Category B (**diclofenac, fenoprofen, flurbiprofen, ibuprofen, indomethacin, ketoprofen, meclofenamate, naproxen, naproxen sodium, sulindac**). *Category C* (**celecoxib, etodolac, ketorolac, mefenamic acid, meloxicam, nabumetone, oxaprozin, piroxicam, tolmetin**). All NSAIDs are *Category D* if used in the third trimester or near delivery. Avoid during pregnancy, especially in the third trimester.

Lactation: Most NSAIDs are excreted in breast milk. In general, do not use in breastfeeding mothers because of effects on the infant's CV system.

Children: **Mefenamic acid** and **meclofenamate** are not recommended in children younger than 14 years of age. **Indomethacin** is not recommended in children 14 years of age and younger, except in circumstances that warrant the risk. Safety and efficacy of **meloxicam** has not been established in children younger than 18 years of age. **Celecoxib**, **tolmetin**, and **naproxen** are the only agents labeled for juvenile RA. Safety and efficacy of tolmetin in infants younger than 2 years of age are not established. Safety and efficacy of other NSAIDs in children are not established.

Elderly: Age appears to increase the possibility of adverse reactions to NSAIDs. The risk of serious ulcer disease is increased; this risk appears to increase with dose. **Ketorolac** is cleared more slowly in the elderly; use caution and reduce dosage.

Monitoring: Assess renal function before and during therapy. Monitor serum creatinine or creatinine clearance.

Drug Interactions

Drugs that affect NSAIDs include bisphosphonates, cholestyramine, cimetidine, colestipol, cyclosporine, diflunisal, dimethyl sulfoxide, fluconazole, ketoconazole, phenobarbital, phenylbutazone, probenecid, rifampin, ritonavir, salicylates, sucralfate.

Drugs that may be affected by NSAIDs include aminoglycosides, anticoagulants, ACE inhibitors, beta blockers, cyclosporine, dextromethorphan, digoxin, dipyridamole, hydantoins, lithium, loop diuretics, methotrexate, penicillamine, potassium-sparing diuretics, sympathomimetics, theophylline, thiazide diuretics.

Drug/Lab test interactions: Naproxen use may result in increased urinary values for 17-ketogenic steroids. Temporarily discontinue naproxen therapy 72 hours before adrenal function tests are performed.

Naproxen – Naproxen may interfere with some urinary assays of 5-hydroxy indoleacetic acid.

Tolmetin – Tolmetin metabolites in urine give positive tests for proteinuria using acid precipitation tests (eg, sulfosalicylic acid).

Mefenamic acid – A false-positive reaction for urinary bile, using the diazo tablet test, may result.

Fenoprofen – *Amerlex-M* kit assay values of total and free triiodothyronine in patients on fenoprofen have been reported as falsely elevated.

Oxaprozin – False-positive urine immunoassay screening tests for benzodiazepines have been reported in patients taking oxaprozin. False-positive test results may be expected for several days following discontinuation of oxaprozin therapy.

NSAIDs can prolong bleeding time by about 3 to 4 minutes by decreasing platelet adhesion and aggregation.

Drug/Food interactions: Administration of **tolmetin** with milk decreased total tolmetin bioavailability by 16%. When tolmetin was taken immediately after a meal, peak plasma concentrations were reduced by 50%, while total bioavailability was again decreased by 16%. Peak concentration of **etodolac** is reduced by about 50% and the time to peak is increased by 1.4 to 3.8 hours following administration with food; however, the extent of absorption is not affected. Food may reduce the rate of absorption of **oxaprozin**, but the extent is unchanged.

Adverse Reactions

Cardiovascular: Arrhythmias; CHF; fluid retention; hypertension (**ketorolac**); hypotension; palpitations; peripheral edema; tachycardia; vasodilation.

CNS: Asthenia (**etodolac, tolmetin**); dizziness (**diclofenac, fenoprofen, flurbiprofen, mefenamic acid, meloxicam, piroxicam**); fatigue (**indomethacin**); headache (**celecoxib, diclofenac, fenoprofen, flurbiprofen, ibuprofen, indomethacin, ketoprofen, ketorolac, meclofenamate, mefenamic acid, meloxicam, nabumetone, naproxen, piroxicam, sulindac, tolmetin**); insomnia (**meloxicam**); malaise (**etodolac**); somnolence/drowsiness (**fenoprofen, naproxen**).

Dermatologic: Alopecia; angioneurotic edema; desquamation; ecchymosis; eczema; hyperpigmentation; peeling; petechiae; pruritus (**nabumetone, naproxen**); purpura; rash/dermatitis, including maculopapular type (**ibuprofen, meclofenamate, mefenamic acid, meloxicam, nabumetone, oxaprozin, sulindac**); skin discoloration; skin eruptions (**naproxen**); skin irritation.

GI: Common GI adverse reactions include abdominal distress/cramps/pain; anorexia; constipation; diarrhea; dyspepsia; flatulence; nausea; stomatitis; vomiting.

Bleeding – Occult blood in the stool (**fenoprofen**).

Hepatic – Elevated liver enzymes (**mefenamic acid, piroxicam**).

Ulcer – Gastric or duodenal ulcer with bleeding or perforation (**mefenamic acid**).

Other – Epigastric pain (**ibuprofen**); gastritis (**etodolac**); GI distress (**tolmetin**); GI pain (**sulindac**); GI tract fullness (**ibuprofen**); gross bleeding (**mefenamic acid**); heartburn (**ibuprofen, meclofenamate, mefenamic acid, naproxen, piroxicam**); indigestion (**ibuprofen**); pyrosis (**meclofenamate**).

Hematologic: Agranulocytosis; aplastic anemia; bruising; ecchymosis, hemolysis (**naproxen**); eosinophilia; epistaxis; granulocytopenia; hemolytic anemia; hemorrhage; leukopenia; menorrhagia; neutropenia; pancytopenia; thrombocytopenia.

Metabolic: Decreased or increased appetite; flushing or sweating; glycosuria; hyperglycemia; hyperkalemia; hypoglycemia; hyponatremia; weight decrease or increase (**tolmetin**).

Renal: Anuria; azotemia; cystitis; dysuria; elevated BUN (**ketoprofen**); hematuria; nocturia; oliguria; polyuria; proteinuria; pyuria; urinary frequency; urinary tract infection (**flurbiprofen, meloxicam**).

Respiratory: Bronchospasm; dyspnea (**naproxen**); pharyngitis; rhinitis; shortness of breath; upper respiratory tract infection (**celecoxib, meloxicam**).

Special senses: Amblyopia; blurred vision; change in taste (metallic or bitter); conjunctivitis; diplopia; ear pain; hearing disturbances or loss; iritis; photophobia; reversible loss of color vision; swollen, dry, or irritated eyes; tinnitus.

Miscellaneous: Breast changes; edema (**flurbiprofen, meloxicam, naproxen**); facial edema; gynecomastia; impotence; influenza-like disease/symptoms (**meloxicam**); menstrual disorders; muscle cramps; pyrexia (fever and chills); sweating; thirst; vaginal bleeding.

AGENTS FOR GOUT

In addition to the agents in this section, sulindac and indomethacin (see Nonsteroidal Anti-inflammatory Agents monograph) and phenylbutazone and oxyphenbutazone (see individual monographs) are indicated for the treatment of gout.

PROBENECID

Tablets: 0.5 g (*Rx*)	Various, *Benemid* (Merck), *Probalan* (Lannett)

Indications

Hyperuricemia: Treatment of hyperuricemia associated with gout and gouty arthritis.

Plasma levels: Adjuvant to therapy with penicillins or cephalosporins, for elevation and prolongation of plasma levels of the antibiotic.

Administration and Dosage

Gout: Do not start therapy until an acute gouty attack has subsided. However, if an acute attack is precipitated during therapy, probenecid may be continued. Give full therapeutic doses of colchicine or other appropriate therapy to control the acute attack.

Adults – 0.25 g twice/day for 1 week; 0.5 g twice/day thereafter. Gastric intolerance may indicate overdosage, and may be reduced by decreasing dosage.

Renal impairment – Some degree of renal impairment may be present in patients with gout. A daily dosage of 1 g may be adequate. However, if necessary, the daily dosage may be increased by 0.5 g increments every 4 weeks within tolerance (usually not more than 2 g/day) if symptoms of gouty arthritis are not controlled or the 24 hour urate excretion is not more than 700 mg. Probenecid may not be effective in chronic renal insufficiency, particularly when the glomerular filtration rate is 30 mL/minute or less.

Urinary alkalinization – Urates tend to crystallize out of an acid urine; therefore, a liberal fluid intake is recommended, as well as sufficient sodium bicarbonate (3 to 7.5 g/day) or potassium citrate (7.5 g/day) to maintain an alkaline urine; continue alkalization until the serum uric acid level returns to normal limits and tophaceous deposits disappear. Thereafter, urinary alkalization and the restriction of purine-producing foods may be relaxed.

Maintenance therapy – Continue the dosage that maintains normal serum uric acid levels. When there have been no acute attacks for 6 months or more and serum uric acid levels have remained within normal limits, decrease the daily dosage by 0.5 g every 6 months. Do not reduce the maintenance dosage to the point where serum uric acid levels increase.

Penicillin or cephalosporin therapy: The PSP excretion test may be used to determine the effectiveness of probenecid in retarding penicillin excretion and maintaining therapeutic levels. The renal clearance of PSP is reduced to about the normal rate when dosage of probenecid is adequate.

Adults – 2 g/day in divided doses. Reduce dosage in older patients in whom renal impairment may be present. Not recommended in conjunction with penicillin or a cephalosporin in the presence of known renal impairment.

Children (2 to 14 years of age) – Initial dose 25 mg/kg or 0.7 g/m^2. Maintenance dose 40 mg/kg/day or 1.2 g/m^2, divided into 4 doses. For children weighing more than 50 kg (110 lb), use the adult dosage. Do not use in children younger than 2 years of age.

Gonorrhea (uncomplicated) – Give probenecid as a single 1g dose immediately before or with 4.8 million units penicillin G procaine, aqueous, divided into at least 2 doses.

Neurosyphilis – Aqueous procaine penicillin G, 2 to 4 million units/day IM plus probenecid 500 mg 4 times/day, both for 10 to 14 days.†

Pelvic inflammatory disease (PID) – Cefoxitin 2 g IM plus probenecid, 1 g orally in a single dose concurrently.

† CDC 1993 Sexually Transmitted Diseases Treatment Guidelines. MMWR. 1993;42 (No. RR-14).

Actions

Pharmacology: A uricosuric and renal tubular blocking agent, probenecid inhibits the tubular reabsorption of urate, thus increasing the urinary excretion of uric acid and decreasing serum uric acid levels.

Probenecid also inhibits the tubular secretion of most penicillins and cephalosporins and usually increases plasma levels by any route the antibiotic is given.

Pharmacokinetics: Probenecid is well absorbed after oral administration and produces peak plasma concentrations in 2 to 4 hours. It is highly protein bound (85% to 95%). Probenecid is excreted in the urine primarily as metabolites.

Contraindications

Hypersensitivity to probenecid; children younger than 2 years of age; blood dyscrasias or uric acid kidney stones. Do not start therapy until an acute gouty attack has subsided.

Warnings/Precautions

Exacerbation of gout: Exacerbation of gout following therapy with probenecid may occur; in such cases, colchicine or other appropriate therapy is advisable.

Salicylates: Use of salicylates is contraindicated in patients on probenecid therapy. Salicylates antagonize probenecid's uricosuric action.

Sulfa drug allergy: Probenecid is a sulfonamide; patients with a history of allergy to sulfa drugs may react to probenecid.

Alkalinization of urine: Hematuria, renal colic, costovertebral pain, and formation of urate stones associated with use in gouty patients may be prevented by alkalization of urine and liberal fluid intake; monitor acid-base balance.

Peptic ulcer history: Use with caution.

Hypersensitivity reactions: Rarely, severe allergic reactions and anaphylaxis have occurred. Most of these occur within several hours after readministration following prior use of the drug.

Renal function impairment: Dosage requirements may be increased in renal impairment. Probenecid may not be effective in chronic renal insufficiency, particularly when the glomerular filtration rate is 30 mL/minute or less. Probenecid is not recommended in conjunction with a penicillin in the presence of known renal impairment.

Pregnancy: Category B.

Children: Do not use in children younger than 2 years of age.

Drug Interactions

Drugs that may affect probenecid include salicylates.

Drugs that may be affected by probenecid include acyclovir; allopurinol; barbiturates; benzodiazepines; clofibrate; dapsone; dyphylline; methotrexate; NSAIDs; pantothenic acid; penicillamine; rifampin; sulfonamides; sulfonylureas; zidovudine; salicylates.

Drug/Lab test interactions: A reducing substance may appear in the urine during therapy. Although this disappears with discontinuation, a false diagnosis of glycosuria may be made. Confirm suspected glycosuria by using a test specific for glucose.

Falsely high determination of **theophylline** has occurred in vitro using the Schack and Waxler technique, when therapeutic concentrations of theophylline and probenecid were added to human plasma.

Probenecid may inhibit the renal excretion of: **Phenolsulfonphthalein (PSP)**, **17-ketosteroids**, and **sulfobromophthalein (BSP)**.

Adverse Reactions

Adverse reactions may include headache; anorexia; nausea; vomiting; urinary frequency; hypersensitivity reactions; sore gums; flushing; dizziness; anemia; hemolytic anemia (possibly related to G-6-PD deficiency); nephrotic syndrome; hepatic necrosis; aplastic anemia; exacerbation of gout; uric acid stones with or without hematuria; renal colic or costovertebral pain.

FEBUXOSTAT

Tablets; oral: 40 and 80 mg (*Rx*) *Uloric* (Takeda Pharmaceuticals America)

Indications

Hyperuricemia: For the chronic management of hyperuricemia in patients with gout.

Administration and Dosage

Testing for the target serum uric acid (SUA) level of less than 6 mg/dL may be performed as early as 2 weeks after initiating febuxostat therapy.

If a gout flare occurs during febuxostat treatment, febuxostat need not be discontinued.

May be taken without regard to food or antacid use.

Hyperuricemia:

Adults – Initial dosage is 40 mg once daily, with the usual dosage in the range of 40 to 80 mg once daily.

For patients who do not achieve a SUA level of less than 6 mg/dL after 2 weeks with 40 mg, febuxostat 80 mg is recommended.

Concomitant therapy: Gout flares may occur after initiation of febuxostat because of changing SUA levels, resulting in mobilization of urate from tissue deposits. Flare prophylaxis with a nonsteroidal anti-inflammatory drug (NSAID) or colchicine is recommended upon initiation of febuxostat. Prophylactic therapy may be beneficial for up to 6 months.

Actions

Pharmacology: Febuxostat, a xanthine oxidase inhibitor, achieves its therapeutic effect by decreasing SUA.

Pharmacokinetics:

Absorption – The absorption of febuxostat following oral dose administration was estimated to be at least 49%. C_{max} of febuxostat occurred between 1 and 1.5 hours postdose.

Distribution – The mean apparent steady-state volume of distribution was approximately 50 L. The plasma protein binding is approximately 99.2%.

Metabolism – Febuxostat is extensively metabolized by both conjugation via UGT enzymes, and oxidation via CYP-450 enzymes.

Excretion – Febuxostat is eliminated by both hepatic and renal pathways. The apparent mean terminal elimination half-life ($t_{½}$) of febuxostat was approximately 5 to 8 hours.

Contraindications

Patients being treated with azathioprine, mercaptopurine, or theophylline.

Warnings/Precautions

Gout flare: After initiation of febuxostat, an increase in gout flares is frequently observed. This increase is caused by reduction in SUA levels, resulting in mobilization of urate from tissue deposits.

In order to prevent gout flares when febuxostat is initiated, concurrent prophylactic treatment with an NSAID or colchicine is recommended.

Cardiovascular events: In the randomized, controlled studies, there was a higher rate of cardiovascular thromboembolic events (cardiovascular deaths, nonfatal myocardial infarctions (MIs), and nonfatal strokes) in patients treated with febuxostat than allopurinol. Monitor for signs and symptoms of MI and stroke.

Liver enzyme elevations: During randomized controlled studies, transaminase elevations greater than 3 times the upper limit of normal (ULN) were observed.

Renal function impairment: Exercise caution in patients with severe renal impairment (CrCl less than 30 mL/min).

Hepatic function impairment: Exercise caution in patients with severe hepatic impairment (Child-Pugh class C).

Special risk: No studies have been conducted in patients with secondary hyperuricemia (including organ transplant recipients); febuxostat is not recommended for use in patients in whom the rate of urate formation is greatly increased (eg, malignant disease and its treatment, Lesch-Nyhan syndrome). The concentration of xanthine in urine could, in rare cases, rise sufficiently to allow deposition in the urinary tract.

Pregnancy: Category C.

Lactation: It is not known whether this drug is excreted in human milk. Exercise caution when febuxostat is administered to a breast-feeding woman.

Children: Safety and effectiveness in children younger than 18 years of age have not been established.

Monitoring: Monitor for signs and symptoms of MI and stroke.

Laboratory assessment of liver function is recommended at, for example, 2 and 4 months following initiation of febuxostat and periodically thereafter.

Drug Interactions

Drugs that may interact with febuxostat include antacids, desipramine, and xanthine oxidase substrate drugs.

Adverse Reactions

The adverse reaction that occurred in 3% or more of patients was liver function abnormalities.

ALLOPURINOL

Tablets: 100 and 300 mg (*Rx*)	Various, *Zyloprim* (Prometheus)

Indications

Gout: Management of signs and symptoms of primary or secondary gout.

Malignancies: Management of patients with leukemia, lymphoma, and malignancies receiving therapy which causes elevations of serum and urinary uric acid. Discontinue allopurinol when the potential for overproduction of uric acid is no longer present.

Calcium oxalate calculi: Management of patients with recurrent calcium oxalate calculi whose daily uric acid excretion exceeds 800 mg/day (males) or 750 mg/day (females). Carefully assess therapy initially and periodically to determine that treatment is beneficial and that the benefits outweigh the risks.

Unlabeled uses: In a limited number of patients, the use of an allopurinol mouthwash (20 mg in 3% methylcellulose; 1 mg/mL) after fluorouracil administration prevented stomatitis, a major dose-limiting toxicity of fluorouracil. However, another report indicated that allopurinol mouthwash is not effective. Further study is needed.

Administration and Dosage

Control of gout and hyperuricemia: The average dose is 200 to 300 mg/day for mild gout and 400 to 600 mg/day for moderately severe tophaceous gout. Divide doses in excess of 300 mg. The minimum effective dose is 100 to 200 mg/day; the maximum recommended dose is 800 mg/day.

Children (6 to 10 years of age) – In secondary hyperuricemia associated with malignancy, give 300 mg/day; those younger than 6 years of age are generally given 150 mg/day. Evaluate response after approximately 48 hours of therapy and adjust dosage if necessary.

Another suggested dose is 1 mg/kg/day divided every 6 hours, to a maximum of 600 mg/day. After 48 hours of treatment, titrate dose according to serum uric acid levels.

Prevention of uric acid nephropathy during vigorous therapy of neoplastic disease: 600 to 800 mg/day for 2 to 3 days together with a high fluid intake. Similar considerations govern dosage regulation for maintenance purposes in secondary hyperuricemia.

To reduce the possibility of flare-up of acute gouty attacks: Start with 100 mg/day and increase at weekly intervals by 100 mg (without exceeding the maximum recommended dosage) until a serum uric acid level of 6 mg/dL or less is attained.

Serum uric acid levels: Normal serum urate levels are usually achieved in 1 to 3 weeks. The upper limit of normal is about 7 mg/dL for men and postmenopausal women and 6 mg/dL for premenopausal women. Do not rely on a single reading since estimation of uric acid may be difficult. By selecting the appropriate dose, and using uricosuric agents in certain patients, it is possible to reduce the serum uric acid level to normal and, if desired, to hold it as low as 2 to 3 mg/dL indefinitely.

Renal impairment: Accumulation of allopurinol and its metabolites can occur in renal failure; consequently, reduce the dose. With a Ccr of 10 to 20 mL/min, 200 mg/day is suitable. When the Ccr is less than 10 mL/min, do not exceed 100 mg/day. With extreme renal impairment (Ccr less than 3 mL/min) the interval between doses may also need to be increased. The correct dosage is best determined by using the serum uric acid level as an index.

Other suggested doses include: Ccr 60 mL/min, 200 mg/day; Ccr 40 mL/min, 15 mg/day; Ccr 20 mL/min, 100 mg/day; Ccr 10 mL/min, 100 mg on alternate days. Ccr less than 10 mL/min, 100 mg 3 times a week.

Concomitant therapy: In patients treated with colchicine or anti-inflammatory agents, continue therapy while adjusting the allopurinol dosage until a normal serum uric acid level and freedom from acute attacks have been maintained for several months.

Replacement therapy: In transferring a patient from a uricosuric agent to allopurinol, gradually reduce the dose of the uricosuric agent over several weeks and gradually increase the dose of allopurinol until a normal serum uric acid level is maintained.

Recurrent calcium oxalate stones: For hyperuricosuric patients, 200 to 300 mg/day in single or divided doses. Adjust dose up or down depending upon the resultant control of the hyperuricosuria based upon subsequent 24 hour urinary urate determinations. Patients may also benefit from dietary changes such as reduction of animal protein, sodium, refined sugars, oxalate-rich foods and excessive calcium intake as well as increase in oral fluids and dietary fiber.

Actions

Pharmacology: Allopurinol inhibits xanthine oxidase, the enzyme responsible for the conversion of hypoxanthine to xanthine to uric acid. Allopurinol acts on purine catabolism, reducing the production of uric acid, without disrupting the biosynthesis of vital purines.

Administration generally results in a fall in both serum and urinary uric acid within 2 to 3 days. The magnitude of this decrease is dose-dependent. One week or more of treatment may be required before the full effects of the drug are manifested; likewise, uric acid may return to pretreatment levels slowly following cessation of therapy.

Pharmacokinetics: Allopurinol is approximately 90% absorbed from the GI tract.

Effective xanthine oxidase inhibition is maintained over 24 hours with single daily doses. Allopurinol is cleared essentially by glomerular filtration; oxipurinol is reabsorbed in the kidney tubules in a manner similar to the reabsorption of uric acid.

Contraindications

Patients who have developed a severe reaction should not be restarted on the drug.

Warnings/Precautions

Asymptomatic hyperuricemia: Generally, do not use to treat asymptomatic hyperuricemia. Treatment should be considered with persistent hyperuricemia characterized by a serum urate concentration of greater than 13 mg/dL. High serum urate may be nephrotoxic.

Hepatotoxicity: A few cases of reversible clinical hepatotoxicity have occurred; in some patients, asymptomatic rises in serum alkaline phosphatase or serum transaminase levels have been observed. If anorexia, weight loss or pruritus develop in patients on allopurinol, evaluation of liver function should be part of their diagnostic workup. Perform periodic liver function tests during early stages of therapy.

Acute attacks of gout: Acute attacks of gout have increased during the early stages of allopurinol administration when normal or subnormal serum uric acid levels have been attained; in general, give maintenance doses of colchicine prophylactically when allopurinol is begun. In addition, start patient at a low dose of allopurinol (100 mg/day) and increase at weekly intervals by 100 mg until a serum uric acid level of 6 mg/dL or less is attained without exceeding the maximum recommended dose. The attacks usually become shorter and less severe after several months of therapy.

Fluid intake: Fluid intake sufficient to yield a daily urinary output of at least 2 L and the maintenance of a neutral or slightly alkaline urine are desirable to avoid the theoretical possibility of formation of xanthine calculi under the influence of allopurinol therapy and to help prevent renal precipitation of urates in patients receiving concomitant uricosurics.

Drowsiness: Drowsiness has occurred occasionally. Patients should observe caution while driving or performing other tasks requiring alertness, coordination, or physical dexterity.

Bone marrow depression: Bone marrow depression has occurred in patients receiving allopurinol, most of whom received concomitant drugs with the potential for causing this reaction. This has occurred as early as 6 weeks to as long as 6 years after the initiation of therapy. Rarely, a patient may develop varying degrees of bone marrow depression, affecting one or more cell lines, while receiving allopurinol alone.

Hypersensitivity reactions: Discontinue at first appearance of skin rash or other signs of allergic reactions. In some instances, rash may be followed by more severe hypersensitivity reactions such as exfoliative, urticarial or purpuric lesions, or Stevens-Johnson syndrome, generalized vasculitis, irreversible hepatotoxicity and rarely, death.

Renal function impairment: Some patients with preexisting renal disease or poor urate clearance have increased BUN during allopurinol administration. Patients with impaired renal function require less drug and careful observation during the early stages of treatment; reduce dosage or discontinue therapy if increased abnormalities in renal function appear and persist.

Renal failure in association with allopurinol has been observed among patients with hyperuricemia secondary to neoplastic diseases. Concurrent conditions such as multiple myeloma and congestive myocardial disease were present. Renal failure is also frequently associated with gouty nephropathy and rarely with allopurinol-associated hypersensitivity reactions. Albuminuria has occurred among patients who developed clinical gout following chronic glomerulonephritis and chronic pyelonephritis.

In patients with severely impaired renal function or decreased urate clearance, the plasma half-life of oxipurinol is greatly prolonged. A dose of 100 mg/day or 300 mg twice a week, or less, may be sufficient to maintain adequate xanthine oxidase inhibition to reduce serum urate levels.

Pregnancy: Category C.

Lactation: Allopurinol and oxipurinol have been found in breast milk. Exercise caution when administering to a nursing woman.

Children: Allopurinol is rarely indicated for use in children, with the exception of those with hyperuricemia secondary to malignancy or to certain rare inborn errors of purine metabolism.

Monitoring: Periodically determine liver and kidney function especially during the first few months of therapy. Perform BUN, serum creatinine, or Ccr and reassess the patient's dosage.

Drug Interactions

Drugs that may affect allopurinol include ACE inhibitors; aluminum salts; thiazide diuretics; uricosuric agents.

Drugs that may be affected by allopurinol include ampicillin; anticoagulants; cyclophosphamide; theophyllines; thiopurines.

Adverse Reactions

Adverse reactions may include skin rash; fever; chills; arthralgias; cholestatic jaundice; eosinophilia; mild leukocytosis; leukopenia; vesicular bullous dermatitis; eczematoid dermatitis; pruritus; urticaria; onycholysis; lichen planus; Stevens-Johnson syndrome; purpura; toxic epidermal necrolysis; nausea; vomiting; diarrhea; intermittent abdominal pain; gastritis; dyspepsia; increased alkaline phosphatase, AST and ALT; hepatomegaly; cholestatic jaundice; granulomatous hepatitis; hepatic necrosis; leukopenia; leukocytosis; eosinophilia; thrombocytopenia; headache; peripheral neuropathy; neuritis; paresthesia; somnolence; arthralgia; acute attacks of gout; ecchymosis; fever; myopathy; epistaxis; taste loss or perversion; renal failure; uremia; alopecia; hypersensitivity vasculitis; necrotizing angiitis.

COLCHICINE

Tablets: 0.6 mg (1/100 g) (*Rx*)	Various, *Colcrys* (AR Scientific)

Indications

Familial Mediterranean fever (Colcrys only): For the treatment of familial Mediterranean fever in adults and children 4 years of age and older.

Gout flares: For the prophylaxis and the treatment of acute gout flares when taken at the first sign of a flare.

Administration and Dosage

Adults:

Familial Mediterranean fever (Colcrys only) – 1.2 to 2.4 mg daily in 1 or 2 divided doses. Increase as needed in increments of 0.3 mg/day to a maximum recommended daily dose to control disease and as tolerated. If intolerable adverse effects develop, the dosage should be decreased in increments of 0.3 mg/day.

Prophylaxis of gout flares – 0.6 mg once or twice daily. The max dose is 1.2 mg/day.

The following dosing information is based on product labeling from non–FDA-approved colchicine products.

Less than 1 attack per year: 0.6 mg/day, 3 or 4 days a week.

More than 1 attack per year: 0.6 mg daily. Severe cases may require 1.2 or 1.8 mg daily.

Surgical patients: 0.6 mg 3 times daily for 3 days before and 3 days after surgery.

Treatment of gout flares – 1.2 mg at the first sign of the flare, followed by 0.6 mg 1 hour later. If also taking colchicine for prophylaxis of gout flares, wait 12 hours after taking the last dose for treatment of the flare, then resume prophylaxis dosage. The max dose is 1.8 mg over a 1-hour period.

The following dosing information is based on product labeling from non–FDA-approved colchicine products.

Initial dosage is 0.6 to 1.2 mg at the first sign of the flare, followed by 0.6 mg every hour or 1.2 mg every 2 hours until pain is relieved or until diarrhea ensues. After the initial dose, it is sometimes sufficient to take 0.6 mg every 2 or 3 hours. The drug should be stopped if there is GI discomfort or diarrhea. An interval of 3 days between colchicine courses is advised in order to minimize the possibility of cumulative toxicity.

Children:

Familial Mediterranean fever (Colcrys only) –

13 years of age and older: See Adults for dosing.

6 to 12 years of age – 0.9 to 1.8 mg daily in 1 or 2 divided doses. Increase as needed in increments of 0.3 mg/day to a maximum daily recommended dose to control disease and as tolerated. If intolerable adverse effects develop, the dosage should be decreased in increments of 0.3 mg/day.

4 to 6 years of age – 0.3 to 1.8 mg daily in 1 or 2 divided doses. Increase as needed in increments of 0.3 mg/day to a maximum daily recommended dose to control disease and as tolerated. If intolerable adverse effects develop, the dosage should be decreased in increments of 0.3 mg/day.

Renal function impairment:

Mild to moderate renal impairment (CrCl 30 to 80 mL/min) –

Familial Mediterranean fever: Dosage adjustment may be necessary. Monitor closely for adverse reactions.

Gout flares: Treatment of gout flares is not recommended in patients with renal impairment who are receiving colchicine for prophylaxis.

Severe renal impairment (CrCl less than 30 mL/min) –

Familial Mediterranean fever: Start with 0.3 mg/day.

Gout flares: Treatment of gout flares is not recommended in patients with renal impairment who are receiving colchicine for prophylaxis.

Prophylaxis – Initially, 0.3 mg/day.

Treatment – Dosage adjustment is not required, but a treatment course should be repeated no more than once every 2 weeks. For patients requiring repeated courses, consider alternate therapy.

Dialysis –

Familial Mediterranean fever: 0.3 g/day. Dosing can be increased with close monitoring.

Gout flares: Treatment of gout flares is not recommended in patients with renal impairment who are receiving colchicine for prophylaxis.

Prophylaxis – 0.3 mg twice a week with close monitoring.

Treatment – Single dose of 0.6 mg. A treatment course should not be repeated more than once every 2 weeks.

Alternative dosing regimen –

Gout flares:

CrCl more than 50 mL/min – 100% of usual daily dose.

CrCl of 10 to 50 mL/min – 50% to 100% of usual daily dose.

CrCl less than 10 mL/min – 25% of usual daily dose.

Peritoneal dialysis – 25% of usual daily dose.

Continuous renal replacement therapy – 50% to 100% of usual daily dose.

Hepatic function impairment:

Familial Mediterranean fever – In patients with severe hepatic impairment, dosage reduction should be considered with careful monitoring as necessary.

Gout flares – Treatment of gout flares is not recommended in patients with hepatic impairment who are receiving colchicine for prophylaxis.

Prophylaxis: Dosage adjustment should be considered in severe hepatic disease.

Treatment: In patients with severe hepatic impairment, carefully monitor and do not repeat the treatment course more than once every 2 weeks. For these patients requiring repeated courses, consideration should be given to alternate therapy.

Concomitant therapy:

Strong CYP3A4 inhibitors (eg, atazanavir, clarithromycin, indinavir, itraconazole, ketoconazole, nefazodone, nelfinavir, ritonavir, saquinavir, telithromycin) –

Familial Mediterranean fever: Maximum daily dose of 0.6 mg. May be given as 0.3 mg twice daily.

Gout flares:

Prophylaxis – If taking 0.6 mg twice daily, decrease dosage to 0.3 mg once daily. If taking 0.6 mg once daily, decrease dosage to 0.3 mg every other day.

Treatment – 0.6 mg as 1 dose at the first sign of attack, followed by 0.3 mg 1 hour later. Dose to be repeated no earlier than 3 days. Use is not recommended in patients receiving prophylactic dose of colchicine and a CYP3A4 inhibitor.

Moderate CYP3A4 inhibitors (amprenavir, aprepitant, diltiazem, erythromycin, fluconazole, fosamprenavir, grapefruit juice, verapamil) –

Familial Mediterranean fever: Maximum daily dose of 1.2 mg. May be given as 0.6 mg twice daily.

Gout flares:

Prophylaxis – If taking 0.6 mg twice daily, decrease dosage to 0.3 mg twice daily. If taking 0.6 mg once daily, decrease dosage to 0.3 mg once daily.

Treatment – 1.2 mg as 1 dose at the first sign of attack. Dose to be repeated no earlier than 3 days. Use is not recommended in patients receiving prophylactic dose of colchicine and CYP3A4 inhibitor.

P-glycoprotein inhibitors (eg, cyclosporine, ranolazine) –

Familial Mediterranean fever: Maximum daily dose of 0.6 mg. May be given as 0.3 mg twice daily.

Gout flares:

Prophylaxis – If taking 0.6 mg twice daily, decrease dosage to 0.3 mg once daily. If taking 0.6 mg once daily, decrease dosage to 0.3 mg every other day.

Treatment – 0.6 mg as 1 dose at the first sign of attack. Dose to be repeated no earlier than 3 days.

Administration: Administer orally without regard to meals.

Actions

Pharmacology: The exact mechanism of action of colchicine in gout is not known.

Colchicine apparently exerts its effect by reducing the inflammatory response to the deposited crystals and also by diminishing phagocytosis. Colchicine diminishes lactic acid production by leukocytes and by diminishing phagocytosis and thereby interrupts the cycle of urate crystal deposition and inflammatory response that sustains the acute attack.

Familial Mediterranean fever – Colchicine may interfere with the intracellular assembly of the inflammasome complex present in neutrophils and monocytes that mediates activation of interleukin-1 beta.

Pharmacokinetics: Colchicine is rapidly absorbed after oral administration (1.81 hours (range, 1 to 2.5 hours); peak plasma concentrations occur. High colchicine concentrations are found in the kidney, liver, and spleen. It is metabolized in the liver. Excretion occurs primarily by biliary and renal routes. Absolute bioavailability is reported to be approximately 45%. Colchicine binding to serum protein is low (39% ± 5%). CYP3A4 is involved in the metabolism of colchicine. The mean elimination half-lives is 26.6 to 31.2 hours.

Contraindications

Hypersensitivity to colchicine; serious GI, renal, hepatic, or cardiac disorders; blood dyscrasias, coadministration with P-glycoprotein or strong CYP3A4 inhibitors in patients with renal or hepatic impairment (*Colcrys* only).

Warnings/Precautions

Fatal overdose: Fatal overdoses, both accidental and intentional, have been reported in adults and children who have ingested colchicine.

Hematologic effects: Myelosuppression, leukopenia, granulocytopenia, thrombocytopenia, pancytopenia, and aplastic anemia with colchicine used in therapeutic doses have been reported.

Neuromuscular toxicity: Colchicine-induced neuromuscular toxicity and rhabdomyolysis have been reported with chronic treatment in therapeutic doses. Patients with renal dysfunction and elderly patients are at increased risk. Concomitant use of atorvastatin, simvastatin, pravastatin, fluvastatin, gemfibrozil, fenofibrate, fenofibric acid, or benzafibrate (themselves associated with myotoxicity), or cyclosporine may potentiate the development of myopathy.

GI effects: If nausea, vomiting, or diarrhea occurs, discontinue the drug.

Prophylaxis of gout flares: See Administration and Dosage.

Adjustment of the recommended dosage is not required; however, monitor patients closely for adverse effects of colchicine. In patients with severe impairment, start the dosage at 0.3 mg/day and make any increase in dosage with close monitoring. For the prophylaxis of gout flares in patients undergoing dialysis, starting doses at 0.3 mg given twice a week with close monitoring.

Treatment of gout flares: For treatment of gout flares in patients with mild (CrCl of 50 to 80 mL/min) to moderate (CrCl of 30 to 50 mL/min) renal impairment, adjustment of the recommended dosage is not required; however, monitor patients closely for adverse effects of colchicine. In patients with severe impairment, while the dosage does not need to be adjusted for the treatment of gout flares, repeat a treatment course no more than once every 2 weeks. For patients with gout flares requiring repeated courses consider alternate therapy. For patients undergoing dialysis, reduce the total recommended dose for the treatment of gout flares to a single dose of 0.6 mg (1 tablet). For these patients, repeat the treatment course no more than once every 2 weeks.

Familial Mediterranean fever: Although pharmacokinetics of colchicine in patients with mild (CrCl of 50 to 80 mL/min) and moderate (CrCl of 30 to 50 mL/min) renal impairment is not known, monitor these patients closely for adverse effects of colchicine. Dosage reduction may be necessary. In patients with severe renal failure (CrCl less than 30 mL/minute) and end-stage renal disease requiring dialysis, colchicine may be started at the dosage of 0.3 mg/day. Any increase in dosage should be done with adequate monitoring of the patient for adverse effects of colchicine.

Hepatic function impairment: See Administration and Dosage.

Increased colchicine toxicity may occur.

Prophylaxis of gout flares – For prophylaxis of gout flares in patients with mild to moderate hepatic impairment, adjustment of the recommended dosage is not required; however, monitor patients closely for adverse effects of colchicine. Consider dosage reduction for the prophylaxis of gout flares in patients with severe hepatic impairment.

Treatment of gout flares – For treatment of gout flares in patients with mild to moderate hepatic impairment, adjustment of the recommended colchicine dosage is not required; however, monitor patients closely for adverse effects of colchicine. For the treatment of gout flares in patients with severe impairment, while the dosage does not need to be adjusted, repeat the treatment course no more than once every 2 weeks. For these patients, requiring repeated courses for the treatment of gout flares, consideration should be given to alternate therapy.

Familial Mediterranean fever – In patients with severe hepatic disease, consider dosage reduction with careful monitoring.

Special risk: Administer with caution to debilitated patients and to those with early manifestations of GI or cardiac disorders.

Pregnancy: Category C.

Lactation: Colchicine is excreted into human milk. Exercise caution when administering colchicine to a nursing woman.

Children: The safety and efficacy of colchicine in children of all ages with familial Mediterranean fever has been evaluated in uncontrolled studies; however, dosing is approved only for children 4 years of age and older. There does not appear to be an adverse effect on growth in children with familial Mediterranean fever treated long-term with colchicine.

Gout is rare in children; safety and effectiveness of colchicine in children have not been established.

Elderly: In general, use caution in dose selection, usually starting at the low end of the dosing range, reflecting the greater frequency of decreased hepatic or renal function, and of concomitant disease or other drug therapy.

Monitoring: Perform periodic blood counts in patients receiving long-term therapy.

Drug Interactions

Drug/Lab test interactions: Decreased **thrombocyte** values may be obtained. Colchicine may cause false-positive results when testing urine for **RBC** or **hemoglobin**. Colchicine therapy may cause elevated alkaline phosphatase and ALT.

Drugs that may affect colchicine include acidifying agents, alkalinizing agents, digoxin, colchicine, cyclosporine, fibric acids, HMG-CoA reductase inhibitors, moderate CYP3A4 inhibitors, P-glycoprotein inhibitors, and strong CYP3A4 inhibitors.

Drugs that may be affected by colchicine include colchicine, digoxin, cyclosporine, fibric acids, HMG-CoA reductase inhibitors, CNS depressants, and sympathomimetics.

Adverse Reactions

Adverse reactions may include bone marrow depression with aplastic anemia, agranulocytosis, or thrombocytopenia (long-term therapy); peripheral neuritis; purpura; myopathy; loss of hair; reversible azoospermia; vomiting; diarrhea; abdominal pain; nausea; elevated alkaline phosphatase; AST; pharyngolaryngeal pain; cramping; abdominal pain; fatigue; vomiting; general disorders and administration-site conditions; and respiratory thoracic mediastinal disorders.

PROBENECID AND COLCHICINE

Tablets: 500 mg probenecid per 0.5 mg colchicine (*Rx*)	Various

For complete prescribing information see the individual probenecid and colchicine monographs.

Indications

For the treatment of chronic gouty arthritis when complicated by frequent, recurrent acute attacks of gout.

Administration and Dosage

Do not start therapy with probenecid and colchicine until an acute gouty attack has subsided. However, if an acute attack is precipitated during therapy, probenecid and colchicine may be continued without changing the dosage and additional colchicine or other appropriate therapy given to control the acute attack.

The recommended adult dosage is 1 tablet/day for 1 week followed by 1 tablet twice daily.

AGENTS FOR MIGRAINE

In addition to the agents on the following pages, **propanolol** and **timolol** are indicated for migraine prophylaxis.

SEROTONIN 5-HT$_1$ RECEPTOR AGONISTS

ALMOTRIPTAN MALATE	
Tablets: 6.25 and 12.5 mg (*Rx*)	*Axert* (Ortho-McNeil)
ELETRIPTAN HBr	
Tablets: 24.2 and 48.5 mg (*Rx*)	*Relpax* (Pfizer)
FROVATRIPTAN SUCCINATE	
Tablets: 2.5 mg (as base) (*Rx*)	*Frova* (Elan)
NARATRIPTAN	
Tablets: 1 and 2.5 mg (as hydrochloride) (*Rx*)	*Amerge* (GlaxoSmithKline)
RIZATRIPTAN BENZOATE	
Tablets: 5 and 10 mg (*Rx*)	*Maxalt* (Merck)
Tablets, orally disintegrating: 5 and 10 mg (*Rx*)	*Maxalt-MLT* (Merck)
SUMATRIPTAN	
Tablets: 25, 50, and 100 mg (as succinate) (*Rx*)	Various, *Imitrex* (GlaxoSmithKline)
Spray, nasal: 5 and 20 mg (*Rx*)	Various, *Imitrex* (GlaxoSmithKline)
Injection: 4 mg per 0.5 mL (as succinate) (*Rx*)	Various, *Imitrex* (GlaxoSmithKline)
6 mg per 0.5 mL (as succinate) (*Rx*)	Various, *Alsuma* (US Worldmeds), *Imitrex* (GlaxoSmithKline), *Sumavel DosePro* (Zogenix)
ZOLMITRIPTAN	
Tablets: 2.5 and 5 mg (*Rx*)	*Zomig* (AstraZeneca)
Tablets, orally disintegrating: 2.5 mg (*Rx*)	*Zomig ZMT* (AstraZeneca)
Spray, nasal: 5 mg (*Rx*)	*Zomig* (AstraZeneca)

Indications

Migraine: Acute treatment of migraine attacks with or without aura.

Cluster headache (sumatriptan injection only): Acute treatment of cluster headache episodes.

Not intended for the prophylactic therapy of migraine or for use in the management of hemiplegic or basilar migraine. Safety and efficacy have not been established for cluster headache, which is present in an older, predominantly male population (**almotriptan, eletriptan, frovatriptan, sumatriptan** tablets and spray, **zolmitriptan**).

Administration and Dosage

ALMOTRIPTAN:

Adults and children 12 to 17 years of age – Doses of 6.25 and 12.5 mg were effective for the acute treatment of migraines in adults, with the 12.5 mg dose tending to be a more effective dose. Individuals may vary in response to doses of almotriptan; therefore, individualize the dosage. Maximum dosage is 25 mg daily.

If the headache returns, the dose may be repeated after 2 hours, but do not give more than 2 doses within a 24-hour period. Controlled trials have not adequately established the efficacy of a second dose if the initial dose is ineffective.

The safety of treating an average of more than 4 headaches in a 30-day period has not been established.

Hepatic function impairment – The maximum decrease expected in the clearance of almotriptan caused by hepatic impairment is 60%. Therefore, do not exceed the maximum daily dose of 12.5 mg over a 24-hour period, and use a starting dose of 6.25 mg.

Renal function impairment – In patients with severe renal impairment, the clearance of almotriptan was decreased. Therefore, do not exceed the maximum daily dose of 12.5 mg over a 24-hour period, and use a starting dose of 6.25 mg.

ELETRIPTAN: Individualize dose. Single doses of 20 and 40 mg were effective for the acute treatment of migraine in adults, with a greater proportion of patients having a response following a 40 mg dose. Individuals may vary in response to doses of eletriptan tablets. An 80 mg dose, although also effective, was associated with an increased incidence of adverse events. Therefore, the maximum recommended single dose is 40 mg.

If, after the initial dose, the headache improves but then returns, a repeat dose may be beneficial. If a second dose is required, it should be taken at least 2 hours after the initial dose. If the initial dose is ineffective, controlled clinical trials have not shown the second dose to be beneficial in treating the same attack. The maximum daily dose should not exceed 80 mg.

The safety of treating an average of more than 3 headaches in a 30-day period has not been established.

Hepatic function impairment – Do not give eletriptan to patients with severe hepatic impairment because the effect of severe hepatic impairment on eletriptan metabolism was not evaluated. No dose adjustment is necessary in mild to moderate impairment.

FROVATRIPTAN: The recommended dosage is a single tablet (2.5 mg) taken orally with fluids.

If the headache recurs after initial relief, a second tablet may be taken, providing there is an interval of 2 or more hours between doses. The total daily dose of frovatriptan should not exceed 3 tablets (3 × 2.5 mg/day).

There is no evidence that a second dose of frovatriptan is effective in patients who do not respond to a first dose of the drug for the same headache.

The safety of treating an average of more than 4 migraine attacks in a 30-day period has not been established.

NARATRIPTAN: Single doses of 1 and 2.5 mg taken with fluid were effective for the acute treatment of migraine in adults. A greater proportion of patients had headache response following a 2.5 mg dose than following a 1 mg dose. Individualize dosage, weighing the possible benefit of the 2.5 mg dose with the potential for a greater risk of adverse events. If the headache returns or if the patient has only partial response, the dose may be repeated once after 4 hours, for a maximum dose of 5 mg in a 24-hour period. There is evidence that doses of 5 mg do not provide a greater effect than 2.5 mg.

Renal/hepatic function impairment – The use of naratriptan is contraindicated in patients with severe renal impairment (CrCl less than 15 mL/min) or severe hepatic impairment (Child-Pugh grade C) because of decreased clearance of the drug. In patients with mild to moderate renal or hepatic impairment, the maximum daily dose should not exceed 2.5 mg over a 24-hour period and a lower starting dose should be considered.

RIZATRIPTAN: Single doses of 5 and 10 mg were effective for the acute treatment of migraines in adults. There is little evidence that the 10 mg dose may provide a greater effect than the 5 mg dose. The choice of dose should be made on an individual basis, weighing the possible benefit of the 10 mg dose with the potential risk for increased adverse events.

Redosing – Doses should be separated by at least 2 hours; no more than 30 mg should be taken in any 24-hour period.

Propranolol patients – In patients receiving propranolol, use the 5 mg dose of rizatriptan benzoate tablets, up to a maximum of 3 doses in 24 hours.

Orally disintegrating tablets – Administration with liquid is not necessary. The orally disintegrating tablet is packaged in a blister within an outer aluminum pouch. Instruct patients not to remove the blister from the outer pouch until just prior to dosing. The blister pack should then be peeled open with dry hands and the orally disintegrating tablet placed on the tongue, where it will dissolve and be swallowed with saliva.

SUMATRIPTAN:

Oral – Single doses of 25, 50, or 100 mg tablets are effective for the acute treatment of migraine in adults. There is evidence that doses of 50 and 100 mg may provide a greater effect than 25 mg. Doses of 100 mg have not been proven to provide a greater effect than 50 mg. Individualize dosage, weighing the possible benefit of a higher dose with the potential for a greater risk of adverse events. If headache returns, or the patient has a partial response to the initial dose, additional doses may be taken at intervals of 2 hours or more up to a daily maximum of 200 mg. If headache returns following an initial treatment with the injection, additional doses of single tablets (up to 100 mg/day) may be given with an interval of 2 hours or more between tablet doses.

Hepatic function impairment: Maximum single dose up to 50 mg.

MAO inhibitors: Because of the potential of MAO-A inhibitors to cause unpredictable elevations in the bioavailability of oral sumatriptan, their combined use is contraindicated.

The safety of treating an average of more than 4 headaches in a 30-day period has not been established.

Injection – The maximum single adult dose is 6 mg injected subcutaneously.

Trials failed to show a clear benefit associated with the administration of a second 6 mg dose in patients who have failed to respond to a first injection. The maximum recommended dose that may be given in 24 hours is two 6 mg injections separated by 1 hour or more. If side effects are dose-limiting, lower doses may be used. In patients receiving doses less than 6 mg, use only the single-dose vial dosage form. An auto-injection device is available for use with 4 or 6 mg prefilled syringes to facilitate self-administration in patients in whom this dose is deemed necessary. With this device, the needle penetrates approximately ¼ inch (5 to 6 mm). Because the injection is intended to be given subcutaneously, intramuscular or intravascular delivery should be avoided. Patients should be directed to use injection sites with an adequate skin and subcutaneous thickness to accommodate the length of the needle.

MAO inhibitors: Consider decreased doses of sumatriptan in patients receiving MAO inhibitors.

Intranasal – A single dose of 5, 10, or 20 mg administered in 1 nostril is effective for the acute treatment of migraine in adults. A greater proportion of patients had headache response following a 20 mg dose than following a 5 to 10 mg dose. Weigh the possible benefit of the 20 mg dose with the potential for a greater risk of adverse events. A 10 mg dose may be achieved by administering a single 5 mg dose in each nostril. There is evidence that doses more than 20 mg do not provide a greater effect than 20 mg. If headache returns, the dose may be repeated once after 2 hours, not to exceed a total daily dose of 40 mg.

The safety of treating an average of more than 4 headaches in a 30-day period has not been established.

ZOLMITRIPTAN: Initial recommended dose is up to 2.5 mg (achieved by manually breaking a 2.5 mg tablet in half). If the headache returns, the dose may be repeated after 2 hours, not to exceed 10 mg within a 24-hour period. Response is greater following the 2.5 or 5 mg dose compared with 1.25 mg, with little added benefit and increased side effects associated with the 5 mg dose.

Orally disintegrating tablets – A single dose of 2.5 mg was effective for the acute treatment of migraines in adults. If the headache returns, the dose may be repeated after 2 hours, not to exceed 10 mg within a 24-hour period. Trials have not adequately established the efficacy of a second dose if the initial dose is ineffective.

Administration with a liquid is not necessary. The orally disintegrating tablet is packaged in a blister. Instruct patients not to remove the tablet from the blister until just prior to dosing. The blister pack should then be peeled open, and the orally disintegrating tablet placed on the tongue, where it will dissolve and be swallowed with the saliva. It is not recommended to break the orally disintegrating tablet.

On average, the safety of treating more than 3 headaches in a 30-day period has not been established.

Nasal spray – Administer 1 dose of 5 mg for the treatment of acute migraine. If the headache returns, the dose may be repeated after 2 hours. Do not exceed a maximum daily dose of 10 mg in any 24-hour period. Individuals may vary in response to zolmitriptan. The pharmacokinetics of a 5 mg nasal spray dose is similar to the 5 mg oral formulations. Doses lower than 5 mg can only be achieved through the use of an oral formulation. Therefore, choose the dose and route of administration on an individual basis. The efficacy of a second dose has not been established in placebo-controlled trials.

The safety of treating an average of more than 4 headaches in a 30-day period has not been established.

Hepatic function impairment – Administer zolmitriptan with caution in patients with liver disease, generally using doses less than 2.5 mg. Patients with moderate to severe hepatic impairment have decreased clearance of zolmitriptan; significant elevation in blood pressure was observed in some patients.

Actions

Pharmacology: **Naratriptan, rizatriptan, sumatriptan, frovatriptan, almotriptan, eletriptan,** and **zolmitriptan** are selective agonists for a vascular 5-hydroxytryptamine$_1$ (serotonin) receptor subtype. Use of 5-HT$_1$ agonists results in cranial vessel constriction and inhibition of pro-inflammatory neuropeptide release, which correlates with the relief of migraine.

Pharmacokinetics:

Pharmacokinetic Parameters of Triptans in Healthy Volunteers and in Patients with Migraine[1]

Drug	Dose and route of administration	T_{max} (h)	C_{max} (mcg/L)	Bioavailability (%)	t½ (h)	AUC (mcg/L•h)	Plasma protein binding (%)
Almotriptan	12.5 mg PO	2.5	49.5	80	3.1	266	≈ 35
	25 mg PO	2.7	64	69	3.6	443	
Eletriptan	20 mg PO	2	–	≈ 50	≈ 4	–	≈ 85
Frovatriptan	2.5 mg PO	3	4.2/7[a]	29.6	25.7	94	≈ 15
	40 mg PO	5	24.7/53.4[a]	17.5	29.7	881	
Naratriptan	2.5 mg PO	2	12.6	74	5.5	98	≈ 28
Rizatriptan	10 mg PO	1, 1.6 to 2.5[b]	19.8	40	2	50	14
Sumatriptan	6 mg SC	0.17	72	96	2	90	14 to 21
	100 mg PO	1.5	54	14	2	158	
	20 mg IN	1.5	13	15.8	1.8	48	
	25 mg PR	1.5	27	19.2	1.8	78	
Zolmitriptan	2.5 mg PO	1.5, 3[b]	3.3/3.8[a]	39	2.3/2.6[a]	18/21[a]	≈ 25
	5 mg PO	1.5, 3[b]	10	46	3	42	
	5 mg IN	3	3.93[c]	102[d]	≈ 3	22.4[c]	

[1] Adapted from *Drugs*. 2000;60:1267.
[a] Value for men and women, respectively.
[b] Orally disintegrating tablets.
[c] Values based on 2.5 mg dose.
[d] Compared with oral tablet.

Injection (Sumatriptan) – Following a 6 mg subcutaneous injection, distribution half-life was 15 minutes, terminal half-life was 115 minutes, and Vd central compartment was 50 L. The T_{max} or amount absorbed were not significantly altered by either the site or technique of injection (deltoid vs thigh).

Contraindications

Injectable preparations used IV, because of the potential to cause coronary vasospasm; patients with ischemic heart disease (angina pectoris, history of MI, silent MI, strokes, transient ischemic attacks [TIAs], or documented silent ischemia); Prinzmetal's variant angina or other significant underlying cardiovascular disease (see Warnings/Precautions); patients with signs or symptoms consistent with ischemic heart disease or coronary artery vasospasm; patients with uncontrolled hypertension; concurrent use of (or use within 24 hours of) ergotamine-containing preparations (or ergot-type medications such as dihydroergotamine or methysergide); concurrent MAO inhibitor therapy (or within 2 weeks of discontinuing an MAOI [except for **eletriptan**]; see Drug Interactions); within 24 hours of another 5-HT$_1$

agonist; hypersensitivity to the product or any of its ingredients; management of hemiplegic or basilar migraine; ischemic bowel disease.

Naratriptan and sumatriptan: Cerebrovascular or peripheral vascular syndromes, severe hepatic impairment (Child-Pugh grade C); severe renal impairment (CrCl less than 15 mL/min) (naratriptan only).

Frovatriptan and eletriptan: Peripheral vascular disease including but not limited to ischemic bowel disease.

Eletriptan: Severe hepatic impairment.

Warnings/Precautions

Use $5\text{-}HT_1$ agonists only where a clear diagnosis of migraine has been established.

Risk of myocardial ischemia or infarction and other adverse cardiac events: Because of the potential of this class of compounds to cause coronary vasospasm, do not give these agents to patients with documented ischemic or vasospastic coronary artery disease (CAD).

It is recommended that patients who are intermittent long-term users of $5\text{-}HT_1$ agonists who have or acquire risk factors predictive of CAD undergo periodic interval cardiovascular evaluation as they continue use.

Zolmitriptan – Patients with symptomatic Wolff-Parkinson-White syndrome or arrhythmias associated with other cardiac accessory conduction pathway disorders should not receive zolmitriptan.

Cardiac events and fatalities associated with $5\text{-}HT_1$ agonists: Serious adverse cardiac events, including acute MI, life-threatening disturbances of cardiac rhythm, and death have been reported within a few hours following the administration of other $5\text{-}HT_1$ agonists.

Cerebrovascular events and fatalities with $5\text{-}HT_1$ agonists: Cerebral hemorrhage, subarachnoid hemorrhage, stroke, and other cerebrovascular events have been reported in patients treated with $5\text{-}HT_1$ agonists, and some have resulted in fatalities. In a number of cases, it appears possible that the cerebrovascular events were primary, the agonist having been administered in the incorrect belief that the symptoms experienced were a consequence of migraine, when they were not. It should be noted that patients with migraine may be at increased risk of certain cerebrovascular events (eg, stroke, hemorrhage, TIA).

CYP3A4 inhibitors: In vitro studies have shown that **eletriptan** is metabolized by the CYP3A4 enzyme. A clinical study has shown that coadministration of eletriptan with ketoconazole, erythromycin, verapamil, and fluconazole increased the C_{max} and AUC of eletriptan 3- and 6-fold, 2- and 4-fold, 2- and 3-fold, and 1.4- and 2-fold, respectively. Do not use eletriptan within 72 hours of taking drugs that have demonstrated potent CYP3A4 inhibition.

Other vasospasm-related events: Peripheral vascular ischemia and colonic ischemia with abdominal pain and bloody diarrhea have been reported with $5\text{-}HT_1$ agonists.

Increases in blood pressure: Significant elevations in systemic blood pressure, including hypertensive crisis, have been reported on rare occasions in patients with and without a history of hypertension treated with $5\text{-}HT_1$ agonists.

Local irritation: Approximately 5% noted irritation in the nose and throat after using **sumatriptan** nasal spray. The symptoms were transient and, in approximately 60% of the cases, resolved in less than 2 hours.

Chest, jaw, or neck tightness: Chest, jaw, or neck tightness is relatively common after $5\text{-}HT_1$ agonist administration, and atypical sensations over the precordium (tightness, pressure, heaviness) have occurred, but have only rarely been associated with ischemic ECG changes.

Seizures: There have been rare reports of seizures following **sumatriptan** use.

Binding to melanin-containing tissues: Accumulation in melanin-rich tissues (such as the eye) could occur over time, raising the possibility that toxicity in these tissues could occur after extended use.

Corneal opacities: **Sumatriptan, eletriptan, naratriptan,** and **almotriptan** cause corneal opacities and defects in dogs, raising the possibility that these changes may occur in humans.

Phenylketonurics: **Rizatriptan** and **zolmitriptan** orally disintegrating tablets contain phenylalanine (a component of aspartame). Each 5 mg rizatriptan orally disintegrating tablet contains 1.05 mg phenylalanine, and each 10 mg orally disintegrating tablet contains 2.1 mg phenylalanine. Each 2.5 mg zolmitriptan orally disintegrating tablet contains 2.81 mg phenylalanine.

Hypersensitivity reactions: Hypersensitivity reactions have occurred on rare occasions, and severe anaphylaxis/anaphylactoid reactions have occurred. Such reactions can be life-threatening or fatal. Refer to Management of Acute Hypersensitivity Reactions.

Renal function impairment: Use **rizatriptan** and **sumatriptan** with caution in dialysis patients because of a decrease in the clearance.

Hepatic function impairment: Administer with caution to patients with diseases that may alter the absorption, metabolism, or excretion of drugs. The bioavailability may be markedly increased in patients with liver disease. No dosage adjustment is necessary when **frovatriptan** or **eletriptan** is given to patients with mild to moderate hepatic impairment. Do not use eletriptan in severe hepatic impairment.

Photosensitivity: Photosensitization may occur. Caution patients to take protective measures against exposure to sunlight or ultraviolet light until tolerance is determined.

Pregnancy: Category C.

Lactation: **Sumatriptan** and **eletriptan** are excreted in breast milk. **Zolmitriptan, naratriptan, almotriptan, frovatriptan,** and **rizatriptan** are excreted in rat milk.

Children: Safety and efficacy in children have not been established. 5-HT_1 receptor agonists are not recommended in patients younger than 18 years of age.

Elderly: Pharmacokinetics in the elderly are similar to those seen in younger adults.

Drug Interactions

Drugs that may affect 5-HT_1 receptor agonists include the following: Cimetidine, ergot-containing drugs, MAO inhibitors, oral contraceptives, potent CYP3A4 inhibitors (eg, ketoconazole), sibutramine, other 5-HT_1 receptor agonists, and propranolol. SSRIs may be affected by 5-HT_1 receptor agonists.

Adverse Reactions

Adverse reactions occurring in 3% or more of patients include the following: asthenia, chest pain/pressure, dizziness, drowsiness, dry mouth, dyspepsia, fatigue, headache, heaviness, miscellaneous CNS effects, miscellaneous sensations, myasthenia, nausea, neck/throat/jaw pain/pressure, pain in specified/unspecified locations, paresthesia, skeletal pain/pressure, somnolence, vertigo, warm/cold sensation, warm/hot sensation.

Zolmitriptan nasal spray: Asthenia, discomfort of the nasal cavity, dizziness, hyperesthesia, nausea, pain, paresthesia, somnolence, throat pain, unusual taste.

ERGOTAMINE DERIVATIVES

DIHYDROERGOTAMINE	
Spray, nasal: 4 mg/mL (*Rx*)	*Migranal* (Valeant)
Injection: 1 mg/mL (*Rx*)	*D.H.E. 45* (Xcel)
ERGOTAMINE TARTRATE	
Tablets, sublingual: 2 mg (*Rx*)	*Ergomar* (Lotus Biochemical)

Warning:

Serious and/or life-threatening peripheral ischemia has been associated with the coadministration of ergotamine with potent CYP 3A4 inhibitors, including protease inhibitors and macrolide antibiotics. Because CYP3A4 inhibition elevates the serum levels of ergotamine, the risk for vasospasm leading to cerebral ischemia and/or ischemia of the extremities is increased. Therefore, concomitant use of these medications is contraindicated.

Indications

Headache: To abort or prevent vascular headaches such as migraine, migraine variant, and cluster headache (histaminic cephalalgia).

Dihydroergotamine: For the acute treatment of migraine headaches with or without aura and the acute treatment of cluster headache episodes (injection only). Dihydroergotamine nasal spray is not intended for the prophylactic therapy of migraine or for the management of hemiplegic or basilar migraine.

Administration and Dosage

DIHYDROERGOTAMINE:

Nasal spray – Start with 1 spray (0.5 mg) in each nostril; repeat in 15 minutes for a total dosage of 4 sprays (2 mg). Studies have shown no additional benefit from acute doses greater than 2 mg for a single migraine administration. The safety of doses greater than 3 mg in a 24-hour period and 4 mg in a 7-day period has not been established. Do not use for chronic daily administration.

Injection – Administer in a dose of 1 mL IV, IM, or subcutaneously; may be repeated as needed at 1-hour intervals to a total dose of 3 mL for IM or subcutaneous delivery or 2 mL for IV delivery in a 24-hour period. Do not exceed a total weekly dosage of 6 mL. Do not use for chronic daily administration.

ERGOTAMINE: Initiate therapy as soon as possible after the first symptoms of an attack. Place 1 tablet under the tongue; take subsequent doses at 30 minute intervals if necessary. Do not exceed 3 tablets/24 hours. Do not exceed 10 mg/week.

Actions

Pharmacology: Ergotamine has partial agonist or antagonist activity against tryptaminergic, dopaminergic and alpha-adrenergic receptors, depending upon their site; it is a highly active uterine stimulant. It constricts peripheral and cranial blood vessels and depresses central vasomotor centers.

Ergotamine reduces extracranial blood flow, causes a decline in the amplitude of pulsation in the cranial arteries and decreases hyperperfusion of the basilar artery territory. Ergotamine is a potent emetic that stimulates the chemoreceptor trigger zone.

Dihydroergotamine, a hydrogenated derivative of ergotamine, differs mainly in its degree of activity. It has less vasoconstrictive action than ergotamine, is 12 times less active as an emetic and has less oxytocic effect.

Pharmacokinetics:

Absorption/Distribution – GI and sublingual absorption of ergotamine is incomplete and erratic; following oral administration, peak blood levels are reached in about 2 hours. Following intranasal administration, however, the mean bioavailability of dihydroergotamine mesylate is 32% relative to the injectable administration.

Onset of action occurs in 15 to 30 minutes following IM administration of dihydroergotamine and persists for 3 to 4 hours.

Metabolism/Excretion – Ergotamine is metabolized by the liver; 90% of the metabolites are excreted in the bile. Although plasma half-life is about 2 hours, ergotamine has long-lasting effects which may be caused by tissue storage.

Contraindications

Pregnancy (ergotamine's powerful uterine stimulant actions may cause fetal harm); hypersensitivity to ergot alkaloids; peripheral vascular disease (eg, thromboangiitis obliterans, leutic arteritis, severe arteriosclerosis, thrombophlebitis, Raynaud's disease); hepatic or renal impairment; severe pruritus; coronary artery disease; hypertension; sepsis. The use of potent CYP3A4 inhibitors (ritonavir, nelfinavir, indinavir, erythromycin, clarithromycin, troleandomycin, ketoconazole, itraconazole) with dihydroergotamine is contraindicated.

Do not give dihydroergotamine to patients with ischemic heart disease (angina pectoris, history of MI, documented silent ischemia) or to patients who have clinical symptoms or findings consistent with coronary artery vasospasm, including Prinzmetal variant angina.

Dihydroergotamine may increase blood pressure; do not give to patients with uncontrolled hypertension.

Do not use dihydroergotamine, 5-HT_1 agonists (eg, sumatriptan), ergotamine-containing or ergot-type medications, or methysergide within 24 hours of each other.

Do not administer dihydroergotamine to patients with hemiplegic or basilar migraine.

Dihydroergotamine should not be used by nursing mothers.

Do not use dihydroergotamine with peripheral and central vasoconstrictors because the combination may result in additive or synergistic elevation of blood pressure.

Warnings/Precautions

CYP3A4 inhibitors (eg, macrolide antibiotics, protease inhibitors): There have been rare reports of serious adverse events in connection with the coadministration.

Fibrotic complications: There have been reports of pleural and retroperitoneal fibrosis in patients following prolonged daily use of injectable dihydroergotamine.

Risk of myocardial ischemia and/or MI and other adverse cardiac events: Do not use dihydroergotamine in patients with documented ischemic or vasospastic coronary artery disease.

Cardiac events and fatalities: Serious adverse cardiac events, including acute MI, life-threatening disturbances of cardiac rhythm, and death have been reported following the administration of dihydroergotamine.

Drug-associated cerebrovascular events and fatalities: Cerebral hemorrhage, subarachnoid hemorrhage, stroke, and other cerebrovascular events have been reported in patients treated with dihydroergotamine; some have resulted in fatalities.

Other vasospasm-related events: Dihydroergotamine, like other ergot alkaloids, may cause vasospastic reactions other than coronary artery vasospasm. Myocardial and peripheral vascular ischemia have been reported with dihydroergotamine.

Increase in blood pressure: Significant elevation in blood pressure has been reported on rare occasions in patients with and without a history of hypertension.

Local irritation: Approximately 30% of patients using dihydroergotamine nasal spray (compared with 9% of placebo patients) have reported irritation in the nose or throat and/or disturbance in taste.

Coronary artery vasospasm: Dihydroergotamine may cause coronary artery vasospasm; patients who experience signs or symptoms suggestive of angina following its administration should, therefore, be evaluated for the presence of CAD or a predisposition to variant angina before receiving additional doses.

Recommended dosage: Exercise care to remain within the limits of recommended dosage.

Drug abuse and dependence: Patients who take ergotamine for extended periods of time may become dependent upon it and require progressively increasing doses for relief of vascular headaches and for prevention of dysphoric effects that follow withdrawal.

Pregnancy: Category X.

Lactation: Ergotamine is secreted into breast milk and has caused symptoms of ergotism (eg, vomiting, diarrhea) in the infant. Excessive dosing or prolonged administration may inhibit lactation.

Children: Safety and efficacy for use in children have not been established.

Drug Interactions

Drugs that may affect ergot alkaloids include beta blockers, CYB3A4 inhibitors (see Contraindications), nicotine, and sibutramine.

Drugs that may be affected by ergot alkaloids include nitrates, $5HT_1$ receptor agonists, and vasoconstrictors.

Adverse Reactions

Dihydroergotamine nasal spray: Adverse reactions occurring in at least 3% of patients include rhinitis, nausea, altered sense of taste, dizziness, vomiting, somnolence, pharyngitis, application site reaction.

Ergotamine tartrate: Nausea and vomiting occur in up to 10% of patients. Numbness and tingling of fingers and toes; muscle pain in the extremities; pulselessness; weakness in the legs; precordial pain; transient tachycardia or bradycardia; localized edema; itching.

Miscellaneous: Numbness and tingling of fingers and toes; muscle pain in the extremities; pulselessness; weakness in the legs; precordial distress and pain; transient tachycardia or bradycardia; localized edema; itching.

Large doses – Large doses raise arterial pressure, produce coronary vasoconstriction, and slow the heart by both a direct action and a vagal effect.

ISOMETHEPTENE MUCATE/DICHLORALPHENAZONE/ACETAMINOPHEN

Capsules: 65 mg isometheptene mucate, 100 mg dichloralphenazone, 325 mg APAP (*c-iv*)	Various, *Midrin* (Caracol), *Epidrin* (Excellium), *Migrazone* (Breckenridge)

Indications

For relief of tension and vascular headaches.

Based on a review of this drug (isometheptene mucate) by the National Academy of Sciences-National Research Council or other information, FDA has classified the other indication as "possibly" effective in the treatment of migraine headache. Final classification of the less-than-effective indication requires further investigation.

Administration and Dosage

Migraine headache: Usual dosage is 2 capsules at once followed by 1 capsule every hour until relieved, up to 5 capsules within a 12 hour period.

Tension headache: Usual dosage is 1 or 2 capsules every 4 hours, up to 8 capsules/day.

Actions

Pharmacology: Isometheptene mucate acts by constricting dilated cranial and cerebral arterioles, thus reducing the stimuli that lead to vascular headaches.

Dichloralphenazone, a mild sedative, reduces the patient's emotional reaction to the pain of both vascular and tension headaches.

Acetaminophen raises the threshold to painful stimuli, thus exerting an analgesic effect against all types of headaches.

Contraindications

Glaucoma; severe cases of renal disease; hypertension; organic heart disease; hepatic disease; MAO inhibitor therapy.

Warnings/Precautions

CNS effects: Because of dichloralphenazone's structural similarity to chloral hydrate, there is a potential for CNS depressant effects.

Observe caution: Observe caution in hypertension, peripheral vascular disease, and after recent cardiovascular attacks.

Drug abuse and dependence: There have been no published reports of withdrawal signs or other signs of abuse. The risk of dependence is increased in patients with a history of alcoholism, drug abuse, or in patients with marked personality disorders.

Drug Interactions

Drugs that may interact include MAO inhibitors.

Adverse Reactions

Adverse reactions may include transient dizziness and skin rash.

CYCLIZINE AND MECLIZINE

CYCLIZINE	
Tablets: 50 mg (as hydrochloride) (*otc*)	*Marezine* (Himmel)
Tablets, chewable; oral: 25 mg (*otc*)	*Bonine for Kids* (Insight Pharm)
MECLIZINE	
Tablets: 12.5, 25, and 50 mg (*Rx*)	Various, *Antivert* (Roerig)
25 mg (otc)	*Dramamine Less Drowsy* (McNeil Consumer), *Medi-Meclizine* (Medique)
Tablets, chewable: 25 mg (*Rx, otc*)	Various, *Bonine* (Pfizer)

Indications

Motion sickness, vestibular system disease: Prevention and treatment of nausea, vomiting, and dizziness of motion sickness.

Meclizine is "possibly effective" for the management of vertigo associated with diseases affecting the vestibular system.

Administration and Dosage

CYCLIZINE:

Marezine –

Adults and children 12 years of age and older: 1 tablet every 4 to 6 hours, not to exceed 4 tablets in 24 hours, or as directed by a doctor.

Children 6 to younger than 12 years of age: ½ tablet every 6 to 8 hours, not to exceed 1 and ½ tablets in 24 hours, or as directed by a doctor.

Do not give to children younger than 6 years of age unless directed by a doctor.

For prevention, take the first dose one-half hour before departure.

Bonine –

Children 6 to younger than 12 years of age: Chew 1 tablet thoroughly every 6 to 8 hours.

Do not exceed 3 tablets in 24 hours or as directed by a doctor.

Dosage should be taken up to 1 hour before travel starts or at onset of symptoms.

MECLIZINE:

Motion sickness – Take an initial dose of 25 to 50 mg, 1 hour prior to travel. May repeat dose every 24 hours for the duration of the journey.

Vertigo – 25 to 100 mg/day in divided doses.

Actions

Pharmacology: Cyclizine and meclizine have antiemetic, anticholinergic, and antihistaminic properties.

Cyclizine and meclizine have an onset of action of 30 to 60 minutes, depending on dosage; their duration of action is 4 to 6 hours and 12 to 24 hours, respectively.

Contraindications

Hypersensitivity to cyclizine or meclizine.

Warnings/Precautions

Hazardous tasks: May produce drowsiness; patients should observe caution while driving or performing other tasks requiring alertness.

Because of the anticholinergic action of these agents, use with caution and with appropriate monitoring in patients with glaucoma, obstructive disease of the GI or GU tract, and in elderly males with possible prostatic hypertrophy. These drugs may have a hypotensive action, which may be confusing or dangerous in postoperative patients.

May have additive effects with alcohol and other CNS depressants (eg, hypnotics, sedatives, tranquilizers, antianxiety agents); use with caution.

Pregnancy: Category B. Meclizine presents the lowest risk of teratogenicity and is the drug of first choice in treating nausea and vomiting during pregnancy.

Lactation: Safety for use in the nursing mother has not been established.

Children: Safety and efficacy for use in children have not been established. Not recommended for use in children younger than 12 years of age.

Adverse Reactions

Adverse reactions include the following: Hypotension; palpitations; tachycardia; drowsiness; restlessness; excitation; nervousness; insomnia; euphoria; blurred vision; diplopia; vertigo; tinnitus; auditory and visual hallucinations (particularly when dosage recommendations are exceeded); urticaria; rash; dry mouth; anorexia; nausea; vomiting; diarrhea; constipation; cholestatic jaundice (cyclizine); urinary frequency; difficult urination; urinary retention; dry nose and throat.

DIMENHYDRINATE

Tablets: 50 mg (*Rx*)	*Dimetabs* (Jones Medical)
50 mg (*otc*)	Various, *Dramamine* (McNeil Consumer), *Triptone Caplets* (Del Pharmaceuticals)
Tablets, chewable: 50 mg (*otc*)	*Dramamine* (McNeil Consumer)
Capsules: 50 mg (*otc*)	*Vertab* (UAD)
Injection: 50 mg/mL (*Rx*)	Various, *Dinate* (Seatrace), *Dramamine* (McNeil Consumer), *Dymenate* (Keene), *Hydrate* (Hyrex)
Liquid: 12.5 mg/4 mL (*otc*)	Various, *Dramamine* (McNeil Consumer)
12.5 mg/5 mL (*otc*)	*Children's Dramamine* (McNeil Consumer)
15.62 mg/5 mL (*Rx*)	*Dramamine* (McNeil Consumer)

Indications

For the prevention and treatment of nausea, vomiting, dizziness, or vertigo of motion sickness.

Administration and Dosage

Adults:

Oral – 50 to 100 mg every 4 to 6 hours. Do not exceed 400 mg in 24 hours.

IM – 50 mg, as needed.

IV – 50 mg in 10 mL Sodium Chloride Injection given over 2 minutes. Do not inject intra-arterially.

Children:

Oral (6 to 12 years of age) – 25 to 50 mg every 6 to 8 hours; do not exceed 150 mg in 24 hours.

Oral (2 to 6 years of age) – Up to 12.5 to 25 mg every 6 to 8 hours; do not exceed 75 mg in 24 hours.

IM – 1.25 mg/kg or 37.5 mg/m^2 4 times/day; do not exceed 300 mg/day.

Children (younger than 2 years of age): Only on advice of a physician.

Actions

Pharmacology: Dimenhydrinate consists of equimolar proportions of diphenhydramine and chlorotheophylline.

Pharmacokinetics: Dimenhydrinate has a depressant action on hyperstimulated labyrinthine function. The precise mode of action is not known. The antiemetic effects are believed to be caused by the diphenhydramine, an antihistamine also used as an antiemetic agent.

Contraindications

Neonates; patients hypersensitive to dimenhydrinate or its components.

Note: Most IV products contain Benzyl Alcohol, which has been associated with a fatal "gasping syndrome" in premature infants and low birth weight infants.

Warnings/Precautions

Use with caution in conditions which might be aggravated by anticholinergic therapy (eg, prostatic hypertrophy, stenosing peptic ulcer, pyloroduodenal obstruction, bladder neck obstruction, narrow angle glaucoma, bronchial asthma, cardiac arrhythmias).

Pregnancy: Category B.

Lactation: Small amounts of dimenhydrinate are excreted in breast milk.

Children: For infants and children especially, an overdose of antihistamines may cause hallucinations, convulsions, or death. Mental alertness may be diminished. In the young child, dimenhydrinate may produce excitation. Do not give to children under 2 years of age unless directed by a physician.

Drug Interactions

Drugs that may interact with dimenhydrinate may include CNS depressants and antibiotics.

Adverse Reactions

Adverse reactions may include drowsiness; confusion; nervousness; restlessness; headache; insomnia (especially in children); tingling, heaviness and weakness of hands; vertigo; dizziness; lassitude; excitation; nausea; vomiting; diarrhea; epigastric distress; constipation; anorexia; blurring of vision; diplopia; palpitations; hypotension; tachycardia; anaphylaxis; photosensitivity; urticaria; drug rash; hemolytic anemia; difficult or painful urination; nasal stuffiness; tightness of chest; wheezing; thickening of bronchial secretions; dryness of mouth, nose, and throat.

SCOPOLAMINE

Tablets: 0.4 mg (*Rx*)	*Scopace* (Hope Pharm.)
Transdermal patch: 1.5 mg (delivers approximately 1 mg over 3 days) (*Rx*)	*Transderm-Scōp* (Baxter)

Indications

Tablets: Used as an anticholinergic CNS depressant; in the symptomatic treatment of postencephalitic parkinsonism and paralysis agitans; in spastic states; and locally as a substitute for atropine in ophthalmology.

Scopolamine inhibits excessive motility and hypertonus of the GI tract in irritable colon syndrome, mild dysentery, diverticulitis, pylorospasm, and cardiospasm.

Transdermal patch: Prevention of nausea and vomiting associated with motion sickness and recovery from anesthesia and surgery in adults.

Administration and Dosage

Tablets: The dosage range is 0.4 to 0.8 mg. The dosage may be cautiously increased in parkinsonism and spastic states.

Transdermal patch:

Initiation of therapy – Apply one system to the postauricular skin (ie, behind the ear) at least 4 hours before the antiemetic effect is required. To prevent postoperative nausea and vomiting, apply the patch the evening before scheduled surgery. To minimize exposure of the newborn baby to the drug, apply the patch 1 hour prior to cesarean section. Scopolamine approximately 1 mg will be delivered over 3 days. Wear only one disc at a time. Do not cut the patch.

For perioperative use, keep patch in place for 24 hours following surgery, then remove and discard.

Handling – After applying the disc on dry skin behind the ear, wash hands thoroughly with soap and water, then dry them. Discard the removed disc and wash the hands and application site thoroughly with soap and water to prevent any traces of scopolamine from coming into direct contact with the eyes.

Continuation of therapy – If the disc is displaced, discard it and place a fresh one on the hairless area behind the other ear. For motion sickness, if therapy is required for more than 3 days, discard the first disc and place a fresh one on the hairless area behind the other ear.

Actions

Pharmacology: The mechanism of action of scopolamine in the CNS is not definitely known but may include anticholinergic effects. The ability of scopolamine to prevent motion-induced nausea is believed to be associated with inhibition of vestibular input to the CNS, which results in inhibition of the vomiting reflex. In addition, scopolamine may have a direct action on the vomiting center within the reticular formation of the brain stem.

Pharmacokinetics: The transdermal system is a 0.2 mm thick film with 4 layers. It is 2.5 cm^2 in area and contains 1.5 mg scopolamine that is gradually released from an adhesive matrix of mineral oil and polyisobutylene following application to the postauricular skin. An initial priming dose released from the system's adhesive layer saturates the skin binding site for scopolamine and rapidly brings the plasma concentration to the required steady-state level. A continuous controlled release of scopolamine flows from the drug reservoir through the rate controlling membrane to maintain a constant plasma level. Antiemetic protection is produced within several hours following application behind the ear.

Contraindications

Hypersensitivity to scopolamine, other belladonna alkaloids, or any component of the product; angle-closure (narrow-angle) glaucoma.

Warnings/Precautions

Potentially alarming idiosyncratic reactions may occur with therapeutic doses.

Use with caution in patients with pyloric obstruction, urinary bladder neck obstruction, and in patients suspected of having intestinal obstruction. Use with special caution in the elderly or in individuals with impaired metabolic, liver, or kidney functions because of the increased likelihood of CNS effects.

Potentially hazardous tasks: May produce drowsiness, disorientation, and confusion. Warn patients against engaging in activities that require mental alertness, such as driving a motor vehicle or operating dangerous machinery.

In patients taking drugs that cause CNS effects, including alcohol, use scopolamine with care.

Drug withdrawal: Dizziness, nausea, vomiting, headache, and disturbances of equilibrium have been reported in a few patients following discontinuation of the use of the transdermal system. This occurred most often in patients who used the system for more than 3 days.

Pregnancy: Category C. Use in pregnancy only if potential benefits justify potential risk to the fetus.

Lactation: Scopolamine is excreted in breast milk. Exercise caution when administering to a nursing woman.

Children: Safety and efficacy have not been established.

Adverse Reactions

Most common: Dry mouth (67%); drowsiness (less than 17%); transient impairment of eye accommodation including blurred vision and dilation of the pupils. Unilateral fixed and dilated pupil has been reported, apparently from accidentally touching one eye after manipulation of the patch.

TRIMETHOBENZAMIDE HYDROCHLORIDE

Capsules: 300 mg (*Rx*)	Various, *Tigan* (Monarch)
Injection: 100 mg/mL (*Rx*)	

Indications

For the treatment of postoperative nausea and vomiting and for nausea associated with gastroenteritis.

Administration and Dosage

Oral:

Adults – 300 mg, 3 or 4 times/day.

Children (30 to 90 lbs; 13.6 to 40.9 kg) – 100 to 200 mg, 3 or 4 times/day.

Injection: For IM use only.

Adults – 200 mg 3 or 4 times/day. Pain, stinging, burning, redness, and swelling may develop at injection site.

Actions

Pharmacokinetics: Mechanism is obscure, but may be mediated through the chemoreceptor trigger zone; direct impulses to vomiting center are not inhibited.

Contraindications

Hypersensitivity to trimethobenzamide, benzocaine or similar local anesthetics; parenteral use in children; suppositories in premature infants or neonates.

Warnings/Precautions

Encephalitides, gastroenteritis, dehydration, electrolyte imbalance (especially in children and the elderly or debilitated), and CNS reactions have occurred when used during acute febrile illness.

Exercise caution when giving the drug with alcohol and other CNS-acting agents such as phenothiazines, barbiturates, and belladonna derivatives.

Pregnancy: Safety for use has not been established.

Lactation: Safety for use in the nursing mother has not been established.

Adverse Reactions

Adverse reactions may include: Hypersensitivity reactions; parkinson-like symptoms; hypotension or pain following IM injection; blood dyscrasias; blurred vision; coma; convulsions; depression; diarrhea; disorientation; dizziness; drowsiness; headache; jaundice; muscle cramps; opisthotonos; allergic-type skin reactions.

DRONABINOL

Gelatin capsules: 2.5, 5, and 10 mg *(c-iii)*	Various, *Marinol* (Unimed Pharmaceuticals)

Indications

Antiemetic: Treatment of nausea and vomiting associated with cancer chemotherapy in patients not responding adequately to conventional antiemetic treatment.

Appetite stimulation: Treating anorexia associated with weight loss in AIDS patients.

Administration and Dosage

Antiemetic: Initially, give 5 mg/m^2 1 to 3 hours prior to the administration of chemotherapy, then every 2 to 4 hours after chemotherapy is given, for a total of 4 to 6 doses/day. If the 5 mg/m^2 dose is ineffective, and there are no significant side effects, increase the dose by 2.5 mg/m^2 increments to a maximum of 15 mg/m^2 per dose. Use caution, however, as the incidence of disturbing psychiatric symptoms increases significantly at this maximum dose. Administration with phenothiazines may improve efficacy (vs either drug alone) without additional toxicity.

Appetite stimulation: Initially, give 2.5 mg twice/day before lunch and supper. For patients who cannot tolerate 5 mg/day, reduce dosage to 2.5 mg/day as a single evening or bedtime dose. When adverse reactions are absent or minimal and further therapeutic effect is desired, increase to 2.5 mg before lunch and 5 mg before supper (or 5 mg at lunch and 5 mg after supper). Although most patients respond to 2.5 mg twice/day, 10 mg twice/day has been tolerated in about 50% of patients. The dosage may be increased to a maximum of 20 mg/day in divided doses. Use caution in escalating the dosage because of the increased frequency of dose-related adverse reactions at higher dosages.

Actions

Pharmacology: Dronabinol is the principal psychoactive substance present in *Cannabis sativa* L (marijuana). The mechanism of action is unknown.

Cannabinoids have complex CNS effects, including central sympathomimetic activity.

Pharmacokinetics:

Absorption/Distribution – Following oral administration, dronabinol is almost completely absorbed (90% to 95%). It has an onset of action of approximately 0.5 to

1 hour and peak effect at 2 to 4 hours. Duration for psychoactive effects is 4 to 6 hours, but the appetite stimulant effect may continue for 24 hours or more after administration.

Metabolism/Excretion – Dronabinol undergoes extensive first-pass hepatic metabolism.

Biliary excretion is the major route of elimination. Extended use at the recommended doses may cause accumulation of toxic amounts of dronabinol and its metabolites.

Contraindications

Hypersensitivity to dronabinol, marijuana, or sesame oil.

Warnings/Precautions

Tolerance: Following 12 days of dronabinol, tolerance to the cardiovascular and subjective effects developed at doses 210 mg/day or less. An initial tachycardia induced by dronabinol was replaced successively by normal sinus rhythm and then bradycardia. A fall in supine blood pressure, made worse by standing, was also observed initially. Within days, these effects disappeared, indicating development of tolerance. Tachyphylaxis and tolerance did not, however, appear to develop to the appetite stimulant effect.

Patient supervision: Because of individual variation, determine clinically the period of patient supervision required.

Hypertension or heart disease: Use with caution since dronabinol may cause a general increase in central sympathomimetic activity.

Psychiatric patients: In manic, depressive, or schizophrenic patients, symptoms of these disease states may be exacerbated by the use of cannabinoids.

Drug abuse and dependence: Dronabinol is highly abusable. Limit prescriptions to the amount necessary for a single cycle of chemotherapy.

A withdrawal syndrome consisting of irritability, insomnia, and restlessness was observed in some subjects within 12 hours following abrupt withdrawal of dronabinol. The syndrome reached its peak intensity at 24 hours when subjects exhibited hot flashes, sweating, rhinorrhea, loose stools, hiccoughs, and anorexia. The syndrome was essentially complete within 96 hours. EEG changes following discontinuation were consistent with a withdrawal syndrome. Several subjects reported impressions of disturbed sleep for several weeks after discontinuing high doses.

Hazardous tasks: Because of its profound effects on mental status, warn patients not to drive, operate complex machinery, or engage in any activity requiring sound judgment and unimpaired coordination while receiving treatment. Effects may persist for a variable and unpredictable period of time.

Pregnancy: *Category B.*

Lactation: Dronabinol is concentrated and excreted in breast milk; nursing mothers should not use dronabinol.

Children: Not recommended for AIDS-related anorexia in children because it has not been studied in this population. Dosage for chemotherapy-induced emesis is the same as in adults. Use caution in children because of the psychoactive effects.

Elderly: Use caution because the elderly are generally more sensitive to the psychoactive effects. In antiemetic studies, no difference in tolerance or efficacy was apparent in patients older than 55 years of age.

Drug Interactions

Drugs that may be affected by dronabinol include amphetamines, cocaine, sympathomimetics, anticholinergics, antihistamines, tricyclic antidepressants, alcohol, sedatives, hypnotics, psychomimetics, disulfiram, fluoxetine, and theophylline.

Adverse Reactions

Adverse reactions occurring in 3% or more of patients include euphoria, nausea, vomiting, dizziness, paranoid reaction, and somnolence.

5-HT_3 RECEPTOR ANTAGONISTS

ALOSETRON HYDROCHLORIDE	
Tablets; oral: 0.5, 1 mg (*Rx*)	*Lotronex* (Prometheus)
DOLASETRON	
Tablets; oral: 50 and 100 mg (*Rx*)	*Anzemet* (Aventis)
Injection, solution: 20 mg/mL (*Rx*)	
GRANISETRON	
Tablets; oral: 1 mg (1.12 mg as hydrochloride) (*Rx*)	Various
Solution; oral: 1 mg per 5 mL (1.12 mg per 5 mL as hydrochloride) (*Rx*)	*Granisol* (Hawthorn), *Kytril* (Roche)
Injection, solution: 0.1 mg/mL (0.112 mg/mL hydrochloride), 1 mg/mL (1.12 mg/mL as hydrochloride) (*Rx*)	Various, *Kytril* (Roche)
Patch; transdermal: 3.1 mg per 24 h (34.3 mg per 52 cm^2) (*Rx*)	*Sancuso* (ProStrakan)
ONDANSETRON	
Tablets; oral: 4, 8, 16, and 24 mg (as hydrochloride) (*Rx*)	Various, *Zofran* (GlaxoSmithKline)
16 mg (as hydrochloride) (*Rx*)	Various
Tablets, orally disintegrating: 4 and 8 mg (*Rx*)	Various, *Zofran ODT* (GlaxoSmithKline)
Solution; oral: 4 mg per 5 mL (as hydrochloride) (*Rx*)	Various, *Zofran* (GlaxoSmithKline)
Injection, solution: 2 mg/mL (*Rx*)	
32 mg per 50 mL (pre-mixed) (as hydrochloride) (*Rx*)	Various
PALONOSETRON HYDROCHLORIDE	
Injection, solution: 0.25 mg per 5 mL (as hydrochloride) (*Rx*)	*Aloxi* (Eisai Inc)

Warning:

Serious GI adverse reactions, some fatal, have been reported with the use of **alosetron**. These events, including ischemic colitis and serious complications of constipation, have resulted in hospitalization, blood transfusion, surgery, and death.

- Only physicians who have enrolled in GlaxoSmithKline's prescribing program for *Lotronex*, based on their attestation of qualifications and acceptance of responsibilities, should prescribe alosetron (see Administration and Dosage).
- Alosetron is indicated only for women with severe diarrhea-predominant irritable bowel syndrome (IBS) who have failed to respond to conventional therapy (see Indications). Less than 5% of IBS is considered severe. Before receiving the initial prescription for alosetron, the patient must read and sign the Patient-Physician Agreement.
- Alosetron should be discontinued immediately in patients who develop constipation or symptoms of ischemic colitis. Instruct patients to immediately report constipation or symptoms of ischemic colitis. Do not resume alosetron in patients who develop ischemic colitis. Instruct patients who report constipation to immediately contact them if the constipation does not resolve after discontinuation of alosetron. Patients with resolved constipation should resume alosetron only on the advice of their treating physician.

Indications

Antiemetic (except alosetron): Prevention of nausea and vomiting associated with initial and repeat courses of emetogenic cancer therapy, including high-dose cisplatin; prevention of postoperative nausea or vomiting (**ondansetron, dolasetron, granisetron** intravenous [IV], and **palonosetron**); for the prevention of nausea and vomiting in patients receiving moderately and/or highly emetogenic chemotherapy regimens of up to 5 consecutive days' duration (**granisetron** transdermal); prevention of nausea and vomiting associated with radiotherapy, including total body irradiation, fractioned abdominal radiation, or daily fractions to the abdomen (oral **ondansetron** and oral **granisetron**); treatment of postoperative nausea or vomiting (**dolasetron** IV and **granisetron** IV); prevention of acute and/or delayed nausea and vomiting associated with initial and repeat courses of emetogenic cancer chemotherapy (**palonosetron**).

IBS (alosetron only): For women with severe diarrhea-predominant IBS who have chronic IBS symptoms (generally lasting 6 months or longer), have had anatomic or biochemical abnormalities of the GI tract excluded, and have not responded adequately to conventional therapy.

Administration and Dosage

ALOSETRON:

Prescribing program – For safety reasons, only health care providers who enroll in the GlaxoSmithKline prescribing program for alosetron should prescribe alosetron.

Adult dosage – To lower the risk of constipation, alosetron should be started at a dosage of 0.5 mg twice a day. Patients well controlled on 0.5 mg twice a day may be maintained on this regimen. If, after 4 weeks, the 0.5 mg twice daily dosage is well tolerated but does not adequately control IBS symptoms, then the dosage can be increased to up to 1 mg twice a day, the dosage used in controlled clinical trials.

Alosetron may be taken with or without food.

Discontinue therapy – Alosetron should be discontinued in patients who have not had adequate control of IBS symptoms after 4 weeks of treatment with 1 mg twice a day.

Alosetron should be discontinued immediately in patients who develop constipation or signs of ischemic colitis. Alosetron should not be restarted in patients who develop ischemic colitis.

Special populations – Clinical trial and postmarketing experience suggest that debilitated patients or patients taking additional medications that decrease GI motility may be at greater risk of serious complications of constipation. Therefore, appropriate caution and follow-up should be exercised if alosetron is prescribed for these patients.

Pharmacists information – Alosetron may be dispensed only on presentation of a prescription for alosetron with a sticker for the prescribing program for alosetron attached. A *MedGuide* for alosetron must be given to the patient each time alosetron is dispensed as required by law. No telephone, facsimile, or computerized prescriptions are permitted with this program. Refills are permitted to be written on prescriptions.

DOLASETRON:

Infusion rate – Dolasetron injection can be safely infused IV as rapidly as 100 mg/30 seconds or diluted in a compatible IV solution to 50 mL and infused over a period of up to 15 minutes.

Chemotherapy-induced nausea and vomiting, prevention –

IV:

Adults – 1.8 mg/kg as a single dose about 30 minutes before chemotherapy. Alternatively, a fixed dose of 100 mg can be administered over 30 seconds.

Children (2 to 16 years of age) – 1.8 mg/kg as a single dose about 30 minutes before chemotherapy, up to a maximum of 100 mg.

Oral:

Adults – 100 mg within 1 hour before chemotherapy.

Children (2 to 16 years of age) – 1.8 mg/kg within 1 hour before chemotherapy, up to a maximum of 100 mg.

Postoperative nausea or vomiting, prevention/treatment –

IV:

Adults – 12.5 mg as a single dose about 15 minutes before the cessation of anesthesia or as soon as nausea or vomiting presents.

Children (2 to 16 years of age) – 0.35 mg/kg as a single dose about 15 minutes before the cessation of anesthesia or as soon as nausea or vomiting presents, up to a maximum of 12.5 mg.

Oral (prevention only) –

Adults: 100 mg 2 hours before surgery.

Children (2 to 16 years of age): 1.2 mg/kg within 2 hours before surgery, up to a maximum of 100 mg.

GRANISETRON:

Oral –

Emetogenic chemotherapy: Adult dosage of 2 mg once daily or 1 mg twice daily. In the 2 mg once-daily regimen, two 1 mg tablets or 10 mL of oral solution are given up to 1 hour before chemotherapy. In the 1 mg twice-daily regimen, give the first 1 mg tablet or 1 teaspoonful (5 mL) of oral solution up to 1 hour before chemotherapy and the second tablet or second teaspoonful (5 mL) of oral solution 12 hours after the first. Administer only on the day(s) chemotherapy is given.

Radiation (total body irradiation or fractionated abdominal radiation): Adult dose of 2 mg once daily. Two 1 mg tablets or 10 mL of oral solution are taken within 1 hour of radiation.

IV –

Prevention of chemotherapy-induced nausea and vomiting:

Infusion preparation – May be administered IV undiluted over 30 seconds, or diluted with 0.9% sodium chloride or 5% dextrose and infused over 5 minutes.

Adults and children 2 years of age and older – 10 mcg/kg administered IV within 30 minutes before initiation of chemotherapy, and only on the day(s) chemotherapy is given. Children younger than 2 years of age have not been studied.

Prevention and treatment of postoperative nausea and vomiting:

Adults –

Prevention: 1 mg undiluted administered IV over 30 seconds, before induction of anesthesia or immediately before reversal of anesthesia.

Treatment: After surgery, 1 mg undiluted administered IV over 30 seconds.

Incompatibilities – As a general precaution, do not mix granisetron injection in a solution with other drugs

Transdermal –

Adults:

Usual dosage – Apply a single patch to the upper outer arm a minimum of 24 hours before chemotherapy. The patch may be applied up to a maximum of 48 hours before chemotherapy as appropriate. Remove the patch a minimum of 24 hours after completion of chemotherapy.

Duration of therapy – The patch can be worn for up to 7 days.

Administration – The transdermal system (patch) should be applied to a clean, dry, intact healthy skin on the upper outer arm. Granisetron should not be placed on skin that is red, irritated, or damaged.

Each patch should be applied directly after the pouch has been opened. The patch should not be cut into pieces.

ONDANSETRON:

Prevention of nausea/vomiting associated with cancer chemotherapy –

Parenteral: Three 0.15 mg/kg doses or a single 32 mg dose. With the 3 dose regimen, the first dose is infused over 15 minutes beginning 30 minutes before the start of emetogenic chemotherapy. Subsequent doses are administered 4 and 8 hours after the first dose. The single 32 mg dose is infused over 15 minutes beginning 30 minutes before the start of emetogenic chemotherapy.

Children (6 months to 18 years of age) – Three 0.15 mg/kg doses (see above). Little information is available about dosage in children 6 months of age or younger.

Oral (moderately emetogenic cancer chemotherapy; patients older than 12 years of age): 8 mg twice/day. Administer the first dose 30 minutes before the start of emetogenic chemotherapy, with a subsequent dose 8 hours after the first dose. Administer 8 mg twice a day (every 12 hours) for 1 to 2 days after completion of chemotherapy.

Children (4 to 11 years of age) – 4 mg 3 times a day. Give the first dose 30 minutes before chemotherapy, with subsequent doses 4 and 8 hours after the first dose. Give 4 mg 3 times a day (every 8 hours) for 1 to 2 days after completion of chemotherapy.

Prevention of nausea and vomiting associated with radiotherapy (oral) – 8 mg 3 times/day.

Total body irradiation: 8 mg 1 to 2 hours before each fraction of radiotherapy administered each day.

Single high-dose fraction radiotherapy to the abdomen: 8 mg 1 to 2 hours before radiotherapy, with subsequent doses every 8 hours after the first dose for 1 to 2 days after completion of radiotherapy.

Daily fractionated radiotherapy to the abdomen: 8 mg 1 to 2 hours before radiotherapy, with subsequent doses every 8 hours after the first dose for each day radiotherapy is given.

Prevention of postoperative nausea or vomiting –

Parenteral: Immediately before induction of anesthesia, or postoperatively if the patient experiences nausea or vomiting shortly after surgery, administer 4 mg undiluted IV in not less than 30 seconds, preferably over 2 to 5 minutes. Alternatively, 4 mg undiluted may be administered IM as a single injection in adults. In patients who do not achieve adequate control, administration of a second IV dose of 4 mg ondansetron postoperatively does not provide additional control of nausea and vomiting.

Children – The recommended IV dosage for pediatric surgical patients (1 month to 12 years of age) is a single 0.1 mg/kg dose for children weighing less than 40 kg, or a single 4 mg dose for patients weighing more than 40 kg. The rate of administration should not be less than 30 seconds, preferably over 2 to 5 minutes, immediately prior to or following anesthesia induction or postoperatively if the patient experiences nausea and/or vomiting occurring shortly after surgery.

Oral: 16 mg given as a single dose 1 hour before induction of anesthesia.

Children: There is no experience in children.

Prevention of nausea and vomiting associated with highly emetogenic cancer chemotherapy (oral) – 24 mg administered 30 minutes before the start of single-day highly emetogenic chemotherapy, including cisplatin greater than 50 mg/m^2.

Hepatic function impairment – Do not exceed an 8 mg oral dose. For IV use, a single maximum daily dose of 8 mg infused over 15 minutes beginning 30 minutes before the start of emetogenic chemotherapy is recommended.

PALONOSETRON:

Adults –

Chemotherapy-induced nausea and vomiting: 0.25 mg administered as a single IV dose administered over 30 seconds approximately 30 minutes before the start of chemotherapy.

Postoperative nausea and vomiting: 0.075 mg IV dose administered over 10 seconds immediately before the induction of anesthesia.

Administration: Flush the infusion line with isotonic sodium chloride solution before and after administration of palonosetron.

Admixture incompatibilities: Palonosetron should not be mixed with other drugs.

Actions

Pharmacology: Selective 5-hydroxytryptamine$_3$ (5-HT$_3$) receptor antagonists are antinauseant, antiemetic, and anti-IBS (**alosetron** only) agents with little or no affinity for other serotonin receptors, alpha- or beta-adrenoreceptors, or for dopamine D$_2$, histamine H$_1$, benzodiazepine, picrotoxin, or opioid receptors.

Pharmacokinetics: The elimination half-lives of these drugs range from 4 to 8 hours. Elimination is primarily via hepatic metabolism. Plasma protein binding is 82% for alosetron, 65% for **granisetron**, and 70% to 76% for **ondansetron**.

Contraindications

Alosetron: Do not initiate in patients with constipation or patients who are unable to comply with or understand the patient-physician agreement for alosetron; coadministration with fluvoxamine; in patients with a history of the following: chronic or severe constipation or sequelae for constipation; intestinal obstruction, stricture, toxic megacolon, GI perforation, and/or adhesions; ischemic colitis, impaired intestinal circulation, thrombophlebitis, or hypercoagulable state; Crohn disease or ulcerative colitis; diverticulitis; severe hepatic function impairment; hypersensitivity to any component of the product.

Dolasetron, granisetron, ondansetron, palonosetron: Hypersensitivity to the drug or any of its components.

Warnings/Precautions

Ischemic colitis: Ischemic colitis has been reported in patients receiving **alosetron**. Immediately discontinue alosetron in patients with signs of ischemic colitis, such as rectal bleeding, bloody diarrhea, or new or worsening abdominal pain. Do not resume alosetron in patients who develop ischemic colitis.

Constipation: Serious complications of constipation, including obstruction, perforation, impaction, toxic megacolon, secondary colonic ischemia, and death have been reported with use of **alosetron**. Immediately discontinue alosetron treatment in patients who develop constipation.

Cardiac effects: Acute, usually reversible, electrocardiogram changes (PR and QTc prolongation; electrocardiograph wave widening) caused by dolasetron have been observed. Dolasetron appears to prolong depolarization and, to a lesser extent, repolarization time. The magnitude and frequency of the ECG changes increased with dose. These ECG interval prolongations usually returned to baseline within 6 to 8 hours but in some patients were present at 24-hour follow-up.

Rarely, and predominantly with **ondansetron** IV, transient ECG changes, including QT interval prolongation, have been reported.

Administer dolasetron and palonosetron with caution in patients who have or may develop cardiac conduction interval prolongation. These include patients with hypokalemia or hypomagnesemia, patients taking diuretics with potential for inducing electrolyte abnormalities, patients with congenital QT syndrome, patients taking antiarrhythmic drugs or other drugs that lead to QT prolongation, and cumulative high-dose anthracycline therapy.

Peristalsis: Ondansetron and granisetron do not stimulate gastric or intestinal peristalsis. Do not use instead of nasogastric suction. Use in abdominal surgery may mask a progressive ileus or gastric distension.

Phenylketonuric patients: Inform phenylketonuric patients that ondansetron orally disintegrating tablets contain phenylalanine (a component of aspartame). Each 4 and 8 mg orally disintegrating tablet contains less that 0.03 mg of phenylalanine.

Benzyl alcohol: Granisetron 1 mg/mL injection contains benzyl alcohol as a preservative. Benzyl alcohol has been associated with a fatal gasping syndrome in premature infants and may cross the placenta of a pregnant woman and reach the fetus. Use granisetron injection in pregnancy only if the benefit outweighs the potential risk.

Hypersensitivity reactions: Rare cases of hypersensitivity reactions, sometimes severe, have occurred.

Hepatic function impairment: Increased exposure to alosetron is likely to occur in patients with hepatic insufficiency.

Pregnancy: Category B.

Lactation: It is not known whether 5-HT_3 antagonists are excreted in breast milk.

Children: Safety and efficacy of alosetron, palonosetron, and oral granisetron in children have not been established.

There is no experience with dolasetron in children younger than 2 years of age.

Safety and efficacy of granisetron injection have not been established in children younger than 2 years of age and have not been established in children for the prevention or treatment of postoperative nausea or vomiting.

Little information is available about oral ondansetron dosage in children 4 years of age or younger. Little information is known about the use of ondansetron injection in pediatric surgical patients younger than 1 month of age or in pediatric cancer patients younger than 6 months of age.

Drug Interactions

Inducers or inhibitors of P-450 enzymes may change the clearance and, hence, the half-life of 5-HT_3 antagonists. No dosage adjustment is recommended for patients on these drugs. **Dolasetron** may be affected by atenolol, cimetidine, rifampin, and ziprasidone. **Ondansetron** may be affected by rifampin, carbamazepine, phenytoin, and rifamycins. Granisetron may be affected by phenobarbital. Alosetron may be affected by CYP 1A2 inhibitors and CYP 3A4 inhibitors. Avoid coadministration of alosetron with fluvoxamine and other CYP 1A2 inhibitors. Dolasetron may affect ziprasidone. Ondansetron may affect cisplatin and cyclophosphamide.

Adverse Reactions

Adverse reactions occurring in at least 3% of patients:

Ondansetron: Abdominal pain; anxiety/agitation; arrhythmias; increased AST and ALT; chills/shivering; constipation; diarrhea; dizziness; drowsiness/sedation; extrapyramidal syndrome; malaise/fatigue; fever/pyrexia; gynecological disorder; headache; hypotension; hypoxia; injection site reaction; musculoskeletal pain; pruritus; urinary retention; wound problem.

Granisetron: Abdominal pain; alopecia; anemia; decreased appetite; increased AST and ALT; asthenia; CNS stimulation; constipation; diarrhea; headache; leukopenia; nausea/vomiting; somnolence; shivers; thrombocytopenia.

Dolasetron: Abdominal pain; increased AST and ALT; bradycardia/tachycardia; dizziness; dyspepsia; fever/pyrexia; headache; hypotension; malaise/fatigue; pruritus.

Alosetron: Abdominal pain; constipation; GI discomfort/pain; nausea.

Palonosetron: Headache; constipation.

APREPITANT

Capsules: 40, 80, and 125 mg (*Rx*) — *Emend* (Merck)

Indications

Prevention of nausea/vomiting associated with highly emetogenic cancer chemotherapy: In combination with other antiemetic agents for the prevention of acute and delayed nausea and vomiting associated with initial and repeat courses of highly emetogenic cancer chemotherapy, including high-dose cisplatin.

Prevention of nausea/vomiting associated with moderately emetogenic cancer chemotherapy: In combination with other antiemetic agents for the prevention of nausea and vomiting associated with initial and repeat courses of moderately emetogenic cancer chemotherapy.

Prevention of postoperative nausea and vomiting: For the prevention of postoperative nausea and vomiting.

Administration and Dosage

Dosage regimen: Aprepitant is given for 3 days as part of a regimen that includes a corticosteroid and a 5-HT$_3$ antagonist. Aprepitant has not been studied for the treatment of established nausea and vomiting.

Chronic continuous administration is not recommended. Aprepitant may be taken with or without food.

Aprepitant Dosage Regimen for Highly Emetogenic Cancer Chemotherapy

Treatment	Day 1	Day 2	Day 3	Day 4
Aprepitant[a]	125 mg	80 mg	80 mg	none
Dexamethasone[b]	12 mg orally	8 mg orally	8 mg orally	8 mg orally
Ondansetron[c]	32 mg intravenous (IV)	none	none	none

[a] Aprepitant was administered orally 1 hour prior to chemotherapy treatment on day 1 and in the morning on days 2 and 3.
[b] Dexamethasone was administered 30 minutes prior to chemotherapy treatment on day 1 and in the morning on days 2 through 4. The dose of dexamethasone was chosen to account for drug interactions.
[c] Ondansetron was administered 30 minutes prior to chemotherapy treatment on day 1.

Aprepitant Dosage Regimen for Moderately Emetogenic Cancer Chemotherapy			
Treatment	Day 1	Day 2	Day 3
Aprepitant[a]	125 mg	80 mg	80 mg
Dexamethasone[b]	12 mg orally	none	none
Ondansetron[c]	8 mg orally × 2	none	none

[a] Aprepitant was administered orally 1 hour prior to chemotherapy treatment on day 1 and in the morning on days 2 and 3.
[b] Dexamethasone was administered 30 minutes prior to chemotherapy treatment on day 1. The dexamethasone dose was chosen to account for drug interactions.
[c] One ondansetron 8 mg capsule was administered 30 to 60 minutes prior to chemotherapy treatment, and a second 8 mg capsule was administered 8 hours after the first dose on day 1.

Concomitant therapy: The oral dexamethasone doses should be reduced by approximately 50% when coadministered with aprepitant.

The IV methylprednisolone dose should be reduced by approximately 25%, and the oral methylprednisolone dose should be reduced by approximately 50% when coadministered with aprepitant.

Actions

Pharmacology: Aprepitant is a selective high-affinity antagonist of human substance P/neurokinin 1 (NK_1) receptors. Aprepitant has little or no affinity for serotonin ($5\text{-}HT_3$), dopamine, and corticosteroid receptors, the targets of existing therapies for chemotherapy-induced nausea and vomiting (CINV).

Studies show that aprepitant augments the antiemetic activity of the $5\text{-}HT_3$-receptor antagonist ondansetron and the corticosteroid dexamethasone and inhibits both the acute and delayed phases of cisplatin-induced emesis.

Pharmacokinetics:

Absorption – The mean absolute oral bioavailability of aprepitant is approximately 60% to 65% and the mean peak plasma concentration (C_{max}) of aprepitant occurred at approximately 4 hours (T_{max}).

Distribution – Aprepitant is greater than 95% bound to plasma proteins. The mean apparent volume of distribution at steady state (Vd_{ss}) is approximately 70 L.

Metabolism – Aprepitant undergoes extensive metabolism. In vitro studies using human liver microsomes indicate that aprepitant is metabolized primarily by CYP3A4 with minor metabolism by CYP1A2 and CYP2C19.

Excretion – Aprepitant is eliminated primarily by metabolism; aprepitant is not renally excreted. The apparent terminal half-life ranged from approximately 9 to 13 hours.

Contraindications

Aprepitant is a moderate CYP3A4 inhibitor. Aprepitant should not be used concurrently with pimozide, terfenadine, astemizole, or cisapride. Inhibition of cytochrome P450 isoenzyme 3A4 (CYP3A4) by aprepitant could result in elevated plasma concentrations of these drugs, potentially causing serious or life-threatening reactions. Aprepitant is contraindicated in patients who are hypersensitive to any component of the product.

Warnings/Precautions

Chronic therapy: Chronic continuous use of aprepitant for prevention of nausea and vomiting is not recommended.

Pregnancy: *Category B.*

Lactation: It is not known whether this drug is excreted in human milk. A decision should be made whether to discontinue nursing or to discontinue the drug, taking into account the importance of the drug to the mother.

Children: Safety and efficacy of aprepitant in children have not been established.

Drug Interactions

Aprepitant is a substrate, a moderate inhibitor, and an inducer of CYP3A4. Aprepitant is also an inducer of CYP2C9. Use aprepitant with caution in patients receiving concomitant medicinal products, including chemotherapy agents that are primarily metabolized through CYP3A4 (docetaxel, paclitaxel, etoposide, irinotecan, ifosfamide, imatinib, vinorelbine, vinblastine, and vincristine).

Drugs that may affect aprepitant include CYP 3A4 inhibitors (eg, clarithromycin, diltiazem, itraconazole, ketoconazole, nefazodone, nelfinavir, ritonavir, troleandomycin), CYP3A4 inducers (eg, carbamazepine, phenytoin, rifampin), and paroxetine.

Aprepitant may be affected by paroxetine, CYP2C9 substrates (eg, phenytoin, tolbutamide, warfarin), CYP3A4 substrates (eg, alprazolam, cisapride, dexamethasone, docetaxel, etoposide, ifosfamide, imatinib, irinotecan, methylprednisolone, midazolam, paclitaxel, pimozide, triazolam, vinblastine, vincristine, vinorelbine), and oral contraceptives.

Adverse Reactions

Adverse reactions occurring in at least 3% of aprepitant patients include the following: Abdominal pain, anorexia, ALT/AST/BUN/Serum creatinine increased, alopecia, asthenia/fatigue, constipation, dehydration, diarrhea, dizziness, epigastric discomfort, gastritis, headache, heartburn, hiccoughs, hot flushes, nausea, neutropenia, proteinuria, stomatitis, tinnitus, vomiting.

FOSAPREPITANT

Injection, lyophilized powder for solution: 115 mg (*Rx*) *Emend* (Merck)

Indications

Prevention of chemotherapy-induced nausea and vomiting: In combination with other antiemetic agents, for the prevention of acute and delayed nausea and vomiting associated with initial and repeat courses of highly and moderately emetogenic cancer chemotherapy, including high-dose cisplatin.

Administration and Dosage

Fosaprepitant injection may be administered with or without food.

Dosing regimen: Fosaprepitant 115 mg may be substituted for aprepitant 125 mg orally 30 minutes prior to chemotherapy, on day 1 only of the chemotherapy-induced nausea and vomiting regimen as an infusion administered over 15 minutes.

Highly emetogenic cancer chemotherapy –

Aprepitant Dosage Regimen for the Prevention of Nausea and Vomiting Associated With Highly Emetogenic Cancer Chemotherapy

	Day 1	Day 2	Day 3	Day 4
Aprepitant[a]	125 mg orally	80 mg orally	80 mg orally	none
Dexamethasone[b]	12 mg orally	8 mg orally	8 mg orally	8 mg orally
Ondansetron[c]	32 mg IV[d]	none	none	none

[a] Aprepitant was administered orally 1 hour prior to chemotherapy treatment on day 1 and in the morning on days 2 and 3.

[b] Dexamethasone was administered 30 minutes prior to chemotherapy treatment on day 1 and in the morning on days 2 through 4. The dose of dexamethasone was chosen to account for drug interactions.

[c] Ondansetron was administered 30 minutes prior to chemotherapy treatment on day 1.

[d] IV = intravenously.

Moderately emetogenic cancer chemotherapy –

Aprepitant Dosage Regimen for the Prevention of Nausea and Vomiting Associated With Moderately Emetogenic Cancer Chemotherapy

	Day 1	Day 2	Day 3
Aprepitant[a]	125 mg orally	80 mg orally	80 mg orally
Dexamethasone[b]	12 mg orally	none	none
Ondansetron[c]	2 × 8 mg orally	none	none

[a] Aprepitant was administered orally 1 hour prior to chemotherapy treatment on day 1 and in the morning on days 2 and 3.
[b] Dexamethasone was administered 30 minutes prior to chemotherapy treatment on day 1. The dose of dexamethasone was chosen to account for drug interactions.
[c] Ondansetron 8 mg capsule was administered 30 to 60 minutes prior to chemotherapy treatment, and one 8 mg capsule was administered 8 hours after the first dose on day 1.

Admixture incompatibilities: Fosaprepitant injection is incompatible with any solutions containing divalent cations (eg, Ca^{2+}, Mg^{2+}), including Ringer's lactate solution and Hartmann's solution.

Actions

Pharmacology: Fosaprepitant is a prodrug of aprepitant and, accordingly, its antiemetic effects are attributable to aprepitant.

Aprepitant is a selective high-affinity antagonist of human substance NK_1 receptors.

Pharmacokinetics:

Distribution – Fosaprepitant is rapidly converted to aprepitant. Aprepitant is more than 95% bound to plasma proteins.

Metabolism – Fosaprepitant IV was rapidly converted to aprepitant within 30 minutes following the end of infusion.

Aprepitant undergoes extensive metabolism. In vitro studies using human liver microsomes indicate that aprepitant is metabolized primarily by cytochrome P-450 isoenzyme 3A4 (CYP3A4), with minor metabolism by CYP1A2 and CYP2C19.

Excretion – The apparent terminal half-life of aprepitant ranged from approximately 9 to 13 hours.

Contraindications

Hypersensitivity to fosaprepitant, aprepitant, polysorbate 80, or any other components of the product; concurrent use with astemizole, cisapride, pimozide, or terfenadine.

Warnings/Precautions

Chronic use: Chronic continuous use of fosaprepitant for prevention of nausea and vomiting is not recommended.

Hepatic function impairment: Exercise caution when fosaprepitant or aprepitant is administered to patients with severe hepatic function impairment (Child-Pugh score higher than 9).

Pregnancy: Category B.

Lactation: It is not known whether this drug is excreted in human milk.

Children: Safety and effectiveness in children have not been established.

Elderly: Greater sensitivity of some older individuals cannot be ruled out. Dosage adjustment in elderly patients is not necessary.

Drug Interactions

Drugs that may be affected by fosaprepitant include astemizole (no longer marketed in the United States), benzodiazepines (eg, alprazolam, midazolam, triazolam), chemotherapy agents (eg, docetaxel, etoposide, ifosfamide, imatinib, irinotecan, paclitaxel, vinblastine, vincristine, vinorelbine), cisapride (available from the manufacturer on a limited access protocol), corticosteroids (eg, dexamethasone, methylprednisolone), CYP2C9 substrates (eg, tolbutamide, warfarin), diltiazem, hormonal contraceptives, paroxetine, pimozide, terfenadine (no longer marketed in the United States).

Drugs that may affect fosaprepitant include CYP3A4 inducers (eg, carbamazepine, phenytoin, rifampin), CYP3A4 inhibitors (eg, clarithromycin, itraconazole, ketoconazole, nefazodone, nelfinavir, ritonavir, troleandomycin [no longer marketed in the United States]), diltiazem, and paroxetine.

Adverse Reactions

Adverse reactions occurring in 3% or more of patients included abdominal pain, alopecia, ALT increased, anorexia, asthenia/fatigue, AST increased, constipation, dehydration, diarrhea, dizziness, dyspepsia, epigastric discomfort, gastritis, headache, heartburn, hiccups, hot flush, infusion-site pain, insomnia, nausea, neutropenia, pharyngolaryngeal pain, proteinuria, serum creatinine increased, serum urea nitrogen increased, stomatitis, tinnitus, vomiting.

NABILONE

Capsules: 1 mg *(c-II)*	*Cesamet* (Valeant Pharmaceuticals International)

Indications

Antiemetic: For the treatment of the nausea and vomiting associated with cancer chemotherapy in patients who have failed to respond adequately to conventional antiemetic treatments. This restriction is required because a substantial proportion of any group of patients treated with nabilone can be expected to experience disturbing psychotomimetic reactions not observed with other antiemetic agents.

Nabilone is intended for use under circumstances that permit close supervision of the patient by a responsible individual, particularly during the initial use of nabilone and during dose adjustments.

Nabilone is not intended for use on an as-needed basis or as the first antiemetic product prescribed for a patient.

Administration and Dosage

Adults: 1 or 2 mg twice a day. On the day of chemotherapy, the initial dose should be given 1 to 3 hours before the chemotherapeutic agent is administered. A dose of 1 or 2 mg the night before may be useful. The maximum recommended daily dose is 6 mg given in divided doses 3 times a day.

Nabilone may be administered 2 or 3 times daily during the entire course of each cycle of chemotherapy and, if needed, for 48 hours after the last dose of each cycle of chemotherapy.

Actions

Pharmacology: Nabilone is an orally active synthetic cannabinoid that has complex effects on the CNS. It has been suggested that the antiemetic effect of nabilone is caused by interaction with the cannabinoid receptor system (the CB 1 receptor), which has been discovered in neural tissues.

Pharmacokinetics:

Absorption/Distribution – Nabilone appears to be completely absorbed from the human GI tract when administered orally. The apparent volume of distribution of nabilone is approximately 12.5 L/kg.

Metabolism – Metabolism of nabilone is extensive, and several metabolites have been identified. Precise information concerning the metabolites that may accumulate is not available.

Excretion – The route and rate of the elimination of nabilone and its metabolites are similar to those observed with other cannabinoids, including delta-9-THC (dronabinol).

Contraindications

History of hypersensitivity to any cannabinoid.

Warnings/Precautions

Duration of effects: The effects of nabilone may persist for a variable and unpredictable period of time following its oral administration. Adverse psychiatric reactions can persist for 48 to 72 hours following cessation of treatment.

CNS effects: Nabilone has the potential to affect the CNS and might manifest itself in dizziness, drowsiness, euphoria ("high"), ataxia, anxiety, disorientation, depression, hallucinations, and psychosis.

Cardiovascular effects: Nabilone can cause tachycardia and orthostatic hypotension.

Close supervision: Because of individual variation in response and tolerance to the effects of nabilone, patients should remain under the supervision of a responsible adult, especially during initial use of nabilone and during dose adjustments.

Special risk: Carefully evaluate the benefit/risk ratio of nabilone use in patients with the following medical conditions because of individual variation in response and tolerance to the effects of nabilone.

- Because nabilone can elevate supine and standing heart rates and cause postural hypotension, use it with caution in the elderly and in patients with hypertension or heart disease.
- Use nabilone with caution in patients with current or previous psychiatric disorders because the symptoms of these disease states may be unmasked by the use of cannabinoids.
- Use nabilone with caution in patients with a history of substance abuse, including alcohol abuse or dependence and marijuana use, because nabilone contains a similar active compound to marijuana.

Drug abuse and dependence: Nabilone, a synthetic cannabinoid pharmacologically related to *Cannabis sativa* L (Marijuana; delta-9-THC) is a highly abusable substance. Nabilone is controlled under schedule II of the Controlled Substances Act.

Abuse – Nabilone was qualitatively and quantitatively similar to approved oral delta-9-THC in the production of cannabis-like effects, demonstrating its potential for abuse.

Dependence – The physical dependence capacity of nabilone is unknown at this time. Patients who participated in clinical trials of up to 5 days' duration evidenced no withdrawal symptoms upon cessation of dosing.

Hazardous tasks: Specifically warn patients receiving nabilone treatment not to drive, operate machinery, or engage in any hazardous activity while receiving nabilone.

Pregnancy: Category C

Lactation: Because many drugs, including some cannabinoids, are excreted in breast milk, it is not recommended that nabilone be given to breast-feeding mothers.

Children: Safety and efficacy have not been established in patients younger than 18 years of age. Caution is recommended in prescribing nabilone to children because of psychoactive effects.

Elderly: Be cautious in dose selection for an elderly patient, usually starting at the low end of the dosing range, reflecting the greater frequency of decreased hepatic, renal, or cardiac function, and of concomitant disease or other drug therapy.

Monitoring: As with all controlled drugs, monitor patients receiving nabilone for signs of excessive use, abuse, and misuse. Patients who may be at increased risk for substance abuse include those with a personal or family history of substance abuse or mental illness.

Drug Interactions

Drugs that affect nabilone include the following: Amphetamines, anticholinergic agents, antihistamines, atropine, barbiturates, benzodiazepines, buspirone, cocaine, CNS depressants, ethanol, lithium, muscle relaxants, naltrexone, opioids, scopolamine, sympathomimetic agents, tricyclic antidepressants.

Drugs that may be affected by nabilone include the following: Amphetamines, anticholinergic agents, antihistamines, antipyrine, atropine, barbiturates, benzodiazepines, buspirone, cocaine, CNS depressants, disulfiram, ethanol, fluoxetine, lithium, muscle relaxants, opioids, scopolamine, sympathomimetic agents, theophylline, tricyclic antidepressants.

Adverse Reactions

Adverse reactions occurring in at least 3% of patients include the following: anorexia, asthenia, ataxia, concentration difficulties, depression, dizziness, drowsiness, dry mouth, dysphoria, euphoria, headache, hypotension, nausea, sedation, sleep disturbance, vertigo, visual disturbances.

MEPROBAMATE

Tablets: 200, 400, and 600 mg (*c-iv*)	Various, *Equanil* (Wyeth-Ayerst), *Miltown* (Wallace)

Indications

Management of anxiety disorders or short-term relief of the symptoms of anxiety.

Administration and Dosage

Adults: 1.2 to 1.6 g/day in 3 to 4 divided doses; do not exceed 2.4 g/day.

Children: 100 to 200 mg 2 or 3 times/day.

Actions

Pharmacology: Meprobamate has selective effects at multiple sites in the CNS, including the thalamus and limbic system. It also appears to inhibit multineuronal spinal reflexes. Meprobamate is mildly tranquilizing, and has some anticonvulsant and muscle relaxant properties.

Pharmacokinetics:

Absorption/Distribution – Meprobamate is well absorbed from the GI tract; peak plasma concentrations are reached within 1 to 3 hours.

Metabolism/Excretion – The liver metabolizes 80% to 92% of the drug; the remainder is excreted unchanged in the urine. Excretion is mainly renal (90%), with less than 10% appearing in feces.

Contraindications

Acute intermittent porphyria; allergic or idiosyncratic reactions to meprobamate or related compounds.

Warnings/Precautions

Epilepsy: May precipitate seizures in epileptic patients.

Hypersensitivity reactions: Usually seen between the first to fourth dose in patients having no previous exposure to the drug.

Renal function impairment: Use with caution to avoid accumulation, since meprobamate is metabolized in the liver and excreted by the kidney.

Drug abuse and dependence: Physical and psychological dependence and abuse may occur.

Abrupt discontinuation after prolonged and excessive use may precipitate a recurrence of pre-existing symptoms or withdrawal syndrome characterized by anxiety, anorexia, insomnia, vomiting, ataxia, tremors, muscle twitching, confusional states, and hallucinations. Generalized seizures occur in about 10% of cases and are more likely to occur in people with CNS damage or preexistent or latent convulsive disorders. Onset of withdrawal symptoms usually occurs within 12 to 48 hours after drug discontinuation; symptoms usually cease in the next 12 to 48 hours.

When excessive dosage has continued for weeks or months, reduce gradually over a period of 1 or 2 weeks rather than stopping abruptly.

Hazardous tasks: May produce drowsiness, dizziness, or blurred vision; patients should observe caution while driving or performing other tasks requiring alertness.

Pregnancy: Category D.

Lactation: Meprobamate is excreted into breast milk at concentrations 2 to 4 times that of maternal plasma.

Children: Do not administer to children younger than 6 years of age. The 600 mg tablet is not intended for use in children.

Elderly: To avoid oversedation, use lowest effective dose.

Drug Interactions

Alcohol: Acute ingestion may result in a decreased clearance of meprobamate through inhibition of hepatic metabolic systems; enhanced CNS depressant effects may occur.

Adverse Reactions

Adverse reactions may include drowsiness; ataxia; dizziness; slurred speech; headache; vertigo; weakness; impairment of visual accommodation; euphoria; overstimulation; paradoxical excitement; nausea; vomiting; diarrhea; palpitations; tachycardia; various arrhythmias; syncope; hypotensive crises; allergic/idiosyncratic reactions; leukopenia; acute nonthrombocytopenic purpura; petechiae; ecchymoses; eosinophilia; peripheral edema; fever; hyperpyrexia; chills; angioneurotic edema; bronchospasm; oliguria; anuria; anaphylaxis; erythema multiforme; exfoliative dermatitis; stomatitis; proctitis; Stevens-Johnson syndrome; bullous dermatitis; paresthesias; agranulocytosis; aplastic anemia; thrombocytopenic purpura.

BENZODIAZEPINES

ALPRAZOLAM	
Tablets; oral: 0.25, 0.5, 1, and 2 mg (*c-iv*)	Various, *Xanax* (Pfizer)
Tablets, extended-release; oral: 0.5, 1, 2, and 3 mg (*c-iv*)	Various, *Xanax XR* (Pfizer)
Tablets, disintegrating; oral: 0.25, 0.5, 1, and 2 mg (*c-iv*)	*Niravam* (Schwarz Pharma)
Solution; oral: 1 mg/mL (*c-iv*)	*Alprazolam Intensol* (Roxane)
CHLORDIAZEPOXIDE	
Capsules; oral: 5, 10, and 25 mg (*c-iv*)	Various
CLONAZEPAM	
Tablets; oral: 0.5, 1, and 2 mg (*c-iv*)	Various, *Klonopin* (Roche)
Tablets, disintegrating; oral: 0.125, 0.25, 0.5, 1, and 2 mg (*c-iv*)	
CLORAZEPATE DIPOTASSIUM	
Tablets; oral: 3.75, 7.5, and 15 mg (*c-iv*)	Various, *Tranxene T-tab* (Ovation)
DIAZEPAM	
Tablets; oral: 2, 5, and 10 mg (*c-iv*)	Various, *Valium* (Roche)
Solution; oral: 5 mg per 5 mL (*c-iv*)	*Diazepam* (Roxane)
Solution, concentrate; oral: 5 mg/mL (*c-iv*)	*Diazepam Intensol* (Roxane)
Gel; rectal: 2.5, 10, and 20 mg (*c-iv*)	*Diastat* (Xcel)
Injection, solution: 5 mg/mL (*c-iv*)	Various
LORAZEPAM	
Tablets; oral: 0.5, 1, and 2 mg (*c-iv*)	Various, *Ativan* (Valeant Pharmaceuticals)
Solution, concentrated; oral: 2 mg/mL (*c-iv*)	Various, *Lorazepam Intensol* (Roxane)
Injection, solution: 2 and 4 mg/mL (*c-iv*)	Various, *Ativan* (Baxter)
OXAZEPAM	
Capsules; oral: 10, 15, and 30 mg (*c-iv*)	Various

Indications

Anxiety: For the management of anxiety disorders or for the short-term relief of the symptoms of anxiety (anxiety associated with depression is also responsive) (**alprazolam** immediate-release and intensol, **clorazepate, chlordiazepoxide, diazepam, lorazepam, oxazepam**); for the management of anxiety, tension, agitation, and irritability in older patients (oxazepam).

Panic disorder: Treatment of panic disorder, with or without agoraphobia (**alprazolam** immediate-release, extended-release, and orally disintegrating; **clonazepam**).

Acute alcohol withdrawal: For the symptomatic relief of acute alcohol withdrawal (**clorazepate, chlordiazepoxide, oxazepam**); may be useful in symptomatic relief of acute agitation, tremor, impending or acute delirium, tremens, and hallucinosis (**diazepam**).

Anticonvulsant: As adjunctive therapy in the management of partial seizures (**clorazepate**); adjunctively in status epilepticus and severe recurrent convulsive seizures (**diazepam IV**); adjunctively in convulsive disorders (**diazepam oral**); for selected refractory patients with epilepsy who are on stable regimens of antiepileptic drugs (AEDs) and require intermittent use of diazepam to control bouts of increased seizure activity (**diazepam rectal**); used alone or as adjunctive treatment of Lennox-Gastaut syndrome (petit mal variant), akinetic, and myoclonic seizures (**clonazepam**; may be useful in patients with absence [petit mal] seizures who have failed to respond to succinimides).

Preoperative: For preoperative apprehension and anxiety (**chlordiazepoxide, diazepam IV**); prior to cardioversion for the relief of anxiety and tension and to diminish patient's recall (diazepam IV); adjunctively prior to endoscopic procedures for apprehension, anxiety, or acute stress reactions and to diminish patient's recall (diazepam IV); for preanesthetic medication to produce sedation, anxiety relief, and a decreased ability to recall surgery-related events (**lorazepam**).

Muscle relaxant: As an adjunct for the relief of skeletal muscle spasm because of reflex spasm caused by local pathology, spasticity caused by uppermotor neuron disorders (eg, cerebral palsy, paraplegia), athetosis, stiff-man syndrome. Used parenterally in the treatment of tetanus (**diazepam**).

Seizure disorder (clonazepam): Alone or as an adjunct in the treatment of the Lennox-Gastaut syndrome (petit mal variant), akinetic, and myoclonic seizures. May be useful in patients with absence seizures (petit mal) who have failed to respond to succinimides (see Anticonvulsant section).

Status epilepticus: For the treatment of status epilepticus (**lorazepam**).

Administration and Dosage

ALPRAZOLAM: Reduce gradually when terminating or decreasing daily dose. Decrease by no more than 0.5 mg every 3 days.

Anxiety disorders (immediate-release and intensol) – Initial dose is 0.25 to 0.5 mg 3 times/day. Titrate to max total dose of 4 mg/day in divided doses at intervals of 3 to 4 days. If side effects occur with starting dose, decrease dose.

Panic disorder (Xanax, Xanax XR, and Niravam) –

Immediate-release tablets: Initial dose is 0.5 mg 3 times/day. Depending on response, increase dose at intervals of 3 to 4 days in increments of no more than 1 mg/day.

Successful treatment has required doses more than 4 mg/day; in controlled studies, doses in the range of 1 to 10 mg/day were used.

Extended-release tablets: Administer once daily, preferably in the morning. Do not chew, crush, or break tablets.

Treatment may be initiated with 0.5 to 1 mg once daily. The suggested total daily dose ranges between 3 and 6 mg/day.

Dose maintenance – Most patients showed efficacy in the range of 3 to 6 mg/day. Occasionally as much as 10 mg/day was required.

Immediate/Extended-release tablets:

Dose titration – The dose may be increased at intervals of 3 to 4 days in increments of no more than 1 mg/day. Slower titration to the dose levels may be advisable.

Switching from immediate-release to extended-release tablets – Patients currently treated with immediate-release tablets (eg, 3 to 4 times/day) may be switched to extended-release tablets at the same total daily dose taken once daily. If response after switching is inadequate, dosage may be titrated as outlined above.

Elderly or debilitated patients –

Immediate release and intensol: 0.25 mg, given 2 or 3 times/day. Gradually increase if needed and tolerated.

Extended-release: 0.5 mg once/day. Gradually increase if needed and tolerated. The elderly may be especially sensitive to the effects of benzodiazepines.

Administration of oral solution – Alprazolam intensol is a concentrated oral solution. The oral solution should be mixed with liquids or semi-solid food such as water, juices, soda or soda-like beverages, applesauce, and puddings. Use only the calibrated dropper provided with this product. The liquid or food should be gently stirred for a few seconds. The patient should consume the entire amount of the mixture of drug and liquid or drug and food immediately and not store it for future use.

Administration of orally disintegrating tablets – Just prior to administration, the tablet should be removed from the bottle and immediately placed on top of the tongue. If only one-half of a scored tablet is used for dosing, discard the unused portion of the tablet immediately.

CHLORDIAZEPOXIDE:

Oral –

Mild to moderate anxiety: 5 or 10 mg 3 or 4 times/day.

Severe anxiety: 20 or 25 mg 3 or 4 times/day.

Geriatric patients or patients with debilitating disease: 5 mg 2 to 4 times/day.

Preoperative apprehension and anxiety: On days preceding surgery, 5 to 10 mg 3 or 4 times/day.

Acute alcohol withdrawal: 50 to 100 mg; repeat as needed (up to 300 mg/day). Parenteral form usually used initially. Reduce to maintenance levels.

Children: Initially, 5 mg 2 to 4 times/day (may be increased in some children to 10 mg 2 or 3 times/day). Not recommended in children under 6 years of age.

A dosage of 0.5 mg/kg/day every 6 to 8 hours in children older than 6 years of age has also been recommended.

CLONAZEPAM:

Panic disorder –

Dosage: Initial dose for adults is 0.25 mg twice daily. An increase to the target dose of 1 mg/day may be made after 3 days. Some individual patients may benefit from doses of up to a maximum dose of 4 mg/day and, in those instances, the dose may be increased in increments of 0.125 to 0.25 mg twice daily every 3 days until panic disorder is controlled or until side effects make further increases undesired.

Discontinuation: Discontinue treatment gradually, with a decrease of 0.125 mg twice daily every 3 days until the drug is completely withdrawn.

Seizure disorders –

Adults: Initial dose should not exceed 1.5 mg/day in 3 divided doses. Increase in increments of 0.5 to 1 mg every 3 days until seizures are adequately controlled or until side effects preclude any further increase. Individualize maintenance dosage. Maximum recommended dosage is 20 mg/day.

Infants and children (10 years of age or younger or 30 kg): To minimize drowsiness, the initial dose should be between 0.01 to 0.03 mg/kg/day, not to exceed 0.05 mg/kg/day, given in 2 or 3 divided doses. Increase dosage by no more than 0.25 to 0.5 mg every third day until a daily maintenance dose of 0.1 to 0.2 mg/kg has been reached, unless seizures are controlled or side effects preclude further increase. When possible, divide the daily dose into 3 equal doses. If doses are not equally divided, give the largest dose at bedtime.

Administration – The patient should swallow the tablet whole with water. Immediately upon opening the blister, the tablet should be removed and placed in the mouth. Tablet disintegration occurs rapidly in saliva so it can be easily swallowed with or without water.

CLORAZEPATE DIPOTASSIUM:

Anxiety – 30 mg/day in divided doses. Adjust gradually within the range of 15 to 60 mg/day. May be administered as a single daily dose of 15 mg initially at bedtime.

Symptomatic relief of acute alcohol withdrawal (immediate-release tablets) –

Day 1: 30 mg initially, followed by 30 to 60 mg in divided doses.

Day 2: 45 to 90 mg in divided doses.

Day 3: 22.5 to 45 mg in divided doses.

Day 4: 15 to 30 mg in divided doses.

Thereafter, gradually reduce the dose to 7.5 to 15 mg once/day. Discontinue drug as soon as patient's condition is stable.

The maximum recommended total daily dose is 90 mg. Avoid excessive reductions in the total amount of drug administered on successive days.

Partial seizures –

Adults and children (older than 12 years of age): The maximum initial dose is 7.5 mg 3 times/day. Increase dosage by 7.5 mg or less every week; do not exceed 90 mg/day.

Children (9 to 12 years of age): Maximum initial dose is 7.5 mg 2 times/day. Increase dosage by 7.5 mg or less every week; do not exceed 60 mg/day. Not recommended in patients younger than 9 years of age.

Elderly or debilitated patients – Initiate treatment at a dose of 7.5 to 15 mg/day.

DIAZEPAM:

Oral –

Management of anxiety disorders and relief of symptoms of anxiety (depending upon severity of symptoms): 2 to 10 mg 2 to 4 times/day.

Acute alcohol withdrawal: 10 mg 3 or 4 times during the first 24 hours; reduce to 5 mg 3 or 4 times/day, as needed.

Adjunct in skeletal muscle spasm: 2 to 10 mg 3 or 4 times/day.

Adjunct in convulsive disorders: 2 to 10 mg 2 to 4 times/day.

Elderly patients or in the presence of debilitating disease: 2 to 2.5 mg 1 or 2 times/day initially; increase gradually as needed and tolerated.

Children: 1 to 2.5 mg 3 or 4 times/day initially; increase gradually as needed and tolerated. Not for use in children under 6 months. For sedation or muscle relaxation, a dosage of 0.12 to 0.8 mg/kg/24 hours divided 3 to 4 times a day has been recommended.

Oral solution: Dosage same as oral tablets.

Intensol – The **Intensol** is a concentrated oral solution as compared to standard oral liquid medications. It is recommended that the **Intensol** be mixed with liquid or semisolid food such as water, juices, soda or soda-like beverages, applesauce, and puddings. Use only the calibrated dropper provided with the product.

Rectal gel –

Dosage: 0.2 to 0.5 mg/kg, depending on age.

The diazepam rectal gel 2.5 mg dose may also be used as a partial replacement dose for patients who may expel a portion of the first dose.

Calculate the recommended dose by rounding upward to the next available unit dose.

Diazepam Rectal Dosing Based on Age

Age (years)	Recommended dose
2 through 5	0.5 mg/kg
6 through 11	0.3 mg/kg
12 and older	0.2 mg/kg

Because diazepam rectal gel is provided as unit doses, the prescribed dose is obtained by rounding upward to the next available dose. For elderly or debilitated patients, adjust dosage downward to reduce ataxia or oversedation.

Diazepam Rectal Dosing Based on Age and Weight

2 to 5 years of age 0.5 mg/kg		6 to 11 years of age 0.3 mg/kg		12 years of age and older 0.2 mg/kg	
Weight (kg)	Dose	Weight (kg)	Dose	Weight (kg)	Dose
6 to 10	5 mg	10 to 16	5 mg	14 to 25	5 mg
11 to 15	7.5 mg	17 to 25	7.5 mg	26 to 37	7.5 mg
16 to 20	10 mg	26 to 33	10 mg	38 to 50	10 mg
21 to 25	12.5 mg	34 to 41	12.5 mg	51 to 62	12.5 mg
26 to 30	15 mg	42 to 50	15 mg	63 to 75	15 mg
31 to 35	17.5 mg	51 to 58	17.5 mg	76 to 87	17.5 mg
36 to 44	20 mg	59 to 74	20 mg	88 to 111	20 mg

Additional dose: A second dose, when required, may be given 4 to 12 hours after the first dose.

Treatment frequency: Do not treat more than 5 episodes per month or more than 1 episode every 5 days.

Parenteral – The IV route is preferred in the convulsing patient. However, if IV administration is impossible, the IM route may be used. Inject deeply into the muscle. Inject IV slowly (at least 1 minute for each 5 mg). Do not use small veins (eg, dorsum of hand or wrist); avoid intra-arterial use and extravasation.

Children: Administer slowly over 3 minutes. Do not exceed 0.25 mg/kg. After an interval of 15 to 30 minutes, the initial dose can be repeated.

Elderly and debilitated patients: Use lower doses (2 to 5 mg) and slow dosage increases for elderly or debilitated patients and when other sedatives are given.

Moderate anxiety disorders and symptoms of anxiety: 2 to 5 mg IM or IV. Repeat in 3 to 4 hours if necessary.

Severe anxiety disorders and symptoms of anxiety: 5 to 10 mg IM or IV. Repeat in 3 to 4 hours if necessary.

Acute alcohol withdrawal: 10 mg IM or IV initially; then 5 to 10 mg in 3 to 4 hours if necessary.

Endoscopic procedures:

IV – 10 mg or less is usually adequate; up to 20 mg may be used, especially when concomitant narcotics are omitted.

IM – 5 to 10 mg 30 minutes prior to procedure if IV route cannot be used.

Muscle spasm: 5 to 10 mg IM or IV initially; then 5 to 10 mg in 3 to 4 hours if necessary. Tetanus may require larger doses.

Status epilepticus and severe recurrent convulsive seizures: The IV route is preferred; administer slowly. Use the IM route if IV administration is impossible.

Adults – Administer 5 to 10 mg initially; repeat if necessary at 10 to 15 minute intervals up to maximum dose of 30 mg. If necessary, repeat therapy in 2 to 4 hours. A dose of 0.2 to 0.5 mg/kg every 15 to 30 minutes for 2 to 3 doses (maximum dose, 30 mg).

Children 5 years of age or older – 1 mg every 2 to 5 minutes up to a maximum of 10 mg. Repeat in 2 to 4 hours if necessary.

Infants (over 30 days of age) and children (under 5 years of age) – Inject 0.2 to 0.5 mg slowly every 2 to 5 minutes up to a maximum of 5 mg; 0.2 to 0.5 mg/kg/dose every 15 to 30 minutes for 2 to 3 doses (maximum dose, 5 mg) has been recommended.

Neonates – 0.3 to 0.75 mg/kg/dose every 15 to 30 minutes for 2 to 3 doses has been suggested.

Preoperative medication: 10 mg IM before surgery.

Cardioversion: 5 to 15 mg IV, 5 to 10 minutes prior to procedure.

Tetanus:

Infants (over 30 days of age) – 1 to 2 mg IM or IV slowly, repeated every 3 to 4 hours as necessary.

Children (5 years of age and older) – 5 to 10 mg repeated every 3 to 4 hours may be required.

Sedation or muscle relaxation:

Children – 0.04 to 0.2 mg/kg/dose every 2 to 4 hours, maximum of 0.6 mg/kg within an 8-hour period.

Adults – 2 to 10 mg/dose every 3 to 4 hours as needed.

Admixture compatibility – Do not mix or dilute with other solutions or drugs in syringe or infusion flask. Diazepam interacts with plastic containers and administration sets, significantly decreasing availability of drug delivered.

LORAZEPAM:

Oral – 2 to 6 mg/day (varies from 1 to 10 mg/day) given in divided doses; take the largest dose before bedtime.

Anxiety: Initial dose, 2 to 3 mg/day given 2 or 3 times/day.

Insomnia caused by anxiety or transient situational stress: 2 to 4 mg at bedtime.

Elderly or debilitated patients: Initial dose, 1 to 2 mg/day in divided doses.

Parenteral –

Status epilepticus: The usual recommended dose is 4 mg given slowly (2 mg/min). If seizures continue or recur after a 10- to 15-minute observation period, an additional 4 mg IV dose may be slowly administered.

Preanesthetic: Reduce the doses of other CNS depressant drugs.

IM – 0.05 mg/kg up to a maximum of 4 mg. For optimum effect, administer at least 2 hours before operative procedure.

IV – Initial dose is 2 mg total or 0.044 mg/kg (0.02 mg/lb), whichever is smaller. This will sedate most adults; ordinarily, do not exceed in patients older than 50 years of age. If a greater lack of recall would be beneficial, doses as high as 0.05 mg/kg up to a total of 4 mg may be given. For optimum effect, give 15 to 20 minutes before the procedure.

Children (younger than 18 years of age) – Parenteral use is not recommended.

OXAZEPAM:

Mild to moderate anxiety, with associated tension, irritability, agitation, or related symptoms of functional origin or secondary to organic disease – 10 to 15 mg 3 or 4 times/day.

Severe anxiety syndromes, agitation, or anxiety associated with depression – 15 to 30 mg 3 or 4 times/day.

Older patients with anxiety, tension, irritability and agitation – Initial dosage is 10 mg 3 times/day. If necessary, increase cautiously to 15 mg 3 or 4 times/day.

Alcoholics with acute inebriation, tremulousness, or anxiety on withdrawal – 15 to 30 mg 3 or 4 times/day.

Children (6 to 12 years of age) – Dosage is not established.

Actions

Pharmacology: Benzodiazepines appear to potentiate the effects of gamma-aminobutyrate (GABA) (ie, they facilitate inhibitory GABA neurotransmission) and other inhibitory transmitters by binding to specific benzodiazepine receptor sites.

Diazepam appears to act on parts of the limbic system, the thalamus and hypothalamus, and induces calming effects. Diazepam has no demonstrable peripheral autonomic blocking action, nor does it produce extrapyramidal adverse reactions.

Pharmacokinetics:

Benzodiazepine Pharmacokinetics

Drug	Dosage range (mg/day)[a]	Peak plasma level (h)[a]	Elimination t½ (h)	Speed of onset[a]	Protein binding
Alprazolam	0.75-4	1-2	6.3-26.9	intermediate	80%
Chlordiazepoxide	15-100	0.5-4	5-30	intermediate	96%
Clonazepam	1.5-20	1-2	18-50	intermediate	97%
Clorazepate	15-60	1-2	40-50	fast	97%-98%
Diazepam	4-40	0.5-2	20-80	very fast	98%
Lorazepam	2-4	2-4	10-20	intermediate	85%
Oxazepam	30-120	2-4	5-20	slow	87%

[a] Oral administration.

Contraindications

Hypersensitivity to benzodiazepines; psychoses; acute narrow-angle glaucoma; patients with clinical or biochemical evidence of significant liver disease; coadministration with ketoconazole and itraconazole caused by inhibition of cytochrome P450 3A; intra-arterial use (lorazepam injection); children younger than 6 months of age (diazepam).

Warnings/Precautions

Administration: Extreme care must be used in administering **diazepam** injection, particularly by the IV route, to the elderly, to very ill patients, and to those with limited pulmonary reserve because of the possibility that apnea and/or cardiac arrest may occur. Concomitant use of barbiturates, alcohol, or other CNS depressants increases depression with increased risk of apnea. Tonic status epilepticus has been precipitated in patients treated with diazepam injection for petit mal status or petit mal variant status.

A significant proportion of patients experience a return to seizure activity, presumable due to the short-lived effect of diazepam after IV administration. Diazepam is not recommended for maintenance.

Psychiatric disorders: These agents are not intended for use in patients with a primary depressive disorder or psychosis, nor in those psychiatric disorders in which anxiety is not a prominent feature.

Worsening of seizures: When **diazepam** is used as an adjunct in treating convulsive disorders, the possibility of an increase in the frequency or severity of grand mal seizures may require an increase in the dosage of standard anticonvulsant medication. Abrupt withdrawal of diazepam may also be associated with a temporary increase in the frequency or severity of seizures.

Special populations: The usual precautions are indicated for severely depressed patients or those in whom there is any evidence of latent depression; particularly the recognition that suicidal tendencies may be present and protective measures may be necessary.

Paradoxical reactions: Excitement, stimulation, and acute rage have occurred in psychiatric patients and hyperactive aggressive children. These reactions may be secondary to relief of anxiety and usually appear in the first 2 weeks of therapy.

Renal function impairment: Observe usual precautions in the presence of impaired renal or hepatic function to avoid accumulation of these agents.

Hepatic function impairment: The usual precautions in treated patients with impaired hepatic function should be observed.

Drug abuse and dependence: Prolonged use of therapeutic doses can lead to dependence. Withdrawal syndrome has occurred after as little as 4 to 6 weeks of treatment. It is more likely if the drug was short-acting (eg, alprazolam), if it was taken regularly for more than 3 months, and if it was abruptly discontinued. Higher dosages may not be a factor affecting withdrawal. Addition-prone individuals (such as drug addicts or alcoholics) should be under careful surveillance when receiving psychotropic agents because of the predisposition of such patients to habituation and dependence.

Parenteral administration – Parenteral (IM or IV) therapy is indicated primarily in acute states. Keep patients under observation, preferably in bed, for up to 3 hours.

Hazardous tasks: These agents may produce drowsiness or dizziness; observe caution while driving or performing other tasks requiring alertness. **Diazepam** injection should not be administered to patients in shock, coma, or in acute alcoholic intoxication with depression of vital signs.

Pregnancy: Category D.

Lactation: Benzodiazepines are excreted in breast milk (**lorazepam** not known). Chronic **diazepam** use in nursing mothers reportedly caused infants to become lethargic and to lose weight; do not give to nursing mothers.

Children:

Chlordiazepoxide – Chlordiazepoxide is not recommended in children younger than 6 years of age (oral) or 12 years of age (injectable).

Alprazolam – Safety and efficacy for use in patients younger than 18 years of age have not been established.

Lorazepam – Do not use in patients younger than 18 years of age (injection); safety and efficacy for use in patients younger than 12 years of age are not established (oral).

Clorazepate – Not recommended for use in patients younger than 9 years of age.

Diazepam – Not for use in children younger than 6 months of age (oral); safety and efficacy have not been established in the neonate (30 days of age or younger; injectable).

Elderly: The initial dose should be small and dosage increments made gradually, in accordance with the response of the patient, to preclude ataxia or excessive sedation.

Monitoring: Because of isolated reports of neutropenia and jaundice, perform periodic blood counts, and liver function tests during long-term therapy.

Drug Interactions

Drugs that may affect benzodiazepines include alcohol, antacids, barbiturates, cimetidine, disulfiram, fluoxetine, isoniazid, ketoconazole, MAOIs, metoprolol, oral contraceptives, narcotics, other depressants, phenothiazines, probenecid, propranolol, ranitidine, rifampin, scopolamine, theophylline, and valproic acid.

Drugs that may be affected by benzodiazepines include digoxin, levodopa, neuromuscular blocking agents, and phenytoin.

Because **diazepam** has a CNS-depressant effect, advise patients against the simultaneous ingestion of alcohol and other CNS-depressant drugs during diazepam therapy. When diazepam is used with a narcotic analgesic, the dosage of the narcotic should be reduced by at least one third and administered in small increments.

Adverse Reactions

Cardiovascular: Bradycardia; cardiovascular collapse; edema; hypertension; hypotension; palpitations; tachycardia.

CNS: Agitation; anterograde amnesia; apathy; ataxia; coma; confusion; crying; depression; delirium; difficulty in concentration; disorientation; dizziness; euphoria; fatigue; headache; hypoactivity; inability to perform complex mental functions; incoordination; irritability; lethargy; lightheadedness; memory impairment; nervousness; neutropenia; restlessness; rigidity; sedation and sleepiness; seizures; slurred speech; sobbing; stupor; syncope; tremor; unsteadiness; vertigo; vivid dreams; weakness.

Dermatologic: Ankle and facial edema; dermatitis; hair loss; hirsutism; pruritus; skin rash; urticaria.

GI: Anorexia; change in appetite; constipation; diarrhea; difficulty in swallowing; dry mouth; gastritis; increased salivation; nausea; sore gums; vomiting.

GU: Changes in libido; incontinence; menstrual irregularities; urinary retention.

Ophthalmic: Diplopia; nystagmus; visual disturbances.

Psychiatric: Behavior problems; hysteria; psychosis; suicidal tendencies.

Respiratory: Nasal congestion; respiratory disturbances.

Miscellaneous: Anemia; auditory disturbances; blood dyscrasias including agranulocytosis; dehydration; depressed hearing; diaphoresis; eosinophilia; fever; galactorrhea; gynecomastia; hiccoughs; increase or decrease in body weight; joint pain; leukopenia; muscular disturbance; paresthesias; phlebitis at injection site; thrombocytopenia; venous thrombosis.

BUSPIRONE HYDROCHLORIDE

Tablets: 5, 7.5, 10, 15, and 30 mg (*Rx*)	Various

Indications

Anxiety disorders: Management of anxiety disorders or short-term relief of symptoms of anxiety.

Administration and Dosage

Initial dose: 15 mg/day (7.5 mg 2 times/day).

To achieve an optimal therapeutic response, increase the dosage 5 mg/day, at intervals of 2 to 3 days, as needed. Do not exceed 60 mg/day. Divided doses of 20 to 30 mg/day have been commonly used.

The bioavailability of buspirone is increased when given with food as compared with the fasted state. Consequently, patients should take buspirone in a consistent manner with regard to the timing of dosing; either always with or always without food.

Concomitant therapy: When buspirone is to be given with a potent inhibitor of CYP3A4, the dosage recommendations described in the Drug Interactions section should be followed.

Actions

Pharmacology: Mechanism of action is unknown. It differs from benzodiazepines in that it does not exert anticonvulsant or muscle relaxant effects. It also lacks prominent sedative effects associated with more typical anxiolytics. Buspirone has effects on serotonin, dopamine, and norephinephrine.

Pharmacokinetics: Buspirone is rapidly absorbed and undergoes extensive first-pass metabolism. Approximately 95% of buspirone is plasma protein bound. In a single dose study, 29% to 63% of the dose was excreted in the urine within 24 hours.

Contraindications

Hypersensitivity to buspirone hydrochloride.

Warnings/Precautions

Buspirone has no established antipsychotic activity; do not employ in lieu of appropriate antipsychotic treatment.

Physical and psychological dependence: Buspirone has shown no potential for abuse or diversion and there is no evidence that it causes tolerance or physical or psychological dependence. However, carefully evaluate patients for a history of drug abuse and follow such patients closely, observing them for signs of misuse or abuse (eg, tolerance, drug-seeking behavior).

Interference with cognitive and motor performance: Buspirone is less sedating than other anxiolytics and does not produce significant functional impairment. However, its CNS effect may not be predictable. Therefore, caution patients about driving or using complex machinery until they are certain that buspirone does not affect them adversely.

Withdrawal reactions: Withdraw patients from their prior treatment gradually before starting buspirone, especially patients who have been using a CNS depressant chronically.

Dopamine receptor binding: Buspirone can bind to central dopamine receptors.

Monitoring: Patients have been treated for several months without ill effect. If used for extended periods, periodically reassess the usefulness of the drug.

Renal/Hepatic function impairment: Because buspirone is metabolized by the liver and excreted by the kidneys, do not use in patients with severe hepatic or renal impairment.

Pregnancy: Category B.

Lactation: The extent of the excretion in breast milk of buspirone or its metabolites is not known.

Children: Safety and efficacy of buspirone were evaluated in 2 placebo-controlled 6-week trials involving a total of 559 pediatric patients (ranging from 6 to 17 years of age) with generalized anxiety disorder (GAD). Doses studied were 7.5 to 30 mg twice/day (15 to 60 mg/day). There were no significant differences between buspirone and placebo with regard to the symptoms of GAD.

Monitoring: Effectiveness for more than 3 to 4 weeks has not been demonstrated in controlled trials. However, patients have been treated for a year without ill effect. If used for extended periods, periodically reassess the usefulness of the drug.

Drug Interactions

CYP450 system: Substances that inhibit CYP3A4, such as ketoconazole or ritonavir, may inhibit buspirone metabolism and increase plasma concentrations of buspirone while substances that induce CYP3A4, such as dexamethasone or certain anticonvulsants (eg, phenytoin, phenobarbital, carbamazepine), may increase the rate of buspirone metabolism. If a patient has been titrated to a stable dosage on buspirone, a dose adjustment of buspirone may be necessary to avoid adverse events attributable to buspirone or diminished anxiolytic activity. Consequently, when administered with a potent inhibitor of CYP3A4, a low dose of buspirone used cautiously is recommended. When used in combination with a potent inducer of CYP3A4 the dosage of buspirone may need adjusting to maintain anxiolytic effect.

Drugs that may interact with buspirone include alcohol, cimetidine, CYP3A4 inhibitors and inducers, diazepam, fluoxetine, haloperidol, nefazodone, monoamine oxidase inhibitors, and trazodone.

Drug/Food interactions: The bioavailability of buspirone is increased when given with food as compared with the fasted state.

Grapefruit juice – Coadministration of buspirone (10 mg as a single-dose) with grapefruit juice (200 mL double-strength twice/day for 2 days) increased plasma buspirone concentrations (4.3-fold increase in C_{max}; 9.2-fold increase in AUC). Advise patients receiving buspirone to avoid drinking large amounts of grapefruit juice.

Adverse Reactions

Adverse reactions occurring in at least 3% of patients include dizziness, drowsiness, dry mouth, fatigue, headache, insomnia, lightheadedness, nausea, nervousness.

ANTIDEPRESSANTS

Antidepressant Pharmacologic and Pharmacokinetic Parameters

0 - none + - slight ++ - moderate +++ - high ++++ - very high +++++ - highest	Major side effects			Amine uptake blocking activity		Half-life (hours)	Therapeutic plasma level (ng/mL)	Time to reach steady state (days)	Dose range (mg/day)
	Anticholinergic	Sedation	Orthostatic hypotension	Norepinephrine	Serotonin				
Tricyclics - Tertiary Amines									
Amitriptyline	++++	++++	++	++	++++	31-46	110-250[a]	4-10	50-300
Clomipramine	+++	+++	++	++	+++++	19-37	80-100	7-14	25-250
Doxepin	++	+++	++	+	++	8-24	100-200[a]	2-8	25-300
Imipramine	++	++	+++	++[b]	++++	11-25	200-350[a]	2-5	30-300
Trimipramine	++	+++	++	+	+	7-30	180[a]	2-6	50-300
Tricyclics - Secondary Amines									
Amoxapine[c]	+++	++	+	+++	++	8[d]	200-500	2-7	50-600
Desipramine	+	+	+	++++	++	12-24	125-300	2-11	25-300
Nortriptyline	++	++	+	++	+++	18-44	50-150	4-19	30-100
Protriptyline	+++	+	+	++++	++	67-89	100-200	14-19	15-60
Tetracyclics									
Maprotiline	++	++	+	+++	0/+	21-25	200-300[a]	6-10	50-225
Mirtazapine	++	+++	++	+++	+++	20-40	-	5	15-45
Triazolopyridine									
Trazodone	+	++++	++	0	+++	4-9	800-1600	3-7	150-600
Aminoketone									
Bupropion[e]	++	++	+	0/+	0/+	8-24	-	1.5-8	200-450
Phenethylamine									
Venlafaxine	0	0	0	+++	+++	5-11[a]	-	3-4	75-375
Phenylpiperazine									
Nefazodone	0/+	++	+	0/+	+++++	2-4	-	4-5	200-600
Selective Serotonin Reuptake Inhibitors									
Citalopram	0/+	0/+	0/+	0/+	++++	33	-	7	20-60
Escitalopram	0/+	0/+	0	0/+	++++	27-32	-	7	10-20
Fluoxetine	0/+	0/+	0/+	0/+	+++++	1-16 days[a]	-	2-4 weeks	20-80
Fluvoxamine	0/+	0/+	0	0/+	+++++	15.6	-	≈ 7	50-300
Paroxetine	0	0/+	0	0/+	+++++	10-24	-	7-14	10-50
Sertraline	0	0/+	0	0/+	+++++	1-4 days[a]	-	7	50-200
Monoamine Oxidase Inhibitors									
Isocarboxazid	0/+	0/+	+	-	-	-	-	-	10-60
Phenelzine	+	+	+	-	-	-	-	-	45-90
Tranylcypromine	+	+	0	-	-	2.4-2.8	-	-	30-60
Serotonin and Norepinephrine Reuptake Inhibitors									
Duloxetine	0/+	+	+	+++	+++	8-17	-	3	40-120
Desvenlafaxine	0	0	0	+++	+++	11-14	-	4-5	50-400

[a] Parent compound plus active metabolite.
[b] Via desipramine, the major metabolite.
[c] Also blocks dopamine receptors.
[d] 30 hours for major metabolite 8-hydroxyamoxapine.
[e] Inhibits dopamine uptake.

TRICYCLIC COMPOUNDS

AMITRIPTYLINE	
Tablets: 10, 25, 50, 75, 100, and 150 mg (*Rx*)	Various, *Elavil* (Zeneca)
AMOXAPINE	
Tablets: 25, 50, 100, and 150 mg (*Rx*)	Various, *Asendin* (Lederle)
CLOMIPRAMINE HYDROCHLORIDE	
Capsules: 25, 50, and 75 mg (*Rx*)	Various, *Anafranil* (Novartis)
DESIPRAMINE HYDROCHLORIDE	
Tablets: 10, 25, 50, 75, 100, and 150 mg (*Rx*)	Various, *Norpramin* (Aventis)
DOXEPIN HYDROCHLORIDE	
Capsules: 10, 25, 50, 75, 100, and 150 mg (*Rx*)	Various, *Sinequan* (Roerig)
Oral concentrate: 10 mg/mL (*Rx*)	Various
IMIPRAMINE HYDROCHLORIDE	
Tablets: 10, 25, and 50 mg (*Rx*)	Various, *Tofranil* (Novartis)
IMIPRAMINE PAMOATE	
Capsules: 75, 100, 125, and 150 mg (as imipramine hydrochloride equivalent) (*Rx*)	Various, *Tofranil-PM* (Novartis)
NORTRIPTYLINE HYDROCHLORIDE	
Capsules: 10, 25, 50, and 75 mg (*Rx*)	Various, *Pamelor* (Mallinckrodt)
Solution: 10 mg (as base) per 5 mL (*Rx*)	Various
PROTRIPTYLINE HYDROCHLORIDE	
Tablets: 5 and 10 mg (*Rx*)	Various, *Vivactil* (Duramed)
TRIMIPRAMINE MALEATE	
Capsules: 25, 50, and 100 mg (*Rx*)	*Surmontil* (Duramed)

Warning:

Suicidality in children and adolescents: Antidepressants increased the risk of suicidal thinking and behavior (suicidality) in short-term studies in children and adolescents with major depressive disorder (MDD) and other psychiatric disorders. Anyone considering the use of amitriptyline or any other antidepressant in a child or adolescent must balance this risk with the clinical need. Patients who are started on therapy should be observed closely for clinical worsening, suicidality, or unusual changes in behavior. Families and caregivers should be advised of the need for close observation and communication with the prescriber. Amitriptyline and desipramine are not approved for use in children.

Pooled analyses of short-term (4 to 16 weeks) placebo-controlled trials of 9 antidepressant drugs (SSRIs and others) in children and adolescents with MDD, obsessive-compulsive disorder (OCD), or other psychiatric disorders (a total of 24 trials involving over 4,400 patients) have revealed a greater risk of adverse reactions representing suicidal thinking or behavior (suicidality) during the first few months of treatment in those receiving antidepressants. The average risk of such reactions in patients receiving antidepressants was 4%, twice the placebo risk of 2%. No suicides occurred in these trials.

Indications

Relief of symptoms of depression (except clomipramine). The activating properties of **protriptyline** make it particularly suitable for withdrawn and anergic patients.

Agents with significant sedative action may be useful in depression associated with anxiety and sleep disturbances. The activating properties of **protriptyline** make it particularly suitable for withdrawn and anergic patients.

Amoxapine: Relief of depressive symptoms in patients with neurotic or reactive depressive disorders and endogenous and psychotic depression; depression accompanied by anxiety or agitation.

Doxepin: Treatment of psychoneurotic patients with depression or anxiety; depression or anxiety associated with alcoholism (not to be taken concomitantly with alcohol); depression or anxiety associated with organic disease (the possibility of drug interaction should be considered if the patient is receiving other drugs concomitantly); psychotic depressive disorders with associated anxiety including involutional depression and manic-depressive disorders. The target symptoms of psychoneurosis that respond particularly well to doxepin include anxiety, tension, depression, somatic symptoms and concerns, sleep disturbances, guilt, lack of energy, fear, apprehension, and worry.

Imipramine: Treatment of enuresis in children 6 years of age or older as temporary adjunctive therapy.

Clomipramine: Only for treatment of Obsessive-Compulsive Disorder (OCD).

Administration and Dosage

Plasma levels: Determination of plasma levels may be useful in identifying patients who appear to have toxic effects and may have excessively high levels, or those in whom lack of absorption or noncompliance is suspected. Make adjustments in dosage according to patient's clinical response and not based on plasma levels.

Adolescent, elderly, and outpatients: Initiate therapy at a low dosage and increase gradually. Most antidepressant drugs have a lag period of 10 days to 4 weeks before a therapeutic response is noted. Increasing the dose will not shorten this period but rather increase the incidence of adverse reactions. Following remission, maintenance medication may be required for a longer time at the lowest dose that will maintain remission. Continue maintenance therapy 3 months or longer to decrease the possibility of relapse.

AMITRIPTYLINE HYDROCHLORIDE:

Outpatients – 75 mg/day in divided doses. May increase to 150 mg/day. Alternatively, initiate therapy with 50 to 100 mg at bedtime. Increase by 25 to 50 mg as necessary, to a total of 150 mg/day.

Hospitalized patients: Hospitalized patients may require 100 mg/day initially. Gradually increase to 200 to 300 mg, if necessary.

Adolescent and elderly patients – 10 mg 3 times a day with 20 mg at bedtime may be satisfactory in adolescent and elderly patients who cannot tolerate higher doses.

Maintenance – 40 to 100 mg/day. Total daily dosage may be given in a single dose, preferably at bedtime.

IM – Do not administer IV. Initially, 20 to 30 mg IM, 4 times a day. The effects may be more rapid with IM than with oral administration.

Children – Not recommended for children younger than 12 years of age.

AMOXAPINE: Amoxapine is not recommended for patients younger than 16 years of age.

Usual effective dose range is 200 to 300 mg/day. If no response is seen at 300 mg, increase dosage, depending upon tolerance, to 400 mg/day. Hospitalized patients refractory to antidepressant therapy and who have no history of convulsive seizures may have dosage cautiously increased up to 600 mg/day in divided doses.

Adults – Initially, 50 mg 2 or 3 times/day. Depending upon tolerance, increase dosage to 100 mg 2 or 3 times/day by the end of the first week. Increase above 300 mg/day only if 300 mg/day has been ineffective for at least 2 weeks. Once an effective dosage is established, the drug may be given in a single bedtime dose (not to exceed 300 mg). If the total daily dosage exceeds 300 mg, give in divided doses.

Elderly patients – Initially, 25 mg 2 or 3 times a day. If tolerated, dosage may be increased by the end of the first week to 50 mg 2 or 3 times a day. Although 100 to 150 mg/day may be adequate for many elderly patients, some may require higher dosage; carefully increase up to 300 mg/day. Once an effective dosage is established, give amoxapine in a single bedtime dose, not to exceed 300 mg.

CLOMIPRAMINE HYDROCHLORIDE: Administer in divided doses with meals to reduce GI side effects. After titration, the total daily dose may be given once/day at bedtime to minimize daytime sedation.

Adults – Initiate at 25 mg/day and gradually increase, as tolerated, to approximately 100 mg during the first 2 weeks. Thereafter, the dosage may be increased gradually over the next several weeks to a maximum of 250 mg/day.

Children and adolescents – Initiate at 25 mg/day and gradually increase during the first 2 weeks, as tolerated, to a daily maximum of 3 mg/kg or 100 mg, whichever is smaller. Thereafter, the dosage may be increased to a daily maximum of 3 mg/kg or 200 mg, whichever is smaller.

DESIPRAMINE HYDROCHLORIDE: Not recommended for use in children.

Adults – 100 to 200 mg/day. Initial therapy may be given in divided doses or as a single daily dose. In more severely ill patients, gradually increase to 300 mg/day, if necessary. Do not exceed 300 mg/day.

Elderly and adolescents – 25 to 100 mg/day. Dosages greater than 150 mg not recommended.

Outpatients – Lower dosages are recommended for outpatients compared with hospitalized patients, who are closely supervised. The dosage should be initiated at a low level and increased according to clinical response and any evidence of tolerance. Following remission, maintenance medication may be required for a period of time and should be given at the lowest dose that will maintain remission.

Dosage adjustments and toxicities – The best available evidence of impending toxicity from very high doses of desipramine is prolongation of the QRS or QT intervals on the ECG. Prolongation of the PR interval is also significant, but less closely correlated with plasma levels. Clinical symptoms of intolerance, especially drowsiness, dizziness, and postural hypotension, also indicate need for reduction in dosage. Plasma desipramine measurement would constitute the optimal guide to dosage monitoring.

DOXEPIN HYDROCHLORIDE: Not recommended for use in children younger than 12 years of age.

Mild to moderate illness – Initially, 75 mg/day. Usual optimum dosage is 75 to 150 mg/day. Alternatively, the total daily dosage, up to 150 mg, may be given at bedtime.

Mild symptomatology or emotional symptoms accompanying organic disease – 25 to 50 mg/day as often as effective.

More severe anxiety or depression – Higher doses (eg, 50 mg 3 times/day) may be required; if necessary, gradually increase to 300 mg/day.

Oral concentrate – Dilute oral concentrate with approximately 120 mL of water, milk or fruit juice prior to administration. Do not mix with carbonated beverages.

IMIPRAMINE HYDROCHLORIDE:

Depression –

Hospitalized patients: Initially, 100 to 150 mg orally in divided doses; gradually increase to 200 mg/day, as required. If no response occurs after 2 weeks, increase to 250 to 300 mg/day. Administer the total daily dosage once/day at bedtime.

Outpatients: Initially, 75 mg/day, increased to 150 mg/day. Do not exceed 200 mg/day. Give once/day, preferably at bedtime.

Maintenance – 50 to 150 mg/day or lowest dose that will maintain remission.

Adolescent and elderly patients: Initially, 30 to 40 mg/day orally; it is generally not necessary to exceed 100 mg/day.

Childhood enuresis (6 years of age or older) – Initially, 25 mg/day 1 hour before bedtime. If no satisfactory response in 1 week, increase up to 50 mg/night if younger than 12 years of age; up to 75 mg/night if older than 12 years of age. A dose more than 75 mg/day does not enhance efficacy and increases side effects. Do not exceed 2.5 mg/kg/day. In early night bedwetters, it may be more effective given earlier and in divided amounts (25 mg midafternoon and bedtime).

IMIPRAMINE PAMOATE:

Hospitalized patients – Initiate therapy at 100 to 150 mg/day; may be increased to 200 mg/day. If there is no response after 2 weeks, increase dosage to 250 to 300 mg/day.

Outpatients – Initiate therapy at 75 mg/day. If necessary, dosage may be increased to 200 mg/day.

Adult maintenance dosage – The usual maintenance dose is 75 to 150 mg/day.

Adolescent and elderly patients – Initiate therapy in these age groups with imipramine hydrochloride at a total daily dosage of 25 to 50 mg because imipramine pamoate does not come in these strengths. Dosage may be increased according to response and tolerance, but it is generally unnecessary to exceed 100 mg/day in these patients. Imipramine pamoate capsules may be used when total daily dosage is established at 75 mg or more.

NORTRIPTYLINE:

Adults – 25 mg 3 or 4 times/day; begin at a low level and increase as required. Total daily dose can be given at bedtime. Doses above 150 mg/day are not recommended.

Elderly and adolescent patients – 30 to 50 mg/day in divided doses or once/day. Not recommended for use in children.

PROTRIPTYLINE HYDROCHLORIDE: Not recommended for use in children.

Adults – 15 to 40 mg/day divided into 3 or 4 doses. May increase to 60 mg/day. Dosages above 60 mg/day are not recommended. Make any increases in the morning dose.

Adolescent and elderly patients – Initially, 5 mg 3 times/day; increase gradually, if necessary. In elderly patients, monitor the cardiovascular system closely if dose exceeds 20 mg/day.

TRIMIPRAMINE MALEATE: Not recommended for use in children.

Adult outpatients – Initially, 75 mg/day in divided doses; increase to 150 mg/day. Do not exceed 200 mg/day. The total dosage requirement may be given at bedtime.

Adult hospitalized patients – Initially, 100 mg/day in divided doses, increased gradually in a few days to 200 mg/day depending upon individual response and tolerance. If improvement does not occur in 2 to 3 weeks, increase to a maximum dose of 250 to 300 mg/day.

Adolescent and elderly patients – Initially, 50 mg/day, with gradual increments up to 100 mg/day.

Maintenance – Maintenance medication may be required at the lowest dose that will maintain remission (range 50 to 150 mg/day). Administer as a single bedtime dose.

Actions

Pharmacology: The tricyclic antidepressants (TCAs), structurally related to the phenothiazine antipsychotic agents, possess 3 major pharmacologic actions in varying degrees: Blocking of the amine pump, sedation, and peripheral and central anticholinergic action. In contrast to phenothiazines, which act on dopamine receptors, TCAs inhibit reuptake of norepinephrine or serotonin (5-hydroxytryptamine, 5-HT) at the presynaptic neuron. Amoxapine, a metabolite of loxapine, retains some of the postsynaptic dopamine receptor-blocking action of neuroleptics.

Other pharmacological effects – Clinical effects, in addition to antidepressant effects, include sedation, anticholinergic effects, mild peripheral vasodilator effects and possible "quinidine-like" actions.

Pharmacokinetics:

Absorption/Distribution – The TCAs are well absorbed from the GI tract with peak plasma concentrations occurring in 2 to 4 hours; they undergo a significant first-pass effect. They are highly bound (more than 90%) to plasma proteins, are lipid soluble and are widely distributed in tissues, including the CNS.

Metabolism/Excretion – Metabolism of TCAs occurs in the liver by demethylation, hydroxylation and glucuronidation, and it varies for each patient. Some intermediate active metabolites include:

Amitriptyline ➡ nortriptyline
Amoxapine ➡ 7 hydroxy and 8 hydroxyamoxapine
Clomipramine ➡ desmethylclomipramine
Doxepin ➡ desmethyldoxepin
Imipramine ➡ desipramine

Because of the long half-life, a single daily dose may be given. Up to 2 to 4 weeks may be required to achieve maximal clinical response.

Contraindications

Prior sensitivity to any tricyclic drug. Not recommended for use during the acute recovery phase following myocardial infarction. Concomitant use of monoamine oxidase inhibitors (MAOIs) is generally contraindicated.

Doxepin: Patients with glaucoma or a tendency for urinary retention.

Cross-sensitivity may occur among the dibenzazepines (**clomipramine**, **desipramine**, **imipramine**, **nortriptyline**, and **trimipramine**). In addition, dibenzoxepines (**doxepin, amoxapine**) may produce cross-sensitivity.

Warnings/Precautions

Tardive dyskinesia: Tardive dyskinesia, a syndrome consisting of potentially irreversible, involuntary, dyskinetic movements may develop in patients treated with neuroleptics (eg, antipsychotics). Amoxapine is not an antipsychotic, but it has substantive neuroleptic activity.

Neuroleptic malignant syndrome (NMS): NMS is a potentially fatal condition reported in association with antipsychotic drugs and with **amoxapine**.

Hyperthermia has occurred with **clomipramine**; most cases occurred when it was used with other drugs (eg, neuroleptics) and may be examples of an NMS.

Seizure disorders: Because TCAs lower the seizure threshold, use with caution in patients with a history of seizures or other predisposing factors (eg, brain damage of varying etiology, alcoholism, concomitant drugs known to lower the seizure threshold). However, seizures have occurred both in patients with and without a history of seizure disorders. Seizure was identified as the most significant risk of **clomipramine** use.

Anticholinergic effects: Use with caution in patients with a history of urinary retention, urethral or ureteral spasm; narrow-angle glaucoma, angle-closure glaucoma, or increased intraocular pressure.

Cardiovascular disorders: Use with extreme caution in patients with cardiovascular disorders because of the possibility of conduction defects, arrhythmias, CHF, sinus tachycardia, MI, strokes, and tachycardia. These patients require cardiac surveillance at all dose levels of the drug. In high doses, TCAs may produce arrhythmias, sinus tachycardia, conduction defects, and prolonged conduction time. Tachycardia and postural hypotension may occur more frequently with **protriptyline**.

Hyperthyroid patients: Hyperthyroid patients or those receiving thyroid medication require close supervision because of the possibility of cardiovascular toxicity, including arrhythmias.

Psychiatric patients: Schizophrenic or paranoid patients may exhibit a worsening of psychosis with TCA therapy, and manic-depressive patients may experience a shift to a hypomanic or manic phase; this may also occur when switching antidepressants and withdrawing them. In overactive or agitated patients, increased anxiety or agitation may occur. Paranoid delusions, with or without associated hostility, may be exaggerated. Reduction of TCA dosage and concomitant antipsychotic therapy may be necessary.

The possibility of suicide in depressed patients remains during treatment and until significant remission occurs. Patients should not have easy access to large quantities of the drug; prescribe small quantities of TCAs.

Mania/Hypomania: Hypomanic or manic episodes may occur, particularly in patients with cyclic disorders. Such reactions may necessitate discontinuation of the drug.

MAOIs: Do not give MAOIs with or immediately following TCAs. Allow at least 14 days to elapse between MAOI discontinuation and TCA institution. Some TCAs have been used safely and successfully with MAOIs. Initiate TCA cautiously with gradual dosage increase until achieving optimum response.

Rash: Antidepressant drugs can cause skin rashes or "drug fever" in susceptible individuals. They are more likely to occur during the first few days of treatment but may also occur later. Discontinue if rash or fever develop.

Electroconvulsive therapy: Electroconvulsive therapy with coadministration of TCAs may increase the hazards of therapy.

Elective surgery: Discontinue therapy for as long as possible before elective surgery.

Blood sugar levels: Elevated and lowered blood sugar levels have occurred.

Sexual dysfunction: Sexual dysfunction was markedly increased in male patients with OCD taking clomipramine (42% ejaculatory failure, 20% impotence) compared to placebo. Sexual dysfunction also occurs with other TCAs.

Weight changes: Weight gain occurred in 18% of patients receiving **clomipramine**. Some patients had weight gain in excess of 25% of their initial body weight. Weight gain also occurs with other TCAs.

Serotonin syndrome: Some TCAs inhibit neuronal reuptake of serotonin and can increase synaptic serotonin levels (eg, **clomipramine, amitriptyline**). Either therapeutic or excessive doses of these drugs, in combination with other drugs that also increase synaptic serotonin levels (such as MAOIs), can cause a serotonin syndrome consisting of tremor, agitation, delirium, rigidity, myoclonus, hyperthermia, and obtundation.

Renal/Hepatic function impairment: Use with caution and in reduced doses in patients with hepatic impairment; metabolism may be impaired, leading to drug accumulation. Use with caution in patients with significantly impaired renal function.

Hazardous tasks: May impair mental or physical abilities required for the performance of potentially hazardous tasks.

Photosensitivity: Photosensitization (photoallergy or phototoxicity) may occur.

Pregnancy: (*Category D* - amitriptyline, imipramine, nortriptyline; *Category* C - amoxapine, clomipramine, desipramine, doxepin, protriptyline, trimipramine).

Lactation: These agents are excreted into breast milk in low concentrations.

Children: Not recommended for patients younger than 12 years of age. Safety and efficacy are not established for **amoxapine** in children younger than 16 years of age or **trazodone** or **clomipramine** in children younger than 10 years of age. The safety and efficacy of **imipramine** as temporary adjunctive therapy for nocturnal enuresis in pediatric patients younger than 6 years of age have not been established. The safety of the drug for long-term, chronic use as adjunctive therapy for nocturnal enuresis in pediatric patients 6 years of age and older has not been established. Safety and efficacy are not established in the pediatric age group for **trimipramine, nortriptyline, protriptyline**, and **desipramine**.

Do not exceed 2.5 mg/kg/day of **imipramine**.

Elderly: Be cautious in dose selection for an elderly patient, usually starting at the low end of the dosing range. Elderly patients may be sensitive to the anticholinergic side effects of TCAs.

Elderly patients taking **amitriptyline** may be at increased risk for falls; start on low doses of amitriptyline and observe closely.

Monitoring: Perform baseline and periodic leukocyte and differential counts and liver function studies. Fever or sore throat may signal serious neutrophil depression; discontinue therapy if there is evidence of pathological neutropenia.

Monitor ECG – Monitor ECG prior to initiation of large doses of TCAs and at appropriate intervals thereafter.

Drug Interactions

P450 system: Concomitant use of TCAs with other drugs metabolized by cytochrome P450 2D6 may require lower doses than those usually prescribed for either the TCA or the other drug.

Drugs that may affect tricyclic compounds include barbiturates, carbamazepine, charcoal, cimetidine, haloperidol, histamine H_2-antagonists, MAO inhibitors, rifamycins, SSRIs, smoking, and valproic acid.

Drugs that may be affected by tricyclic compounds include anticholinergics, carbamazepine, clonidine, dicumarol, grepafloxacin, guanethidine, levodopa, quinolones, sparfloxacin, and sympathomimetics.

Adverse Reactions

Sedation and anticholinergic effects are reported most frequently.

Withdrawal symptoms – Although not indicative of addiction, abrupt cessation after prolonged therapy may produce nausea, headache, vertigo, nightmares, and malaise. Gradual dosage reduction may produce, within 2 weeks, transient symptoms including irritability, restlessness, dreams, and sleep disturbance.

Enuretic children – Consider adverse reactions reported with adult use. Most common are nervousness, sleep disorders, tiredness, and mild GI disturbances. These usually disappear with continued therapy or dosage reduction.

Cardiovascular:

General – Arrhythmias; changes in AV conduction; ECG changes (most frequently with toxic doses); flushing; heart block; hot flushes; hypertension; hypotension; orthostatic hypotension; palpitations; precipitation of CHF; premature ventricular contractions; stroke; sudden death; syncope; tachycardia.

Desipramine – Hypertensive episodes during surgery. There have been reports of sudden death in children.

CNS:

General – Agitation; akathisia; alterations in EEG patterns; anxiety; ataxia; coma; confusion (especially in the elderly); disorientation; disturbed concentration; dizziness; drowsiness; dysarthria; exacerbation of psychosis; excitement; excessive appetite; extrapyramidal symptoms including abnormal involuntary movements and tardive dyskinesia; fatigue; hallucinations; delusions; headache; hyperthermia; hypomania; incoordination; insomnia; mania; nervousness; neuroleptic malignant syndrome; nightmares; numbness; panic; paresthesias of extremities; peripheral neuropathy; restlessness; tremors; seizures; tingling; weakness.

GU: Gynecomastia and testicular swelling in the male; breast enlargement, menstrual irregularity and galactorrhea in the female; increased or decreased libido; painful ejaculation; impotence; nocturia; urinary frequency.

GI: Nausea and vomiting; anorexia; epigastric distress; diarrhea; flatulence; dysphagia; increased salivation; stomatitis; glossitis; parotid swelling; abdominal cramps; pancreatitis; black tongue.

Hematologic: Bone marrow depression including agranulocytosis; eosinophilia; purpura; thrombocytopenia; leukopenia.

Clomipramine – Anemia; leukemoid reaction; lymphadenopathy; lymphoma-like disorder.

Hypersensitivity:

General – Cross-sensitivity with other TCAs; drug fever; edema (general or of face and tongue); itching; petechiae; photosensitization; pruritus; rash; urticaria; vasculitis.

Respiratory:

General – Exacerbation of asthma.

Special senses: Tinnitus; abnormal lacrimation.

Miscellaneous:

General – Alopecia; fever; hyperthermia; hyperpyrexia; local edema; nasal stuffiness; increased perspiration; proneness to falling; weight gain or loss.

Clomipramine – Abnormal skin odor; arthralgia; back pain; chest pain; chills; dependent edema; general edema; fever; halitosis; increased susceptibility to infection; malaise; muscle weakness; myalgia; pain; thirst; withdrawal syndrome.

TETRACYCLIC COMPOUNDS

MAPROTILINE	
Tablets; oral: 25, 50, and 75 mg (*Rx*)	Various
MIRTAZAPINE	
Tablets; oral: 7.5, 15, 30, and 45 mg (*Rx*)	Various, *Remeron* (Organon)
Tablets, orally disintegrating: 15, 30, and 45 mg (*Rx*)	Various, *Remeron SolTab* (Organon)

Warning:

Suicidality and antidepressant drugs: Antidepressants increased the risk compared with placebo of suicidal thinking and behavior (suicidality) in children, adolescents, and young adults in short-term studies of major depressive disorder (MDD) and other psychiatric disorders. Anyone considering the use of maprotiline, mirtazapine, or any other antidepressant in a child, adolescent, or young adult must balance this risk with the clinical need. Short-term studies did not show an increase in the risk of suicidality with antidepressants compared with placebo in adults older than 24 years of age; there was a reduction in risk with antidepressants compared with placebo in adults 65 years of age and older. Depression and certain other psychiatric disorders are associated with increases in suicide risk. Appropriately monitor and closely observe patients of all ages who are started on antidepressant therapy for clinical worsening, suicidality, or unusual changes in behavior. Advise families and caregivers of the need for close observation and communication with the prescriber. Maprotiline and mirtazapine are not approved for use in children.

Indications

Maprotiline hydrochloride: For the treatment of depressive illness in patients with depressive neurosis (dysthymic disorder) and manic-depressive illness, depressed type (MDD); also effective for the relief of anxiety associated with depression.

Mirtazapine: Mirtazapine tablets are indicated for the treatment of MDD.

Administration and Dosage

MAPROTILINE HYDROCHLORIDE: May be given as a single daily dose or in divided doses. Therapeutic effects are sometimes seen within 3 to 7 days, although as long as 2 to 3 weeks are usually necessary.

Initial adult dosage –

Mild to moderate depression: 75 mg/day. In some patients, an initial dose of 25 mg/day may be used. Maintain initial dosage for 2 weeks. Gradually increase the dosage in 25 mg increments, as required and tolerated. A maximum daily dose of 150 mg/day.

Severe depression: Give hospitalized patients an initial daily dose of 100 to 150 mg, which may be gradually increased as required and tolerated. Most hospitalized patients respond to a daily dosage of 150 mg, although doses as high as 225 mg may be required. Do not exceed 225 mg/day.

Maintenance – Dosage may be reduced to 75 to 150 mg/day with adjustment depending on therapeutic response.

Elderly – Lower doses are recommended for patients older than 60 years of age. An initial dose of 25 mg/day may be used. Doses of 50 to 75 mg/day are satisfactory as maintenance therapy for elderly patients who do not tolerate higher amounts.

MIRTAZAPINE:

Initial treatment – The recommended starting dose for mirtazapine is 15 mg/day administered in a single dose, preferably in the evening prior to sleep. The effective dose range is generally 15 to 45 mg/day.

Discontinuation of therapy – A gradual reduction in the dose over several weeks, rather than abrupt cessation, is recommended whenever possible.

Administration of orally disintegrating tablets – Open tablet blister pack with dry hands and place tablet on tongue. The tablet will disintegrate rapidly on the tongue and can be swallowed with saliva. Use the tablet immediately after removal from the blister; it cannot be stored. No water is needed. Do not attempt to split the tablet.

Actions

Pharmacology: Tetracyclics enhance central noradrenergic and serotonergic activity. Maprotiline blocks reuptake of norepinephrine at nerve endings.

Mirtazapine is a potent antagonist of 5-HT_2 and 5-HT_3 receptors. It is a potent antagonist of histamine (H_1) receptors and a moderate antagonist at muscarinic receptors.

Pharmacokinetics:

Maprotiline – The mean time to peak is 12 hours. The elimination half-life averages 43 hours. Binding to serum proteins is approximately 88%. Maprotiline is metabolized in the liver and excreted via the bile.

Mirtazapine – Mirtazapine is rapidly and completely absorbed following oral administration and has a half-life of approximately 20 to 40 hours, with females of all ages exhibiting significantly longer elimination half-lives than males (37 vs 26 hours). Steady-state plasma levels of mirtazapine are attained within 5 days. Mirtazapine is approximately 85% bound to plasma protein.

Metabolism/Excretion: Mirtazapine has an absolute bioavailability of approximately 50%. It is eliminated predominantly via urine (75%), with 15% in feces.

Contraindications

Hypersensitivity to maprotiline or mirtazapine; coadministration with MAOIs.

Maprotiline: Known or suspected seizure disorders; during acute phase of myocardial infarction (MI).

Warnings/Precautions

Clinical worsening and suicide risk: Adults and children with MDD may experience worsening of their depression and/or the emergence of suicidal ideation and behavior (suicidality) or unusual changes in behavior, whether or not they are taking antidepressant medications, and this risk may persist until significant remission occurs.

Anticholinergic properties: Administer maprotiline with caution in patients with increased intraocular pressure, history of urinary retention, or history of narrow-angle glaucoma because of the drug's anticholinergic properties.

Monoamine oxidase inhibitors: Do not give tetracyclics with MAOIs. Allow a minimum of 14 days to elapse after discontinuation of MAOIs before starting a tetracyclic.

Screening for bipolar disorder: A major depressive episode may be the initial presentation of bipolar disorder. It is generally believed that treating such an episode with an antidepressant alone may increase the likelihood of precipitation of a mixed/manic episode in patients at risk for bipolar disorder.

Seizures: Seizures have been associated with the use of **maprotiline**. Most of the seizures have occurred in patients without a known history of seizures.

Cardiovascular: Use with caution in patients with a history of MI and angina because of the possibility of conduction defects, arrhythmia, MI, strokes, and tachycardia. Use with caution in patients predisposed to hypotension.

Electroshock therapy: Avoid concurrent administration of maprotiline with electroshock therapy because of the lack of experience in this area.

Agranulocytosis: In clinical trials, 2 patients treated with mirtazapine developed agranulocytosis and a third patient developed severe neutropenia. All 3 patients recovered after mirtazapine was stopped.

Somnolence: Somnolence was reported in 54% of patients treated with mirtazapine.

Dizziness: Dizziness was reported in 7% of patients treated with mirtazapine.

Increased appetite/weight gain: Appetite increase was reported in 17% of patients treated with mirtazapine. In some trials, weight gain of 7% or more of body weight occurred in 7.5% of patients treated.

Cholesterol/Triglycerides: Nonfasting cholesterol increases to 20% or more above the upper limit of normal (ULN) and nonfasting triglyceride increases to 500 mg/dL or more were observed.

Transaminase levels: Clinically significant ALT elevations (at least 3 times the ULN range) were observed in 2% of patients exposed to **mirtazapine**.

Mania/Hypomania: Use carefully in patients with a history of mania/hypomania.

Elective surgery: Prior to elective surgery, discontinue **maprotiline** for as long as possible, because little is known about the interaction between maprotiline and general anesthetics.

Orthostatic hypotension: Orthostatic hypotension was infrequently observed in clinical trials with depressed patients.

Renal/Hepatic function impairment: Use mirtazapine with caution in patients with impaired renal and hepatic function.

Special risk: Administer **maprotiline** with caution in patients with increased intraocular pressure, history of urinary retention, or history of narrow-angle glaucoma because of the drug's anticholinergic properties. Exercise caution when administering maprotiline to hyperthyroid patients because of enhanced potential for cardiovascular toxicity of maprotiline. Exercise extreme caution when administering maprotiline to patients with a history of MI and with a history or presence of cardiovascular disease because of the possibility of conduction defects, arrhythmia, MI, stroke, and tachycardia.

Hazardous tasks: Caution patients about engaging in hazardous activities until they are reasonably certain that tetracyclics do not adversely affect their ability to engage in such activities.

Pregnancy: Category B (maprotiline); *Category* C (mirtazapine).

Lactation:

Maprotiline – Maprotiline is excreted in breast milk. At steady state, the concentration in milk corresponds closely to the concentrations in whole blood.

Mirtazapine – It is not known if mirtazapine is excreted in breast milk.

Children: Safety and efficacy in children have not been established.

Elderly: Oral clearance was reduced in elderly patients compared with the younger patients. Caution is indicated in administering mirtazapine to elderly patients.

Lab test abnormalities: Clinically significant ALT elevations (3 times or more the ULN range) were observed in 2% of patients exposed to mirtazapine.

Monitoring: Discontinue **maprotiline** if there is evidence of pathological neutrophil depression. Perform leukocyte and differential counts in patients who develop fever and sore throat during therapy.

Drug Interactions

Drugs that may affect maprotiline include alcohol, anticholinergics, benzodiazepines, cisapride, CYP inducers and inhibitors, MAOIs, phenothiazines, SSRIs, and sympathomimetics. Drugs that may be affected by mirtazapine include alcohol, anticholinergics, benzodiazepines, cisapride, guanethidine, MAOIs, sympathomimetics, and thyroid hormones.

QT prolongation: An additive effect of **maprotiline** with other drugs that prolong the QT interval cannot be excluded.

Adverse Reactions

Adverse reactions include abnormal dreams, abnormal thinking, anxiety, asthenia, blurred vision, constipation, dizziness, drowsiness, dry mouth, flu syndrome, headache, increased appetite, nervousness, somnolence, tremor, weakness and fatigue, weight gain.

TRAZODONE HYDROCHLORIDE

Tablets; oral: 50, 100, 150, and 300 mg (*Rx*)	Various
Tablets, extended-release; oral: 150 and 300 mg (*Rx*)	*Oleptro* (Labopharm)

Warning:

Suicidality and antidepressant drugs: Antidepressants increase the risk, compared with placebo, of suicidal thinking and behavior (suicidality) in children, adolescents, and young adults in short-term studies of major depressive disorder (MDD) and other psychiatric disorders. Anyone considering the use of trazodone or any other antidepressant in a child, adolescent, or young adult must balance the risk with the clinical need. Short-term studies did not show an increase in the risk of suicidality with antidepressants compared with placebo in adults older than 24 years of age; there was a reduction in risk with antidepressants compared with placebo in adults 65 years of age and older. Depression and certain other psychiatric disorders are themselves associated with increases in the risk of suicide. Appropriately monitor patients of all ages who are started on antidepressant therapy and observe them closely for clinical worsening, suicidality, or unusual changes in behavior. Advise families and caregivers of the need for close observation and communication with the prescriber. Trazodone is not approved for use in children.

Indications

Depression: For the treatment of depression (immediate release) and MDD in adults (extended release [ER]).

Administration and Dosage

Immediate-release tablets:

Adults – An initial dosage is 150 mg/day in divided doses. This may be increased by 50 mg/day every 3 to 4 days. The maximum dosage for outpatients usually should not exceed 400 mg/day in divided doses. Inpatients or more severely depressed subjects may be given up to 600 mg/day in divided doses.

Maintenance: Keep dosage at the lowest effective level. Once an adequate response has been achieved, dosage may be gradually reduced depending on response.

Administration: Drowsiness may require the administration of a major portion of the daily dose at bedtime or a reduced dosage. Take shortly after a meal or light snack.

Extended-release tablets:

Adults – An initial dosage is 150 mg once daily. Increase by 75 mg/day every 3 days (ie, start 225 mg on day 4 of therapy). Maximum dose is 375 mg/day.

Maintenance: Patients should be maintained on the lowest effective dose and periodically reassessed to determine the continued need for maintenance treatment.

Dosage adjustment: Once an adequate response has been achieved, the dosage may be gradually reduced, with subsequent adjustment depending on therapeutic response.

Discontinuation of therapy: Patients should be monitored for withdrawal symptoms when discontinuing treatment with trazodone. The dose should be gradually reduced whenever possible.

Administration: Trazodone ER should be taken at the same time every day in the late evening, preferably at bedtime, on an empty stomach. Can be swallowed whole or administered as a half tablet by breaking the tablet along the score line. Breaking the tablet in half does not affect the controlled-release properties. In order to maintain its controlled-release properties, trazodone ER should not be chewed or crushed.

Actions

Pharmacology: Trazodone selectively inhibits neuronal reuptake of serotonin and acts as an antagonist at 5-HT-2A/2C serotonin receptors.

Pharmacokinetics:

Absorption/Distribution – Trazodone is well absorbed after oral administration. Peak plasma levels of trazodone immediate-release tablets occur in approximately 1 hour when taken on an empty stomach or in 2 hours when taken with food. Trazodone is 89% to 95% protein bound.

Metabolism/Excretion – Trazodone is extensively metabolized in the liver and is a CYP3A4 substrate. Following single-dose administration of trazodone 300 mg ER tablets, a mean apparent terminal half-life of 10 hours was reported.

Contraindications

Hypersensitivity to trazodone.

Warnings/Precautions

Clinical worsening and suicide risk: Patients with MDD, adult and pediatric, may experience worsening of their depression and/or the emergence of suicidal ideation and behavior (suicidality) or unusual changes in behavior, whether or not they are taking antidepressant medications, and this risk may persist until significant remission occurs. Antidepressants increased the risk of suicidality in short-term studies in children and adolescents with MDD and other psychiatric disorders.

Closely observe all children being treated with antidepressants for any indication of clinical worsening, suicidality, or unusual changes in behavior, especially during the initial few months of a course of drug therapy, or at times of dose changes (either increases or decreases).

Serotonin syndrome/neuroleptic malignant syndrome–like reactions: The development of potentially life-threatening serotonin syndrome or neuroleptic malignant syndrome–like reactions have been reported with antidepressants alone and may occur with trazodone treatment, but particularly with concomitant use of other serotonergic drugs (including selective serotonin reuptake inhibitors [SSRIs], serotonin-norepinephrine reuptake inhibitors, and triptans) and with drugs that impair metabolism of serotonin (including monoamine oxidase inhibitors [MAOIs]), or with antipsychotics or other dopamine antagonists.

Bipolar disorder: It is generally believed that treating such an episode with an antidepressant alone may increase the likelihood of precipitation of a mixed/manic episode in patients at risk for bipolar disorder. Prior to initiating treatment with an antidepressant, adequately screen patients with depressive symptoms to determine if they are at risk for bipolar disorder.

Cardiac effects:

QT prolongation and risk of sudden death – Trazodone is known to prolong the QT/QTc interval. Some drugs that prolong the QT/QTc interval can cause torsades de pointes with sudden, unexplained death.

Preexisting cardiac disease – Not recommended for use during the initial recovery phase of MI. Trazodone may be arrhythmogenic in some patients.

Hypotension – Hypotension, including orthostatic hypotension and syncope, has occurred.

Abnormal bleeding: Postmarketing data have shown an association between the use of drugs that interfere with serotonin reuptake and the occurrence of GI bleeding. While no association between trazodone and bleeding events, in particular GI bleeding, was shown, caution patients about the potential risk of bleeding associated with the concomitant use of trazodone and nonsteroidal anti-inflammatory drugs (NSAIDs), aspirin, or other drugs that affect coagulation or bleeding.

Priapism: Instruct patients with prolonged or inappropriate penile erection to discontinue use immediately and consult a health care provider or go to an emergency room.

Hyponatremia: Hyponatremia may occur as a result of treatment with antidepressants.

Elective surgery: There is little known about the interaction between trazodone and general anesthetics; therefore, prior to elective surgery, discontinue trazodone for as long as clinically feasible.

Electroconvulsive therapy: Avoid concurrent administration with electroconvulsive therapy because of the absence of experience in this area.

Hematological effects: Occasional low white blood cell (WBC) and neutrophil counts have been noted in patients receiving trazodone. Discontinue the drug in any patient whose WBC count or absolute neutrophil count falls below normal levels.

Renal/Hepatic function impairment: Use trazodone with caution in patients with renal or hepatic function impairment.

Hazardous tasks: Antidepressants may impair the mental or physical abilities required for the performance of potentially hazardous tasks.

Pregnancy: Category C.

Lactation: The drug may be excreted in breast milk.

Children: Safety and efficacy in children have not been established.

Anyone considering the use of trazodone immediate-release tablets in a child or adolescent must balance the potential risks with the clinical need. Do not use trazodone ER tablets in children or adolescents.

Elderly: Antidepressants have been associated with cases of clinically significant hyponatremia in elderly patients who may be at greater risk for this adverse reaction.

Monitoring: Appropriately monitor all patients being treated with antidepressants for any indication and closely observe for clinical worsening, suicidality, and unusual changes in behavior, especially during the initial few months of a course of drug therapy or at times of dosage changes, either increases or decreases.

WBC and differential counts are recommended for patients who develop fever and sore throat (or other signs of infection) during therapy. Closely monitor patients with preexisting cardiac disease.

Drug Interactions

Drugs that may affect trazodone include alcohol, antihypertensives, azole antifungals, barbiturates, carbamazepine, CNS depressants, delavirdine, *Ginkgo biloba*, macrolide antibiotics, MAOIs, phenothiazines, protease inhibitors, serotonergic drugs, sodium oxybate, and SSRI antidepressants. Drugs that may be affected by trazodone include alcohol, antihypertensives, barbiturates, CNS depressants, carbamazepine, digoxin, MAOIs, NSAIDS, phenytoin, salicylates, serotonergic drugs, sodium oxybate, and warfarin.

Adverse Reactions

Adverse reactions occurring in 3% or more of patients include: abdominal/gastric disorder, aches/pains, allergic skin condition/edema, anger/hostility, blurred vision, confusion, constipation, decreased appetite, diarrhea, dizziness/light-headedness, drowsiness, dry mouth, excitement, fatigue, headache, hypotension, incoordination, insomnia, nasal/sinus congestion, nausea/vomiting, nervousness, nightmares/vivid dreams, syncope, tachycardia/palpitations, tremors, weight gain/loss.

BUPROPION

Tablets: 75 and 100 mg (as hydrochloride) (*Rx*)	Various, *Wellbutrin* (GlaxoSmithKline)
Tablets, extended-release: 150 mg (as hydrochloride) (*Rx*)	*Zyban* (GlaxoSmithKline)
Tablets, extended-release: 174, 348, and 522 mg (as hydrobromide) (*Rx*)	*Aplenzin* (Sanofi-Aventis)
Tablets, extended-release (12-hour): 100, 150, and 200 mg (as hydrochloride) (*Rx*)	Various, *Budeprion SR* (Teva), *Wellbutrin SR* (GlaxoSmithKline)
Tablets, extended-release (24-hour): 150 mg (as hydrochloride) (*Rx*)	Various, *Wellbutrin XL* (Biovail)
Tablets, extended-release (24-hour): 300 mg (as hydrochloride) (*Rx*)	*Budeprion XL* (Teva), *Wellbutrin XL* (GlaxoSmithKline

Warning:

Suicidality in children and adolescents: Although *Zyban* is not indicated for treatment of depression, it contains the same active ingredient as the antidepressant bupropion medications *Wellbutrin*, *Wellbutrin SR*, and *Wellbutrin XL*.

Antidepressants increased the risk of suicidal thinking and behavior (suicidality) in short-term studies in children and adolescents with major depressive disorder (MDD) and other psychiatric disorders. Bupropion is not approved for use in children.

Short-term studies did not show an increase in the risk of suicidality with antidepressants compared with placebo in adults older than 24 years of age; there was a reduction in risk with antidepressants compared with placebo in adults 65 years of age and older. Depression and certain other psychiatric disorders are themselves associated with increases in suicide risk. Appropriately monitor patients of all ages who are started on antidepressant therapy and closely observe them for clinical worsening, suicidality, or unusual changes in behavior. Advise families and caregivers of the need for close observation and communication with the prescriber.

Indications

MDD: Immediate-release (IR), and extended-release (XL) bupropion are indicated for the treatment of MDD.

Seasonal affective disorder (Wellbutrin XL only): For the prevention of seasonal major depressive episodes in patients with a diagnosis of seasonal affective disorder.

Smoking cessation (Zyban only): Indicated as an aid to smoking-cessation treatment.

Administration and Dosage

General: It is particularly important to administer bupropion in a manner most likely to minimize the risk of seizure (see Warnings/Precautions). Gradual escalation of dosage also is important to minimize agitation, motor restlessness, and insomnia often seen during the initial days of treatment. If necessary, these effects may be managed by temporary reduction of dose or the short-term administration of an intermediate- to long-acting sedative-hypnotic. A sedative-hypnotic usually is not required beyond the first week of treatment. Insomnia also may be minimized by avoiding bedtime doses. If distressing, untoward effects supervene, stop dose escalation.

Bupropion hydrochloride:

Bupropion IR – Increases in dose should not exceed 100 mg/day in a 3-day period. No single dose of bupropion should exceed 150 mg. Administer 3 times/day, preferably with at least 6 hours between successive doses.

Adults: 300 mg/day, given 3 times/day. Begin dosing at 200 mg/day, given as 100 mg twice/day. Based on clinical response, this dose may be increased to 300 mg/day, given as 100 mg 3 times/day no sooner than 3 days after beginning therapy.

Increasing the dosage above 300 mg/day: An increase in dosage up to a maximum of 450 mg/day given in divided doses of not more than 150 mg each may be considered for patients in whom no clinical improvement is noted after several weeks of treatment at 300 mg/day. Dosing above 300 mg/day may be accomplished using the 75 or 100 mg tablets. The 100 mg tablets must be administered 4 times/day with at least 4 hours between successive doses in order not to exceed the limit of 150 mg in a single dose. Discontinue in patients who do not demonstrate an adequate response after an appropriate period of 450 mg/day.

Bupropion ER – The usual adult target dosage is 300 mg/day, given as 150 mg twice/day. Begin dosing with 150 mg/day, given as a single daily dose in the morning. If the 150 mg initial dose is adequately tolerated, increase to 300 mg/day, given as 150 mg twice/day as early as day 4 of dosing. Allow at least 8 hours between successive doses. Swallow whole; do not crush, divide, or chew.

Increasing the dosage above 300 mg/day: As with other antidepressants, the full antidepressant effect of the SR formula may not be evident until 4 weeks of treatment or longer. Consider an increase in dosage to the maximum of 400 mg/day, given as 200 mg twice/day, for patients in whom no clinical improvement is noted after several weeks of 300 mg/day treatment.

Bupropion XL – May be taken without regard to meals. The usual adult target dose is 300 mg/day, given once daily in the morning. Dosing should begin at 150 mg/day, given as a single daily dose in the morning. If the 150 mg initial dose is adequately tolerated, an increase to the 300 mg/day target dose, given once daily, may be made as early as day 4 of dosing. There should be an interval of at least 24 hours between successive doses. Swallow whole; do not crush, divide, or chew.

Increasing the dosage above 300 mg/day: As with other antidepressants, the full antidepressant effect of the XL formula may not be evident until 4 weeks of treatment or longer. An increase in dosage to the maximum of 450 mg/day, given as a single dose, may be considered for patients in whom no clinical improvement is noted after several weeks of treatment at 300 mg/day.

Switching to Bupropion XL: When switching patients from bupropion tablets to XL tablets or from SR tablets to XL tablets, give the same total daily dose when possible. Patients who are currently being treated with bupropion IR tablets at 300 mg/day (eg, 100 mg 3 times/day) may be switched to XL tablets 300 mg once daily. Patients who are currently being treated with SR tablets at 300 mg/day (eg, 150 mg twice daily) may be switched to XL tablets 300 mg once daily.

Seasonal affective disorder (Wellbutrin XL only) – For the prevention of seasonal major depressive episodes associated with seasonal affective disorder, *Wellbutrin XL* should generally be initiated in the autumn prior to the onset of depressive symptoms. Treatment should continue through the winter season and should be tapered and discontinued in early spring. The timing of initiation and duration of treatment should be individualized based on the patient's historical pattern of seasonal major depressive episodes. Patients whose seasonal depressive episodes are infrequent or not associated with significant impairment should not generally be treated prophylactically.

Initial dose: Dosing should begin at 150 mg/day given as a single daily dose in the morning. If the 150 mg initial dose is adequately tolerated, the dose should be increased to the 300 mg/day dose after 1 week. If the 300 mg dose is not adequately tolerated, the dose can be reduced to 150 mg/day. The usual adult target dose is 300 mg/day, given once daily in the morning.

Discontinuation of treatment: For patients taking 300 mg/day during the autumn-winter season, the dose should be tapered to 150 mg/day for 2 weeks prior to discontinuation

Maximum dosage: Doses above 300 mg/day have not been studied for the prevention of seasonal major depressive episodes.

Maintenance – Use the lowest dose that maintains remission. Although it is not known how long the patient should remain on bupropion, acute episodes of depression generally require several months or longer of treatment.

Zyban –

Usual dosage for adults: The recommended and maximum dose of *Zyban* is 300 mg/day, given as 150 mg twice daily. Dosing should begin at 150 mg/day, given every day for the first 3 days, followed by a dose increase for most patients to the recommended usual dose of 300 mg/day. There should be an interval of at least 8 hours between successive doses. Doses above 300 mg/day should not be used. *Zyban* should be swallowed whole; do not crushed, divided, or chewed.

Treatment with *Zyban* should be initiated while the patient is still smoking, because approximately 1 week of treatment is required to achieve steady-state blood levels of bupropion. Treatment with *Zyban* should be continued for 7 to 12 weeks. If a patient has not made significant progress towards abstinence by the seventh week of therapy with *Zyban*, it is unlikely that he or she will quit during that attempt, and treatment should probably be discontinued. Dose tapering of *Zyban* is not required when discontinuing treatment.

Maintenance: Systematic evaluation of *Zyban* 300 mg/day for maintenance therapy demonstrated that treatment for up to 6 months was efficacious. Whether to continue treatment with *Zyban* for periods longer than 12 weeks for smoking cessation must be determined for individual patients.

Combination treatment with Zyban and a nicotine transdermal system (NTS): Combination treatment with *Zyban* and NTS may be prescribed for smoking cessation.

Monitoring for treatment-emergent hypertension in patients treated with the combination of *Zyban* and NTS is recommended.

Hepatic function impairment – Use bupropion with extreme caution in patients with severe hepatic cirrhosis. The dose should not exceed 75 mg once/day (100 mg every day or 150 mg every other day for bupropion SR; 150 mg every other day for XL) in these patients.

Renal function impairment – Use bupropion with caution in patients with renal function impairment and consider a reduced frequency or dose.

Bupropion hydrobromide:

MDD – 348 mg/day (equivalent to bupropion hydrochloride 300 mg/day) given once daily in the morning. Swallow whole and do not crush, divide, or chew tablets. May be taken without regard to meals.

Maximum dose: 522 mg/day.

Initial dose: 174 mg/day (equivalent to 150 mg/day) given as a single daily dose in the morning.

Dosage titration: If the 174 mg initial dose is adequately tolerated, an increase to the 348 mg/day target dosage, given once daily, may be made as early as day 4 of dosing. There should be an interval of at least 24 hours between successive doses. An increase in dosage to the maximum of 522 mg/day, given as a single dose, may be considered for patients in whom no clinical improvement is noted after several weeks of treatment at 348 mg/day.

Maintenance dosage: Patients should be periodically reassessed to determine the need for maintenance treatment and the appropriate dose for such treatment.

Conversion: When switching patients from bupropion hydrochloride to bupropion hydrobromide, give the equivalent total daily dose when possible (bupropion hydrobromide 522 mg is equivalent to bupropion hydrochloride 450 mg; bupropion hydrobromide 348 mg is equivalent to bupropion hydrochloride 300 mg; bupropion hydrobromide 174 mg is equivalent to bupropion hydrochloride 150 mg). Patients who are currently being treated with bupropion hydrochloride tablets at 300 mg/day (eg, 100 mg 3 times a day) may be switched to bupropion hydrobromide 348 mg once daily. Patients who are currently being treated with bupropion hydrochloride tablets at 300 mg/day (eg, 150 mg twice daily) may be switched to bupropion hydrobromide 348 mg once daily.

Elderly – Care should be taken in dose selection, and it may be useful to monitor renal function.

Renal function impairment – Use with caution in patients with renal impairment and a reduced frequency and/or dose should be considered.

Hepatic function impairment – Use with extreme caution in patients with severe hepatic cirrhosis. The dose should not exceed 174 mg every other day in these patients. Bupropion should be used with caution in patients with hepatic impairment (including mild to moderate hepatic cirrhosis) and a reduced frequency and/or dose should be considered in patients with mild to moderate hepatic cirrhosis.

Actions

Pharmacology: Bupropion is a weak blocker of the neuronal uptake of serotonin and norepinephrine.

Pharmacokinetics:

Absorption/Distribution – Following oral administration, peak plasma concentrations usually are achieved within 2 hours for bupropion, 3 hours for bupropion SR, and 5 hours for bupropion XL, followed by a biphasic decline. The half-life of the second (postdistributional) phase of bupropion ranges 8 to 24 hours; mean elimination half-life for bupropion SR is 21 hours.

Metabolism/Excretion – Bupropion is extensively metabolized in the liver. Steady-state plasma concentrations of bupropion and its metabolites are reached within 5 and 8 days, respectively.

Contraindications

Hypersensitivity to the drug; seizure disorder; current or prior diagnosis of bulimia or anorexia nervosa; coadministration of a monoamine oxidase inhibitor (MAOI) (at least 14 days should elapse between discontinuation of an MAOI and initiation of treatment with bupropion); in patients being treated with other bupropion products (eg, for smoking cessation); in patients undergoing abrupt discontinuation of alcohol or sedatives (including benzodiazepines).

Warnings/Precautions

Clinical worsening and suicide risk: See Warning Box.

Screening patients for bipolar disorder: Prior to initiating treatment with an antidepressant, adequately screen patients with depressive symptoms to determine if they are at risk for bipolar disorder.

Other bupropion medications: Do not use bupropion in combination with *Zyban* or any other medications that contain bupropion.

Seizures: Bupropion is associated with a dose-related risk of seizures. Discontinue bupropion and do not restart in patients who experience a seizure while on treatment. Use extreme caution when bupropion is administered to patients with a history of seizure, cranial trauma, or other predisposition(s) toward seizure, or prescribed with other agents (eg, antipsychotics, other antidepressants, theophylline, systemic steroids) that lower seizure threshold.

CNS symptoms: A substantial proportion of patients experience some degree of increased restlessness, agitation, anxiety, and insomnia, especially shortly after initiation of treatment.

Altered appetite and weight: A weight loss of more than 5 pounds occurred in 28% of patients treated with bupropion IR and in at least 14% of patients treated with bupropion SR.

Cardiac effects: Hypertension, in some cases severe, requiring acute treatment, has been reported in patients receiving bupropion alone and in combination with nicotine replacement therapy. Exercise care if bupropion is used in patients with a recent history of MI or unstable heart disease.

Activation of psychosis and/or mania: Antidepressants can precipitate manic episodes in bipolar disorder patients during the depressed phase of their illness and may activate latent psychosis in other susceptible patients. Bupropion is expected to pose similar risks.

Hypersensitivity reactions: Anaphylactoid reactions characterized by symptoms such as pruritus, urticaria, angioedema, and dyspnea requiring medical treatment have been reported. In addition, there have been rare spontaneous postmarketing reports of erythema multiforme, Stevens-Johnson syndrome, and anaphylactic shock associated with bupropion.

Tartrazine sensitivity: Some of these products contain tartrazine, which may cause allergic-type reactions (including bronchial asthma) in susceptible individuals.

Renal function impairment: Use bupropion with caution in patients with renal function impairment and consider a reduced frequency or dose.

Hepatic function impairment: Use bupropion with extreme caution in patients with severe hepatic cirrhosis. In these patients, a reduced dose or frequency is required. Do not exceed 75 mg once a day (100 mg every day or 150 mg every other day for bupropion SR; 150 mg every other day for bupropion XL) in these patients.

Drug abuse and dependence: Studies in healthy volunteers, subjects with a history of multiple drug abuse, and depressed patients showed some increase in motor activity and agitation/excitement. In individuals experienced with drugs of abuse, a single dose of 400 mg bupropion produced mild amphetamine-like activity as compared with placebo.

Photosensitivity: Photosensitization may occur; therefore, caution patients to take protective measures (ie, sunscreens, protective clothing) against exposure to ultraviolet light or sunlight until tolerance is determined.

Pregnancy: Category C.

Pregnancy registry – To monitor fetal outcomes of pregnant women exposed to bupropion, GlaxoSmithKline maintains a Bupropion Pregnancy Registry. Health care providers are encouraged to register patients by calling (800) 336-2176.

Lactation: Bupropion and its metabolites are secreted in breast milk. Decide whether to discontinue breast-feeding or the drug.

Children: Safety and efficacy in children have not been established.

Elderly: Because elderly patients are more likely to have decreased renal function, take care in dose selection; it may be useful to monitor renal function (see Precautions, Administration and Dosage).

Monitoring: Closely monitor all patients with hepatic function impairment. Monitoring of blood pressure is recommended in patients who receive the combination of bupropion and nicotine replacement.

Drug Interactions

Drugs that may affect bupropion include amantadine, levodopa, carbamazepine, MAOIs, nicotine replacement, ritonavir, clopidogrel, phenobarbital, phenytoin, cimetidine, ticlopidine, and drugs that lower the seizure threshold.

Drugs that may be affected by bupropion include alcohol, drugs metabolized by CYP-450 2D6, warfarin, guanfacine, linezolid, MAOIs, antiarrhythmics, antipsychotics, cyclosporine, SSRIs, and TCAs.

Use caution during coadministration of bupropion and agents (eg, antipsychotics, other antidepressants, theophylline, systemic steroids) or treatment regimens (eg, abrupt discontinuation of benzodiazepines) that lower seizure threshold. Use low initial dosing and small gradual dose increases.

Adverse Reactions

Adverse reactions occurring in at least 3% of patients include abdominal pain; agitation; akinesia/bradykinesia; amblyopia; anorexia; anxiety; appetite increase; arthralgia; arthritis; asthenia; auditory disturbance; blurred vision; cardiac arrythmias; chest pain; confusion; constipation; decreased libido; diarrhea; disturbed concentration; dizziness; dream abnormality; dry mouth; dyspepsia; excessive sweating; fatigue; flushing; gustatory disturbance; hostility; headache/migraine; hot flashes; hypertension; impaired sleep quality; impotence; infection; insomnia; irritability; memory decreased; menstrual complaints; myalgia; nausea/vomiting; nervousness; pain; palpitations; pharyngitis; pruritus; rash; sedation; sensory disturbance; sinusitis; somnolence; sweating; tachycardia; taste perversion; tinnitus; tremor; upper respiratory complaints; urinary frequency; weight loss/gain.

NEFAZODONE HYDROCHLORIDE

Tablets: 50, 100, 150, 200, and 250 mg (*Rx*) Various

Warning:

Cases of life-threatening hepatic failure have been reported in patients treated with nefazodone. The reported rate in the United States is about 1 case of liver failure resulting in death or transplant per 250,000 to 300,000 patient-years of nefazodone treatment.

Ordinarily, do not initiate treatment with nefazodone in individuals with active liver disease or with elevated baseline serum transaminases. There is no evidence that preexisting liver disease increases the likelihood of developing liver failure; however, baseline abnormalities can complicate patient monitoring.

Advise patients to be alert for signs and symptoms of liver dysfunction (eg, jaundice, anorexia, GI complaints, malaise) and to report them to their doctor immediately if they occur.

Discontinue nefazodone if clinical signs or symptoms suggest liver failure. Patients who develop evidence of hepatocellular injury such as increased serum AST or serum ALT levels at least 3 times the upper limit of normal while on nefazodone should be withdrawn from the drug. These patients should be presumed to be at increased risk for liver injury if nefazodone is reintroduced. Accordingly, do not consider such patients for retreatment.

Suicidality in children and adolescents: Antidepressants increased the risk of suicidal thinking and behavior (suicidality) in short-term studies in children and adolescents with major depressive disorder (MDD) and other psychiatric disorders. Anyone considering the use of nefazodone or any other antidepressant in a child or adolescent must balance this risk with the clinical need. Patients who are started on therapy should be observed closely for clinical worsening, suicidality, or unusual changes in behavior.

Indications

Depression: Treatment of depression.

Administration and Dosage

Initial treatment: Recommended starting dose is 200 mg/day, administered in 2 divided doses. In clinical trials, the effective dose range was generally 300 to 600 mg/day. Increase doses in increments of 100 to 200 mg/day, again on a twice/day schedule, at intervals of no less than 1 week.

Elderly/Debilitated patients: The recommended initial dose is 100 mg/day on a twice/day schedule.

Maintenance/Continuation/Extended treatment: There is no evidence to indicate how long the depressed patient should be treated with nefazodone. However, it is generally agreed that pharmacologic treatment for acute episodes of depression should continue for at least 6 months. Whether the dose of antidepressant needed to induce remission is identical to the dose needed to maintain euthymia is unknown. In clinical trials, more than 250 patients were treated for at least 1 year.

Switching to or from a monoamine oxidase inhibitor (MAOI): At least 14 days should elapse between discontinuation of an MAOI and initiation of therapy with nefazodone. In addition, wait at least 7 days after stopping nefazodone before starting an MAOI.

Actions

Pharmacology: Nefazodone is an antidepressant with a chemical structure unrelated to available antidepressant agents. The mechanism of action is unknown. Nefazodone inhibits neuronal uptake of serotonin and norepinephrine.

Pharmacokinetics:

Absorption/Distribution – Nefazodone is rapidly and completely absorbed. Its absolute bioavailability is low (about 20%) and variable. Food delays absorption of nefazodone and decreases the bioavailability about 20%. Peak plasma concentrations occur at about 1 hour.

Metabolism/Excretion – Nefazodone is extensively metabolized after oral administration by less than 1% is excreted unchanged in urine. The mean half-life ranged between 11 and 24 hours. Nefazodone is extensively (more than 99%) bound to human plasma proteins in vitro.

Contraindications

Coadministration with cisapride, pimozide, or carbamazepine (see Warnings and Drug Interactions); patients who were withdrawn from nefazodone because of evidence of liver injury (see Warning box, Warnings); hypersensitivity to nefazodone or other phenylpiperazine antidepressants.

Coadministration of triazolam and nefazodone causes a significant increase in the plasma level of triazolam; a 75% reduction in the initial triazolam dosage is recommended. Avoid the coadministration of triazolam and nefazodone for most patients, including the elderly.

Warnings/Precautions

Clinical worsening and suicide risk: See Warning box. Patients with MDD, both adult and pediatric, may experience worsening of their depression and/or the emergence of suicidal ideation and behavior (suicidality) or unusual changes in behavior, whether or not they are taking antidepressant medications, and this risk may persist until significant remission occurs. Antidepressants increased the risk of suicidal thinking and behavior (suicidality) in short-term studies in children and adolescents with MDD and other psychiatric disorders.

Closely observe all pediatric patients being treated with antidepressants for any indication for clinical worsening, suicidality, and unusual changes in behavior, especially during the initial few months of a course of drug therapy, or at times of dose changes, either increases or decreases. Such observation would generally include at least weekly face-to-face contact with patients or their family members or caregivers during the first 4 weeks of treatment, then every-other-week visits for the next 4 weeks, then at 12 weeks, and as clinically indicated beyond 12 weeks. Additional contact by telephone may be appropriate between face-to-face visits.

If the decision has been made to discontinue treatment, taper medication as rapidly as is feasible, but with recognition that abrupt discontinuation can be associated with certain symptoms.

Screening patients for bipolar disorder: A major depressive episode may be the initial presentation of bipolar disorder. It is generally believed that treating such an episode with an antidepressant alone may increase the likelihood of precipitation of a mixed/manic episode in patients at risk for bipolar disorder. Prior to initiating treatment with an antidepressant, adequately screen patients with depressive symptoms to determine if they are at risk for bipolar disorder.

Hepatotoxicity: See Warning box. Cases of life-threatening hepatic failure have been reported in patients treated with nefazodone. The time to liver injury resulting in death or transplant generally ranged from 2 weeks to 6 months on nefazodone therapy. Advise patients to be alert for signs and symptoms of liver dysfunction (eg, jaundice, anorexia, GI complaints, malaise) and to report them to their doctor immediately if they occur. Discontinue nefazodone if clinical signs or symptoms suggest liver failure. Patients who develop evidence of hepatocellular injury such as increased serum AST or serum ALT levels 3 times or more the upper limit of normal, while on nefazodone should be withdrawn from the drug. Such patients should not be considered for retreatment.

Serious interactions:

MAOIs – Because nefazodone is an inhibitor of both serotonin and norepinephrine reuptake, it is recommended that nefazodone not be used in combination with an MAOI, or within 14 days of discontinuing treatment with an MAOI. Allow at least 1 week after stopping nefazodone before starting an MAOI.

Triazolobenzodiazepines – Triazolam and alprazolam, metabolized by cytochrome P-450 3A4, have increased plasma concentrations when administered concomitantly with nefazodone. If triazolam is coadministered with nefazodone, a 75% reduction in the initial triazolam dosage is recommended. It is recommended that triazolam not be used in combination with nefazodone. No dosage adjustment is required for nefazodone.

Antihistamines, nonsedating/Cisapride/Pimozide – Cisapride and pimozide are metabolized by the cytochrome P-450 3A4 isozyme; inhibitors of 3A4 can block the metabolism of these drugs, resulting in increased plasma concentrations of parent drug, which is associated with QT prolongation and with rare cases of serious cardiovascular adverse events, including death, because of ventricular tachycardia of the torsades de pointes type. In vitro, nefazodone inhibits 3A4. It is recommended that nefazodone not be used in combination with cisapride or pimozide.

Use in patients with concomitant illness: Sinus bradycardia, defined as heart rate up to 50 bpm and a decrease of at least 15 bpm from baseline, was observed in 1.5% of nefazodone-treated patients compared with 0.4% of placebo-treated patients ($P \leq 0.05$). Treat patients with a recent history of MI or unstable heart disease with caution.

Postural hypotension: Use nefazodone with caution in patients with known cardiovascular or cerebrovascular disease that could be exacerbated by hypotension and conditions that would predispose patients to hypotension.

Mania/Hypomania: As with all antidepressants, use nefazodone cautiously in patients with a history of mania.

Seizures: Rare occurrences of convulsions (including grand mal seizures) following nefazodone administration have been reported since market introduction. A causal relationship to nefazodone has not been established.

Priapism: If patients present with prolonged or inappropriate erections, they should discontinue therapy immediately and consult their physicians.

Hepatic cirrhosis: In patients with cirrhosis of the liver, the AUC values of nefazodone and its metabolite HO-NEF were increased by about 25%.

Visual disturbances: There have been reports of visual disturbances associated with the use of nefazodone, including blurred vision, scotoma, and visual trails.

Drug abuse and dependence: Carefully evaluate patients for a history of drug abuse and follow such patients closely, observing them for signs of misuse or abuse of nefazodone.

Hazardous tasks: Caution patients about operating hazardous machinery, including automobiles, until they are reasonably certain that nefazodone therapy does not adversely affect their ability to engage in such activities.

Photosensitivity: Photosensitization (photoallergy or phototoxicity) may occur; therefore, caution patients to take protective measures (ie, sunscreens, protective clothing) against exposure to sunlight or ultraviolet light (eg, tanning beds) until tolerance is determined.

Pregnancy: Category C.

Lactation: It is not known whether nefazodone or its metabolites are excreted in breast milk.

Children: Safety and efficacy have not been established.

Elderly: Initiate treatment at 50% of the usual dose, but titrate upward over the same range as in younger patients. Observe the usual precautions in elderly patients who have concomitant medical illnesses or who are receiving concomitant drugs.

Drug Interactions

Drugs that affect nefazodone include general anesthetics, sibutramine, sumatriptan, buspirone, carbamazepine, and propranolol. Drugs that may be affected by nefazodone include alcohol, benzodiazepines, buspirone, carbamazepine, cisapride, digoxin, haloperidol, HMG-CoA reductase inhibitors, MAOIs, propranolol, St. John's wort, cyclosporine, and tacrolimus.

Potential interaction with drugs that inhibit or are metabolized by cytochrome P-450 (3A4 and 2D6) isozymes: Caution is indicated in the combined use of nefazodone with any drugs known to be metabolized by the 3A4 isozyme (in particular, cisapride or pimozide).

Drugs highly bound to plasma protein: Administration to a patient taking another drug that is highly protein bound may cause increased free concentrations of the other drug, potentially resulting in adverse events. Conversely, adverse effects could result from displacement of nefazodone by other highly bound drugs.

Drug/Food interactions: Food delays absorption of nefazodone and decreases the bioavailability by about 20%.

Adverse Reactions

Adverse reactions occurring in at least 3% of patients include abnormal dreams, abnormal vision, asthenia, blurred vision, confusion, constipation, cough, decreased concentration, diarrhea, dizziness, dry mouth, dyspepsia, flu syndrome, headache, increased appetite, infection, insomnia, lightheadedness, memory impairment, nausea, paresthesia, peripheral edema, pharyngitis, postural hypotension, somnolence, vasodilation.

DULOXETINE HYDROCHLORIDE

Capsules, delayed-release[a]; oral: 20, 30, and 60 mg (*Rx*) *Cymbalta* (Eli Lilly)

[a] Contains enteric-coated pellets.

Warning:

Suicidality in children and adolescents: Antidepressants increased the risk of suicidal thinking and behavior (suicidality) in short-term studies in children and adolescents with major depressive disorder (MDD) and other psychiatric disorders. Anyone considering the use of duloxetine or any other antidepressant in a child or adolescent must balance this risk with the clinical need. Patients who are started on therapy should be observed closely for clinical worsening, suicidality, or unusual changes in behavior. Duloxetine is not approved for use in children.

Indications

Diabetic peripheral neuropathic (DPN) pain: For the management of neuropathic pain associated with DPN.

Fibromyalgia: For the management of fibromyalgia.

Generalized anxiety disorder (GAD): For the treatment of GAD.

MDD: For the treatment of MDD as defined in the *Diagnostic and Statistical Manual of Mental Disorders, Fourth Edition.*

Unlabeled uses: Stress urinary incontinence.

Administration and Dosage

Swallow capsules whole; do not chew or crush. The contents should not be sprinkled on food or mixed with liquids.

DPN pain:

Initial treatment – Administer as a total dose of 60 mg/day given once daily without regard to meals.

Maintenance/Continuation/Extended treatment – Because the progression of DPN is highly variable and management of pain is empirical, assess the effectiveness of duloxetine individually. Efficacy beyond 12 weeks has not been studied.

Fibromyalgia:

Initial dose – 30 mg once daily for 1 week and then increase to 60 mg once daily. Some patients may respond to the starting dose.

GAD:

Initial dose – 60 mg once daily. For some patients, it may be desirable to start at 30 mg once daily for 1 week to allow patients to adjust to the medication before increasing to 60 mg once daily.

Dosage adjustment – While a 120 mg once-daily dosage was shown to be effective, there is no evidence that dosages of more than 60 mg once daily confer additional benefit.

Maintenance/Continuation/Extended treatment – GAD is generally recognized as a chronic condition. The efficacy of duloxetine in long-term use for GAD, that is, for more than 10 weeks, has not been systematically evaluated.

MDD:

Initial dose – For some patients, it may be desirable to start at 30 mg once daily for 1 week to allow patients to adjust to the medication before increasing to 60 mg once daily.

Maintenance dosage – 40 mg/day (given as 20 mg twice daily) to 60 mg/day (given once a day or as 30 mg twice daily).

Duration of therapy – It is generally agreed that acute episodes of major depression require several months or longer of sustained pharmacologic therapy. Patients should be periodically reassessed to determine the need for maintenance treatment and the appropriate dose for such treatment.

Switching patients to or from a monoamine oxidase inhibitor (MAOI) – At least 14 days should elapse between discontinuation of an MAOI and initiation of therapy with duloxetine. In addition, at least 5 days should be allowed after stopping duloxetine before starting an MAOI.

Actions

Pharmacology: Although the mechanism of the antidepressant and central pain inhibitory action of duloxetine in humans is unknown, it is believed to be related to its potentiation of serotonergic and noradrenergic activity in the CNS. Preclinical studies have shown that duloxetine is a potent inhibitor of neuronal serotonin and norepinephrine reuptake and a less potent inhibitor of dopamine reuptake. Duloxetine has no significant affinity for dopaminergic, adrenergic, cholinergic, histaminergic, opioid, glutamate, and gamma-aminobutyric acid (GABA) receptors in vitro and does not inhibit MAO.

Pharmacokinetics:

Absorption/Distribution – Orally administered duloxetine is well absorbed. There is a median 2-hour lag until absorption begins, with maximum plasma concentration (C_{max}) occurring 6 hours postdose. Food does not affect the C_{max} of duloxetine but delays the time to reach peak concentration from 6 to 10 hours. The apparent volume of distribution averages approximately 1,640 L. Duloxetine is highly bound (more than 90%) to proteins in human plasma, binding primarily to albumin and α_1-acid glycoprotein. Steady-state plasma concentrations are typically achieved after 3 days of dosing.

Metabolism/Excretion – Duloxetine undergoes extensive metabolism and has an elimination half-life of approximately 12 hours (range, 8 to 17 hours). Elimination is mainly through hepatic metabolism involving two P450 isozymes, CYP2D6 and CYP1A2.

Contraindications

Concomitant use in patients taking MAOIs; use in patients with uncontrolled narrow-angle glaucoma.

Warnings/Precautions

Abnormal bleeding: SSRIs and SNRIs, including duloxetine, may increase the risk of bleeding events. Bleeding events related to SSRI and SNRI use have ranged from ecchymoses, hematomas, epistaxis, and petechiae to life-threatening hemorrhages.

Blood pressure (BP) effects: In clinical trials, duloxetine treatment was associated with mean increases in BP, averaging 2 mm Hg systolic and 0.5 mm Hg diastolic and an increase in the incidence of at least 1 measurement of systolic BP over 140 mm Hg compared with placebo. Measure BP prior to initiating treatment and periodically throughout treatment.

Clinical worsening and suicide risk: See Warning box. Patients with MDD, both adult and pediatric, may experience worsening of their depression and/or the emergence of suicidal ideation and behavior (suicidality) or unusual changes in behavior, whether or not they are taking antidepressant medications, and this risk may persist until significant remission occurs. Antidepressants increased the risk of suicidal thinking and behavior (suicidality) in short-term studies in children and adolescents with MDD and other psychiatric disorders.

Closely observe all pediatric patients being treated with antidepressants for any indication for clinical worsening, suicidality, and unusual changes in behavior, especially during the initial few months of a course of drug therapy, or at times of dose changes, either increases or decreases. Such observation would generally include at least weekly face-to-face contact with patients or their family members or caregivers during the first 4 weeks of treatment, then every-other-week visits for the next 4 weeks, then at 12 weeks, and as clinically indicated beyond 12 weeks. Additional contact by telephone may be appropriate between face-to-face visits.

If the decision has been made to discontinue treatment, taper medication as rapidly as is feasible, but with recognition that abrupt discontinuation can be associated with certain symptoms.

Discontinuation of treatment: Symptoms associated with discontinuation of duloxetine and other SSRIs and SNRIs have been reported. Monitor patients for symptoms including dizziness, nausea, headache, paresthesia, vomiting, irritability, and nightmares when discontinuing treatment.

A gradual reduction in the dose rather than abrupt cessation is recommended whenever possible. If intolerable symptoms occur following a decrease in the dose or discontinuation of treatment, resuming the previously prescribed dose may be considered. Subsequently, the physician may continue decreasing the dose, but at a more gradual rate.

Hyponatremia: Cases of hyponatremia (some with serum sodium less than 110 mmol/L) have been reported and appeared to be reversible when duloxetine was discontinued.

Orthostatic hypotension and syncope: Orthostatic hypotension and syncope have been reported with therapeutic doses of duloxetine.

Screening patients for bipolar disorder: A major depressive episode may be the initial presentation of bipolar disorder. It is generally believed that treating such an episode with an antidepressant alone may increase the likelihood of precipitation of a mixed/manic episode in patients at risk for bipolar disorder. Prior to initiating treatment with an antidepressant, adequately screen patients with depressive symptoms to determine if they are at risk for bipolar disorder.

Serotonin syndrome: The development of a potentially life-threatening serotonin syndrome may occur with selective norepinephrine reuptake inhibitors (SNRIs) and selective serotonin reuptake inhibitors (SSRIs), including duloxetine treatment, particularly with concomitant use of serotonergic drugs (including triptans) and with drugs that impair metabolism of serotonin (including MAOIs).

Urinary effects: Duloxetine is in a class of drugs known to affect urethral resistance. If symptoms of urinary hesitation develop during treatment with duloxetine, consider the possibility that they might be drug-related.

Renal function impairment: Increased plasma concentrations of duloxetine, and especially of its metabolites, occur in patients with end-stage renal disease (ESRD) and severe renal impairment (creatinine clearance less than 30 mL/min). Duloxetine is not recommended for patients with ESRD.

Hepatic function impairment:

Hepatotoxicity – Duloxetine increases the risk of elevation of serum transaminase levels. The combination of transaminase elevations and elevated bilirubin, without evidence of obstruction, is generally recognized as an important predictor of severe liver injury. Because it is possible that duloxetine and alcohol may interact to cause liver injury, duloxetine should ordinarily not be prescribed to patients with substantial alcohol use.

Do not administer duloxetine to patients with hepatic insufficiency; markedly increased exposure occurs.

Special risk:

Mania/Hypomania activation – In placebo-controlled trials in patients with MDD, activation of mania or hypomania was reported in 0.1% of duloxetine-treated patients and 0.1% of placebo-treated patients. Use cautiously in patients with a history of mania.

Seizures – In placebo-controlled clinical trials in patients with MDD, seizures occurred in 0.1% of patients treated with duloxetine and 0% of patients treated with placebo. Prescribe duloxetine with care in patients with a history of a seizure disorder.

Controlled narrow-angle glaucoma – In clinical trials, duloxetine was associated with an increased risk of mydriasis; therefore, use cautiously in patients with controlled narrow-angle glaucoma.

Gastric motility alteration – Duloxetine is rapidly hydrolyzed in acidic media to naphthol; use caution in patients with conditions that may slow gastric emptying.

Diabetes – In clinical trials, small increases in fasting blood glucose were observed in duloxetine-treated patients; however, overall diabetic control did not worsen as evidenced by stable glycosylated hemoglobin values.

Hazardous tasks: Caution patients about operating hazardous machinery, including automobiles, until they are reasonably certain that duloxetine therapy does not adversely affect their ability to engage in such activities.

Pregnancy: *Category C*; *Category D* if taken in the second half of pregnancy.

Lactation: It is unknown whether or not duloxetine and/or its metabolites are excreted into human milk. Breast-feeding while taking duloxetine is not recommended.

Children: Safety and efficacy have not been established.

Monitoring: Monitor patients for the emergence of agitation, irritability, and other symptoms, as well as the emergence of suicidality; monitor BP prior to initiation and periodically during treatment.

Drug Interactions

Drugs that may affect duloxetine include inhibitors of CYP1A2 (eg, fluvoxamine, quinolone antibiotics), inhibitors of CYP2D6 (eg, fluoxetine, quinidine, paroxetine), alcohol. linezolid, MAOIs, methylene blue, serotonergic drugs, St. John's wort, triptans, CNS-acting drugs.

Drugs that may be affected by duloxetine include drugs extensively metabolized by CYP2D6 (eg, flecainide, phenothiazines, propafenone, tricyclic antidepressants, thioridazine), alcohol, antiarrhythmics, aspirin, beta-blockers, CNS-acting drugs, linezolid, MAOIs, methylene blue, NSAIDs, phenothiazines, serotonergic drugs, St. John's wort, sympathomimetics, TCAs, triptans, drugs highly bound to plasma proteins (eg, warfarin).

Adverse Reactions

Small mean increases from baseline to end point in ALT, AST, creatine phosphokinase, and alkaline phosphatase have occurred.

Duloxetine is in a class of drugs known to affect urethral resistance.

MDD: Adverse reactions occurring in at least 3% of patients include the following: abnormal orgasm, anxiety, blurred vision, constipation, decreased appetite/anorexia, decreased libido, delayed ejaculation, diarrhea, dizziness, dry mouth, ejaculatory dysfunction, erectile dysfunction, fatigue, increased sweating, insomnia, nausea, somnolence, tremor, vomiting.

DPN pain: Adverse reactions occurring in at least 3% of patients include the following: anorexia, asthenia, constipation, cough, decrease appetite, diarrhea, dizziness, dry mouth, dyspepsia, erectile dysfunction, fatigue, headache, hyperhydrosis, insomnia, loose stools, muscle cramp, myalgia, nasopharyngitis, nausea, pharyngolaryngeal pain, pollakiuria, pyrexia, somnolence, tremor, vomiting.

VENLAFAXINE

Tablets: 25, 37.5, 50, 75, and 100 mg (*Rx*)	Various
Tablets, extended-release: 37.5, 75, 150, and 225 mg (*Rx*)	Teva pharmaceuticals USA
Capsules, extended-release: 37.5, 75, and 150 mg (*Rx*)	*Effexor XR* (Wyeth Pharmaceuticals, Upstate Pharma)

Warning:

Suicidality and antidepressant drugs: Antidepressants increased the risk of suicidal thinking and behavior (suicidality) compared with placebo in short-term studies in children, adolescents, and young adults with major depressive disorder (MDD) and other psychiatric disorders. Anyone considering the use of venlafaxine or any other antidepressant in a child, adolescent, or young adult must balance this risk with the clinical need. Short-term studies did not show an increase in the risk of suicidality with antidepressants compared with placebo in adults older than 24 years of age; there was a reduction in risk with antidepressants compared with placebo in adults 65 years of age and older. Depression and certain other psychiatric disorders are themselves associated with increases in the risk of suicide. Closely observe and appropriately monitor patients of all ages who are started on antidepressant therapy for clinical worsening, suicidality, or unusual changes in behavior. Advise families and caregivers of the need for close observation and communication with the prescriber. Venlafaxine is not approved for use in children.

Indications

MDD: Treatment of MDD.

Anxiety: Treatment of generalized anxiety disorder (GAD) and social anxiety disorder (SAD) (extended-release only).

Panic disorder (extended-release capsules only): For the treatment of panic disorder, with or without agoraphobia.

Administration and Dosage

Venlafaxine immediate-release:

MDD –

Initial treatment: 75 mg/day, administered in 2 or 3 divided doses taken with food. Depending on tolerability and the need for further clinical effect, the dose may be increased to 150 mg/day. If needed, further increase the dose to 225 mg/day. When increasing the dose, make increments of up to 75 mg/day at intervals of at least 4 days. Certain patients, including more severely depressed patients, may respond more to higher doses, up to a maximum of 375 mg/day, generally in 3 divided doses.

Venlafaxine extended-release: Administer in a single dose with food either in the morning or in the evening at approximately the same time each day. Swallow each capsule whole with fluid; do not divide, crush, chew, or place in water. Capsules may be administered by carefully opening the capsule and sprinkling the entire contents onto a spoonful of applesauce. Swallow this drug/food mixture immediately without chewing and follow with a glass of water to ensure complete swallowing of the pellets.

Bioequivalency – Equal doses of venlafaxine ER tablets are bioequivalent (but not AB rated) to *Effexor XR* capsules when administered under fed conditions.

MDD –

Initial treatment: 75 mg/day, administered in a single dose. For some new patients, it may be desirable to start at 37.5 mg/day for 4 to 7 days. Patients not responding to the initial 75 mg/day dosage may benefit from dose increases to a maximum of approximately 225 mg/day. Dose increases should be in increments of up to 75 mg/day as needed and should be made at intervals of at least 4 days.

Generalized anxiety disorder (ER capsules)/social anxiety disorder (ER capsules or tablets) – 75 mg/day, administered in a single dose. For some patients, it may be desirable to start at 37.5 mg/day for 4 to 7 days before increasing to 75 mg/day. Certain patients not responding to the initial 75 mg/day dose may benefit from dose increases to a maximum of approximately 225 mg/day. Dose increases should be in increments of up to 75 mg/day, as needed, and should be made at intervals of not less than 4 days.

Panic disorder (ER capsules only) – 37.5 mg/day for 7 days. Initial doses of 37.5 mg/day for 7 days can be followed by doses of 75 mg/day and subsequent weekly dose increases of 75 mg/day to a maximum dose of 225 mg/day. Dose increases should be in increments of up to 75 mg/day, as needed, and should be made at intervals of no less than 7 days. Depressed patients who are currently being treated at a therapeutic dose with venlafaxine may be switched to venlafaxine ER at the nearest equivalent dose (mg/day) (ie, venlafaxine 37.5 mg 2 times daily to venlafaxine ER 75 mg once daily). However, individual dosage adjustments may be necessary.

Social anxiety disorder – 75 mg/day as a single dose.

Discontinuation: Monitor patients for associated symptoms when discontinuing treatment. A gradual reduction in the dose rather than abrupt cessation is recommended whenever possible.

Hepatic function impairment: It is recommended that the total daily dose be reduced by 50% in patients with mild to moderate hepatic impairment. It may be necessary to reduce the dose more than 50%.

Renal function impairment: It is recommended that the total daily dose be reduced by 25% to 50% in patients taking ER formulation with mild to moderate renal function impairment. Reduce the total daily dose by 25% in patients taking immediate release formulations. The dose be withheld until the dialysis treatment is completed (4 hours) in patients undergoing hemodialysis

Switching patients from immediate-release to extended-release venlafaxine: Patients may be switched to the extended-release form at the nearest equivalent dose (mg/day; eg, venlafaxine 37.5 mg 2 times/day to venlafaxine extended-release 75 mg once daily). However, individual dosage adjustments may be necessary.

Switching patients to or from a monoamine oxidase inhibitor: At least 14 days should elapse between discontinuation of an monoamine oxidase inhibitor (MAOI) and initiation of therapy with venlafaxine. In addition, allow at least 7 days after stopping venlafaxine before starting an MAOI.

Actions

Pharmacology: Venlafaxine and its active metabolite, O-desmethylvenlafaxine, are potent inhibitors of neuronal serotonin and norepinephrine reuptake and weak inhibitors of dopamine reuptake.

Pharmacokinetics:

Absorption/Distribution –

Immediate-release: Venlafaxine is minimally bound to plasma proteins (27%).

Extended-release: Venlafaxine is well absorbed (at least 92%) and extensively metabolized in the liver. O-desmethylvenlafaxin is the only major active metabolite. Venlafaxine extended-release provides a slower rate of absorption but the same extent of absorption compared with the immediate-release tablet.

Administration of venlafaxine extended-release generally resulted in later time to maximum plasma concentration (T_{max}) (5.5 hours) than for immediate-release venlafaxine (T_{max} was 2 hours).

Metabolism/Excretion – Renal elimination of venlafaxine and its metabolites is the primary route of excretion. Venlafaxine undergoes extensive presystemic metabolism in the liver by CYP2D6.

Contraindications

Hypersensitivity to venlafaxine or any ingredients of the product; concomitant use in patients taking MAOIs or in patients who have taken MAOIs within the preceding 14 days.

Warnings/Precautions

Clinical worsening and suicide risk: See Warning box. Patients with MDD, both adults and children, may experience worsening of their depression and/or the emergence of suicidal ideation and behavior (suicidality) or unusual changes in behavior, whether or not they are taking antidepressant medications, and this risk may persist until significant remission occurs.

Closely monitor and observe all patients being treated with antidepressants for any indication for clinical worsening, suicidality, and unusual changes in behavior, especially during the initial few months of a course of drug therapy or at times of dose changes, either increases or decreases.

If the decision has been made to discontinue treatment, taper medication as rapidly as is feasible, but with recognition that abrupt discontinuation can be associated with certain symptoms.

Bipolar disorder: A major depressive episode may be the initial presentation of bipolar disorder. It is generally believed that treating such an episode with an antidepressant alone may increase the likelihood of precipitation of a mixed/manic episode in patients at risk for bipolar disorder. Prior to initiating treatment with an antidepressant, adequately screen patients with depressive symptoms to determine if they are at risk for bipolar disorder.

Monoamine oxidase inhibitors: Because venlafaxine is an inhibitor of norepinephrine and serotonin reuptake, it is recommended that venlafaxine not be used in combination with an MAOI or within 14 days of discontinuing treatment with an MAOI. Allow at least 7 days after stopping venlafaxine before starting an MAOI.

Serotonin syndrome or neuroleptic malignant syndrome-like reactions: The development of a potentially life-threatening serotonin syndrome or neuroleptic malignant syndrome (NMS)-like reactions have been reported with SNRI and SSRIs alone, including venlafaxine treatment, particularly with concomitant use of serotonergic drugs (including triptans) with drugs that impair metabolism of serotonin (including MAOIs), or with antipsychotics or other dopamine antagonists. Serotonin syndrome symptoms may include mental status changes (eg, agitation, hallucinations, coma), autonomic instability (eg, tachycardia, labile blood pressure, hyperthermia), neuromuscular aberrations (eg, hyperreflexia, incoordination), and/or GI symptoms (eg, nausea, vomiting, diarrhea).

Sustained hypertension: Venlafaxine treatment is associated with sustained hypertension (defined as treatment-emergent supine diastolic blood pressure [SDBP] 90 mm Hg or higher and 10 mm Hg or higher above baseline for 3 consecutive on-therapy visits.

Discontinuation of treatment: Abrupt discontinuation or dose reduction of venlafaxine at various doses has been associated with the appearance of new symptoms, the frequency of which increased with increased dose level and with longer duration of treatment. Reported symptoms include agitation, anorexia, anxiety, confusion, impaired coordination and balance, diarrhea, dizziness, dry mouth, dysphoric mood, fasciculation, fatigue, flu-like syndrome, headaches, hypomania, insomnia, nausea, nervousness, nightmares, sensory disturbances (including shock-like electrical sensations), somnolence, sweating, tremor, vertigo, and vomiting. A gradual reduction in the dose rather than abrupt cessation is recommended whenever possible.

Pregnant women during the third trimester: Neonates exposed to serotonin-norepinephrine reuptake inhibitors (SNRIs), or SSRIs late in the third trimester have developed complications requiring prolonged hospitalizations, respiratory support, and tube feeding. When treating pregnant women with venlafaxine during the third trimester, carefully consider the potential risk and benefits of treatment. Consider tapering venlafaxine in the third trimester.

Changes in height (children): In open-label studies, children and adolescents had height increases that were less than expected based on data from age- and sex-matched peers. The difference between observed and expected growth rates was larger for children younger than 12 years of age than for adolescents older than 12 years of age.

CNS effects: Anxiety, nervousness, and insomnia were reported for venlafaxine-treated patients.

Appetite/Weight changes: A dose-dependent weight loss was noted in patients treated for several weeks.

Mania/Hypomania: Activation of mania/hypomania has been reported in a small proportion of patients with major affective disorder who were treated with other marketed antidepressants. As with all antidepressants, use venlafaxine cautiously in patients with a history of mania.

Seizures: Use venlafaxine cautiously in patients with a history of seizures.

Serum cholesterol elevation: Clinically relevant increases in serum cholesterol were recorded in venlafaxine-treated patients in placebo-controlled trials. Consider measurement of serum cholesterol levels during long-term treatment.

Abnormal bleeding: SSRIs and SNRIs, including venlafaxine, may increase the risk of bleeding reactions.

Interstitial lung disease and eosinophilic pneumonia: Interstitial lung disease and eosinophilic pneumonia associated with venlafaxine therapy have been rarely reported.

Cardiac patients: Venlafaxine has not been evaluated in patients with a recent history of myocardial infarction or unstable heart disease.

Electroconvulsive therapy: There are no clinical data establishing the benefit of electroconvulsive therapy combined with venlafaxine treatment.

Renal/Hepatic function impairment: In patients with renal impairment (glomular filtration rate, 10 to 70 mL/min) or cirrhosis of the liver, a lower dose may be necessary.

Pregnancy: Category C.

Lactation: Venlafaxine and O-desmethylvenlafaxin are excreted in breast milk.

Children: Safety and efficacy have not been established.

Monitoring: Monitor all patients for clinical worsening, suicidality, and unusual changes in behavior. Monitor patients for adverse reactions during discontinuation of therapy. Monitor sodium levels periodically during venlafaxine therapy. Consider measurement of serum cholesterol levels during long-term treatment. Monitor blood pressure and heart rate regularly during venlafaxine treatment. Monitor patients with raised intraocular pressure or who are at risk of acute narrow-angle glaucoma (angle-closure glaucoma).

Drug Interactions

QT prolongation: An additive effect of venlafaxine with other drugs that prolong the QT interval cannot be excluded. The following drugs may prolong the QT interval and increase the risk of life-threatening cardiac arrhythmias, including torsades de pointes: antiarrhythmic agents (eg, amiodarone, bretylium, disopyramide, dofetilide, procainamide, quinidine, sotalol), arsenic trioxide, chlorpromazine, cisapride, dolasetron, droperidol, mefloquine, mesoridazine, moxifloxacin, pentamidine, pimozide, tacrolimus, thioridazine, and ziprasidone.

Drugs that may affect venlafaxine include aspirin, NSAIDs, azole antifungals, bupropion, cimetidine, cyproheptadine, fenfluramine, lithium, MAOIs, methylene blue, methylphenidate, nefazodone, opioid analgesics (eg, meperidine), propafenone, rasagiline, sour date nut, terbinafine, and L-tryptophan.

Drugs that may be affected by venlafaxine include bupropion, clozapine, dextromethorphan, fenfluramine, haloperidol, indinavir, lithium, methylphenidate, metoprolol, nefazodone, opioid analgesics (eg, meperidine), propafenone, rasagiline selective serotonin reuptake inhibitors or selective norepinephrine reuptake inhibitors, serotonergic drugs (sibutramine, tramadol, trazodone), St. John's wort, sympathomimetics, TCAs, triptans, L-tryptophan, and warfarin.

Drug/Lab test interactions: Venlafaxine may reduce uptake and diagnostic efficacy of lobenguane. False-negative lobenguane imaging test may result.

Adverse Reactions

Adverse reactions occurring in at least 3% of patients include abdominal pain, abnormal dreams, abnormal ejaculation/orgasm, abnormality of accommodation, abnormal vision, accidental injury, agitation, anorexia, anorgasmia (women), anxiety, asthenia, chills, constipation, decreased libido, depression, diarrhea, dizziness, dry mouth, dyspepsia, flatulence, headache, hypertonia, impotence, increased blood pressure/hypertension, infection, insomnia, nausea, nervousness, palpitation, paresthesia, pharyngitis, somnolence, sweating, tremor, twitching, vasodilation, vomiting, weight loss, yawning.

DESVENLAFAXINE

Tablets, extended-release: 50 and 100 mg (*Rx*)	*Pristiq* (Wyeth)

Warning:

Suicidality and antidepressant drugs: Antidepressants increased the risk compared with placebo of suicidal thinking and behavior (suicidality) in children, adolescents, and young adults in short-term studies of major depressive disorder and other psychiatric disorders. Anyone considering the use of desvenlafaxine or any other antidepressant in a child, adolescent, or young adult must balance this risk with the clinical need. Short-term studies did not show an increase in the risk of suicidality with antidepressants compared with placebo in adults beyond 24 years of age; there was a reduction in risk with antidepressants compared with placebo in adults 65 years of age and older. Depression and certain other psychiatric disorders are associated with increases in the risk of suicide. Monitor patients of all ages who are started on antidepressant therapy appropriately and observe closely for clinical worsening, suicidality, or unusual changes in behavior. Advise families and caregivers of the need for close observation and communication with the prescriber. Desvenlafaxine is not approved for use in children.

Indications

Major depressive disorder: For the treatment of major depressive disorder.

Administration and Dosage

Desvenlafaxine should be taken at approximately the same time each day. Tablets must be swallowed whole with fluid and not divided, crushed, chewed, or dissolved.

Initial treatment: 50 mg once daily, with or without food.

Discontinuation: A gradual reduction in the dose (by giving desvenlafaxine 50 mg less frequently) rather than abrupt cessation is recommended whenever possible. If intolerable symptoms occur following a decrease in the dose or upon discontinuation of treatment, then resuming the previously prescribed dose may be considered. Subsequently, continue decreasing the dose, but at a more gradual rate.

Renal function impairment: The recommended dose in patients with moderate renal function impairment (24-hour CrCl = 30 to 50 mL/min) is 50 mg/day. The recommended dose in patients with severe renal function impairment (24-hour CrCl less than 30 mL/min) or end-stage renal disease (ESRD) is 50 mg every other day. Supplemental doses should not be given to patients after dialysis.

Hepatic function impairment: No adjustment of the starting dosage is necessary for patients with hepatic function impairment. However, dose escalation above 100 mg/day is not recommended.

Pregnancy: When treating pregnant women with desvenlafaxine during the third trimester, carefully consider the potential risks and benefits of treatment. Consider tapering desvenlafaxine in the third trimester.

Switching patients to or from a monoamine oxidase inhibitor (MAOI): At least 14 days must elapse between discontinuation of an MAOI and initiation of therapy with desvenlafaxine. In addition, at least 7 days must be allowed after stopping desvenlafaxine before starting an MAOI.

Actions

Pharmacology: Desvenlafaxine is an extended-release tablet for oral administration that contains desvenlafaxine succinate, a structurally novel SNRI for the treatment of major depressive disorder.

Pharmacokinetics:

Absorption/Distribution – With once-daily dosing, steady-state plasma concentrations are achieved within approximately 4 to 5 days.

The absolute oral bioavailability after oral administration is approximately 80%. Mean time to peak plasma concentrations (T_{max}) is about 7.5 hours after oral administration. The plasma protein binding of desvenlafaxine is low (30%).

Metabolism/Excretion – CYP3A4 is the cytochrome P450 isozyme mediating the oxidative metabolism of desvenlafaxine. Approximately 45% of desvenlafaxine is excreted unchanged in urine at 72 hours after oral administration. The mean terminal half-life is approximately 11 hours.

Contraindications

Hypersensitivity to desvenlafaxine, venlafaxine, or to any excipients in the desvenlafaxine formulation; concomitant use in patients taking MAOIs.

Warnings/Precautions

Clinical worsening and suicide risk: Adults and children with major depressive disorder may experience worsening of their depression and/or the emergence of suicidal ideation and behavior (suicidality) or unusual changes in behavior, whether or not they are taking antidepressant medications.

Screening patients for bipolar disorder: A major depressive episode may be the initial presentation of bipolar disorder. It is generally believed (though not established in controlled studies) that treating such an episode with an antidepressant alone may increase the likelihood of precipitation of a mixed/manic episode in patients at risk for bipolar disorder.

Serotonin syndrome: The development of a potentially life-threatening serotonin syndrome may occur with desvenlafaxine treatment, particularly with concomitant use of other serotonergic drugs (including SSRIs, SNRIs, and triptans) and with drugs that impair metabolism of serotonin (including MAOIs).

Elevated blood pressure: Regularly monitor blood pressure of patients receiving desvenlafaxine because sustained increases in blood pressure were observed in clinical studies.

Abnormal bleeding: SSRIs and SNRIs, including desvenlafaxine, may increase the risk of bleeding events. Concomitant use of aspirin, nonsteroidal anti-inflammatory drugs (NSAIDs), warfarin, and other anticoagulants may add to this risk.

Narrow-angle glaucoma: Mydriasis has been reported in association with desvenlafaxine; therefore, monitor patients with raised intraocular pressure or those at risk of acute narrow-angle glaucoma (angle-closure glaucoma).

Mania/Hypomania activation: During all major depressive disorder and vasomotor symptoms phase 2 and 3 studies, mania was reported for approximately 0.1% of patients treated with desvenlafaxine.

Cardiovascular/Cerebrovascular disease: Caution is advised in administering desvenlafaxine to patients with cardiovascular, cerebrovascular, or lipid metabolism disorders.

Serum cholesterol and triglyceride elevation: Dose-related elevations in fasting serum total cholesterol, low-density lipoprotein (LDL) cholesterol, and triglycerides were observed in the controlled studies. Consider measurement of serum lipids during treatment with desvenlafaxine.

Discontinuation of treatment: A gradual reduction in the dose rather than abrupt cessation is recommended whenever possible.

Seizure: Cases of seizure have been reported in premarketing clinical studies with desvenlafaxine.

Hyponatremia: Hyponatremia may occur as a result of treatment with SSRIs and SNRIs, including desvenlafaxine.

Interstitial lung disease and eosinophilic pneumonia: Interstitial lung disease and eosinophilic pneumonia associated with venlafaxine (the parent drug of desvenlafaxine) therapy have been rarely reported.

Renal function impairment: In patients with moderate or severe renal function impairment or ESRD, the clearance of desvenlafaxine was decreased, thus prolonging the elimination half-life of the drug.

Hepatic function impairment: No adjustment in starting dosage is necessary for patients with hepatic function impairment.

Pregnancy: Category C.

Lactation: Desvenlafaxine (O-desmethylvenlafaxine) is excreted in human milk.

Children: Safety and effectiveness in children have not been established.

Elderly: Of the 3,292 patients in clinical studies with desvenlafaxine, 5% were 65 years of age and older. No overall differences in safety or efficacy were observed between these patients and younger patients; however, in the short-term, placebo-controlled studies, there was a higher incidence of systolic orthostatic hypotension in patients 65 years of age or older compared with patients younger than 65 years of age treated with desvenlafaxine. For elderly patients, consider possible reduced renal clearance of desvenlafaxine when determining dose. If desvenlafaxine is poorly tolerated, every other day dosing can be considered.

SSRIs and SNRIs, including desvenlafaxine, have been associated with cases of clinically significant hyponatremia in elderly patients, who may be at greater risk for this adverse reaction.

Greater sensitivity of some older patients cannot be ruled out.

Monitoring: Measure serum lipids during desvenlafaxine treatment. Appropriately monitor all patients being treated with antidepressants for any indication and observe closely for clinical worsening, suicidality, and unusual changes in behavior, especially during the initial few months of a course of drug therapy, or at times of dose changes, either increases or decreases. Regularly monitor blood pressure. Monitor patients with raised intraocular pressure or those at risk of acute narrow-angle glaucoma (angle-closure glaucoma). Carefully evaluate patients for a history of drug abuse and follow such patients closely, observing them for signs of misuse or abuse of desvenlafaxine (eg, development of tolerance, incrementation of dose, drug-seeking behavior). Monitor patients for the emergence of serotonin-syndrome or NMS-like signs and symptoms.

Monitor patients for symptoms (eg, agitation, anxiety, confusion, headache, hypomania, insomnia, lethargy, seizures) when discontinuing desvenlafaxine treatment.

Drug Interactions

Drugs that may affect desvenlafaxine include CNS acting drugs (eg, alcohol), CYP3A4 inhibitors (eg, ketoconazole), MAOIs, and serotonergic drugs.

Drugs that may be affected by desvenlafaxine include aspirin, CNS acting drugs (eg, alcohol), desipramine, lithium, MAOIs, midazolam, NSAIDs, serotonergic drugs, St. John's wort, tryptophan, and warfarin.

Adverse Reactions

Adverse reactions occurring in at least 3% of patients include abnormal dreams, anxiety, chills, constipation, decreased appetite, diarrhea, dizziness, dry mouth, fasting triglycerides abnormal (fasting: 327 mg/dL or higher), fatigue, feeling jitery, headache, hyperhidrosis, insomnia, mydriasis, nausea, palpitations, paresthesia, proteinuria, somnolence, total cholesterol abnormal (increase of ≥ 50 mg/dL and an absolute value of 261 mg/dL or more), tremor, vision blurred, vomiting, yawning.

Men: Anorgasmia, ejaculation delayed, ejaculation disorder, ejaculation failure, erectile dysfunction, libido decreased, orgasm abnormal, sexual dysfunction.

Women: Anorgasmia.

MILNACIPRAN HYDROCHLORIDE

Tablets; oral: 12.5, 25, 50, and 100 mg (*Rx*) *Savella* (Forest)

Warning:

Suicidality and antidepressant drugs: Milnacipran is a selective serotonin and norepinephrine reuptake inhibitor (SNRI), similar to some drugs used for the treatment of depression and other psychiatric disorders. Antidepressants increased the risk, compared with placebo, of suicidal thinking and behavior (suicidality) in children, adolescents, and young adults in short-term studies of major depressive disorder (MDD) and other psychiatric disorders. Anyone considering the use of such drugs in a child, adolescent, or young adult must balance this risk with the clinical need. Short-term studies did not show an increase in the risk of suicidality with antidepressants compared with placebo in adults older than 24 years of age; there was a reduction in risk with antidepressants compared with placebo in adults 65 years of age and older. Depression and certain other psychiatric disorders are themselves associated with increases in the risk of suicide. Appropriately monitor patients of all ages who are started on milnacipran and observe closely for clinical worsening, suicidality, or unusual changes in behavior. Advise families and caregivers of the need for close observation and communication with the prescriber. Milnacipran is not approved for use in the treatment of MDD. Milnacipran is not approved for use in children.

Indications

Fibromyalgia: For the management of fibromyalgia.

Administration and Dosage

Adults: Administer 50 mg twice daily: 12.5 mg once on day 1, 12.5 mg twice daily on days 2 and 3, 25 mg twice daily on days 4 to 7, and 50 mg twice daily after day 7.

May increase to 100 mg twice daily (maximum doses) based on individual response.

Milnacipran is given orally with or without food.

Taking milnacipran with food may improve the tolerability of the drug.

Concomitant therapy – At least 14 days should elapse between discontinuation of a monoamine oxidase inhibitor (MAOI) and initiation of therapy with milnacipran. In addition, at least 5 days should be allowed after stopping milnacipran before starting a MAOI.

Discontinuation of therapy – Milnacipran should be tapered and not abruptly discontinued after extended use.

Renal function impairment – Milnacipran should be used with caution in patients with moderate renal impairment. For patients with severe renal impairment (indicated by an estimated creatinine clearance [CrCl] of 5 to 29 mL/min), the maintenance dosage should be reduced by 50% to 25 mg twice daily. Milnacipran is not recommended for patients with end-stage renal disease.

Actions

Pharmacology: Preclinical studies have shown that milnacipran is a potent inhibitor of neuronal norepinephrine and serotonin reuptake.

Pharmacokinetics:

Absorption/Distribution – Milnacipran is absorbed following oral administration with maximum concentrations (C_{max}) reached within 2 to 4 hours postdose. The absolute bioavailability is approximately 85% to 90%. Steady-state levels are reached within 36 to 48 hours. Plasma protein binding is 13%.

Metabolism/Excretion – Milnacipran and its metabolites are eliminated primarily by renal excretion. Milnacipran has a terminal elimination half-life of about 6 to 8 hours.

Contraindications

Concomitant use in patients taking MAOIs or within 14 days of discontinuing treatment with an MAOI, and with uncontrolled narrow-angle glaucoma.

Warnings/Precautions

Suicide risk: Refer to the Black Box Warning.

Serotonin syndrome or neuroleptic malignant syndrome-like reactions: The development of a potentially life-threatening serotonin syndrome may occur with agents that inhibit serotonin reuptake, including milnacipran, particularly with concomitant use of serotonergic drugs (including triptans) and drugs that impair metabolism of serotonin (including MAOIs) or with antipsychotic or other dopamine antagonists.

Cardiovascular effects:

Blood pressure – SNRIs, including milnacipran, have been associated with reports of increase in blood pressure.

Heart rate – SNRIs have been associated with reports of increase in heart rate.

Seizures: Seizures have been reported infrequently in patients treated with milnacipran for disorders other than fibromyalgia. Prescribe milnacipran with care in patients with a history of a seizure disorder.

Hepatotoxicity: In the placebo-controlled fibromyalgia trials, increases in the number of patients treated with milnacipran with mild elevations of ALT or AST (1 to 3 times the upper limit of normal [ULN]) were observed.

Discontinue milnacipran in patients who develop jaundice or other evidence of liver dysfunction. Do not resume treatment with milnacipran unless another cause can be established.

Ordinarily, do not prescribe milnacipran to patients with substantial alcohol use or evidence of chronic liver disease.

Discontinuation of treatment: Withdrawal symptoms have been observed in clinical trials following discontinuation of milnacipran, as with other SNRIs and SSRIs.

The adverse reactions included agitation, anxiety, confusion, dizziness, dysphoric mood, emotional lability, headache, hypomania, insomnia, irritability, lethargy, sensory disturbances (eg, paresthesias such as electric shock sensations), seizures, and tinnitus.

Hyponatremia: Hyponatremia may occur as a result of treatment with SSRIs and SNRIs, including milnacipran. In many cases, this hyponatremia appears to be the result of the syndrome of inappropriate antidiuretic hormone secretion (SIADH).

Abnormal bleeding: SSRIs and SNRIs, including milnacipran, may increase the risk of bleeding events. Concomitant use of aspirin, nonsteroidal anti-inflammatory drugs (NSAIDs), warfarin, and other anticoagulants may add to this risk.

Activation of mania: Use milnacipran cautiously in patients with a history of mania.

GU effects: Because of their noradrenergic effect, SNRIs, including milnacipran, can affect urethral resistance and micturition.

Glaucoma: Mydriasis has been reported in association with SNRIs and milnacipran; therefore, use milnacipran cautiously in patients with controlled narrow-angle glaucoma.

Drug abuse and dependence: Milnacipran produces physical dependence, as evidenced by the emergence of withdrawal symptoms following drug discontinuation, similar to other SNRIs and SSRIs. These withdrawal symptoms can be severe; thus, taper milnacipran and do not abruptly discontinue after extended use.

Hazardous tasks: Caution patients about operating machinery or driving motor vehicles until they are reasonably certain that milnacipran treatment does not affect their ability to engage in such activities.

Pregnancy: Category C.

Lactation: Because the safety of milnacipran in infants is not known, breast-feeding while on milnacipran is not recommended.

Children: Safety and effectiveness of milnacipran in children younger than 17 years of age with fibromyalgia have not been established. The use of milnacipran is not recommended in children.

Elderly: Consider renal function prior to use of milnacipran in elderly patients.

SNRIs, SSRIs, and milnacipran have been associated with cases of clinically significant hyponatremia in elderly patients, who may be at greater risk for this adverse reaction.

Monitoring: Measure heart rate and blood pressure prior to initiating treatment and periodically measure throughout milnacipran treatment. Monitor patients for withdrawal symptoms when discontinuing treatment with milnacipran. Advise family and caregivers to monitor patients for the emergence of agitation, irritability, unusual changes in behavior, and the other symptoms, as well as the emergence of suicidality, and to report such symptoms immediately.

Monitor patients for the emergence of serotonin syndrome or NMS-like signs and symptoms.

Drug Interactions

Drugs that may affect milnacipran include alcohol, antipsychotic agents (eg, risperidone), clomipramine, CNS drugs, cyclobenzaprine, dopamine antagonists (eg, metaclopramide), lithium, MAOIs, L-tryptophan, methylene blue, and serotonergic drugs.

Drugs that may be affected by milnacipran include clonidine, CNS drugs, cyclobenzaprine, digoxin, drugs that interfere with hemostasis, epinephrine, MAOIs (eg, phenelzine, rasagiline), norepinephrine, and serotonergic drugs.

Adverse Reactions

Adverse reactions occurring in at least 3% of patients include the following: abdominal pain, anxiety, chest discomfort, chest pain, chills, constipation, decreased appetite, dizziness, dry mouth, dyspnea, flushing, headache, hot flush, hyperhidrosis, hypertension, hypesthesia, increased blood pressure and heart rate, insomnia, migraine, nausea, palpitations, paresthesia, pruritus, rash, tachycardia, tension headache, tremor, upper respiratory tract infection, vision blurred, vomiting.

SELECTIVE SEROTONIN REUPTAKE INHIBITORS

CITALOPRAM HBr	
Tablets; oral: 10, 20, 40 mg (as base) (*Rx*)	Various, *Celexa* (Forest)
Solution; oral: 10 mg (as base) per 5 mL (*Rx*)	
ESCITALOPRAM OXALATE	
Tablets; oral: 5, 10, 20 mg (as base) (*Rx*)	*Lexapro* (Forest)
Solution; oral: 5 mg (as base) per 5 mL (*Rx*)	
FLUOXETINE HYDROCHLORIDE	
Tablets; oral: 10, 15, and 20 mg (as base) (*Rx*)	Various, *Sarafem* (Warner Chilcott)
Capsules; oral: 10, 20, and 40 mg (as base) (*Rx*)	Various, *Prozac Pulvules* (Eli Lilly/Dista), *Sarafem Pulvules* (Warner Chilcott), *Selfemra* (Teva)
Capsules, delayed-release; oral: 90 mg (as base) (*Rx*)	*Prozac Weekly* (Eli Lilly/Dista)
Solution; oral: 20 mg (as base) per 5 mL (*Rx*)	Various, *Prozac* (Eli Lilly/Dista)
FLUVOXAMINE MALEATE	
Tablets; oral: 25, 50, and 100 mg (*Rx*)	Various, *Luvox* (Jazz Pharmaceuticals)
Capsules, extended-release; oral: 100 and 150 mg (*Rx*)	*Luvox CR* (Jazz Pharmaceuticals)
PAROXETINE	
Tablets; oral: 10, 20, 30, and 40 mg (as hydrochloride) (*Rx*)	Various, *Paxil* (Apotex)
10, 20, 30, and 40 mg (as mesylate) (*Rx*)	*Pexeva* (Synthon)
Tablets, controlled-release; oral: 12.5, 25, and 37.5 mg (as hydrochloride) (*Rx*)	Various, *Paxil CR* (Apotex)
Suspension; oral: 10 mg (as hydrochloride) per 5 mL (*Rx*)	Various, *Paxil* (Apotex)

SERTRALINE HYDROCHLORIDE

Tablets; oral: 25, 50, and 100 mg (as base) (*Rx*)	Various, *Zoloft* (Pfizer)
Solution, concentrate; oral: 20 mg (as base)/mL (*Rx*)	

Warning:

Suicidality in children and adolescents:

Suicidality and antidepressant drugs – Antidepressants increased the risk compared with placebo of suicidal thinking and behavior (suicidality) in children, adolescents, and young adults in short-term studies of major depressive disorder (MDD) and other psychiatric disorders. Anyone considering the use of escitalopram or any other antidepressant in a child, adolescent, or young adult must balance this risk with the clinical need. Short-term studies did not show an increase in the risk of suicidality with antidepressants compared with placebo in adults beyond 24 years of age; there was a reduction in risk with antidepressants compared with placebo in adults 65 years of age and older. Depression and certain other psychiatric disorders are themselves associated with increases in the risk of suicide. Appropriately monitor patients of all ages who are started on antidepressant therapy and closely observe for clinical worsening, suicidality, or unusual changes in behavior. Advise families and caregivers of the need for close observation and communication with the prescriber.

Citalopram, **escitalopram**, and **paroxetine** are not approved for use in children. **Fluoxetine** is approved for use in children with MDD and obsessive-compulsive disorder (OCD). **Sertraline** is not approved for use in children except for patients with OCD. **Fluvoxamine** is not approved for use in children except for patients with OCD.

Pooled analyses of short-term (4 to 16 weeks), placebo-controlled trials of 9 antidepressant drugs (SSRIs and others) in children and adolescents with MDD, OCD, or other psychiatric disorders (a total of 24 trials involving over 4,400 patients) have revealed a greater risk of adverse reactions representing suicidal thinking or behavior (suicidality) during the first few months of treatment in those receiving antidepressants. The average risk of such reactions in patients receiving antidepressants was 4%, twice the placebo risk of 2%. No suicides occurred in these trials.

Indications

Bulimia nervosa: Fluoxetine.

Depression: Citalopram, escitalopram, fluoxetine, paroxetine (immediate- and controlled-release), sertraline.

Depressive episodes associated with bipolar I disorder: Fluoxetine and olanzapine in combination.

OCD: Fluoxetine, fluvoxamine (immediate- and extended-release), paroxetine (immediate-release), sertraline.

Panic disorder: Paroxetine (immediate- and controlled-release), sertraline, fluoxetine.

Posttraumatic stress disorder (PTSD): Paroxetine (immediate-release; except *Pexeva*), sertraline.

Premenstrual dysphoric disorder (PMDD): Fluoxetine (*Sarafem* only), paroxetine (controlled-release), sertraline.

Social anxiety disorder/generalized anxiety disorder (GAD): Paroxetine (immediate-release; except *Pexeva*), sertraline, escitalopram.

Treatment-resistant depression: Fluoxetine and olanzapine.

Administration and Dosage

Pregnancy: Neonates exposed to selective serotonin reuptake inhibitors (SSRIs) or serotonin and norepinephrine reuptake inhibitors (SNRIs) late in the third trimester have developed complications requiring prolonged hospitalization, respiratory support, and tube feeding. When treating pregnant women with SSRIs during the third trimester, carefully consider the potential risks and benefits of treatment. Consider tapering SSRIs in the third trimester.

Discontinuation of treatment: Symptoms associated with discontinuation of SSRIs and SNRIs have been reported. Monitor patients for these symptoms when discontinuing treatment. A gradual reduction in the dose rather than abrupt cessation is recommended whenever possible.

Switching patients to or from a monoamine oxidase inhibitor (MAOI): Allow at least 14 days to elapse between discontinuation of an MAOI and initiation of SSRI therapy. Similarly, allow at least 14 days (at least 5 weeks for **fluoxetine**) after stopping an SSRI before starting an MAOI.

CITALOPRAM HBr:

Warnings – See Warning Box at the beginning of the monograph.

Initial therapy – 20 mg once/day in the morning or evening with or without food. Dose increases usually should occur in increments of 20 mg at intervals of no less than 1 week. Doses greater than 40 mg/day are not recommended.

Elderly/Hepatic function impairment – 20 mg/day is the recommended dose for most elderly patients and patients with hepatic function impairment, with titration to 40 mg/day only for nonresponding patients.

Renal function impairment – Use with caution in patients with severe renal function impairment.

ESCITALOPRAM OXALATE:

Warnings – See Warning Box at the beginning of the monograph.

Administer once daily in the morning or evening, with or without food. Dose increases should occur after a minimum of 1 week.

GAD –

Initial therapy: 10 mg once daily. Dose may be increased to 20 mg/day after a minimum of 1 week.

MDD –

Initial therapy:

Adults and children 12 to 17 years of age – 10 mg once daily. Dose may be increased to 20 mg/day after a minimum of 1 week. Maximum dose is 20 mg once daily.

Elderly/Hepatic function impairment – 10 mg/day is the recommended dose for most elderly patients and patients with hepatic function impairment.

Renal function impairment – Use with caution in patients with severe renal function impairment.

FLUOXETINE HYDROCHLORIDE:

Warnings – See Warning Box at the beginning of the monograph.

Consider a dose increase after several weeks if no clinical improvement is observed. Administer doses greater than 20 mg/day on a once (morning) or twice (eg, morning and noon) daily schedule. Do not exceed a maximum dose of 80 mg/day.

Depression –

Initial:

Adults – 20 mg/day in the morning.

Children (8 to up to 18 years of age) – Initiate treatment with a dose of 10 or 20 mg/day. After 1 week at 10 mg/day, increase the dose to 20 mg/day. However, because of higher plasma levels in lower weight children, the starting and target dose in this group may be 10 mg/day. A dose increase to 20 mg/day may be considered after several weeks if insufficient clinical improvement is observed.

Weekly dosing: Initiate *Prozac Weekly* 7 days after the last 20 mg/day dose. If satisfactory response is not maintained, consider re-establishing a daily dosing regimen.

OCD –

Initial:

Adults – 20 mg/day in the morning. A dose range of 20 to 60 mg/day is recommended; however, doses of up to 80 mg/day have been well tolerated.

Children (7 to 18 years of age) – In adolescents and higher weight children, initiate treatment with a dose of 10 mg/day. After 2 weeks, increase the dose to 20 mg/day. A dose range of 20 to 60 mg/day is recommended.

In lower weight children, initiate treatment with a dose of 10 mg/day. Additional dose increases may be considered after several more weeks if insufficient clinical improvement is observed. A dose range of 20 to 30 mg/day is recommended. Experience with daily doses greater than 20 mg is very minimal; there is no experience with doses greater than 60 mg.

Bulimia nervosa –

Initial: 60 mg/day administered in the morning. It may be advisable to titrate up to this target dose over several days.

Panic disorder –

Initial: 10 mg/day. After 1 week, increase the dose to 20 mg/day. **Fluoxetine** doses above 60 mg/day have not been evaluated.

PMDD (Sarafem) –

Initial: 20 mg/day given continuously (every day of the menstrual cycle) or intermittently (defined as starting a daily dose 14 days prior to the anticipated onset of menstruation through the first full day of menses and repeating with each new cycle).

Depressive episodes associated with bipolar I disorder (in combination with olanzapine) – Once daily in the evening without regard to meals, generally beginning with oral olanzapine 5 mg and fluoxetine 20 mg. Dosage adjustments, if indicated, can be made according to efficacy and tolerability within dose ranges of fluoxetine 20 to 50 mg and oral olanzapine 5 to 12.5 mg.

Treatment-resistant depression (in combination with olanzapine) – Once daily in the evening without regard to meals, generally beginning with oral olanzapine 5 mg and fluoxetine 20 mg. Dosage adjustments, if indicated, can be made according to efficacy and tolerability within dose ranges of fluoxetine 20 to 50 mg and oral olanzapine 5 to 20 mg.

Hepatic function impairment – Use a lower or less frequent dosage.

Special risk patients – Consider a lower or less frequent dosage for patients, such as the elderly, with concurrent disease or on multiple medications.

Switching patients to a tricyclic antidepressant (TCA) – Dosage of TCA may need to be reduced, and plasma TCA concentrations may need to be monitored temporarily when fluoxetine is coadministered or has been recently discontinued.

Thioridazine – Do not administer thioridazine with fluoxetine or within a minimum of 5 weeks after fluoxetine has been discontinued.

FLUVOXAMINE MALEATE:

Warnings – See Warning Box at the beginning of the monograph.

Tablets –

Initial therapy: 50 mg as a single bedtime dose. Increase dose in 50 mg increments every 4 to 7 days, as tolerated, until maximum therapeutic benefit is achieved, not to exceed 300 mg/day. It is advisable to give total daily doses greater than 100 mg in 2 divided doses; if doses are unequal, give larger dose at bedtime.

Pediatric therapy (8 to 17 years of age): 25 mg as a single daily dose at bedtime. The maximum dose in children up to 11 years of age should not exceed 200 mg/day. Increase the dose in 25 mg increments every 4 to 7 days as tolerated until maximum therapeutic benefit is achieved (not to exceed 300 mg/day). Divide total daily doses greater than 50 mg into 2 doses. If the doses are not equal, give the larger dose at bedtime.

Extended-release capsules – The recommended starting dose in adults is 100 mg once per day. The dose should be increased in 50 mg increments every week, as tolerated, until maximum therapeutic benefit is achieved, not to exceed 300 mg/day. Fluvoxamine extended-release capsules should be administered with or without food as a single daily dose at bedtime. Capsules should not be crushed or chewed.

Elderly/Hepatic function impairment – These patients have been observed to have decreased fluvoxamine clearance. It may be appropriate to modify initial dose and subsequent titration.

PAROXETINE:

Warnings – See Warning Box at the beginning of the monograph.

May be taken with or without food. Swallow controlled-release tablets whole; do not chew or crush. Administer as a single daily dose, usually in the morning. Dose changes should occur at intervals of at least 1 week.

Depression –

Initial dose:

Immediate-release – 20 mg/day. Usual range is 20 to 50 mg/day, up to a maximum of 50 mg/day.

Controlled-release – 25 mg/day. Administer as a single daily dose with or without food, usually in the morning. Usual range is 25 to 62.5 mg/day, up to a maximum of 62.5 mg/day.

OCD (immediate-release) –

Initial: 40 mg/day. Start on 20 mg/day and increase dose in 10 mg/day increments. Usual range is 20 to 60 mg/day. Maximum dose should not exceed 60 mg/day.

Panic disorder –

Initial:

Immediate-release – 10 mg/day; the recommended target dose is 40 mg/day. Dose changes should occur in 10 mg/day increments. Usual range is 10 to 60 mg/day. The maximum dosage should not exceed 60 mg/day.

Controlled-release – 12.5 mg/day. Dose changes occur in 12.5 mg/day increments. Usual range is 12.5 to 75 mg/day. Do not exceed the maximum dosage of 75 mg/day.

Social anxiety disorder –

Immediate-release: 20 mg/day. Usual range is 20 to 60 mg/day.

Controlled-release: 12.5 mg/day. Usual range is 12.5 to 37.5 mg/day, up to a maximum of 37.5 mg/day.

GAD (immediate-release) –

Initial: 20 mg/day. Usual range is 20 to 50 mg/day. Dose changes should occur in 10 mg/day increments.

PTSD (immediate-release) –

Initial: 20 mg/day. Usual range is 20 to 50 mg/day. Dose changes should occur in 10 mg/day increments.

PMDD (controlled-release) –

Initial: 12.5 mg/day. Paroxetine CR may be administered either daily throughout the menstrual cycle or limited to the luteal phase of the menstrual cycle.

Elderly or debilitated or patients with severe renal or hepatic function impairment – The recommended initial dose is 10 mg/day (immediate-release) or 12.5 mg/day (controlled-release). Increases may be made if indicated. Do not exceed 40 mg/day (immediate-release) or 50 mg/day (controlled-release).

Administration of suspension – Shake suspension well before using.

Discontinuation of treatment – Symptoms associated with discontinuation of paroxetine have been reported. There have been spontaneous reports of adverse reactions upon the discontinuation of paroxetine (particularly when abrupt), including the following: dizziness, sensory disturbances (eg, paresthesias, such as electric shock sensations), agitation, anxiety, nausea, and sweating. These reactions are generally self-limiting. A gradual reduction in the dose rather than abrupt cessation is recommended whenever possible.

SERTRALINE HYDROCHLORIDE:

Warnings – See Warning Box at the beginning of the monograph.

Adults –

Initial treatment:

Depression and OCD – 50 mg once/day.

Panic disorder, social anxiety disorder, and PTSD – 25 mg once/day. After 1 week, increase the dose to 50 mg once/day.

Usual range of 50 to 200 mg/day. Dose changes should not occur at intervals of less than 1 week.

PMDD – 50 mg/day, either daily throughout the menstrual cycle or limited to the luteal phase of the menstrual cycle.

Patients not responding to 50 mg/day may benefit from dose increases (at 50 mg increments/menstrual cycle) up to 150 mg/day when dosing daily throughout the menstrual cycle, or 100 mg/day when dosing during the luteal phase of the menstrual cycle. If a 100 mg/day dose has been established with luteal phase dosing, utilize a 50 mg/day titration step for 3 days at the beginning of each luteal phase dosing period.

Children –

OCD: 25 mg once/day for children (6 to 12 years of age) and 50 mg once/day in adolescents (13 to 17 years of age) in the morning or evening. Patients not responding to an initial dose of 25 or 50 mg/day may benefit from dose increases up to a maximum of 200 mg/day. For children, take into account the generally lower body weights when increasing the dose to avoid excess dosing. Dose changes should not occur at intervals of less than 1 week.

Hepatic function impairment – Give a lower or less-frequent dosage in patients with hepatic function impairment. Use with caution in these patients.

Oral concentrate – Dilute prior to use with 4 oz (½ cup) of water, ginger ale, lemon/lime soda, lemonade, or orange juice only. Administer the dose immediately after mixing; do not mix in advance.

Actions

Pharmacology: These agents are potent and selective inhibitors of neuronal serotonin reuptake, and they also have a weak effect on norepinephrine and dopamine neuronal reuptake.

Pharmacokinetics:

SSRI Pharmacokinetics

SSRIs	Time to peak plasma concentration (h)	Half-life (h)	Protein binding (%)	Time to reach steady state (days)	Primary route of elimination	Bioavailability (%)
Citalopram	≈ 4	≈ 35	≈ 80	≈ 7	20% renal, fecal	≈ 80
Escitalopram	5	27 to 32	≈ 56	≈ 7	7% renal	80[a]
Fluoxetine	6 to 8	24 to 384[b]	≈ 94.5	≈ 28	hepatic	nd[c]
Fluvoxamine	3 to 8	13.6 to 15.6	≈ 80	≈ 7	≈ 94% renal	53
Paroxetine	5.2	21	≈ 93 to 95	≈10	64% renal, 36% fecal	100
Paroxetine CR	6 to 10	15 to 20		14		
Sertraline	4.5 to 8.4	26 to 104[b]	98	≈ 7	40% to 45% renal, 40% to 45% fecal	nd

[a] Based on citalopram data.
[b] t½ includes the active metabolite.
[c] nd = No data.

Contraindications

Hypersensitivity to SSRIs; in combination with an MAOI, or within 14 days of discontinuing an MAOI; administration of **thioridazine** with **fluoxetine** or within a minimum of 5 weeks after **fluoxetine** has been discontinued; coadministration of **fluvoxamine** with **cisapride, thioridazine,** or **pimozide**; concomitant use of **thioridazine** with **paroxetine**; concomitant use of **pimozide** with **sertraline**; coadministration of **sertraline** oral concentrate and **disulfiram**.

Warnings/Precautions

Long-term use: The effectiveness of long-term use of SSRIs for OCD, panic disorder, and bulimia has not been systematically evaluated. However, the long-term use of SSRIs for depression has been evaluated and demonstrated to maintain antidepressant response for up to 1 year.

MAOIs: It is recommended that SSRIs not be used in combination with an MAOI or within 14 days of discontinuing treatment with an MAOI. Allow at least 2 weeks after stopping the SSRIs before starting an MAOI.

Platelet function: Altered platelet function or abnormal results from laboratory studies have occurred in patients taking **fluoxetine**, **paroxetine**, or **sertraline**.

Suicide risk: The possibility of a suicide attempt is inherent in depression. Patients with major depressive disorder, both adult and pediatric, may experience worsening of their depression and/or the emergence of suicidal ideation and behavior (suicidality), whether or not they are taking antidepressant medications, and this risk may persist until significant remission occurs.

Rash and accompanying events: Seven percent of patients taking **fluoxetine** have developed a rash or urticaria. Several other patients have had systemic syndromes suggestive of serum sickness.

Systemic events, possibly related to vasculitis, have developed in patients with rash. Although rare, these reactions may be serious, involving lung, kidney, or liver. Death has been associated with these reactions.

Anxiety, nervousness, and insomnia: Anxiety, nervousness, and insomnia occurred in 2% to 22% of patients treated with an SSRI.

Altered appetite and weight: Significant weight loss, especially in underweight depressed patients, has occurred. Approximately 3% to 17% of patients treated with an SSRI experienced anorexia during initial therapy.

Abnormal bleeding: Altered platelet function and/or abnormal results from laboratory studies in patients taking **fluoxetine**, **paroxetine**, or **sertraline** have occurred. There have been reports of abnormal bleeding or purpura in several patients; it is unclear whether the SSRIs had a causative role.

Mania/Hypomania: Activation of mania/hypomania occurred infrequently in about 0.1% to 2.2% of patients taking SSRIs. Use cautiously in patients with a history of mania.

Seizures: Seizures have occurred with **citalopram** (0.3%), **fluvoxamine** (0.2%), **sertraline** (0.2%), **fluoxetine** (0.1%), and**paroxetine** (0.1%). Use with care in patients with history of seizures.

Concomitant illness: Use caution in patients with diseases or conditions that could affect metabolism or hemodynamic responses.

Cardiac effects: SSRIs have not been systematically evaluated in patients with a recent history of myocardial infarction or unstable heart disease. The ECGs of patients who received SSRIs in clinical trials were evaluated and the data indicate that they are not associated with the development of clinically significant ECG abnormalities.

Fluoxetine dose changes: The long elimination half-life of **fluoxetine** and **norfluoxetine** means that changes in dose will not be fully reflected in plasma for several weeks, affecting titration to final dose and withdrawal from treatment.

Glaucoma: A few cases of acute angle-closure glaucoma associated with **paroxetine** therapy have been reported in the literature. Use caution when SSRIs are prescribed for patients with narrow-angle glaucoma.

Effects of smoking: Smokers had a 25% increase in the metabolism of **fluvoxamine** compared with nonsmokers.

Electroconvulsive therapy (ECT): There are no clinical studies establishing the benefit of the combined use of ECT and SSRIs. Rare prolonged seizure in patients on **fluoxetine** has occurred.

Hyponatremia: Several cases of SSRI-induced hyponatremia (some with serum sodium less than 110 mmol/L) have occurred.

Diabetes: **Fluoxetine** may alter glycemic control. The dosage of insulin or the sulfonylurea may need to be adjusted when fluoxetine is started or discontinued.

Uricosuric effect: **Sertraline** is associated with a mean decrease in serum uric acid of about 7%. The clinical significance of this weak uricosuric effect is unknown.

Discontinuation of SSRIs: During marketing of SSRIs and SNRIs, there have been spontaneous reports of adverse reactions occurring upon discontinuation of these drugs, particularly when abrupt, including the following: agitation, anxiety, confusion, dizziness, dysphoric mood, emotional lability, headache, hypomania, insomnia, irritability, lethargy, and sensory disturbances (eg, paresthesias such as electric shock sensations). While these reactions are generally self-limiting, there have been reports of serious discontinuation symptoms.

Renal function impairment: No dose adjustment of **citalopram, fluoxetine,** or **fluvoxamine** in patients with renal function impairment is routinely necessary.

Reduce the initial dosage of **paroxetine** in patients with severe renal function impairment.

Use **sertraline** and **escitalopram** with caution in patients with severe renal function impairment.

Hepatic function impairment: SSRIs are metabolized extensively by the liver. Use with caution in patients with severe liver function impairment.

In subjects with hepatic function impairment, clearance of racemic citalopram was decreased and plasma concentrations were increased. The recommended dose of **escitalopram** in patients with hepatic function impairment is 10 mg/day.

Drug abuse and dependence: Before starting an SSRI, carefully evaluate patients for history of drug abuse and follow such patients closely, observing them for signs of misuse or abuse.

Hazardous tasks: SSRIs may cause dizziness or drowsiness. Instruct patients to observe caution while driving or performing tasks requiring alertness, coordination, or physical dexterity.

Photosensitivity: Photosensitization may occur.

Pregnancy: Category C.

Lactation: **Escitalopram, fluoxetine, fluvoxamine, citalopram,** and **paroxetine** are excreted in breast milk. It is not known whether **sertraline** or its metabolites are excreted in breast milk.

Children: Safety and efficacy in children (younger than 18 years of age) have not been established.

The efficacy of **sertraline** for the treatment of OCD was demonstrated in a 12-week, multicenter, placebo-controlled study with 187 outpatients 6 to 17 years of age.

The efficacy of **fluvoxamine** for the treatment of OCD was demonstrated in a 10-week, multicenter, placebo-controlled study with 120 outpatients 8 to 17 years of age.

Elderly: Clearance of **fluvoxamine** is decreased by about 50% in elderly patients. A lower starting dose of **paroxetine** is recommended. **Sertraline** plasma clearance may be lower. In 2 pharmacokinetic studies, **citalopram** AUC was increased by 23% and 30%, respectively, in elderly subjects as compared with younger subjects, and its half-life was increased by 30% and 50%, respectively. In 2 pharmacokinetic studies, **escitalopram** half-life was increased by approximately 50% in elderly subjects as compared with young subjects, and C_{max} was unchanged.

Drug Interactions

Drugs highly bound to plasma protein: Because SSRIs are highly bound to plasma protein, administration to a patient taking another drug that is highly protein-bound may cause increased free concentrations of the other drug, potentially resulting in adverse reactions. Conversely, adverse reactions could result from displacement of SSRIs by other highly bound drugs.

CYP-450 system: Concomitant use of SSRIs with drugs metabolized by CYP-450 2D6 may require lower doses than usually prescribed for either **paroxetine** or the other drug because paroxetine may significantly inhibit the activity of this isozyme.

Hepatic metabolism of **citalopram** and **escitalopram** occurs primarily through CYP-450 3A4 and 2C19 isoenzymes. Inhibitors of 3A4 (eg, azole antifungals, macrolide antibiotics) and 2C19 (eg, **omeprazole**) would be expected to increase plasma **citalopram** levels. Inducters of 3A4 (eg, **carbamazepine**) would be expected to decrease **citalopram** and **escitalopram** levels.

Serotonin syndrome: The serotonin syndrome is a rare complication of therapy with serotonergic drugs. When this problem occurs with SSRIs, it is most commonly in the setting of other concurrent medications that increase serotonin by different mechanisms.

Drugs that may affect SSRIs: Drugs that may affect SSRIs include azole antifungals, barbiturates, carbamazepine, cimetidine, cyproheptadine, lithium, macrolides, MAOIs, metoclopramide, phenytoin, sibutramine, smoking, St. John's wort, tramadol, linezolid, L-tryptophan.

Drugs that may be affected by SSRIs: Drugs that may be affected by SSRIs include alcohol, benzodiazepines, beta blockers, buspirone, carbamazepine, cisapride, clozapine, cyclosporine, digoxin, diltiazem, haloperidol, hydantoins, lithium, methadone, mexiletine, nonsedating antihistamines, NSAIDs, olanzapine, phenothiazines, phenytoin, pimozide, procyclidine, ritonavir, ropivacaine, sumatriptan, sulfonylureas, sympathomimetics, tacrine, theophylline, tolbutamide, tricyclic antidepressants, and warfarin.

Drug/Food interactions: In one study following a single dose of **sertraline** with and without food, sertraline AUC was slightly increased and C_{max} was 25% greater. Time to reach peak plasma level decreased from 8 hours post-dosing to 5.5 hours.

Food does not appear to affect systemic bioavailability of **fluoxetine**, although it may delay absorption. **Fluvoxamine** and **citalopram** bioavailability is not affected by food. Thus, **fluoxetine**, **fluvoxamine**, and **citalopram** may be given with or without food.

Adverse Reactions

Adverse reactions occurring in at least 3% of patients include the following: abnormal dreams/thinking, abnormal ejaculation, abdominal pain, accidental injury/trauma, agitation, anorexia, anxiety, asthenia, back pain, concentration decreased/impaired, constipation, decreased appetite, diarrhea/loose stools, dizziness, dry mouth, dyspepsia, fatigue, fever, flatulence, flu syndrome, headache, increased appetite, insomnia, libido decreased, male/female genital disorders, myalgia, nausea, nervousness, pain, paresthesia, pharyngitis, rash, respiratory disorder, rhinitis, sexual dysfunction/impotence/anorgasmia, sinusitis, somnolence, sweating increased, tremor, vasodilation, vision disturbances/blurred vision/abnormal vision, vomiting, upper respiratory tract infection, yawning.

MONOAMINE OXIDASE INHIBITORS

ISOCARBOXAZID	
Tablets: 10 mg (*Rx*)	*Marplan* (Validus)
PHENELZINE	
Tablets: 15 mg (as base) (*Rx*)	*Nardil* (Parke-Davis)
TRANYLCYPROMINE	
Tablets: 10 mg (as sulfate) (*Rx*)	Various, *Parnate* (GlaxoSmithKline)

Warning:

Suicidality in children and adolescents: Antidepressants increased the risk of suicidal thinking and behavior (suicidality) in short-term studies in children, adolescents, and young adults with Major Depressive Disorder (MDD) and other psychiatric disorders. Anyone considering the use of phenelzine, tranylcypromine, or any other antidepressant in a child or adolescent must balance this risk with the clinical need. Closely observe patients who are started on therapy for clinical worsening, suicidality, or unusual changes in behavior. Advise families and caregivers of the need for close observation and communication with the prescriber. Neither phenelzine nor tranylcypromine are approved for use in pediatric patients. Safety and efficacy in the pediatric population have not been established.

Short-term studies did not show an increase in the risk of suicidality with antidepressants compared with placebo in adults older than 24 years of age; there was a reduction in risk with antidepressants compared with placebo in adults 65 years of age and older. Depression and certain other psychiatric disorders are associated with increases in the risk of suicide. Closely observe and appropriately monitor patients of all ages who are started on antidepressant therapy for clinical worsening, suicidality, or unusual changes in behavior. Advise families and caregivers of the need for close observation and communication with the health care provider. Tranylcypromine is not approved for use in children.

Pooled analyses of short-term (4 to 16 weeks) placebo-controlled trials of 9 antidepressant drugs (SSRIs and others) in children and adolescents with MDD, obsessive compulsive disorder (OCD), or other psychiatric disorders (a total of 24 trials involving over 4,400 patients) have revealed a greater risk of adverse reactions representing suicidal thinking or behavior (suicidality) during the first few months of treatment in those receiving antidepressants. The average risk of such events in patients receiving antidepressants was 4%, twice the placebo risk of 2%. No suicides occurred in these trials.

Indications

Depression: In general, the MAOIs are indicated in patients with atypical (exogenous) depression, and in some patients unresponsive to other antidepressive therapy. They are not a drug of first choice.

Major depression (tranylcypromine): For the treatment of a major depressive episode without melancholia.

Administration and Dosage

ISOCARBOXAZID:

Initial dosage – 10 mg twice daily. Increase dosage by 10 mg every 2 to 4 days to achieve a dosage of 40 mg by the end of the first week. Increase by up to 20 mg/week, to a maximum of 60 mg/day. Daily dosage should be divided into 2 to 4 doses.

Maintenance dosage – After maximum clinical response is achieved, attempt to reduce the dosage slowly over a period of several weeks without jeopardizing therapeutic response. Beneficial effect may not be seen in some patients for 3 to 6 weeks. If no response is obtained by then, discontinue therapy.

Because of the limited experience with patients receiving 60 mg/day, caution is indicated when a dose of 40 mg/day is exceeded.

PHENELZINE:

Initial dose – 15 mg 3 times/day.

Early phase treatment – Increase dosage to 60 mg/day as tolerated. It may be necessary to increase dosage up to 90 mg/day to obtain sufficient MAO inhibition. A clinical response may not be seen until treatment at 60 mg has been continued for at least 4 weeks.

Maintenance dose – After maximum benefit is achieved, reduce dosage slowly over several weeks. Maintenance dose may be as low as 15 mg/day or every other day; continue for as long as required.

TRANYLCYPROMINE: The usual effective dosage is 30 mg/day in divided doses. If there is no improvement after 2 weeks, increase dosage in 10 mg/day increments of 1 to 3 weeks. Maximum of 60 mg/day. Withdrawal from tranylcypromine should be gradual.

Actions

Pharmacology: These drugs are non-selective MAOIs and cause an increase in the concentration of endogenous epinephrine, norepinephrine, and serotonin (5HT) in storage sites throughout the nervous system.

Pharmacokinetics: Phenelzine and tranylcypromine are well absorbed orally. The clinical effects of phenelzine may continue for up to 2 weeks after discontinuation of therapy. When tranylcypromine is withdrawn, MAO activity is recovered in 3 to 5 days (possibly up to 10 days), although the drug is excreted in 24 hours.

Contraindications

Hypersensitivity to these agents; pheochromocytoma; CHF; a history of liver disease or abnormal liver function tests; severe impairment of renal function; confirmed or suspected cerebrovascular defect; cardiovascular disease; hypertension; history of headache; in patients over 60 because of the possibility of existing cerebral sclerosis with damaged vessels; coadministration with other MAOIs; dibenzazepine-related agents including tricyclic antidepressants, carbamazepine, and cyclobenzaprine; bupropion; SSRIs; buspirone; sympathomimetics; meperidine; dextromethorphan; anesthetic agents; CNS depressants; antihypertensives; caffeine; cheese or other foods with high tyramine content (see Warnings and Drug Interactions).

Warnings/Precautions

Hypertensive crises: The most serious reactions involve changes in blood pressure; it is inadvisable to use these drugs in elderly or debilitated patients or in the presence of hypertension, cardiovascular, or cerebrovascular disease. Not recommended in patients with frequent or severe headaches because headache during therapy may be the first symptom of a hypertensive reaction.

Warning to the patient – Warn all patients against eating foods with high tyramine or tryptophan content and for 2 weeks after discontinuing MAOIs. Also warn patients against drinking alcoholic beverages and against self-medication with certain proprietary agents such as cold, hay fever, or weight reduction preparations containing sympathomimetic amines while undergoing therapy. Instruct patients not to consume excessive amounts of caffeine in any form and to report promptly the occurrence of headache or other unusual symptoms.

Concomitant antidepressants: In patients receiving a selective serotonin reuptake inhibitor (SSRIs) in combination with an MAOI, there have been reports of serious, sometimes fatal, reactions including hyperthermia, rigidity, myoclonus, autonomic instability with possible rapid fluctuations of vital signs, and mental status changes that include extreme agitation progressing to delirium and coma. It is recommended that SSRIs not be used in combination with an MAOI, or within 14 days of an MAOI. Allow 2 weeks or longer after stopping the SSRIs before starting an MAOI. Allow 5 weeks or longer after stopping fluoxetine before starting an MAOI.

MAOIs should not be administered together with or immediately following tricyclic antidepressants (TCAs). At least 14 days should elapse between the discontinuation of the MAOIs and the institution of a TCA. Some TCAs have been used safely and successfully in combination with MAOIs.

Withdrawal: Withdrawal may be associated with nausea, vomiting, and malaise.

Coexisting symptoms: **Tranylcypromine** and **isocarboxazid** may aggravate coexisting symptoms in depression, such as anxiety and agitation.

Hypotension: Follow all patients for symptoms of postural hypotension. Blood pressure usually returns to pretreatment levels rapidly when the drug is discontinued or the dosage is reduced.

Hypomania: Hypomania has been the most common severe psychiatric side effect reported. This has been largely limited to patients in whom disorders characterized by hyperkinetic symptoms coexist with, but are obscured by, depressive affect.

Diabetes: There is conflicting evidence as to whether MAOIs affect glucose metabolism or potentiate hypoglycemic agents.

Epilepsy: The effect of MAOIs on the convulsive threshold may vary. Do not use with metrizamide; discontinue MAOI 48 hours or more prior to myelography and resume at least 24 hours postprocedure.

Hepatic complications: Perform periodic liver function tests, such as bilirubins, alkaline phosphatase, or transaminases during therapy; discontinue at the first sign of hepatic dysfunction or jaundice.

Myocardial ischemia: MAOIs may suppress anginal pain that would otherwise serve as a warning of myocardial ischemia.

Hyperthyroid patients: Use **tranylcypromine** and **isocarboxazid** cautiously because of increased sensitivity to pressor amines.

Switching MAOIs: In several case reports, hypertensive crisis, cerebral hemorrhage and death have possibly resulted from switching from one MAOI to another without a waiting period. However, in other patients no adverse reactions occurred. Nevertheless, a waiting period of 10 to 14 days is recommended when switching from one MAOI to another.

Renal function impairment: Observe caution in patients with impaired renal function because there is a possibility of cumulative effects in such patients.

Drug abuse and dependence: There have been reports of drug dependency in patients using doses of **tranylcypromine** and **isocarboxazid** significantly in excess of the therapeutic range.

Pregnancy: Category C.

Lactation: Safety for use during lactation has not been established. **Tranylcypromine** is excreted in breast milk.

Children: Not recommended for patients younger than 16 years of age.

Elderly: Older patients may suffer more morbidity than younger patients during and following an episode of hypertension or malignant hyperthermia with MAOI use. Use with caution in the elderly.

Drug Interactions

Drugs that may affect MAOIs include dibenzazepine-related entities, disulfiram, methylphenidate, metrizamide, and sulfonamide.

Drugs that may be affected by MAOIs include anesthetics, antidepressants, antidiabetic agents, barbiturates, beta blockers, bupropion, buspirone, carbamazepine, cyclobenzapine, dextromethorphan, guanethidine, levodopa, meperidine, methyldopa, rauwolfia alkaloids, sulfonamide, sumatriptan, sympathomimetics, thiazide diuretics, and L-tryptophan.

Drug/Food interactions: Warn all patients against eating foods with a high **tyramine** content. Hypertensive crisis may result (see Warnings/Precautions).

Adverse Reactions

Cardiovascular: Orthostatic hypotension, associated in some patients with falling; disturbances in cardiac rate and rhythm.

CNS: Dizziness; vertigo; headache; overactivity; hyperreflexia; tremors; muscle twitching; mania; hypomania; jitteriness; confusion; memory impairment; sleep disturbances including hypersomnia and insomnia; weakness; myoclonic movements; fatigue; drowsiness; restlessness; overstimulation including increased anxiety, agitation and manic symptoms.

GI: Constipation; nausea; diarrhea; abdominal pain.

Miscellaneous: Edema; dry mouth; blurred vision; hyperhidrosis; elevated serum transaminases; minor skin reactions such as skin rashes; anorexia; weight changes.

ANTIPSYCHOTIC AGENTS

Warning:

Increased mortality in elderly patients with dementia-related psychosis: Elderly patients with dementia-related psychosis treated with atypical antipsychotic drugs are at an increased risk of death compared with placebo. Although the causes of death were varied, most of the deaths appeared to be either cardiovascular (eg, heart failure, sudden death) or infectious (eg, pneumonia) in nature. Atypical antipsychotics are not approved for the treatment of patients with dementia-related psychosis.

Agranulocytosis: Because of a significant risk of agranulocytosis, a potentially life-threatening adverse reaction, reserve **clozapine** use 1) in the treatment of severely ill patients with schizophrenia who fail to show an acceptable response to adequate courses of standard antipsychotic drug treatment, or 2) for reducing the risk of recurrent suicidal behavior in patients with schizophrenia or schizoaffective disorder who are judged to be at risk of reexperiencing suicidal behavior. Patients being treated with clozapine must have a baseline white blood cell (WBC) and differential count before initiation of treatment, as well as regular WBC counts during treatment and for 4 weeks after discontinuation of treatment. Clozapine is available only through a distribution system that ensures monitoring of WBC counts according to the schedule described below, prior to delivery of the next supply of medication.

Seizures: Seizures have been associated with the use of **clozapine**. Dose appears to be an important seizure predictor, with a greater likelihood at higher **clozapine** doses. Use caution when administering **clozapine** to patients with a history of seizures or other predisposing factors. Advise patients not to engage in any activity where sudden loss of consciousness could cause serious risk to themselves or others.

Myocarditis: Analyses of postmarketing safety databases suggest **clozapine** is associated with an increased risk of fatal myocarditis, especially during, but not limited to, the first month of therapy. In patients in whom myocarditis is suspected, discontinue clozapine treatment promptly.

Other adverse cardiovascular and respiratory effects: Orthostatic hypotension, with or without syncope, can occur with **clozapine** treatment. Rarely, collapse can be profound and accompanied by respiratory and/or cardiac arrest. Orthostatic hypotension is more likely to occur during initial titration in association with rapid dose escalation. In patients who have had even a brief interval off clozapine, start treatment with 12.5 mg once or twice daily. Because collapse, respiratory arrest, and cardiac arrest during initial treatment have occurred in patients receiving benzodiazepines or other psychotropic drugs, caution is advised when clozapine is initiated in patients taking a benzodiazepine or any other psychotropic drug.

Mesoridazine, thioridazine: Some antipsychotics have been shown to prolong the QTc interval in a dose-related manner, and drugs with this potential, including **mesoridazine** and **thioridazine**, have been associated with torsade-de-pointes-type arrhythmias and sudden death.

Indications

Antipsychotics — Summary of Indications[a]

Indications ✓ = labeled	Aripiprazole	Chlorpromazine	Clozapine	Fluphenazine	Haloperidol	Iloperidone	Loxapine	Mesoridazine	Olanzapine	Paliperidone	Perphenazine	Pimozide	Prochlorperazine	Quetiapine	Risperidone	Thioridazine	Thiothixene	Trifluoperazine	Ziprasidone
Acute agitation associated with bipolar I mania	✓ (IM)[b]								✓ (IM)[b]										
Acute agitation in schizophrenia	✓ (IM)[b]								✓ (IM)[b]										✓ (IM)[b]
Acute intermittent porphyria		✓																	
Acute manic and/or mixed episodes associated with bipolar disorder	✓	✓							✓					✓[c]	✓				✓
Hyperactivity (pediatric patients)		✓			✓														
Intractable hiccoughs		✓																	
Nausea/ Vomiting		✓									✓		✓						
Nonpsychotic anxiety													✓					✓	
Presurgical apprehension/ restlessness		✓																	
Psychotic disorders				✓	✓						✓								
Recurrent suicidal behavior			✓																
Schizophrenia	✓	✓	✓	✓		✓	✓	✓	✓	✓	✓		✓	✓	✓	✓	✓	✓	✓
Severe behavioral problems (pediatric patients)		✓			✓														
Tetanus		✓ (IM)[b]	✓																
Tourette disorder					✓							✓							

[a] For more detailed information, see the following information and individual drug monographs.
[b] IM = intramuscular.
[c] Immediate-release only.

Actions

Pharmacology:

Antipsychotic Receptor Affinity	
Antipsychotic agent	Receptor affinity
Conventional agents	
Chlorpromazine	**High** — adrenergic **Weak** — peripheral anticholinergic, histaminergic, serotonergic
Fluphenazine	Dopamine D_2, histamine H_1, alpha-adrenergic, serotonin 5-HT_2
Haloperidol	Dopamine D_2, alpha-adrenergic, serotonin 5-HT_2
Loxapine	Dopamine D_2, histamine H_1, alpha-adrenergic, muscarinic M_1
Mesoridazine	Dopamine D_2, histamine H_1, alpha-adrenergic, muscarinic M_1
Perphenazine	Dopamine D_2, histamine H_1, alpha-adrenergic
Pimozide	Dopamine D_2, alpha-adrenergic, serotonin 5-HT_2
Prochlorperazine	Dopamine D_2, histamine H_1, alpha-D_2 adrenergic, serotonin 5-HT_2
Promethazine[a]	Histamine H_1, muscarinic, some serotonin
Thioridazine	Dopamine D_2, histamine H_1, alpha-adrenergic, muscarinic M_1, serotonin 5-HT_2
Thiothixene	**High** — dopamine D_2 **Low** — histamine H_1, alpha-adrenergic
Trifluoperazine	Dopamine D_2, histamine H_1, alpha-adrenergic, muscarinic M_1, serotonin 5-HT_2
Atypical agents	
Aripiprazole	**High** — dopamine D_2[b] D_3, serotonin 5-HT_{1A}[b], 5-HT_{2A} **Moderate** — dopamine D_4, 5-HT_{2C}, 5-HT_7, $alpha_1$-adrenergic, histamine H_1
Clozapine	**High** — dopamine D_4 Other receptors — dopamine D_1, D_2, D_3, D_5, adrenergic, cholinergic, histaminergic, serotonergic
Iloperidone	**High**—Serotonin 5-HT_{2A}, Dopamine D_2 and D_3, **Moderate**—Dopamine D_4, Serotonin 5-HT_6, 5-HT_7, Norepinephrine $NE_{\alpha\text{-}1}$ **Low**—Serotonin 5-HT_{1A}, Dopamine D_1, Histamine H_1
Olanzapine	**High** — serotonin 5-HT_{2A}, 5-HT_{2C}, dopamine D_1, D_2, D_3, D_4, muscarinic M_1, M_2, M_3, M_4, M_5, histamine H_1, $alpha_1$-adrenergic **Weak** — $GABA_A$, benzodiazepine receptor, beta-adrenergic
Paliperidone	**High** — Dopamine D_2, serotonin $5Ht_{2A}$; **Low to moderate** — alpha adrenergic, histamine H_1
Quetiapine	Serotonin 5-HT_{1A}, 5-HT_2, dopamine D_1, D_2, $alpha_1$ and $_2$-adrenergic, histamine H_1
Risperidone	**High** — dopamine D_2, serotonin 5-HT_2 **Low to moderate** — 5-HT_{1C}, 5-HT_{1D}, 5-HT_{1A}, histamine H_1, alpha-adrenergic **Weak** — D_1, haloperidol-sensitive sigma site
Ziprasidone	**High** — dopamine D_2, D_3, 5-HT_{2A}, 5-HT_{2C}, 5-HT_{1A}, 5-HT_{1D}, $alpha_1$-adrenergic **Moderate** — histamine H_1

[a] Promethazine is classified as a phenothiazine but not indicated as an antipsychotic.
[b] Partial agonist activity.

Pharmacological Parameters of Antipsychotics

Antipsychotic agent	Approx. equiv. dose (mg)	Usual oral adult daily dose range (mg)	Sedation	EPS	Anticholinergic effects	Orthostatic hypotension	Weight gain
Phenothiazines							
Aliphatic							
Chlorpromazine	100	30 to 800	+++	++	++	+++	
Piperazine							
Fluphenazine	2	1 to 40	+	++++	+	+	
Perphenazine	10	12 to 64	++	++	+	+	
Prochlorperazine		15 to 150					
Trifluoperazine	5	2 to 15	+	+++	+	+	
Piperidines							
Mesoridazine	50	100 to 400	+++	+	+++	++	
Thioridazine	100	150 to 800	+++	+	+++	+++	
Thioxanthenes							
Thiothixene	4	6 to 60	+	+++	+	+	
Phenylbutylpiperadines							
Butyrophenone							
Haloperidol	2	1 to 100	+	++++	+	+	
Diphenylbutylpiperadine							
Pimozide		1 to 10	+	+++	++	+	
Dibenzepines							
Dibenzoxazepines							
Loxapine	10	20 to 250	+	++	+	+	
Dibenzodiazepine							
Clozapine	50	300 to 900	+++	0	+++	+++	++++
Thienbenzodiazepine							
Olanzapine		5 to 20	++	+	++	++	++++
Dibenzothiazepine							
Quetiapine		50 to 800	++	0	0-+	++	+++
Benzisoxazole							
Iloperidone		12 to 24	++	+	+	++	+
Paliperidone		3 to 12	+		0-+		
Risperidone		4 to 16	+	++	0-+	++	+++
Ziprasidone		40 to 200	++	++	+	++	+
Quinolinone							
Aripiprazole		10 to 30	+	0	0-+	+	+

++++ = Very high incidence of side effects; +++ = high incidence of side effects; ++ = moderate incidence of side effects; + = low incidence of side effects.

The exact mechanism of action of the antipsychotic agents is unknown; however, it is thought to be because of their antagonistic actions on the receptors of several neurotransmitters.

Pharmacokinetics:

Antipsychotic Pharmacokinetics					
Drug	Bioavailability	T_{max}	Protein bound (%)	Routes of metabolism	t½
Conventional agents					
Chlorpromazine	20% to 40%	1 to 4 h	92% to 97%	—	24 h
Fluphenazine	2.7% (oral); 3.4% (IM/ subcutaneous)	≈ 2.8 h (oral); 24 to 48 h (IM/ subcutaneous)	—	—	18 h (oral)
Haloperidol	60% to 65% (oral)	6 days (decanoate)	≈ 92%	—	≈ 18 h (oral); ≈ 3 wk (decanoate)
Loxapine	≈ 100%	—	—	—	8 h
Mesoridazine	—	—	—	—	30 h
Perphenazine	20%	1 to 3 h	—	Sulfoxidation, hydroxylation, dealkylation, and glucuronidation by CYP2D6	9 to 12 h
Pimozide	> 50%	4 to 12 h	99%	N-dealkylation by CYP3A and CYP1A2 to a lesser extent	≈ 55 h
Prochlorperazine	—	—	—	—	3 to 5 h (oral); 6.9 h (IV)
Promethazine[a]	—	2 to 3 h	76% to 80%	N-demethylation and sulfoxidation	5 to 14 h
Thioridazine	—	—	99%	—	24 h
Thiothixene	—	—	—	—	34 h
Trifluoperazine	—	—	—	—	18 h
Atypical agents					
Aripiprazole	87%	3 to 5 h	> 99%[b]	Dehydrogenation, hydroxylation, and N-dealkylation by CYP3A4 and CYP2D6	75[c] to 146[d] h
Clozapine	27% to 47%	2.5 h	≈ 97%	Demethylation, hydroxylation, and N-oxidation	8 h[e]; 12 h[f]
Iloperidone	96%	2 to 4 h	≈ 95%	Carbonyl reduction, hydroxylation, and o-demethylation by CYP2D6 and CYP3A4	≈ 18 h[d] ≈ 33 h[e]
Olanzapine	≈ 60%	≈ 6 h	93% over a concentration range of 7 to 1,100 ng/mL	Glucuronidation and oxidation by CYP1A2 and CYP2D6	21 to 54 h
Paliperidone	28%	24 h	74%	Dealkylation, hydroxylation, dehydrogenation, benzisoxazole scission	23 h
Quetiapine	≥ 73%	1.5 h	83%[a]	Sulfoxidation and oxidation by CYP3A4	≈ 6 h
Risperidone	70%	≈ 1 h	90%	Hydroxylation by CYP2D6 and N-dealkylation	3[c] to 20[d] h

Antipsychotic Pharmacokinetics					
Drug	Bioavailability	T_{max}	Protein bound (%)	Routes of metabolism	t½
Ziprasidone	≈ 60% (oral); 100% (IM)	6 to 8 h (oral); ≈ 60 min (IM)	> 99%	Reduction by aldehyde oxidase, methylation, and oxidation by CYP3A4 and CYP1A2 to a lesser extent	≈ 7 h (oral); 2 to 5 h (IM)

[a] Promethazine is classified as a phenothiazine but not indicated as an antipsychotic.
[b] At therapeutic concentrations.
[c] Extensive metabolizers.
[d] Poor metabolizers.
[e] Single dose.
[f] At steady state.

Contraindications

Hypersensitivity to the drug or any other component of the product (cross-sensitivity between phenothiazines may occur); comatose or greatly depressed states caused by CNS depressants or from any other cause (phenothiazines, **clozapine**, **loxapine**, **pimozide**, **haloperidol**); coadministration with other drugs that prolong the QT interval and in patients with congenital long QT syndrome or a history of cardiac arrhythmias (**mesoridazine**, **thioridazine**, **pimozide**, **ziprasidone**).

Clozapine: Myeloproliferative disorders; uncontrolled epilepsy; history of clozapine-induced agranulocytosis or severe granulocytopenia; do not use with other agents having a well-known potential to cause agranulocytosis or suppress bone marrow function.

Haloperidol: Parkinson disease.

Paliperidone: Hypersensitivity to **risperidone**.

Phenothiazines: Suspected or established subcortical brain damage (**fluphenazine**); blood dyscrasias (**perphenazine**, **trifluoperazine**, **fluphenazine**); bone marrow depression (**perphenazine**, **trifluoperazine**, **fluphenazine**); preexisting liver damage (**perphenazine**, **trifluoperazine**, **fluphenazine**); pediatric surgery (**prochlorperazine**); hypertensive or hypotensive heart disease of extreme degree (**thioridazine**).

Pimozide: Treatment of simple tics or tics other than those associated with Tourette disorder; in combination with drugs (eg, pemoline, methylphenidate, amphetamines) that may cause motor or phonic tics until it is determined whether or not the drugs, rather than Tourette disorder, are responsible for the tics.

Thiothixene: Circulatory collapse; blood dyscrasias.

Ziprasidone: Recent acute myocardial infarction (MI); uncompensated heart failure.

Warnings/Precautions

Tardive dyskinesia: Tardive dyskinesia (TD), a syndrome consisting of potentially irreversible, involuntary dyskinetic movements, may develop in patients treated with antipsychotic drugs. Both the risk of developing TD and the likelihood that it will become irreversible are increased as duration of treatment and total cumulative dose administered increase.

Extrapyramidal symptoms: Dystonic reactions develop primarily with the use of traditional antipsychotics. Extrapyramidal symptoms (EPS) have occurred during the administration of **haloperidol** and **pimozide** frequently, often during the first few days of treatment.

Neuroleptic malignant syndrome: A potentially fatal symptom complex sometimes referred to as Neuroleptic malignant syndrome (NMS) has been reported in association with administration of antipsychotic drugs. Clinical manifestations of NMS are hyperpyrexia, muscle rigidity, altered mental status, and evidence of autonomic instability (irregular pulse or blood pressure, tachycardia, diaphoresis, cardiac dysrhythmia). Additional signs may include elevated creatine phosphokinase, rhabdomyolysis, and acute renal failure.

CNS effects: These agents may impair mental or physical abilities, especially during the first few days. Caution patients against activities requiring alertness (ie, operating vehicles or machinery).

Encephalopathic syndrome – An encephalopathic syndrome (characterized by weakness, lethargy, fever, tremulousness, confusion, EPS, leukocytosis, elevated serum enzymes, blood urea nitrogen, fasting blood sugar) has occurred in some patients treated with lithium plus an antipsychotic (**haloperidol**).

Cardiovascular: Use with caution in patients with cardiovascular disease, cerebrovascular disease, conditions that would predispose patients to hypotension, or mitral insufficiency. Increased pulse rates occur in most patients.

ECG changes – A minority of **clozapine** patients experience ECG repolarization changes similar to those seen with other antipsychotic drugs, including S-T segment depression and flattening or inversion of T waves, which all normalize after discontinuation of clozapine.

Paliperidone, iloperidone, ziprasidone, pimozide, mesoridazine, and **thioridazine** have been shown to prolong the QT interval, and drugs with this potential have been associated with torsade de pointes-type arrhythmias and sudden death. Perform a baseline ECG and measure serum potassium and magnesium before initiation of treatment and periodically during treatment, especially during a period of dose adjustment. Do not give mesoridazine or thioridazine to patients with QT interval over 450 msec. Avoid ziprasidone in patients with histories of significant cardiovascular illness (eg, QT prolongation, recent acute MI, uncompensated heart failure, cardiac arrhythmia). Discontinue treatment if the QT interval is over 500 msec. Patients who experience symptoms that may be associated with the occurrence of torsade de pointes (eg, dizziness, palpitations, syncope) may warrant further cardiac evaluation; in particular, consider Holter monitoring.

Nonspecific ECG changes, usually reversible Q- and T-wave distortions, have been observed in some patients receiving phenothiazines. Nonspecific ECG changes have been observed in some patients receiving **thiothixene**.

Haloperidol has been associated with ECG changes, including QT interval prolongation and ECG pattern changes compatible with the polymorphous configuration of torsade de pointes.

Prolongation of the QT interval and torsade de pointes have been reported with **risperidone** overdoses.

Myocarditis – Postmarketing **clozapine** surveillance data from 4 countries revealed cases of myocarditis, some which were fatal.

Cardiomyopathy – Cases of cardiomyopathy have been reported in patients treated with **clozapine**.

Pulmonary embolism – Consider the possibility of pulmonary embolism in patients receiving **clozapine** who present with deep vein thrombosis, acute dyspnea, chest pain, or with other respiratory signs and symptoms.

Hypotension – Orthostatic hypotension with or without syncope can occur, especially during initial titration in association with rapid dose escalation, and may represent a continuing risk in some patients. Carefully watch those undergoing surgery and those who are on large doses of phenothiazines for hypotensive phenomena. The hypotensive effects may occur after the first injection of the antipsychotic, occasionally after subsequent injections, and rarely after the first oral dose.

Tachycardia – Tachycardia, which may be sustained, also has been observed in approximately 25% of patients taking **clozapine**.

Cerebrovascular effects: Cerebrovascular adverse reactions (eg, stroke, transient ischemic attack), including fatalities, were reported in patients (mean age, 85 years; range, 73 to 97 years) in trials of **risperidone** in elderly patients with dementia-related psychosis.

Sudden death: Previous brain damage or seizures may be predisposing factors; avoid high doses in known seizure patients.

Priapism: Rare cases of priapism have been associated with **risperidone, ziprasidone, quetiapine, aripiprazole**, and **olanzapine**.

Hyperprolactinemia: Antipsychotic drugs elevate prolactin levels; the elevation persists during chronic administration.

Hyperglycemia and diabetes mellitus: Hyperglycemia, in some cases extreme and associated with ketoacidosis or hyperosmolar coma or death, has been reported in patients treated with atypical antipsychotics.

Regularly monitor patients with an established diagnosis of diabetes mellitus who are started on atypical antipsychotics for worsening of glucose control. Patients with risk factors for diabetes mellitus (eg, obesity, family history of diabetes) who are starting treatment with atypical antipsychotics should undergo fasting blood glucose testing at baseline and periodically during treatment. Monitor any patient treated with atypical antipsychotics for symptoms of hyperglycemia, including polydipsia, polyuria, polyphagia, and weakness. Patients who develop symptoms of hyperglycemia during treatment with atypical antipsychotics should undergo fasting blood glucose testing.

Antiemetic effects: Drugs with antiemetic effects can obscure signs of toxicity of other drugs or mask symptoms of disease (eg, brain tumor, intestinal obstruction, Reye syndrome). They can suppress the cough reflex; aspiration is possible.

Pulmonary: Cases of bronchopneumonia (some fatal) have followed the use of antipsychotic agents. Lethargy and decreased sensation of thirst may lead to dehydration, hemoconcentration, and reduced pulmonary ventilation.

GI effects: Because the **paliperidone** tablet is nondeformable and does not appreciably change in shape in the GI tract, do not ordinarily administer **paliperidone** to patients with pre-existing severe GI narrowing (pathologic or iatrogenic). Only use **Paliperidone** in patients who are able to swallow the tablet whole.

Agranulocytosis: Agranulocytosis, defined as an ANC of less than 500/mm^3, occurs in association with **clozapine** use at a cumulative incidence at 1 year of about 1.3%. This reaction could prove fatal if not detected early and therapy interrupted.

Ophthalmic: Use with caution in patients with a history of glaucoma. During prolonged therapy, ocular changes may occur; these include particle deposition in the cornea and lens, progressing in more severe cases to star-shaped lenticular opacities. Pigmentary retinopathy occurs most frequently in patients receiving **thioridazine** dosages more than 1 g/day.

Cataracts – Lens changes also have been observed in patients taking **quetiapine** during long-term treatment. Examination of the lens by methods adequate to detect cataract formation, such as slit-lamp exam, is recommended at initiation of treatment or shortly thereafter and at 6-month intervals.

Seizure disorders: These drugs can lower the convulsive threshold and may precipitate seizures. Use cautiously in patients with a history of epilepsy and only when absolutely necessary.

Pigmentary retinopathy: Observe carefully for pigmentary retinopathy and lenticular pigmentation.

GI dysmotility: Esophageal dysmotility and aspiration have been associated with antipsychotic drug use. Use **quetiapine, ziprasidone, risperidone, olanzapine, aripiprazole**, and others cautiously in patients at risk for aspiration pneumonia.

Anticholinergic effects: Most antipsychotic agents are associated with constipation, dry mouth, and tachycardia, all adverse reactions possibly related to cholinergic antagonism. Anticholinergic effects of **clozapine** are very potent. Use caution in patients with clinically significant prostatic hypertrophy, narrow-angle glaucoma, or a history of paralytic ileus.

Cholesterol: Decreased serum cholesterol has occurred with some agents; however, **quetiapine** may raise plasma cholesterol and triglycerides.

Concomitant conditions: Use with caution in the following: patients exposed to extreme heat or phosphorus insecticides; atropine or related drugs, because of additive anticholinergic effects; those in a state of alcohol withdrawal; those with dermatoses or other allergic reactions to phenothiazine derivatives because of the possibility of cross-sensitivity; those who have exhibited idiosyncrasy to other centrally-acting drugs.

Hematologic: Various blood dyscrasias have occurred.

Myelography: Discontinue phenothiazines at least 48 hours before myelography because of the possibility of seizures; do not resume therapy for at least 24 hours postprocedure.

Thrombotic thrombocytopenic purpura: A single case of thrombotic thrombocytopenic purpura was reported with **risperidone**. The relationship to therapy is unknown.

Parkinson disease/Dementia: Patients with Parkinson disease or dementia with Lewy bodies are reported to have an increased sensitivity to antipsychotic medication.

Thyroid: Severe neurotoxicity (rigidity, inability to walk or talk) may occur in patients with thyrotoxicosis who are also receiving antipsychotics.

Hypothyroidism – **Quetiapine** demonstrated a dose-related decrease in total and free thyroxine (T_4) of approximately 20% at the higher end of the therapeutic dose range that was maximal in the first 2 to 4 weeks of treatment and maintained without adaptation or progression during more chronic therapy.

Hyperpyrexia: A significant, not otherwise explained rise in body temperature may indicate intolerance to antipsychotics.

Abrupt withdrawal: These drugs are not known to cause psychic dependence and do not produce tolerance or addiction. However, following abrupt withdrawal of high-dose therapy, symptoms such as gastritis, nausea, vomiting, dizziness, headache, tachycardia, insomnia, and tremulousness have occurred. These symptoms can be reduced by gradual reduction of the dosage or by continuing antiparkinson agents for several weeks after the antipsychotic is withdrawn.

Suicide: Suicide possibility in depressed patients remains during treatment and until significant remission occurs. Do not allow this type of patient to have access to large quantities of the drug.

Cutaneous pigmentation changes: Rare instances of skin pigmentation have occurred, primarily in women on long-term, high-dose therapy. These changes, restricted to exposed areas of skin, range from almost imperceptible darkening to a slate gray color, sometimes with a violet hue. Pigmentation may fade following drug discontinuation.

Phenylketonurics: Inform phenylketonuric patients that some of these products contain phenylalanine.

Benzyl alcohol: Some of these products contain benzyl alcohol, which has been associated with a fatal "gasping syndrome" in premature infants.

Hypersensitivity reactions: Patients who have demonstrated a hypersensitivity reaction (eg, blood dyscrasias, jaundice) with a phenothiazine should not be re-exposed to any phenothiazine unless the potential benefits of treatment outweigh the possible hazards.

Sulfite sensitivity: Some of these products contain sulfites that may cause allergic-type reactions, including anaphylactic symptoms and life-threatening or less severe asthmatic episodes in certain susceptible persons.

Renal function impairment: Administer cautiously to those with diminished renal function.

Hepatic function impairment: Use with caution in patients with impaired hepatic function. Patients with a history of hepatic encephalopathy caused by cirrhosis have increased sensitivity to the CNS effects of antipsychotic drugs (ie, impaired cerebration and abnormal slowing of the EEG). Dosage adjustments may be necessary in patients receiving **quetiapine** who are hepatically impaired.

Drug abuse and dependence: Evaluate patients for a history of drug abuse, and observe such patients closely for signs of misuse or abuse (eg, development of tolerance, increases in dose, drug-seeking behavior).

Photosensitivity: Because photosensitivity has been reported (rarely with **thioridazine**), instruct patients to avoid undue exposure to the sun during phenothiazine treatment.

Carcinogenesis: Antipsychotic drugs (except **promazine**) elevate prolactin levels that persist during chronic use. Tissue culture experiments indicate approximately one-third of human breast cancers are prolactin-dependent in vitro, a factor of potential importance if use of these drugs is contemplated in a patient with previously detected breast cancer.

Pregnancy: *Category* C. (*Category* B, **clozapine**).

Lactation: Decide whether to discontinue breast-feeding or the drug, taking into account the importance of the drug to the mother.

Children: In general, these products are not recommended for children younger than 12 years of age. Children seem more prone to develop extrapyramidal reactions, even at moderate doses. Therefore, use the lowest effective dosage.

Elderly: Dosages in the lower range are sufficient for most elderly patients. Monitor response and adjust dosage accordingly. Increase dosage gradually in elderly patients.

Drug Interactions

Antipsychotics and Enzymes Involved With Metabolism

Antipsychotic agent	Enzyme(s)
Aripiprazole	CYP3A4, 2D6
Clozapine	CYP1A2, 2D6, 3A4
Iloperidone	CYP3A4, 2D6
Olanzapine	CYP1A2, 2D6
Perphenazine	CYP2D6
Pimozide	CYP3A, 1A2
Quetiapine	CYP3A4
Risperidone	CYP2D6
Thioridazine	CYP2D6
Ziprasidone	Aldehyde oxidase, CYP3A4, 1A2

Antipsychotic Drug Contraindications

Antipsychotic	Contraindicated with
Clozapine	Drugs having a well known potential to cause agranulocytosis or suppress bone marrow function
Phenothiazines	Cisapride or sparfloxacin because of possible additive QT interval prolongation
Mesoridazine Ziprasidone	Drugs that prolong the QT interval[a]
Pimozide	Drugs that prolong the QT interval[a]; CYP3A inhibitors (eg, clarithromycin, dirithromycin, erythromycin, itraconazole, ketoconazole, nefazodone, protease inhibitors, sertraline, telithromycin, troleandomycin, voriconazole)
Thioridazine	Drugs that prolong the QT interval[a]; CYP2D6 inhibitors (eg, fluoxetine, fluvoxamine, paroxetine, pindolol, propranolol)

[a] The following drugs may prolong the QT interval and increase the risk of life-threatening cardiac arrhythmias, including torsade de pointes: antiarrhythmic agents (eg, amiodarone, bretylium, disopyramide, dofetilide, iloperidone, procainamide, quinidine, sotalol), arsenic trioxide, chlorpromazine, cisapride, dolasetron mesylate, droperidol, gatifloxacin, halofantrine, levomethadyl acetate, mefloquine, mesoridazine, moxifloxacin, pentamidine, pimozide, probucol, sparfloxacin, tacrolimus, thioridazine, ziprasidone.

Drugs that may affect phenothiazines include anticholinergics, beta-blockers, meperidine, paroxetine, ritonavir, and thiazide diuretics.

Drugs that may be affected by phenothiazines include anticholinergics, beta-blockers, dofetilide, guanethidine, meperidine, oral anticoagulants, phenytoin, and thiazide diuretics.

Drugs that may interact with antipsychotics include alcohol, antihypertensive agents, charcoal, CNS depressants, dopamine, and epinephrine.

Drugs that may interact with the atypical antipsychotics include the following: carbamazepine, cimetidine, CYP1A2 inducers/inhibitors, CYP3A4 inhibitors, dopamine agonists, famotidine, levodopa, lorazepam, phenytoin, quinidine, ritonavir, SSRIs, thioridazine, and valproate.

Drugs that may interact with clozapine include benzodiazepines, caffeine, CYP1A2 induces/inhibitors, CYP3A4 inhibitors, phenobarbital, risperidone, ritonavir, and SSRIs.

Drugs that may interact with haloperidol include anticholinergic agents, azole antifungal agents, carbamazepine, fluoxetine, lithium, and rifamycins.

Drug/Lab test interactions: Phenothiazines may produce false-positive phenylketonuria test results. Phenothiazines may cause false-positive pregnancy test results.

Adverse Reactions

Adverse reactions occurring in 3% or more of patients include the following:

Typical antipsychotic agents:

CNS – Akathesia, akinesia, asthenia, bizarre dreams, depression, drowsiness, EPS, headache, hyperkinesia, insomnia, NMS, somnolence.

GI – Appetite increased, constipation, diarrhea, dry mouth, dysphagia, polydipsia, salivation, taste altered.

Miscellaneous – Muscle rigidity, myalgia, rash, rigidity, torticollis.

Atypical antipsychotic agents:

Cardiovascular – Hypertension, hypotension, tachycardia.

CNS – Agitation, akathesia, akinesia, anxiety, asthenia, confusion, convulsions, dizziness, drowsiness, dystonia, EPS, gait abnormal, headache, hypokinesia, insomnia, libido decreased, light-headedness, restlessness, somnolence, syncope, tardive dystonia, tremor, vertigo.

Dermatologic – Ecchymosis, eczema, rash.

GI – Abdominal pain/discomfort, appetite increased, constipation, diarrhea, dry mouth, dyspepsia, gastroesophageal reflux, nausea, salivation, vomiting, weight gain.

GU – Ejaculation disorders, impotence, menorrhagia.

Respiratory – Coughing, pharyngitis, rhinitis.

Special senses – Abnormal vision, blurred vision, visual disturbances.

Miscellaneous – Accidental injury, arthralgia, back/chest pain, diaphoresis, edema (peripheral), fever, hypertonia, joint pain, leukopenia, myalgia, rigidity.

PHENOTHIAZINE AND THIOXANTHENE DERIVATIVES

PHENOTHIAZINE DERIVATIVES	
CHLORPROMAZINE HYDROCHLORIDE	
Tablets; oral: 10, 25, 50, 100, and 200 mg (*Rx*)	Various
Injection: 25 mg/mL (*Rx*)	Various
FLUPHENAZINE	
Tablets; oral: 1, 2.5, 5, and 10 mg (*Rx*)	Various
Elixir; oral: 2.5 mg per 5 mL (*Rx*)	
Solution, concentrate; oral: 5 mg/mL (*Rx*)	
Injection: 2.5 mg/mL; 25 mg/mL (as decanoate) (*Rx*)	
PERPHENAZINE	
Tablets; oral: 2, 4, 8, and 16 mg (*Rx*)	Various

PROCHLORPERAZINE	
Tablets; oral: 5 and 10 mg (as maleate) (*Rx*)	Various
Suppositories: 25 mg (*Rx*)	Various, *Compro* (Paddock)
Injection: 5 mg/mL (as edisylate) (*Rx*)	Various
THIORIDAZINE	
Tablets; oral: 10, 15, 25, 50, 100, 150, 200 mg (*Rx*)	Various
THIOXANTHENE DERIVATIVES	
THIOTHIXENE	
Capsules; oral: 1, 2, 5, 10, and 20 mg (*Rx*)	Various, *Navane* (Pfizer)

Warning:

Increased mortality in elderly patients with dementia-related psychosis: Elderly patients with dementia-related psychosis treated with antipsychotic drugs are at an increased risk of death. Analyses of 17 placebo-controlled trials (modal duration of 10 weeks), largely in patients taking atypical antipsychotic drugs, revealed a risk of death in drug-treated patients of between 1.6 and 1.7 times the risk of death in placebo-treated patients. Over the course of a typical 10-week controlled trial, the rate of death in drug-treated patients was about 4.5%, compared with a rate of about 2.6% in the placebo group. Although the causes of death were varied, most of the deaths appeared to be cardiovascular (eg, heart failure, sudden death) or infectious (eg, pneumonia) in nature. Observational studies suggest that, similar to atypical antipsychotic drugs, treatment with conventional antipsychotic drugs may increase mortality. The extent to which the findings of increased mortality in observational studies may be attributed to the antipsychotic drug as opposed to some characteristic(s) of the patients is not clear. Thiothixene is not approved for the treatment of patients with dementia-related psychosis.

Thioridazine: Thioridazine has been shown to prolong the QTc interval in a dose-related manner. Drugs with this potential, including thioridazine, have been associated with torsade de pointes-type arrhythmias and sudden death. Because of its potential for significant, possibly life-threatening, proarrhythmic effects, reserve thioridazine use in the treatment of schizophrenic patients who fail to show an acceptable response to adequate courses of treatment with other antipsychotic drugs, either because of insufficient effectiveness or the inability to achieve an effective dose because of intolerable adverse effects from those drugs.

Indications

Chlorpromazine hydrochloride:

Behavioral problems – For the treatment of severe behavioral problems in children 1 to 12 years of age marked by combativeness and/or explosive hyperexcitable behavior (out of proportion to immediate provocations).

Emesis/Hiccoughs – For the control of nausea and vomiting and relief of intractable hiccoughs.

Hyperactivity – For the short-term treatment of hyperactive children who show excessive motor activity with accompanying conduct disorders consisting of some or all of the following symptoms: impulsivity, difficulty sustaining attention, aggressivity, mood lability, and poor frustration tolerance.

Manic-depressive illness – For the control of manifestations of the manic type of manic-depressive illness.

Porphyria, acute intermittent – For the treatment of acute intermittent porphyria.

Schizophrenia – For the treatment of schizophrenia.

Surgery – Relief of restlessness and apprehension prior to surgery.

Tetanus – An adjunct in treatment of tetanus.

Fluphenazine:

Psychotic disorders – For the management of manifestations of psychotic disorders; esterified formulations (decanoate) are indicated for patients requiring prolonged and parenteral neuroleptic therapy (eg, chronic schizophrenic patients).

Perphenazine:

Emesis – To control severe nausea and vomiting and intractable hiccoughs.

Psychotic disorders – For the treatment of schizophrenia.

Prochlorperazine:

Emesis – To control severe nausea and vomiting. (*Compro* is only indicated for severe nausea and vomiting in adults.)

Nonpsychotic anxiety – Short-term treatment of generalized nonpsychotic anxiety; however, prochlorperazine is not the first drug of choice for this indication.

Schizophrenia – For the treatment of schizophrenia.

Trifluoperazine hydrochloride:

Nonpsychotic anxiety – Short-term treatment of nonpsychotic anxiety (not the drug of choice in most patients).

Schizophrenia – For the management of schizophrenia.

Thioridazine hydrochloride:

Schizophrenia – For the management of schizophrenic patients who fail to respond adequately to treatment with other antipsychotic drugs. Before initiating treatment with thioridazine, it is strongly recommended that a patient be given at least 2 trials, each with a different antipsychotic drug product, at an adequate dose and for an adequate duration.

Thiothixene:

Schizophrenia – For the management of schizophrenia.

Administration and Dosage

CHLORPROMAZINE: Increase dosage until symptoms are controlled, then gradually reduce dosage to the lowest effective maintenance level. Increase parenteral dosage only if hypotension has not occurred.

Injection – Subcutaneous administration is not advised. Inject IM slowly, deep into upper outer quadrant of buttock. Because of possible hypotensive effects, reserve for bedfast patients or for acute ambulatory cases and keep patient recumbent for at least a half hour after injection. If irritation is a problem, dilute injection with saline or 2% procaine; do not mix with other agents in the syringe. Avoid injecting undiluted into vein. Use the IV route only for severe hiccoughs, surgery, and tetanus. Slight yellowing will not alter potency. Discard if markedly discolored.

Because of the possibility of contact dermatitis, avoid getting solution on hands or clothing.

Psychotic disorders – Maximum improvement may not be seen for weeks or even months. Continue optimum dosage for 2 weeks, then gradually reduce to lowest effective maintenance level; 200 mg/day is not unusual. Some patients require higher dosages (eg, 800 mg/day is not uncommon in discharged mental patients).

Hospitalized patients:

Acute schizophrenic or manic states –

IM: 25 mg initially. If necessary, give an additional 25 to 50 mg injection in 1 hour. Increase gradually over several days (up to 400 mg every 4 to 6 hours in exceptionally severe cases) until patient is controlled. Patient usually becomes quiet and cooperative within 24 to 48 hours. Substitute oral dosage and increase until the patient is calm; 500 mg/day is usually sufficient. While gradual increases to 2,000 mg or more/day may be necessary, little therapeutic gain is achieved by exceeding 1,000 mg/day for extended periods.

Less acutely disturbed –

Oral: 25 mg 3 times/day. Increase gradually until effective dose is reached, usually 400 mg/day.

Outpatients:

Oral – Initial oral dose is 10 mg 3 or 4 times/day or 25 mg 2 or 3 times/day.

More severe cases:

Oral – Give 25 mg 3 times/day. After 1 or 2 days, daily dosage may be increased by 20 to 50 mg at semiweekly intervals until patient becomes calm and cooperative.

Prompt control of severe symptoms:

IM – 25 mg; if necessary, repeat in 1 hour. Give subsequent doses orally, 25 to 50 mg 3 times/day.

Behavioral disorders/Hyperactivity – Generally, do not use chlorpromazine in children younger than 6 months of age except where potentially lifesaving. It should not be used in conditions for which specific children's dosages have not been established.

Outpatients:

Oral – 0.5 mg/kg (0.25 mg/lb) every 4 to 6 hours, as needed.

IM – 0.5 mg/kg (0.25 mg/lb) every 6 to 8 hours, as needed.

Hospitalized patients:

Oral – Start with low doses and increase gradually. In severe behavior disorders, 50 to 100 mg/day, or in older children, 200 mg/day or more may be necessary. There is little evidence that improvement in severely disturbed mentally retarded patients is enhanced by doses beyond 500 mg/day.

IM –

5 years of age or younger or 50 lbs: Do not exceed 40 mg/day.

5 to 12 years of age or 50 to 100 lbs: Do not exceed 75 mg/day, except in unmanageable cases.

Nausea and vomiting –

Adults:

Oral – 10 to 25 mg every 4 to 6 hours, as needed; increase if necessary.

IM – 25 mg. If no hypotension occurs, give 25 to 50 mg every 3 to 4 hours, as needed, until vomiting stops. Then switch to oral dosage.

Children:

Oral – 0.25 mg/lb (0.55 mg/kg) every 4 to 6 hours.

IM – 0.25 mg/lb (0.55 mg/kg) every 6 to 8 hours, as needed.

Maximum IM dosage –

Children up to 5 years of age: 40 mg/day.

Children 5 to 12 years of age: 75 mg/day, except in severe cases.

Intractable hiccoughs –

Adults: Orally, 25 to 50 mg 3 or 4 times/day. If symptoms persist 2 to 3 days, give 25 to 50 mg IM. If still persistent, use slow IV infusion with patient flat in bed. Give 25 to 50 mg in 500 to 1,000 mL saline. Monitor blood pressure.

Surgery –

Adults:

Preoperative apprehension – 25 to 50 mg orally 2 to 3 hours before surgery or 12.5 to 25 mg IM 1 to 2 hours before surgery.

Intraoperative (to control acute nausea/vomiting) –

IM: 12.5 mg. Repeat in a half hour if necessary and if no hypotension occurs.

IV: 2 mg per fractional injection at 2-minute intervals. Do not exceed 25 mg (dilute 1 mg/mL with saline).

Children:

Preoperative apprehension – 0.5 mg/kg (0.25 mg/lb) orally 2 to 3 hours before operation or 0.5 mg/kg (0.25 mg/lb) IM 1 to 2 hours before operation.

Intraoperative (to control acute nausea/vomiting) –

IM: 0.25 mg/kg (0.125 mg/lb); repeat in a half hour if needed and if no hypotension occurs.

IV: 1 mg per fractional injection at 2-minute intervals; do not exceed IM dosage. Always dilute to 1 mg/mL with saline.

Tetanus –

Adults: 25 to 50 mg IM 3 or 4 times/day, usually with barbiturates. For IV use, 25 to 50 mg diluted to at least 1 mg/mL and administered at a rate of 1 mg/min.

Children: 0.5 mg/kg (0.25 mg/lb) IM or IV every 6 to 8 hours. When given IV, dilute to at least 1 mg/mL and administer at a rate of 1 mg per 2 minutes. In children up to 23 kg (50 lbs), do not exceed 40 mg/day; 23 to 45 kg (50 to 100 lbs), do not exceed 75 mg/day, except in severe cases.

Acute intermittent porphyria (adults) – 25 to 50 mg orally 3 or 4 times/day or 25 mg IM 3 or 4 times/day until patient can take oral therapy.

Elderly/Debilitated/Emaciated – Lower initial doses and more gradual adjustments are recommended.

FLUPHENAZINE HYDROCHLORIDE: The oral dose is approximately 2 to 3 times the parenteral dose. Institute treatment with a low initial dosage; increase as necessary. Therapeutic effect is often achieved with doses less than 20 mg/day. However, daily doses of up to 40 mg may be needed.

Oral –

Adults: Initially administer 2.5 to 10 mg/day in divided doses at 6-hour to 8-hour intervals. When symptoms are controlled, reduce dosage gradually to daily maintenance doses of 1 or 5 mg, often given as a single daily dose.

Elderly – Initially, 1 to 2.5 mg/day, adjusted according to response.

For psychotic patients stabilized on a fixed daily dosage of orally administered fluphenazine, conversion from oral therapy to the long-acting injectable fluphenazine decanoate may be indicated.

Injection –

Hydrochloride formulation: Administer IM. Average starting dose for adults is 1.25 mg (0.5 mL) IM. Initial total daily dose may range from 2.5 to 10 mg and should be divided and given at 6-hour to 8-hour intervals. Use dosages exceeding 10 mg per day with caution. When symptoms are controlled, oral maintenance therapy can generally be instituted, often with single daily doses.

Decanoate formulation: Administer IM or subcutaneously with a minimum 21-gauge needle. A wet needle or syringe may cause the solution to become cloudy. Initiate with 12.5 to 25 mg (0.5 to 1 mL). The onset of action generally appears between 24 and 72 hours after injection, and the effects of the drug on psychotic symptoms become significant within 48 to 96 hours. When administered as maintenance therapy, a single injection may be effective in controlling schizophrenic symptoms for up to 4 weeks or longer. The response to a single dose has been found to last as long as 6 weeks in a few patients on maintenance therapy.

Initially, treat patients who have never taken phenothiazines with a shorter-acting form of the drug before administering the decanoate. This helps to determine the response to fluphenazine and to establish appropriate dosage.

No precise formula can be given to convert to fluphenazine decanoate use. However, in a controlled, multicenter study, oral fluphenazine hydrochloride 20 mg/day was equivalent to fluphenazine decanoate 25 mg every 3 weeks. This is an approximate conversion ratio of decanoate 0.5 mL (12.5 mg) every 3 weeks for every fluphenazine hydrochloride 10 mg daily. Do not exceed 100 mg. If doses greater than 50 mg are needed, increase succeeding doses cautiously in 12.5 mg increments.

Severely agitated patients – Initially treat with a rapid-acting phenothiazine. When acute symptoms subside, administer fluphenazine decanoate 25 mg; adjust subsequent dosage as necessary.

"Poor risk" patients – In "poor risk" patients (known phenothiazine hypersensitivity or with disorders predisposing to undue reactions), cautiously initiate oral or parenteral fluphenazine. When appropriate dosage is established, give equivalent dose of fluphenazine decanoate.

PERPHENAZINE:

Moderately disturbed nonhospitalized patients with schizophrenia – 4 to 8 mg 3 times/day; reduce as soon as possible to minimum effective dosage.

Hospitalized patients with schizophrenia – 8 to 16 mg 2 to 4 times/day; avoid dosages of more than 64 mg/day.

Reserve prolonged administration of doses exceeding 24 mg/day for hospitalized patients or patients under continued observation for early detection and management of adverse reactions. An antiparkinsonian agent, such as trihexyphenidyl hydrochloride or benztropine mesylate, is valuable in controlling drug-induced extrapyramidal symptoms.

Nausea/Vomiting/Intractable hiccoughs – 8 to 16 mg daily in divided doses; occasionally, 24 mg may be necessary. Early dosage reduction is desirable.

Children – Not recommended for children younger than 12 years of age.

Elderly – Geriatric patients are particularly sensitive to the side effects of antipsychotics. Start on lower doses and observe closely.

PROCHLORPERAZINE: Do not crush or chew sustained-release preparations.

Adults – Increase dosage more gradually in debilitated or emaciated patients.

Control of severe nausea and vomiting:

Oral – Usually, 5 or 10 mg 3 or 4 times/day; *sustained-release* —15 mg on arising or 10 mg every 12 hours.

Rectal – 25 mg twice/day.

IM – Initially, 5 to 10 mg. If necessary, repeat every 3 or 4 hours. Do not exceed 40 mg/day.

Subcutaneous – Do not administer subcutaneously because of local irritation.

Adult surgery — control of severe nausea and vomiting: Total parenteral dosage should not exceed 40 mg/day. Hypotension may occur if the drug is given IV or by infusion.

IM – 5 to 10 mg 1 to 2 hours before induction of anesthesia (may repeat once in 30 minutes), or to control acute symptoms during and after surgery (may repeat once).

IV injection – 5 to 10 mg 15 to 30 minutes before induction of anesthesia or to control acute symptoms during or after surgery. Repeat once if necessary. Prochlorperazine may be administered either undiluted or diluted in isotonic solution, but do not exceed 10 mg in a single dose of the drug. Do not exceed 5 mg/mL/min. Do not use bolus injection.

IV infusion – 20 mg/L of isotonic solution. Do not dilute in less than 1 L of isotonic solution. Add to IV infusion 15 to 30 minutes before induction.

Schizophrenia: Adjust dosage in adult psychiatric disorders to the response of the individual and according to the severity of the condition. Begin with the lowest recommended dose. Although response is ordinarily seen within 1 or 2 days, longer treatment is usually required before maximal improvement is seen.

Oral –

Mild conditions: 5 or 10 mg 3 or 4 times/day.

Moderate to severe conditions: 10 mg 3 or 4 times/day. Gradually Increase dosage until symptoms are controlled or side effects become bothersome. When dosage is increased by small increments over 2 or 3 days, side effects either do not occur or are easily controlled. Some patients respond satisfactorily on 50 to 75 mg/day.

Severe conditions: 100 to 150 mg/day.

IM – Subcutaneous administration is not advisable because of local irritation.

Inject an initial dose of 10 to 20 mg (2 to 4 mL) deeply into the upper outer quadrant of the buttock. Many patients respond shortly after the first injection. Repeat the initial dose every 2 to 4 hours (or, in resistant cases, every hour) to gain control of the patient, if necessary. More than 3 or 4 doses are seldom necessary. After control is achieved, switch patient to an oral form of the drug at the same dosage levels or higher. If, in rare cases, parenteral therapy is needed for a prolonged period, give 10 to 20 mg (2 to 4 mL) every 4 to 6 hours.

Nonpsychotic anxiety in adults:

Oral – 5 mg 3 to 4 times/day; by spansule capsule, usually one 15 mg capsule on arising or one 10 mg capsule every 12 hours. Do not administer in doses of more than 20 mg/day or for longer than 12 weeks.

Children – Do not use in pediatric patients under 20 lb or younger than 2 years of age. Do not use in conditions for which children's dosages have not been established.

Children seem more prone to develop extrapyramidal reactions, even on moderate doses. Use the lowest effective dose. Occasionally the patients may react to the drug with signs of restlessness and excitement. Do not administer additional doses if this occurs. Take particular precaution in administering the drug to children with acute illnesses or dehydration.

Adjust dosage and frequency of administration according to the severity of the symptoms and the response of the patient. The duration of activity following IM administration may last for up to 12 hours. Subsequent doses may be given by the same route, if necessary.

Control of severe nausea and vomiting:

Oral or rectal – More than 1 day of therapy is seldom necessary.

9.1 to 13.2 kg: 2.5 mg 1 or 2 times/day (not to exceed 7.5 mg/day).

13.6 to 17.7 kg: 2.5 mg 2 or 3 times/day (not to exceed 10 mg/day).

18.2 to 38.6 kg: 2.5 mg 3 times/day or 5 mg twice/day (not to exceed 15 mg/day).

IM – 0.06 mg/lb (0.132 mg/kg). Give by deep IM injection. Control is usually obtained with 1 dose. Duration of action may be 12 hours. Subsequent doses may be given if necessary.

Schizophrenia in children:

Oral or rectal – For children 2 to 12 years of age, starting dosage is 2½ mg 2 or 3 times/day. Do not give more than 10 mg on the first day. Then increase dosage according to the patient's response. When writing a prescription for the 2½ mg size suppository, write "2½", not "2.5". This will help avoid confusion with the 25 mg adult size.

Children (2 to 5 years of age): Usual total daily dose does not exceed 20 mg.

Children (6 to 12 years of age): Usual total daily dose does not exceed 25 mg.

IM – For ages under 12, calculate the dose on the basis of 0.06 mg/lb of body weight; give by deep IM injection. Control is usually obtained with 1 dose. After control is achieved, switch the patient to an oral form of the drug at the same dosage level or higher.

Elderly – Dosages in the lower range are sufficient for most elderly patients. Because they appear to be more susceptible to hypotension and neuromuscular reactions, observe patients closely. Tailor dosage to the individual, carefully monitor response, and adjust dose accordingly. Increase dosage more gradually in elderly patients.

Compatibility – Do not mix prochlorperazine injection with other agents in the syringe.

THIORIDAZINE: Dosage must be individualized and the smallest effective dosage should be determined for each patient.

Adults – Starting dose is 50 to 100 mg 3 times/day, with a gradual increment to a maximum of 800 mg/day, if necessary. Once effective control of symptoms has been achieved, the dosage may be reduced gradually to determine the minimum maintenance dose. The total daily dosage ranges from 200 to 800 mg, divided into 2 to 4 doses.

Children – For patients unresponsive to other agents, the recommended initial dose is 0.5 mg/kg/day given in divided doses. Dosage may be increased gradually until optimum therapeutic effect is obtained or the maximum dose of 3 mg/kg/day has been reached.

Oral concentrate – Concentrate may be diluted with distilled or acidified tap water or suitable juices. Dilute each dose just prior to administration; preparation and storage of bulk dilutions is not recommended.

TRIFLUOPERAZINE: Increase dosage more gradually in debilitated or emaciated patients. When maximum response is achieved, reduce dosage gradually to a maintenance level. Use the lowest effective dosage. Patients may be controlled with once- or twice-daily administration.

Schizophrenia –

Oral:

Adults – 2 to 5 mg orally twice daily. Start small or emaciated patients on the lower dosage. Most patients will show optimum response with 15 or 20 mg/day, although a few may require 40 mg/day or more. Optimum therapeutic dosage levels should be reached within 2 or 3 weeks.

Children (6 to 12 years of age) – Adjust dosage to the weight of the child and severity of the symptoms. These dosages are for children 6 to 12 years of age who are hospitalized or under close supervision. Initial dose is 1 mg once or twice daily. Dosage may be increased gradually until symptoms are controlled or until side effects become troublesome. While it is usually not necessary to exceed 15 mg/day, older children with severe symptoms may require higher doses.

Nonpsychotic anxiety – 1 or 2 mg twice daily. Do not administer more than 6 mg/day or for longer than 12 weeks because trifluoperazine use at higher doses or for longer intervals may cause persistent tardive dyskinesia that may prove irreversible.

Elderly patients – Usually, lower dosages are sufficient. The elderly appear more susceptible to hypotension and neuromuscular reactions; observe closely and increase dosage gradually.

THIOTHIXENE: Not recommended in children younger than 12 years of age.

Mild conditions – Initially, 2 mg 3 times/day. If indicated, an increase to 15 mg/day is often effective.

Severe conditions – Initially, 5 mg twice per day. Optimal is 20 to 30 mg/day. If indicated, 60 mg/day is often effective. Exceeding 60 mg/day rarely increases response.

PHENYLBUTYLPIPERADINE DERIVATIVES

HALOPERIDOL	
Tablets: 0.5, 1, 2, 5, 10, and 20 mg (*Rx*)	Various
Oral concentrate: 2 mg/mL (as lactate) (*Rx*)	Various
Injection: 5 mg/mL (as lactate) (*Rx*)	Various, *Haldol* (Janssen)
50 and 100 mg/mL (as decanoate) (*Rx*)	Various, *Haldol Decanoate* (Janssen)
PIMOZIDE	
Tablets: 1 and 2 mg (*Rx*)	*Orap* (Gate)

Indications

Haloperidol:

Psychotic disorder – For use in the management of manifestations of psychotic disorders.

Behavioral problems – For the treatment of behavioral problems in children with combative, explosive hyperexcitability that cannot be accounted for by immediate provocation. Reserve for use in these children only after failure to respond to psychotherapy or medications other than antipsychotics.

Hyperactivity – For short-term treatment of hyperactive children who show excessive motor activity with accompanying conduct disorders consisting of impulsivity, difficulty sustaining attention, aggression, mood lability, or poor frustration tolerance. Reserve for use in these children only after failure to respond to psychotherapy or medications other than antipsychotics.

Tourette disorder – For the control of tics and vocal utterances in Tourette disorder.

Pimozide:

Tourette disorder – For suppression of motor and phonic tics in patients with Tourette disorder who have failed to respond satisfactorily to standard treatment. Pimozide is not intended as a treatment of first choice, nor is it intended for the treatment of tics that are merely annoying or cosmetically troublesome. Reserve for use in Tourette disorder patients whose development or daily life function is severely compromised by the presence of motor and phonic tics.

Administration and Dosage

HALOPERIDOL: Individualize dosage. Children, debilitated, or geriatric patients and those with a history of adverse reactions to neuroleptic drugs may require less haloperidol.

Psychotic disorders –

Adults: Initial dosage: Moderate symptoms or geriatric or debilitated patients: 0.5 to 2 mg given 2 or 3 times per day; severe symptoms or chronic or resistant patients: 3 to 5 mg 2 or 3 times per day. To achieve prompt control, higher doses may be required.

Patients who remain severely disturbed or inadequately controlled may require dosage adjustment. Daily doses up to 100 mg may be necessary. Infrequently, doses more than 100 mg have been used for severely resistant patients; however, safety of prolonged administration of such doses has not been demonstrated.

Children (3 to 12 years of age; 15 to 40 kg): Do not use in children younger than 3 years of age. Initial dosage is 0.5 mg/day. If required, increase in 0.5 mg increments each 5 to 7 days until therapeutic effect is obtained. Total dose may be divided and given 2 or 3 times per day. Maintenance dosage is 0.05 to 0.15 mg/kg/day given in 2 to 3 divided doses. Upon achieving a satisfactory therapeutic response, dosage should then be gradually reduced to the lowest effective maintenance level.

IM administration: Haloperidol lactate 2 to 5 mg for prompt control of the acutely agitated patient with moderately severe to very severe symptoms. Depending on response, administer subsequent doses as often as every 60 minutes, although 4- to 8-hour intervals may be satisfactory.

The safety and efficacy of IM administration in children have not been established.

The oral form should replace the injectable as soon as it is feasible. For an approximation of the total daily dose required, use the parenteral dose administered in the preceding 24 hours; carefully monitor the patient for the first several days. Give the first oral dose within 12 to 24 hours following the last parenteral dose.

Tourette disorder –

Adults: See Psychotic disorders.

Children (3 to 12 years of age; 15 to 40 kg): See Behavioral disorders/hyperactivity.

Behavioral disorders/hyperactivity –

Children (3 to 12 years of age; 15 to 40 kg): Initial dose is 0.5 mg/day. If required, increase in 0.5 mg increments each 5 to 7 days until therapeutic effect is obtained. Maintenance dosage is 0.05 to 0.075 mg/kg/day given in 2 to 3 divided doses. Upon achieving a satisfactory therapeutic response, dosage should then be gradually reduced to the lowest effective maintenance level.

In severely disturbed, nonpsychotic children or in hyperactive children with conduct disorders, short-term administration may suffice. There is little evidence that behavior improvement is further enhanced by dosages more than 6 mg/day.

Haloperidol decanoate injection – Individualize dosage and provide close clinical supervision during initiation and stabilization of therapy. The recommended interval between doses is monthly or every 4 weeks. However, variation in patient response may dictate a need for adjustment of the dosing interval, as well as the dose. To determine the minimum effective dose, begin with lower initial doses and adjust the dose upward as needed.

Intended for use in chronic psychotic patients who require prolonged parenteral antipsychotic therapy. These patients should be previously stabilized on antipsychotic medication and should have been treated with, and well-tolerated on, short-acting haloperidol in order to exclude the possibility of an unexpected adverse sensitivity to haloperidol. Close clinical supervision is required during the initial period of dose adjustment in order to minimize the risk of overdosage or reappearance of psychotic symptoms before the next injection. During dose adjustment or episodes of exacerbation of psychotic symptoms, haloperidol decanoate therapy can be supplemented with short-acting forms of haloperidol.

Haloperidol Decanoate Dosing Recommendations[a]		
Patients	1st Month[b]	Monthly maintenance
Stabilized on low daily oral doses (≤ 10 mg/day)	10 to 15 × daily oral dose	10 to 15 × previous daily oral dose
Elderly or debilitated		
Stabilized on higher doses; risk of relapse	20 × daily oral dose	10 to 15 × previous daily oral dose
Tolerant to oral haloperidol		

[a] Clinical experience with doses greater than 450 mg/month has been limited.
[b] Initial dose should not exceed 100 mg. See below.

Initial dosage: The initial dose should not exceed 100 mg regardless of previous antipsychotic dose requirements. If the conversion requires more than haloperidol decanoate 100 mg as an initial dose, administer that dose in 2 injections (maximum of 100 mg initially followed by the balance in 3 to 7 days).

Maintenance dosage: Individualize with titration upward or downward based on therapeutic response.

Administration: Administer by deep IM injection. A 21-gauge needle is recommended. The maximum volume per injection site should not exceed 3 mL. Do not administer intravenously.

Elderly/Debilitated – Lower initial doses and more gradual adjustments are recommended.

PIMOZIDE: Introduce the drug slowly and gradually. Perform electrocardiogram at baseline and periodically thereafter, especially during dosage adjustment.

Tourette disorder –

Adults:

Initial dose – 1 to 2 mg/day in divided doses. Thereafter, increase dose every other day.

Maintenance dose – Less than 0.2 mg/kg/day or 10 mg/day, whichever is less. Do not exceed 0.2 mg/kg/day or 10 mg/day.

Children: Although Tourette disorder most often has its onset between the ages of 2 and 15 years, information on the use and efficacy of pimozide in patients younger than 12 years of age is limited.

Initiate at a dose of 0.05 mg/kg, preferably taken once at bedtime; the dose may be increased every third day to a maximum of 0.2 mg/kg, not to exceed 10 mg/day.

Gradual withdrawal – Periodically attempt to reduce dosage to see if tics persist. Increases of tic intensity and frequency may represent a transient, withdrawal-related phenomenon rather than a return of symptoms. Allow 1 or 2 weeks to elapse before concluding that an increase in tic manifestations is caused by the underlying disease rather than drug withdrawal. A gradual withdrawal is recommended in any case.

ATYPICAL ANTIPSYCHOTICS

BENZISOXAZOLE DERIVATIVES

ILOPERIDONE

Tablets; oral: 1, 2, 4, 6, 8, 10, and 12 mg (***Rx***)	*Fanapt* (Vanda Pharmaceuticals Inc)

PALIPERIDONE

Tablets, extended-release; oral: 1.5, 3, 6, and 9 mg (***Rx***)	*Invega* (Janssen)
Injection, suspension, extended-release: 39, 78, 117, 156, and 234 mg (***Rx***)	*Invega Sustenna* (Janssen)

RISPERIDONE

Tablets; oral: 0.25, 0.5, 1, 2, 3, and 4 mg (***Rx***)	Various, *Risperdal* (Janssen)
Tablets, orally disintegrating; oral: 0.5, 1, 2, 3, and 4 mg (***Rx***)	*Risperdal* M-TAB (Janssen)
Solution; oral: 1 mg/mL (***Rx***)	*Risperdal* (Janssen)
Injection, powder for solution, extended-release: 12.5, 25, 37.5, and 50 mg (***Rx***)	*Risperdal Consta* (Janssen)

ZIPRASIDONE	
Capsules; oral: 20, 40, 60, and 80 mg (as hydrochloride) (*Rx*)	*Geodon* (Pfizer)
Injection, powder for solution: 20 mg (as mesylate)/mL (*Rx*)	
BENZOISOTHIAZOL DERIVATIVES	
LURASIDONE	
Tablets; oral: 40 and 80 mg (*Rx*)	*Latuda* (Sunovion)
DIBENZAPINE DERIVATIVES	
ASENAPINE	
Tablets; sublingual: 5 and 10 mg (*Rx*)	*Saphris* (Organon)
CLOZAPINE	
Tablets; oral: 12.5 mg (*Rx*)	Various
25, 50, 100, and 200 mg (*Rx*)	Various, *Clozaril* (Novartis)
Tablets, orally disintegrating; oral: 12.5, 25, 50, and 100 mg (*Rx*)	*FazaClo* (Azur)
LOXAPINE	
Capsules; oral: 5 mg (6.8 mg as loxapine succinate), 10 mg (13.6 mg as loxapine succinate), 25 mg (34 mg as loxapine succinate), and 50 mg (68.1 mg loxapine succinate) (*Rx*)	Various, *Loxitane* (Watson)
OLANZAPINE	
Tablets; oral: 2.5, 5, 7.5, 10, 15, and 20 mg (*Rx*)	*Zyprexa* (Eli Lilly)
Tablets, orally disintegrating; oral: 5, 10, 15, and 20 mg (*Rx*)	*Zyprexa Zydis* (Eli Lilly)
Injection, powder for solution: 10 mg (*Rx*)	*Zyprexa IntraMuscular* (Eli Lilly)
Injection, powder for suspension, extended-release: 210 (as pamoate monohydrate 483 mg), 300 (as pamoate monohydrate 690 mg), and 405 mg (as pamoate monohydrate 931 mg) (*Rx*)	*Zyprexa Relprevv* (Eli Lilly)
QUETIAPINE FUMARATE	
Tablets; oral: 25, 50, 100, 200, 300, and 400 mg (as quetiapine fumarate) (*Rx*)	*Seroquel* (AstraZeneca)
Tablets, extended-release; oral: 50 (equiv. to 58 mg quetiapine fumarate), 150 (equiv. to quetiapine fumarate 173 mg), 200 (equiv. to 230 mg quetiapine fumarate), 300 (equiv. to 345 mg quetiapine fumarate), and 400 mg (equiv. to 461 mg quetiapine fumarate) (*Rx*)	*Seroquel XR* (AstraZeneca)
QUINOLINONE DERIVATIVES	
ARIPIPRAZOLE	
Tablets; oral: 2, 5, 10, 15, 20, and 30 mg (*Rx*)	*Abilify* (Otsuka America)
Tablets, orally disintegrating; oral: 10 and 15 mg (*Rx*)	*Abilify Discmelt* (Otsuka America)
Solution; oral: 1 mg/mL (*Rx*)	*Abilify* (Otsuka America)
Injection, solution: 7.5 mg/mL (*Rx*)	*Abilify* (Otsuka America)

Warning:

Increased mortality in elderly patients with dementia-related psychosis: Elderly patients with dementia-related psychosis treated with atypical antipsychotic drugs are at an increased risk of death. Analyses of 17 placebo-controlled trials (modal duration of 10 weeks), largely in patients taking atypical antipsychotic drugs, revealed a risk of death in the drug-treated patients between 1.6 and 1.7 times that seen in placebo-treated patients. Over the course of a typical 10-week controlled trial, the rate of death in drug-treated patients was about 4.5%, compared with a rate of about 2.6% in the placebo group. Although the causes of death were varied, most of the deaths appeared to be either cardiovascular (eg, heart failure, sudden death) or infectious (eg, pneumonia) in nature.

continued on next page

Warning: (cont.)

Observational studies suggest that, similar to atypical antipsychotic drugs, treatment with conventional antipsychotic drugs may increase mortality. The extent to which the findings of increased mortality in observational studies may be attributed to the antipsychotic drug as opposed to some characteristic(s) of the patient is not clear. Atypical antipsychotics are not approved for the treatment of patients with dementia-related psychosis.

Suicidality and antidepressant drugs: Antidepressants increased the risk compared with placebo of suicidal thinking and behavior (suicidality) in children, adolescents, and young adults in short-term studies of major depressive disorder (MDD) and other psychiatric disorders. Anyone considering the use of any antidepressant in a child, adolescent, or young adult must balance this risk with the clinical need.

Short-term studies did not show an increase in the risk of suicidality with antidepressants compared with placebo in adults older than 24 years of age; there was a reduction in risk with antidepressants compared with placebo in adults 65 years of age and older. Depression and certain other psychiatric disorders are themselves associated with increases in the risk of suicide. Patients of all ages who are started on antidepressant therapy should be monitored appropriately and observed closely for clinical worsening, suicidality, or unusual changes in behavior. Families and caregivers should be advised of the need for close observation and communication with the prescriber. Atypical antipsychotic agents are not approved for use in children.

Clozapine:

Agranulocytosis – Because of a significant risk of agranulocytosis, a potentially life-threatening adverse reaction, reserve clozapine for use in the treatment of severely ill patients with schizophrenia who fail to show an acceptable response to adequate courses of standard antipsychotic drug treatment or for reducing the risk of recurrent suicidal behavior in patients with schizophrenia or schizoaffective disorder who are judged to be at risk of reexperiencing suicidal behavior.

Patients being treated with clozapine must have a baseline white blood cell (WBC) count and absolute neutrophil count (ANC) before initiation of treatment as well as regular WBC counts and ANCs during treatment and for at least 4 weeks after discontinuation of treatment.

Clozapine is available only through a distribution system that ensures monitoring of WBC counts and ANCs according to the following schedule prior to delivery of the next supply of medication.

Seizures – Seizures have been associated with the use of clozapine. Dose appears to be an important predictor of seizure, with a greater likelihood at higher clozapine doses. Use caution when administering clozapine to patients who have a history of seizures or other predisposing factors. Advise patients not to engage in any activity in which sudden loss of consciousness could cause serious risk to themselves or others.

Myocarditis – Analyses of postmarketing safety databases suggest that clozapine is associated with an increased risk of fatal myocarditis, especially during, but not limited to, the first month of therapy. In patients in whom myocarditis is suspected, promptly discontinue clozapine treatment.

Other adverse cardiovascular and respiratory reactions – Orthostatic hypotension, with or without syncope, can occur with clozapine treatment. Rarely, collapse can be profound and be accompanied by respiratory and/or cardiac arrest. Orthostatic hypotension is more likely to occur during initial titration in association with rapid dose escalation. In patients who have had even a brief interval off clozapine (2 or more days since the last dose), start treatment with 12.5 mg once or twice daily.

continued on next page

Warning: (cont.)

Because collapse, respiratory arrest, and cardiac arrest during initial treatment have occurred in patients who were being administered benzodiazepines or other psychotropic drugs, caution is advised when clozapine is initiated in patients taking a benzodiazepine or any other psychotropic drug.

Olanzapine:

Postinjection delirium/sedation syndrome – Adverse reactions with signs and symptoms consistent with olanzapine overdose, in particular, sedation (including coma) and/or delirium, have been reported following injections of olanzapine extended release (ER). Olanzapine ER must be administered in a registered health care facility with ready access to emergency response services. After each injection, patients must be observed at the health care facility by a health care provider for at least 3 hours. Because of this risk, olanzapine ER is available only through a restricted distribution program called *Zyprexa Relprevv* Patient Care Program, and requires health care provider, health care facility, patient, and pharmacy enrollment.

Indications

Aripiprazole:

Bipolar mania –

Monotherapy: For the acute and maintenance treatment of manic and mixed episodes associated with bipolar I disorder with or without psychotic features in adults and children 10 to 17 years of age.

Adjunctive therapy: As adjunctive therapy to either lithium or valproate for the acute treatment of manic and mixed episodes associated with bipolar I disorder with or without psychotic features in adults and children 10 to 17 years of age.

Irritability – For the treatment of irritability associated with autistic disorder in children 6 to 17 years of age.

Major depressive disorder, adjunctive treatment – For use as an adjunctive treatment to antidepressants for the treatment of major depressive disorder in adults.

Schizophrenia –

Adults: For the acute and maintenance treatment of schizophrenia.

Adolescents: For the treatment of schizophrenia in adolescents 13 to 17 years of age.

Agitation associated with schizophrenia or bipolar mania (injection only) – For the treatment of agitation associated with schizophrenia or bipolar disorder, manic or mixed in adults.

Asenapine:

Schizophrenia – For the acute treatment of schizophrenia in adults.

Bipolar disorder – For the acute treatment of manic or mixed episodes associated with bipolar I disorder; as adjunctive therapy with lithium or valproate for the acute treatment of manic or mixed episodes associated with bipolar I disorder.

Clozapine:

Recurrent suicidal behavior (except orally disintegrating tablets) – For reducing the risk of recurrent suicidal behavior in patients with schizophrenia or schizoaffective disorder who are judged to be at chronic risk for reexperiencing suicidal behavior. Continue clozapine treatment for at least 2 years.

Schizophrenia – For the management of severely ill schizophrenic patients who fail to respond adequately to standard antipsychotic drug treatment.

Iloperidone:

Schizophrenia – For the acute treatment of adults with schizophrenia.

Loxapine:

Schizophrenia – For the treatment of schizophrenia.

Lurasidone:

Schizophrenia – For the treatment of patients with schizophrenia.

Olanzapine:

Oral –

Bipolar disorder:

Monotherapy – For the treatment of acute mixed or manic episodes associated with bipolar I disorder and for the maintenance monotherapy of bipolar disorder.

Adjunctive therapy with lithium or valproate – As an adjunct to lithium or valproate for the treatment of mixed or manic episodes associated with bipolar I disorder.

Depressive episodes associated with bipolar I disorder – In combination with fluoxetine for the treatment of depressive episodes associated with bipolar I disorder, based on clinical studies in adult patients.

Treatment-resistant depression: In combination with fluoxetine for the treatment of treatment-resistant depression (major depressive disorder in patients who do not respond to 2 separate trials of different antidepressants of adequate dose and duration in the current episode), based on clinical studies in adult patients.

Schizophrenia: For the treatment of schizophrenia.

Children: For pediatric schizophrenia and bipolar I disorder.

Injection –

Agitation associated with schizophrenia and bipolar I mania: For the treatment of agitation associated with schizophrenia and bipolar I mania.

Pamoate injection –

Schizophrenia: For the treatment of schizophrenia.

Paliperidone:

Schizoaffective disorder – For the acute treatment of schizoaffective disorder as monotherapy or as an adjunct to mood stabilizers and/or antidepressants (oral only).

Schizophrenia – For the acute and maintenance treatment of schizophrenia (oral and injectable).

Quetiapine fumarate:

Adjunctive treatment of major depressive disorder (extended-release only) – For use as adjunctive therapy to antidepressants for the treatment of MDD.

Bipolar disorder – For treatment of acute manic episodes associated with bipolar I disorder, as monotherapy or adjunct therapy to lithium or divalproex.

Quetiapine ER is indicated for the acute treatment of manic or mixed episodes associated with bipolar I disorder, both as monotherapy and as an adjunct to lithium or divalproex.

Depressive episodes: For the treatment of depressive episodes associated with bipolar disorder.

Maintenance of bipolar I disorder: For the maintenance of bipolar I disorder as adjunct therapy to lithium or divalproex.

Schizophrenia – For the treatment of schizophrenia. Quetiapine ER is indicated for the acute and maintenance treatment of schizophrenia.

Risperidone:

Bipolar mania –

Monotherapy: For the short-term treatment of acute manic or mixed episodes associated with bipolar I disorder in adults and in children and adolescents 10 to 17 years of age.

Combination therapy (adults): The combination of risperidone with lithium or valproate is indicated for the short-term treatment of adults with acute manic or mixed episodes associated with bipolar I disorder.

Irritability associated with autistic disorder – For the treatment of irritability associated with autistic disorder in children and adolescents 5 to 16 years of age, including symptoms of aggression towards others, deliberate self-injuriousness, temper tantrums, and quickly changing moods.

Schizophrenia –

Adults: For the acute and maintenance treatment of schizophrenia. For the treatment of schizophrenia.

Adolescents: For the treatment of schizophrenia in adolescents 13 to 17 years of age.

Ziprasidone:

Acute agitation (injection only) – For the treatment of acute agitation in schizophrenic patients who need intramuscular (IM) antipsychotic medication for rapid control of the agitation.

Bipolar mania (oral only) – For the treatment of acute manic or mixed episodes associated with bipolar disorder, with or without psychotic features.

Schizophrenia (oral only) – For the treatment of schizophrenia.

Administration and Dosage

ARIPIPRAZOLE: The maximum dose is 30 mg/day.

The oral solution can be substituted for tablets on a mg-per-mg basis up to the 25 mg dose level. Patients receiving 30 mg tablets should receive 25 mg of the solution. The dosing for aripiprazole orally disintegrating tablets is the same as for the oral tablets.

Bipolar disorder –

Adults:

Acute treatment – The recommended starting and target dose is 15 mg as monotherapy or as adjunctive therapy with lithium or valproate given once daily, without regard to meals. The dose can be increased to 30 mg/day based on clinical response.

Maintenance treatment – 15 or 30 mg/day.

Children (10 to 17 years of age):

Acute treatment – The recommended target dose of aripiprazole is 10 mg/day as monotherapy or as adjunctive therapy with lithium or valproate. The starting daily dose was 2 mg/day, which was titrated to 5 mg/day after 2 days and to the target dose of 10 mg/day after 2 additional days. Subsequent dose increases should be administered in 5 mg/day increments.

Maintenance treatment – 10 or 30 mg/day.

Irritability associated with autistic disorder –

Children (6 to 17 years of age): The initial dosage is 2 mg/day increased to 5 mg/day with subsequent increases to 10 to 15 mg/day, if needed. Dosage adjustments of up to 5 mg/day should occur gradually at intervals of no less than 1 week.

Major depressive disorder, adjunctive treatment –

Adults:

Acute treatment – The recommended starting dose for aripiprazole as adjunctive treatment for patients already taking an antidepressant is 2 to 5 mg/day. Dose adjustments of up to 5 mg/day should occur gradually, at intervals of no less than 1 week.

Maintenance treatment – 2 to 15 mg/day.

Schizophrenia –

Adults:

Usual dose – 10 or 15 mg once daily without regard to meals. Dosage increases should not be made before 2 weeks.

Maintenance dose – 10 to 30 mg/day when administered as the tablet formulation.

Adolescents (13 to 17 years of age):

Usual dose – Starting with an initial dosage of 2 mg/day, titrate to 5 mg after 2 days and to the target dose of 10 mg/day after 2 additional days. Subsequent dose increases should be administered in 5 mg increments.

Maintenance dose – 10 to 30 mg/day. The 30 mg/day dosage was not shown to be more effective than the 10 mg/day dosage.

Switching from other antipsychotics: While immediate discontinuation of the previous antipsychotic treatment may be acceptable for some patients with schizophrenia, gradual discontinuation may be more appropriate for others. In all cases, minimize the period of overlapping antipsychotic administration.

Major depressive disorder –

Adults:

Usual dose – Starting dose is 2 to 5 mg/day with a usual dose range of 2 to 15 mg/day. Dose adjustments of up to 5 mg/day should occur gradually, at intervals of no less than 1 week.

Orally disintegrating tablets – Do not open the blister until ready to administer. It is recommended that orally disintegrating tablets be taken without liquid. However, if needed, it can be taken with liquid. Do not attempt to split the tablet.

Oral solution – The oral solution can be given on a mg-per-mg basis in place of the 5, 10, 15, or 20 mg tablet strengths. Patients receiving 30 mg tablets should receive 25 mg of the solution.

IM injection –

Agitation associated with schizophrenia or bipolar mania: The recommended dose is 9.75 mg. The efficacy of aripiprazole injection in controlling agitation associated with schizophrenia and bipolar mania was demonstrated over a dose range of 5.25 to 15 mg. No additional benefit was demonstrated for 15 mg compared with 9.75 mg. If agitation warranting a second dose persists following the initial dose, cumulative doses up to a total of 30 mg/day may be given.

If ongoing aripiprazole therapy is indicated, oral aripiprazole in a range of 10 to 30 mg/day should replace aripiprazole injection as soon as possible.

Administration: Aripiprazole injection is intended for IM use only.

Concomitant use with potential CYP3A4 inhibitors – During coadministration with strong CYP3A4 inhibitors (eg, clarithromycin, ketoconazole), reduce the aripiprazole dose to one-half of the usual dose.

Concomitant use with potential CYP2D6 inhibitors – During coadministration with quinidine, fluoxetine, or paroxetine, reduce the aripiprazole dose to at least one-half of its normal dose.

Concomitant use with potential CYP3A4 inducers – When a potential CYP3A4 inducer such as carbamazepine is added to aripiprazole, double the aripiprazole dose to 20 to 30 mg. Base additional dose increases on clinical evaluation. When carbamazepine is withdrawn, reduce the aripiprazole dose to 10 to 15 mg.

ASENAPINE:

Schizophrenia – 5 mg twice daily increasing up to 10 mg twice daily after 1 week based on tolerability.

Bipolar disorder – 10 mg twice daily. The dose can be decreased to 5 mg twice daily if there are adverse effects.

Adjunctive therapy: 5 mg twice daily increasing to 10 mg twice daily depending on the clinical response and tolerabilty. Administer with lithium or valproate.

Hepatic function impairment – Asenapine is not recommended in patients with severe hepatic impairment.

Switching from other antipsychotics – While immediate discontinuation of the previous antipsychotic treatment may be acceptable for some patients with schizophrenia, more gradual discontinuation may be most appropriate for others. In all cases, the period of overlapping antipsychotic administration should be minimized.

Administration – For sublingual use only. Instruct patients to place the tablet under the tongue and allow it to dissolve completely. The tablet will dissolve in saliva within seconds. The tablet should not be crushed, chewed, or swallowed. Patients should be instructed to not eat or drink for 10 minutes after administration and to handle the tablets with dry hands.

CLOZAPINE:

Initial treatment – Begin treatment with a 12.5 mg dose once or twice daily. If a half-tablet of the orally disintegrating tablet is used to achieve the 12.5 mg dose, the remaining one-half tablet should be destroyed. Continue with daily dosage increments of 25 to 50 mg/day to achieve a target dose of 300 to 450 mg/day by the end of 2 weeks. Subsequent dosage increments should be made no more than once or twice weekly, in increments not to exceed 100 mg.

Maximum dosage – Dosing should not exceed 900 mg/day.

Discontinuation – Gradual reduction in dose is recommended over a 1- to 2-week period. However, if a patient's medical condition requires abrupt discontinuation (eg, leukopenia), observe the patient for the recurrence of psychotic symptoms and symptoms related to cholinergic rebound, such as headache, nausea, vomiting, and diarrhea.

Reinitiation of treatment – When restarting patients who have had even a brief interval off clozapine (ie, 2 days or more since the last dose), treatment should be reinitiated with a 12.5 mg dose once or twice daily. If a half-tablet is used to achieve the 12.5 mg dose, the remaining one-half tablet should be destroyed. If that dose is well tolerated, it may be feasible to titrate patients back to a therapeutic dose more quickly than is recommended for initial treatment. However, any patient who has previously experienced respiratory or cardiac arrest with initial dosing, but was then able to be successfully titrated to a therapeutic dose, should be retitrated with extreme caution even after 24 hours of discontinuation.

Patients discontinued for WBC counts less than 2,000/mm^3 or an ANC less than 1,000/mm^3 must not be restarted on clozapine.

Recurrent suicidal behavior (except orally disintegrating tablets) – The dosage and administration recommendations outlined previously regarding the use of clozapine in patients with treatment-resistant schizophrenia should also be followed when treating patients with schizophrenia or schizoaffective disorder at risk for recurrent suicidal behavior.

Orally disintegrating tablets – Just prior to use, instruct patient to remove the orally disintegrating tablet, immediately place the tablet in the mouth, and allow it to disintegrate.

ILOPERIDONE: Iloperidone must be titrated slowly to avoid orthostatic hypotension because of its alpha-adrenergic blocking properties.

Maximum dose – 12 mg twice daily (24 mg/day).

Initial dosage – 1 mg twice daily on day 1.

Dosage titration – 2, 4, 6, 8, 10, and 12 mg twice daily on days 2, 3, 4, 5, 6, and 7, respectively. Control of symptoms may be delayed during the first 1 to 2 weeks of treatment.

Maintenance dosage – 6 to 12 mg twice daily.

Concomitant therapy –

CYP2D6 inhibitors: Reduce iloperidone dose by one-half when coadministered with strong CYP2D6 inhibitors such as fluoxetine or paroxetine.

CYP3A4 inhibitors: Reduce iloperidone dose by one-half when coadministered with strong CYP3A4 inhibitors such as ketoconazole or clarithromycin.

Elderly – Exercise vigilance when electing to treat elderly patients.

Hepatic function impairment – Iloperidone is not recommended.

Reinitiation of treatment in patients previously discontinued – It is recommended that the initiation titration schedule be followed whenever patients have had an interval of more than 3 days off iloperidone.

Switching from other antipsychotics – The period of overlapping antipsychotic administration should be minimized.

Poor metabolizers of CYP2D6 – Have higher exposure to iloperidone compared with extensive metabolizers.

Administration – Can be administered without regard to meals.

LOXAPINE: Administer 2 to 4 times/day in divided doses.

Initial dosage – 10 mg twice/day. In severely disturbed patients, up to 50 mg/day may be desirable. Increase dosage rapidly over 7 to 10 days until symptoms are controlled.

Maintenance – The usual range is 60 to 100 mg/day. Dosage higher than 250 mg/day is not recommended.

LURASIDONE: Take with food (at least 350 calories).

Schizophrenia – 40 to 80 mg/day with a maximum dose of 80 mg/day.

Cytochrome P450 3A4 inhibitors: When coadministration with a moderate cytochrome P450 3A4 (CYP3A4) inhibitor such as diltiazem is considered, the dosage should not exceed 40 mg/day. Do not use in combination with a strong CYP3A4 inhibitor (eg, ketoconazole).

CYP3A4 inducers: Do not use in combination with a strong CYP3A4 inducer (eg, rifampin).

Moderate to severe renal impairment – Do not exceed 40 mg/day.

Moderate to severe hepatic impairment – Do not exceed 40 mg/day.

OLANZAPINE: Oral formulation may be taken without regard to meals.

Adults –

Bipolar mania:

Monotherapy – Initial dose is 10 to 15 mg/day without regard to meals. Adjust dosage at 5 mg increments in intervals of not less than 24 hours. Maintenance dose is 5 to 20 mg/day.

Adjunctive therapy – When coadministered with lithium or valproate, generally begin with 10 mg once daily without regard to meals; the usual dose is 5 to 20 mg/day.

Depressive episodes associated with bipolar I disorder – Olanzapine 5 mg and fluoxetine 20 mg once daily in the evening, without regard to meals. Dosage adjustments, if indicated, can be made according to efficacy and tolerability within dose ranges of oral olanzapine 5 to 12.5 mg and fluoxetine 20 to 50 mg.

Treatment-resistant depression: Olanzapine 5 mg and fluoxetine 20 mg once daily in the evening, without regard to meals. Dosage adjustments, if indicated, can be made according to efficacy and tolerability within dose ranges of olanzapine 5 to 12.5 mg and fluoxetine 20 to 50 mg.

Schizophrenia:

Oral – Initial dose is 5 to 10 mg once daily without regard to meals, with a target dose of 10 mg/day within several days of initiation. Adjust dosage at 5 mg/day increments in intervals not less than 1 week. Maintenance dosage is between 10 to 20 mg/day.

Extended-release injection – Be aware that there are 2 olanzapine intramuscular (IM) formulations with different dosing schedules. Olanzapine short-acting (10 mg/vial) formulation should not be confused with olanzapine ER.

Establish tolerability with oral olanzapine prior to initiating treatment with olanzapine ER.

The usual dosage is 150 to 300 mg every 2 weeks or 405 mg every 4 weeks.

Recommended Dosing for Extended-Release Olanzapine Based on Correspondence to Oral Olanzapine Doses

Target oral olanzapine dosage	Dosing of olanzapine ER during the first 8 weeks	Maintenance dose after 8 weeks of olanzapine ER treatment
10 mg/day	210 mg per 2 weeks or 405 mg per 4 weeks	150 mg per 2 weeks or 300 mg per 4 weeks
15 mg/day	300 mg per 2 weeks	210 mg per 2 weeks or 405 mg per 4 weeks
20 mg/day	300 mg per 2 weeks	300 mg per 2 weeks

Olanzapine ER injection is intended for deep IM gluteal injection only. Do not administer either formulations intravenously or subcutaneously.

Agitation associated with schizophrenia and bipolar I mania (IM): Usual dose is 10 mg. A lower dose of 5 or 7.5 mg may be considered. Subsequent doses up to 10 mg may be given. Maximal dosing of IM olanzapine (eg, 3 doses of 10 mg given 2 to 4 hours apart) may be associated with significant orthostatic hypotension.

If ongoing olanzapine therapy is indicated, oral olanzapine may be initiated in a range of 5 to 20 mg/day as soon as clinically appropriate.

Children –

13 years of age and older (oral):

Bipolar I disorder – 2.5 or 5 mg without regard to meals, with a maintenance dosage of 10 mg/day. Dose increments/decrements of 2.5 to 5 mg are recommended.

Schizophrenia – 2.5 or 5 mg without regard to meals, with a maintenance dosage of 10 mg/day. Dose increments/decrements of 2.5 to 5 mg are recommended.

Elderly – Consider a lower starting dose for any elderly patient if factors are present that might decrease pharmacokinetic clearance or increase the pharmacodynamic response to olanzapine.

Special populations – The recommended starting dose for schizophrenia is 5 mg in patients who are debilitated, who have a predisposition to hypotensive reactions, who exhibit a combination of factors that may result in slower metabolism of olanzapine (eg, nonsmoking women 65 years of age and older), or who may be more sensitive to olanzapine.

Immediate-release injection: A lower dose of 2.5 mg per injection should be considered for patients who otherwise might be debilitated, predisposed to hypotensive reactions, or more pharmocodynamically sensitive to olanzapine.

Extended-release injection: The recommended starting dose is 150 mg per 4 weeks in patients who are debilitated, who have a predisposition to hypotensive reactions, who otherwise exhibit a combination of factors that may result in slower metabolism of olanzapine (eg, nonsmoking women 65 years of age and older), or who may be more pharmacodynamically sensitive to olanzapine. Dose escalation should be undertaken with caution in these patients.

Administration of orally disintegrating tablets – Peel back foil on blister. Using dry hands, remove and place the entire tablet in the mouth. The tablet will disintegrate rapidly in saliva so it can be easily swallowed with or without liquid.

Admixture compatibility – Olanzapine injection should be reconstituted only with sterile water for injection. Olanzapine injection should not be combined in a syringe with diazepam injection. Lorazepam injection should not be used to reconstitute olanzapine injection. Olanzapine injection should not be combined in a syringe with haloperidol injection.

Olanzapine ER must be suspended using only the diluent provided in the convenience kit.

PALIPERIDONE:

Oral –

Dosage: 6 mg once daily, administered in the morning. Dose increases more than 6 mg/day should be made only after clinical reassessment and generally should occur at intervals of more than 5 days in increments of 3 mg/day. The maximum recommended dose is 12 mg/day (usual range, 3 to 12 mg/day).

Administration: Paliperidone can be taken with or without food.

Paliperidone must be swallowed whole with the aid of liquids. Tablets should not be chewed, divided, or crushed. The medication is contained within a nonabsorbable shell designed to release the drug at a controlled rate. The tablet shell, along with insoluble core components, is eliminated from the body.

Special populations:

Renal function impairment – For patients with mild renal function impairment (creatinine clearance [CrCl] 50 to less than 80 mL/min), the maximum recommended dose is 6 mg once daily. For patients with moderate to severe renal function impairment (CrCl 10 to less than 50 mL/min), the maximum recommended dose is 3 mg once daily.

Injection –

Recommended dosing: For patients who have never taken oral paliperidone or oral or injectable risperidone, it is recommended to establish tolerability with oral paliperidone or oral risperidone prior to initiating treatment with paliperidone injection.

Recommended initiation is with a dose of 234 mg on treatment day 1 and 156 mg one week later, both administered in the deltoid muscle. The recommended monthly maintenance dose is 117 mg; some patients may benefit from lower or higher maintenance doses within the recommended range of 39 to 234 mg based on individual patient tolerability and/or efficacy. Following the second dose, monthly maintenance doses can be administered in either the deltoid or gluteal muscle.

Adjustment of the maintenance dose may be made monthly.

Maintenance therapy: It is recommended that responding patients be continued on treatment at the lowest effective dose needed. Patients should be periodically reassessed to determine the need for continued treatment.

Switching from other antipsychotics:

Switching from oral antipsychotics – Previous oral antipsychotics can be discontinued at the time of initiation of treatment with paliperidone injection, Patients previously stabilized on different doses of paliperidone extended-release tablets can attain similar paliperidone steady-state exposure during maintenance treatment with paliperidone injection monthly doses as depicted in the following table.

Doses of Oral Paliperidone and IM Paliperidone Needed to Attain Similar Paliperidone Exposure at Steady-State

Formulation	Paliperidone extended-release tablets	Paliperidone injection
Dosing frequency	Once daily	Once every 4 weeks
Dose (mg)	12	234
	6	117
	3	39 to 78

Switching from long-acting antipsychotics – When switching patients from previous long-acting injectable antipsychotics, initiate paliperidone injection in place of the next scheduled injection. Paliperidone should then be continued at monthly intervals. The 1-week initiation dosing regimen as described in Recommended Dosing is not required.

Missed doses:

Avoiding missed doses – It is recommended that the second initiation dose of paliperidone be given 1 week after the first dose. Similarly, the third and subsequent injections after the initiation regimen are recommended to be given monthly.

To avoid a missed dose, patients may be given the second dose 2 days before or after the 1-week time point. To avoid a missed monthly dose, patients may be given the injection up to 7 days before or after the monthly time point.

Missed dose (1 month to 6 weeks) – After initiation, the recommended injection cycle of paliperidone is monthly.

If less than 6 weeks have elapsed since the last injection, the previously stabilized dose should be administered as soon as possible, followed by injections at monthly intervals.

Missed dose (more than 6 weeks to 6 months) – If more than 6 weeks have elapsed since the last injection of paliperidone, resume the same dose the patient was previously stabilized on (unless the patient was stabilized on a dose of 234 mg, then the first 2 injections should each be 156 mg) in the following manner: 1) a deltoid injection as soon as practically possible, followed by 2) another deltoid injection (same dose) 1 week later, and 3) resumption of either deltoid or gluteal dosing at monthly intervals.

Missed dose (more than 6 months) – If more than 6 months have elapsed since the last injection of paliperidone, initiate dosing as described in Recommended Dosing.

Elderly: In general, recommended dosing of paliperidone for elderly patients with healthy renal function is the same as for younger adult patients with healthy renal function.

Renal function impairment: For patients with mild renal impairment (CrCl of at least 50 mL/min to less than 80 mL/min), recommended initiation of paliperidone is with a dose of 156 mg on treatment day 1 and 117 mg 1 week later, both administered in the deltoid muscle. Thereafter, follow with monthly injections of 78 mg in either the deltoid or gluteal muscle.

Paliperidone is not recommended in patients with moderate or severe renal impairment (CrCl less than 50 mL/min).

Hepatic function impairment: Paliperidone has not been studied in patients with hepatic function impairment.

Administration: Paliperidone injection is intended for IM use only. Inject slowly, deep into the muscle. Do not administer the dose in divided injections. Do not administer intravascularly or subcutaneously.

Concomitant medications – Because paliperidone is the major active metabolite of risperidone, consideration should be given to the additive paliperidone exposure if risperidone is coadministered with paliperidone.

QUETIAPINE FUMARATE:

Adults –

Immediate-release: Quetiapine immediate release can be taken with or without food.

Bipolar disorder –

Depressive episodes: Administer once daily at bedtime to reach 300 mg/day by day 4. The dosing schedule is 50, 100, 200, and 300 mg/day for days 1 through 4.

Acute manic episodes: Initiate in twice-daily doses totaling 100 mg/day on day 1, increased to 400 mg/day on day 4 in increments of up to 100 mg/day in twice-daily doses. Further dosage adjustments up to 800 mg/day by day 6 should be in increments of no more than 200 mg/day. Dosages more than 800 mg/day have not been evaluated.

Maintenance: Maintenance of efficacy in bipolar I disorder was demonstrated with quetiapine (administered twice daily totaling 400 to 800 mg/day) as adjunct therapy to lithium or divalproex.

Schizophrenia –

Usual dose: Initial dose of 25 mg twice/day, with increases in increments of 25 to 50 mg 2 or 3 times/day on the second and third day to a target dose range of 300 to 400 mg/day by the fourth day. Dose increments/decrements of 25 to 50 mg twice/day at intervals of at least 2 days are recommended. Dosages more than 800 mg/day have not been evaluated.

ER: Quetiapine ER tablets should be swallowed whole and not split, chewed, or crushed. It is recommended that quetiapine ER be taken without food or with a light meal.

Bipolar disorder –

Acute manic episodes: Initial dosage is 300 mg on day 1 and 600 mg on day 2, once daily in the evening. Dose may be adjusted between 400 and 800 mg beginning on day 3, depending on the response and tolerance of the individual patient.

Depressive episodes: 50 mg on day 1; 100 mg on day 2; 200 mg on day 3; 300 mg on day 4 given once daily in the evening.

Major depressive disorder, adjunctive therapy with antidepressants – 50 mg once daily in the evening. On day 3, the dose can be increased to 150 mg once daily in the evening. Dosages above 300 mg/day were not studied.

Schizophrenia – 300 mg/day once daily, preferably in the evening. Dose increases can be made at intervals as short as 1 day and in increments of 300 mg/day. Patients should be titrated within a dose range of 400 to 800 mg/day.

Children –

Immediate release:

Bipolar I disorder, acute manic episodes (10 to 17 years of age) – Efficacy was demonstrated at 400 and 600 mg.

Initial dosage: The total daily dose for the initial 5 days of therapy is 50 (day 1), 100 (day 2), 200 (day 3), 300 (day 4), and 400 mg (day 5).

Dosage adjustment: After day 5, the dose should be adjusted within the recommended dosage range of 400 to 600 mg/day, based on response and tolerability. Dosage adjustments should be in increments of no greater than 100 mg/day.

Schizophrenia (13 to 17 years of age) –

Initial dosage: The total daily dose for the initial 5 days of therapy is 50 (day 1), 100 (day 2), 200 (day 3), 300 (day 4), and 400 mg (day 5). The usual dosage is 400 to 800 mg/day.

Dosage adjustment: After day 5, the dose should be adjusted within the recommended dosage range of 400 to 800 mg/day based on response and tolerability. Dosage adjustments should be in increments of no greater than 100 mg/day.

Maintenance dosage – It is generally recommended that responding patients be continued at the lowest dose needed to maintain remission.

Elderly and debilitated patients – Consider a slower rate of dose titration and a lower target dose. When indicated, dose escalation should be performed with caution in these patients.

Start elderly patients on quetiapine ER 50 mg/day; the dosage can be increased in increments of 50 mg/day, depending on the response and tolerance.

Hepatic function impairment –

Immediate release: Start patients on quetiapine immediate release 25 mg/day. Increase daily dosage in increments of 25 to 50 mg/day to an effective dosage, depending on the clinical response and tolerability.

Extended release: Start patients on quetiapine ER 50 mg/day. Increase daily dosage in increments of 50 mg/day to an effective dosage, depending on the clinical response and tolerance.

Reinitiation of treatment – When restarting patients who have discontinued quetiapine ER for an interval of less than 1 week, titration of quetiapine is not required and the maintenance dose may be reinitiated. When restarting therapy for patients who have discontinued quetiapine immediate release for longer than 1 week, the initial titration schedule should be followed.

Switching patients from IR to ER tablets – Schizophrenic patients who are currently being treated with divided doses of quetiapine IR may be switched to quetiapine ER at the equivalent total daily dose taken once daily.

Switching from other antipsychotics – The period of overlapping antipsychotic administration should be minimized. When switching patients with schizophrenia from depot antipsychotics, initiate quetiapine therapy in place of the next scheduled injection.

Coadministration with enzyme inducers – The elimination of quetiapine was enhanced in the presence of phenytoin. Higher maintenance doses may be required when it is coadministered with phenytoin and other enzyme inducers such as carbamazepine and phenobarbital.

RISPERIDONE:

Bipolar mania –

Oral:

Adults – Administer on a once-daily schedule, starting with 2 to 3 mg/day. Adjust dosage at intervals of not less than 24 hours and in increments/decrements of 1 mg/day. Doses higher than 6 mg/day were not studied.

Children – Initiate at 0.5 mg once daily, as a once-daily dose in either the morning or evening. Dosage adjustments should occur at intervals of not less than 24 hours in increments of 0.5 or 1 mg/day, as tolerated, to a recommended dose of 2.5 mg/day. Doses higher than 6 mg/day have not been studied.

Patients experiencing persistent somnolence may benefit from administering half the daily dose twice daily.

Injection: 25 mg IM every 2 weeks. Some patients may benefit from a higher dose of 37.5 or 50 mg.

Irritability associated with autistic disorder (oral) –

Oral: Initiate at 0.25 mg/day for patients weighing less than 20 kg and 0.5 mg/day for patients at least 20 kg. After a minimum of 4 days from treatment initiation, the dose may be increased to the recommended dose of 0.5 mg/day for patients weighing less than 20 kg and 1 mg/day for patients at least 20 kg. This dose should be maintained for a minimum of 14 days. In patients not achieving sufficient clinical response, dose increases may be considered at intervals of at least 2 weeks in increments of 0.25 mg/day for patients weighing less than 20 kg or 0.5 mg/day for patients at least 20 kg. Caution should be exercised with dosage for smaller children who weigh less than 15 kg.

Patients experiencing persistent somnolence may benefit from a once-daily dose administered at bedtime, administering half the daily dose twice daily, or a reduction of the dose.

Schizophrenia –

Oral:

Adults –

Usual initial dose: Administer once or twice daily. Initial dosing is generally 2 mg/day. Dose increases should then occur at intervals not less than 24 hours, in increments of 1 to 2 mg/day to a recommended dose of 4 to 8 mg/day. In some patients, slower titration may be appropriate. Doses above 6 mg/day for twice-daily dosing were associated with more extrapyramidal symptoms and other adverse reactions, and are generally not recommended. The safety of doses more than 16 mg/day has not been evaluated.

Adolescents – Initiate at 0.5 mg once daily, administered as a once-daily dose in either the morning or evening. Dosage adjustments, if indicated, should occur at intervals not less than 24 hours in increments of 0.5 or 1 mg/day, as tolerated, to a recommended dose of 3 mg/day. Doses higher than 6 mg/day have not been studied.

Patients experiencing persistent somnolence may benefit from administering half the daily dose twice daily.

Reinitiation of treatment – When restarting patients who have had an interval off risperidone, follow the initial titration schedule.

Special populations – Recommended initial oral dose is 0.5 mg twice daily in patients who are elderly, debilitated, have severe renal or hepatic function impairment, are predisposed to hypotension, or in whom hypotension would pose a risk. Adjust oral dose at increments of no more than 0.5 mg twice daily. Increase to dosages above 1.5 mg twice daily at intervals of at least 1 week. Slower titration may be appropriate.

Once-daily oral dosing in the elderly or debilitated may occur after titration on a twice-daily regimen for 2 to 3 days at the target dose.

Injection: 25 mg IM every 2 weeks.

Maintenance treatment – Once sufficient clinical response has been achieved and maintained, consideration should be given to gradually lowering the dose to achieve the optimal balance of efficacy and safety.

Oral solution administration – The oral solution can be mixed with water, coffee, orange juice, or low-fat milk; it is not compatible with cola or tea.

Orally disintegrating tablet administration – Remove the tablet from the blister unit, and immediately place the entire tablet on the tongue. Consume the tablet immediately; swallow with or without liquid. Do not split or chew the tablet.

Injection – For patients who have never taken oral risperidone, establish tolerability with oral risperidone prior to initiating treatment with injectable risperidone.

The recommended dose is 25 mg IM every 2 weeks. The maximum dose should not exceed risperidone 50 mg injection every 2 weeks.

Give oral risperidone or another antipsychotic medication with the first risperidone injection and continue for 3 weeks (then discontinue) to ensure that adequate therapeutic plasma concentrations are maintained prior to the main release phase of risperidone.

Dose adjustments: Do not make upward dosage adjustments more frequently than every 4 weeks.

Administration of IM: Administer risperidone injection every 2 weeks by deep IM gluteal injection. Alternate injections between buttocks. Do not administer IV.

Do not combine 2 different dosage strengths of risperidone injection in a single administration.

Renal/Hepatic function impairment: The starting dose is oral risperidone 0.5 mg twice daily during the first week, increased to 1 mg twice daily or 2 mg once daily during the second week. If at least 2 mg of oral risperidone is well tolerated, an injection of risperidone 25 mg can be administered every 2 weeks. Continue oral supplementation for 3 weeks after the first injection until the main release of risperidone injection.

Concomitant therapy: Coadministration of carbamazepine and other enzyme inducers (eg, phenytoin, rifampin, phenobarbital) with risperidone would be expected to cause decreases in the plasma concentrations of risperidone, which could lead to decreased efficacy of risperidone treatment. The dose of risperidone needs to be titrated accordingly for patients receiving these enzyme inducers, especially during initiation or discontinuation of therapy with these inducers.

Fluoxetine and paroxetine have been shown to increase the plasma concentration of risperidone. When initiation of fluoxetine or paroxetine is considered, patients may be placed on a lower dose of risperidone between 2 to 4 weeks before the planned start of fluoxetine or paroxetine therapy.

Patients who have a history of poor tolerability to psychotropic medications: A lower initial dose of 12.5 mg IM may be appropriate.

Switching from other antipsychotic agents –

Oral: Immediate discontinuation of the previous antipsychotic treatment may be acceptable for some patients; gradual discontinuation may be more appropriate. In all cases, minimize the period of overlapping antipsychotic administration. When switching patients from a depot antipsychotic, initiate risperidone therapy in place of the next scheduled injection.

Injection: Previous antipsychotics should be continued for 3 weeks after the first injection of risperidone to ensure that therapeutic concentrations are maintained until the main release phase of risperidone from the injection site has begun. For schizophrenic patients who have never taken oral risperidone, it is recommended to establish tolerability with oral risperidone prior to initiating treatment with risperidone injection. As recommended with other antipsychotic medications, the need for continuing existing extrapyramidal symptom medication should be reevaluated periodically.

ZIPRASIDONE:

Bipolar mania –

Initial treatment: 40 mg twice/day with food. Increase to 60 or 80 mg twice/day on the second day. Usual dose range 40 to 80 mg twice/day.

Schizophrenia –

Initial treatment: 20 mg twice/day with food. Daily dosage may be adjusted up to 80 mg twice/day. Dosage adjustments should occur at intervals of not less than 2 days. Doses more than 80 mg twice daily are not recommended. The safety of doses more than 100 mg twice daily has not been evaluated.

Acute agitation – 10 to 20 mg administered as required up to a maximum dose of 40 mg/day. Doses of 10 mg may be administered every 2 hours; doses of 20 mg may be administered every 4 hours up to a maximum of 40 mg/day. IM administration of ziprasidone for more than 3 consecutive days has not been studied.

If long-term therapy is indicated, oral ziprasidone capsules should replace IM administration as soon as possible.

Coadministration of ziprasidone IM to schizophrenic patients already taking oral ziprasidone is not recommended.

Contraindications

Clozapine: Hypersensitivity to clozapine or any other component of the drug; uncontrolled epilepsy; myeloproliferative disorders; history of clozapine-induced agranulocytosis or severe granulocytopenia; simultaneous administration with other agents having a well-known potential to cause agranulocytosis or otherwise suppress bone marrow function; severe CNS depression or comatose states from any cause. Causative factors of agranulocytosis may interact synergistically to increase the risk or severity of bone marrow suppression.

LITHIUM

Capsules: 150 mg lithium carbonate (4.06 mEq lithium) (*Rx*)	*Lithium Carbonate* (Roxane)
300 mg lithium carbonate (8.12 mEq lithium) (*Rx*)	Various, *Eskalith* (SKB), *Lithonate* (Solvay Pharm.)
600 mg lithium carbonate (16.24 mEq lithium) (*Rx*)	*Lithium Carbonate* (Roxane)
Tablets: 300 mg lithium carbonate (8.12 mEq lithium) (*Rx*)	Various, *Lithane* (Miles Pharm.), *Lithotabs* (Solvay Pharm.)
Tablets, slow release: 300 mg lithium carbonate (8.12 mEq lithium) (*Rx*)	*Lithobid* (Noven Therapeutics)
Syrup: 8 mEq lithium (as citrate equivalent to 300 mg lithium carbonate) per 5 mL (*Rx*)	Various

Warning:
Toxicity is closely related to serum lithium levels and can occur at therapeutic doses. Facilities for serum lithium determinations are required to monitor therapy.

Indications

Mania: For the treatment of manic episodes of manic-depressive illness. Maintenance therapy prevents or diminishes the frequency and intensity of subsequent manic episodes in those manic-depressive patients with a history of mania.

Unlabeled uses: Lithium carbonate (300 to 1,000 mg/day) has improved the neutrophil count in patients with cancer chemotherapy-induced neutropenia, in children with chronic neutropenia, and in AIDS patients receiving zidovudine.

Administration and Dosage

Individualize dosage according to both serum levels and clinical response.

Serum lithium levels: Draw blood samples immediately prior to the next dose (8 to 12 hours after the previous dose) when lithium concentrations are relatively stable. Do not rely on serum levels alone.

Acute mania: Optimal patient response is usually established and maintained with 600 mg 3 times/day or 900 mg twice/day for the slow release form. Such doses normally produce an effective serum lithium level ranging between 1 and 1.5 mEq/L.

Determine serum levels twice weekly during the acute phase, and until the serum level and clinical condition of the patient have been stabilized.

Long-term use: The desirable serum levels are 0.6 to 1.2 mEq/L. Dosage will vary, but 300 mg 3 to 4 times/day will usually maintain this level. Monitor serum levels in uncomplicated cases on maintenance therapy during remission every 2 to 3 months.

Actions

Pharmacology: Lithium alters sodium transport in nerve and muscle cells, and effects a shift toward intraneuronal catecholamine metabolism. The specific mechanism in mania is unknown, but it affects neurotransmitters associated with affective disorders. Its antimanic effects may be the result of increases in norepinephrine reuptake and increased serotonin receptor sensitivity.

Pharmacokinetics:

Absorption/Distribution – Lithium is readily absorbed from the GI tract. Peak serum levels occur in 0.5 to 3 hours and absorption is complete within 8 hours. Onset of action is slow (5 to 14 days). Until the desired therapeutic effect is attained, maintain a steady-state serum level of 0.8 to 1.4 mEq/L, then slowly decrease the lithium dose to a maintenance level. The therapeutic serum level range is from 0.4 to 1 mEq/L.

Excretion – About 95% of the lithium dose is eliminated by the kidney.

Warnings/Precautions

High-risk patients: The risk of lithium toxicity is very high in patients with significant renal or cardiovascular disease, severe debilitation, dehydration, or sodium depletion, or in patients receiving diuretics. Undertake treatment with extreme caution.

Encephalopathic syndrome: Encephalopathic syndrome has occurred in a few patients given lithium plus a neuroleptic. In some instances, irreversible brain damage occurred. Monitor closely for evidence of neurologic toxicity.

Infection: Concomitant infection with elevated temperature may necessitate a temporary reduction or cessation of medication.

Hazardous tasks: Observe caution while driving or performing other tasks requiring alertness.

Tolerance of lithium: Tolerance of lithium is greater during the acute manic phase and decreases when manic symptoms subside.

Hypothyroidism: Hypothyroidism may occur with long-term lithium administration. Patients may develop enlargement of thyroid gland and increased thyroid-stimulating hormone levels.

Sodium depletion: Lithium decreases renal sodium reabsorption, which could lead to sodium depletion. Therefore, the patient must maintain a normal diet (including salt) and an adequate fluid intake (2,500 to 3,000 mL).

Parameters to monitor: Perform the following laboratory tests prior to and periodically during lithium therapy: Serum creatinine; complete blood count; urinalysis; sodium and potassium; fasting glucose; electrocardiogram; and thyroid function tests. Check lithium serum levels twice weekly until dosage is stabilized. Once steady state has been reached, monitor the level weekly. Once the patient is on maintenance therapy, the level may be checked every 2 to 3 months.

Renal function impairment: Morphologic changes with glomerular and interstitial fibrosis and nephron atrophy have occurred in patients on chronic lithium therapy. The relationship between such changes and renal function has not been established.

Acquired nephrogenic diabetes insipidus – Acquired nephrogenic diabetes insipidus unresponsive to vasopressin has been associated with chronic lithium administration. Polydipsia and polyuria occur frequently. The mechanism is thought to be the decreased response of the renal tubules to the antidiuretic hormone causing decreased reabsorption of water. Impairment of the concentrating ability of the kidneys is reversed when lithium therapy is discontinued. Management may involve decreasing the dose, discontinuing lithium, or the cautious use of a thiazide diuretic or amiloride. Monitor the patient's renal status.

Pregnancy: *Category D.*

Lactation: Lithium is excreted in breast milk. Do not nurse during lithium therapy.

Children: Safety and efficacy for use in children younger than 12 years of age have not been established.

Elderly: The decreased rate of excretion in the elderly contributes to a high incidence of toxic effects. Use lower doses and more frequent monitoring.

Drug Interactions

Drugs that may affect lithium include acetazolamide, carbamazepine, fluoxetine, haloperidol, loop diuretics, methyldopa, NSAIDs, osmotic diuretics, theophyllines, thiazide diuretics, urinary alkalinizers, and verapamil.

Drugs that may be affected by lithium include phenothiazines, sympathomimetics, iodide salts, neuromuscular blocking agents, and tricyclic antidepressants.

Adverse Reactions

Adverse reactions may include arrhythmia; hypotension; peripheral circulatory collapse; bradycardia; sinus node dysfunction with severe bradycardia; ECG changes; tremor; muscle hyperirritability; ataxia; choreoathetotic movements; hyperactive deep tendon reflexes; pseudotumor cerebri; euthyroid goiter; hypothyroidism; EEG changes; blackout spells; epileptiform seizures; slurred speech; dizziness; vertigo; incontinence of urine or feces; somnolence; psychomotor retardation; restlessness; confusion; stupor; coma; acute dystonia; downbeat nystagmus; blurred vision; startled response; hypertonicity; slowed intellectual functioning; hallucinations; poor memory; tongue movements; tics; tinnitus; cog wheel rigidity; anorexia; nausea; vomiting; diarrhea; dry mouth; gastritis; salivary gland swelling; abdominal pain; excessive salivation; flatulence; indigestion; albuminuria; oliguria; glycosuria; decreased Ccr; symptoms of nephrogenic diabetes; drying and thinning of hair; anesthesia of skin; chronic folliculitis; xerosis cutis; alopecia; exacerbation of psoriasis; acne; angioedema; fatigue; lethargy; sleepiness; dehydration; weight loss; transient scotomata; impotence; sexual dysfunction; dysgeusia; taste distortion; tightness in chest; hypercalcemia; hyperparathyroidism; salty taste; swollen lips; swollen, painful joints; fever; polyarthralgia; dental caries; leukocytosis; headache; transient hyperglycemia; generalized pruritus with or without rash; cutaneous ulcers; worsening of organic brain syndromes; excessive weight gain; edematous swelling of ankles or wrists; thirst or polyuria, sometimes resembling diabetes insipidus; metallic taste; painful discoloration of fingers and toes and coldness of the extremities.

MEMANTINE

Tablets: 5 and 10 mg (*Rx*)	*Namenda* (Forest Laboratories)
Oral solution: 2 mg/mL (*Rx*)	
Capsules, extended-release: 7, 14, 21, and 28 mg (*Rx*)	*Namenda XR* (Forest Laboratories)

Indications

Alzheimer disease: For the treatment of moderate to severe dementia of the Alzheimer type.

Administration and Dosage

Memantine can be taken with or without food.

Dosage: The starting dose is 5 mg once daily. The recommended target dose is 20 mg/day. Increase the dose in 5 mg increments to 10 mg/day (5 mg twice daily), 15 mg/day (5 mg and 10 mg as separate doses), and 20 mg/day (10 mg twice daily). The minimum recommended interval between dose increases is 1 week.

Extended release: The usual dosage is 28 mg once daily. The maximum dose is 28 mg once daily. The initial dosage is 7 mg once daily. Dosage is increased in 7 mg increments to 28 mg once daily. The minimum recommended interval between dose increases is 1 week. Patients taking 10 mg immediate-release tablets twice daily may switch to 28 mg extended-release (ER) capsules once daily.

Renal function impairment:

Severe renal impairment (creatinine clearance [CrCl] 5 to 29 mL/min) – A target dosage of 5 mg twice daily is recommended. Patients taking the 5 mg tablet twice daily may switch to the 14 mg ER capsule once daily the day following the last dose of an immediate-release 5 mg tablet.

Administration: Capsules can be taken intact or may be opened, sprinkled on applesauce, and thereby swallowed. The entire contents of each capsule should be consumed; the dose should not be divided. The capsules should be swallowed whole and not be divided, chewed, or crushed.

Actions

Pharmacology: Persistent activation of CNS N-methyl-D-aspartate (NMDA) receptors by the excitatory amino acid glutamate has been hypothesized to contribute to the symptomatology of Alzheimer disease. Memantine is an NMDA receptor antagonist.

Pharmacokinetics:

Absorption/Distribution – Memantine is highly absorbed with peak concentrations reached in approximately 3 to 7 hours. After multiple dose administration of memantine ER, memantine peak concentrations occur around 9 to 12 hours post-dose. The mean volume of distribution is 9 to 11 L/kg and the plasma protein binding is low (45%).

Metabolism/Excretion – Memantine undergoes partial hepatic metabolism; about 48% of administered drug is excreted unchanged in urine. Memantine has a terminal elimination half-life of about 60 to 80 hours. Renal clearance involves active tubular secretion.

Contraindications

Known hypersensitivity to memantine or to any excipients used in the formulation.

Warnings/Precautions

GU conditions: Conditions that raise urine pH may decrease the urinary elimination of memantine, resulting in increased plasma levels of memantine.

Seizures: Memantine has not been systematically evaluated in patients with a seizure disorder.

Renal function impairment: See Administration and Dosage for more information.

Pregnancy: Category B.

Lactation: It is not known whether memantine is excreted in human breast milk.

Children: There are no adequate and well-controlled trials documenting the safety and efficacy of memantine in any illness occurring in children.

Drug Interactions

Drugs that may interact with memantine include NMDA antagonists, urinary alkalinizers and thiazide diuretics.

Adverse Reactions

Adverse reactions occurring in at least 3% of patients include the following: back pain, confusion, constipation, coughing, dizziness, hallucination, headache, hypertension, pain, somnolence, vomiting.

DEXMETHYLPHENIDATE HYDROCHLORIDE

Tablets: 2.5, 5, and 10 mg *(c-ii)*	Various, *Focalin* (Novartis)
Capsules, extended-release: 5, 10, 15, 20, and 30 mg *(c-ii)*	*Focalin XR* (Novartis)

Warning:

Drug dependence: Give dexmethylphenidate cautiously to patients with a history of drug dependence or alcoholism. Chronic, abusive use can lead to marked tolerance and psychological dependence with varying degrees of abnormal behavior. Frank psychotic episodes can occur, especially with parenteral abuse. Careful supervision is required during drug withdrawal from abusive use because severe depression may occur. Withdrawal following chronic therapeutic use may unmask symptoms of the underlying disorder that may require follow-up.

Indications

Attention deficit hyperactivity disorder (ADHD): For the treatment of ADHD in patients 6 years of age and older. Dexmethylphenidate is indicated as an integral part of a total treatment program for ADHD that may include other measures (eg, psychological, educational, social) for patients with this syndrome. Drug treatment may not be indicated for all patients. Stimulants are not intended for use in the patient who exhibits symptoms secondary to environmental factors or other primary psychiatric disorders, including psychosis.

The effectiveness of dexmethylphenidate for longer than 6 weeks (immediate release [IR]) or for more than 7 weeks (extended release [ER]) has not been systematically evaluated in controlled trials. Therefore, the health care provider who elects to use dexmethylphenidate for extended periods should periodically reevaluate the long-term usefulness of the drug for the individual patient.

Administration and Dosage

Dexmethylphenidate ER capsules are for oral administration once daily in the morning. Capsules may be swallowed whole or, alternatively, may be administered by sprinkling the capsule contents on a small amount of applesauce.

Administer IR tablets twice/day, at least 4 hours apart, with or without food.

Individualize dosage according to the needs and responses of the patient.

Patients new to methylphenidate: The recommended starting dose of dexmethylphenidate for patients who are not currently taking racemic methylphenidate or for patients who are on stimulants other than methylphenidate is the following:

ER – 5 mg/day for children and 10 mg/day for adult patients. Dosage may be adjusted in 5 mg increments to a maximum of 30 mg/day for children and in 10 mg/day increments to a maximum of 40 mg/day for adult patients. In general, dosage adjustments may proceed at approximately weekly intervals.

IR – 5 mg/day (2.5 mg twice/day, IR). Dosage may be adjusted in 2.5 to 5 mg increments to a maximum of 20 mg/day (10 mg twice/day). In general, dosage adjustments may proceed at approximately weekly intervals.

Patients currently using methylphenidate: For patients currently using methylphenidate, the recommended starting dose of dexmethylphenidate IR or ER is half the dose of racemic methylphenidate. The maximum recommended dose is 20 mg/day (10 mg twice/day, IR).

Dose reduction and discontinuation: If paradoxical aggravation of symptoms or other adverse events occur, reduce the dosage, or, if necessary, discontinue the drug.

If improvement is not observed after appropriate dosage adjustment over a 1-month period, discontinue the drug.

Actions

Pharmacology: Dexmethylphenidate hydrochloride is a CNS stimulant. It is the more pharmacologically active enantiomer of the *d-* and *l-*enantiomers and is thought to block the reuptake of norepinephrine and dopamine into the presynaptic neuron and increase the release of these monoamines into the extraneuronal space.

Pharmacokinetics:

Absorption –

ER: Dexmethylphenidate ER produces a bimodal plasma-concentration profile when orally administered to healthy adults. The initial rate of absorption for dexmethylphenidate ER is similar to that of dexmethylphenidate IR tablets. The mean time to interpeak minimum (T_{minip}) is slightly shorter, and time to second peak (T_{max2}) is slightly longer for dexmethylphenidate ER given once daily compared with dexmethylphenidate IR tablets given in 2 doses 4 hours apart, although the ranges observed are greater for dexmethylphenidate ER.

Dexmethylphenidate ER given once daily exhibits a lower second peak concentration (C_{max2}), higher interpeak minimum concentrations (C_{minip}), and less peak and trough fluctuations than dexmethylphenidate tablets given in 2 doses 4 hours apart. This is because of an earlier onset and more prolonged absorption from the delayed-release beads.

IR: Dexmethylphenidate hydrochloride is readily absorbed following oral administration. In patients with ADHD, plasma dexmethylphenidate concentrations increase rapidly, reaching a maximum in the fasted state at approximately 1 to 1.5 hours postdose.

Distribution –

ER: The plasma protein binding of dexmethylphenidate is not known; racemic methylphenidate is bound to plasma proteins by 12% to 15%, independent of concentration. Dexmethylphenidate shows a volume of distribution of 2.65 ± 1.11 L/kg. Plasma dexmethylphenidate concentrations decline monophasically following oral administration of dexmethylphenidate ER.

IR: Plasma dexmethylphenidate concentrations in children decline exponentially following oral administration.

Metabolism –

ER and IR: Dexmethylphenidate is metabolized primarily to *d*-α-phenylpiperidine acetic acid (also known as *d*-ritalinic acid) by de-esterification. This metabolite has little or no pharmacological activity.

In vitro studies showed that dexmethylphenidate did not inhibit CYP-450 isoenzymes.

Excretion –

ER: The mean terminal elimination half-life of dexmethylphenidate was just over 3 hours in healthy adults. Children tend to have a slightly shorter half-lives, with means of 2 to 3 hours.

IR: The mean plasma elimination half-life of dexmethylphenidate is approximately 2.2 hours.

Contraindications

Patients with marked anxiety, tension, and agitation, because the drug may aggravate these symptoms; hypersensitivity to methylphenidate or other components of the product; patients with glaucoma, motor tics, or a family history or diagnosis of Tourette's syndrome; during treatment with monoamine oxidase inhibitors (MAOIs), and also within a minimum of 14 days following discontinuation of an MAOI (hypertensive crises may result).

Warnings/Precautions

Cardiovascular effects:

Sudden death and preexisting structural cardiac abnormalities –

Children and adolescents: Sudden death has been reported in association with CNS stimulant treatment at usual doses in children and adolescents with structural cardiac abnormalities or other serious heart problems.

Adults: Sudden death, stroke, and myocardial infarction have been reported in adults taking stimulant drugs at the usual doses for ADHD.

Hypertension and other cardiovascular conditions – Use cautiously in patients with hypertension. Monitor blood pressure at appropriate intervals in all patients taking dexmethylphenidate, especially those with hypertension. Caution is indicated in treating patients whose underlying medical conditions might be compromised by increases in blood pressure or heart rate (eg, pre-existing hypertension, heart failure, recent MI, hyperthyroidism).

Stimulant medications cause a modest increase in average blood pressure and average heart rate, and individuals may have larger increases.

Assessing cardiovascular status in patients being treated with stimulant medications – Children, adolescents, or adults who are being considered for treatment with stimulant medications should have a careful history and physical exam to assess for the presence of cardiac disease, and should receive further cardiac evaluation if findings suggest such disease. Patients who develop symptoms, such as exertional chest pain, unexplained syncope, or other symptoms suggestive of cardiac disease during stimulant treatment, should undergo a prompt cardiac evaluation.

Psychiatric effects:

Psychosis – Administration of stimulants may exacerbate symptoms of behavior disturbance and thought disorder in patients with preexisting psychotic disorder.

Bipolar illness – Take particular care in using stimulants to treat ADHD in patients with comorbid bipolar disorder because of concern for possible induction of a mixed/manic episode in such patients.

Emergence of new psychotic or manic symptoms – Treatment-emergent psychotic or manic symptoms in children and adolescents without a prior history of psychotic illness or mania can be caused by stimulants at usual doses.

Aggression – Aggressive behavior or hostility is often observed in children and adolescents with ADHD and has been reported in clinical trials and the postmarketing experience of some medications indicated for the treatment of ADHD.

Long-term suppression of growth: Although a causal relationship has not been established, suppression of growth (eg, weight gain, height) has been reported with long-term stimulant use in children. Monitor growth during treatment with stimulants; patients who are not growing or gaining height or weight as expected may need to have their treatment interrupted.

Seizures: Methylphenidate may lower the convulsive threshold in patients with history of seizures, in patients with prior EEG abnormalities in the absence of a history of seizures, and, very rarely, in the absence of a history of seizures and no prior EEG evidence of seizures. In the presence of seizures, discontinue the drug.

Visual disturbance: Difficulties with accommodation and blurring of vision have been reported.

Carcinogenesis: In a lifetime carcinogenicity study carried out in B6C3F1 mice, racemic methylphenidate caused an increase in hepatocellular adenomas and, in males only, an increase in hepatoblastomas at a daily dose of approximately 60 mg/kg/day. The significance to these results to humans is unknown.

Pregnancy: Category C.

Lactation: It is not known whether dexmethylphenidate is excreted in human milk.

Children: The safety and efficacy of dexmethylphenidate in children younger than 6 years of age have not been established.

Monitoring: Periodic CBC, differential, and platelet counts are advised during prolonged therapy.

Drug Interactions

Drugs that may be affected by dexmethylphenidate or racemic methylphenidate include antihypertensive agents, pressor agents, coumarin anticoagulants, anticonvulsants, tricyclic antidepressants, selective serotonin reuptake inhibitors, and clonidine. Drugs that may affect dexmethylphenidate include MAOIs.

Adverse Reactions

ER: Adverse reactions occurring in 5% or more of patients include anxiety, decreased appetite, dry mouth, dyspepsia, headache, and pharyngolaryngeal pain.

IR: Adverse reactions occurring in 5% or more of patients include abdominal pain, anorexia, fever, and nausea.

Adverse reactions with other methylphenidate hydrochloride products: Nervousness and insomnia are the most common adverse reactions reported with other methylphenidate products. In children, loss of appetite, abdominal pain, weight loss during prolonged therapy, insomnia, and tachycardia may occur more frequently; however, any of the other adverse reactions listed also may occur.

METHYLPHENIDATE HYDROCHLORIDE

Tablets: 5, 10, and 20 mg (*c-ii*)	Various, *Ritalin* (Novartis), *Methylin* (Mallinckrodt)
Tablets, chewable: 2.5, 5, and 10 mg (*c-ii*)	*Methylin* (Alliant)
Tablets, extended-release: 10 mg (*c-ii*)	*Metadate ER* (Celltech), *Methylin ER* (Alliant)
18 mg (*c-ii*)	*Concerta* (McNeil)
20 mg (*c-ii*)	Various, *Metadate ER* (Celltech), *Methylin ER* (Alliant)
27, 36, and 54 mg (*c-ii*)	*Concerta* (McNeil)
Tablets, sustained-release: 20 mg (*c-ii*)	*Ritalin-SR* (Novartis)
Capsules, extended-release: 10, 20, and 30 mg (*c-ii*)	*Metadate CD* (Celltech), *Ritalin LA* (Novartis)
40 mg (*c-ii*)	*Ritalin LA* (Novartis)
Oral solution: 5 and 10 mg per 5 mL (*c-ii*)	*Methylin* (Alliant)
Patch, transdermal: 10, 15, 20, and 30 mg (*c-ii*)	*Daytrana* (Shire)

Warning:

Drug dependence: Give methylphenidate cautiously to emotionally unstable patients, such as those with a history of drug dependence or alcoholism, because such patients may increase dosage on their own initiative.

Chronic abuse can lead to marked tolerance and psychological dependence with varying degrees of abnormal behavior. Frank psychotic episodes can occur, especially with parenteral abuse. Careful supervision is required during drug withdrawal because severe depression, as well as the effects of chronic overactivity, can be unmasked. Long-term follow-up may be required because of the patient's basic personality disturbances.

Indications

Attention deficit disorder (ADD)/Attention deficit hyperactivity disorder (ADHD): As an integral part of a total treatment program that typically includes other remedial measures (eg, psychological, educational, social) for a stabilizing effect in children with a behavioral syndrome characterized by the following group of developmentally inappropriate symptoms: moderate to severe distractibility, short attention span, hyperactivity, emotional lability, and impulsivity.

Narcolepsy (except Concerta, Metadate CD, and Ritalin LA): Treatment of narcolepsy.

Administration and Dosage

Adults (immediate-release [IR] tablets, chewable tablets, and oral solution): Individualize dosage. Administer in divided doses 2 or 3 times/day, preferably 30 to 45 minutes before meals. Average dose is 20 to 30 mg/day. Dosage ranges from 10 to 15 mg/day to 40 to 60 mg/day. Patients who are unable to sleep if medication is taken late in the day should take the last dose before 6 pm.

Children (6 years of age and older): Start with small doses (eg, 5 mg before breakfast and lunch) with gradual increments of 5 to 10 mg/wk (IR tablets, chewable tablets, and oral solution). Daily dosage above 60 mg is not recommended. If improvement is not observed after dosage adjustment over 1 month, discontinue use. If paradoxical aggravation of symptoms or other adverse effects occurs, reduce dosage or discontinue the drug.

Discontinue periodically to assess condition. Improvement may be sustained when the drug is temporarily or permanently discontinued. Drug treatment should not be indefinite and usually may be discontinued after puberty.

All patients: Instruct patients to take methylphenidate chewable tablets with at least 240 mL (8 ounces) of water or other fluid. Taking this product without enough liquid may cause choking.

Sustained-release (SR) and extended-release (ER) tablets have a duration of approximately 8 hours and may be used in place of regular tablets when the 8-hour dosage of the SR tablets and ER tablets corresponds to the titrated 8-hour dosage of the regular tablets. SR and ER tablets must be swallowed whole, never crushed or chewed.

Maintenance/Extended treatment: Discontinue periodically to assess condition. Improvement may be sustained when the drug is either temporarily or permanently discontinued. Drug treatment should not and need not be indefinite and usually may be discontinued after puberty.

Dose reduction and discontinuation: If paradoxical aggravation of symptoms or other adverse events occur, reduce dosage or discontinue the drug.

If improvement is not observed after appropriate dosage adjustment over a 1-month period, discontinue the drug.

Concerta: Administer orally once/day in the morning with or without food. Advise patients to swallow the capsules whole with the aid of liquids and not to chew, divide, or crush them. Doses may be increased at weekly intervals. The tablet shell, along with insoluble core components, is eliminated from the body.

Patients new to methylphenidate – The recommended starting dose for patients who are not currently taking methylphenidate or for patients who are on stimulants other than methylphenidate is 18 mg once/day. Dosage may be adjusted in 18 mg increments at weekly intervals to a maximum of 54 mg/day taken once/day in the morning for children 6 to 12 years of age, and a maximum of 72 mg/day (not to exceed 2 mg/kg/day) for adolescents 13 to 17 years of age.

Patients currently using methylphenidate – The recommended dosage of *Concerta* for patients who are currently taking methylphenidate 2 or 3 times daily at dosages of 10 to 45 mg/day is provided in the following table. Initial conversion dosage should not exceed 54 mg/day. After conversion, dosages may be adjusted to a maximum of 72 mg/day taken once daily in the morning.

In general, dosage adjustment may proceed at approximately weekly intervals.

Recommended Dose Conversion from Methylphenidate Regimens to *Concerta*

Previous methylphenidate daily dosage	Recommended *Concerta* starting dose
Methylphenidate 5 mg 2 or 3 times daily	18 mg every morning
Methylphenidate 10 mg 2 or 3 times daily	36 mg every morning
Methylphenidate 15 mg 2 or 3 times daily	54 mg every morning

A 27 mg dosage strength is available for physicians who wish to prescribe between the 18 and 36 mg dosages.

ER capsules (Ritalin LA, Metadate CD): Administer once daily in the morning before breakfast. The capsules may be swallowed whole with the aid of liquids or may be opened and the capsule contents sprinkled onto a small amount (tablespoon) of applesauce and given immediately; do not store for future use. The capsules and the capsule contents must not be crushed or chewed.

Sprinkle administration – The capsules may be carefully opened and the beads sprinkled over a spoonful of applesauce. The applesauce should not be warm because it could affect the modified release properties of *Ritalin LA*. The mixture of drug and applesauce should be consumed immediately in its entirety. Drinking some fluids (eg, water) should follow the intake of the sprinkles with applesauce. The drug and applesauce mixture should not be stored for future use.

Metadate CD –

Initial treatment: 20 mg once/day. Adjust dosage in weekly 10 to 20 mg increments to a maximum of 60 mg/day taken once/day in the morning, depending upon tolerability and degree of efficacy. Daily dosage above 60 mg is not recommended.

Ritalin LA: Individualize dosage.

Initial treatment – The recommended starting dose is 20 mg once/day. Dosage may be adjusted in weekly 10 mg increments to a maximum of 60 mg/day taken once/day in the morning, depending on tolerability and degree of efficacy observed. Daily dosage above 60 mg is not recommended. When a lower initial dose is appropriate, patients may begin treatment with *Ritalin LA* 10 mg.

Patients currently using methylphenidate – The recommended dosage of *Ritalin LA* for patients currently taking methylphenidate twice daily or SR is provided in the following table. For other methylphenidate regimens, use clinical judgment when selecting a starting dosage.

Previous Methylphenidate Dosage	Recommended *Ritalin LA* Dosage
Methylphenidate 5 mg twice daily	10 mg once daily
Methylphenidate 10 mg twice daily or methylphenidate SR 20 mg	20 mg once daily
Methylphenidate 15 mg twice daily	30 mg once daily
Methylphenidate 20 mg twice daily or methylphenidate SR 40 mg	40 mg once daily
Methylphenidate 30 mg twice daily or methylphenidate SR 60 mg	60 mg once daily

Daytrana:

Recommended dose – It is recommended that methylphenidate be applied to the hip area 2 hours before an effect is needed and should be removed 9 hours after application. Dosage should be titrated to effect. The recommended dose titration schedule is shown below. Dose titration, final dosage, and wear time should be individualized according to the needs and response of the patient.

Methylphenidate Transdermal Recommended Titration Schedule (Patients New to Methylphenidate)				
Upward titration, if response is not maximized				
	Week 1	Week 2	Week 3	Week 4
Patch size	12.5 cm^2	18.75 cm^2	25 cm^2	37.5^2
Nominal delivered dose* (mg/9 hrs)	10 mg	15 mg	20 mg	30 mg
Delivery rate*	(1.1 mg/h)*	(1.6 mg/h)*	(2.2 mg/h)*	(3.3 mg/h)*

* Nominal in vivo delivery rate in pediatric subjects aged 6-12 when applied to the hip, based on a 9-hour wear period.

Conversion – Patients converting from another formulation of methylphenidate should follow the above titration schedule due to differences in bioavailability of methylphenidate transdermal compared to other products.

The adhesive side of the patch should be placed on a clean, dry area of the hip. The area selected should not be oily, damaged, or irritated. Apply patch to the hip area. Avoid the waistline, since clothing may cause the patch to rub off. When applying the patch the next morning, place on the opposite hip at a new site if possible.

Disposal – Upon removal, used patches should be folded so that the adhesive side of the patch adheres to itself and should be flushed down the toilet or disposed of in an appropriate lidded container. If the patient stops using the prescription, each unused patch should be removed from its pouch, separated from the protective liner, folded onto itself, and flushed down the toilet or disposed of in an appropriate lidded container.

Dose/Wear time reduction and discontinuation – The patch may be removed earlier than 9 hours if a shorter duration of effect is desired or late day side effects appear. Plasma concentrations of d-methylphenidate generally begin declining when the patch is removed, although absorption may continue for several hours.

Actions

Pharmacology: Methylphenidate is a CNS stimulant. The exact mechanism of action is not fully understood. Methylphenidate is thought to block the reuptake of norepinephrine and dopamine into the presynaptic neuron and increase the release of these monoamines into the extraneuronal space.

Pharmacokinetics:

Absorption – Rapidly and well absorbed from the GI tract, methylphenidate achieves peak blood levels in 1 to 3 hours. Peak plasma levels occur in children in 4.7 hours for the SR tablets and 1.9 hours for the regular tablets. Mean times to reach peak plasma concentrations across all doses of *Concerta* occurred between 6 and 10 hours. Plasma half-life for *Metadate CD* is reportedly 6.8 hours. SR and ER tablets are more slowly but as extensively absorbed as regular tablets.

Chewable tablets and oral solution: Peak plasma concentrations are achieved at approximately 1 to 2 hours.

Metadate CD: The early peak concentrations (median) were reached approximately 1.5 hours after dose intake, and the second peak concentrations (median) were reached approximately 4.5 hours after dose intake.

Ritalin LA: Ritalin LA produces a bimodal plasma concentration-time profile (2 distinct peaks approximately 4 hours apart) when orally administered.

Distribution – Binding to plasma proteins is low (10% to 33%), and the apparent distribution volume at steady state with IV administration has been reported to be approximately 6 L/kg.

Metabolism – Methylphenidate is metabolized rapidly primarily via deesterification to alpha-phenyl-piperidine acetic acid (PPA or ritalinic acid). The metabolite has little or no pharmacologic activity.

Excretion – The mean half-life for the various dosage forms range from 2.7 to 3.5 hours in adults. The half-life in children for the IR tablets is 2.5 hours. The half-life of ritalinic acid is approximately 3 to 4 hours.

Contraindications

Marked anxiety, tension, and agitation (the drug may aggravate these symptoms); hypersensitivity to methylphenidate or other components of the product; glaucoma; motor tics or a family history or diagnosis of Tourette syndrome.

Concurrent treatment with monoamine oxidase inhibitors (MAOIs) and within a minimum of 14 days following discontinuation of an MAOI (hypertensive crisis may result).

Warnings/Precautions

Seizure disorders: Methylphenidate may lower the seizure threshold in patients with a history of seizures, with prior EEG abnormalities in absence of seizures, and, very rarely, in the absence of history of seizures and no prior EEG evidence of seizures. If seizures occur, discontinue the drug.

GI obstruction (Concerta only): Because the *Concerta* tablet is nondeformable and does not appreciably change shape in the GI tract, do not administer to patients with pre-existing severe GI narrowing (eg, small bowel inflammatory disease, "short gut" syndrome because of adhesions or decreased transit time, history of peritonitis, cystic fibrosis, chronic intestinal pseudo-obstruction, Meckel's diverticulum). Because of the controlled-release design of the tablet, only use *Concerta* in patients who are able to swallow the tablet whole.

Hypertension: Use cautiously; monitor blood pressure in all patients, especially those with hypertension.

Depression: Do not use methylphenidate to treat severe depression of exogenous or endogenous origin.

Fatigue: Do not use methylphenidate for the prevention or treatment of normal fatigue states.

Long-term suppression of growth: Suppression of growth has been reported with long-term use in children. Interrupt treatment for patients who are not growing or gaining weight as expected.

Psychosis: Methylphenidate may exacerbate symptoms of behavior disturbances and thought disorder.

Visual disturbances: Visual disturbances have been encountered rarely. Difficulties with accommodation and blurring of vision have been reported.

Phenylketonurics: Each 2.5 mg chewable tablet contains 0.42 mg phenylalanine; each 5 mg chewable tablet contains 0.84 mg phenylalanine; and each 10 mg chewable tablet contains 1.68 mg phenylalanine.

Agitation: Patients with an element of agitation may react adversely; discontinue therapy if necessary.

Prescribing: Drug treatment is not indicated in all cases of this behavioral syndrome. The decision to prescribe methylphenidate should depend on chronicity and severity of symptoms and appropriateness for age.

Acute stress: When symptoms are associated with acute stress reactions, treatment with methylphenidate usually is not indicated.

Drug abuse and dependence: Give cautiously to emotionally unstable patients, such as those with a history of drug dependence or alcoholism, because they may increase dosage on their own initiative (see Warning Box).

Pregnancy: Category C.

Lactation: The amount of methylphenidate excreted in breast milk is unknown.

Children: Do not use in children under 6 years of age because safety and efficacy have not been established.

Safety and efficacy of long-term use in children are not established. Although a causal relationship has not been established, suppression of growth (eg, weight gain or height) has been reported with long-term use of stimulants in children. Carefully monitor patients on long-term therapy.

Monitoring: Perform periodic CBC, differential, and platelet counts during prolonged therapy.

Drug Interactions

Drugs that may affect methylphenidate include MAOIs. Drugs that may be affected by methylphenidate hydrochloride include guanethidine, anticonvulsants (eg, phenytoin, phenobarbital, primidone), selective serotonin reuptake inhibitors, coumarin anticoagulants, and tricyclic antidepressants.

Antacids/Acid suppressants (Ritalin LA only): Because the modified release characteristics of *Ritalin LA* capsules are pH dependent, the coadministration of antacids or acid suppressants could alter the release of methylphenidate.

Clonidine: Serious adverse reactions have been reported in concomitant use with clonidine, although no causality for the combination has been established.

Adverse Reactions

Adverse reactions may include the following: Skin rash; urticaria; fever; arthralgia; exfoliative dermatitis; erythema multiforme with necrotizing vasculitis; thrombocytopenic purpura; dizziness; headache; dyskinesia; drowsiness; Tourette syndrome; toxic psychosis; blood pressure and pulse changes; tachycardia; angina; cardiac arrhythmias; palpitations; anorexia; nausea; abdominal pain; weight loss; nervousness; insomnia; leukopenia; anemia; hair loss; loss of appetite; abdominal pain; vomiting, upper respiratory tract infection; cough increased; pharyngitis; sinusitis.

TACRINE HYDROCHLORIDE (Tetrahydroaminoacridine; THA)

Capsules: 10, 20, 30, and 40 mg (*Rx*)	Cognex (Parke-Davis)

Indications

Alzheimer disease: Treatment of mild to moderate dementia of the Alzheimer type.

Administration and Dosage

The rate of dose escalation may be slowed if a patient is intolerant to the recommended titration schedule. However, it is not advisable to accelerate the dose incrementation plan. Following initiation of therapy, or any dosage increase, observe patients carefully for adverse effects. Take between meals whenever possible; however, if minor GI upset occurs, take with meals to improve tolerability. Taking tacrine with meals can be expected to reduce plasma levels approximately 30% to 40%.

Initiation of treatment: The initial dose of tacrine is 40 mg/day (10 mg 4 times/day). Maintain this dose for 4 weeks or more with every other week monitoring of transaminase levels beginning at week 4 of therapy. It is important that the dose not be increased during this period because of the potential for delayed onset of transaminase elevations.

Dose titration: Following 4 weeks of treatment at 40 mg/day (10 mg 4 times/day), increase the dose to 80 mg/day (20 mg 4 times/day), providing there are no significant transaminase elevations and the patient is tolerating treatment. Titrate patients to higher doses (120 and 160 mg/day in divided doses on a 4 times/day schedule) at 4-week intervals on the basis of tolerance.

Dose adjustment: Monitor serum transaminase levels (specifically ALT) every other week from at least week 4 to week 16 following initiation of treatment, after which monitoring may be decreased to every 3 months. For patients who develop ALT elevations more than 2 times the upper limit of normal (ULN), the dose and monitoring regimen should be modified as described in the table below.

A full monitoring and dose titration sequence must be repeated in the event that a patient suspends treatment with tacrine for more than 4 weeks.

Recommended Tacrine Dose and Monitoring Regimen Modification in Response to Transaminase Elevations	
Transaminase levels	Treatment and monitoring regimen
≤ 2 × ULN	Continue treatment according to recommended titration and monitoring schedule.
> 2 to ≤ 3 × ULN	Continue treatment according to recommended titration. Monitor transaminase levels weekly until levels return to normal limits.
> 3 to ≤ 5 × ULN	Reduce the daily dose by 40 mg/day. Monitor ALT levels weekly. Resume dose titration and every other week monitoring when transaminase levels return to within normal limits.
> 5 × ULN	Stop treatment. Monitor the patient closely for signs and symptoms associated with hepatitis and follow transaminase levels until within normal limits (see Rechallenge).

Experience is limited in patients with ALT more than 10 × ULN. The risk of rechallenge must be considered against demonstrated clinical benefit. Patients with clinical jaundice confirmed by a significant elevation in total bilirubin (more than 3 mg/dL) or those exhibiting clinical signs or symptoms of hypersensitivity (eg, rash or fever) in association with ALT elevations should immediately and permanently discontinue tacrine and not be rechallenged.

Rechallenge: Patients who are required to discontinue treatment because of transaminase elevations may be rechallenged once transaminase levels return to within normal limits. Rechallenge of patients exposed to transaminase elevations less than 10 × ULN has not resulted in serious liver injury. However, because experience in the rechallenge of patients who had elevations greater than 10 × ULN is limited, the risks associated with the rechallenge of these patients are not well characterized. Carefully and frequently (weekly) monitor serum ALT when rechallenging such patients. If rechallenged, give patients an initial dose of 40 mg/day (10 mg 4 times/day) and monitor transaminase levels weekly. If, after 6 weeks on 40 mg/day, the patient is tolerating the dosage with no unacceptable elevations in transaminases, recommended dose titration and transaminase monitoring may be resumed.

Continue weekly monitoring of ALT levels for a total of 16 weeks, after which monitoring may be decreased to monthly for 2 months and every 3 months thereafter.

Actions

Pharmacology: Tacrine is a centrally acting reversible cholinesterase inhibitor, commonly referred to as THA.

Pharmacokinetics:

Absorption – Maximal plasma concentrations occur within 1 to 2 hours.

Distribution – Mean volume of distribution of tacrine is approximately 349 L. Tacrine is approximately 55% bound to plasma proteins.

Metabolism – Tacrine is extensively metabolized by the cytochrome P450 system.

Excretion – The elimination half-life is approximately 2 to 4 hours.

Contraindications

Hypersensitivity to tacrine or acridine derivatives; patients previously treated with tacrine who developed treatment-associated jaundice; a serum bilirubin greater than 3 mg/dL; signs or symptoms of hypersensitivity (eg, rash or fever) in association with ALT elevations.

Warnings/Precautions

Anesthesia: Tacrine is likely to exaggerate succinylcholine-type muscle relaxation during anesthesia.

Cardiovascular conditions: Tacrine may have vagotonic effects on the heart rate.

GI disease/dysfunction: Tacrine is an inhibitor of cholinesterase and may be expected to increase gastric acid secretion caused by increased cholinergic activity. Therefore, closely monitor patients at increased risk for developing ulcers for symptoms of active or occult GI bleeding.

Hepatic effects: Prescribe with care in patients with current evidence or history of abnormal liver function indicated by significant abnormalities in serum transaminase, bilirubin, and gamma-glutamyl transpeptidase levels.

The incidence of transaminase elevations is higher among females. There are no other known predictors of the risk of hepatocellular injury.

GU effects: Cholinomimetics may cause bladder outflow obstruction.

Neurological conditions:

Seizures – Cholinomimetics are believed to have some potential to cause generalized convulsions; however, seizure activity may also be a manifestation of Alzheimer disease.

Cognitive function – Worsening of cognitive function has been reported following abrupt discontinuation of tacrine or after a large reduction in total daily dose (80 mg/day or more).

Pulmonary conditions: Because of its cholinomimetic action, use tacrine with care in patients with a history of asthma.

Hepatic disease: Although studies in patients with liver disease have not been done, it is likely that functional hepatic impairment will reduce the clearance of tacrine and its metabolites.

Hematology: Decreased absolute neutrophil counts (ANC) less than 500 to 1500/mcL have been reported rarely. The total clinical experience in more than 12,000 patients does not indicate a clear association between tacrine treatment and serious white blood cell abnormalities.

Pregnancy: Category C.

Lactation: It is not known whether this drug is excreted in breast milk.

Children: There are no adequate and well controlled trials to document the safety and efficacy of tacrine in any dementing illness occurring in children.

Monitoring: Monitor serum transaminase levels (specifically ALT) every other week from at least week 4 to week 16 following initiation of treatment, after which monitoring may be decreased to every 3 months. Repeat a full monitoring sequence in the event that a patient suspends treatment with tacrine for more than 4 weeks. If transaminase elevations occur, modify the dose (see Administration and Dosage).

Continue to monitor ALT levels weekly for a total of 16 weeks, then decrease to monthly for 2 months and to every 3 months thereafter.

Drug Interactions

Drugs that may be affected by tacrine include anticholinergics, cholinomimetics, cholinesterase inhibitors, and theophylline.

Drugs that may affect tacrine include cimetidine.

Tacrine is primarily eliminated by hepatic metabolism via cytochrome P450 drug metabolizing enzymes. Drug interactions may occur when it is given concurrently with agents such as theophylline that undergo extensive metabolism via cytochrome P450 IA2.

Adverse Reactions

Adverse reactions occurring in 3% or more of patients include elevated transaminases; nausea; vomiting; diarrhea; dyspepsia; myalgia; headache; fatigue; chest pain; weight decrease; agitation; depression; abnormal thinking; anxiety; anorexia; abdominal pain; flatulence; constipation; dizziness; confusion; ataxia; insomnia; somnolence; urinary incontinence; urinary tract infection; urination frequency; rash; facial flushing; coughing; upper respiratory tract infection; rhinitis.

RIVASTIGMINE

Capsules, oral: 1.5, 3, 4.5, 6 mg (as tartrate) (*Rx*)	Various, *Exelon* (Novartis)
Solution, oral: 2 mg/mL (as tartrate) (*Rx*)	*Exelon* (Novartis)
Patch, transdermal: 4.6 mg/24 h, 9.5 mg/24 h (*Rx*)	

Indications

Alzheimer dementia: For the treatment of mild to moderate dementia of the Alzheimer type.

Dementia associated with Parkinson disease: For the treatment of mild to moderate dementia associated with Parkinson disease.

Administration and Dosage

Capsules and oral solution:

Alzheimer dementia – 1.5 mg twice a day. If dose is well tolerated, after a minimum of 2 weeks of treatment, increase to 3 mg twice a day. Increases to 4.5 and 6 mg twice/day should be attempted after a minimum of 2 weeks at the previous dose. If adverse reactions (eg, nausea, vomiting, abdominal pain, loss of appetite) cause intolerance during treatment, discontinue treatment for several doses and then restart at the same or next lower dose level. If treatment is interrupted for longer than several days, reinitiate treatment with the lowest daily dose and titrate as previously described. The maximum dose is 6 mg twice/day.

Take with food in divided doses in the morning and evening.

Dementia associated with Parkinson disease – The dose of rivastigmine shown to be effective is 3 to 12 mg/day given as twice-daily dosing (daily doses of 1.5 to 6 mg twice daily). The starting dose of rivastigmine is 1.5 mg twice daily; subsequently, the dose may be increased to 3 mg twice daily and further to 4.5 mg twice daily and 6 mg twice daily, based on tolerability, with a minimum of 4 weeks at each dose.

Oral solution – Each dose may be swallowed directly from the syringe or first mixed with a small glass of water, cold fruit juice, or soda. Instruct patients to stir and drink the mixture.

Rivastigmine oral solution and capsules may be interchanged at equal doses.

Transdermal patch:

Initial dose – Treatment is started with rivastigmine 4.6 mg/24 h transdermal patch. After a minimum of 4 weeks of treatment and if well tolerated, the dose should be increased to rivastigmine 9.5 mg/24 h transdermal patch, which is the recommended effective dose.

Maintenance dose – The maximum recommended effective dose is 9.5 mg/24 h. If adverse reactions cause intolerance during treatment, the patient should be instructed to discontinue treatment for several days and then restart at the same or next lower dose level. If treatment is interrupted for longer than several days, reinitiate with the lowest daily dose and titrate as previously described.

Low body weight (below 50 kg) – Particular caution should be exercised in titrating these patients above the recommended maintenance dose of rivastigmine 9.5 mg/24 h transdermal patch.

Switching from capsules or oral solution – A patient who is on a total daily dose of less than 6 mg of oral rivastigmine can be switched to the rivastigmine 4.6 mg/24 h transdermal patch.

A patient who is on a total daily dose of 6 to 12 mg of oral rivastigmine may be directly switched to the rivastigmine 9.5 mg/24 h transdermal patch.

Apply the first transdermal patch on the day following the last oral dose.

Administration – Apply once daily to clean, dry, hairless, intact healthy skin in a place that will not be rubbed by tight clothing. The upper or lower back is recommended as the site of application because the transdermal patch is less likely to be removed by the patient; the transdermal patch can also be applied to the upper arm or chest. Do not apply to skin that is red, irritated, or cut. Change the site of application daily to avoid potential irritation. Consecutive patches can be can be applied to the same anatomic site (eg another spot on the upper back). The same site should not be used within 14 days. The transdermal patch should be replaced with a new patch every 24 hours.

Storage/Stability: When rivastigmine oral solution is combined with cold fruit juice or soda, the mixture is stable at room temperature for up to 4 hours.

Actions

Pharmacology: While the precise mechanism of rivastigmine's action is unknown, it is postulated to enhance cholinergic function by increasing the concentration of acetylcholine through reversible inhibition of its hydrolysis by cholinesterase. If this proposed mechanism is correct, rivastigmine's effect may lessen as the disease process advances and fewer cholinergic neurons remain functionally intact.

Pharmacokinetics:

Absorption – Rivastigmine is rapidly and completely absorbed with an absolute bioavailability of approximately 40% (3 mg dose). Peak plasma concentrations are reached in approximately 1 hour.

Distribution – Rivastigmine is widely distributed throughout the body with a volume of distribution in the range of 1.8 to 2.7 L/kg. Rivastigmine is about 40% bound to plasma proteins.

Metabolism – Rivastigmine is rapidly and extensively metabolized, primarily via cholinesterase-mediated hydrolysis.

Excretion – The elimination half-life is approximately 1.5 hours, with most elimination as metabolites via the urine.

Contraindications

Hypersensitivity to rivastigmine, other carbamate derivatives, or other components of the formulation.

Warnings/Precautions

Gastrointestinal (GI) effects: Rivastigmine is associated with significant GI adverse reactions, including anorexia, nausea and vomiting, and weight loss.

Weight loss: In the controlled trials, approximately 26% of women on high doses of rivastigmine (more than 9 mg/day) had weight loss of 7% or more of their baseline weight compared with 6% in the placebo-treated patients. Approximately 18% of the men in the high dose group experienced a similar degree of weight loss compared with 4% in placebo-treated patients. It is not clear how much of the weight loss was associated with anorexia, nausea, vomiting, and diarrhea associated with drug administration.

Anorexia: In the controlled clinical trials, of the patients treated with a rivastigmine dose of 6 to 12 mg/day, 17% developed anorexia compared with 3% of the placebo patients.

Nausea and vomiting: In the controlled clinical trials, 47% of patients treated with a rivastigmine dose in the therapeutic range of 6 to 12 mg/day developed nausea compared with 12% for placebo. A total of 31% of rivastigmine-treated patients developed at least 1 episode of vomiting compared with 6% for placebo. The rates were higher in women than in men. Five percent of patients discontinued for vomiting compared with less than 1% of patients on placebo. The rate of nausea and vomiting was higher during the titration phase than in the maintenance phase.

Peptic ulcers/GI bleeding: Monitor patients closely for symptoms of active or occult GI bleeding, especially those at increased risk for developing ulcers (eg, those with a history of ulcer disease or those receiving concurrent nonsteroidal anti-inflammatory drugs).

Anesthesia: Rivastigmine, as a cholinesterase inhibitor, is likely to exaggerate succinylcholine-type muscle relaxation during anesthesia.

Cardiovascular effects: Drugs that increase cholinergic activity may have vagotonic effects on heart rates (eg, bradycardia). The potential for this action may be particularly important in patients with "sick sinus syndrome" or other supraventricular cardiac conduction conditions.

Urinary obstruction: Drugs that increase cholinergic activity may cause urinary obstruction.

Seizures: Drugs that increase cholinergic activity are believed to have some potential for causing seizures. However, seizure activity also may be a manifestation of Alzheimer disease.

Pulmonary effects: Like other drugs that increase cholinergic activity, use with care in patients with a history of asthma or obstructive pulmonary disease.

Pregnancy: Category B.

Lactation: It is not known whether rivastigmine is excreted in breast milk.

Children: There are no adequate and well-controlled trials documenting the safety and efficacy of rivastigmine in any illness occurring in children.

Drug Interactions

Drugs that may interact with rivastigmine include anticholinergics and cholinomimetics and other cholinesterase inhibitors.

Adverse Reactions

Adverse reactions occurring in 3% or more of patients include dizziness, headache, insomnia, confusion, depression, anxiety, somnolence, hallucination, nausea, vomiting, diarrhea, anorexia, abdominal pain, dyspepsia, constipation, accidental trauma, fatigue, urinary tract infection, rhinitis.

GALANTAMINE HBr

Tablets: 4, 8, and 12 mg (*Rx*)	Various, *Razadyne* (Janssen)
Capsules, extended-release: 8, 16, 24 mg (*Rx*)	Various, *Razadyne ER* (Janssen)
Oral solution: 4 mg/mL (*Rx*)	*Razadyne* (Janssen)

Indications

Alzheimer disease: Treatment of mild to moderate dementia of the Alzheimer type.

Administration and Dosage

Dosage: Starting dose is 4 mg twice/day (8 mg/day). After a minimum of 4 weeks, increase the dose to 8 mg twice/day. Increase to 12 mg twice/day only after a minimum of 4 weeks at the previous dose.

16 to 24 mg/day given twice/day with morning and evening meals.

If therapy has been interrupted for several days or longer, the patient should be restarted at the lowest dose and the dose escalated to the current dose.

Extended-release (ER): 16 to 24 mg/day.

Starting dose is 8 mg/day. Increase to 16 mg/day after a minimum of 4 weeks. Attempt an increase to 24 mg/day after a minimum of 4 weeks of 16 mg/day.

Administer once daily in the morning, preferably with food.

Actions

Pharmacology: Galantamine is a competitive and reversible inhibitor of acetylcholinesterase. While the precise mechanism is unknown, it may exert its therapeutic effect by enhancing cholinergic function.

Pharmacokinetics:

Absorption/Distribution – Galantamine is rapidly and completely absorbed with time-to-peak concentration in about 1 hour. Galantamine has an absolute oral bioavailability of about 90%. The plasma protein binding of galantamine is 18%.

Galantamine 24 mg ER capsules administered once daily under fasting conditions are bioequivalent to galantamine 12 mg tablets twice daily with respect to AUC_{24h} and minimum drug concentrations (C_{min}).

Metabolism/Excretion – Galantamine is metabolized by hepatic CYP-450 CYP 2D6 and CYP 3A4 enzymes, glucuronidated, and excreted unchanged in the urine.

Galantamine has a terminal elimination half-life of approximately 7 hours.

Special populations –

Gender: Galantamine clearance is about 20% lower in women than in men (explained by lower body weight in women).

Contraindications

Known hypersensitivity to galantamine or to any excipients used in the formulation.

Warnings/Precautions

Renal function impairment: For patients with moderate renal function impairment, the dose generally should not exceed 16 mg/day. In patients with severe renal function impairment (Ccr less than 9 mL/min), the use of galantamine is not recommended.

Hepatic function impairment: In patients with moderately impaired hepatic function, the dose generally should not exceed 16 mg/day. The use of galantamine in patients with severe hepatic impairment is not recommended.

Special risk:

Anesthesia – Galantamine is likely to exaggerate the neuromuscular blockade effects of succinylcholine-type and similar neuromuscular blocking agents during anesthesia.

Cardiovascular conditions – Cholinesterase inhibitors have vagotonic effects on the sinoatrial and atrioventricular nodes, leading to bradycardia and AV block.

GI conditions – Cholinomimetics may increase gastric acid secretion because of increased cholinergic activity. Therefore, monitor patients closely for symptoms of active or occult GI bleeding, especially those with an increased risk for developing ulcers.

Galantamine has been shown to produce nausea, vomiting, diarrhea, anorexia, and weight loss. In patients who experienced nausea, the median duration was 5 to 7 days.

GU – Although this was not observed in clinical trials with galantamine, cholinomimetics may cause bladder outflow obstruction.

Pulmonary conditions – Prescribe galantamine with care to patients with a history of severe asthma or obstructive pulmonary disease.

Seizures – Cholinesterase inhibitors are believed to have some potential to cause generalized convulsions.

Pregnancy: Category B.

Lactation: It is not known whether galantamine is excreted in breast milk. Galantamine has no indication for use in breast-feeding mothers.

Children: Safety and efficacy of galantamine in children have not been established.

Monitoring: Monitor patients for symptoms of active or occult GI bleeding, especially those with increased risk of developing ulcers (eg, history of ulcer disease).

Drug Interactions

Drugs that may affect galantamine include succinylcholine, bethanechol, and other cholinesterase inhibitors, cimetidine, CYP2D6 or CYP3A4 inhibitors, erythromycin, ketoconazole, and paroxetine. Drugs that may be affected by galantamine include succinylcholine, bethanechol, and other cholinesterase inhibitors, cimetidine, ketoconazole, paroxetine, erythromycin, anticholinergics, neuromuscular-blocking agents, and NSAIDs.

Adverse Reactions

The most frequent adverse reactions leading to discontinuation of galantamine therapy included nausea, dizziness, vomiting, anorexia, and syncope.

Adverse reactions occurring in at least 5% of galantamine patients and at least 2 times placebo include anorexia, diarrhea, nausea, vomiting, and weight decrease. Other adverse reactions occurring in at least 3% of patients receiving galantamine include abdominal pain, anemia, anorexia, dizziness, depression, diarrhea, dyspepsia, fatigue, headache, hematuria, insomnia, nausea, rhinitis, somnolence, tremor, urinary tract infection, vomiting, and weight decrease.

DONEPEZIL HYDROCHLORIDE

Tablets: 5, 10, and 23 mg (*Rx*)	Various, *Aricept* (Eisai)
Tablets, orally disintegrating: 5 and 10 mg (*Rx*)	Various, *Aricept ODT* (Eisai)

Indications

Alzheimer disease: For the treatment of dementia of the Alzheimer type.

Administration and Dosage

Mild to moderate Alzheimer disease: 5 or 10 mg once daily.

The higher dose of 10 mg did not provide a statistically significant clinical benefit greater than that of 5 mg. Do not increase to 10 mg until patients have been on a daily dose of 5 mg for 4 to 6 weeks.

Severe Alzheimer disease: 10 mg administered once daily.

Take donepezil in the evening, just prior to retiring.

Donepezil may be taken with or without food; allow donepezil orally disintegrating tablets to dissolve on the tongue and follow with water.

Bioequivalence: Donepezil orally disintegrating tablets are bioequivalent to donepezil tablets and can be taken without regard to meals.

Actions

Pharmacology: Donepezil enhances cholinergic function by increasing the concentration of acetylcholine through reversible inhibition of its hydrolysis by acetylcholinesterase (AChE). Donepezil's effect may lessen as the disease process advances and fewer cholinergic neurons remain functionally intact.

Pharmacokinetics:

Absorption – Donepezil is well absorbed with a relative oral bioavailability of 100% and reaches peak plasma concentrations in 3 to 4 hours.

Distribution – Following multiple-dose administration, steady state is reached within 15 days. Donepezil is approximately 96% bound to human plasma proteins.

Metabolism – Donepezil is excreted in urine. It is metabolized by CYP-450 isoenzyme 2D6 and 3A4, and undergoes glucuronidation.

Excretion – The elimination half-life of donepezil is approximately 70 hours and the mean apparent plasma clearance is 0.13 L/h/kg.

Contraindications

Hypersensitivity to donepezil or to piperidine derivatives.

Warnings/Precautions

Anesthesia: Donepezil, as a cholinesterase inhibitor, is likely to exaggerate succinylcholine-type muscle relaxation during anesthesia.

Cardiovascular: Cholinesterase inhibitors may have vagotonic effects on the sinoatrial and atrioventricular nodes. This effect may manifest as bradycardia or heart block in patients with and without known underlying cardiac conduction abnormalities. Syncopal episodes have been reported in association with the use of donepezil.

GI: Cholinesterase inhibitors may be expected to increase gastric acid secretion because of increased cholinergic activity. Monitor patients closely for symptoms of active or occult GI bleeding, especially those at increased risk for developing ulcers.

GU: Cholinomimetics may cause bladder outflow obstruction.

Seizures: Cholinomimetics may have some potential to cause generalized convulsions. However, seizure activity also may be a manifestation of Alzheimer disease.

Pulmonary: Prescribe cholinesterase inhibitors with care for patients with a history of asthma or obstructive pulmonary disease.

Hepatic function impairment: In a study of 10 patients with stable alcoholic cirrhosis, the clearance of donepezil was decreased 20% relative to 10 healthy age- and sex-matched subjects.

Pregnancy: Category C.

Lactation: It is not known whether donepezil is excreted in breast milk.

Children: There are no adequate and well controlled trials to document the safety and efficacy of donepezil in any illness occurring in children.

Drug Interactions

Drugs that may affect donepezil are CYP-450 3A4 and 2D6 inhibitors (eg, ketoconazole, quinidine) and CYP-450 3A4 and 2D6 inducers (eg, carbamazepine, dexamethasone, phenobarbital, phenytoin, rifampin). Drugs that may be affected by donepezil include anticholinergics, cholinomimetics/cholinesterase inhibitors, and NSAIDs.

Adverse Reactions

Adverse reactions that may occur in 3% or more of patients include abnormal dreams, accident, anorexia, depression, diarrhea, dizziness, ecchymosis, fatigue, headache, insomnia, muscle cramps, nausea, pain, vomiting, and weight decrease.

ERGOLOID MESYLATES (Dihydrogenated Ergot Alkaloids, Dihydroergotoxine)

Tablets, oral: 0.5 and 1 mg (*Rx*)	Various, *Gerimal* (Rugby), *Hydergine* (Sandoz)
Tablets, sublingual: 0.5 and 1 mg (*Rx*)	Various, *Gerimal* (Rugby), *Hydergine* (Sandoz)
Liquid: 1 mg/mL (*Rx*)	*Hydergine* (Sandoz)

Indications

Age-related mental capacity decline: Individuals older than 60 years of age who manifest signs and symptoms of an idiopathic decline in mental capacity. Patients who respond suffer from some process related to aging or have some underlying dementing condition.

Administration and Dosage

The usual starting dose is 1 mg 3 times/day. Alleviation of symptoms usually is gradual; results may not be observed for 3 to 4 weeks. Doses up to 4.5 to 12 mg/day have been used. Up to 6 months of treatment may be necessary to determine efficacy, using doses of 6 mg/day or more. Do not chew or crush sublingual tablets.

Actions

Pharmacology: Ergoloid mesylates contain equal proportions of dihydroergocornine mesylate, dihydroergocristine mesylate, and dihydroergocryptine mesylate.

The mechanism by which ergoloid mesylates produce mental effects is unknown.

Pharmacokinetics: Ergoloid mesylates are rapidly absorbed from the GI tract; peak plasma concentrations are achieved within 0.6 to 3 hours. The liquid capsule has a 12% greater bioavailability than the oral tablet. The mean half-life of unchanged ergoloid in plasma is about 2.6 to 5.1 hours.

Contraindications

Hypersensitivity to ergoloid mesylates.

Acute or chronic psychosis, regardless of etiology.

Warnings/Precautions

Before prescribing: Before prescribing ergoloid mesylates, exclude the possibility that the patient's signs and symptoms arise from a potentially reversible and treatable condition. Exclude delirium and dementiform illness secondary to systemic disease, primary neurological disease, or primary disturbance of mood.

Reassessment: Periodically reassess the diagnosis and the benefit of current therapy to the patient.

Adverse Reactions

Adverse reactions may include sublingual irritation; transient nausea and GI disturbances.

ATOMOXETINE HYDROCHLORIDE

Capsules; oral: 10, 18, 25, 40, 60, 80, and 100 mg (as base) (*Rx*)	*Strattera* (Eli Lilly)

Warning:

Suicidal ideation in children and adolescents: Atomoxetine increased the risk of suicidal ideation in short-term studies in children and adolescents with attention deficit hyperactivity disorder (ADHD). Anyone considering the use of atomoxetine in a child or adolescent must balance this risk with the clinical need. Closely monitor patients who are started on therapy for suicidality (suicidal thinking and behavior), clinical worsening, or unusual changes in behavior. Advise families and caregivers of the need for close observation and communication with the prescribing health care provider. Atomoxetine is approved for ADHD in children and adults. Atomoxetine is not approved for major depressive disorder (MDD).

Pooled analysis of short-term (6- to 18-week), placebo-controlled trials of atomoxetine in children and adolescents (12 trials involving more than 2,200 patients, including 11 trials in ADHD and 1 trial in enuresis) has revealed a greater risk of suicidal ideation early during treatment in those receiving atomoxetine compared with placebo. The average risk of suicidal ideation in patients receiving atomoxetine was 0.4% (5/1,357 patients), compared with none in placebo-treated patients (0/851 patients). No suicides occurred in these trials.

Indications

Attention deficit hyperactivity disorder: For the treatment of ADHD.

Administration and Dosage

The safety of single doses above 120 mg and total daily doses above 150 mg have not been systematically evaluated.

Initial treatment:

Children up to 70 kg – Initiate at a total daily dose of approximately 0.5 mg/kg and increase after a minimum of 3 days to a target total daily dose of approximately 1.2 mg/kg administered as a single daily dose in the morning or as evenly divided doses in the morning and late afternoon/early evening. No additional benefit has been demonstrated for doses higher than 1.2 mg/kg/day. The total daily dose in children and adolescents should not exceed 1.4 mg/kg or 100 mg, whichever is less.

Adults and children over 70 kg – Initiate at a total daily dose of 40 mg and increase after a minimum of 3 days to a target total daily dose of approximately 80 mg administered as a single daily dose in the morning or as evenly divided doses in the morning and late afternoon/early evening. After 2 to 4 additional weeks, the dose may be increased to a maximum of 100 mg in patients who have not achieved an optimal response. There are no data that support increased efficacy at higher doses. The maximum recommended total daily dose in children over 70 kg and adults is 100 mg.

Maintenance/Extended treatment: It is generally agreed that pharmacological treatment of ADHD may be needed for extended periods. The health care provider who elects to use atomoxetine for extended periods should periodically reevaluate the long-term usefulness of the drug for the individual patient.

Hepatic function impairment: For patients with moderate hepatic function impairment (Child-Pugh class B), reduce initial and target doses to 50% of the normal dose. For patients with severe hepatic function impairment (Child-Pugh class C), reduce initial and target doses to 25% of normal.

Concomitant use: In children up to 70 kg body weight administered strong CYP2D6 inhibitors, initiate atomoxetine at 0.5 mg/kg/day and only increase to the usual target dose of 1.2 mg/kg/day if symptoms fail to improve after 4 weeks and the initial dose is well-tolerated.

In children over 70 kg body weight and adults administered strong CYP2D6 inhibitors, initiate atomoxetine at 40 mg/day and only increase to the usual target dose of 80 mg/day if symptoms fail to improve after 4 weeks and the initial dose is well-tolerated.

Discontinuation: Atomoxetine can be discontinued without being tapered.

Actions

Pharmacology: Atomoxetine is a selective norepinephrine reuptake inhibitor. The precise mechanism by which it produces its therapeutic effects in ADHD is unknown, but it is thought to be related to selective inhibition of the presynaptic norepinephrine transporter, as determined in ex vivo uptake and neurotransmitter depletion studies.

Pharmacokinetics:

Absorption/Distribution – Atomoxetine is well absorbed after oral administration and is minimally affected by food. It is rapidly absorbed after oral administration, with absolute bioavailability of about 63% in extensive metabolizers (EMs) and 94% in poor metabolizers (PMs). Maximal plasma concentrations (C_{max}) are reached approximately 1 to 2 hours after dosing. At therapeutic concentrations, 98% of atomoxetine in plasma is bound to protein, primarily albumin.

Metabolism/Excretion – Atomoxetine is metabolized primarily through the CYP2D6 enzymatic pathway. In adult EMs, mean half-life is 5.2 hours. In PMs, mean half-life is 21.6 hours.

Atomoxetine is excreted primarily as 4-hydroxyatomoxetine-O-glucuronide, mainly in the urine (greater than 80%) and to a lesser extent in the feces (less than 17%).

Special populations –

Hepatic function impairment: Atomoxetine exposure area under the curve is increased, compared with normal subjects, in EM subjects with moderate (Child-Pugh class B; 2-fold increase) and severe (Child-Pugh class C; 4-fold increase) hepatic insufficiency. Dosage adjustment is recommended for patients with moderate or severe hepatic insufficiency.

Contraindications

Patients known to be hypersensitive to atomoxetine or other constituents of the product; with a monoamine oxidase inhibitor (MAOI) or within 2 weeks after discontinuing an MAOI; narrow angle glaucoma.

Warnings/Precautions

Suicidal ideation: Atomoxetine increased the risk of suicidal ideation in short-term studies in children and adolescents with ADHD. Pooled analysis of short-term (6- to 18-week), placebo-controlled trials of atomoxetine in children and adolescents have revealed a greater risk of suicidal ideation early during treatment in those receiving atomoxetine. A similar analysis in adult patients treated with atomoxetine for either ADHD or major depressive disorder did not reveal an increased risk of suicidal ideation or behavior in association with the use of atomoxetine.

The following symptoms have been reported with atomoxetine: aggressiveness, agitation, akathisia (eg, psychomotor restlessness), anxiety, hostility, hypomania, insomnia, irritability, impulsivity, mania, and panic attacks. Although a casual link between the emergence of such symptoms and the emergence of suicidal impulses has not been established, there is a concern that such symptoms may represent precursors to emerging suicidality.

Give consideration to changing the therapeutic regimen, including possibly discontinuing the medication, in patients who are experiencing emerging suicidality or symptoms that might be precursors to emerging suicidality, especially if these symptoms are severe or abrupt in onset or were not part of the patient's presenting symptoms.

Screening patients for bipolar disorder: In general, take particular care in treating ADHD in patients with comorbid bipolar disorder because of concern for possible induction of a mixed/manic episode in patients at risk for bipolar disorder.

Hepatic effects: Postmarketing reports indicate that atomoxetine can cause severe liver injury in rare cases. Although no evidence of liver injury was detected in clinical trials of about 6,000 patients, there have been 2 reported cases of markedly elevated hepatic enzymes and bilirubin, in the absence of other obvious explanatory factors, out of more than 2 million patients during the first 2 years of postmarketing experience.

Discontinue atomoxetine in patients with jaundice or laboratory evidence of liver injury and do not restart.

Emergence of new psychotic or manic symptoms: Treatment-emergent psychotic or manic symptoms (eg, delusional thinking, hallucinations, mania) in children and adolescents without a prior history of psychotic illness or mania can be caused by atomoxetine at usual doses.

Narrow-angle glaucoma: In clinical trials, atomoxetine use was associated with an increased risk of mydriasis; therefore, its use is not recommended in patients with narrow-angle glaucoma.

Priapism: Rare postmarketing cases of priapism, defined as painful and nonpainful penile erection lasting more than 4 hours, have been reported for children and adults treated with atomoxetine.

Growth: Monitor growth during treatment with atomoxetine. In general, the weight and height gain of children treated with atomoxetine lags behind that predicated by normative population data for about the first 9 to 12 months of treatment. Subsequently, weight gain rebounds and, at about 3 years of treatment, patients treated with atomoxetine have gained 17.9 kg on average, 0.5 kg more than predicted by their baseline data. After about 12 months, gain in height stabilizes and, at 3 years, patients treated with atomoxetine have gained 19.4 cm on average, 0.4 cm less than predicted by their baseline data. This growth pattern was generally similar regardless of pubertal status at the time of treatment initiation.

Cardiovascular effects:

Sudden death and other serious heart problems –

Children and adolescents: Sudden death has been reported in association with atomoxetine treatment at usual doses in children and adolescents with structural cardiac abnormalities or other serious heart problems.

Adults: Sudden death, stroke, and myocardial infarction have been reported in adults taking atomoxetine at usual doses for ADHD. Although the role of atomoxetine in these adult cases is also unknown, adults have a greater likelihood than children of having serious structural cardiac abnormalities, cardiomyopathy, serious heart rhythm abnormalities, coronary artery disease, or other serious cardiac problems. Consider not treating adults with clinically significant cardiac abnormalities.

Assessing cardiovascular status – Children, adolescents, or adults who are being considered for treatment with atomoxetine should have a careful history (including assessment for a family history of sudden death or ventricular arrhythmia) and physical exam to assess for the presence of cardiac disease, and should receive further cardiac evaluation if findings suggest such disease (eg, echocardiogram, electrocardiogram).

Blood pressure and heart rate effects – Use atomoxetine with caution in patients with hypertension, tachycardia, or cardiovascular or cerebrovascular disease because it can increase blood pressure and heart rate. Measure pulse and blood pressure at baseline, following dose increases, and periodically while on therapy.

Peripheral vascular effects – There have been spontaneous postmarketing reports of Raynaud phenomenon (new onset and exacerbation of preexisting condition).

Urinary retention/hesitancy: In adult ADHD controlled trials, the rates of urinary retention and urinary hesitation (3%, 7/269) were increased among atomoxetine subjects compared with placebo subjects (0%, 0/263). Consider a complaint of urinary retention or urinary hesitancy to be potentially related to atomoxetine.

Aggressive behavior or hostility: Aggressive behavior or hostility is often observed in children and adolescents with ADHD and has been reported in clinical trials and the postmarketing experience of some medications indicated for the treatment of ADHD. Monitor patients beginning treatment for ADHD for the appearance of or worsening of aggressive behavior or hostility.

Hypersensitivity reactions: Although uncommon, allergic reactions (eg, angioneurotic edema, rash, urticaria) have been reported in patients taking atomoxetine.

Hazardous tasks: Advise patients to use caution when driving a car or operating hazardous machinery until they are reasonably certain that their performance is not affected by atomoxetine.

Pregnancy: Category C.

Lactation: Atomoxetine and/or its metabolites were excreted in the milk of rats. It is not known if atomoxetine is excreted in human milk. Exercise caution if atomoxetine is administered to a breast-feeding woman.

Children: The safety and efficacy of atomoxetine in children younger than 6 years of age have not been established.

Drug Interactions

Drugs that may interact with atomoxetine include albuterol, CYP2D6 inhibitors, MAOIs, and pressor agents.

Adverse Reactions

Children and adolescents:

Commonly observed adverse reactions – The most commonly observed adverse reactions in patients treated with atomoxetine were the following: abdominal pain, decreased appetite, dizziness, fatigue, headache, irritability, nausea, somnolence, vomiting, weight decreased.

Other adverse reactions (at least 3%) – Adverse reactions observed in at least 3% of patients in child and adolescent trials included the following: abdominal pain upper, appetite decreased, constipation, cough, dermatitis, diarrhea, dizziness (excluding vertigo), dyspepsia, ear infection, fatigue, headache, influenza, irritability, rhinorrhea, somnolence, vomiting.

Poor CYP2D6 metabolizers – The following adverse reactions occurred in at least 2% of PM patients and were twice as frequent or statistically significantly more frequent in PM patients compared with EM patients: decreased appetite, depression, early morning awakening, insomnia, mydriasis, pruritus, sedation, tremor.

Adults: Adverse reactions observed in at least 3% of patients in adult trials included the following: abnormal dreams, appetite decreased, constipation, dizziness, dry mouth, dysmenorrhea, dyspepsia, ejaculation failure and/or ejaculation disorder, erectile disturbance, fatigue and/or lethargy, headache, hot flushes, impotence, insomnia and/or middle insomnia, libido decreased, menstrual disorder, myalgia, nausea, palpitations, paresthesia, prostatitis, pyrexia, rigors, sinus headache, sinusitis, sleep disorder, sweating increased, urinary hesitation and/or urinary retention and/or difficulty in micturition.

OLANZAPINE AND FLUOXETINE HYDROCHLORIDE

Capsules: 3 mg olanzapine/25 mg fluoxetine, 6 mg olanzapine/25 mg fluoxetine, 6 mg olanzapine/50 mg fluoxetine, 12 mg olanzapine/25 fluoxetine, 12 mg olanzapine/ 50 mg fluoxetine (*Rx*)	*Symbyax* (Eli Lilly)

Warning:

Suicidality and antidepressant drugs: Antidepressants increased the risk compared with placebo of suicidal thinking and behavior (suicidality) in children, adolescents, and young adults in short-term studies of major depressive disorder (MDD) and other psychiatric disorders. Anyone considering the use of olanzapine/fluoxetine or any other antidepressant in a child, adolescent, or young adult must balance this risk with clinical need. Short-term studies did not show an increase in the risk of suicidality with antidepressants compared with placebo in adults older than 24 years of age; there was a reduction in risk with antidepressants compared with placebo in adults 65 years of age and older. Depression and certain other psychiatric disorders are themselves associated with increases in the risk of suicide. Patients of all ages who are started on antidepressant therapy should be monitored appropriately and observed closely for clinical worsening, suicidality, or unusual changes in behavior. Families and caregivers should be advised of the need for close observation and communication with the health care provider. Olanzapine/fluoxetine is not approved for use in children.

Increased mortality in elderly patients with dementia-related psychosis: Elderly patients with dementia-related psychosis treated with antipsychotic drugs are at an increased risk of death. Analyses of 17 placebo-controlled trials (modal duration of 10 weeks), largely in patients taking atypical antipsychotic drugs, revealed a risk of death in drug-treated patients of between 1.6 and 1.7 times the risk of death in placebo-treated patients. Over the course of a typical 10-week controlled trial, the rate of death in drug-treated patients was approximately 4.5% compared with a rate of approximately 2.6% in the placebo group. Although the causes of death were varied, most of the deaths appeared to be either cardiovascular (eg, heart failure, sudden death) or infectious (eg, pneumonia) in nature. Observational studies suggest that, similar to atypical antipsychotic drugs, treatment with conventional antipsychotic drugs may increase mortality. The extent to which the findings of increased mortality in observational studies may be attributed to the antipsychotic drug may be attributed to the antipsychotic drug, as opposed to some characteristic(s) of patients, is not clear. Olanzapine/fluoxetine is not approved for the treatment of patients with dementia-related psychosis.

Indications

Bipolar I disorder: For the treatment of depressive episodes associated with bipolar I disorder.

Treatment-resistent depression: For the acute treatment of treatment-resistent depression (MDD in adults who do not respond to 2 separate trials of different antidepressants of adequate dose and duration in the current episode).

Administration and Dosage

Bipolar I disorder:

Maximum dosage – The safety of doses above olanzapine 18 mg/fluoxetine 75 mg has not been evaluated in clinical studies.

Initial dose – Olanzapine 6 mg/fluoxetine 25 mg capsule once daily in the evening.

Dosage adjustments – Dosage adjustments, if indicated, can be made according to efficacy and tolerability. Antidepressant efficacy was demonstrated with olanzapine/fluoxetine in a dose range of olanzapine 6 to 12 mg and fluoxetine 25 to 50 mg.

Treatment-resistent depression –

Initial dosage: Olanzapine 6 mg/fluoxetine 25 mg capsule once daily in the evening.

Usual dose: Olanzapine 6 to 18 mg/fluoxetine 25 to 50 mg.

Maximum dosage: Olanzapine 18 mg/fluoxetine 75 mg.

Special populations: Use a starting dose of 6 mg/25 mg for patients with a predisposition to hypotensive reactions, patients with hepatic impairment, or patients who exhibit a combination of factors that may slow the metabolism of olanzapine/fluoxetine (eg, female gender, elderly, nonsmoking status). When indicated, perform dose escalation with caution in these patients. Olanzapine/fluoxetine has not been systemically studied in patients older than 65 years of age or in patients younger than 18 years of age.

Treatment of pregnant women during the third trimester: Neonates exposed to fluoxetine and other selective serotonin reuptake inhibitors (SSRIs) or selective norepinephrine reuptake inhibitors (SNRIs) late in the third trimester have developed complications requiring prolonged hospitalization, respiratory support, and tube feeding. When treating pregnant women with fluoxetine during the third trimester, carefully consider the potential risks and benefits of treatment. Consider using a lower dose of fluoxetine in the third trimester.

SEDATIVES/HYPNOTICS, NONBARBITURATE

To facilitate comparison, the products are divided into the following 2 groups: Miscellaneous nonbarbiturates and benzodiazepines. Although sedative doses can be given, these agents primarily are intended to be hypnotics.

In the table below, some pharmacokinetic properties of the nonbarbiturate sedative/hypnotics are compared. Do not use this table to predict exact duration of effect, but use as a guide in drug selection.

Nonbarbiturate Sedative/Hypnotics Pharmacokinetic Parameters

Drug	Adult oral dose		Onset (min)	Duration of action (h)	Half-life (h)	Protein binding (%)	Urinary excretion, unchanged (%)
	Hypnotic	Sedative					
Miscellaneous nonbarbiturates							
Chloral hydrate	0.5 to 1 g	250 mg tid pc	30	nd	7 to 10[a]	35-41	nd
Ethchlorvynol	500 mg	100 to 200 mg bid or tid	15 to 60	5	10 to 20[b]	nd	40[c]
Paraldehyde	10 to 30 mL	5 to 10 mL	10 to 15	8 to 12	3.4 to 9.8	nd	small
Propiomazine	nd	10 to 20 mg	nd	nd	nd	nd	nd
Benzodiazepines							
Estazolam	1 to 2 mg	na[d]	nd[e]	nd	10 to 24	93	< 5
Flurazepam	15 to 30 mg	na	17	7 to 8	150 to 100[f]	97	< 1[f]
Quazepam	15 mg	na	nd	nd	25 to 41	> 95	trace
Temazepam	15 to 30 mg	na	nd	nd	10 to 17	98	1.5
Triazolam	0.125 to 0.5 mg	na	nd	nd	1.5 to 5.5	90	2

[a] Trichloroethanol, the principal metabolite.
[b] In acute use, half-life of the distribution phase (1 to 3 hours) is more appropriate.
[c] Free and conjugated forms of the major metabolite, secondary alcohol of ethchlorvynol.
[d] na = Not applicable.
[e] nd = No data.
[f] Active metabolite, desalkylflurazepam.

ZOLPIDEM TARTRATE

Tablets; oral: 5 and 10 mg (*c-iv*) — Various, *Ambien* (Sanofi-Aventis)
Tablets, extended release; oral: 6.25 and 12.5 mg (*c-iv*) — Various, *Ambien CR* (Sanofi-Aventis)
Tablets; sublingual: 5 and 10 mg (*Rx*) — *Edluar* (Meda Pharmaceuticals)
Spray, solution; lingual: 5 mg/actuation (*Rx*) — *Zolpimist* (NovaDel Pharma)

Indications

Insomnia: For the short-term treatment of insomnia, characterized by difficulties with sleep onset and/or sleep maintenance (as measured by wake time after sleep onset).

Administration and Dosage

Adults:

Immediate-release, sublingual tablets, and oral spray – 10 mg immediately before bedtime. The total dose should not exceed 10 mg.

Downward dosage adjustment may be necessary when zolpidem is administered with agents having known CNS-depressant effects because of the potentially additive effects.

The orally disintegrating tablet may be taken with or without water. Do not chew, break, or split the orally disintegrating tablet. The orally disintegrating tablet should not be administered with or immediately after a meal.

Extended-release – 12.5 mg immediately before bedtime. Extended-release tablets should be swallowed whole and not divided, crushed, or chewed.

The effect of the extended-release tablets may be slowed by ingestion with or immediately after a meal.

Elderly or debilitated patients, hepatic function impairment: 5 mg of the immediate-release tablet or 6.25 mg of the extended-release tablet taken immediately before bedtime. Elderly or debilitated patients may be especially sensitive to the effects of zolpidem.

Actions

Pharmacology: Zolpidem is a nonbenzodiazepine hypnotic. While zolpidem is a hypnotic agent with a chemical structure unrelated to benzodiazepines, barbiturates, or other drugs with known hypnotic properties, it interacts with a GABA-BZ receptor complex and shares some of the pharmacological properties of the benzodiazepines.

Pharmacokinetics:

Absorption/Distribution – Total protein binding is approximately 92%.

Immediate-release and orally disintegrating tablets: For 5 and 10 mg tablets, mean peak concentrations (C_{max}) were 59 and 121 ng/mL, respectively, and time to reach maximum plasma concentration (T_{max}) was 1.6 hours for both.

Results of a food effect study suggest that, for faster sleep onset, zolpidem should not be administered with, or immediately after, a meal.

Extended-release: Extended-release tablets have a T_{max} of 1.5 hours.

Results of a food effect study suggest that, for faster sleep onset, zolpidem should not be administered with, or immediately after, a meal.

Metabolism/Excretion – Zolpidem is converted to inactive metabolites that are eliminated primarily by renal excretion.

Immediate-release: The mean zolpidem elimination half-life was 2.5 and 2.6 hours for the 5 and 10 mg tablets, respectively.

Extended-release: The mean zolpidem elimination half-life was 2.8 hours.

Contraindications

Known hypersensitivity to zolpidem or to any of the inactive ingredients in the formulation.

Warnings/Precautions

Psychiatric/Physical disorder: Because sleep disturbances may be the presenting manifestation of a physical or psychiatric disorder, initiate symptomatic treatment of insomnia only after a careful evaluation of the patient.

CNS effects: A variety of abnormal thinking and behavior changes have been reported to occur in association with the use of sedative/hypnotics. Some of these changes may be characterized by decreased inhibition, similar to effects produced by alcohol and other CNS depressants. Visual and auditory hallucinations as well as behavioral changes have been reported. Amnesia, anxiety, and other neuropsychiatric symptoms may occur unpredictably. In primarily depressed patients, worsening of depression, including suicidal thinking, has been reported.

Abrupt discontinuation: Following the rapid dose decrease or abrupt discontinuation of sedative-hypnotics, there have been reports of signs and symptoms similar to those associated with withdrawal from other CNS-depressant drugs.

Concomitant illness: Use zolpidem with caution in patients with diseases or conditions that could effect metabolism or hemodynamic responses. Observe caution if zolpidem is prescribed to patients with compromised respiratory function, since sedative/hypnotics have the capacity to depress respiratory drive.

Depression: Administer zolpidem with caution to patients exhibiting signs or symptoms of depression. Suicidal tendencies may be present in such patients and protective measures may be required. Intentional overdosage is more common in this group of patients; therefore, prescribe the least amount of drug that is feasible for the patient at any one time.

Hypersensitivity reactions: Rare cases of angioedema involving the glottis, larynx, or tongue have been reported in patients after taking the first or subsequent doses of sedative-hypnotics, including zolpidem. Patients who develop angioedema after treatment with zolpidem should not be rechallenged with the drug.

Renal/Hepatic function impairment: Closely monitor patients with renal and hepatic function impairment.

Drug abuse and dependence: Sedative/hypnotics have produced withdrawal signs and symptoms following abrupt discontinuation. These reported symptoms range from mild dysphoria and insomnia to a withdrawal syndrome that may include abdominal and muscle cramps, vomiting, sweating, tremors, and convulsions. Zolpidem does not reveal any clear evidence for withdrawal syndrome.

Because individuals with a history of psychiatric disorders or addiction to, or abuse of, drugs or alcohol are at risk of misuse and abuse of and addiction to zolpidem, monitor these patients carefully when administering zolpidem or any other hypnotic.

Hazardous tasks: Zolpidem should only be ingested immediately prior to going to bed. Caution patients against engaging in hazardous occupations requiring complete mental alertness or motor coordination and inform them of the potential impairment of the performance of such activities that may occur the day following ingestion of zolpidem. Zolpidem showed additive effects when combined with alcohol and should not be taken with alcohol. Also caution patients about possible combined effects with other CNS-depressant drugs. Dosage adjustments may be necessary when zolpidem is administered with such agents because of potentially additive effects.

Pregnancy: Category C.

Lactation: The use of zolpidem in breast-feeding mothers is not recommended.

Children: Safety and efficacy in children younger than 18 years of age have not been established.

Elderly: Closely monitor these patients. Impaired motor or cognitive performance after repeated exposure or unusual sensitivity to sedative/hypnotic drugs is a concern in the treatment of elderly or debilitated patients.

Drug Interactions

Drugs that may affect zolpidem include azole antifungals, chlorpromazine, flumazenil, imipramine, rifamycins, selective serotonin reuptake inhibitors, CNS depressants, and ritonavir.

Drugs that zolpidem may affect include chlorpromazine, imipramine, and CNS depressants.

Drug/Food interactions: For faster sleep onset, do not administer with or immediately after a meal.

Adverse Reactions

Adverse reactions occurring in 3% or more of patients include allergy; anxiety; arthralgia; back pain; diarrhea; disorientation; dizziness; drowsiness; drugged feelings; dry mouth, dyspepsia; fatigue; hallucinations; headache; influenza; lethargy; memory disorders; myalgia; nausea; nasopharyngitis; pharyngitis; sinusitis; somnolence; upper respiratory tract infection; visual disturbance.

ZALEPLON

Capsules: 5 and 10 mg (*c-iv*)	Various, *Sonata* (Wyeth-Ayerst)

Indications

Insomnia: For the short-term treatment of insomnia.

Administration and Dosage

The recommended dose of zaleplon for most nonelderly adults is 10 mg. For certain low-weight individuals, 5 mg may be a sufficient dose. Although the risk of certain adverse events associated with zaleplon appears to be dose dependent, the 20 mg dose has been shown to be adequately tolerated and may be considered for the occasional patient who does not benefit from a trial of a lower dose. Doses greater than 20 mg have not been adequately evaluated and are not recommended.

Hypnotics should generally be limited to 7 to 10 days of use, and re-evaluation of the patient is recommended if they are to be taken for longer than 2 to 3 weeks.

Take zaleplon immediately before bedtime or after going to bed and experiencing difficulty falling asleep. Taking it with or immediately after a heavy, high-fat meal results in slower absorption and would be expected to reduce the effect of zaleplon on sleep latency.

Elderly/Debilitated: Elderly and debilitated patients appear to be more sensitive to the effects of hypnotics; therefore, the recommended dose for these patients is 5 mg. Doses larger than 10 mg are not recommended.

Hepatic function impairment: Treat patients with mild to moderate hepatic impairment with zaleplon 5 mg because of reduced clearance. Do not use in patients with severe hepatic impairment.

Renal function impairment: No dose adjustment is necessary in patients with mild to moderate renal impairment.

Concomitant cimetidine – Give an initial dose of 5 mg to patients concomitantly taking cimetidine (see Drug Interactions).

Actions

Pharmacology: Zaleplon is a nonbenzodiazepine hypnotic. Zaleplon has a chemical structure unrelated to benzodiazepines, barbiturates, or other drugs with known hypnotic properties.

Zaleplon binds selectively to the brain omega$_1$ receptor situated on the alpha subunit of the GABA$_A$ receptor complex and potentiates t-butyl-bicyclophosphorothionate (TBPS) binding.

Pharmacokinetics:

Absorption – Zaleplon is rapidly and almost completely absorbed following oral administration. Peak plasma concentrations are attained within approximately 1 hour after oral administration.

Distribution – Zaleplon is a lipophilic compound with a volume of distribution of approximately 1.4 L/kg following IV administration, indicating substantial distribution into extravascular tissues.

Metabolism – After oral administration, zaleplon is extensively metabolized with less than 1% of the dose excreted unchanged in urine.

Excretion – Following oral or IV administration, zaleplon is rapidly eliminated with a mean half-life of approximately 1 hour.

Contraindications

None known.

Warnings/Precautions

Duration of therapy: Because sleep disturbances may be the presenting manifestation of a physical or psychiatric disorder, initiate symptomatic treatment of insomnia only after careful evaluation of the patient. The failure of insomnia to remit after 7 to 10 days of treatment may indicate the need for evaluation of a primary psychiatric or medical illness. Do not prescribe zaleplon in quantities exceeding a 1-month supply.

Abnormal thinking/behavior changes: A variety of abnormal thinking and behavior changes have been reported to occur in association with the use of sedatives/hypnotics.

Rapid dose decrease/discontinuation: Following rapid dose decrease or abrupt discontinuation of sedatives/hypnotics, there have been reports of signs and symptoms similar to those associated with withdrawal from other CNS-depressant drugs.

CNS effects: Zaleplon, like other hypnotics, has CNS-depressant effects. Caution patients receiving zaleplon against engaging in hazardous occupations requiring complete mental alertness or motor coordination (eg, operating machinery or driving a motor vehicle) after ingesting the drug, including potential impairment of the performance of such activities that may occur the day following zaleplon ingestion. Zaleplon, as well as other hypnotics, may produce additive CNS-depressant effects when coadministered with other psychotropic medications, anticonvulsants, antihistamines, ethanol, and other drugs that produce CNS depression. Do not take zaleplon with alcohol.

Timing of drug administration: Take zaleplon immediately before bedtime or after going to bed and experiencing difficulty falling asleep. As with all sedatives/hypnotics, taking zaleplon while ambulatory may result in short-term memory impairment, hallucinations, impaired coordination, dizziness, and lightheadedness.

Respiratory effects: Although preliminary studies did not reveal respiratory depressant effects at hypnotic doses of zaleplon in healthy subjects, observe caution if zaleplon is prescribed to patients with compromised respiratory function because sedatives/hypnotics have the capacity to depress respiratory drive.

Depression: As with other sedative/hypnotic drugs, administer zaleplon with caution to patients exhibiting signs or symptoms of depression. Suicidal tendencies may be present in such patients and protective measures may be required. Intentional overdosage is more common in this group of patients; therefore, prescribe the least amount of the drug that is feasible for the patient at any one time.

Hepatic function impairment: Zaleplon is metabolized primarily by the liver and undergoes significant presystemic metabolism. Consequently, the oral clearance of zaleplon was reduced by 70% and 87% in compensated and decompensated cirrhotic patients, respectively.

Drug abuse and dependence:

Abuse – Two studies assessed the abuse liability of zaleplon at doses of 25, 50, and 75 mg in subjects with known histories of sedative drug abuse. The results of these studies indicate that zaleplon has an abuse potential similar to benzodiazepine and benzodiazepine-like hypnotics.

Pregnancy: Category C.

Lactation: Because the effects of zaleplon on a nursing infant are not known, it is recommended that nursing mothers not take zaleplon.

Children: The safety and efficacy have not been established.

Elderly: Impaired motor or cognitive performance after repeated exposure or unusual sensitivity to sedative/hypnotic drugs is a concern in the treatment of elderly or debilitated patients.

Drug Interactions

Drugs that induce CYP3A4: CYP3A4 is a minor metabolizing enzyme of zaleplon. The CYP3A4-inducer rifampin reduced zaleplon C_{max} and AUC by approximately 80%.

Cimetidine: Cimetidine inhibits aldehyde oxidase and CYP3A4, the primary and secondary enzymes, respectively, responsible for zaleplon metabolism. Use an initial dose of 5 mg for patients concomitantly treated with cimetidine.

Drug/Food interactions: The effects of zaleplon on sleep onset may be reduced if it is taken with or immediately after a high-fat/heavy meal.

Adverse Reactions

Adverse effects occurring in 3% or more of patients include the following: Amnesia; anxiety; dizziness; paresthesia; somnolence; dyspepsia; nausea; eye pain; abdominal pain; asthenia; headache; myalgia; dysmenorrhea.

RAMELTEON

Tablets: 8 mg (Rx)	*Rozerem* (Takeda Pharmaceutical)

Indications

Insomnia: For the treatment of insomnia characterized by difficulty with sleep onset.

Administration and Dosage

Dosage: The recommended dose of ramelteon is 8 mg taken within 30 minutes of going to bed. It is recommended that ramelteon not be taken with or immediately after a high-fat meal. After taking ramelteon, patients should confine their activities to those necessary to prepare for bed.

Actions

Pharmacology: Ramelteon is a melatonin receptor agonist with high affinity for melatonin MT_1 and MT_2 receptors and selectivity over the MT_3 receptor.

The activity of ramelteon at the MT_1 and MT_2 receptors is believed to contribute to its sleep-promoting properties, as these receptors, acted upon by endogenous melatonin, are thought to be involved in the maintenance of the circadian rhythm underlying the normal sleep-wake cycle.

Pharmacokinetics:

Absorption – Ramelteon is absorbed rapidly, with median peak concentrations occurring at approximately 0.75 hours (range, 0.5 to 1.5 hours) after fasted oral administration. Although the total absorption of ramelteon is at least 84%, the absolute oral bioavailability is only 1.8% because of extensive first-pass metabolism.

Distribution – Protein binding of ramelteon is approximately 82% and 70% of the drug is bound in human serum albumin.

Ramelteon has a mean volume of distribution after intravenous (IV) administration of 73.6 L, suggesting substantial tissue distribution.

Metabolism – Ramelteon undergoes rapid, high first-pass metabolism, and exhibits linear pharmacokinetics. Several metabolites have been identified in human serum and urine.

Metabolism of ramelteon consists primarily of oxidation to hydroxyl and carbonyl derivatives, with secondary metabolism producing glucuronide conjugates. CYP1A2 is the major isozyme involved in the hepatic metabolism of ramelteon; the CYP2C subfamily and CYP3A4 isozymes also are involved to a minor degree.

Excretion – 84% of total radioactivity is excreted in urine and approximately 4% in feces, resulting in a mean recovery of 88%. Less than 0.1% of the dose was excreted in urine and feces as the parent compound. Elimination was essentially complete by 96 hours postdose.

The half-life of the principle metabolite M-II is 2 to 5 hours and is independent of dose.

Contraindications

Hypersensitivity to ramelteon or any components of the ramelteon formulation.

Warnings/Precautions

Psychiatric/Physical disorder: Because sleep disturbances may be the presenting manifestation of a physical and/or psychiatric disorder, initiate symptomatic treatment of insomnia only after a careful evaluation of the patient.

Hepatic function impairment: Do not use ramelteon in patients with severe hepatic function impairment. Use with caution in patients with moderate hepatic function.

Special risk: Ramelteon has not been studied in subjects with severe sleep apnea or severe COPD and is not recommended for use in those populations. Advise patients to exercise caution if they consume alcohol in combination with ramelteon.

Hazardous tasks: Avoid engaging in hazardous activities that require concentration (eg, operating a motor vehicle or heavy machinery) after taking ramelteon.

Pregnancy: Category C.

Lactation: Ramelteon is secreted into the milk of lactating rats. It is not known whether this drug is excreted in human milk.

Children: Safety and efficacy of ramelteon in children have not been established.

Monitoring: For patients presenting with unexplained amenorrhea, galactorrhea, decreased libido, or problems with fertility, consider assessment of prolactin levels and testosterone levels as appropriate.

Drug Interactions

CYP1A2 inhibitors: Administer ramelteon with caution to patients taking less strong CYP1A2 inhibitors.

Ramelteon is affected by alcohol, azole antifungals, fluvoxamine, and rifampin.

Drug/Food interactions: Ramelteon should not be taken with or immediately after a high-fat meal.

Adverse Reactions

The most frequent adverse reactions leading to discontinuation were somnolence (0.8%), dizziness (0.5%), nausea (0.3%), fatigue (0.3%), headache (0.3%), and insomnia (0.3%).

Other adverse reactions occurring in 3% or more of patients receiving ramelteon include dizziness, fatigue, headache, exacerbated insomnia, somnolence, nausea, and upper respiratory tract infection.

BENZODIAZEPINES

ESTAZOLAM **Tablets:** 1 and 2 mg (*c-iv*)	*Estazolam* (Zenith-Goldline), *ProSom* (Abbott)
FLURAZEPAM HYDROCHLORIDE **Capsules:** 15 and 30 mg (*c-iv*)	Various
QUAZEPAM **Tablets:** 7.5 and 15 mg (*c-iv*)	*Doral* (Questcor)
TEMAZEPAM **Capsules:** 7.5, 15, 22.5, and 30 mg (*c-iv*)	Various, *Restoril* (Mallinckrodt)
TRIAZOLAM **Tablets:** 0.125 and 0.25 mg (*c-iv*)	Various, *Halcion* (Upjohn)

Indications

Insomnia: Insomnia characterized by difficulty in falling asleep, frequent nocturnal awakenings, or early morning awakening. Can be used for recurring insomnia or poor sleeping habits and in acute or chronic medical situations requiring restful sleep.

Administration and Dosage

ESTAZOLAM:

Adults – 1 mg at bedtime; however, some patients may need a 2 mg dose.

Elderly – If healthy, 1 mg at bedtime; initiate increases with particular care.

Debilitated or small elderly patients – Consider a starting dose of 0.5 mg, although this is only marginally effective in the overall elderly population.

FLURAZEPAM:

Adults – 30 mg before bedtime. In some patients, 15 mg may suffice.

Elderly or debilitated – Initiate with 15 mg until individual response is determined.

QUAZEPAM:

Adults – Initiate at 15 mg until individual responses are determined; may reduce to 7.5 mg in some patients.

Elderly or debilitated – Attempt to reduce nightly dosage after the first 1 or 2 nights.

TEMAZEPAM:

Adults – Give 15 to 30 mg before bedtime.

Elderly or debilitated – Initiate with 7.5 to 15 mg until individual response is determined.

TRIAZOLAM:

Adults – 0.125 to 0.5 mg before bedtime.

Elderly or debilitated – 0.125 to 0.25 mg. Initiate with 0.125 mg until individual response is determined.

Actions

Pharmacology: **Estazolam, flurazepam, quazepam, temazepam,** and **triazolam** are benzodiazepine derivatives useful as hypnotics. Benzodiazepines are believed to potentiate gamma-aminobutyric acid (GABA) neuronal inhibition.

Pharmacokinetics:

Select Benzodiazepine (Hypnotic) Pharmacokinetic Parameters

Drug	Usual adult oral dose (mg)	Time to peak plasma levels (h)	Half-life (h)	Protein binding (%)	Urinary excretion, unchanged (%)
Estazolam	1 to 2	2	8 to 28	93	< 5
Flurazepam	15 to 30	0.5 to 1 (7.6 to 13.6)[a]	2 to 3 (47 to 100)[a]	97	< 1
Quazepam	7.5 to 15	2 (1 to 2)	41 (47 to 100)[a]	> 95	trace
Temazepam	15 to 30	1.2 to 1.6	3.5 to 18.4 (9 to 15)	96	0.2
Triazolam	0.125 to 0.5	1 to 2	1.5 to 5.5	78 to 89	2

[a] N-desalkylflurazepam, active metabolite.

Contraindications

Hypersensitivity to other benzodiazepines; pregnancy (see Warnings); established or suspected sleep apnea (**quazepam**).

Concurrent use with ketoconazole, itraconazole, and nefazodone, medications that significantly impair the oxidative metabolism of **triazolam** mediated by cytochrome P-450 3A (CYP3A).

Warnings/Precautions

Anterograde amnesia: Anterograde amnesia of varying severity and paradoxical reactions has occurred following therapeutic doses of **triazolam**. Although this effect generally occurred with a dose of 0.5 mg, it has also been reported with 0.125 and 0.25 mg doses. This effect may occur with some other benzodiazepines, but data suggest that it may occur at a higher rate with triazolam. Cases of "traveler's amnesia" have been reported by individuals who have taken triazolam to induce sleep while traveling.

Depression: Administer with caution in severely depressed patients or in those in whom there is evidence of latent depression or suicidal tendencies. Signs or symptoms of depression may be intensified by hypnotic drugs.

Sleep disorder: Rebound sleep disorder, which is characterized by recurrence of insomnia to levels worse than before treatment began, may occur following abrupt withdrawal of **triazolam**, usually during the first 1 to 3 nights. Gradual rather than abrupt discontinuation of the drug may help avoid this syndrome.

Nocturnal sleep: Disturbed nocturnal sleep may occur for the first or second night after discontinuing use.

Morning insomnia: Early morning insomnia, or early morning awakenings, appears to be more common with the use of short half-life agents (**temazepam, triazolam**) than agents with intermediate or long half-lives (**estazolam, flurazepam, quazepam**). Daytime sleepiness appears to be more prevalent with the long half-life agents.

Respiratory depression and sleep apnea: Observe caution. In patients with compromised respiratory function, respiratory depression and sleep apnea have occurred.

Renal/Hepatic function impairment: Observe usual precautions under these conditions.

Abnormal liver function tests as well as blood dyscrasias have been reported with benzodiazepines.

Drug abuse and dependence: Withdrawal symptoms following abrupt discontinuation of benzodiazepines have occurred in patients receiving excessive doses over extended periods of time. Gradual withdrawal is preferred.

Hazardous tasks: Observe caution while driving or performing tasks requiring alertness.

Pregnancy: Category X (**estazolam, flurazepam, quazepam, temazepam, triazolam**).

Lactation: Safety for use in the breast-feeding mother has not been established.

Children:

Estazolam, quazepam, temazepam, triazolam – Not for use in children younger than 18 years of age.

Flurazepam – Not for use in children younger than 15 years of age.

Elderly: The risk of developing oversedation, dizziness, confusion, or ataxia increases substantially with larger doses of benzodiazepines in elderly and debilitated patients. Initiate with lowest effective dose.

Monitoring: When **triazolam** or **estazolam** treatment is protracted, obtain periodic blood counts, urinalysis, and blood chemistry analyses.

Drug Interactions

Drugs that may affect benzodiazepines include alcohol/CNS depressants, cimetidine, oral contraceptives, disulfiram, isoniazid, probenecid, rifampin, smoking, theophyllines, and macrolides.

Drugs that may be affected by benzodiazepines include digoxin, neuromuscular blocking agents (nondepolarizing), and phenytoin.

Adverse Reactions

Adverse reactions include the following: anorexia, apprehension, body/joint pain, chest pains, confusion, confusional states/memory impairment, congestion, constipation, coordination disorders, cramps/pain, depression, diarrhea, dreaming/nightmares, dry mouth, dysesthesia, euphoria, GI pain, GU complaints, headache, heartburn, insomnia, irritability, lack of concentration, nausea, nervousness, palpitations, paresthesia, relaxed feeling, restlessness, tachycardia, taste alterations, tinnitus, tiredness, tremor, vomiting, weakness.

Estazolam: Other adverse reactions reported only for estazolam include the following: somnolence (42%); asthenia (11%); hypokinesia (8%); hangover (3%); cold symptoms, lower extremity/back/abdominal pain (1% to 3%).

ESZOPICLONE

Tablets: 1, 2, and 3 mg (*c-iv*)	*Lunesta* (Sepracor)

Indications

Insomnia: For the treatment of insomnia.

Administration and Dosage

Adults: The recommended starting dose for eszopiclone is 2 mg immediately before bedtime. Dosing can be initiated at or raised to 3 mg if clinically indicated for sleep maintenance.

Elderly: The recommended starting dose for elderly patients whose primary complaint is difficulty falling asleep is 1 mg immediately before bedtime. The dose may be increased to 2 mg if clinically indicated. For elderly patients whose primary complaint is difficulty staying asleep, the recommended dose is 2 mg immediately before bedtime.

Administration: Taking eszopiclone with or immediately after a heavy, high-fat meal results in slower absorption and would be expected to reduce the effect of eszopiclone on sleep latency.

Hepatic function impairment: The starting dose should be 1 mg in patients with severe hepatic impairment.

Coadministration with CYP3A4 inhibitors: Do not exceed a 1 mg starting dose in patients coadministered eszopiclone with potent CYP3A4 inhibitors (eg, ketoconazole). If needed, the dose can be raised to 2 mg.

Actions

Pharmacology: Eszopiclone is a nonbenzodiazepine hypnotic. The precise mechanism of action of eszopiclone as a hypnotic is unknown, but its effect is believed to result from its interaction with gamma-aminobutyric acid (GABA)-receptor complexes at binding domains located close to or allosterically coupled to benzodiazepine receptors.

Pharmacokinetics:

Absorption/Distribution – Eszopiclone is rapidly absorbed, with a time to peak concentration (T_{max}) of approximately 1 hour. Eszopiclone is weakly bound to plasma protein (52% to 59%). The large free fraction suggests that eszopiclone disposition should not be affected by drug-drug interactions caused by protein binding.

Metabolism – Eszopiclone is extensively metabolized by oxidation and demethylation. In vitro studies have shown that CYP3A4 and CYP2E1 enzymes are involved in the metabolism of eszopiclone.

Excretion – Eszopiclone is eliminated with a mean t½ of approximately 6 hours. Up to 75% of an oral dose of racemic zopiclone is excreted in the urine, primarily as metabolites. Less than 10% of the oral eszopiclone dose is excreted in the urine as parent drug.

Warnings/Precautions

Psychiatric/Physical disorder: Because sleep disturbances may be the presenting manifestation of a physical and/or psychiatric disorder, initiate symptomatic treatment of insomnia only after careful evaluation of the patient. Because some of the important adverse effects of eszopiclone appear to be dose-related, it is important to use the lowest possible effective dose, especially in the elderly.

Abnormal thinking and behavioral changes – A variety of abnormal thinking and behavioral changes have been reported to occur in association with the use of sedative/hypnotic drugs. Some of these changes may be characterized by decreased inhibition similar to effects produced by alcohol and other CNS depressants. Other reported behavioral changes have included agitation, bizarre behavior, depersonalization, and hallucinations. Complex behaviors, such as sleep-driving, have been reported. These reactions can occur in sedative/hypnotic-naive and sedativ/hypnotic-experienced people.

Rapid dose decrease/discontinuation: Following rapid dose decrease or abrupt discontinuation of the use of sedative/hypnotics, there have been reports of signs and symptoms similar to those associated with withdrawal from other CNS-depressant drugs.

CNS effects: Because of the rapid onset of action, eszopiclone should only be ingested immediately prior to going to bed or after the patient has gone to bed and has experienced difficulty falling asleep. Eszopiclone may produce additive CNS-depressant effects when coadministered with other psychotropic medications, anticonvulsants, antihistamines, ethanol, and other drugs that produce CNS depression. Eszopiclone should not be taken with alcohol. Dose adjustment may be necessary when eszopiclone is administered with other CNS-depressant agents because of the potentially additive effects.

Timing of drug administration: Eszopiclone should be taken immediately before bedtime. Taking a sedative/hypnotic while still ambulatory may result in short-term memory impairment, hallucinations, impaired coordination, dizziness, and light-headedness.

Hypersensitivity reactions: Rare cases of angioedema involving the tongue, glottis, or larynx have been reported in patients after taking the first or subsequent doses of sedative/hypnotic drugs, including eszopiclone.

Hepatic function impairment: Reduce the dose of eszopiclone to 1 mg in patients with severe hepatic impairment.

Special risk:

Elderly/Debilitated patients – Subjects 65 years of age and older had an increase of 41% in total exposure (AUC) and a slightly prolonged elimination of eszopiclone (t½ approximately 9 hours). Decrease the starting dose of eszopiclone to 1 mg. The dose should not exceed 2 mg.

Impaired motor and/or cognitive performance or unusual sensitivity to sedative/hypnotic drugs is a concern in the treatment of elderly and/or debilitated patients.

Patients with concomitant illness – Use eszopiclone with caution in patients with diseases or conditions that could affect metabolism or hemodynamic responses. Caution is advised if eszopiclone is prescribed to patients with compromised respiratory function.

Depression – Administer sedative/hypnotic drugs with caution to patients exhibiting signs and symptoms of depression.

Drug abuse and dependence: In a study of abuse liability conducted in individuals with known histories of benzodiazepine abuse, doses of eszopiclone 6 and 12 mg produced euphoric effects similar to those of diazepam 20 mg.

Hazardous tasks: Caution patients receiving eszopiclone against engaging in hazardous occupations requiring complete mental alertness or motor coordination after ingesting the drug, and caution them about potential impairment of the performance of such activities on the day following ingestion of eszopiclone.

Pregnancy: Category C.

Lactation: It is not known whether eszopiclone is excreted in human milk.

Children: Safety and efficacy of eszopiclone in children younger than 18 years of age have not been established.

Drug Interactions

Drugs that may interact with eszopiclone include CYP3A4 inducers, CYP3A4 inhibitors, and ethanol.

Drug/Food interactions: The effects of eszopiclone on sleep onset may be reduced if it is taken with or immediately after a high-fat/heavy meal.

Adverse Reactions

Adverse reactions occurring in 3% or more of patients include anxiety, confusion, depression, dizziness, dry mouth, dysmenorrhea, dyspepsia, gynecomastia, hallucinations, headache, infection, libido decreased, nausea, nervousness, rash, somnolence, unpleasant taste, viral infection, vomiting.

Adverse reactions occurring in 3% or more of elderly patients include abnormal dreams, accidental injury, diarrhea, dizziness, dry mouth, dyspepsia, headache, neuralgia, pain, pruritus, unpleasant taste, urinary tract infection.

SEDATIVES AND HYPNOTICS, BARBITURATE

AMOBARBITAL SODIUM	
Powder for injection: (*c-ii*)	*Amytal Sodium* (Lilly)
APROBARBITAL	
Elixir: 40 mg per 5 mL (*c-iii*)	*Alurate* (Roche)
BUTABARBITAL SODIUM	
Tablets: 30 and 50 mg (*c-iii*)	*Butisol Sodium* (Meda Pharmaceuticals)
Elixir: 30 mg per 5 mL (*c-iii*)	
MEPHOBARBITAL	
Tablets: 32, 50, and 100 mg (*c-iv*)	*Mebaral* (Sanofi Winthrop)
PENTOBARBITAL SODIUM	
Capsules: 50 and 100 mg (*c-ii*)	Various, *Nembutal Sodium* (Abbott)
Suppositories: 30, 60, 120, and 200 mg (*c-iii*)	*Nembutal Sodium* (Abbott)
Injection: 50 mg/mL (*c-ii*)	*Pentobarbital Sodium* (Wyeth-Ayerst), *Nembutal Sodium* (Abbott)
PHENOBARBITAL	
Tablets: 15, 16, 30, 60, and 100 mg (*c-iv*)	Various, *Solfoton* (ECR Pharm.)
Capsules: 16 mg (*c-iv*)	*Solfoton* (ECR Pharm.)
Elixir: 15 mg per 5 mL and 20 mg per 5 mL (*c-iv*)	Various
Injection: 30, 60, 65, and 130 mg/mL (*c-iv*)	Various, *Luminal Sodium* (Sanofi Winthrop)
SECOBARBITAL SODIUM	
Capsules: 100 mg (*c-ii*)	Various, *Seconal Sodium Pulvules* (Marathon)
Injection: 50 mg/mL (*c-ii*)	*Secobarbital Sodium* (Wyeth-Ayerst)

The following general discussion of the barbiturates refers to their use as sedative-hypnotic agents and as anticonvulsants.

Indications

Acute convulsive episodes: Emergency control of certain acute convulsive episodes (eg, those associated with status epilepticus, cholera, eclampsia, meningitis, tetanus, and toxic reactions to strychnine or local anesthetics).

Anticonvulsant (mephobarbital, phenobarbital): Treatment of partial and generalized tonic-clonic and cortical focal seizures.

Hypnotic: Short-term treatment of insomnia, because barbiturates appear to lose their effectiveness in sleep induction and maintenance after 2 weeks. If insomnia persists, seek alternative therapy (including nondrug) for chronic insomnia.

Preanesthetic: Used as preanesthetic sedatives.

Sedation: Although traditionally used as nonspecific CNS depressants for daytime sedation, the barbiturates have generally been replaced by the benzodiazepines.

Administration and Dosage

IM injection: IM injection of the sodium salts should be made deeply into a large muscle. Do not exceed 5 mL at any one site because of possible tissue irritation. Monitor patient's vital signs.

IV: Restrict to conditions in which other routes are not feasible, either because the patient is unconscious or resists, or because prompt action is imperative. Slow IV injection is essential; observe patients carefully during administration.

Rectal administration: Rectally administered barbiturates are absorbed from the colon and are used occasionally in infants for prolonged convulsive states, or when oral or parenteral administration may be undesirable.

Elderly/Debilitated: Reduce dosage because these patients may be more sensitive to barbiturates.

Hepatic/Renal function impairment: Reduce dosage.

AMOBARBITAL SODIUM: The maximum single dose for an adult is 1 g.

Sedative – The usual adult dosage is 30 to 50 mg 2 or 3 times/day.

Hypnotic – The usual adult dose is 65 to 200 mg.

IM – The average IM dose ranges from 65 to 500 mg.

IV – Do not exceed the rate of 50 mg/min. Ordinarily, 65 to 500 mg may be given to a child 6 to 12 years of age.

APROBARBITAL:

Sedative – 40 mg 3 times/day.

Mild insomnia – 40 to 80 mg before retiring.

Pronounced insomnia – 80 to 160 mg before retiring.

BUTABARBITAL SODIUM:

Adults –

Daytime sedation: 15 to 30 mg 3 or 4 times/day.

Bedtime hypnotic: 50 to 100 mg

Preoperative sedation: 50 to 100 mg, 60 to 90 minutes before surgery.

Children –

Preoperative sedation: 2 to 6 mg/kg/day (maximum 100 mg).

MEPHOBARBITAL:

Sedative –

Adults: 32 to 100 mg 3 or 4 times/day. Optimum dose is 50 mg 3 or 4 times/day.

Children: 16 to 32 mg 3 or 4 times/day.

Epilepsy –

Adults: Average dose is 400 to 600 mg/day.

Children (younger than 5 years of age): 16 to 32 mg 3 or 4 times/day.

Children (older than 5 years of age): 32 to 64 mg 3 or 4 times/day.

Take at bedtime if seizures generally occur at night, and during the day if attacks are diurnal. Start treatment with a small dose and gradually increase over 4 or 5 days until optimum dosage is determined.

Combination drug therapy – May be used in combination with phenobarbital, in alternating courses or concurrently. When the two are used at the same time, the dose should be approximately ½ the amount of each used alone. The average daily dose for an adult is 50 to 100 mg phenobarbital and 200 to 300 mg mephobarbital. May also be used with phenytoin. When used concurrently, a reduced dose of phenytoin is advisable, but the full dose of mephobarbital may be given. Satisfactory results have been obtained with an average daily dose of 230 mg phenytoin plus about 600 mg mephobarbital.

PENTOBARBITAL SODIUM:

Oral –

Adults:

Sedation – 20 mg 3 or 4 times/day.

Hypnotic – 100 mg at bedtime.

Children:

Sedation/Preanesthetic – 2 to 6 mg/kg/day (maximum 100 mg), depending on age, weight, and degree of sedation desired.

Hypnotic – Base dosage on age and weight.

Rectal – Do not divide suppositories.

Adults: 120 to 200 mg.

Children:

12 to 14 years of age (36.4 to 50 kg; 80 to 110 lbs) – 60 or 120 mg.

5 to 12 years of age (18.2 to 36.4 kg; 40 to 80 lbs) – 60 mg.

1 to 4 years of age (9 to 18.2 kg; 20 to 40 lbs) – 30 or 60 mg.

2 months to 1 year of age (4.5 to 9 kg; 10 to 20 lbs) – 30 mg.

Parenteral –

IV: Initially administer 100 mg in the 70 kg adult. Reduce dosage proportionally for pediatric or debilitated patients. At least 1 minute is necessary to determine the full effect. If needed, additional small increments of the drug may be given to a total of 200 to 500 mg for healthy adults.

IM: The usual adult dosage is 150 to 200 mg; children's dosage frequently ranges from 2 to 6 mg/kg as a single IM injection, not to exceed 100 mg.

PHENOBARBITAL:

Anticonvulsant – In infants and children, a loading dose of 15 to 20 mg/kg produces blood levels of ≈ 20 mcg/mL shortly after administration.

Oral –

Adults:

Sedation – 30 to 120 mg/day in 2 to 3 divided doses. A single dose of 30 to 120 mg may be given at intervals; frequency is determined by response. It is generally considered that no more than 400 mg should be given during a 24-hour period.

Hypnotic – 100 to 200 mg.

Anticonvulsant – 60 to 100 mg/day.

Children:

Anticonvulsant – 3 to 6 mg/kg/day.

Sedation – 8 to 32 mg.

Hypnotic – Determined by age and weight.

Parenteral –

Adults:

Sedation – 30 to 120 mg/day IM or IV in 2 to 3 divided doses.

Preoperative sedation – 100 to 200 mg, IM only, 60 to 90 minutes before surgery.

Hypnotic – 100 to 320 mg IM or IV.

Acute convulsions – 200 to 320 mg IM or IV, repeat 6 hours as necessary.

Children:

Preoperative sedation – 1 to 3 mg/kg IM or IV.

Anticonvulsant – 4 to 6 mg/kg/day for 7 to 10 days to blood level of 10 to 15 mcg/mL, or 10 to 15 mg/kg/day, IV or IM.

Status epilepticus – 15 to 20 mg/kg IV over 10 to 15 minutes. It is imperative to achieve therapeutic levels as rapidly as possible. When given IV, it may require 15 minutes or longer to attain peak levels in the brain.

SECOBARBITAL SODIUM:

Oral –

Adults:

Preoperative sedation – 200 to 300 mg 1 to 2 hours before surgery.

Bedtime hypnotic – 100 mg.

Children: For preoperative sedation, 2 to 6 mg/kg (maximum 100 mg).

Parenteral –

Adults:

Hypnotic – Usual dose is 100 to 200 mg IM or 50 to 250 mg IV.

Preoperative sedation – For light sedation, 1 mg/kg (0.5 to 0.75 mg/lb) IM, 10 to 15 minutes before procedure.

Dentistry – In patients who are to receive nerve blocks, 100 to 150 mg IV.

Children:

Preoperative sedation – 4 to 5 mg/kg IM.

Status epilepticus – 15 to 20 mg/kg IV over 15 minutes.

Actions

Pharmacology: These agents depress the sensory cortex, decrease motor activity, alter cerebellar function, and produce drowsiness, sedation, and hypnosis.

Barbiturates have little analgesic action at subanesthetic doses and may increase the reaction to painful stimuli. All barbiturates exhibit anticonvulsant activity in anesthetic doses. However, only phenobarbital and mephobarbital are effective as oral anticonvulsants in subhypnotic doses.

Pharmacokinetics:

Pharmacokinetics of Sedatives and Hypnotic Barbiturates

	Barbiturate	Half-Life (h) Range	Half-Life (h) Mean	Oral dosage range (mg) Sedative[a]	Oral dosage range (mg) Hypnotic	Onset (minutes)	Duration (hours)
Long-acting	Mephobarbital	11 to 67	34	32 to 200	—	30 to ≥ 60	10 to 16
	Phenobarbital	53 to 118	79	30 to 120	100 to 320		
Intermediate	Amobarbital[b]	16 to 40	25	—	—	45 to 60	6 to 8
	Aprobarbital	14 to 34	24	120	40 to 160		
	Butabarbital	66 to 140	100	45 to 120	50 to 100		
Short-acting	Pentobarbital	15 to 50	†[c]	40 to 120	100	10 to 15	3 to 4
	Secobarbital	15 to 40	28	—	100		

[a] Total daily dose; administered in 2 to 4 divided doses.
[b] Available as injection only.
[c] May follow dose-dependent kinetics. Mean $t_{1/2}$ is 50 hours for 50 mg and 22 hours for 100 mg.

Contraindications

Barbiturate sensitivity; manifest or latent porphyria; marked impairment of liver function; severe respiratory disease when dyspnea or obstruction is evident; nephritic patients; patients with respiratory disease where dyspnea or obstruction is present; intra-arterial administration; subcutaneous administration; previous addiction to the sedative/hypnotic group.

Warnings/Precautions

Habit forming: Tolerance or psychological and physical dependence may occur with continued use. Administer with caution, if at all, to patients who are mentally depressed, have suicidal tendencies or a history of drug abuse. Limit prescribing and dispensing to the amount required for the interval until the next appointment.

Withdrawal symptoms – Withdrawal symptoms can be severe and may cause death.

Treatment of dependence – Treatment of dependence consists of cautious and gradual withdrawal of the drug that takes an extended period of time.

IV administration: Too rapid administration may cause respiratory depression, apnea, laryngospasm, or vasodilation with fall in blood pressure. Parenteral solutions of barbiturates are highly alkaline. Therefore, use extreme care to avoid perivascular extravasation or intra-arterial injection.

Phenobarbital sodium – Phenobarbital sodium may be administered IM or IV as an anticonvulsant for emergency use. When administered IV, it may require 15 minutes or more before reaching peak concentrations in the brain.

Pain: Exercise caution when administering to patients with acute or chronic pain, because paradoxical excitement could be induced or important symptoms could be masked.

Seizure disorders: Status epilepticus may result from abrupt discontinuation, even when administered in small daily doses in the treatment of epilepsy.

Effects on vitamin D: Barbiturates may increase vitamin D requirements, possibly by increasing the metabolism of vitamin D via enzyme induction.

Monitoring: During prolonged therapy, perform periodic laboratory evaluation of organ systems, including hematopoietic, renal, and hepatic systems.

Special risk patients: Untoward reactions may occur in the presence of fever, hyperthyroidism, diabetes mellitus, and severe anemia. Use with caution.

Use **mephobarbital** with caution in myasthenia gravis and myxedema.

Renal function impairment: Barbiturates are excreted either partially or completely unchanged in the urine and are contraindicated in impaired renal function.

Hepatic function impairment: Barbiturates are metabolized primarily by hepatic microsomal enzymes. Administer with caution and initially in reduced doses.

Pregnancy: Category D.

Lactation: Exercise caution when administering to the nursing mother because small amounts are excreted in breast milk.

Children: In some people, especially children, barbiturates repeatedly produce excitement rather than depression. Barbiturates may produce irritability, excitability, inappropriate tearfulness, and aggression in children. Safety and efficacy of amobarbital (children younger than 6 years of age) and aprobarbital have not been established.

Elderly: May produce marked excitement, depression, and confusion.

Drug Interactions

Drugs that may affect barbiturates include alcohol, charcoal, chloramphenicol, MAO inhibitors, rifampin, and valproic acid. Drugs that may be affected by barbiturates include acetaminophen, anticoagulants, beta blockers, carbamazepine, chloramphenicol, clonazepam, oral contraceptives, corticosteroids, digitoxin, doxorubicin, doxycycline, felodipine, fenoprofen, griseofulvin, hydantoins, methoxyflurane, metronidazole, narcotics, phenmetrazine, phenylbutazone, quinidine, theophylline, and verapamil.

Adverse Reactions

Adverse reactions may include somnolence; agitation; confusion; hyperkinesia; ataxia; CNS depression; nightmares; nervousness; psychiatric disturbance; hallucinations; insomnia; anxiety; dizziness; abnormal thinking; headache; fever (especially with chronic phenobarbital use); hypoventilation; apnea; bradycardia; hypotension; syncope; nausea; vomiting; constipation; liver damage, particularly with chronic phenobarbital use; skin rashes; angioedema (particularly following chronic phenobarbital use).

ANTICONVULSANTS

Anticonvulsants: Indications and Pharmacokinetics						
	Drug	Labeled indications	Protein binding (%)	Metabolism/ Excretion	t½ (h)	Therapeutic serum levels (mcg/mL)
Barbiturates	Phenobarbital[a] (PB)	Status epilepticus Epilepsy, all forms Tonic-clonic	40 to 60	Liver; 25% eliminated unchanged in urine	53 to 140	15 to 40
Hydantoins	Phenytoin	Tonic-clonic Psychomotor	≈ 90	Liver; renal excretion. < 5% excreted unchanged	Dose-dependent[b]	5 to 20
Hydantoins	Mephenytoin	Tonic-clonic Psychomotor Focal Jacksonian	nd	Liver	95 (active metabolite)	nd
Hydantoins	Ethotoin	Tonic-clonic Psychomotor	nd	Liver; renal excretion of metabolites	3 to 9[c]	15 to 50
Succinimides	Ethosuximide	Absence	0	Liver; 25% excreted unchanged in urine	30 (children 7 to 9 yrs) 40 to 60 (adults)	40 to 100
Succinimides	Methsuximide	Absence	nd	Liver; < 1% excreted unchanged in urine	< 2 (40, active metabolite)	nd
Succinimides	Phensuximide	Absence	nd	Urine, bile	8 (active metabolite)	nd
Sulfonamides	Zonisamide	Partial[d]	40	Acetylation and reduction; excreted in urine	63	nd
Oxazolidinediones	Trimethadione	Absence	0	Demethylated to dimethadione; 3% excreted unchanged	6 to 13 days (dimethadione)	≥ 700 (dimethdione)
Benzodiazepines	Clonazepam	Absence Myoclonic Akinetic	50 to 85	5 metabolites identified; urine is major excretion route	18 to 60	20 to 80 ng/mL
Benzodiazepines	Clorazepate	Partial[d]	97	Hydrolyzed in stomach to desmethyldiazepam (active); metabolized in liver, renally excreted	30 to 100	nd
Benzodiazepines	Diazepam	Status epilepticus[d] Epilepsy, all forms[d]	97 to 99	Liver, active metabolites	20 to 50	nd

Anticonvulsants: Indications and Pharmacokinetics

	Drug	Labeled indications	Protein binding (%)	Metabolism/ Excretion	t½ (h)	Therapeutic serum levels (mcg/mL)
Miscellaneous	Primidone	Tonic-clonic Psychomotor Focal	20 to 25	Metabolized to PB and PEMA, both active	5 to 15 (primidone) 10 to 18 (PEMA) 53 to 140 (PB)	5 to 12 (primidone) 15 to 40 (PB)
	Valproic acid	Absence	80 to 94	Liver; excreted in urine	5 to 20	50 to 150
	Carbamazepine	Tonic-clonic Mixed Psychomotor	≈ 75	Liver to active 10, 11-epoxide. 72% excreted in urine, 28% in feces	18 to 54 (initial) 10 to 20[e] ≈ 6 (10, 11-epoxide)	4 to 12
	Phenacemide	Severe mixed psychomotor	nd	Liver	nd	nd
	Felbamate[f]	Partial (adults) Partial/generalized assoc. with Lennox-Gastaut syndrome (children)	22 to 25	40% to 50% unchanged in urine, 40% as unidentified metabolites and conjugates	20 to 23	nd[g]
	Oxcarbazepine	Partial	40	Reduced to 10-monohydroxy metabolite (active); excreted in urine (80%)	2; 9 (MHD)	nd[g]
	Lamotrigine	Partial (adults)	≈ 55	Glucuronic acid conjugation to inactive metabolites; 94% excreted in urine, 2% in feces	≈ 33[e]	nd

[a] Other barbiturates are also used as anticonvulsants. See Sedatives/Hypnotics section.
[b] Exhibits dose-dependent, nonlinear pharmacokinetics.
[c] Below 8 mcg/mL; > 8 mcg/mL, t½ not defined because of dose-dependent, nonlinear pharmacokinetics.
[d] Recommended for adjunctive use.
[e] Undergoes autoinduction. Half-life after repeated doses.
[f] Because of cases of aplastic anemia, it has been recommended that the use of this drug be discontinued unless, in the judgment of the physician, continued therapy is warranted.
[g] Value of monitoring blood levels not established.

HYDANTOINS

ETHOTOIN

Tablets: 250 mg (*Rx*) — *Peganone* (Ovation)

FOSPHENYTOIN SODIUM

Injection: 75 mg/mL (equiv. to phenytoin sodium 50 mg/mL) (*Rx*) — Various, *Cerebyx* (Parke-Davis)

PHENYTOIN

Tablets, chewable: 50 mg (*Rx*) — *Dilantin Infatab* (Kabivitrum)

Suspension; oral: 125 mg per 5 mL (*Rx*) — Various, *Dilantin* (Kabivitrum)

PHENYTOIN SODIUM

Capsules, extended-release; oral: 30 and 100 mg (*Rx*) — Various, *Dilantin* (Kabivitrum)

200 and 300 mg (*Rx*) — Various, *Phenytek* (Mylan)

Injection: 50 mg/mL (*Rx*) — Various

Indications

Refer to individual product monographs for specific indications.

Hydantoins: Summary of Indications

FDA-approved indication	Ethotoin	Fosphenytoin[a]	Phenytoin Chewable tablets	Phenytoin ER[b] capsules	Phenytoin Oral suspension	Phenytoin Injection
Complex partial seizures[c]	✓		✓	✓	✓	
Generalized tonic-clonic seizures	✓		✓	✓	✓	
Prevent/Treat seizures during or following neurosurgery		✓	✓	✓		✓
Status epilepticus		✓				✓ (IV)

[a] May be substituted short-term for oral phenytoin when other means of phenytoin administration are unavailable, inappropriate, or deemed less advantageous.
[b] ER = extended-release.
[c] Also called psychomotor or temporal lobe seizures.

Administration and Dosage

ETHOTOIN: Administer in 4 to 6 divided doses/day. Take after food; space doses as evenly as practical.

Adults – The initial daily dose should be 1 g or less, with subsequent gradual dosage increases over several days. The usual adult maintenance dose is 2 to 3 g/day; less than 2 g/day is ineffective in most adults.

Pediatric – Initial dose should not exceed 750 mg/day. The usual maintenance dose in children ranges from 500 mg to 1 g/day, although occasionally 2 g or rarely 3 g/day may be necessary.

FOSPHENYTOIN: The dose, concentration in dosing solutions and infusion rate of IV fosphenytoin is expressed as phenytoin sodium equivalents (PE) to avoid the need to perform molecular weight-based adjustments when converting between fosphenytoin and phenytoin sodium doses. Prescribe and dispense fosphenytoin in PEs.

Dilute fosphenytoin in 5% Dextrose or 0.9% Saline Solution for Injection to a concentration ranging from 1.5 to 25 mg PE/mL.

Status epilepticus – The loading dose 15 to 20 mg PE/kg administered at 100 to 150 mg PE/min.

Because the full antiepileptic effect of phenytoin, whether given as fosphenytoin or parenteral phenytoin, is not immediate, other measures, including concomitant administration of an IV benzodiazepine, will usually be necessary for control of status epilepticus.

Nonemergent and maintenance dosing –

Loading dose: 10 to 20 mg PE/kg given IV or IM.

Maintenance dose: 4 to 6 mg PE/kg/day.

IM or IV substitution for oral phenytoin therapy: Fosphenytoin IM or IV can be substituted for oral phenytoin therapy at the same total daily dose.

Phenytoin, supplied as fosphenytoin, is 100% bioavailable by the IM and IV routes. Plasma phenytoin concentrations may increase modestly when IM or IV fosphenytoin is substituted for oral phenytoin therapy.

In controlled trials, IM fosphenytoin was administered as a single daily dose utilizing either 1 or 2 injection sites. Some patients may require more frequent dosing.

Because if the risk of hypotension, administer at a rate of 150 mg PE/min or less.

Continuously monitor the electrocardiogram, blood pressure, and respiratory function and observe the patient throughout the period of maximal serum phenytoin concentrations, approximately 10 to 20 minutes after the end of the infusion.

Renal/Hepatic function impairment – Because of an increased fraction of unbound phenytoin in patients with renal or hepatic disease, or in those with hypoalbuminemia, interpret total phenytoin plasma concentrations with caution. Unbound phenytoin concentrations may be more useful in these patients.

Elderly – Phenytoin clearance is decreased slightly in elderly patients and lower or less frequent dosing may be required.

PHENYTOIN:

Dosage – The clinically effective serum level is usually 10 to 20 mcg/mL. With recommended dosage, a period of 7 to 10 days may be required to achieve steady-state blood levels with phenytoin, and changes in dosage (increase or decrease) should not be carried out at intervals shorter than 7 to 10 days.

Adults – Adults who have received no previous treatment may be started on 100 mg (125 mg suspension) 3 times/day. Satisfactory maintenance dosage is 300 to 400 mg/day. An increase to 600 mg/day (625 mg/day suspension) may be necessary.

Children – Initially, 5 mg/kg/day in 2 or 3 equally divided doses, with subsequent dosage individualized to a maximum of 300 mg daily. The recommended daily maintenance dose is usually 4 to 8 mg/kg. Children older than 6 years of age and adolescents may require the minimum adult dose (300 mg/day).

If the daily dosage cannot be divided equally, the larger dose should be given before retiring.

Administration – Tablets are not for once-daily dosing.

Tablets can be chewed thoroughly before swallowing or swallowed whole.

PHENYTOIN SODIUM:

Oral –

Loading dose: Initially, 1 g of phenytoin capsules is divided into 3 doses (400 mg, 300 mg, 300 mg) and administered at intervals of 2 hours. Normal maintenance dosage is then instituted 24 hours after the loading dose, with frequent serum level determinations. This dosing regimen should be reserved for patients in a clinical or hospital setting where phenytoin serum levels can be closely monitored. Patients with a history of renal or liver disease should not receive the oral loading regimen.

Divided daily dosage: 100 mg extended-release capsule 3 times daily. For most adults, the satisfactory maintenance dosage will be 1 capsule 3 to 4 times a day. An increase of up to 200 mg 3 times a day may be made if necessary.

Pediatric: Initially, 5 mg/kg/day in 2 or 3 equally divided doses with subsequent dosage individualized to a maximum of 300 mg/day. Daily maintenance dosage is 4 to 8 mg/kg. Children over 6 years may require the minimum adult dose (300 mg/day).

Single daily dosage: In adults, if seizure control is established with divided doses of three 100 mg extended phenytoin sodium capsules daily, once/day dosage with 300 mg may be considered.

Bioavailability: Because of the potential bioavailability differences between products, brand interchange is not recommended. Only extended phenytoin sodium capsules are recommended once/day.

When a change in the dosage form or brand is prescribed, carefully monitor phenytoin serum levels.

Phenytoin sodium extended-release capsules are formulated with the sodium salt of phenytoin. The free acid form of phenytoin is used in phenytoin suspensions and tablets. Because there is an approximate 8% increase in drug content with the free acid form compared with the sodium salt, dosage adjustments and serum level monitoring may be necessary when switching from a product formulated with the free acid to a product formulated with the sodium salt and vice versa.

Injection –

Warning: This drug must be administered slowly. In adults, do not exceed 50 mg per minute IV. In neonates, administer the drug at a rate not exceeding 1 to 3 mg/kg/min.

Loading dose: The loading dose for obese patients may be calculated using an adjusted body weight based on the following formula:

Dosing weight (kg) = ideal body weight (IBW) + 1.33 × (measured weight – IBW)

Conversion: An IM dose of 50% more than the oral dose is necessary to maintain these levels. When returned to oral administration, the dose should be reduced by 50% of the original oral dose for 1 week to prevent excessive plasma levels caused by sustained release from IM tissue sites.

Status epilepticus: In adults, administer loading dose of 10 to 15 mg/kg slowly. Follow by maintenance doses of 100 mg orally or IV every 6 to 8 hours. For neonates and children, IV loading dose is 15 to 20 mg/kg injected slowly IV at a rate not exceeding 1 to 3 mg/kg/min.

Neurosurgery (prophylactic dosage): 100 to 200 mg IM at approximately 4 hour intervals during surgery and the postoperative period.

Administration: Inject phenytoin slowly and directly into a large vein through a large-gauge needle or IV catheter. Each injection of IV phenytoin should be followed by an injection of sterile saline through the same needle or catheter to avoid local venous irritation due to the alkalinity of the solution. Continuous infusion should be avoided.

Incompatibilities: The addition of phenytoin injection solution to IV fluids is not recommended because of the lack of solubility and likelihood of precipitation

Actions

Pharmacology: The primary site of action of hydantoins appears to be the motor cortex, where spread of seizure activity is inhibited. Possibly by promoting sodium efflux from neurons, hydantoins tend to stabilize the threshold against hyperexcitability.

Pharmacokinetics:

Absorption/Distribution – Phenytoin is slowly absorbed from the small intestine. Rate and extent of absorption varies and is dependent on the product formulation. Bioavailability may differ among products of different manufacturers. Administration IM results in precipitation of phenytoin at the injection site, resulting in slow and erratic absorption, which may continue for up to 5 days or more. Plasma protein binding is 87% to 93% and is lower in uremic patients and neonates. Volume of distribution averages 0.6 L/kg.

Phenytoin's therapeutic plasma concentration is 10 to 20 mcg/mL, although many patients achieve complete seizure control at lower serum concentrations.

Metabolism/Excretion – Phenytoin is metabolized in the liver and excreted in the urine. Elimination is exponential (first-order) at plasma concentrations less than 10 mcg/mL, and plasma half-life ranges from 6 to 24 hours.

Contraindications

Hypersensitivity to hydantoins; hepatic abnormalities or hematologic disorders (ethotoin only).

Because of the effect of parenteral phenytoin on ventricular automaticity, parenteral phenytoin and fosphenytoin are contraindicated in patients with sinus bradycardia, sinoatrial block, second- and third-degree AV block, or in patients with Adams-Stokes syndrome.

Warnings/Precautions

Administration: The IM route is not recommended for the treatment of status epilepticus because blood levels of phenytoin in the therapeutic range cannot be readily achieved with doses and methods of administration ordinarily employed.

Local effects: Soft tissue irritation and inflammation have occurred at the site of injection with and without extravasation of IV phenytoin.

Withdrawal: Abrupt withdrawal in epileptic patients may precipitate increased seizure frequency, including status epilepticus.

Cardiovascular: Hypotension may occur, especially after IV administration of phenytoin and fosphenytoin at high doses and high rates of administration. Use with caution in hypotension and severe myocardial insufficiency.

Lymphadenopathy: There have been a number of reports that have suggested a relationship between hydantoins and the development of lymphadenopathy (local or generalized).

Dermatologic effects: Discontinue these drugs if a skin rash appears. If the rash is exfoliative, purpuric, or bullous, do not resume use.

Hepatic effects: Cases of acute hepatotoxicity, including infrequent cases of acute hepatic failure, have been reported with phenytoin.

Hematologic effects: Hemopoietic complications have occasionally been reported in association with phenytoin. Blood dyscrasias have been reported in patients receiving ethotoin.

Sensory disturbances: Severe burning, itching, and/or paresthesia were reported following administration of IV fosphenytoin.

The occurrence and intensity of the discomfort can be lessened by slowing or temporarily stopping the infusion.

Phosphate load: Consider the phosphate load provided by fosphenytoin (0.0037 mmol of phosphate/mg phenytoin equivalent) when treating patients who require phosphate restriction.

Slow metabolism: A small percentage of individuals treated with phenytoin have been shown to metabolize the drug slowly.

Acute intermittent porphyria: Administer hydantoins cautiously to patients with acute intermittent porphyria.

Hyperglycemia: Hyperglycemia, resulting from the drug's inhibitory effect on insulin release, has occurred. Hydantoins also may raise blood sugar levels in hyperglycemic people.

Other seizures: Hydantoins are not indicated in seizures caused by hypoglycemia or other metabolic causes. Hydantoins are not indicated for the treatment of absence seizures. If tonic-clonic and absence seizures are present, combined drug therapy is needed.

Folate levels: Phenytoin has the potential to lower serum folate levels.

Osteomalacia: Osteomalacia has been associated with phenytoin therapy.

Hypersensitivity reactions: Hydantoins are contraindicated in patients who have experienced phenytoin hypersensitivity. Additionally, exercise caution if using structurally similar drugs (eg, barbiturates, oxazolidinediones, succinimides, and other related compounds) in these same patients.

Renal/Hepatic function impairment: After IV administration to patients with renal and/or hepatic disease, or those with hypoalbuminemia, fosphenytoin clearance to phenytoin may be increased without a similar increase in phenytoin clearance.

The liver is the primary site of biotransformation of phenytoin; patients with hepatic function impairment, elderly patients, or patients who are gravely ill may show early signs of toxicity.

Pregnancy: Category D.

Lactation: According to manufacturers, breast-feeding is not recommended for women receiving phenytoin or fosphenytoin. However, the American Academy of Pediatrics considers phenytoin to be compatible with breast-feeding.

Ethotoin is excreted in breast milk. Because of the potential for serious adverse reactions in breast-feeding infants from ethotoin, decide whether to discontinue breast-feeding or the drug, taking into account the importance of the drug to the mother.

Children: Phenytoin and ethotoin are approved for use in children. The safety of fosphenytoin in children has not been established.

Elderly: Phenytoin clearance tends to decrease with increasing age. The liver is the primary site of biotransformation of phenytoin; patients with hepatic function impairment, elderly patients, or patients who are gravely ill may show early signs of toxicity.

Lab test abnormalities: Phenytoin may cause increased serum concentrations of alkaline phosphatase, gamma glutamyl transpeptidase (GGT), and glucose.

Monitoring: Perform liver function tests if clinical evidence suggests the possibility of hepatic function impairment.

Phenytoin – Continuous monitoring of the ECG, blood pressure, and respiratory function is essential. Also observe for signs of respiratory depression.

Fosphenytoin – It is recommended that phenytoin concentrations not be monitored until conversion to phenytoin is essentially complete (approximately 2 hours after the end of IV infusion and 4 hours after IM injection).

Ethotoin – Blood cell counts and urinalyses be performed when therapy is begun and at monthly intervals for several months thereafter.

Drug Interactions

Drugs that may affect hydantoins include alcohol, amiodarone, antacids, anticoagulants, antineoplastic agents, azole antifungals, barbiturates, benzodiazepines, carbamazepine, chloral hydrate, chloramphenicol, cimetidine, contraceptives (hormonal), diazoxide, disulfiram, estrogens, felbamate, folic acid, halothane, ibuprofen, isoniazid, methylphenidate, metronidazole, omeprazole, phenacemide, phenothiazines, phenylbutazone, protease inhibitors, reserpine, rifamycins, salicylates, SSRIs, succinimides, sucralfate, sulfonamides, tacrolimus, ticlopidine, theophylline, tolbutamide, topiramate, trazodone, trimethoprim, valproic acid.

Drugs that may be affected by hydantoins include acetaminophen, amiodarone, anticoagulants, azole antifungals, barbiturates, benzodiazepines, carbamazepine, contraceptives (hormonal), corticosteroids, cyclosporine, digoxin, disopyramide, dopamine, doxycycline, estrogens, felbamate, felodipine, haloperidol, levodopa, loop diuretics, methadone, metyrapone, mexiletine, mirtazapine, nisoldipine, nondepolarizing muscle relaxants, phenothiazines, praziquantel, primidone, progestins, protease inhibitors, quetiapine, quinidine, rifamycins, SSRIs, tacrolimus, theophylline, tolbutamide, topiramate, valproic acid, vitamin D.

Drug/Lab test interactions: Phenytoin may decrease serum concentrations of T_4. It may also produce artificially low results in dexamethasone or metyrapone tests.

Take care when using immunoanalytical methods to measure plasma phenytoin concentrations following fosphenytoin administration.

Drug/Food interactions: Phenytoin should not be coadministered with an enteral feeding preparation. More frequent phenytoin level monitoring may be necessary in these patients.

Adverse Reactions

Adverse reactions occurring in at least 3% of patients include the following: accidental injury; agitation; asthenia; ataxia; diplopia; dizziness; dry mouth; ecchymosis; extrapyramidal syndrome; headache; hypotension; incoordination; nausea; nystagmus; pelvic pain; paresthesia; pruritus; somnolence; stupor; taste perversion; tinnitus; tongue disorder; tremor; vasodilation; vomiting.

ZONISAMIDE

Capsules: 25, 50, and 100 mg (*Rx*)	Various, *Zonegran* (Eisai)

Indications

Epilepsy: Adjunctive therapy in the treatment of partial seizures in adults with epilepsy.

Administration and Dosage

Adults older than 16 years of age: The initial dose is 100 mg daily. The dose may be increased 400 mg/day at least 2 week intervals. Doses of 100 to 600 mg/day are effective, but there is no suggestion of increasing response above 400 mg/day.

Zonisamide may be taken with or without food. Swallow the capsules whole. Use caution in patients with renal or hepatic disease.

Discontinuation of therapy: Abrupt withdrawal of zonisamide in patients with epilepsy may precipitate increased seizure frequency or status epilepticus. Gradually reduce dose.

Actions

Pharmacology: The precise mechanism(s) of action is unknown. In vitro pharmacological studies suggest that zonisamide blocks sodium channels and reduces voltage-dependent, transient inward currents, stabilizing neuronal membranes and suppressing neuronal hypersynchronization. Zonisamide does not appear to potentiate the synaptic activity of GABA. In vivo studies demonstrated that zonisamide facilitates dopaminergic and serotonergic neurotransmission.

Pharmacokinetics: Peak plasma concentrations (range, 2 to 5 mcg/mL) in healthy volunteers occur within 2 to 6 hours. The apparent volume of distribution is approximately 1.45 L/kg. At concentrations of 1 to 7 mcg/mL, it is approximately 40% bound to human plasma proteins. The elimination half-life in plasma is approximately 63 hours. The elimination half-life in red blood cells is approximately 105 hours. Zonisamide is excreted primarily in urine.

Contraindications

Hypersensitivity to sulfonamides or zonisamide.

Warnings/Precautions

Oligohydrosis and hyperthermia in children: Oligohydrosis, sometimes resulting in heat stroke and hospitalization, is associated with zonisamide in children.

Decreased sweating and elevated body temperature characterized these cases. Many cases were reported after exposure to elevated environmental temperatures. Heat stroke, requiring hospitalization, was diagnosed in some cases. There have been no reported deaths.

Children appear to be at an increased risk for zonisamide-associated oligohydrosis and hyperthermia. Closely monitor patients, especially children, treated with zonisamide for evidence of decreased sweating and increased body temperature, particularly in warm or hot weather. Use caution when zonisamide is prescribed with other drugs that predispose patients to heat-related disorders (eg, carbonic anhydrase inhibitors, drugs with anticholinergic activity).

Cognitive/Neuropsychiatric adverse events: Use of zonisamide was frequently associated with the following CNS-related adverse events: 1) Psychiatric symptoms, including depression and psychosis; 2) psychomotor slowing, difficulty with concentration, and speech or language problems, in particular, word-finding difficulties; and 3) somnolence or fatigue.

Potentially fatal reactions to sulfonamides: Fatalities have occurred, although rarely, as a result of severe reactions to sulfonamides (eg, zonisamide), including Stevens-Johnson syndrome, toxic epidermal necrolysis, fulminant hepatic necrosis, agranulocytosis, aplastic anemia, and other blood dyscrasias.

Serious skin reactions: Discontinue zonisamide in patients who develop an otherwise unexplained rash or observe them frequently.

Serious hematological events: Two confirmed cases of aplastic anemia and 1 confirmed case of agranulocytosis were reported in the first 11 years of marketing in Japan.

Seizures on withdrawal: Abrupt withdrawal of zonisamide in patients with epilepsy may precipitate increased seizure frequency or status epilepticus. Dose reduction or discontinuation of zonisamide should be done gradually.

Cognitive/neuropsychiatric adverse reactions: Use of zonisamide was frequently associated with central nervous system-related adverse reactions. The most significant of these can be classified into 3 general categories:

1.) Psychiatric symptoms, including depression and psychosis.
2.) Psychomotor slowing, difficulty with concentration, and speech or language problems, in particular, word-finding difficulties.
3.) Somnolence or fatigue.

Creatine phosphokinase (CPK) elevation and pancreatitis: If patients develop severe muscle pain and/or weakness, either in the presence or absence of a fever, markers of muscle damage should be assessed, including serum CPK and aldolase levels.

Patients taking zonisamide that manifest clinical signs and symptoms of pancreatitis should have pancreatic lipase and amylase levels monitored. If pancreatitis is evident, in the absence of another obvious cause, tapering and/or discontinuation of zonisamide should be considered and appropriate treatment initiated.

Kidney stones: An increased risk of kidney stone formation in patients treated with zonisamide has been reported.

Sudden unexplained death in epilepsy: During the development of zonisamide, 9 sudden unexplained deaths occurred among 991 patients with epilepsy receiving zonisamide for whom accurate exposure data are available. This represents an incidence of 7.7 deaths per 1000 patient years. Some of the deaths could represent seizure-related deaths in which the seizure was not observed.

Status epilepticus: Among patients treated with zonisamide across all epilepsy studies, 1% of patients had an event reported as status epilepticus.

Renal/Hepatic function impairment: Zonisamide is metabolized by the liver and eliminated by the kidneys; caution should therefore be exercised when administering zonisamide to patients with hepatic and renal dysfunction.

Hazardous tasks: Zonisamide may produce drowsiness, especially at higher doses. Advise patients not to drive a car or operate other complex machinery until the effect of zonisamide is known.

Pregnancy: Category C. Advise women of childbearing potential who are given zonisamide to use effective contraception.

Lactation: It is not known whether zonisamide is excreted in breast milk.

Children: Safety and efficacy of zonisamide in patients younger than 16 years of age have not been established. Zonisamide is not approved for pediatric use.

Elderly: Use caution in selecting a dose for an elderly patient, usually starting at the low end of the dosing range.

Drug Interactions

CYP 450: Drugs that induce liver enzymes (eg, phenytoin, carbamazepine, phenobarbital) increase the metabolism and clearance of zonisamide and decrease its half-life. Concurrent medication with drugs that induce or inhibit CYP3A4 would be expected to alter serum concentrations of zonisamide. Zonisamide is not expected to interfere with the metabolism of other drugs that are metabolized by cytochrome P450 isozymes.

Drug/Food interactions: The time to maximum concentration of zonisamide is delayed in the presence of food, but no effect on bioavailability occurs.

Adverse Reactions

The most commonly observed adverse events associated with the use of zonisamide were agitation/irritability, anorexia, dizziness, headache, nausea, and somnolence.

The adverse events most commonly associated with discontinuation were somnolence, fatigue, or ataxia (6%); anorexia (3%); difficulty concentrating (2%); difficulty with memory, mental slowing, nausea/vomiting (2%); and weight loss (1%). Many of these adverse events were dose-related.

Adverse reactions occurring in at least 3% of patients include the following: Abdominal pain, agitation/irritability, anorexia, anxiety, ataxia, confusion, depression, diarrhea, difficulty concentrating, difficulty with memory, diplopia, dizziness, dyspepsia, fatigue, flu syndrome, headache, insomnia, mental slowing, nausea, nystagmus, paresthesia, rash, somnolence, speech abnormalities, tiredness, weight loss.

LAMOTRIGINE

Tablets; oral: 25, 50, 100, 150, 200, and 250 mg (*Rx*)	Various, *Lamictal* (GlaxoSmithKline)
Tablets, chewable/dispersible; oral: 2, 5, and 25 mg (*Rx*)	Various, *Lamictal* (GlaxoSmithKline)
Tablets, orally disintegrating; oral: 25, 50, 100, and 200 mg (*Rx*)	*Lamictal ODT*, *Lamictal ODT Patient Titration Kit* (GlaxoSmithKline)
Tablets, extended-release; oral: 25, 50, 100, and 200 mg (*Rx*)	*Lamictal XR*, *Lamictal XR Patient Titration Kit* (GlaxoSmithKline)

Warning:

Serious rashes requiring hospitalization and discontinuation of treatment have been reported in association with lamotrigine use. The incidence of these rashes, which include Stevens-Johnson syndrome, is approximately 1% in pediatric patients (younger than 16 years of age) and 0.3% in adults.

In clinical trials of bipolar and other mood disorders, the rate of serious rash was 0.08% in adult patients receiving lamotrigine as initial monotherapy and 0.13% in adult patients receiving lamotrigine as adjunctive therapy.

Rare cases of toxic epidermal necrolysis or rash-related death have occurred, but their numbers are too few to permit a precise estimate of the rate.

Because the rate of serious rash is greater in pediatric patients than in adults, it bears emphasis that lamotrigine is approved only for use in pediatric patients younger than 16 years of age who have seizures associated with the Lennox-Gastaut syndrome or in patients with partial seizures.

Other than age, no factors have been identified that are known to predict the risk of occurrence or the severity of rash associated with lamotrigine. It is suggested, yet to be proven, that the risk of rash may also be increased by 1) coadministration of lamotrigine with valproic acid (VPA), 2) exceeding the recommended initial dose of lamotrigine, or 3) exceeding the recommended dose escalation for lamotrigine. However, cases have been reported in the absence of these factors.

Nearly all cases of life-threatening rashes associated with lamotrigine have occurred within 2 to 8 weeks of treatment initiation. However, isolated cases have been reported after prolonged treatment (eg, 6 months). Accordingly, duration of therapy cannot be relied upon as a means to predict the potential risk heralded by the first appearance of a rash.

Although benign rashes also occur with lamotrigine, it is not possible to predict reliably which rashes will prove to be life-threatening. Accordingly, discontinue lamotrigine at the first sign of rash, unless the rash is clearly not drug-related. Discontinuation of treatment may not prevent a rash from becoming life-threatening or permanently disabling or disfiguring.

Indications

Bipolar disorder (immediate release only): For the maintenance treatment of Bipolar I Disorder to delay the time to occurrence of mood episodes (eg, depression, mania, hypomania, mixed episodes) in patients treated for acute mood episodes with standard therapy.

Epilepsy:

Adjunctive therapy – Adjunctive therapy for partial seizures, in the generalized seizures of Lennox-Gastaut syndrome, and primary generalized tonic-clonic seizures in children (at least 2 years of age) and adults (immediate release); for partial-onset seizures with or without secondary generalization in patients 13 years of age and older (ER).

Monotherapy (immediate release) – Indicated for conversion to monotherapy in adults (16 years of age and older) with partial seizures who are receiving treatment with carbamazepine, phenytoin, phenobarbital, primidone, or valproate as the single antiepileptic drug (AED).

Administration and Dosage

General dosing considerations: To avoid an increased risk of rash, the recommended initial dose and subsequent dose escalations of lamotrigine should not be exceeded.

Lamotrigine starter kits, lamotrigine orally disintegrating tablet titration kits, and lamotrigine ER titration kits provide lamotrigine at doses consistent with the recommended titration schedule for the first 5 weeks of treatment, based on concomitant medication, and are intended to help reduce the potential for rash. The use of these kits is recommended for appropriate patients who are starting or restarting lamotrigine.

It is recommended that lamotrigine not be restarted in patients who discontinued therapy because of rash associated with prior treatment with lamotrigine, unless the potential benefits clearly outweigh the risks. If the decision is made to restart a patient who has discontinued lamotrigine, the need to restart with the initial dosing recommendations should be assessed. The greater the interval of time since the previous dose, the greater the consideration should be given to restarting with the initial dosing recommendations. If a patient has discontinued lamotrigine for a period of more than 5 half-lives, it is recommended that initial dosing recommendations and guidelines be followed. The half-life of lamotrigine is affected by other concomitant medications.

For patients receiving lamotrigine in combination with other AEDs, a reevaluation of all AEDs in the regimen should be considered if a change in seizure control or an appearance or worsening of adverse reactions is observed.

Adults:

Bipolar disorder – For dosing guidelines below, enzyme-inducing antiepileptic drugs (EIAEDs) include phenytoin, carbamazepine, phenobarbital, and primidone.

To avoid an increased risk of rash, the recommended initial dose and subsequent dose escalations of lamotrigine should not be exceeded.

Lamotrigine Immediate Release Escalation Regimen for Bipolar Disorder Patients[a]

	For patients not taking carbamazepine, phenytoin,[b] phenobarbital, primidone,[b] or valproate[c]	For patients taking valproate[c]	For patients taking carbamazepine, phenytoin,[b] phenobarbital, primidone,[b] and not taking valproate[c]
Weeks 1 and 2	25 mg/day	25 mg every other day	50 mg/day
Weeks 3 and 4	50 mg/day	25 mg/day	100 mg/day in divided doses
Week 5	100 mg/day	50 mg/day	200 mg/day in divided doses
Week 6	200 mg/day	100 mg/day	300 mg/day in divided doses
Week 7	200 mg/day	100 mg/day	Up to 400 mg/day in divided doses

[a] See Drug Interactions for a description of known drug interactions.

[b] These drugs induce lamotrigine glucuronidation and increase clearance. Other drugs that have similar effects include estrogen-containing oral contraceptives. Patients taking rifampin, or other drugs that induce lamotrigine glucuronidation and increase clearance, should follow the same dosing titration/maintenance regimen as that used with anticonvulsants that have this effect.

[c] Valproate has been shown to inhibit glucuronidation and decrease the apparent clearance of lamotrigine.

Dose adjustment: If other psychotropic medications are withdrawn following stabilization, the dose of lamotrigine should be adjusted. For patients discontinuing valproate, the dose of lamotrigine should be doubled over a 2-week period in equal weekly increments. For patients discontinuing carbamazepine, phenytoin, phenobarbital, primidone, or rifampin, the dose of lamotrigine should remain constant for the first week and then should be decreased by half over a 2-week period in equal weekly decrements (see the following table). The dose of lamotrigine may then be further adjusted to the target dose (200 mg) as clinically indicated.

If other drugs are subsequently introduced, the dose of lamotrigine may need to be adjusted. In particular, the introduction of valproate requires reduction in the dose of lamotrigine.

Adjustments to Lamotrigine Dosing for Patients With Bipolar Disorder Following Discontinuation of Psychotropic Medications			
	Discontinuation of psychotropic drugs (excluding carbamazepine, phenytoin, phenobarbital, primidone,[a] and valproate[b])	After discontinuation of valproate[b]	After discontinuation of carbamazepine, phenytoin, phenobarbital, or primidone[a]
		Current lamotrigine dose 100 mg/day	Current lamotrigine dose 400 mg/day
Week 1	Maintain current lamotrigine dose	150 mg/day	400 mg/day
Week 2	Maintain current lamotrigine dose	200 mg/day	300 mg/day
Week 3 onward	Maintain current lamotrigine dose	200 mg/day	200 mg/day

[a] These drugs induce lamotrigine glucuronidation and increase clearance. Other drugs that have similar effects include estrogen-containing oral contraceptives. Patients taking rifampin, or other drugs that induce lamotrigine glucuronidation and increase clearance, should follow the same dosing titration/maintenance regimen as that used with anticonvulsants that have this effect.

[b] Valproate has been shown to inhibit glucuronidation and decrease the apparent clearance of lamotrigine.

Usual maintenance dose – In patients receiving multidrug regimens employing carbamazepine, phenytoin, phenobarbital, or primidone without valproate, maintenance doses of adjunctive lamotrigine immediate release as high as 700 mg/day have been used. In patients receiving valproate alone, maintenance doses of adjunctive lamotrigine immediate release as high as 200 mg/day have been used.

Discontinuation strategy – As with other AEDs, lamotrigine should not be abruptly discontinued.

If a decision is made to discontinue therapy with lamotrigine, a stepwise reduction of dose over 2 weeks or more (approximately 50% per week) is recommended unless safety concerns require a more rapid withdrawal (see Precautions).

Epilepsy –

Lamotrigine Immediate Release Escalation Regimen in Patients > 12 Years of Age With Epilepsy			
	For patients taking valproate[a]	For patients not taking carbamazepine, phenytoin, phenobarbital, primidone,[b] or valproate[a]	For patients taking carbamazepine, phenytoin, phenobarbital, or primidone[b] (without valproate[a])
Weeks 1 and 2	25 mg every other day	25 mg/day	50 mg/day
Weeks 3 and 4	25 mg/day	50 mg/day	100 mg/day in 2 divided doses
Weeks 5 onwards to maintenance	Increase by 25 to 50 mg/day every 1 to 2 weeks	Increase by 50 mg/day every 1 to 2 weeks	Increase by 100 mg/day every 1 to 2 weeks

Lamotrigine Immediate Release Escalation Regimen in Patients > 12 Years of Age With Epilepsy			
	For patients taking valproate[a]	For patients not taking carbamazepine, phenytoin, phenobarbital, primidone,[b] or valproate[a]	For patients taking carbamazepine, phenytoin, phenobarbital, or primidone[b] (without valproate[a])
Usual maintenance dose	100 to 400 mg/day with valproate and other drugs that induce glucuronidation. 100 to 200 mg/day with valproate alone (1 or 2 divided doses)	225 to 375 mg/day (in 2 divided doses)	300 to 500 mg/day (in 2 divided doses)

[a] Valproate has been shown to inhibit glucuronidation and decrease the apparent clearance of lamotrigine.

[b] These drugs induce glucuronidation and increase clearance. Other drugs that have similar effects include estrogen-containing oral contraceptives. Patients taking rifampin, or other drugs that induce lamotrigine glucuronidation and increase clearance, should follow the same dosing titration/ maintenance regimen as that used with anticonvulsants that have this effect.

ER:

Lamotrigine ER Escalation Regimen			
	Patients taking valproate[a]	Patients not taking carbamazepine, phenytoin, phenobarbital, primidone,[b] or valproate[a]	Patients taking carbamazepine, phenytoin, phenobarbital, or primidone,[b] and not taking valproate[a]
Weeks 1 and 2	25 mg every other day	25 mg/day	50 mg/day
Weeks 3 and 4	25 mg/day	50 mg/day	100 mg/day
Week 5	50 mg/day	100 mg/day	200 mg/day
Week 6	100 mg/day	150 mg/day	300 mg/day
Week 7	150 mg/day	200 mg/day	400 mg/day
Maintenance range (week 8 and onward)	200 to 250 mg/day[c]	300 to 400 mg/day[c]	400 to 600 mg/day[c]

[a] Valproate has been shown to inhibit glucuronidation and decrease the apparent clearance of lamotrigine.

[b] These drugs induce glucuronidation and increase clearance. Other drugs that have similar effects include estrogen-containing oral contraceptives. Dosing recommendations for oral contraceptives can be found in Concomitant Therapy. Patients on rifampin, or other drugs that induce glucuronidation and increase clearance, should follow the same dosing titration/maintenance regimen as that used with anticonvulsants that have this effect.

[c] Dose increases at week 8 or later should not exceed 100 mg daily at weekly intervals.

Conversion from adjunctive therapy with carbamazepine, phenytoin, phenobarbital, or primidone to monotherapy with lamotrigine – After achieving a dosage of 500 mg/day of lamotrigine according to the guidelines in the previous table, the concomitant AED should be withdrawn by 20% decrements each week over a 4-week period.

Conversion from adjunctive therapy with valproate to monotherapy with lamotrigine immediate release –

Conversion from Adjunctive Therapy with Valproate to Monotherapy with Lamotrigine Immediate Release in Patients 16 Years of Age and Older With Epilepsy		
	Lamotrigine immediate release	Valproate
Step 1	Achieve a dosage of 200 mg/day (if not already on 200 mg/day) according to escalation regimen	Maintain previous stable dose.
Step 2	Maintain at 200 mg/day	Decrease to 500 mg/day by decrements no greater than 500 mg/day. Maintain the dose of 500 mg/day for 1 week.
Step 3	Increase to 300 mg/day and maintain for 1 week	Simultaneously decrease to 250 mg/day and maintain for 1 week.
Step 4	Increase by 100 mg/day every week to achieve maintenance dose of 500 mg/day	Discontinue.

Children 2 to 12 years of age:

Epilepsy, adjunctive therapy –

Lamotrigine Immediate Release Escalation Regimen in Patients 2 to 12 Years of Age With Epilepsy[a]			
	For patients taking valproate[b]	For patients not taking carbamazepine, phenytoin, phenobarbital, primidone,[c] or valproate[b]	For patients taking carbamazepine, phenytoin, phenobarbital, or primidone[c] (without valproate)[b]
Weeks 1 and 2	0.15 mg/kg/day in 1 or 2 divided doses, rounded down to the nearest whole tablet	0.3 mg/kg/day in 1 or 2 divided doses, rounded down to the nearest whole tablet	0.6 mg/kg/day in 2 divided doses, rounded down to the nearest whole tablet
Weeks 3 and 4	0.3 mg/kg/day in 1 or 2 divided doses, rounded down to the nearest whole tablet	0.6 mg/kg/day in 2 divided doses, rounded down to the nearest whole tablet	1.2 mg/kg/day in 2 divided doses, rounded down to the nearest whole tablet
Weeks 5 onwards to maintenance	The dose should be increased every 1 to 2 weeks as follows: Calculate 0.3 mg/kg/day, round this amount down to the nearest whole tablet, and add this amount to the previously administered daily dose	The dose should be increased every 1 to 2 weeks as follows: Calculate 0.6 mg/kg/day, round this amount down to the nearest whole tablet, and add this amount to the previously administered daily dose	The dose should be increased every 1 to 2 weeks as follows: Calculate 1.2 mg/kg/day, round this amount down to the nearest whole tablet, and add this amount to the previously administered daily dose

Lamotrigine Immediate Release Escalation Regimen in Patients 2 to 12 Years of Age With Epilepsy[a]			
	For patients taking valproate[b]	For patients not taking carbamazepine, phenytoin, phenobarbital, primidone,[c] or valproate[b]	For patients taking carbamazepine, phenytoin, phenobarbital, or primidone[c] (without valproate)[b]
Usual maintenance dose	1 to 5 mg/kg/day (maximum 200 mg/day in 1 or 2 divided doses) 1 to 3 mg/kg/day with valproate alone	4.5 to 7.5 mg/kg/day (maximum 300 mg/day in 2 divided doses)	5 to 15 mg/kg/day (maximum 400 mg/day in 2 divided doses)
Maintenance doses in patients weighing less than 30 kg	May need to be increased by as much as 50%, based on clinical response	May need to be increased by as much as 50%, based on clinical response	May need to be increased by as much as 50%, based on clinical response

[a] Note: Only whole tablets should be used for dosing.

[b] Valproate has been shown to inhibit glucuronidation and decrease the apparent clearance of lamotrigine.

[c] These drugs induce glucuronidation and increase the clearance. Other drugs that have similar effects include estrogen-containing oral contraceptives. Patients taking rifampin, or other drugs that induce lamotrigine glucuronidation and increase clearance, should follow the same dosing titration/maintenance regimen as that used with anticonvulsants that have this effect.

Initial Lamotrigine Immediate Release Weight-Based Dosing Guide for Patients 2 to 12 Years of Age Taking Valproate			
If the patient's weight is		Give this daily dose, using the most appropriate combination of lamotrigine 2 mg and 5 mg tablets	
Greater than	And less than	Weeks 1 and 2	Weeks 3 and 4
6.7 kg	14 kg	2 mg every other day	2 mg/day
14.1 kg	27 kg	2 mg/day	4 mg/day
27.1 kg	34 kg	4 mg/day	8 mg/day
34.1 kg	40 kg	5 mg/day	10 mg/day

The smallest available strength of lamotrigine chewable tablets is 2 mg, and only whole tablets should be administered. If the calculated dose cannot be achieved using whole tablets, the dose should be rounded down to the nearest whole tablet.

Conversion: Patients may be converted directly from immediate-release to ER tablets. The initial dose of lamotrigine ER should match the total daily dose of immediate-release lamotrigine; however, some subjects on concomitant enzyme-inducing agents may have lower plasma levels of lamotrigine on conversion and should be monitored.

Following conversion to lamotrigine ER, all patients (but especially those on drugs that induce lamotrigine glucuronidation) should be closely monitored for seizure control. Depending on the therapeutic response after conversion, the total daily dose may need to be adjusted within the recommended dosing instructions.

Discontinuation of therapy: Lamotrigine should not be abruptly discontinued. A step-wise reduction of dose over at least 2 weeks (approximately 50% per week) is recommended unless safety concerns require a more rapid withdrawal.

Adjustments to the maintenance dose of lamotrigine:

Taking or starting oral contraceptives – For women not taking carbamazepine, phenytoin, phenobarbital, primidone, or rifampin, the maintenance dose of lamotrigine may need to be increased by as much as 2 fold over the recommended target maintenance dose.

Stopping oral contraceptives – For women not taking carbamazepine, phenytoin, phenobarbital, primidone, or rifampin, the maintenance dose of lamotrigine may need to be decreased by as much as 50% of the maintenance dose with concurrent oral contraceptives.

Renal function impairment: Initial doses of lamotrigine should be based on patients' concomitant medications; reduced maintenance doses may be effective for patients with significant renal impairment.

Hepatic function impairment: Escalation and maintenance doses should be adjusted according to clinical response.

Moderate and severe hepatic impairment (without ascites) – Reduce initial, escalation, and maintenance doses by approximately 25%.

Severe hepatic impairment – Reduce initial, escalation, and maintenance doses by 50%.

Administration:

Chewable dispersible tablets – Swallow lamotrigine chewable dispersible tablets whole, chewed, or dispersed in water or diluted fruit juice. If chewed, consume a small amount of water or diluted fruit juice to aid in swallowing.

To disperse chewable dispersible tablets, add the tablets to a small amount of liquid (5 mL or enough to cover the medication). Approximately 1 minute later, when the tablets are completely dispersed, swirl the solution and consume the entire quantity immediately. Do not attempt to administer partial quantities of the dispersed tablets.

Orally disintegrating tablets – Lamotrigine orally disintegrating tablets should be placed on the tongue and moved around in the mouth. The tablet will disintegrate rapidly, can be swallowed with or without water, and can be taken with our without food.

Extended-release tablets – ER tablets should be taken once daily, with or without food. Tablets must be swallowed whole and not chewed, crushed, or divided.

Actions

Pharmacology: Lamotrigine is chemically unrelated to existing AEDs. In vitro studies suggest that lamotrigine inhibits voltage-sensitive sodium channels, thereby stabilizing neuronal membranes and consequently modulating presynaptic transmitter release of excitatory amino acids.

Pharmacokinetics:

Absorption/Distribution – Lamotrigine is rapidly and completely absorbed after oral administration. Absolute bioavailability is 98%. Peak plasma concentrations occur anywhere from 1.4 to 4.8 hours following drug administration. Lamotrigine chewable/dispersible tablets were found to be equivalent, whether they were administered as dispersed in water, chewed and swallowed, or swallowed as whole, to lamotrigine compressed tablets in terms of rate and extent of absorption.

Estimates of the mean apparent volume of distribution (Vd/F) of lamotrigine following oral administration ranged from 0.9 to 1.3 L/kg. Vd/F is independent of dose and is similar following single and multiple doses in patients with epilepsy and in healthy volunteers.

Metabolism/Excretion – Lamotrigine is approximately 55% bound to human plasma proteins. Following multiple administrations to healthy volunteers taking no other medications, lamotrigine induced its own metabolism resulting in a 25% decrease in half-life and a 37% increase in plasma clearance.

Because the half-life of lamotrigine following administration of single doses of lamotrigine immediate release is comparable with that observed following administration of lamotrigine ER, similar changes in the half-life of lamotrigine would be expected for lamotrigine ER.

Contraindications

Hypersensitivity to the drug or its components.

Warnings/Precautions

Withdrawal seizures: Do not abruptly discontinue AEDs because of the possibility of increasing seizure frequency in patients with epilepsy and seizures in bipolar patients. Unless safety concerns require a more rapid withdrawal, taper the dose of lamotrigine over a period of at least 2 weeks.

Acute multiorgan failure: Fatalities associated with multiorgan failure and various degrees of hepatic failure have been reported. Most cases occurred in association with other serious events (eg, status epilepticus, overwhelming sepsis), making it impossible to identify the initiating cause.

Hematologic effects: There have been reports of blood dyscrasias that may or may not be associated with the hypersensitivity syndrome.

Suicidal behavior and ideation: AEDs, including lamotrigine, increase the risk of suicidal thoughts or behavior in patients taking these drugs for any indication. Patients treated with any AED for any indication should be monitored for the emergence or worsening of depression, suicidal thoughts or behavior, and/or any unusual changes in behavior.

Bipolar disorder – Patients with bipolar disorder may experience worsening of their depressive symptoms and/or the emergence of suicidal ideation and behaviors (suicidality) whether or not they are taking medications for bipolar disorder.

Addition of lamotrigine to a multidrug regimen that includes valproic acid: Because valproic acid reduces the clearance of lamotrigine, the dosage of lamotrigine in the presence of valproic acid is less than half of that required in its absence.

Dermatologic: See Warning Box.

Serious rashes associated with hospitalization and discontinuation of lamotrigine have been reported. It is recommended that lamotrigine not be restarted in patients who discontinued use due to rash associated with prior treatment with lamotrigine unless the potential benefits clearly outweigh the risks. If the decision is made to restart a patient who has discontinued lamotrigine, assess the need to restart with the initial dosing recommendations (See Administration and Dosage).

Sudden unexplained death in epilepsy (SUDEP): During premarketing development, 20 sudden and unexplained deaths were recorded among 4700 patients with epilepsy (5747 patient-years of exposure). Some of these could represent seizure-related deaths in which the seizure was not observed (eg, at night).

Status epilepticus: Valid estimates of the incidence of treatment-emergent status epilepticus among lamotrigine-treated patients are difficult to obtain. At a minimum, 7 of 2343 adult patients had episodes that could unequivocally be described as status epilepticus. In addition, variably defined episodes of seizure exacerbation (eg, seizure clusters, seizure flurries) were reported.

Clinical worsening and suicide risk: Treatment with antidepressants is associated with an increased risk of suicidal thinking and behavior in children and adolescents with major depressive disorder and other psychiatric disorders. It is not known whether lamotrigine is associated with a similar risk in this population.

Patients with bipolar disorder may experience worsening of their depressive symptoms and/or the emergence of suicidal ideation and behaviors (suicidality) whether or not they are taking medications for bipolar disorder.

Melanin-containing tissues: Lamotrigine binds to melanin and may cause toxicity in these tissues after extended use. Be aware of the possibility of long-term ophthalmologic effects.

Hypersensitivity reactions: Hypersensitivity reactions, some fatal or life-threatening, also have occurred. Some reactions have included clinical features of multiorgan dysfunction such as hepatic abnormalities and evidence of disseminated intravascular coagulation. It is important to note that early manifestations of hypersensitivity (eg, fever, lymphadenopathy) may be present even though a rash is not evident.

Renal function impairment: Administer a reduced maintenance dose for patients with significant impairment.

Hepatic function impairment: Reduce initial, escalation, and maintenance doses by approximately 50% in patients with moderate (Child Pugh grade B) and 75% in patients with severe (Child Pugh grade C) hepatic impairment.

Pregnancy: Category C.

Nonteratogenic effects – There have been reports of decreased lamotrigine concentrations during pregnancy and restoration of prepartum concentrations after delivery. Dosage adjustments may be necessary to maintain clinical response.

Pregnancy exposure registry – To facilitate monitoring fetal outcomes of pregnant women exposed to lamotrigine, health care providers are encouraged to register patients, before fetal outcome (eg, ultrasound, results of amniocentesis, birth) is known, and can obtain information by calling the pregnancy registry at 1-800-336-2176 (toll-free). Patients can enroll themselves in the North American Antiepileptic Drug Pregnancy Registry by calling 1-888-233-2334.

Lactation: Preliminary data indicate that lamotrigine passes into breast milk. Breastfeeding while taking lamotrigine is not recommended.

Children: Lamotrigine is indicated as adjunctive therapy for partial seizures for the generalized seizures of Lennox-Gastaut syndrome, and for primary generalized tonic-clonic seizures in patients older than 2 years of age. Safety and efficacy in patients younger than the age of 18 years with bipolar disorder have not been established. Safety and effectiveness of lamotrigine ER for any use in patients younger than 13 years of age have not been established.

Elderly: Exercise caution in dose selection for elderly patients.

Monitoring: The value of monitoring plasma concentrations of lamotrigine has not been established. Because of the possible pharmacokinetic interactions between lamotrigine and other AEDs being taken concomitantly, monitoring of the plasma levels of lamotrigine and concomitant AEDs may be indicated, particularly during dosage adjustments.

Drug Interactions

Drugs that may affect lamotrigine include acetaminophen, carbamazepine, hormonal contraceptives, orlistat, oxcarbazepine, phenobarbital, phenytoin, primidone, protease inhibitors, rifamycins, sertraline, succinimides, and valproic acid.

Drugs that may be affected by lamotrigine include carbamazepine, hormonal contraceptives, clozapine, topiramate, and valproic acid.

Adverse Reactions

Adverse reactions occurring in 3% or more of patients include the following: abdominal pain, accidental injury, anxiety, asthenia, ataxia, blurred vision, bronchitis, chest pain, constipation, convulsion, cough increased, depression, diarrhea, diplopia, dizziness, dysmenorrhea, dyspepsia, emotional lability, fever, flu syndrome, gait abnormality, headache, incoordination, infection, insomnia, irritability, nausea, pain, pharyngitis, pruritus, rash, rhinitis, somnolence, speech disorder, thinking abnormality, tooth disorder, tremor, urinary tract infection, vaginitis, vision abnormality, vomiting, weight decrease.

RUFINAMIDE

Tablets, oral: 200 mg, 400 mg (*Rx*)	*Banzel* (Novartis Pharma AG)

Indications

Seizures: For adjunctive treatment of seizures associated with Lennox-Gastaut syndrome in adults and children 4 years of age and older.

Administration and Dosage

Tablets may be split or crushed. It is not known whether doses lower than the target doses are effective.

Adults:

Maximum dosage – 3,200 mg/day in 2 equally divided doses.

Initial dosage – 400 to 800 mg/day in 2 equally divided doses.

Dosage titration – Increase the dose by 400 to 800 mg/day every 2 days until a maximum daily dose of 3,200 mg/day, administered in 2 equally divided doses is reached.

Maintenance dosage – 3,200 mg/day.

Children 4 years of age and older:

Initial dosage – Approximately 10 mg/kg/day, administered in 2 equally divided doses.

Dosage titration – Increase the dose by approximately 10 mg/kg increments every other day to a target dose of 45 mg/kg/day or 3,200 mg/day (whichever is less) administered in 2 equally divided doses.

Maintenance dosage – 45 mg/kg/day or 3,200 mg/day (whichever is less) administered in 2 equally divided doses.

Renal function impairment: Hemodialysis may reduce exposure by approximately 30%. Consider adjusting the rufinamide dose during the dialysis process.

Hepatic function impairment: Use of rufinamide in patients with hepatic impairment has not been studied. Therefore, use in patients with severe hepatic impairment is not recommended.

Discontinuation: Withdraw rufinamide gradually to minimize the risk of precipitating seizures, seizure exacerbation, or status epilepticus. If abrupt discontinuation of the drug is medically necessary, the transition to another antiepileptic drug (AED) should be made under close medical supervision. In clinical trials, rufinamide discontinuation was achieved by reducing the dose by approximately 25% every 2 days.

Actions

Pharmacology: The results of in vitro studies suggest that the principal mechanism of action of rufinamide is modulation of the activity of sodium channels and, in particular, prolongation of the inactive state of the channel.

Pharmacokinetics:

Absorption/Distribution – Rufinamide is well absorbed after oral administration. Following oral administration of rufinamide, peak plasma concentrations occur between 4 and 6 hours both under fed and fasted conditions. Only a small fraction of rufinamide (34%) is bound to human serum proteins, predominantly to albumin (27%).

Metabolism/Excretion – Rufinamide is extensively metabolized but has no active metabolites. Plasma half-life of rufinamide is approximately 6 to 10 hours.

Contraindications

Patients with familial short QT syndrome.

Warnings/Precautions

Suicidal behavior and ideation: AEDs increase the risk of suicidal thoughts or behavior in patients taking these drugs for any indication.

CNS reactions: Use of rufinamide has been associated with CNS-related adverse reactions. The most significant of these can be classified into 2 general categories: somnolence or fatigue and coordination abnormalities, dizziness, gait disturbances, and ataxia.

QT interval: Formal cardiac electrocardiographic studies demonstrated shortening of the QT interval (up to 20 msec) with rufinamide treatment.

Status epilepticus: Estimates of the incidence of treatment-emergent status epilepticus among patients treated with rufinamide are difficult because standard definitions were not employed. In all controlled trials that included patients with different epilepsies, 0.9% of rufinamide-treated patients had episodes that could be described as status epilepticus compared with none of 635 placebo-treated patients

Hypersensitivity reactions: Multiorgan hypersensitivity syndrome has occurred in association with rufinamide therapy in clinical trials.

Pregnancy: Category C.

Lactation: Rufinamide is likely to be excreted in breast milk.

Children: The safety and effectiveness in patients with Lennox-Gastaut syndrome have not been established in children younger than 4 years of age.

Elderly: In general, use caution in dose selection for an elderly patient, usually starting at the low end of the dosing range, reflecting the greater frequency of decreased hepatic, renal, or cardiac function, and of concomitant disease or other drug therapy in elderly patients.

Monitoring: Monitor patients treated with any AED for any indication for the emergence or worsening of depression, suicidal thoughts or behavior, or any unusual changes in mood or behavior.

Drug Interactions

Drugs that may affect rufinamide include carbamazepine, phenobarbital, phenytoin, primidone, and valproate.

Drugs that may be affected by rufinamide include carbamazepine, hormonal contraceptives, lamotrigine, phenobarbital, phenytoin, and triazolam.

Adverse Reactions

Adverse reactions occurring in at least 3% of adults treated with rufinamide include abdominal pain upper, aggression, anxiety, ataxia, back pain, bronchitis, constipation, decreased appetite, diplopia, disturbance in attention, dizziness, dyspepsia, ear infection, fatigue, gait disturbance, headache, influenza, nasopharyngitis, nausea, nystagmus, pruritus, psychomotor hyperactivity, rash, sinusitis, somnolence, tremor, vertigo, vision blurred, vomiting.

Adverse reactions occurring in at least 3% of children treated with rufinamide include abdominal pain upper, aggression, ataxia, bronchitis, decreased appetite, diplopia, disturbance in attention, dizziness, ear infection, fatigue, headache, influenza, nasopharyngitis, nausea, pruritus, psychomotor hyperactivity, rash, sinusitis, somnolence, vomiting.

LEVETIRACETAM

Tablets; oral: 250, 500, and 750 mg (*Rx*)	Various, *Keppra* (UCB)
1,000 mg (*Rx*)	*Keppra* (UCB)
Tablets, extended-release; oral: 500 and 750 mg (*Rx*)	*Keppra* XR (UCB)
Solution; oral: 100 mg/mL (*Rx*)	Various, *Keppra* (UCB)
Injection, solution, concentrate: 100 mg/mL (*Rx*)	*Keppra* (UCB)

Indications

Myoclonic seizures: Adjunctive therapy in the treatment of myoclonic seizures in adults and adolescents 12 years of age and older with juvenile myoclonic epilepsy.

Partial-onset seizures:

Immediate-release tablets/oral solution – Adjunctive therapy in the treatment of partial-onset seizures in adults and children 4 years of age and older with epilepsy.

Extended-release (ER) tablets – Adjunctive therapy in the treatment of partial-onset seizures in adults and adolescents 16 years of age and older with epilepsy.

Primary generalized tonic-clonic seizures: Adjunctive therapy in the treatment of primary generalized tonic-clonic seizures in adults and children 6 years of age and older with idiopathic generalized epilepsy (immediate-release tablets/oral solution).

Administration and Dosage

Treatment can be initiated with either intravenous (IV) or oral therapy.

Oral therapy: Give orally with or without food. Only whole tablets should be administered.

Maximum dose – 3,000 mg/day, but may differ depending on indication.

Myoclonic seizures (immediate-release tablets/oral solution) – Initiate treatment at 1,000 mg/day, given as twice-daily dosing (500 mg twice daily). Increase by 1,000 mg/day every 2 weeks to the recommended daily dose of 3,000 mg.

Partial-onset seizures –

Adults (16 years of age and older):

Immediate-release tablets/oral solution – Initiate treatment at 1,000 mg/day, given as twice-daily dosing (500 mg twice daily). Additional dosing increments may be given (additional 1,000 mg/day every 2 weeks) to a maximum recommended daily dose of 3,000 mg.

ER tablets – Initiate dosage with 1,000 mg once daily. The daily dosage may be adjusted in increments of 1,000 mg every 2 weeks to a maximum recommended daily dose of 3,000 mg.

Children (4 to younger than 16 years of age):

Immediate-release tablets/oral solution – Initiate with a daily dose of 20 mg/kg in 2 divided doses (10 mg/kg twice daily). Increase every 2 weeks by increments of 20 mg/kg to the recommended daily dose of 60 mg/kg (30 mg/kg twice daily). If a patient cannot tolerate a daily dose of 60 mg/kg, the daily dose may be reduced. Patients with body weight of 20 kg or less should be dosed with oral solution.

Immediate-release tablets:

Levetiracetam Weight-Based Dosing Guide for Children			
	Daily dose		
Patient weight	20 mg/kg/day (twice-daily dosing)	40 mg/kg/day (twice-daily dosing)	60 mg/kg/day (twice-daily dosing)
20.1 to 40 kg	500 mg/day (1 × 250 mg tablet twice daily)	1,000 mg/day (1 × 500 mg tablet twice daily)	1,500 mg/day (1 × 750 mg tablet twice daily)
> 40 kg	1,000 mg/day (1 × 500 mg tablet twice daily)	2,000 mg/day (2 × 500 mg tablets twice daily)	3,000 mg/day (2 × 750 mg tablets twice daily)

Oral solution: The following calculation should be used to determine the appropriate daily dose of oral solution for children based on a daily dose of 20, 40, or 60 mg/kg/day: Total daily dose (mL/day) = (daily dose [mg/kg/day] × patient weight [kg]) ÷ 100 mg/mL.

Primary generalized tonic-clonic seizures (immediate-release tablets and oral solution) –

Adults (16 years of age and older): Initiate with a dose of 1,000 mg/day, given as twice-daily dosing (500 mg twice daily). Increase by 1,000 mg/day every 2 weeks to the recommended daily dose of 3,000 mg.

Children (6 to younger than 16 years of age): Initiate with a daily dose of 20 mg/kg in 2 divided doses (10 mg/kg twice daily). Increase every 2 weeks by increments of 20 mg/kg to the recommended daily dose of 60 mg/kg (30 mg/kg twice daily). Patients with a body weight of 20 kg or less should be dosed with oral solution. Patients with a body weight greater than 20 kg can be dosed with tablets or oral solution. See the previous table for tablet dosing based on weight during titration to 60 mg/kg/day.

IV replacement therapy: When switching from oral levetiracetam, the initial total daily IV dose of levetiracetam should be equivalent to the total daily dosage and frequency of oral levetiracetam and should be administered as a 15-minute IV infusion following dilution in 100 mL of a compatible diluent. At the end of the IV treatment period, the patient may be switched to levetiracetam oral administration at the equivalent daily dosage and frequency of the IV administration.

Preparation/Administration – Levetiracetam injection is for IV use only and must be diluted in 100 mL of a compatible diluent and administered IV as a 15-minute IV infusion. Any unused portion of the vial contents should be discarded. Product with particulate matter or discoloration should not be used.

Admixture compatibility – Levetiracetam was found to be physically compatible and chemically stable when mixed with the following diluents and antiepileptic drugs (AEDs) for at least 24 hours and stored in polyvinyl chloride bags at controlled room temperature, 15° to 30°C (59° to 86°F).

Levetiracetam is compatible with the following diluents: sodium chloride 0.9% injection, dextrose 5% injection, and Ringer's lactate injection. Levetiracetam is compatible with the following AEDs: lorazepam, diazepam, and valproate sodium. There are no data to support the physical compatibility of levetiracetam with antiepileptic drugs that are not listed.

Renal function impairment: Individualize dosing according to the patient's renal function status. Recommended doses and adjustment for dose are shown in the following table.

Immediate-release tablets/oral solution –

Levetiracetam Dosing Adjustment Regimen for Patients with Impaired Renal Function			
Group	CrCl (mL/min)	Dosage (mg)	Frequency
Healthy	> 80	500 to 1,500	every 12 h
Mild	50 to 80	500 to 1,000	every 12 h
Moderate	30 to 50	250 to 750	every 12 h
Severe	< 30	250 to 500	every 12 h
ESRD patients using dialysis	—	500 to 1,000[a]	every 24 h

[a] Following dialysis, a 250 to 500 mg supplemental dose is recommended.

ER tablets –

Levetiracetam ER Tablets Dosage for Adult With Renal Function Impairment			
Renal function status	CrCl (mL/min per 1.73 m^2)	Dosage (mg)	Frequency
Healthy	> 80	1,000 to 3,000	Every 24 h
Mild	50 to 80	1,000 to 2,000	Every 24 h
Moderate	30 to 50	500 to 1,500	Every 24 h
Severe	< 30	500 to 1,000	Every 24 h

Actions

Pharmacology: Levetiracetam is chemically unrelated to other antiepileptic drugs. The precise mechanism by which levetiracetam exerts its antiepileptic effect is unknown.

Pharmacokinetics:

Immediate-release tablets/oral solution – Absorption is rapid, with peak plasma concentrations occurring in approximately 1 hour following oral administration in fasted subjects. Steady state is achieved after 2 days of multiple twice/day dosing. Levetiracetam is not extensively metabolized. The plasma half-life in adults is approximately 7 hours. Levetiracetam is eliminated from the systemic circulation by renal excretion.

The oral bioavailability of levetiracetam tablets is 100% and the tablets and oral solution are bioequivalent in rate and extent of absorption. Levetiracetam and its major metabolite are less than 10% bound to plasma proteins. The volume of distribution of levetiracetam is close to the volume of intracellular and extracellular water.

ER tablets – Levetiracetam ER peak plasma concentrations occur in about 4 hours. The time to peak plasma concentrations is about 3 hours longer with levetiracetam ER than with immediate-release tablets. Plasma half-life of levetiracetam ER is approximately 7 hours.

Contraindications

Hypersensitivity to the drug or any of its ingredients.

Warnings/Precautions

Partial onset seizures in adults:

Dizziness – Dizziness was reported in 5.2% of levetiracetam ER–treated patients compared with 2.5% of placebo-treated patients.

Somnolence – In controlled trials of patients with epilepsy, 14.8% of immediate-release levetiracetam-treated patients reported somnolence compared with 8.4% of placebo patients and 7.8% of ER levetiracetam-treated patients experienced somnolence compared with 2.5% of placebo patients.

Asthenia – In controlled trials of patients with epilepsy, 14.7% of levetiracetam-treated patients reported asthenia vs 9.1% with placebo.

Coordination difficulties – A total of 3.4% of levetiracetam-treated patients experienced coordination difficulties (reported as either ataxia, abnormal gait, or incoordination) vs 1.6% with placebo.

Somnolence, asthenia, and coordination difficulties occurred most frequently within the first 4 weeks of treatment.

Psychotic symptoms – In controlled trials of patients with epilepsy, 5 (0.7%) of levetiracetam-treated patients experienced psychotic symptoms compared with 1 (0.2%) placebo patient. A total of 13.3% of levetiracetam patients experienced other behavioral symptoms (eg, aggression, agitation, anger, hostility, irritability, anxiety, apathy, emotional lability, depersonalization, depression) compared with 6.2% of placebo patients.

In addition, 4 (0.5%) levetiracetam-treated patients attempted suicide vs 0% with placebo.

ER tablets: A total of 6.5% of levetiracetam ER–treated patients experienced nonpsychotic behavioral disorders (reported as irritability and aggression) compared with 0% of placebo-treated patients. Irritability was reported in 6.5% of levetiracetam ER–treated patients. Aggression was reported in 1.3% of levetiracetam ER–treated patients.

Hematologic symptoms –

Immediate-release tablets/oral solution: Minor but statistically significant decreases compared with placebo in WBC and neutrophil counts, total mean RBC count ($0.03 \times 10^6/mm^2$), mean hemoglobin (0.09 g/dL), and mean hematocrit (0.38%), were seen in levetiracetam-treated patients in controlled trials.

Partial-onset seizures in children: In children experiencing partial-onset seizures, levetiracetam is associated with somnolence, fatigue, and behavioral abnormalities.

Somnolence – In the double-blind, controlled trial in children with epilepsy experiencing partial-onset seizures, 22.8% of levetiracetam-treated patients experienced somnolence, compared with 11.3% of placebo patients.

Asthenia – Asthenia was reported in 8.9% of levetiracetam-treated patients, compared with 3.1% of placebo patients.

Behavioral symptoms – A total of 37.6% of the levetiracetam-treated patients experienced behavioral symptoms (eg, agitation, anxiety, apathy, depersonalization, depression, emotional lability, hostility, hyperkinesia, nervousness, neurosis, personality disorder), compared with 18.6% of placebo patients. Hostility was reported in 11.9% of levetiracetam-treated patients, compared with 6.2% of placebo patients. Nervousness was reported in 9.9% of levetiracetam-treated patients, compared with 2.1% of placebo patients. Depression was reported in 3% of levetiracetam-treated patients, compared with 1% of placebo patients. One levetiracetam-treated patient experienced suicidal ideation.

Psychotic symptoms – A total of 3% of levetiracetam-treated patients discontinued treatment because of psychotic and nonpsychotic adverse reactions, compared with 4.1% of placebo patients.

Hematologic symptoms – Minor, but statistically significant, decreases in WBC and neutrophil counts were seen in levetiracetam-treated children compared with placebo.

Myoclonic seizures:

Somnolence – In the double-blind, controlled trial in adults and adolescents with juvenile myoclonic epilepsy who were experiencing myoclonic seizures, 11.7% of levetiracetam-treated patients experienced somnolence, compared with 1.7% of placebo patients.

Behavioral symptoms – Nonpsychotic behavioral disorders (reported as aggression and irritability) occurred in 5% of levetiracetam-treated patients, compared with 0% of placebo patients. Nonpsychotic mood disorders (reported as depressed mood, depression, and mood swings) occurred in 6.7% of levetiracetam-treated patients, compared with 3.3% of placebo patients.

Primary generalized tonic-clonic seizures:

Behavioral symptoms – In patients 6 years of age and older nonpsychotic behavioral disorders (reported as abnormal behavior, aggression, conduct disorder, and irritability) occurred in 11.4% of the levetiracetam-treated patients, compared with 3.6% of placebo patients.

Psychotic symptoms – In the double-blind, controlled trial in patients with idiopathic generalized epilepsy experiencing primary generalized tonic-clonic seizures, irritability was the most frequently reported psychiatric adverse reaction occurring in 6.3% of levetiracetam-treated patients, compared with 2.4% of placebo patients. Nonpsychotic mood disorders (ie, anger, apathy, depression, mood alterations/swings, negativism, suicidal ideation, tearfulness) occurred in 12.7% of levetiracetam-treated patients, compared with 8.3% of placebo patients.

Withdrawal seizure: Withdraw levetiracetam gradually to minimize the potential of increased seizure frequency.

Renal function impairment: Reduce dosage in patients with impaired renal function receiving immediate-release levetiracetam, and give supplemental doses to patients after dialysis (see Actions and Administration and Dosage).

The effect of levetiracetam ER on renally impaired patients was not assessed. However, it is expected that the effect on levetiracetam ER–treated patients would be similar to the effect seen in levetiracetam immediate-release tablets.

Hepatic function impairment: There were no meaningful changes in mean liver function tests in the levetiracetam ER controlled trial.

Hazardous tasks: Patients should use caution while driving or performing other tasks requiring alertness, coordination or physical dexterity.

Pregnancy: Category C.

Lactation: Levetiracetam is excreted in breast milk. Because of the potential for serious adverse reactions in nursing infants, decide whether to discontinue nursing or discontinue the drug, taking into account the importance of the drug to the mother.

Children: Safety and efficacy in patients younger than 4 years of age have not been established.

Safety and effectiveness of levetiracetam ER in patients younger than 16 years of age have not been established.

Elderly: Levetiracetam is known to be substantially excreted by the kidney, and the risk of adverse reactions to this drug may be greater in patients with renal function impairment. Because elderly patients are more likely to have decreased renal function, take care in dose selection; it may be useful to monitor renal function.

Drug Interactions

Levetiracetam may cause carbamazepine toxicity and may be affected by probenecid.

Drug/Food interactions: Food does not affect the extent of absorption of levetiracetam, but it decreases C_{max} by 20% and delays T_{max} by 1.5 hours.

Adverse Reactions

The most frequently reported adverse events associated with the use of levetiracetam in combination with other AEDs were asthenia, dizziness, infection, and somnolence.

Adverse reactions occurring in at least 3% of children administered levetiracetam include the following: accidental injury, agitation, albuminuria, anorexia, asthenia, conjunctivitis, constipation, depression, diarrhea, dizziness, ecchymosis, emotional lability, flu syndrome, gastroenteritis, hostility, increased cough, nervousness, pain, personality disorder, pharyngitis, rhinitis, somnolence, vertigo, vomiting,

Adverse reactions occurring in at least 3% of adults taking levetiracetam include the following: Anorexia, asthenia, ataxia, depression, dizziness, headache, influenza, infection, nervousness, pain, pharyngitis, rhinitis, somnolence, vertigo.

PRIMIDONE

Tablets; oral: 50 mg (*Rx*)	Various, *Mysoline* (Xcel Pharm.)
250 mg (*Rx*)	

Indications

Epilepsy: Primidone, used alone or concomitantly with other anticonvulsants, is indicated in the control of grand mal, psychomotor, and focal epileptic seizures. It may control grand mal seizures refractory to other anticonvulsant therapy.

Administration and Dosage

Individualize dosage.

Adults and children (older than 8 years of age): Patients who have received no previous treatment may be started on primidone according to the following regimen:

Days 1 to 3 – 100 to 125 mg at bedtime.
Days 4 to 6 – 100 to 125 mg twice/day (morning and evening).
Days 7 to 9 – 100 to 125 mg 3 times/day (morning, noon, and evening).
Day 10 to maintenance – 250 mg 3 times a day (morning, noon, and evening).

For most adults and children 8 years of age and over, the usual maintenance dosage is 250 mg 3 or 4 times daily. If required, an increase to five or six 250 mg tablets daily may be made, but daily doses should not exceed 500 mg 4 times daily.

Serum blood level determinations of primidone may be necessary for optimal dosage adjustment. The clinically effective serum level for primidone is between 5 to 12 mcg/mL.

Children (younger than 8 years of age): The following regimen may be used to initiate therapy:

Days 1 to 3 – 50 mg at bedtime.
Days 4 to 6 – 50 mg twice/day.
Days 7 to 9 – 100 mg twice/day.
Day 10 – maintenance – 125 to 250 mg 3 times/day.

For children younger than 8 years of age, the usual maintenance dosage is 125 to 250 mg 3 times daily or 10 to 25 mg/kg/day in divided doses.

Patients already receiving other anticonvulsants: Start primidone at 100 to 125 mg at bedtime; gradually increase to maintenance level as the other drug is gradually decreased. When therapy with primidone alone is the objective, the transition should not be completed in less than 2 weeks.

Actions

Pharmacology: Primidone's mechanism of antiepileptic action is not known.

Primidone and its 2 metabolites, phenobarbital and phenylethylmalonamide have anticonvulsant activity.

Contraindications

Porphyria; hypersensitivity to phenobarbital, a metabolite of primidone.

Warnings/Precautions

Status epilepticus: Abrupt withdrawal of antiepileptic medication may precipitate status epilepticus.

Therapeutic efficacy: Therapeutic efficacy of a dosage regimen takes several weeks to assess.

Hazardous tasks: Patients should use caution while driving or performing other tasks requiring alertness, coordination, or physical dexterity.

Pregnancy: Category D.

Lactation: It is suggested that the presence of undue somnolence and drowsiness in nursing newborns of primidone-treated mothers be taken as an indication that nursing should be discontinued.

Monitoring: Because therapy generally extends over prolonged periods, perform complete blood counts and a sequential multiple analysis test every 6 months.

Drug Interactions

Drugs that may affect primidone include carbamazepine, hydantoins, succinimides, and valproic acid.

Drugs that may be affected by primidone include anticoagulants, beta blockers, carbamazepine, corticosteroids, doxycycline, estrogens, ethanol, felodipine, methadone, metronidazole, nifedipine, oral contraceptives, quinidine, theophylline.

Adverse Reactions

Adverse reactions may include anorexia, ataxia, diplopia, drowsiness, emotional disturbances, fatigue, hyperirritability, impotence, morbilliform skin eruptions, nausea, nystagmus, vertigo, vomiting.

VIGABATRIN

Tablets; oral: 500 mg (*Rx*)	*Sabril* (Lundbeck)
Powder for solution; oral:500 mg (*Rx*)	

Warning:

Vision loss: Vigabatrin causes permanent vision loss in infants, children, and adults. Because assessing vision loss is difficult in children, the frequency and extent of vision loss in infants and children is poorly characterized. For this reason, the following data are primarily based on the adult experience.

In adults, vigabatrin causes permanent bilateral concentric visual field constriction in 30% or more of patients; it ranges in severity from mild to severe, including tunnel vision to within 10 degrees of visual fixation, and can result in disability. In some cases, vigabatrin also can damage the central retina and may decrease visual acuity.

The onset of vision loss from vigabatrin is unpredictable, and can occur within weeks of starting treatment or sooner, or at any time during treatment, even after months or years.

The risk of vision loss increases with increasing dose and cumulative exposure, but there is no dose or exposure known to be free of risk of vision loss.

Vision testing at baseline (no later than 4 weeks after starting vigabatrin) and at least every 3 months during therapy is required for adults on vigabatrin. In infants and children, vision loss may not be detected until it is severe. Nonetheless, assess vision to the extent possible at baseline (no later than 4 weeks after starting vigabatrin) and at least every 3 months during therapy. Vision testing is also required about 3 to 6 months after the discontinuation of vigabatrin therapy. Once detected, vision loss caused by vigabatrin is not reversible. It is expected that, even with frequent monitoring, some patients will develop severe vision loss.

It is possible that vision loss can worsen despite discontinuing vigabatrin.

Because of the risk of vision loss, withdraw vigabatrin from patients who fail to show substantial clinical benefit within 2 to 4 weeks of initiation when used in children or within 3 months when used in adults, or sooner if treatment failure becomes obvious. Periodically reassess patient response to and continued need for vigabatrin.

continued on next page

Warning: (cont.)

Symptoms of vision loss from vigabatrin are unlikely to be recognized by the parent or caregiver before vision loss is severe. Vision loss of milder severity, although unrecognized by the caregiver, may still adversely affect function.

Do not use vigabatrin in patients with, or at high risk of, other types of irreversible vision loss unless the benefits of treatment clearly outweigh the risks. The interaction of other types of irreversible vision damage with vision damage from vigabatrin has not been well characterized, but is likely adverse.

Do not use vigabatrin with other drugs associated with serious adverse ophthalmic effects such as retinopathy or glaucoma unless the benefits clearly outweigh the risks.

Use the lowest dose and shortest exposure to vigabatrin that is consistent with clinical objectives.

The possibility that vision loss from vigabatrin may be more common, more severe, or have more severe functional consequences in infants and children than in adults cannot be excluded.

Because of the risk of permanent vision loss, vigabatrin is available only through a special restricted distribution program called SHARE, by calling 1-888-457-4273. Only prescribers and pharmacies registered with SHARE may prescribe and distribute vigabatrin. In addition, vigabatrin may be dispensed only to patients who are enrolled in and meet all conditions of SHARE.

Indications

Infantile spasms (1 month to 2 years of age): As monotherapy for infants and children with infantile spasms for whom the potential benefits outweigh the potential risk of vision loss.

Refractory complex partial seizures: As adjunctive therapy for adults with refractory complex partial seizures who have inadequately responded to several alternative treatments and for whom the potential benefits outweigh the risk of vision loss.

Administration and Dosage

Monitoring of vigabatrin concentrations to optimize therapy is not helpful.

Vigabatrin should be given as twice-daily oral administration with or without food.

Adults:

Refractory complex partial seizures – Initial dosage is 1 g/day (500 mg twice daily), with a usual dosage of 3 g/day (1.5 g twice daily) and a maximum dosage of 6 g/day. Increase total daily dose in 500 mg increments at weekly intervals depending on response.

Tapering: Vigabatrin should be withdrawn gradually. In controlled clinical studies, vigabatrin was tapered by decreasing the daily dose 1 g/day on a weekly basis until discontinued.

Children:

Infantile spasms (1 month to 2 years of age) – Initial dosage is 50 mg/kg/day given in 2 divided doses, with a maximum dosage of 150 mg/kg/day. Titrate by 25 to 50 mg/kg/day increments every 3 days, up to a maximum of 150 mg/kg/day.

Vigabatrin Infant Dosing Table

Weight (kg)	Starting dose 50 mg/kg/day	Maximum dose 150 mg/kg/day
3	1.5 mL twice daily	4.5 mL twice daily
4	2 mL twice daily	6 mL twice daily
5	2.5 mL twice daily	7.5 mL twice daily
6	3 mL twice daily	9 mL twice daily
7	3.5 mL twice daily	10.5 mL twice daily
8	4 mL twice daily	12 mL twice daily

Vigabatrin Infant Dosing Table		
Weight (kg)	Starting dose 50 mg/kg/day	Maximum dose 150 mg/kg/day
9	4.5 mL twice daily	13.5 mL twice daily
10	5 mL twice daily	15 mL twice daily
11	5.5 mL twice daily	16.5 mL twice daily
12	6 mL twice daily	18 mL twice daily
13	6.5 mL twice daily	19.5 mL twice daily
14	7 mL twice daily	21 mL twice daily
15	7.5 mL twice daily	22.5 mL twice daily
16	8 mL twice daily	24 mL twice daily

Tapering: In a controlled clinical study, vigabatrin was tapered by decreasing the dose at a rate of 25 to 50 mg/kg every 3 to 4 days.

Refractory complex seizures –

16 years of age and older: See Adults for dosing.

Younger than 16 years of age: Safety and efficacy in children younger than 16 years of age with complex partial seizures have not been established.

Renal function impairment: Information about how to adjust the dose in children with renal impairment is unavailable.

Mild renal impairment (creatinine clearance greater than 50 to 80 mL/min) – Decrease the dose by 25%.

Moderate renal impairment (creatinine clearance greater than 30 to 50 mL/min) – Decrease the dose by 50%.

Severe renal impairment (creatinine clearance greater than 10 to less than 30 mL/min) – Decrease the dose by 75%.

Actions

Pharmacology: The precise mechanism of vigabatrin's antiseizure effect is unknown, but it is believed to be the result of its action as an irreversible inhibitor of gamma-aminobutyric acid transaminase (GABA-T), the enzyme responsible for the metabolism of the inhibitory neurotransmitter GABA. This action results in increased levels of GABA in the CNS.

Pharmacokinetics:

Absorption – Following oral administration, vigabatrin is essentially completely absorbed.

Time to maximum concentration (T_{max}) is approximately 2.5 hours in infants and approximately 1 hour in children and adults following a single dose.

Bioequivalence: Bioequivalence has been established between the oral solution and tablet formulations.

Distribution – Vigabatrin does not bind to plasma proteins.

Metabolism/Excretion – Vigabatrin is not significantly metabolized; it is eliminated primarily through renal excretion. The half-life of vigabatrin in adults is approximately 7.5 hours and approximately 5.7 hours in infants. Vigabatrin induces CYP2C9, but does not induce other hepatic cytochrome P450 enzyme systems.

Warnings/Precautions

Vision loss: Withdraw the patient who fails to show substantial clinical benefit within 2 to 4 weeks of initiation of treatment for infants and children and within 3 months for adults from vigabatrin.

Monitoring of vision – Indirect ophthalmoscopy of the retina must be performed at baseline (no later than 4 weeks after starting vigabatrin) and at least every 3 months while on therapy. Vision testing is also required about 3 to 6 months after the discontinuation of vigabatrin therapy. Ensure that this assessment includes visual acuity and visual field whenever possible.

Distribution program: Vigabatrin is available only under a special restricted distribution program called the SHARE program. Under the SHARE program, only prescribers and pharmacies registered with the program are able to prescribe and distribute vigabatrin. In addition, vigabatrin may be dispensed only to patients who are enrolled in and meet all conditions of SHARE. Contact the SHARE program at 1-888-457-4273. To enroll in SHARE, prescribers must understand the risks of vigabatrin and complete the SHARE Prescriber Enrollment and Agreement Form indicating agreement to:

- Enroll all patients in SHARE.
- Review the vigabatrin Medication Guide with every patient and/or caregiver.
- Educate caregiver(s) and patients on the risks of vigabatrin, including the risk of vision loss.
- Arrange for visual field and retinal exam by an expert examiner and review visual evaluation prior to initiation of vigabatrin treatment and every 3 months during therapy.
- Remove patients from vigabatrin therapy if the patients do not experience a meaningful reduction in seizures.
- Counsel caregiver(s) and patients who fail to comply with the program requirements.
- Remove patients who fail to comply, or whose caregiver(s) fail to comply, with the program requirements after appropriate counseling from vigabatrin therapy.

Magnetic resonance imaging: Abnormal magnetic resonance imaging (MRI) signal changes characterized by increased T2 signal and restricted diffusion in a symmetric pattern involving the thalamus, basal ganglia, brain stem, and cerebellum have been observed in some infants treated for infantile spasms with vigabatrin.

Neurotoxicity: Vacuolization, characterized by fluid accumulation and separation of the outer layers of myelin, has been observed in brain white matter tracts in adult animals following administration of vigabatrin.

Suicidal behavior and ideation: Antiepileptic drugs (AEDs), including vigabatrin, increase the risk of suicidal thoughts or behavior in patients taking these drugs for any indication.

Anemia: In controlled trials in adults, 5.7% of patients receiving vigabatrin and 1.6% of patients receiving placebo had adverse events of anemia and/or met criteria for potentially clinically important hematology changes involving hemoglobin, hematocrit, and/or red blood cell indices.

Peripheral neuropathy: Vigabatrin has been shown to cause symptoms of peripheral neuropathy in adults.

Weight gain: Vigabatrin has been shown to cause weight gain in adults.

Edema: Vigabatrin has been shown to cause edema in adults.

Renal function impairment: In adults, dose adjustment, including initiating treatment with a lower dose, is necessary in patients with mild (CrCl greater than 50 to 80 mL/min), moderate (CrCl greater than 30 to 50 mL/min), and severe (CrCl greater than 10 to 30 mL/min) renal impairment.

Hazardous tasks: Vigabatrin causes somnolence and fatigue. Advise patients not to drive a car or operate other complex machinery until they are familiar with the effects of vigabatrin on their ability to perform such activities.

Pregnancy: Category C.

Lactation: Vigabatrin is excreted in human milk. Because of the potential for serious adverse reactions from vigabatrin in breast-feeding infants, decide whether to discontinue breast-feeding or the drug, taking into account the importance of the drug to the mother.

Children: The safety and efficacy of vigabatrin in children younger than 16 years of age with complex partial seizures have not been established.

Elderly: Because elderly patients are more likely to have decreased renal function, exercise care in dose selection; it may be useful to monitor renal function.

Consider adjustment of dose or frequency of administration. Such patients may respond to a lower maintenance dose.

Monitoring: Monitoring of vision by an ophthalmic professional with expertise in visual field interpretation and the ability to perform dilated indirect ophthalmoscopy of the retina must be performed at baseline (no later than 4 weeks after starting vigabatrin) and at least every 3 months while on therapy. Vision testing is also required about 3 to 6 months after the discontinuation of vigabatrin therapy. Ensure that this assessment includes visual acuity and visual field whenever possible.

Monitor patients for the emergence or worsening of the signs and symptoms of depression, any unusual changes in mood or behavior, or the emergence of suicidal thoughts, behavior, or thoughts about self-harm.

Drug Interactions

Drugs that may interact with vigabatrin include clonazepam, hydantoins, phenobarbital, primidone, valproic acid, and drugs associated with serious adverse ophthalmic effects such as retinopathy (eg, hydroxychloroquine) or glaucoma (eg, corticosteroids [open-angle], tricyclic antidepressants [closed-angle]).

Drug/Lab test interactions: Vigabatrin suppresses ALT and AST enzyme activity in up to 90% of patients. The suppression of ALT and AST activity may preclude the use of these markers to detect early hepatic injury.

Vigabatrin may increase the amount of amino acids in the urine, possibly leading to a false-positive test for certain rare genetic metabolic diseases.

Adverse Reactions

Adults (refractory complex partial seizures): Adverse reactions occurring in 3% or more of patients include abdominal pain, abdominal pain upper, abnormal behavior, abnormal dreams, anxiety, arthralgia, asthenia, back pain, bronchitis, chest pain, confusional state, constipation, contusion, coordination abnormal, cough, depressed mood, depression, diarrhea, diplopia, disturbance in attention, dizziness, dysarthria, dysmenorrhea, dyspepsia, erectile dysfunction, expressive language disorder, eye pain, fatigue, fever, gait disturbance, headache, hypesthesia, hyperreflexia, hyporeflexia, increased appetite, influenza, irritability, lethargy, malaise, memory impairment, muscle spasms, muscle twitching, myalgia, nasopharyngitis, nausea, nervousness, nystagmus, pain in extremity, paresthesia, peripheral edema, pharyngolaryngeal pain, pulmonary congestion, postictal state, rash, sedation, sensory disturbance, sensory loss, sinus headache, somnolence, status epilepticus, stomach discomfort, thinking abnormal, toothache, tremor, upper respiratory tract infection, urinary tract infection, vertigo, vision blurred, vomiting, weight increased,

Children (infantile spasms): Adverse reactions occurring in at least 3% of patients include the following: candidiasis, conjunctivitis, constipation, convulsions, cough, croup infectious, decreased appetite, diarrhea, ear infection, fever, gastroenteritis viral, hypotonia, influenza, insomnia, irritability, lethargy, nasal congestion, otitis media, pneumonia, rash, sedation, sinusitis, somnolence, status epilepticus, strabismus, urinary tract infection, upper respiratory tract infection, viral infection, vomiting,

VALPROIC ACID and DERIVATIVES

Tablets, delayed-release; oral: 125, 250, and 500 mg (as divalproex sodium) (*Rx*)	Various, *Depakote* (Abbott)
Tablets, extended-release; oral: 250 and 500 mg (as divalproex sodium) (*Rx*)	*Depakote ER* (Abbott)
Capsules; oral: 250 mg (*Rx*)	Various, *Depakene* (Abbott)
Capsules, sprinkle; oral: 125 mg (as divalproex sodium) (*Rx*)	*Depakote* (Abbott)
Syrup; oral: 250 mg per 5 mL (*Rx*)	Various, *Depakene* (Abbott)
Injection, concentrate: 100 mg/mL (*Rx*)	Various, *Depacon* (Abbott)

Warning:

Hepatotoxicity: Hepatic failure resulting in fatalities has occurred in patients receiving valproic acid and its derivatives. Children under 2 years of age are at a considerably increased risk of developing fatal hepatotoxicity, especially those on multiple anticonvulsants and those with congenital metabolic disorders, severe seizure disorders accompanied by mental retardation, and organic brain disease. In this patient group, use with extreme caution and as a sole agent. Weigh benefits of seizure control against risks. Above this age group, the incidence of fatal hepatotoxicity decreases considerably in progressively older patient groups. These incidents usually have occurred during the first 6 months of treatment. Serious or fatal hepatotoxicity may be preceded by nonspecific symptoms such as loss of seizure control, malaise, weakness, lethargy, facial edema, anorexia, jaundice, and vomiting. Monitor patients closely for appearance of these symptoms. Perform liver function tests prior to therapy and at frequent intervals thereafter, especially during the first 6 months.

Teratogenicity: Valproate can produce teratogenic effects such as neural tube defects (eg, spina bifida). The use of divalproex sodium in women of childbearing potential requires that the benefits of its use be weighed against the risk of injury to the fetus. This is especially important when the treatment of a spontaneously reversible condition ordinarily not associated with permanent injury or risk of death (eg, migraine) is contemplated (see Warnings and Patient Information). An information sheet describing the teratogenic potential of valproate is available for patients.

Pancreatitis: Cases of life-threatening pancreatitis have been reported in children and adults receiving valproate. Some of the cases have been described as hemorrhagic with a rapid progression from initial symptoms to death. Cases have been reported shortly after initial use as well as after several years of use. Warn patients and guardians that abdominal pain, nausea, vomiting, or anorexia can be symptoms of pancreatitis that require prompt medical evaluation. If pancreatitis is diagnosed, discontinue valproate. Initiate alternative treatment for the underlying medical condition as clinically indicated.

Indications

Epilepsy: For use as sole and adjunctive therapy in the treatment of simple and complex absence seizures and adjunctively in patients with multiple seizure types that include absence seizures; as monotherapy and adjunctive therapy in the treatment of patients with complex partial seizures that occur in isolation or in association with other types of seizures.

Valproate sodium injection is indicated as an IV alternative in patients for whom oral administration of valproate products is temporarily not feasible.

Mania (divalproex sodium delayed-release and extended-release [ER] tablets): For the treatment of manic episodes (delayed-release) and acute manic or mixed episodes, with or without psychotic features (ER), associated with bipolar disorder.

Migraine (divalproex sodium delayed-release and ER tablets): As prophylaxis of migraine headaches in adults.

Administration and Dosage

Oral products: Bedtime administration may minimize effects of CNS depression. GI irritation may be minimized by taking with food or by slowly increasing the dose. Delayed-release divalproex sodium may reduce the incidence of irritative GI effects. Swallow the ER tablets whole; do not crush or chew. Swallow the valproic acid capsules without chewing to avoid local irritation of the mouth and throat.

Sprinkle capsules: Capsules may be swallowed whole or opened and the entire contents sprinkled on a small amount (teaspoonful) of soft food such as applesauce or pudding. Swallow drug/food mixture immediately; do not chew. Do not store for future use.

Valproic acid syrup or capsule dosing: The following table is a guide for the initial daily dose of valproic acid (15 mg/kg/day) syrup and capsules.

Valproic Acid Syrup and Capsule Initial Dosing Guide					
Weight		Total daily dose (mg)	Number of capsules or teaspoonfuls of syrup		
kg	lb		Dose 1	Dose 2	Dose 3
10 to 24.9	22 to 54.9	250	0	0	1
25 to 39.9	55 to 87.9	500	1	0	1
40 to 59.9	88 to 131.9	750	1	1	1
60 to 74.9	132 to 164.9	1,000	1	1	2
75 to 89.9	165 to 197.9	1,250	2	1	2

Injection: For IV use only. Administer as a 60-minute infusion (but not more than 20 mg/min) with the same frequency as the oral products. Use of valproate sodium injection for periods of more than 14 days has not been studied. Switch patients to oral valproate products as soon as it is clinically feasible.

Rapid infusion of IV valproate sodium has been associated with an increase in adverse events.

Conversion from oral products to injection: When switching from oral products, the total daily dose of valproate sodium injection should be equivalent to the total daily dose of the oral product. Closely monitor patients receiving doses near the maximum recommended daily dose of 60 mg/kg/day, particularly those not receiving enzyme-inducing drugs. If the total daily dose exceeds 250 mg, give in a divided regimen.

Younger children: Younger children, especially those receiving enzyme-inducing drugs, will require larger maintenance doses to attain targeted valproic acid concentrations.

Elderly: Reduce the starting dose because of a decrease in unbound clearance of valproate and a greater sensitivity to somnolence; base therapeutic dose on clinical response.

Dose-related adverse reactions: Because the frequency of adverse effects (particularly elevated liver enzymes and thrombocytopenia) may be dose-related, weigh the benefit of improved therapeutic effect with higher doses against the possibility of a greater incidence of adverse reactions. The probability of thrombocytopenia appears to increase significantly at total valproate concentrations of 110 mcg/mL or more (females) or 135 mcg/mL or more (males).

Complex partial seizures:

Monotherapy – Adults and children 10 years of age or older.

Initiate therapy at 10 to 15 mg/kg/day; increase by 5 to 10 mg/kg/wk to achieve optimal clinical response. Ordinarily, optimal clinical response is achieved at daily doses below 60 mg/kg/day. If satisfactory clinical response has not been achieved, measure plasma levels to determine whether they are in the usually accepted therapeutic range (50 to 100 mcg/mL).

Conversion to monotherapy: Initiate therapy at 10 to 15 mg/kg/day. Increase the dosage by 5 to 10 mg/kg/wk to achieve optimal clinical response. Ordinarily, optimal clinical response is achieved at daily doses less than 60 mg/kg/day. If satisfactory clinical response has not been achieved, measure plasma levels to determine whether they are in the usually accepted therapeutic range (50 to 100 mcg/mL). Concomitant antiepilepsy drug (AED) dosage ordinarily can be reduced by about 25% every 2 weeks. This reduction may be started at initiation of therapy or delayed by 1 to 2 weeks if there is a concern that seizures are likely to occur. Monitor patients closely during this period for increased seizure frequency.

Adjunctive therapy – Divalproex sodium or valproic acid may be added to the patient's regimen at a dosage of 10 to 15 mg/kg/day. The dosage may be increased by 5 to 10 mg/kg/wk to achieve optimal clinical response. Ordinarily, optimal clinical response is achieved at daily doses less than 60 mg/kg/day. If satisfactory clinical response has not been achieved, measure plasma levels to determine whether they are in the usually accepted therapeutic range (50 to 100 mcg/mL). If the total daily dose exceeds 250 mg, administer in divided doses.

Simple and complex absence seizures: The recommended initial dose is 15 mg/kg/day; increase at 1-week intervals by 5 to 10 mg/kg/day until seizures are controlled or side effects preclude further increase. The maximum recommended dosage is 60 mg/kg/day. If the total daily dose is more than 250 mg, give in divided doses.

In epileptic patients previously receiving valproic acid therapy, initiate divalproex sodium at the same daily dose and dosing schedule. After the patient is stabilized on divalproex tablets, a dosing schedule of 2 or 3 times/day may be elected in selected patients.

Conversion from Depakote to Depakote ER: In adult and pediatric patients 10 years of age and older, patients with epilepsy previously receiving *Depakote*, *Depakote ER* should be administered once daily using a dose 8% to 20% higher than the total daily dose of *Depakote*. For patients whose *Depakote* total daily dose cannot be directly converted to *Depakote ER*, consideration may be given at the clinician's discretion to increase the patient's *Depakote* total daily dose to the next higher dosage before converting to the appropriate total daily dose of *Depakote ER*.

Dose Conversion from *Depakote* to *Depakote ER*

Depakote total daily dose (mg)	*Depakote ER* (mg)
500[a] to 625	750
750[a] to 875	1,000
1,000[a] to 1,125	1,250
1,250 to 1,375	1,500
1,500 to 1,625	1,750
1,750	2,000
1,875 to 2,000	2,250
2,125 to 2,250	2,500
2,375	2,750
2,500 to 2,750	3,000
2,875	3,250
3,000 to 3,125	3,500

[a] These total daily doses of *Depakote* cannot be directly converted to an 8% to 20% higher total daily dose of *Depakote ER* because the required dosing strengths of *Depakote ER* are not available. Consideration may be given at the clinician's discretion to increase the patient's *Depakote* total daily dose to the next higher dosage before converting to the appropriate total daily dose of *Depakote ER*.

Mania:

Divalproex sodium delayed-release tablets – 750 mg/day in divided doses; increase as rapidly as possible to achieve the lowest therapeutic dose that produces the desired clinical effect or the desired range of plasma concentrations (trough plasma concentrations 50 to 125 mcg/mL). Maximum concentrations generally were achieved within 14 days. Maximum recommended dosage is 60 mg/kg/day.

Divalproex sodium ER – The recommended initial dose is 25 mg/kg/day given once daily. The dose should be increased as rapidly as possible to achieve the lowest therapeutic dose that produces the desired clinical effect or the desired range of plasma concentrations. The maximum recommended dose is 60 mg/kg/day.

Migraine:

Divalproex sodium delayed-release tablets – The starting dose is 250 mg orally twice/day. Some patients may benefit from doses up to 1,000 mg/day. There is no evidence that higher doses lead to greater efficacy.

Divalproex sodium ER tablets – The recommended starting dose is 500 mg once daily for 1 week, thereafter increasing to 1,000 mg once daily. Although doses other than 1,000 mg once daily have not been evaluated in patients with migraines, the effective dose range of delayed-released tablets in these patients is 500 to 1,000 mg/day. As with other valproate products, individualize doses of the ER tablets and adjust the dose as necessary. When ER tablets are given in doses 8% to 20% higher than the total daily dose of the delayed-release tablets, the two formulations are bioequivalent. If a patient requires smaller dose adjustments than that available with the ER tablets, use the delayed-release tablets instead.

Therapeutic serum levels: Therapeutic serum levels for most patients with seizures will range from 50 to 100 mcg/mL; however, a good correlation has not been established between daily dose, serum level, and therapeutic effect.

Actions

Pharmacology: This group includes valproic acid, sodium valproate (the sodium salt), and divalproex sodium (a compound containing equal proportions of valproic acid and sodium valproate). Regardless of form, dosage is expressed as valproic acid equivalents.

Valproic acid is chemically unrelated to other drugs used to treat seizure disorders. Although the mechanism of action is not established, its activity may be related to increased brain levels of gamma-aminobutyric acid (GABA).

Pharmacokinetics:

Absorption – Valproic acid is rapidly and almost completely absorbed from the GI tract. Absorption of the drug is delayed but not decreased by administration with meals; administration of the drug with milk products does not affect the rate or degree of absorption. The bioavailability of valproate from divalproex sodium delayed-release tablets and capsules containing coated particles has been shown to be equivalent to that of valproic acid capsules.

The absolute bioavailability of divalproex ER tablets administered as a single dose after a meal was approximately 90% relative to IV infusion. The ER tablet produced an average bioavailability of 89% relative to divalproex delayed-release tablets given 2, 3, or 4 times daily. Maximum valproate plasma concentrations in these studies were achieved on average 4 to 17 hours after the ER dose intake. The ER tablets are not bioequivalent to the delayed-release tablets.

Distribution – Valproic acid is rapidly distributed. Volume of distribution of total or free valproic acid is 11 or 92 L/1.73 m^2, respectively. Valproic acid has been detected in CSF (approximately 10% of total concentrations) and milk (about 1% to 10% of serum concentrations). Therapeutic range is commonly considered to be 50 to 100 mcg/mL of total valproate. The plasma protein binding of valproate is concentration-dependent. Protein binding of valproate is reduced in the elderly, in patients with chronic hepatic diseases, in patients with renal impairment, and in the presence of other drugs (eg, aspirin). Conversely, valproate may displace certain protein-bound drugs (eg, phenytoin, carbamazepine, warfarin, tolbutamide).

Metabolism/Excretion – Primarily metabolized in liver. Mean terminal half-life for valproate monotherapy ranges from 9 to 16 hours. Half-lives in the lower part of the range usually are found in patients taking other enzyme-inducing antiepileptic drugs.

Contraindications

Hepatic disease or significant hepatic dysfunction; hypersensitivity to valproic acid; known urea cycle disorders (see Warnings).

Warnings/Precautions

Pancreatitis: Cases of life-threatening pancreatitis have been reported in children and adults receiving valproate. Some of the cases have been described as hemorrhagic with rapid progression from initial symptoms to death. Some cases have occurred shortly after initial use as well as after several years of use. Warn patients and guardians that abdominal pain, nausea, vomiting, or anorexia can be symptoms of pancreatitis that require prompt medical evaluation. See Warning Box.

Urea cycle disorders (UCDs): Hyperammonemic encephalopathy, sometimes fatal, has been reported following initiation of valproate therapy in patients with UCDs, a group of uncommon genetic abnormalities, particularly ornithine transcarbamylase deficiency. Patients who develop symptoms of unexplained hyperammonemic encephalopathy while receiving valproate therapy should receive prompt treatment (including discontinuation of valproate therapy) and be evaluated for underlying urea cycle disorders (see Contraindications).

Thrombocytopenia: The frequency of thrombocytopenia may be dose-related. The probability of thrombocytopenia increases significantly at total trough valproate plasma concentrations greater than or equal to 110 mcg/mL in females and 135 mcg/mL in males.

Multiorgan hypersensitivity reaction: Multiorgan hypersensitivity reactions have been rarely reported in close temporal association to the initiation of valproate therapy in adults and children (median time to detection, 21 days; range, 1 to 40 days). Patients typically, although not exclusively, presented with fever and rash associated with other organ system involvement.

HIV: There are in vitro studies that suggest valproate stimulates the replication of the HIV and cytomegalovirus (CMV) under certain experimental conditions. The clinical consequence, if any, is not known.

Acute head injuries: A study evaluating the effect of IV valproate in the prevention of posttraumatic seizures in patients with acute head injuries found a higher incidence of death in valproate treatment groups compared with the IV phenytoin treatment group. Until further information is available, it seems prudent not to use valproate sodium injection in patients with acute head trauma for the prophylaxis of posttraumatic seizures.

Hepatotoxicity: See Warning Box.

Long-term use: Safety and effectiveness for long-term use in mania (more than 3 weeks) have not been systematically evaluated in clinical trials.

Discontinuation: Do not abruptly discontinue in patients with major seizures because of the strong possibility of precipitating status epilepticus with hypoxia and threat to life.

Hematologic effects: Thrombocytopenia, inhibition of the secondary phase of platelet aggregation, and abnormal coagulation parameters have occurred; determine platelet counts and bleeding time before initiating therapy, at periodic intervals, and prior to surgery.

Hyperammonemia: Hyperammonemia has been reported and may be present despite normal liver function tests. In patients who develop unexplained lethargy and vomiting or changes in mental status, measure an ammonia level.

Suicidal ideation: Suicidal ideation may be a manifestation of certain psychiatric disorders and may persist until significant remission of symptoms occurs.

Hepatic function impairment: Observe caution when administering divalproex, valproate, and valproic acid to patients with a history of hepatic function impairment.

Hazardous tasks: Patients should use caution while driving or performing other tasks requiring alertness, coordination, or physical dexterity.

Pregnancy: Category D.

Lactation: Concentrations of valproic acid in breast milk are 1% to 10% of serum concentrations. Consider discontinuing nursing when valproate products are administered to a nursing woman.

Children: See Warning Box. The safety and efficacy of divalproex sodium for the treatment of acute mania has not been studied in individuals younger than 18 years of age. Divalproex sodium ER tablets are not recommended in children. Use of valproate sodium injection has not been studied in children below 2 years of age.

Migraine – The safety and efficacy of divalproex sodium for the prophylaxis of migraines has not been studied in individuals under 16 years of age.

Elderly: In elderly patients, increase dosage more slowly and with regular monitoring for fluid and nutritional intake, dehydration, somnolence, and other adverse events. Consider dose reductions or discontinuation of valproate in patients with decreased food or fluid intake and in patients with excessive somnolence. A reduced starting dose is recommended (see Administration and Dosage).

Monitoring: Perform liver function tests prior to therapy and at frequent intervals thereafter, especially during the first 6 months. Platelet counts and coagulation tests are recommended before initiating therapy and at periodic intervals.

Drug Interactions

Drugs that may affect valproic acid include carbapenem antibiotics, barbiturates, carbamazepine, chlorpromazine, cholestyramine, ethosuximide, felbamate, lamotrigine, phenytoin, rifampin, salicylates, and topiramate. Drugs that may be affected by valproic acid include barbiturates, carbamazepine, clonazepam, diazepam, ethosuximide, lamotrigine, phenobarbital, phenytoin, tolbutamide, topiramate, tricyclic antidepressants, warfarin, and zidovudine.

Drug/Lab test interactions: Valproic acid is partially eliminated in the urine as a keto-metabolite, which may lead to a false interpretation of the urine ketone test. There have been reports of altered thyroid function tests associated with valproic acid.

Adverse Reactions

Adverse reactions in at least 3% of patients include the following: Asthenia, somnolence, dizziness, tremor, ataxia, emotional lability, abnormal thinking, amnesia, euphoria, hypesthesia, nervousness, paresthesia, insomnia, depression, nausea, dyspepsia, diarrhea, vomiting, abdominal pain, increased appetite, constipation, anorexia, thrombocytopenia, ecchymosis, flu syndrome, infection, bronchitis, rhinitis, pharyngitis, dyspnea, nystagmus, diplopia, amblyopia/blurred vision, taste perversion, tinnitus, weight gain, back pain, alopecia, fever, weight loss, headache, peripheral edema, infection, rash.

CARBAMAZEPINE

Tablets: 200 mg (*Rx*)	Various, *Epitol* (Teva), *Tegretol* (Novartis)
Tablets, chewable: 100 mg (*Rx*)	Various, *Tegretol* (Novartis)
Tablets, extended release: 100, 200, and 400 mg (*Rx*)	*Tegretol-XR* (Novartis)
Capsules, extended release: 100, 200, and 300 mg (*Rx*)	*Carbatrol* (Shire), *Equetro* (Shire)
Suspension: 100 mg per 5 mL (*Rx*)	Various, *Tegretol* (Novartis)

Warning:

Aplastic anemia and agranulocytosis have been reported in association with the use of carbamazepine. Data from a population-based, case-control study demonstrate that the risk of developing these reactions is 5 to 8 times greater than in the general population. However, the overall risk of these reactions in the untreated general population is low, approximately 6 patients per 1 million population per year for agranulocytosis and 2 patients per 1 million population per year for aplastic anemia.

continued on next page

Warning: (cont.)

Although reports of transient or persistent decreased platelet or white blood cell counts are not uncommon in association with the use of carbamazepine, data are not available to accurately estimate their incidence or outcome. However, the vast majority of the cases of leukopenia have not progressed to the more serious conditions of aplastic anemia or agranulocytosis.

Because of the very low incidence of agranulocytosis and aplastic anemia, the vast majority of minor hematological changes observed while monitoring patients on carbamazepine are unlikely to signal the occurrence of either abnormality. Nonetheless, obtain complete pretreatment hematological testing as a baseline. If a patient in the course of treatment exhibits low or decreased white blood cell or platelet counts, monitor the patient closely. Consider discontinuation of the drug if any evidence of significant bone marrow depression develops.

Indications

Bipolar disorder (Equetro only): For the treatment of acute manic and mixed episodes associated with bipolar I disorder.

Epilepsy (except Equetro): For the treatment of partial seizures with complex symptoms. Also for generalized tonic-clonic seizures, mixed seizure patterns, or other partial or generalized seizures.

Trigeminal neuralgia (except Equetro): For the treatment of pain associated with true trigeminal neuralgia and glossopharyngeal neuralgia.

Administration and Dosage

Tablets: Take with meals.

Conversion from conventional tablets to extended-release tablets: Extended-release carbamazepine is for twice daily administration. When converting patients from conventional tablets to extended-release tablets, administer the same total daily mg dose of extended-release carbamazepine. Swallow extended-release tablets whole; never crush or chew. Inspect extended-release tablets for chips or cracks; do not consume damaged tablets. Extended-release tablet coating is not absorbed and is excreted in the feces; these coatings may be noticeable in the stool.

Conversion from tablets to suspension: Convert by administering the same number of milligrams per day in smaller, more frequent doses (ie, twice-daily tablets to 3-times-daily suspension).

Capsules, extended-release: Extended-release capsules may be opened and the beads sprinkled over food (eg, teaspoon of applesauce or other similar food products). Do not crush or chew the capsules or their contents. Extended-release capsules can be taken with or without meals.

Suspension: Do not administer carbamazepine suspension with other liquid medications or diluents.

Bipolar disorder (Equetro only): The initial dosage is 200 mg twice daily. Adjust in 200 mg daily increments to achieve optimal clinical response. Doses greater than 1,600 mg/day have not been studied.

Epilepsy (except Carbatrol):

Initial –

Adults and children (older than 12 years of age): 200 mg twice/day (100 mg 4 times/day of suspension). Increase at weekly intervals by 200 mg/day or less using a 3 or 4 times/day regimen (2 times/day with extended-release formulations) until the best response is obtained. Generally, do not exceed 1,000 mg/day in children 12 to 15 years of age or 1,200 mg/day in patients older than 15 years of age. Doses 1,600 mg/day or less have been used in adults.

Children (6 to 12 years of age): 100 mg twice/day (50 mg 4 times/day of suspension). Increase at weekly intervals gradually by adding 100 mg/day or less using a

3 or 4 times/day regimen (2 times/day with extended-release formulations) until the best response is obtained. Generally, do not exceed 1,000 mg/day.

Children (younger than 6 years of age): 10 to 20 mg/kg/day 2 or 3 times/day (4 times/day with suspension). Increase weekly to achieve optimal clinical response administered 3 or 4 times/day.

Maintenance –

Adults and children (older than 12 years of age): Adjust to minimum effective level, usually 800 to 1,200 mg/day.

Children (6 to 12 years of age): Adjust to minimum effective level, usually 400 to 800 mg/day.

Children (younger than 6 years of age): Optimal clinical response is achieved at daily doses of less than 35 mg/kg. If satisfactory clinical response has not been achieved, measure plasma levels to determine whether or not they are in the therapeutic range. No recommendation regarding the safety of carbamazepine for use at doses greater than 35 mg/kg per 24 hours can be made.

Combination therapy – When adding to existing anticonvulsant therapy, do so gradually while other anticonvulsants are maintained or gradually decreased, except phenytoin, which may have to be increased.

Epilepsy (Carbatrol only):

Adults and children older than 12 years of age –

Initial: 200 mg twice daily. Increase at weekly intervals by adding up to 200 mg/day until the optimal response is obtained. Dosage generally should not exceed 1,000 mg/day in children 12 to 15 years of age and 1,200 mg daily in patients older than 15 years of age. Doses of up to 1,600 mg daily have been used in adults.

Maintenance: Adjust dosage to the minimum effective level, usually 800 to 1,200 mg/day.

Children younger than 12 years of age – Total daily doses of immediate-release carbamazepine 400 mg or more may be converted to the same total daily dose of carbamazepine extended-release capsules using a twice-daily regimen. Ordinarily, optimal clinical response is achieved at daily doses of less than 35 mg/kg. If satisfactory clinical response has not been achieved, plasma levels should be measured to determine whether they are in the therapeutic range. No recommendation regarding the safety of carbamazepine for use at doses of more than 35 mg/kg per 24 hours can be made.

Trigeminal neuralgia (except Carbatrol):

Initial – 100 mg twice/day on the first day (50 mg 4 times/day of suspension; one 200 mg *Carbatrol* capsule). May increase by up to 200 mg/day using 100 mg increments every 12 hours (50 mg 4 times/day of suspension; 200 mg *Carbatrol* capsule) as needed. Do not exceed 1,200 mg/day.

Maintenance – Control of pain can usually be maintained with 400 to 800 mg/day (range, 200 to 1,200 mg/day). Attempt to reduce the dose to the minimum effective level or to discontinue the drug at least once every 3 months.

Trigeminal neuralgia (Carbatrol only):

Initial – On the first day, start with one 200 mg capsule. This daily dose may be increased by up to 200 mg/day every 12 hours, only as needed to achieve freedom from pain. Do not exceed 1,200 mg daily.

Maintenance – Control of pain can be maintained in most patients with 400 to 800 mg daily. However, some patients may be maintained on as little as 200 mg daily, while others may require as much as 1,200 mg daily. At least once every 3 months throughout the treatment period, attempts should be made to reduce the dose to the minimum effective level or even discontinue the drug.

Carbamazepine Dosage Information

Indication	Initial dose				Subsequent dose				Maximum daily dose			
	Extended-release capsules	Tablets[a]	Extended-release tablets	Suspension	Extended-release capsules	Tablets[a]	Extended-release tablets	Suspension	Extended-release capsules	Tablets[a]	Extended-release tablets	Suspension
Bipolar I disorder (*Equetro* only)												
	200 mg twice daily (400 mg/day)				Adjust in 200 mg daily increments to achieve optimal clinical response				1,600 mg per 24 h			
Epilepsy												
< 6 years of age		10 to 20 mg/kg/day twice daily or 3 times daily		10 to 20 mg/kg/day 4 times daily		Increase weekly to achieve optimal clinical response, 3 or 4 times daily		Increase weekly to achieve optimal clinical response, 3 or 4 times daily		35 mg/kg per 24 h		35 mg/kg per 24 h
6 to 12 years of age		100 mg twice daily (200 mg/day)	100 mg twice daily (200 mg/day)	2.5 mL 4 times daily (200 mg/day)		Add up to 100 mg/day at weekly intervals, 3 or 4 times daily	Add 100 mg/day at weekly intervals, twice daily	Add up to 5 mL (100 mg)/ day at weekly intervals, 3 or 4 times daily		1,000 mg per 24 h		

Carbamazepine Dosage Information

Indication	Initial dose				Subsequent dose				Maximum daily dose			
	Extended-release capsules	Tablets[a]	Extended-release tablets	Suspension	Extended-release capsules	Tablets[a]	Extended-release tablets	Suspension	Extended-release capsules	Tablets[a]	Extended-release tablets	Suspension
Children < 12 years of age					Convert children taking at least 400 mg daily of immediate-release carbamazepine to the same total daily dosage of extended-release capsule using a twice daily regimen.					35 mg/kg per 24 h		
> 12 years of age		200 mg twice daily (400 mg/day)	200 mg twice daily (400 mg/day)	5 mL 4 times daily (400 mg/day)		Add up to 200 mg/day at weekly intervals, 3 or 4 times daily	Add up to 200 mg/ day at weekly intervals, twice daily	Add up to 10 mL (200 mg)/ day at weekly intervals, 3 or 4 times daily		1,000 mg per 24 h (12 to 15 years of age); 1,200 mg per 24 h (> 15 years of age); 1,600 mg per 24 h (adults, in rare instances)		
Adults and children > 12 years of age	200 mg twice daily				Add up to 200 mg/ day at weekly intervals							

Carbamazepine Dosage Information

Indication	Initial dose				Subsequent dose				Maximum daily dose			
	Extended-release capsules	Tablets[a]	Extended-release tablets	Suspension	Extended-release capsules	Tablets[a]	Extended-release tablets	Suspension	Extended-release capsules	Tablets[a]	Extended-release tablets	Suspension
Trigeminal neuralgia												
		100 mg twice daily (200 mg/day)	100 mg twice daily (200 mg/day)	2.5 mL 4 times daily (200 mg/day)		Add up to 200 mg/day in increments of 100 mg every 12 hours	Add up to 200 mg/day in increments of 100 mg every 12 hours	Add up to 10 mL (200 mg/day) in increments of 50 mg (2.5 mL) 4 times daily		1,200 mg per 24 h		

[a] Tablet = chewable or conventional tablets.

Actions

Pharmacology: Carbamazepine's mechanism of action is unknown. It appears to act by reducing polysynaptic responses and blocking the posttetanic potentiation.

Pharmacokinetics:

Absorption/Distribution – Both the suspension and tablet deliver equivalent amounts of drug to the systemic circulation; however, the suspension is absorbed somewhat faster than the tablet. Following chronic oral administration of suspension, plasma levels peak at approximately 1.5 hours, compared with 4 to 5 hours after administration of conventional carbamazepine tablets, and 3 to 12 hours after administration of extended-release carbamazepine tablets. Carbamazepine is 76% bound to plasma proteins.

Metabolism/Excretion – Carbamazepine is metabolized in the liver by CYP-450 3A4. It induces its own metabolism. Initial half-life ranges from 25 to 65 hours and decreases to 12 to 17 hours with repeated doses.

Contraindications

History of bone marrow depression; acute intermittent porphyria; hypersensitivity to carbamazepine and tricyclic antidepressants; concomitant use of monoamine oxidase inhibitors (MAOIs). Discontinue MAOIs for a minimum of 14 days before carbamazepine administration.

Warnings/Precautions

Minor pain: This drug is not a simple analgesic. Do not use for the relief of minor aches or pains.

Dermatologic: Severe dermatologic reactions, including toxic epidermal necrolysis (Lyell syndrome) and Stevens-Johnson syndrome, have been reported with carbamazepine. These reactions have been extremely rare; however, a few fatalities have been reported.

Discontinuation: In patients with seizure disorder, do not discontinue carbamazepine abruptly because of the strong possibility of precipitating status epilepticus with attendant hypoxia and threat to life.

Hematologic: Patients with a history of adverse hematologic reaction to any drug may be particularly at risk.

Hepatic effects: Hepatic effects, ranging from slight elevations in liver enzymes to rare cases of hepatic failure have been reported. In some cases, hepatic effects may progress despite discontinuation of the drug.

Anticholinergic effects: Carbamazepine has shown mild anticholinergic activity; therefore, use with caution in patients with increased intraocular pressure.

CNS effects: Because of the drug's relationship to other tricyclic compounds, the possibility of activating latent psychosis, confusion, or agitation in elderly patients may occur.

Hepatic porphyria (Tegratol only): Avoid the use of *Tegratol* in patients with a history of hepatic porphyria (eg, acute intermittent porphyria, porphyria cutanea tarda, variegate porphyria).

Hyponatremia: Hyponatremia has been reported in association with carbamazepine use, either alone or in combination with other drugs.

Suicide (Equetro only): The possibility of suicide attempt is inherent in bipolar disorder and close supervision of high risk patients should accompany drug therapy. Write prescriptions for carbamazepine for the smallest quantity consistent with good patient management in order to reduce the risk of overdosage.

Absence seizures: Use carbamazepine with caution in patients with a mixed seizure disorder that includes atypical absence seizures, since in these patients carbamazepine has been associated with increased frequency of generalized convulsions.

Hypersensitivity reactions: Hypersensitivity reactions to carbamazepine have been reported in patients who previously experienced this reaction to anticonvulsants, including phenytoin and phenobarbital. Consider discontinuation of carbamazepine if any evidence of hypersensitivity develops.

Special risk: Prescribe carbamazepine only after benefit-to-risk appraisal in patients with a history of the following: cardiac, hepatic, or renal damage; adverse hematologic reaction to other drugs; interrupted courses of therapy with the drug.

Hazardous tasks: May produce drowsiness, dizziness, or blurred vision; patients should observe caution while driving or performing other tasks requiring alertness.

Pregnancy: *Category D.*

Lactation: Carbamazepine and its epoxide metabolite are transferred into breast milk. Because of the potential for serious adverse reactions, decide whether to discontinue breast-feeding or to discontinue the drug, taking into account the importance of the drug to the mother.

Children: The safety of carbamazepine in children has been studied up to 6 months of age.

Elderly: Because of the relationship of the drug to other tricyclic compounds, keep in mind the possibility of activation of a latent psychosis and, in elderly patients, confusion or agitation.

Monitoring: Obtain complete pretreatment blood counts as a baseline. Monitoring of blood levels may be useful in cases of dramatic increase in seizure frequency, for verification of drug compliance, assessing safety, and determining the cause of toxicity. If a patient in the course of treatment exhibits low or decreased white blood cell or platelet counts, monitor the patient closely. Consider discontinuation of the drug if any evidence of significant bone marrow depression develops.

Baseline and periodic evaluations of liver function, particularly in patients with histories of liver disease, must be performed during treatment. Discontinue carbamazepine if indicated by newly occurring or worsening clinical or laboratory evidence of liver dysfunction or hepatic damage, or in the case of active liver disease.

Baseline and periodic eye examinations, including slit-lamp, funduscopy, and tonometry, are recommended because many phenothiazines and related drugs have been shown to cause eye changes.

Baseline and periodic complete urinalysis and blood urea nitrogen (BUN) determinations are recommended for patients treated with this agent because of observed renal dysfunction.

Increases in total cholesterol, low-density lipoprotein, and high-density lipoprotein have been observed in some patients taking anticonvulsants. Therefore, periodic evaluation of these parameters is also recommended.

Drug Interactions

Drugs that can increase carbamazepine serum levels include acetazolamide, antipsychotics, azole antifungals, barbiturates, cimetidine, dalfopristin, danazol, delavirdine, diltiazem, isoniazid, macrolides, MAOIs, nefazodone, niacin, nonsedating antihistamines, protease inhibitors, quinine, quinupristin, selective serotonin reuptake inhibitors (SSRIs), theophylline, tricyclic antidepressants, valproate, verapamil, zileuton.

Drugs that can decrease carbamazepine serum levels include antimalarials, azole antifungals, cisplatin, doxorubicin, felbamate, MAOIs, rifampin, phenytoin, primidone, succinimides, and theophylline.

The serum levels of the following may be lowered by carbamazepine: acetaminophen, anticoagulants, atypical antipsychotics, benzodiazepines, bupropion, buspirone, calcium channel blockers, cyclosporine, delavirdine, doxycycline, felodipine, glucocorticoids, haloperidol, HMG-CoA reductase inhibitors, hydantoins, lamotrigine, levothyroxine, methadone, mirtazepine, nefazodone, nondepolarizing muscle relaxants, oral contraceptives, oxcarbazepine, praziquantel, primidone, protease inhibitors, SSRIs, succinimides, theophylline, tiagabine, topiramate, tramadol, trazodone, triazole, tricyclic antidepressants, valproic acid, and zonisamide.

Serum levels of the following may be increased by carbamazepine: clomipramine, hydantoins, isoniazid, lithium, and theophylline.

Drug/Lab test interactions:

Thyroid function – Thyroid function tests show decreased values with carbamazepine.

Pregnancy tests – Interference with some pregnancy tests has been reported.

Drug/Food interactions: Avoid coadministration of carbamazepine with grapefruit products. Serum carbamazepine levels may be elevated.

Adverse Reactions

Adverse reactions occurring in 3% or more of patients include accidental injury, amblyopia, amnesia, anxiety, asthenia, ataxia, back pain, chest pain, constipation, depression, diarrhea, dizziness, drowsiness, dry mouth, dyspepsia, headache, infection, manic depressive reaction, nausea, pain, pruritus, rash, somnolence, speech disorder, unsteadiness, and vomiting.

GABAPENTIN

Tablets: 100, 300, and 400 mg (*Rx*)	Various, *Gabarone* (Ivax)
600 and 800 mg (*Rx*)	Various, *Neurontin* (Parke-Davis)
Capsules: 100, 300, and 400 mg (*Rx*)	Various, *Neurontin* (Parke-Davis)
Solution, oral: 250 mg/5 mL (*Rx*)	*Neurontin* (Parke-Davis)

Indications

Epilepsy: Adjunctive therapy in the treatment of partial seizures with and without secondary generalization in patients more than 12 years of age with epilepsy. Also indicated as adjunctive therapy for partial seizures in children 3 to 12 years of age.

Postherpetic neuralgia: For management of postherpetic neuralgia in adults.

Administration and Dosage

Take with or without food.

Postherpetic neuralgia: In adults with postherpetic neuralgia, gabapentin therapy may be initiated as a single 300 mg dose on day 1, 600 mg/day on day 2 (divided twice daily), and 900 mg/day on day 3 (divided 3 times daily). The dose can subsequently be titrated up as needed for pain relief to a daily dose of 1800 mg (divided 3 times daily).

Epilepsy: Recommended for add-on therapy in patients 3 years of age or older.

Patients more than 12 years of age – The effective dose is 900 to 1800 mg/day in divided doses (3 times/day) using 300 or 400 mg capsules or 600 or 800 mg tablets. The starting dose is 300 mg 3 times/day. If necessary, the dose may be increased using 300 or 400 mg capsules or 600 or 800 mg tablets 3 times/day up to 1800 mg/day. Dosages up to 2400 mg/day have been well tolerated in long-term clinical studies. Doses of 3600 mg/day also have been administered to a small number of patients for a relatively short duration, and have been well tolerated. The maximum time between doses in the 3 times/day schedule should not exceed 12 hours.

Pediatric patients 3 to 12 years of age – The starting dose should range from 10 to 15 mg/kg/day in 3 divided doses, and the effective dose reached by upward titration over a period of about 3 days. The effective dose of gabapentin in patients 5 years of age or older is 25 to 35 mg/kg/day and given in divided doses (3 times/day). The effective dose in pediatric patients 3 and 4 years of age is 40 mg/kg/day and given in divided doses (3 times/day). Gabapentin may be administered as the oral solution, capsule, tablet, or using combinations of these formulations. Dosages up to 50 mg/kg/day have been well tolerated in a long-term clinical study. The maximum time interval between doses should not exceed 12 hours.

It is not necessary to monitor gabapentin plasma concentrations to optimize therapy. Further, because there are no significant pharmacokinetic interactions with other commonly used anti-epileptic drugs, the addition of gabapentin does not alter the plasma levels of these drugs appreciably.

If gabapentin is discontinued or an alternate anticonvulsant medication is added to the therapy, this should be done gradually over a minimum of 1 week.

Renal function impairment:

Gabapentin Dosage Based on Renal Function in Patients ≥ 12 Years of Age						
Creatinine clearance (mL/min)	Total daily dose range (mg/day)	Dose regimen (mg)				
≥ 60	900 to 3600	300 tid[a]	400 tid	600 tid	800 tid	1200 tid
> 30 to 59	400 to 1400	200 bid[a]	300 bid	400 bid	500 bid	700 bid
> 15 to 29	200 to 700	200 qd[a]	300 qd	400 qd	500 qd	700 qd
15[b]	100 to 300	100 qd	125 qd	150 qd	200 qd	300 qd
Posthemodialysis supplemental dose (mg)[c]						
Hemodialysis		125	150	200	250	350

[a] tid = 3 times daily; bid = twice daily; qd = once daily.

[b] For patients with creatinine clearance (Ccr) < 15 mL/min, reduce daily dose in proportion to Ccr (eg, patients with a Ccr of 7.5 mL/min should receive one-half the daily dose that patients with a Ccr of 15 mL/min receive.

[c] Patients on hemodialysis should receive maintenance doses based on estimates of Ccr as indicated in the upper portion of the table and a supplemental posthemodialysis dose administered after each 4 hours of hemodialysis as indicated in the lower portion of the table.

Use of gabapentin in patients under 12 years of age with compromised renal function has not been studied.

Actions

Pharmacology: Gabapentin is an oral antiepileptic agent. The mechanism by which it exerts its anticonvulsant and analgesic actions is unknown.

Pharmacokinetics: Gabapentin bioavailability is not dose-proportional. It circulates largely unbound (less than 3%) to plasma protein and is eliminated from the systemic circulation by renal excretion as unchanged drug; it is not appreciably metabolized.

Contraindications

Hypersensitivity to the drug or its ingredients.

Warnings/Precautions

Neuropsychiatric adverse events (3 to 12 years of age): Gabapentin use in pediatric patients with epilepsy 3 to 12 years of age is associated with the occurrence of CNS-related adverse events.

Among the gabapentin-treated patients, most of the events were mild to moderate in intensity.

Withdrawal-precipitated seizure: Antiepileptic drugs should not be abruptly discontinued because of the possibility of increasing seizure frequency.

Status epilepticus: In the placebo controlled studies, the incidence of status epilepticus in patients receiving gabapentin was 0.6% vs 0.5% with placebo.

Sudden and unexplained deaths: During the course of premarketing development of gabapentin, 8 sudden and unexplained deaths were recorded among 2203 patients.

Pregnancy: Category C.

Lactation: Gabapentin is secreted into breast milk.

Children: Safety and efficacy in children less than 3 years of age has not been established.

Elderly: No systematic studies in geriatric patients have been conducted. Adverse clinical events reported among 59 gabapentin-exposed patients more than 65 years of age did not differ in kind from those reported for younger individuals.

Drug Interactions

Drugs that may affect gabapentin include antacids, cimetidine, hydrocodone, and morphine. Drugs that may be affected by gabapentin include oral contraceptives and hydrocodone.

Drug/Lab test interactions: Because false-positive readings were reported with the *Ames N-Multistix SG* dipstick test for urinary protein when gabapentin was added to other antiepileptic drugs, the more specific sulfosalicylic acid precipitation procedure is recommended to determine the presence of urine protein.

Adverse Reactions

Adverse reactions occurring in at least 3% of patients include somnolence, weight gain, hostility, emotional lability, nausea/vomiting, bronchitis, viral infections, fever, dizziness, ataxia, fatigue, nystagmus, rhinitis, diplopia, amblyopia, tremor, asthenia, headache, peripheral edema, diarrhea, constipation, dry mouth.

PREGABALIN

Capsules; oral: 25, 50, 75, 100, 150, 200, 225, and 300 mg *(c-v)*	*Lyrica* (Pfizer)
Solution; oral: 20 mg/mL *(c-v)*	

Indications

Neuropathic pain associated with diabetic peripheral neuropathy: For management of neuropathic pain associated with diabetic peripheral neuropathy.

Partial-onset seizures: As adjunctive therapy for adult patients with partial-onset seizures.

Postherpetic neuralgia: For the management of postherpetic neuralgia.

Fibromyalgia: For the management of fibromyalgia.

Administration and Dosage

Pregabalin is given orally with or without food. Maximum dosage is 600 mg/ day. When discontinuing pregabalin, taper gradually over a minimum of 1 week.

Neuropathic pain associated with diabetic peripheral neuropathy: The maximum recommended dose of pregabalin is 100 mg 3 times a day (300 mg/day) in patients with creatinine clearance (CrCl) of at least 60 mL/min. Dosing should begin at 50 mg 3 times a day (150 mg/day) and may be increased to 300 mg/day within 1 week based on efficacy and tolerability.

Partial-onset seizures: Pregabalin, at doses of 150 to 600 mg/day, has been shown to be effective as adjunctive therapy in the treatment of partial-onset seizures in adults. The total daily dose should be divided and given 2 or 3 times daily. The efficacy and adverse reaction profiles of pregabalin have been shown to be dose related. In general, it is recommended that patients be started on a total daily dose no greater than 150 mg/day (75 mg 2 times a day, or 50 mg 3 times a day). Based on individual patient response and tolerability, the dose may be increased to a maximum dose of 600 mg/day.

Postherpetic neuralgia: The recommended dose of pregabalin is 75 to 150 mg 2 times a day, or 50 to 100 mg 3 times a day (150 to 300 mg/day) in patients with CrCl of at least 60 mL/min. Dosing should begin at 75 mg 2 times a day, or 50 mg 3 times a day (150 mg/day) and may be increased to 300 mg/day within 1 week based on efficacy and tolerability.

Dosing above 300 mg/day should be reserved only for those patients who have ongoing pain and are tolerating 300 mg daily.

Fibromyalgia: 300 to 450 mg/day. Dosing should begin at 75 mg 2 times a day (150 mg/ day) and may be increased to 150 mg 2 times a day (300 mg/day) within 1 week, based on efficacy and tolerability. Patients who do not experience sufficient benefit with 300 mg/day may be further increased to 225 mg 2 times a day (450 mg/ day). Treatment with doses higher than 450 mg/day is not recommended.

Renal function impairment: Dosage adjustment in patients with renal impairment should be based on CrCl, as indicated in the following table. Estimate CrCl using the Cockcroft and Gault equation.

For patients undergoing hemodialysis, pregabalin daily dose should be adjusted based on renal function. In addition to the daily dose adjustment, a supplemental dose should be given immediately following every 4-hour hemodialysis treatment (see the following table).

Pregabalin Dosage Based on Renal Function					
CrCl (mL/min)	Total pregabalin daily dose (mg/day)[a]				Dose regimen
≥ 60	150	300	450	600	2 divided doses or 3 divided doses
30 to 60	75	150	225	300	2 divided doses or 3 divided doses
15 to 30	25 to 50	75	100 to 150	150	Single daily dose or 2 divided doses
< 15	25	25 to 50	50 to 75	75	Single daily dose
Supplementary dosage following hemodialysis (mg)[b]					
Patients on the 25 mg single daily dose regimen: Take 1 supplemental dose of 25 or 50 mg.					
Patients on the 25 to 50 mg single daily dose regimen: Take 1 supplemental dose of 50 or 75 mg.					
Patients on the 50 to 75 mg single daily dose regimen: Take 1 supplemental dose of 75 or 100 mg.					
Patients on the 75 mg single daily dose regimen: Take 1 supplemental dose of 100 or 150 mg.					

[a] Total daily dose (mg/day) should be divided as indicated by dose regimen to provide mg/dose.
[b] Supplementary dose is a single additional dose.

Actions

Pharmacology: Pregabalin binds with high affinity to the alpha$_2$-delta site (an auxiliary subunit of voltage-gated calcium channels) in CNS tissues. Although the mechanism of action of pregabalin is unknown, results with genetically modified mice and with compounds structurally related to pregabalin (such as gabapentin) suggest that binding to the alpha$_2$-delta subunit may be involved in pregabalin's antinociceptive and antiseizure effects in animal models. In vitro, pregabalin reduces the calcium-dependent release of several neurotransmitters, possibly by modulation of calcium channel function.

While pregabalin is a structural derivative of the inhibitory neurotransmitter gamma-aminobutyric acid (GABA), it does not bind directly to $GABA_A$, $GABA_B$, or benzodiazepine receptors, does not augment $GABA_A$ responses in cultured neurons, does not alter rat brain GABA concentration or have acute effects on GABA uptake or degradation.

Pharmacokinetics:

Absorption/Distribution – Pregabalin is well absorbed after oral administration, is eliminated largely by renal excretion, and has an elimination half-life of approximately 6 hours.

Pregabalin does not bind to plasma proteins. The apparent volume of distribution of pregabalin following oral administration is approximately 0.5 L/kg. Pregabalin is a substrate for system L transporter, which is responsible for the transport of large amino acids across the blood-brain barrier.

Metabolism/Excretion – Pregabalin undergoes negligible metabolism in humans.

Pregabalin is eliminated from the systemic circulation primarily by renal excretion as unchanged drug, with a mean elimination half-life of 6.3 hours in subjects with normal renal function. Mean renal clearance was estimated to be 67 to 80.9 mL/min in young healthy subjects. Because pregabalin is not bound to plasma proteins, this clearance rate indicates that renal tubular reabsorption is involved. Pregabalin elimination is nearly proportional to CrCl.

Special populations –

Elderly: Pregabalin oral clearance tended to decrease with increasing age. This decrease in pregabalin oral clearance is consistent with age-related decreases in CrCl. Reduction of pregabalin dose may be required in patients who have age-related compromised renal function.

Contraindications

Hypersensitivity to pregabalin or any of its components.

Warnings/Precautions

Angioedema: There have been postmarketing reports of angioedema in patients during initial and chronic treatment with pregabalin. Specific symptoms included swelling of the face, mouth (gums, lips, and tongue), and neck (larynx and throat). There were reports of life-threatening angioedema with respiratory compromise requiring emergency treatment. Discontinue pregabalin immediately in patients with these symptoms.

Discontinuation: Withdraw pregabalin gradually to minimize the potential of increased seizure frequency in patients with seizure disorders. If pregabalin is discontinued, this should be done gradually over a minimum of 1 week.

Suicidal behavior and ideation: AEDs, including pregabalin, increase the risk of suicidal thoughts or behavior in patients taking these drugs for any indication. Monitor patients treated with any AED for any indication for the emergence of worsening of depression, suicidal thoughts or behavior, and any unusual changes in mood or behavior.

Peripheral edema: Pregabalin treatment may cause peripheral edema.

CNS effects: Pregabalin may cause dizziness and somnolence.

Weight gain: Pregabalin treatment may cause weight gain. Pregabalin-associated weight gain was related to dose and duration of exposure but did not appear to be associated with baseline body mass index, gender, or age. Weight gain was not limited to patients with edema.

Ophthalmological effects: In controlled studies, a higher proportion of patients treated with pregabalin reported blurred vision (7%) than patients treated with placebo (2%), which resolved in a majority of cases with continued dosing. Less than 1% of patients discontinued pregabalin treatment because of vision-related reactions (primarily blurred vision).

Congestive heart failure (CHF): Because there are limited data on CHF patients with New York Heart Association class III or IV cardiac status, use pregabalin with caution in these patients.

Creatine kinase elevations, decreased platelet count, PR interval prolongation: Pregabalin treatment was associated with creatine kinase elevations, a decrease in platelet count, and mild PR interval prolongation.

Hypersensitivity reactions: There have been postmarketing reports of hypersensitivity in patients shortly after initiation of treatment with pregabalin. Adverse reactions included blisters, dyspnea, hives, rash, skin redness, and wheezing. Discontinue pregabalin immediately in patients with these symptoms.

Drug abuse and dependence: Pregabalin is a schedule V controlled substance. Pregabalin is not known to be active at receptor sites associated with drugs of abuse.

Pregnancy: Category C.

Lactation: It is not known if pregabalin is excreted in human milk; it is, however, present in the milk of rats.

Children: The safety and efficacy of pregabalin in children have not been established.

Drug Interactions

Concomitant thiazolidinedione administration: Because the thiazolidinedione class of antidiabetic drugs can cause weight gain and/or fluid retention, possibly exacerbating or leading to heart failure, take care when coadministering pregabalin and these agents.

Oxycodone/Lorazepam/Ethanol: Multiple oral doses of pregabalin were coadministered with oxycodone, lorazepam, or ethanol. Although no pharmacokinetic interactions were seen, additive effects on cognitive and gross motor functioning were seen when pregabalin was coadministered with those drugs.

Adverse Reactions

Adverse reactions most commonly leading to discontinuation: Adverse reactions most frequently leading to discontinuation were dizziness (4%) and somnolence (3%). Other adverse reactions that led to discontinuation were asthenia, ataxia, blurred vision, confusion, incoordination, peripheral edema, and thinking abnormal (1% each).

Most common adverse reactions in all controlled clinical studies: Blurred vision, dizziness, dry mouth, edema, somnolence, thinking abnormal (primarily difficulty with concentration/attention), and weight gain were more commonly reported by subjects treated with pregabalin.

TIAGABINE HYDROCHLORIDE

Tablets: 2, 4, 12, and 16 mg (*Rx*) *Gabitril* (Cephalon)

Indications

Partial seizures: As adjunctive therapy in adults and children at least 12 years of age in the treatment of partial seizures.

Administration and Dosage

All patients: The following dosing recommendations apply to all patients taking tiagabine:

- Tiagabine is given orally and should be taken with food.
- Do not use a loading dose of tiagabine.
- Dose titration: Rapid escalation and/or large dose increments of tiagabine should not be used.
- Dosage adjustment of tiagabine should be considered whenever a change in patient's enzyme-inducing status occurs as a result of the addition, discontinuation, or dose change of the enzyme-inducing agent.

Patients taking enzyme-inducing antiepilepsy drugs (AEDs): The following dosing recommendations apply to patients who are already taking enzyme-inducing AEDs (eg, carbamazepine, phenytoin, primidone, phenobarbital).

Children (12 to 18 years of age) – Initiate tiagabine at 4 mg once/day. The total daily dose of tiagabine may be increased by 4 mg at the beginning of week 2. Thereafter, the total daily dose of may be increased by 4 to 8 mg at weekly intervals until clinical response is achieved or up to 32 mg/day. Give the total daily dose in 2 to 4 divided doses.

Adults older than 18 years of age – Initiate tiagabine at 4 mg once/day. The total daily dose of tiagabine may be increased by 4 to 8 mg at weekly intervals until clinical response is achieved or up to 56 mg/day. Give the total daily dose in 2 to 4 divided doses. Usual adult maintenance dosage is 32 to 56 mg/day in 2 to 4 divided doses.

Patients not taking an enzyme-inducing AED (12 years of age and older): Following a given dose of tiagabine, the estimated plasma concentration in the noninduced patients is more than twice that in patients receiving enzyme-inducing agents. Use in noninduced patients requires lower doses of tiagabine. These patients may also require a slower titration of tiagabine compared with that of induced patients.

Discontinuation of therapy: Do not abruptly discontinue tiagabine. Withdraw gradually to minimize the potential for increased seizure frequency, unless safety concerns require a more rapid withdrawal.

Actions

Pharmacology: The precise mechanism by which tiagabine exerts its antiseizure effect is unknown, although it is believed that it blocks GABA uptake into presynaptic neurons, permitting more GABA to be available for receptor binding on the surfaces of postsynaptic cells.

Pharmacokinetics:

Absorption/Distribution – Tiagabine is 96% bound to human plasma proteins. Tiagabine is nearly completely absorbed (more than 95%), with an absolute oral bioavailability of about 90%. Food slows the absorption rate but does not altering the extent of absorption. Absorption is rapid, with peak plasma concentrations occurring at approximately 45 minutes after an oral dose. Steady state is achieved within 2 days.

Metabolism/Excretion – Tiagabine is likely to be metabolized primarily by the P-450 3A (CYP3A) isoform, although contributions to the metabolism of tiagabine from CYP 1A2, CYP 2D6, or CYP 2C19 have not been excluded. Approximately 2%

of an oral dose of tiagabine is excreted unchanged, with 25% and 63% of the remaining dose excreted into the urine and feces, respectively, primarily as metabolites. The average elimination half-life for tiagabine in healthy subjects ranged from 7 to 9 hours. The elimination half-life decreased 50% to 65% in hepatic enzyme-induced patients (2 to 5 hours).

Contraindications

Hypersensitivity to the drug or its ingredients.

Warnings/Precautions

Seizures in patients without epilepsy: Postmarketing reports have shown that tiagabine use has been associated with new onset seizures and status epilepticus in patients without epilepsy.

Suicidal behavior and ideation: AEDs, including tiagabine, increase the risk of suicidal thoughts or behavior in patients taking these drugs for any indication.

Withdrawal seizures: Do not abruptly discontinue antiepilepsy drugs (AEDs) because of the possibility of increasing seizure frequency. Withdraw tiagabine gradually to minimize the potential for increased seizure frequency, unless safety concerns require a more rapid withdrawal.

Cognitive/Neuropsychiatric adverse reactions: Adverse reactions most often associated with the use of tiagabine were related to the CNS.

1.) Impaired concentration, speech or language problems, and confusion (effects on thought processes).
2.) Somnolence and fatigue (effects on level of consciousness).

The majority of these reactions were mild to moderate.

Additionally, there have been postmarketing reports cognitive/neuropsychiatric symptoms, some accompanied by EEG abnormalities such as generalized spike and wave activity, that have been reported as nonconvulsant status epilepticus.

Status epilepticus: Among the patients treated with tiagabine across all epilepsy studies (controlled and uncontrolled), 5% had some form of status epilepticus. Of the 5%, 57% of patients experienced complex partial status epilepticus. A critical risk factor for status epilepticus was the presence of the condition history; 33% of patients with a history of status epilepticus had recurrence during tiagabine treatment.

Sudden unexpected death in epilepsy (SUDEP): There have been as many as 10 cases of SUDEP during the clinical development of tiagabine among 2531 patients with epilepsy (3831 patient-years of exposure).

The rate is within the range of estimates for the incidence of SUDEP not receiving tiagabine. The estimated SUDEP rates in patients receiving tiagabine are similar to those observed in patients receiving other AEDs, chemically unrelated to tiagabine, who underwent clinical testing in similar populations at about the same time. This evidence suggests that the SUDEP rates reflect population rates, not a drug effect.

Concomitant EIAED: Blood levels of tiagabine obtained depend on whether the patient also is receiving a drug that induces the metabolism of tiagabine. The presence of an inducer means that the attained blood level will be substantially reduced. Dosing should take the presence of concomitant medications into account.

Generalized weakness: Moderately severe to incapacitating generalized weakness has been reported following administration of tiagabine in approximately 1% of patients with epilepsy. The weakness resolved in all cases after a reduction in dose or discontinuation of tiagabine.

Ophthalmic effects: Although no specific recommendations for periodic ophthalmologic monitoring exists, be aware of the possibility of long-term ophthalmologic effects.

Serious rash: Four patients treated with tiagabine during premarketing clinical testing developed what were considered to be serious rashes. In 2 patients, the rash was described as maculopapular; in 1 it was described as vesiculobullous; and in the fourth case, a diagnosis of Stevens-Johnson syndrome was made. Drug associated rash can, if extensive and serious, cause irreversible morbidity, even death.

Hepatic function impairment: Because the clearance of tiagabine is reduced in patients with liver disease, dosage reduction or longer dosing intervals may be necessary in these patients.

Hazardous tasks: Advise patients that tiagabine may cause dizziness, somnolence, and other symptoms and signs of CNS depression. Because of the possible additive depressive effects, use caution when patients are taking other CNS depressants in combination with tiagabine.

Pregnancy: Category C.

Lactation: Tiagabine and/or its metabolites are excreted in the milk of rats. Use in women who are nursing only if the benefits clearly outweigh the risks.

Children: Safety and efficacy in children younger than 12 years of age have not been established.

Lab test abnormalities:

EEG abnormalities – Patients with a history of spike and wave discharges on EEG have been reported to have exacerbations of their EEG abnormalities associated with cognitive/neuropsychiatric events. In the documented cases of spike and wave discharges on EEG with cognitive/neuropsychiatric reactions, patients usually continued tiagabine, but required dosage adjustment.

Monitoring: Monitor patients treated with any AED for any indication for the emergence of worsening of depression, suicidal thoughts or behavior, and/or any unusual changes in mood or behavior.

A therapeutic range for tiagabine plasma concentrations has not been established. Because of the potential for pharmacokinetic interactions between tiagabine and drugs that induce or inhibit hepatic metabolizing enzymes, it may be useful to obtain plasma levels of tiagabine before and after changes are made in the therapeutic regimen.

Drug Interactions

Interaction of tiagabine with highly protein-bound drugs: Tiagabine is 96% bound to human plasma protein and therefore has the potential to interact with other highly protein-bound compounds. Such an interaction can potentially lead to higher free fractions of either tiagabine or the competing drug.

Drugs that may affect tiagabine include bupropion, carbamazepine, gemfibrozil, highly protein-bound drugs, phenobarbital, phenytoin, primidone, tramadol, and valproate.

Drugs that may be affected by tiagabine include highly protein-bound drugs and valproate.

Drug/Food interactions: A high-fat meal decreases the rate, but not the extent (AUC), of tiagabine absorption.

Adverse Reactions

Adverse reactions that occurred in 3% or more of patients include the following: abnormal gait, abdominal pain, accidental injury, amblyopia, asthenia, ataxia, confusion, cough increased, depression, diarrhea, difficulty with concentration/attention, difficulty with memory, dizziness, ecchymosis, emotional lability, flu syndrome, hostility, infection, insomnia, myalgia, nausea, nervousness, paresthesia, pain (unspecified), pharyngitis, rash, somnolence, speech disorder, tremor, urinary tract infection, vomiting.

TOPIRAMATE

Tablets: 25, 50, 100, and 200 mg (*Rx*)	Various, *Topamax* (Janssen)
Capsules, sprinkle: 15 and 25 mg (*Rx*)	Various, *Topamax* (Janssen)

Indications

Epilepsy, monotherapy: As initial monotherapy in patients 10 years of age and older with partial onset or primary generalized tonic-clonic seizures.

Epilepsy, adjunctive therapy: As adjunctive therapy for adults and children 2 to 16 years of age with partial onset seizures or primary generalized tonic-clonic seizures and in patients 2 years of age and older with seizures associated with Lennox-Gastaut syndrome.

Migraine: As prophylaxis of migraine headache in adults. The usefulness of topiramate in the acute treatment of migraine headache has not been studied.

Administration and Dosage

It is not necessary to monitor topiramate plasma concentrations to optimize therapy.

Because of the bitter taste, do not break tablets.

Topiramate can be taken without regard to meals.

Epilepsy, monotherapy: The recommended dosage for topiramate monotherapy in adults and children 10 years of age and older is 400 mg/day in 2 divided doses. The dosage should be achieved by titrating according to the following schedule:

	Morning dose	Evening dose
Week 1	25 mg	25 mg
Week 2	50 mg	50 mg
Week 3	75 mg	75 mg
Week 4	100 mg	100 mg
Week 5	150 mg	150 mg
Week 6	200 mg	200 mg

Epilepsy, adjunctive therapy:

Adults (17 years of age and older): partial seizures, primary generalized tonic-clonic seizures, or Lennox-Gastaut syndrome – The recommended total daily dosage of topiramate as adjunctive therapy in adults with partial seizures is 200 to 400 mg/day in 2 divided doses, and 400 mg/day in 2 divided doses as adjunctive treatment in adults with primary generalized tonic-clonic seizures. It is recommended that therapy be initiated at 25 to 50 mg/day followed by titration to an effective dosage in increments of 25 to 50 mg/week. Titrating in increments of 25 mg/week may delay the time to reach an effective dosage. Daily doses above 1,600 mg have not been studied.

In a study of primary generalized tonic-clonic seizures, the initial titration rate was slower than in previous studies; the assigned dose was reached at the end of 8 weeks.

Children (2 to 16 years of age): partial seizures, primary generalized tonic-clonic seizures, or Lennox-Gastaut syndrome – The recommended total daily dose as adjunctive therapy is approximately 5 to 9 mg/kg/day in 2 divided doses. Begin titration at or below 25 mg (based on a range of 1 to 3 mg/kg/day) nightly for the first week. Then increase the dosage at 1- or 2-week intervals by increments of 1 to 3 mg/kg/day (administered in 2 divided doses) to achieve optimal clinical response. Guide dose titration by clinical outcome.

Migraine: The recommended total daily dose is 100 mg/day administered in 2 divided doses. The recommended titration rate 100 mg/day is:

	Morning dose	Evening dose
Week 1	None	25 mg
Week 2	25 mg	25 mg
Week 3	25 mg	50 mg
Week 4	50 mg	50 mg

Guide dose titration rate by clinical outcome. If required, longer intervals between dose adjustments can be used.

Concomitant therapy: On occasion, the addition of topiramate to phenytoin may require an adjustment of the dose of phenytoin to achieve optimal clinical outcome. The addition or withdrawal of phenytoin and/or carbamazepine during adjunctive therapy with topiramate may require adjustment of the dose of topiramate.

Sprinkle capsules: Swallow whole or administer by carefully opening the capsule and sprinkling the entire contents on a small amount (teaspoon) of soft food. Swallow this drug/food mixture immediately; do not chew. Do not store for future use.

Hepatic function impairment: In hepatically impaired patients, topiramate plasma concentrations may be increased. Administer with caution.

Renal function impairment: In renally impaired subjects (Ccr less than 70 mL/min/1.73 m^2), 50% of the usual adult dose is recommended. Such patients will require a longer time to reach steady state at each dose.

Hemodialysis: Topiramate is cleared by hemodialysis 4 to 6 times greater than in a healthy individual; a prolonged period of dialysis may cause topiramate levels to fall below that required to maintain an antiseizure effect. To avoid rapid drops in topiramate plasma concentration during hemodialysis, a supplemental dose of topiramate may be required. The actual adjustment should take into account 1) the duration of the dialysis period, 2) the clearance rate of the dialysis system being used, and 3) the effective renal clearance of topiramate in the patient being dialyzed.

Actions

Pharmacology: The precise mechanism by which topiramate exerts its anticonvulsant and migraine prophylaxis effects are unknown. Topiramate, at pharmacologically relevant concentrations, blocks voltage-dependent sodium channels, augments the activity of the neurotransmitter gamma-aminobutyrate at some subtypes of the GABA-A receptor, antagonizes the AMPA/kainate subtype of the glutamate receptor, and inhibits the carbonic anhydrase enzyme, particularly isozymes II and IV.

Pharmacokinetics:

Absorption/Distribution – Absorption of topiramate is rapid, with peak plasma concentrations occurring at approximately 2 hours following a 400 mg oral dose. The relative bioavailability of topiramate from the tablet formulation is approximately 80% compared with a solution. The bioavailability of topiramate is not affected by food.

Steady state is reached in approximately 4 days in patients with normal renal function. Topiramate is 15% to 41% bound to human plasma proteins over the concentration range of 0.5 to 250 mcg/mL.

Metabolism/Excretion – Topiramate is not extensively metabolized and is primarily eliminated unchanged in the urine (approximately 70% of an administered dose). The mean plasma elimination half-life is 21 hours after single or multiple doses. Overall, plasma clearance is approximately 20 to 30 mL/min following oral administration.

Bioequivalency – The sprinkle formulation is bioequivalent to the immediate-release tablet formulation and, therefore, may be substituted as therapeutically equivalent.

Contraindications

A history of hypersensitivity to any component of this product.

Warnings/Precautions

Acute myopia and secondary-angle closure glaucoma: A syndrome consisting of acute myopia associated with secondary-angle closure glaucoma has been reported in pediatric and adult patients receiving topiramate. Symptoms include acute onset of decreased visual acuity or ocular pain. Ophthalmologic findings can include myopia, anterior chamber shallowing, ocular hyperemia (redness), and increased intraocular pressure. Mydriasis may or may not be present. Symptoms typically occur within 1 month of initiating topiramate therapy. The primary treatment to reverse symptoms is discontinuation of topiramate as rapidly as possible, according to the judgment of the treating physician.

Metabolic acidosis: Hyperchloremic, nonanion gap, metabolic acidosis is associated with topiramate treatment. This metabolic acidosis is caused by renal bicarbonate loss because of the inhibitory effect of topiramate on carbonic anhydrase. Generally, topiramate-induced metabolic acidosis occurs early in treatment, although cases can occur at any time during treatment. Bicarbonate decrements usually are mild to moderate; rarely, patients can experience severe decrements to values below 10 mEq/L. Conditions or therapies that predispose to acidosis may be additive to the bicarbonate lowering effects of topiramate. If metabolic acidosis develops and persists, consider reducing the dose or discontinuing topiramate.

Oligohydrosis and hyperthermia: Oligohydrosis (decreased sweating), infrequently resulting in hospitalization, has been reported in association with topiramate use. Decreased sweating and an elevation in body temperature above normal characterized these cases. The majority of the reports have been in children.

Closely monitor patients, especially pediatric patients, treated with topiramate for evidence of decreased sweating and increased body temperature, especially in hot weather. Use caution when topiramate is prescribed with other drugs that predispose patients to heat-related disorders; these drugs include, but are not limited to, other carbonic anhydrase inhibitors and drugs with anticholinergic activity.

Withdrawal: Withdraw antiepileptic drugs, including topiramate, gradually to minimize the potential of increased seizure frequency.

CNS-effects:

Adults – Adverse reactions most often associated with the use of topiramate were related to the CNS and were observed in both the epilepsy and migraine populations. In adults, the most frequent of these can be classified into 3 general categories:

1.) Cognitive-related dysfunction (eg, confusion; psychomotor slowing; difficulty with concentration/attention; difficulty with memory; speech or language problems, particularly word-finding difficulties).
2.) Psychiatric/behavioral disturbances (eg, depression, mood problems).
3.) Somnolence or fatigue.

Children – The incidences of cognitive/neuropsychiatric adverse reactions in children generally were lower than previously observed in adults. These events included psychomotor slowing, difficulty with concentration/attention, speech disorders/related speech problems, and language problems. The most frequently reported neuropsychiatric events in this population were somnolence and fatigue.

Sudden unexplained death in epilepsy: Sudden and unexplained deaths were recorded among a cohort of treated patients (2,796 subject years of exposure). This represents an incidence of 0.0035 deaths per patient year.

Hyperammonemia and encephalopathy associated with concomitant valproic acid use: Administration of topiramate and valproic acid has been associated with hyperammonemia with or without encephalopathy in patients who have tolerated either drug alone. In most cases, symptoms and signs abated with discontinuation of either drug.

In patients who develop unexplained lethargy, vomiting, or changes in mental status, consider hyperammonemic encephalopathy and measure an ammonia level.

Kidney stones: A total of 1.5% patients exposed to topiramate during its development reported the occurrence of kidney stones; an incidence approximately 2 to 4 times that expected in a similar, untreated population. Kidney stones also have been reported in pediatric patients.

An explanation for the association of topiramate and kidney stones may lie in the fact that topiramate is a weak carbonic anhydrase inhibitor. Carbonic anhydrase inhibitors (eg, acetazolamide, dichlorphenamide) promote stone formation by reducing urinary citrate excretion and by increasing urinary pH. The concomitant use of topiramate with other carbonic anhydrase inhibitors or potentially in patients on a ketogenic diet may create a physiological environment that increases the risk of kidney stone formation and should be avoided.

Increased fluid intake increases urinary output, lowering substance concentration involved in stone formation. Hydration is recommended to reduce new stone formation.

Paresthesia: Paresthesia, an effect associated with the use of other carbonic anhydrase inhibitors, appears to be a common effect of topiramate.

Renal function impairment: The major route of elimination of unchanged topiramate and its metabolites is via the kidney. Dosage adjustment may be required.

Hepatic function impairment: In hepatically impaired patients, administer topiramate with caution because clearance may be decreased.

Carcinogenesis: An increase in urinary bladder tumors was observed in mice given topiramate (20, 75, and 300 mg/kg) for 21 months. The relevance of this finding to human carcinogenic risk is uncertain.

Pregnancy: Category C.

Lactation: Topiramate is excreted in the milk of lactating rats. Limited observations in patients suggest an extensive secretion of topiramate into breast milk. Weigh the potential benefit to the mother against the potential risk to the infant.

Children: Safety and efficacy in children younger than 2 years of age have not been established.

Elderly: No age-related difference in efficacy or adverse effects were evident. However, clinical studies of topiramate did not include sufficient numbers of subjects 65 years of age and older to determine whether they respond differently than younger subjects.

Monitoring: Measurement of baseline and periodic serum bicarbonate during topiramate treatment is recommended.

Drug Interactions

Topiramate may affect alcohol, amitriptyline, carbonic anhydrase inhibitors, CNS depressants, lithium, oral contraceptives, pioglitazone, digoxin, estrogens, hydantoins, metformin, risperidone, and valproic acid.

Topiramate may be affected by carbamazepine, hydantoins, metformin, valproic acid, carbonic anhydrase inhibitors, hydrochlorothiazide, lamotrigine, and pioglitazone.

Adverse Reactions

Epilepsy – Adverse reactions occurring in at least 3% of adult patients include abdominal pain, abnormal coordination, abnormal gait, abnormal vision, aggressive reaction, agitation, allergy, anorexia, apathy, asthenia, ataxia, back pain, breast pain, chest pain, cognitive problems, confusion, constipation, depression, difficulty with concentration/attention, difficulty with memory, diplopia, dizziness, dry mouth, dyspepsia, emotional lability, fatigue, influenza-like symptoms, language problems, leg pain, mood problems, nausea, nervousness, nystagmus, paresthesia, pharyngitis, psychomotor slowing, rhinitis, sinusitis, somnolence, speech disorders/related speech problems, taste perversion, tremor, urinary tract infection, weight decrease.

Adverse reactions occurring in at least 3% of pediatric patients include abnormal gait, aggressive reaction, anorexia, ataxia, confusion, constipation, difficulty with concentration/attention, difficulty with memory, dizziness, epistaxis, fatigue, gastroenteritis, hyperkinesia, increased saliva, injury, insomnia, nausea, nervousness, personality disorder (behavior problems), pneumonia, psychomotor slowing, purpura, skin disorder, somnolence, speech disorders/related speech problems, urinary incontinence, viral infection, weight decrease.

Migraine – Adverse reactions occurring in at least 3% of patients include the following: abdominal pain, anorexia, anxiety, arthralgia, blurred vision, bronchitis, confusion, coughing, depression, diarrhea, difficulty with memory, difficulty concentrating, dizziness, dyspepsia, dyspnea, dry mouth, ejaculation premature, fatigue, gastroenteritis, hypoesthesia, injury, insomnia, involuntary muscle contractions, language problems, menstrual disorder, mood problems, nausea, nervousness, paresthesia, pharyngitis, psychomotor slowing, pruritus, sinusitis, somnolence, taste perversion, upper respiratory infection, urinary tract infection, viral infection, vomiting, weight decrease.

OXCARBAZEPINE

Tablets: 150, 300, and 600 mg (*Rx*) **Suspension**: 300 mg/5 mL (*Rx*)	*Trileptal* (Novartis)

Indications

Epilepsy: For use as monotherapy or adjunctive therapy in the treatment of partial seizures in adults and as monotherapy in the treatment of partial seizures in children 4 years of age and older with epilepsy, and as adjunctive therapy in children 2 years of age and older with epilepsy.

Administration and Dosage

Oxcarbazepine may be taken with or without food.

Withdrawal of antiepileptic drugs (AEDs): Withdraw gradually to minimize the potential of increased seizure frequency.

Adults:

Adjunctive therapy – Initiate treatment with a dose of 600 mg/day as a twice-daily regimen. If clinically indicated, the dose may be increased by a maximum of 600 mg/day at approximately weekly intervals; the recommended daily dose is 1200 mg/day. Daily doses more than 1200 mg/day show somewhat greater effectiveness in controlled trials, but most patients were not able to tolerate the 2400 mg/day dose, primarily because of CNS effects. Observe and monitor closely the plasma levels of the concomitant AEDs during the period of oxcarbazepine titration, especially at oxcarbazepine doses more than 1200 mg/day.

Conversion to monotherapy (600 mg/day twice/day) – Patients receiving concomitant AEDs may be converted to monotherapy by initiating treatment with oxcarbazepine at 300 mg twice daily while simultaneously initiating the reduction of the concomitant AED dose. Withdraw the concomitant AEDs over 3 to 6 weeks, while reaching the maximum dose of oxcarbazepine in approximately 2 to 4 weeks. Oxcarbazepine may be increased as clinically indicated by a maximum increment of 600 mg/day at approximate weekly intervals to achieve the recommended daily dose of 2400 mg/day. A daily dose of 1200 mg/day has been shown in 1 study to be effective in patients in whom monotherapy has been initiated with oxcarbazepine.

Initiation of monotherapy (600 mg/day twice/day) – Increase by 300 mg/day every third day to a dose of 1200 mg/day. Controlled trials in these patients examined the effectiveness of a 1200 mg/day dose; a dose of 2400 mg/day has been shown to be effective in patients converted from other AEDs to oxcarbazepine monotherapy.

Pediatric patients 2 to 16 years of age:

Adjunctive therapy – In children 4 to 16 years of age, initiate treatment at a daily dose of 8 to 10 mg/kg, generally not to exceed 600 mg/day, given as a twice-daily regimen. Achieve the target maintenance dose of oxcarbazepine over 2 weeks, according to patient weight, using the following table.

Oxcarbazepine Target Maintenance Doses for Pediatric Patients

Patient weight (kg)	Target maintenance dose (mg/day)
20 to 29	900
29.1 to 39	1200
> 39	1800

In the clinical trial, in which the intention was to reach these target doses, the median daily dose was 31 mg/kg with a range of 6 to 51 mg/kg.

In children 2 to 4 years of age, treatment also should be initiated at a daily dose of 8 to 10 mg/kg, generally not to exceed 600 mg/day, given as a twice-daily regimen. For patients weighing less than 20 kg, a starting dose of 16 to 20 mg/kg may be considered. The maximum maintenance dose of oxcarbazepine should be achieved over 2 to 4 weeks and should not exceed 60 mg/kg/day as a twice-daily regimen.

Conversion to monotherapy (4 to 16 years of age): Patients receiving concomitant AEDs may be converted to monotherapy by initiating treatment at approximately 8 to 10 mg/

kg/day given in a twice-daily regimen, while simultaneously initiating the reduction of the dose of the concomitant AEDs. The concomitant AEDs can be completely withdrawn over 3 to 6 weeks, while oxcarbazepine may be increased as clinically indicated by a maximum increment of 10 mg/kg/day at approximately weekly intervals to achieve the recommended daily dose.

Initiation of monotherapy (4 to 16 years of age): Patients not currently being treated with antiepileptic drugs may have monotherapy initiated with oxcarbazepine. Initiate at a dose of 8 to 10 mg/kg/day given in a twice-daily regimen. Increase the dose by 5 mg/kg/day every third day to the recommended daily dose shown in the table below.

Maintenance Doses of Oxcarbazepine for Children During Monotherapy		
Weight (kg)	From	To
20	600 mg/day	900 mg/day
25	900 mg/day	1,200 mg/day
30	900 mg/day	1,200 mg/day
35	900 mg/day	1,500 mg/day
40	900 mg/day	1,500 mg/day
45	1,200 mg/day	1,500 mg/day
50	1,200 mg/day	1,800 mg/day
55	1,200 mg/day	1,800 mg/day
60	1,200 mg/day	2,100 mg/day
65	1,200 mg/day	2,100 mg/day
70	1,500 mg/day	2,100 mg/day

Renal function impairment (Ccr less than 30 mL/min): Initiate therapy at ½ the usual starting dose (300 mg/day) and increase slowly to achieve the desired clinical response.

Actions

Pharmacology: Oxcarbazepine activity is primarily exerted through the 10-monohydroxy metabolite (MHD) of oxcarbazepine. The precise mechanism by which oxcarbazepine and MHD exert their antiseizure effect is unknown.

Pharmacokinetics:

Absorption – Following oral administration of oxcarbazepine, it is completely absorbed and extensively metabolized to its pharmacologically active MHD metabolite.

Distribution – Approximately 40% of MHD is bound to serum proteins, predominantly to albumin.

Metabolism – Oxcarbazepine is rapidly reduced by cytosolic enzymes in the liver to its MHD, which is primarily responsible for the pharmacological effect of oxcarbazepine. MHD is metabolized further by conjugation with glucuronic acid.

Excretion – The half-life of the parent drug is approximately 2 hours, while the half-life of MHD is approximately 9 hours.

Contraindications

Known hypersensitivity to oxcarbazepine or any of its components.

Warnings/Precautions

Hyponatremia: Clinically significant hyponatremia generally occurred during the first 3 months of treatment with oxcarbazepine, although there were patients who first developed a serum sodium less than 125 mmol/L greater than 1 year after initiation of therapy. Most patients who developed hyponatremia were asymptomatic, but patients in the clinical trials were frequently monitored and some had their oxcarbazepine dose reduced or discontinued or had their fluid intake restricted for hyponatremia. When oxcarbazepine was discontinued, normalization of serum sodium generally occurred within a few days without additional treatment.

Measure serum sodium levels for patients during maintenance treatment with oxcarbazepine.

Serious dermatological reactions: Serious dermatological reactions, including Stevens-Johnson syndrome and toxic epidermal necrolysis, have been reported in children and adults in association with oxcarbazepine use. The median time of onset for reported cases was 19 days. Such serious skin reactions may be life-threatening, and some patients have required hospitalization with very rare reports of fatal outcome. Recurrence of serious skin reactions following rechallenge with oxcarbazepine has also been reported.

If a patient develops a skin reaction while taking oxcarbazepine, consider discontinuing oxcarbazepine use and prescribing another AED.

History of hypersensitivity reaction to carbamazepine: Approximately 25% to 30% of patients who have had hypersensitivity reactions to carbamazepine will experience a hypersensitivity reaction with oxcarbazepine.

CNS effects: Psychomotor slowing, difficulty with concentration, and speech or language problems; somnolence or fatigue; and coordination abnormalities, including ataxia and gait disturbances.

Withdrawal of AEDs: Withdraw gradually to minimize the potential of increased seizure frequency.

Multiorgan hypersensitivity: Multiorgan hypersensitivity reactions have occurred in close temporal association (median time to detection, 13 days; range, 4 to 60) to the initiation of oxcarbazepine therapy in adults and children. Although there have been a limited number of reports, many of these cases resulted in hospitalization and some were considered life-threatening. Signs and symptoms of this disorder were diverse; however, patients typically, although not exclusively, presented with fever and rash associated with other organ system involvement. Other associated manifestations included arthralgia, asthenia, hematological abnormalities (eg, eosinophilia, neutropenia, thrombocytopenia), hepatitis, hepatorenal syndrome, liver function test abnormalities, lymphadenopathy, nephritis, oliguria, and pruritus. Because the disorder is variable in its expression, other organ system symptoms and signs not noted here may occur. If this reaction is suspected, discontinue oxcarbazepine and start an alternative treatment.

Renal function impairment: Initiate oxcarbazepine therapy at one half the usual starting dose and increase, if necessary, at a slower than usual rate until the desired clinical response is achieved.

Hepatic function impairment: The pharmacokinetics of oxcarbazepine and MHD have not been evaluated in severe hepatic impairment. Adjust dose in renally impaired patients.

Carcinogenesis: In mice, a dose-related increase in the incidence of hepatocellular adenomas was observed with oxcarbazepine.

There was an increase in the incidence of benign testicular interstitial cell tumors and granular cell tumors in the cervix and vagina in rats.

Mutagenesis: Oxcarbazepine increased mutation frequencies in the Ames test in vitro in the absence of metabolic activation in 1 of 5 bacterial strains. Oxcarbazepine and MHD produced increases in chromosomal aberrations and polyploidy in the Chinese hamster ovary assay in vitro in the absence of metabolic activation.

Fertility impairment: In a fertility study in rats, estrous cyclicity was disrupted and numbers of corpora lutea, implantations, and live embryos were reduced in females receiving the highest dose (approximately 2 times the maximum recommended human dose on a mg/m^2 basis).

Pregnancy: Category C.

Lactation: Oxcarbazepine and its active metabolite MHD are excreted in human breast milk.

Children: Oxcarbazepine is indicated for use as adjunctive therapy for partial seizures in patients 2 to 16 years of age. Oxcarbazepine is also indicated as monotherapy for partial seizures in patients 4 to 16 years of age. Oxcarbazepine has been given to

898 patients between 1 month and 17 years of age in controlled clinical trials (332 treated as monotherapy) and about 677 patients between the 1 month and 17 years of age in other trials.

Elderly: Following administration of single (300 mg) and multiple (600 mg/day) doses of oxcarbazepine to elderly volunteers (60 to 82 years of age), the maximum plasma concentrations and AUC values of MHD were 30% to 60% higher than in younger volunteers (18 to 32 years of age).

Lab test abnormalities: Serum sodium levels less than 125 mmol/L have been observed in patients treated with oxcarbazepine. Experience from clinical trials indicates that serum sodium levels return toward normal when the oxcarbazepine dosage is reduced or discontinued or when the patient was treated conservatively (eg, fluid restriction).

Laboratory data from clinical trials suggest that oxcarbazepine use was associated with decreases in T_4, without changes in T_3 or TSH.

Monitoring: It is recommended that the patient be closely observed and plasma levels of the concomitant AEDs be monitored during the period of oxcarbazepine titration, as these plasma levels may be altered, especially at oxcarbazepine doses above 1,200 mg/day.

Consider measurement of serum sodium levels for patients during maintenance treatment with oxcarbazepine, particularly if the patient is receiving other medications known to decrease serum sodium levels (eg, drugs associated with inappropriate antidiuretic hormone secretion) or if symptoms possibly indicating hyponatremia develop (eg, confusion, headache, increase in seizure frequency or severity, lethargy, malaise, nausea, obtundation).

Drug Interactions

Drugs that may be affected by oxcarbazepine include felodipine, lamotrigine, oral contraceptives, phenobarbital, and phenytoin. Drugs that may affect oxcarbazepine include carbamazepine, phenobarbital, phenytoin, valproic acid, and verapamil.

Cytochrome P450: Oxcarbazepine inhibits CYP2C19 and induces CYP3A4/5 with potentially important effects on plasma concentrations of other drugs.

Strong inducers of cytochrome P450 enzymes (ie, carbamazepine, phenytoin, phenobarbital) have been shown to decrease the plasma levels of MHD (29% to 40%).

Cimetidine, erythromycin, and dextropropoxyphene had no effect on the pharmacokinetics of MHD. Results with warfarin show no evidence of interaction with either single or repeated doses of oxcarbazepine.

Adverse Reactions

Adverse reactions that occurred in 3% or more of patients were as follows: Headache; dizziness; somnolence; anxiety; ataxia; nystagmus; abnormal gait; insomnia; tremor; amnesia; convulsions aggravated; emotional lability; hypoesthesia; nervousness; abnormal coordination; speech disorder; confusion; dysmetria; abnormal thinking; rash; nausea; vomiting; abdominal pain; anorexia; dry mouth; diarrhea; dyspepsia; constipation; urinary tract infection; hyponatremia; back pain; rhinitis; upper respiratory tract infection; coughing; bronchitis; pharyngitis; epistaxis; chest infection; sinusitis; diplopia; vertigo; taste perversion; abnormal vision; fatigue; fever; asthenia; falling down (nos); infection viral.

Adjunctive therapy/monotherapy in adults previously treated with other AEDs – The most commonly observed (5% or more) adverse experiences seen in association with oxcarbazepine and substantially more frequent than in placebo-treated patients were the following: Dizziness, somnolence, diplopia, fatigue, nausea, vomiting, ataxia, abnormal vision, abdominal pain, tremor, dyspepsia, abnormal gait.

Approximately 23% of these 1537 adult patients discontinued treatment because of an adverse experience. The adverse experiences most commonly associated with discontinuation were the following: Dizziness (6.4%), diplopia (5.9%), ataxia (5.2%), vomiting (5.1%), nausea (4.9%), somnolence (3.8%), headache (2.9%), fatigue (2.1%), abnormal vision (2.1%), tremor (1.8%), abnormal gait (1.7%), rash (1.4%), hyponatremia (1%).

Adjunctive therapy/monotherapy in pediatric patients 4 years of age and older previously treated with other AEDs – The most commonly observed (5% or more) adverse experiences seen in association with oxcarbazepine in pediatric patients were similar to those seen in adults.

Approximately 11% of the 456 pediatric patients discontinued treatment because of an adverse experience. The adverse experiences most commonly associated with discontinuation were the following: Somnolence (2.4%); vomiting (2%); ataxia (1.8%); diplopia, dizziness (1.3%); fatigue, nystagmus (1.1%).

Monotherapy in adults not previously treated with other AEDs – Approximately 9% of 295 adult patients discontinued treatment because of an adverse experience. The adverse experiences most commonly associated with discontinuation were the following: Dizziness, nausea, rash (1.7%); headache (1.4%).

Monotherapy in pediatric patients 4 years of age and older not previously treated with other AEDs – Approximately 9.2% of 152 pediatric patients discontinued treatment because of an adverse experience. The adverse experiences most commonly associated (at least 1%) with discontinuation were rash (5.3%) and maculopapular rash (1.3%).

Adjunctive therapy/monotherapy in children 1 month to younger than 4 years of age previously treated or not previously treated with other AEDs: The most commonly observed (at least 5%) adverse reactions seen in association with oxcarbazepine in these patients were similar to those seen in older children and adults except for infections and infestations, which were more frequently seen in these younger children.

Approximately 11% of these 241 children discontinued treatment because of an adverse reaction. The adverse reactions most commonly associated with discontinuation were convulsions (3.7%), ataxia (1.2%), and status epilepticus (1.2%).

LACOSAMIDE

Tablets, oral: 50 mg, 100 mg, 150 mg, 200 mg (*Rx*)	*Vimpat* (UCB)
Solution, oral: 10 mg/mL (*Rx*)	
Injection, solution: 10 mg/mL (*Rx*)	

Indications

Partial-onset seizures: As adjunctive therapy in the treatment of partial-onset seizures in patients 17 years of age and older with epilepsy. Injection is indicated when oral administration is temporarily not feasible.

Administration and Dosage

Adults:

Initial dosage – 50 mg twice daily (100 mg/day).

Dosage titration – Increase at weekly intervals by 100 mg/day given as 2 divided doses, up to the recommended maintenance dosage of 200 to 400 mg/day. In clinical trials, the 600 mg daily dose was not more effective than the 400 mg daily dose and was associated with a substantially higher rate of adverse reactions.

Maintenance dosage – 200 to 400 mg/day.

Conversion – When switching from oral lacosamide, the initial total daily IV dosage of lacosamide should be equivalent to the total daily dosage and frequency of oral lacosamide and should be infused IV over a period of 30 to 60 minutes. There is experience with twice-daily IV infusion for up to 5 days.

The patient may be switched to oral administration at the equivalent daily dosage and frequency of the IV administration.

Renal function impairment: A maximum dosage of 300 mg/day is recommended for patients with severe renal function impairment (CrCl of 30 mL/min or less) and in patients with end-stage renal disease.

Lacosamide is effectively removed from plasma by hemodialysis. Dosage supplementation of up to 50% should be considered.

Hepatic function impairment: A maximum dosage of 300 mg/day is recommended for patients with mild or moderate hepatic function impairment. Use is not recommended in patients with severe hepatic function impairment.

Discontinuation: As with all antiepileptic drugs (AEDs), gradually withdraw lacosamide (over a minimum of 1 week) to minimize the potential of increased seizure frequency in patients with seizure disorders.

Preparation for administration: Lacosamide injection can be administered IV without further dilution or may be mixed with diluents.

Admixture compatibility: Lacosamide injection was found to be physically compatible and chemically stable when mixed with sodium chloride injection 0.9%, dextrose injection 5%, and Ringer's lactate injection for at least 24 hours and stored in glass or polyvinyl chloride bags at ambient room temperature, 15° to 30°C (59° to 86°F).

The stability of lacosamide injection in other infusion solutions has not been evaluated.

Administration: Lacosamide may be taken with or without food.

Actions

Pharmacology: In vitro electrophysiological studies have shown that lacosamide selectively enhances slow inactivation of voltage-gated sodium channels, resulting in stabilization of hyperexcitable neuronal membranes and inhibition of repetitive neuronal firing.

Pharmacokinetics:

Absorption/Distribution – Lacosamide is completely absorbed after oral administration with negligible first-pass effect, with a high absolute bioavailability of approximately 100%. The maximum lacosamide plasma concentrations occur approximately 1 to 4 hours postdose after oral dosing. Steady-state plasma concentrations are achieved after 3 days of twice-daily repeated administration.

After IV administration, maximal drug concentration is reached at the end of infusion. The 30- and 60-minute IV infusions are bioequivalent to the oral tablet.

Lacosamide is less than 15% bound to plasma proteins.

Metabolism/Excretion – The elimination half-life is approximately 13 hours

Lacosamide is a CYP2C19 substrate.

Lacosamide is primarily eliminated from the systemic circulation by renal excretion and biotransformation.

Contraindications

None well documented.

Warnings/Precautions

Suicidal behavior and ideation: AEDs, including lacosamide, increase the risk of suicidal thoughts or behavior in patients taking these drugs for any indication.

CNS effects: In patients with partial-onset seizures taking 1 to 3 concomitant AEDs, dizziness was experienced by 25% of patients and was the adverse reaction most frequently leading to discontinuation (3%). Ataxia was experienced by 6%. The onset of dizziness and ataxia was most commonly observed during titration. There was a substantial increase in these adverse reactions at dosages higher than 400 mg/day.

Cardiovascular effects: Dose-dependent prolongations in PR interval with lacosamide have been observed in clinical studies in patients and in healthy volunteers.

In the short-term investigational trials of lacosamide in epilepsy patients, there were no cases of atrial fibrillation or flutter. In patients with diabetic neuropathy, 0.5% of patients treated with lacosamide experienced an adverse reaction of atrial fibrillation or atrial flutter.

In the short-term controlled trials of lacosamide in epilepsy patients with no significant system illnesses, there was no increase in syncope compared with placebo. In the short-term controlled trials of lacosamide in patients with diabetic neuropathy, 1.2% of patients who were treated with lacosamide reported an adverse reaction of syncope or loss of consciousness.

Discontinuation of therapy: As with all AEDs, gradually withdraw lacosamide (over a minimum of 1 week) to minimize the potential of increased seizure frequency in patients with seizure disorders.

Phenylketonurics: Lacosamide oral solution contains aspartame, a source of phenylalanine. A dose of lacosamide 200 mg oral solution (equivalent to 20 mL) contains phenylalanine 0.32 mg.

Hypersensitivity reactions: One case of symptomatic hepatitis and nephritis was observed among 4,011 subjects exposed to lacosamide during clinical development. Multiorgan hypersensitivity reactions have been reported with other anticonvulsants and typically, although not exclusively, present with fever and rash associated with other organ system involvement that may or may not include eosinophilia, hepatitis, nephritis, lymphadenopathy, and/or myocarditis.

Renal function impairment: A maximum dosage of 300 mg/day is recommended for patients with severe renal impairment and in patients with end-stage renal disease. Lacosamide is effectively removed from plasma by hemodialysis. Following a 4-hour hemodialysis treatment, AUC of lacosamide is reduced by approximately 50%. Therefore, consider dosage supplementation of up to 50% following hemodialysis. In all renally impaired patients, perform dosage titration with caution.

Hepatic function impairment: Closely observe patients with mild to moderate hepatic impairment during dose titration. A maximum dosage of 300 mg/day is recommended for patients with mild to moderate hepatic impairment. The pharmacokinetics of lacosamide have not been evaluated in severe hepatic impairment. Lacosamide use is not recommended in patients with severe hepatic impairment.

Drug abuse and dependence: The rate of euphoria reported as an adverse reaction in the lacosamide development program at therapeutic doses was less than 1%. Abrupt termination of lacosamide in clinical trials produced no signs or symptoms that are associated with a withdrawal syndrome indicative of physical dependence. However, psychological dependence cannot be excluded because of the ability of lacosamide to produce euphoria-type adverse reactions.

Hazardous tasks: Advise patients that lacosamide may cause dizziness and ataxia. Accordingly, advise them not to drive a car or operate other complex machinery until they are familiar with the effects of lacosamide on their ability to perform such activities.

Pregnancy: Category C. The manufacturer has established the UCB AED Pregnancy Registry to advance scientific knowledge about safety and outcomes in pregnant women being treated with lacosamide. To ensure broad program access and reach, initiate enrollment by calling 888-537-7734.

Lactation: It is not known whether lacosamide is excreted in human milk. Because many drugs are excreted into human milk, decide whether to discontinue breast-feeding or lacosamide, taking into account the importance of the drug to the mother.

Children: The safety and effectiveness of lacosamide in children younger than 17 years of age have not been established.

Elderly: No dose adjustment based on age is considered necessary. Exercise caution for dose titration in elderly patients.

Monitoring: Monitor patients treated with any AED for any indication for the emergence or worsening of depression, suicidal thoughts or behavior, and/or any unusual changes in mood or behavior. Obtain an electrocardiogram before beginning therapy and after lacosamide is titrated to steady state in patients with known conduction problems or severe cardiac disease. Closely monitor patients with coexisting hepatic and renal function impairment during dose titration.

Drug Interactions

Drugs that may interact with lacosamide include AEDs, omeprazole, and hormonal contraceptives.

Adverse Reactions

Adverse reactions occurring in at least 3% of patients treated with lacosamide include asthenia, ataxia, balance disorder, contusion, diarrhea, diplopia, dizziness, fatigue, gait disturbance, headache, memory impairment, nausea, nystagmus, pruritus, skin laceration, somnolence, tremor, vertigo, vision blurred, and vomiting.

BACLOFEN

Tablets: 10 and 20 mg (*Rx*)	Various, *Lioresal* (Novartis)
Tablets, orally disintegrating: 10 and 20 mg (*Rx*)	*Kemstro* (Schwarz)
Intrathecal: 0.5 mg/mL (50 mcg/mL), 10 mg per 20 mL (500 mcg/mL), and 10 mg per 5 mL (2,000 mcg/mL) (*Rx*)	*Lioresal* (Medtronic)

Warning:

Abrupt discontinuation of intrathecal baclofen, regardless of the cause, has resulted in sequelae that include high fever, altered mental status, exaggerated rebound spasticity, and muscle rigidity, which in rare cases has advanced to rhabdomyolysis, multiple organ-system failure, and death.

Prevention of abrupt discontinuation of intrathecal baclofen requires careful attention to programming and monitoring of the infusion system, refill scheduling and procedures, and pump alarms. Advise patients and caregivers of the importance of keeping scheduled refill visits and educate them on the early symptoms of baclofen withdrawal. Give special attention to patients at apparent risk (eg, spinal cord injuries at T-6 or above, communication difficulties, history of withdrawal symptoms from oral or intrathecal baclofen). Consult the technical manual of the implantable infusion system for additional postimplant clinician and patient information (see Warnings).

Indications

Oral: Alleviation of signs and symptoms of spasticity resulting from multiple sclerosis, particularly for the relief of flexor spasms and concomitant pain, clonus, and muscular rigidity. Patients should have reversible spasticity so that treatment will aid in restoring residual function.

Oral baclofen may be of some value in patients with spinal cord injuries and other spinal cord diseases.

Intrathecal: For use in the management of severe spasticity. Patients should first respond to a screening dose of intrathecal baclofen prior to consideration for long-term infusion. For spasticity of spinal cord origin, chronic infusion of baclofen intrathecal injection should be reserved for patients unresponsive to oral baclofen therapy, or those who experience intolerable CNS side effects at effective doses. Patients with spasticity due to traumatic brain injury should wait at least 1 year after the injury before consideration of long-term intrathecal baclofen therapy.

Administration and Dosage

Oral: Individualize dosage. Start at a low dosage and increase gradually until the optimum effect is achieved (usually 40 to 80 mg/day).

The following dosage schedule is suggested: 5 mg 3 times/day for 3 days; 10 mg 3 times/day for 3 days; 15 mg 3 times/day for 3 days; 20 mg 3 times/day for 3 days. Thereafter, additional increases may be necessary, but the total daily dose should not exceed 80 mg/day (20 mg 4 times/day).

The lowest effective dose is recommended. If benefits are not evident after a reasonable trial period, withdraw the drug slowly.

Intrathecal: Refer to the manufacturer's manual for the implantable intrathecal infusion pump for specific instructions and precautions for programming the pump or refilling the reservoir.

Consult complete *Drug Facts and Comparisons* monograph and/or manufacturer product information for full intrathecal dosing information.

Dilution instructions –

Screening: Use the 1 mL screening ampule only (50 mcg/mL) for bolus injection into the subarachnoid space. For a 50 mcg bolus dose, use 1 mL of the screening ampule. Use 1.5 mL of 50 mcg/mL baclofen intrathecal for a 75 mcg bolus dose. For the maximum screening dose of 100 mcg, use 2 mL of 50 mcg/mL baclofen intrathecal (2 screening ampules).

Maintenance: For patients who require concentrations other than 500 or 2,000 mcg/mL, baclofen intrathecal must be diluted with sterile, preservative free Sodium Chloride for Injection, USP.

Delivery regimen – Baclofen intrathecal is most often administered in a continuous infusion mode immediately following implant. For those patients implanted with programmable pumps who have achieved relatively satisfactory control on continuous infusion, further benefit may be attained using more complex schedules of delivery.

Actions

Pharmacology: The precise mechanism of action is not known. Baclofen can inhibit mono- and polysynaptic reflexes at the spinal level, possibly by decreasing excitatory neurotransmitter release from primary afferent terminals, although actions at supraspinal sites also may contribute to its clinical effect. Baclofen has CNS-depressant properties.

Pharmacokinetics:

Oral – Baclofen is rapidly and extensively absorbed and eliminated. Absorption may be dose-dependent, being reduced with increasing doses. Baclofen is excreted primarily by the kidney in unchanged form and there is relatively large intersubject variation in absorption and/or elimination.

Intrathecal –

Bolus: The onset of action is generally 0.5 to 1 hour after an intrathecal bolus dose. Peak spasmolytic effect is seen at about 4 hours after dosing and effects may last 4 to 8 hours. After a bolus lumbar injection of 50 to 100 mcg baclofen intrathecal injection, the average CSF elimination half-life was 1.51 hours over the first 4 hours.

Continuous infusion: The antispastic action is first seen at 6 to 8 hours after initiation of continuous infusion. Maximum activity is observed in 24 to 48 hours. Concurrent plasma concentrations of baclofen during intrathecal administration are expected to be low (0 to 5 ng/mL).

Contraindications

Hypersensitivity to baclofen.

Oral: Treatment of skeletal muscle spasm resulting from rheumatic disorders; stroke, cerebral palsy, and Parkinson's disease.

Intrathecal: IV, IM, subcutaneous, or epidural administration.

Warnings/Precautions

Intrathecal administration: Because of the possibility of potentially life-threatening CNS depression, cardiovascular collapse, or respiratory failure, physicians must be adequately trained and educated in chronic intrathecal infusion therapy.

Extreme caution must be used when filling an FDA-approved implantable pump. Such pumps should only be refilled through the reservoir refill septum. However, some pumps are also equipped with a catheter access port that allows direct access to the intrathecal catheter. Direct injection into this catheter access port may cause a life-threatening overdose.

Infection: Patients should be infection-free prior to the screening trial with baclofen injection because the presence of a systemic infection may interfere with an assessment of the patient's response.

Patients should be infection-free prior to pump implantation because the presence of infection may increase the risk of surgical complications. Moreover, a systemic infection may complicate attempts to adjust the pump's dosing rate.

Abrupt drug withdrawal:

Oral – Hallucinations and seizures have occurred on abrupt withdrawal. An isolated case of manic psychosis has been reported. Except in cases of serious adverse reactions, reduce dose slowly when drug is discontinued.

Intrathecal – Early symptoms of baclofen withdrawal may include return of baseline spasticity, pruritus, hypotension, and paresthesias. Some clinical characteristics of the advanced intrathecal baclofen withdrawal syndrome may resemble autonomic dysreflexia, infection (sepsis), malignant hyperthermia, neuroleptic-malignant syndrome, or other conditions associated with a hypermetabolic state or widespread rhabdomyolysis.

The suggested treatment for intrathecal baclofen withdrawal is the restoration of intrathecal baclofen at or near the same dosage as before therapy was interrupted. If restoration of intrathecal delivery is delayed, treatment with GABA-ergic agonist drugs, such as oral or enteral baclofen, or oral, enteral, or IV benzodiazepines may prevent potentially fatal sequelae.

Hallucinations: Hallucinations have occurred after abrupt withdrawal of baclofen intrathecal injection.

Seizures: Seizures have been reported during overdose and with withdrawal from baclofen intrathecal injection and in patients maintained on therapeutic doses of baclofen intrathecal injection.

Fatalities:

Spasticity of spinal cord origin – There were 16 deaths reported among the 576 US patients treated with baclofen intrathecal injection in pre- and postmarketing studies evaluated as of December 1992. Because these patients were treated under uncontrolled clinical settings, it is impossible to determine definitively what role, if any, baclofen intrathecal injection played in their deaths.

Spasticity of cerebral origin – There were 3 deaths occurring among the 211 patients treated with baclofen intrathecal in premarketing studies as of March 1996. These deaths were not attributed to the therapy.

Need for spasticity: Use with caution where spasticity is used to sustain upright posture and balance in locomotion or whenever spasticity is utilized to obtain increased function.

Ovarian cysts: Ovarian cysts have been found by palpation in about 4% of multiple sclerosis patients treated with baclofen for up to 1 year. In most cases, these cysts disappeared spontaneously while patients continued to receive the drug. Ovarian cysts are estimated to occur spontaneously in about 1% to 5% of the normal female population.

Psychotic disorders: Cautiously treat patients suffering from psychotic disorders, schizophrenia, or confusional states and keep under careful surveillance because exacerbations of these conditions have been observed with oral administration.

Autonomic dysreflexia: Use baclofen intrathecal injection with caution in patients with a history of autonomic dysreflexia. The presence of nociceptive stimuli or abrupt withdrawal of baclofen intrathecal may cause an autonomic dysreflexic episode.

Renal function impairment: Because baclofen is primarily excreted unchanged through the kidneys, administer with caution to patients with impaired renal function. Dosage reduction may be necessary.

Hazardous tasks: Because of the possibility of sedation, patients should observe caution while driving or performing other tasks requiring alertness, coordination, or physical dexterity.

Pregnancy: Category C.

Lactation: In mothers treated with oral baclofen in therapeutic doses, the active substance passes into the breast milk. It is not known whether detectable levels of drug are present in breast milk of nursing mothers receiving intrathecal baclofen.

Children:

Oral – Safety for use in children younger than 12 years of age has not been established. Oral baclofen is not recommended for use in children.

Intrathecal – Safety in children younger than 4 years of age has not been established.

Drug Interactions

Alcohol and other CNS depressants: Patients should also be cautioned that the CNS depressant effects of baclofen intrathecal injection may be additive to those of alcohol and other CNS depressants.

Adverse Reactions

Adverse reactions occurring in at least 3% of patients included the following:

Oral: Blurred vision, confusion, coma, constipation, dizziness/lightheadedness, drowsiness, headache, hypotension, hypotonia, insomnia, lethargy/fatigue, nausea/vomiting, numbness/itching/tingling, seizures, slurred speech, urinary frequency, weakness of extremities.

Intrathecal: Accidental injury, constipation, convulsion, death, dizziness, dry mouth, headache, hypertonia, hypotonia, hypoventilation, nausea, pain, paresthesia, peripheral edema, pruritus, somnolence, speech disorder, urinary retention, vomiting.

CARISOPRODOL

Tablets; oral: 250 mg (*Rx*) 350 mg (*Rx*)	Various, *Soma* (MedPointe)

Indications

Musculoskeletal conditions: For the relief of discomfort associated with acute, painful musculoskeletal conditions in adults.

Administration and Dosage

Dosage: 250 to 350 mg 3 times a day and at bedtime. The recommended maximum duration of carisoprodol use is up to 2 or 3 weeks.

Actions

Pharmacology: The mode of action has not been clearly identified, but may be related to its sedative properties. Carisoprodol produces muscle relaxation in animals by blocking interneuronal activity in the descending reticular formation and spinal cord.

Pharmacokinetics: The onset of action is rapid (30 minutes) and effects last 4 to 6 hours.

Contraindications

Acute intermittent porphyria as well as allergic or idiosyncratic reactions to carisoprodol or related compounds such as meprobamate, mebutamate or tybamate.

Warnings/Precautions

Hypersensitivity reactions: Rarely, the first dose of carisoprodol has been followed by idiosyncratic symptoms appearing within minutes or hours. Symptoms reported include extreme weakness, transient quadriplegia, dizziness, ataxia, temporary loss of vision, diplopia, mydriasis, dysarthria, agitation, euphoria, confusion, and disorientation. Symptoms usually subside over the next several hours.

Renal/Hepatic function impairment: To avoid excess accumulation, caution should be exercised in administration to patients with compromised liver or kidney function.

Drug abuse and dependence: In clinical use, psychological dependence and abuse have been rare, and there have been no reports of significant abstinence signs. Nevertheless, the drug should be used with caution in addiction-prone individuals.

Hazardous tasks: Carisoprodal may impair the mental or physical abilities required for the performance of potentially hazardous tasks such as driving a motor vehicle or operating machinery.

Pregnancy: Category C.

Lactation: Safe usage of this drug in lactation has not been established. Therefore, use of this drug in nursing mothers requires that the potential benefits of the drug be weighed against the potential hazards to mother and child

Children: Because of limited clinical experience, carisoprodol is not recommended for use in patients less than 12 years of age.

Drug Interactions

CNS agents: Because the effects of carisoprodol and alcohol or carisoprodol and other CNS depressants or psychotropic drugs may be additive, appropriate caution should be exercised with patients who take more than one of these agents simultaneously.

Adverse Reactions

Allergic: Allergic or idiosyncratic reactions occasionally develop. Skin rash, erythema multiforme, pruritus, eosinophilia, and fixed drug eruption with cross reaction to meprobamate have been reported with carisoprodol. Severe reactions have been manifested by asthmatic episodes, fever, weakness, dizziness, angioneurotic edema, smarting eyes, hypotension, and anaphylactoid shock.

Cardiovascular: Tachycardia, postural hypotension, and facial flushing.

CNS: Drowsiness and other CNS effects, dizziness, vertigo, ataxia, tremor, agitation, irritability, headache, depressive reactions, syncope, insomnia

GI: Nausea, vomiting, hiccup, and epigastric distress.

Hematologic: Leukopenia, in which other drugs or viral infection may have been responsible, and pancytopenia, attributed to phenylbutazone, have been reported.

CHLORZOXAZONE

Tablets: 250 mg (*Rx*)	Various, *Paraflex* (McNeil), *Remular-S* (Inter. Ethical)
500 mg (*Rx*)	Various, *Parafon Forte DSC* (NcNeil)

Indications

Musculoskeletal conditions: As an adjunct to rest, physical therapy, and other measures for the relief of discomfort associated with acute, painful musculoskeletal conditions.

Administration and Dosage

Usual adult dose:

Tablets (500 mg) – 1 tablet 3 or 4 times daily. If adequate response is not obtained, increase to 1 ½ tablets (750 mg) 3 or 4 times daily. As improvement occurs, reduce dosage.

Tablets (250 mg) – 1 tablet (250 mg) 3 or 4 times daily. Initial dosage for painful musculoskeletal conditions should be 2 tablets (500 mg) 3 or 4 times daily. If adequate response is not obtained, increase to 3 tablets (750 mg) 3 or 4 times daily. As improvement occurs, reduce dosage.

Actions

Pharmacology: Chlorzoxazone is a centrally acting agent that acts primarily at the level of the spinal cord and subcortical areas of the brain where it inhibits multisynaptic reflex arcs involved in producing and maintaining skeletal muscle spasm. The clinical result is a reduction of the skeletal muscle spasm with relief of pain and increased mobility of the involved muscles.

Pharmacokinetics:

Absorption – Blood levels of chlorzoxazone can be detected during the first 30 minutes and peak levels may be reached in about 1 to 2 hours after oral administration of chlorzoxazone.

Metabolism/Excretion – Chlorzoxazone is rapidly metabolized and is excreted in the urine, primarily in a conjugated form as the glucuronide. Less than 1% of a chlorzoxazone dose is excreted unchanged in the urine in 24 hours.

Contraindications

Intolerance to the drug.

Warnings/Precautions

Hepatotoxicity: Serious (including fatal) hepatocellular toxicity has been reported rarely.

Hypersensitivity reactions: Use with caution in patients with known allergies or with a history of allergic reactions to drugs.

Pregnancy: Category C.

Drug Interactions

The concomitant use of alcohol or other CNS depressants with chlorzoxazone may have an additive effect.

Adverse Reactions

Dizziness, drowsiness, GI disturbances, lightheadedness, malaise, overstimulation.

CYCLOBENZAPRINE HYDROCHLORIDE

Tablets: 5 and 10 mg (*Rx*)	Various, *Flexeril* (McNeil)
7.5 mg (*Rx*)	Various, *Fexmid* (Victory)
Capsules, extended-release: 15 and 30 mg (*Rx*)	*Amrix* (ECR)

Indications

Musculoskeletal conditions: Adjunct to rest and physical therapy for relief of muscle spasm associated with acute painful musculoskeletal conditions.

Administration and Dosage

Tablets: Give 5 mg 3 times/day; may be increased to 7.5 or 10 mg 3 times/day. Do not use longer than 2 or 3 weeks.

Extended-release capsules: 15 mg capsule taken once daily. Some patients may require up to 30 mg/day. Instruct patients to take doses at approximately the same time each day. Do not use longer than 2 to 3 weeks.

Actions

Pharmacology: Cyclobenzaprine relieves skeletal muscle spasm of local origin without interfering with muscle function. It is ineffective in muscle spasm caused by CNS disease.

Pharmacokinetics:

Absorption/Distribution –

Tablets: Mean oral bioavailability of cyclobenzaprine range from 33% to 55%. It is highly bound to plasma proteins. Drug accumulates when dosed 3 times a day, reaching steady state within 3 to 4 days.

Capsules: For the cyclobenzaprine 15 mg capsule, the time to maximum concentration is about 8 hours and the half-life is about 33 hours.

Metabolism/Excretion – Cyclobenzaprine is extensively metabolized, and is excreted primarily as glucuronides via the kidney. Cyclobenzaprine has an elimination half-life of 18 hours (tablets) and 32 hours (capsules).

Contraindications

Hypersensitivity to any component of this product; acute recovery phase of myocardial infarction; arrhythmias; heart block or conduction disturbances; congestive heart failure; hyperthyroidism. Concomitant use of monoamine oxidase inhibitors (MAOIs) or within 14 days after their discontinuation. Hyperpyretic crisis seizures, and deaths have occurred in patients receiving cyclobenzaprine (or structurally similar TCAs) concomitantly with MAOIs.

Warnings/Precautions

Spasticity: Cyclobenzaprine is not effective in the treatment of spasticity associated with cerebral or spinal cord disease, or in children with cerebral palsy.

Duration: Use only for short periods (up to 2 or 3 weeks); effectiveness for more prolonged use is not proven.

Similarity to TCAs: Cyclobenzaprine is closely related to the TCAs. In short-term studies for indications other than muscle spasm associated with acute musculoskeletal conditions, and usually at doses greater than those recommended, some of the more serious CNS reactions noted with the TCAs have occurred.

Anticholinergic effects: Because of its anticholinergic action, use with caution in patients with a history of urinary retention, angle-closure glaucoma, and increased intraocular pressure.

Hepatic function impairment: The plasma concentration of cyclobenzaprine is increased in patients with hepatic function impairment.

Use cyclobenzaprine tablets with caution in patients with mild hepatic function impairment starting with a 5 mg dose and titrating slowly upward. Use of cyclobenzaprine capsules is not recommended in subjects with mild, moderate, or severe hepatic function impairment.

Drug abuse and dependence: Similarities among the tricyclic drugs require that certain withdrawal symptoms be considered when cyclobenzaprine is administered. Abrupt cessation of treatment after prolonged administration may rarely produce nausea, headache, and malaise.

Hazardous tasks: May impair mental or physical abilities required for performance of hazardous tasks; patients should observe caution while driving or performing other tasks requiring alertness, coordination, and physical dexterity.

Pregnancy: Category B.

Lactation: It is not known whether cyclobenzaprine is excreted in breast milk.

Children: Safety and efficacy in children younger than 15 years of age have not been established.

Elderly:

Tablets – Use cyclobenzaprine only if clearly needed. In such patients, initiate cyclobenzaprine with a 5 mg dose and titrate slowly upward.

Capsules – The plasma concentration and half-life of cyclobenzaprine are substantially increased in elderly patients; do not use cyclobenzaprine capsules in elderly patients.

Drug Interactions

Drugs that may interact with cyclobenzaprine include MAOIs, CNS depressants, guanethidine, and tramadol.

Drug/Food interactions: A single dose of cyclobenzaprine 30 mg demonstrated a statistically significant increase in bioavailability when given with food relative to the fasted state. There was a 35% increase in peak plasma cyclobenzaprine concentration and a 20% increase in exposure in the presence of food.

Adverse Reactions

Adverse reactions occurring in 3% or more of patients include acne, blurred vision, drowsiness, dizziness, fatigue, headache, dry mouth/throat, constipation, disturbance in attention, dysgeusia, dyspepsia, nausea, palpitations, somnolence, and tremor.

METAXALONE

Tablets; oral: 800 mg (*Rx*)	*Skelaxin* (King)

Indications

Musculoskeletal conditions: As an adjunct to rest, physical therapy, and other measures for the relief of discomforts associated with acute, painful musculoskeletal conditions.

Administration and Dosage

Adults: One 800 mg tablet 3 to 4 times a day.

Actions

Pharmacology: The mechanism of action in humans has not been established but may be due to general CNS depression.

Pharmacokinetics:

Absorption/Distribution – The absolute bioavailability of metaxalone is not known. Peak plasma concentrations of metaxalone occur approximately 3 hours after a 400 mg oral dose under fasted conditions. Doubling the dose of metaxalone from 400 to 800 mg results in a roughly proportional increase in metaxalone exposure, as indicated by peak plasma concentrations and area under the curve.

Mean (% CV) Metaxalone Pharmacokinetic Parameters[a]					
Dose (mg) (ng/mL)	C_{max}	T_{max} (h)	AUC_{∞} (ng•h/mL)	Half-life (h)	CL/F (L/h)
400[b]	983 (53)	3.3 (35)	7,479 (51)	9 (53)	68 (50)
800[c]	1,816 (43)	3 (39)	15,044 (46)	8 (58)	66 (51)

[a] CV = coefficient of variation; C_{max} = peak plasma concentrations; T_{max} = time to maximum concentration; AUC = area under the curve; CL/F = apparent oral clearance.

[b] Subjects received 1 × 400 mg tablet under fasted conditions (n= 42).

[c] Subjects received 2 × 400 mg tablets under fasted conditions (n= 59).

Compared with fasted conditions, the presence of a high-fat meal at the time of drug administration increased C_{max} by 177.5% and increased AUC (AUC_{0-t}, AUC_8) by 123.5% and 115.4%, respectively. T_{max} was also delayed (4.3 vs 3.3 h) and terminal half-life was decreased (2.4 vs 9 h) under fed conditions compared with the fasted state.

Metabolism/Excretion – Metaxalone is metabolized by the liver and excreted in the urine as unidentified metabolites.

Contraindications

Hypersensitivity to the drug; tendency to drug-induced, hemolytic, or other anemias; significant renal or hepatic function impairment.

Warnings/Precautions

CNS effects: Taking metaxalone with food may enhance general CNS depression; elderly patients may be especially susceptible to this CNS effect.

Hepatic function impairment: Administer metaxalone with great care to patients with preexisting liver damage. Perform serial liver function studies in these patients.

Hazardous tasks: Metaxalone may impair the mental or physical abilities required for performance of hazardous tasks, such as operating machinery or driving a motor vehicle, especially when used with alcohol or other CNS depressants.

Pregnancy: Safe use of metaxalone has not been established with regard to possible adverse reactions on fetal development. Do not use metaxalone tablets in women who are or may become pregnant and particularly during early pregnancy unless in the judgment of the health care provider the potential benefits outweigh the possible hazards.

Lactation: It is not known whether this drug is secreted in human milk.

Children: Safety and efficacy in children 12 years of age and younger have not been established.

Drug Interactions

CNS depressants: Metaxalone may enhance the effects of alcohol, barbiturates, and other CNS depressants.

Drug/Lab test interactions: False-positive Benedict test.

Adverse Reactions

Adverse reactions that may occur during treatment include the following: Dizziness, drowsiness, GI upset, headache, hemolytic anemia, hypersensitivity reaction, irritability, jaundice, leukopenia, nausea, nervousness, rash with or without pruritus, vomiting.

METHOCARBAMOL

Tablets; oral: 500 and 750 mg (*Rx*) Various, *Robaxin* (Schwarz Pharma)
Injection solution: 100 mg/mL (*Rx*)

Indications

As an adjunct to rest, physical therapy, and other measures for the relief of discomfort associated with acute, painful musculoskeletal conditions.

Administration and Dosage

Oral:

500 mg tablets – Initial dosage is 3 tablets 4 times a day, and maintenance dosage is 2 tablets 4 times a day.

750 mg tablets – Initial dosage is 2 tablets 4 times a day and maintenance dosage is 1 tablet every 4 hours, or 2 tablets 3 times a day.

6 g/day is recommended for the first 48 to 72 hours of treatment (for severe conditions 8 g/day may be administered). Thereafter, the dosage usually can be reduced to approximately 4 g/day.

Injection: For IV and IM use only. Total adult dosage should not exceed 30 mL (3 vials) a day for more than 3 consecutive days except in the treatment of tetanus. A like course may be repeated after a lapse of 48 hours if the condition persists.

For the relief of symptoms of moderate degree, 10 mL (1 vial) may be adequate. Ordinarily this injection need not be repeated, as the administration of the oral form will usually sustain the relief initiated by the injection. For the severest cases or in postoperative conditions in which oral administration is not feasible, 20 to 30 mL (2 to 3 vials) may be required.

Directions for IV use – May be administered undiluted directly into the vein at a maximum rate of 3 mL/min. It may also be added to an IV drip of sodium chloride injection (sterile isotonic sodium chloride solution for parenteral use) or 5% dextrose injection (sterile 5% dextrose solution); 1 vial given as a single dose should not be diluted to more than 250 mL for IV infusion. Care should be exercised to avoid vascular extravasation of this hypertonic solution. It is preferable that the patient be in a recumbent position during and for at least 10 to 15 minutes following the injection.

Directions for IM use – When the IM route is indicated, not more than 5 mL (one-half vial) should be injected into each gluteal region. The injections may be repeated at 8 hour intervals, if necessary.

Not recommended for subcutaneous administration.

Special directions for use in tetanus – There is clinical evidence which suggests that methocarbamol may have a beneficial effect in the control of the neuromuscular manifestations of tetanus. It does not, however, replace the usual procedure of debridement, tetanus antitoxin, penicillin, tracheotomy, attention to fluid balance, and supportive care. Methocarbamol should be added to the regimen as soon as possible.

For adults: Inject 1 or 2 vials directly into the tubing of the previously inserted indwelling needle. An additional 10 mL or 20 mL may be added to the infusion bottle so that a total of up to 30 mL (3 vials) is given as the initial dose. Rate of injection should not exceed 3 mL/min. Since methocarbamol injectable is hypertonic, vascular extravasation must be avoided. A recumbent position will reduce the likelihood of side reactions. This procedure should be repeated every 6 hours until conditions allow for the insertion of a nasogastric tube. Crushed methocarbamol tablets suspended in water or saline may then be given through this tube. Total daily oral doses up to 24 g may be required

For children: A minimum initial dose of 15 mg/kg is recommended. This dosage may be repeated every 6 hours as indicated. The maintenance dosage may be given by injection into tubing or by IV infusion with an appropriate quantity of fluid. See directions for IV use.

Actions

Pharmacology: The mechanism of action of methocarbamol in humans has not been established, but may be due to CNS depression.

Pharmacokinetics:

Absorption – Methocarbamol has an onset of action of 30 minutes. Peak plasma levels occur approximately 2 hours after administration.

Metabolism/Excretion – The half-life is from 1 to 2 hours; inactive metabolites are excreted in the urine and small amounts in the feces.

Contraindications

Hypersensitivity to any of the ingredients or to any of the injection components; known or suspected renal pathology. This caution is necessary because of the presence of polyethylene glycol 300 in the vehicle.

Warnings/Precautions

Administration: Rate of injection should not exceed 3 mL/min, (one 10 mL vial in approximately 3 minutes). Since methocarbamol injectable is hypertonic, vascular extravasation must be avoided. A recumbent position will reduce the likelihood of side reactions.

Special risk: Caution should be observed in using the injectable form in patients with suspected or known seizure disorders.

Hazardous tasks: Methocarbamol may impair mental or physical abilities required for performance of hazardous tasks, such as operating machinery or driving a motor vehicle. Caution patients about operating machinery, including automobiles, until they are reasonably certain that methocarbamol therapy does not adversely affect their ability to engage in such activities.

Pregnancy: Category C.

Lactation: It is not known whether methocarbamol or its metabolites are excreted in human milk.

Children: Safety and efficacy of methocarbamol in children younger than 16 years of age have not been established. Safety and effectiveness of methocarbamol injection in children have not been established except in tetanus.

Drug Interactions

Drugs that may interact with methocarbamol include pyridostigmine and CNS agents.

Drug/Lab test interactions: Methocarbamol may cause a color interference in certain screening tests for 5-hydroxyindoleacetic acid (5-HIAA) using nitrosonaphthol reagent and in screening tests for urinary vanillylmandelic acid (VMA) using the Gitlow method.

Adverse Reactions

Adverse reactions that may occur during treatment include the following: amnesia, anaphylactic reaction, angioneurotic edema, blurred vision, conjunctivitis, bradycardia, confusion, diplopia, dizziness or light-headedness, drowsiness, dyspepsia, fever, flushing, headache, hypersensitivity reactions, hypotension, insomnia, jaundice (including cholestatic jaundice), leukopenia, metallic taste, mild muscular incoordination, nasal congestion, nausea, nystagmus, pruritus, rash, sedation, seizures (including grand mal), syncope, thrombophlebitis, urticaria, vertigo, vomiting.

ORPHENADRINE CITRATE

Tablets; oral: 100 mg (*Rx*)	Various
Tablets, sustained release; oral: 100 mg (*Rx*)	*Orphenadrine* (Apothecon)
Injection solution: 30 mg/mL (*Rx*)	Various, *Banflex* (Forest Pharm.), *Flexon* (Various), *Norflex* (3M Pharm)

Indications

As an adjunct to rest, physical therapy, and other measures for the relief of discomfort associated with acute painful musculoskeletal conditions.

Administration and Dosage

Oral: 100 mg in the morning and 100 mg in the evening.

Injection: 60 mg IV or IM; may be repeated every 12 hours. Relief may be maintained by 1 orphenadrine extended-release tablet twice daily.

Actions

Pharmacology: The mode of therapeutic action has not been clearly identified, but may be related to its analgesic properties. Orphenadrine also possesses anticholinergic actions.

Pharmacokinetics:

Absorption – Peak plasma levels occur 2 hours after administration; duration of action is 4 to 6 hours.

Metabolism/Excretion – The half-life is approximately 14 hours for the parent drug and 2 to 25 hours for metabolites. Excretion is via urine and feces.

Contraindications

Glaucoma, pyloric or duodenal obstruction, stenosing peptic ulcers, prostatic hypertrophy or obstruction of the bladder neck, cardiospasm (megaesophagus) and myasthenia gravis; hypersensitivity to the drug.

Warnings/Precautions

Long-term therapy: Safety of continuous long-term therapy has not been established. If orphenadrine is prescribed for prolonged use, periodic monitoring of blood, urine, and liver function values is recommended.

Cardiac disease: Use with caution in patients with tachycardia, cardiac decompensation, coronary insufficiency, cardiac arrhythmias.

Sulfite sensitivity: Orphenadrine injection contains sodium bisulfite, a sulfite that may cause allergic-type reactions including anaphylactic symptoms and life-threatening or less severe asthmatic episodes in certain susceptible people. Sulfite sensitivity is seen more frequently in asthmatic than nonasthmatic people.

Hazardous tasks: Orphenadrine may impair the ability of the patient to engage in potentially hazardous activities such as operating machinery or driving a motor vehicle; ambulatory patients should therefore be cautioned accordingly.

Pregnancy: Category C.

Children: Safety and efficacy in children have not been established.

Drug Interactions

Drugs that may interact with orphenadrine include amantadine, haloperidol, and phenothiazines.

Adverse Reactions

Adverse reactions that may occur during treatment include the following: agitation, blurred vision, constipation, dilation of pupils, dizziness, drowsiness, dryness of the mouth, gastric irritation, hallucinations, headache, hypersensitivity reactions, increased ocular tension, mental confusion, nausea, palpitation, pruritus, tachycardia, tremor, urinary hesitancy or retention, vomiting, weakness.

TIZANIDINE HYDROCHLORIDE

Tablets: 2 and 4 mg (as base) (*Rx*)	Various, *Zanaflex* (Acorda Therapeutics)
Capsules: 2, 4, and 6 mg (as base) (*Rx*)	*Zanaflex* (Acorda Therapeutics)

Indications

Muscle spasticity: For the management of spasticity.

Administration and Dosage

Dosage: A single oral dose of tizanidine 8 mg reduces muscle tone in patients with spasticity for a period of several hours. The effect peaks at approximately 1 to 2 hours and dissipates between 3 and 6 hours. Effects are dose related.

Although single doses of less than 8 mg have not been determined to be effective in controlled clinical studies, the dose-related nature of tizanidine's common adverse reactions makes it prudent to begin therapy with single oral doses of 4 mg. Increase the dose gradually (2 to 4 mg steps) to achieve optimal effect.

Repeat dose at 6– to 8–hour intervals, as needed, to a maximum of 3 doses in 24 hours. Do not exceed 36 mg/day.

Experience with single doses exceeding 8 mg and daily doses exceeding 24 mg is limited. There is essentially no experience with repeated, single, daytime doses greater than 12 mg or total daily doses greater than 36 mg.

Administration: Food has complex effects on tizanidine pharmacokinetics, which differ with the different formulations.

Actions

Pharmacology: Tizanidine is an agonist at alpha-2 adrenergic receptor sites and presumably reduces spasticity by increasing presynaptic inhibition of motor neurons.

Pharmacokinetics:

Absorption/Distribution – Following oral administration, tizanidine is essentially completely absorbed. Tizanidine is extensively distributed throughout the body, with a mean steady-state volume of distribution of 2.4 L/kg. Tizanidine is approximately 30% bound to plasma proteins.

Tizanidine tablets and capsules are bioequivalent to each other under fasted conditions but not under fed conditions.

Following oral administration of the tablet or capsule (in the fasted state), tizanidine peak plasma concentrations occur 1 hour after dosing, with a half-life of approximately 2 hours.

When two 4 mg tablets are administered with food, the mean maximal plasma concentration (C_{max}) is increased approximately 30%, and the median time to peak plasma concentration is increased from 25 minutes to 1 hour and 25 minutes.

In contrast, when two 4 mg capsules are administered with food, the mean C_{max} is decreased 20%, and the median time to peak plasma concentration is increased from 2 hours to 3 hours. Consequently, the C_{max} for the capsule when administered with food is approximately two-thirds the C_{max} for the tablet when administered with food.

Food also increases the extent of absorption for tablets and capsules. The increase with the tablet (approximately 30%) is significantly greater than with the capsule (approximately 10%). Consequently, when each is administered with food, the amount absorbed from the capsule is about 80% of the amount absorbed from the tablet. Administration of the capsule contents on applesauce results in a 15% to 20% increase in C_{max} and AUC of tizanidine compared with administration of an intact capsule while fasting and a 15-minute decrease in the median lag time and time to C_{max}.

Metabolism/Excretion – The absolute oral bioavailability of tizanidine is approximately 40% (CV = 24%), due to extensive first-pass metabolism in the liver; approximately 95% of an administered dose is metabolized. Tizanidine metabolites are not known to be active; their half-lives range from 20 to 40 hours.

Special populations –

Age: Cross-study comparison of pharmacokinetic data following single-dose administration of tizanidine 6 mg showed that younger subjects cleared the drug 4 times faster than the elderly subjects.

Hepatic function impairment: Because tizanidine is extensively metabolized in the liver, hepatic function impairment would be expected to have significant effects on the pharmacokinetics of tizanidine. Ordinarily, avoid tizanidine use or use it with extreme caution in this patient population.

Renal function impairment: Tizanidine clearance is reduced by greater than 50% in elderly patients with renal insufficiency (creatinine clearance less than 25 mL/min) compared with healthy elderly subjects; this would be expected to lead to a longer duration of clinical effect. Use tizanidine with caution in patients with renal function impairment.

Contraindications

Known hypersensitivity to tizanidine or its ingredients; concomitant use of tizanidine with fluvoxamine, a potent inhibitor of CYP-450 1A2, is contraindicated.

Warnings/Precautions

Long-term use: Clinical experience with long-term use of tizanidine at doses of 8 to 16 mg single doses or total daily doses of 24 to 36 mg is limited.

Hypotension: Tizanidine is an alpha-2 adrenergic agonist (eg, clonidine) and can produce hypotension. The hypotensive effect is dose related and has been measured following single doses of greater than or equal to 2 mg.

Sedation: In the multiple-dose, controlled clinical studies, 48% of patients receiving any dose of tizanidine reported sedation as an adverse event.

The effect appears to be dose related.

Hallucinosis/psychotic-like symptoms: Tizanidine use has been associated with hallucinations. Formed visual hallucinations or delusions have been reported.

Cardiovascular: Prolongation of the QT interval and bradycardia were noted in chronic toxicity studies in dogs at doses equal to the maximum human dose on a mg/m^2 basis.

Ophthalmic: Dose-related retinal degeneration and corneal opacities have been found in animal studies at doses equivalent to approximately the maximum recommended dose on a mg/m^2 basis.

Discontinuing therapy: If therapy needs to be discontinued, especially in patients who have been receiving high doses for long periods, decrease the dose slowly to minimize the risk of withdrawal and rebound hypertension, tachycardia, and hypertonia.

Renal function impairment: Use tizanidine with caution in patients with renal insufficiency (creatinine clearance less than 25 mL/min), as clearance is reduced by greater than 50%.

Hepatic function impairment: Monitoring of aminotransferase levels is recommended during the first 6 months of treatment (eg, baseline, 1, 3 and 6 months) and periodically thereafter, based on clinical status. Avoid the drug or use with extreme caution in patients with hepatic function impairment.

Risk of liver injury – Tizanidine occasionally causes liver injury, most often hepatocellular in type.

Drug abuse and dependence: Tizanidine is closely related to clonidine, which is often abused in combination with narcotics and is known to cause symptoms of rebound upon abrupt withdrawal. Case reports suggest that patients experiencing this were also misusing narcotics. Withdrawal symptoms included hypertension, tachycardia, hypertonia, tremor, and anxiety. Withdrawal is expected to be more likely in cases in which high doses are used, especially for prolonged periods.

Pregnancy: Category C.

Lactation: It is not known whether tizanidine is excreted in human milk; although, as a lipid-soluble drug, it might be expected to pass into breast milk.

Children: There are no adequate and well-controlled studies to document the safety and efficacy of tizanidine in children.

Elderly: Use tizanidine with caution in elderly patients because clearance is decreased 4-fold.

Monitoring: Monitoring of aminotransferase levels is recommended during the first 6 months of treatment (eg, baseline, 1, 3, and 6 months) and periodically thereafter. Because of the potential toxic hepatic effect of tizanidine, use the drug with extreme caution in patients with hepatic function impairment.

Drug Interactions

Drugs that may affect tizanidine include acyclovir, alcohol, antiarrhythmics, cimetidine, oral contraceptives, famotidine, fluoroquinolones, fluvoxamine, rofecoxib, ticlopidine, and zileuton.

Drugs that may be affected by tizanidine include acetaminophen and antihypertensives.

Adverse Reactions

The adverse reactions most frequently leading to withdrawal of tizanidine-treated patients in the controlled clinical studies were asthenia (eg, weakness, fatigue, tiredness) (3%), somnolence (3%), dry mouth (3%), increased spasm or tone (2%), and dizziness (2%).

Adverse reactions experienced in at least 3% of patients include the following: amblyopia, ALT increased, asthenia, bradycardia, constipation, dizziness, dry mouth, dyskinesia, flu syndrome, hypotension, infection, liver function tests abnormal, nervousness, pharyngitis, rhinitis, somnolence, speech disorder, urinary frequency, urinary tract infection, vomiting.

DANTROLENE SODIUM

Capsules: 25, 50, and 100 mg (*Rx*)	Various, *Dantrium* (Procter & Gamble)
Powder for injection: 20 mg/vial (approximately 0.32 mg/mL after reconstitution) (*Rx*)	*Dantrium Intravenous* (Procter & Gamble)

Warning:

Dantrolene has a potential for hepatotoxicity. Do not use in conditions other than those recommended. Symptomatic hepatitis (fatal and nonfatal) has been reported at various dose levels of the drug. The incidence of symptomatic hepatitis (fatal and nonfatal) reported in patients taking up to 400 mg/day is much lower than in those taking 800 mg/day or more. Even sporadic short courses of these higher dose levels within a treatment regimen markedly increased the risk of serious hepatic injury. Liver dysfunction, as evidenced by liver enzyme elevations, has been observed in patients exposed to the drug for varying periods of time. Overt hepatitis has been most frequently observed between the third and twelfth months of therapy. Risk of hepatic injury appears to be greater in females, in patients older than 35 years of age, and in patients taking other medications in addition to dantrolene. Use dantrolene only in conjunction with appropriate monitoring of hepatic function including frequent determination of AST and ALT.

If no observable benefit is derived from therapy after 45 days, discontinue use.

Use the lowest possible effective dose for each patient.

Indications

Spasticity:

Oral – For the control of clinical spasticity resulting from upper motor neuron disorders such as spinal cord injury, stroke, cerebral palsy, or multiple sclerosis.

Malignant hyperthermia (MH):

IV – Management of the fulminant hypermetabolism of skeletal muscle characteristic of MH crisis, along with appropriate supportive measures.

Preoperatively, and sometimes postoperatively, to prevent or attenuate the development of clinical and laboratory signs of MH in individuals judged to be susceptible to MH.

Oral – Preoperatively to prevent or attenuate the development of signs of MH in susceptible patients who require anesthesia or surgery. Currently accepted clinical practices in the management of such patients must still be adhered to (careful monitoring for early signs of MH, minimizing exposure to triggering mechanisms, and prompt use of IV dantrolene and indicated supportive measures if signs of MH appear).

Following a MH crisis to prevent recurrence of MH.

Administration and Dosage

Exercise caution at meals on the day of administration because difficulty swallowing and choking has been reported.

Chronic spasticity: In view of the potential for liver damage in long-term use, discontinue therapy if benefits are not evident within 45 days.

Adults – Maintain each dosage level for 7 days to determine the patient's response. If no further benefit is observed at the next higher dose, decrease the dosage to the previous lower dose. Begin with 25 mg once daily for 7 days; then increase to 25 mg 3 times daily for 7 days; then increase to 50 mg 3 times daily for 7 days with a final dosage of 100 mg 3 times daily.

Therapy with a dose 4 times daily may be necessary for some individuals. Do not use doses higher than 100 mg 4 times daily.

Children – Maintain each dosage level for 7 days to determine the patient's response. If no further benefit is observed at the next higher dose, decrease the dosage to the previous lower dose. Start with 0.5 mg/kg once daily for 7 days; then increase to 0.5 mg/kg 3 times daily for 7 days; then increase to 1 mg/kg 3 times daily for 7 days with a final dosage of 2 mg/kg 3 times daily. Therapy with a dose 4 times daily may be necessary for some individuals.

Do not use doses higher than 100 mg 4 times daily.

MH:

Preoperative prophylaxis – Dantrolene may be given orally or IV to patients judged susceptible to MH as part of the overall patient management to prevent or attenuate development of clinical and laboratory signs of MH.

Oral – Give 4 to 8 mg/kg/day orally in 3 or 4 divided doses for 1 or 2 days prior to surgery, with last dose given approximately 3 to 4 hours before scheduled surgery with a minimum of water. This dosage usually will be associated with skeletal muscle weakness and sedation (sleepiness or drowsiness); adjust within the recommended dosage range to avoid incapacitation or excessive GI irritation.

IV – 2.5 mg/kg, starting approximately 1 hour and 15 minutes before anticipated anesthesia and infused over approximately 1 hour.

Additional dantrolene IV may be indicated because of the appearance of early clinical and/or blood gas signs of malignant hyperthermia or because of prolonged surgery.

Treatment – As soon as the MH reaction is recognized, discontinue all anesthetic agents. Use of 100% oxygen is recommended. Administer dantrolene by continuous rapid IV push beginning at a minimum dose of 1 mg/kg, and continuing until symptoms subside or a maximum cumulative dose of 10 mg/kg has been reached. If the physiologic and metabolic abnormalities reappear, repeat the regimen. Administration should be continuous until symptoms subside.

Children – Dose is the same as for adults.

Postcrisis follow-up – Following a MH crisis, give 4 to 8 mg/kg/day orally, in 4 divided doses for 1 to 3 days to prevent recurrence. IV dantrolene may be used when oral administration is not practical. The IV dose must be individualized, starting with 1 mg/kg or more as the clinical situation dictates.

Actions

Pharmacology: In isolated nerve-muscle preparation, dantrolene produced relaxation by affecting contractile response of the skeletal muscle at a site beyond the myoneural junction and directly on the muscle itself. In skeletal muscle, the drug dissociates the excitation-contraction coupling, probably by interfering with the release of calcium from the sarcoplasmic reticulum.

MH – Dantrolene may prevent changes within the muscle cell that result in MH syndrome by interfering with calcium release from the sarcoplasmic reticulum to the myoplasm.

Pharmacokinetics:

Absorption/Distribution – Absorption after oral administration is incomplete and slow but consistent, and dose-related blood levels are obtained.

Metabolism – Dantrolene is found in measurable amounts in blood and urine. Mean half-life in adults is 9 hours after a 100 mg dose. Because it is probably metabolized by hepatic microsomal enzymes, metabolism enhancement by other drugs is possible.

Contraindications

Oral: Active hepatic disease, such as hepatitis and cirrhosis; where spasticity is used to sustain upright posture and balance in locomotion or to obtain or maintain increased function.

Warnings/Precautions

Hepatic effects: Fatal and nonfatal liver disorders of an idiosyncratic or hypersensitivity type may occur. At the start of therapy, perform baseline liver function studies. If abnormalities exist, the potential for hepatotoxicity could be enhanced.

Perform liver function studies at appropriate intervals during therapy. If such studies reveal abnormal values, generally discontinue therapy. Some laboratory values may return to normal with continued therapy; others may not.

If symptoms of hepatitis accompanied by liver function test abnormalities or jaundice appear, discontinue therapy. If caused by dantrolene and detected early, abnormalities may revert to normal when the drug is discontinued. See Warning Box.

Long-term use: Safety and efficacy have not been established.

MH: IV use is not a substitute for previously known supportive measures. These measures include discontinuing the suspect triggering agents, attending to increased oxygen requirements, managing the metabolic acidosis, instituting cooling when necessary, attending to urinary output, and monitoring electrolyte imbalance.

Extravasation: Because of the high pH of the IV formulation, prevent extravasation into the surrounding tissues.

Mannitol: When mannitol is used for prevention or treatment of late renal complications of malignant hyperthermia, the 3 g of mannitol needed to dissolve each 20 mg vial of IV dantrolene should be taken into consideration.

Hepatic function impairment: Fatal and nonfatal liver disorders of an idiosyncratic or hypersensitivity type may occur with dantrolene therapy.

Special risk: Use with caution in patients with impaired pulmonary function, particularly those with obstructive pulmonary disease; severely impaired cardiac function caused by myocardial disease; history of previous liver disease or dysfunction.

Hazardous tasks: Patients should use caution while driving or performing other tasks requiring alertness, coordination or physical dexterity.

Photosensitivity: Caution patients about exposure to sunlight while taking dantrolene.

Pregnancy: Category C (parenteral).

Lactation: Do not use in women who are breast-feeding.

Children: The long-term safety of dantrolene in children younger than 5 years of age has not been established.

Elderly: In general, dose selection for an elder patient should be cautious reflecting the greater frequency of decreased hepatic, renal, or cardiac function, and of concomitant disease or other drug therapy.

Drug Interactions

Drugs that may interact with dantrolene include calcium channel blockers, clofibrate, estrogens, vecuronium, and warfarin.

Avoid alcohol and other CNS depressants.

Adverse Reactions

Adverse reactions may include the following: abdominal cramps, abnormal hair growth, acne-like rash, anaphylaxis, anorexia, aplastic anemia, backache, chills, confusion, constipation, crystalluria, diarrhea, difficult erection, diplopia, drooling, drowsiness, dizziness, dysuria, eczematoid eruption, erratic blood pressure, excessive tearing, fatigue, feeling of suffocation, fever, gastric irritation, general malaise, headache, heart failure, hematuria, hepatitis, increased nervousness, increased urinary frequency, insomnia, GI bleeding, leukopenia, lightheadedness, lymphocytic lymphoma, mental depression, myalgia, nausea, nocturia, phlebitis, pleural effusion with pericarditis, pruritus, respiratory depression, seizure, speech disturbance, swallowing difficulty, sweating, tachycardia, taste alteration, thrombocytopenia, thrombophlebitis following IV dantrolene, urinary incontinence, urinary retention, urticaria, visual disturbance, vomiting, weakness.

PARKINSON DISEASE

Parkinsonism is a neurological disease with a variety of origins characterized by tremor, rigidity, akinesia, and disorders of posture and equilibrium. The onset is slow and progressive, with symptoms advancing over months to years.

Drug Therapy for Parkinsonism

Drugs	Indications					Usual daily dose range (mg)
	Post-encephalitic	Arterio-sclerotic	Idiopathic	Drug/ chemical induced	Adjunct to Levodopa/ carbidopa	
Anticholinergics						
Procyclidine	✓	✓	✓	✓		7.5 to 20
Trihexyphenidyl	✓	✓	✓	✓	✓	1 to 15
Benztropine	✓	✓	✓	✓		0.5 to 6.5
Biperiden	✓	✓	✓	✓		2 to 8
Ethopropazine	✓	✓	✓	✓		50 to 600
Diphenhydramine	✓	✓	✓	✓		10 to 400
Dopaminergic Agents						
Carbidopa/ Levodopa	✓		✓	✓[a]		10/100 to 200/2,000
Amantadine	✓	✓	✓	✓		200 to 400
Bromocriptine	✓		✓			12.5 to 100
Pergolide					✓	1 to 5
Selegiline					✓	10
Pramipexole			✓			0.375 to 4.5
Ropinirole			✓			0.75 to 3

[a] Not effective in drug-induced extrapyramidal symptoms.

ANTICHOLINERGICS

BENZTROPINE MESYLATE	
Tablets: 0.5, 1, and 2 mg (*Rx*)	Various, *Cogentin* (Merck)
Injection: 1 mg/mL (*Rx*)	*Cogentin* (Merck)
ETHOPROPAZINE HYDROCHLORIDE	
Tablets: 10 and 50 mg (*Rx*)	*Parsidol* (Parke-Davis)
TRIHEXYPHENIDYL HYDROCHLORIDE	
Tablets: 2 and 5 mg (*Rx*)	Various, *Artane* (Lederle)
Capsules, sustained release: 5 mg (*Rx*)	*Artane Sequels* (Lederle)
Elixir: 2 mg/5 mL (*Rx*)	*Artane* (Lederle)

Indications

Adjunctive therapy in all forms of parkinsonism (postencephalitic, arteriosclerotic and idiopathic) and in the control of drug-induced extrapyramidal disorders.

Administration and Dosage

Give before or after meals, as determined by patient's reaction. Postencephalitic patients (more prone to excessive salivation) may prefer to take it after meals and may, in addition, require small amounts of atropine. If the mouth dries excessively, take before meals, unless it causes nausea. If taken after meals, thirst can be allayed by mint candies, chewing gum, or water.

BENZTROPINE MESYLATE: Because there is not significant difference in onset of action after IV or IM injection, there is usually no need to use the IV route. In emergency situations, when the condition of the patients is alarming, 1 to 2 mL will normally provide quick relief.

Dosage titration – Because of cumulative action, initiate therapy with a low dose, increase in increments of 0.5 mg gradually at 5 or 6 day intervals to the smallest amount necessary for optimal relief. Maximum daily dose is 6 mg.

Dose intervals – Some patients experience greatest relief by taking the entire dose at bedtime; others react more favorably to divided doses, 2 to 4 times/day.

Parkinsonism – 1 to 2 mg/day, with a range of 0.5 to 6 mg/day, orally or parenterally.

Idiopathic parkinsonism: Start with 0.5 to 1 mg at bedtime; 4 to 6 mg/day may be required.

Postencephalitic parkinsonism: 2 mg/day in 1 dose or more. In highly sensitive patients, begin therapy with 0.5 mg at bedtime; increase as necessary.

Drug-induced extrapyramidal disorders – Administer 1 to 4 mg once or twice/day.

Acute dystonic reactions: 1 to 2 mL IM or IV usually relieves the condition quickly. After that, 1 to 2 mL orally 2 times/day usually prevents recurrence.

Extrapyramidal disorders which develop soon after initiating treatment with neuroleptic drugs are likely to be transient. A dosage of 1 to 2 mg orally 2 or 3 times a day usually provides relief within 1 or 2 days. After 1 or 2 weeks, withdraw drug to determine its continued need. If such disorders recur, reinstitute benztropine.

ETHOPROPAZINE:

Initially – 50 mg once or twice/day; increase gradually, if necessary.

Mild to moderate symptoms – 100 to 400 mg/day.

Severe cases – Gradually increase to 500 or 600 mg or more daily.

DIPHENHYDRAMINE: For complete prescribing information and product availability, see the Antihistamines group monograph.

Oral –

Adults: 25 to 50 mg 3 to 4 times/day.

Children more than 20 lbs (9 kg): 12.5 to 25 mg 3 or 4 times/day or 5 mg/kg/day. Do not exceed 300 mg/day or 150 mg/m^2/day.

Parenteral – Administer IV or deeply IM.

Adults: 10 to 50 mg; 100 mg if required. Maximum daily dosage is 400 mg.

Children: 5 mg/kg/day or 150 mg/m^2/day.

TRIHEXYPHENIDYL HYDROCHLORIDE:

Parkinsonism – Initially, administer 1 to 2 mg the first day; increase by 2 mg increments at intervals of 3 to 5 days, until a total of 6 to 10 mg is given daily. Many patients derive maximum benefit from a total daily dose of 6 to 10 mg; however, postencephalitic patients may require a total daily dose of 12 to 15 mg. Trihexyphenidyl is tolerated best if divided into 3 doses and taken at mealtimes. High doses may be divided into 4 parts, administered at mealtimes and at bedtime.

Concomitant use with levodopa: Trihexyphenidyl 3 to 6 mg/day in divided doses is usually adequate.

Drug-induced extrapyramidal disorders – Start with a single 1 mg dose. Daily dosage usually ranges between 5 to 15 mg, although reactions have been controlled on as little as 1 mg/day.

Sustained release – Do not use for initial therapy. Once patients are stabilized on conventional dosage forms, they may be switched to sustained release capsules on a milligram per milligram of total daily dose basis. Administer as a single dose after breakfast or in 2 divided doses 12 hours apart.

Actions

Pharmacology: Anticholinergic agents reduce the incidence and severity of akinesia, rigidity, and tremor by approximately 20%; secondary symptoms such as drooling are also reduced. In addition to suppressing central cholinergic activity, these agents also may inhibit the reuptake and storage of dopamine at central dopamine receptors, thereby prolonging the action of dopamine.

Pharmacokinetics:

Various Antiparkinson Anticholinergic Pharmacokinetic Parameters

Anticholinergic	Time to peak concentration (h)	Peak concentration (mcg/L)	Half-life (h)	Oral bioavailability (%)
Benztropine[a]				
Diphenhydramine	2 to 4	65 to 90	4 to 15	50 to 72
Ethopropazine[a]				
Trihexyphenidyl	1 to 1.3	87.2	5.6 to 10.2	≈ 100

[a] No data available.

Contraindications

Hypersensitivity to any component; glaucoma, particularly angle-closure glaucoma; pyloric or duodenal obstruction; stenosing peptic ulcers; prostatic hypertrophy or bladder neck obstructions; achalasia (megaesophagus); myasthenia gravis; megacolon.

Benztropine: Children younger than 3 years of age; use with caution in older children.

Warnings/Precautions

Ophthalmic: Incipient narrow-angle glaucoma may be precipitated by these drugs.

Concomitant conditions: Use caution in patients with tachycardia, cardiac arrhythmias, hypertension, hypotension, prostatic hypertrophy (particularly in the elderly), or any tendency toward urinary retention, liver or kidney disorders, and obstructive disease of the GI or GU tract.

CNS: When used to treat extrapyramidal reactions resulting from phenothiazines in psychiatric patients, antiparkinson agents may exacerbate mental symptoms and precipitate a toxic psychosis.

In addition, 19% to 30% of patients given anticholinergics develop depression, confusion, delusions, or hallucinations.

Tardive dyskinesia – Tardive dyskinesia may appear in some patients on long-term therapy with phenothiazines and related agents, or may occur after therapy has been discontinued.

Dry mouth: If dry mouth is so severe that swallowing or speaking is difficult, or if loss of appetite and weight occurs, reduce dosage or discontinue drug temporarily.

Abuse potential: Some patients may use these agents for mood elevations or psychedelic experiences. Cannabinoids, barbiturates, opiates, and alcohol may have additive effects with anticholinergics.

Hazardous tasks: May impair mental or physical abilities; patients should observe caution while driving or performing other tasks requiring alertness.

Pregnancy: Category C.

Lactation: An inhibitory effect on lactation may occur.

Children: Safety and efficacy for use in children have not been established.

Elderly: Geriatric patients, particularly older than 60 years of age, frequently develop increased sensitivity to anticholinergic drugs and require strict dosage regulation. Occasionally, mental confusion and disorientation may occur; agitation, hallucinations, and psychotic-like symptoms may develop.

Drug Interactions

Drugs that may interact with anticholinergic antiparkinson agents include amantadine, digoxin, haloperidol, levodopa, and phenothiazines.

Adverse Reactions

Adverse reactions include the following: Tachycardia; palpitations; hypotension; disorientation; confusion; memory loss; hallucinations; psychoses; agitation; nervousness; delusions; delirium; paranoia; euphoria; excitement; lightheadedness; dizziness; headache; listlessness; depression; drowsiness; weakness; giddiness; paresthesia; heaviness of the limbs; dry mouth; nausea; vomiting; epigastric distress; constipation; development of duodenal ulcer; skin rash; urticaria; other dermatoses; blurred vision; mydriasis; diplopia; increased intraocular tension; angle-closure glaucoma;

dilation of pupils; muscular weakness; muscular cramping; urinary retention; urinary hesitancy; dysuria; elevated temperature; flushing; numbness of fingers; decreased sweating, hyperthermia, heat stroke; difficulty in achieving or maintaining an erection.

AMANTADINE HYDROCHLORIDE

Capsules: 100 mg (*Rx*)	Various, *Symadine* (Solvay), *Symmetrel* (DuPont)
Syrup: 50 mg per 5 mL (*Rx*)	*Symmetrel* (DuPont)

This is an abbreviated monograph. For full prescribing information, refer to the Antiviral Agents monograph.

Indications

Parkinson's disease/syndrome and drug-induced extrapyramidal reactions: Idiopathic Parkinson's disease (paralysis agitans); postencephalitic parkinsonism; arteriosclerotic parkinsonism; drug-induced extrapyramidal reactions; symptomatic parkinsonism following injury to the nervous system by carbon monoxide intoxication.

Administration and Dosage

Parkinson's disease: 100 mg twice/day when used alone. Onset of action is usually within 48 h. Initial dose is 100 mg/day for patients with serious associated medical illnesses or those receiving high doses of other antiparkinson drugs. After one to several weeks at 100 mg once/day, increase to 100 mg twice/day, if necessary. Patients whose responses are not optimal at 200 mg/day may occasionally benefit from an increase up to 400 mg/day in divided doses; supervise closely. Patients initially benefiting from amantadine often experience decreased efficacy after a few months. Benefit may be regained by increasing to 300 mg/day, or by temporary discontinuation for several weeks. Other antiparkinson drugs may be necessary.

Concomitant therapy – When amantadine and levodopa are initiated concurrently, the patient can exhibit rapid therapeutic benefits. Maintain the dose at 100 mg/day or twice/day, while levodopa is gradually increased to optimal benefit.

Renal function impairment: The following table is designed to yield steady-state plasma concentrations of 0.7 to 1 mcg/mL.

Suggested Dosage Guidelines for Amantadine in Impaired Renal Function

Ccr (mL/min/1.73 m^2)	Estimated half-life (hours)	Suggested maintenance regimen[a]
100	11	100 mg twice a day or 200 mg/day
80	14	100 mg twice a day
60	19	200 mg alternated with 100 mg/day
50	23	100 mg/day
40	29	100 mg/day
30	40	200 mg twice weekly
20	66	100 mg 3 times weekly
10	178	200 mg alternated with 100 mg every 7 days
3 times weekly chronic hemodialysis	199	200 mg alternated with 100 mg every 7 days

[a] Loading dose on first day of 200 mg. Reproduced with permission from Horadam VW, Sharp JG, Smilack JD, et al. Pharmacokinetics of amantadine hydrochloride in subjects with normal and impaired renal function. *Ann Intern Med.* 1981;94:454-458.

Drug-induced extrapyramidal reactions: 100 mg twice/day. Patients with suboptimal responses may benefit from 300 mg/day in divided doses.

Actions

Pharmacology: The exact mechanism of action is unknown, but amantadine is thought to release dopamine from intact dopaminergic terminals that remain in the substantia nigra of parkinson patients.

BROMOCRIPTINE MESYLATE

Tablets; oral: 0.8 mg (*Rx*)	*Cycloset* (Patheon)
2.5 mg (*Rx*)	Various, *Parlodel SnapTabs* (Novartis)
Capsules; oral: 5 mg (*Rx*)	Various, *Parlodel* (Novartis)

Indications

Hyperprolactinemia (associated dysfunctions) (except Cycloset): For the treatment of dysfunctions associated with hyperprolactinemia including amenorrhea with or without galactorrhea, infertility, or hypogonadism in patients with prolactin-secreting adenomas.

Acromegaly (except Cycloset): For the treatment of acromegaly.

Parkinson disease (except Cycloset): For the treatment signs and symptoms of idiopathic or postencephalitic Parkinson disease; as adjunctive treatment to levodopa (alone or with a peripheral decarboxylase inhibitor).

Type 2 diabetes mellitus (Cycloset only): As an adjunct to diet and exercise to improve glycemic control in adults with type 2 diabetes mellitus.

Administration and Dosage

It is recommended that bromocriptine be taken with food. Patients should be evaluated frequently during dose escalation to determine the lowest dosage that produces a therapeutic response.

Hyperprolactinemia: The initial dosage is ½ to one 2.5 mg tablet daily. An additional 2.5 mg tablet may be added to the treatment regimen as tolerated every 2 to 7 days until an optimal therapeutic response is achieved. The therapeutic dosage range is from 2.5 to 15 mg daily in adults.

Acromegaly: The initial recommended dosage is ½ to one 2.5 mg tablet on retiring (with food) for 3 days. An additional ½ to 1 tablet should be added to the treatment regimen as tolerated every 3 to 7 days until optimal therapeutic benefit. The therapeutic dosage range varies from 20 to 30 mg/day, not to exceed 100 mg/day.

Parkinson disease: The dosage of levodopa during this introductory period should be maintained, if possible. The initial dose of bromocriptine is ½ of a 2.5 mg tablet twice daily with meals. Assessments are advised at 2-week intervals during dosage titration. The dosage may be increased every 14 to 28 days by 2.5 mg/day with meals.

The safety of bromocriptine has not been demonstrated in dosages exceeding 100 mg/day.

Type 2 diabetes mellitus (Cycloset only): Initially, 0.8 mg (usual dose is 1.6 to 4.8 mg) orally once daily administered within 2 hours after waking in the morning. Increase by one tablet per week until a maximum daily dose of 6 tablets (4.8 mg) or until the maximal tolerated number of tablets between 2 and 6 per day is reached.

Children:

Hyperprolactinemia (except Cycloset) –

11 to 15 years of age: Based on limited data, the initial dosage is one-half to one 2.5 mg tablet daily.

Dosing may need to be increased as tolerated until a therapeutic response is achieved. The therapeutic dosage ranged from 2.5 to 10 mg daily in children with prolactin-secreting pituitary adenomas.

Actions

Pharmacology: Bromocriptine is a dopamine receptor agonist and a nonhormonal, nonestrogenic agent that inhibits the secretion of prolactin in humans with little or no effect on other pituitary hormones, except in patients with acromegaly, where it lowers elevated blood levels of growth hormone in the majority of patients.

Bromocriptine, a dopamine receptor agonist produces its therapeutic effect in the treatment of Parkinson disease by directly stimulating the dopamine receptors in the corpus striatum.

Pharmacokinetics:

Absorption/Distribution – Twenty-eight percent of an oral dose was absorbed from the GI tract and was 90% to 96% bound to serum albumin. The absorption half-life is 0.2 to 0.5 hours, and the peak plasma levels of bromocriptine are reached within 1 to 3 hours.

Metabolism/Excretion – Bromocriptine was completely metabolized prior to excretion. The major route of excretion of absorbed drug was via the bile. Only 2.5% to 5.5% of the dose was excreted in the urine. Bromocriptine shows a high affinity for CYP3A and is also a potent inhibitor of CYP3A4. The elimination half life is approximately 6 hours.

Contraindications

Hypersensitivity to bromocriptine or any component of the product; hypersensitivity to ergot alkaloids or ergot-related drugs; women who are breast-feeding, may inhibit lactation and potential for increased risk of stroke.

Parlodel: Uncontrolled hypertension; pregnancy (risk to benefit evaluation must be performed in women who become pregnant during treatment for acromegaly, prolactinoma, or Parkinson disease; hypertension during treatment should generally result in efforts to withdraw); postpartum period in women with a history of coronary artery disease or severe cardiovascular conditions unless withdrawal is medically contraindicated.

Cycloset: Syncopal migraine because of increased risk of hypotensive episodes.

Warnings/Precautions

Pituitary tumors: Because hyperprolactinemia with amenorrhea/galactorrhea and infertility has been found in patients with pituitary tumors, a complete evaluation of the pituitary is indicated before treatment with bromocriptine mesylate.

Hypotension: Symptomatic hypotension can occur in patients treated with bromocriptine for any indication. In postpartum studies, decreases in supine systolic and diastolic pressures of greater than 20 mm Hg and 10 mm Hg, respectively, have been observe in almost 30% of patients receiving bromocriptine.

Seizures have been reported with and without the prior development of hypertension. Cases of stroke have been reported mostly in postpartum patients whose prenatal and obstetric courses had been uncomplicated.

Use of bromocriptine for the prevention of physiological lactation or in patients with uncontrolled hypertension is not recommended. Periodic monitoring of the blood pressure, particularly during the first weeks of therapy is prudent.

Pulmonary effects: Among patients on bromocriptine, particularly on long-term and high-dose treatment, pleural and pericardial effusions, as well as pleural and pulmonary fibrosis and constrictive pericarditis, have occasionally been reported. Once treatment was terminated, the changes slowly reverted toward normal.

Hyperprolactinemic states: Monitoring of visual fields in patients with macroprolactinoma is therefore recommended for an early recognition of secondary field loss due to chiasmal herniation and adaptation of drug dosage.

Acromegaly: Cold-sensitive digital vasospasm has been observed in some acromegalic patients treated with bromocriptine. Cases of severe GI bleeding from peptic ulcers have been reported, some fatal.

Possible tumor expansion while receiving therapy has been reported. Carefully monitor all patients and discontinue treatment if necessary.

Parkinson disease: Safety during long-term use for more than 2 years at the doses required for parkinsonism has not been established.

CNS effects: High doses of bromocriptine may be associated with confusion and mental disturbances. Because parkinsonian patients may manifest mild degrees of dementia, caution should be used when treating such patients. Bromocriptine administered alone or concomitantly with levodopa may cause hallucinations (visual or auditory). Hallucinations usually resolve with dosage reduction; occasionally, discontinuation of bromocriptine is required.

Somnolence – Bromocriptine has been associated with somnolence, and episodes of sudden sleep onset, particularly in patients with Parkinson disease. Sudden onset of sleep during daily activities, in some cases without awareness or warning signs, has been reported very rarely.

Retroperitoneal fibrosis: Retroperitoneal fibrosis has been reported in a few patients receiving long-term therapy (2 to 10 years) with bromocriptine in doses ranging from 30 to 140 mg daily.

Ophthalmic effects: Monitoring of visual fields in patients with macroprolactinoma is therefore recommended for an early recognition of secondary field loss caused by chiasmal herniation and adaptation of drug dosage.

Syncopal migraine: Bromocriptine is contraindicated in patients with syncopal migraine.

Galactose intolerance/Malabsorption: Advise patients with rare hereditary problems of galactose intolerance, the severe lactase deficiency or glucose-galactose malabsorption to not take this medicine.

Cerebrospinal fluid rhinorrhea: In some patients with prolactin-secreting adenomas treated with bromocriptine, cerebrospinal fluid rhinorrhea has been observed.

Special risk: As with levodopa, caution should be exercised when administering bromocriptine to patients with a history of myocardial infarction who have a residual atrial, nodal, or ventricular arrhythmia.

Exercise care when administering bromocriptine concomitantly with other medications known to lower blood pressure.

Use with caution in patients with a history of psychosis or cardiovascular disease. If acromegalic patients with prolactinoma or Parkinson disease are being treated with bromocriptine during pregnancy, they should be cautiously observed, particularly during the postpartum period if they have a history of cardiovascular disease.

Hazardous tasks: Because hypotensive reactions may occasionally occur and result in reduced alertness especially during the first days of treatment, exercise particular care when driving a vehicle or operating machinery.

Carcinogenesis: Malignant uterine tumors, endometrial and myometrial, were found in rats as follows: 0 out of 50 control females, 2 out of 50 females given 1.7 mg/kg daily, 7 out of 49 females given 9.8 mg/kg daily, and 9 out of 50 females given 44 mg/kg daily. The occurrence of these neoplasms is probably attributable to the high estrogen/progesterone ratio which occurs in rats as a result of the prolactin-inhibiting action of bromocriptine.

Fertility impairment: Increased perinatal loss was produced in the subgroups of female rats, sacrificed on day 21 postpartum after mating with males treated with the highest dose (50 mg/kg).

Pregnancy: *Category B* Because the studies in humans cannot rule out the possibility of harm, use bromocriptine during pregnancy only if clearly needed.

Lactation: Bromocriptine is contraindicated in women who are breast-feeding . Do not use bromocriptine during lactation in postpartum women.

Children: The safety and effectiveness of bromocriptine for the treatment of prolactin-secreting pituitary adenomas have been established in patients age 16 years to adult. Safety and effectiveness of bromocriptine in pediatric patients have not been established for any other indication listed.

Elderly: In general, be cautious in dose selection for an elderly patient, starting at the lower end of the dose range, reflecting the greater frequency of decreased hepatic, renal or cardiac function, and of concomitant disease or other drug therapy in this population.

Monitoring: Monitoring of visual fields in patients with macroprolactinoma is recommended for an early recognition of secondary field loss caused by chiasmal herniation and adaptation of drug dosage.

As with any chronic therapy, periodic evaluation of hepatic, hematopoietic, cardiovascular, and renal function is recommended.

Closely monitor patients closely throughout pregnancy for signs and symptoms that may signal the enlargement of a previously undetected or existing prolactin-secreting tumor.

Periodic monitoring of the blood pressure, particularly during the first weeks of therapy is prudent.

Drug Interactions

Drugs that may affect bromocriptine include alcohol, haloperidol, dopamine receptor antagonists, macrolide antibiotics, metoclopramide, phenothiazines, pimozide, protease inhibitors, sympathomimetics, and triptans.

Drugs that may be affected by bromocriptine include chloramphenicol, dopamine receptor antagonists, ergot drugs, octreotide, probenecid, methyldopa, salicylates, sulfonamides, and triptans.

Adverse Reactions

Adverse reactions occurring in at least 3% of patients are listed in the following categories.

Acromegaly: Anorexia, constipation, digital vasospasm, drowsiness/tiredness, dry mouth/nasal stuffiness, indigestion/dyspepsia, nausea, postural/orthostatic hypotension.

Hyperprolactinemia (associated dysfunctions): Abdominal cramps, constipation, diarrhea, dizziness, drowsiness, fatigue, headache, light-headedness, nasal congestion, nausea, vomiting.

Parkinson disease: Abdominal discomfort, abnormal involuntary movements, asthenia, ataxia, confusion, constipation, depression, dizziness, drowsiness, faintness/fainting, hallucinations, hypotension, insomnia, nausea, "on-off" phenomenon, shortness of breath, vertigo, vomiting, visual disturbance.

Postpartum patients: Decrease in blood pressure, dizziness, headache, nausea, vomiting.

Type 2 diabetes (Cycloset only): Amblyopia, anorexia, asthenia, cold, constipation, diarrhea, dizziness, dyspepsia, fatigue, flu syndrome, headache, infection, nausea, rhinitis, sinusitis, somnolence, vomiting,

CARBIDOPA

Tablets; oral: 25 mg (*Rx*)	*Lodosyn*[a] (Bristol-Myers Squibb Company)

[a] Most patients may be maintained on carbidopa/levodopa combination products. *Lodosyn* is available to physicians for use in patients requiring individual titration of carbidopa and levodopa.

Indications

Parkinsonism: For use with carbidopa-levodopa or with levodopa in the treatment of the symptoms of idiopathic Parkinson's disease (paralysis agitans), postencephalitic parkinsonism, and symptomatic parkinsonism which may follow injury to the nervous system by carbon monoxide intoxication and/or manganese intoxication.

For use with carbidopa-levodopa in patients for whom the dosage of carbidopa-levodopa provides less than adequate daily dosage (usually 70 mg daily) of carbidopa.

For use with levodopa in the occasional patient whose dosage requirement of carbidopa and levodopa necessitates separate titration of each entity.

Carbidopa is used with carbidopa-levodopa or with levodopa to permit the administration of lower doses of levodopa with reduced nausea and vomiting, more rapid dosage titration, and with a somewhat smoother response. However, patients with markedly irregular ("on-off") responses to levodopa have not been shown to benefit from the addition of carbidopa.

Administration and Dosage

Because carbidopa prevents the reversal of levodopa effects caused by pyridoxine, supplemental pyridoxine (vitamin B_6), can be given to patients when they are receiving carbidopa and levodopa concomitantly or as carbidopa-levodopa.

Administer with food to reduce GI upset.

Adults:

Parkinsonism –

Adding carbidopa to carbidopa-levodopa: When patients are taking carbidopa-levodopa 10-100 (which contains 10 mg of carbidopa and 100 mg of levodopa), 25 mg of carbidopa may be given with the first dose of carbidopa-levodopa each day. Additional doses of 12.5 mg or 25 mg may be given during the day with each dose of carbidopa-levodopa. When patients are taking carbidopa-levodopa 25-250 (which contains 25 mg of carbidopa and 250 mg of levodopa) or carbidopa-levodopa 25-100 (which contains 25 mg of carbidopa and 100 mg of levodopa), 25 mg of carbidopa may be given with any dose of carbidopa-levodopa as required for optimum therapeutic response.

Individual titration of carbidopa and levodopa: Initiate at 25 mg 3 or 4 times a day. The 2 drugs should be given at the same time, starting with no more than one-fifth (20%) to one-fourth (25%) of the previous or recommended daily dosage of levodopa when given without carbidopa. In patients already receiving levodopa therapy, at least 12 hours should elapse between the last dose of levodopa and initiation of therapy with carbidopa and levodopa. A convenient way to initiate therapy in these patients is in the morning following a night when the patient has not taken levodopa for at least 12 hours.

Maximum dosage: 200 mg/day given as carbidopa and carbidopa-levodopa.

Dosage adjustment: Dosage of carbidopa may be adjusted by adding or omitting one-half or one tablet a day.

Concomitant therapy: Other standard antiparkinsonian drugs may be continued while carbidopa and levodopa are being administered. However, the dosage of such other standard antiparkinsonian drugs may require adjustment.

Discontinuation of therapy: Patients should be observed carefully if abrupt reduction or discontinuation of carbidopa-levodopa or carbidopa-levodopa sustained-release is required, especially if the patient is receiving neuroleptics.

Interruption of therapy: If general anesthesia is required, therapy may be continued as long as the patient is permitted to take fluids and medication by mouth. When therapy is interrupted temporarily, the patient should be observed for symptoms resembling NMS, and the usual daily dosage may be resumed as soon as the patient is able to take medication orally.

Actions

Pharmacology: Levodopa, the metabolic precursor of dopamine, does cross the blood-brain barrier, and presumably is converted to dopamine in the brain. This is thought to be the mechanism whereby levodopa relieves symptoms of Parkinson's disease. Carbidopa inhibits decarboxylation of peripheral levodopa.

Pharmacokinetics: Carbidopa reduces the amount of levodopa required to produce a given response by about 75% and, when administered with levodopa, increases both plasma levels and the plasma half-life of levodopa.

Supplemental pyridoxine (vitamin B_6) can be given to patients when they are receiving carbidopa and levodopa concomitantly or as carbidopa-levodopa sustained-release or carbidopa-levodopa. The introduction of carbidopa to levodopa therapy, which inhibits the peripheral decarboxylation of levodopa to dopamine, counteracts the metabolic-enhancing effect of pyridoxine.

Contraindications

Hypersensitivity to any component of this drug.

Nonselective monoamine oxidase (MAO) inhibitors are contraindicated for use with levodopa or carbidopa-levodopa combination products with or without carbidopa. These inhibitors must be discontinued at least 2 weeks prior to initiating therapy with levodopa. Carbidopa-levodopa or levodopa may be administered concomitantly with the manufacturer's recommended dose of an MAO inhibitor with selectivity for MAO type B (eg, selegiline HCl).

Levodopa or carbidopa-levodopa products, with or without carbidopa, are contraindicated in patients with narrow-angle glaucoma.

Because levodopa or carbidopa-levodopa products, with or without carbidopa, may activate a malignant melanoma, they should not be used in patients with suspicious, undiagnosed skin lesions or a history of melanoma.

Warnings/Precautions

Use with levodopa: Carbidopa has no antiparkinsonian effect when given alone. It is indicated for use with carbidopa-levodopa or levodopa. Carbidopa does not decrease adverse reactions due to central effects of levodopa.

Although the administration of carbidopa permits control of parkinsonism and Parkinson's disease with much lower doses of levodopa, there is no conclusive evidence at present that this is beneficial other than in reducing nausea and vomiting, permitting more rapid titration, and providing a somewhat smoother response to levodopa.

In considering whether to give carbidopa with carbidopa-levodopa or with levodopa to patients who have nausea or vomiting, the physician should be aware that, while many patients may be expected to improve, some may not. This can only be determined by a trial of therapy.

CNS effects: Concomitant administration of carbidopa and levodopa may cause involuntary movements and mental disturbances. All patients should be observed carefully for the development of depression with concomitant suicidal tendencies. The occurrence of dyskinesias may require levodopa dosage reduction.

Neuroleptic malignant syndrome (NMS): Sporadic cases of a symptom complex resembling NMS have been reported in association with dose reductions or withdrawal of certain antiparkinsonian agents such as levodopa, carbidopa-levodopa or carbidopa-levodopa sustained-release. Therefore, patients should be observed carefully when the dosage of levodopa is reduced abruptly or discontinued, especially if the patient is receiving neuroleptics.

Special risk: Patients with chronic wide-angle glaucoma may be treated cautiously with carbidopa and levodopa or carbidopa-levodopa, or any combination of these drugs, just as with levodopa alone, provided the intraocular pressure is well controlled and the patient is monitored carefully for changes in intraocular pressure during therapy.

Pregnancy: Category C.

Lactation: It is not known whether carbidopa is excreted in human milk. Because many drugs are excreted in human milk, a decision should be made whether to discontinue nursing or to discontinue the drug.

Children: Safety and effectiveness in pediatric patients have not been established, and use of the drug in patients below the age of 18 is not recommended.

Lab test abnormalities: Abnormalities in laboratory tests may include elevations of liver function tests such as alkaline phosphatase, AST, ALT, lactic dehydrogenase, and bilirubin. Abnormalities in blood urea nitrogen and positive Coombs test have also been reported.

Monitoring: Periodic evaluations of hepatic, hematopoietic, cardiovascular, and renal function are recommended.

Drug Interactions

Antihypertensive agents: Symptomatic postural hypotension has occurred when carbidopa, given with levodopa or carbidopa-levodopa combination products, was added to the treatment of a patient receiving antihypertensive drugs.

Monoamine oxidase inhibitors: Concomitant therapy with selegiline and carbidopa-levodopa may be associated with severe orthostatic hypotension not attributable to carbidopa-levodopa alone.

Tricyclic antidepressants: There have been rare reports of adverse reactions, including hypertension and dyskinesia, resulting from the concomitant use of tricyclic antidepressants and carbidopa-levodopa preparations.

Dopamine D_2 receptor antagonists and isoniazid: Dopamine D_2 receptor antagonists (eg, phenothiazines, butyrophenones, risperidone) and isoniazid may reduce the therapeutic effects of levodopa.

Iron salts: Iron salts may reduce the bioavailability of carbidopa and levodopa.

Metoclopramide: Although metoclopramide may increase the bioavailability of levodopa by increasing gastric emptying, metoclopramide may also adversely affect disease control by its dopamine receptor antagonistic properties.

Drug/Lab test interactions: Levodopa and carbidopa-levodopa combination products may cause a false-positive reaction for urinary ketone bodies. This reaction will not be altered by boiling the urine specimen. False-negative tests may result with the use of glucose-oxidase methods of testing for glucosuria.

Adverse Reactions

The most common adverse reactions have included dyskinesias such as choreiform, dystonic, and other involuntary movements, and nausea; psychotic episodes including delusions, hallucinations, paranoid ideation, depression with or without development of suicidal tendencies, and dementia.

LEVODOPA AND CARBIDOPA

Tablets: 10 mg carbidopa and 100 mg levodopa, 25 mg carbidopa and 100 mg levodopa, 25 mg carbidopa and 250 mg levodopa (*Rx*)	Various, *Sinemet* (Bristol-Myers Squibb)
Tablets, extended-release: 25 mg carbidopa and 100 mg levodopa, 50 mg carbidopa and 200 mg levodopa (*Rx*)	Various, *Sinemet CR* (Bristol-Myers Squibb)
Tablets, orally-disintegrating: 10 mg carbidopa and 100 mg levodopa, 25 mg carbidopa and 100 mg levodopa, 25 mg carbidopa and 250 mg levodopa (*Rx*)	Various, *Parcopa* (Schwarz Pharma)

Indications

Treatment of symptoms of idiopathic Parkinson's disease (paralysis agitans), postencephalitic parkinsonism, and sympathetic parkinsonism that may follow injury to the nervous system by carbon monoxide and manganese intoxication.

Administration and Dosage

Patients not receiving levodopa:

Immediate-release tablets – 1 tablet of carbidopa 25 mg/levodopa 100 mg 3 times/day or carbidopa 10 mg/levodopa 100 mg 3 or 4 times/day. Dosage may be increased by 1 tablet every day or every other day, as necessary, until a dosage of 8 tablets a day is reached.

Tablets of the 2 ratios (eg, 1:4, 25/100 or 1:10, 10/100 and 25/250) may be given separately or combined as needed to provide the optimum dosage.

Provide at least 70 to 100 mg carbidopa per day. When more carbidopa is required, substitute one 25/100 tablet for each 10/100 tablet. When more levodopa is required, substitute the 25/250 tablet for the 25/100 or 10/100 tablet.

Extended-release tablets – 1 tablet (usually 50/200 mg tablet) twice/day at intervals of not less than 6 hours. Doses and dosing intervals may be increased or decreased based on response. Most patients have been adequately treated with 2 to 8 tablets (400 to 1600 mg of levodopa) per day (divided doses) at intervals of 4 to 8 hours while awake. Higher doses (12 tablets or more per day, 2400 mg or more levodopa/day) and intervals of less than 4 hours have been used but are not usually recommended. If an interval of less than 4 hours is used or if the divided doses are not equal, give the smaller doses at the end of the day.

Extended-release tablets may be administered as whole or half tablets which should not be crushed or chewed.

Patients currently treated with levodopa: Levodopa must be discontinued at least 12 hours before therapy with levodopa/carbidopa. Substitute the combination drug at a dosage that will provide about 25% of the previous levodopa dosage.

Immediate-release – Suggested starting dosage is 1 tablet of carbidopa 25 mg/levodopa 250 mg 3 or 4 times/day for patients taking more than 1500 mg levodopa or carbidopa 25 mg/levodopa 100 mg for patients taking less than 1500 mg levodopa.

Extended-release – In patients with mild to moderate disease, the initial dose is usually one 50/200 extended-release tablet twice daily.

Patients currently treated with conventional carbidopa/levodopa preparations: Substitute dosage with extended-release tablets at an amount that provides about 10% more levodopa per day, although this may need to be increased to a dosage that provides up to 30% more levodopa per day. Use intervals of 4 to 8 hours while awake.

Guidelines for Initial Conversion From Immediate-Release to Extended-Release (50/100 mg Tablets)

Immediate-release total daily levodopa dose (mg)	Extended-release (50/100 mg tablets) suggested dosage regimen
300 to 400	200 mg twice daily
500 to 600	300 mg twice daily or 200 mg 3 times/day
700 to 800	Total of 800 mg in 3 or more divided doses (eg, 300 mg am, 300 mg early pm, and 200 mg later pm)
900 to 1,000	Total of 1,000 mg in 3 or more divided doses (eg, 400 mg am, 400 mg early pm, and 200 mg later pm)

Combination therapy: Other antiparkinson drugs can be given concurrently; dosage adjustment may be necessary.

Immediate-release tablets – Immediate-release tablets (25/100 or 10/100) can be added to the dosage regimen of extended-release tablets in selected patients with advanced disease who need additional levodopa.

Administration of orally disintegrating tablets: Just prior to administration, gently remove the tablet from the bottle with dry hands. Immediately place the tablet on top of the tongue where it will dissolve in seconds, then swallow with saliva. Administration with liquid is not necessary.

Actions

Pharmacology: These agents are used in combination because carbidopa inhibits decarboxylation of levodopa and makes more levodopa available for transport to the brain. There is less variation in plasma levodopa levels than with the conventional formulation. However, the extended-release form is less systemically bioavailable (70% to 75%) and may require increased daily doses to achieve the same level of symptomatic relief.

Pharmacokinetics: The half-life of levodopa may be prolonged following the extended-release form because of continuous absorption. In elderly subjects, the mean time to peak levodopa concentration was 2 hours for extended-release vs 0.5 hours for conventional. The maximum concentration following the extended-release form was about 35% of the conventional form.

Warnings/Precautions

CNS effects: Certain adverse CNS effects (eg, dyskinesias) will occur at lower dosages and sooner during therapy with levodopa and carbidopa than with levodopa alone.

Drug Interactions

Drug/Food interactions: Administration of a single dose of the extended-release form with food increased the extent of levodopa availability by 50% and increased peak levodopa concentrations by 25%.

Adverse Reactions

In clinical trials, the adverse reaction profile of the extended-release form did not differ substantially from that of the conventional form.

ENTACAPONE

Tablets: 200 mg (*Rx*)	*Comtan* (Novartis)

Indications

Parkinson's disease: As an adjunct to levodopa/carbidopa to treat patients with idiopathic Parkinson's disease who experience the signs and symptoms of end-of-dose "wearing-off." The effectiveness of entacapone has not been systematically evaluated in patients with idiopathic Parkinson's disease who do not experience end-of-dose "wearing-off."

Administration and Dosage

The recommended dose of entacapone is one 200 mg tablet administered concomitantly with each levodopa/carbidopa dose to a maximum of 8 times/day (200 mg $\times$ 8 = 1600 mg/day). Clinical experience with daily doses greater than 1600 mg is limited.

Always administer entacapone in combination with levodopa/carbidopa. Entacapone has no antiparkinsonian effect of its own.

In clinical trials, the majority of patients required a decrease in daily levodopa dose if their daily dose of levodopa had been 800 mg or more, or if they had moderate or severe dyskinesias prior to treatment with entacapone.

Reducing the daily levodopa dose or extending the interval between doses may be necessary to optimize patient response. In clinical trials, the average reduction in the daily levodopa dose was approximately 25% in those patients requiring a levodopa dose reduction. (More than 58% of patients with levodopa doses more than 800 mg daily required such a reduction.)

Entacapone can be combined with the immediate- and sustained-release formulations of levodopa/carbidopa.

Entacapone may be taken with or without food.

Withdrawing patients from entacapone: Rapid withdrawal or abrupt reduction in the entacapone dose could lead to emergence of signs and symptoms of Parkinson's disease and may lead to hyperpyrexia and confusion, a symptom complex resembling neuroleptic malignant syndrome (see Precautions). Consider this syndrome in the differential diagnosis for any patient who develops a high fever or severe rigidity. If a decision is made to discontinue treatment with entacapone, monitor patients closely and adjust other dopaminergic agents as needed. Although tapering entacapone has not been evaluated, it seems reasonable to withdraw patients slowly if the decision to discontinue treatment is made.

Actions

Pharmacology: Entacapone is a selective and reversible inhibitor of catechol-O-methyltransferase (COMT), which alters the plasma pharmacokinetics of levodopa. When entacapone is given in conjunction with levodopa and an aromatic amino acid decarboxylase inhibitor (such as carbidopa), plasma levels of levodopa are greater and more sustained than after administration of levodopa and an aromatic amino acid decarboxylase inhibitor alone.

Pharmacokinetics: Entacapone is rapidly absorbed, with a T_{max} of approximately 1 hour. The absolute bioavailability following oral administration is 35%. The plasma protein binding of entacapone is 98%, mainly to serum albumin. Entacapone is almost completely metabolized prior to excretion, with only a small amount (0.2% of dose) excreted in the urine.

Contraindications

Hypersensitivity to the drug or any of its ingredients.

Warnings/Precautions

Hypotension/Syncope: Dopaminergic therapy in patients with Parkinson's disease has been associated with orthostatic hypotension. Entacapone enhances levodopa bioavailability and, therefore, might be expected to increase the occurrence of orthostatic hypotension. However, in entacapone clinical trials, no differences from placebo were seen for measured orthostasis or symptoms of orthostasis.

Diarrhea: In clinical trials, diarrhea developed in 10% and 4% of patients treated with 200 mg entacapone and placebo, respectively, and was regarded as severe in 1.3% of patients.

Hallucinations: Dopaminergic therapy in Parkinson's disease patients has been associated with hallucinations. In clinical trials, hallucinations developed in approximately 4% of patients treated with 200 mg entacapone or placebo.

Dyskinesia: Entacapone may potentiate the dopaminergic side effects of levodopa and may cause or exacerbate pre-existing dyskinesia.

Dopaminergic therapy reactions: The events listed below are rare events known to be associated with the use of drugs that increase dopaminergic activity, although they are most often associated with the use of direct dopamine agonists:

Rhabdomyolysis – Cases of severe rhabdomyolysis have been reported with entacapone use. The complicated nature of these cases makes it impossible to determine what role, if any, entacapone played in their pathogenesis.

Hyperpyrexia and confusion –

Tapering of dose: Cases of a symptom complex resembling neuroleptic malignant syndrome characterized by elevated temperature, muscular rigidity, altered consciousness, and elevated creatine phosphokinase (CPK) have been reported in association with the rapid dose reduction or withdrawal of other dopaminergic drugs.

Prescribers should exercise caution when discontinuing entacapone treatment. When considered necessary, withdrawal should proceed slowly. Consider this syndrome in the differential diagnosis for any patient who develops a high fever or severe rigidity.

Fibrotic complications – Cases of retroperitoneal fibrosis, pulmonary infiltrates, pleural effusion, and pleural thickening have been reported in some patients treated with ergot-derived dopaminergic agents. Although these adverse events are believed to be related to the ergoline structure of these compounds, whether other nonergot-derived drugs (eg, entacapone) that increase dopaminergic activity can cause them is unknown.

Renal toxicity: In a 1-year toxicity study, entacapone (plasma exposure 20 times that in humans receiving the MRDD of 1600 mg) caused an increased incidence of nephrotoxicity in male rats.

Biliary excretion: As most entacapone excretion is via the bile, exercise caution when drugs known to interfere with biliary excretion, glucuronidation, and intestinal beta-glucuronidase are given concurrently with entacapone (see Drug Interactions).

Lab test abnormalities: Entacapone is an iron chelator. The impact of entacapone on the body's iron stores is unknown; however, a tendency towards decreasing serum iron concentrations was noted in clinical trials. In a controlled clinical study, serum ferritin levels (as a marker of iron deficiency and subclinical anemia) were not changed with entacapone compared with placebo after 1 year of treatment and there was no difference in rates of anemia or decreased hemoglobin levels.

Hepatic function impairment: Treat hepatically impaired patients with caution. The AUC and C_{max} of entacapone approximately doubled in patients with documented liver disease compared with controls.

Carcinogenesis: An increased incidence of renal tubular adenomas and carcinomas was found in male rats treated with the highest dose of entacapone.

Mutagenesis: Entacapone was mutagenic and clastogenic in the in vitro mouse lymphoma/thymidine kinase assay in the presence and absence of metabolic activation, and was clastogenic in cultured human lymphocytes in the presence of metabolic activation.

Pregnancy: Category C.

Lactation: It is not known whether entacapone is excreted in human breast milk.

Children: There is no identified potential use of entacapone in pediatric patients.

Drug Interactions

Entacapone inhibited the CYP isoenzymes 1A2, 2A6, 2C9, 2C19, 2D6, 2E1, and 3A only at very high concentrations and would not be expected to be inhibited in clinical use.

Monoamine oxidase (MAO) inhibitors: MAO and COMT are the 2 major enzyme systems involved in the metabolism of catecholamines. Do not treat patients concomitantly with entacapone and a nonselective MAO inhibitor.

Entacapone can be taken concomitantly with a selective MAO-B inhibitor (eg, selegiline).

Drugs metabolized by COMT: Administer drugs known to be metabolized by COMT (ie, isoproterenol, epinephrine, norepinephrine, dopamine, dobutamine, methyldopa, apomorphine, isoetherine, bitolterol) with caution in patients receiving entacapone regardless of the route of administration (including inhalation), as their interaction may result in increased heart rates, arrhythmias, and excessive changes in blood pressure.

Drugs that interfere with biliary excretion of glucuronidation (erythromycin, rifampin, cholestyramine) might decrease entacapone elimination.

Drug/Food interactions: Food does not affect the pharmacokinetics of entacapone.

Adverse Reactions

Adverse reactions that occur in 3% or more of patients include the following: Dyskinesias; dizziness; nausea; diarrhea; abdominal pain; urine discoloration; hyper- and hypokinesia; constipation; vomiting; dry mouth; back pain; fatigue; dyspnea.

SELEGILINE HYDROCHLORIDE (L-Deprenyl)

Tablets: 5 mg (*Rx*)	Various
Tablets, orally disintegrating: 1.25 mg (*Rx*)	*Zelapar* (Valeant Pharmaceuticals)
Capsules: 5 mg (*Rx*)	Various, *Eldepryl* (Somerset)
Transdermal: 6 mg per 24 h (20 mg per 20 cm^2), 9 mg per 24 h (30 mg per 30 cm^2), 12 mg per 24 h (40 mg per 40 cm^2) (*Rx*)	*Emsam* (Dey)

Warning:

Suicidality and antidepressant drugs: Antidepressants increased the risk compared with placebo of suicidal thinking and behavior (suicidality) in children, adolescents, and young adults in short-term studies of major depressive disorder (MDD) and other psychiatric disorders. Anyone considering the use of selegiline or any other antidepressant in a child, adolescent, or young adult must balance this risk with the clinical need. Short-term studies did not show an increase in the risk of suicidality with antidepressants compared with placebo in adults 24 years of age and older; there was a reduction in risk with antidepressants compared with placebo in adults 65 years of age and older. Depression and certain other psychiatric disorders are themselves associated with increases in the risk of suicide. Patients of all ages who are started on antidepressant therapy should be monitored appropriately and observed closely for clinical worsening, suicidality, or unusual changes in behavior. Families and caregivers should be advised for the need for close observation and communication with the prescriber. Selegiline is not approved for use in children. Furthermore, selegiline at any dose should not be used in children younger than 12 years of age, even when administered with dietary modifications.

Indications

Parkinson disease (oral): Adjunct in the management of parkinsonian patients being treated with levodopa/carbidopa who exhibit deterioration in the quality of their response to this therapy.

MDD (transdermal): For the treatment of MDD.

Administration and Dosage

Tablets/capsules: 10 mg/day administered as divided doses of 5 mg taken at breakfast and lunch.

After 2 to 3 days of treatment, attempt to reduce the dose of levodopa/carbidopa. A reduction of 10% to 30% appears typical. Further reductions of levodopa/carbidopa may be possible during continued selegiline therapy.

Orally disintegrating tablets: Initiate with 1.25 mg given once a day for at least 6 weeks. After 6 weeks, the dose may be increased to 2.5 mg given once a day. Tablets should be taken in the morning before breakfast, without liquid.

Patients should not attempt to push selegiline orally disintegrating tablets through the foil backing. Patients should peel back the backing of 1 or 2 blisters (as prescribed) with dry hands and gently remove the tablet(s). Patients should immediately place the selegiline orally disintegrating tablets on top of the tongue, where it will disintegrate in seconds. Patients should avoid ingesting food or liquids for 5 minutes before and after taking selegiline orally disintegrating tablets.

MDD (transdermal):

Administration – Apply to dry, intact skin on the upper torso (below the neck and above the waist), upper thigh, or the outer surface of the upper arm once every 24 hours.

Initial treatment – The recommended starting dosage and target dosage is 6 mg per 24 hours. It has been systematically evaluated and shown to be effective in a dose range of 6 mg per 24 hours to 12 mg per 24 hours.

Dose adjustments – If dose increases are indicated, they should occur in dose increments of 3 mg per 24 hours (up to a maximum dose of 12 mg per 24 hours) at intervals of no less than 2 weeks.

Food/drug interactions – Inform patients that they should avoid tyramine-rich foods and beverages beginning on the first day of 9 mg per 24 hours or 12 mg per 24 hours treatment and continue to avoid these foods and beverages for 2 weeks after a dose reduction to 6 mg per 24 hours or following the discontinuation of 9 mg per 24 hours or 12 mg per 24 hours treatment.

Elderly – The recommended dosage for patients 65 years of age or older is 6 mg per 24 hours daily. Patients should be closely observed for postural changes in blood pressure throughout treatment.

Actions

Pharmacology: Selegiline is an irreversible inhibitor of MAO. The mechanisms accounting for selegiline's beneficial adjunctive action in the treatment of Parkinson disease are not fully understood. Inhibition of monoamine oxidase type B (mao-B), activity is generally considered to be of primary importance. It is important to be aware that selegiline may have pharmacological effects unrelated to MAO-B inhibition. As previously noted, there is some evidence that it may increase dopaminergic activity by other mechanisms, including interfering with dopamine reuptake at the synapse.

Pharmacokinetics:

Absorption/Distribution – The bioavailability of selegiline is increased 3- to 4-fold when it is taken with food.

Following dermal application of selegiline to humans, 25% to 30% of the selegiline content on average is delivered systemically over 24 hours. Transdermal dosing results in substantially higher exposure to selegiline and lower exposure to metabolites, compared with oral dosing, where extensive first-pass metabolism occurs. Steady-state selegiline plasma concentrations were achieved within 5 days of daily dosing. Selegiline is approximately 90% bound to plasma protein. On a dose-normalized basis, the relative bioavailability of selegiline from orally disintegrating tablets is greater than from the swallowed formulation.

Upon repeat dosing, accumulation in the plasma concentration of selegiline is observed both with selegiline orally disintegrating tablets and the swallowed 5 mg tablet. Steady state is achieved after 8 days.

Up to 85% of plasma selegiline is reversibly bound to proteins.

Metabolism – Selegiline undergoes extensive metabolism.

Transdermally absorbed selegiline is not metabolized in human skin and does not undergo extensive first-pass metabolism. Selegiline is extensively metabolized by several CYP-450–dependent enzyme systems.

Excretion – Following a single oral dose, the mean elimination half-life of selegiline is 2 hours (1.3 hours at the 1.25 mg orally disintegrating dose). Under steady-state conditions, the elimination half-life increases to 10 hours. The mean half-lives of selegiline and its 3 metabolites ranged from 18 to 25 hours.

Contraindications

Oral: Hypersensitivity to any formulation of selegiline or any of the active ingredients in the formulation; use with dextromethorphan, other MAO inhibitors (MAOIs), meperidine, methadone, and tramadol.

Transdermal: Pheochromocytoma; tyramine-rich foods (see Warnings/Precautions); known hypersensitivity to selegiline or to any componenet of the patch; concomitant use with selective serotonin reuptake inhibitors (SSRIs) (eg, fluoxetine, sertraline, paroxetine); dual serotonin and norepinephrine reuptake inhibitors (SNRIs) (eg, duloxetine, venlafaxine); tricyclic antidepressants (TCAs) (eg, amitriptyline, imipramine); bupropion; meperidine and analgesic agents such as tramadol, and methadone; dextromethorphan; St. John's wort; mirtazapine; cyclobenzaprine; carbamazepine; oxcarbazepine; and sympathomimetic amines, including amphetamines as well as cold products and weight-reducing preparations that contain vasoconstrictors (eg, pseudoephedrine, phenylephrine, phenylpropanolamine, ephedrine); oral selegiline or other MAO inhibitors (MAOIs) (eg, isocarboxazid, phenelzine, tranylcypromine). Patients should not undergo elective surgery requiring general anesthesia; they should not be given cocaine or local anesthesia containing sympathomimetic vasoconstrictors. Discontinue selegiline at least 10 days prior to elective surgery. If surgery is necessary sooner, benzodiazepines, mivacurium, rapacuronium, fentanyl, morphine, and codeine may be used cautiously.

Warnings/Precautions

Clinical worsening and suicide risk: Patients with MDD, both adults and children, may experience worsening of their depression and/or the emergence of suicidality or unusual changes in behavior, whether or not they are taking antidepressant medications, and this risk may persist until significant remission occurs.

Activation of mania/hypomania: During phase 3 trials, a manic reaction occurred in 0.4% patients treated with selegiline. As with all antidepressants, use selegiline cautiously in patients with a history of mania.

Buccal mucosa irritation: Selegiline orally disintegrating tablet patients also showed an increased frequency of mild oropharyngeal abnormality (eg, swallowing pain, mouth pain, discrete areas of focal reddening, multiple foci of reddening, edema, and/or ulceration).

CNS toxicity: Severe CNS toxicity associated with hyperpyrexia and death has been reported with the combination of tricyclic antidepressants and nonselective MAOIs (phenelzine, tranylcypromine).

Serious, sometimes fatal reactions with signs and symptoms that may include hyperthermia, rigidity, myoclonus, autonomic instability with rapid fluctuations of the vital signs, and mental status changes have been reported in patients receiving a combination of selective serotonin reuptake inhibitors (SSRIs).

Dyskinesia: Selegiline orally disintegrating tablets may potentiate the dopaminergic adverse reactions of levodopa and may cause or exacerbate preexisting dyskinesia.

Elective surgery: As with other MAOIs, patients taking selegiline should not undergo elective surgery requiring general anesthesia. They also should not be given cocaine or local anesthesia containing sympathomimetic vasoconstrictors. Discontinue selegiline at least 10 days prior to elective surgery.

External heat: Advise patients to avoid exposing the selegiline application site to external sources of direct heat, such as heating pads or electric blankets, heat lamps, saunas, hot tubs, heated water beds, and prolonged direct sunlight.

Hypertensive crisis: MAOIs have been associated with hypertensive crises caused by the ingestion of foods with a high concentration of tyramine. Hypertensive crises, which in some cases may be fatal, are characterized by some or all of the following symptoms: occipital headache (which may radiate frontally), palpitation, neck stiffness or soreness, nausea, vomiting, sweating (sometimes with fever and sometimes with cold, clammy skin), dilated pupils, and photophobia. Either tachycardia or bradycardia may be present and can be associated with constricting chest pain. Intracranial bleeding has been reported in association with the increase in blood pressure.

If a hypertensive crisis occurs, discontinue selegiline immediately. Phentolamine 5 mg or labetalol 20 mg administered slowly IV is the recommended therapy to control hypertension. Alternately, nitroprusside delivered by continuous IV infusion may be used. Manage fever by means of external cooling.

Hypotension: As with other MAOIs, postural hypotension, sometimes with orthostatic symptoms, can occur with selegiline therapy.

Levodopa: Some patients given selegiline may experience an exacerbation of levodopa-associated side effects, presumably due to the increased amounts of dopamine with super-sensitive, postsynaptic receptors. These effects may often be mitigated by reducing the dose of levodopa/carbidopa by approximately 10% to 30%.

Maximum dose: 10 mg/day (capsules/tablets) or 2.5 mg/day (orally disintegrating tablets).

Melanoma: Epidemiological studies have shown that patients with Parkinson disease have a higher risk (2- to approximately 6-fold higher) of developing melanoma.

Phenylketonurics: Each orally disintegrating tablet contains phenylalanine 1.25 mg (a component of aspartame). Patients taking the 2.5 mg dose of orally disintegrating tablets will receive phenylalanine 2.5 mg.

Screening patients for bipolar disorder: Prior to initiating treatment with an antidepressant, adequately screen patients with depressive symptoms to determine if they are at risk for bipolar disorder; such screening should include a detailed psychiatric history, including a family history of suicide, bipolar disorder, and depression.

Serotonin syndrome: Serious, sometimes fatal, CNS toxicity referred to as the "serotonin syndrome" has been reported with the combination of nonselective MAOIs with certain other drugs, including TCAs or SSRI antidepressants, amphetamines, meperidine, or pentazocine. Serotonin syndrome is characterized by signs and symptoms that may include hyperthermia, rigidity, myoclonus, autonomic instability with rapid fluctuations of the vital signs, and mental status changes that include extreme agitation progressing to delirium and coma. Concomitant use of selegiline with buspirone is not advised.

Special risk patients: Clinical experience with selegiline in patients with certain concomitant systemic illnesses is limited. Caution is advised when using selegiline in patients with disorders or conditions that can produce altered metabolism or hemodynamic responses.

Required dietary modifications: Patients should avoid the following foods and beverages beginning on the first day of selegiline 9 mg per 24 hours or 12 mg per 24 hours treatment and should continue to avoid them for 2 weeks after a dosage reduction to selegiline 6 mg per 24 hours or following the discontinuation of selegiline 9 mg per 24 hours or 12 mg per 24 hours.

Acceptable and Unacceptable Tyramine-Containing Foods/Beverages When Taking Selegiline		
Class of food and beverage	Tyramine-rich foods and beverages to avoid	Acceptable foods, containing no or little tyramine
Meat, poultry, and fish	Air-dried, aged, and fermented meats, sausages, and salamis (including cacciatore, hard salami, and mortadella); pickled herring; any spoiled or improperly stored meat, poultry, or fish (eg, foods that have undergone changes in colorationor odor, or become moldy); spoiled or improperly stored animal livers	Fresh meat, poultry, and fish, including fresh, processed meats (eg, lunch meats; hot dogs; breakfast sausage; cooked, sliced ham)
Vegetables	Broad bean pods (fava bean pods)	All other vegetables
Dairy	Aged cheeses	Processed cheeses, mozzarella, ricotta cheese, cottage cheese, yogurt
Beverages	All varieties of tap beer and beers that have not been pasteurized so as to allow for ongoing fermentation	Concomitant use of alcohol with selegiline transdermal is not recommended. (Bottled and canned beers and wines contain little or no tyramine.)
Miscellaneous	Concentrated yeast extract (eg, *Marmite*), sauerkraut, most soybean products (including soy sauce and tofu), nonprescription supplements containing tyramine	Brewer's yeast, baker's yeast, soy milk, commercial chain restaurant pizzas prepared with cheeses low in tyramine

Renal function impairment: Use selegiline orally disintegrating tablets with caution in patients with a history of, suspected, or known renal function impairment.

Hepatic function impairment: Use selegiline orally disintegrating tablets with caution in patients with a history of, suspected, or known hepatic impairment, particularly if the patient has an increased prothrombin time or increased serum bilirubin or decreased serum albumin.

Hazardous tasks: Caution patients about operating hazardous machinery, including automobiles, until they are reasonably certain that selegiline therapy does not impair their ability to engage in such activities.

Pregnancy: Category C.

Lactation: It is not known whether selegiline is excreted in breast milk.

Children: Safety and efficacy in children have not been established. Anyone considering the use of selegiline in a child or adolescent must balance the potential risks with the clinical need. The effects of selegiline orally disintegrating tablets in children younger than 16 years of age have not been evaluated.

Elderly: In short-term, placebo-controlled depression trials, patients 50 years of age and older appeared to be at higher risk for rash than younger patients.

Monitoring: Observe patients closely for atypical responses.

Monitor for melanomas frequently and on a regular basis when using selegiline for any indication.

Closely observe all patients being treated with antidepressants for any indication for clinical worsening, suicidality, and unusual changes in behavior, especially during the initial few months of a course of drug therapy, or at times of dose changes, either increases or decreases.

Closely monitor elderly patients treated with selegiline for postural changes in blood pressure throughout treatment.

Evaluate patients for a history of drug abuse, and closely observe such patients for signs of selegiline misuse or abuse (eg, development of tolerance, increase in dose, drug-seeking behavior).

Drug Interactions

Drugs that may affect selegiline include apraclonidine, buspirone, CNS stimulants (eg, atomoxetine, amphetamine, dexmethylphenidate, methylphenidate, sibutramine), hormonal contraceptives, linezolid, tetrabenazine, MAOIs (eg, isocarboxazid, other selegiline products, phenelzine, tranylcypromine), serotonin reuptake inhibitors (eg, citalopram, duloxetine, fluoxetine, fluvoxamine, nefazodone, paroxetine, sertraline, venlafaxine).

Drugs that may be affected by selegiline include CNS stimulants (eg, atomoxetine, amphetamine, dexmethylphenidate, methylphenidate, sibutramine), tetrabenazine, alcohol, analgesics (eg, meperidine, methadone, tramadol), anesthetics, bupropion, cyclobenzaprine, dextromethorphan, ginseng, insulin, MAOIs (eg, isocarboxazid, other selegiline products, phenelzine, tranylcypromine), maprotiline, meglitinide antidiabetic agents (eg, nateglinide, repaglinide), serotonin reuptake inhibitors (eg, citalopram, duloxetine, fluoxetine, fluvoxamine, nefazodone, paroxetine, sertraline, venlafaxine), sulfonylureas, sympathomimetic agents (eg, ephedrine, phenylephrine, pseudoephedrine), tricyclic antidepressants (eg, amitriptyline, protriptyline).

Adverse Reactions

Oral: Adverse reactions occurring in 3% or more of patients include nausea, dizziness, lightheadedness, fainting, abdominal pain, confusion, hallucinations, depression, loss of balance, insomnia, orthostatic hypotension, increased akinetic involuntary movements, agitation, arrhythmias, bradykinesia, chorea, delusions, hypertension, new or increased angina pectoris, syncope, and dry mouth.

Orally disintegrating: Adverse reactions occurring in 3% or more of patients include ataxia, back pain, constipation, dyskinesia, dyspepsia, dyspnea, headache, leg cramps, myalgia, pain, pharyngitis, rash, rhinitis, skin disorders, somnolence, tremor, vomiting

Transdermal: Application site reaction, diarrhea, dry mouth, dyspepsia, headache, insomnia, orthostatic changes in blood pressure, pharyngitis, rash, sinusitis, weight changes

RASAGILINE

Tablets: 0.5 mg and 1 mg (*Rx*)	*Azilect* (Teva)

Indications

Parkinson disease: For the treatment of the signs and symptoms of idiopathic Parkinson disease as initial monotherapy and as adjunct therapy to levodopa.

Administration and Dosage

Tyramine-rich foods, beverages, or dietary supplements and amines (from nonprescription cough/cold medications) should be avoided to prevent a possible hypertensive crisis/"cheese reaction" during rasagiline treatment.

Monotherapy: 1 mg administered once daily.

Adjunctive therapy: The recommended initial dosage is 0.5 mg administered once daily. If a sufficient clinical response is not achieved, the dosage may be increased to 1 mg administered once daily.

Change of levodopa dose in adjunct therapy – When rasagiline is used in combination with levodopa, a reduction of the levodopa dosage may be considered based upon individual response.

Hepatic function impairment: Patients with mild hepatic function impairment should use rasagiline 0.5 mg/day. Rasagiline should not be used in patients with moderate or severe hepatic function impairment.

Concomitant ciprofloxacin and other CYP1A2 inhibitors: Patients taking concomitant ciprofloxacin or other CYP1A2 inhibitors should use rasagiline 0.5 mg/day.

Actions

Pharmacology: Rasagiline is an irreversible monoamine oxidase (MAO) inhibitor indicated for the treatment of idiopathic Parkinson disease.

Pharmacokinetics:

Absorption – Rasagiline is rapidly absorbed, reaching peak plasma concentration (C_{max}) in approximately 1 hour. The absolute bioavailability of rasagiline is about 36%.

Rasagiline can be administered with or without food.

Distribution – The mean volume of distribution at steady state is 87 L. Plasma protein-binding ranges from 88% to 94%.

Metabolism/Excretion – Rasagiline undergoes almost complete biotransformation in the liver prior to excretion. CYP1A2 is the major isoenzyme involved in rasagiline metabolism. Glucuronide conjugation of rasagiline and its metabolites, with subsequent urinary excretion, is the major elimination pathway. Less than 1% of rasagiline was excreted as unchanged drug in urine. Its mean steady-state half-life is 3 hours.

Contraindications

Hypersensitivity to the drug; pheochromocytoma; coadministration with meperidine, methadone, tramadol, dextromethorphan, St. John's wort, mirtazapine, cyclobenzaprine, sympathomimetic amines (including amphetamines, nasal and oral decongestants, cold products, and weight-reducing preparations), other MAO inhibitors, cocaine, and local or general anesthetic agents.

Warnings/Precautions

Hypertensive crisis: Rasagiline treatment at any dose may be associated with a hypertensive crisis/cheese reaction if the patient ingests tyramine-rich foods, beverages, or dietary supplements or amines (from nonprescription medications).

Melanoma: Patients and doctors are advised to monitor for melanomas frequently and on a regular basis. Ideally, periodic skin examinations should be performed by appropriately qualified individuals (eg, dermatologists).

Dyskinesia caused by levodopa treatment: When used as an adjunct to levodopa, rasagiline may potentiate dopaminergic side effects and exacerbate preexisting dyskinesia. Decreasing the dose of levodopa may ameliorate this side effect.

Postural hypotension: When used as monotherapy, postural hypotension was reported in approximately 3% of patients treated with rasagiline 1 mg and 5% of patients treated with placebo. Postural hypotension occurs most frequently in the first 2 months of rasagiline treatment and tends to decrease over time.

Hallucinations: In the monotherapy study, hallucinations were reported as an adverse reaction in 1.3% of patients treated with rasagiline 1 mg and in 0.7% of patients treated with placebo.

When used as an adjunct to levodopa, hallucinations were reported as an adverse reaction in approximately 5% of patients treated with 0.5 mg/day, 4% of patients treated with rasagiline 1 mg/day, and 3% of patients treated with placebo. Caution patients of the possibility of developing hallucinations and instruct patients to report them to their health care provider promptly if they develop.

Hepatic function impairment: Rasagiline plasma concentration may increase in patients with mild (up to 2-fold; Child-Pugh score 5 to 6), moderate (up to 7-fold; Child-Pugh score 7 to 9), and severe (Child-Pugh score 10 to 15) hepatic function impairment. Give patients with mild hepatic function impairment the dose of 0.5 mg/day. Do not use rasagiline in patients with moderate or severe hepatic function impairment.

Carcinogenesis: In mice, there was an increase in lung tumors (combined adenomas/carcinomas) at 15 and 45 mg/kg in males and females.

Pregnancy: Category C.

Lactation: In rats, rasagiline was shown to inhibit prolactin secretion and it may inhibit milk secretion in females. Exercise caution when rasagiline is administered to a breast-feeding woman.

Children: The safety and efficacy of rasagiline in children have not been studied.

Monitoring: Patients and doctors are advised to monitor for melanomas frequently and on a regular basis. Qualified individuals (eg, dermatologist) should perform periodic skin examinations.

Drug Interactions

Rasagiline may affect anesthetics, antidepressants, cyclobenzaprine, dextromethorphan, levodopa, MAO inhibitors, meperidine, St. John's wort, and sympathomimetics.

Rasagiline may be affected by ciprofloxacin and CYP1A2 inhibitors.

Adverse Reactions

The most commonly observed adverse reactions that occurred in at least 5% of patients receiving rasagiline were arthralgia, depression, dyspepsia, fall, and flu syndrome.

DOPAMINE RECEPTOR AGONISTS, NON-ERGOT

APOMORPHINE HYDROCHLORIDE	
Injection; solution: 10 mg/mL (*Rx*)	*Apokyn* (Vernalis)
PRAMIPEXOLE	
Tablets; oral: 0.125, 0.25, 0.5, 0.75, 1, and 1.5 mg (*Rx*)	*Mirapex* (Boehringer Ingelheim)
Tablets, extended-release; oral: 0.375, 0.75, 1.5, 3, and 4.5 mg (*Rx*)	*Mirapex XR* (Boehringer Ingelheim)
ROPINIROLE	
Tablets; oral: 0.25, 0.5, 1, 2, 3, 4, and 5 mg (*Rx*)	Various, *Requip* (GlaxoSmithKline)
Tablets, extended-release; oral: 2, 4, and 8 mg (*Rx*)	*Requip XL* (GlaxoSmithKline)

Indications

Parkinson disease: For the treatment of the signs and symptoms of idiopathic Parkinson disease.

Apomorphine – For the acute, intermittent treatment of hypomobility, "off" episodes ("end-of-dose wearing off" and unpredictable "on/off" episodes) associated with advanced Parkinson disease.

Restless legs syndrome (ropinirole [immediate-release only], pramipexole [immediate-release only]): For the treatment of moderate to severe primary restless legs syndrome (RLS).

Administration and Dosage

APOMORPHINE: Doses greater than 0.6 mL (6 mg) are not recommended.

For subcutaneous administration only.

Concomitant medication – Do not initiate apomorphine without the use of a concomitant antiemetic. Start trimethobenzamide (300 mg 3 times daily orally) 3 days prior to the initial dose of apomorphine and continue during at least the first 2 months of therapy.

Dosage – Titrate the dose of apomorphine starting at 0.2 mL (2 mg) and up to a maximum recommended dose of 0.6 mL (6 mg) as follows:

Give patients in an "off" state a 0.2 mL (2 mg) test dose where blood pressure can be closely monitored. Check supine and standing blood pressure predose and at 20, 40, and 60 minutes postdose. Do not consider patients who develop clinically significant orthostatic hypotension as candidates for treatment. If the patient tolerates the 0.2 mL (2 mg) dose and responds, use the starting dose of 0.2 mL (2 mg) on an as-needed basis to treat existing "off" episodes. If needed, the dose can be increased in 0.1 mL (1 mg) increments every few days on an outpatient basis.

Generally, the test dose is to determine a dose (0.3 or 0.4 mL) that the patient will tolerate under monitored conditions, and then begin an outpatient dosing trial using a dose 0.1 mL (1 mg) lower than the tolerated test dose.

- For patients who tolerate the test dose of 0.2 mL (2 mg) but achieve no response, a dose of 0.4 mL (4 mg) may be administered at the next observed "off" period, but no sooner than 2 hours after the initial test dose. Check supine and standing blood pressure predose and at 20, 40, and 60 minutes postdose.
- If the patient tolerates a test dose of 0.4 mL (4 mg), the starting dose should be 0.3 mL (3 mg) used on an as-needed basis to treat existing "off" episodes. If needed, the dose can be increased in 0.1 mL (1 mg) increments every few days on an outpatient basis.
- If a patient does not tolerate a test dose of 0.4 mL (4 mg), a test dose of 0.3 mL (3 mg) may be administered during a separate "off" period, no sooner than 2 hours after the test dose. Check supine and standing blood pressure predose and at 20, 40, and 60 minutes postdose.
- If the patient tolerates the 0.3 mL (3 mg) test dose, the starting dose should be 0.2 mL (2 mg) used on an as-needed basis to treat existing "off" episodes. If needed, and the 0.2 mL (2 mg) dose is tolerated, the dose can be increased to 0.3 mL (3 mg) after a few days. In such a patient, the dose should ordinarily not be increased to 0.4 mL (4 mg) on an outpatient basis.

Most patients studied responded to 3 to 6 mg. The average frequency of dosing was 3 times per day.

If a single dose of apomorphine is ineffective for a particular "off" period, do not give a second dose for that "off" episode.

Interruption of therapy – Patients who have an interruption in therapy (more than a week) should be restarted on a 0.2 mL (2 mg) dose and gradually titrated to effect.

Hepatic function impairment – For patients with mild and moderate hepatic function impairment, exercise caution because of the increased maximal plasma concentration and area under the curve in these patients.

Renal function impairment – For patients with mild and moderate renal function impairment, reduce the testing dose and subsequent starting dose to 0.1 mL (1 mg).

PRAMIPEXOLE: May take with food to reduce the occurrence of nausea.

Parkinson disease –

Immediate-release tablets:

Initial treatment – Increase gradually from a starting dose of 0.375 mg/day given in 3 divided doses every 5 to 7 days to 4.5 mg/day.

Ascending Dose Schedule of Pramipexole Immediate Release for Parkinson Disease

Week	Dosage	Total daily dose
1	0.125 mg 3 times daily	0.375 mg
2	0.25 mg 3 times daily	0.75 mg
3	0.5 mg 3 times daily	1.5 mg
4	0.75 mg 3 times daily	2.25 mg
5	1 mg 3 times daily	3 mg
6	1.25 mg 3 times daily	3.75 mg
7	1.5 mg 3 times daily	4.5 mg

Maintenance treatment – Pramipexole is effective and well tolerated over a dosage range of 1.5 to 4.5 mg/day administered in equally divided doses 3 times per day with or without concomitant levodopa (approximately 800 mg/day). When pramipexole is used in combination with levodopa, consider a reduction of the levodopa dosage.

Discontinuation – Discontinue over a period of 1 week.

Extended-release tablets:

Maximum dose – 4.5 mg/day.

Initial dose – 0.375 mg once per day.

Dosage titration – Based on efficacy and tolerability, dosages may be increased gradually, not more frequently than every 5 to 7 days, first to 0.75 mg/day and then by 0.75 mg increments up to a maximum recommended dosage of 4.5 mg/day.

Discontinuation of therapy – Taper the dose gradually over a period of 1 week.

Dosing in patients with renal function impairment:

Immediate-release tablets –

Pramipexole Immediate-Release Dose in Parkinson Patients With Renal Function Impairment		
Renal status	Starting dosage	Maximum dosage
Healthy function to mild impairment (CrCl[a] > 60 mL/min)	0.125 mg 3 times a day	1.5 mg 3 times a day
Moderate impairment (CrCl = 35 to 59 mL/min)	0.125 mg twice a day	1.5 mg twice a day
Severe impairment (CrCl = 15 to 34 mL/min)	0.125 mg once daily	1.5 mg once daily
Very severe impairment (CrCl < 15 mL/min and hemodialysis patients)	The use of pramipexole has not been adequately studied in this group of patients.	

[a] CrCl = creatinine clearance.

Extended-release tablets – In patients with moderate renal impairment (CrCl between 30 and 50 mL/min), pramipexole extended release should initially be taken every other day. Caution should be exercised and careful assessment of therapeutic response and tolerability should be made before increasing to daily dosing after 1 week and before any additional titration in 0.375 mg increments up to 2.25 mg/day. Dose adjustment should occur no more frequently than at weekly intervals.

Pramipexole extended-release tablets have not been studied in patients with severe renal impairment (CrCl less than 30 mL/min) or patients on hemodialysis and are not recommended in these patients.

RLS –

Immediate-release tablets: 0.125 mg taken once daily 2 to 3 hours before bedtime. For patients requiring additional symptomatic relief, the dose may be increased every 4 to 7 days.

Ascending Dose Schedule of Pramipexole Immediate Release for RLS		
Titration step	Duration	Dose to be taken once daily 2 to 3 hours before bedtime
1	4 to 7 days	0.125 mg
2 (if needed)	4 to 7 days	0.25 mg
3 (if needed)	4 to 7 days	0.5 mg

Discontinuation – No taper of pramipexole required when treating RLS.

Patients with renal function impairment: The duration between titration steps should be increased to 14 days in patients with RLS with severe and moderate renal impairment (CrCl 20 to 60 mL/min).

Switching from immediate-release to extended-release tablets – Patients may be switched overnight from pramipexole immediate release to pramipexole extended release at the same daily dose. When switching between extended-release and immediate-release tablets, patients should be monitored to determine if dosage adjustment is necessary.

Administration – Take with or without food. Extended-release tablets should not be chewed, crushed, or divided.

ROPINIROLE: Ropinirole can be taken with or without food. Patients may be advised that taking ropinirole with food may reduce the occurrence of nausea; however, this has not been established in controlled clinical trials. If a significant interruption in therapy with ropinirole has occurred, retitration of therapy may be warranted. Extended-release tablets must be swallowed whole and must not be chewed, crushed, or divided.

Parkinson disease –

Immediate-release tablets: 0.25 mg 3 times per day, with or without food. Taking ropinirole with food may reduce the occurrence of nausea.

Based on individual patient response, dosage should then be titrated in weekly increments. After week 4, if necessary, daily dosage may be increased by 1.5 mg/day on a weekly basis up to a dose of 9 mg/day, and then by 3 mg/day or less weekly to a total dose of 24 mg/day.

Ascending-Dose Schedule of Ropinirole

Week	Dosage	Total daily dose
1	0.25 mg 3 times per day	0.75 mg
2	0.5 mg 3 times per day	1.5 mg
3	0.75 mg 3 times per day	2.25 mg
4	1 mg 3 times per day	3 mg

Extended-release tablets: The starting dosage is 2 mg once daily for 1 to 2 weeks, followed by increases of 2 mg/day at 1-week or longer intervals, up to a maximum recommended dose of 24 mg/day.

Switching from ropinirole immediate release to extended release: Patients may be switched directly from ropinirole immediate release to extended release. The initial dose of ropinirole extended release should most closely match the total daily dose of the immediate-release formulation, as shown in the following table. Following conversion to extended release, the dose may be adjusted depending on therapeutic response and tolerability.

Conversion From Ropinirole Immediate Release to Extended Release

Immediate-release total daily dose	Extended-release total daily dose
0.75 to 2.25 mg	2 mg
3 to 4.5 mg	4 mg
6 mg	6 mg
7.5 to 9 mg	8 mg
12 mg	12 mg
15 to 18 mg	16 mg
21 mg	20 mg
24 mg	24 mg

When ropinirole is administered as adjunct therapy to levodopa, the concurrent dose of levodopa may be decreased gradually as tolerated.

Restless legs syndrome (immediate release only) – RLS is 0.25 mg once daily 1 to 3 hours before bedtime with or without food. After 2 days, the dosage can be increased to 0.5 mg once daily, then increased as shown in the following table as needed to achieve efficacy. For RLS, the safety and efficacy of doses greater than 4 mg once daily have not been established.

Dose Titration Schedule of Ropinirole for RLS

Day/Week	Dosage to be taken once daily 1 to 3 hours before bedtime
Days 1 and 2	0.25 mg
Days 3 to 7	0.5 mg
Week 2	1 mg
Week 3	1.5 mg
Week 4	2 mg
Week 5	2.5 mg
Week 6	3 mg
Week 7	4 mg

Elderly – Pharmacokinetic studies demonstrated a reduced clearance of ropinirole in the elderly. Dose adjustment is not necessary because the dose is individually titrated to clinical response.

Hepatic function impairment – Because patients with hepatic impairment may have higher plasma levels and lower clearance, ropinirole should be titrated with caution in these patients.

Discontinuation – Immediate release should be discontinued gradually over a 7-day period. The frequency of administration should be reduced from 3 times daily to twice daily for 4 days. For the remaining 3 days, the frequency should be reduced to once daily prior to complete withdrawal.

Extended-release tablets should be discontinued gradually over a 7-day period.

In clinical trials of patients being treated for RLS with dosages of up to 4 mg once daily, ropinirole was discontinued without a taper.

Actions

Pharmacology: **Apomorphine, pramipexole,** and **ropinirole** are non-ergot dopamine agonists for Parkinson disease with high specificity at the D_2 subfamily of dopamine receptors, binding with higher affinity to D_3 than to D_2 or D_4 receptor subtypes.

The mechanism of action is believed to be related to its ability to stimulate dopamine receptors in the striatum.

Pharmacokinetics: Non-ergot dopamine agonists are rapidly absorbed. The absolute bioavailability is more than 90%. Steady-state concentrations are achieved within 2 days of dosing. Terminal half-life is approximately 8 hours (approximately 40 minutes for **apomorphine**) in young healthy volunteers and approximately 12 hours in elderly volunteers. Urinary excretion is the major route of elimination.

Contraindications

Hypersensitivity to the drug or any components of the product; concomitant use of **apomorphine** with drugs of the 5-HT_3 antagonist class (eg, ondansetron, granisetron, dolasetron, palonosetron, alosetron) due to reports of profound hypotension and loss of consciousness with ondansetron.

Warnings/Precautions

Intravenous administration: Avoid intravenous (IV) administration with **apomorphine**. Serious adverse events (such as IV crystallization of apomorphine leading to thrombus formation and pulmonary embolism) have followed IV administration.

Nausea and vomiting: At the recommended doses of **apomorphine**, severe nausea and vomiting can be expected. There was no experience with antiemetics other than trimethobenzamide. Some antiemetics with antidopaminergic actions have the potential to worsen the clinical state of patients with Parkinson disease and should be avoided.

QT prolongation and potential for proarrhythmic effects: In single-dose studies of **apomorphine**, changes in QTc ranging from 0 to 7 msec were reported. Some drugs that prolong the QT/QTc interval have been associated with the occurrence of torsades de pointes and sudden unexplained death.

Symptomatic hypotension: Patients require careful monitoring for signs and symptoms of orthostatic hypotension while being treated with dopaminergic agonists, especially during dose escalation. The effects of **apomorphine** on blood pressure may be increased by the concomitant use of alcohol, antihypertensive medications, and vasodilators (especially nitrates).

Falls: Patients with Parkinson disease are at risk of falling due to the underlying postural instability and concomitant autonomic instability from syncope caused by the blood pressure–lowering effects of the drugs used to treat Parkinson disease. Subcutaneous **apomorphine** might increase the risk of falling by simultaneously lowering blood pressure and altering mobility.

Hallucinations: Hallucinations were observed in a greater number of patients receiving dopaminergics than placebo. Age appears to increase the risk of hallucination attributable to dopaminergics.

Sleepiness during daily activities: Somnolence is commonly associated with **apomorphine**.

Coronary events: Angina, myocardial infarction, cardiac arrest, and/or sudden death have been reported during clinical trials with **apomorphine**. Use extra caution in prescribing apomorphine for patients with known cardiovascular and cerebrovascular disease.

Sulfite: Apokyn (**apomorphine**) contains metabisulfite, a sulfite that may cause allergic-type reactions, including anaphylactic symptoms and life-threatening or less severe asthmatic episodes.

Injection-site reactions: Injection-site reactions, including bruising, granuloma, and pruritus, were reported with **apomorphine**.

Dyskinesia: Dopamine receptor agonists may potentiate the dopaminergic adverse effects of levodopa and may cause or exacerbate pre-existing dyskinesia. Decreasing the dose of levodopa may ameliorate this adverse effect.

CNS effects: Use concomitant CNS depressants with caution because of the possible additive sedative effects.

Binding to melanin: Ropinirole binds to melanin-containing tissues in pigmented rats.

Priapism: **Apomorphine** may cause prolonged painful erections in some patients.

Renal function impairment: Exercise caution when prescribing to patients with renal insufficiency. The starting dose may need to be reduced.

Hepatic function impairment: Exercise caution when administrating **apomorphine** to patients with mild and moderate hepatic impairment.

Drug abuse and dependence: There are rare reports of **apomorphine** abuse by patients with Parkinson disease. These cases are characterized by increasingly frequent dosing leading to hallucinations, dyskinesia, and abnormal behavior.

Pregnancy: Category C.

Lactation: It is not known whether these drugs are excreted in breast milk.

Children: Safety and efficacy have not been established.

Elderly: **Pramipexole** total oral clearance was approximately 30% lower in subjects older than 65 years of age compared with younger subjects because of a decline in pramipexole renal clearance. The incidence of confusion and hallucinations appears to increase with age. Serious adverse events were more common in older patients (ie, falling, cardiovascular events, respiratory disorders, GI events).

Monitoring: Monitor for signs and symptoms of orthostatic hypotension.

Drug Interactions

5-HT_3 antagonist use is contraindicated with **apomorphine**. Drugs that may affect dopamine receptors agonists include cimetidine; estrogen; ciprofloxacin; drugs eliminated via renal excretion; inhibitors of CYP1A2 and dopamine antagonists; dopamine agonists, such as neuroleptics (eg, phenothiazines, butyrophenones, thioxanthenes) or metoclopramide. Drugs that may be affected by dopamine receptor agonists include levodopa. Use caution when prescribing apomorphine concomitantly with drugs that prolong the QT/QTc interval.

Drug/Food interactions: **Pramipexole** and **ropinirole** time to maximal plasma concentration are increased by approximately 1 and 2.5 hours, respectively, when taken with food, although the extent of absorption is not affected.

Adverse Reactions

Adverse reactions occurring in at least 3% of patients with early Parkinson disease (without levodopa) included the following: abdominal pain; abnormal vision; amnesia; angina; anorexia; anxiety; arthralgia; asthenia; back pain; bronchitis; chest pain; confusion; congestive heart failure; constipation; dehydration; depression; diarrhea; dizziness; drowsiness; dry mouth; dyskinesias; dyspepsia; dyspnea; ecchymosis; edema; eye abnormality; fall; fatigue; flatulence; flushing; hallucinations; headache; hypertension; hypesthesia; impotence; increased alkaline phosphatase; increased sweating; injection-site complaint (**apomorphine**); insomnia; limb pain;

malaise; nausea; orthostatic symptoms; pain; palpitations; Parkinson disease aggravated; peripheral edema; peripheral ischemia; pharyngitis; pneumonia; postural hypotension; rhinitis; rhinorrhea; sinusitis; somnolence; syncope; urinary tract infection; viral infection; vomiting; weakness; yawning.

Adverse reactions occurring in at least 3% of patients with advanced Parkinson disease (with levodopa) included the following: abdominal pain; accidental injury; accommodation abnormalities; akathisia; amnesia; arthritis; asthenia; chest pain; confusion; constipation; diarrhea; dizziness; dream abnormalities; dry mouth; dyskinesia; dyspnea; dystonia; extrapyramidal syndrome; falls; flushing; gait abnormalities/hypokinesia; general edema; hallucinations; headache; hypertonia; increased drug level; increased sweating; insomnia; malaise; nausea; nervousness; pain; pallor; paresis; paresthesia; pneumonia; postural hypotension; rhinitis; rhinorrhea; somnolence; syncope; thinking abnormalities; tremor/twitching; urinary frequency; urinary tract infection; vision abnormalities; vomiting; yawning.

CARBIDOPA, LEVODOPA, AND ENTACAPONE

Tablets: carbidopa 12.5 mg/levodopa 50 mg/entacapone 200 mg (*Rx*)	*Stalevo 50* (Novartis)
carbidopa 18.75 mg/levodopa 75 mg/entacapone 200 mg (*Rx*)	*Stalevo 75* (Novartis)
carbidopa 25 mg/levodopa 100 mg/entacapone 200 mg (*Rx*)	*Stalevo 100* (Novartis)
carbidopa 31.25 mg/levodopa 125 mg/entacapone 200 mg (*Rx*)	*Stalevo 125* (Novartis)
carbidopa 37.5 mg/levodopa 150 mg/entacapone 200 mg (*Rx*)	*Stalevo 150* (Novartis)
carbidopa 50 mg/levodopa 200 mg/entacapone 200 mg (*Rx*)	*Stalevo 200* (Novartis)

Indications

Parkinson disease: To treat patients with idiopathic Parkinson disease; to substitute (with equivalent strength of each of the 3 components) for immediate release carbidopa/levodopa and entacapone previously administered as individual products; to replace immediate release carbidopa/levodopa therapy (without entacapone) when patients experience the signs and symptoms of end-of-dose "wearing-off" (only for patients taking a total daily dose of levodopa of 600 mg or less and not experiencing dyskinesias).

Administration and Dosage

Do not fractionate individual tablets and administer only 1 tablet at each dosing interval. Individualize therapy and adjust according to the desired therapeutic response.

Use carbidopa, levodopa, and entacapone combination as a substitute for patients already stabilized on equivalent doses of carbidopa/levodopa and entacapone. Some patients who have been stabilized on a given dose of carbidopa/levodopa may be treated with carbidopa, levodopa, and entacapone combination if a decision has been made to add entacapone.

The optimum daily dosage of carbidopa, levodopa, and entacapone combination must be determined by careful titration in each patient. Carbidopa, levodopa, and entacapone combination tablets are available in 6 strengths, each in a 1:4 ratio of carbidopa to levodopa and combined with 200 mg of entacapone in a standard release formulation.

Transferring patients currently treated with carbidopa/levodopa and entacapone to carbidopa, levodopa, and entacapone combination tablet:

Carbidopa/levodopa – There is no experience in transferring patients currently treated with formulation of carbidopa/levodopa other than immediate release carbidopa/levodopa with a 1:4 ratio (controlled release formulations, or standard release presentations with a 1:10 ratio of carbidopa/levodopa) and entacapone to carbidopa, levodopa, and entacapone combination.

Entacapone – Patients who are currently treated with entacapone 200 mg tablet with each dose of standard release carbidopa/levodopa, can be directly switched to the corresponding strength of carbidopa, levodopa, and entacapone combination containing the same amounts of levodopa and carbidopa.

Transferring patients not currently treated with entacapone tablets from carbidopa/levodopa to carbidopa, levodopa, and entacapone combination tablets: In patients with Parkinson disease who experience the signs and symptoms of end-of-dose "wearing-off" on their current standard release carbidopa/levodopa treatment, clinical experience shows that patients with a history of moderate or severe dyskinesias or taking more than 600 mg/day of levodopa are likely to require a reduction in daily levodopa dose when entacapone is added to their treatment.

Maintenance therapy: Individualize therapy and adjust for each patient according to the desired therapeutic response.

When less levodopa is required, reduce the total daily dosage of carbidopa/levodopa by decreasing the strength of carbidopa, levodopa, and entacapone combination at each administration or by decreasing the frequency of administration by extending the time between doses.

When more levodopa is required, take the next higher strength of carbidopa, levodopa, and entacapone combination and/or increase the frequency of doses, up to a maximum of 8 times daily and not to exceed the maximum daily dose recommendations as outlined above.

Maximum dose: Clinical experience with daily doses above entacapone 1,600 mg is limited. It is recommended that no more than 1 carbidopa/levodopa/entacapone combination tablet be taken at each dosing administration. Thus, the maximum recommended daily dose of carbidopa 12.5 mg, levodopa 50 mg, and entacapone 200 mg combination; carbidopa 18.75 mg, levodopa 75 mg, and entacapone 200 mg combination; carbidopa 25 mg, levodopa 100 mg, and entacapone 200 mg combination; carbidopa 31.25 mg, levodopa 125 mg, and entacapone 200 mg combination; and carbidopa 37.5 mg, levodopa 150 mg, and entacapone 200 mg combination, defined by the maximum daily dose of entacapone, is 8 tablets/day. Because there is limited experience with total daily doses of carbidopa greater than 300 mg, the maximum recommended daily dose of the carbidopa 50 mg, levodopa 200 mg, and entacapone 200 mg combination is 6 tablets/day.

Addition of other antiparkinsonian medications: Standard drugs for Parkinson disease may be used concomitantly while carbidopa, levodopa, and entacapone combination is being administered, although dosage adjustments may be required.

Interruption of therapy: Sporadic cases of a symptom complex resembling Neuroleptic Malignant Syndrome (NMS) have been associated with dose reductions and withdrawal of levodopa preparations.

Hepatic function impairment: Treat patients with hepatic impairment with caution. The AUC and C_{max} of entacapone approximately doubled in patients with documented liver disease, compared with controls.

DISULFIRAM

Tablets: 250 and 500 mg (*Rx*)	Various, *Antabuse* (Duramed)

Warning:

Never give disulfiram to a patient in a state of alcohol intoxication or without the patient's full knowledge. Instruct the patient's relatives accordingly.

Indications

An aid in the management of selected chronic alcoholics who want to remain in a state of enforced sobriety so that supportive and psychotherapeutic treatment may be applied to best advantage.

Administration and Dosage

Do not administer until the patient has abstained from alcohol for at least 12 hours.

Initial dosage schedule: Administer a maximum of 500 mg/day in a single dose for 1 to 2 weeks. If a sedative effect is experienced, take at bedtime or decrease dosage.

Maintenance regimen: The average maintenance dose is 250 mg/day (range, 125 to 500 mg), not to exceed 500 mg/day. Maintenance therapy may be required for months or even years.

Actions

Pharmacology: Disulfiram produces a sensitivity to alcohol that results in a highly unpleasant reaction when the patient under treatment ingests even small amounts of alcohol. Disulfiram blocks oxidation of alcohol at the acetaldehyde stage by inhibiting aldehyde dehydrogenase. Accumulation of acetaldehyde produces the disulfiram-alcohol reaction. This reaction persists as long as alcohol is being metabolized. Disulfiram does not influence alcohol elimination. Prolonged administration of disulfiram does not produce tolerance; the longer a patient remains on therapy, the more sensitive the patient becomes to alcohol.

Pharmacokinetics: Disulfiram is slowly absorbed from the GI tract and eliminated slowly from the body. The average time to reach maximum plasma concentrations were 8 to 10 hours for disulfiram and its metabolites. Disulfiram is metabolized to diethyldithiocarbamate, which is oxidized to carbon disulfide and diethylamine. The metabolites are primarily excreted in the urine and carbon disulfide is exhaled in the breath. Ingestion of alcohol may produce unpleasant symptoms for 1 to 2 weeks after the last dose of disulfiram.

Contraindications

Severe myocardial disease or coronary occlusion; psychoses; hypersensitivity to disulfiram or to other thiuram derivatives used in pesticides and rubber vulcanization; patients receiving or who have recently received metronidazole, paraldehyde, alcohol, or alcohol-containing preparations.

Warnings/Precautions

Hepatic Toxicity: Hepatic toxicity including hepatic failure resulting in transplantation or death has been reported. Severe and sometimes fatal hepatitis associated with disulfiram therapy may develop even after many months of therapy. Hepatic toxicity has occurred in patients with or without prior history of abnormal liver function. Advise patients to immediately notify their physician of any early symptoms of hepatitis (eg, fatigue, weakness, malaise, anorexia, nausea, vomiting, jaundice, dark urine).

Administration: Never administer to an intoxicated patient or without the patient's knowledge (see Warning Box). The patient must be fully informed of the disulfiram-alcohol reaction. The patient must be strongly cautioned against surreptitious drinking while taking the drug, and fully aware of the possible consequences. Warn patient to avoid alcohol in disguised forms (eg, in sauces, vinegars, cough mixtures, aftershave lotions, back rubs). Also, warn that reactions may occur with alcohol up to 14-days after ingesting disulfiram.

Disulfiram-alcohol reaction: Disulfiram plus alcohol, even small amounts, produces flushing, throbbing in head and neck, throbbing headaches, respiratory difficulty, nausea, copious vomiting, sweating, thirst, chest pain, palpitations, dyspnea, hyperventilation, tachycardia, hypotension, syncope, marked uneasiness, weakness, vertigo, blurred vision, and confusion. In severe reactions there may be respiratory depression, cardiovascular collapse, arrhythmias, MI, acute CHF, unconsciousness, convulsions, and death. The intensity of the reaction is proportional to the amounts of disulfiram and alcohol ingested. The duration of the reaction varies from 30 to 60 minutes to several hours.

Concomitant conditions: Because of the possibility of an accidental reaction, use with caution in patients with diabetes mellitus, hypothyroidism, epilepsy, cerebral damage, chronic and acute nephritis, or hepatic cirrhosis or insufficiency.

Dependence and addiction: Alcoholism may accompany or be followed by dependence on narcotics or sedatives. Barbiturates have been coadministered with disulfiram without untoward effects, but consider the possibility of initiating a new abuse.

Ethylene dibromide: Do not expose patients to ethylene dibromide or its vapors. This precaution is based on preliminary results of animal research which suggest a toxic interaction between inhaled ethylene dibromide and ingested disulfiram results in a higher incidence of tumors and mortality in rats.

Ethylene dibromide: Patients should not be exposed to ethylene dibromide or its vapors.

Hypersensitivity reactions: Evaluate patients with a history of rubber contact dermatitis for hypersensitivity to thiuram derivatives before administering disulfiram.

Pregnancy: Category C.

Lactation: It is not known whether this drug is excreted in human milk. Do not give disulfiram to breastfeeding mothers.

Children: Safety and efficacy in pediatric patients have not been established.

Monitoring: Perform baseline and follow-up LFTs (10 to 14 days) to detect hepatic dysfunction resulting from therapy. Perform a CBC and serum chemistries.

Drug Interactions

Drugs that may interact with disulfiram include alcohol, benzodiazepines, caffeine, chlorzoxazone, cocaine, hydantoins, isoniazid, metronidazole, theophylline, tricyclic antidepressants, and warfarin.

Adverse Reactions

Adverse reactions may include acneiform eruptions; allergic dermatitis; arthropathy; multiple cases of cholestatic and fulminant hepatitis; drowsiness; fatigue; headache; hepatotoxicity resembling viral or alcoholic hepatitis; impotence; metallic or garlic-like aftertaste; peripheral neuropathy; polyneuritis; optic or retrobulbar neuritis; restlessness; occasional skin eruptions.

ACAMPROSATE CALCIUM

Tablets, delayed release: 333 mg (*Rx*)	*Campral* (Forest)

Indications

For maintenance of abstinence from alcohol in patients with alcohol dependence who are abstinent at treatment initiation. Treatment with acamprosate should be part of a comprehensive management program that includes psychosocial support.

The efficacy of acamprosate in promoting abstinence has not been demonstrated in subjects who have not undergone detoxification and not achieved alcohol abstinence prior to beginning acamprosate treatment. The efficacy of acamprosate in promoting abstinence from alcohol in polysubstance abusers has not been adequately assessed.

Administration and Dosage

The recommended dose is two 333 mg tablets (total dose, 666 mg) taken 3 times daily. Although dosing may be done without regard to meals, dosing with meals was employed during clinical trials and is suggested as an aid to compliance in those patients who regularly eat 3 meals daily. A lower dose may be effective in some patients.

Initiate treatment with acamprosate as soon as possible after the period of alcohol withdrawal, when the patient has achieved abstinence, and maintain treatment if the patient relapses.

Renal function impairment: For patients with moderate renal impairment (Ccr 30 to 50 mL/min), a starting dose of one 333 mg tablet taken 3 times daily is recommended. Do not give acamprosate to patients with severe renal impairment (Ccr 30 mL/min or less).

Actions

Pharmacology: Acamprosate is a synthetic compound with a chemical structure similar to that of the endogenous amino acid homotaurine, which is a structural analogue of the amino acid neurotransmitter γ-aminobutyric acid and the amino acid neuromodulator taurine.

The mechanism of action of acamprosate in the maintenance of alcohol abstinence is not completely understood. Chronic alcohol exposure is hypothesized to alter the normal balance between neuronal excitation and inhibition. Studies suggest acamprosate may interact with glutamate and gamma-aminobutyric acid (GABA) neurotransmitter systems centrally, and have led to the hypothesis that acamprosate restores this balance.

Acamprosate is not known to cause alcohol aversion and does not cause a disulfiram-like reaction as a result of ethanol ingestion.

Pharmacokinetics:

Absorption – The absolute bioavailability of acamprosate is approximately 11%. Steady-state plasma concentrations are reached within 5 days of dosing. Steady-state peak plasma concentrations after acamprosate doses of two 333 mg tablets 3 times daily average 350 ng/mL and occur at 3 to 8 hours postdose.

Distribution – Plasma protein binding of acamprosate is negligible.

Metabolism – Acamprosate does not undergo metabolism.

Excretion – After oral dosing of two 333 mg acamprosate tablets, the terminal half-life ranges from approximately 20 to 33 hours. The major route of excretion is via the kidneys as acamprosate.

Contraindications

Patients who have previously exhibited hypersensitivity to acamprosate or any of its components; patients with severe renal impairment (Ccr 30 mL/min or less).

Warnings/Precautions

Withdrawal symptoms: Use of acamprosate does not eliminate or diminish withdrawal symptoms.

Suicide: In controlled clinical trials of acamprosate, adverse events of a suicidal nature (eg, suicidal ideation, suicide attempts, completed suicides) were more common in acamprosate-treated patients than in patients treated with placebo (1.4% vs 0.5% in studies of 6 months or less; 2.4% vs 0.8% in year-long studies). Completed suicides occurred in 3 of 2,272 (0.13%) patients in the pooled acamprosate group from all controlled studies and 2 of 1,962 patients (0.1%) in the placebo group. Monitor alcohol-dependent patients, including those patients being treated with acamprosate, for the development of symptoms of depression or suicidal thinking. Alert families and caregivers of patients being treated with acamprosate of the need to monitor patients for the emergence of symptoms of depression or suicidality, and to report such symptoms to the patient's health care provider.

Renal function impairment: Treatment with acamprosate in patients with moderate renal impairment (Ccr 30 to 50 mL/min) requires a dose reduction. Do not give acamprosate to patients with severe renal impairment (Ccr 30 mL/min or less).

Pregnancy: Category C.

Lactation: It is not known whether acamprosate is excreted in human milk. Exercise caution when acamprosate is administered to a woman who is breastfeeding.

Children: Safety and efficacy have not been established.

Elderly: Because elderly patients are more likely to have decreased renal function, use care in dose selection.

Adverse Reactions

Adverse reactions occurring in at least 3% of patients include the following: accidental injury, anorexia, anxiety, asthenia, depression, diarrhea, dizziness, dry mouth, flatulence, insomnia, nausea, pain, paresthesia, pruritus, sweating.

NICOTINE

NICOTINE TRANSDERMAL	
Transdermal Systems (*otc*)	Various, *Habitrol* (Basel Pharm.), *Nicoderm CQ* (GlaxoSmithKline Consumer), *Nicotrol* (Pharmacia)
NICOTINE LOZENGE	
Nicotine lozenge: 2 and 4 mg nicotine (as polacrilex) (*otc*)	*Commit* (GlaxoSmithKline Consumer)
NICOTINE POLACRILEX	
Lozenge; oral: 2 and 4 mg (otc)	*Nicorette* (GlaxoSmithKline Consumer)
Chewing gum: 2 and 4 mg nicotine (as polacrilex) (*otc*)	Various, *Nicorette* (GlaxoSmithKline Consumer), *Thrive* (Novartis)
NICOTINE INHALATION SYSTEM	
Inhaler: 4 mg delivered (10 mg/cartridge) (*Rx*)	*Nicotrol Inhaler* (Pharmacia)
NICOTINE NASAL SPRAY	
Spray pump: 0.5 mg nicotine/actuation (10 mg/mL) (*Rx*)	*Nicotrol NS* (Pharmacia)

Indications

As an aid to smoking cessation for the relief of nicotine withdrawal symptoms. Use as part of a comprehensive behavioral smoking-cessation program.

Administration and Dosage

Nicotine Replacement Pharmacotherapy

Type of therapy	Dosage	Duration	Availability
Gum	Less than 24 cigarettes/day: 2 mg gum up to 24 pieces/day	up to 12 weeks	*otc*
	More than 25 cigarettes/day: 4 mg gum up to 24 pieces/day		
Inhaler	6 to 16 cartridges/day	up to 6 months	*Rx* only
Transdermal patch	21 mg/24 h 14 mg/24 h 7 mg/24 h	4 to 6 weeks then 2 weeks then 2 weeks	*otc*
	15 mg/16 h	6 weeks	
Nasal spray	8 to 40 doses/day	3 months	*Rx* only

NICOTINE TRANSDERMAL SYSTEM:

Recommended Dosing Schedule of Transdermal Nicotine for Healthy Patients

Dose	Duration: Per strength of patch	Duration: Entire course of therapy
Nicoderm[a]		
21 mg/day	First 6 weeks	8 to 10 weeks
14 mg/day	Next 2 weeks	
7 mg/day	Last 2 weeks	
Nicotrol		
15 mg/16 h	First 6 weeks	10 weeks
10 mg/16 h	Next 2 weeks	
5 mg/16 h	Last 2 weeks	

[a] Start with 14 mg/day for 6 weeks for patients who smoke less than 10 cigarettes/day. Decrease dose to 7 mg/day for the final 2 weeks.

Nicoderm – After 16 or 24 hours, remove the used system and apply a new system to an alternate skin site. Skin sites should not be reused for at least a week. Caution patients not to continue to use the same system for more than 24 hours.

Nicotrol – Each day apply a new system upon waking and remove at bedtime.

NICOTINE POLACRILEX (GUM): Advise patient to stop smoking completely when beginning to use the gum. If the patient smokes less than 25 cigarettes/day, start with the 2 mg nicotine gum. If the patient smokes more than 25 cigarettes/day, use according to the following 12-week schedule:

Nicotine Polacrilex Dosing Schedule		
Weeks 1 to 6	Weeks 7 to 9	Weeks 10 to 12
1 piece of gum or lozenge every 1 to 2 hours	1 piece of gum or lozenge every 2 to 4 hours	1 piece of gum or lozenge every 4 to 8 hours

Instruct patient to chew the gum slowly until it tingles, then park it between the cheek and gum. When the tingle is gone, instruct patient to begin chewing again until the tingle returns. Repeat the process until most of the tingle is gone (approximately 30 minutes).

Advise patient not to eat or drink for 15 minutes before chewing the nicotine gum or while chewing a piece. To improve the chances of quitting, chew at least 9 pieces/day for the first 6 weeks. If there are strong and frequent cravings, use a second piece within the hour. However, do not continuously use 1 piece after another since this may cause hiccoughs, heartburn, nausea, or other side effects.

Do not use more than 24 pieces/day. Stop using the nicotine gum at the end of 12 weeks. If there is still a need to use nicotine gum, have the patient contact a physician.

NICOTINE POLACRILEX (LOZENGE): If the patient smokes his/her first cigarette more than 30 minutes after waking up, start with the 2 mg nicotine lozenge. If the patient smokes their first cigarette within 30 minutes of waking up, start with the 4 mg nicotine lozenge. Refer to the dosing schedule in the table above.

Instruct the patient to place the lozenge in the mouth and allow it to slowly dissolve (about 20 to 30 minutes). Minimize swallowing. Advise the patient not to chew or swallow the lozenge. The patient may feel a warm or tingling sensation. Advise the patient to occasionally move the lozenge from one side of the mouth to the other until completely dissolved.

Advise the patient not to eat or drink 15 minutes before using or while the lozenge is in the mouth. To improve the chances of quitting, use at least 9 lozenges/day for the first 6 weeks. Do not use more than 1 lozenge at a time or continuously use 1 lozenge after another because this may cause hiccoughs, heartburn, nausea, or other side effects.

Advise the patient not to use more than 5 lozenges in 6 hours or more than 20 lozenges/day and to stop using the nicotine lozenge at the end of 12 weeks. If there is still a need to use the nicotine lozenge, have the patient contact a physician.

NICOTINE INHALATION SYSTEM: Patients should be encouraged to use at least 6 cartridges/day at least for the first 3 to 6 weeks of treatment. Additional doses may be needed to control the urge to smoke with a maximum of 16 cartridges/day for up to 12 weeks. The safety and efficacy of the continued use of the nicotine inhaler for periods more than 6 months have not been studied and such use is not recommended.

NICOTINE NASAL SPRAY: Instruct patients to stop smoking completely when using the product. Instruct them not to sniff, swallow, or inhale through the nose as the spray is being administered. Advise patients to administer the spray with the head tilted back slightly.

Dosage – Each actuation of the nasal spray delivers a metered 50 mcL spray containing 0.5 mg nicotine. One dose is 1 mg of nicotine (2 sprays, 1 in each nostril). Start patients with 1 or 2 doses per hour, which may be increased up to a maximum recommended dose of 40 mg (80 sprays, somewhat less than ½ of the bottle) per day. For best results, encourage patients to use at least the recommended minimum of 8 doses/day, as less is unlikely to be effective.

Nicotine Nasal Spray Dosing Recommendations			
Maximum recommended duration of treatment	Recommended doses/h	Maximum doses/h	Maximum doses/day
3 months	1 to 2[a]	5	40

[a] One dose = 2 sprays (1 in each nostril). One dose delivers 1 mg of nicotine to the nasal mucosa.

Individualization of dosage – The goal of the nasal spray therapy is complete abstinence. If a patient is unable to stop smoking by the fourth week of therapy, discontinue treatment. Regular use of the spray during the first week of treatment may help patients adapt to the irritant effects of the spray. Patients who are successfully abstinent on the nasal spray should be treated at the selected dosage for up to 8 weeks, following which use of the spray should be discontinued over the next 4 to 6 weeks. Some patients may not require gradual reduction of dosage and may abruptly stop treatment successfully. Treatment with the nasal spray for longer periods has not been shown to improve outcome, and the safety of use for periods longer than 6 months has not been established.

Actions

Pharmacology: Nicotine, the chief alkaloid in tobacco products, binds stereo-selectively to acetylcholine receptors at the autonomic ganglia, in the adrenal medulla, at neuromuscular junctions, and in the brain.

Pharmacokinetics:

Nicotine Pharmacokinetics

Parameter	Smoking	Gum	Transdermal	Nasal spray	Inhaler
Time to peak levels (hours)	ND[a]	0.25 to 0.5	2 to 12	0.25	0.25
Peak plasma level (ng/mL)	44	5 to 10	5 to 17	12	6
Half-life (hours)	15 to 20[b]	3 to 4	3 to 4	1 to 2	ND[a]

[a] No data.
[b] Refers to cotinine, the primary plasma metabolite of nicotine.

Contraindications

Hypersensitivity to nicotine or any components of the products, including menthol.

Warnings/Precautions

Nicotine risks: Nicotine from any source can be toxic and addictive. Smoking causes lung disease, cancer, and heart disease, and may adversely affect pregnant women or the fetus.

General: Urge the patient to stop smoking completely when initiating nicotine replacement therapy. Inform patients that if they continue to smoke while using the product, they may experience adverse effects because of peak nicotine levels higher than those experienced from smoking alone. If there is a clinically significant increase in cardiovascular or other effects attributable to nicotine, the treatment should be discontinued. Physicians should anticipate that concomitant medications may need dosage adjustment (see Drug Interactions). Sustained use (older than 6 months) of inhaler or nasal spray by patients who stop smoking has not been studied and is not recommended (see Drug Abuse and Dependence).

Bronchospastic disease: The **inhaler** and **nasal spray** have not been specifically studied in asthma or chronic pulmonary disease. Nicotine is an airway irritant and might cause bronchospasm.

Use of the **nasal spray** or **inhaler** in patients with severe reactive airway disease is not recommended.

Nasal disorders: Use of the **nasal spray** is not recommended in patients with known chronic nasal disorders (eg, allergy, rhinitis, nasal polyps, sinusitis) because such use has not been adequately studied.

Cardiovascular: Specifically, screen and evaluate patients with coronary heart disease, serious cardiac arrhythmias or vasospastic diseases before nicotine is prescribed. There have been occasional reports of tachyarrhythmias associated with nicotine use; therefore, if an increase in cardiovascular symptoms occurs, discontinue the drug.

Accelerated hypertension – Nicotine therapy constitutes a risk factor for development of malignant hypertension in patients with accelerated hypertension. **Inhaler** therapy should be used with caution in these patients and only when the benefits of including nicotine replacement in a smoking cessation program outweigh the risks.

Endocrine: Because of the action of nicotine on the adrenal medulla, use with caution in patients with hyperthyroidism, pheochromocytoma or insulin-dependent diabetes.

Oral/GI: Use caution in patients with oral or pharyngeal inflammation and in those with history of esophagitis or active or inactive peptic ulcer.

Dental problems: Dental problems might be exacerbated by chewing nicotine gum.

Renal/Hepatic function impairment: Anticipate some influence of hepatic impairment on drug kinetics (reduced clearance). Only severe renal impairment should affect clearance of nicotine or its metabolites from circulation.

Drug abuse and dependence: Urge patients to stop smoking completely when initiating therapy. If patients smoke while using nicotine, they may experience adverse effects because of peak nicotine levels higher than those caused by smoking alone.

The nicotine **inhaler** is likely to have a low abuse potential based on slower absorption, smaller fluctuations, and lower blood levels of nicotine when compared with cigarettes. Nicotine **nasal spray** has a dependence potential intermediate between other nicotine-based therapies and cigarettes. To minimize risk of dependence, encourage patients to gradually withdraw or stop gum and inhaler usage at 3 months, transdermal nicotine after 4 to 8 weeks. Chronic consumption is toxic and addicting.

Pregnancy: Category D (**inhaler, spray, transdermal patch**); *Category* C (**gum**). Nicotine is contraindicated in women who are or may become pregnant; advise patients to use contraceptive measures.

Lactation: Nicotine passes freely into breast milk and has the potential for serious adverse reactions in nursing infants.

Children: Safety and efficacy in children/adolescents younger than 18 years of age who smoke are not evaluated.

Elderly: Nicotine **inhaler** therapy appeared to be as effective in elderly patients 60 years of age or older as in younger smokers.

Drug Interactions

Smoking cessation, with or without nicotine substitutes, may alter response to concomitant medication in ex-smokers. Smoking may affect alcohol, benzodiazepines, beta-adrenergic blockers, caffeine, clozapine, fluvoxamine, olanzapine, tacrine, theophylline, clorazepate, lidocaine (oral), estradiol, flecanide, imipramine, heparin, insulin, mexiletine, opioids, propranolol, catecholamines, and cortisol.

Nasal spray: The extent of absorption and peak plasma concentration is slightly reduced in patients with the common cold/rhinitis. In addition, the time to peak concentration is prolonged. The use of a nasal vasoconstrictor such as xylometazoline in patients with rhinitis will further prolong the time to peak.

Adverse Reactions

Inhaler – Local irritation (mouth, throat); coughing; rhinitis; dyspepsia; headache; taste complaints; pain in jaw and neck; tooth disorders; sinusitis; influenza-like symptoms; pain; back pain; allergy; paresthesia; flatulence; fever; dizziness; anxiety; sleep disorder; depression; withdrawal syndrome; drug dependence; fatigue; myalgia; nausea; diarrhea; hiccough; chest discomfort; bronchitis; hypertension.

Nasal spray – Runny nose; throat irritation; watering eyes; sneezing; cough; nasal congestion; subjective comments related to the taste or usage of the dosage form; sinus irritation; transient epistaxis; eye irritation; transient changes in sense of smell; pharyngitis; paresthesias of the nose, mouth, or head; numbness of the nose or mouth; burning of the nose or eyes; earache; facial flushing; transient changes in sense of taste; hoarseness; nasal ulcer or blister; headache; back pain; dyspnea; nausea; arthralgia; menstrual disorder; palpitation; flatulence; tooth disorder; gum disorder; myalgia; abdominal pain; confusion; acne; dysmenorrhea.

Gum – Injury to mouth, teeth, or dental work; belching; increased salivation; mild jaw muscle ache; sore mouth or throat.

Transdermal – Erythema, pruritus, and burning at the application site.

BUPROPION HYDROCHLORIDE

Tablets, sustained release: 150 mg (*Rx*)	*Zyban* (GlaxoSmithKline)

Indications

Smoking cessation: An aid to smoking cessation treatment.

Administration and Dosage

The recommended and maximum dose of bupropion is 300 mg/day, given as 150 mg twice/day. Begin dosing at 150 mg/day given every day for the first 3 days, followed by a dose increase for most patients to the recommended usual dose of 300 mg/day. There should be an interval of 8 hours or more between successive doses. Do not give doses greater than 300 mg/day.

Initiate treatment with bupropion while the patient is still smoking because approximately 1 week of treatment is required to achieve steady-state blood levels of bupropion. Patients should set a "target quit date" within the first 2 weeks of treatment with bupropion, generally in the second week. Continue treatment for 7 to 12 weeks; base duration of treatment on the relative benefits and risks for individual patients. If a patient has not made significant progress toward abstinence by week 7 of therapy with bupropion, it is unlikely that he or she will quit during that attempt; discontinue treatment. Dose tapering of bupropion is not required when discontinuing treatment. It is important that patients continue to receive counseling and support throughout treatment with bupropion and for a period of time thereafter.

Maintenance: Nicotine dependence is a chronic condition. Some patients may need continuous treatment. Systematic evaluation of bupropion 300 mg/day for maintenance therapy demonstrated that treatment for up to 6 months was effective. Whether to continue treatment with bupropion for periods longer than 12 weeks for smoking cessation must be determined for individual patients.

Combination treatment: Combination treatment with bupropion and nicotine transdermal system (NTS) may be prescribed for smoking cessation.

Hepatic function impairment: Use extreme caution in patients with severe hepatic cirrhosis. The dose should not exceed 150 mg every other day in these patients. Use bupropion with caution in patients with hepatic impairment (including mild to moderate hepatic cirrhosis) and consider a reduced frequency of dosing in patients with mild to moderate hepatic cirrhosis (see Warnings).

Renal function impairment: Use caution in patients with renal impairment and consider a reduced frequency of dosing (see Warnings).

Actions

Pharmacology: Bupropion is a nonnicotine aid to smoking cessation. The mechanism by which bupropion enhances the ability of patients to abstain from smoking is unknown. However, it is presumed that this action is mediated by noradrenergic or dopaminergic mechanisms.

Pharmacokinetics: Following oral administration to healthy volunteers, mean peak plasma concentrations were achieved within 3 hours. Bupropion is 84% bound to human plasma proteins in vitro. Bupropion is extensively metabolized with a mean elimination half-life of approximately 21 hours.

Contraindications

Coadministration with a monoamine oxidase (MAO) inhibitor, *Wellbutrin*, *Wellbutrin SR* or any medications that contain bupropion; current or prior diagnosis of bulimia or anorexia nervosa, seizure disorders; patients who have shown an allergic response to bupropion or other ingredients in the formulation; patients undergoing abrupt discontinuation of alcohol or sedatives (including benzodiazepines).

Warnings/Precautions

Antidepressants: Bupropion is the active ingredient found in *Wellbutrin* and *Wellbutrin SR* used to treat depression. Do not use in combination with *Wellbutrin*, *Wellbutrin SR* or any other medication that contains bupropion.

Anorexia nervosa/bulimia: Do not give with current or prior diagnosis of bulimia or anorexia nervosa because of a higher incidence of seizures noted in patients treated for bulimia with the immediate-release formulation of bupropion.

Seizures: Because the use of bupropion is associated with a dose-dependent risk of seizures, do not prescribe doses greater than 300 mg/day for smoking cessation. The seizure rate associated with doses of sustained —release bupropion 300 mg/day or less is approximately 0.1%.

Concomitant medications – Many medications (eg, antipsychotics, antidepressants, theophylline, systemic steroids) and treatment regimens (eg, abrupt discontinuation of benzodiazepines) are known to lower seizure threshold.

Reducing the risk of seizures – Retrospective analysis suggests that the risk of seizures may be minimized if the total daily dose of bupropion does not exceed 300 mg (the maximum recommended dose) and no single dose exceeds 150 mg.

Insomnia: In one trial, 29% of patients treated with 150 mg/day and 35% of patients treated with 300 mg/day experienced insomnia vs 21% with placebo.

Psychosis or mania: Antidepressants can precipitate manic episodes in bipolar disorder patients during the depressed phase of their illness and may activate latent psychosis in other susceptible individuals. The sustained-release formulation of bupropion is expected to pose similar risks. There were no reports of activation of psychosis or mania in clinical trials conducted in nondepressed smokers.

Cardiac effects: Hypertension, in some cases severe, requiring acute treatment, has been reported in patients receiving bupropion alone and in combination with nicotine replacement therapy. These events have been observed in both patients with and without evidence of pre-existing hypertension.

Use caution in patients with a recent history of MI or unstable heart disease. Bupropion was well tolerated in depressed patients who had previously developed orthostatic hypotension while receiving tricyclic antidepressants and was generally well tolerated in depressed patients with stable CHF. Bupropion was associated with a rise in supine blood pressure in the study of patients with CHF, resulting in discontinuation of treatment in 2 patients for exacerbation of baseline hypertension.

Hypersensitivity reactions: Anaphylactoid reactions characterized by symptoms such as pruritus, urticaria, angioedema, and dyspnea requiring medical treatment have been reported at a rate of approximately 1 to 3 per thousand in clinical trials of bupropion. In addition, there have been rare spontaneous postmarketing reports of erythema multiformes, Stevens-Johnson syndrome, and anaphylactic shock associated with bupropion.

Renal function impairment: Use bupropion with caution in patients with renal impairment and consider a reduced frequency of dosing as bupropion and its metabolites may accumulate in such patients to a greater extent than usual.

Hepatic function impairment: Use with extreme caution in patients with severe hepatic cirrhosis. In these patients, a reduced frequency of dosing is required, as peak bupropion levels are substantially increased and accumulation is likely to occur in such patients to a greater extent than usual. The dose should not exceed 150 mg every other day.

Use with caution in patients with hepatic impairment (including mild to moderate hepatic cirrhosis) and consider reduced frequency of dosing in patients with mild to moderate hepatic cirrhosis.

Drug abuse and dependence: Bupropion is likely to have a low abuse potential. There have been a few reported cases of drug dependence and withdrawal symptoms associated with the immediate-release formulation of bupropion.

Pregnancy: Category B.

To monitor fetal outcomes of pregnant women exposed to bupropion, the manufacturer maintains a bupropion pregnancy registry. Health care providers are encouraged to register patients by calling (800) 336-2176.

Lactation: Bupropion and its metabolites are secreted in breast milk.

Children: Safety and efficacy in patients younger than 18 years of age has not been established.

Drug Interactions

Because bupropion is extensively metabolized, the coadministration of other drugs may affect its clinical activity. In particular, certain drugs may induce the metabolism of bupropion (eg, carbamazepine, phenobarbital, phenytoin) while other drugs may inhibit the metabolism of bupropion (eg, cimetidine, ritonavir).

Drugs that may increase the effects or side effects of bupropion include levodopa, MAOIs, ritonavir, antidepressants, antipsychotics, beta blockers, type IC antiarrhythmics.

Drugs that lower seizure threshold: Concurrent administration of bupropion and agents (eg, antipsychotics, antidepressants, theophylline, systemic steroids) or treatment regimens (eg, abrupt discontinuation of benzodiazepines) that lower seizure threshold should be undertaken only with extreme caution.

Drug/Food interactions: Food increased the C_{max} by 11%, the extent of absorption (AUC) by 17% and the mean time to peak concentration of bupropion.

Adverse Reactions

Adverse reactions occurring in 3% or more of patients include: Abdominal pain; insomnia; dream abnormality; anxiety; disturbed concentration; dizziness; nervousness; application site reaction; rash; pruritus; nausea; dry mouth; constipation; diarrhea; anorexia; myalgia; arthralgia; rhinitis; increased cough; pharyngitis; taste perversion.

VARENICLINE TARTRATE

Tablets: 0.5 mg, 1 mg (as base) (*Rx*)	*Chantix* (Pfizer)

Warning:

Serious neuropsychiatric events, including but not limited to depression, suicidal ideation, suicide attempt, and completed suicide, have been reported in patients taking **varenicline**. Some reported cases may have been complicated by symptoms of nicotine withdrawal in patients who stopped smoking. Depressed mood may be a symptom of nicotine withdrawal. Observe all patients being treated with **varenicline** for neuropsychiatric symptoms, including changes in behavior, hostility, agitation, depressed mood, and suicide-related events, including ideation, behavior, and attempted suicide. These symptoms, as well as worsening of preexisting psychiatric illness and completed suicide, have been reported in some patients attempting to quit smoking while taking **varenicline**

Indications

Smoking cessation: An aid to smoking cessation treatment.

Administration and Dosage

Adults: The patient should set a date to stop smoking. Varenicline dosing should start 1 week before this date.

Varenicline should be taken after eating and with a full glass of water.

The recommended dosage is 1 mg twice daily, following a 1-week titration as follows: days 1 through 3: 0.5 mg once daily; days 4 through 7: 0.5 mg twice daily; day 8 through end of treatment: 1 mg twice daily.

Patients who cannot tolerate the adverse reactions of varenicline may have the dose lowered temporarily or permanently.

Duration of therapy – Patients should be treated with varenicline for 12 weeks. For patients who have successfully stopped smoking at the end of 12 weeks, an additional course of 12 weeks of treatment with varenicline is recommended to further increase the likelihood of long-term abstinence.

Relapse of therapy – Patients who do not succeed in stopping smoking during 12 weeks of initial therapy or who relapse after treatment should be encouraged to make another attempt once factors contributing to the failed attempt have been identified and addressed.

Renal function impairment: For patients with severe renal function impairment, the recommended starting dosage is 0.5 mg once daily. Patients may then titrate as needed to a maximum dosage of 0.5 mg twice daily. For patients with end-stage renal disease undergoing hemodialysis, a maximum dosage of 0.5 mg once daily may be administered if well tolerated.

Actions

Pharmacology: Varenicline binds with high affinity and selectivity at nicotinic acetylcholine receptors. The efficacy in smoking cessation is believed to be the result of varenicline's activity at a subtype of the nicotinic receptor, where its binding produces agonist activity while simultaneously preventing nicotine binding to nicotine receptors.

Pharmacokinetics:

Absorption/Distribution – Maximum plasma concentrations of varenicline typically occur within 3 to 4 hours after oral administration. Following administration of multiple oral doses of varenicline, steady-state conditions were reached within 4 days.

Oral bioavailability of varenicline is unaffected by food or time-of-day dosing. Plasma protein-binding of varenicline is low (20% or less).

Metabolism/Excretion – The elimination half-life of varenicline is approximately 24 hours. Varenicline undergoes minimal metabolism, with 92% excreted unchanged in the urine. Renal elimination of varenicline is primarily through glomerular filtration along with active tubular secretion.

Warnings/Precautions

Neuropsychiatric symptoms: Serious neuropsychiatric symptoms have occurred in patients being treated with varenicline. Some cases may have been complicated by the symptoms of nicotine withdrawal in patients who have stopped smoking; however, some of these symptoms have occurred in patients who continued to smoke. Observe all patients being treated with varenicline for neuropsychiatric symptoms, including changes in behavior, agitation, depressed mood, suicidal ideation, and suicidal behavior. Alert patients attempting to quit smoking with varenicline and their families and caregivers about the need to monitor for these symptoms and to report such symptoms immediately to the patient's health care provider.

Skin reactions: There have been postmarketing reports of rare but serious skin reactions, including Stevens-Johnson syndrome and erythema multiforme, in patients using varenicline.

Drug abuse and dependence: Abrupt discontinuation of varenicline was associated with an increase in irritability and sleep disturbances in up to 3% of patients. In some patients, varenicline may produce mild physical dependence, which is not associated with addiction.

GI effects: Nausea was the most common adverse reaction associated with varenicline treatment.

Hypersensitivity reactions: There have been postmarketing reports of hypersensitivity reactions, including angioedema, in patients treated with varenicline. Clinical signs included swelling of the face, mouth (tongue, lips, and gums), extremities, and neck (throat and larynx).

Hazardous tasks: There have been postmarketing reports of traffic accidents, near-miss incidents in traffic, or other accidental injuries in patients taking varenicline. In some cases, patients reported somnolence, dizziness, loss of consciousness, or difficulty concentrating that resulted in impairment or concern about potential impairment while driving or operating machinery.

Pregnancy: Category C.

Lactation: Because many drugs are excreted in human milk and because of the potential for serious adverse reactions in breast-feeding infants from varenicline, decide whether to discontinue breast-feeding or the drug, taking into account the importance of the drug to the mother.

Children: Safety and efficacy of varenicline in children have not been established. Varenicline is not recommended for use in patients younger than 18 years of age.

Elderly: Because elderly patients are more likely to have decreased renal function, take care in dose selection; it may be useful to monitor renal function.

Drug Interactions

Effect of smoking cessation: Physiological changes resulting from smoking cessation may alter the pharmacokinetics or pharmacodynamics of some drugs, for which dosage adjustment may be necessary (eg, insulin, theophylline, warfarin).

Drugs that may interact with varenicline include cimetidine and transdermal nicotine.

Adverse Reactions

Nausea was the most common adverse reaction associated with varenicline treatment. Nausea was generally described as mild or moderate and often transient. Nausea was reported by approximately 30% of patients.

Adverse reactions that occurred in 3% or more of patients were as follows: abdominal pain, abnormal dreams, constipation, dry mouth, dysgeusia, dyspepsia, fatigue/malaise/asthenia, flatulence, headache, increased appetite, insomnia, nausea, rash, sleep disorder, somnolence, upper respiratory tract disorder, vomiting.

DALFAMPRIDINE

Tablets, extended-release; oral: 10 mg (*Rx*)	*Ampyra* (Acorda)

Indications

Multiple sclerosis: To improve walking in patients with multiple sclerosis (MS).

Administration and Dosage

Multiple sclerosis:

Usual dosage – 10 mg twice daily.

Maximum dose – 20 mg/day.

Renal function impairment – The risk of seizures in patients with mild renal impairment (creatinine clearance [CrCl] 51 to 80 mL/min) is unknown, but dalfampridine plasma exposure in these patients may approach that seen at a dosage of 15 mg twice daily, a dose that may be associated with an increased risk of seizures.

Dalfampridine is contraindicated in patients with moderate or severe renal impairment.

Administration: May be taken with or without food; doses should be taken approximately 12 hours apart.

Tablets should only be taken whole; do not divide, crush, chew, or dissolve.

Actions

Pharmacology: Dalfampridine is a broad-spectrum potassium channel blocker.

Pharmacokinetics:

Absorption/Distribution – Relative bioavailability is 96%. Single dalfampridine tablet 10 mg doses administered to healthy patients in a fasted state gave peak concentrations occurring 3 to 4 hours postadministration.

Dalfampridine is largely unbound to plasma proteins (97% to 99%).

Metabolism/Excretion – Dalfampridine and its metabolites' elimination is nearly complete after 24 hours, with 95.9% of the dose recovered in urine and 0.5% recovered in feces.

The elimination half-life of dalfampridine following administration of the extended-release tablet formulation of dalfampridine is 5.2 to 6.5 hours.

In vitro studies with human liver microsomes indicate that CYP2E1 was the major enzyme responsible for the 3-hydroxylation of dalfampridine.

Contraindications

History of seizure; moderate or severe renal impairment.

Warnings/Precautions

Seizures: Dalfampridine is contraindicated in patients with a history of seizures.

Dalfampridine should be discontinued and not restarted in patients who experience a seizure while on treatment.

Urinary tract infections: Urinary tract infections (UTIs) were reported more frequently as adverse reactions in controlled studies in patients receiving dalfampridine 10 mg twice daily compared with placebo.

Renal function impairment: Dalfampridine is eliminated through the kidneys primarily as unchanged drug.

Because patients with renal impairment would require a dosage lower than 10 mg twice daily and no strength smaller than 10 mg is available, dalfampridine is contraindicated in patients with moderate to severe renal impairment (CrCl 50 mL/min or less).

Pregnancy: Category C.

Lactation: It is not known whether dalfampridine is excreted in human milk. Because many drugs are excreted in human milk. Decide whether to discontinue breastfeeding or to discontinue the drug.

Children: Safety and effectiveness of dalfampridine in patients younger than 18 years of age have not been established.

Elderly: Dalfampridine is known to be substantially excreted by the kidney, and the risk of adverse reactions, including seizures, is greater with increasing exposure of dalfampridine. Because elderly patients are more likely to have decreased renal function, it is particularly important to know the estimated CrCl in these patients.

Drug Interactions

Coadministration with other forms of 4-aminopyridine: Do not administer dalfampridine with other forms of 4-aminopyridine (4-AP, fampridine) because the active ingredient is the same.

Adverse Reactions

Adverse reactions that occurred in at least 2% of patients included asthenia, back pain, balance disorder, constipation, dizziness, headache, insomnia, MS relapse, nasopharyngitis, nausea, paresthesia, and UTI.

BOTULINUM TOXIN TYPE A

Powder for injection (vacuum-dried): 50, 100, and 200 units of vacuum-dried *Clostridium botulinum* toxin type A neurotoxin complex[a] (*Rx*)	*Botox* (Allergan), *Botox Cosmetic* (Allergan), *Dysport* (Tercica), *Xeomin* (Merz Pharma

[a] One unit corresponds to the calculated median lethal intraperitoneal dose (LD_{50}) in mice.

Warning:

Postmarketing reports indicate that the effects of all botulinum toxin products may spread from the area of injection to produce symptoms consistent with botulinum toxin effects. These may include asthenia, generalized muscle weakness, diplopia, blurred vision, ptosis, dysphagia, dysphonia, dysarthria, urinary incontinence, and breathing difficulties. These symptoms have been reported hours to weeks after injection. Swallowing and breathing difficulties can be life-threatening, and there have been reports of death. The risk of symptoms is probably greatest in children treated for spasticity, but symptoms can also occur in adults treated for spasticity and other conditions, particularly in those patients who have underlying conditions that would predispose them to these symptoms. In unapproved uses, including spasticity in children and adults, and in approved indications, cases of spread of effect have been reported at doses comparable with those used to treat cervical dystonia and at lower doses.

Indications

Blepharospasm (Xeomin only): For the treatment of adults with blepharospasm who were previously treated with *Botox*.

Cervical dystonia (CD) (Botox, Dysport, and Xeomin): For the treatment of CD in adults to decrease the severity of abnormal head position and neck pain in botulinum toxin-naive and previously treated patients.

Chronic migraine (Botox only): For the prophylaxis of headaches in adult patients with chronic migraine (at least 15 days per month with headache lasting 4 hours a day or longer).

Safety and effectiveness have not been established for the prophylaxis of episodic migraine (14 headache days or fewer per month) in 7 placebo-controlled studies.

Glabellar lines (Botox Cosmetic and Dysport only): For the temporary improvement in the appearance of moderate to severe glabellar lines associated with corrugator or procerus muscle activity in adult patients 65 years of age or younger.

Axillary hyperhidrosis (Botox only): For the treatment of severe primary axillary hyperhidrosis that is inadequately managed with topical agents.

Strabismus and blepharospasm associated with dystonia (Botox only): For the treatment of strabismus and blepharospasm associated with dystonia, including benign essential blepharospasm or VII nerve disorders in patients 12 years of age and older.

Upper limb spasticity (Botox only): For the treatment of upper limb spasticity in adults, to decrease the severity of increased muscle tone in elbow flexors (biceps), wrist flexors (flexor carpi radialis and flexor carpi ulnaris), and finger flexors (flexor digitorum profundus and flexor digitorum sublimis).

Safety and effectiveness of *Botox* have not been established for the treatment of other upper limb muscle groups, or for the treatment of lower limb spasticity. Safety and effectiveness of *Botox* have not been established for the treatment of spasticity in children younger than 18 years of age. *Botox* has not been shown to improve upper extremity functional abilities or range of motion at a joint affected by a fixed contracture. Treatment with *Botox* is not intended to substitute for usual standard of care rehabilitation regimens.

Administration and Dosage

The potency units of botulinum toxin type A products are specific to the preparation not interchangeable with other preparations of botulinum toxin products;

therefore, units of biological activity of *Dysport, Botox, Botox Cosmetic,* and *Xeomin* cannot be compared with or converted into units of any other botulinum toxin products.

The initial effect of the injections is seen within 3 days and reaches a peak at 1 to 2 weeks posttreatment. Each treatment lasts approximately 3 months.

Dose may be increased up to 2-fold if the response from the initial treatment is considered insufficient (usually defined as an effect that does not last longer than 2 months). There appears to be little benefit obtainable from injecting more than 5 units per site. Some tolerance may be found if treatments are given any more frequently than every 3 months; it is rare to have the effect be permanent.

Glabellar lines (Botox Cosmetic only): Inject IM only.

Reconstitute with 0.9% sterile, nonpreserved saline (100 units in 2.5 mL saline) prior to IM injection. The resulting formulation will be 4 units/0.1 mL and a total treatment dose of 20 units in 0.5 mL. The duration of activity of botulinum toxin type A for glabellar lines is approximately 3 to 4 months. Injection intervals should be no more frequent than every 3 months and should be performed using the lowest effective dose. The safety and efficacy of more frequent dosing have not been clinically evaluated; more frequent dosing is not recommended.

Cervical dystonia (Botox): 50 units per site.

Botulinum toxin-experienced patients – The mean dose administered to patients in the phase 3 study was 236 units. Dose was divided among the affected muscles. Tailor dosing in initial and sequential treatment sessions to the individual patient.

Botulinum toxin-naive patients – The initial dose should be at a lower dose, with subsequent dosing adjusted based on individual response. Limiting the total dose injected into the sternocleidomastoid muscles to 100 units or less may decrease the occurrence of dysphagia.

Clinical improvement generally begins within the first 2 weeks after injection, with maximum clinical benefit at approximately 6 weeks postinjection.

The usual dosage is 155 units administered intramuscularly (IM) as 0.1 mL (5 units) injections per each site.

Botox Recommended Dose by Muscle for Chronic Migraine

Head/Neck area	Recommended dose (number of sites[a])
Frontalis[b]	20 units divided in 4 sites
Corrugator[b]	10 units divided in 2 sites
Procerus	5 units in 1 site
Occipitalis[b]	30 units divided in 6 sites
Temporalis[b]	40 units divided in 8 sites
Trapezius[b]	30 units divided in 6 sites
Cervical paraspinal muscle group[b]	20 units divided in 4 sites
Total dose	155 units divided in 31 sites

[a] Each IM injection site = 0.1 mL = 5 units *Botox.*
[b] Dose distributed bilaterally.

The recommended re-treatment schedule is every 12 weeks.

Primary axillary hyperhidrosis (Botox only): 50 units per axilla. Define the hyperhidrotic area to be injected using standard staining techniques (eg, Minor's Iodine-Starch Test). 50 units of botulinum toxin type A (2 mL) is injected intradermally in 0.1 to 0.2 mL aliquots to each axilla evenly distributed in multiple sites (10 to 15) approximately 1 to 2 cm apart.

Administer repeat injections for hyperhidrosis when the clinical effect of a previous injection diminishes.

The maximum dose is 25 units for any 1 muscle as a single injection.

Vertical muscles, and for horizontal strabismus of less than 20 prism diopters – 1.25 to 2.5 units in any 1 muscle.

Horizontal strabismus of 20 to 50 prism diopters – 2.5 to 5 units in any 1 muscle.

Persistent VI nerve palsy of 1 month or longer duration – 1.25 to 2.5 units in the medial rectus muscle.

Duration of activity – The initial doses create paralysis of injected muscles beginning 1 to 2 days after injection that increases in intensity during the first week. The paralysis lasts for 2 to 6 weeks and gradually resolves over a similar time period.

Subsequent doses for residual or recurrent strabismus – Patients should be reexamined 7 to 14 days after each injection to assess the effect of that dose. Patients experiencing adequate paralysis of the target muscle should receive a dose comparable with the initial dose. Subsequent doses for patients experiencing incomplete paralysis may be increased up to 2-fold. Do not administer subsequent injections until the effects of the previous dose have dissipated.

Upper limb spasticity:

***Botox* Recommended Dose Ranges Per Muscle**	
	Total dosage (number of sites)
Biceps brachii	100 to 200 units divided in 4 sites
Flexor carpi radialis	12.5 to 50 units in 1 site
Flexor carpi ulnaris	12.5 to 50 units in 1 site
Flexor digitorum profundus	30 to 50 units in 1 site
Flexor digitorum sublimis	30 to 50 units in 1 site

50 units per site.

Use the lowest recommended starting dose.

Repeat botulinum toxin type A treatment may be administered generally no sooner than 12 weeks after the previous injection.

Botox Cosmetic:

Glabellar lines – Inject 0.1 mL into each of 5 sites, 2 in each corrugator muscle and 1 in the procerus muscle for a total dose of 20 units.

Duration of activity: Typically, the initial doses induce a chemical denervation of the injected muscles 1 to 2 days after injection, increasing in intensity during the first week. Duration of activity is approximately 3 to 4 months; more frequent dosing is not recommended.

Dysport:

Cervical dystonia – 250 to 1,000 units IM every 12 weeks or longer.

The initial dose is 500 units IM as a divided dose among affected muscles in patients with or without a history of treatment with botulinum toxin.

Make dosage adjustments in 250 unit steps according to the patient's response, with re-treatment every 12 weeks or longer as necessary.

Duration of activity: Clinical studies suggest peak effect occurs between 2 and 4 weeks after injection.

Glabellar lines – 50 units IM in 5 equal aliquots of 10 units each.

Duration of activity: Up to 4 months.

Subsequent doses: Repeat-dose clinical studies demonstrated continued efficacy with up to 4 repeated administrations. Administer no more frequently than every 3 months.

Blepharospasm (Botox and Xeomin): The recommended initial total dose should be the same dose as the patient's previous treatment of *Botox*. If the previous dose of *Botox* is not known, the initial dose should be between 1.25 to 2.5 units per injection site (0.05 to 0.1 mL volume at each site) injected into the medial and lateral pretarsal orbicularis oculi of the upper lid and into the lateral pretarsal orbicularis oculi of the lower lid.

The total initial dose in both eyes should not exceed 70 units (35 units per eye).

The median first onset of effect occurs within 7 days after injection. Typical duration of effect of each treatment is up to 3 months.

Subsequent dosing should be tailored to the individual patient up to a maximum dose of 35 units per eye. The frequency of repeat treatments should generally be no more frequent than every 12 weeks.

Cervical dystonia (Xeomin): The frequency of repeat treatments should generally be no more frequent than every 12 weeks.

The median first onset of effect occurs within 7 days after injection. Typical duration of effect of each treatment is up to 3 months.

Children:

Botox –

Blepharospasm: See Adults for dosing for children 12 years of age and older.

Cervical dystonia: See Adults for dosing for children 16 years of age and older

Strabismus: See Adults for dosing for children 12 years of age and older.

Botulinum toxin assay: The method utilized for performing the potency assay is specific to the manufacturer's botulinum toxin type A. Because of specific details of this assay, such as the vehicle, dilution scheme, and laboratory protocols for the various potency assays, units of biological activity of botulinum toxin type A cannot be compared with nor converted into units of any other botulinum toxin or any toxin assessed with any other specific assay method. Therefore, differences in species sensitivities to different botulinum neurotoxin serotypes precludes extrapolation of animal dose-activity relationships to human dose relationships.

Administration:

Botox –

Blepharospasm: For IM injection only. Inject reconstituted toxin using a sterile, 27- to 30-gauge needle without EMG guidance. Avoiding injection near the levator palpebrae superioris may reduce the complication of ptosis. Avoiding medial lower lid injections may reduce the complication of diplopia. Ecchymosis occurs easily in the soft eyelid tissues. This can be prevented by applying pressure at the injection site immediately after the injection.

Cervical dystonia: For IM injection only. A 25- to 30-gauge needle may be used for superficial muscles, and a longer 22-gauge needle may be used for deeper musculature.

Chronic migraine: Use a sterile 30-gauge, 0.5 inch needle as 0.1 mL (5 units) injections per each site. A 1-inch needle may be needed in the neck region for patients with thick neck muscles. With the exception of the procerus muscle, which should be injected at 1 site (midline), all muscles should be injected bilaterally.

Primary axillary hyperhidrosis: Use a 30-gauge needle. Each dose is injected to a depth of approximately 2 mm and at a 45-degree angle to the skin surface, with the bevel side up to minimize leakage and to ensure the injections remain intradermal.

Strabismus: For IM injection only. Injection without surgical exposure or EMG guidance should not be attempted. It is recommended that several drops of a local anesthetic and an ocular decongestant be given several minutes prior to injection. The volume injected for treatment of strabismus should be between 0.05 to 0.15 mL per muscle.

Upper limb spasticity: For IM injection only. An appropriately sized needle (eg, 25- to 30-gauge) may be used for superficial muscles, and a longer 22-gauge needle may be used for deeper musculature.

Botox Cosmetic – For IM injection only; use a 30- to 33-gauge needle. To reduce the complication of ptosis avoid injection near the levator palpebrae superioris; place lateral corrugator injections at least 1 cm above the bony supraorbital ridge; do not inject toxin closer than 1 cm above the central eyebrow.

Dysport –

Cervical dystonia: For IM injection. A sterile 23- or 25-gauge needle should be used for administration. Limiting the dose injected into the sternocleidomastoid muscle may reduce the occurrence of dysphagia.

Glabellar lines: Advance the needle through the skin into the underlying muscle while applying finger pressure on the superior medial orbital rim. Using a 30-gauge needle, inject 10 units into 5 sites, 2 in each corrugator muscle and 1 in the procerus muscle.

To reduce the complication of ptosis, avoid injection near the levator palpebrae superioris; medial corrugator injections should be placed at least 1 cm above the bony supraorbital ridge; and do not inject closer than 1 cm above the central eyebrow.

Xeomin – For IM injection only. A suitable sterile needle (eg, 26-gauge [0.45 mm diameter], 37 mm length for superficial muscles; or 22-gauge [0.7 mm diameter], 75 mm length for injections into deeper muscles) should be used.

Usually injected into the sternocleidomastoid, levator scapulae, splenius capitis, scalenus, and/or the trapezius muscle(s) for the treatment of cervical dystonia.

Admixture compatibility: Reconstitute with sterile, nonpreserved sodium chloride only.

Actions

Pharmacology: Botulinum toxin type A blocks neuromuscular conduction by binding to receptor sites on motor nerve terminals, entering the nerve terminals, and inhibiting the release of acetylcholine. When injected IM at therapeutic doses, botulinum toxin type A produces a partial chemical denervation of the muscle, resulting in a localized reduction in muscle activity. In addition, the muscle may atrophy, axonal sprouting may occur, and extrajunctional acetylcholine receptors may develop, thus, slowly reversing muscle denervation produced by botulinum toxin type A. When injected intradermally, botulinum toxin type A produces temporary chemical denervation of the sweat gland, resulting in local reduction in sweating.

Contraindications

Presence of infection at the proposed injection site(s); hypersensitivity to any botulinum toxin preparation including cow's milk protein (*Dysport* only).

Warnings/Precautions

Lack of interchangeability: The potency units of botulinum toxin type A are specific to the preparation and assay method used. They are not interchangeable with other preparations of botulinum toxin products.

Neuropathic disorders: Closely monitor individuals with peripheral motor neuropathic diseases (eg, amyotrophic lateral sclerosis) or neuromuscular junctional disorders (eg, myasthenia gravis, Lambert-Eaton syndrome). Patients with neuromuscular disorders may be at increased risk of clinically significant systemic effects including severe dysphagia and respiratory compromise from typical doses of botulinum toxin type A.

Dysphagia: Treatment with botulinum toxin type A and other botulinum toxin products can result in swallowing or breathing difficulties.

Facial anatomy in the treatment of glabellar lines: Exercise caution when administering botulinum toxin type A to patients with surgical alterations to the facial anatomy, excessive weakness or atrophy in the target muscle(s), marked facial asymmetry, inflammation at the injection site(s), ptosis, excessive dermatochalasis, deep dermal scarring, thick sebaceous skin, or the inability to substantially lessen glabellar lines by physically spreading them apart.

Albumin: This product contains albumin, a derivative of human blood. Based on effective donor screening and product manufacturing processes, it carries an extremely remote risk for transmission of viral diseases. A theoretical risk for transmission of Creutzfeldt-Jakob disease (CJD) also is considered extremely remote. No cases of transmission of viral diseases or CJD have ever been identified for albumin.

Administration: Botox and *Botox Cosmetic* contain the same active ingredient in the same formulation. Adverse reactions observed with the use of *Botox* also have the potential to be associated with the use of *Botox Cosmetic*. Do not exceed the recommended dosage and frequency of administration for botulinum toxin type A.

Cardiovascular events: There have been reports following administration of botulinum toxin type A of adverse events involving the cardiovascular system, including arrhythmia and MI, some with fatal outcomes. Some of these patients had risk factors including pre-existing cardiovascular disease.

Safe and effective use: Safe and effective use of botulinum toxin type A depends upon proper storage of the product, selection of the correct dose, and proper reconstitution and administration techniques. Physicians administering botulinum toxin type A must understand the relevant neuromuscular or orbital anatomy of the area involved and any alterations to the anatomy caused by prior surgical procedures.

Retrobulbar hemorrhages: During the administration of botulinum toxin type A for the treatment of strabismus, retrobulbar hemorrhages sufficient to compromise retinal circulation have occurred. It is recommended that appropriate instruments to decompress the orbit be accessible.

Administration: Inject botulinum toxin type A (cosmetic) no more frequently than every 3 months and perform using the lowest effective dose.

Injection site: Use caution when botulinum toxin type A treatment is used in the presence of inflammation at the proposed injection site(s) or when excessive weakness or atrophy is present in the target muscle(s).

Corneal exposure and ulceration: Reduced blinking from botulinum toxin type A injection of the orbicularis muscle can lead to corneal exposure, persistent epithelial defect, and corneal ulceration, especially in patients with VII nerve disorders.

Immunogenicity: Treatment with botulinum toxin type A may result in the formation of neutralizing antibodies that may reduce the effectiveness of subsequent treatments with botulinum toxin type A treatment by inactivating the biological activity of the toxin.

The results from some studies suggest that botulinum toxin type A injections at more frequent intervals or at higher doses may lead to greater incidence of antibody formation. The potential for antibody formation may be minimized by injecting with the lowest effective dose given at the longest feasible intervals between injections.

Race: Exploratory analyses in trials for glabellar lines in black subjects with Fitzpatrick skin types IV, V, or VI and in Hispanic subjects suggested that response rates at day 30 were comparable with and no worse than the overall population

Respiratory effects: Closely monitor patients with compromised respiratory status treated with *Botox* for upper limb spasticity.

Hypersensitivity reactions: Serious and/or immediate hypersensitivity reactions have been rarely reported. These reactions include anaphylaxis, serum sickness, urticaria, soft tissue edema, and dyspnea.

Pregnancy: Category C.

Administration of *Botox Cosmetic* is not recommended during pregnancy.

Lactation: It is not known whether this drug is excreted in breast milk. Exercise caution when botulinum toxin type A is administered to a nursing woman.

Children:

Botox – Safety and effectiveness in children younger than 12 years of age have not been established for blepharospasm or strabismus, or younger than 16 years of age for cervical dystonia or 18 years of age for axillary hyperhidrosis, spasticity, or chronic migraine.

Botox Cosmetic – Use of botulinum toxin type A (cosmetic) is not recommended in children.

Dysport –

Cervical dystonia: Safety and effectiveness in children have not been established.

Glabellar lines: Botulinum toxin type A is not recommended for use in children younger than 18 years of age.

Xeomin – Safety and effectiveness in patients younger than 18 years of age have not been established.

Elderly: In general, be cautious in dose selection for an elderly patient, usually starting at the low end of the dosing range, reflecting the greater frequency of decreased hepatic, renal, or cardiac function, and of concomitant disease or other drug therapy.

Monitoring: Closely monitor patients with peripheral motor neuropathic diseases, amyotrophic lateral sclerosis, or neuromuscular junction disorders (eg, myasthenia gravis, Lambert-Eaton syndrome) when they are given botulinum toxin.

Closely monitor patients with compromised respiratory status treated with *Botox* for upper limb spasticity.

Drug Interactions

The effect of administering different botulinum neurotoxin serotypes at the same time or within several months of each other may exacerbate excessive neuromuscular weakness. Use with caution.

Drugs that may interact with botulinum toxin type A include aminoglycosides, muscle relaxants, and nondepolarizing muscle relaxants and other agents interfering with neuromuscular transmission.

Adverse Reactions

In general, adverse events occur within the first week following injection of botulinum toxin type A and, while generally transient, may have a duration of several months.

Cervical dystonia: Adverse reactions in at least 3% of patients include dysphagia, upper respiratory infection, neck pain, headache, dyspnea, increased cough, flu syndrome, back pain, rhinitis, dizziness, hypertonia, injection site soreness, asthenia, oral dryness, speech disorder, fever, nausea, and drowsiness, and dysphagia (19%), upper respiratory tract infection (12%), headache (11%), and neck pain (11%).

Adverse reactions include dry mouth, injection-site discomfort, musculoskeletal pain, nervous system disorders, respiratory, thoracic and mediastinal disorders, dysphonia, eye disorders, infections and infestations, and facial paresis.

Primary axillary hyperhidrosis: Adverse events (in at least 3% of patients) included injection site pain and hemorrhage, nonaxillary sweating, infection, pharyngitis, flu syndrome, headache, fever, neck or back pain, pruritus, and anxiety. Adverse events in 3% to 10% included anxiety, fever, flu syndrome, headache, infection, injection-site pain and hemorrhage, neck or back pain, nonaxillary sweating, pharyngitis, and pruritus.

Blepharospasm: The most frequently reported treatment-related adverse reactions were diarrhea, visual impairment, respiratory tract infection ptosis (20.8%), superficial punctate keratitis (6.3%), and eye dryness (6.3%), and ptosis (21%), eye dryness (6%), and superficial punctate keratitis (6%).

Strabismus: Extraocular muscles adjacent to the injection site can be affected, causing vertical deviation (17%), ptosis, vertical deviation, spatial disorientation, double vision, or past-pointing, especially with higher doses of botulinum toxin type A. Ptosis has been reported in 16% after horizontal rectus injections and 38% after superior rectus injections.

Upper limb spasticity: Adverse reactions include muscle weakness (4%), pain in extremity (5%), and bronchitis, fatigue, and nausea (3%).

Glabellar lines: Adverse reactions in at least 3% of patients include headache, infection, injection-site reaction, nasopharyngitis, blepharoptosis, and nausea.

Chapter 8
GASTROINTESTINAL AGENTS

ANTACIDS

ALUMINUM HYDROXIDE GEL	
Suspension; oral: 320 mg per 5 mL (*otc*)	Various
600 mg per 5 mL (*otc*)	Various, *AlternaGEL* (J & J-Merck)
MAGALDRATE	
Suspension; oral: 540 mg per 5 mL (*otc*)	*Riopan* (Whitehall)
Liquid; oral: 540 mg per 5 mL (*otc*)	Various, *Iosopan* (Goldline)
MAGNESIA (Magnesium Hydroxide)	
Tablets, chewable; oral: 311 mg (*otc*)	*Phillips' Chewable* (Bayer Consumer)
400 mg (*otc*)	*Pedia-Lax* (Fleet)
Liquid; oral: 400 mg per 5 mL (otc)	Various, *Phillips' Milk of Magnesia* (Sterling Health), *Dulcolax* (Boehringer Ingelheim)
Liquid, concentrate; oral: 800 mg per 5 mL (*otc*)	*Phillips' Concentrated Milk of Magnesia* (Sterling Health)
1,200 mg per 5 mL (otc)	Various
SODIUM BICARBONATE	
Tablets; oral: 325 and 650 mg (*otc*)	Various
SODIUM CITRATE	
Solution; oral: 450 mg per 5 mL (*otc*)	*Citra pH* (ValMed)

Indications

Hyperacidity: Symptomatic relief of upset stomach associated with hyperacidity (heartburn, gastroesophageal reflux, acid indigestion, and sour stomach); hyperacidity associated with peptic ulcer and gastric hyperacidity.

Administration and Dosage

ALUMINUM HYDROXIDE GEL:

Suspension – 5 to 30 mL as needed between meals and at bedtime or as directed.

MAGALDRATE (*aluminum magnesium hydroxide sulfate*):

Suspension/Liquid – 5 to 10 mL between meals and at bedtime.

MAGNESIA (*magnesium hydroxide*):

Adults and children older than 12 years of age –

Tablets: 622 mg to 1244 mg up to 4 times daily.

Liquid: 5 to 15 mL up to 4 times daily with water.

Liquid, concentrated: 2.5 to 7.5 mL up to 4 times daily with water.

SODIUM BICARBONATE: 0.3 to 2 g 1 to 4 times daily.

SODIUM CITRATE: 30 mL daily.

Actions

Pharmacology: Antacids neutralize gastric acidity, resulting in an increase in the pH of the stomach and duodenal bulb. Additionally, by increasing the gastric pH above 4, they inhibit the proteolytic activity of pepsin. Antacids do not "coat" the mucosal lining, but may have a local astringent effect. Antacids also increase the lower esophageal sphincter tone. Aluminum ions inhibit smooth muscle contraction, thus inhibiting gastric emptying.

Acid neutralizing capacity (ANC) – ANC is a consideration in selecting an antacid. It varies for commercial antacid preparations and is expressed as mEq/mL. Milliequivalents of ANC is defined by the mEq of hydrochloride required to keep an antacid suspension at pH 3.5 for 10 minutes in vitro. An antacid must neutralize at least 5 mEq/dose. Also, any ingredient must contribute at least 25% of the total ANC of a given product to be considered an antacid.

Aluminum hydroxide and calcium-containing antacids may reduce LDL cholesterol and increase the HDL/LDL ratio.

Warnings/Precautions

Sodium content: Sodium content of antacids may be significant. Patients with hypertension, CHF, marked renal failure, or those on restricted or low-sodium diets should use a low sodium preparation.

"Acid rebound": Antacids may cause dose-related rebound hyperacidity because they may increase gastric secretion or serum gastrin levels.

Milk-alkali syndrome: Milk-alkali syndrome, an acute illness with symptoms of headache, nausea, irritability, and weakness, or a chronic illness with alkalosis, hypercalcemia and, possibly, renal impairment, has occurred following the concurrent use of high-dose calcium carbonate and sodium bicarbonate.

Hypophosphatemia: Prolonged use of aluminum-containing antacids may result in hypophosphatemia in normophosphatemic patients if phosphate intake is not adequate.

GI hemorrhage: Use aluminum hydroxide with care in patients who have recently suffered massive upper GI hemorrhage.

Renal function impairment: Use magnesium-containing products with caution, particularly when more than 50 mEq magnesium is given daily. Hypermagnesemia and toxicity may occur because of decreased clearance of the magnesium ion.

Prolonged use of aluminum-containing antacids in patients with renal failure may result in or worsen dialysis osteomalacia.

Pregnancy: If pregnant, consult a physician before using.

Drug Interactions

Drugs that may be affected by antacids include allopurinol, amphetamines, benzodiazepines, captopril, chloroquine, corticosteroids, dicumarol, diflunisal, digoxin, ethambutol, flecainide, fluoroquinolones, histamine H_2 antagonists, hydantoins, iron salts, isoniazid, ketoconazole, levodopa, lithium, methenamine, methotrexate, nitrofurantoin, penicillamine, phenothiazines, quinidine, salicylates, sodium polystyrene sulfonate, sulfonylureas, sympathomimetics, tetracyclines, thyroid hormones, ticlopidine, and valproic acid.

Adverse Reactions

Magnesium-containing antacids – Laxative effect as saline cathartic, may cause diarrhea; hypermagnesemia in renal failure patients.

Aluminum-containing antacids – Constipation (may lead to intestinal obstruction); aluminum-intoxication; osteomalacia and hypophosphatemia; accumulation of aluminum in serum, bone, and the CNS (aluminum accumulation may be neurotoxic); encephalopathy.

Antacids – Dose-dependent rebound hyperacidity and milk-alkali syndrome.

SUCRALFATE

Tablets: 1 g (*Rx*)	Various, *Carafate* (Aventis)
Suspension: 1 g per 10 mL (*Rx*)	*Carafate* (Aventis)

Indications

Duodenal ulcer: Short-term treatment (up to 8 weeks) of active duodenal ulcer.

Maintenance therapy (tablets only): Duodenal ulcer patients at reduced dosage after healing of acute ulcers.

Administration and Dosage

Active duodenal ulcer:

Adults – 1 g 4 times daily on an empty stomach (1 hour before meals and at bedtime).

Take antacids as needed for pain relief but not within ½ hour before or after sucralfate.

While healing with sucralfate may occur within the first 2 weeks, continue treatment for 4 to 8 weeks unless healing is demonstrated by X-ray or endoscopic examination.

Maintenance therapy (tablets only):

Adults – 1 g twice daily.

Actions

Pharmacology: Sucralfate does not affect gastric acid output or concentration. It rapidly reacts with hydrochloric acid in the stomach to form a condensed, viscous, adhesive, paste-like substance with the capacity to buffer acid and binds to the surface of gastric and duodenal ulcers.

The barrier formed at the ulcer site protects the ulcer from the potential ulcerogenic properties of pepsin, acid, and bile, thus allowing the ulcer to heal.

Pharmacokinetics: Sucralfate is minimally absorbed from the GI tract following an oral dose. The duration of action depends on the time that the drug is in contact with this site. Binding to the ulcer site has been shown for up to 6 hours. Approximately 95% of the dose remains in the GI tract.

Warnings/Precautions

Chronic renal failure/dialysis: During sucralfate administration, small amounts of aluminum are absorbed. Concomitant use with other aluminum-containing products may increase the total body burden of aluminum. Patients with chronic renal failure or receiving dialysis have impaired excretion of absorbed aluminum, and aluminum is not dialyzed. Aluminum accumulation and toxicity have occurred.

Ulcer recurrence: Duodenal ulcer is a chronic recurrent disease. While short-term treatment can completely heal the ulcer, do not expect a successful course to alter posthealing frequency or severity of duodenal ulceration.

Pregnancy: Category B.

Lactation: It is not known whether this drug is excreted in breast milk.

Children: Safety and efficacy in children have not been established.

Drug Interactions

Drugs that may be affected by sucralfate include aluminum-containing antacids, anticoagulants, diclofenac, digoxin, histamine H_2 antagonists (eg, cimetidine, ranitidine), hydantoins, ketoconazole, levothyroxine, penicillamine, quinidine, quinolones, tetracycline, and theophylline.

Adverse Reactions

Adverse reactions in clinical trials were minor and rarely led to drug discontinuation. Constipation was the most frequent complaint (2%).

GASTROINTESTINAL ANTICHOLINERGICS/ANTISPASMODICS

ANISOTROPINE METHYLBROMIDE	
Tablets: 50 mg (*Rx*)	Various
ATROPINE SULFATE	
Injection: 0.05, 0.1, 0.3, 0.4, 0.5, 0.8, and 1 mg/mL (*Rx*)	Various
0.5, 1, and 2 mg (*Rx*)	*Atro-Pen* (Meridian Medical Technologies)
Tablets: 0.4 mg (*Rx*)	*Sal-Tropine* (Hope)
DICYCLOMINE HYDROCHLORIDE	
Capsules: 10 and 20 mg (*Rx*)	Various, *Bentyl* (Lakeside Pharm.), *Byclomine* (Major), *Di-Spaz* (Vortech)
Tablets: 20 mg (*Rx*)	Various, *Bentyl* (Lakeside Pharm.), *Byclomine* (Major)
Syrup: 10 mg per 5 mL (*Rx*)	Various, *Bentyl* (Lakeside Pharm.)
Injection: 10 mg/mL (*Rx*)	Various, *Bentyl* (Lakeside Pharm.), *Dilomine* (Kay Drug), *Di-Spaz* (Vortech), *Or-Tyl* (Ortega)
GLYCOPYRROLATE	
Tablets: 1 and 2 mg (*Rx*)	Various, *Robinul* (Robins)
Injection: 0.2 mg/mL (*Rx*)	Various, *Robinul* (Robins)
LEVOROTATORY ALKALOIDS OF BELLADONNA	
Tablets: 0.25 mg (*Rx*)	*Bellafoline* (Sandoz)
L-HYOSCYAMINE SULFATE	
Tablets: 0.125 mg (*Rx*)	Various, *Levsin* (Alaven)
0.15 mg (*Rx*)	*Cystospaz* (PolyMedica)
Tablets, chewable: 125 mg (*Rx*)	*HyoMax-FT* (Aristos Pharmaceutical)
Tablets, sublingual: 0.125 mg (*Rx*)	Various, *Levsin/SL* (Alaven), *Symax-SL* (Capellon)
Tablets, extended release: 0.25 mg (0.125 mg immediate-release) (*Rx*)	*Hyoscyamine Sulfate* (River's Edge)
0.375 mg (*Rx*)	Various, *Levbid* (Alaven)
0.375 mg (0.125 mg immediate-release, 0.25 mg extended-release) (*Rx*)	*Symax Duotab* (Capellon)
Tablets, sustained release: 0.375 mg (*Rx*)	*Symax-SR* (Capellon)
Tablets, disintegrating: 0.125 mg (*Rx*)	Various, *Neosol* (Breckenridge), *NuLev* (Schwarz Pharma), *Symax FasTab* (Capellon)
0.25 mg (*Rx*)	*Mar-Spas* (Marnel)
Capsules, timed release: 0.375 mg (*Rx*)	Various, *Levsinex Timecaps* (Schwarz Pharma)
Capsules, extended release: 0.375 mg (*Rx*)	*Hyoscyamine Sulfate* (Ethex)
Solution, oral: 0.125 mg/mL (*Rx*)	*Hyoscyamine Sulfate* (Goldline)
Oral spray: 0.125 mg/mL (0.125 mg/spray) (*Rx*)	*IB-Stat* (InKine)
Injection: 0.5 mg/mL (*Rx*)	*Levsin* (Alaven)
METHSCOPOLAMINE BROMIDE	
Tablets: 2.5 and 5 mg (*Rx*)	Various, *Pamine* (Kenwood/Bradley)
MEPENZOLATE BROMIDE	
Tablets: 25 mg (*Rx*)	*Cantil* (Aventis)
METHANTHELINE BROMIDE	
Tablets: 50 mg (*Rx*)	*Banthine* (Schiapparelli Searle)
OXYPHENCYCLIMINE HYDROCHLORIDE	
Tablets: 10 mg (*Rx*)	*Daricon* (GlaxoSmithKline)
PROPANTHELINE BROMIDE	
Tablets: 7.5 and 15 mg (*Rx*)	Various
SCOPOLAMINE HBr (Hyoscine HBr)	
Injection: 0.3, 0.4, 0.86, and 1 mg/mL (*Rx*)	Various
Tablets, soluble: 0.4 mg (*Rx*)	*Scopace* (Hope Pharm)
TRIDIHEXETHYL CHLORIDE	
Tablets: 25 mg (*Rx*)	*Pathilon* (Lederle)

Indications

Peptic ulcer: Adjunctive therapy for peptic ulcer. These agents suppress gastric acid secretion.

Other GI conditions: Functional GI disorders (diarrhea, pylorospasm, hypermotility, neurogenic colon), irritable bowel syndrome (spastic colon, mucous colitis), acute enterocolitis, ulcerative colitis, diverticulitis, mild dysenteries, pancreatitis, splenic flexure syndrome, and infant colic.

Biliary tract: For spastic disorders of the biliary tract. Given in conjunction with a narcotic analgesic.

Urogenital tract: Uninhibited hypertonic neurogenic bladder.

Bradycardia: **Atropine** is used in the suppression of vagally mediated bradycardias.

Preoperative medication: **Atropine, scopolamine, hyoscyamine,** and **glycopyrrolate** are used as preanesthetic medication to control bronchial, nasal, pharyngeal, and salivary secretions and to block cardiac vagal inhibitory reflexes during induction of anesthesia and intubation. Scopolamine is used for preanesthetic sedation and for obstetric amnesia.

Antidotes for poisoning by cholinergic drugs: Atropine is used for poisoning by organophosphorus insecticides, chemical warfare nerve gases, and as an antidote for mushroom poisoning caused by muscarine in certain species, such as *Amanita muscaria.*

Miscellaneous uses: Calming delirium; motion sickness (**scopolamine**); parkinsonism.

Unlabeled uses:

Bronchial asthma – Atropine and related agents are effective in some patients with cholinergic-mediated bronchospasm.

Glycopyrrolate may be effective in the treatment of bronchial asthma.

Administration and Dosage

ANISOTROPINE METHYLBROMIDE: 50 mg 3 times daily.

ATROPINE SULFATE:

Adults – 0.4 to 0.6 mg.

Children –

Atropine Dosage Recommendations in Children

Weight		Dose
lb	kg	mg
7 to 16	3.2 to 7.3	0.1
16 to 24	7.3 to 10.9	0.15
24 to 40	10.9 to 18.1	0.2
40 to 65	18.1 to 29.5	0.3
65 to 90	29.5 to 40.8	0.4
> 90	40.8	0.4 to 0.6

Hypotonic radiography – 1 mg IM.

Surgery – Give subcutaneously, IM, or IV. The average adult dose is 0.5 mg (range, 0.4 to 0.6 mg). In children, it has been suggested to use a dose of 0.01 mg/kg to a maximum of 0.4 mg, repeated every 4 to 6 hours as needed. A recommended infant dose is 0.04 mg/kg (infants less than 5 kg) or 0.03 mg/kg (infants more than 5 kg), repeated every 4 to 6 hours as needed.

Bradyarrhythmias – The usual IV adult dosage ranges from 0.4 to 1 mg every 1 to 2 hours as needed; larger doses, up to a maximum of 2 mg, may be required. In children, IV dosage ranges from 0.01 to 0.03 mg/kg.

Poisoning – In anticholinesterase poisoning from exposure to insecticides, give large doses of at least 2 to 3 mg parenterally; repeat until signs of atropine intoxication appear.

Atro-Pen – Primary protection against exposure to chemical nerve agent and insecticide poisoning is the wearing of protective garments including masks, designed specifically for this use.

The *AtroPen* Auto-injector should be administered as soon as symptoms of organophosphorus. or carbamate poisoning appear (eg, usually tearing, excessive oral secretions, wheezing, muscle fasciculations). In moderate to severe poisoning, the administration of more than 1 *AtroPen* may be required until atropinization is achieved (flushing, mydriasis, tachycardia, dryness of the mouth and nose).

No more than 3 *AtroPen* injections should be used unless the patient is under the supervision of a trained medical provider. Different dose strengths of the *AtroPen* are available depending on the recipient's age and weight.

AtroPen Dosing

Patient group	Dose strength
Adults and children weighing more than 90 lbs (generally over 10 years of age)	2 mg
Children weighing 40 to 90 lbs (generally 4 to 10 years of age)	1 mg
Children weighing 15 to 40 lbs (generally 6 months to 4 years of age)[a]	0.5 mg

[a] Children weighing less than 15 lbs (generally younger than 6 months of age) should ordinarily not be treated with the *AtroPen* auto-injector. Atropine doses for these children should be individualized at doses of 0.05 mg/kg.

DICYCLOMINE HYDROCHLORIDE:

Oral –

Adults: The only oral dose shown to be effective is 160 mg/day in 4 equally divided doses. However, because of side effects, begin with 80 mg/day (in 4 equally divided doses). Increase dose to 160 mg/day unless side effects limit dosage.

Parenteral – IM only. Not for IV use.

Adults: 80 mg/day in 4 divided doses.

GLYCOPYRROLATE: Not recommended for children younger than 12 years of age for the management of peptic ulcer.

Oral – 1 mg 3 times daily or 2 mg 2 to 3 times daily.

Maintenance: 1 mg 2 times daily.

Parenteral –

Peptic ulcer: 0.1 to 0.2 mg IM or IV 3 or 4 times daily.

Preanesthetic medication: 0.002 mg/lb (0.004 mg/kg) IM, 30 minutes to 1 hour prior to anesthesia. Children younger than 2 years of age may require up to 0.004 mg/lb. Children younger than 12 years of age, give 0.002 to 0.004 mg/lb IM.

Intraoperative medication: Adults, 0.1 mg IV. Repeat as needed at 2- to 3-minute intervals. Children, give 0.002 mg/lb (0.004 mg/kg) IV, not to exceed 0.1 mg in a single dose; may be repeated at 2- to 3-minute intervals.

Reversal of neuromuscular blockade: Adults and children, 0.2 mg for each 1 mg neostigmine or 5 mg pyridostigmine. Administer IV simultaneously.

L-HYOSCYAMINE SULFATE:

Oral –

Adults: 0.125 to 0.25 mg 3 or 4 times/day orally or sublingually; or 0.375 to 0.75 mg in sustained release form every 12 hours.

Children: Individualize dosage according to weight.

Parenteral – 0.25 to 0.5 mg subcutaneously, IM, or IV, 2 to 4 times daily, as needed.

LEVOROTATORY ALKALOIDS OF BELLADONNA:

Oral –

Adults: 0.25 to 0.5 mg 3 times daily.

Children (older than 6 years of age): 0.125 to 0.25 mg 3 times daily.

MEPENZOLATE BROMIDE:

Adults – 25 to 50 mg 4 times daily with meals and at bedtime.

Children – Safety and efficacy have not been established.

METHANTHELINE BROMIDE:

Adults – 50 to 100 mg every 6 hours.

Pediatric –

Newborns: 12.5 mg 2 times daily, then 12.5 mg 3 times daily.

Infants (1 to 12 months of age): 12.5 mg 4 times daily, increased to 25 mg 4 times daily.

Children (older than 1 year of age): 12.5 to 50 mg 4 times daily.

METHSCOPOLAMINE BROMIDE: 2.5 mg 30 minutes before meals and 2.5 to 5 mg at bedtime.

OXPHENCYCLIMINE HYDROCHLORIDE:

Adults – 5 to 10 mg 2 or 3 times daily, preferably in the morning and at bedtime. Some respond to 5 mg 2 times/day, while some may require higher dosage 3 times/day.

Children – Not for use in children younger than 12 years of age.

PROPANTHELINE BROMIDE:

Adults – 15 mg 30 minutes before meals and 30 mg at bedtime. For patients with mild manifestations, geriatric patients, or those of small stature, take 7.5 mg 3 times daily.

Children –

Peptic ulcer: Safety and efficacy have not been established.

Antisecretory: 1.5 mg/kg/day divided 3 to 4 times daily.

Antispasmodic: 2 to 3 mg/kg/day divided every 4 to 6 hours and at bedtime.

SCOPOLAMINE HBr (Hyoscine HBr): Give subcutaneously or IM; may give IV after dilution with Sterile Water for Injection.

Adults – 0.32 to 0.65 mg.

Children – 0.006 mg/kg. Maximum dosage, 0.3 mg.

Tablets – 0.4 to 0.8 mg. Dosage may be cautiously increased in parkinsonism and spastic states.

TRIDIHEXETHYL CHLORIDE: 25 to 50 mg 3 or 4 times daily before meals and at bedtime. Bedtime dose, 50 mg.

Actions

Pharmacology: GI anticholinergics are used primarily to decrease motility (smooth muscle tone) in GI, biliary, and urinary tracts and for antisecretory effects. Antispasmodics, related compounds, decrease GI motility by acting on smooth muscle.

These agents inhibit the muscarinic actions of acetylcholine at postganglionic parasympathetic neuroeffector sites including smooth muscle, secretory glands, and CNS sites. Large doses may block nicotinic receptors at the autonomic ganglia and at the neuromuscular junction.

Pharmacokinetics:

Belladonna alkaloids – Belladonna alkaloids are rapidly absorbed after oral use. They readily cross the blood-brain barrier and affect the CNS.

Atropine – Atropine has a half-life of approximately 2.5 hours; 94% of a dose is eliminated through the urine in 24 hours.

Quaternary anticholinergics – Synthetic or semisynthetic derivatives structurally related to the belladonna alkaloids, they are poorly and unreliably absorbed orally. Because they do not cross the blood-brain barrier, CNS effects are negligible. Duration of action is more prolonged than alkaloids.

Contraindications

Hypersensitivity: Hypersensitivity to anticholinergic drugs. Patients hypersensitive to belladonna or to barbiturates may be hypersensitive to **scopolamine**.

Ocular: Narrow-angle glaucoma; adhesions (synechiae) between the iris and lens.

Cardiovascular: Tachycardia; unstable cardiovascular status in acute hemorrhage; myocardial ischemia.

GI: Obstructive disease (eg, achalasia, pyloroduodenal stenosis or pyloric obstruction, cardiospasm); paralytic ileus; intestinal atony of the elderly or debilitated; severe ulcerative colitis; toxic megacolon complicating ulcerative colitis; hepatic disease.

GU: Obstructive uropathy (eg, bladder neck obstruction caused by prostatic hypertrophy); renal disease.

Musculoskeletal: Myasthenia gravis.

Atropine: Atropine is contraindicated in asthma patients.

Dicyclomine: Dicyclomine is contraindicated in infants younger than 6 months of age.

Warnings/Precautions

Heat prostration: Heat prostration can occur with anticholinergic drug use (fever and heat stroke caused by decreased sweating) in the presence of a high environmental temperature.

Diarrhea: Diarrhea may be an early symptom of incomplete intestinal obstruction, especially in patients with ileostomy or colostomy. Treatment of diarrhea with these drugs is inappropriate and possibly harmful.

Anticholinergic psychosis: Anticholinergic psychosis has been reported in sensitive individuals given anticholinergic drugs.

Gastric ulcer: Gastric ulcer may produce a delay in gastric emptying time and may complicate therapy (antral stasis).

Use with caution in the following:

Ocular – Glaucoma; light irides. Use caution in the elderly because of increased incidence of glaucoma.

GI – Hepatic disease; early evidence of ileus, as in peritonitis; ulcerative colitis; hiatal hernia associated with reflux esophagitis.

GU – Renal disease; prostatic hypertrophy.

Cardiovascular – Coronary heart disease; CHF; cardiac arrhythmias; tachycardia; hypertension.

Pulmonary – Debilitated patients with chronic lung disease; reduction in bronchial secretions can lead to inspissation and formation of bronchial plugs.

Miscellaneous – Autonomic neuropathy; hyperthyroidism.

Special risk: Use cautiously in infants, small children, and people with Down syndrome, brain damage, or spastic paralysis.

Hazardous tasks: May produce drowsiness, dizziness, or blurred vision; observe caution while driving or performing other tasks requiring alertness.

Pregnancy: Category B (glycopyrrolate, parenteral); *Category* C (hyoscyamine, atropine, scopolamine, propantheline, methantheline).

Lactation: **Hyoscyamine** is excreted in breast milk; other anticholinergics (especially **atropine**) may be excreted in milk, causing infant toxicity, and may reduce milk production.

Children: Safety and efficacy are not established. **Hyoscyamine** has been used in infant colic. Safety and efficacy of **glycopyrrolate** in children younger than 12 years of age are not established for peptic ulcer. **Dicyclomine** is contraindicated in infants younger than 6 months of age.

Elderly: Elderly patients may react with excitement, agitation, drowsiness, and other untoward manifestations to even small doses of anticholinergic drugs.

Drug Interactions

Drugs that may interact with GI anticholinergics include amantadine, atenolol, digoxin, phenothiazines, and tricyclic antidepressants.

Adverse Reactions

Xerostomia; altered taste perception; nausea; vomiting; dysphagia; heartburn; constipation; bloated feeling; paralytic ileus; urinary hesitancy and retention; impotence; blurred vision; mydriasis; photophobia; cycloplegia; increased intraocular pressure; dilated pupils; palpitations; tachycardia (after higher doses); headache; flushing; nervousness; drowsiness; weakness; dizziness; confusion; insomnia; fever (especially in children); mental confusion or excitement; CNS stimulation (restlessness, tremor with large doses); severe allergic reactions including anaphylaxis, urticaria and other dermal manifestations; nasal congestion; decreased sweating.

HISTAMINE H_2 ANTAGONISTS

CIMETIDINE	
Tablets: 200 mg (*otc*)	Various, *Tagamet HB* (GlaxoSmithKline)
200, 300, 400, and 800 mg (*Rx*)	Various, *Tagamet* (GlaxoSmithKline)
Oral solution: 300 mg (as hydrochloride) per 5 mL (*Rx*)	Various, *Cimetidine* (Roxane)
Injection: 150 mg (as hydrochloride) per mL (*Rx*)	Various, *Cimetidine* (Hospira)
Injection (premixed): 6 mg (as hydrochloride) per mL (*Rx*)	*Cimetidine* (Hospira)
FAMOTIDINE	
Tablets: 10 mg (*otc*)	Various, *Pepcid AC* (J & J Merck)
20 mg (*otc*)	Various, *Pepcid AC Maximum Strength* (J & J Merck)
20 and 40 mg (*Rx*)	Various, *Pepcid* (Merck)
Gelcaps: 10 mg (*otc*)	*Pepcid AC* (J & J Merck)
Tablets, chewable: 10 mg (*otc*)	*Pepcid AC* (J & J Merck)
20 mg (*otc*)	*Pepcid AC Maximum Strength EZ Chews* (J & J Merck)
Tablets, orally disintegrating: 20 and 40 mg (*Rx*)	*Pepcid RPD* (Merck)
Powder for oral suspension: 40 mg per 5 mL when reconstituted (*Rx*)	*Pepcid* (Merck)
Injection: 10 mg/mL (*Rx*)	Various
Injection, premixed: 20 mg per 50 mL (*Rx*)	Various
NIZATIDINE	
Tablets: 75 mg (*otc*)	*Axid AR* (Wyeth Consumer)
Capsules: 150 and 300 mg (*Rx*)	Various, *Axid Pulvules* (Reliant)
Oral solution: 15 mg/mL (*Rx*)	*Axid* (Braintree)
RANITIDINE	
Tablets: 75 mg (*otc*)	*Zantac 75* (Pfizer Consumer Healthcare)
150 and 300 mg (as hydrochloride) (*Rx*)	Various, *Zantac* (GlaxoSmithKline)
Tablets, effervescent: 25 mg (*Rx*)	*Zantac EFFERdose* (GlaxoSmithKline)
Capsules: 150 and 300 mg (*Rx*)	Various
Syrup: 15 mg (as base) per mL (*Rx*)	Various, *Zantac* (GlaxoSmithKline)
Injection: 25 mg (as hydrochloride)/mL (*Rx*)	Various, *Zantac* (GlaxoSmithKline)
HISTAMINE H_2 ANTAGONIST COMBINATIONS	
Tablets, chewable: 10 mg famotidine, 800 mg calcium carbonate, 165 mg magnesium hydroxide (*otc*)	*Pepcid Complete* (J & J Merck), *Dual Action Complete* (Major), *Tums Dual Action* (GlaxoSmithKline)

Indications

Histamine H_2 Antagonists: Summary of Indications				
	Cimetidine	Famotidine	Nizatidine	Ranitidine
Benign gastric ulcer				
Treatment	✔	✔	✔	✔
Maintenance				✔
Duodenal ulcer				
Treatment	✔	✔	✔	✔
Maintenance	✔	✔	✔	✔
Erosive esophagitis, maintenance				✔
GERD (including erosive esophagitis)	✔	✔	✔	✔
Pathological hypersecretory conditions	✔	✔		✔
Prevent upper GI bleeding	✔ (IV)			
Relieve and prevent heartburn/acid indigestion/sour stomach	✔[a]	✔[a]	✔[b]	✔[a]

[a] Relief of symptoms only.
[b] OTC use only.

Administration and Dosage

CIMETIDINE:

Duodenal ulcer –

Short-term treatment: 800 mg at bedtime. Alternate regimens are 300 mg 4 times/day with meals and at bedtime, or 400 mg twice/day.

Maintenance therapy: 400 mg at bedtime.

Benign gastric ulcer – For short-term treatment, 800 mg at bedtime or 300 mg 4 times/day with meals and at bedtime.

Erosive GERD –

Adults: 800 mg twice daily or 400 mg 4 times/day for 12 weeks. Use longer than 12 weeks has not been established.

Heartburn, acid indigestion, and sour stomach (otc only) – 200 mg (1 tablet) with water as symptoms occur or as directed, up to twice daily (up to 2 tablets in 24 hours).

Pathological hypersecretory conditions – 300 mg 4 times/day with meals and at bedtime. If necessary, give 300 mg doses more often. Do not exceed 2,400 mg/day.

Severely impaired renal function – 300 mg every 12 hours orally or IV has been recommended. Dosage frequency may be increased to every 8 hours or even further with caution.

Parenteral – The usual dose is 300 mg IM or IV every 6 to 8 hours. If it is necessary to increase dosage, do so by more frequent administration of a 300 mg dose, not to exceed 2400 mg/day.

Prevention of upper GI bleeding: Continuous IV infusion of 50 mg/h. Patients with Ccr less than 30 mL/min should receive half the recommended dose. Treatment longer than 7 days has not been studied.

FAMOTIDINE:

Duodenal ulcer –

Acute therapy: 40 mg/day at bedtime or 20 mg twice/day.

Maintenance therapy: 20 mg once a day at bedtime.

Benign gastric ulcer –

Acute therapy: 40 mg once a day at bedtime.

Pathological hypersecretory conditions – 20 mg every 6 hours.

GERD – 20 mg twice daily for up to 6 weeks. For esophagitis including erosions and ulcerations, 20 or 40 mg twice daily for up to 12 weeks.

Renal function impairment – To avoid excess accumulation of the drug in patients with moderate (Ccr less than 50 mL/min) or severe renal insufficiency (Ccr less than 10 mL/min), the dose may be reduced to half the dose or the dosing interval may be prolonged to 36 to 48 hours, as indicated.

Parenteral –

IV: Give famotidine IV 20 mg every 12 hours.

Children –

Peptic ulcer: 0.5 mg/kg/day orally at bedtime or divided twice daily up to 40 mg/day.

GERD with or without esophagitis including erosions and ulcerations: 1 mg/kg/day orally divided twice daily up to 40 mg twice daily.

Heartburn, acid indigestion, and sour stomach (OTC only) –

Acute therapy: 10 mg with water.

Prevention: 10 mg 15 minutes before eating food or drinking a beverage that is expected to cause symptoms.

Use: Can be used up to twice daily (up to 2 tablets in 24 hours). Do not take maximum dose for more than 2 weeks continuously unless otherwise directed by a physician.

Children: Do not give to children under 12 years of age unless otherwise directed.

NIZATIDINE:

Active duodenal ulcer – 300 mg once daily at bedtime or 150 mg twice daily.

Maintenance of healed duodenal ulcer – 150 mg once daily at bedtime.

GERD – 150 mg twice daily.

Benign gastric ulcer – 150 mg twice daily or 300 mg once daily at bedtime.

Heartburn, acid indigestion, and sour stomach (OTC only) – Can be used up to twice daily (up to 2 tablets in 24 hours).

Relief: For relief of symptoms, take 1 tablet with a full glass of water.

Prevention: For prevention of symptoms, take 1 tablet with a full glass of water right before eating or up to 60 minutes before consuming food and beverages that cause heartburn.

Moderate to severe renal insufficiency –

Nizatidine Dosage in Renal Insufficiency		
	Dosage	
Ccr	Active duodenal ulcer	Maintenance therapy
20 to 50 mL/min	150 mg/day	150 mg every other day
< 20 mL/min	150 mg every other day	150 mg every 3 days

Children – Each mL of the oral solution contains 15 mg of nizatidine. For children 12 years of age and older, the dosage is 150 mg twice daily (10 mL [2 teaspoons] twice daily).

Erosive esophagitis: For children 12 years of age and older, the dosage is 150 mg twice daily (300 mg/day). The maximum daily dose for nizatidine oral is 300 mg/day. The dosing duration may be up to 8 weeks.

GERD: For children 12 years of age and older, the dosage is 150 mg twice daily (300 mg/day). The maximum daily dose for nizatidine oral is 300 mg/day. The dosing duration may be up to 8 weeks.

RANITIDINE:

Duodenal ulcer –

Short-term treatment of active duodenal ulcer: 150 mg orally twice daily. 300 mg once daily at bedtime.

Maintenance therapy: 150 mg at bedtime.

Pathological hypersecretory conditions – 150 mg orally twice a day. More frequent doses may be necessary. Doses up to 6 g/day have been used.

GERD – 150 mg twice daily.

Benign gastric ulcer –

Treatment: 150 mg twice daily.

Maintenance: 150 mg at bedtime.

Erosive esophagitis –

Treatment: 150 mg 4 times daily.

Maintenance: 150 mg twice daily.

Heartburn (OTC only) –

Treatment: For relief of symptoms, swallow 1 tablet with a glass of water.

Prevention: To prevent symptoms, swallow 1 tablet with a glass of water 30 to 60 minutes before eating food or drinking beverages that cause heartburn.

Maintenance: Can be used up to twice daily (up to 2 tablets in 24 hours).

Children – Do not give OTC ranitidine to children younger than 12 years of age unless directed by health care provider.

Active duodenal and gastric ulcers:

Treatment – 2 to 4 mg/kg/day twice daily to a maximum of 300 mg/day.

Maintenance – 2 to 4 mg/kg once daily to a maximum of 150 mg/day.

GERD and erosive esophagitis: 5 to 10 mg/kg/day, usually given as 2 divided doses.

Zantac 25 EFFERdose tablets – Dissolve 1 tablet in no less than 5 mL (1 teaspoonful) of water. Wait until the tablet is completely dissolved before administering the solution to the infant/child. The solution may be administered by medicine dropper for infants.

Zantac 150 EFFERdose tablets – Dissolve each dose in approximately 6 to 8 oz of water before drinking.

Renal impairment (Ccr less than 50 mL/min) – 150 mg orally every 24 hours or 50 mg parenterally every 18 to 24 hours. The frequency of dosing may be increased to every 12 hours or further with caution.

Parenteral –

IM: 50 mg (2 mL) every 6 to 8 hours.

IV injection: 50 mg (2 mL) every 6 to 8 hours; do not exceed 400 mg/day.

Children – The recommended dose is for a total daily dose of 2 to 4 mg/kg, to be divided and administered every 6 to 8 hours up to a maximum of 50 mg given every 6 to 8 hours. Limited data in neonatal patients (under 1 month of age) receiving extracorporeal-membrane oxygenation (ECMO) have shown that a dose of 2 mg/kg is usually sufficient to increase gastric pH to greater than 4 for at least 15 hours. Therefore, consider doses of 2 mg/kg given every 12 to 24 hours or as a continuous infusion.

Actions

Pharmacology: Histamine H_2 antagonists are reversible competitive blockers of histamine at the H_2 receptors. They also inhibit fasting and nocturnal secretions, and secretions stimulated by food, insulin, caffeine, pentagastrin, and betazole. **Cimetidine, ranitidine,** and **famotidine** have no effect on gastric emptying, and cimetidine and famotidine have no effect on lower esophageal sphincter pressure. Ranitidine, **nizatidine**, and famotidine have little or no effect on fasting or postprandial serum gastrin.

Pharmacokinetics:

Pharmacokinetic Properties of Histamine H_2 Antagonists

H_2 receptor antagonist	Bioavailability (%)	T_{max} (h)[a]	Peak plasma concentration[b] (mcg/mL)	Half-life (h)	Protein binding (%)	Volume of distribution (L/kg)	Elimination (%) Urine, unchanged Oral	IV
Cimetidine	≈ 60 (oral)	0.75 to 1.5 (oral)	2 to 3 (400 mg oral dose)	≈ 2[c]	13 to 25	≈ 1	48	75
Famotidine	40 to 45 (oral)	1 to 3	–	2.5 to 3.5[d]	15 to 20	≈ 1.3	25 to 30	65 to 70
Nizatidine	> 70	0.5 to 3	0.7 to 1.8/ 1.4 to 3.6 (150/300 mg dose)	1 to 2[d]	≈ 35	0.8 to 1.5	60	NA[e]
Ranitidine	50 (oral) (90 to 100 IM)[f]	2 to 3 (oral) (0.25 IM)	0.44 to 0.55 (oral) (0.58 IM)	2.5 to 3 (oral)[d] 2 to 2.5 (IV)[d]	15	1.3	30	≈70

[a] T_{max} = time to maximum concentration.
[b] Dose-dependent.
[c] Increased in patients with renal and hepatic function impairment and in elderly patients.
[d] Increased in patients with renal function impairment.
[e] NA = not applicable.
[f] IM = intramuscular. Additional pharmacokinetic data for these agents are discussed individually.

Contraindications

Hypersensitivity to individual agents or to other H_2-receptor antagonists.

Warnings/Precautions

Benzyl alcohol: Benzyl alcohol, contained in some of these products as a preservative, has been associated with a fatal "gasping syndrome" in premature infants.

Phenylketonuria: Inform patients with phenylketonuria that some of these products contain phenylalanine.

Gastric malignancy: Symptomatic response to these agents does not preclude gastric malignancy.

CNS effects: Reversible CNS effects (eg, mental confusion, agitation, psychosis, depression, anxiety, hallucinations, disorientation) have occurred. Advancing age (50 years of age and older) and preexisting liver and/or renal disease appear to be contributing factors.

Hepatic effects: Occasionally, reports of hepatocellular, cholestatic, or mixed hepatitis, with or without jaundice, have occurred with ranitidine. Rare cases of hepatic failure have also been reported.

Laboratory test monitoring – Laboratory test monitoring for liver abnormalities is appropriate.

Porphyria: Rare reports suggest that **ranitidine** may precipitate acute porphyric attacks in patients with acute porphyria. Avoid using ranitidine in patients with a history of acute porphyria.

Rapid IV administration: Rapid IV administration of cimetidine has been followed by rare instances of cardiac arrhythmias and hypotension. Bradycardia, tachycardia, and premature ventricular beats in association with rapid administration of IV ranitidine may occur rarely, usually in patients predisposed to cardiac rhythm disturbances.

Antiandrogenic effect: Cimetidine has a weak antiandrogenic effect in animals. Gynecomastia in patients treated for at least 1 month may occur.

Immunocompromised patients: Decreased gastric acidity, including that produced by acid-suppressing agents such as H_2 antagonists, may increase the possibility of strongyloidiasis.

Hypersensitivity reactions: Rare cases of anaphylaxis have occurred as well as rare episodes of hypersensitivity (eg, bronchospasm, laryngeal edema, rash, eosinophilia).

Renal function impairment: Because these agents are excreted primarily via the kidneys, decreased clearance may occur; reduced dosage may be necessary.

Hepatic function impairment: Observe caution. Decreased clearance may occur; these agents are partly metabolized in the liver.

Pregnancy: Category B.

Lactation:

Cimetidine – Cimetidine is excreted in breast milk with milk:plasma ratios of about 5:1 to 12:1. Potential daily infant ingestion is about 6 mg. Do not breast-feed.

Famotidine – Famotidine is excreted in the breast milk of rats. It is not known whether it is excreted in human breast milk. Decide whether to discontinue breast-feeding or to discontinue the drug, taking into account the importance of the drug to the mother.

Nizatidine – Nizatidine is excreted in breast milk. Decide whether to discontinue breast-feeding or discontinue the drug, taking into account the importance of the drug to the mother.

Ranitidine – Ranitidine is excreted in breast milk. Exercise caution when administering to a breast-feeding mother.

Children:

Cimetidine – Safety and efficacy are limited. Cimetidine is not recommended for children younger than 16 years of age, unless anticipated benefits outweigh potential risks. OTC use is not recommended in children younger than 12 years of age.

Famotidine – Efficacy has been established. See individual monograph for suggested dosages.

Nizatidine – Efficacy in patients younger than 12 years of age has not been established.

Ranitidine – Safety and efficacy of ranitidine have been established in infants and children from 1 month to 16 years of age for treatment of duodenal and gastric ulcers, GERD, and erosive esophagitis; and for the maintenance of healed duodenal and gastric ulcer. Safety and efficacy in neonates (younger than 1 month of age) have not been established.

Elderly: Safety and efficacy appear similar to those of younger age; however, the elderly may have reduced renal function.

Drug Interactions

Ranitidine, famotidine, and nizatidine do not inhibit the CYP-450–linked oxygenase enzyme system in the liver.

Drugs that may be affected by H_2 antagonists include: amiodarone, benzodiazepines, beta-blockers (ie, metoprolol, propranolol, timolol), calcium channel blockers (ie, diltiazem, nifedipine), carbamazepine, carmustine, cephalosporins (ie, cefpodoxime, cefuroxime, cephalexin), chloroquine, cofetilide, ethanol, hydantoins (eg, phenytoin), iron salts, ketoconazole, lidocaine, metformin, metronidazole, moricizine, pentoxifylline, praziquantel, procainamide, quinidine, salicylates, sildenafil, selective serotonin reuptake inhibitors, St. John's wort, sulfonylureas, theophyllines, tricyclic antidepressants, warfarin.

Drug/Lab test interactions: False-positive tests for urobilinogen with *Multistix* may occur during nizatidine therapy. False-positive tests for urine protein with *Multistix* may occur during ranitidine therapy; testing with sulfosalicylic acid is recommended.

Drug/Food interactions: Food may increase bioavailability of famotidine and nizatidine; this is of no clinical consequence.

Adverse Reactions Adverse reactions may include headache, dizziness, diarrhea, and gynecomastia.

MISOPROSTOL

Tablets: 100 and 200 mcg (*Rx*) — Various, *Cytotec* (Pfizer)

Warning:

Misoprostol administration in pregnant women can cause abortion, premature birth, or birth defects. Uterine rupture has been reported when misoprostol was administered in pregnant women to induce labor or to induce abortion beyond the eighth week of pregnancy. Misoprostol should not be taken by pregnant women to reduce the risk of ulcers induced by nonsteroidal anti-inflammatory drugs (NSAIDs).

Advise patients of the abortifacient property and warn them not to give the drug to others.

Misoprostol should not be used for reducing the risk of NSAID-induced ulcers in women of childbearing potential unless the patient is at high risk of developing complications from gastric ulcers associated with NSAIDs or of developing gastric ulceration. In such patients, misoprostol may be prescribed if the patient:

- Has had a negative serum pregnancy test within 2 weeks prior to beginning therapy;
- is capable of complying with effective contraceptive measures;
- has received both oral and written warnings of the hazards of misoprostol, the risk of possible contraception failure, and the danger to other women of childbearing potential should the drug be taken by mistake; and
- will begin misoprostol only on the second or third day of the next normal menstrual period.

Indications

Gastric ulcers: To reduce the risk of NSAID- (including aspirin) induced gastric ulcers in patients at high risk of complications from a gastric ulcer (eg, the elderly, patients with concomitant debilitating disease), as well as patients at high risk of developing gastric ulceration, such as patients with a history of ulcer. Take misoprostol for the duration of NSAID therapy.

Unlabeled uses:

Pregnancy termination – Misoprostol has been used in combination with mifepristone for pregnancy termination. Patients taking mifepristone must take 400 mcg misoprostol orally 2 days after taking mifepristone unless a complete abortion has already been confirmed before that time.

Chronic, idiopathic constipation – Short-term trials have shown an acceleration of intestinal transit in healthy individuals and in those with chronic constipation. Improvement in stool frequency in patients with chronic constipation has been seen with treatment doses of 200 mcg 2 to 4 times/day.

Administration and Dosage

Adults: 200 mcg 4 times daily with food. If this dose cannot be tolerated, 100 mcg may be used. Take misoprostol for the duration of NSAID therapy as prescribed. Take with meals, with the last dose of the day taken at bedtime.

Actions

Pharmacology: Misoprostol, a synthetic prostaglandin E_1 analog, inhibits gastric acid secretion. NSAIDs inhibit prostaglandin synthesis; a deficiency of prostaglandins within the gastric mucosa may lead to diminishing bicarbonate and mucous secretion and may contribute to the mucosal damage caused by these agents. Misoprostol can increase bicarbonate and mucus production.

Pharmacokinetics: Misoprostol is extensively absorbed, with a time-to-reach peak concentration of misoprostol acid of 12 minutes and a terminal half-life of 20 to 40 minutes. Plasma steady-state was achieved within 2 days. The serum protein binding of misoprostol acid is less than 90%.

Contraindications

History of allergy to prostaglandins; pregnancy.

Warnings/Precautions

Cardiovascular: Use caution when administering misoprostol to patients with pre-existing cardiovascular disease.

Duodenal ulcers: Misoprostol does not prevent duodenal ulcers in patients on NSAIDs.

Women of childbearing potential: Advise women of childbearing potential that they must not be pregnant when misoprostol therapy is initiated and that they must use an effective contraception method while taking misoprostol.

Diarrhea: Diarrhea (13% to 40%) is dose-related, usually develops early in the course of therapy (after 13 days), and usually is self-limiting (often resolving after 8 days), but requires discontinuation of misoprostol in some of patients. The incidence of diarrhea can be minimized by administering after meals and at bedtime and by avoiding coadministration of misoprostol with magnesium-containing antacids.

Renal function impairment: No routine dosage adjustment is recommended, but dosage may need to be reduced if usual dose is not tolerated.

Fertility impairment: Results of animal studies suggest the possibility of a general adverse effect on fertility in males and females.

Pregnancy: Category X.

Labor and delivery – Misoprostol can induce or augment uterine contractions. A major adverse effect of the obstetrical use of misoprostol is hyperstimulation of the uterus, which may progress to uterine tetany with marked impairment of uteroplacental blood flow, uterine rupture (requiring surgical repair, hysterectomy, and/or salpingo-oophorectomy), or amniotic fluid embolism. Pelvic pain, retained placenta, severe genital bleeding, shock, fetal bradycardia, and fetal and maternal death have been reported.

Lactation: It is not known if misoprostol acid is excreted in breast milk. Do not administer to nursing mothers because the potential excretion of misoprostol acid could cause significant diarrhea in nursing infants.

Children: Safety and efficacy in children less than 18 years of age have not been established.

Elderly: No routine dosage adjustment is recommended. Reduce the dose if the usual dose is not tolerated.

Drug Interactions

Antacids: Antacids reduce the total availability of misoprostol acid, but this does not appear clinically important.

Drug/Food interactions: Maximum plasma concentrations of misoprostol acid are diminished when taken with food.

Adverse Reactions

Adverse reactions associated with misoprostol may include abdominal pain (7% to 20%), diarrhea (13% to 40%), and nausea (3%).

PROTON PUMP INHIBITORS

DEXLANSOPRAZOLE	
Capsules, delayed-release; oral: 30 and 60 mg (*Rx*)	*Kapidex* (Takeda Pharmaceuticals America)
ESOMEPRAZOLE	
Capsules, delayed-release; oral[a]: 20 and 40 mg (as esomeprazole magnesium) (*Rx*)	*Nexium* (AstraZeneca)
Powder for suspension, delayed-release; oral: 10, 20, and 40 mg (as esomeprazole magnesium) (*Rx*)	
Injection, powder or cake for solution: 20 and 40 mg (as esomeprazole sodium) (*Rx*)	*Nexium I.V.* (AstraZeneca)
LANSOPRAZOLE	
Capsules, delayed-release; oral: 15 mg (*otc*)	Various, *Prevacid 24 Hour* (Novartis)
30 mg (*Rx*)	Various
Tablets, orally disintegrating, delayed-release; oral: 15 and 30 mg (*Rx*)	*Prevacid* (Takeda Pharmaceuticals)
Capsules, delayed-release; oral: 15 and 30 mg (*Rx*)	
Granules for suspension, delayed-release; oral: 15 and 30 mg (*Rx*)	
OMEPRAZOLE	
Tablets, delayed-release; oral: 20 mg (as omeprazole magnesium) (*otc*)	*Prilosec OTC* (Procter & Gamble)
Capsules, delayed-release; oral: 10, 20, and 40 mg (*Rx*)	Various, *Prilosec* (AstraZeneca)
Suspension, delayed release; oral: 2.5 mg (equiv. to omeprazole magnesium 2.8 mg) and 10 mg (equiv. to omeprazole magnesium 11.2 mg) (*Rx*)	*Prilosec* (AstraZeneca)
PANTOPRAZOLE	
Tablets, delayed-release; oral: 20 and 40 mg (*Rx*)	Various, *Protonix* (Wyeth-Ayerst)
Granules for suspension, delayed-release; oral: 40 mg (*Rx*)	*Protonix* (Wyeth-Ayerst)
Injection, lyophilized powder for solution: 40 mg (*Rx*)	*Protonix I.V.* (Wyeth-Ayerst)
RABEPRAZOLE	
Tablets, delayed-release; oral: 20 mg (*Rx*)	*Aciphex* (Eisai)
PROTON PUMP INHIBITOR COMBINATIONS	
Capsules, immediate-release; oral: omeprazole 20 mg/sodium bicarbonate 1,100 mg (*otc*)	*Zegerid OTC* (Santarus)
omeprazole 40 mg/sodium bicarbonate 1,100 mg (*Rx*)	*Zegerid* (Santarus)
Powder for suspension; oral: omeprazole 20 mg/sodium bicarbonate 1,680 mg and omeprazole 40 mg/sodium bicarbonate 1,680 mg (*Rx*)	

Indications

Proton Pump Inhibitors - Summary of Indications[a]

Indication ✓ = Labeled	Dexlansoprazole	Esomeprazole	Lansoprazole	Omeprazole	Pantoprazole	Rabeprazole	Omeprazole/ Sodium bicarbonate
Duodenal ulcer			✓[b]	✓[c]		✓	✓
Duodenal ulcer associated with *Helicobacter pylori* (in combination with antibiotics)		✓[b]	✓[b]	✓[d]		✓	
Gastric ulcer			✓[b]	✓[c]			✓
Erosive esophagitis	✓	✓[b]	✓	✓[c]	✓	✓	✓
GERD[e] in adults	✓	✓[b]	✓[b]	✓[c]	✓	✓	✓
GERD with a history of erosive esophagitis		✓				✓	
H. pylori gastritis in children[f]							
Hypersecretory conditions (eg, Zollinger-Ellison syndrome)		✓[b]	✓	✓[d]	✓	✓	
Reduction of risk of upper GI bleeding				✓[g]			✓

Proton Pump Inhibitors - Summary of Indications[a]

Indication ✓ = Labeled	Dexlansoprazole	Esomeprazole	Lansoprazole	Omeprazole	Pantoprazole	Rabeprazole	Omeprazole/ Sodium bicarbonate
Reduction of risk of NSAID[h]-associated gastric ulcer		✓[b]					
Maintenance of healing of erosive esophagitis	✓	✓[b]					✓
Heartburn		✓	✓[i]	✓[i]			

[a] For more detailed information, see the information below and the individual drug monographs.
[b] Oral only.
[c] Prescription only.
[d] Except omeprazole oral suspension.
[e] Gastroesophageal reflux disease.
[f] In combination with amoxicillin and clarithromycin.
[g] *Zegerid* only.
[h] NSAID = nonsteroidal anti-inflammatory drug.
[i] OTC only.

Duodenal ulcer associated with H. pylori infection: For treatment of patients with *H. pylori* infection and duodenal ulcer to eradicate *H. pylori.*

Dual therapy – In combination with clarithromycin (**omeprazole**) or amoxicillin (**lansoprazole**).

Triple therapy (esomeprazole, lansoprazole, omeprazole, rabeprazole) – In combination with clarithromycin and amoxicillin.

NSAID-associated gastric ulcers: **Lansoprazole** also is indicated for the healing and reducing the risk of NSAID-associated gastric ulcers in patients who continue NSAID use.

Administration and Dosage

DEXLANSOPRAZOLE:

Gastroesophageal reflux disease –

Healing of erosive esophagitis: 60 mg once daily with 30 mg once daily as maintenance therapy for up to 8 weeks.

Symptomatic nonerosive gastroesophageal reflux disease: 30 mg once daily for 4 weeks.

Administration – Can be taken without regard to food. Dexlansoprazole should be swallowed whole. Alternatively, dexlansoprazole capsules can be opened and administered as follows: open capsule, sprinkle intact granules on 1 tablespoon of applesauce, and swallow immediately.

Hepatic function impairment – Consider a maximum daily dose of 30 mg for patients with moderate hepatic impairment (Child-Pugh class B). No studies have been conducted in patients with severe hepatic impairment (Child-Pugh class C).

ESOMEPRAZOLE:

Delayed-release capsules – Swallow capsules whole. Take at least 1 hour before eating.

Difficulty swallowing: 1 tablespoon of applesauce can be added to an empty bowl and the esomeprazole capsule opened and the pellets inside carefully emptied onto the applesauce. The pellets should be mixed with the applesauce and swallowed immediately. The applesauce should not be hot and should be soft enough to swallow without chewing. Do not chew or crush the pellets. Do not store the pellet/applesauce mixture for future use.

Administration per nasogastric tube: For patients who have a nasogastric (NG) tube, esomeprazole capsules can be opened and the intact granules emptied into a 60 mL syringe and mixed with 50 mL of water. Replace the plunger and shake the syringe vigorously for 15 seconds. Hold the syringe with the tip up and check for granules remaining in the tip. Attach the syringe to a NG tube and deliver the contents of the syringe through the NG tube into the stomach. After administering the granules, the NG tube should be flushed with additional water. Do not administer the pellets if they have dissolved or disintegrated.

The suspension must be used immediately after preparation.

Esomeprazole Adult Dosage Schedule		
Indication	Dose	Frequency
GERD		
Healing of erosive esophagitis	20 or 40 mg	Once daily for 4 to 8 weeks[a]
Maintenance of healing of erosive esophagitis	20 mg	Once daily[b]
Pathological hypersecretory conditions, including Zollinger-Ellison syndrome	40 mg	Twice daily[g]
Symptomatic GERD	20 mg	Once daily for 4 weeks[c]
Risk reduction of NSAID-associated gastric ulcer	20 or 40 mg	Once daily for up to 6 months[b]
H. pylori eradication to reduce the risk of duodenal ulcer recurrence		
Triple therapy		
Esomeprazole	40 mg	Once daily for 10 days
Amoxicillin	1,000 mg	Twice daily for 10 days
Clarithromycin	500 mg	Twice daily for 10 days
Children (12 to 17 years of age)		
Short-term treatment of GERD	20 or 40 mg	Once daily for up to 8 weeks
Pathological hypersecretory conditions	40 mg[d]	Twice daily[e]
Children 1 to 11 years of age[f]		
Healing of erosive esophagitis (weight ≥ 20 kg)	10 or 20 mg	Once daily for 8 weeks
Healing of erosive esophagitis (weight < 20 kg)	10 mg	Once daily for 8 weeks
Short-term treatment of symptomatic GERD	10 mg	Once daily for up to 8 weeks

[a] The majority of patients are healed within 4 to 8 weeks. For patients who do not heal after 4 to 8 weeks, consider an additional 4 to 8 weeks of treatment.
[b] Controlled studies did not extend beyond 6 months.
[c] If symptoms do not resolve completely after 4 weeks, consider an additional 4 weeks of treatment.
[d] The dosage of esomeprazole in patients with pathological hypersecretory conditions varies with the individual patient. Dosage regimens should be adjusted to individual patient needs.
[e] Doses of up to 240 mg daily have been administered.
[f] Dosages of > 1 mg/kg/day have not been studied.
[g] Dosages vary with the individual patient. Doses of up to 240 mg daily have been administered.

Delayed-release oral suspension –

Esomeprazole Administration Options		
Type	Route	Options
Delayed-release capsule	Oral	Capsule can be swallowed whole or opened and mixed with applesauce.
Delayed-release capsule	NG tube	Capsule can be opened and the intact granules emptied into a syringe and delivered through the NG tube.
Delayed-release oral suspension	Oral	Mix contents of 10, 20, or 40 mg packet with 1 tablespoon (15 mL) of water, then leave 2 to 3 minutes to thicken, then stir and drink within 30 minutes.
Delayed-release oral suspension	NG or gastric tube	Add 15 mL of water to a syringe and then add contents of 10, 20, or 40 mg packet. Shake the syringe, leave 2 to 3 minutes to thicken. Shake the syringe and inject through NG or gastric tube within 30 minutes.

IV – The recommended adult dose is esomeprazole 20 or 40 mg given once daily by IV injection (no less than 3 minutes) or IV infusion (10 to 30 minutes).

Duration of treatment: Discontinue treatment with esomeprazole IV as soon as the patient is able to resume treatment with esomeprazole delayed-release capsule.

Hepatic function impairment – For patients with severe liver impairment (Child Pugh class C), do not exceed a dose of 20 mg.

Administration/Preparation for IV use –

IV injection (20 or 40 mg) over no less than 3 minutes: Reconstitute the freeze-dried powder with 5 mL of 0.9% sodium chloride injection. Withdraw 5 mL of the reconstituted solution and administer as an IV injection over no less than 3 minutes.

Store the reconstituted solution at room temperature up to 30°C (86°F) and administer within 12 hours after reconstitution. No refrigeration is required.

IV infusion (20 or 40 mg) over 10 to 30 minutes: Do not administer esomeprazole IV concomitantly with any other medications through the same IV site and/or tubing. Always flush the IV line with 0.9% sodium chloride injection, lactated Ringer's injection, or 5% dextrose injection, both prior to and after administration of esomeprazole IV.

LANSOPRAZOLE: Take before meals. Do not crush or chew lansoprazole oral products.

Duodenal ulcer –

Short-term treatment: 15 mg once/day for 4 weeks.

Maintenance: 15 mg once/day to maintain healing of duodenal ulcers.

Associated with H. pylori:

Dual therapy – 30 mg lansoprazole plus 1 g amoxicillin both taken 3 times/day for 14 days for patients intolerant or resistant to clarithromycin.

Triple therapy – 30 mg lansoprazole plus 500 mg clarithromycin and 1 g amoxicillin all taken twice/day for 10 to 14 days.

Gastric ulcer –

Short-term treatment: 30 mg once/day for up to 8 weeks.

Associated with NSAIDs:

Healing – 30 mg once/day for 8 weeks.

Risk reduction – 15 mg once/day for up to 12 weeks.

GERD –

Adults and children 12 to 17 years of age: 15 mg once/day for up to 8 weeks.

Children 1 to 11 years of age (short-term treatment):

30 kg or less – 15 mg/day for up to 12 weeks.

Over 30 kg – 30 mg/day for up to 12 weeks.

Erosive esophagitis –

Adults and children 12 to 17 years of age:

Short-term treatment – 30 mg/day for up to 8 weeks. For patients who do not heal within 8 weeks, give an additional 8 weeks of treatment. If there is a recurrence of erosive esophagitis, consider an additional 8-week course.

Maintenance (adults) – 15 mg once/day to maintain healing of erosive esophagitis.

Children 1 to 11 years of age (short-term treatment):

30 kg or less – 15 mg/day for up to 12 weeks.

Over 30 kg – 30 mg/day for up to 12 weeks.

Heartburn –

Adults: 1 capsule with a glass of water before eating in the morning, taken every day for 14 days. A 14-day course may be repeated every 4 months.

Patients should not take more than 1 capsule per day. Instruct patients not to use for longer than 14 days unless directed by their health care provider.

Hypersecretory conditions including Zollinger-Ellison syndrome – The recommended starting dose is 60 mg/day. Dosages of up to 90 mg twice/day have been administered. Administer daily dosages of greater than 120 mg in divided doses.

Hepatic function impairment – Consider dosage adjustment in patients with severe liver disease.

Difficulty swallowing – Lansoprazole capsules can be opened and the intact granules sprinkled on 1 tablespoon of applesauce, *Ensure* pudding, cottage cheese, yogurt, or strained pears and swallowed immediately. The delayed-release capsules may be emptied into a small volume of either orange juice or tomato juice (60 mL; approximately 2 oz), mixed briefly, and swallowed immediately. To ensure complete delivery of the dose, rinse the glass with 2 or more volumes of juice (apple, cranberry, grape, orange, pineapple, prune, tomato, or V-8 vegetable juice). Do not chew or crush the granules.

Oral suspension: Empty packet contents into 2 tablespoons of water. Do not use other liquids or foods. Stir well and drink immediately. If any material remains after drinking, add more water, stir, and drink immediately. Do not give through enteral administration tubes.

Orally disintegrating tablets: Place the tablet on the tongue. Allow it to disintegrate with or without water until the particles can be swallowed. *SoluTabs* are not designed to be swallowed intact or chewed.

For administration via oral syringe, place a 15 mg tablet in an oral syringe and draw up approximately 4 mL of water, or place a 30 mg tablet in oral syringe and draw up approximately 10 mL of water. Shake gently to allow for a quick dispersal. After the tablet has dispersed, administer the contents within 15 minutes. Refill the syringe with approximately 2 mL (5 mL for the 30 mg tablet) of water, shake gently, and administer any remaining contents.

Administration: An in-line filter must be used. Administer over 30 minutes. A dedicated line is not required; however, flush the IV line before and after administration with 0.9% sodium chloride injection, lactated Ringer's injection, or 5% dextrose injection. Do not administer with other drugs or diluents, as this may cause incompatibilities.

NG tube –

Tablets: Lansoprazole can be opened and the intact granules mixed in 40 mL of apple juice and injected through the NG tube into the stomach. After administering the granules, flush the NG tube with additional apple juice to clear the tube.

Orally disintegrating tablets: For administration via NG tube, place a 15 mg tablet in a syringe and draw up 4 mL water, or place a 30 mg tablet in a syringe and draw up 10 mL water. Shake gently to allow for a quick dispersal. After the tablet has dispersed, inject through the NG tube into the stomach within 15 minute. Refill the syringe with approximately 5 mL of water, shake gently, and flush the NG tube.

OMEPRAZOLE: Take on an empty stomach at least 1 hour before a meal. Administer daily doses more than 80 mg in divided doses. Do not open, crush, or chew the capsule; swallow whole.

Duodenal ulcer –

Treatment: 20 mg/day for 4 to 8 weeks.

Associated with H. pylori:

Triple therapy (omeprazole/clarithromycin/amoxicillin) – Omeprazole 20 mg plus clarithromycin 500 mg plus amoxicillin 1,000 mg each given twice/day for 10 days. If an ulcer is present at the initiation of therapy, continue omeprazole 20 mg for an additional 18 days.

Dual therapy (omeprazole/clarithromycin) – Omeprazole 40 mg once/day plus clarithromycin 500 mg 3 times/day for 14 days. If an ulcer is present at the initiation of therapy, continue omeprazole 20 mg for an additional 14 days.

Gastric ulcer, treatment – 40 mg once/day for 4 to 8 weeks.

Erosive esophagitis –

Treatment: 20 mg/day for 4 to 8 weeks.

Maintenance: 20 mg/day.

Children: On a per kg basis, the doses of omeprazole required to heal erosive esophagitis are greater than those for adults.

20 kg or more – 20 mg daily.

10 to 20 kg – 10 mg daily.

5 to 10 kg – 5 mg daily.

GERD –

GERD without esophageal lesions: 20 mg/day for up to 4 weeks.

GERD with erosive esophagitis: 20 mg/day for 4 to 8 weeks.

Children:

20 kg or more – 20 mg daily.

10 to 20 kg – 10 mg daily.

5 to 10 kg – 5 mg daily.

Pathological hypersecretory conditions – Initial adult dose is 60 mg/day. Doses up to 120 mg 3 times/day have been administered. Administer daily dosages greater than 80 mg in divided doses.

Heartburn (nonprescription) – Usual dose is 20 mg daily for 14 days. Maximum dose is 20 mg daily.

It may take 1 to 4 days for full effect, although some patients get complete relief within 24 hours. The 14-day course may be repeated every 4 months.

Difficulty swallowing – For patients who have difficulty swallowing capsules, add 1 tablespoon of applesauce to an empty bowl, open the omeprazole capsule, and empty the pellets onto the applesauce. Mix the pellets with the applesauce and swallow immediately. Do not heat or chew the applesauce. Do not chew or crush the pellets. Do not store the pellet/applesauce mixture for future use.

Administration – Prescription capsules should be taken on an empty stomach at least 1 hour before a meal. The capsule should not be crushed or chewed; swallow whole.

Nonprescription tablets should be swallowed with a glass of water once daily in the morning before eating. The tablets should not be chewed or crushed.

Oral suspension: Empty the contents of a 2.5 mg packet into a container containing 5 mL of water, or empty the contents of a 10 mg packet into a container containing 15 mL of water. Stir. Leave 2 to 3 minutes to thicken. Stir and drink within 30 minutes. If any material remains after drinking, add more water, stir, and drink immediately.

For patients with a NG or gastric tube: Add 5 mL of water to a catheter tipped syringe and then add the contents of a 2.5 mg packet (or 15 mL of water for the 10 mg packet). It is important to only use a catheter tipped syringe when administering omeprazole through a nasogastric tube or gastric tube. Immediately shake the syringe and leave 2 to 3 minutes to thicken. Shake the syringe and inject through the nasogastric or gastric tube, French size 6 or larger, into the stomach within 30 minutes. Refill the syringe with an equal amount of water. Shake and flush any remaining contents from the nasogastric tube into the stomach.

PANTOPRAZOLE:

Oral – Administer without regard to meals, but administer with food if GI upset occurs.

May be used concomitantly with antacids.

Erosive esophagitis associated with GERD:

Treatment – 40 mg once/day for up to 8 weeks. For those patients who have not healed after 8 weeks, consider an additional 8-week course.

Maintenance – 40 mg once/day.

Pathological hypersecretory conditions, including Zollinger-Ellison syndrome: The recommended adult starting dose is 40 mg twice daily. Doses of up to 240 mg/day have been administered. Some patients have been treated continuously for more than 2 years.

Administration: Swallow tablets whole, with or without food. Do not chew, crush, or split.

Delayed-release oral suspension – Delayed-release oral suspension should be administered in applesauce or apple juice approximately 30 minutes prior to a meal. Patients should be cautioned that the granules for delayed-release oral suspension should not be split, chewed, or crushed.

Delayed-release oral suspension should only be administered in apple juice or applesauce, not in water or other liquids or foods.

Oral administration in applesauce – Open the packet. Sprinkle intact granules on 1 teaspoonful of applesauce. Swallow within 10 minutes of preparation.

Oral administration in apple juice – Empty intact granules into a small cup containing 5 mL of apple juice (approximately 1 teaspoonful). Stir for 5 seconds and swallow immediately. To ensure complete delivery of the dose, rinse the container once or twice with apple juice to remove any remaining granules and swallow immediately.

NG tube administration: Separate the plunger from the barrel of a 2 oz (60 mL) catheter tip syringe. Connect the catheter tip of the syringe to a 16 French (or larger) NG tube. Hold the syringe attached to the tubing as high as possible during application steps. Empty the contents of the packet into the barrel of the syringe. Add 10 mL of apple juice and gently tap and/or shake the barrel of the syringe to help empty the syringe. Add an additional 10 mL of apple juice and gently tap and/or shake the barrel of the syringe to help rinse the syringe and NG tube. Repeat with at least 2 additional 10 mL aliquots of apple juice. No granules should remain in the syringe. Make sure the nasogastric tube is not clogged to ensure that the patient receives the full dose.

IV – Discontinue treatment with IV pantoprazole as soon as the patient is able to resume treatment with pantoprazole delayed-release tablets.

GERD associated with a history of erosive esophagitis: Administer pantoprazole 40 mg once daily by infusion for 7 to 10 days. Safety and efficacy of IV pantoprazole as a treatment for GERD in patients with a history of erosive esophagitis for more than 10 days have not been demonstrated.

Pathological hypersecretion associated with Zollinger-Ellison syndrome: The recommended adult dosage is 80 mg every 12 hours. In those patients who need a higher dosage, 80 mg every 8 hours is expected to maintain acid output below 10 mEq/h. Daily doses higher than 240 mg or administered for more than 6 days have not been studied. Perform transition from oral to IV and from IV to oral formulations of gastric acid inhibitors in such a manner to ensure continuity of effect of suppression of acid secretion.

Administration: May be administered as a 2-minute or 15-minute infusion.

Compatibility: When administered through a Y-site, pantoprazole IV is compatible with the following solutions: dextrose 5% injection, sodium chloride 0.9% injection, or Ringer's lactate injection.

Incompatibilities: Midazolam has been shown to be incompatible with Y-site administration of pantoprazole injection, and pantoprazole may not be compatible with products containing zinc. Immediately stop use if precipitation or discoloration occurs.

RABEPRAZOLE: Swallow tablets whole, with or without food. Do not chew, crush, or split.

Duodenal ulcer – 20 mg once/day after the morning meal for a period of up to 4 weeks.

Erosive or ulcerative GERD –

Treatment: 20 mg once/day for 4 to 8 weeks. For those patients not healed after 8 weeks of treatment, consider an additional 8-week course.

Maintenance: 20 mg once/day.

GERD –

Adults: 20 mg once/day for 4 weeks. If symptoms do not resolve completely after 4 weeks, an additional course of treatment may be considered.

Adolescents (12 years of age and older): 20 mg once daily for up to 8 weeks.

Hypersecretory conditions, including Zollinger-Ellison syndrome – Start dosing at 60 mg once/day. Dosing may be divided. Doses of up to 100 mg/day and 60 mg twice/day have been administered. Continue for as long as clinically indicated. Some patients with Zollinger-Ellison syndrome have been treated continuously with rabeprazole for up to 1 year.

H. pylori eradication to reduce risk of duodenal ulcer recurrence – Rabeprazole 20 mg, amoxicillin 1,000 mg, and clarithromycin 500 mg twice daily for 7 days with the morning and evening meals.

OMEPRAZOLE/SODIUM BICARBONATE: 20 and 40 mg capsule and oral suspension packets contain the same amount of sodium bicarbonate. Two packets or 2 capsules are not equivalent to one 40 mg capsule or packet.

Recommended Doses of Omeprazole/Sodium Bicarbonate for Adults 18 Years of Age and Older		
Indication	Recommended dose	Frequency
Active duodenal ulcer	20 mg	Once daily for 4 weeks[a]
Benign gastric ulcer	40 mg	Once daily for 4 to 8 weeks
GERD		
Symptomatic GERD (with no esophageal erosions)	20 mg	Once daily for up to 4 weeks
Erosive esophagitis	20 mg	Once daily for 4 to 8 weeks
Maintenance of healing of erosive esophagitis	20 mg	Once daily
Reduction of risk of upper GI bleeding in critically ill patients (40 mg oral suspension only)	40 mg	40 mg initially followed by 40 mg 6 to 8 hours later and 40 mg daily thereafter for 14 days

[a] Most patients heal within 4 weeks. Some patients may require an additional 4 weeks of therapy.

Administration of capsules – Swallow intact with water. Do not use other liquids. Do not open capsule and sprinkle contents onto food.

Preparation and administration of oral suspension – Take on an empty stomach 1 hour before a meal. The powder for oral suspension is supplied as unit-dose packets containing an immediate-release formulation of omeprazole.

Directions for use: Empty packet contents into a small cup containing 1 to 2 tablespoons of water. Do not use other liquids or foods. Stir well and drink immediately. Refill cup with water and drink.

For patients receiving continuous NG/orogastric (OG) tube feeding, enteral feeding should be suspended approximately 3 hours before and 1 hour after administration of *Zegerid*. If *Zegerid* is to be administered through a NG or OG tube, constitute the suspension with approximately 20 mL of water. Do not use other liquids or foods. Stir well and administer immediately. Use an appropriately sized syringe to instill the suspension in the tube. Wash the suspension through the tube with 20 mL of water.

Hepatic function impairment/race – Consider dose adjustment, particularly where maintenance of healing of erosive esophagitis is indicated, for hepatically impaired and Asian patients.

Actions

Pharmacology: These agents have been characterized as gastric acid pump inhibitors; they block the final step of acid production. Proton pump inhibitors do not exhibit anticholinergic or H_2 histamine antagonistic properties.

Pharmacokinetics:

Absorption/Distribution – Most of these oral agents contain enteric-coated granules. Absorption of these agents is rapid and begins only after the granules leave the stomach.

Metabolism/Excretion – These agents are extensively metabolized by the liver. The plasma elimination half-life is less than 2 hours, while the acid inhibitory effect lasts more than 24 hours. When the drug is discontinued, secretory activity returns over 1 to 5 days.

Proton Pump Inhibitors Pharmacokinetics					
Parameter	Esomeprazole	Lansoprazole	Omeprazole[a]	Pantoprazole	Rabeprazole
Bioavailability (%)	64 to 90	> 80	30 to 40	≈ 77 (oral)	≈ 52
T_{max}[b] (h)	≈ 1.5	1.7	0.5 to 3.5	≈ 2.5 (oral)	2 to 5
Protein binding (%)	97	97	≈ 95	≈ 98	96.3

Proton Pump Inhibitors Pharmacokinetics

Parameter	Esomeprazole	Lansoprazole	Omeprazole[a]	Pantoprazole	Rabeprazole
Half-life (h)	≈ 1 to 1.5	≈ 1.5 (oral)	0.5 to 1	≈ 1	1 to 2
Onset (h)		1 to 3	≤ 1		≤ 1
Duration (h)		> 24	72	> 24	

[a] Capsules.
[b] T_{max} = time to maximal concentration.

Contraindications

Hypersensitivity to any component of the formulation; substituted benzimidazoles (**rabeprazole, esomeprazole**).

Warnings/Precautions

Gastritis: Atrophic gastritis has been noted occasionally in gastric corpus biopsies from patients treated long-term with **omeprazole** and **esomeprazole**.

Patients with healed GERD were treated for up to 40 months with **rabeprazole** and monitored with serial gastric biopsies. Approximately 4% of patients had intestinal metaplasia at some point during follow-up, but no consistent changes were seen.

Hepatic effects: In patients with various degrees/types of hepatic disease, the area under the curve (AUC) was prolonged (**lansoprazole, esomeprazole, rabeprazole, pantoprazole**), half-life was prolonged (**lansoprazole, omeprazole, rabeprazole, pantoprazole**), increased bioavailability was observed (**omeprazole**), decreased clearance with **rabeprazole** and increased maximum **pantoprazole** concentrations.

Gastric malignancy: Symptomatic response to therapy with proton pump inhibitors does not preclude gastric malignancy.

Vitamin B_{12} deficiency: Generally, daily treatment with any acid-suppressing medications over a long period of time may lead to malabsorption of cyanocobalamin (vitamin B_{12}).

Hypersensitivity reactions: Anaphylaxis has been reported with the use of IV **pantoprazole**. This may require emergency medical treatment.

Pregnancy: Category C (**omeprazole**); *Category* B (**lansoprazole, rabeprazole, pantoprazole, esomeprazole**).

Lactation: Omeprazole has been measured in the breast milk. Because of the potential for serious adverse reactions in breast-feeding infants, decide whether to discontinue breast-feeding or the drug, taking into account the importance of the drug to the mother.

Children: The safety and efficacy of **esomeprazole, pantoprazole**, and **rabeprazole** in children have not been established. The safety and efficacy of **lansoprazole** in patients younger than 1 year of age have not been established. The safety and efficacy of **omeprazole** have not been established for children younger than 2 years of age.

Elderly: The elimination rate of **omeprazole** was somewhat decreased in the elderly and the bioavailability increased.

The clearance of **lansoprazole** is decreased in the elderly, with an approximately 50% to 100% increase of elimination half-life.

AUC values and maximum concentration of **esomeprazole, rabeprazole**, and oral **pantoprazole** were increased in elderly subjects compared with healthy controls, but no dosage adjustment is recommended.

Drug Interactions

Drugs that may be affected by proton pump inhibitors include azole antifungal agents (eg, itraconazole, ketoconazole), benzodiazepines, cilostazol, clarithromycin, digoxin, phenytoin, salicylates, sulfonylureas, and warfarin. Drugs that may affect proton pump inhibitors include clarithromycin and sucralfate.

Proton pump inhibitors cause a profound and long-lasting inhibition of gastric acid secretion; therefore, proton pump inhibitors may interfere with the absorption of drugs where gastric pH is an important determinant of bioavailability (eg, ampicillin, cyanocobalamin, digoxin, iron salts, ketoconazole).

CYP-450 system: Drugs that may be affected by proton pump inhibitors include azole antifungal agents, benzodiazepines, cilostazol, clarithromycin, cyclosporine, digoxin, disulfiram, hydantoins, salicylates, sulfonylureas, and warfarin.

Drugs that affect proton pump inhibitors include clarithromycin and sucralfate.

Adverse Reactions

The most common adverse effects (greater than 3%) of proton pump inhibitors include diarrhea and headache.

ORLISTAT

Capsules: 60 mg (*otc*)	*Alli* (GlaxoSmithKline)
120 mg (*Rx*)	*Xenical* (Roche)

Indications

Obesity management:

Rx – For management of obesity, including weight loss and weight maintenance, when used in conjunction with a reduced-calorie diet. Orlistat also is indicated to reduce the risk for weight regain after prior weight loss. Orlistat is indicated for obese patients with an initial body mass index (BMI) of 30 kg/m^2 or more, or 27 kg/m^2 or more in the presence of other risk factors (eg, diabetes, dyslipidemia, hypertension).

OTC – For weight loss in overweight adults 18 years of age and older, when used along with a reduced-calorie and low-fat diet.

Administration and Dosage

Rx: The recommended dose of orlistat is one 120 mg capsule 3 times a day with each main meal containing fat (during or up to 1 hour after the meal).

Place the patient on a nutritionally-balanced, reduced-calorie diet that contains approximately 30% of calories from fat. Distribute the daily intake of fat, carbohydrate, and protein over 3 main meals. If a meal is occasionally missed or contains no fat, the dose of orlistat can be omitted.

Because orlistat reduces the absorption of some fat-soluble vitamins and beta-carotene, counsel patients to take a multivitamin containing fat-soluble vitamins to ensure adequate nutrition. Instruct the patient to take the supplement once a day, at least 2 hours before or after the administration of orlistat, such as at bedtime.

Doses greater than 120 mg 3 times a day have not been shown to provide additional benefit.

Based on fecal fat measurements, the effect of orlistat is seen as soon as 24 to 48 hours after dosing. Upon discontinuation of therapy, fecal fat content usually returns to pretreatment levels within 48 to 72 hours.

Safety and effectiveness beyond 2 years have not been determined at this time.

OTC: The recommended dose of orlistat is one 60 mg capsule with each meal containing fat. Dosage should not exceed 3 capsules a day.

Orlistat should be taken with a reduced-calorie, low-fat diet and exercise program until patient's weight-loss goal is reached. Most weight loss occurs in the first 6 months.

If discontinuing orlistat, a diet and exercise program should be continued.

If weight gain occurs after discontinuation of orlistat, orlistat therapy may be restarted along with a diet and exercise program.

Because orlistat has been shown to reduce the absorption of some vitamins, patients should be instructed to take a multivitamin once a day at bedtime.

Actions

Pharmacology: Orlistat is a reversible lipase inhibitor for obesity management that acts by inhibiting the absorption of dietary fats. It exerts its therapeutic activity in the lumen of the stomach and small intestine.

Pharmacokinetics:

Absorption – Systemic exposure to orlistat is minimal. Peak plasma concentrations occurred at approximately 8 hours following oral dosing with 360 mg of orlistat; plasma concentrations of intact orlistat were near the limits of detection (less than 5 ng/mL).

Distribution – In vitro orlistat was greater than 99% bound to plasma proteins (lipoproteins and albumin were major binding proteins). Orlistat minimally partitioned into erythrocytes.

Metabolism – It is likely that the metabolism of orlistat occurs mainly within the GI wall. In obese patients, 2 metabolites, M1 (4-member lactone ring hydrolyzed) and M3 (M1 with N-formyl leucine moiety cleaved), accounted for approximately 42% in plasma.

Excretion – Fecal excretion was the major route of elimination following a single oral dose of orlistat 360 mg in healthy and obese subjects. Orlistat and its M1 and M3 metabolites also underwent biliary excretion. Approximately 97% was excreted in feces; 83% of that was found to be unchanged orlistat. The cumulative renal excretion was less than 2%. Based on limited data, the half-life of the absorbed drug is in the range of 1 to 2 hours.

Contraindications

Chronic malabsorption syndrome or cholestasis; hypersensitivity to orlistat or to any component of this product.

Warnings/Precautions

Causes of obesity: Exclude organic causes of obesity (eg, hypothyroidism) before prescribing orlistat.

Diet: Advise patients to adhere to dietary guidelines. GI events may increase when orlistat is taken with a diet high in fat (more than 30% total daily calories from fat). The daily intake of fat should be distributed over 3 main meals. If orlistat is taken with any 1 meal that is very high in fat, the possibility of GI effects increases.

Multivitamin supplement: Counsel patients to take a multivitamin supplement that contains fat-soluble vitamins to ensure adequate nutrition because orlistat reduces the absorption of some fat-soluble vitamins and beta-carotene. Instruct patients to take the supplement once a day at least 2 hours before or after the administration of orlistat, such as at bedtime.

Urinary oxalate: Some patients may develop increased levels of urinary oxalate following treatment. Exercise caution in patients with a history of hyperoxaluria or calcium oxalate nephrolithiasis.

Diabetic patients: Weight-loss induction by orlistat may be accompanied by improved metabolic control in diabetic patients, which might require a reduction in the dose of oral hypoglycemic medication (eg, sulfonylureas, metformin) or insulin.

Misuse potential: As with any weight-loss agent, the potential exists for misuse of orlistat in inappropriate patient populations (eg, patients with anorexia nervosa or bulimia).

Pregnancy: Category B.

Lactation: It is not known if orlistat is secreted in breast milk.

Children: The safety and efficacy of orlistat have been evaluated in obese adolescent patients 12 to 16 years of age. Orlistat has not been studied in children younger than 12 years of age.

Drug Interactions

Drugs that may interact with orlistat include cyclosporine, fat-soluble vitamins, pravastatin, and warfarin.

Adverse Reactions

Adverse reactions occurring in at least 3% of patients include the following:

GI: Oily spotting; flatus with discharge; fecal urgency; fatty/oily stool; oily evacuation; increased defecation; fecal incontinence.

Miscellaneous: Abdominal pain/discomfort; anxiety; arthritis; back pain; depression; dizziness; fatigue; gingival disorder; headache; infectious diarrhea; influenza; lower extremity pain; menstrual irregularity; myalgia; nausea; otitis; rash; rectal pain/discomfort; sleep disorder; tooth disorder; upper/lower respiratory tract infection; urinary tract infection; vaginitis; vomiting.

METOCLOPRAMIDE

Tablets; oral: 5 and 10 mg (*Rx*)	Various, *Reglan* (Alaven)
Tablets, disintegrating; oral 5 and 10 mg (*Rx*)	*Metozolv ODT* (Salix)
Syrup; oral: 5 mg per 5 mL (*Rx*)	Various
Injection: 5 mg/mL (*Rx*)	Various, *Reglan* (Wyeth-Ayerst)

Warning:

Treatment with metoclopramide can cause tardive dyskinesia, a serious movement disorder that is often irreversible. The risk of developing tardive dyskinesia increases with duration of treatment and total cumulative dose.

Discontinue metoclopramide therapy in patients who develop signs or symptoms of tardive dyskinesia. There is no known treatment for tardive dyskinesia. In some patients, symptoms lessen or resolve after metoclopramide treatment is stopped.

Avoid treatment with metoclopramide for longer than 12 weeks in all but rare cases in which therapeutic benefit is thought to outweigh the risk of developing tardive dyskinesia.

Indications

Oral:

Symptomatic gastroesophageal reflux – Short-term (4 to 12 weeks) therapy for adults with symptomatic documented gastroesophageal reflux who fail to respond to conventional therapy.

Parenteral: For prevention of nausea and vomiting associated with emetogenic cancer chemotherapy.

Prophylaxis of postoperative nausea and vomiting when nasogastric suction is undesirable.

Single doses may facilitate small bowel intubation when the tube does not pass the pylorus with conventional maneuvers.

Stimulates gastric emptying and intestinal transit of barium in cases where delayed emptying interferes with radiological examination of the stomach or small intestine.

Administration and Dosage

For adults, if extrapyramidal symptoms occur, inject diphenhydramine 50 mg intramuscularly (IM) and symptoms usually subside.

Discontinue metoclopramide therapy in patients who develop signs or symptoms of tardive dyskinesia. There is no known treatment for tardive dyskinesia. In some patients, symptoms may lessen or resolve after metoclopramide treatment is stopped.

Prolonged treatment (longer than 12 weeks) with metoclopramide should be avoided in all but rare cases in which therapeutic benefit is thought to outweigh the risks to the patient of developing tardive dyskinesia.

Diabetic gastroparesis: 10 mg 30 minutes before each meal and at bedtime for 2 to 8 weeks. Duration of therapy should not exceed 12 weeks (oral).

Administer 10 mg IV over 1 to 2 minutes. Parenteral administration up to 10 days may be required before symptoms subside, then oral administration may be instituted.

Symptomatic gastroesophageal reflux: 10 to 15 mg orally up to 4 times daily 30 minutes before each meal and at bedtime. If symptoms occur only intermittently or at specific times of the day, single doses up to 20 mg prior to the provoking situation may be preferred rather than continuous treatment.

Prolonged treatment (longer than 12 weeks) with metoclopramide should be avoided in all but rare cases in which therapeutic benefit is thought to outweigh the risks to the patient of developing tardive dyskinesia.

Prevention of postoperative nausea and vomiting: Inject IM near the end of surgery. The usual adult dose is 10 mg; however, doses of 20 mg may be used.

Prevention of chemotherapy-induced emesis: Infuse slowly 30 minutes before beginning cancer chemotherapy; repeat every 2 hours for 2 doses, then every 3 hours for 3 doses.

The initial 2 doses should be 2 mg/kg if highly emetogenic drugs such as cisplatin or dacarbazine are used alone or in combination. For less emetogenic regimens, 1 mg/kg/dose may be adequate.

If extrapyramidal symptoms occur, administer 50 mg diphenhydramine IM.

Elderly: Occasionally, patients who are more sensitive to the therapeutic or adverse effects of metoclopramide will require 5 mg/dose.

IV admixture: When diluted in a parenteral solution, administer IV slowly over a period of not less than 15 minutes.

Direct IV injection: Inject undiluted metoclopramide slowly IV allowing 1 to 2 minutes for 10 mg.

Facilitation of small bowel intubation – If the tube has not passed the pylorus with conventional maneuvers in 10 minutes, administer a single undiluted dose slowly IV over 1 to 2 minutes.

Recommended single dose –

Adults: 10 mg (2 mL).

Children (6 to 14 years of age): 2.5 to 5 mg (0.5 to 1 mL).

Children (younger than 6 years of age): 0.1 mg/kg.

Radiological examinations – In patients where delayed gastric emptying interferes with radiological examination of the stomach or small intestine, a single dose may be administered slowly IV over 1 to 2 minutes.

Renal/Hepatic function impairment: Because metoclopramide is excreted principally through the kidneys, in those patients whose Ccr is less than 40 mL/min, initiate therapy at approximately½ the recommended dosage. Depending on clinical efficacy and safety considerations, the dosage may be increased or decreased as appropriate.

Administration: Give 30 minutes before meals and at bedtime.

Orally disintegrating tablets – Take on an empty stomach at least 30 minutes before eating. Do not repeat dose if inadvertently taken with food.

Because the tablet absorbs moisture rapidly, only remove each dose from the packaging just prior to taking. Handle the tablet with dry hands and place on the tongue. If the tablet should break or crumble while handling, discard and remove a new tablet.

Admixture compatibilities/incompatibilities:

Physically and chemically compatible up to 48 hours – Cimetidine; mannitol; potassium acetate; potassium chloride; potassium phosphate.

Physically compatible up to 48 hours – Ascorbic acid; benztropine; cytarabine; dexamethasone sodium phosphate; diphenhydramine; doxorubicin; heparin sodium; hydrocortisone sodium phosphate; lidocaine; multivitamin infusion (must be refrigerated) vitamin B complex with ascorbic acid.

Physically compatible up to 24 hours (do not use if precipitation occurs) – Clindamycin phosphate, cyclophosphamide, insulin.

Conditionally compatible (use within 1 hour after mixing or may be infused directly into the same running IV line) – Ampicillin, cisplatin, erythromycin lactobionate, methotrexate, penicillin G potassium, tetracycline.

Incompatible – Cephalothin; chloramphenicol; sodium bicarbonate.

Actions

Pharmacology: Metoclopramide stimulates motility of the upper GI tract without stimulating gastric, biliary, or pancreatic secretions. Its mode of action is unclear.

Pharmacokinetics:

Absorption/Distribution – Metoclopramide is rapidly and well absorbed. Onset of action is 1 to 3 minutes following an IV dose, 10 to 15 minutes following IM administration, and 30 to 60 minutes following an oral dose. Effects persist for 1 to 2 hours.

Relative to an IV dose of 20 mg, the absolute oral bioavailability of metoclopramide is approximately 80%. Peak plasma concentrations occur at approximately 1 to 2 hours after a single oral dose. The drug is not extensively bound to plasma proteins (about 30%).

Metabolism/Excretion – Approximately 85% of an orally administered dose appears in the urine within 72 hours. Of the 85% eliminated in the urine, about one-half is present as free or conjugated metoclopramide. The average elimination half-life in individuals with normal renal function is 5 to 6 hours.

Contraindications

When stimulation of GI motility might be dangerous (eg, in the presence of GI hemorrhage, mechanical obstruction, or perforation); pheochromocytoma; sensitivity or intolerance to metoclopramide; epileptics or patients receiving drugs likely to cause extrapyramidal reactions.

Warnings/Precautions

Depression: Depression has occurred in patients with and without a history of depression. Give metoclopramide to patients with a prior history of depression only if the expected benefits outweigh the potential risks.

Extrapyramidal symptoms: Extrapyramidal symptoms, manifested primarily as acute dystonic reactions, occur in approximately 0.2% to 1% of patients treated with the usual adult dosages of 30 to 40 mg/day. These usually are seen during the first 24 to 48 hours of treatment, occur more frequently in children and young adults, and are even more frequent at the higher doses used in prophylaxis of vomiting caused by cancer chemotherapy. If symptoms occur, they usually subside following 50 mg diphenhydramine IM. Benztropine 1 to 2 mg IM may also be used to reverse these reactions.

Parkinson-like symptoms: Parkinson-like symptoms have occurred, more commonly within the first 6 months after beginning treatment with metoclopramide but occasionally after longer periods. Give metoclopramide cautiously, if at all, to patients with preexisting Parkinson disease.

Tardive dyskinesia: Tardive dyskinesia may develop in patients treated with metoclopramide. Metoclopramide itself, however, may suppress (or partially suppress) the signs of tardive dyskinesia, thereby masking the underlying disease process. Therefore, the use of metoclopramide for the symptomatic control of tardive dyskinesia is not recommended.

Hypertension: In one study of hypertensive patients, IV metoclopramide released catecholamines. Use caution in hypertensive patients.

Anastomosis or closure of the gut: Giving a promotility drug such as metoclopramide could theoretically put increased pressure on suture lines following a gut anastomosis or closure.

Hypoglycemia: Gastroparesis (gastric stasis) may be responsible for poor diabetic control. Exogenously administered insulins may act before food has left the stomach, leading to hypoglycemia.

Special risk: Because metoclopramide produces a transient increase in plasma aldosterone, certain patients, especially those with cirrhosis or congestive heart failure, may be at risk of developing fluid retention and volume overload.

Patients with NADH-cytochrome b_5 reductase deficiency are at an increased risk of developing methemoglobinemia or sulfhemoglobinemia when metoclopramide is administered. In patients with glucose-6-phosphate dehydrogenase deficiency who experience metoclopramide-induced methemoglobinemia, methylene blue treatment is not recommended.

Hazardous tasks: May cause drowsiness; observe caution while driving or performing other tasks requiring alertness, coordination or physical dexterity.

Pregnancy: Category B.

Lactation: Metoclopramide is excreted into breast milk.

Children: Safety and effectiveness in children have not been established except to facilitate small bowel intubation.

Drug Interactions

Drugs that may affect metoclopramide include levodopa, anticholinergics, and narcotic analgesics. Drugs that may be affected by metoclopramide include alcohol, cimetidine, cyclosporine, digoxin, levodopa, MAO inhibitors, and succinylcholine.

Adverse Reactions

Adverse reactions occurring in at least 3% of patients include restlessness; drowsiness; fatigue; lassitude; akathisia; dizziness; anxiety; dystonia; insomnia; headache; myoclonus; confusion; convulsive seizures; hallucinations; nausea; bowel disturbances, primarily diarrhea.

LAXATIVES

BISACODYL	
Tablets: 5 mg (*otc*)	*Dulcolax Bowel Prep Kit* (Boehringer Ingelheim)
Tablets, enteric-coated: 5 mg (*otc*)	Various, *Alophen* (Numark), *Bisa-Lax* (Bergen Brunswig), *Dulcolax* (Boehringer Ingelheim), *Ex-Lax Ultra* (Novartis Consumer Health), *Fleet Laxative* (Fleet), *Modane* (Savage), *Bisac-Evac* (G & W), *Caroid* (Metholatum Co.), *Correctol* (Schering-Plough), *Feen-a-mint* (Schering-Plough)
Tablets, delayed-release: 10 mg	*Doxidan* (Pharmacia)
Suppositories: 10 mg (*otc*)	Various, *Bisacodyl Uniserts* (Upsher-Smith), *Bisa-Lax* (Bergen Brunswig), *Bisac-Evac* (G & W), *Dulcolax* (Boehringer Ingelheim), *Dulcolax Bowel Prep Kit* (Boehringer Ingelheim), *Fleet Laxative* (Fleet)
CASCARA SAGRADA	
Capsules: 450 mg (*otc*)	Various
Fluid extract; oral: 1 g/mL, 325 mg per 5 mL (*otc*)	*Cascara Sagrada Aromatic Fluid Extract* (Various)
CASTOR OIL	
Liquid: 95% castor oil (*otc*)	Various, *Purge* (Fleming)
Emulsion: 95% castor oil with emulsifying agents (*otc*)	*Emulsoil* (Paddock)
36.4% castor oil with 0.1% sodium benzoate, 0.2% potassium sorbate (*otc*)	*Neoloid* (Kenwood)
CO_2 RELEASING SUPPOSITORIES	
Suppositories: Sodium bicarbonate and potassium bitartrate in a water soluble polyethylene glycol base (*otc*)	*Ceo-Two* (Beutlich)
DOCUSATE CALCIUM (DIOCTYL CALCIUM SULFOSUCCINATE)	
Capsules: 240 mg (*otc*)	Various, *DC Softgels* (Goldline), *Stool Softener* (Apothecary), *Stool Softener DC* (Rugby), *Surfak Liquigels* (Pharmacia)
DOCUSATE SODIUM (DIOCTYL SODIUM SULFOSUCCINATE; DSS)	
Tablets: 100 mg (*otc*)	*ex-lax Stool Softener* (Novartis Consumer)
Capsules: 50 and 100 mg (*otc*)	Various, *Colace* (Roberts), *D-S-S* (Magno-Humphries), *Non-Habit Forming Stool Softener*, *Stool Softener* (Rugby)
250 mg (*otc*)	Various, *Stool Softener* (Rugby)
Capsules, soft gel: 50, 100, and 250 mg (*otc*)	Various, *Dulcolax* (Boehringer Ingelheim), *D.O.S.*, *Phillip's Liqui-Gels* (Bayer Consumer), *Stool Softener* (Rugby)
Liquid: 10 mg/mL (*otc*)	*Silace* (Silarx)
Syrup: 50, 60, 150 mg per 15 mL; 20 mg per 5 mL; 100 mg per 30 mL (*otc*)	Various, *Colace* (Roberts), *Diocto* (Various), *Docu* (Hi-Tech Pharmacal), *Silace* (Silax)
GLYCERIN	
Suppositories: Glycerin (*otc*)	Various, *Sani-Supp* (G & W), *Colace* (Roberts)
Liquid: 4 mL/applicator (*otc*)	*Fleet Babylax* (Fleet)
LACTULOSE	
Solution; oral: 10 g per 15 mL (< 1.6 g galactose, < 1.2 g lactose, and ≤ 1.2 g of other sugars) (*Rx*)	Various, *Cephulac* (Hoechst-Marion Roussel), *Constulose* (Alpharma), *Enulose* (Alpharma)
Solution; oral or rectal: 10 g per 15 mL (*Rx*)	*Generiac* (Morton Groves Pharmaceuticals)
Solution, crystals; oral: Lactulose (< galactose 0.3 g and lactose/10 g) (*Rx*)	*Kristalose* (Bertek)
MINERAL OIL	
Liquid: Mineral oil (*otc*)	Various
Emulsion: Mineral oil with an emulsifier (*otc*)	*Kondremul Plain* (Heritage Consumer)
POLYCARBOPHIL	
Tablets: 500 and 625 mg (*otc*)	*FiberNorm* (G & W), *Konsyl Fiber* (Konsyl)
625 mg (as calcium) (*otc*)	*Bulk Forming Fiber Laxative* (Goldline Consumer), *Fiber-Lax* (Rugby), *FiberCon* (Lederle)
Tablets, chewable: 625 mg (as calcium) (*otc*)	*Equalactin* (Numark), *Mitrolan* (Whitehall-Robins)

PSYLLIUM	
Powder: Psyllium (*otc*)	Various, *Fiberall Tropical Fruit Flavor, Fiberall Orange Flavor* (Heritage Consumer), *Genfiber, Genfiber, Orange Flavor* (Goldline Consumer), *Hydrocil Instant* (Numark), *Konsyl, Konsyl-D, Konsyl-Orange, Konsyl Easy Mix Formula* (Konsyl Pharm.), *Metamucil, Metamucil Sugar Free, Metamucil Orange Flavor* (Procter & Gamble), *Natural Fiber Laxative* (Apothecary), *Reguloid, Reguloid, Orange, Reguloid, Sugar Free Orange* (Rugby), *Syllact* (Wallace)
Wafers: Psyllium (*otc*)	*Metamucil* (Procter & Gamble)
Granules: Psyllium (*otc*)	*Serutan* (Menley & James)
SALINE LAXATIVES	
Granules: Magnesium sulfate (*otc*)	*Epsom Salt* (Various)
Suspension: Magnesium hydroxide (*otc*)	*Milk of Magnesia, Milk of Magnesia, Concentrated* (*Various*), *Phillips' Milk of Magnesia, Phillips' Milk of Magnesia, Concentrated* (Bayer)
Solution: Magnesium citrate (*otc*)	*Magnesium Citrate Solution* (Humco)
Sodium phosphates (*otc*)	Various
SENNOSIDES	
Tablets: 6 mg (*otc*)	*Black Draught* (Lee Pharmaceuticals)
8.6 mg (*otc*)	*Dr. Edward's Olive* (Oakhurst), *Senexon* (Rugby), *Senna-Gen* (Zenith-Goldline), *Senokot* (Purdue Fredrick)
15 mg (*otc*)	*ex•lax, ex•lax chocolated* (Novartis Consumer), *Lax-Pills* (G & W Labs), *Senna Smooth* (Novartis Consumer)
17 mg (*otc*)	*SenokotXTRA* (Purdue Fredrick)
25 mg (*otc*)	*Lax-Pills* (G & W Labs), *Maximum Relief ex•lax* (Novartis Consumer)
Tablets, chewable: 10 mg (*otc*)	*Black Draught, Evac-u-gen* (Lee Pharmaceuticals)
Granules: 15 mg/5 mL	*Senokot* (Purdue Frederick)
20 mg/5 mL	*Black-Draught* (Lee Pharmaceuticals)
Liquid: 8.8 mg per 5 mL	*Senexon* (Rugby)
33.3 mg/mL senna concentrate (*otc*)	*Fletcher's Castoria* (Mentholatum)
Syrup: 8.8 mg per 5 mL sennosides (*otc*)	*Senokot* (Purdue Frederick)
176 mg per 5 mL senna leaf extract	*Senna* (Pharmaceutical Associates)
Drops: 8.8 mg/ mL sennosides (*otc*)	*Little Tummys Laxative Drops* (Vetco Inc)
ENEMAS	
Disposable enemas	*Fleet, Fleet Bisacodyl, Fleet Mineral Oil* (Fleet), *Therevac-SB, Therevac-Plus* (Jones Medical)
LAXATIVE COMBINATIONS	
Tablets: 50 mg docusate sodium, 8.6 mg senna concentrate (*otc*)	*Senokot-S* (Purdue Frederick), *Senna Plus* (Contract Pharmacal), *Senna-S* (Akyma), *Peri-Colace* (Perdue)
150 mg cascara sagrada (*otc*)	*Nature's Remedy* (Block Drug)
Capsules: 100 mg docusate sodium, 30 mg casanthranol (*otc*)	Various, *DSS 100 Plus* (Magno-Humphries), *Peri-Dos Softgels* (Goldline)
Liquids, syrups, emulsions, suspensions: 60 mg docusate sodium and 30 mg casanthranol per 15 mL (*otc*)	*Diocto C* (Various)
90 mg per 15 mL casanthranol with senna extract, rhubarb, methyl salicylate, and menthol (*otc*)	*Black-Draught* (Monticello)
30 mg casanthranol, 60 mg docusate sodium per 15 mL (*otc*)	*Silace-C* (Silarx)
Mineral oil in emulsifying base (*otc*)	*Liqui-Doss* (Ferndale)
≈ 900 mg magnesium hydroxide and 3.75 mL mineral oil per 15 mL (*otc*)	*Haley's M-O* (Bayer)
Solution: 70% w/w D-sorbitol (*otc*)	Various
MISCELLANEOUS BOWEL EVACUANTS	
Liquid; oral: magnesium citrate 19 g (*otc*)	*Tridate Bowel Cleansing System*[a] (Lafayette)
Liquid; oral: monobasic sodium phosphate 21.6 g and dibasic sodium phosphate 8.1g (*otc*)	*Fleet Prep Kit 3*[b] (Fleet)

Tablets; oral: sodium phosphate monobasic monohydrate 1.102 g, sodium phosphate dibasic anhydrous 0.398 g (*Rx*)	*Visicol* (Salix), *OsmoPrep* (Salix)
Solution, powder for reconstitution; oral: 210 g of PEG 3350, sodium chloride 5.6 g, sodium bicarbonate 2.86 g, potassium chloride 0.74 g (*Rx*)	*HalfLytely*[c] (Braintree)
MISCELLANEOUS BULK-PRODUCING LAXATIVES	
Tablets; oral: 500 mg methylcellulose (*otc*)	*Citrucel* (GlaxoSmithKline)
Fiber 1 g (*otc*)	*Benefiber Ultra* (Novartis), *Benefiber Plus Heart* (Novartis)
Tablets, chewable; oral Fiber 1 g (*otc*)	*Benefiber* (Novartis), *Benefiber Plus Calcium* (Novartis)
Powder: 2 g methylcellulose per heaping tbsp (*otc*)	*Citrucel*, *Citrucel Sugar Free*[d] (GlaxoSmithKline)
Powdered cellulose (*otc*)	*Unifiber* (Niche)
8 g malt soup extract/scoop (*otc*)	*Maltsupex* (Wallace)
Fiber 1.5 g per teaspoon	*Benefiber* (Novartis), *Benefiber for Children* (Novartis), *Benefiber Plus Heart Health* (Novartis)
Fiber 3 g per tbsp/packet	*Benefiber Plus Calcium* (Novartis), *Benefiber Sticks* (Novartis), *Benefiber Drink Mix* (Novartis)

[a] With 3 bisacodyl 5 mg tablets and 1 bisacodyl 10 mg suppository.
[b] With 4 bisacodyl 5 mg enteric-coated tablets and one 30 mL bisacodyl 10 mg enema.
[c] With 4 bisacodyl 5 mg delayed-release, enteric-coated tablets.
[d] With 52 mg phenylalanine per dose.

Warning:

There have been rare but serious reports of acute phosphate nephropathy in patients who received oral **sodium phosphate** products for colon cleansing prior to colonoscopy. Some cases have resulted in permanent impairment of renal function, and some patients required long-term dialysis. While some cases have occurred in patients without identifiable risk factors, patients at increased risk of acute phosphate nephropathy may include those with increased age, hypovolemia, increased bowel transit time (such as bowel obstruction), active colitis, or baseline kidney disease, and those using medicines that affect renal perfusion or function (such as diuretics, angiotensin-converting enzyme inhibitors, angiotensin receptor blockers, and possibly nonsteroidal anti-inflammatory drugs).

It is important to use the dose and dosing regimen as recommended (PM/AM split dose).

Indications

Constipation: Treatment of constipation.

Rectal/Bowel examinations: Certain stimulant, lubricant, and saline laxatives are used to evacuate the colon for rectal and bowel examinations.

Prophylaxis: Laxatives, generally **fecal softeners** or **mineral oil**, are useful prophylactically in patients who should not strain during defecation (ie, following anorectal surgery, myocardial infarction).

Lactulose (certain brands): Prevention and treatment of portal-systemic encephalopathy, including the stages of hepatic precoma and coma.

Psyllium: Useful in patients with irritable bowel syndrome and diverticular disease.

Polycarbophil: For constipation or diarrhea associated with conditions such as irritable bowel syndrome and diverticulosis; acute nonspecific diarrhea.

Sodium phosphate: For cleansing of the colon as a preparation for colonoscopy in adults 18 years of age and older.

Mineral oil (enema): Relief of fecal impaction.

Docusate sodium: Prevention of dry, hard stools.

Administration and Dosage

BISACODYL: Swallow whole; do not chew. Do not take within 1 hour of antacids or milk.

Tablets –

Adults and children 12 years of age and older: 10 to 15 mg (usually 10 mg) in a single dose once daily.

Children (6 to 11 years of age): 5 mg once daily.

Suppositories –

Adults: 10 mg once daily.

Children (6 to 11 years of age): 5 mg once daily.

CASCARA SAGRADA:

Tablets – 1 tablet at bedtime.

Liquid – 5 mL.

CASTOR OIL:

Liquid –

Adults: Daily dose range, 15 to 60 mL.

Children (2 to 12 years of age): 5 to 15 mL.

Infants: 2.5 to 7.5 mL.

Emulsion –

Adults: 67%, 15 to 60 mL; 95%, 45 mL (should be mixed with ½ to 1 glass liquid).

Children (2 to 12 years of age): 67%, 15 mL; 95%, 5 to 10 mL (should be mixed with ½ to 1 glass liquid).

DOCUSATE CALCIUM *(Dioctyl calcium sulfosuccinate):*

Adults and children 12 years of age and older – 240 mg daily until bowel movements are normal.

DOCUSATE SODIUM *(Dioctyl sodium sulfosuccinate; DSS):* Administer in milk, fruit juice, or infant formula to mask taste. In enemas, add 50 to 100 mg (5 to 10 mL liquid) to a retention or flushing enema.

Adults and older children – 50 to 500 mg.

Children (6 to 12 years of age) – 40 to 120 mg.

Children (3 to 6 years of age) – 20 to 60 mg.

Children (younger than 3 years of age) – 10 to 40 mg.

GLYCERIN:

Suppositories – Insert 1 suppository high in the rectum and retain 15 to 30 minutes; it need not melt to produce laxative action.

Rectal liquid – With gentle, steady pressure, insert stem with tip pointing towards navel. Squeeze unit until nearly all the liquid is expelled, then remove. A small amount of liquid will remain in unit.

LACTULOSE:

Chronulac, Constilac, Duphalac, Constulose –

Treatment of constipation: 15 to 30 mL (lactulose 10 to 20 g) daily, increased to 60 mL/day, if necessary.

Cephulac, Cholac, Enulose – Prevent and treat portal-systemic encephalopathy

Oral:

Adults – 30 to 45 mL 3 or 4 times daily. Adjust dosage every day or 2 days to produce 2 or 3 soft stools daily. Hourly doses of 30 to 45 mL may be used to induce rapid laxation in the initial phase of therapy. When the laxative effect has been achieved, reduce dosage to recommended daily dose. Improvement may occur within 24 hours, but may not begin before 48 hours or later. Continuous long-term therapy is indicated to lessen severity and prevent recurrence of portal-systemic encephalopathy.

Children – Recommended initial daily oral dose in infants is 2.5 to 10 mL in divided doses. For older children and adolescents, the total daily dose is 40 to 90 mL. If the initial dose causes diarrhea, reduce immediately. If diarrhea persists, discontinue use.

May be more palatable when mixed with fruit juice, water, or milk.

Rectal: Administer to adults during impending coma or coma stage of portal-systemic encephalopathy when the danger of aspiration exists or when endoscopic or intubation procedures interfere with oral administration. The goal of treatment is reversal of the coma stage so the patient can take oral medication. Reversal of coma may occur within 2 hours of the first enema. Start recommended oral doses before enema is stopped entirely.

Lactulose may be given as a retention enema via a rectal balloon catheter. Do not use cleansing enemas containing soap suds or other alkaline agents.

Mix lactulose 300 mL with 700 mL of water or physiologic saline and retain for 30 to 60 minutes. The enema may be repeated every 4 to 6 hours. If the enema is inadvertently evacuated too promptly, it may be repeated immediately.

MINERAL OIL:

Dose –

Adults and children 12 years of age and older: 15 to 45 mL, take at bedtime; *Kondremul,* 30 to 75 mL.

Children 6 to 11 years of age: 5 to 15 mL; *Kondremul,* 10 to 25 mL.

POLYCARBOPHIL:

Adults and children 12 years of age and older – 1 g 1 to 4 times daily or as needed. Do not exceed 4 g in 24 hours.

Children 6 to 11 years of age – 500 mg no more than 4 times daily or as needed. Do not exceed 2 g/day.

Children younger than 6 years of age – Products vary. Consult product labeling for specific guidelines.

For severe diarrhea, repeat dose every 30 minutes; do not exceed maximum daily dose.

When using as a laxative, drink 8 oz water or other liquid with each dose.

PSYLLIUM: Refer to respective package inserts for particular dosing.

SALINE LAXATIVES:

Magnesium sulfate –

Adults: 10 to 15 g in glass of water.

Children: 5 to 10 g in glass of water.

Magnesium hydroxide –

Adults: Recommended dosage varies from product to product, ranging from 10 to 60 mL/day. See individual package labeling for specific dosing information.

Children (2 years of age and older): 5 to 30 mL, depending on age (must be at least 2 years of age).

Magnesium citrate –

Adults: 1 glassful (approximately 240 mL) as needed.

Children: ½ the adult dose as needed; repeat if necessary.

Sodium phosphates –

Adults: 20 to 30 mL mixed with ½ glass cool water.

Children: 5 to 15 mL.

SENNOSIDES: The following dosages are for senna concentrate only. For other forms of senna, consult labeling. Dosages are different.

Tablets (6 and 8.6 mg) –

Adults: 2 tablets, up to 8 per day.

Children: 1 tablet, up to 4 per day.

Tablets (15 mg) –

Adults: 1 tablet at bedtime, up to 4 per day.

Granules –

Adults: 1 tsp, up to 4 tsp/day.

Children: ½ tsp, up to 2 tsp/day.

Suppositories –

Adults: 1 at bedtime; repeat in 2 hours if necessary.

Children: ½ suppository at bedtime.

Liquid –

Adults: 15 to 30 mL with or after meals or at bedtime.

Children (6 to 15 years of age): 10 to 15 mL at bedtime.

Children (2 to 5 years of age): 5 to 10 mL at bedtime.

Syrup –

Adults: 10 to 15 mL at bedtime (up to 30 mL/day).

Children (5 to 15 years of age): 5 to 10 mL at bedtime (up to 20 mL/day).

Children (1 to 5 years of age): 2.5 to 5 mL at bedtime (up to 10 mL/day).

Children (1 month to 1 year of age): 1.25 to 2.5 mL at bedtime (up to 5 mL/day).

Miscellaneous BOWEL EVACUANTS:

Colon cleansing –

OsmoPrep: 32 tablets (sodium phosphate 48 g) with a total of 2 quarts of clear liquids in the following manner: the evening before the procedure, take 4 tablets with 8 oz of clear liquids every 15 minutes for a total of 20 tablets. On the day of the procedure, starting 3 to 5 hours before the procedure, take 4 tablets with 8 oz of clear liquids every 15 minutes for a total of 12 tablets.

Visicol: 40 tablets (sodium phosphate 60 g) with a total of 3.6 quarts of clear liquids in the following manner: the evening before the procedure, take 3 tablets (the last dose will be 2 tablets) with 8 oz of clear liquids every 15 minutes for a total of 20 tablets. On the day of the procedure, starting 3 to 5 hours before the procedure, take 3 tablets (the last dose will be 2 tablets) with 8 oz of clear liquids every 15 minutes for a total of 20 tablets.

Miscellaneous BULK-PRODUCING LAXATIVES:

Citrucel –

Adults and children 12 years of age and older: 1 heaping tbsp (19 g) in 8 oz cold water 1 to 3 times daily.

Children (6 to 11 years of age): ½ the adult dose in 8 oz cold water once daily.

Unifiber – Dose is 1 tbsp in 3 or 4 oz of fruit juice, milk, or water, or mix with soft foods, such as applesauce, mashed potatoes, or pudding. Can be taken up to 3 times daily if needed or as recommended by a doctor.

Maltsupex –

Tablets: Adults, 12 to 36 g/day. Initially, 4 tablets 4 times daily (meals and bedtime).

Powder: 16 g equals 1 heaping tablespoon.

Adults, up to 32 g twice daily for 3 or 4 days, then 16 to 32 g at bedtime. Children 6 to 12 years of age, up to 16 g twice daily for 3 or 4 days; 2 to 6 years of age, 8 g twice daily for 3 or 4 days. For infants younger than 2 years of age, consult a doctor.

Liquid: Adults, 2 tbsp twice daily for 3 or 4 days, then 1 to 2 tbsp at bedtime. Children 6 to 12 years of age, 1 tbsp twice daily for 3 or 4 days; 2 to 6 years of age, ½ tbsp twice daily for 3 or 4 days. For infants younger than 2 years of age, consult a doctor.

Actions

Pharmacology:

Pharmacologic Actions of Laxatives

	Laxatives	Onset of action (h)	Site of action	Mechanism of action	Comments
Saline	Dibasic sodium phosphate[a,b] Magnesium citrate Magnesium hydroxide Magnesium sulfate Monobasic sodium phosphate[a,b] Sodium biphosphate[a]	0.5 to 3	Small & large intestine	Attract/Retain water in intestinal lumen increasing intraluminal pressure; cholecystokinin release	May alter fluid and electrolyte balance. Sulfate salts are considered the most potent.
Stimulant/Irritant	Cascara	6 to 8	Colon	Direct action on intestinal mucosa or nerve plexus, alters water and electrolyte secretion	May prefer castor oil when more complete evacuation is required.
	Bisacodyl tablets Casanthranol Senna	6 to 10			
	Bisacodyl suppository	0.25 to 1			

Pharmacologic Actions of Laxatives					
	Laxatives	Onset of action (h)	Site of action	Mechanism of action	Comments
Bulk-Producing	Methylcellulose Polycarbophil Psyllium	12 to 72	Small & large intestine	Holds water in stool to increase bulk-stimulating peristalsis; forms emollient gel	Safe; minimal side effects. Take with plenty of water (240 mL/dose).
Emollient	Mineral oil	6 to 8	Colon	Retards colonic absorption of fecal water; softens stool	May decrease absorption of fat-soluble vitamins.
Fecal Softeners/ Surfactants	Docusate[c]	12 to 72	Small & large intestine	Facilitates admixture of fat and water to soften stool	Beneficial in anorectal conditions where passage of a firm stool is painful.
Hyperosmotic	Glycerin suppository	0.25 to 1	Colon	Local irritation; hyperosmotic action	Sodium stearate in preparation causes the local irritation.
Hyperosmotic	Lactulose	24 to 48	Colon	Osmotic effect retains fluid in the colon, lowering the pH and increasing colonic peristalsis	Also indicated in portal-systemic encephalopathy.
Miscellaneous	Castor oil	2 to 6	Small intestine	Direct action on intestinal mucosa or nerve plexus, alters water and electrolyte secretion	Castor oil is converted to ricinoleic acid (active component) in the gut.

[a] Onset of action for rectal preparations is 2 to 15 minutes.
[b] Colon is site of action for rectal preparations.
[c] Site of action for potassium salt is in the colon.

Contraindications

Hypersensitivity to any ingredient; nausea, vomiting, or other symptoms of appendicitis; fecal impaction; intestinal obstruction; undiagnosed abdominal pain; patients who require a low galactose diet (**lactulose**).

Do not give **docusate sodium** if **mineral oil** is being given.

Warnings/Precautions

Fluid and electrolyte balance: Excessive laxative use may lead to significant fluid and electrolyte imbalance. Monitor patients periodically.

Preparations containing sodium should be used cautiously by individuals on a sodium-restricted diet and in the presence of edema, congestive heart failure (CHF), renal failure, or borderline hypertension.

Hydration: It is recommended that patients receiving **sodium phosphate** be advised to adequately hydrate before, during, and after the use of the medicine.

Cardiovascular effects: Use with considerable caution in patients with CHF or unstable angina.

QT prolongation – Prolongation of the QT interval has been observed in some patients who were dosed with **sodium phosphate**.

Cardiac arrhythmias – There have been rare but serious reports of arrhythmias associated with the use of **sodium phosphate** products.

Cardiac surgery – Because *Visicol* was not studied in patients who recently had cardiac surgery, use with caution in these patients.

Bulimia: Laxatives and purgatives have the potential for abuse by bulimia nervosa patients who frequently binge eat and vomit.

GI effects: Use with considerable caution in patients with ascites, gastric retention, ileus, acute bowel obstruction, pseudo-obstruction of the bowel, severe chronic constipation, bowel perforation, acute colitis, toxic megacolon, gastric bypass or stapling surgery, or hypomotility syndrome.

Aphthous ulcers – Administration of **sodium phosphate** tablets may induce colonic mucosal aphthous ulcerations.

Inflammatory bowel disease – Use **sodium phosphate** with caution in patients with inflammatory bowel disease.

Seizures: There have been rare reports of generalized tonic-clonic seizures and/or loss of consciousness associated with use of **sodium phosphate** products in patients with no prior history of seizures.

Dysphagia: Patients with a history of swallowing difficulties or anatomic narrowing of the esophagus may have difficulty swallowing *Visicol* tablets. Undigested or partially digested tablets from other medications may be seen in the stool or during colonoscopy.

Megacolon, bowel obstruction, imperforate anus, or congestive heart failure: Do not use **sodium phosphate** and **sodium biphosphate** in these patients; hypernatremic dehydration may occur.

Abuse/Dependency: Chronic use of laxatives, particularly stimulants, may lead to laxative dependency, which in turn may result in fluid and electrolyte imbalances, steatorrhea, osteomalacia, vitamin and mineral deficiencies, and a poorly functioning colon. Also known as laxative abuse syndrome, it is difficult to diagnose.

Cathartic colon: Cathartic colon, a poorly functioning colon, results from the chronic abuse of stimulant cathartics.

Melanosis coli: Melanosis coli is a darkened pigmentation of the colonic mucosa resulting from chronic use of anthraquinone derivatives (**casanthrol**, **cascara sagrada**, **senna**).

Lipid pneumonitis: Lipid pneumonitis may result from oral ingestion and aspiration of mineral oil, especially when the patient reclines. The young, elderly, debilitated, and dysphagic are at greatest risk.

Electrocautery procedures: A theoretical hazard may exist for patients being treated with **lactulose** who may undergo electrocautery procedures during proctoscopy or colonoscopy. Accumulation of H_2 gas in significant concentration in the presence of an electrical spark may result in an explosion. Although this complication has not been reported with **lactulose**, patients should have a thorough bowel cleansing with a nonfermentable solution.

Diabetic patients: **Lactulose** syrup contains galactose (less than 1.6 g per 15 mL) and lactose (less than 1.2 g per 15 mL). Use with caution in diabetic patients.

Concomitant laxative use: Do not use other laxatives, especially during the initial phase of therapy for portal-systemic encephalopathy; the resulting loose stools may falsely suggest adequate **lactulose** dosage.

Rectal bleeding or response failure: Rectal bleeding or failure to respond to therapy may indicate a serious condition that may require further medical attention.

Discoloration: Discoloration of acid urine to yellow-brown or black may occur with **cascara sagrada** or **senna**. Pink-red, red-violet, or red-brown discoloration of alkaline urine may occur with **phenolphthalein**, **cascara sagrada**, or **senna**.

Impaction or obstruction: Impaction or obstruction may be caused by bulk-forming agents if temporarily arrested in their passage through the alimentary canal (eg, patients with esophageal strictures). Administer bulk-forming agents with at least 240 mL fluid.

Renal function impairment: Up to 20% of the magnesium in magnesium salts may be absorbed. Do not use products containing phosphate, sodium, magnesium, or potassium salts in the presence of renal dysfunction.

Pregnancy: Category B (**Lactulose, magnesium sulfate**). *Category C* (**Casanthranol, cascara sagrada, danthron, docusate sodium, docusate calcium, docusate potassium, mineral oil, senna, sodium phosphate**). Do not use **castor oil** during pregnancy; its irritant effect may induce premature labor. Mineral oil may decrease absorption of fat-soluble vitamins. Improper use of saline cathartics can lead to dangerous electrolyte imbalance. If needed, limit use to bulk-forming or surfactant laxatives.

Lactation: Anthraquinone derivatives (eg, **casanthranol, cascara sagrada, danthron**) are excreted in breast milk, resulting in a potential increased incidence of diarrhea in the breast-feeding infant. *Sennosides* A and B (eg, **senna**) are not excreted in breast milk. It is not known whether **docusate calcium, docusate potassium, docusate sodium, lactulose**, and **mineral oil** are excreted in breast milk.

Children: Physical manipulation of a glycerin suppository in infants often initiates defecation; hence, adverse effects are minimal. Do not administer enemas to children younger than 2 years of age.

Monitoring: In the overall management of portal-systemic encephalopathy, there is serious underlying liver disease with complications, such as electrolyte disturbance (eg, hypokalemia, hypernatremia), which may require other specific therapy. Elderly, debilitated patients who receive **lactulose** for longer than 6 months should have serum electrolytes (potassium, chloride) and carbon dioxide measured periodically.

Drug Interactions

Medications administered in close proximity to **sodium phosphate** may not be absorbed from the GI tract because of the rapid intestinal peristalsis and watery diarrhea induced by the purgative agent.

An additive effect of **sodium phosphate** with other drugs that prolong the QT interval cannot be excluded.

Drugs that may interact with laxatives include H_2 antagonists, lipid soluble vitamins (A, D, E, and K), milk or antacids, mineral oil, proton pump inhibitors, and tetracycline.

Adverse Reactions

abdominal cramps, abdominal pain; bloating; excessive bowel activity (griping, diarrhea, nausea, vomiting); dizziness; fainting; flatulence; palpitations; perianal irritation; sweating; weakness.

Esophageal, gastric, small intestinal, and rectal obstruction caused by the accumulation of mucilaginous components of bulk laxatives have occurred.

Large doses of mineral oil may cause anal seepage, resulting in itching (pruritus ani), irritation, hemorrhoids, and perianal discomfort.

Lactulose – Gaseous distention with flatulence, belching, abdominal discomfort such as cramping (approximately 20%); nausea; vomiting. Excessive dosage can lead to diarrhea.

POLYETHYLENE GLYCOL-ELECTROLYTE SOLUTION (PEG-ES)

Powder for oral solution: 1 gal: PEG 3350 227.1 g, sodium sulfate 21.5 g, sodium bicarb 6.36 g, NaCl 5.53 g, KCl 2.82 g (*Rx*) 4 L: PEG 3350 240 g, sodium sulfate 22.72 g, sodium bicarb 6.72 g, NaCl 5.84 g, KCl 2.98 g (*Rx*)	*CoLyte* (Alaven)
Powder for oral solution: PEG 3350 236 g, sodium sulfate 22.74 g, sodium bicarb 6.74 g, NaCl 5.86 g, KCl 2.97 g; PEG 3350 227.1 g, sodium sulfate 21.5 g, sodium bicarb 6.36 g, NaCl 5.53 g, KCl 2.82 g (*Rx*)	*GoLYTELY* (Braintree Labs)
Powder for oral solution: PEG 3350 100 g, sodium sulfate 7.5 g, NaCl 2.691 g, KCl 1.015 (*Rx*)	*MoviPrep* (Salix)

Powder for oral solution: PEG 3350 420 g, sodium bicarb 5.72 g, NaCl 11.2 g, KCl 1.48 g (*Rx*)	*NuLytely* (Braintree), *TriLyte* (Alaven)
Powder for oral solution: PEG 3350 240 g, sodium bicarbonate 6.72 g, sodium chloride 5.84 g, sodium sulfate 22.72 g, potassium chloride 2.98 g (*Rx*)	*GaviLyte-C* (Gavis)
Powder for oral solution: PEG 3350 236 g, sodium bicarbonate 6.74 g, sodium chloride 5.86 g, sodium sulfate 22.74 g, potassium chloride 2.97 g (*Rx*)	*GaviLyte-G* (Gavis)
Oral solution: NaCl 146 mg, sodium bicarb 168 mg, sodium sulfate decahydrate 1.29 g, KCl 75 mg, PEG 3350 6 g, polysorbate-80 30 mg per 100 mL (*Rx*)	*OCL* (Abbott)

Indications

For bowel cleansing prior to GI examination.

Unlabeled uses: PEG electrolyte solutions are useful in the management of acute iron overdose in children.

Administration and Dosage

The patient should fast approximately 3 to 4 hours prior to ingestion of the solution; solid foods should never be given less than 2 hours before solution is administered.

One method is to schedule patients for midmorning exam, allowing 3 hours for drinking and 1 hour to complete bowel evacuation. Another method is to give the solution the evening before the exam, particularly if the patient is to have a barium enema. No foods except clear liquids are permitted after solution administration.

Adult dosage: Adult dosage is 4 L orally of solution prior to GI exam. May be given via a nasogastric tube to patients unwilling or unable to drink the preparation. Drink 240 mL every 10 minutes until 4 L are consumed or until the rectal effluent is clear. Rapid drinking of each portion is preferred to drinking small amounts continuously. Nasogastric tube administration is at the rate of 20 to 30 mL/min (1.2 to 1.8 L/hour). The first bowel movement should occur in approximately 1 hour.

Actions

Pharmacology: Oral solution induces diarrhea (onset, 30 to 60 minutes) that rapidly cleanses the bowel, usually within 4 hours. Polyethylene glycol 3350 (PEG 3350), a nonabsorbable solution, acts as an osmotic agent.

Contraindications

GI obstruction; gastric retention; bowel perforation; toxic colitis, megacolon, or ileus.

Warnings/Precautions

Regurgitation/Aspiration: Observe unconscious or semiconscious patients with impaired gag reflex and those who are otherwise prone to regurgitation or aspiration during use, especially if given via a nasogastric tube. If GI obstruction or perforation is suspected, rule out these contraindications before administration.

Severe bloating: If a patient experiences severe bloating, distention, or abdominal pain, slow or temporarily discontinue administration until symptoms abate.

Severe ulcerative colitis: Use with caution.

Pregnancy: *Category C.*

Children: Safety and efficacy for use in children have not been established.

Several studies in infants and children ranging in age from 3 to 14 years of age showed that the use of PEG-electrolyte solutions are safe and effective in bowel evacuation.

Drug Interactions

Oral medication given within 1 hour of start of therapy may be flushed from the GI tract and not absorbed.

Adverse Reactions

Nausea, abdominal fullness, bloating (50% or less); abdominal cramps, vomiting, anal irritation (less frequent).

POLYETHYLENE GLYCOL (PEG) SOLUTION

Powder for oral solution: PEG 3350 17 g (*Rx*)	*GlycoLax* (Kremers Urban)
PEG 3350 17 g (*otc*)	*GaviLAX* (Gavis), *MiraLax* (Schering-Plough)
PEG 3350 119, 238, and 510 g (*otc*)	*MiraLax* (Schering-Plough)
PEG 3350 255 g (*Rx*)	Various, *GlycoLax* (Kremers Urban)
PEG 3350 527 g (*Rx*)	Various

For complete prescribing information, refer to the Laxatives group monograph.

Indications

For the treatment of occasional constipation. Do not use for more than 2 weeks.

Administration and Dosage

The usual dose is 17 g of powder/day in 8 ounces of water. Each bottle is supplied with a measuring cap marked to contain 17 g of laxative powder when filled to the indicated line.

Two to 4 days (48 to 96 hours) may be required to produce a bowel movement.

DIFENOXIN HYDROCHLORIDE WITH ATROPINE SULFATE

Tablets: 1 mg difenoxin (as hydrochloride) and 0.025 mg atropine sulfate (*c-iv*)	*Motofen* (Valeant)

Indications

Adjunctive therapy in management of acute nonspecific diarrhea and acute exacerbations of chronic functional diarrhea.

Administration and Dosage

Adults: Recommended starting dose: 2 tablets, then 1 tablet after each loose stool; 1 tablet every 3 to 4 hours as needed. The total dosage during any 24-hour treatment period should not exceed 8 tablets. For diarrhea in which clinical improvement is not observed in 48 hours, continued administration is not recommended. For acute diarrhea and acute exacerbations of functional diarrhea, treatment beyond 48 hours is usually not necessary.

Actions

Pharmacology: Difenoxin is an antidiarrheal agent chemically related to meperidine. Atropine sulfate is present to discourage deliberate overdosage.

Difenoxin manifests its antidiarrheal effect by slowing intestinal motility. The mechanism of action is by a local effect on the GI wall.

Difenoxin is the principal active metabolite of diphenoxylate and is effective at one-fifth the dosage of diphenoxylate.

Pharmacokinetics: Difenoxin is rapidly and extensively absorbed orally. Mean peak plasma levels occur within 40 to 60 minutes. Plasma levels decline to less than 10% of their peak values within 24 hours and to less than 1% of their peak values within 72 hours. This decline parallels the appearance of difenoxin and its metabolites in the urine. Difenoxin is metabolized to an inactive hydroxylated metabolite. The drug and its metabolites are excreted, mainly as conjugates, in urine and feces.

Contraindications

Diarrhea associated with organisms that penetrate the intestinal mucosa (eg, toxigenic *Escherichia coli*, *Salmonella* sp., *Shigella*;) and pseudomembranous colitis associated with broad-spectrum antibiotics. Antiperistaltic agents may prolong or worsen diarrhea.

Children: Children less than 2 years of age because of the decreased margin of safety of drugs in this class in younger age groups.

Hypersensitivity to difenoxin, atropine, or any of the inactive ingredients; jaundice.

Warnings/Precautions

Difenoxin hydrochloride with atropine sulfate is not innocuous; strictly adhere to dosage recommendations. Overdosage may result in severe respiratory depression and coma, possibly leading to permanent brain damage or death.

Fluid and electrolyte balance: The use of this drug does not preclude the administration of appropriate fluid and electrolyte therapy. Dehydration, particularly in children, may further influence the variability of response and may predispose to delayed difenoxin intoxication. Drug-induced inhibition of peristalsis may result in fluid retention in the colon, and this may further aggravate dehydration and electrolyte imbalance.

Ulcerative colitis: Agents that inhibit intestinal motility or delay intestinal transit time have induced toxic megacolon. Consequently, carefully observe patients with acute ulcerative colitis.

Liver and kidney disease: Use with extreme caution in patients with advanced hepatorenal disease and in all patients with abnormal liver function tests because hepatic coma may be precipitated.

Atropine: A subtherapeutic dose of atropine has been added to difenoxin to discourage deliberate overdosage. A recommended dose is not likely to cause prominent anticholinergic side effects, but avoid in patients in whom anticholinergic drugs are contraindicated. In children, signs of atropinism may occur even with recommended doses, particularly in patients with Down Syndrome.

Drug abuse and dependence: Addiction to (dependence on) difenoxin is theoretically possible at high dosage. Therefore, do not exceed recommended dosage.

Pregnancy: Category C.

Lactation: Decide whether to discontinue nursing or to discontinue the drug, taking into account the importance of the drug to the mother.

Children: Contraindicated in children under 2 years of age. Safety and efficacy in children below the age of 12 have not been established.

Drug Interactions

Drugs that may interact include MAO inhibitors, barbiturates, tranquilizers, narcotics, and alcohol.

Adverse Reactions

Adverse reactions may include nausea, dry mouth, dizziness, lightheadedness, and drowsiness.

DIPHENOXYLATE HYDROCHLORIDE WITH ATROPINE SULFATE

Tablets: 2.5 mg diphenoxylate hydrochloride and 0.025 mg atropine sulfate (*c-v*)	Various, *Logen* (Goldline), *Lomotil* (Searle), *Lonox* (Sandoz)
Liquid: 2.5 mg diphenoxylate hydrochloride and 0.025 mg atropine sulfate per 5 mL (*c-v*)	Various, *Lomotil* (Searle)

Indications

Adjunctive therapy in the management of diarrhea.

Administration and Dosage

Adults: Individualize dosage. Initial dose is 5 mg 4 times/day.

Children: In children 2 to 12 years of age, use liquid form only. The recommended initial dosage is 0.3 to 0.4 mg/kg daily, in 4 divided doses.

Diphenoxylate w/Atropine Pediatric Dosage

Age (years)	Approximate weight kg	Approximate weight lb	Dosage (mL) (4 times daily)
2	11-14	24-31	1.5-3
3	12-16	26-35	2-3
4	14-20	31-44	2-4
5	16-23	35-51	2.5-4.5
6-8	17-32	38-71	2.5-5
9-12	23-55	51-121	3.5-5

Reduce dosage: Reduce dosage as soon as initial control of symptoms is achieved. Maintenance dosage may be as low as ¼ of the initial daily dosage. Do not exceed recommended dosage. Clinical improvement of acute diarrhea is usually observed within 48 hours. If clinical improvement of chronic diarrhea is not seen within 10 days after a maximum daily dose of 20 mg, symptoms are unlikely to be controlled by further use.

Actions

Pharmacology: Diphenoxylate, a constipating meperidine congener, lacks analgesic activity. High doses cause opioid activity.

Pharmacokinetics: Bioavailability of tablet vs liquid is approximately 90%. Diphenoxylate is rapidly, extensively metabolized to diphenoxylic acid (difenoxine), the active major metabolite. Elimination half-life is approximately 12 to 14 hours. An average of 14% of drug and metabolites are excreted over 4 days in urine, 49% in feces. Urinary excretion of unmetabolized drug is less than 1%; difenoxine plus its glucuronide conjugate constitutes approximately 6%.

Contraindications

Children younger than 2 years of age because of greater variability of response; hypersensitivity to diphenoxylate or atropine; obstructive jaundice; diarrhea associated with pseudomembranous enterocolitis or enterotoxin-producing bacteria.

Warnings/Precautions

Diarrhea: Diphenoxylate may prolong or aggravate diarrhea associated with organisms that penetrate intestinal mucosa (ie, toxigenic *Escherichia coli*, *Salmonella*, *Shigella*) or in pseudomembranous enterocolitis associated with broad-spectrum antibiotics. Do not use diphenoxylate in these conditions. In some patients with acute ulcerative colitis, diphenoxylate may induce toxic megacolon.

Fluid/Electrolyte balance: Dehydration, particularly in younger children, may influence variability of response and may predispose to delayed diphenoxylate intoxication. Inhibition of peristalsis may result in fluid retention in the intestine, which may further aggravate dehydration and electrolyte imbalance.

Hepatic function impairment: Use with extreme caution in patients with advanced hepatorenal disease or abnormal liver function; hepatic coma may be precipitated.

Drug abuse and dependence: In recommended doses, diphenoxylate has not produced addiction and is devoid of morphine-like subjective effects. At high doses, it exhibits codeine-like subjective effects; therefore, addiction to diphenoxylate is possible. A subtherapeutic dose of atropine may discourage deliberate abuse.

Pregnancy: Category C.

Lactation: Diphenoxylic acid may be excreted in breast milk and atropine is excreted in breast milk.

Children: Use with caution; signs of atropinism may occur with recommended doses, particularly in Down syndrome patients. Use with caution in young children because of variable response. Not recommended in children less than 2 years of age.

Drug Interactions

Drugs that may interact include MAO inhibitors, barbiturates, tranquilizers, and alcohol.

Adverse Reactions

Adverse reactions may include dry skin and mucous membranes, flushing, hyperthermia, tachycardia, urinary retention (especially in children), pruritus, gum swelling, angioneurotic edema, urticaria, anaphylaxis, dizziness, drowsiness, sedation, headache, malaise, lethargy, restlessness, euphoria, depression, numbness of extremities, confusion, anorexia, nausea, vomiting, abdominal discomfort, toxic megacolon, and pancreatitis.

LOPERAMIDE HYDROCHLORIDE

Tablets: 2 mg (*otc*)	Various, *Imodium A-D Caplets* (McNeil-CPC), *Kaopectate II Caplets* (Upjohn)
Capsules: 2 mg (*Rx*)	Various, *Imodium* (Janssen)
Liquid: 1 mg per 5 mL, 1 mg per 7.5 mL (*otc*)	Various, *Imodium A-D* (McNeil Consumer)
1 mg/mL (*otc*)	*Pepto Diarrhea Control* (Procter & Gamble)

Indications

Rx: Control and symptomatic relief of acute nonspecific diarrhea and of chronic diarrhea associated with inflammatory bowel disease.

For reducing the volume of discharge from ileostomies.

OTC: Control of symptoms of diarrhea, including traveler's diarrhea.

Administration and Dosage

Rx:

Acute diarrhea –

Adults: 4 mg followed by 2 mg after each unformed stool. Do not exceed 16 mg/day. Clinical improvement is usually observed within 48 hours.

Children:

Loperamide Pediatric Dosage (First Day Schedule)			
Age (years)	Weight (kg)	Doseform	Amount
2-5	13-20	liquid	1 mg tid
6-8	20-30	liquid or capsule	2 mg bid
8-12	> 30	liquid or capsule	2 mg tid

Subsequent doses: Administer 1 mg per 10 kg only after a loose stool. Total daily dosage should not exceed recommended dosages for the first day.

Chronic diarrhea –

Adults: 4 mg followed by 2 mg after each unformed stool until diarrhea is controlled. When optimal daily dosage (average, 4 to 8 mg) has been established, administer as a single dose or in divided doses.

If clinical improvement is not observed after treatment with 16 mg/day for at least 10 days, symptoms are unlikely to be controlled by further use.

Children – Dose has not been established.

OTC:

Acute diarrhea, including traveler's diarrhea –

Adults: 4 mg after first loose bowel movement followed by 2 mg after each subsequent loose bowel movement but no more than 8 mg/day for no more than 2 days.

Children:

9 to 11 years of age (60 to 95 lbs) – 2 mg after first loose bowel movement followed by 1 mg after each subsequent loose bowel movement but no more than 6 mg/day for no more than 2 days.

6 to 8 years of age (48 to 59 lbs) – 1 mg after first loose bowel movement followed by 1 mg after each subsequent loose bowel movement but no more than 4 mg/day for no more than 2 days.

Younger than 6 years of age (up to 47 lbs) – Consult physician (not for use in children younger than 6 years of age).

Actions

Pharmacology: Loperamide slows intestinal motility and affects water and electrolyte movement through the bowel. It inhibits peristalsis by a direct effect on the circular and longitudinal muscles of the intestinal wall. It reduces daily fecal volume, increases viscosity and bulk density and diminishes the loss of fluid and electrolytes.

Pharmacokinetics:

Absorption/Distribution – Loperamide is 40% absorbed after oral administration and does not penetrate well into the brain. Peak plasma levels occur approximately 5 hours after capsule administration, 2.5 hours after liquid administration and are similar for both formulations.

Metabolism/Excretion – The apparent elimination half-life is 10.8 hours (range, 9.1 to 14.4 hours). Of a 4 mg oral dose, 25% is excreted unchanged in the feces, and 1.3% is excreted in the urine as free drug and glucuronic acid conjugate within 3 days.

Contraindications

Hypersensitivity to the drug and in patients who must avoid constipation.

OTC use: Bloody diarrhea; body temperature greater than 101°F.

Warnings/Precautions

Diarrhea: Do not use loperamide in acute diarrhea associated with organisms that penetrate the intestinal mucosa (enteroinvasive *Escherichia coli*, *Salmonella*, and *Shigella*) or in pseudomembranous colitis associated with broad-spectrum antibiotics.

Acute ulcerative colitis: In some patients with acute ulcerative colitis, agents that inhibit intestinal motility or delay intestinal transit time may induce toxic megacolon.

Fluid/electrolyte depletion: Fluid/electrolyte depletion may occur in patients who have diarrhea. Loperamide use does not preclude administration of appropriate fluid and electrolyte therapy.

Acute diarrhea: If clinical improvement is not observed in 48 hours, discontinue use.

Hepatic dysfunction: Monitor patients with hepatic dysfunction closely for signs of CNS toxicity because of the apparent large first-pass biotransformation.

Pregnancy: Category B.

Lactation: It is not known whether loperamide is excreted in breast milk.

Children: Not recommended for use in children younger than 2 years of age. Use special caution in young children because of the greater variability of response in this age group. Dehydration may further influence variability of response. Dosage has not been established for children in treatment of chronic diarrhea.

Adverse Reactions

Adverse reactions may include abdominal pain, distention, or discomfort; constipation; dry mouth; nausea; vomiting; tiredness, drowsiness, or dizziness; hypersensitivity reactions (including skin rash).

BISMUTH SUBSALICYLATE (BSS)

Tablets: 262 mg (*otc*)	*Kaopectate* (Pfizer Consumer Health)
Tablets, chewable: 262 mg (*otc*)	*Bismatrol* (Major), *Peptic Relief* (Rugby), *Pepto-Bismol* (Procter & Gamble)
Liquid: 87 mg per 5 mL (*otc*)	*Kaopectate Children's* (Pharmacia)
130 mg per 15 mL (*otc*)	Various
262 mg per 15 mL (*otc*)	Various, *Kao-Tin* (Major), *Kaopectate* (Pharmicia), *Peptic Relief* (Rugby), *Pepto-Bismol* (Procter & Gamble)
524 mg per 15 mL (*otc*)	*Pepto-Bismol Maximum Strength* (Procter & Gamble)
525 mg per 15 mL (*otc*)	*Kaopectate Extra Strength* (Pharmicia)
Suspension: 525 mg per 15 mL (*otc*)	*Maalox Total Stomach Relief Liquid* (Novartis)

Indications

To control diarrhea, gas, upset stomach, indigestion, heartburn, nausea; reduce number of bowel movements; help firm stool.

Administration and Dosage

Adults and children 12 years of age and older: 2 tablets or 30 mL.

Children: 9 to 11 years of age – 1 tablet or 15 mL.
6 to 8 years of age – ⅔ tablet or 10 mL.
3 to 5 years of age – ⅓ tablet or 5 mL.
Younger than 3 years of age – Consult physician.

Repeat dosage every 30 minutes to 1 hour, as needed, up to 8 doses in 24 hours.

Actions

Pharmacology: BSS appears to have antisecretory and antimicrobial effects in vitro and may have some anti-inflammatory effects. The salicylate moiety provides the antisecretory effect, while the bismuth moiety may exert direct antimicrobial effects against bacterial and viral enteropathogens.

Pharmacokinetics: BSS undergoes chemical dissociation in the GI tract. Two BSS tablets yield 204 mg salicylate. Following ingestion, salicylate is absorbed, with greater than 90% recovered in the urine; plasma levels are similar to levels achieved after a comparable dose of aspirin. Absorption of bismuth is negligible.

Warnings/Precautions

Impaction: Impaction may occur in infants and debilitated patients.

Radiologic examinations: May interfere with radiologic examinations of GI tract. Bismuth is radiopaque.

Drug Interactions

Drugs that may be affected by bismuth include aspirin and tetracyclines.

Adverse Reactions

May cause a harmless darkening of the tongue or stool.

MESALAMINE (5-aminosalicylic acid, 5-ASA)

Tablets, delayed-release; oral: 1.2 g (*Rx*)	*Lialda* (Shire US)
400 mg (*Rx*)	*Asacol* (Procter & Gamble)
Capsules, controlled-release; oral: 250 and 500 mg (*Rx*)	*Pentasa* (Shire US)
Capsules,[a] extended-release; oral: 375 mg (*Rx*)	*Apriso* (Salix)
Suppositories; rectal: 1,000 mg (*Rx*)	*Canasa* (Axcan Scandipharm)
Enema; rectal: 4 g per 60 mL (*Rx*)	Various, *Rowasa* (Alaven)

[a] Capsule is a delayed- and extended-release dosage form.

Indications

Ulcerative colitis:

Asacol – For the treatment of mildly to moderately active ulcerative colitis and for the maintenance of remission of ulcerative colitis.

Apriso – For the maintenance of remission of ulcerative colitis in patients 18 years of age and older.

Lialda – For the induction of remission in patients with active, mild to moderate ulcerative colitis.

Pentasa – For the induction of remission and for the treatment of patients with mildly to moderately active ulcerative colitis.

Administration and Dosage

Monitor renal function in all patients prior to initiation and periodically while on mesalamine therapy. Closely monitor blood cell counts during drug therapy.

Adults:

Induction of remission in patients with active, mild to moderate ulcerative colitis –

Lialda: Two to four 1.2 g tablets taken once daily with food for a total daily dose of 2.4 or 4.8 g for up to 8 weeks.

Pentasa: 1 g (four 250 mg capsules or two 500 mg capsules) 4 times daily for a total dose of 4 g for up to 8 weeks.

Maintenance of remission of ulcerative colitis –

Apriso: 1.5 g (4 capsules) orally once daily in the morning. May be taken without regard to meals for 6 months. Mesalamine should not be coadministered with antacids.

Asacol: 1.6 g daily in divided doses for 6 months.

Treatment of mildly to moderately active ulcerative colitis –

Asacol: Two 400 mg tablets to be taken 3 times daily for a total daily dose of 2.4 g for a duration of 6 weeks.

Pentasa: 1 g (four 250 mg capsules or two 500 mg capsules) 4 times daily for a total dose of 4 g for up to 8 weeks.

Administration: Swallow tablets whole, taking care not to break the outer coating. Take *Lialda* with food.

Actions

Pharmacology: Sulfasalazine is split by bacterial action in the colon into sulfapyridine and mesalamine (5-ASA).

The mechanism of action of mesalamine (and sulfasalazine) is unknown, but appears to be topical rather than systemic, and it is possible that mesalamine diminishes inflammation by blocking cyclooxygenase and inhibiting prostaglandin production in the colon.

Pharmacokinetics:

Absorption/Distribution –

Oral:

Asacol – Mesalamine tablets are coated with an acrylic-based resin that delays release of mesalamine until it reaches the terminal ileum and beyond. Approximately 28% is absorbed after oral ingestion, leaving the remainder available for topical action and excretion in the feces. Mesalamine from oral mesalamine tablets appears to be more extensively absorbed than that released from sulfasalazine.

Lialda – The total absorption of mesalamine from *Lialda* 2.4 or 4.8 g given once daily for 14 days to healthy volunteers was found to be approximately 21% or 22% of the administered dose.

Pentasa – Mesalamine capsules are designed to release therapeutic quantities of the drug throughout the GI tract; 20% to 30% of mesalamine is absorbed. Plasma mesalamine concentration peaked at approximately 1 mcg/mL 3 hours after administration of a 1 g dose and declined in a biphasic manner. Mean terminal half-life was 42 minutes after IV administration.

Suppository: Absorbed mesalamine does not accumulate in the plasma. Mesalamine administered as rectal suppositories distributes in rectal tissue to some extent.

Suspension: Mesalamine administered rectally as a suspension enema is poorly absorbed from the colon and is excreted principally in the feces during subsequent bowel movements. At steady state, approximately 10% to 30% of the daily 4 g dose can be recovered in cumulative 24-hour urine collections.

Metabolism/Excretion –

Oral:

Asacol – Following oral administration, the absorbed mesalamine is rapidly acetylated in the gut mucosal wall and by the liver. It is excreted mainly by the kidneys as N-acetyl-5-ASA. The half-lives of elimination for mesalamine and the metabolite are usually approximately 12 hours, but are variable ranging from 2 to 15 hours.

Lialda – There is limited excretion of the parent drug in the urine. The apparent terminal half-life for mesalamine and its major metabolite after administration of *Lialda* 2.4 and 4.8 g were, on average, 7 to 9 hours and 8 to 12 hours, respectively.

Pentasa – Elimination of free mesalamine and salicylates in feces increased proportionately with the dose. N-acetyl-5-ASA was the primary compound excreted in the urine (19% to 30%).

Suppository: The mean elimination half-life was 5 hours for 5-aminosalicylic acid and 6 hours for mesalamine following the initial dose. At steady state, the mean elimination half-life was 7 hours for both mesalamine and N-acetyl-5-ASA.

Suspension: Whatever the metabolic site, most absorbed mesalamine is excreted in urine as the N-acetyl-5-ASA metabolite. While the elimination half-life of mesalamine is short (0.5 to 1.5 hours), the acetylated metabolite exhibits a half-life of 5 to 10 hours.

Contraindications

Hypersensitivity to mesalamine, salicylates, or any component of the formulation (ie, suppository vehicle of vegetable fatty acid esters).

Warnings/Precautions

Cardiac hypersensitivity: Mesalamine-induced cardiac hypersensitivity reactions (myocarditis and pericarditis) have been reported with mesalamine medications. Take caution in prescribing mesalamine to patients with conditions predisposing to the development of myocarditis or pericarditis.

Pyloric stenosis: Patients with pyloric stenosis may have prolonged gastric retention of mesalamine delayed-release tablets, which could delay the release of mesalamine in the colon.

Intolerance/Colitis exacerbation: Mesalamine has been implicated in the production of an acute intolerance syndrome or exacerbation of colitis characterized by cramping, acute abdominal pain and bloody diarrhea, and occasionally fever, headache, malaise, pruritus, conjunctivitis, and rash. Symptoms usually abate when mesalamine is discontinued.

Pancolitis: While using mesalamine, some patients have developed pancolitis.

Hypersensitivity reactions: Most patients who were hypersensitive to sulfasalazine were able to take mesalamine enemas without evidence of any allergic reaction. Nevertheless, exercise caution when mesalamine is initially used in patients known to be allergic to sulfasalazine.

Renal function impairment: Renal impairment, including minimal change nephropathy, nephrotic syndrome, acute and chronic interstitial nephritis, and, rarely, renal failure, has occurred.

Pregnancy: Category B. Mesalamine is known to cross the placental barrier.

Lactation: Low concentrations of mesalamine and higher concentrations of N-acetyl-5-ASA have been detected in breast milk.

Children: Safety and efficacy for use in children 18 years of age and younger have not been established.

Elderly: In general, dose selection for an elderly patient should be cautious, usually starting at the low end of the dosing range, reflecting the greater frequency of decreased hepatic, renal, or cardiac function, and of concomitant disease or other drug therapy in elderly patients.

Drug Interactions

Drugs that may interact with mesalamine include azathioprine, mercaptopurine, nephrotoxic drugs (eg, NSAIDs), and warfarin.

Adverse Reactions

Adverse reactions may include abdominal pain/cramps/discomfort; colitis exacerbation; constipation; diarrhea; dyspepsia; eructation; flatulence/gas; nausea; vomiting; asthenia; chills; dizziness; fever; headache; malaise/fatigue/weakness; sweating; pharyngitis; rhinitis; pruritus; rash/spots; arthralgia; back pain; hypertonia; myalgia; chest pain; dysmenorrhea; edema; flu syndrome; pain.

OLSALAZINE SODIUM

Capsules: 250 mg (*Rx*)	*Dipentum* (UCB Pharma)

Indications

Maintenance of remission of ulcerative colitis in patients intolerant of sulfasalazine.

Administration and Dosage

1 g/day in 2 divided doses.

Actions

Pharmacology: Olsalazine sodium is a sodium salt of a salicylate compound that is effectively bioconverted to 5-aminosalicylic acid (mesalamine; 5-ASA), which has anti-inflammatory activity in ulcerative colitis. Approximately 98% to 99% of an oral dose will reach the colon, where each molecule is rapidly converted into 2 molecules of 5-ASA by colonic bacteria. The liberated 5-ASA is absorbed slowly, resulting in very high local concentrations in the colon.

Mechanism of action of mesalamine is unknown, but appears topical rather than systemic. It may diminish colonic inflammation by blocking cyclooxygenase and inhibiting colon prostaglandin production in bowel mucosa.

Pharmacokinetics: After oral administration approximately 2.4% of a single 1 g oral dose is absorbed. Maximum serum concentrations appear after approximately 1 hour, and are low even after a single 1 g dose. Olsalazine has a very short serum half-life of approximately 0.9 hours and is greater than 99% bound to plasma proteins. Urinary recovery is less than 1%. Total oral olsalazine recovery ranges from 90% to 97%.

Serum concentrations of 5-ASA are detected after 4 to 8 hours. Of the total urinary 5-ASA, greater than 90% is in the form of N-acetyl-5-ASA (Ac-5-ASA).

Contraindications

Hypersensitivity to salicylates.

Warnings/Precautions

Diarrhea: About 17%, resulting in drug withdrawal in 6%; appears dose-related, but may be difficult to distinguish from underlying disease symptoms.

Colitis symptoms: Exacerbation of the symptoms of colitis thought to have been caused by mesalamine or sulfasalazine has been noted.

Renal abnormalities: Renal abnormalities were not reported in clinical trials with olsalazine; however, the possibility of renal tubular damage caused by absorbed mesalamine or its n-acetylated metabolite must be kept in mind, particularly in pre-existing renal disease.

Pregnancy: Category C.

Lactation: It is not known whether this drug is excreted in breast milk.

Children: Safety and efficacy in children have not been established.

Adverse Reactions

Adverse reactions may include headache; diarrhea; pain/cramps; nausea; dyspepsia; arthralgia.

BALSALAZIDE DISODIUM

Capsules, oral: 750 mg (*Rx*)	Various, *Colazal* (Salix)

Indications

Active ulcerative colitis: Treatment of mildly to moderately active ulcerative colitis in patients 5 yr of age and older. Safety and efficacy of balsalazide beyond 8 weeks in children 5 to 17 yr of age and beyond 12 weeks in adults have not been established.

Administration and Dosage

Dosage:

Adults – The usual dosage is 3 capsules 3 times daily (6.75 g/day) for up to 8 weeks. Some patients in the adult clinical trials required treatment for up to 12 weeks.

Children – In children 5 to 17 years of age, the usual dosage is either 3 capsules 3 times daily (6.75 g/day) for up to 8 weeks, or 1 capsule 3 times daily (2.25 g/day) for up to 8 weeks.

Administration: For patients who have difficulty swallowing, administer by carefully opening the capsule and sprinkling the contents on applesauce. The entire drug/applesauce mixture should be swallowed immediately; the contents may be chewed, if necessary, because they are not coated beads/granules. Do not store the drug/applesauce mixture for future use.

If the capsules are opened for sprinkling, color variation of the powder inside the capsules ranges from orange to yellow and is expected because of color variation of the active pharmacological ingredient.

Teeth and/or tongue staining may occur in some patients who sprinkle balsalazide on applesauce.

Actions

Pharmacology: Balsalazide is delivered intact to the colon where it is cleaved by bacterial azoreduction to release equimolar quantities of mesalamine. The recommended dose of 6.75 g/day for the treatment of active disease provides 2.4 g of free 5-aminosalicylic acid (5-ASA) to the colon.

Pharmacokinetics:

Absorption – In healthy individuals, the systemic absorption of intact balsalazide was very low and variable. Balsalazide is insoluable in acid and is designed to be delivered to the colon as the intact prodrug.

Distribution – Balsalazide binding to human plasma proteins was at least 99%.

Metabolism – The products of the azoreduction of this compound, 5-ASA and 4-aminobenzoyl-β-alanine, and their N-acetylated metabolites have been identified in plasma, urine, and feces.

Excretion – Less than 1% of an oral dose was recovered as parent compound, 5-ASA, or 4-aminobenzoyl-β-alanine in the urine of healthy subjects.

Contraindications

Hypersensitivity to salicylates or any of the components of balsalazide capsules or balsalazide metabolites.

Warnings/Precautions

Exacerbation of symptoms: Exacerbation of the symptoms of colitis has been reported.

Pyloric stenosis: Patients with pyloric stenosis may have prolonged gastric retention of balsalazide.

Renal function impairment: Renal toxicity has been observed in animals and patients given other mesalamine products. Exercise caution when administering balsalazide to patients with known renal function impairment or history of renal disease.

Pregnancy: Category B.

Lactation: It is not known whether balsalazide is excreted in breast milk. Exercise caution when administering to a breast-feeding woman.

Children: Safety and efficacy of balsalazide in children younger than 5 yr of age have not been established. Based on limited data available in patients 5 to 17 yr of age, dosing can be initiated at either 6.75 or 2.25 g/day.

Monitoring: Monitor colitis symptoms, including rectal bleeding, stool frequency and character, abdominal pain, and overall status.

Drug Interactions

None known.

Adverse Reactions

Adverse reactions occurring in at least 3% of adults include abdominal pain; arthralgia; diarrhea and nausea; headache; respiratory infection; vomiting.

Adverse reactions occurring in at least 3% of children include abdominal pain; cough; diarrhea; dysmenorrhea; fatigue; headache; hematochezia; influenza; nasopharyngitis; nausea; pharyngolaryngeal pain; pyrexia; stomatitis; ulcerative colitis; upper abdominal pain; vomiting.

SULFASALAZINE

Tablets: 500 mg (*Rx*)	Various, *Azulfidine* (Pfizer)
Tablets, delayed-release: 500 mg (*Rx*)	Various, *Azulfidine EN-tabs* (Pfizer)

Indications

Ulcerative colitis: In the treatment of mild to moderate ulcerative colitis and as adjunctive therapy in severe ulcerative colitis; for the prolongation of the remission period between acute attacks of ulcerative colitis.

Rheumatoid arthritis (RA; delayed-release tablets): In the treatment of patients with RA who have responded inadequately to salicylates or other nonsteroidal anti-inflammatory drugs (NSAIDs).

Juvenile rheumatoid arthritis (JRA; delayed-release tablets): In the treatment of pediatric patients with polyarticular-course JRA who have responded inadequately to salicylates or other NSAIDs.

Administration and Dosage

Adjust dosage to individual response and tolerance. Instruct patients to take sulfasalazine tablets in evenly divided doses, preferably after meals, and to swallow the tablets whole.

Some patients may be sensitive to treatment with sulfasalazine. Various desensitization-like regimens have been reported to be effective. These regimens suggest starting with a total daily dose of 50 to 250 mg initially, and doubling it every 4 to 7 days until the desired therapeutic level has been achieved. If the symptoms of sensitivity recur, discontinue sulfasalazine. Do not attempt desensitization in patients who have a history of agranulocytosis, or who have experienced an anaphylactoid reaction while previously receiving sulfasalazine.

Ulcerative colitis:

Initial therapy –

Adults: 3 to 4 g daily in evenly divided doses with intervals not exceeding 8 hours. It may be advisable to initiate therapy with a lower dosage (eg, 1 to 2 g daily), to reduce possible GI intolerance.

Children 6 years of age and older: 40 to 60 mg/kg in each 24-hour period, divided into 3 to 6 doses.

Maintenance therapy –

Adults: 2 g daily.

Children 6 years of age and older: 30 mg/kg in each 24-hour period, divided into 4 doses.

It is often necessary to continue medication even when clinical symptoms, including diarrhea, have been controlled. When endoscopic examination confirms satisfactory improvement, reduce dosage to a maintenance level. If diarrhea recurs, increase dosage to previously effective levels.

Gastric intolerance: If symptoms of gastric intolerance (eg, anorexia, nausea, vomiting) occur after the first few doses of sulfasalazine, they are probably caused by increased serum levels of total sulfapyridine and may be alleviated by halving the daily dose of sulfasalazine and subsequently increasing it gradually over several days. If gastric intolerance continues, stop the drug for 5 to 7 days, then reintroduce at a lower daily dose.

Sulfasalazine enteric-coated delayed-release tablets are particularly indicated in patients who cannot take uncoated sulfasalazine tablets because of GI intolerance (eg, anorexia, nausea).

Adult RA:

Delayed-release tablets – 2 g daily in 2 evenly divided doses. It is advisable to initiate therapy with a lower dosage (eg, 0.5 to 1 g daily) to reduce possible GI intolerance.

Suggested Dosing Schedule for Adult RA		
	Number of sulfasalazine delayed-release tablets	
Week of treatment	Morning	Evening
1	-	1
2	1	1
3	1	2
4	2	2

A therapeutic response has been observed as early as 4 weeks after starting treatment with sulfasalazine delayed-release tablets, but treatment for 12 weeks may be required before clinical benefit is noted. Consideration can be given to increasing the daily dose of sulfasalazine delayed-release tablets to 3 g if the clinical response after 12 weeks is inadequate. Careful monitoring is recommended for doses over 2 g/day.

JRA (polyarticular course):

Delayed-release tablets – Children 6 years of age and older should take 30 to 50 mg/kg of body weight daily in 2 evenly divided doses. Typically, the maximum dose is 2 g/day. Begin with a quarter to a third of the planned maintenance dose and increase weekly until reaching the maintenance dose at 1 month.

Actions

Pharmacology: The mode of action of sulfasalazine or its metabolites may be related to the anti-inflammatory or immunomodulatory properties. In ulcerative colitis, the major therapeutic action may reside in the 5-aminosalicylic acid (5-ASA) moiety.

Pharmacokinetics:

Absorption – The absolute bioavailability of oral sulfasalazine is less than 15% for parent drug. In the intestine, sulfasalazine is metabolized by intestinal bacteria to sulfapyridine (SP) and 5-ASA. Peak plasma levels of both occur approximately 10 hours after dosing.

Distribution – Sulfasalazine is highly bound to albumin (greater than 99.3%), while SP is only approximately 70% bound to albumin.

Metabolism – The observed plasma half-life for IV sulfasalazine is 7.6 hours. The primary route of metabolism is acetylation. In fast acetylators, the mean plasma half-life of SP is 10.4 hours, while in slow acetylators it is 14.8 hours.

Excretion – Absorbed SP and 5-ASA and their metabolites are primarily eliminated in the urine either as free metabolites or as glucuronide conjugates. Renal clearance was estimated to account for 37% of total clearance.

Contraindications

Intestinal or urinary obstruction; hypersensitivity to sulfasalazine, its metabolites, salicylates, or sulfonamides.

Warnings/Precautions

Porphyria: Patients with porphyria should not receive sulfonamides as these drugs have been reported to precipitate an acute attack.

Deaths: Deaths associated with the administration of sulfasalazine have been reported from hypersensitivity reactions, agranulocytosis, aplastic anemia, other blood dyscrasias, renal and liver damage, irreversible neuromuscular and CNS changes, and fibrosing alveolitis. If toxic or hypersensitivity reactions occur, discontinue sulfasalazine immediately.

Undisintegrated tablets: Isolated instances have been reported when sulfasalazine delayed-release tablets have passed undisintegrated. If this is observed, discontinue the administration of sulfasalazine delayed-release tablets immediately.

Hypersensitivity reactions: Give sulfasalazine with caution to patients with severe allergy or bronchial asthma. Adequate fluid intake must be maintained in order to prevent crystalluria and stone formation. Observe patients with glucose-6-phosphate dehydrogenase deficiency closely for signs of hemolytic anemia.

Renal/Hepatic function impairment: Only after critical appraisal should sulfasalazine be given to patients with hepatic or renal damage.

Fertility impairment: Oligospermia and infertility have been observed in men treated with sulfasalazine. Withdrawal of the drug appears to reverse these effects.

Pregnancy: Category B.

Lactation: Sulfonamides are excreted in breast milk. In newborns, they compete with bilirubin for binding sites on the plasma proteins and may cause kernicterus.

Children: The safety and efficacy of sulfasalazine in pediatric patients younger than 2 years of age with ulcerative colitis have not been established.

Delayed-release tablets – The frequency of adverse reactions in patients with systemic-course of juvenile arthritis is high. Use in children with systemic-course JRA has frequently resulted in a serum sickness-like reaction. Treatment of systemic-course JRA with sulfasalazine is not recommended.

Monitoring: Perform complete blood counts, including differential white cell count and liver function tests before starting sulfasalazine and every second week during the first 3 months of therapy. During the second 3 months, perform the same tests once monthly and, thereafter, once every 3 months and as clinically indicated. Also perform urinalysis and assess renal function periodically during treatment.

The determination of serum sulfapyridine levels may be useful because concentrations greater than 50 mcg/mL appear to be associated with an increased incidence of adverse reactions.

Drug Interactions

Drugs that may be affected by sulfasalazine include cyclosporine, digoxin, folic acid, methotrexate, sulfonylureas, thiopurines, and warfarin.

Adverse Reactions

Adverse events occurring in at least 3% of patients with ulcerative colitis include the following: Anorexia; headache; nausea; vomiting; gastric distress; reversible oligospermia.

May produce an orange-yellow discoloration of the urine or skin.

Delayed-release tablets (RA): Abdominal pain, abnormal LFTs, dizziness, dyspepsia, fever, headache, leukopenia, nausea, pruritus, rash, stomatitis, vomiting.

LUBIPROSTONE

Capsules: 24 and 8 mcg (*Rx*)	*Amitza* (Sucampo Pharm/Takeda Pharm)

Indications

Chronic idiopathic constipation: For the treatment of chronic idiopathic constipation in adults.

Irritable bowel syndrome (IBS) with constipation: For the treatment of IBS with constipation in adults.

Administration and Dosage

Chronic idiopathic constipation: 24 mcg taken twice daily orally with food and water..

IBS with constipation: 8 mcg taken twice daily orally with food and water.

Actions

Pharmacology: Lubiprostone is a locally acting chloride channel activator that enhances a chloride-rich intestinal fluid secretion without altering sodium and potassium concentrations in the serum. By increasing intestinal fluid secretion, lubiprostone increases motility in the intestine, thereby increasing the passage of stool and alleviating symptoms associated with chronic idiopathic constipation.

Pharmacokinetics:

Absorption – Lubiprostone has low systemic availability following oral administration. Peak plasma levels occur at approximately 1 hour.

Distribution – Lubiprostone is approximately 94% bound to human plasma proteins.

Metabolism – Lubiprostone is rapidly and extensively metabolized by reduction and oxidation. These biotransformations are not mediated by the hepatic CYP-450 system.

Excretion – Lubiprostone has a half-life ranging from 0.9 to 1.4 hours.

Contraindications

Known hypersensitivity to the drug or any of its excipients; in patients with a history of mechanical GI obstruction.

Warnings/Precautions

Dyspnea: There were reports of dyspnea in clinical trials conducted to study lubiprostone. Some patients discontinued treatment because of this reaction.

GI obstruction: Evaluate patients with symptoms suggestive of mechanical GI obstruction prior to initiating lubiprostone treatment.

GI effects: Lubiprostone may cause nausea. If this occurs, coadministration of food with lubiprostone may reduce symptoms of nausea. Do not administer lubiprostone to patients that have severe diarrhea.

Pregnancy: Category C.

Lactation: It is not known whether lubiprostone is excreted in human milk. Because many drugs are excreted in human milk, decide whether to discontinue breastfeeding or the drug, taking into account the importance of the drug to the mother.

Children: Lubiprostone has not been studied in children.

Drug Interactions

None known.

Adverse Reactions

Adverse reactions occurring in more than 3% of patients taking lubiprostone include dizziness, headache, hypesthesia, abdominal discomfort, abdominal distension, abdominal pain, diarrhea, flatulence, loose stools, nausea, dyspnea, chest discomfort, edema, vomiting.

HELICOBACTER PYLORI AGENTS

Helicobacter pylori: H. *pylori* is found in approximately 100% of chronic active antral gastritis cases, 90% to 95% of duodenal ulcer patients, and 50% to 80% of gastric ulcer patients. The treatment of documented H. *pylori* infection in patients with confirmed peptic ulcer on first presentation or recurrence has been recommended by the National Institutes for Health in a 1994 Consensus Conference. Once H. *pylori* eradication has been achieved, reinfection rates are less than 0.5% per year, and ulcer recurrence rates are dramatically reduced.

Numerous clinical trials have been performed to determine the optimal regimen for H. *pylori* eradication, but there remains no gold standard of therapy to date. When selecting a regimen, take into account efficacy, tolerability, compliance, and cost. H. *pylori* is easily suppressed but, to ensure successful eradication, requires the use of 2 antimicrobial agents with either a bismuth compound, an antisecretory agent, or both. These combinations have been shown to enhance H. *pylori* cure, shorten the duration of treatment, and decrease treatment failure caused by antimicrobial resistance.

Double antimicrobial therapy plus an antisecretory drug:

Regimens Used in the Eradication of *H. pylori*[a]			
Regimen	Dosing	Duration	Eradication
Metronidazole	500 mg twice daily with meals	1 week	87% to 91%
Omeprazole	20 mg twice daily with meals		
Clarithromycin	500 mg twice daily with meals		
Amoxicillin	1 g twice daily with meals	1 to 2 weeks	77% to 83%
Omeprazole	20 mg twice daily before meals		
Clarithromycin	500 mg twice daily with meals		
Metronidazole	500 mg twice daily with meals	1 to 2 weeks	77% to 83%
Omeprazole	20 mg twice daily before meals		
Amoxicillin	1 g twice daily with meals		

[a] Extending therapy to 10 to 14 days in the previous regimens may provide additional benefit. H_2 blockers may be used with 2 antibiotics, but a longer treatment course (10 to 14 days), higher antibiotic doses, and 3 times daily administration are required.

Triple-therapy regimens: These regimens have proven to be very effective in eradicating H. *pylori*. The primary disadvantage of these regimens is compliance because of the variety and number of medications used. Likewise, adverse effects are more common in patients taking these regimens compared with alternatives.

Regimens Used in the Eradication of *H. pylori*[a]			
Regimen	Dosing	Duration	Eradication
Bismuth subsalicylate	525 mg 4 times daily with meals and at bedtime	2 weeks 1 week	88% to 90% 86% to 90%
Metronidazole	250 mg 4 times daily with meals and at bedtime		
Tetracycline	500 mg 4 times daily		
Bismuth subsalicylate	525 mg 4 times daily with meals and at bedtime	1 week	94% to 98%
Metronidazole	250 mg 4 times daily with meals and at bedtime		
Tetracycline	500 mg 4 times daily		
Omeprazole	20 mg 2 times daily before meals		

Regimens Used in the Eradication of *H. pylori*[a]			
Regimen	Dosing	Duration	Eradication
Bismuth subsalicylate	525 mg 4 times daily with meals and at bedtime	2 weeks 1 week	80% to 86% 75% to 81%
Metronidazole	250 mg 4 times daily with meals and at bedtime		
Amoxicillin	500 mg 4 times daily with meals and at bedtime		

[a] One week of 4 times daily therapy may be sufficient in the absence of antibiotic resistance. Adding a proton pump inhibitor facilitates shorter treatment periods. Until more data is available, the use of H_2 antagonists or proton pump inhibitors with the previous regimens is appropriate to enhance ulcer healing and provide symptomatic relief.

Quadruple therapy regimens (2 antibiotics, bismuth, antisecretory agent): Like triple therapy regimens, these have proven to be effective in *H. pylori* eradication. The primary disadvantage of these regimens is compliance. In addition, because of the variety and number of medications used, adverse reactions are more common in patients taking these regimens compared with alternatives.

FDA-Approved Regimens for the Eradication of *H. pylori*			
Regimen	Dosing	Eradication	Comments
Omeprazole Clarithromycin	40 mg once daily followed by a 2-week course of 20 mg once daily 500 mg 3 times daily for 2 weeks	64% to 74%	The American College of Gastroenterology recommends that either tetracycline or amoxicillin be added to this regimen.
Ranitidine bismuth citrate Clarithromycin	400 mg twice daily for 4 weeks 500 mg 3 times daily for 2 weeks	82%	The American College of Gastroenterology recommends that either tetracycline or amoxicillin be added to this regimen.
Metronidazole Tetracycline hydrochloride Bismuth subsalicylate	250 mg 4 times daily at meals and bedtime 500 mg 4 times daily at meals and bedtime 525 mg 4 times daily at meals and bedtime	82%	*Helidac* and *Pylera* therapy combines bismuth, metronidazole, and tetracycline in a consumer-tested, patient-friendly kit.

Practice Guidelines from the American College of Gastroenterology: In the 1996 Consensus Statement on Medical Treatment of Peptic Ulcer Disease, the American College of Gastroenterology does not recommend single-antibiotic combinations of either clarithromycin or amoxicillin with proton pump inhibitors because efficacy is less than 70% (cure), and a high-dose, 2-week treatment period is required. The Consensus Statement recommends a 2-antibiotic combination of clarithromycin, metronidazole, or amoxicillin in regimens that do not employ a bismuth compound. In addition, the American College of Gastroenterology suggests adding either tetracycline or amoxicillin to the recently approved ranitidine-bismuth citrate-clarithromycin combination to enhance successful *H. pylori* eradication. Combining a proton pump inhibitor, either omeprazole or lansoprazole, with 2 antibiotics is thought to enhance effectiveness and allow for a shorter duration of treatment.

There are a number of factors that limit the effectiveness of regimens designed to eradicate *H. pylori*. The first, antibiotic resistance, is seen with metronidazole and clarithromycin but has not been reported with bismuth, amoxicillin, or tetracycline.

The second, mild adverse reactions (eg, diarrhea, metallic taste, black stools), occur in approximately 30% to 50% of patients. Therefore, shorter treatment periods in this group of patients may be better tolerated.

Finally, patient compliance is often a problem because of cumbersome regimens and adverse reactions.

Maintenance therapy with antisecretory agents: Currently, it is advisable to continue maintenance until *H. pylori* cure has been confirmed in patients with a history of complications, frequent or troublesome recurrences, or refractory ulcers.

Successful eradication: Confirming successful eradication is important in patients with a history of complicated or refractory ulcers but is controversial in those with uncomplicated ulcers who remain asymptomatic after therapy.

Refractory ulcers: Refractory ulcers in patients receiving antibiotic therapy for *H. pylori* eradication is often because of failure to successfully eradicate *H. pylori* infection. Resistance patterns, as well as noncompliance and concurrent NSAID use, may play a role in refractory cases.

PILOCARPINE HYDROCHLORIDE

Tablets: 5 and 7.5 mg (*Rx*) Various, *Salagen* (Eisai)

Indications

Xerostomia: Treatment of symptoms of xerostomia from salivary gland hypofunction caused by radiotherapy for cancer of the head and neck.

Administration and Dosage

The recommended dose for the initiation of treatment is 5 mg 3 times/day. Titration up to 10 mg 3 times/day may be considered for patients who have not responded adequately and who can tolerate lower doses. The incidence of the most common adverse events increases with dose. Use the lowest dose that is tolerated and effective for maintenance.

Actions

Pharmacology: Pilocarpine is a cholinergic parasympathomimetic agent exerting a broad spectrum of pharmacologic effects with predominant muscarinic action. Pilocarpine can increase secretion by the exocrine glands, can stimulate intestinal tract smooth muscle (dose-related), and may increase bronchial smooth muscle tone. The tone and motility of urinary tract, gallbladder, and biliary duct smooth muscle may be enhanced. Pilocarpine may have paradoxical effects on the cardiovascular system. The expected effect of a muscarinic agonist is vasodepression, but administration of pilocarpine may produce hypertension after a brief episode of hypotension. Bradycardia and tachycardia have been reported with use of pilocarpine.

Pharmacokinetics: Following single 5 and 10 mg oral doses, unstimulated salivary flow was time-related with an onset at 20 minutes and a peak at 1 hour with a duration of 3 to 5 hours.

Following 2 days of 5 or 10 mg oral pilocarpine given at 8 am, noon, and 6 pm, the mean elimination half-life was 0.76 and 1.35 hours for the 5 and 10 mg doses, respectively. T_{max} was 1.25 and 0.85 hours and C_{max} was 15 and 41 ng/mL, respectively. The AUC was 33 and 108 h•ng/mL, respectively, following the last 6-hour dose.

Inactivation of pilocarpine is thought to occur at neuronal synapses and probably in plasma. Pilocarpine and its minimally active or inactive degradation products, including pilocarpic acid, are excreted in the urine.

Contraindications

Uncontrolled asthma; hypersensitivity to pilocarpine; when miosis is undesirable.

Warnings/Precautions

Cardiovascular disease: Patients with significant cardiovascular disease may be unable to compensate for transient changes in hemodynamics or rhythm induced by pilocarpine. Pulmonary edema has been reported as a complication of pilocarpine toxicity from high ocular doses given for acute angle-closure glaucoma. Administer pilocarpine with caution and under close medical supervision in patients with cardiovascular disease.

The dose-related cardiovascular effects of pilocarpine include hypotension, hypertension, bradycardia, and tachycardia.

Ocular effects: Carefully examine the fundus prior to initiating therapy with pilocarpine. An association of ocular pilocarpine use and retinal detachment in patients with preexisting retinal disease has been reported. The systemic blood level that is associated with this finding is not known.

Ocular formulations of pilocarpine have caused visual blurring that may result in decreased visual acuity, especially at night and in patients with central lens changes, and impairment of depth perception. Advise caution while driving at night or performing hazardous activities in reduced lighting.

Pulmonary disease: Pilocarpine has been reported to increase airway resistance, bronchial smooth muscle tone, and bronchial secretions. Administer with caution and under close medical supervision in patients with controlled asthma, chronic bronchitis, or chronic obstructive pulmonary disease.

Toxicity: Toxicity is characterized by an exaggeration of parasympathomimetic effects which may include the following: Headache; visual disturbance; lacrimation; sweating; respiratory distress; GI spasm; nausea; vomiting; diarrhea; AV block; tachycardia; bradycardia; hypotension; hypertension; shock; mental confusion; cardiac arrhythmia; tremors.

Biliary tract: Administer with caution to patients with known or suspected cholelithiasis or biliary tract disease. Contractions of the gallbladder or biliary smooth muscle could precipitate complications including cholecystitis, cholangitis, and biliary obstruction.

Renal colic: Pilocarpine may increase ureteral smooth muscle tone and could theoretically precipitate renal colic (or "ureteral reflux"), particularly in patients with nephrolithiasis.

Psychiatric disorder: Cholinergic agonists may have dose-related CNS effects. Consider this when treating patients with underlying cognitive or psychiatric disturbances.

Pregnancy: Category C.

Lactation: It is not known whether this drug is excreted in breast milk.

Children: Safety and efficacy in children have not been established.

Elderly: Adverse events reported by those older than 65 years of age and those 65 years of age and younger were comparable. Elderly women volunteers had a higher C_{max} and AUC than elderly men.

Drug Interactions

Drugs that may interact with pilocarpine include beta blockers and anticholinergics.

Drug/Food interactions: The rate of absorption of pilocarpine is decreased when taken with a high-fat meal. Maximum concentration is decreased and time to reach maximum concentration is increased.

Adverse Reactions

The most frequent adverse experiences associated with pilocarpine were a consequence of the expected pharmacologic effects. Adverse reactions occurring in at least 3% of patients include the following: Sweating, nausea, rhinitis, chills, flushing, urinary frequency, dizziness, asthenia, headache, dyspepsia, lacrimation, diarrhea, edema, abdominal pain, amblyopia, vomiting, pharyngitis, and hypertension.

AMLEXANOX

Paste: 5% (*Rx*)	*Aphthasol* (Discus Dental)

Indications

Aphthous ulcers: Treatment of aphthous ulcers in people with healthy immune systems.

Administration and Dosage

Apply 4 times/day beginning as soon as symptoms occur. Use after oral hygiene. With gentle pressure, dab paste onto each ulcer in mouth. Use until ulcer heals. If significant healing or pain reduction has not occurred in 10 days, consult a dentist or physician.

Actions

Pharmacology: The mechanism of action is unknown.

Contraindications

Hypersensitivity to amlexanox or other ingredients in the formulation.

Warnings/Precautions

Local irritation: In the event that rash or contact mucositis occurs, discontinue use.

Pregnancy: Category B.

Lactation: Exercise caution when administering amlexanox oral paste to a nursing woman.

Children: Safety and efficacy in pediatric patients have not been established.

Adverse Reactions

Transient pain, stinging, or burning at the site of application (1% to 2%).

SULFURIC ACID/SULFONATED PHENOLICS

Liquid: 30% sulfuric acid and 22% sulfonated phenolics (*Rx*)	*Debacterol* (Henry Schein/Sullivan-Schein Dental)

Indications

Ulcerating lesions: Topical treatment of ulcerating lesions of the oral cavity, such as recurrent aphthous stomatitis (canker sores).

Not intended for the treatment of vesicular lesions, such as cold sores or fever blisters.

Administration and Dosage

Dry the ulcerated area of oral mucosa using a sterile cotton-tipped applicator or some similar method. After drying the lesion, hold swab with the colored ring end up. Bend the colored ring tip gently to the side until it snaps to release the liquid inside. Then apply the coated applicator directly to the dried ulcer bed. Hold applicator in contact with the ulcer for at least 5 seconds while rolling to thoroughly coat the entire ulcer bed, the ulcer rim, and the surrounding halo of normal mucosa. Do not hold the applicator on the ulcer for more than 10 seconds. Thoroughly rinse out the mouth with water and spit out the rinse water. The stinging sensation and ulcer pain will subside almost immediately after the water rinse.

One application per ulcer treatment is usually sufficient. If the ulcer pain returns shortly after rinsing with water, some part of the ulcer was not covered. Then apply a second application to the ulcer immediately until it remains pain-free after rinsing. It is not recommended that more than 1 treatment session be performed on any individual mucosal ulcer. Do not reapply the product to the same lesion after it is free of pain.

Actions

Pharmacology: The liquid contains sulfonated phenolics, which are antiseptic agents with topical analgesic properties, and sulfuric acid, which is a tissue denaturant and sterilizing agent.

Contraindications

Known allergy to sulfonated phenolics.

Warnings/Precautions

Keep out of the reach of children. Do not use if allergic to sulfonated phenolics.

Prolonged use: Prolonged use on normal tissue should be avoided. Prolonged use will eventually necrotize and slough all tissue to which it is applied in sufficient volume; apply carefully.

External use only: Avoid eye contact.

Pregnancy: Category C.

Children: Safety and efficacy in children under 12 years of age have not been established.

Adverse Reactions

May cause local irritation upon administration. If excess irritation occurs, a rinse with sodium bicarbonate (baking soda) solution will neutralize the reaction (use 2.5 mL in 120 mL of water).

Chapter 9

SYSTEMIC ANTI-INFECTIVE AGENTS

PENICILLINS

AMOXICILLIN	
Tablets; oral: 500 and 875 mg (*Rx*)	Various, *Amoxil* (GlaxoSmithKline)
Tablets, chewable; oral: 125, 200, 250, and 400 mg (*Rx*)	Various
Tablets for suspension; oral: 200 and 400 mg (*Rx*)	*DisperMox* (Ranbaxy)
Tablets, extended-release; oral: 775 mg (*Rx*)	*Moxatag* (Middlebrook)
Capsules; oral: 250 and 500 mg (*Rx*)	Various, *Amoxil* (GlaxoSmithKline)
Powder for suspension; oral: 125, 200, 250, and 400 mg per 5 mL when reconstituted (*Rx*)	Various
AMOXICILLIN AND POTASSIUM CLAVULANATE	
Tablets; oral: amoxicillin 250, 500, or 875 mg and clavulanic acid 125 mg (*Rx*)	Various, *Augmentin* (GlaxoSmithKline)
Tablets, extended-release; oral: amoxicillin 1,000 mg and clavulanic acid 62.5 mg (*Rx*)	*Augmentin XR* (GlaxoSmithKline)
Tablets, chewable; oral: amoxicillin 200 mg and clavulanic acid 28.5 mg; amoxicillin 400 mg and clavulanic acid 57 mg (*Rx*)	Various, *Augmentin* (GlaxoSmithKline)
Powder for suspension; oral: amoxicillin 125 mg and clavulanic acid 31.25 mg per 5 mL; amoxicillin 250 mg and clavulanic acid 62.5 mg per 5 mL (after reconstitution) (*Rx*)	*Augmentin* (GlaxoSmithKline)
amoxicillin 200 mg and clavulanic acid 28.5 mg per 5 mL (*Rx*)	Various, *Amoclan* (West-Ward)
amoxicillin 400 mg and clavulanic acid 57 mg per 5 mL (after reconstitution) (*Rx*)	Various, *Amoclan* (West-Ward), *Augmentin* (GlaxoSmithKline)
amoxicillin 600 mg and clavulanic acid 42.9 mL per 5 mL (after reconstitution) (*Rx*)	Various, *Augmentin ES-600* (GlaxoSmithKline)
AMPICILLIN	
Capsules; oral: 250 and 500 mg (as trihydrate or anhydrous) (*Rx*)	Various, *Principen* (Geneva)
Powder for suspension; oral: 125 and 250 mg per 5 mL (as trihydrate) when reconstituted (*Rx*)	*Principen* (Geneva)
AMPICILLIN SODIUM, PARENTERAL	
Injection, powder for solution: 250 and 500 mg and 1 and 2 g (*Rx*)	Various
AMPICILLIN SODIUM AND SULBACTAM SODIUM	
Injection, powder for solution: 1.5 g (ampicillin sodium 1 g/sulbactam sodium 0.5 g), 3 g (ampicillin sodium 2 g/sulbactam sodium 1 g), 15 g (ampicillin sodium 10 g/sulbactam sodium 5 g) (*Rx*)	Various, *Unasyn* (Roerig)
DICLOXACILLIN SODIUM	
Capsules; oral: 250 and 500 mg (*Rx*)	Various
NAFCILLIN SODIUM	
Injection, powder for solution: 1 and 2 g (*Rx*)	Various
OXACILLIN SODIUM, PARENTERAL	
Injection, powder for solution: 1, 2, and 10 g/mL (*Rx*)	Various
PENICILLIN G (AQUEOUS)	
Injection, premixed, frozen: 1, 2, and 3 million units (*Rx*)	*Penicillin G Potassium* (Baxter)
Injection, powder for solution: 5 and 20 million units/vial (*Rx*)	Various, *Pfizerpen* (Roerig)
PENICILLIN G BENZATHINE, IM	
Injection: 600,000 units, 1,200,000, and 2,400,000 units/dose (*Rx*)	*Bicillin L-A* (Wyeth-Ayerst), *Permapen* (Roerig)
PENICILLIN G PROCAINE, IM	
Injection: 600,000 and 1,200,000 units/vial (*Rx*)	*Wycillin* (Wyeth-Ayerst)
PENICILLIN G BENZATHINE AND PROCAINE COMBINED, IM	
Injection: 300,000 units/mL; 600,000, 1,200,000, and 2,400,000 units/dose; 900,000 units penicillin G benzathine and 300,000 units penicillin G procaine/dose (*Rx*)	*Bicillin C-R*, *Bicillin C-R 900/300* (Monarch)
PENICILLIN V (PHENOXYMETHYL PENICILLIN)	
Tablets; oral: 250 and 500 mg (*Rx*)	Various, *Veetids* (Geneva)
Powder for solution; oral: 125 or 250 mg per 5 mL when reconstituted (*Rx*)	Various, *Veetids* (Geneva)

PIPERACILLIN SODIUM	
Injection, powder for solution: 2, 3, 4, and 40 g (*Rx*)	Various
PIPERACILLIN SODIUM AND TAZOBACTAM SODIUM	
Injection, powder for solution: piperacillin 2 g/tazobactam 0.25 g; piperacillin 3 g/tazobactam 0.375 g; piperacillin 4 g/tazobactam 0.5 g; piperacillin 36 g/tazobactam 4.5 g (*Rx*)	*Zosyn* (Wyeth)
Injection, solution: piperacillin 2 g/tazobactam 0.25 g; piperacillin 3 g/tazobactam 0.375 g; piperacillin 4 g/tazobactam 0.5 g (*Rx*)	*Zosyn* (Wyeth)
TICARCILLIN AND CLAVULANATE POTASSIUM	
Injection, powder for reconstitution: ticarcillin 3 g (as disodium) and clavulanic acid 0.1 g (as potassium) (*Rx*)	*Timentin* (GlaxoSmithKline)
Injection, solution: ticarcillin 3 g (as disodium) and clavulanic acid 0.1 g (as potassium) per 100 mL (*Rx*)	*Timentin* (GlaxoSmithKline)

Indications

Oral: Penicillins generally are indicated in the treatment of mild to moderately severe infections caused by penicillin-sensitive microorganisms.

Penicillinase-resistant penicillins: The percentage of staphylococcal isolates resistant to **penicillin G** outside the hospital is increasing, approximating the high percentage found in the hospital. Therefore, use a penicillinase-resistant penicillin as initial therapy for any suspected staphylococcal infection until culture and sensitivity results are known.

When treatment is initiated before definitive culture and sensitivity results are known, consider that these agents are only effective in the treatment of infections caused by pneumococci, group A beta-hemolytic streptococci, and penicillin G-resistant and penicillin G-sensitive staphylococci.

Parenteral: In patients with severe infection or when there is nausea, vomiting, gastric dilatation, cardiospasm, or intestinal hypermotility.

Administration and Dosage

Therapy may be initiated prior to obtaining results of bacteriologic studies when there is reason to believe the causative organisms may be susceptible. Once results are known, adjust therapy.

Continue treatment of all infections for a minimum of 48 to 72 hours beyond the time that the patient becomes asymptomatic or evidence of bacterial eradication has been obtained, unless single-dose therapy is employed.

AMOXICILLIN:

Capsules, chewable tablets, and oral suspension – Amoxicillin capsules, chewable tablets, and oral suspensions may be given without regard to meals. The 400 mg suspension, 400 mg chewable tablet, and 875 mg tablet have been studied only when administered at the start of a light meal. However, food-effect studies have not been performed with the 200 and 500 mg formulations.

Neonates and infants 12 weeks (3 months) of age and younger – Because of incompletely developed renal function affecting elimination of amoxicillin, the recommended upper dose of amoxicillin is 30 mg/kg/day divided every 12 hours.

Amoxicillin Dosing in Adults and Pediatric Patients > 3 Months of Age

Infection	Severity[a]	Usual adult dose	Usual dose for children > 3 months[b,c]
Ear/nose/throat	Mild/moderate	500 mg every 12 h or 250 mg every 8 h	25 mg/kg/day in divided doses every 12 h or 20 mg/kg/day in divided doses every 8 h
	Severe	875 mg every 12 h or 500 mg every 8 h or extended-release 775 mg every 24 h	45 mg/kg/day in divided doses every 12 h or 40 mg/kg/day in divided doses every 8 h

Amoxicillin Dosing in Adults and Pediatric Patients > 3 Months of Age

Infection	Severity[a]	Usual adult dose	Usual dose for children > 3 months[b,c]
Gonorrhea, acute uncomplicated (anogenital and urethral infections) in males and females		3 g as single oral dose	Prepubertal children: 50 mg/kg amoxicillin, combined with 25 mg/kg probenecid as a single dose. Note: Probenecid is contraindicated in children < 2 years of age; do not use this regimen in these cases.
GU tract	Mild/moderate	500 mg every 12 h or 250 mg every 8 h	25 mg/kg/day in divided doses every 12 h or 20 mg/kg/day in divided doses every 8 h
	Severe	875 mg every 12 h or 500 mg every 8 h	45 mg/kg/day in divided doses every 12 h or 40 mg/kg/day in divided doses every 8 h
Lower respiratory tract	Mild/moderate or severe	875 mg every 12 h or 500 mg every 8 h	45 mg/kg/day in divided doses every 12 h or 40 mg/kg/day in divided doses every 8 h
Skin/skin structure	Mild/moderate	500 mg every 12 h or 250 mg every 8 h	25 mg/kg/day in divided doses every 12 h or 20 mg/kg/day in divided doses every 8 h
	Severe	875 mg every 12 h or 500 mg every 8 h	45 mg/kg/day in divided doses every 12 h or 40 mg/kg/day in divided doses every 8 h

[a] Dosing for infections caused by less susceptible organisms should follow the recommendations for severe infections.
[b] The children's dose is intended for individuals who weigh < 40 kg. Children weighing ≥ 40 kg should be dosed according to the adult recommendations.
[c] Each strength of the suspension of amoxicillin is available as a chewable tablet for use by older children.

H. pylori eradication to reduce the risk of duodenal ulcer recurrence (adults) –

Dual therapy (amoxicillin/lansoprazole): Amoxicillin 1 g and lansoprazole 30 mg, each given 3 times daily (every 8 hours) for 14 days.

Triple therapy (amoxicillin/clarithromycin/lansoprazole): Amoxicillin 1 g, clarithromycin 500 mg, and lansoprazole 30 mg, all given twice daily (every 12 hours) for 14 days.

Renal function impairment – Severely impaired patients with a glomerular filtration rate (GFR) of less than 30 mL/min should not receive the 875 mg tablet. Patients with a GFR of 10 to 30 mL/min should receive 500 or 250 mg every 12 hours. Patients with a less than 10 mL/min GFR should receive 500 or 250 mg every 24 hours.

Hemodialysis patients should receive 500 or 250 mg every 24 hours. They should receive an additional dose both during and at the end of dialysis.

There are currently no dosing recommendations for children with impaired renal function.

Extended-release tablets – 775 mg once daily taken within 1 hour of finishing a meal for 10 days.

AMOXICILLIN AND POTASSIUM CLAVULANATE:

Usual dose –

Adults: One 250 mg tablet every 8 hours or one 500 mg tablet every 12 hours.

Suspension – Adults who have difficulty swallowing may be given the 125 mg/5 mL or 250 mg/5 mL suspension in place of the 500 mg tablet, or give 200 mg/5 mL or 400 mg/5 mL suspension in place of the 875 mg tablet.

Severe infections and respiratory tract infections – One 500 mg tablet every 8 hours or one 875 mg tablet every 12 hours.

Renal function impairment – Severely impaired patients with a GFR of less than 30 mL/min should not receive the 875 mg tablet. Give patients with a GFR of 10 to 30 mL/min 500 or 250 mg every 12 hours, depending on the severity of infection. Give patients with a GFR less than 10 mL/min 500 or 250 mg every 24 hours, depending on severity of infection. Give hemodialysis patients 500 or 250 mg every 24 hours and an additional dose during and at the end of dialysis.

Hepatic function impairment – Dose with caution and monitor hepatic function.

Children:

Younger than 3 months of age – 30 mg/kg/day divided every 12 hours, based on the amoxicillin component. Use of the 125 mg/5 mL oral suspension is recommended.

3 months of age or older – Children's dose is based on amoxicillin content. Refer to the following table. Because of the different amoxicillin to clavulanic acid ratios in the 250 mg tablets (250/125) versus the 250 mg chewable tablets (250/62.5), do not use the 250 mg tablet until the child weighs 40 kg or more.

40 kg or more – Dose according to adult recommendations.

Amoxicillin/Potassium Clavulanate Dosing in Children ≥ 3 Months of Age

Infections	Dosing regimen	
	200 mg/5 mL or 400 mg/5 mL (every 12 h)[a,b]	125 mg/5 mL or 250 mg/5 mL (every 8 h)[b]
Otitis media,[c] sinusitis, lower respiratory tract infections, severe infections	45 mg/kg/day	40 mg/kg/day
Less severe infections	25 mg/kg/day	20 mg/kg/day

[a] The every-12-hour regimen is associated with significantly less diarrhea; however, the 200 and 400 mg formulations (suspension and chewable tablets) contain aspartame and should not be used by phenylketonurics.
[b] Each strength of the suspension is available as a chewable tablet for use by older children.
[c] Recommended duration is 10 days.

Augmentin ES-600 – *Augmentin ES-600* 600 mg/5 mL does not contain the same amount of clavulanic acid (as the potassium salt) as any of the other *Augmentin* suspensions. Do not substitute *Augmentin* 200 and 400 mg/5 mL suspensions for *Augmentin ES-600*, as they are not interchangeable.

Dosage:

Children 3 months of age and older – Based on the amoxicillin component (600 mg/5 mL), the recommended dose of *Augmentin ES-600* is 90 mg/kg/day divided every 12 hours, administered for 10 days (see the following table).

Recommended Dose of *Augmentin ES-600*

Body weight (kg)	Volume of *Augmentin* ES-600 providing 90 mg/kg/day
8	3 mL twice daily
12	4.5 mL twice daily
16	6 mL twice daily
20	7.5 mL twice daily
24	9 mL twice daily
28	10.5 mL twice daily
32	12 mL twice daily
36	13.5 mL twice daily

Children weighing 40 kg or more – Experience with *Augmentin ES-600* in this group is not available.

Adults – Experience with *Augmentin ES-600* in adults is not available. Adults who have difficulty swallowing should not be given *Augmentin ES-600* in place of the *Augmentin* 500 or 875 mg tablet.

Hepatic function impairment – Dose patients with hepatic function impairment with caution and monitor hepatic function at regular intervals.

Augmentin XR – The recommended dose is 4,000 mg/250 mg daily according to the following table.

Augmentin XR Dosing		
Indication	Dose	Duration
Acute bacterial sinusitis	2 tablets every 12 h	10 days
Community-acquired pneumonia	2 tablets every 12 h	7 to 10 days

The scored extended-release tablets are available for adults who have difficulty swallowing. The scored tablet may be broken in half at the score line.

Renal function impairment: Augmentin XR is contraindicated in severely impaired patients with a creatinine clearance (CrCl) of less than 30 mL/min and in hemodialysis patients.

Hepatic function impairment: Dose patients with hepatic function impairment with caution and monitor hepatic function at regular intervals.

Children: Safety and efficacy in children under 16 years of age have not been established.

Interchangeability –

Tablets: Because the 250 and 500 mg tablets contain the same amount of clavulanic acid (125 mg as potassium salt), two 250 mg tablets are not equivalent to one 500 mg tablet. In addition, the 250 mg tablet and 250 mg chewable tablet do not contain the same amount of clavulanate potassium; do not substitute them for each other. Amoxicillin/clavulanate potassium tablets (250 or 500 mg) cannot be used to provide the same dosages as amoxicillin/clavulanate potassium extended-release tablets. In addition, the extended-release tablet provides an extended time course of plasma amoxicillin concentrations compared with immediate-release tablets.

Suspensions: Amoxicillin/clavulanate potassium *ES-600* suspension 600 mg per 5 mL does not contain the same amount of clavulanic acid (as the potassium salt) as any of the other amoxicillin/clavulanate potassium suspensions.

Administration – Amoxicillin/clavulanate potassium (tablets, chewable tablets, and standard and *ES-600* suspensions) may be taken without regard to meals; however, absorption of clavulanate potassium is enhanced when amoxicillin/clavulanate potassium is administered at the start of a meal. To minimize the potential for GI intolerance, amoxicillin/clavulanate potassium should be taken at the start of a meal.

Amoxicillin/clavulanate potassium should be taken at the start of a meal to enhance the absorption of amoxicillin and minimize the potential for GI intolerance. Absorption of the amoxicillin component is decreased when amoxicillin/clavulanate potassium is taken on an empty stomach.

AMPICILLIN:

Ampicillin Uses and Dosages	
Organisms/Infections	Dosage
Enterococcal endocarditis	12 g/day IV either continuously or in equally divided doses every 4 h plus 1 mg/kg IM or IV gentamicin every 8 h for 4 to 6 wk
Respiratory tract and soft tissue infections	*Parenteral:* Patients ≥ 40 kg – 250 to 500 mg every 6 h; < 40 kg – 25 to 50 mg/kg/day in equally divided doses at 6- to 8-h intervals *Oral:* Patients > 20 kg – 250 mg every 6 h; ≤ 20 kg – 50 mg/kg/day in equally divided doses at 6- to 8-h intervals
Bacterial meningitis	Adults/Children: 150 to 200 mg/kg/day in equally divided doses every 3 to 4 h. Initial treatment is usually by IV, followed by IM injections.
Septicemia	Adults/Children: 150 to 200 mg/kg/day. Give IV at least 3 days; continue IM every 3 to 4 h.

Ampicillin Uses and Dosages	
Organisms/Infections	Dosage
GI and GU infections: Other than *N. gonorrhoeae*[a]	*Oral:* Adults/Children > 20 kg – 500 mg orally every 6 h. Use larger doses for severe or chronic infections, if needed. Children ≤ 20 kg – 100 mg/kg/day every 6 h
N. gonorrhoeae	*Oral:* Single dose of 3.5 g administered simultaneously with 1 g probenecid *Parenteral:* Adults/children ≥ 40 kg – 500 mg IV or IM every 6 h Children < 40 kg – 50 mg/kg/day IV or IM in equally divided doses at 6- to 8-h intervals
Urethritis caused by *N. gonorrhoeae* in men	*Parenteral:* Adult men – Two 500 mg doses, IV or IM, at an interval of 8 to 12 h. Treatment may be repeated if necessary or extended if required. In complicated gonorrheal urethritis (eg, prostatitis, epididymitis), prolonged and intensive therapy is recommended.

[a] Ampicillin is not included in the 2002 CDC recommendations for the treatment of gonorrhea.

Renal function impairment – Increase dosing interval to 6 to 12 hours in moderate renal function impairment (CrCl 10 to 50 mL/min) and 12 to 24 hours in severe renal function impairment (CrCl less than 10 mL/min).

AMPICILLIN SODIUM AND SULBACTAM SODIUM: Give IV or IM. The recommended adult dosage is 1.5 (1 g ampicillin plus 0.5 g sulbactam) to 3 g (2 g ampicillin plus 1 g sulbactam) every 6 hours. Do not exceed sulbactam 4 g/day.

Renal function impairment – In patients with renal function impairment, give as follows:

Ampicillin/Sulbactam Dosage Guide For Patients With Renal Function Impairment		
CrCl (mL/min/1.72 m²)	Half-life (h)	Recommended dosage
≥ 30	1	1.5 to 3 g every 6 to 8 h
15 to 29	5	1.5 to 3 every 12 h
5 to 14	9	1.5 to 3 g every 24 h

Children – Do not routinely exceed 14 days of IV therapy. Safety and efficacy of IM administration have not been established.

Children 1 year of age and older (less than 40 kg): 300 mg/kg/day IV (200 mg ampicillin/100 mg sulbactam) in divided doses every 6 hours.

Children 40 kg or more: Dose according to adult recommendations; total sulbactam dose should not exceed 4 g/day.

The safety and efficacy of ampicillin/sulbactam sodium has not been established for children for intra-abdominal infections.

DICLOXACILLIN SODIUM:

For mild to moderate upper respiratory and localized skin and soft tissue infections –

Adults and children (40 kg or more): 125 mg every 6 hours.

Children (less than 40 kg): 12.5 mg/kg/day in equal doses every 6 hours.

For more severe infections, such as lower respiratory tract or disseminated infections –

Adults and children (40 kg or more): 250 mg every 6 hours.

Children (less than 40 kg): 25 mg/kg/day in equally divided doses every 6 hours.

Use in newborns is not recommended.

NAFCILLIN SODIUM:

Adults – 500 mg IV every 4 hours. For severe infections, 1 g every 4 hours is recommended. Administer slowly over at least 30 to 60 minutes to minimize the risk of vein irritation and extravasation.

Duration – Duration of therapy varies with the type and severity of infection as well as the overall condition of the patient. In severe staphylococcal infections, continue nafcillin therapy for at least 14 days. The treatment of endocarditis and osteomyelitis may require a longer duration of therapy.

OXACILLIN SODIUM:

Oxacillin Dosage		
Indication	Adults	Children (< 40 kg)
Parenteral (IM or IV)		
Mild to moderate infection	250 to 500 mg IM or IV every 4 to 6 h	50 mg/kg/day IM or IV every 6 h
Severe infection	1 g IM or IV every 4 to 6 h	100 mg/kg/day IM or IV every 4 to 6 h. **Premature/Neonates:** 25 mg/kg/day IM or IV

PENICILLIN G (AQUEOUS):

Infants – Preferably administered IV as 15- to 30-minute infusions.

Older than 7 days of age: 75,000 units/kg/day in divided doses every 8 hours (meningitis, 200,000 to 300,000 units/kg/day every 6 hours).

Younger than 7 days of age: 50,000 units/kg/day in divided doses every 12 hours (group B streptococcus, 100,000 units/kg/day; meningitis, 100,000 to 150,000 units/kg/day).

Administer penicillin G injection by IV infusion.

Parenteral Penicillin G Use and Dosages in Adults	
Indications	Adult dosage
Meningococcal meningitis/septicemia	24 million units/day; 1 to 2 million units IM every 2 h; or 20 to 30 million units/day continuous IV drip for 14 days or until afebrile for 7 days; or 200,000 to 300,000 units/kg/day every 2 to 4 h in divided doses for a total of 24 doses
Actinomycosis:	
For cervicofacial cases	1 to 6 million units/day
For thoracic and abdominal disease	10 to 20 million units/day IV every 4 to 6 h for 6 wk. May be followed by oral penicillin V, 500 mg 4 times daily for 2 to 3 mo
Clostridial infections:	
Botulism (adjunctive therapy to antitoxin), gas gangrene and tetanus (adjunctive therapy to human tetanus immune globulin)	20 million units/day every 4 to 6 h as adjunct to antitoxin
Fusospirochetal infections: Severe infections of oropharynx, lower respiratory tract, and genital area	5 to 10 million units/day every 4 to 6 h
Rat-bite fever (Spirillum minus, Streptobacillus moniliformis), Haverhill fever	12 to 20 million units/day every 4 to 6 h for 3 to 4 wk
Listeria infections (Listeria monocytogenes):	
Meningitis (adults)	15 to 20 million units/day every 4 to 6 h for 2 wk
Endocarditis (adults)	15 to 20 million units/day every 4 to 6 h for 4 wk
Pasteurella infections (Pasteurella multocida): Bacteremia and meningitis	4 to 6 million units/day every 4 to 6 h for 2 wk
Erysipeloid (Erysipelothrix rhusiopathiae): Endocarditis	12 to 20 million units/day every 4 to 6 h for 4 to 6 wk
Diphtheria: Adjunct to antitoxin to prevent carrier state	2 to 3 million units/day in divided doses every 4 to 6 h for 10 to 12 days
Anthrax: (*Bacillus anthracis* is often resistant)	Minimum 5 million units/day; 12 to 20 million units/day have been used
Serious streptococcal infections (S. pneumoniae):	
Empyema, pneumonia, pericarditis, endocarditis, meningitis	5 to 24 million units/day in divided doses every 4 to 6 h
Syphilis:	
Neurosyphilis	18 to 24 million units/day IV (3 to 4 million units every 4 h) for 10 to 14 days. Many recommend benzathine penicillin G 2.4 million units/wk IM for 3 wk following the completion of this regimen

Parenteral Penicillin G Use and Dosages in Adults	
Indications	Adult dosage
Disseminated gonococcal infections: (eg, meningitis, endocarditis, arthritis)	10 million units/day every 4 to 6 h, with the exception of meningococcal meningitis/septicemia (ie, every 2 h)

Children –

Parenteral Penicillin G Use and Dosages in Children	
Indications	Pediatric dosage
Serious streptococcal infections, such as pneumonia and endocarditis (*S. pneumoniae*) and meningococcus	150,000 units/kg/day divided in equal doses every 4 to 6 h
Meningitis caused by susceptible strains of pneumococcus and meningococcus	250,000 units/kg/day divided in equal doses every 4 h for 7 to 14 days (maximum dose, 12 to 20 million units/day)
Disseminated gonococcal infections (penicillin-susceptible strains):	*Weight < 45 kg:*
Arthritis	100,000 units/kg/day in 4 equally divided doses for 7 to 10 days
Meningitis	250,000 units/kg/day in equal doses every 4 h for 10 to 14 days
Endocarditis	250,000 units/kg/day in equal doses every 4 h for 4 wk
	Weight ≥ 45 kg:
Arthritis, meningitis, endocarditis	10 million units/day in 4 equally divided doses
Syphilis (congenital and neurosyphilis) after the newborn period:	200,000 to 300,000 units/kg/day (administered as 50,000 units/kg every 4 to 6 h) for 10 to 14 days
Congenital syphilis: symptomatic or asymptomatic infants	*Infants:* 50,000 units/kg/dose IV every 12 h the first 7 days, thereafter every 8 h for a total of 10 days. *Children:* 50,000 units/kg every 4 to 6 h for 10 days
Diphtheria (adjunctive therapy to antitoxin and for prevention of carrier state)	150,000 to 250,000 units/kg/day every 6 h for 7 to 10 days
Rat-bite fever; Haverhill fever (with endocarditis caused by S. moniliformis)	150,000 to 250,000 units/kg/day every 4 h for 4 wk

PENICILLIN G BENZATHINE, IM: Administer by deep IM injection in the upper outer quadrant of the buttock. In neonates, infants, and small children, the midlateral aspect of the thigh may be preferable. When doses are repeated, rotate the injection site. Do not administer IV.

Penicillin G Benzathine Uses and Dosages	
Organisms/Infections	Dosage
Streptococcal (group A): Upper respiratory tract infections	*Adults:* 1.2 million units IM as a single injection *Older children:* 900,000 units IM as a single injection *Infants and children (< 60 lbs; 27 kg):* 300,000 to 600,000 units
Syphilis:[a] *Early syphilis* - Primary, secondary, or latent syphilis	*Adults:* 2.4 million units IM in single dose *Children:* 50,000 units/kg IM, up to adult dosage
Gummas and cardiovascular syphilis[a] - Latent	*Adults:* 2.4 million units IM once per wk for 3 wk *Children:* 50,000 units/kg IM, up to adult dosage

Penicillin G Benzathine Uses and Dosages	
Organisms/Infections	Dosage
Neurosyphilis[a]	Aqueous penicillin G, 18 to 24 million units/day IV (3 to 4 million units every 4 h) for 10 to 14 days. Many recommend benzathine penicillin G, 2.4 million IM units once per wk for up to 3 wk following completion of this regimen. or Procaine penicillin G 2.4 million units/day IM *plus* probenecid 500 mg orally 4 times/day, both for 10 to 14 days. Many recommend benzathine penicillin G 2.4 million units IM once per wk for up to 3 wk following completion of this regimen.
Syphilis in pregnancy[a]	Dosage schedule appropriate for stage of syphilis recommended for nonpregnant patients.
Congenital syphilis	*Children < 2 years of age:* 50,000 units/kg/body weight *Children 2 to 12 years of age:* Adjust dosage based on adult dosage schedule.
Yaws, bejel, and pinta	1.2 million units IM in a single dose
Prophylaxis for rheumatic fever and glomerulonephritis	Following an acute attack, may be given IM in doses of 1.2 million units once per mo or 600,000 units every 2 wk

[a] CDC 2002 Sexually Transmitted Diseases Treatment Guidelines. MMWR *Morbid Mortal Wkly Rept*. 2002;51(RR-6):1-82.

PENICILLIN G PROCAINE, IM: Administer by deep IM injection only into the upper outer quadrant of the buttock. In infants and small children, the midlateral aspect of the thigh may be preferable. When doses are repeated, rotate the injection site. Do not administer IV.

Newborns – Avoid use in these patients because sterile abscesses and procaine toxicity are of much greater concern than in older children.

Penicillin G Procaine Uses and Dosages	
Organisms/Infections	Dosage
Pneumococcal infections: Moderately severe upper respiratory tract infections	*Adults:* 600,000 to 1 million units/day IM *Children (< 60 lbs, 27 kg):* 300,000 units/day IM
Streptococcal infections (group A): Moderately severe to severe tonsillitis, erysipelas, scarlet fever, upper respiratory tract, and skin and soft tissue infections	*Adults:* 600,000 to 1 million units/day IM for a minimum of 10 days *Children (< 60 lbs, 27 kg):* 300,000 units/day IM
Bacterial endocarditis – Only in extremely sensitive infections (Group A streptococci)	600,000 to 1 million units/day IM
Staphylococcal infections: Moderately severe infections of the skin and soft tissue	*Adults:* 600,000 to 1 million units/day IM *Children (< 60 lbs, 27 kg):* 300,000 units/day
Diphtheria: Adjunctive therapy with antitoxin	300,000 to 600,000 units/day IM for 14 days
Carrier state	300,000 units/day IM for 10 days
Anthrax: Cutaneous	600,000 to 1 million units/day IM. Continue prophylaxis until exposure to *Bacillus anthracis* has been excluded. If exposure is confirmed and vaccine is available, continue prophylaxis for 4 weeks and until 3 doses of vaccine have been administered, or for 30 to 60 days if vaccine is not available.
Vincent's gingivitis and pharyngitis (fusospirochetosis)	600,000 to 1 million units/day IM. Obtain necessary dental care in infections involving gum tissue.
Erysipeloid	600,000 to 1 million units/day IM
Rat-bite fever (Streptobacillus moniliformis and *Spirillum minus)*	600,000 to 1 million units/day IM

Penicillin G Procaine Uses and Dosages	
Organisms/Infections	Dosage
Syphilis: primary, secondary, and latent with a negative spinal fluid (adults and children > 12 years of age)	600,000 units/day IM for 8 days; total, 4.8 million units
Late (tertiary, neurosyphilis, and latent syphilis with positive spinal fluid examination or no spinal fluid examination)	600,000 units/day IM for 10 to 15 days; total, 6 to 9 million units
Neurosyphilis[a] (as an alternative to the recommended regimen of penicillin G aqueous)	2.4 million units/day IM plus probenecid 500 mg orally 4 times/day, both for 10 to 14 days; many recommend benzathine penicillin G 2.4 million/units IM following the completion of this regimen
Congenital syphilis[a]	*Children < 70 lb (32 kg)*: 50,000 units/kg/day (administered as a single IM dose) for 10 to 14 days.
Yaws, bejel, and pinta	Treat same as syphilis in corresponding stage of disease

[a] CDC 2002 Sexually Transmitted Diseases Treatment Guidelines. *MMWR Morbid Mortal Wkly Rept.* 2002;51(RR-6):1-82.

PENICILLIN G BENZATHINE AND PROCAINE COMBINED, IM: For IM use only. Do not inject IV or admix with other IV solutions. There have been reports of inadvertent IV administration of penicillin G benzathine, which has been associated with cardio-respiratory arrest and death. Prior to administration of this drug, carefully read the labeling.

Administer by deep IM injection in the upper outer quadrant of the buttock. In infants, neonates, and small children, the midlateral aspect of the thigh may be preferable. When doses are repeated, rotate the injection site.

Streptococcal infections group A: Infections of the upper respiratory tract, skin and soft-tissue infections, scarlet fever, and erysipelas.

Bicillin C-R 900/300 – A single injection of *Bicillin C-R 900/300* is usually sufficient for the treatment of group A streptococcal infections in children.

Bicillin C-R – Treatment is usually given at a single session using multiple IM sites when indicated.

1.) Adults and children (over 60 lbs [27 kg]): 2,400,000 units
2.) Children (30 to 60 lbs [14 to 27 kg]): 900,000 to 1,200,000 units
3.) Children (under 30 lbs [14 kg]): 600,000 units

Alternative dosing – An alternative dosage schedule may be used, giving one-half the total dose on day 1 and one-half on day 3. This will also ensure the penicillinemia required over a 10-day period; however, this alternate schedule should be used only when the health care provider can be assured of the patient's cooperation.

Pneumococcal infections (except pneumococcal meningitis):

Bicillin C-R – The dose should be repeated every 2 or 3 days until the temperature is normal for 48 hours. Other forms of penicillin may be necessary for severe cases.

1.) Adults: 1,200,000 units IM
2.) Children: 600,000 units IM

Bicillin C-R 900/300 – One *Tubex* cartridge of *Bicillin C-R 900/300* repeated at 2- or 3-day intervals until the temperature is normal for 48 hours. Other forms of penicillin may be necessary for severe cases.

PENICILLIN V (PHENOXYMETHYL PENICILLIN): 250 mg equals 400,000 units.

Adults – 125 to 500 mg 4 times/day; in renal function impairment (CrCl 10 mL/min or less) - Do not exceed 250 mg every 6 hours.

Children – 25 to 50 mg/kg/day in divided doses every 6 to 8 hours.

Penicillin V Uses and Dosages for Adults and Children > 12 Years of Age	
Organisms/Infections	Dosage
Streptococcal infections: Mild to moderately severe infections of the upper respiratory tract, including scarlet fever and mild erysipelas	125 to 250 mg orally every 6 to 8 h for 10 days
Pharyngitis in children	25 to 50 mg/kg/day divided every 6 h for 10 days
Pneumococcal infections: Mild to moderately severe respiratory tract infections including otitis media	250 to 500 mg orally every 6 h until afebrile at least 2 days
Staphylococcal infections: Mild infections of skin and soft tissue	250 to 500 mg orally every 6 to 8 h
Fusospirochetosis (Vincent's infection) of the oropharynx: Mild to moderately severe infections	250 to 500 mg orally every 6 to 8 h
For prevention of recurrence following rheumatic fever or chorea	125 to 250 mg orally 2 times/day on a continuing basis
Unlabeled uses:	
Prophylactic treatment of children with sickle cell anemia or splenectomy: To reduce the incidence of S. *pneumoniae* septicemia	*3 months to 5 years of age:* 125 mg orally 2 times/day *> 5 years of age:* 250 mg twice daily
Actinomycosis	Penicillin G 10 to 20 mg/day IV for 4 to 6 weeks, then Penicillin V 2 to 4 g/day for 6 to 12 months
Early Lyme disease (Borrelia burgdorferi): Erythema migrans	500 mg orally 4 times a day for 10 to 20 days
Anthrax: postexposure prophylaxis - Confirmed or suspected exposure to *Bacillus anthracis*	*Adults:* 7.5 mg/kg orally 4 times/day *Children < 9 years of age:* 50 mg/kg/day orally divided 4 times/day Continue prophylaxis until exposure to B. *anthracis* has been excluded. If exposure is confirmed and vaccine is available, continue prophylaxis for 4 weeks and until 3 doses of vaccine have been administered or for 30 to 60 days if vaccine is not available.

PIPERACILLIN SODIUM: Administer IM or IV. For serious infections, give 3 to 4 g every 4 to 6 hours as a 20- to 30-minute IV infusion. Maximum daily dose is 24 g/day, although higher doses have been used. Limit IM injections to 2 g/site.

Hemodialysis – Maximum dose is 6 g/day (2 g every 8 hours). Hemodialysis removes 30% to 50% of piperacillin in 4 hours; administer an additional 1 g after dialysis.

Infants and children younger than 12 years of age – Dosages have not been established; however, the following doses have been suggested:

Neonates:

Younger than 36 weeks of age – 75 mg/kg IV every 12 hours in the first week of life, then every 8 hours in the second week.

Full-term – 75 mg/kg IV every 8 hours the first week of life, then every 6 hours thereafter.

Other conditions, 200 to 300 mg/kg/day, up to a maximum of 24 g/day divided every 4 to 6 hours.

Piperacillin Uses and Dosages	
Organisms/Infections	Dosage
Serious infections: Septicemia, nosocomial pneumonia, intra-abdominal infections, aerobic and anaerobic gynecologic infections, and skin and soft tissue infections:	12 to 18 g/day IV (200 to 300 mg/kg/day) in divided doses every 4 to 6 h
Renal function impairment – CrCl	
20 to 40 mL/min	12 g/day; 4 g every 8 h

Piperacillin Uses and Dosages	
Organisms/Infections	Dosage
< 20 mL/min	8 g/day; 4 g every 12 h
Urinary tract infections: Complicated (normal renal function)	8 to 16 g/day IV (125 to 200 mg/kg/day) in divided doses every 6 to 8 h
Renal function impairment – CrCl	
20 to 40 mL/min	9 g/day; 3 g every 8 h
< 20 mL/min	6 g/day; 3 g every 12 h
Uncomplicated UTI and most community-acquired pneumonia (normal renal function)	6 to 8 g/day IM or IV (100 to 125 mg/kg/day) in divided doses every 6 to 12 h
Uncomplicated UTI with renal function impairment – CrCl < 20 mL/min	6 g/day; 3 g every 12 h
Uncomplicated gonorrhea infections	2 g IM in a single dose with 1 g probenecid ½ h prior to injection
Prophylaxis: Intra-abdominal surgery	2 g IV just prior to anesthesia; 2 g during surgery; 2 g every 6 h post-op for no more than 24 h
Vaginal hysterectomy	2 g IV just prior to anesthesia; 2 g 6 h after initial dose; 2 g 12 h after first dose
Cesarean section	2 g IV after cord is clamped; 2 g 4 h after initial dose; 2 g 8 h after first dose
Abdominal hysterectomy	2 g IV just prior to anesthesia; 2 g on return to recovery room; 2 g after 6 h

PIPERACILLIN SODIUM AND TAZOBACTAM SODIUM:

Adults – 3.375 g every 6 hours for 7 to 10 days.

Children –

9 months of age and older with appendicitis and/or peritonitis, weighing up to 40 kg, and with healthy renal function: 100 mg of piperacillin per 12.5 mg of tazobactam per kilogram of body weight, every 8 hours.

Between 2 and 9 months of age: 80 mg of piperacillin per 10 mg of tazobactam per kilogram of body weight, every 8 hours.

Nosocomial pneumonia – 4.5 g every 6 hours plus an aminoglycoside for 7 to 14 days. Continue the aminoglycoside in patients from whom *P. aeruginosa* is isolated.

Concurrent aminoglycoside administration – Because of in vitro inactivation of the aminoglycoside by beta-lactam antibiotics, piperacillin/tazobactam and the aminoglycoside are recommended for separate administration.

Vials/Bulk containers:

Piperacillin/Tazobactam + Aminoglycoside Compatibility				
Aminoglycosides	Piperacillin/tazobactam dose (g)	Piperacillin/tazobactam diluent volume (mL)	Aminoglycoside concentration range[a] (mg/mL)	Acceptable diluents
Amikacin	2.25, 3.375, 4.5	50, 100, 150	1.75 to 7.5	Sodium chloride 0.9% or dextrose 5%
Gentamicin	2.25, 3.375, 4.5	100, 150	0.7, 3.32	Sodium chloride 0.9%

[a] The concentration ranges in this table are based on administration of the aminoglycoside in divided doses (10 to 15 mg/kg/day in 2 daily doses for amikacin and 3 to 5 mg/kg/day in 3 daily doses for gentamicin). Administration of amikacin or gentamicin in a single daily dose or in doses exceeding those previously stated via Y-site with piperacillin/tazobactam containing EDTA has not been evaluated. See the individual monographs for each aminoglycoside for complete dosage and administration instructions.

Galaxy containers:

Piperacillin/Tazobactam + Aminoglycoside Compatibility			
Aminoglycosides	Piperacillin/ tazobactam (g)	Aminoglycoside concentration range[a] (mg/mL)	Acceptable diluents
Amikacin	2.25, 3.375, 4.5	1.75 to 7.5	Sodium chloride 0.9% or dextrose 5%
Gentamicin	2.25 or 4.5	0.7 to 3.32	Sodium chloride 0.9%

[a] The concentration ranges in this table are based on administration of the aminoglycoside in divided doses (10 to 15 mg/kg/day in 2 daily doses for amikacin and 3 to 5 mg/kg/day in 3 daily doses for gentamicin). Administration of amikacin or gentamicin in a single daily dose or in doses exceeding those stated above via Y-site with piperacillin/tazobactam containing EDTA has not been evaluated. See the individual monographs for each aminoglycoside for complete dosage and administration instructions.

Renal function impairment –

Piperacillin/Tazobactam Dosage Recommendations for Renal Function Impairment[a]		
CrCl (mL/min)	All indications (except nosocomial pneumonia)	Nosocomial pneumonia
> 40	3.375 g every 6 hours	4.5 g every 6 hours
20 to 40[b]	2.25 g every 6 hours	3.375 g every 6 hours
< 20[b]	2.25 g every 8 hours	2.25 g every 6 hours
Hemodialysis[c]	2.25 g every 12 hours	2.25 g every 8 hours
CAPD[d]	2.25 g every 12 hours	2.25 g every 8 hours

[a] Dosage provided is "total" combined piperacillin/tazobactam.
[b] CrCl for patients not receiving hemodialysis.
[c] Administer 0.75 g following each hemodialysis session on hemodialysis days.
[d] CAPD = continuous ambulatory peritoneal dialysis.

Hemodialysis – The maximum dosage is 2.25 g every 12 hours for all indications other than nosocomial pneumonia and 2.25 g every 8 hours for nosocomial pneumonia. Because hemodialysis removes 30% to 40% of a dose, give 1 additional dose of 0.75 g following each dialysis period. No additional dosage of piperacillin/tazobactam is necessary for CAPD patients.

Compatible IV solutions – These include sodium chloride 0.9% for injection, sterile water for injection (maximum recommended volume per dose is 50 mL), dextrose 5%, dextran 6% in saline, and Ringer's lactate solution (only with piperacillin/tazobactam containing EDTA).

Incompatible admixtures – Do not add supplementary medications to the *Galaxy* container.

Piperacillin/tazobactam should not be mixed with other drugs in a syringe or infusion bottle. Piperacillin/tazobactam is not chemically stable in solutions that contain only sodium bicarbonate and solutions that significantly alter the pH. Piperacillin/tazobactam should not be added to blood products or albumin hydrolysates.

ADD-Vantage system admixtures – These include dextrose 5% in water (50 or 100 mL) and sodium chloride 0.9% (50 or 100 mL).

Administration – Administer by infusion over a period of at least 30 minutes. During infusion, it is desirable to discontinue the primary infusion solution.

TICARCILLIN AND CLAVULANATE POTASSIUM: Administer by IV infusion over 30 minutes.

Adults –

Ticarcillin/Clavulanate Potassium Administration in Adults			
	Systemic and urinary tract infections	Gynecological infections	
		Moderate	Severe
Adults ≥ 60 kg	3.1 g every 4 to 6 h	200 mg/kg/day every 6 h	300 mg/kg/day every 4 h
Adults < 60 kg	200 to 300 mg/kg/day every 4 to 6 h		

Children –

Dosage Guidelines for Ticarcillin/Clavulanate Potassium in Children ≥ 3 months of age		
	Mild to moderate infections	Severe infections
Children ≥ 60 kg	3.1 g every 6 h	3.1 g every 4 h
Children < 60 kg (dosed at 50 mg/kg/dose)	200 mg/kg/day every 6 h	300 mg/kg/day every 4 h

Renal function impairment –

Dosage of Ticarcillin/Clavulanate Potassium in Renal Function Impairment[a]	
CrCl (mL/min)	Dosage
> 60	3.1 g every 4 h
30 to 60	2 g every 4 h
10 to 30	2 g every 8 h
< 10	2 g every 12 h
< 10 with hepatic function impairment	2 g every 24 h
Patients on peritoneal dialysis	3.1 g every 12 h
Patients on hemodialysis	2 g every 12 h supplemented with 3.1 g after each dialysis

[a] Initial loading dose is 3.1 g. Follow with doses based on CrCl and type of dialysis.

Actions

Pharmacology: Penicillins inhibit the biosynthesis of cell wall mucopeptide. They are bactericidal against sensitive organisms when adequate concentrations are reached and most effective during the stage of active multiplication. Inadequate concentrations may produce only bacteriostatic effects.

Penicillins					
	Routes of administration	Penicillinase-resistant	Acid stable	% Protein bound	May be taken with meals
Natural penicillins					
Penicillin G	IM-IV	no	†[a]	60	†[a]
Penicillin V	Oral	no	yes	80	yes
Penicillinase-resistant					
Dicloxacillin	Oral	yes	yes	98	no
Nafcillin	IM-IV-Oral	yes	yes	87 to 90	no
Oxacillin	IM-IV	yes	yes	94	no
Aminopenicillins					
Amoxicillin	Oral	no	yes	20	yes
Amoxicillin/potassium clavulanate	Oral	yes	yes	18/25	yes
Ampicillin	IM-IV-Oral	no	yes	20	no
Ampicillin/sulbactam	IM-IV	yes	†[a]	28/38	†[a]

Penicillins					
	Routes of administration	Penicillinase-resistant	Acid stable	% Protein bound	May be taken with meals
Extended-spectrum					
Piperacillin	IM-IV	no	†[a]	16	†[a]
Piperacillin/ Tazobactam sodium	IV	yes	†[a]	30/30	†[a]
Ticarcillin/ Potassium clavulanate	IV	yes	†[a]	45/9	†[a]

[a] Available only for IM or IV use.

Pharmacokinetics:

Absorption – Peak serum levels occur approximately 1 hour after oral use. Parenteral **penicillin G** (sodium and potassium) gives rapid and high but transient blood levels; derivatives provide prolonged penicillin blood levels with IM use.

Distribution – Penicillins are bound to plasma proteins, primarily albumin, in varying degrees. They diffuse readily into most body tissues and fluids.

Excretion – Penicillins are excreted largely unchanged in the urine by glomerular filtration and active tubular secretion. Nonrenal elimination includes hepatic inactivation and excretion in bile; this is only a minor route for all penicillins except **nafcillin** and **oxacillin**. Excretion by renal tubular secretion can be delayed by coadministration of probenecid. Elimination half-life of most penicillins is short (no more than 1.5 hours). Renal function impairment prolongs the serum half-life of penicillins eliminated primarily by renal excretion.

Contraindications

History of hypersensitivity to penicillins, cephalosporins, or imipenem.

Do not treat severe pneumonia, empyema, bacteremia, pericarditis, meningitis, or purulent or septic arthritis with an oral penicillin during the acute stage.

Warnings/Precautions

Bleeding abnormalities: **Piperacillin** may induce hemorrhagic manifestations associated with abnormalities of coagulation tests.

Cystic fibrosis: Cystic fibrosis patients have a higher incidence of adverse reactions (eg, fever, rash) when treated with extended-spectrum penicillins (eg, **piperacillin**).

Streptococcal infections: Therapy must be sufficient to eliminate the organism (minimum, 10 days); otherwise, sequelae (eg, endocarditis, rheumatic fever) may occur.

Sexually transmitted diseases: When treating gonococcal infections in which primary and secondary syphilis are suspected, perform proper diagnostic procedures, including darkfield examinations and monthly serological tests for at least 4 months.

Resistance: The number of strains of staphylococci resistant to penicillinase-resistant penicillins has been increasing; widespread use of penicillinase-resistant penicillins may result in an increasing number of resistant staphylococcal strains.

Pseudomembranous colitis: Pseudomembranous colitis has occurred with the use of broad-spectrum antibiotics caused by overgrowth of clostridia; therefore, it is important to consider its diagnosis in patients who develop diarrhea in association with antibiotic use.

Procaine sensitivity: If sensitivity to the procaine in **penicillin G procaine** is suspected, inject 0.1 mL of a 1% to 2% procaine solution intradermally. Development of erythema, wheal, flare, or eruption indicates procaine sensitivity; treat by the usual methods.

Parenteral administration: Inadvertent intravascular administration, including direct intra-arterial injection or injection immediately adjacent to arteries, has resulted in severe neurovascular damage, including transverse myelitis with permanent paralysis, gangrene requiring amputation of digits and more proximal portions of extremities, and necrosis and sloughing at and surrounding the injection site.

Electrolyte imbalance: Patients given continuous IV therapy with **potassium penicillin G** in high dosage (more than 10 million units daily) may suffer severe or even fatal potassium poisoning, particularly if renal function impairment is present. High dosages of **sodium salts of penicillins** may result in or aggravate CHF caused by high sodium intake. Individuals with liver disease or those receiving cytotoxic therapy or diuretics rarely demonstrated a decrease in serum potassium concentrations with high doses of **piperacillin. Sodium penicillin G** contains 2 mEq sodium per million units; **potassium penicillin G** contains 1.7 mEq potassium and 0.3 mEq sodium per million units. The sodium content of other IV penicillin derivatives is listed as follows.

Sodium Content of IV Penicillins			
Penicillin	Maximum recommended daily dose (g)	Sodium content (mEq/g)[a]	Sodium (mEq/day)[a,b]
Ampicillin sodium	14	2.9 to 3.1	40.6 to 43.4
Nafcillin sodium	6	2.9	17.4
Oxacillin sodium	6	2.5 to 3.1	15 to 18.6
Piperacillin sodium	24	1.85	44.4
Piperacillin/Tazobactam sodium	12	2.35	28.2

[a] 1 mEq sodium equals 23 mg.
[b] Based on maximum daily dose.

Hypokalemia – Hypokalemia has occurred in some patients receiving **piperacillin.**

Hypersensitivity reactions: Serious and occasionally fatal immediate-hypersensitivity reactions have occurred. The incidence of anaphylactic shock is between 0.015% and 0.04%. Anaphylactic shock resulting in death has occurred in approximately 0.002% of the patients treated. These reactions are likely to be immediate and severe in penicillin-sensitive individuals with a history of atopic conditions.

Hypersensitivity myocarditis – Hypersensitivity myocarditis is not dose-dependent and may occur at any time during treatment.

An urticarial rash, not representing a true penicillin allergy, occasionally occurs with **ampicillin** (9%). Typically, the rash appears 7 to 10 days after the start of oral ampicillin therapy and remains for a few days to a week after drug discontinuance. In most cases, the rash is maculopapular, pruritic, and generalized.

Cross-allergenicity with cephalosporins: Individuals with a history of penicillin hypersensitivity have experienced severe reactions when treated with a cephalosporin. The incidence of cross-allergenicity between penicillins and cephalosporins is estimated to range from 5% to 16%; however, it is possible the incidence is much lower, possibly 3% to 7%.

Pregnancy: *Category* B. Penicillins cross the placenta.

Lactation: Penicillins are excreted in breast milk in low concentrations; use may cause diarrhea, candidiasis, or allergic response in the breast-feeding infant.

Children: Safety and efficacy of **piperacillin** and the β-lactamase inhibitor/penicillin combinations have not been established in infants and children younger than 12 years of age. Use caution in administering to newborns, and evaluate organ system function frequently.

Monitoring: Obtain blood cultures, white blood cell counts, and differential cell counts prior to initiation of therapy and at least weekly during therapy with penicillinase-resistant penicillins. Measure AST and ALT during therapy to monitor for liver function abnormalities.

Perform periodic urinalysis, BUN, and creatinine determinations during therapy with penicillinase-resistant penicillins, and consider dosage alterations if these values become elevated.

Monitoring is particularly important in newborns and infants and when high dosages are used.

Drug Interactions

Drugs that may affect penicillins include allopurinol, aminoglycosides (parenteral), aspirin, beta blockers, chloramphenicol, erythromycin, ethacrynic acid, furosemide, indomethacin, phenylbutazone, probenecid, sulfonamides, tetracycline, and thiazide diuretics.

Drugs that may be affected by penicillins include aminoglycosides (parenteral), anticoagulants, beta blockers, chloramphenicol, cyclosporine, erythromycin, heparin, oral contraceptives, and vecuronium.

Drug/Lab test interactions: False-positive **urine glucose** reactions may occur with penicillin therapy if *Clinitest*, *Benedict's Solution*, or *Fehling's Solution* are used. It is recommended that enzymatic glucose oxidase tests (such as *Clinistix* or *Tes-Tape*) be used. Positive Coombs' tests have occurred. High urine concentrations of some penicillins may produce false-positive protein reactions (pseudoproteinuria) with the following methods: sulfosalicylic acid and boiling test, acetic acid test, biuret reaction, and nitric acid test. The bromphenol blue (*Multi-Stix*) reagent strip test has been reported to be reliable.

Drug/Food interactions: Absorption of most penicillins is affected by food; these medications are best taken on an empty stomach, 1 hour before or 2 hours after meals. **Penicillin V** may be given with meals; however, blood levels may be slightly higher when taken on an empty stomach. **Amoxicillin** and **amoxicillin/potassium clavulanate** tablets may be given without regard to meals.

Adverse Reactions

CNS: Penicillins have caused neurotoxicity (manifested as lethargy, neuromuscular irritability, hallucinations, convulsions, and seizures) when given in large IV doses, especially in patients with renal failure.

GI: Abdominal pain or cramp; abnormal taste sensation; black "hairy" tongue; diarrhea or bloody diarrhea; dry mouth; enterocolitis; epigastric distress; flatulence; furry tongue; glossitis; gastritis; nausea; pseudomembranous colitis; rectal bleeding; sore mouth or tongue; stomatitis; vomiting.

Hematologic/Lymphatic: Agranulocytosis; anemia; bone marrow depression; decrease in white blood cell count and lymphocyte counts; eosinophilia; granulocytopenia; hemolytic anemia; increase in lymphocytes, monocytes, basophils, and platelets; leukopenia; neutropenia; prolongation of bleeding and prothrombin time; reduction of hemoglobin or hematocrit; thrombocytopenia; thrombocytopenic purpura.

Hypersensitivity: Adverse reactions (estimated incidence, 1% to 10%) are more likely to occur in individuals with previously demonstrated hypersensitivity. In penicillin-sensitive individuals with a history of allergy, asthma, or hay fever, the reactions may be immediate and severe.

Allergic symptoms include angioneurotic edema; bronchospasm; death; erythema multiforme; hypotension; laryngeal edema; laryngospasm; maculopapular to exfoliative dermatitis; prostration; reactions resembling serum sickness (eg, arthralgia, arthritis, chills, edema, fever, malaise); skin rashes; urticaria; vascular collapse; vesicular eruptions.

Lab test abnormalities: Elevations of AST, ALT, bilirubin, and lactate dehydrogenase have been noted in patients receiving semisynthetic penicillins (particularly **oxacillin**); such reactions are more common in infants. Elevations of serum alkaline phosphatase and hypernatremia and reduction in serum potassium, albumin, total proteins, and uric acid may occur.

Local: Deep vein thrombosis; ecchymosis; hematomas; pain (accompanied by induration) at the site of injection.

Miscellaneous: Anorexia; vaginitis.

CEPHALOSPORINS AND RELATED ANTIBIOTICS

CEFACLOR	
Capsules; oral: 250 and 500 mg (*Rx*)	Various, *Ceclor Pulvules* (Eli Lilly)
Tablets; oral: 125, 187, 250, and 375 mg (*Rx*)	*Raniclor* (Ranbaxy)
Tablets, extended release; oral: 375 and 500 mg (*Rx*)	Various
Powder for suspension; oral: 125, 187, 250, and 375 mg per 5 mL (*Rx*)	Various, *Ceclor* (Eli Lilly)
CEFADROXIL	
Capsules; oral: 500 mg (as monohydrate) (*Rx*)	Various
Tablets; oral: 1 g (as monohydrate) (*Rx*)	
Powder for suspension; oral: 125, 250, and 500 mg per 5 mL (*Rx*)	
CEFAZOLIN SODIUM	
Injection, powder for solution: 500 mg and 1, 5, 10, and 20 g (*Rx*)	Various
CEFDINIR	
Capsules; oral: 300 mg (*Rx*)	*Omnicef* (Abbott)
Suspension; oral: 125 mg and 5 mL, 250 mg per 5 mL (*Rx*)	Various, *Omnicef* (Abbott)
CEFDITOREN PIVOXIL	
Tablets; oral: 200 mg (*Rx*)	*Spectracef* (Purdue)
CEFEPIME HYDROCHLORIDE	
Injection, powder for solution: 500 mg and 1 and 2 g (*Rx*)	Various, *Maxipime* (Dura)
CEFIXIME	
Powder for suspension; oral: 100 and 200 mg per 5 mL (*Rx*)	*Suprax* (Lupin Pharma)
CEFOTAXIME SODIUM	
Injection, powder for solution: 500 mg, 1, 2, and 10 g (*Rx*)	Various, *Claforan* (Hoechst Marion Roussel)
Injection: 1 and 2 g (*Rx*)	
CEFOTETAN DISODIUM	
Injection, powder for solution: 1, 2, and 10 g (*Rx*)	Various
CEFOXITIN SODIUM	
Injection, powder for solution: 1, 2, and 10 g (*Rx*)	Various
CEFPODOXIME PROXETIL	
Tablets; oral: 100 and 200 mg (*Rx*)	Various, *Vantin* (Pharmacia & Upjohn)
Suspension, granules; oral: 50 and 100 mg per 5 mL (*Rx*)	Various
CEFPROZIL	
Tablets; oral: 250 and 500 mg (as anhydrous) (*Rx*)	Various
Powder for suspension; oral: 125 and 250 mg (as anhydrous) per 5 mL (*Rx*)	
CEFTAROLINE FOSAMIL	
Injection, powder for solution: 400 and 600 mg	*Teflaro* (Forest Pharmaceuticals)
CEFTAZIDIME	
Injection, powder for solution: 500 mg, 1, 2, and 6 g (*Rx*)	Various, *Fortaz* (GlaxoWellcome), *Tazidime* (Eli Lilly), *Ceptaz* (GlaxoWellcome), *Tazicef* (Hospira)
Injection: 1 and 2 g (*Rx*)	*Fortaz* (GlaxoWellcome), *Tazicef* (Hospira)
CEFTIBUTEN	
Capsules; oral: 400 mg (*Rx*)	*Cedax* (Shionogi)
Powder for suspension; oral: 90 mg per 5 mL (*Rx*)	
CEFTIZOXIME SODIUM	
Injection, powder for solution: 500 mg, 1, 2, and 10 g (as sodium) (*Rx*)	*Cefizox* (Fujisawa)
Injection: 1 and 2 g (as sodium) (*Rx*)	
CEFTRIAXONE SODIUM	
Injection, powder for solution: 250 and 500 mg, 1, 2, and 10 g (*Rx*)	Various, *Rocephin* (Roche)

CEFUROXIME	
Tablets; oral: 125, 250, and 500 mg (as axetil) (*Rx*)	Various, *Ceftin* (GlaxoWellcome)
Suspension; oral: 125 and 250 mg (as axetil) per 5 mL (when reconstituted) (*Rx*)	
Injection, powder for solution: 750 mg, 1.5 and 7.5 g (as sodium)/vial (*Rx*)	Various, *Zinacef* (GlaxoWellcome)
Injection: 750 mg and 1.5 g (as sodium) (*Rx*)	*Zinacef* (GlaxoWellcome)
CEPHALEXIN	
Capsules; oral: 250, 333, 500, and 750 mg (*Rx*)	Various, *Keflex* (Advancis)
Tablets; oral: 250 and 500 mg and 1 g (*Rx*)	Various
Powder for suspension; oral: 125 and 250 mg per 5 mL (*Rx*)	Various, *Keflex* (Advancis)

Indications

For approved indications, refer to the Administration and Dosage section.

Administration and Dosage

CEFACLOR:

Adults – Usual dosage is 250 mg every 8 hours. In severe infections or those caused by less susceptible organisms, dosage may be doubled.

Capsules: Food does not affect the extent of absorption.

Tablets, extended release: Administer with food to enhance absorption. Do not cut, crush, or chew.

Equivalence – 500 mg twice daily of cefaclor extended-release tablets is clinically equivalent to 250 mg 3 times daily of cefaclor immediate-release capsules.

Acute bacterial exacerbations of chronic bronchitis – 500 mg every 12 hours for 7 days.

Secondary bacterial infection of acute bronchitis – 500 mg every 12 hours for 7 days.

Pharyngitis or tonsillitis – 375 mg every 12 hours for 10 days.

Uncomplicated skin and skin structure infections – 375 mg every 12 hours for 7 to 10 days.

Children – Give 20 mg/kg/day in divided doses every 8 hours. In more serious infections, otitis media, and infections caused by less susceptible organisms, administer 40 mg/kg/day, with a maximum dosage of 1 g/day.

Twice-daily treatment option: For otitis media and pharyngitis, the total daily dosage may be divided and administered every 12 hours.

CEFADROXIL: Can be given without regard to meals.

Urinary tract infections – For uncomplicated lower urinary tract infection (eg, cystitis), the usual dosage is 1 or 2 g/day in single doses or 2 divided doses. For all other urinary tract infections, the usual dosage is 2 g/day in 2 divided doses.

Skin and skin structure infections – 1 g/day in single doses or 2 divided doses.

Pharyngitis and tonsillitis –

Group A β-hemolytic streptococci: 1 g/day in single doses or 2 divided doses for 10 days.

Children –

Urinary tract infections, skin and skin structure infections: 30 mg/kg/day in divided doses every 12 hours.

Pharyngitis, tonsillitis: 30 mg/kg/day in single doses or 2 divided doses. For β-hemolytic streptococcal infections, continue treatment for at least 10 days.

Renal function impairment –

Initial adult dose: 1 g: 500 mg at the intervals below.

Cefadroxil Dosage in Renal Function Impairment

CrCl[a] (mL/min)	Dosage interval (hours)
0 to 10	36
10 to 25	24
25 to 50	12
> 50	No adjustment

[a] CrCl = creatinine clearance.

CEFAZOLIN SODIUM: Total daily dosages are the same for intramuscular (IM) and intravenous (IV) administration.

Mild infections caused by susceptible gram-positive cocci – 250 to 500 mg every 8 hours.

Moderate-to-severe infections – 500 mg to 1 g every 6 to 8 hours.

Pneumococcal pneumonia – 500 mg every 12 hours.

Severe, life-threatening infections (eg, endocarditis, septicemia) – 1 to 1.5 g every 6 hours. Rarely, 12 g/day have been used.

Acute uncomplicated urinary tract infections – 1 g every 12 hours.

Perioperative prophylaxis –

Preoperative: 1 g IV or IM, ½ to 1 hour prior to surgery.

Intraoperative (at least 2 h): 0.5 to 1 g IV or IM during surgery at appropriate intervals.

Postoperative: 0.5 to 1 g IV or IM every 6 to 8 hours for 24 hours after surgery.

Renal function impairment – All reduced dosage recommendations apply after an initial loading dose appropriate to the severity of the infection.

Cefazolin Dosage in Renal Function Impairment

Serum Creatinine (mg %)	CrCl (mL/min)	Dose		Dosage interval (h)
		≤ 1.5	≥ 55	
≤ 1.5	≥ 55	250 to 500	500 to 1000	6 to 8
1.6 to 3	35 to 54	250 to 500	500 to 1000	≥ 8
3.1 to 4.5	11 to 34	125 to 250	250 to 500	12
≥ 4.6	≤ 10	125 to 250	250 to 500	18 to 24

Children –

Mild to moderately severe infections: A total daily dosage of 25 to 50 mg/kg (approximately 10 to 20 mg/lb) in 3 or 4 equal doses.

Severe infections: Total daily dosage may be increased to 100 mg/kg (45 mg/lb).

CEFDINIR:

Adults/Adolescents – Capsules may be taken without regard to meals.

Cefdinir Dosage in Adults and Adolescents (≥ 13 years of age)

Type of infection	Dosage	Duration
Community-acquired pneumonia	300 mg q 12 h	10 days
Acute exacerbations of chronic bronchitis	300 mg q 12 h or 600 mg q 24 h	5 to 10 days 10 days
Acute maxillary sinusitis	300 mg q 12 h or 600 mg q 24 h	10 days 10 days
Pharyngitis/Tonsillitis	300 mg q 12 h or 600 mg q 24 h	5 to 10 days 10 days
Uncomplicated skin and skin structure infections	300 mg q 12 h	10 days

Children (6 months to 12 years of age) – The recommended dosage in children is 14 mg/kg, up to a maximum dose of 600 mg/day. Once daily dosing for 10 days is as effective as twice-daily dosing. Once-daily dosing has not been studied in skin infections; therefore, administer oral suspension twice daily in this infection. Oral suspension may be administered without regard to meals.

Cefdinir Dosage in Children (6 Months Through 12 Years of Age)

Type of infection	Dosage	Duration
Acute bacterial otitis media	7 mg/kg q 12 h or 14 mg/kg q 24 h	5 to 10 days 10 days
Acute maxillary sinusitis	7 mg/kg q 12 h or 14 mg/kg q 24 h	10 days 10 days

Cefdinir Dosage in Children (6 Months Through 12 Years of Age)		
Type of infection	Dosage	Duration
Pharyngitis/Tonsillitis	7 mg/kg q 12 h or 14 mg/kg q 24 h	5 to 10 days 10 days
Uncomplicated skin and skin structure infections	7 mg/kg q 12 h	10 days

Cefdinir for Oral Suspension Pediatric Dosage Chart			
Weight			
kg	lb	125 mg per 5 mL	250 mg per 5 mL
9	20	2.5 mL (½ tsp) q 12 h or 5 mL (1 tsp) q 24 h	use 125 mg per 5 mL product
18	40	5 mL (1 tsp) q 12 h or 10 mL (2 tsp) q 24 h	2.5 mL q 12 h or 5 mL q 24 h
27	60	7.5 mL (1½ tsp) q 12 h or 15 mL (3 tsp) q 24 h	3.75 mL q 12 h or 7.5 mL q 24 h
36	80	10 mL (2 tsp) q 12 h or 20 mL (4 tsp) q 24 h	5 mL q 12 h or 10 mL q 24 h
≥ 43[a]	95	12 mL (2½ tsp) q 12 h or 24 mL (5 tsp) q 24 h	6 mL q 12 h or 12 mL q 24 h

[a] Children who weigh at least 43 kg should receive the maximum daily dose of 600 mg.

Renal function impairment – For adult patients with CrCl less than 30 mL/min, the dose of cefdinir should be 300 mg given once daily.

For children with a CrCl of less than 30 mL/min/1.73 m^2, the dose of cefdinir should be 7 mg/kg (300 mg or less) given once daily.

Hemodialysis – The recommended initial dosage regimen is a 300 mg or 7 mg/kg dose every other day. At the conclusion of each hemodialysis session, give 300 mg (or 7 mg/kg). Subsequent doses (300 mg or 7 mg/kg) are then administered every other day.

CEFDITOREN PIVOXIL: Take cefditoren with meals.

Cefditoren Dosage and Administration in Adults and Adolescents ≥ 12 Years of Age[a]		
Type of infection	Dosage	Duration (days)
Community-acquired pneumonia	400 mg twice daily	14
Acute bacterial exacerbation of chronic bronchitis	400 mg twice daily	10
Pharyngitis/Tonsillitis	200 mg twice daily	
Uncomplicated skin and skin structure infections		

[a] Take with meals.

Renal function impairment – It is recommended that 200 mg or less twice daily be administered to patients with moderate renal function impairment (CrCl 30 to 49 mL/min/1.73 m^2) and 200 mg every day be administered to patients with severe renal function impairment (CrCl < 30 mL/min/1.73 m^2).

CEFEPIME:

Recommended Dosage Schedule for Cefepime			
Site and type of infection	Dose	Frequency	Duration (days)
Mild to moderate uncomplicated or complicated urinary tract infections, including pyelonephritis, caused by *Escherichia coli*, *Klebsiella pneumoniae*, or *Proteus mirabilis*.[a]	0.5 to 1 g IV/IM[b]	q 12 h	7 to 10
Severe uncomplicated or complicated urinary tract infections, including pyelonephritis, caused by *E. coli* or *K. pneumoniae*.[a]	2 g IV	q 12 h	10
Moderate to severe pneumonia caused by *Streptococcus pneumoniae*,[a] *Pseudomonas aeruginosa*, *K. pneumoniae*, or *Enterobacter* sp.	1 to 2 g IV	q 12 h	10
Moderate to severe uncomplicated skin and skin structure infections caused by *Staphylococcus aureus* or *Streptococcus pyogenes*.	2 g IV	q 12 h	10
Empiric therapy for febrile neutropenic patients.	2 g IV	q 8 h	7[c]
Complicated intra-abdominal infections (used in combination with metronidazole) caused by *E. coli*, viridans group streptococci, *P. aeruginosa*, *K. pneumoniae*, *Enterobacter* species, or *Bacteroides fragilis*.	2 g IV	q 12 h	7 to 10

[a] Including cases associated with concurrent bacteremia.

[b] IM route of administration is indicated only for mild to moderate, uncomplicated, or complicated urinary tract infections caused by *E. coli* when the IM route is a more appropriate route of drug administration.

[c] Or until resolution of neutropenia. In patients whose fever resolves but who remain neutropenic for more than 7 days, frequently re-evaluate the need for continued antimicrobial therapy.

Children (2 months to 16 years of age) – Treatment of uncomplicated and complicated urinary tract infections (including pyelonephritis), uncomplicated skin and skin structure infections, pneumonia, and as empiric therapy for febrile neutropenic patients.

Complicated intra-abdominal infections – In combination with metronidazole for complicated intra-abdominal infections.

Empiric therapy for febrile neutropenic patients – As monotherapy for empiric treatment of febrile neutropenic patients. In patients at high risk for severe infection, antimicrobial monotherapy may not be appropriate. Insufficient data exist to support the efficacy of cefepime monotherapy in such patients.

Renal function impairment – In patients with renal function impairment (CrCl less than 60 mL/min), adjust the dose of cefepime to compensate for the slower rate of renal elimination. The recommended initial dose should be the same as patients with healthy renal function except in patients undergoing hemodialysis.

<table>
<tr><th colspan="5">Recommended Dosing Schedule for Cefepime in Adults by Renal Function</th></tr>
<tr><th>CrCl (mL/min)</th><th colspan="4">Recommended maintenance schedule</th></tr>
<tr><td>> 60
normal recommended dosing schedule</td><td>500 mg q 12 h</td><td>1 g q 12 h</td><td>2 g q 12 h</td><td>2 g q 8 h</td></tr>
<tr><td>30 to 60</td><td rowspan="2">500 mg q 24 h</td><td>1 g q 24 h</td><td>2 g q 24 h</td><td>2 g q 12 h</td></tr>
<tr><td>11 to 29</td><td>500 mg q 24 h</td><td>1 g q 24 h</td><td>2 g q 24 h</td></tr>
<tr><td>< 11</td><td>250 mg q 24 h</td><td>250 mg q 24 h</td><td>500 mg q 24 h</td><td>1 g q 24 h</td></tr>
<tr><td>CAPD[a]</td><td>500 mg q 48 h</td><td>1 g q 48 h</td><td>2 g q 48 h</td><td>2 g q 48 h</td></tr>
<tr><td>Hemodialysis[b]</td><td colspan="3">1 g on day 1, then 500 mg q 24 h thereafter</td><td>1 g q 24 h</td></tr>
</table>

[a] CAPD = Continuous ambulatory peritoneal dialysis.

[b] On hemodialysis days, cefepime should be administered following hemodialysis. Whenever possible, cefepime should be administered at the same time each day.

IV administration – Administer over approximately 30 minutes. Reconstitute with 50 or 100 mL of a compatible IV fluid. Cefepime is compatible at concentrations of 1 to 40 mg/mL with 0.9% sodium chloride Injection, 5% and 10% dextrose injection, M/6 sodium lactate injection, 5% dextrose and 0.9% sodium chloride injection, lactated ringers and 5% dextrose injection, *Normosol-R* or *Normosol-M* in 5% dextrose injection.

Cefepime Admixture Stability

Cefepime concentration (mg/mL)	Admixture and concentration	IV Infusion solutions	Stability time for RT/L[a] (20° to 25°C) (hours)	Stability time for refrigeration (2° to 8°C)
40	Amikacin 6 mg/mL	NS[b] or D5W[c]	24	7 days
40	Ampicillin 1 mg/mL	D5W[c]	8	8 h
40	Ampicillin 10 mg/mL	D5W[c]	2	8 h
40	Ampicillin 1 mg/mL	NS[b]	24	48 h
40	Ampicillin 10 mg/mL	NS[b]	8	48 h
4	Ampicillin 40 mg/mL	NS[b]	8	8 h
4 to 40	Clindamycin phosphate 0.25 to 6 mg/mL	NS[b] or D5W[c]	24	7 days
4	Heparin 10 to 50 units/mL	NS[b] or D5W[c]	24	7 days
4	Potassium chloride 10 to 40 mEq/L	NS[b] or D5W[c]	24	7 days
4	Theophylline 0.8 mg/mL	D5W[c]	24	7 days
1 to 4	na	*Aminosyn II* 4.25% with electrolytes and calcium	8	3 days
0.125 to 0.25	na	*Inpersol* with 4.25% dextrose	24	7 days

[a] Ambient room temperature and light.
[b] 0.9% sodium chloride injection.
[c] 5% dextrose injection.

Admixture compatibility/incompatibility: Solutions of cefepime should not be added to metronidazole, vancomycin, gentamicin, tobramycin, netilmicin sulfate, or aminophylline.

IM administration: Reconstitute cefepime with the following diluents: sterile water for injection, 0.9% sodium chloride, 5% dextrose injection, 0.5% or 1% lidocaine hydrochloride, or sterile bacteriostatic water for injection with parabens or benzyl alcohol.

Pediatric dosing: The usual recommended daily dosage in children up to 40 kg in weight is 50 mg/kg/dose administered every 12 hours (every 8 hours for febrile neutropenic patients), for 7 to 10 days, depending on the indication and severity of infection. The maximum dose for children (2 months to 16 years of age) should not exceed the recommended adult dose.

Renal function impairment – Data in children with renal function impairment are not available; however, because cefepime pharmacokinetics are similar in adult and children, changes in dosing regimen similar to those in adults are recommended for children.

CEFIXIME:

Adults – 400 mg daily. For the treatment of uncomplicated cervical/urethral gonococcal infections, a single oral dose of 400 mg is recommended.

Children – The recommended dose is 8 mg/kg/day of the suspension. This may be administered as a single daily dose or may be given in 2 divided doses, as 4 mg/kg every 12 hours.

Pediatric Dosage Chart					
		100 mg per 5 mL suspension		200 mg per 5 mL suspension	
Patient weight (kg)	Dose/day (mg)	Dose/day (mL)	Dose/day (5 mL of suspension)	Dose/day (mL)	Dose/day (5 mL of suspension)
6.25	50	2.5	0.5	1.25	0.25
12.5	100	5	1	2.5	0.5
18.75	150	7.5	1.5	3.75	0.75
25	200	10	2	5	1
31.25	250	12.5	2.5	6.25	1.25
37.5	300	15	3	7.5	1.5

Children weighing more than 50 kg or older than 12 years of age should be treated with the recommended adult dose.

In the treatment of infections due to *S. pyogenes*, a therapeutic dosage of cefixime should be administered for at least 10 days.

Renal function impairment –

Cefixime Dosage in Renal Function Impairment	
CrCl (mL/min)	Dosage
> 60	standard
21 to 60 or renal hemodialysis	75% of standard
< 20 or continuous ambulatory peritoneal dialysis	50% of standard

Neither hemodialysis nor peritoneal dialysis removes significant amounts of drug from the body.

CEFOTAXIME SODIUM:

Adults –

Cefotaxime Dosage Guidelines for Adults		
Type of infection	Daily dosage (g)	Frequency and route
Gonococcal urethritis/ cervicitis in men and women	0.5	0.5 g IM (single dose)
Rectal gonorrhea in women	0.5	0.5 g IM (single dose)
Rectal gonorrhea in men	1	1 g IM (single dose)
Uncomplicated infections	2	1 g every 12 h IM or IV
Moderate to severe infections	3 to 6	1 to 2 g every 8 h IM or IV
Infections commonly needing higher dosage (eg, septicemia)	6 to 8	2 g every 6 to 8 h IV
Life-threatening infections	≤ 12	2 g every 4 h IV

Premixed injection: Premixed cefotaxime injection is intended for IV administration after thawing.

Powder for injection: Cefotaxime sterile powder for injection may be administered IM or IV after reconstitution.

Perioperative prophylaxis: 1 g IV or IM, 30 to 90 minutes prior to surgery.

Cesarean section: Administer the first 1 g dose IV as soon as the umbilical cord is clamped. Administer the second and third doses as 1 g IV or IM at 6- and 12-hour intervals after the first dose.

Children –

Cefotaxime Dosage Guidelines in Children			
Age	Weight (kg)	Dosage schedule	Route
0 to 1 week	-	50 mg/kg every 12 h	IV
1 to 4 weeks	-	50 mg/kg every 8 h	IV
1 month to 12 years	< 50[a]	50 to 180 mg/kg/day in 4 to 6 divided doses[b]	IV or IM

[a] For children at least 50 kg, use adult dosage.
[b] Use higher doses for more severe or serious infections including meningitis.

Renal function impairment – In patients with estimated CrCl less than 20 mL/min/1.73 m^2, reduce dosage by 50%.

The serum creatinine should represent steady-state renal function.

CDC-recommended treatment schedules for gonorrhea –

Uncomplicated gonococcal infections of the cervix, urethra, and rectum: 500 mg IM.

Disseminated gonococcal infection: 1 g IV every 8 hours.

Disseminated gonococcal infection and gonococcal scalp abscesses in newborns: 25 mg/kg IV or IM every 12 hours for 7 days, with a duration of 10 to 14 days if meningitis is documented.

Administration –

Intermittent IV: A solution containing 1 or 2 g in 10 mL of sterile water for injection can be injected over a period of 3 to 5 minutes.

Duration of treatment – A minimum of 10 days of treatment is recommended for infections caused by group A beta-hemolytic streptococci.

Admixture incompatibility – Solution of cefotaxime must not be admixed with aminoglycoside solutions.

CEFOTETAN DISODIUM:

Adults – The usual dosage is 1 or 2 g IV or IM or cefotetan injection in the *Galaxy* plastic container (PL 2040) administered IV every 12 hours for 5 to 10 days. Determine proper dosage and route of administration by the condition of the patient, severity of the infection, and susceptibility of the causative organism.

General Cefotetan Dosage Guidelines		
Type of infection	Daily dose	Frequency and route
Urinary tract	1 to 4 g	500 mg every 12 h IV or IM
Skin/Skin structure		2 g q 24 h IV
Mild to moderate[a]	2 g	1 g q 12 h IV or IM
Severe	4 g	2 g q 12 h IV
Other sites	2 to 4 g	1 or 2 g every 12 h IV or IM
Severe	4 g	2 g every 12 h IV
Life-threatening	6 g[b]	3 g every 12 h IV

[a] Treat *K. pneumoniae* skin and skin structure infections with 1 or 2 g every 12 hours IV or IM.
[b] Maximum daily dosage should not exceed 6 g.

Prophylaxis – To prevent postoperative infection in clean contaminated or potentially contaminated surgery in adults, give a single 1 or 2 g IV dose 30 to 60 minutes prior to surgery. In patients undergoing cesarean section, give the dose as soon as the umbilical cord is clamped.

Renal function impairment – Reduce the dosage schedule using the following guidelines:

Cefotetan Dosage in Renal Function Impairment		
CrCl (mL/min)	Dose	Frequency
> 30	Usual recommended dose[a]	Every 12 h
10 to 30	Usual recommended dose[a]	Every 24 h
< 10	Usual recommended dose[a]	Every 48 h

[a] Dose determined by the type and severity of infection and susceptibility of the causative organism.

Alternatively, the dosing interval may remain constant at 12-hour intervals, but reduce dose by ½ for patients with a CrCl of 10 to 30 mL/min, and by ¼ for patients with a CrCl less than 10 mL/min.

Dialysis – Cefotetan is dialyzable; for patients undergoing intermittent hemodialysis, give ¼ of the usual recommended dose every 24 hours on days between dialysis and ½ of the usual recommended dose on the day of dialysis.

IV administration – The IV route is preferable for patients with bacteremia, bacterial septicemia, or other severe or life-threatening infections, or for patients who may be risks because of lowered resistance resulting from such debilitating conditions as malnutrition, trauma, surgery, diabetes, heart failure, or malignancy, particularly if shock is present or impending.

Intermittent IV administration: 3 to 5 minutes.

Galaxy containers: 20 to 60 minutes.

Admixture incompatibility – Solutions of cefotetan must not be admixed with solutions containing aminoglycosides. Do not add supplementary medications.

CEFOXITIN SODIUM:

Adult – Adult dosage range is 1 to 2 g every 6 to 8 hours.

Cefoxitin Dosage Guidelines

Type of infection	Daily dosage	Frequency and route
Uncomplicated (pneumonia, urinary tract, cutaneous)[a]	3 to 4 g	1 g every 6 to 8 h IV or IM
Moderately severe or severe	6 to 8 g	1 g every 4 h or 2 g every 6 to 8 h IV
Infections commonly requiring higher dosage (eg, gas gangrene)	12 g	2 g every 4 h or 3 g every 6 h IV

[a] Including patients in whom bacteremia is absent or unlikely.

Streptococcal infections – Antibiotic therapy for group A beta-hemolytic streptococcal infections should be maintained for at least 10 days.

Prophylactic use, surgery – Administer 2 g IV or IM 30 to 60 minutes prior to surgery followed by 2 g every 6 hours after the first dose for no more than 24 hours.

Prophylactic use, cesarean section – Administer 2 g IV as soon as the umbilical cord is clamped. If a 3-dose regimen is used, give the second and third 2 g dose IV, 4 and 8 hours after the first dose.

Administration – 3 to 5 minutes.

Admixture incompatibilities – Should not be added to aminoglycoside solutions.

Renal function impairment –

Adults: Initial loading dose is 1 to 2 g. Maintenance doses:

Maintenance Cefoxitin Dosage in Renal Function Impairment

Renal function	CrCl (mL/min/1.73 m^2)	Dose (g)	Frequency (h)
Mild impairment	30 to 50	1 to 2	8 to 12
Moderate impairment	10 to 29	1 to 2	12 to 24
Severe impairment	5 to 9	0.5 to 1	12 to 24
Essentially no function	< 5	0.5 to 1	24 to 48

Hemodialysis – Administer a loading dose of 1 to 2 g after each hemodialysis. Give the maintenance dose as indicated in the previous table.

Infants and children 3 months of age and older: 80 to 160 mg/kg/day divided every 4 to 6 hours. Use higher dosages for more severe or serious infections. Do not exceed 12 g/day.

Prophylactic use (at least 3 months) – 30 to 40 mg/kg/dose every 6 hours.

Renal function impairment – Modify consistent with recommendation for adults.

CEFPODOXIME PROXETIL: Administer with food.

Cefpodoxime Dosing in Adults and Adolescents (12 Years of Age and Older)			
Type of infection	Total daily dose	Dose frequency	Duration
Pharyngitis and/or tonsillitis	200 mg	100 mg every 12 h	5 to 10 days
Acute community-acquired pneumonia	400 mg	200 mg every 12 h	14 days
Uncomplicated gonorrhea (men and women) and rectal gonococcal infections (women)	200 mg	single dose	
Skin and skin structure	800 mg	400 mg every 12 h	7 to 14 days
Acute maxillary sinusitis	400 mg	200 mg every 12 h	10 days
Uncomplicated urinary tract infection	200 mg	100 mg every 12 h	7 days
Infants and children (2 months through 12 years of age):			
Acute otitis media	10 mg/kg/day (max 400 mg/day)	5 mg/kg every 12 hours (max 200 mg dose)	5 days
Pharyngitis and/or tonsillitis	10 mg/kg/day (max 200 mg/day)	5 mg/kg/dose every 12 hours (max 100 mg/dose)	5 to 10 days
Acute maxillary sinusitis	10 mg/kg/day (max 400 mg/day)	5 mg/kg every 12 hours (max 200 mg/dose)	10 days

Renal function impairment – For patients with severe renal function impairment (CrCl less than 30 mL/min), increase the dosing intervals to every 24 hours. In patients maintained on hemodialysis, use a frequency of 3 times per week after hemodialysis.

CEFPROZIL:

Cefprozil Dosage and Duration		
Population/Infection	Dosage (mg)	Duration (days)
Adults (≥ 13 years of age)		
Pharyngitis/Tonsillitis	500 q 24 h	10[a]
Acute sinusitis (use higher dose for moderate to severe infections)	250 q 12 h or 500 q 12 h	10
Secondary bacterial infection of acute bronchitis and acute bacterial exacerbation of chronic bronchitis	500 q 12 h	10
Uncomplicated skin and skin structure infections	250 q 12 h, 500 q 24 h, or 500 q 12 h	10
Children (2 to 12 years of age)[b]		
Pharyngitis/Tonsillitis	7.5 mg/kg q 12 h	10[a]
Uncomplicated skin and skin structure infections	20 mg/kg q 24 h	10
Infants and children (6 months to 12 years of age)[b]		
Otitis media	15 mg/kg q 12 h	10
Acute sinusitis (use higher dose for moderate to severe infections)	7.5 mg/kg q 12 h or 15 mg/kg q 12 h	10

[a] For infections caused by *S. pyogenes*, administer for at least 10 days.
[b] Not to exceed adult recommended doses.

Renal function impairment – For CrCl of 30 to 120 mL/min, use standard dosage and dosing interval. For CrCl less than 30 mL/min, use a dosage 50% of standard at the standard dosing interval.

Cefprozil is in part removed by hemodialysis; therefore, administer after the completion of hemodialysis.

CEFTAROLINE FOSAMIL:

Acute bacterial skin and skin structure infection – 600 mg intravenous (IV) every 12 hours for 5 to 14 days.

Community-acquired bacterial pneumonia – 600 mg IV every 12 hours for 5 to 7 days.

Elderly – Dosage adjustment should be based on renal function.

Renal function impairment –

Ceftaroline Fosamil Injection Dosage in Renal Impairment	
Estimated CrCl[a] (mL/min)	Ceftaroline fosamil recommended dosage regimen
> 50 mL/min	No dosage adjustment necessary
> 30 to ≤ 50 mL/min	400 mg IV every 12 hours
≥ 15 to ≤ 30 mL/min	300 mg IV every 12 hours
ESRD including hemodialysis[b]	200 mg IV every 12 hours[c]

[a] Creatinine clearance (CrCl) estimated using the Cockcroft-Gault formula.
[b] End-stage renal disease (ESRD) is defined as CrCl < 15 mL/min.
[c] Ceftaroline fosamil is hemodialyzable; therefore, ceftaroline should be administered after hemodialysis on hemodialysis days.

Administration – Administer by IV infusion over 1 hour.

Admixture compatibility – Ceftaroline fosamil should not be mixed with or physically added to solutions containing other drugs.

CEFTAZIDIME:

Ceftazidime Dosage Guidelines		
Patient/Infection site	Dose	Frequency
Adults		
Usual recommended dose	1 g IV or IM	q 8 to 12 h
Uncomplicated urinary tract infections	250 mg IV or IM	q 12 h
Complicated urinary tract infections	500 mg IV or IM	q 8 to 12 h
Uncomplicated pneumonia; mild skin and skin structure infections	500 mg to 1 g IV or IM	q 8 h
Bone and joint infections	2 g IV	q 12 h
Serious gynecological and intra-abdominal infections		
Meningitis	2 g IV	q 8 h
Very severe life-threatening infections, especially in immunocompromised patients		
Pseudomonal lung infections in cystic fibrosis patients with normal renal function[a]	30 to 50 mg/kg IV up to 6 g/day	q 8 h
Neonates (0 to 4 weeks)	30 mg/kg IV	q 12 h
Infants and children (1 month to 12 years of age)	30 to 50 mg/kg IV up to 6 g/day[b]	q 8 h

[a] Although clinical improvement has been shown, bacteriological cures cannot be expected in patients with chronic respiratory disease and cystic fibrosis.
[b] Reserve the higher dose for immunocompromised children or children with cystic fibrosis or meningitis.

Renal function impairment – In patients with suspected renal function impairment, give an initial loading dose of 1 g.

Ceftazidime Dosage in Renal Function Impairment		
CrCl (mL/min)	Recommended unit dose of ceftazidime	Frequency of dosing
31 to 50	1 g	q 12 h
16 to 30	1 g	q 24 h
6 to 15	500 mg	q 24 h
≤ 5	500 mg	q 48 h

In patients with severe infections who would normally receive 6 g ceftazidime daily were it not for renal function impairment, the unit dose given in the previous table may be increased by 50% or the dosing frequency increased appropriately.

Dialysis –

Hemodialysis: 1 g loading dose, followed by 1 g after each hemodialysis period.

CAPD and Intraperitoneal dialysis: 1 g loading dose followed by 500 mg every 24 hours. In addition to IV use, ceftazidime can be incorporated in the dialysis fluid at a concentration of 250 mg per 2 L of dialysis fluid.

IM administration – Constitute with one of the following diluents: sterile water for injection, bacteriostatic water for injection, or 0.5% or 1% lidocaine hydrochloride injection.

Intermittent IV administration: 3 to 5 minutes.

Intermittent IV infusion: Discontinue the other solution.

Admixture incompatibility – Do not add to solutions of aminoglycoside antibiotics.

CEFTIBUTEN: Ceftibuten suspension must be administered at least 2 hours before or 1 hour after a meal.

Ceftibuten Dosage and Duration

Type of infection	Daily maximum dose	Dose and frequency	Duration
Adults ≥ 12 years of age			
Acute bacterial exacerbations of chronic bronchitis caused by *H. influenzae, M. catarrhalis,* or *Streptococcus pneumoniae*	400 mg	400 mg/day	10 days
Pharyngitis and tonsillitis caused by *S. pyogenes*			
Acute bacterial otitis media caused by *H. influenzae, M. catarrhalis,* or *S. pyogenes*			
Children			
Pharyngitis and tonsillitis caused by *S. pyogenes*	400 mg	9 mg/kg/day	10 days
Acute bacterial otitis media caused by *H. influenzae, M. catarrhalis,* or *S. pyogenes*			

Ceftibuten Oral Suspension Pediatric Dosage Chart[a]

Weight (kg)	Weight (lb)	90 mg/5 mL
10	22	5 mL (1 tsp)/day
20	44	10 mL (2 tsp)/day
40	88	20 mL (4 tsp)/day

[a] Children greater than 45 kg should receive the maximum daily dose of 400 mg.

Renal function impairment – Ceftibuten may be given at normal doses in patients with renal function impairment with CrCl of at least 50 mL/min. Dosing recommendations for patients with varying degrees of renal function impairment are presented in the following table.

Ceftibuten Dosage in Renal Function Impairment

CrCl (mL/min)	Recommended dosing schedules
> 50	9 mg/kg or 400 mg q 24 h (normal dosing schedule)
30 to 49	4.5 mg/kg or 200 mg q 24 h
5 to 29	2.25 mg/kg or 100 mg q 24 h

Hemodialysis patients – In patients undergoing hemodialysis 2 or 3 times weekly, a single 400 mg dose of ceftibuten capsules or a single dose of 9 mg/kg (maximum of 400 mg) oral suspension may be given at the end of each hemodialysis session.

CEFTIZOXIME SODIUM:

Adults – Usual dosage is 1 or 2 g every 8 to 12 hours.

Ceftizoxime Dosage Guidelines in Adults		
Type of infection	Daily dose (g)	Frequency and route
Uncomplicated urinary tract	1	500 mg every 12 h IM or IV
Pelvic inflammatory disease (PID)[a]	6	2 g every 8 h IV
Other sites	2 to 3	1 g every 8 to 12 h IV or IM
Severe or refractory	3 to 6	1 g every 8 hours IM or IV 2 g every 8 to 12 h IM [a] or IV
Life-threatening[b]	9 to 12	3 to 4 g every 8 h IV

[a] Dosages up to 2 g every 4 hours have been given.
[b] Divide 2 g IM doses and give in different large muscle masses.

Urinary tract infections – Because of the serious nature of urinary tract infections caused by *P. aeruginosa* and because many strains of *Pseudomonas* species are only moderately susceptible to ceftizoxime, higher dosage is recommended.

Gonorrhea, uncomplicated – A single 1 g IM injection is the usual dose.

Life-threatening infections – The IV route may be preferable for patients with bacterial septicemia, localized parenchymal abscesses, peritonitis, or other severe or life-threatening infections.

In conditions such as bacterial septicemia, 6 to 12 g/day IV may be given initially for several days, and the dosage gradually reduced according to clinical response and laboratory findings.

Renal function impairment – Following an initial loading dose of 500 mg to 1 g IM or IV, use the maintenance dosing schedule in the following table.

Hemodialysis: No additional supplemental dosing is required following hemodialysis; give the dose (according to the following table) at the end of dialysis.

Ceftizoxime Dosage in Adults with Renal Function Impairment			
Renal function	CrCl (mL/min)	Less severe infections	Life-threatening infections
Mild impairment	50 to 79	500 mg q 8 h	750 mg to 1.5 g q 8 h
Moderate to severe impairment	5 to 49	250 to 500 mg q 12 h	500 mg to 1 g q 12 h
Dialysis patients	0 to 4	500 mg q 48 h or 250 mg q 24 h	500 mg to 1 g q 48 h or 500 mg q 24 h

Pediatric –

Children (6 months of age and older): 50 mg/kg every 6 to 8 hours. Dosage may be increased to 200 mg/kg/day. Do not exceed the maximum adult dose for serious infection.

Compatibility –

IV administration: Slowly over 3 to 5 minutes. 50 to 100 mL of 1 of the following solutions: sodium chloride injection, 5% or 10% dextrose injection, 5% dextrose and 0.9%, 0.45%, or 0.2% sodium chloride injection, ringer's injection, lactated ringer's injection, invert sugar 10% in sterile water for injection, 5% sodium bicarbonate in sterile water for injection, 5% dextrose in lactated Ringer's injection (only when reconstituted with 4% sodium bicarbonate injection).

CEFTRIAXONE SODIUM:

Administration – Administer IV or IM.

IV: Administer IV by infusion over a period of 30 minutes.

Admixture incompatibility – Ceftriaxone has been shown to be compatible with metronidazole hydrochloride injection. No compatibility studies have been conducted with the *Flagyl IV RUT* (metronidazole) formulation or using other diluents. Metronidazole at concentrations greater than 8 mg/mL will precipitate.

Vancomycin and fluconazole are physically incompatible with ceftriaxone in admixtures.

Adults – Usual daily dosage is 1 to 2 g once a day (or in equally divided doses twice a day) depending on type and severity of infection. Do not exceed a total daily dose of 4 g.

Uncomplicated gonococcal infections: Give a single IM dose of 250 mg.

Surgical prophylaxis: Give a single 1 g dose ½ to 2 hours before surgery.

Children – For serious infections other than meningitis, administer 50 to 75 mg/kg/day (not to exceed 2 g) every 12 hours.

Meningitis: 100 mg/kg/day (not to exceed 4 g). Thereafter, a total daily dose of 100 mg/kg/day (not to exceed 4 g/day) is recommended. May give daily dose once per day or in divided doses every 12 hours. Usual duration is 7 to 14 days.

Skin and skin structure infections: Give 50 to 75 mg/kg once daily (or in divided doses twice daily), not to exceed 2 g.

Streptococcal infections: When treating infections caused by *S. pyogenes*, therapy should be continued for at least 10 days.

CEFUROXIME:

Oral – Tablets and suspension are not bioequivalent and not substitutable on a mg/mg basis.

Tablets: Tablets may be given without regard to meals.

Suspension: Administer with food.

Dosage for Cefuroxime Axetil Tablets

Population/Infection	Dosage	Duration (days)
Adults (≥ 13 years of age)		
Pharyngitis/Tonsillitis	250 mg twice daily	10
Acute bacterial maxillary sinusitis	250 mg twice daily	10
Acute bacterial exacerbations of chronic bronchitis[a]	250 or 500 mg twice daily	10
Secondary bacterial infections of acute bronchitis	250 or 500 mg twice daily	5 to 10
Uncomplicated skin and skin structure infections	250 or 500 mg twice daily	10
Uncomplicated urinary tract infections	250 mg twice daily	7 to 10
Uncomplicated gonorrhea	1,000 mg once	single dose
Early Lyme disease	500 mg twice daily	20
Children who can swallow tablets whole[b]		
Acute otitis media	250 mg twice daily	10
Acute bacterial maxillary sinusitis	250 mg twice daily	10

[a] Safety and efficacy of drug administered less than 10 days in patients with acute exacerbations of chronic bronchitis have not been established.

[b] Do not exceed adult recommended doses.

Dosage for Cefuroxime Axetil Suspension

Population/Infection	Dosage	Daily maximum dose	Duration (days)
Infants and children (3 months to 12 years of age)			
Pharyngitis/Tonsillitis	20 mg/kg/day divided twice daily	500 mg	10
Acute otitis media	30 mg/kg/day divided twice daily	1,000 mg	10
Acute bacterial maxillary sinusitis	30 mg/kg/day divided twice daily	1,000 mg	10
Impetigo	30 mg/kg/day divided twice daily	1,000 mg	10

Renal failure: Because cefuroxime is renally eliminated, its half-life will be prolonged in patients with renal failure.

Parenteral –

Dosage:

Adults – 750 mg to 1.5 g IM or IV every 8 hours, usually for 5 to 10 days.

Cefuroxime Dosage Guidelines		
Type of infection	Daily dosage (g)	Frequency
Uncomplicated urinary tract, skin and skin structure, disseminated gonococcal, uncomplicated pneumonia	2.25	750 mg every 8 h
Severe or complicated	4.5	1.5 g every 8 h
Bone and joint	4.5	1.5 g every 8 h
Life-threatening or caused by less susceptible organisms	6	1.5 g every 6 h
Bacterial meningitis	9	≤ 3 g every 8 h
Uncomplicated gonococcal	1.5 g IM[a]	single dose

[a] Administered at 2 different sites together with 1 g oral probenecid.

Preoperative prophylaxis: For clean-contaminated or potentially contaminated surgical procedures, administer 1.5 g IV prior to surgery (approximately ½ to 1 hour before). Thereafter, give 750 mg IV or IM every 8 hours when the procedure is prolonged.

For preventative use during open heart surgery, give 1.5 g IV at the induction of anesthesia and every 12 hours thereafter for a total of 6 g.

Renal function impairment: Reduce dosage.

Parenteral Cefuroxime Dosage in Renal Function Impairment (Adults)	
CrCl (mL/min)	Dose and frequency
> 20	750 mg to 1.5 g every 8 h
10 to 20	750 mg every 12 h
< 10	750 mg every 24 h [a]

[a] Because cefuroxime is dialyzable, give patients on hemodialysis a further dose at the end of the dialysis.

Infants and children (3 months of age and older) – 50 to 100 mg/kg/day in equally divided doses every 6 to 8 hours. Use 100 mg/kg/day (not to exceed the maximum adult dose) for more severe or serious infections.

Bone and joint infections: 150 mg/kg/day (not to exceed maximum adult dose) in equally divided doses every 8 hours.

Bacterial meningitis: Initially, 200 to 240 mg/kg/day IV in divided doses every 6 to 8 hours.

In renal function impairment, modify dosage frequency per adult guidelines.

CEPHALEXIN:

Adults – 1 to 4 g/day in divided doses.

Usual dose: 250 mg every 6 hours.

Streptococcal pharyngitis, skin and skin structure infections, uncomplicated cystitis in patients older than 15 years of age: 500 mg every 12 hours.

May need larger doses for more severe infections or less susceptible organisms. If dose is greater than 4 g/day, use parenteral drugs.

Children – Do not exceed adult recommended doses.

Monohydrate: 25 to 50 mg/kg/day in divided doses. For streptococcal pharyngitis in patients older than 1 year of age and for skin and skin structure infections, divide total daily dose and give every 12 hours. In severe infections, double the dose.

Otitis media – 75 to 100 mg/kg/day in 4 divided doses.

β-hemolytic streptococcal infections – Continue treatment for at least 10 days.

Actions

Pharmacology: Cephalosporins are structurally and pharmacologically related to penicillins. **Cefoxitin** and **cefotetan** (cephamycins) are included because of their similarity.

Cephalosporins inhibit mucopeptide synthesis in the bacterial cell wall, making it defective and osmotically unstable. The drugs are usually bactericidal, depending on organism susceptibility, dose, tissue concentrations, and the rate at which organisms are multiplying. They are more effective against rapidly growing organisms forming cell walls.

Pharmacokinetics:

Pharmacokinetic Parameters of Cephalosporins

			Half-Life						
	Drug	Routes	Normal renal function (minutes)	ESRD[a] (hours)	Hemodialysis (hours)	Protein bound (%)	Recovered unchanged in urine (%)	Peak serum level 1 g IV dose (mcg/mL)	Sodium (mEq/g)
First	Cefadroxil	Oral	78-96	20-25	3-4	20	> 90	—	—
	Cefazolin	IM-IV	90–120	3-7	9-14	80-86	60-80	185	2-2.1
	Cephalexin	Oral	50-80	19-22	4-6	10	> 90	—	—
Second	Cefaclor	Oral	35-54	2-3	1.6-2.1	25	60-85	—	—
	Cefotetan	IM-IV	180-276	13-35	5	88-90	51-81	158	3.5
	Cefoxitin	IV	40-60	20	4	73	85	110	2.3
	Cefprozil	Oral	78	5.2-5.9	decreased	36	60	—	—
	Cefuroxime	Oral/IM-IV	80	16-22[b]	3.5	50	66-100	100[c]	2.4[b]
Third	Cefdinir	Oral	100	16	3.2	60-70	12-18	—	—
	Cefepime	IM-IV	102-138	17-21	11-16	20	85	79	—
	Cefotaxime	IM-IV	60	3-11	2.5	30-40	60	42-102	2.2
	Cefpodoxime[d]	Oral	120-180	9.8	—	21-29	29-33	—	—
	Ceftazidime	IM-IV	114-120	14-30	—	< 10	80-90	69-90	2.3
	Ceftibuten	Oral	144	13.4-22.3	2-4	65	56	—	—
	Ceftizoxime	IM-IV	102	25-30	6	30	80	60-87	2.6
	Ceftriaxone	IM-IV	348-522	15.7	14.7	85-95	33-67	151	3.6

[a] ESRD = End stage renal disease (CrCl < 10 mL/min/1.73 m^2).
[b] Injection only.
[c] Following 1.5 g IV dose.
[d] Extended spectrum agent.

Cephalexin, cefaclor, cefprozil, cefadroxil, and **ceftibuten** are well absorbed from the GI tract. Cephalosporins are widely distributed to most tissues and fluids. First and second generation agents do not readily enter cerebrospinal fluid (CSF), except **cefuroxime**, even when meninges are inflamed. Third generation compounds readily diffuse into the CSF of patients with inflamed meninges. Most cephalosporins and metabolites are primarily excreted renally.

Microbiology:

Organisms Generally Susceptible to Cephalosporins

✓ = generally susceptible
‡ = demonstrated in vitro activity

	Organisms	First generation			Second generation					Third generation								Organisms
		Cefadroxil	Cefazolin	Cephalexin	Cefaclor	Cefoxitin	Cefuroxime	Cefotetan	Cefprozil	Cefdinir	Cefepime[a]	Cefotaxime	Cefpodoxime[b]	Ceftazidime	Ceftibuten	Ceftizoxime	Ceftriaxone	
Gram-positive	*Staphylococci*[c]	✓	✓	✓[d]	✓[d]	✓	✓	✓	✓	✓[e]	✓[f]	✓[e]	✓[d]	✓		✓	✓	*Staphylococci*[c]
	Staphylococcus aureus									✓[e]								*Staphylococcus aureus*
	Staphylococcus epidermidis						‡			‡[f]								*Staphylococcus epidermidis*
	Staphylococcus saprophyticus						‡											*Staphylococcus saprophyticus*
	Streptococci, beta-hemolytic	✓	✓	✓	✓	✓	✓	✓	✓		‡	✓	✓	✓		✓	✓	*Streptococci*, beta-hemolytic
	Streptococcus agalactiae						‡			‡								*Streptococcus agalactiae*
	Streptococcus bovis																	*Streptococcus bovis*
	Streptococcus pneumoniae	✓	✓	✓	✓	✓	✓	✓	✓	✓[g]	✓	✓	✓	✓	✓[g]	✓	✓	*Streptococcus pneumoniae*
	Streptococcus pyogenes				✓		✓	✓	✓	✓	✓[h]	✓	✓	✓	✓	✓	✓	*Streptococcus pyogenes*
	Streptococcus viridans									‡								*Streptococcus viridans*
Gram-negative	*Acinetobacter* sp.										‡	✓		‡		✓	‡	*Acinetobacter* sp
	Citrobacter sp.						✓[d]	‡	‡	‡	‡	✓	‡	✓		‡	‡	*Citrobacter* sp
	Enterobacter sp.		✓[d]				✓[d]	✓			✓	✓		✓		✓	✓	*Enterobacter* sp
	Escherichia coli	✓	✓	✓	✓	✓	✓	✓	‡	‡	✓	✓	✓	✓		✓	✓	*Escherichia coli*
	Haemophilus influenzae		✓	✓	✓[e]	✓[e]	✓[e]	✓[e]	✓[e]	✓[e]	‡[e]	✓[e]	✓[e]	✓[e]	✓[e]	✓[e]	✓[e]	*Haemophilus influenzae*
	Haemophilus parainfluenzae				‡		‡			✓[e]		✓	‡	‡			✓	*Haemophilus parainfluenzae*
	Hafnia alvei										‡							*Hafnia alvei*
	Klebsiella sp.	✓	✓	✓	✓	✓	✓	✓	‡	‡	✓	✓	✓	✓		✓	✓	*Klebsiella* sp
	Klebsiella pneumoniae				‡													*Klebsiella pneumoniae*
	Moraxella (Branhamella) catarrhalis	‡		‡	✓[e]		‡	‡	✓[e]	✓[e]	‡[e]		✓	✓	✓[e]	‡		*Moraxella (Branhamella) catarrhalis*
	Morganella (Proteus) morganii					✓	✓[d]	✓			‡	✓		‡		✓	✓	*Morganella (Proteus) morganii*

Organisms Generally Susceptible to Cephalosporins																			
Organisms		First generation			Second generation					Third generation								Organisms	
✓ = generally susceptible ‡ = demonstrated in vitro activity		Cefadroxil	Cefazolin	Cephalexin	Cefaclor	Cefoxitin	Cefuroxime	Cefotetan	Cefprozil	Cefdinir	Cefepime[a]	Cefotaxime	Cefpodoxime[b]	Ceftazidime	Ceftibuten	Ceftizoxime	Ceftriaxone	✓ = generally susceptible ‡ = demonstrated in vitro activity	
Gram-negative (con't)	*Neisseria catarrhalis*			✓														*Neisseria catarrhalis*	Gram-negative (con't)
	Neisseria gonorrhoeae				‡	✓	✓	‡	‡			✓	✓[d]	‡		✓	✓	*Neisseria gonorrhoeae*	
	Neisseria meningitidis						✓					✓		✓		‡	✓	*Neisseria meningitidis*	
	Pasteurella multocida																	*Pasteurella multocida*	
	Proteus inconstans						‡											*Proteus inconstans*	
	Proteus mirabilis	✓	✓	✓	✓	✓	✓	✓	‡	‡	✓	✓	✓	✓		✓	✓	*Proteus mirabilis*	
	Proteus vulgaris					✓		✓			‡	✓	‡	✓		✓	✓	*Proteus vulgaris*	
	Providencia sp.					✓	✓	✓			‡	‡		‡		‡	‡	*Providencia* sp	
	Providencia rettgeri					✓	✓	✓			‡	✓	‡	‡		✓	‡	*Providencia rettgeri*	
	Pseudomonas aeruginosa										✓	✓[d]		✓		✓[d]	✓[d]	*Pseudomonas aeruginosa*	
	Salmonella sp.						✓	‡	‡			‡		‡		‡	‡	*Salmonella* sp	
	Salmonella typhi											‡				‡	‡	*Salmonella typhi*	
	Serratia sp.							‡			‡	✓		✓		✓	✓	*Serratia* sp	
	Shigella sp.						✓	‡	‡			‡		‡		‡	‡	*Shigella* sp	
	Yersinia enterocolitica							✓										*Yersinia enterocolitica*	

Organisms Generally Susceptible to Cephalosporins

Organisms		First generation			Second generation					Third generation								Organisms	
✓ = generally susceptible ‡ = demonstrated in vitro activity		Cefadroxil	Cefazolin	Cephalexin	Cefaclor	Cefoxitin	Cefuroxime	Cefotetan	Cefprozil	Cefdinir	Cefepime[a]	Cefotaxime	Cefpodoxime[b]	Ceftazidime	Ceftibuten	Ceftizoxime	Ceftriaxone	✓ = generally susceptible ‡ = demonstrated in vitro activity	
Anaerobes	*Bacteroides* sp.				✓	✓	✓	✓[d]	‡			✓		✓[d]		‡	✓	*Bacteroides* sp	Anaerobes
	Bacteroides fragilis					✓		✓				✓				✓	‡	*Bacteroides fragilis*	
	Clostridium sp.					✓	✓	✓	‡			✓		‡		‡	‡	*Clostridium* sp	
	Clostridium difficile							‡	‡									*Clostridium difficile*	
	Eubacterium sp.																‡	*Eubacterium* sp	
	Fusobacterium sp.						✓	✓	‡			✓				‡	‡	*Fusobacterium* sp	
	Peptococcus sp.				‡	✓	✓	✓				✓		‡		✓	‡	*Peptococcus* sp	
	Peptococcus niger				‡													*Peptococcus niger*	
	Peptostreptococcus sp.				‡	✓	✓	✓	‡			✓	‡	‡		✓	‡	*Peptostreptococcus* sp	
	Porphyromonas asaccharolytica							‡										*Porphyromonas asaccharolytica*	
	Prevotella bivia							✓										*Prevotella bivia*	
	Prevotella digiens							✓										*Prevotella digiens*	
	Prevotella melaninogenica							‡										*Prevotella melaninogenica*	
	Prevotella oralis							‡										*Prevotella oralis*	
	Propionibacterium acnes				‡													*Propionibacterium acnes*	
	Propionibacterium sp.							‡										*Propionibacterium* sp	
	Veillonella sp.							‡										*Veillonella* sp	
Other	*Borrelia burgdorferi*						✓											*Borrelia burgdorferi*	Other

[a] Extended spectrum agent.
[b] Some other references consider this fourth generation.
[c] Coagulase-positive, coagulase-negative and penicillinase-producing.
[d] Some strains are resistant.
[e] Including some β-lactamase-producing strains.
[f] Methicillin-susceptible strains only.
[g] Penicillin-susceptible strains only.
[h] Lancefield's Group A streptococci.

Contraindications

Hypersensitivity to cephalosporins or related antibiotics.

Cefditoren: Cefditoren is contraindicated in patients with carnitine deficiency or inborn errors of metabolism that may result in clinically significant carnitine deficiency because use of cefditoren causes renal excretion of carnitine.

Cefditoren contains sodium caseinate, a milk protein. Do not administer cefditoren to patients with milk protein hypersensitivity (not lactose intolerance).

Warnings/Precautions

Cross-allergenicity with penicillin: Administer cautiously to penicillin-sensitive patients. There is evidence of partial cross-allergenicity; cephalosporins cannot be assumed to be an absolutely safe alternative to penicillin in the penicillin-allergic patient. The estimated incidence of cross-sensitivity is 5% to 16%; however, it is possibly as low as 3% to 7%.

Serum sickness-like reactions: Erythema multiforme or skin rashes accompanied by polyarthritis, arthralgia and, frequently, fever have been reported; these reactions usually occurred following a second course of therapy. Signs and symptoms occur after a few days of therapy and resolve a few days after drug discontinuation with no serious sequelae.

Seizures: Several cephalosporins have been implicated in triggering seizures, particularly in patients with renal function impairment when the dosage was not reduced.

Coagulation abnormalities: **Cefotetan** and **ceftriaxone** may be associated with a fall in prothrombin activity. Those at risk include patients with renal function impairment, cancer, impaired vitamin K synthesis, or low vitamin K stores (eg, chronic hepatic disease or malnutrition), as well as patients receiving a protracted course of antimicrobial therapy. Monitor prothrombin time for patients at risk and administer exogenous vitamin K as indicated. Vitamin K administration may be necessary if the prothrombin time is prolonged before therapy.

Pseudomembranous colitis: Pseudomembranous colitis occurs with the use of cephalosporins (and other broad spectrum antibiotics); therefore, consider its diagnosis in patients who develop diarrhea with antibiotic use.

Immune hemolytic anemia: Immune hemolytic anemia has been observed in patients receiving cephalosporin class antibiotics.

Parenteral use: Inject IM preparations deep into musculature; properly dilute IV preparations and administer over an appropriate time interval.

Gonorrhea: In the treatment of gonorrhea, all patients should have a serologic test for syphilis. Patients with incubating syphilis (seronegative without clinical signs of syphilis) are likely to be cured by the regimens used for gonorrhea.

Hypersensitivity reactions: Reactions range from mild to life-threatening. Before therapy is instituted, inquire about previous hypersensitivity reactions to cephalosporins and penicillins.

Renal function impairment: Cephalosporins may be nephrotoxic; use with caution in the presence of markedly impaired renal function (CrCl less than 50 mL/min/1.73 m^2).

Superinfection: Use of antibiotics (especially prolonged or repeated therapy) may result in bacterial or fungal overgrowth of nonsusceptible organisms. Such overgrowth may lead to a secondary infection. Take appropriate measures if superinfection occurs.

Pregnancy: Category B. These agents cross the placenta.

Lactation: Most of these agents are excreted in breast milk in small quantities.

Children: When using cephalosporins in infants, consider the relative benefit to risk. In neonates, accumulation of cephalosporin antibiotics (with resulting prolongation of drug half-life) has occurred.

Safety and efficacy in children younger than 1 month of age (**cefazolin** and **cefaclor** capsule and suspension), younger than 3 months of age (**cefuroxime**, and

cefoxitin), younger than 5 months of age (**cefpodoxime**), younger than 6 months of age (**cefdinir**, **ceftozoxime**, and **cefprozil**), and younger than 1 year of age (**cefepime**) have not been established.

Safety and efficacy of **cefaclor** extended-release tablets in children younger than 16 years of age have not been established.

Safety and efficacy of **cephalexin** and **cefotetan** in children have not been established.

Drug Interactions

Agents that may interact with cephalosporins include ethanol, aminoglycosides, anticoagulants, polypeptide antibiotics, probenecid, antacids, H_2 antagonists, iron supplements, and loop diuretics.

Drug/Lab test interactions: A false-positive reaction for **urine glucose** may occur with *Benedict's* solution, *Fehling's* solution, or with *Clinitest* tablets, but not with enzyme-based tests such as *Clinistix* and *Tes-Tape*.

Cefuroxime may cause a false-negative reaction in the ferricyanide test for blood glucose.

Cefdinir may cause a false-positive reaction for ketones in urine when measured using nitroprusside but not nitroferricynide.

A false-positive direct *Coombs' test* has occurred in some patients receiving cephalosporins.

Cephalosporins may falsely elevate *urinary 17-ketosteroid* values.

High concentrations of **cefoxitin** (greater than 100 mcg/mL) may interfere with measurement of creatinine levels by the Jaffe reaction and produce false results. **Cefotetan** may also affect these measurements.

Drug/Food interactions: Food increases absorption of **cefpodoxime** and oral **cefuroxime**.

Adverse Reactions

Most common – candidal overgrowth consisting of oral candidiasis, vaginitis, genital moniliasis, vaginal discharge, and genito-anal pruritus; confusion; dizziness; dyspnea; fever; GI disturbances (diarrhea, nausea, vomiting); hypersensitivity phenomena (most common); hypertonia; hypotension; insomnia; nervousness; somnolence.

CNS: Confusion; diaphoresis; dizziness; fatigue; flushing; headache; lethargy; paresthesia.

Hematologic: Agranulocytosis; anemia; aplastic anemia; bone marrow depression; decreased platelet function; eosinophilia; granulocytopenia; hemolytic anemia; hemorrhage; leukocytosis; leukopenia; pancytopenia; thrombocythemia; thrombocytopenia; transient neutropenia.

Hepatic: Elevated AST, ALT, GGTP, total bilirubin, alkaline phosphatase, lactate dehydrogenase; hepatitis.

Local: IM administration commonly results in induration, pain, temperature elevation, and tenderness.

Renal: Transitory elevations in serum urea nitrogen with and without elevated serum creatinine (frequency increases in patients older than 50 years of age and in children younger than 3 years of age).

MEROPENEM

Powder for injection: 500 mg and 1 g (*Rx*) *Merrem IV* (AstraZeneca)

Indications

Intra-abdominal infections: Complicated appendicitis and peritonitis caused by viridans group streptococci, *Escherichia coli*, *Klebsiella pneumoniae*, *Pseudomonas aeruginosa*, *Bacterioides fragilis*, *Bacterioides thetaiotaomicron*, and *Peptostreptococcus* sp.

Bacterial meningitis (pediatric patients 3 months of age or older only): Bacterial meningitis caused by *Streptococcus pneumoniae*, *Haemophilus influenzae* (β-lactamase and non-β-lactamase-producing strains), and *Neisseria meningitidis*.

Skin and skin structure infections (SSSIs): Complicated SSSIs caused by *Staphylococcus aureus* (β-lactamase and non-β-lactamase-producing, methicillin-susceptible isolates only), *Streptococcus pyogenes*, *Streptococcus agalactiae*, viridans group streptococci, *Enterococcus faecalis* (excluding vancomycin-resistant isolates), *P. aeruginosa*, *E. coli*, *Proteus mirabilis*, *B. fragilis*, and *Peptostreptococcus* species.

Administration and Dosage

Administer by intravenous (IV) infusion over 15 to 30 minutes. Doses of 1 g may also be administered as an IV bolus (5 to 20 mL) over 3 to 5 minutes.

Adults:

SSSIs – 500 mg given every 8 hours.

Intra-abdominal infections – 1 g given every 8 hours.

Renal function impairment –

Recommended Meropenem IV Dosage Schedule for Adults with Impaired Renal Function

CrCl[a] (mL/min)	Dose	Dosing interval
≥ 51	500 mg complicated SSSI and 1 g intra-abdominal	every 8 hours
26 to 50	500 mg complicated SSSI and 1 g intra-abdominal	every 12 hours
10 to 25	½ recommended dose	every 12 hours
< 10	½ recommended dose	every 24 hours

[a] CrCl = creatinine clearance.

Children: For children 3 months of age and older, the dose is 20 or 40 mg/kg every 8 hours (maximum dose, 2 g every 8 hours), depending on the type of infection. Give over approximately 15 to 30 minutes or as an IV bolus injection (5 to 20 mL) over approximately 3 to 5 minutes.

Recommended Meropenem IV Dosage Schedule for Children with Healthy Renal Function

Type of infection	Dose (mg/kg)	Up to a maximum dose	Dosing interval
Complicated SSSI	10	500 mg	every 8 hours
Intra-abdominal	20	1 g	every 8 hours
Meningitis	40	2 g	every 8 hours

Children (more than 50 kg) –

SSSIs: 500 mg every 8 hours or complicated SSSIs.

Intra-abdominal infections: 1 g every 8 hours for intra-abdominal infections.

Meningitis: 2 g every 8 hours for meningitis.

Renal function impairment – There is no experience in children with renal function impairment.

Compatibility and stability: Compatibility of meropenem with other drugs has not been established. Meropenem should not be mixed with or physically added to solutions containing other drugs.

Freshly prepared solutions of meropenem should be used whenever possible. However, constituted solutions of meropenem maintain satisfactory potency at controlled room temperature 15° to 25°C (59° to 77°F) or under refrigeration at 4°C (39°F) as described below. Solutions of meropenem should not be frozen.

Actions

Pharmacology: Meropenem is a broad-spectrum carbapenem antibiotic. The bactericidal activity of meropenem results from the inhibition of cell-wall synthesis. Meropenem readily penetrates the cell wall of most gram-positive and gram-negative bacteria to reach penicillin-binding-protein (PBP) targets.

Pharmacokinetics: In subjects with normal renal function, the elimination half-life of meropenem is approximately 1 hour.

Plasma protein binding of meropenem is approximately 2%. The volume of meropenem distribution is 15.7 to 26.68 L. Meropenem penetrates well into most body fluids and tissues, including cerebrospinal fluid, achieving concentrations matching or exceeding those required to inhibit most susceptible bacteria.

Approximately 70% of the IV dose is recovered as unchanged meropenem in the urine.

Contraindications

Hypersensitivity to any component of this product or to other drugs in the same class or in patients who have demonstrated anaphylactic reactions to β-lactams.

Warnings/Precautions

Clostridium difficile–associated diarrhea: Clostridium difficile–associated diarrhea (CDAD) has been reported with use of nearly all antibacterial agents, including meropenem, and may range in severity from mild diarrhea to fatal colitis. Treatment with antibacterial agents alters the normal flora of the colon and may permit overgrowth of C. *difficile*.

C. *difficile* produces toxins A and B, which contribute to the development of CDAD. Hypertoxin-producing strains of C. *difficile* cause increased morbidity and mortality because these infections can be refractory to antimicrobial therapy and may require colectomy. CDAD must be considered in all patients who present with diarrhea following antibiotic use. Careful medical history is necessary because CDAD has been reported to occur more than 2 months after the administration of antibacterial agents.

If CDAD is suspected or confirmed, ongoing antibiotic use not directed against C. *difficile* may need to be discontinued. Institute appropriate fluid and electrolyte management, protein supplementation, antibiotic treatment of C. *difficile*, and surgical evaluation as clinically indicated.

Seizures: Seizures and other CNS adverse experiences have been reported during treatment with meropenem. These adverse experiences have occurred most commonly in patients with CNS disorders (eg, brain lesions or history of seizures) or with bacterial meningitis or compromised renal function.

Hypersensitivity reactions: Serious and occasionally fatal hypersensitivity (anaphylactic) reactions have been reported in patients receiving therapy with β-lactams. These reactions are more likely to occur with a history of sensitivity to multiple allergens.

There have been reports of individuals with a history of penicillin hypersensitivity who have experienced severe hypersensitivity reactions when treated with other β-lactams.

Renal function impairment: Dosage should be reduced in patients with a CrCl less than 51 mL/min.

Superinfection: As with other broad-spectrum antibiotics, prolonged use of meropenem may result in overgrowth of nonsusceptible organisms.

Pregnancy: Category B.

Lactation: It is not known whether this drug is excreted in breast milk.

Children: The safety and efficacy of meropenem have not been established for children younger than 3 months of age.

Elderly: Of the total number of subjects in clinical studies of meropenem, approximately 1,100 (30%) were 65 years of age and older, while 400 (11%) were 75 years of age and older. Additionally, in a study of 511 patients with complicated SSSIs, 93 (18%) were 65 years of age and older, while 38 (7%) were 75 years of age and older. No overall differences in safety or efficacy were observed between these subjects and younger subjects; spontaneous reports and other reported clinical experience have not identified differences in responses between the elderly and younger patients, but greater sensitivity of some older individuals cannot be ruled out.

A pharmacokinetic study with meropenem in elderly patients with renal insufficiency has shown a reduction in plasma clearance of meropenem that correlates with age-associated reduction in CrCl.

Meropenem is known to be substantially excreted by the kidney, and the risk of toxic reactions to this drug may be greater in patients with impaired renal function. Because elderly patients are more likely to have decreased renal function, take care in dose selection; it may be useful to monitor renal function.

Monitoring: Periodic assessment of organ system functions, including renal, hepatic, and hematopoietic is advisable during prolonged therapy.

Drug Interactions

Probenecid: Probenecid competes with meropenem for active tubular secretion and thus inhibits the renal excretion of meropenem. This led to statistically significant increases in the elimination half-life (38%) and in the extent of systemic exposure (56%). Therefore, the coadministration of probenecid with meropenem is not recommended.

Valproic acid: Meropenem may reduce serum levels of valproic acid to subtherapeutic levels.

Adverse Reactions

Adverse reactions occurring in at least 3% of patients include anemia, constipation, headache, inflammation at the injection site, diarrhea, nausea, pain, and vomiting.

Adverse reactions occurring in at least 3% of pediatric patients include diarrhea, vomiting, and rash (mostly diaper-area moniliasis).

IMIPENEM-CILASTATIN

Powder for injection: 250 and 500 mg imipenem equivalent and cilastatin equivalent (*Rx*)	*Primaxin I.V.* (Merck), *Primaxin I.M.* (Merck)

Indications

Intravenous (IV): Treatment of serious infections caused by susceptible strains of the designated microorganisms in the conditions listed below:

Lower respiratory tract infections – *Staphylococcus aureus* (penicillinase-producing), *Escherichia coli*, *Klebsiella* sp., *Enterobacter* sp., *Haemophilus influenzae*, *Haemophilus parainfluenzae*, *Acinetobacter* sp., *Serratia marcescens*.

Urinary tract infections (complicated and uncomplicated) – *Enterococcus faecalis*, *S. aureus* (penicillinase-producing), *E. coli*, *Klebsiella* sp., *Enterobacter* sp., *Proteus vulgaris*, *Providencia rettgeri*, *Morganella morganii*, *Pseudomonas aeruginosa*.

Intra-abdominal infections – *Enterococcus faecalis*, *S. aureus* (penicillinase-producing), *Staphylococcus epidermidis*, *E. coli*, *Klebsiella* sp., *Enterobacter* sp., *Proteus* sp., *M. morganii*, *P. aeruginosa*, *Citrobacter* sp., *Clostridium* sp., *Bacteroides* sp. including *Bacteroides fragilis*, *Fusobacterium* sp.; *Peptococcus* sp., *Peptostreptococcus* sp., *Eubacterium* sp., *Propionibacterium* sp., *Bifidobacterium* sp.

Gynecologic infections – *E. faecalis*; *S. aureus* (penicillinase-producing), *S. epidermidis*, *Streptococcus agalactiae* (group B streptococcus), *E. coli*, *Klebsiella* sp., *Proteus* sp., *Enterobacter* sp., *Bifidobacterium* sp., *Bacteroides* sp. including *B. fragilis*, *Gardnerella vaginalis*; *Peptococcus* sp., *Peptostreptococcus* sp., *Propionibacterium* sp.

Bacterial septicemia – *E. faecalis*, *S. aureus* (penicillinase-producing), *E. coli*, *Klebsiella* sp., *P. aeruginosa*, *Serratia* sp., *Enterobacter* sp., *Bacteroides* sp.

Bone and joint infections – *E. faecalis*; *S. aureus* (penicillinase-producing), *S. epidermidis*, *Enterobacter* sp., *P. aeruginosa*.

Skin and skin structure infections – *E. faecalis*, *S. aureus* (penicillinase-producing), *S. epidermidis*, *E. coli*, *Klebsiella* sp., *Enterobacter* sp., *P. vulgaris*, *P. rettgeri*, *M. morganii*,

P. aeruginosa, *Serratia* sp., *Citrobacter* sp., *Acinetobacter* sp., *Bacteroides* sp., *Fusobacterium* sp.; *Peptococcus* sp., *Peptostreptococcus* sp.

Endocarditis – *S. aureus* (penicillinase-producing).

Polymicrobic infections – Polymicrobic infections, including those in which *S. pneumoniae* (pneumonia, septicemia), *S. pyogenes* (skin and skin structure) or nonpenicillinase-producing *S. aureus* is one of the causative organisms. However, these monobacterial infections usually are treated with narrower spectrum antibiotics (eg, penicillin G). Although clinical improvement has been observed in patients with cystic fibrosis, chronic pulmonary disease, and lower respiratory tract infections caused by *P. aeruginosa*, bacterial eradication may not be achieved.

Intramuscular (IM): Treatment of serious infections of mild to moderate severity where IM therapy is appropriate. Not intended for severe or life-threatening infections, including bacterial sepsis or endocarditis, or in major physiological impairments (eg, shock).

Lower respiratory tract infections – Lower respiratory tract infections, including pneumonia and bronchitis as an exacerbation of COPD, caused by *S. pneumoniae* and *H. influenzae*.

Intra-abdominal infections – Intra-abdominal infections, including acute gangrenous or perforated appendicitis and appendicitis with peritonitis, caused by group D streptococcus including *E. faecalis*; *Streptococcus* (*viridans* group); *E. coli*; *Klebsiella pneumoniae*; *P. aeruginosa*; *Bacteroides* sp. including *B. fragilis*, *B. distasonis*, *B. intermedius*, and *B. thetaiotaomicron*; *Fusobacterium* sp.; *Peptostreptococcus* sp.

Skin and skin structure infections – Skin and skin structure infections, including abscesses, cellulitis, infected skin ulcers, and wound infections caused by *S. aureus* (including penicillinase-producing strains); *Streptococcus pyogenes*; group D streptococcus including *E. faecalis*; *Acinetobacter* sp. including *A. calcoaceticus*; *Citrobacter* sp.; *E. coli*; *Enterobacter cloacae*; *K. pneumoniae*; *P. aeruginosa*; *Bacteroides* sp. including *B. fragilis*.

Gynecologic infections – Gynecologic infections, including postpartum endomyometritis, caused by group D streptococcus such as *E. faecalis*; *E. coli*; *K. pneumoniae*; *B. intermedius*; *Peptostreptococcus* sp.

Infections resistant to other antibiotics (eg, cephalosporins, penicillins, aminoglycosides) have responded to treatment with imipenem.

Administration and Dosage

Dosage recommendations represent the quantity of imipenem to be administered. An equivalent amount of cilastatin is also present in the solution.

IV:

Adults – Give a 125, 250, or 500 mg dose by IV infusion over 20 to 30 minutes. Infuse a 750 or 1 g dose over 40 to 60 minutes. In patients who develop nausea, slow the infusion rate.

Because of high antimicrobial activity, do not exceed 50 mg/kg/day or 4 g/day, whichever is lower.

Imipenem-Cilastatin IV Dosing Schedule for Adults with Normal Renal Function

Type or severity of infection	Fully susceptible organisms[a]	Total daily dose	Moderately susceptible organisms, primarily some strains of *P. aeruginosa*	Total daily dose
Mild	250 mg q 6 h	1 g	500 mg q 6 h	2 g
Moderate	500 mg q 8 h or 500 mg q 6 h	1.5 or 2 g	500 mg q 6 h or 1 g q 8 h	2 or 3 g
Severe, life-threatening	500 mg q 6 h	2 g	1 g q 8 h or 1 g q 6 h	3 or 4 g
Uncomplicated UTI	250 mg q 6 h	1 g	250 mg q 6 h	1 g
Complicated UTI	500 mg q 6 h	2 g	500 mg q 6 h	2 g

[a] Including gram-positive and -negative aerobes and anaerobes

Children –

Pediatric Dosing Guidelines (≥ 3 months old)
≥ 3 months old (non-CNS infections)
15 to 25 mg/kg/dose every 6 hours
Maximum daily dose for fully susceptible organisms is 2 g/day, and for infections with moderately susceptible organisms (primarily some strains of *P. aeruginosa*) is 4 g/day (based on adults studies).
Higher doses (≤ 90 mg/kg/day in older children) have been used in cystic fibrosis patients.

Pediatric Dosing Guidelines (≤ 3 months old)
≤ 3 months old (weighing ≥ 1500 g; non-CNS infections)
< 1 week old: 25 mg/kg every 12 hours
1 to 4 weeks old: 25 mg/kg every 8 hours
4 weeks to 3 months old: 25 mg/kg every 6 hours

Give doses less than or equal to 500 mg by IV infusion over 15 to 30 minutes. Give doses greater than 500 mg by IV infusion over 40 to 60 minutes.

Imipenem-cilastatin IV is not recommended in pediatric patients with CNS infections because of the risk of seizures and in pediatric patients less than 30 kg with impaired renal function, as no data are available.

Renal function impairment –

Reduced IV Dosage in Adult Patients with Impaired Renal Function or Body Weight < 70 kg					
Body weight	≥ 70 kg	60 kg	50 kg	40 kg	30 kg
CrCl[a] (mL/min/1.73 m^2)	If total daily dose for normal renal function is 1 g/day, use:				
≥ 71	250 q 6 h	250 q 8 h	125 q 6 h	125 q 6 h	125 q 8 h
41 to 70	250 q 8 h	125 q 6 h	125 q 6 h	125 q 8 h	125 q 8 h
21 to 40	250 q 12 h	250 q 12 h	125 q 8 h	125 q 12 h	125 q 12 h
6 to 20	250 q 12 h	125 q 12 h	125 q 12 h	125 q 12 h	125 q 12 h
	If total daily dose for normal renal function is 1.5 g/day, use:				
≥ 71	500 q 8 h	250 q 6 h	250 q 6 h	250 q 8 h	125 q 6 h
41 to 70	250 q 6 h	250 q 8 h	250 q 8 h	125 q 6 h	125 q 8 h
21 to 40	250 q 8 h	250 q 8 h	250 q 12 h	125 q 8 h	125 q 8 h
6 to 20	250 q 12 h	250 q 12 h	250 q 12 h	125 q 12 h	125 q 12 h
	If total daily dose for normal renal function is 2 g/day, use:				
≥ 71	500 q 6 h	500 q 8 h	250 q 6 h	250 q 6 h	250 q 8 h
41 to 70	500 q 8 h	250 q 6 h	250 q 6 h	250 q 8 h	125 q 6 h
21 to 40	250 q 6 h	250 q 8 h	250 q 8 h	250 q 12 h	125 q 8 h
6 to 20	250 q 12 h	250 q 12 h	250 q 12 h	250 q 12 h	125 q 12 h
	If total daily dose for normal renal function is 3 g/day, use:				
≥ 71	1000 q 8 h	750 q 8 h	500 q 6 h	500 q 8 h	250 q 6 h
41 to 70	500 q 6 h	500 q 8 h	500 q 8 h	250 q 6 h	250 q 8 h
21 to 40	500 q 8 h	500 q 8 h	250 q 6 h	250 q 8 h	250 q 8 h
6 to 20	500 q 12 h	500 q 12 h	250 q 12 h	250 q 12 h	250 q 12 h
	If total daily dose for normal renal function is 4 g/day, use:				
≥ 71	1000 q 6 h	1000 q 8 h	750 q 8 h	500 q 6 h	500 q 8 h
41 to 70	750 q 8 h	750 q 8 h	500 q 6 h	500 q 8 h	250 q 6 h
21 to 40	500 q 6 h	500 q 8 h	500 q 8 h	250 q 6 h	250 q 8 h
6 to 20	500 q 12 h	500 q 12 h	500 q 12 h	250 q 12 h	250 q 12 h

[a] CrCl = creatinine clearance.

IM: Total daily IM dosages greater than 1500 mg/day are not recommended.

Administer by deep IM injection into a large muscle mass (such as the gluteal muscles or lateral part of the thigh) with a 21-gauge 2" needle.

Imipenem-Cilastatin IM Dosage Guidelines		
Type/Location of infection	Severity	Dosage regimen
Lower respiratory tract Skin and skin structure Gynecologic	Mild/Moderate	500 or 750 mg q 12 h depending on the severity of infection
Intra-abdominal	Mild/Moderate	750 mg q 12 h

Hemodialysis – Imipenem-cilastatin is cleared by hemodialysis. The patient should receive imipenem-cilastatin after hemodialysis and at 12-hour intervals timed from the end of that dialysis session.

Actions

Pharmacology: This product is a formulation of imipenem, a thienamycin antibiotic, and cilastatin sodium, the inhibitor of the renal dipeptidase, dehydropeptidase-1, which is responsible for the extensive metabolism of imipenem when it is administered alone. Cilastatin prevents the metabolism of imipenem, increasing urinary recovery and decreasing possible renal toxicity. The bactericidal activity of imipenem results from the inhibition of cell-wall synthesis, related to binding to penicillin-binding proteins (PBP).

Pharmacokinetics:

Absorption/Distribution –

IV: IV infusion over 20 minutes results in peak plasma levels of imipenem antimicrobial activity that range from 14 to 83 mcg/mL, depending on the dose. Plasma levels declined to 1 mcg/mL or less in 4 to 6 hours. Peak plasma levels of cilastatin following a 20-minute IV infusion range from 15 to 88 mcg/mL, depending on the dose. The plasma half-life of each component is approximately 1 hour. Protein binding is 20% for imipenem and 40% for cilastatin.

IM: Following IM administration of 500 or 750 mg doses, peak plasma levels of imipenem antimicrobial activity occur within 2 hours and average 10 and 12 mcg/mL, respectively. When compared with IV administration, imipenem is approximately 75% bioavailable following IM administration, while cilastatin is approximately 95% bioavailable. The prolonged absorption of imipenem following IM use results in an effective plasma half-life of approximately 2 to 3 hours and plasma levels that remain greater than 2 mcg/mL for at least 6 or 8 hours following a 500 or 750 mg dose, respectively. This plasma profile for imipenem permits IM administration every 12 hours with no accumulation of cilastatin and only slight accumulation of imipenem.

Imipenem urine levels remain above 10 mcg/mL for the 12-hour dosing interval following IM administration of 500 or 750 mg doses. Total urinary excretion of imipenem and cilastatin averages 50% and 75%, respectively, following either dose.

Metabolism/Excretion – Cilastatin prevents renal metabolism of imipenem. The protein binding of imipenem and cilastatin is approximately 20% and 40%, respectively. Approximately 70% of imipenem and cilastatin is recovered in urine within 10 hours of administration.

Microbiology: Imipenem-cilastatin has a high degree of stability in the presence of β-lactamases, including penicillinases and cephalosporinases produced by gram-negative and gram-positive bacteria.

Contraindications

Hypersensitivity to any component of this product.

IM: Hypersensitivity to local anesthetics of the amide type and in patients with severe shock or heart block due to the use of lidocaine hydrochloride diluent.

IV: Patients with meningitis (safety and efficacy have not been established).

Warnings/Precautions

Resistance: As with other β-lactam antibiotics, some strains of *P. aeruginosa* may develop resistance fairly rapidly during treatment with imipenem-cilastatin.

Pseudomembranous colitis: Pseudomembranous colitis has occurred with virtually all antibiotics.

CNS adverse experiences: CNS adverse experiences have occurred with the IV formulation, especially when recommended dosages were exceeded. They are most common in patients with CNS disorders who also have compromised renal function and are rare when no underlying CNS disorder exists (continue anticonvulsants in patients with a known seizure disorder). If focal tremors, myoclonus, or seizures occur, neurologically evaluate the patient, institute anticonvulsants, re-examine the dose, and determine whether to decrease dosage or discontinue the drug. If these effects occur with the IM formulation, discontinue the drug.

Hypersensitivity reactions: Serious and occasionally fatal hypersensitivity reactions have occurred in patients receiving therapy with β-lactams. They are more apt to occur in people with a history of sensitivity to multiple allergens. Patients with a history of penicillin hypersensitivity have experienced severe reactions when treated with another β-lactam.

Renal function impairment: Do not give imipenem-cilastatin IV to patients with CrCl less than or equal to 5 mL/min/1.73 m^2, unless hemodialysis is instituted within 48 hours. For patients on hemodialysis, imipenem-cilastatin IV is recommended only when the benefit outweighs the potential risk of seizures.

Pregnancy: Category C.

Lactation: It is not known whether this drug is excreted in breast milk.

Children:

IM – Safety and efficacy for use in children younger than 12 years of age are not established for IM use.

IV – Use of IV in neonates to 16 years of age (with non-CNS infections) is supported by evidence from adequate and well-controlled studies. IV use is not recommended in pediatric patients with CNS infections because of the risk of seizures, or in pediatric patients less than 30 kg with impaired renal function as no data are available.

Monitoring: Periodically assess organ system function during prolonged therapy.

Drug Interactions

Drugs that may interact with imipenem-cilastatin include ganciclovir, probenecid, and cyclosporine.

Adverse Reactions

Adverse reactions occurring in at least 3% of patients include phlebitis and thrombophlebitis; in newborn patients to 3 months of age and older, diarrhea and convulsions have occurred.

ERTAPENEM

Injection, lyophilized powder for solution: 1 g (equivalent to ertapenem sodium 1.046 g) (*Rx*)	*Invanz* (Merck)

Indications

Complicated intra-abdominal infections (IAIs): Caused by *Escherichia coli, Clostridium clostridioforme, Eubacterium lentum, Peptostreptococcus* sp., *Bacteroides fragilis, B. distasonis, B. ovatus, B. thetaiotaomicron*, or *B. uniformis*.

Complicated skin and skin structure infections (SSSI): Including diabetic foot infections without osteomyelitis caused by *Staphylococcus aureus* (methicillin-susceptible isolates only), *S. agalactiae, Streptococcus pyogenes, E. coli, Klebsiella pneumoniae, Proteus mirabilis, B. fragilis, Peptostreptococcus* species, *P. asaccharolytica*, or *P. bivia*.

Community-acquired pneumonia: Caused by *Streptococcus pneumoniae* (penicillin-susceptible strains only), including cases with concurrent bacteremia, *Haemophilus influenzae* (beta-lactamase-negative strains only), or *Moraxella catarrhalis*.

Complicated urinary tract infections, including pyelonephritis: Caused by *E. coli*, including cases with concurrent bacteremia, or *Klebsiella pneumoniae*.

Acute pelvic infections, including postpartum endomyometritis, septic abortion, and postsurgical gynecologic infections: Caused by *Streptococcus agalactiae*, *E. coli*, *B. fragilis*, *Porphyromonas asaccharolytica*, *Peptostreptococcus* sp., or *Prevotella bivia*.

Prophylaxis:

Colorectal surgery – For the prophylaxis of surgical-site infection following elective colorectal surgery in adults.

Administration and Dosage

Adults and children 13 years of age and older: 1 g given once a day.

Children 3 months to 12 years of age: 15 mg/kg twice daily (not to exceed 1 g/day).

Administer by intravenous (IV) infusion up to 14 days or intramuscular (IM) injection up to 7 days. Infuse IV over 30 minutes.

Do not mix or infuse ertapenem with other medications. Do not use diluents containing dextrose.

Ertapenem Dosage Guidelines for Adults and Children with Healthy Renal Function[a] and Body Weight

Infection[b]	Daily dose (IV or IM) in adults and children 13 years of age and older	Daily dose (IV or IM) in children 3 months to 12 years of age	Recommended duration of total antimicrobial treatment
Complicated IAI	1 g	15 mg/kg twice daily[c]	5 to 14 days
Complicated SSSIs, including diabetic foot infections[d]	1 g	15 mg/kg twice daily[c]	7 to 14 days[e]
CAP	1 g	15 mg/kg twice daily[c]	10 to 14 days[f]
Complicated UTIs, including pyelonephritis	1 g	15 mg/kg twice daily[c]	10 to 14 days[f]
APIs, including postpartum endomyometritis, septic abortion, and postsurgical gynecologic infections	1 g	15 mg/kg twice daily[c]	3 to 10 days

[a] Defined as creatinine clearance (CrCl) greater than 90 mL/min/1.73 m^2.
[b] Caused by the designated pathogens.
[c] Not to exceed 1 g/day.
[d] Ertapenem has not been studied in diabetic foot infections with concomitant osteomyelitis.
[e] Adult patients with diabetic foot infections received up to 28 days of treatment (parenteral or parenteral plus oral switch therapy).
[f] Duration includes a possible switch to an appropriate oral therapy, after at least 3 days of parenteral therapy, once clinical improvement has been demonstrated.

The following table presents prophylaxis guidelines for ertapenem.

Prophylaxis Dosage Guidelines for Adults

Indication	Daily dose (IV) adults	Recommended duration of total antimicrobial treatment
Prophylaxis of surgical-site infection following elective colorectal surgery	1 g	Single IV dose given 1 hour prior to surgical incision

Renal insufficiency: Patients with advanced renal insufficiency (CrCl less than or equal to 30 mL/min/1.73 m^2) and end-stage renal insufficiency (CrCl less than or equal to 10 mL/min/1.73 m^2) should receive 500 mg daily.

Hemodialysis: When the recommended daily dose of 500 mg of ertapenem within 6 hours prior to hemodialysis, a supplementary dose of 150 mg is recommended following hemodialysis. If ertapenem is given at least 6 hours prior to hemodialysis, no supplementary dose is needed. There are no data in patients undergoing peritoneal dialysis or hemofiltration.

Admixture incompatibility: Do not mix or co-infuse ertapenem with other medications. Do not use diluents containing dextrose (α-D-glucose).

Actions

Pharmacology: Ertapenem is structurally related to beta-lactam antibiotics. The bactericidal activity of ertapenem results from the inhibition of cell wall synthesis.

Pharmacokinetics:

Absorption – The mean bioavailability is approximately 90%. Following IM administration, mean peak plasma concentrations are achieved in approximately 2.3 hours.

Distribution – Ertapenem is highly bound to human plasma proteins, primarily albumin. The apparent volume of distribution at steady state of ertapenem is approximately 8.2 L.

Metabolism – In vitro studies in human liver microsomes indicate that ertapenem does not inhibit metabolism mediated by any of the following cytochrome P450 (CYP) isoforms: 1A2, 2C9, 2C19, 2D6, 2E1, and 3A4.

Excretion – Ertapenem is eliminated primarily by the kidneys. The mean plasma half-life in healthy young adults is approximately 4 hours.

Following the administration of intravenous (IV) radiolabeled ertapenem 1 g to healthy young adults, approximately 80% is recovered in urine and 10% in feces.

Contraindications

Known hypersensitivity to any component of this product or to other drugs in the same class or in patients who have demonstrated anaphylactic reactions to beta-lactams; known hypersensitivity to local anesthetics of the amide type (IM use only).

Warnings/Precautions

Clostridium difficile-associated diarrhea: Clostridium difficile-associated diarrhea has been reported and may range in severity from mild to life-threatening.

IM administration: Use caution when administering ertapenem IM to avoid inadvertent injection into a blood vessel. Lidocaine is the diluent for IM administration of ertapenem.

Drug resistance: Prescribing ertapenem in the absence of a proven or strongly suspected bacterial infection or a prophylactic indication is unlikely to provide benefit to the patient and increases the risk of the development of drug-resistant bacteria.

Seizures: Seizures and other CNS adverse reactions have been reported during treatment with ertapenem.

Hypersensitivity reactions: Serious and occasionally fatal hypersensitivity (anaphylactic) reactions have been reported in patients receiving therapy with beta-lactams. These reactions are more likely to occur in individuals with a history of sensitivity to multiple allergens. There have been reports of individuals with a history of penicillin hypersensitivity who have experienced severe hypersensitivity reactions when treated with another beta-lactam.

Superinfection: Use of antibiotics (especially prolonged or repeated therapy) may result in bacterial or fungal overgrowth of nonsusceptible organisms. Such overgrowth may lead to a secondary infection. Take appropriate measures if superinfection occurs.

Pregnancy: *Category B.*

Lactation: Ertapenem is excreted in breast milk. Exercise caution when ertapenem is administered to a nursing woman. Administer ertapenem to nursing mothers only when the expected benefit outweighs the risk.

Children: Ertapenem is not recommended in infants younger than 3 months of age; no data are available.

Ertapenem is not recommended in the treatment of meningitis in the pediatric population because of a lack of sufficient cerebrospinal fluid penetration.

Elderly: This drug is known to be substantially excreted by the kidney, and the risk of toxic reactions to this drug may be greater in patients with impaired renal function. Because elderly patients are more likely to have decreased renal function, take care in dose selection; it may be useful to monitor renal function.

Monitoring: While ertapenem possesses toxicity similar to the beta-lactam group of antibiotics, periodic assessment of organ system function, including renal, hepatic, and hematopoietic, is advisable during prolonged therapy.

Drug Interactions

Drugs that may interact with ertapenem include probenecid and valproic acid.

Adverse Reactions

The most common drug-related adverse experiences in patients treated with ertapenem, including those who were switched to therapy with an oral antimicrobial, were diarrhea, infused vein complication, nausea, headache, vaginitis, phlebitis/thrombophlebitis, and vomiting.

Adverse reactions occurring in at least 3% of adults included the following: abdominal pain, altered mental status, anemia, atelectasis, constipation, diarrhea, edema/swelling, fever, headache, infused vein complication, insomnia, nausea, urinary tract infection, vaginitis, vomiting, wound infection.

Adverse reactions occurring in at least 3% of children include the following: abdominal pain, cough, diaper dermatitis, diarrhea, headache, infusion site erythema and pain, pyrexia, and vomiting.

Drug-related laboratory adverse experiences that were reported during therapy in at least 3% of patients treated with ertapenem in clinical studies were ALT increased, AST increased, hematocrit decreased, hemoglobin decreased, neutrophil count decreased, platelet count increased, serum alkaline phosphatase increased.

DORIPENEM

Injection, powder for solution, concentrate: 500 mg (*Rx*) *Doribax* (Ortho-McNeil)

Indications

Complicated intra-abdominal infections: As a single agent for the treatment of complicated intra-abdominal infections caused by *Escherichia coli, Klebsiella pneumoniae, Pseudomonas aeruginosa, Bacteroides caccae, Bacteroides fragilis, Bacteroides thetaiotaomicron, Bacteroides uniformis, Bacteroides vulgatus, Streptococcus intermedius, Streptococcus constellatus*, and *Peptostreptococcus micros*.

Complicated urinary tract infections (UTIs), including pyelonephritis: As a single agent for the treatment of complicated UTIs, including pyelonephritis, caused by *E. coli*, including cases with concurrent bacteremia, *K. pneumoniae, Proteus mirabilis, P. aeruginosa*, and *Acinetobacter baumannii*.

Administration and Dosage

Dosage:

Doripenem Dosage by Infection

Infection	Dosage	Frequency	Infusion time (h)	Duration
Complicated intraabdominal infection	500 mg	every 8 h	1	5 to 14 days[a]
Complicated UTIs, including pyelonephritis	500 mg	every 8 h	1	10 days[a,b]

[a] Duration includes a possible switch to an appropriate oral therapy, after at least 3 days of parenteral therapy, once clinical improvement has been demonstrated.

[b] Duration can be extended up to 14 days in patients with concurrent bacteremia.

Renal function impairment:

Doripenem Dosage in Patients With Renal Function Impairment	
Estimated CrCl[a] (mL/min)	Recommended dosage regimen of doripenem
> 50	No dosage adjustment necessary
≥ 30 to ≤ 50	250 mg IV (over 1 h) every 8 h
> 10 to < 30	250 mg IV (over 1 h) every 12 h

[a] CrCl = creatinine clearance.

Doripenem is hemodialyzable; however, there is insufficient information to make dose adjustment recommendations in patients on hemodialysis.

Admixture compatibility/incompatibility: Doripenem should not be mixed with or physically added to solutions containing other drugs.

Actions

Pharmacology: Doripenem belongs to the carbapenem class of antimicrobials. Doripenem exerts its bactericidal activity by inhibiting bacterial cell wall biosynthesis.

Pharmacokinetics:

Distribution – The average binding of doripenem to plasma proteins is approximately 8.1%.

Excretion – Doripenem is primarily eliminated unchanged by the kidneys. The mean plasma terminal elimination half-life is approximately 1 hour.

Special populations –

Renal function impairment: Following a single 500 mg dose of doripenem, the mean AUC of doripenem in subjects with mild (CrCl 50 to 79 mL/min), moderate (CrCl 31 to 50 mL/min), and severe renal function impairment (CrCl 30 mL/min or less) was 1.6, 2.8, and 5.1 times that of age-matched healthy subjects with healthy renal function (CrCl 80 mL/min or more), respectively. Dosage adjustment is necessary in patients with moderate and severe renal function impairment.

A single 500 mg dose of doripenem was administered to subjects with end-stage renal disease 1 hour prior to or 1 hour after hemodialysis. The mean doripenem AUC following the posthemodialysis infusion was 7.8 times that of healthy subjects with healthy renal function. The mean total recovery of doripenem and doripenem-M1 in the dialysate following a 4-hour hemodialysis session was 231 and 28 mg, respectively, or a total of 259 mg (52% of the dose). There is insufficient information to make dose adjustment recommendations in patients on hemodialysis.

Contraindications

Known serious hypersensitivity to doripenem or other drugs in the same class or in patients who have demonstrated anaphylactic reactions to beta-lactams.

Warnings/Precautions

Clostridium difficile–associated diarrhea: *C. difficile*–associated diarrhea has been reported with nearly all antibacterial agents and may range in severity from mild diarrhea to fatal colitis.

Drug-resistant bacteria: Prescribing doripenem in the absence of a proven or strongly suspected bacterial infection is unlikely to provide benefit to the patient and increases the risk of the development of drug-resistant bacteria.

Pneumonitis with inhalational use: When doripenem has been used investigationally via inhalation, pneumonitis has occurred. Do not administer doripenem by this route.

Hypersensitivity reactions: Serious and occasionally fatal hypersensitivity (anaphylactic) and serious skin reactions have been reported in patients receiving beta-lactam antibiotics.

Renal function impairment: See Administration and Dosage for more information.

Pregnancy: Category B.

Lactation: It is not known whether this drug is excreted in human milk. Because many drugs are excreted in human milk, exercise caution when doripenem is administered to a breast-feeding woman.

Children: Safety and effectiveness in children have not been established.

Elderly: Clinical cure rates in complicated intra-abdominal and complicated UTIs were slightly lower in patients 65 years of age and older and also in the subgroup of patients 75 years of age and older versus patients younger than 65 years of age. These results were similar between doripenem and comparator treatment groups.

Elderly subjects had greater doripenem exposure relative to nonelderly subjects; however, this increase in exposure was mainly attributed to age-related changes in renal function.

Doripenem is known to be excreted substantially by the kidney, and the risk of adverse reactions to this drug may be greater in patients with renal function impairment or prerenal azotemia.

Monitoring: Monitor renal function in patients with moderate to severe renal function impairment.

Drug Interactions

Drugs that may interact with doripenem include probenecid and valproic acid.

Adverse Reactions

Adverse reactions occurring in 3% or more of patients include anemia, diarrhea, headache, nausea, phlebitis, pruritus, and rash.

AZTREONAM

Powder for injection (lyophilized cake): 500 mg, 1 g, and 2 g (*Rx*)	Various, *Azactam* (Squibb)
Powder for solution, lyophilized; inhalation: 75 mg (*Rx*)	*Cayston* (Gilead Sciences)

Indications

Urinary tract infections: Urinary tract infections (complicated and uncomplicated), including pyelonephritis and cystitis (initial and recurrent) caused by *Escherichia coli, Klebsiella pneumoniae, Proteus mirabilis, Pseudomonas aeruginosa, Enterobacter cloacae, Klebsiella oxytoca, Citrobacter* sp., and *Serratia marcescens.*

Lower respiratory tract infections: Lower respiratory tract infections, including pneumonia and bronchitis caused by *E. coli, K. pneumoniae, P. aeruginosa, Haemophilus influenzae, P. mirabilis, Enterobacter* sp. and *S. marcescens.*

Septicemia: Septicemia caused by *E. coli, K. pneumoniae, P. aeruginosa, P. mirabilis, S. marcescens,* and *Enterobacter* sp.

Skin and skin structure infections: Skin and skin structure infections, including those associated with postoperative wounds, ulcers, and burns caused by *E. coli, P. mirabilis, S. marcescens, Enterobacter* sp., *P. aeruginosa, K. pneumoniae,* and *Citrobacter* sp.

Intra-abdominal infections: Intra-abdominal infections, including peritonitis caused by *E. coli, Klebsiella* sp. including *K. pneumoniae, Enterobacter* sp. including *E. cloacae,* and *P. aeruginosa, Citrobacter* sp. including *C. freundii,* and *Serratia* sp. including *S. marcescens.*

Gynecologic infections: Gynecologic infections, including endometritis and pelvic cellulitis caused by *E. coli, K. pneumoniae, Enterobacter* sp. including *E. cloacae,* and *P. mirabilis.*

Surgery: For adjunctive therapy to surgery to manage infections caused by susceptible organisms.

Concurrent initial therapy: Concurrent initial therapy with other antimicrobials and aztreonam is recommended before the causative organism(s) is known in seriously ill patients who also are at risk of having an infection caused by gram-positive aerobic pathogens. If anaerobic organisms are also suspected, initiate therapy concurrently with aztreonam.

Cystic fibrosis (inhalation only): To improve respiratory symptoms in patients with cystic fibrosis with *P. aeruginosa.*

Unlabeled uses: 1 g intramuscular (IM) may be beneficial for acute uncomplicated gonorrhea in patients with penicillin-resistant gonococci, as an alternative to spectinomycin.

Administration and Dosage

Give IM or intravenously (IV).

Aztreonam Dosage Guide (Adults)

Type of infection	Dose[a]	Frequency (hours)
Urinary tract infection	500 mg or 1 g	8 or 12
Moderately severe systemic infections	1 or 2 g	8 or 12
Severe systemic or life-threatening infections	2 g	6 or 8

[a] Maximum recommended dose is 8 g/day.

Aztreonam Dosage Guide (Children)

Type of infection	Dose[a]	Frequency (hours)
Mild to moderate infections	30 mg/kg	8
Moderate to severe infections	30 mg/kg	6 or 8

[a] Maximum recommended dose is 120 mg/kg/day.

IV route: IV route is recommended for patients requiring single doses greater than 1 g or those with bacterial septicemia, localized parenchymal abscess (eg, intra-abdominal abscess), peritonitis, or other severe systemic or life-threatening infections. For infections due to *P. aeruginosa*, a dosage of 2 g every 6 or 8 hours is recommended, at least upon initiation of therapy.

Duration: Duration of therapy depends on the severity of infection. Generally, continue aztreonam for at least 48 hours after the patient becomes asymptomatic or evidence of bacterial eradication has been obtained. Persistent infections may require treatment for several weeks.

Children: Administer aztreonam IV to children with normal renal function. There are insufficient data regarding IM administration to children or dosing in children with renal impairment.

Renal function impairment: Reduce dosage by 50% in patients with estimated creatinine clearance (CrCl) between 10 and 30 mL/min/1.73 m^2 after an initial loading dose of 1 or 2 g.

In patients with severe renal failure, give 500 mg, 1 or 2 g initially. The maintenance dose should be 25% of the usual initial dose given at the usual fixed interval of 6, 8, or 12 hours. For serious or life-threatening infections, in addition to the maintenance doses, give 12.5% of the initial dose after each hemodialysis session.

Elderly: Obtain estimates of CrCl and make appropriate dosage modifications.

IV: Bolus injection may be used to initiate therapy. Slowly inject directly into a vein or into the tubing of a suitable administration set over 3 to 5 minutes.

IM: Inject deeply in large muscle mass.

Cystic fibrosis (inhalation only):

Adults and children 7 years of age and older – 75 mg 3 times a day. Doses should be taken at least 4 hours apart for 28 days (followed by 28 days off aztreonam therapy).

Concomitant therapy – Patients should use a bronchodilator before administration. Short-acting bronchodilators can be taken between 15 minutes and 4 hours prior to each dose of aztreonam. Alternatively, long-acting bronchodilators can be taken between 30 minutes and 12 hours prior to administration of aztreonam. For patients taking multiple inhaled therapies, the recommended order of administration is as follows: bronchodilator, mucolytics, and, lastly, aztreonam

Administration – For inhalation use only; not for IV or IM administration. Aztreonam is administered by inhalation using an *Altera Nebulizer System.* Aztreonam should not be administered with any other nebulizer. Aztreonam should not be mixed with any other drugs in the *Altera Nebulizer Handset.*

Actions

Pharmacology: Aztreonam, a synthetic bactericidal antibiotic, is the first of a class identified as monobactams. The monobactams have a monocyclic β-lactam nucleus. Aztreonam's bactericidal action results from the inhibition of bacterial cell wall synthesis because of a high affinity of aztreonam for penicillin-binding protein 3 (PBP3).

Pharmacokinetics:

Absorption/Distribution – Following single IM injections of 500 mg and 1 g, maximum serum concentrations occur at about 1 hour.

The serum half-life averaged 1.7 hours in subjects with normal renal function. In healthy subjects, the serum clearance was 91 mL/min and renal clearance was 56 mL/min; the apparent mean volume of distribution at steady state averaged 12.6 L.

Metabolism/Excretion – In healthy subjects, aztreonam is excreted in the urine about equally by active tubular secretion and glomerular filtration. Approximately 60% to 70% of an IV or IM dose was recovered in the urine by 8 hours; recovery was complete by 12 hours.

Administration IV or IM of a single 500 mg or 1 g dose every 8 hours for 7 days to healthy subjects produced no apparent accumulation; serum protein binding averaged 56% and was independent of dose.

Contraindications

Hypersensitivity to aztreonam or any other component in the formulation.

Warnings/Precautions

Pseudomembranous colitis: Pseudomembranous colitis has been reported with nearly all antibacterial agents, including aztreonam, and may range in severity from mild to life-threatening.

Epidermal necrolysis: Epidermal necrolysis rarely has been reported in association with aztreonam in patients undergoing bone marrow transplant with multiple risk factors.

Bronchospasm (inhalation only): Bronchospasm is a complication associated with nebulized therapies, including aztreonam.

Hypersensitivity reactions: Make careful inquiry for a history of hypersensitivity reactions. Monitor patients who have had immediate hypersensitivity reactions to penicillins or cephalosporins. If an allergic reaction occurs, discontinue the drug and institute supportive treatment. Cross-sensitivity with other penicillins or beta-lactam antibiotics is rare.

Renal/Hepatic function impairment: Appropriate monitoring is recommended.

In patients with impaired renal function, the serum half-life is prolonged.

Pregnancy: Category B. Aztreonam crosses the placenta and enters fetal circulation.

Lactation: Aztreonam is excreted in breast milk in concentrations that are less than 1% of maternal serum. Consider temporary discontinuation of breast-feeding.

Children: Safety and efficacy of IV aztreonam have been established in children 9 months to 16 years of age. Sufficient data are not available for children younger than 9 months of age or for treatment of the following indications/pathogens: septicemia and skin and skin-structure infections (where the skin infection is caused by *H. influenzae* type b). In children with cystic fibrosis, higher doses of aztreonam may be warranted.

Drug Interactions

Drugs that may interact with aztreonam include other beta-lactamase–inducing antibiotics and aminoglycosides.

Adverse Reactions

Adults: No adverse reactions have been reported in at least 3% of adults.

Children: In patients younger than 2 years of age receiving 30 mg/kg every 6 hours, 11.6% experienced neutropenia; in patients older than 2 years of age receiving 50 mg/kg every 6 hours, 15% to 20% had elevations of AST and ALT more than 3 times the upper limit of normal. The increased frequency of these reported laboratory adverse events may be caused by increased severity of illness treated or higher doses of aztreonam administered.

Adults and children receiving inhalation therapy: Abdominal pain, bronchospasm, chest discomfort, cough, nasal congestion, pharyngolaryngeal pain, pyrexia, vomiting, and wheezing.

FLUOROQUINOLONES

CIPROFLOXACIN	
Tablets; oral: 100, 250, 500, and 750 mg (*Rx*)	Various, *Cipro* (Schering-Plough)
Tablets, extended-release; oral: 500 and 1,000 mg (*Rx*)	Various, *Cipro XR* (Schering-Plough), *Proquin XR* (Esprit)
Powder for suspension; oral: 250 mg per 5 mL (5%) and 500 mg per 5 mL (10%) (when reconstituted) (*Rx*)	*Cipro* (Schering-Plough)
Injection, solution, concentrate: 200 and 400 mg (*Rx*)	Various, *Cipro* (Schering-Plough)
Injection: 200 and 400 mg (*Rx*)	Various, *Cipro IV* (Schering-Plough)
GEMIFLOXACIN MESYLATE	
Tablets; oral: 320 mg (as base) (*Rx*)	*Factive* (Oscient)
LEVOFLOXACIN	
Tablets; oral: 250, 500, and 750 mg (*Rx*)	*Levaquin* (Ortho-McNeil)
Solution; oral: 25 mg/mL (*Rx*)	
Injection (concentrate) (single-use vials): 500 mg (25 mg/mL) and 750 mg (25 mg/mL) (*Rx*)	
Injection (premix): 250 (5 mg/mL), 500 mg (5 mg/mL), and 750 mg (5 mg/mL) (*Rx*)	
MOXIFLOXACIN HYDROCHLORIDE	
Tablets; oral: 400 mg (*Rx*)	*Avelox* (Schering-Plough)
Injection (premix): 400 mg (*Rx*)	*Avelox IV* (Schering-Plough)
NORFLOXACIN	
Tablets; oral: 400 mg (*Rx*)	*Noroxin* (Merck)
OFLOXACIN	
Tablets; oral: 200, 300, and 400 mg (*Rx*)	*Floxin* (Various)

Warning:

Fluoroquinolones, including ciprofloxacin hydrochloride, are associated with an increased risk of tendinitis and tendon rupture in all ages. This risk is further increased in older patients usually older than 60 years of age, in patients taking corticosteroid drugs, and in patients with kidney, heart, or lung transplants.

Indications

For specific approved indications, refer to the Administration and Dosage section.

Administration and Dosage

CIPROFLOXACIN:

IR tablets and oral suspension –

Adults:

Ciprofloxacin Dosage Guidelines for Adults				
Infection	Severity	Dose	Frequency	Usual duration[a]
Acute sinusitis	Mild/Moderate	500 mg	Every 12 h	10 days
Bone and joint	Mild/Moderate	500 mg	Every 12 h	≥ 4 to 6 weeks
	Severe/Complicated	750 mg	Every 12 h	≥ 4 to 6 weeks
Chronic bacterial prostatitis	Mild/Moderate	500 mg	Every 12 h	28 days
Infectious diarrhea	Mild/Moderate/Severe	500 mg	Every 12 h	5 to 7 days
Inhalational anthrax (postexposure)[b]		500 mg	Every 12 h	60 days
Intra-abdominal[c]	Complicated	500 mg	Every 12 h	7 to 14 days
Lower respiratory tract	Mild/Moderate	500 mg	Every 12 h	7 to 14 days
	Severe/Complicated	750 mg	Every 12 h	7 to 14 days
Skin and skin structure	Mild/Moderate	500 mg	Every 12 h	7 to 14 days
	Severe/Complicated	750 mg	Every 12 h	7 to 14 days
Typhoid fever	Mild/Moderate	500 mg	Every 12 h	10 days

Ciprofloxacin Dosage Guidelines for Adults				
Infection	Severity	Dose	Frequency	Usual duration[a]
Urethral and cervical gonococcal infections	Uncomplicated	250 mg	Single dose	Single dose
Urinary tract infection (UTI)	Acute uncomplicated	250 mg	Every 12 h	3 days
	Mild/Moderate	250 mg	Every 12 h	7 to 14 days
	Severe/Complicated	500 mg	Every 12 h	7 to 14 days

[a] Generally, ciprofloxacin should be continued for at least 2 days after the signs and symptoms of infection have disappeared, except for inhalational anthrax (postexposure).
[b] Drug administration should begin as soon as possible after suspected or confirmed exposure. This indication is based on a surrogate end point, ciprofloxacin serum concentrations achieved in humans, reasonably likely to predict clinical benefit.
[c] Used in conjunction with metronidazole.

Children:

Ciprofloxacin Dosing Guidelines for Children				
Infection	Route of administration	Dose (mg/kg)	Frequency	Total duration
Complicated UTI of pyelonephritis (patients 1 to 17 years of age)	Oral	10 to 20 mg/kg (maximum 750 mg/dose; not to be exceeded even in patients weighing > 51 kg)	Every 12 h	10 to 21 days[a]
Inhalational anthrax (postexposure)[b]	Oral	15 mg/kg (maximum 500 mg/dose)	Every 12 h	60 days

[a] The total duration of therapy for complicated UTIs and pyelonephritis in the clinical trial was determined by the health care provider. The mean duration of treatment was 11 days (range, 10 to 21 days).
[b] Drug administration should begin as soon as possible after suspected of confirmed exposure to *B. anthracis* spores. This indication is based on a surrogate end point, ciprofloxacin serum concentration achieved in humans, reasonably likely to predict clinical benefit.

Administer ciprofloxacin at least 2 hours before or 6 hours after magnesium/aluminum antacids, sucralfate, didanosine chewable/buffered tablets or pediatric powder for oral solution, or other products containing calcium, iron, or zinc.

ER tablets –

Ciprofloxacin ER Tablets			
Indication	Dose	Frequency	Usual duration
Acute uncomplicated pyelonephritis	1,000 mg	Every 24 h	7 to 14 days
Complicated UTIs	1,000 mg	Every 24 h	7 to 14 days
Uncomplicated UTIs (acute cystitis)	500 mg	Every 24 h	3 days

No dosage adjustment is required for patients with uncomplicated UTIs receiving ciprofloxacin XR 500 mg. In patients with complicated urinary tract infections and acute uncomplicated pyelonephritis who have a creatinine clearance (CrCl) of less than 30 mL/min, reduce the dose of ER tablets from 1,000 to 500 mg/day. For patients on hemodialysis or peritoneal dialysis, administer ER tablets after dialysis.

ER and IR tablets are not interchangeable.

ER tablets may be taken with meals that include milk; however, avoid coadministration with dairy products alone or with calcium-fortified products. A 2-hour window between substantial calcium intake (more than 800 mg) and dosing with ER tablets is recommended. Swallow the ER tablet whole; do not split, crush, or chew.

Proquin XR: Proquin XR and other oral formulations of ciprofloxacin are not interchangeable. *Proquin XR* should be administered orally as 500 mg once daily for 3 days with a main meal of the day, preferably the evening meal. *Proquin XR* should be administered at least 4 hours before or 2 hours after antacids containing magnesium or aluminum, sucralfate, *Videx* (didanosine) chewable/buffered tablets or pediatric powder, metal cations such as iron, and multivitamin preparations containing zinc. *Proquin XR* tablets should be taken whole and never split, crushed, or chewed.

IV – Administer by IV infusion over 60 minutes.

Admixture compatibility: Sodium chloride 0.9% injection, dextrose 5% injection, sterile water for injection, dextrose 10% for injection, dextrose 5% and sodium chloride 0.225% for injection, dextrose 5% and sodium chloride 0.45% for injection, or Ringer's lactate for injection are compatible IV solutions for diluting ciprofloxacin in vials. If the Y-type or the piggyback method of administration is used, it is advisable to temporarily discontinue the administration of any other solutions during the infusion of ciprofloxacin.

Adults:

Ciprofloxacin IV Dosage Guidelines for Adults

Infection[a]	Severity	Dose	Frequency	Usual duration
Acute sinusitis	Mild/Moderate	400 mg	Every 12 h	10 days
Bone and joint	Mild/Moderate	400 mg	Every 12 h	≥ 4 to 6 weeks
	Severe/Complicated	400 mg	Every 8 h	≥ 4 to 6 weeks
Chronic bacterial prostatitis	Mild/Moderate	400 mg	Every 12 h	28 days
Empirical therapy in febrile neutropenic patients	Severe	Ciprofloxacin 400 mg	Every 8 h	7 to 14 days
		Piperacillin 50 mg/kg, not to exceed 24 g/day	Every 4 h	
Inhalational anthrax (postexposure)[b]		400 mg	Every 12 h	60 days
Intra-abdominal[c]	Complicated	400 mg	Every 12 h	7 to 14 days
Lower respiratory tract	Mild/Moderate	400 mg	Every 12 h	7 to 14 days
	Severe/Complicated	400 mg	Every 8 h	7 to 14 days
Nosocomial pneumonia	Mild/Moderate/Severe	400 mg	Every 8 h	10 to 14 days
Skin and skin structure	Mild/Moderate	400 mg	Every 12 h	7 to 14 days
	Severe/Complicated	400 mg	Every 8 h	7 to 14 days
UTI	Mild/Moderate	200 mg	Every 12 h	7 to 14 days
	Severe/Complicated	400 mg	Every 12 h	7 to 14 days

[a] Caused by the designated pathogens.

[b] Drug administration should begin as soon as possible after suspected or confirmed exposure. This indication is based on a surrogate end point, ciprofloxacin serum concentrations achieved in humans, reasonably likely to predict clinical benefit. Total duration of ciprofloxacin administration (IV or oral) for inhalational anthrax (postexposure) is 60 days.

[c] Used in conjunction with metronidazole.

Conversion from IV to oral dosing in adults –

Equivalent AUC Dosing Regimens

Ciprofloxacin oral dosage[a]	Equivalent ciprofloxacin IV dosage
250 mg tablet every 12 h	200 mg IV every 12 h
500 mg tablet every 12 h	400 mg IV every 12 h
750 mg tablet every 12 h	400 mg IV every 8 h

[a] IR tablets and oral suspension only.

Children: See Indications for more information.

Ciprofloxacin Dosing Guidelines for Children				
Infection	Route of administration	Dose (mg/kg)	Frequency	Total duration
Complicated UTI of pyelonephritis (patients 1 to 17 years of age)	IV	6 to 10 mg/kg (maximum 400 mg/dose; not to be exceeded even in patients weighing > 51 kg)	Every 8 h	10 to 21 days[a]
Inhalational anthrax (postexposure)[b]	IV	10 mg/kg (maximum 400 mg/dose)	Every 12 h	60 days

[a] The total duration of therapy for complicated UTIs and pyelonephritis in the clinical trial was determined by the health care provider. The mean duration of treatment was 11 days (range, 10 to 21 days).

[b] Drug administration should begin as soon as possible after suspected or confirmed exposure to *B. anthracis* spores. This indication is based on surrogate end point ciprofloxacin serum concentrations achieved in humans reasonably likely to predict clinical benefit.

Renal function impairment –

Ciprofloxacin Oral Dosage in Adults With Renal Function Impairment	
CrCl (mL/min)	Dose
> 50	See usual dosage
30 to 50	250 to 500 mg every 12 h
5 to 29	250 to 500 mg every 18 h
Patients on hemodialysis or peritoneal dialysis	250 to 500 mg every 24 h (after dialysis)

In patients with severe infections and severe renal function impairment, 750 mg may be administered orally at the intervals noted in the previous table.

Ciprofloxacin IV Dosage in Adults With Renal Function Impairment	
CrCl (mL/min)	Dose
> 30	Usual dosage
5 to 29	200 to 400 mg every 18 to 24 h

GEMIFLOXACIN: Gemifloxacin can be taken with or without food and should be swallowed whole with a liberal amount of liquid.

Gemifloxacin Dosage Guidelines		
Indication	Dose (mg)	Duration (days)
Acute bacterial exacerbation of chronic bronchitis	320 mg once daily	5
Community-acquired pneumonia (of mild to moderate severity)		
Due to known or suspected *S. pneumoniae*, *H. influenzae*, *M. pneumoniae*, or *C. pneumoniae* infection	320 mg once daily	5
Due to known or suspected MDRSP, *K. pneumoniae*, or *M. catarrhalis* infection	320 mg once daily	7

Renal function impairment –

Recommended Doses for Patients With Renal Function Impairment	
Creatinine clearance (mL/min)	Dose
> 40	See usual dosage
≤ 40, hemodialysis, CAPD[a]	160 mg every 24 h

[a] CAPD = continuous ambulatory peritoneal dialysis.

LEVOFLOXACIN: Levofloxacin tablets can be administered without regard to food. It is recommended that levofloxacin oral solution be taken 1 hour before or 2 hours after eating.

Administer oral doses at least 2 hours before or 2 hours after antacids containing magnesium or aluminum, as well as sucralfate, metal cations such as iron, and multivitamin preparations with zinc, or didanosine (chewable/buffered tablets or pediatric powder for oral solution).

Levofloxacin Dosage in Patients With Healthy Renal Function (CrCl ≥ 50 mL/min)		
Type of infection[a]	Dosed every 24 hours	Duration (days)[b]
Acute bacterial exacerbation of chronic bronchitis	500 mg	7
Acute bacterial sinusitis	750 mg	5
	500 mg	10 to 14
Chronic bacterial prostatitis	500 mg	28
Community-acquired pneumonia[c]	500 mg	7 to 14
Community-acquired pneumonia[d]	750 mg	5
Complicated skin and skin structure infections	750 mg	7 to 14
Complicated UTI or acute pyelonephritis[e]	750 mg	5
Complicated UTI or acute pyelonephritis[f]	250 mg	10
Inhalational anthrax (postexposure), adult[g,h]	500 mg	60
Nosocomial pneumonia	750 mg	7 to 14
Uncomplicated skin and skin structure infections	500 mg	7 to 10
Uncomplicated UTI	250 mg	3

[a] Due to the designated pathogens.
[b] Sequential therapy (IV to oral) may be instituted at the discretion of the health care provider.
[c] Due to methicillin-susceptible *S. aureus*, *S. pneumoniae* (including multidrug-resistant strains), *H. influenzae*, *H. parainfluenzae*, *K. pneumoniae*, *M. catarrhalis*, *C. pneumoniae*, *L. pneumophila*, or *M. pneumoniae*.
[d] Due to *S. pneumoniae* (excluding multidrug-resistant strains), *H. influenzae*, *H. parainfluenzae*, *M. pneumoniae*, or *C. pneumoniae*.
[e] This regimen is indicated for complicated UTIs caused by *E. coli*, *K. pneumoniae*, *P. mirabilis*, and acute pyelonephritis caused by *E. coli*, including cases with concurrent bacteremia.
[f] This regimen is indicated for complicated UTIs caused by *E. faecalis*, *E. cloacae*, *E. coli*, *K. pneumoniae*, *P. mirabilis*, *P. aeruginosa*; and for acute pyelonephritis caused by *E. coli*.
[g] Drug administration should begin as soon as possible after suspected or confirmed exposure to aerosolized *B. anthracis*. This indication is based on a surrogate end point. Levofloxacin plasma concentrations achieved in humans are reasonably likely to predict clinical benefit.
[h] The safety of levofloxacin in adults for durations of therapy beyond 28 days has not been studied. Prolonged levofloxacin therapy in adults should only be used when the benefit outweighs the risk.

Levofloxacin Dosage in Children 6 Months of Age and Older			
Type of infection[a]	Dose	Frequency	Duration (days)[b]
Inhalational anthrax (postexposure)[c,d]			
> 50 kg	500 mg	Once every 24 h	60
< 50 kg	8 mg/kg (not to exceed 250 mg/dose)	Once every 12 h	60

[a] Due to *B. anthracis*.
[b] Sequential therapy (IV to oral) may be instituted at the discretion of the health care provider.
[c] Drug administration should begin as soon as possible after suspected or confirmed exposure to aerosolized *B. anthracis*. This indication is based on a surrogate end point. Levofloxacin plasma concentrations achieved in humans are reasonably likely to predict clinical benefit.
[d] The safety of levofloxacin in pediatric patients for durations of therapy beyond 14 days has not been studied. An increased incidence of musculoskeletal adverse reactions compared with controls has been observed in children. Prolonged levofloxacin therapy should only be used when the benefit outweighs the risk.

Levofloxacin Dosage in Patients With Renal Function Impairment (CrCl < 50 mL/min)			
Dosage in healthy renal function every 24 hours	CrCl 20 to 49 mL/min	CrCl 10 to 19 mL/min	Hemodialysis or chronic ambulatory peritoneal dialysis (CAPD)
750 mg	750 mg every 48 hours	750 mg initial dose, then 500 mg every 48 hours	750 mg initial dose, then 500 mg every 48 hours

Levofloxacin Dosage in Patients With Renal Function Impairment (CrCl < 50 mL/min)			
Dosage in healthy renal function every 24 hours	CrCl 20 to 49 mL/min	CrCl 10 to 19 mL/min	Hemodialysis or chronic ambulatory peritoneal dialysis (CAPD)
500 mg	500 mg initial dose, then 250 mg every 24 hours	500 mg initial dose, then 250 mg every 48 hours	500 mg initial dose, then 250 mg every 48 hours
250 mg	No dosage adjustment required	250 mg every 48 hours. If treating uncomplicated UTI, no dosage adjustment is required.	No information on dosing adjustment is available.

IV administration – Administer by IV infusion only, slowly over a period of 60 minutes or more (750 mg over 90 minutes). Avoid rapid or bolus IV infusion. Do not administer by IM, intrathecal, intraperitoneal, or subcutaneous routes. Single-use vials require dilution prior to administration.

Compatible IV solutions – sodium chloride 0.9% injection, dextrose 5% (D5W) injection, D5W/sodium chloride 0.9% injection, D5W in Ringer's lactate, *Plasma-Lyte 56*/D5W injection, D5W, sodium chloride 0.45%, and potassium chloride 0.15% injection, sodium lactate injection (M/6)

MOXIFLOXACIN HYDROCHLORIDE: The dose of moxifloxacin is 400 mg (orally or as an IV infusion) once every 24 hours.

Moxifloxacin Dosage Guidelines (IV and Oral)		
Infection[a]	Daily dose (mg)	Duration (days)
Acute bacterial sinusitis	400	10
Acute bacterial exacerbation of chronic bronchitis	400	5
Community-acquired pneumonia	400	7 to 14
Complicated intra-abdominal infections[b]	400 mg	5 to 14
Complicated skin and skin structure infections	400 mg	7 to 21
Uncomplicated skin and skin structure infections	400	7

[a] Caused by the designated pathogens (see Indications).
[b] For complicated intra-abdominal infections, therapy should be initiated with the IV formulation.

Administer oral doses of moxifloxacin at least 4 hours before or 8 hours after antacids containing magnesium or aluminum, sucralfate, metal cations such as iron, multivitamin preparations with zinc, or didanosine (chewable/buffered tablets or pediatric powder for oral solution).

Moxifloxacin may be administered without regard to food.

Switching from IV to oral dosing – When switching from IV to oral dosage administration, no dosage adjustment is necessary.

IV – Administer IV moxifloxacin by IV infusion only. It is not intended for IM, intrathecal, intra-arterial, intraperitoneal, or subcutaneous administration.

Administer by IV infusion over a period of 60 minutes by direct infusion or through a Y-type IV infusion set. Rapid or bolus IV infusion must be avoided.

Do not add additives or other medications to IV moxifloxacin or infuse simultaneously through the same IV line. If the same IV line is used for sequential infusion of other drugs, or if the "piggyback" method of administration is used, flush the line before and after infusion of moxifloxacin IV with a compatible solution.

Moxifloxacin IV is compatible with the following IV solutions at ratios from 1:10 to 10:1: sodium chloride 0.9% injection, sodium chloride 1M injection, dextrose 5% injection, sterile water for injection, dextrose 10% for injection, lactated Ringer's solution for injection.

NORFLOXACIN: Take 1 hour before or 2 hours after meals or dairy products and with a glass of water. Patients should be well hydrated.

Recommended Norfloxacin Dosage

Infection	Description	Dose	Frequency	Duration
UTIs	Uncomplicated (cystitis) caused by *E. coli*, *Klebsiella pneumoniae*, or *Proteus mirabilis*	400 mg	Every 12 h	3 days
	Uncomplicated caused by other organisms	400 mg	Every 12 h	7 to 10 days
	Complicated	400 mg	Every 12 h	10 to 21 days
Sexually transmitted diseases	Uncomplicated gonorrhea	800 mg	Single dose	1 day
Prostatitis	Acute or chronic	400 mg	Every 12 h	28 days

Renal function impairment ($CrCl$ 30 mL/min/1.73 m² or less) – Administer 400 mg once daily for the duration given above.

CDC-recommended treatment schedules for gonorrhea –

Gonococcal infections, uncomplicated: 800 mg as a single dose (alternative regimen to **ciprofloxacin** or **ofloxacin**).

OFLOXACIN: Usual daily dose is 200 to 400 mg every 12 hours as described in the following table:

Ofloxacin Dosage Guidelines (Oral and IV)[a]

Infection	Description	Dose	Frequency	Duration
Lower respiratory tract	Exacerbation of chronic bronchitis	400 mg	Every 12 h	10 days
	Community acquired pneumonia	400 mg	Every 12 h	10 days
Sexually transmitted diseases	Acute, uncomplicated urethral and cervical gonorrhea	400 mg	Single dose	1 day
	Cervicitis/Urethritis caused by *Chlamydia trachomatis*	300 mg	Every 12 h	7 days
	Cervicitis/Urethritis caused by *C. trachomatis* and *Neisseria gonorrhoeae*	300 mg	Every 12 h	7 days
	Acute pelvic inflammatory disease	400 mg	Every 12 h	10 to 14 days
Skin and skin structure	Uncomplicated	400 mg	Every 12 h	10 days
Urinary tract	Uncomplicated cystitis caused by *E. coli* or *K. pneumoniae*	200 mg	Every 12 h	3 days
	Uncomplicated cystitis caused by other organisms	200 mg	Every 12 h	7 days
	Complicated UTIs	200 mg	Every 12 h	10 days
Prostatitis	Caused by *E. coli*	300 mg	Every 12 h	6 weeks[b]

[a] Caused by the designated pathogens (see Indications).

[b] Because there are no safety data presently available to support the use of the IV formulation for more than 10 days, switch to oral or other appropriate therapy after 10 days.

Do not take antacids containing calcium, magnesium, or aluminum; sucralfate; divalent or trivalent cations such as iron; multivitamins containing zinc; or didanosine (chewable/buffered tablets or pediatric powder for oral solution) 2 hours before or 2 hours after taking ofloxacin.

Renal function impairment – After a usual initial dose, adjust the dosing interval as follows:

Ofloxacin Dosage in Impaired Renal Function		
CrCl (mL/min)	Maintenance dose	Frequency
20 to 50	usual dose	Every 24 h
< 20	½ usual dose	Every 24 h

Chronic hepatic function impairment (cirrhosis) – The excretion of ofloxacin may be reduced in patients with severe liver function disorders (eg, cirrhosis with or without ascites). Do not exceed a maximum dose of 400 mg/day.

CDC-recommended treatment schedules for chlamydia, epididymitis, pelvic inflammatory disease (PID), and gonorrhea – CDC 1998 Sexually Transmitted Diseases Treatment Guidelines. MMWR. 1998;47(RR-1):1-118.

Chlamydia: 300 mg orally 2 times/day for 7 days (alternative regimen).

Epididymitis: 300 mg orally 2 times/day for 10 days.

PID, outpatient: 400 mg orally 2 times/day for 14 days plus metronidazole.

Gonococcal infections, uncomplicated: 400 mg orally in a single dose plus doxycycline or azithromycin.

Actions

Pharmacology: The fluoroquinolones are synthetic, broad-spectrum antibacterial agents that inhibit DNA gyrase and topoisomerase IV. DNA gyrase is an essential enzyme that is involved in the replication, transcription, and repair of bacterial DNA. Topoisomerase IV is an enzyme known to play a key role in the partitioning of the chromosomal DNA during bacterial cell division.

Pharmacokinetics:

Pharmacokinetics of Fluoroquinolones[a,b]			
Fluoroquinolone	Bioavailability (%)	Protein binding (%)	t½ (h)
Ciprofloxacin Oral	≈ 70 to 80	20 to 40	≈ 4
IV			≈ 5 to 6
Levofloxacin	≈ 99	≈ 24 to 38	≈ 6.3 to 8.8
Moxifloxacin	≈ 90	≈ 50	≈ 12
Norfloxacin	30 to 40	10 to 15	3 to 4
Ofloxacin Oral	≈ 98	≈ 32	≈ 9
IV		≈ 32	5 to 10

[a] Single dose: AUC (0-∞); Multiple dose: AUC (0-24).
[b] t½ = terminal half life; AUC = area under the curve.

Ciprofloxacin – Ciprofloxacin is rapidly and well absorbed from the GI tract after oral administration with no substantial loss by first-pass metabolism. When given concomitantly with food, there is a delay in the absorption of the drug; however, the overall absorption is not substantially affected. Maximum serum concentrations are attained 1 to 2 hours after oral dosing. The drug diffuses into the cerebrospinal fluid (CSF); however, CSF concentrations are generally less than 10% of peak serum concentrations. Active tubular secretion plays a significant role in clearance; only a small amount is recovered from the bile. In patients with reduced renal function, the half-life is slightly prolonged; dosage adjustments may be required.

Levofloxacin – Levofloxacin is rapidly and completely absorbed after oral administration. Peak plasma concentrations are usually attained 1 to 2 hours after oral dosing. Steady-state is reached within 48 hours. Levofloxacin tablets can be administered without regard to food. The oral and IV routes of administration can be considered interchangeable. Levofloxacin also penetrates well into the lung tissues. Levofloxacin undergoes limited metabolism and is primarily excreted as unchanged drug in the urine. Renal clearance in excess of the glomerular filtration rate suggest the tubular secretion of levofloxacin occurs in addition to glomerular filtration.

Moxifloxacin – Moxifloxacin is well absorbed from the GI tract. The maximal drug concentration (C_{max}) is attained 1 to 3 hours after oral dosing. Steady state is achieved after 3 days or more. Moxifloxacin is widely distributed throughout the body. Moxifloxacin is metabolized via glucuronide and sulfate conjugation.

Norfloxacin – Absorption is rapid. Food or dairy products may decrease absorption. Steady-state norfloxacin levels will be attained within 2 days of dosing. Norfloxacin is eliminated through metabolism, biliary excretion, and renal excretion. Renal excretion occurs by glomerular filtration and tubular secretion. In healthy elderly volunteers, norfloxacin is eliminated more slowly because of decreased renal function. In patients with CrCl rates of 30 mL/min/1.73 m^2 or less, the renal elimination decreases so that the effective serum half-life is 6.5 hours; dosage alteration is necessary.

Ofloxacin – Maximum serum concentrations are achieved 1 to 2 hours after an oral dose. Steady-state concentrations are achieved after 4 doses. Ofloxacin is widely distributed to body tissues and fluids. Elimination is mainly by renal excretion; 4% to 8% is excreted in the feces. A longer plasma half-life of about 6.4 to 7.4 hours was observed in elderly subjects, compared with 4 to 5 hours for young subjects. Dosage adjustment is necessary for patients with renal function impairment (CrCl of 50 mL/min or less).

Contraindications

Hypersensitivity to fluoroquinolones or the quinolone group; tendinitis or tendon rupture associated with quinolone use; patients receiving disopyramide and amiodarone or other QT_c-prolonging antiarrhythmic drugs reported to cause torsade de pointes, such as class IA antiarrhythmic agents (eg, quinidine, procainamide) and class III antiarrhythmic agents (eg, sotalol).

Warnings/Precautions

Phototoxicity: Moderate to severe phototoxic reactions have occurred in patients exposed to direct or indirect sunlight or to artificial ultraviolet light (eg, sunlamps) during or following treatment with **ofloxacin**.

Cardiac toxicity: **Moxifloxacin** has been shown to prolong the QT interval of the electrocardiogram in some patients. Avoid in patients with known prolongation of the QT interval, patients with uncorrected hypokalemia, and patients receiving class IA (eg, quinidine, procainamide) or class III (eg, amiodarone, sotalol) antiarrhythmic agents.

Avoid the concomitant prescription of medications known to prolong the QT_c interval (eg, erythromycin, cisapride, pentamidine, tricyclic antidepressants, some antipsychotics including phenothiazines).

Tendon rupture/tendinitis: Ruptures of the shoulder, hand, and Achilles tendons that required surgical repair or resulted in prolonged disability have been reported with fluoroquinolone antimicrobials.

Seizures: Increased intracranial pressure, convulsions, and toxic psychosis have occurred. CNS stimulation also may occur and may lead to tremor, restlessness, lightheadedness, confusion, dizziness, depression, hallucinations, and rarely, suicidal thoughts or acts.

Syphilis: **Ciprofloxacin**, **norfloxacin**, and **ofloxacin** are not effective for syphilis. High doses of antimicrobial agents for short periods of time to treat gonorrhea may mask or delay symptoms of incubating syphilis. All patients should have a serologic test for syphilis at the time of gonorrhea diagnosis. Patients treated with ciprofloxacin, norfloxacin, and ofloxacin should have a follow-up serologic test after 3 months.

Pseudomembranous colitis: Pseudomembranous colitis has been reported with nearly all antibacterial agents, including fluoroquinolones, and may range from mild to life-threatening in severity.

Crystalluria: Needle-shaped crystals were found in the urine of some volunteers who received either placebo or **norfloxacin**. Do not exceed the daily recommended dosage. The patient should drink sufficient fluids to ensure proper hydration and adequate urinary output.

Hemolytic reactions: Rarely, hemolytic reactions have been reported in patients with latent or actual defects in glucose-6-phosphate dehydrogenase activity who take quinolone antibacterial agents, including **norfloxacin**.

Myasthenia gravis: Quinolones may exacerbate the signs of myasthenia gravis and lead to life-threatening weakness of the respiratory muscles. Exercise caution when using quinolones in patients with myasthenia gravis.

Blood glucose abnormalities: Disturbances of blood glucose, including symptomatic hyper- and hypoglycemia, have been reported, usually in diabetic patients receiving concomitant treatment with an oral hypoglycemic agent or with insulin.

Hypersensitivity reactions: Hypersensitivity reactions, serious and occasionally fatal, have occurred in patients receiving quinolone therapy, some following the first dose. Refer to Management of Acute Hypersensitivity Reactions.

Renal function impairment: Alteration in dosage regimen is necessary. See Administration and Dosage.

Hepatic function impairment: There are no data in patients with severe cirrhosis. Dosage adjustment is recommended in patients with mild to moderate cirrhosis.

Pregnancy: Category C.

Lactation: Because of the potential for serious adverse reactions in breast-feeding infants, decide whether to discontinue breast-feeding or to discontinue the drug, taking into account the importance of the drug to the mother.

Children: Safety and efficacy of **levofloxacin**, **moxifloxacin**, **norfloxacin**, and **ofloxacin** in children younger than 18 years of age have not been established.

Elderly: **Norfloxacin** is eliminated more slowly because of decreased renal function. The apparent half-life of **ofloxacin** is 6 to 8 hours, compared with approximately 5 hours in younger adults.

Monitoring: Periodic assessment of organ system functions, including renal, hepatic, and hematopoietic, is advisable during prolonged therapy.

Drug Interactions

Drugs that may affect fluoroquinolones include antacids, azlocillin, bismuth subsalicylate, cimetidine, cisapride, didanosine, iron salts, morphine, nitrofurantoin, nonsteroidal anti-inflammatory drugs (NSAIDs), probenecid, and sucralfate.

Drugs that may be affected by fluoroquinolones include antiarrhythmic agents, anticoagulants, bepridil, caffeine, cyclosporine, digoxin, erythromycin, phenothiazine, procainamide, tricyclic antidepressants, and theophylline.

Drug/Food interactions: Refer to the Administration and Dosage section.

Adverse Reactions

Adverse reactions occurring in at least 3% of patients are in the following table.

Fluoroquinolone Adverse Reactions (≥ 3%)

	Adverse reaction	Ciprofloxacin[a]	Levofloxacin	Moxifloxacin	Norfloxacin[b]	Ofloxacin[a]
CNS	Headache	1.2	0.1 to 6.4	2	2 to 2.8	1 to 9
	Dizziness	< 1	0.3 to 2.7	3	1.7 to 2.6	1 to 5
	Insomnia	< 1	0.5 to 4.6	> 0.05 to < 1	0.3 to 1	3 to 7
GI	Nausea	5.2	1.3 to 7.2	8	2.6 to 4.2	3 to 10
	Diarrhea	2.3	1 to 5.6	6	0.3 to 1	1 to 4
	Vomiting	≤ 1 to 2	0.2 to 2.3	2	0.3 to 1	1 to 4
	Constipation	< 1	0.1 to 3.2	> 0.05 to < 1	0.3 to 1	1 to 3
	Flatulence	< 1	0.4 to 1.5		0.3 to 1	1 to 3
Miscellaneous	Visual disturbances	< 1			0.1 to 0.2	1 to 3
	Vaginitis	< 1	0.7 to 1.8	> 0.05 to < 1		1 to 5
	Pruritus	< 1	0.4 to 1.3	> 0.05 to < 1	0.3 to 1	1 to 3

[a] Includes data for oral and IV formulations.
[b] From single- and multiple-dose studies.

TETRACYCLINES

DEMECLOCYCLINE HYDROCHLORIDE	
Tablets; oral: 150 and 300 mg (*Rx*)	*Declomycin* (Lederle)
DOXYCYCLINE	
Tablets; oral: 20 mg (as hyclate) (*Rx*)	Various, *Alodox Convenience Kit* (OcuSoft), *Periostat* (CollaGenex)
50, 75, and 100 mg (as monohydrate) (*Rx*)	Various, *Adoxa* (Doak)
100 mg (as hyclate) (*Rx*)	Various, *Vibra-Tabs* (Pfizer)
150 mg (as monohydrate) (*Rx*)	Various, *Adoxa, Adoxa TT Kit* (Doak)
Tablets, delayed release; oral: 75, 100, and 150 mg (as hyclate) (*Rx*)	*Doryx* (Warner Chilcott)
Capsules; oral: 20 mg (as hyclate) (*Rx*)	*Oraxyl* (E5 Pharma)
40 mg (30 mg immediate release, 10 mg delayed release) (*Rx*)	*Oracea* (Galderma)
75 mg (as monohydrate) (*Rx*)	*NutriDox* (Advanced Vision Research)
50 and 100 mg (as monohydrate) (*Rx*)	Various, *Monodox* (Oclassen)
50 and 100 mg (as hyclate) (*Rx*)	Various, *Vibramycin* (Pfizer)
150 mg (as monohydrate) (*Rx*)	*Adoxa, Adoxa CK Kit* (Doak)
Capsules, coated pellets; oral: 75 and 100 mg (as hyclate) (*Rx*)	Various, *Doryx* (Warner Chilcott)
Syrup; oral: 50 mg (as calcium) per 5 mL (*Rx*)	*Vibramycin* (Pfizer)
Powder for suspension; oral: 25 mg (as monohydrate) per 5 mL (*Rx*)	Various, *Vibramycin* (Pfizer)
Injection: 42.5 mg (10%) (as hyclate) (*Rx*)	*Atridox* (CollaGenex)
Injection, lyophilized powder: 100 and 200 mg (as hyclate) (*Rx*)	Various, *Doxy 100, Doxy 200* (APP)
MINOCYCLINE	
Tablets; oral 50, 75, and 100 mg (as hydrochloride) (*Rx*)	Various, *Cleervue-M* (Stonebridge), *Dynacin* (Medicis), *Myrac* (Glades)
Tablets, extended-release; oral 45, 65, 90, 115, and 135 mg (as hydrochloride) (*Rx*)	Various, *Solodyn* (Medicis)
Capsules; oral 50, 75, and 100 mg (as hydrochloride) (*Rx*)	Various, *Dynacin* (Medicis)
Capsules, pellet-filled; oral 50 and 100 mg (as hydrochloride) (*Rx*)	*Minocin* (Lederle)
Suspension; oral: 50 mg (as hydrochloride) per 5 mL (*Rx*)	
Injection, powder for reconstitution: 100 mg (as hydrochloride)/vial (*Rx*)	*Minocin* (Triax)
TETRACYCLINE HYDROCHLORIDE	
Capsules; oral: 250 and 500 mg (*Rx*)	Various, *Sumycin 250, Sumycin 500* (Par)
Suspension; oral: 125 mg/5 mL (*Rx*)	Various, *Sumycin Syrup* (Par)

Indications

Gram-negative organisms (not extended release): *Haemophilus ducreyi* (chancroid); *Francisella tularensis* (tularemia); *Yersinia pestis* (plague); *Bartonella bacilliformis* (bartonellosis); *Campylobacter fetus*; *Vibrio cholerae* (cholera); *Brucella* sp. (brucellosis, may be in conjunction with streptomycin); *Calymmatobacterium granulomatis* (granuloma inguinale); *Neisseria gonorrhoeae* (uncomplicated urethritis in men).

Infections caused by the following miscellaneous microorganisms (not extended release): *Rickettsiae* (Rocky Mountain spotted fever, typhus fever and the typhus group, Q fever, rickettsialpox, and tick fevers); *Mycoplasma pneumoniae* (respiratory tract infections); *Chlamydia trachomatis* (lymphogranuloma venereum, trachoma [infectious agent not always eliminated], inclusion conjunctivitis, uncomplicated urethral, endocervical, or rectal infections); *Chlamydia psittaci* (psittacosis [ornithosis]); *Borrelia recurrentis* (relapsing fever); *Ureaplasma urealyticum* (nongonococcal urethritis).

Following susceptibility testing (resistance has been documented): *Escherichia coli*; *Enterobacter aerogenes*; *Acinetobacter* and *Shigella* sp.; *Haemophilus influenzae* (respiratory tract infections); *Klebsiella* sp. (respiratory and urinary infections); *Streptococcus pneumoniae* (upper respiratory tract infections); *Staphylococcus aureus* (skin and skin structure infections).

Alternative therapy for the following infections when penicillin is contraindicated (not extended release): *Neisseria gonorrhoeae* infections; syphilis due to *Treponema pallidum*; yaws due to *T. pertenue*; listeriosis caused by *Listeria monocytogenes*; anthrax due to *Bacillus anthracis*; Vincent infection due to *Fusobacterium fusiforme*; actinomycosis due to *Actinomyces israelii*; infections caused by *Clostridium* sp.

Acute intestinal amebiasis (minocycline; not extended release): As adjunct to amebicides.

Rosacea: For the treatment of only inflammatory lesions (papules and pustules) of rosacea in adult patients (**doxycycline** [*Oracea*]).

Severe acne (tetracycline, doxycycline, minocycline only): As adjunctive therapy.

Anthrax, including inhalational anthrax (doxycycline only): To reduce the incidence or progression of disease following exposure to aerosolized *Bacillus anthracis*.

Malaria (doxycycline only): Prophylaxis of malaria due to *Plasmodium falciparum* in short-term travelers (less than 4 months) to areas with chloroquine and/or pyrimethamine-sulfadoxine resistant strains.

Adult periodontitis: For use as an adjunct to scaling and root planing to promote attachment level gain and to reduce pocket depth in patients with adult periodontitis (**doxycycline** [*Periostat*]); as an adjunct to scaling and root planing procedures for reduction of pocket depth in patients with adult periodontitis and may be used as part of a periodontal maintenance program that includes good oral hygiene and scaling and root planing (**minocycline** [Arestin]).

Neisseria meningitidis (minocycline; not extended release): Treatment of asymptomatic meningococcal carriers of *N. meningitidis*.

Note: Do not use tetracyclines for streptococcal disease unless organism has been shown to be susceptible. Tetracyclines are not the drugs of choice in treatment of any type of staphylococcal infection.

Administration and Dosage

Avoid rapid IV administration. Thrombophlebitis may result from prolonged IV therapy.

Continue therapy at least 24 to 48 hours after symptoms and fever subside. Treat all infections caused by group A β-hemolytic streptococci for at least 10 days.

Take on an empty stomach, at least 2 hours before or after meals. Absorption and peak plasma levels may be reduced when administered with meals or with dairy products, including milk.

Antacids containing aluminum, calcium, magnesium, sodium bicarbonate, and iron-containing preparations should not be given to patients using oral tetracyclines.

DEMECLOCYCLINE HYDROCHLORIDE:

Adults –

Daily dose: 4 divided doses of 150 mg each or 2 divided doses of 300 mg each.

Children (over 8 years of age) –

Usual daily dose: 3 to 6 mg/lb (6.6 to 13.2 mg/kg), depending upon the severity of the disease, divided into 2 or 4 doses.

Gonorrhea patients sensitive to penicillin – Initially, 600 mg; follow with 300 mg every 12 hours for 4 days to a total of 3 g.

Streptococcal infections – Treat streptococcal infections for at least 10 days.

Concomitant therapy – Absorption is impaired by antacids containing aluminum, calcium, or magnesium, and by preparations containing iron. Take demeclocycline at least 1 hour before or 2 hours after these products.

DOXYCYCLINE:

Oral – When used in streptococcal infections, continue therapy for 10 days. Take with plenty of fluids.

Adults:

Usual dose – 200 mg (100 mg every 12 hours) on the first day of treatment followed with a maintenance dose of 100 mg/day administered as a single dose or as 50 mg every 12 hours.

More severe infections (particularly chronic urinary tract infections) – 100 mg every 12 hours.

Children (older than 8 years of age):

100 lbs or less (less than 45 kg) – 2 mg/lb (4.4 mg/kg) divided into 2 doses on the first day of treatment; follow with 1 mg/lb (2.2 mg/kg) given as a single daily dose or divided into 2 doses on subsequent days.

More severe infections – Up to 2 mg/lb (4.4 mg/kg) may be used.

More than 100 lbs (45 kg) – Use the usual adult dose.

Uncomplicated gonococcal infection in adults (except anorectal infections in men): 100 mg twice daily for 7 days.

Single visit dose – Administer 300 mg immediately followed in 1 hour by a second 300 mg dose.

Nongonococcal urethritis caused by C. trachomatis or U. urealyticum: 100 mg twice daily for 7 days.

Syphilis:

Early (except Adoxa, Doryx, Monodox) – Patients allergic to penicillins should be treated with 100 mg twice daily for 2 weeks.

More than 1 year duration (except Adoxa, Doryx, Monodox) – Patients allergic to penicillins should be treated with 100 mg twice daily for 4 weeks.

Primary and secondary (Adoxa, Doryx, Monodox only) – 300 mg/day in divided doses for at least 10 days.

Uncomplicated urethral, endocervical or rectal infections in adults caused by C. trachomatis: 100 mg twice daily for at least 7 days.

Acute epididymo-orchitis caused by N. gonorrhoeae or C. trachomatis: 100 mg twice daily for at least 10 days.

Malaria prophylaxis (except Adoxa, Doryx, Monodox): Begin prophylaxis 1 to 2 days prior to travel to an endemic area, continue during travel and for 4 weeks after returning from travel.

Adults – 100 mg/day.

Children (older than 8 years of age) – 2 mg/kg once daily up to 100 mg/day.

Inhalation anthrax (postexposure):

Adults and children (100 lb [45 kg] or more) – 100 mg twice daily for 60 days.

Children (weighing less than 100 lb [45 kg]) – 1 mg/lb (2.2 mg/kg) of body weight twice a day for a 60 days.

Rosacea: Exceeding the recommended doxycycline dosage may result in an increased incidence of side effects including the development of resistant microorganisms.

One *Oracea* capsule (40 mg) should be taken once daily in the morning on an empty stomach, preferably at least 1 hour prior to or 2 hours after a meal. Administration of adequate amounts of fluid along with the capsules is recommended to wash down the capsule to reduce the risk of esophageal irritation and ulceration.

Coated pellets:

Primary and secondary syphilis – 300 mg/day in divided doses for at least 10 days.

Sprinkling the capsule contents (coated pellets) on applesauce – Doxycycline hyclate coated pellet capsules may also be administered by sprinkling the capsule contents onto a spoonful of applesauce. The applesauce should be swallowed immediately without chewing and followed with a cool 240 mL glass of water. The applesauce should not be hot, and it should be just enough to be swallowed without chewing. In the event that a prepared dose cannot be taken immediately, the mixture should be discarded and not stored for later use.

Adult periodontitis: Periostat 20 mg twice daily as an adjunct following scaling and root planing may be administered for up to 9 months; it should be taken at 12-hour intervals in the morning and evening. Patients should allow at least 1 hour prior to or 2 hours after meals when taking *Periostat*.

Parenteral – Do not inject IM or subcutaneously. Avoid rapid administration. Switch to oral therapy as soon as possible. The duration of IV infusion may vary with the dose (100 to 200 mg/day), but is usually 1 to 4 hours. A recommended minimum infusion time for 100 mg of a 0.5 mg/mL solution is 1 hour.

Adults: The usual dosage is 200 mg IV on the first day of treatment, administered in 1 or 2 infusions. Subsequent daily dosage is 100 to 200 mg, depending upon the severity of infection, with 200 mg administered in 1 or 2 infusions.

Primary and secondary syphilis – 300 mg/day for at least 10 days.

Children (older than 8 years of age):

Up to 100 lb (45 kg) – Give 2 mg/lb (4.4 mg/kg) on the first day of treatment, in 1 or 2 infusions. Subsequent daily dosage is 1 to 2 mg/lb (2.2 to 4.4 mg/kg) given as 1 or 2 infusions, depending on the severity of the infection.

Over 100 lb (45 kg) – Use the usual adult dose.

MINOCYCLINE:

Adults –

Immediate release:

Usual dose – 200 mg initially, followed by 100 mg every 12 hours. If more frequent doses are preferred, give 100 or 200 mg initially; follow with 50 mg 4 times/day.

Syphilis – 200 mg initially, followed by 100 mg every 12 hours for 10 to 15 days. Close follow-up, including laboratory tests, is recommended.

Uncomplicated urethral infections in adults caused by C. trachomatis *or Ureaplasma urealyticum* – 100 mg every 12 hours for at least 7 days.

Uncomplicated gonococcal urethritis in men – 100 mg every 12 hours for 5 days.

Uncomplicated gonococcal infections except urethritis and anorectal infections in men – 200 mg initially, followed by 100 mg every 12 hours for at least 4 days, with posttherapy cultures within 2 to 3 days.

Meningococcal carrier state – 100 mg every 12 hours for 5 days.

Extended-release, tablets:

Acne vulgaris – 1 mg/kg/day for 12 weeks.

Minocycline Extended Release Dosing

Patients weight (lbs)	Patients weight (kg)	Tablet strength (mg)	Actual mg/kg dose
99 to 131	45 to 59	45	1 to 0.76
132 to 199	60 to 90	90	1.5 to 1
200 to 300	91 to 136	135	1.48 to 0.99

Renal function impairment – In patients with renal impairment, the total dosage should be decreased by either reducing the recommended individual doses and/or by extending the time intervals between doses.

Parenteral: Administer diluted injections immediately. Avoid rapid administration. Switch to oral therapy as soon as possible.

Adults – 200 mg followed by 100 mg every 12 hours; do not exceed 400 mg in 24 hours.

Children (older than 8 years of age) – Initially, usual pediatric dose is 4 mg/kg, followed by 2 mg/kg every 12 hours, not to exceed the usual adult dose.

Incompatibilities – Do not mix IV minocycline before or during administration with any solutions containing the following: Adrenocorticotropic hormone (ACTH), aminophylline, amobarbital sodium, amphotericin B, bicarbonate infusion mixtures, calcium gluconate or chloride, carbenicillin, cephalothin sodium, cefazolin sodium, chloramphenicol succinate, colistin sulfate, heparin sodium, hydrocortisone sodium succinate, iodine sodium, methicillin sodium, novobiocin, penicillin, pentobarbital, phenytoin sodium, polymyxin, prochlorperazine, sodium ascorbate, sulfadiazine, sulfisoxazole, thiopental sodium, vitamin K (sodium bisulfate or sodium salt), whole blood.

Children (older than 8 years of age) –

Immediate release: Initially, 4 mg/kg; follow with 2 mg/kg every 12 hours.

Extended release: See Adults for dosing for children 12 years of age and older.

Renal function impairment – Decrease the recommended dosage and/or increase the dosing intervals in patients with renal impairment. Do not exceed 200 mg *Minocin* in 24 hours in patients with renal impairment.

Administration – Take minocycline with plenty of fluids. Capsules and extended-release tablets may be taken with or without food.

Take minocycline tablets and pellet-filled capsules 1 hour before or 2 hours after a meal.

Capsules should be swallowed whole.

TETRACYCLINE HYDROCHLORIDE:

Adults –

Usual dose: 1 to 2 g/day in 2 or 4 equal doses.

Mild to moderate infections: 500 mg 2 times/day or 250 mg 4 times/day.

Severe infections: 500 mg 4 times/day.

Children (older than 8 years of age) – Daily dose is 10 to 20 mg/lb (25 to 50 mg/kg) in 4 equal doses.

Brucellosis – 500 mg 4 times/day for 3 weeks, accompanied by 1 g streptomycin IM twice/day the first week, and once daily the second week.

Syphilis –

Sumycin only: A total of 30 to 40 g in equally divided doses over 10 to 15 days. Perform close follow-up and laboratory tests.

All except Sumycin:

Early (less than 1 year) – 500 mg 4 times/day for 15 days.

More than 1 year duration – 500 mg 4 times/day for 30 days.

Uncomplicated gonorrhea – 500 mg every 6 hours for 7 days.

Uncomplicated urethral, endocervical, or rectal infections caused by Chlamydia trachomatis – 500 mg 4 times/day for at least 7 days.

Severe acne (long-term therapy) – Initially, 1 g/day in divided doses. For maintenance, give 125 to 500 mg/day.

Streptococcal infections – Treat streptococcal infections for at least 10 days.

Concomitant therapy – Absorption is impaired by antacids containing aluminum, calcium, or magnesium, and preparations containing iron, zinc, or sodium bicarbonate.

Actions

Pharmacology: The tetracyclines are bacteriostatic. They exert their antimicrobial effect by inhibition of protein synthesis. Tetracyclines are active against a wide range of gram-positive and gram-negative organisms.

Pharmacokinetics:

Tetracycline Pharmacokinetics

Tetracyclines	Absorption (%)	C_{max} (mcg/mL)	T_{max} (h)	Protein binding (%)	Serum half-life (h)
Demeclocycline	60 to 80	1.5 to 1.7[a]	3 to 4[a]	35 to 90	16
Doxycycline	90 to 100	2.6 (hyclate)[b] 3.61 (monohydrate)[b] 3.6 (IV)[c]	2 (hyclate)[b] 2.6 (monohydrate)[b]	80 to 95	18 to 22
Minocycline	90 to 100	2.1 to 5.1[d]	1 to 4	75	11 to 22 (oral) 15 to 23 (IV)
Tetracycline	60 to 80	nd[e]	2 to 4	20 to 65	6 to 12

[a] 300 mg single oral dose.
[b] 200 mg single oral dose.
[c] 200 mg administered IV over 2 hours.
[d] Single oral dose of two 100 mg pellet-filled capsules.
[e] nd = no data

Contraindications

Hypersensitivity to any of the tetracyclines.

Warnings/Precautions

Malaria prophylaxis (doxycycline only): **Doxycycline** offers substantial but not complete suppression of the asexual stages of *Plasmodium* strains. Advise patients taking doxycycline for malaria prophylaxis of when prophylaxis should begin and end; that no present-day antimalarial, including doxycycline, guarantees protection against malaria; and to avoid being bitten by mosquitos by wearing protective clothing, using effective insect-repellent, mosquito nets, etc.

Pseudomembranous colitis: Treatment with antibacterial agents alters the normal flora of the colon and may permit overgrowth of clostridia. Pseudomembranous colitis has been reported with nearly all antibacterial agents.

Parenteral therapy: Reserve for situations in which oral therapy is not indicated. Institute oral therapy as soon as possible. If given IV over prolonged periods, thrombophlebitis may result. IM use produces lower blood levels than recommended oral dosages.

Nephrogenic diabetes insipidus: Administration of **demeclocycline** has resulted in appearance of the diabetes insipidus syndrome (polyuria, polydipsia, and weakness) in some patients on long-term therapy.

Pseudotumor cerebri: Pseudotumor cerebri (benign intracranial hypertension) in adults has been associated with tetracycline use.

Outdated products: Under no circumstances should outdated tetracyclines be administered; the degradation products of tetracyclines are highly nephrotoxic and have, on occasion, produced a Fanconi-like syndrome.

Hypersensitivity reactions: Sensitivity reactions are more likely to occur on patients with a history of allergy, asthma, hay fever, or urticaria.

Renal function impairment: If renal impairment exists, even usual doses may lead to excessive systemic accumulation of the tetracyclines (with the exception of doxycycline and minocycline) and possible liver toxicity. Use lower than usual doses and/or extend the dosing interval.

Hepatic function impairment: Doses more than 2 g/day IV can be extremely dangerous. In the presence of renal dysfunction, and particularly in pregnancy, IV tetracycline more than 2 g/day has been associated with death secondary to liver failure. Hepatotoxicity has been reported with **minocycline**. Administer with caution; reduce the recommended dosage and/or extend the dosing interval.

Hazardous tasks: Lightheadedness, dizziness or vertigo may occur with tetracyclines. Patients should observe caution while driving or performing other tasks requiring alertness.

Superinfection: Use of antibiotics (especially prolonged or repeated therapy) may result in bacterial or fungal overgrowth of nonsusceptible organisms.

Photosensitivity: Photosensitivity manifested by an exaggerated sunburn reaction has been observed in some individuals taking tetracyclines. Advise patients who are apt to be exposed to direct sunlight or ultraviolet light that this reaction can occur with tetracycline drugs, and discontinue treatment at the first evidence of skin erythema.

Phototoxic reactions are most frequent with demeclocycline, and occur less frequently with the other tetracyclines; minocycline is least likely to cause phototoxic reactions.

Carcinogenesis: There has been evidence of oncogenic activity in studies with **minocycline** (thyroid tumors) in rats and dogs.

Mutagenesis: **Tetracycline** has produced positive mutagenic results in mammalian cell assays in vitro.

Fertility impairment: **Minocycline** has been shown to impair fertility in male rats.

Pregnancy: *Category D.*

Lactation: Tetracyclines are excreted in breast milk.

Children: Tetracyclines generally should not be used in children less than 8 years of age (except for anthrax, including inhalational) unless other drugs are not likely to be effective or are contraindicated.

Teeth – The use of tetracyclines during the period of tooth development may cause permanent discoloration of deciduous and permanent teeth.

Bone – Tetracycline forms a stable calcium complex in any bone-forming tissue. Decreased fibula growth rate occurred in premature infants given 25 mg/kg oral tetracycline every 6 hours.

Monitoring: In sexually transmitted diseases when coexistent syphilis is suspected, perform darkfield examination before starting treatment and repeat the blood serology monthly for at least 4 months.

In long-term therapy, perform periodic laboratory evaluation of organ systems, including hematopoietic, renal, and hepatic studies.

Drug Interactions

Drugs that may affect tetracyclines include antacids containing aluminum, calcium, or magnesium; iron salts; zinc salts; barbiturates; bismuth salts; carbamazepine; cholestyramine; colestipol; phenytoin; rifamycins; urinary alkalinizers (eg, sodium lactate, potassium citrate).

Drugs that may be affected by tetracyclines include oral anticoagulants, digoxin, insulin, isotretinoin, methoxyflurane, oral contraceptives, penicillins, and theophyllines.

Drug/Lab test interactions: The antianabolic action of tetracyclines may cause an increase in blood urea nitrogen. During **doxycycline** or **minocycline** therapy, false elevations of urinary catecholamine levels may occur.

Drug/Food interactions: The administration of **demeclocycline** and **tetracycline** with milk and dairy products forms poorly absorbed chelates. Administer the interacting tetracyclines at least 2 hours before or after meals. The inhibitory effect of food and milk on the absorption of **doxycycline** and **minocycline** is considerably less than that observed with the other tetracycline derivatives. These 2 drugs are often administered without regard to meals; but the potential risk of decreased drug efficacy must be weighed against the benefit of treating the infection.

Adverse Reactions

The following adverse reactions have been reported with the tetracyclines.

CNS: Bulging fontanel, convulsions, dizziness, headache, hypesthesia, paresthesia, pseudotumor cerebri, sedation, vertigo.

Dermatologic: Alopecia, balanitis, erythema multiforme, erythema nodosum, fixed drug eruptions, hyperpigmentation of the nails, injection site erythema and injection site pain, maculopapular and erythematous rashes, photosensitivity, pruritus, skin and mucus membrane pigmentation, Stevens-Johnson syndrome, toxic epidermal necrolysis, vasculitis.

GI: Anorexia, diarrhea, dyspepsia, dysphagia, enamel hypoplasia, enterocolitis, esophageal ulcerations, esophagitis, glossitis, inflammatory lesions (with monilial overgrowth) in the anogenital region, nausea, pancreatitis, pseudomembranous colitis, stomatitis, vomiting; black hairy tongue, bulky loose stools, hoarseness, sore throat (**tetracycline**).

Hematologic: Agranulocytosis, anemia, eosinophilia, hemolytic anemia, leukopenia, neutropenia, pancytopenia, thrombocytopenia.

Hepatic: Hepatic cholestasis, hepatic toxicity, hepatitis, hyperbilirubinemia, increased liver enzymes, jaundice, liver failure.

Hypersensitivity: Anaphylactoid purpura, anaphylaxis, angioneurotic edema, myocarditis, pericarditis, polyarthralgia, pulmonary infiltrates with eosinophilia, systemic lupus erythematous exacerbation, urticaria; hypersensitivity syndrome (cutaneous reaction, eosinophilia, and one or more of the following: Hepatitis, pneumonitis, nephritis, myocarditis, pericarditis, fever, lymphadenopathy).

Musculoskeletal: Arthralgia, arthritis, bone discoloration, joint stiffness and swelling, myalgia, polyarthralgia.

Renal: Acute renal failure, dose-related increase in BUN, interstitial nephritis; nephrogenic diabetes insipidus (**demeclocycline**).

Respiratory: Asthma exacerbation, bronchospasm, cough, dyspnea.

Miscellaneous: Brown-black microscopic discoloration of thyroid glands (prolonged therapy), decreased hearing, fever, lupus-like syndrome, secretion discoloration, serum sickness-like syndrome, tinnitus, tooth discoloration, vulvovaginitis.

TIGECYCLINE

Powder for injection, lyophilized: 50 mg (*Rx*)	*Tygacil* (Wyeth)

Indications

For the treatment of infections in patients 18 years of age and older caused by susceptible strains of the designated microorganisms in the following conditions:

Community-acquired bacterial pneumonia: Caused by *Streptococcus pneumoniae* (penicillin-susceptible isolates), including cases with concurrent bacteremia, *Haemophilus influenzae* (beta-lactamase negative isolates), and *Legionella pneumophila.*

Complicated skin and skin structure infections: Complicated skin and skin structure infections caused by *Escherichia coli, Enterococcus faecalis* (vancomycin-susceptible isolates only), *Staphylococcus aureus* (methicillin-susceptible and methicillin-resistant isolates), *Streptococcus agalactiae, Streptococcus anginosus* group (includes *S. anginosus, Streptococcus intermedius,* and *Streptococcus constellatus*), *Streptococcus pyogenes,* and *Bacteroides fragilis.*

Complicated intraabdominal infections: Complicated intraabdominal infections caused by *Citrobacter freundii, Enterobacter cloacae, E. coli, Klebsiella oxytoca, Klebsiella pneumoniae, E. faecalis* (vancomycin-susceptible isolates only), *S. aureus* (methicillin-susceptible isolates only), *S. anginosus* group (includes *S. anginosus, S. intermedius,* and *S. constellatus*), *B. fragilis, Bacteroides thetaiotaomicron, Bacteroides uniformis, Bacteroides vulgatus, Clostridium perfringens,* and *Peptostreptococcus micros.*

Administration and Dosage

Community-acquired bacterial pneumonia: Initial dosage is 100 mg intravenous (IV) administered over approximately 30 to 60 minutes. Maintenance dosage is 50 mg IV every 12 hours administered over approximately 30 to 60 minutes. Duration is 7 to 14 days.

Complicated intra-abdominal infections: Initial dosage is 100 mg IV administered over approximately 30 to 60 minutes. Maintenance dosage is 50 mg IV every 12 hours administered over approximately 30 to 60 minutes. Duration is 5 to 14 days.

Complicated skin and skin structure infections: Initial dosage is 100 mg IV administered over approximately 30 to 60 minutes. Maintenance dosage is 50 mg IV every 12 hours administered over approximately 30 to 60 minutes. Duration is 5 to 14 days.

Hepatic function impairment: For patients with severe hepatic function impairment, the initial dose is 100 mg IV, and the maintenance dosage is 25 mg every 12 hours.

Admixture compatibility: Compatible IV solutions include sodium chloride 0.9% injection, dextrose 5% injection, and Ringer's lactate injection. When administered through a Y-site, tigecycline is compatible with the following drugs or diluents when used with either sodium chloride 0.9% injection or dextrose 5% injection: amikacin, dobutamine, dopamine hydrochloride, gentamicin, haloperidol, lidocaine hydrochloride, metoclopramide, morphine, norepinephrine, piperacillin/tazobactam (EDTA formulation), potassium chloride, propofol, ranitidine hydrochloride, Ringer's lactate, theophylline, and tobramycin.

Incompatibility: The following drugs should not be administered simultaneously through the same Y-site with tigecycline: amphotericin B, amphotericin B complex, diazepam, esomeprazole, and omeprazole.

Actions

Pharmacology: Tigecycline, a glycylcycline, inhibits protein translation in bacteria by binding to the 30S ribosomal subunit and blocking entry of amino-acyl tRNA molecules into the A site of the ribosome. This prevents incorporation of amino acid residues into elongating peptide chains.

Glycylcycline class antibiotics are structurally similar to tetracycline class antibiotics and may have similar adverse reactions.

Pharmacokinetics: The in vitro plasma protein binding of tigecycline ranges from approximately 71% to 89% at concentrations observed in clinical studies. The steady-state volume of distribution of tigecycline averaged 500 to 700 L (7 to 9 L/kg), indicating tigecycline is extensively distributed beyond the plasma volume and into the tissues.

Tigecycline is not extensively metabolized.

The primary route of elimination for tigecycline is biliary excretion of unchanged tigecycline and its metabolites.

Contraindications

Known hypersensitivity to tigecycline.

Warnings/Precautions

All-cause mortality: In a pooled analysis of Phase 3 and 4 clinical trials, an adjusted risk difference of all-cause mortality was 0.6% between tigecycline and comparator-treated patients. The cause of this increase has not been established. This increase in all-cause mortality should be considered when selecting among treatment options.

Ventilator-associated pneumonia: A trial of patients with hospital-acquired pneumonia failed to demonstrate the efficacy of tigecycline. Patients with ventilator-associated pneumonia who received tigecycline had lower cure rates.

Pancreatitis: Acute pancreatitis, including fatal cases, has occurred in association with tigecycline treatment. Cases have been reported in patients without known risk factors for pancreatitis. consider discontinuation of tigecycline in patients suspected of having developed pancreatitis.

Tooth discoloration: The use of tigecycline during tooth development (last half of pregnancy, infancy, and childhood until the age of 8 years) may cause permanent discoloration of the teeth (yellow-gray-brown).

Ventilator-associated pneumonia: A study of patients with hospital acquired pneumonia failed to demonstrate the efficacy of tigecycline.

Clostridium difficile–associated diarrhea: C. *difficile* associated diarrhea has been reported with use of nearly all antibacterial agents, including tigecycline, and may range in severity from mild diarrhea to fatal colitis. Treatment with antibacterial agents alters the flora of the colon, leading to overgrowth of C. *difficile.*

Intestinal perforation: Exercise caution when considering tigecycline monotherapy in patients with complicated intra-abdominal infections secondary to clinically apparent intestinal perforation.

Tetracycline class antibiotics: Glycylcycline class antibiotics are structurally similar to tetracycline class antibiotics and may have similar adverse effects. Such effects may include photosensitivity, pseudotumor cerebri, and antianabolic action (which has led to increased serum urea nitrogen [BUN], azotemia, acidosis, and hypophosphatemia).

Resistance: Prescribing tigecycline in the absence of a proven or strongly suspected bacterial infection is unlikely to provide benefit to the patient and increases the risk of the development of drug-resistant bacteria.

Hypersensitivity reactions: Administer tigecycline with caution to patients with known hypersensitivity to tetracycline class antibiotics.

Hepatic function impairment: In patients with severe hepatic impairment (Child-Pugh class C), the initial dose of tigecycline should be 100 mg followed by a reduced maintenance dosage of 25 mg every 12 hours. Treat patients with severe hepatic impairment with caution and monitor them for treatment response.

Special risk: Exercise caution when considering tigecycline monotherapy in patients with complicated intraabdominal infections secondary to clinically apparent intestinal perforation.

Superinfection: As with other antibacterial drugs, use of tigecycline may result in overgrowth of nonsusceptible organisms, including fungi. Carefully monitor patients during therapy. If superinfection occurs, take appropriate measures.

Pregnancy: Category D.

Lactation: It is not known whether this drug is excreted in human milk. Because many drugs are excreted in human milk, exercise caution when tigecycline is administered to a breast-feeding woman.

Children: Safety and efficacy in pediatric patients younger than 18 years of age have not been established. Because of the effects on tooth development, use in patients younger than 8 years of age is not recommended.

Monitoring: Monitor prothrombin time or other suitable anticoagulation test if tigecycline is administered with warfarin. Monitor patients for superinfection during therapy. Monitor patients who develop abnormal liver function tests during tigecycline therapy for evidence of worsening hepatic function and evaluate for risk/benefit of continuing tigecycline therapy.

Drug Interactions

Warfarin: Monitor prothrombin time or other suitable anticoagulation test if tigecycline is administered with warfarin.

Oral contraceptives: Concurrent use of antibacterial drugs with oral contraceptives may render oral contraceptives less effective.

Adverse Reactions

Adverse reactions include abdominal pain, abnormal healing, abscess, alkaline phosphatase increased, ALT increased, amylase increased, anemia, asthenia, AST increased, BUN increased, diarrhea, dizziness, headache, hypoproteinemia, infection, nausea, phlebitis, rash, vomiting.

MACROLIDES

AZITHROMYCIN	
Tablets; oral: 250, 500, and 600 mg (*Rx*)	Various,[a,b] *Zithromax*[a] (Pfizer)
Powder for suspension; oral: 100 and 200 mg per 5 mL, 1 g/packet (*Rx*)	
167 mg per 5 mL when reconstituted (*Rx*)	*Zmax*[a] (Pfizer)
Injection, lyophilized, powder for solution: 500 mg (*Rx*)	Various, *Zithromax*[a] (Pfizer)
CLARITHROMYCIN	
Tablets; oral: 250 and 500 mg (*Rx*)	Various, *Biaxin* (Abbott)
Tablets, extended-release; oral: 500 (*Rx*)	Various, *Biaxin XL* (Abbott)
Granules for suspension; oral: 125 and 250 mg per 5 mL when reconstituted (*Rx*)	Various, *Biaxin* (Abbott)
ERYTHROMYCIN BASE	
Tablets, delayed-release; oral: 250 mg (*Rx*)	*Ery-Tab* (Abbott)
333 and 500 mg (*Rx*)	*Ery-Tab* (Abbott), *PCE Dispertab* (Abbott)
Tablets, film-coated; oral: 250 and 500 mg (*Rx*)	*Erythromycin Filmtabs* (Abbott)
Capsules, delayed-release; oral: 250 mg (*Rx*)	Various
ERYTHROMYCIN LACTOBIONATE	
Injection, lyophilized powder for solution: 500 mg and 1 g (as lactobionate) (*Rx*)	*Erythrocin Lactobionate* (Hospira)
ERYTHROMYCIN ETHYLSUCCINATE	
Tablets; oral: 400 mg of erythromycin activity[c] (*Rx*)	*Erythromycin Ethylsuccinate* (Abbott), *E.E.S. 400 Filmtab* (Abbott)
Suspension; oral: 200 mg of erythromycin activity[d] per 5 mL (*Rx*)	*Erythromycin Ethylsuccinate* (Abbott)
400 mg of erythromycin activity[c] per 5 mL (*Rx*)	*Erythromycin Ethylsuccinate* (Abbott), *E.E.S. 400 Liquid* (Abbott)
Powder for suspension; oral: 100 mg of erythromycin activity[e] per 2.5 mL (after reconstitution) (*Rx*)	*EryPed Drops* (Abbott)
200 mg of erythromycin activity[d] per 5 mL (after reconstitution) (*Rx*)	*EryPed 200* (Abbott)
400 mg of erythromycin activity[c] per 5 mL (after reconstitution) (*Rx*)	*EryPed 400* (Abbott)
Granules for suspension; oral: 200 mg of erythromycin activity[d] per 5 mL (after reconstitution) (*Rx*)	*E.E.S. Granules* (Abbott)
ERYTHROMYCIN STEARATE	
Tablets; oral: 250 mg (*Rx*)	*Erythrocin Stearate* (Abbott)

[a] Supplied as azithromycin dihydrate.
[b] Supplied as azithromycin monohydrate.
[c] Equivalent to 250 mg of erythromycin activity as the stearate or base.
[d] Equivalent to 125 mg of erythromycin activity as the stearate or base.
[e] Equivalent to 62.5 mg of erythromycin activity as the stearate or base.

Indications

For specific approved indications, refer to the Administration and Dosage sections.

Administration and Dosage

AZITHROMYCIN: Azithromycin tablets and oral suspension (except *Zmax*) can be taken with or without food; however, increased tolerability has been observed when tablets are taken with food. It is recommended that *Zmax* be taken on an empty stomach (at least 1 hours before or 2 hours following a meal). Single-dose 1 g packets are not for pediatric use.

Adults –

Mild to moderate acute bacterial exacerbations of chronic obstructive pulmonary disease (COPD): 500 mg/day for 3 days or 500 mg as a single dose on the first day followed by 250 mg once daily on days 2 through 5.

Community-acquired pneumonia of mild severity, pharyngitis/tonsillitis (as second-line therapy), and uncomplicated skin and skin structure infections: 500 mg as a single dose on the first day followed by 250 mg once daily on days 2 through 5. For community-acquired pneumonia, a single 2 g dose of *Zmax* may be given.

Acute bacterial sinusitis: 500 mg/day for 3 days or 2 g as a single dose of *Zmax*.

Genital ulcer disease caused by Haemophilus ducreyi (chancroid): Single 1 g dose.

Nongonococcal urethritis/cervicitis caused by Chlamydia trachomatis: Single 1 g dose.

Gonococcal urethritis/cervicitis caused by Neisseria gonorrhoeae: Single 2 g dose.

Prevention of disseminated Mycobacterium avium complex (MAC) infections: 1,200 mg taken once weekly.

Treatment of disseminated MAC infections: 600 mg/day in combination with ethambutol at the recommended daily dose of 15 mg/kg.

Children (6 months of age and older) –

Acute otitis media: The recommended dose of azithromycin oral suspension is 30 mg/kg given as a single dose or 10 mg/kg once daily for 3 days or 10 mg/kg as a single dose on the first day (not to exceed 500 mg/day), followed by 5 mg/kg on days 2 through 5 (not to exceed 250 mg/day).

Acute bacterial sinusitis: 10 mg/kg oral suspension once daily for 3 days.

Community-acquired pneumonia: 10 mg/kg oral suspension as a single dose on the first day followed by 5 mg/kg on days 2 through 5.

Azithromycin Pediatric Dosage Guidelines for Otitis Media and Community-Acquired Pneumonia (≥ 6 months of age) 5-Day Regimen[a,b]

Weight		Amount of 100 mg/5 mL suspension		Amount of 200 mg/5 mL suspension		Total mL per treatment course	Total mg per treatment course
kg	lbs	Day 1	Days 2 to 5	Day 1	Days 2 to 5		
5	11	2.5 mL	1.25 mL			7.5 mL	150 mg
10	22	5 mL	2.5 mL			15 mL	300 mg
20	44			5 mL	2.5 mL	15 mL	600 mg
30	66			7.5 mL	3.75 mL	22.5 mL	900 mg
40	88			10 mL	5 mL	30 mL	1,200 mg
≥ 50	≥ 110			12.5 mL	6.25 mL	37.5 mL	1,500 mg

[a] Dosing calculated on 10 mg/kg on day 1, followed by 5 mg/kg on days 2 to 5.
[b] Efficacy of the 1- or 3-day regimen in children with community-acquired pneumonia has not been established.

Azithromycin Pediatric Dosage Guidelines for Otitis Media and Acute Bacterial Sinusitis: 3-Day Regimen[a]

Weight		Amount of 100 mg/5 mL suspension	Amount of 200 mg/5 mL suspension	Total mL per treatment course	Total mg per treatment course
kg	lbs	Day 1 to 3	Day 1 to 3		
5	11	2.5 mL		7.5 mL	150 mg
10	22	5 mL		15 mL	300 mg
20	44		5 mL	15 mL	600 mg
30	66		7.5 mL	22.5 mL	900 mg
40	88		10 mL	30 mL	1,200 mg
≥ 50	≥ 110		12.5 mL	37.5 mL	1,500 mg

[a] Dosing calculated on 10 mg/kg/day.

Azithromycin Pediatric Dosage Guidelines for Otitis Media: 1-Day Regimen[a]

Weight		Amount of 200 mg/5 mL suspension	Total mL per treatment course	Total mg per treatment course
kg	lbs	Day 1		
5	11	3.75 mL	3.75 mL	150 mg
10	22	7.5 mL	7.5 mL	300 mg
20	44	15 mL	15 mL	600 mg
30	66	22.5 mL	22.5 mL	900 mg
40	88	30 mL	30 mL	1,200 mg
≥ 50	≥ 110	37.5 mL	37.5 mL	1,500 mg

[a] Dosing calculated on 30 mg/kg as a single dose.

Pharyngitis/Tonsillitis: The recommended dose for children is 12 mg/kg once daily for 5 days (not to exceed 500 mg/day). See the following table.

Pediatric Dosage Guidelines for Pharyngitis/Tonsillitis (≥ 2 years of age)				
Dosing calculated on 12 mg/kg once daily on days 1 through 5				
Weight		Amount of 200 mg/5 mL suspension	Total mL per treatment course	Total mg per treatment course
kg	lbs	Days 1 to 5		
8	18	2.5 mL	12.5 mL	500 mg
17	37	5 mL	25 mL	1,000 mg
25	55	7.5 mL	37.5 mL	1,500 mg
33	73	10 mL	50 mL	2,000 mg
40	88	12.5	62.5 mL	2,500 mg

Parenteral – Infuse injections over a period of longer than 60 minutes. Do not administer azithromycin for injection as a bolus or IM injection. IV azithromycin is not for use in children younger than 16 years of age.

Community-acquired pneumonia: 500 mg as a single daily dose IV for at least 2 days. Follow IV therapy by the oral route at a single daily dose of 500 mg to complete a 7- to 10-day course of therapy.

Pelvic inflammatory disease (PID): 500 mg as a single daily dose for 1 or 2 days. Follow IV therapy by the oral route at a single daily dose of 250 mg to complete a 7-day course of therapy.

The concentration and rate of infusion for azithromycin for injection should be either 1 mg/mL over 3 hours or 2 mg/mL over 1 hour.

CLARITHROMYCIN: Clarithromycin may be given with or without meals. Take the extended-release tablets with food. Swallow the extended-release tablets whole and not chewed, broken, or crushed.

Adults –

Clarithromycin Dosage Guidelines				
	Tablets		Extended-release tablets	
Infection	Dosage (every 12 h)	Duration (days)	Dosage (every 24 h)	Duration (days)
Pharyngitis/Tonsillitis	250 mg	10	—	—
Acute maxillary sinusitis	500 mg	14	1,000 mg	14
Acute exacerbation of chronic bronchitis caused by:				
Haemophilus parainfluenzae	500 mg	7	1,000 mg	7
Streptococcus pneumoniae	250 mg	7 to 14	1,000 mg	7
Moraxella catarrhalis	250 mg	7 to 14	1,000 mg	7
Haemophilus influenzae	500 mg	7 to 14	1,000 mg	7
Community-acquired pneumonia caused by:				
S. pneumoniae	250 mg	7 to 14	1,000 mg	7
Mycoplasma pneumoniae	250 mg	7 to 14	1,000 mg	7
H. influenzae	250 mg	7	1,000 mg	7
H. parainfluenzae	—	—	1,000 mg	7
M. catarrhalis	—	—	1,000 mg	7
Chlamydia pneumoniae	250 mg	7 to 14	1,000 mg	7
Uncomplicated skin and skin structure infection	250 mg	7 to 14	—	—

H. pylori eradication to reduce the risk of duodenal ulcer recurrence –

Triple therapy:

Clarithromycin/Lansoprazole/Amoxicillin – 500 mg clarithromycin, 30 mg lansoprazole, and 1 g amoxicillin every 12 hours for 10 or 14 days.

Clarithromycin/Omeprazole/Amoxicillin – 500 mg clarithromycin, 20 mg omeprazole, and 1 g amoxicillin every 12 hours for 10 days. In patients with an ulcer present at the time of initiation of therapy, an additional 18 days of omeprazole 20 mg once daily is recommended for ulcer healing and symptom relief.

Dual therapy:

Clarithromycin/Omeprazole – 500 mg clarithromycin 3 times/day (every 8 hours), and 40 mg omeprazole once daily (every morning) for 14 days. An additional 14 days of 20 mg omeprazole once daily is recommended for ulcer healing and symptom relief.

Clarithromycin/Ranitidine bismuth citrate – 500 mg clarithromycin 2 times/day (every 12 hours) or 3 times/day (every 8 hours), and 400 mg ranitidine bismuth citrate given 2 times/day (every 12 hours) for 14 days. An additional 14 days of ranitidine bismuth citrate 2 times/day is recommended for ulcer healing and symptom relief. This combination is not recommended in patients with a creatinine clearance (CrCl) less than 25 mL/min.

Mycobacterial infections – Recommended as the primary agent for the treatment of disseminated MAC. Use in combination with other antimycobacterial drugs that have shown in vitro activity against MAC. Continue therapy for life if clinical and mycobacterial improvements are observed.

Dosage for mycobacterial infection:

Adults – 500 mg twice daily.

Children – 7.5 mg/kg twice daily up to 500 mg twice daily. Refer to the Pediatric Dosing table.

Children – Usual recommended daily dosage is 15 mg/kg/day divided every 12 hours for 10 days.

Pediatric Dosage Guidelines (Based on Body Weight)

Dosing calculated on 7.5 mg/kg every 12 h

Weight kg	Weight lb	Dose (every 12 h)	125 mg/5 mL (every 12 h)	250 mg/5 mL (every 12 h)
9	20	62.5 mg	2.5 mL	1.25 mL
17	37	125 mg	5 mL	2.5 mL
25	55	187.5 mg	7.5 mL	3.75 mL
33	73	250 mg	10 mL	5 mL

Renal/Hepatic function impairment – In the presence of severe renal impairment (CrCl less than 30 mL/min) with or without coexisting hepatic impairment, halve the dose or double the dosing interval.

ERYTHROMYCIN IV: Erythromycin IV is indicated when oral use is impossible, or when severity of the infection requires immediate high serum levels. Replace IV therapy with oral as soon as possible.

Continuous infusion is preferable, but intermittent infusion in 20- to 60-minute periods at intervals of up to 6 hours is also effective. Because of irritative properties of erythromycin, IV push is unacceptable.

Adults and children – 15 to 20 mg/kg/day given IV. Higher dosages, up to 4 g/day, may be given for severe infections.

Acute pelvic inflammatory disease – 500 mg IV every 6 hours for 3 days, followed by 500 mg orally every 12 hours, 333 mg orally every 8 hours, or 250 mg orally every 6 hours for 7 days.

Legionnaire disease – Although optimal dosage has not been established, doses utilized in reported clinical data were 1 to 4 g daily in divided doses.

Streptococcal infections – In the treatment of streptococcal infections of the upper respiratory tract (eg, tonsillitis, pharyngitis), the therapeutic dosage of erythromycin should be administered for at least 10 days.

ERYTHROMYCIN, ORAL: Dosages and product strengths are expressed as erythromycin base equivalents (400 mg erythromycin ethylsuccinate produces the same free erythromycin serum levels as 250 mg of erythromycin base or stearate).

Optimal serum levels of erythromycin are reached when erythromycin base or stearate is taken in the fasting state or immediately before meals. Erythromycin ethylsuccinate, estolate, and enteric-coated erythromycin may be administered without regard to meals.

Usual dosage –

Adults: 250 mg (or 400 mg ethylsuccinate) every 6 hours, or 500 mg every 12 hours, or 333 mg every 8 hours. May increase up to at least 4 g/day, according to severity of infection. If twice-daily dosage is desired, the recommended dose is 500 mg every 12 hours. Twice-daily dosing is not recommended when doses larger than 1 g daily are administered.

Children: 30 to 50 mg/kg/day in divided doses.

Erythromycin Uses and Dosages[a]		
Indication	Dosage (stated as erythromycin base)	Duration of treatment
Labeled uses:		
Conjunctivitis of the newborn *C. trachomatis*	50 mg/kg/day in 4 divided doses	≥ 14 days
Pneumonia of infancy *C. trachomatis*	50 mg/kg/day in 4 divided doses	≥ 21 days (14 days per CDC)[b]
Urogenital infections during pregnancy *C. trachomatis*	500 mg 4 times/day or two 333 mg tablets (666 mg) every 8 hours (For women who are unable to tolerate this regimen, give 250 mg every 6 h or 333 mg every 8 h or 500 mg every 12 hours for ≥ 14 days)	≥ 7 days
Diphtheria *C. diphtheriae*	500 mg 4 times/day[c]	14 days[c] (7 days for cutaneous diphtheria and carriers)[c]
Erythrasma *C. minutissimum*	250 mg every 6 h[d]	14 days[d]
Intestinal amebiasis *E. histolytica*	*Adults:* 250 mg (or 400 mg as ethylsuccinate) every 6 h or 333 mg every 8 h or 500 mg every 12 h *Children:* 30 to 50 mg/kg/day in equally divided doses.	10 to 14 days
Legionnaire disease *L. pneumophila*	1 to 4 g in divided doses	
Nongonococcal urethritis *U. urealyticum*	500 mg 4 times/day or two 333 mg tablets (666 mg) every 8 hours or 800 mg (as ethylsuccinate) every 8 h	≥ 7 days
Pelvic inflammatory disease (acute) *N. gonorrhoeae*	500 mg IV every 6 h for 3 days followed by 250 mg orally every 6 h or 333 mg every 8 h for 7 days or 500 mg orally every 12 h	10 days
Pertussis (whooping cough) *B. pertussis*	40 to 50 mg/kg/day, given in divided doses	5 to 14 days
Primary syphilis *T. pallidum*	30 to 40 grams (or 48 to 64 g as ethylsuccinate) given in divided doses over 10 to 15 days	10 to 15 days
Respiratory tract infections *M. pneumoniae*	*Adults:* 250 to 500 mg every 6 h[c] *Children:* 20 to 50 mg/kg/day in 3 or 4 divided doses[c]	14 to 21 days[c]
Rheumatic fever, prevention of initial attack	400 mg every 6 h	10 days
Rheumatic fever, prevention of recurrent attacks	250 mg (or 400 mg as ethylsuccinate) twice daily	Continuous
Uncomplicated urethral, endocervical, or rectal infections *C. trachomatis*	Adults: 500 mg 4 times/day or two 333 mg tablets (666 mg) every 8 h or 800 mg (as ethylsuccinate) 4 times/day[b]	≥ 7 days
	Children (≤ 45 kg): 50 mg/kg/day in 4 divided doses[b]	14 days[b]

Erythromycin Uses and Dosages[a]		
Indication	Dosage (stated as erythromycin base)	Duration of treatment
Upper respiratory tract infections of mild to moderate severity *S. pyogenes* *S. pneumoniae* *H. influenzae*	*Adults:* 250 mg every 6 h or 333 mg every 8 h or 500 mg every 12 h. Max dose is 4 g/day. *Children:* 30 to 50 mg/kg/day in equally divided doses. Max dose is 4 g/day. *H. influenzae* infections should be treated concomitantly with a sulfonamide.	≥ 10 days (for streptococcal infections)
Unlabeled uses:		
Acne vulgaris	250 to 1,000 mg/day[c]	
Bacillary angiomatosis (immunocompromised patients):[d] *Bartonella henselae* or *B. quintana*	500 mg 4 times/day	
Campylobacter enteritis[c] *C. jejuni*	*Adults:* 250 mg 4 times/day *Children:* 30 to 50 mg/kg/day in divided doses	5 to 7 days
Chancroid[b] *H. ducreyi*	500 mg 3 times/day	7 days
Granuloma inguinale (Donavanosis)[b] *C. granulomatis*	500 mg 4 times/day	≥ 21 days
Inclusion conjunctivitis (adults) *C. trachomatis*	250 mg 4 times/day	1 to 3 weeks
Leptospirosis[c] *Leptospira* species	500 mg IV 4 times/day	7 days
Lyme disease[c] *B. burgdorferi*	250 mg 4 times/day	
Lymphogranuloma venereum[b] *C. trachomatis*	500 mg 4 times/day	21 days
Relapsing fever[c]	*Louse-borne:* 500 mg (single dose)	Single dose
	Tick-borne: 500 mg every 6 h	7 days

[a] Dosages are for adults unless otherwise specified.
[b] CDC 2002 *Sexually Transmitted Diseases Treatment Guidelines.*
[c] *Harrison's Principles of Internal Medicine,* 14th ed.
[d] *The Sanford Guide to Antimicrobial Therapy* 2004.

Actions

Pharmacology: Macrolide antibiotics reversibly bind to the P site of the 50S ribosomal subunit of susceptible organisms and inhibit RNA-dependent protein synthesis. They may be bacteriostatic or bactericidal, depending on such factors as drug concentration.

Pharmacokinetics:

Macrolides — Summary of Pharmacokinetics[a]

Macrolide	Oral bioavailability	C_{max} (mcg/mL)	T_{max}	Protein binding	Volume of distribution	Effect of food	Half-life	Metabolism	Elimination
Azithromycin		0.5 mcg/mL (single 500 mg dose)	≈ 2 to 2.5 h (≈ 5 h for ER oral suspension)	51% (at 0.02 mcg/mL); 7% (at 2 mcg/mL)	31.1 L/kg = (oral); 33.3 L/kg (IV)	*Tablets and oral suspension*: Take with or without food. Food increased C_{max} by 23% (tablets) and by 56% (oral suspension); no effect on AUC. *ER oral suspension*: Take on an empty stomach (≥ 1 h before or 2 h following a meal). Administration with food increased C_{max} by 115% to 119% and the AUC by 12% to 23%.	68[b] h	Some hepatic metabolism to inactive metabolites	Primarily excreted unchanged in bile; ≈ 6% of dose is excreted unchanged in urine
Clarithromycin	≈ 50% (tablets)	1 to 2 mcg/mL (after doses of 250 mg every 12 h); 3 to 4 mcg/mL (after doses of 500 mg every 8 to 12 h)	*Tablets*: 2 to 3 h *Oral suspension*: ≈ 3 h *ER tablets*: 5 to 8 h	40% to 70%		*Tablets and oral suspension*: Take without regard to food. Food slightly delays onset of absorption; does not affect extent of bioavailability. *ER tablets*: Administer with food. Administration under fasting conditions lowers clarithromycin AUC by ≈ 30%.	3 to 7[c] h (5 to 9[c] h for 14-OH clarithromycin)	Metabolized in the liver to active metabolite (14-OH clarithromycin)	Renal clearance approximates the normal GFR. *Tablets*: ≈ 20% to 30% of dose is excreted in urine as clarithromycin and ≈ 10% to 15% as 14-OH clarithromycin. *Oral suspension*: ≈ 40% of dose is excreted in urine as clarithromycin.
Erythromycin		*Base*: 0.3 to 1.9 mcg/mL *Ethylsuccinate*: 1.5 mcg/mL *IV*: 10 mcg/mL	*Base*: 4 h *Ethylsuccinate*: 1 to 2 h *IV*: 1 h	70% to 80%		*Erythromycin base film-coated tablets and delayed-release capsules and erythromycin stearate*: Take on an empty stomach. *Erythromycin base delayed-release tablets and erythromycin ethylsuccinate*: Take without regard to food.	1.6 h[d]	Metabolized in the liver to inactive metabolites	< 5% (oral) and 12% to 15% (IV) excreted unchanged in urine; significant quantity excreted in bile

[a] C_{max} = maximum plasma concentration; T_{max} = time to reach maximum concentration; AUC = area under the curve; GFR = glomerular filtration rate; IV = intravenous.
[b] Terminal elimination half-life.
[c] Elimination half-life.
[d] Serum half-life.

Contraindications

Hypersensitivity to any of the macrolide antibiotics.

Azithromycin is also contraindicated in patients with a hypersensitivity to a ketolide antibiotic (eg, telithromycin).

Clarithromycin is contraindicated in patients receiving any of the following drugs: cisapride, pimozide, astemizole, terfenadine, and ergotamine or dihydroergotamine.

Erythromycin is contraindicated in patients receiving any of the following drugs: cisapride, pimozide, astemizole, or terfenadine.

Warnings/Precautions

Clostridium difficile-associated diarrhea: Pseudomembranous colitis has occurred with nearly all antibacterial agents and may range in severity from mild to life-threatening.

Acute porphyria: Do not use **clarithromycin** in combination with ranitidine bismuth citrate in patients with a history of acute porphyria.

Pneumonia: Do not use oral **azithromycin** in patients with pneumonia who are judged to be inappropriate for oral therapy because of moderate to severe illness or risk factors such as any of the following: nosocomially acquired infections; known or suspected bacteremia; conditions requiring hospitalization; cystic fibrosis; significant underlying health problems that may compromise patients' ability to respond to their illness (including immunodeficiency or functional asplenia); elderly or debilitated patients.

Cardiac effects: Ventricular arrhythmias in individuals with prolonged QT intervals have occurred with macrolide products.

Hepatic effects: There have been reports of hepatic function impairment, including increased liver enzymes, and hepatocellular and/or cholestatic hepatitis, with or without jaundice, occurring in patients receiving oral **erythromycin**.

Syphilis: There have been reports suggesting that **erythromycin** does not reach the fetus in adequate concentration to prevent congenital syphilis. Use an appropriate penicillin regimen to treat infants born to women treated with oral erythromycin during pregnancy for early syphilis.

Myasthenia gravis: There have been reports that **erythromycin** may aggravate the weakness of patients with myasthenia gravis.

Drug-resistant bacteria: Prescribing macrolides in the absence of a proven or strongly suspected bacterial infection or a prophylactic indication is unlikely to provide benefit to the patient and increases the risk of the development of drug-resistant bacteria.

Superinfection: Prolonged or repeated use of macrolides may result in an overgrowth of nonsusceptible bacteria or fungi. If superinfection occurs, discontinue the macrolide and institute appropriate therapy.

Infantile hypertrophic pyloric stenosis: There have been reports of infantile hypertrophic pyloric stenosis (IHPS) occurring in infants following **erythromycin** therapy. Because erythromycin may be used in the treatment of conditions in infants that are associated with significant mortality or morbidity (such as pertussis or neonatal *C. trachomatis* infections), the benefit of erythromycin therapy needs to be weighed against the potential risk of developing IHPS. Inform parents to contact their health care provider if vomiting or irritability with feeding occurs.

Local IV-site reactions: Local IV-site reactions have been reported with the IV administration of **azithromycin**.

Hypersensitivity reactions: Rare serious allergic reactions, including angioedema, anaphylaxis, and dermatologic reactions including Stevens-Johnson syndrome and toxic epidermal necrolysis have occurred in patients on **azithromycin** therapy.

Allergic reactions ranging from urticaria and mild skin eruptions to rare cases of anaphylaxis, Stevens-Johnson syndrome, and toxic epidermal necrolysis have occurred with **clarithromycin**.

Allergic reactions ranging from urticaria to anaphylaxis have occurred with **erythromycin**. Skin reactions ranging from mild eruptions to erythema multiforme, Stevens-Johnson syndrome, and toxic epidermal necrolysis have been reported rarely.

Renal/Hepatic function impairment: Because **azithromycin** is principally eliminated via the liver, exercise caution when administering to patients with hepatic function impairment. Because of the limited data in subjects with GFR less than 10 mL/min, exercise caution when prescribing azithromycin to these patients.

Clarithromycin is principally excreted via the liver and kidney, and may be administered without dosage adjustment to patients with hepatic function impairment and healthy renal function. However, in the presence of severe renal function impairment (CrCl less than 30 mL/min) with or without coexisting hepatic function impairment, the dosage should be halved or the dosing intervals doubled.

Erythromycin is principally excreted by the liver. Exercise caution in administering to patients with hepatic function impairment. There have been isolated reports of reversible hearing loss occurring chiefly in patients with renal function impairment and in patients receiving high doses of erythromycin.

Pregnancy: Category B (**azithromycin, erythromycin**); *Category* C (**clarithromycin**).

Lactation:

Clarithromycin and azithromycin – It is not known whether these agents are excreted in breast milk.

Erythromycin – Erythromycin is excreted in breast milk, and may concentrate (observed milk:plasma ratio of 0.5 to 3). Erythromycin is considered compatible with breast-feeding by the American Academy of Pediatrics.

Children:

Azithromycin – Safety and efficacy in children younger than 6 months of age (acute otitis media, community-acquired pneumonia) or younger than 2 years of age (pharyngitis/tonsillitis) have not been established.

IV use: Safety and efficacy of azithromycin for IV injection in children or adolescents younger than 16 years of age have not been established.

Clarithromycin – Safety and efficacy in children younger than 6 months of age have not been established.

Elderly:

Clarithromycin – Studies show age-related decreases in renal function. Consider dosage adjustment in elderly patients with severe renal impairment.

Drug Interactions

Azithromycin: Drugs that may affect azithromycin include antacids, antiarrhythmic agents, fluoroquinolones, and nelfinavir.

Drugs that may be affected by azithromycin include antiarrhythmic agents, fluoroquinolones, theophyllines, benzodiazepines, cyclosporine, digoxin, ergot derivatives, hexobarbital, HMG-CoA reductase inhibitors, phenytoin, pimozide, ranolazine, valproic acid, and warfarin.

Clarithromycin: Drugs that may affect clarithromycin include antiarrhythmic agents, cimetidine, diltiazem, fluconazole, fluoroquinolones, proton pump inhibitors, rifamycins, ritonavir, and verapamil.

Drugs that may be affected by clarithromycin include alfentanil, antiarrhythmic agents, antihistamines, benzodiazepines, bromocriptine, buspirone, cabergoline, carbamazepine, cilostazol, cisapride, clopidogrel, clozapine, colchicine, conivaptan, cyclosporine, digoxin, eletriptan, eplerenone, ergot derivatives, fluoroquinolones, HMG-CoA reductase inhibitors, lapatinib, methylprednisolone, phenytoin, pimozide, proton pump inhibitors, quetiapine, ranolazine, repaglinide, rifamycins, sildenafil, tacrolimus, theophyllines, valproic acid, verapamil, warfarin, and zidovudine.

Erythromycin: Drugs that may affect erythromycin include alcohol, antiarrhythmic agents, diltiazem, fluoroquinolones, rifamycins, theophyllines, and verapamil.

Drugs that may be affected by erythromycin include alfentanil, antiarrhythmic agents, antihistamines, benzodiazepines, bromocriptine, buspirone, cabergoline, carbamazepine, cilostazol, cisapride, clopidogrel, clozapine, colchicine, cyclosporine, digoxin, eletriptan, ergot derivatives, felodipine, fluoroquinolones, hexobarbital, HMG-CoA reductase inhibitors, methylprednisolone, phenytoin, pimozide, quetiapine, ranolazine, repaglinide, rifamycins, sildenafil, tacrolimus, theophyllines, valproic acid, vinblastine, verapamil, and warfarin.

Drug/Food interactions: Grapefruit juice may inhibit the metabolism of **clarithromycin** and **erythromycin**, resulting in elevated plasma levels of the macrolide. Avoid coadministration.

Azithromycin tablets and oral suspension can be taken with or without food. Following administration of azithromycin extended-release oral suspension with food, the C_{max} increased by 115% to 119%, and the AUC increased by 12% to 23%. Advise patient to only take the extended-release oral suspension on an empty stomach (at least 1 hour before or 2 hours following a meal).

Antimicrobial effectiveness of **erythromycin** stearate and certain formulations of erythromycin base may be reduced when taken with food. Erythromycin ethylsuccinate and the base in a delayed release tablet form may be administered without regard to meals (See Patient Information).

Adverse Reactions

Azithromycin: Adverse reactions occurring in at least 3% of patients include abdominal pain, diarrhea/loose stools, increased ALT and AST, increased bilirubin, increased serum creatinine, nausea, and vomiting.

Clarithromycin: Adverse reactions occurring in at least 3% of patients include abdominal pain, abnormal taste, decreased hemoglobin, diarrhea, increased BUN, nausea, rash, and vomiting.

Erythromycin: Adverse reactions occurring in at least 3% of patients include abdominal pain/discomfort, diarrhea/loose stools, headache, increased platelet count, and nausea.

Local: Venous irritation and phlebitis have occurred with parenteral administration, but the risk of such reactions may be reduced if the infusion is given slowly, in dilute solution, by continuous IV infusion, or intermittent infusion over 20 to 60 minutes.

TELITHROMYCIN

Tablets; oral: 300 and 400 mg (*Rx*) — *Ketek* (Aventis)

Warning:
Telithromycin is contraindicated in patients with myasthenia gravis. There have been reports of fatal and life-threatening respiratory failure in patients with myasthenia gravis associated with the use of telithromycin.

Indications

Community-acquired pneumonia (CAP) (of mild to moderate severity): Due to *Streptococcus pneumoniae* (including multidrug-resistant *S. pneumoniae* [MDRSP] isolates, including isolates known as penicillin-resistant *S. pneumoniae* [PRSP], and are isolates resistant to 2 or more of the following antibiotics: penicillin, second-generation cephalosporins [eg, cefuroxime], macrolides, tetracyclines, and trimethoprim/sulfamethoxazole), *Haemophilus influenzae, Moraxella catarrhalis, Chlamydophila pneumoniae*, or *Mycoplasma pneumoniae*.

Administration and Dosage

The dose of telithromycin tablets is 800 mg taken orally once every 24 hours for 7 to 10 days. Telithromycin can be administered with or without food.

Renal function impairment: In the presence of severe renal function impairment (creatinine clearance [CrCl] less than 30 mL/min), including patients who need dialysis, the dosage should be reduced to telithromycin 600 mg once daily. In patients undergoing hemodialysis, telithromycin should be given after the dialysis session on dialysis days.

In the presence of severe renal function impairment (CrCl less than 30 mL/min) with coexisting hepatic function impairment, the dosage should be reduced to telithromycin 400 mg once daily.

Actions

Pharmacology: Telithromycin belongs to the ketolide class of antibacterials and is structurally related to the macrolide family of antibiotics. Telithromycin blocks protein synthesis by binding to domains II and V of 23S rRNA of the 50S ribosomal subunit.

Pharmacokinetics:

Absorption/Distribution – Following oral administration, telithromycin reached maximal concentration at about 1 hour.

Mean Telithromycin Pharmacokinetic Parameters

Parameter	Single dose (n = 18)	Multiple dose (n = 18)
C_{max} (mcg/mL)	1.9	2.27
T_{max} (hr; median value)	1	1
$AUC_{(0\ to\ 24)}$ (mcg•h/mL)	8.25	12.5
Terminal $t_{1/2}$ (h)	7.16	9.81
C_{24h}[a] (mcg/mL)	0.03	0.07

[a] C_{24h} = Plasma concentration at 24 hours postdose

In a patient population, mean peak and trough plasma concentrations were 2.9 mcg/mL (n = 219) and 0.2 mcg/mL (n = 204), respectively, after 3 to 5 days of 800 mg telithromycin once daily.

Total in vitro protein binding is approximately 60% to 70% and is primarily caused by human serum albumin. The volume of distribution of telithromycin after IV infusion is 2.9 L/kg.

Metabolism/Excretion – Metabolism accounts for approximately 70% of the dose. It is estimated that approximately 50% of its metabolism is mediated by CYP-450 3A4 and the remaining 50% is CYP-450-independent. Seven percent of the dose is excreted unchanged in feces; 13% is excreted unchanged in urine; and 37% of the dose is metabolized by the liver. The mean terminal elimination half-life is 10 hours.

Contraindications

A history of hypersensitivity to telithromycin and/or any components of the product or any macrolide antibiotic; in patients with myasthenia gravis; previous history of hepatitis and/or jaundice associated with the use of telithromycin, or any macrolide antibiotic. Coadministration of telithromycin with cisapride or pimozide is contraindicated.

Warnings/Precautions

Hepatotoxicity: Acute hepatic failure and severe liver injury, in some cases fatal, have been reported in patients treated with telithromycin.

Cardiac effects: Telithromycin has the potential to prolong the QTc interval in some patients. QTc prolongation may lead to an increased risk for ventricular arrhythmias, including torsades de pointes.

Myasthenia gravis: Exacerbations of myasthenia gravis have been reported in patients with myasthenia gravis treated with telithromycin. This has sometimes occurred within a few hours after intake of the first dose of telithromycin. Reports have included life-threatening acute respiratory failure with a rapid onset. Telithromycin is not recommended in patients with myasthenia gravis unless no other therapeutic alternatives are available.

Hepatic effects: Hepatic dysfunction including increased liver enzymes and hepatitis, with or without jaundice, has been reported with the use of telithromycin.

Loss of consciousness: There have been postmarketing adverse reaction reports of transient loss of consciousness, including some cases associated with vagal syndrome.

Clostridium difficile– associated diarrhea: *Clostridium difficile*– associated diarrhea has been reported with nearly all antibacterial agents, including telithromycin, and may range in severity from mild diarrhea to fatal colitis.

Visual disturbances: Telithromycin may cause visual disturbances particularly in slowing the ability to accommodate and the ability to release accommodation. Most visual adverse events (65%) occurred following the first or second dose. Visual disturbances included blurred vision, difficulty focusing, and diplopia.

Renal/Hepatic function impairment: In the presence of severe renal function impairment (CrCl less than 30 mL/min), a reduced dosage of telithromycin is recommended. Telithromycin may be administered without dosage adjustment in the presence of hepatic function impairment.

Hazardous tasks: Caution patients about the potential effects of visual disturbances and syncope on driving a vehicle, operating machinery, or engaging in other potentially hazardous activities.

Superinfection: Prescribing telithromycin in the absence of a proven or strongly suspected bacterial infection or a prophylactic indication is unlikely to benefit the patient and increases the risk of the development of drug-resistant bacteria.

Pregnancy: Category C.

Lactation: Exercise caution when telithromycin is given to a breast-feeding mother.

Children: The safety and effectiveness of telithromycin in children has not been established.

Elderly: Efficacy and safety in elderly patients 65 years of age or older were generally similar to those observed in younger patients. No dosage adjustment is required based on age alone.

Monitoring: Monitor for the appearance of signs or symptoms of hepatitis such as fatigue, malaise, anorexia, nausea, jaundice, bilirubinuria, acholic stools, liver tenderness, or hepatomegaly.

Drug Interactions

Drugs that may affect telithromycin include itraconazole, ketoconazole, rifampin, phenytoin, phenobarbital, carbamazepine.

Drugs that may be affected by telithromycin include antiarrhythmic agents, carbamazepine, cisapride, colchicine, cyclosporine, CYP3A4 inhibitors, digoxin, ergot alkaloids, HMG-CoA reductase inhibitors, metoprolol, midazolam, oral anticoagulants, oral contraceptives, phenytoin, pimozide, sirolimus, sotalol, tacrolimus, theophylline, and verapamil.

CYP-450: Telithromycin is a strong inhibitor of the CYP-450 3A4 system.

Adverse Reactions

Adverse reactions occurring in at least 3% of patients include the following: diarrhea, dizziness (excluding vertigo), headache, nausea, vomiting.

DAPTOMYCIN

Powder for injection, lyophilized: 500 mg (*Rx*) *Cubicin* (Cubist)

Indications

Complicated skin and skin structure infections (cSSSIs): For the treatment of complicated skin and skin structure infections caused by susceptible strains of the following gram-positive microorganisms: *Staphylococcus aureus* (including methicillin-resistant strains), *Streptococcus pyogenes*, *Streptococcus agalactiae*, *Streptococcus dysgalactiae* subsp. *equisimilis*, and *Enterococcus faecalis* (vancomycin-susceptible strains only). Combination therapy may be clinically indicated if the documented or presumed pathogens include gram-negative or anaerobic organisms.

Staphylococcus aureus bloodstream infections: For the treatment of *S. aureus* bloodstream infections (bacteremia), including those with right-sided infective endocarditis, caused by methicillin-susceptible and methicillin-resistant isolates.

Combination therapy may be clinically indicated if the documented or presumed pathogens include gram-negative or anaerobic organisms.

Administration and Dosage

cSSSIs: Administer daptomycin 4 mg/kg over a 30-minute period by IV infusion once every 24 hours for 7 to 14 days.

S. aureus bloodstream infections (bacteremia), including those with right-sided endocarditis, caused by methicillin-susceptible and methicillin-resistant strains: Daptomycin 6 mg/kg should be administered over a 30-minute period by IV infusion once every 24 hours for a minimum of 2 to 6 weeks.

Renal function impairment: Because daptomycin is eliminated primarily by the kidney, a dosage modification is recommended for patients with creatinine clearance (CrCl) less than 30 mL/min, including patients receiving hemodialysis or continuous ambulatory peritoneal dialysis (CAPD). When possible, administer daptomycin following hemodialysis on hemodialysis days.

Daptomycin Dosage in Adult Patients with Renal Impairment

Creatinine clearance	Dosage regimen (cSSSI)	Dosage regimen (*S. aureus* bloodstream infections)
≥ 30 mL/min	4 mg/kg once every 24 h	6 mg/kg once every 24 hours
< 30 mL/min, including hemodialysis or CAPD	4 mg/kg once every 48 h	6 mg/kg once every 48 hours

Incompatibilities: Daptomycin is not compatible with dextrose-containing diluents. Do not add additives or other medications to daptomycin single-use vials or infuse simultaneously through the same IV line.

Admixture compatibility: Daptomycin is compatible with 0.9% sodium chloride injection and Ringer's lactate injection.

Actions

Pharmacology: Daptomycin is an antibacterial agent of a new class of antibiotics, the cyclic lipopeptides. Daptomycin binds to bacterial membranes and causes a rapid depolarization of membrane potential. Daptomycin exhibits rapid, concentration-dependent bactericidal activity against gram-positive organisms in vitro. Daptomycin retains potency against antibiotic-resistant gram-positive bacteria, including isolates resistant to methicillin, vancomycin, and linezolid.

Pharmacokinetics:

Absorption – The mean pharmacokinetic parameters of daptomycin on day 7 following the IV administration of 4, 6, and 8 mg/kg once daily to healthy young adults (mean age, 35.8 years) are summarized in the following table.

Mean (SD) Daptomycin Pharmacokinetic Parameters in Healthy Volunteers at Steady State[a]					
Dose[b]	AUC_{0-24} (mcg•h/mL)	t½ (h)	V_{ss} (L/kg)	CL_T (mL/h/kg)	C_{max} (mcg/mL)
4 mg/kg (n = 6)	494 (75)	8.1 (1)	0.096 (0.009)	8.3 (1.3)	57.8 (3)
6 mg/kg (n = 6)	632 (78)	7.9 (1)	0.101 (0.007)	9.1 (1.5)	93.9 (6)
8 mg/kg (n = 6)	858 (213)	8.3 (2.2)	0.101 (0.013)	9 (3)	123.3 (16)
10 mg/kg (n = 9)	1,039 (178)	7.9 (0.6)	0.098 (0.017)	8.8 (2.2)	141.1 (24)
12 mg/kg (n = 9)	1,277 (253)	7.7 (1.1)	0.097 (0.018)	9 (2.8)	183.7 (25)

[a] AUC_{0-24} = area under the concentration time-curve from 0 to 24 hours; t½ = terminal elimination half-life; V_{ss} = volume of distribution at steady state; CL_T = plasma clearance; C_{max} = maximum plasma concentration

[b] Doses of daptomycin in excess of 6 mg/kg have not been approved.

Daptomycin pharmacokinetics are nearly linear and time-independent at doses up to 6 mg/kg administered once daily for 7 days. Steady-state concentrations are achieved by the third daily dose.

Distribution – Daptomycin is reversibly bound to human plasma proteins, primarily to serum albumin. The mean serum protein binding of daptomycin was approximately 92% in healthy adults.

Metabolism – It is unlikely that daptomycin will inhibit or induce the metabolism of drugs metabolized by the CYP 450 system.

Excretion – Daptomycin is excreted primarily by the kidney.

Contraindications

Known hypersensitivity to daptomycin.

Warnings/Precautions

Pseudomembranous colitis: Pseudomembranous colitis has been reported with nearly all antibacterial agents, including daptomycin, and may range in severity from mild to life-threatening. Therefore, it is important to consider this diagnosis in patients who present with diarrhea subsequent to the administration of any antibacterial agent.

Skeletal muscle effects: Monitor patients receiving daptomycin for the development of muscle pain or weakness, particularly of the distal extremities. Monitor CPK levels weekly in patients who receive daptomycin. Monitor patients who develop unexplained elevations in CPK while receiving daptomycin more frequently.

Neuropathy: Administration of daptomycin was associated with decreases in nerve conduction velocity and with adverse events (eg, paresthesias, Bell palsy), possibly reflective of peripheral or cranial neuropathy. Nerve conduction deficits were also detected in a similar number of comparator subjects in these studies.

Persisting or relapsing S. aureus infection – Patients with persisting or relapsing *S. aureus* infection or poor clinical response should have repeat blood cultures. If a culture is positive for *S. aureus*, perform minimum inhibitory concentration susceptibility testing of the isolate using a standardized procedure, as well as diagnostic evaluation to rule out sequestered foci of infection. Appropriate surgical intervention and/or consideration of a change in antibiotic regimen may be required.

Superinfection: The use of antibiotics may promote the overgrowth of nonsusceptible organisms. Should superinfection occur during therapy, take appropriate measures.

Pregnancy: Category B.

Lactation: It is not known if daptomycin is excreted in human milk. Exercise caution when administering daptomycin to nursing women.

Children: Safety and efficacy of daptomycin in patients younger than 18 years of age have not been established.

Elderly: In the two phase 3 clinical studies in patients with complicated skin and skin structure infections (cSSSI), lower clinical success rates were seen in patients 65 years of age and older compared with those younger than 65 years of age. In addition, treatment-emergent adverse events were more common in patients 65 years of age and older than in patients younger than 65 years of age in both cSSSI studies.

Monitoring: Monitor CPK levels weekly in patients who receive daptomycin. Monitor patients who develop unexplained elevations in CPK while receiving daptomycin more frequently.

Drug Interactions

Although no specific drug-drug interactions have been documented, exercise caution when using daptomycin in patients receiving warfarin (monitor INR) or HMG-CoA reductase inhibitors (may cause myopathy and increase CPK levels).

Adverse Reactions

Adverse drug reactions occurring in at least 3% of patients receiving daptomycin include the following: abdominal pain, abnormal liver function tests, acute renal failure, anemia, anxiety, arthralgia, asthenia, back pain, bacteremia, blood CPK increased, chest pain, constipation, cough, diarrhea, dizziness, dyspepsia, dyspnea, edema, erythema, headache, hyperkalemia, hypokalemia, hypertension, hypotension, injection-site reactions, insomnia, lab test abnormalities, loose stools, nausea, osteomyelitis, pain in extremity, pharyngolaryngeal pain, pleural effusion, pneumonia, pruritus, pyrexia, rash, renal failure, sweating increased, urinary tract infection, vomiting.

VANCOMYCIN

Capsules; oral: 125 mg and 250 mg (*Rx*)	*Vancocin* (ViroPharm)
Powder for injection: 500 mg, 750 mg, 1, 5, and 10 g (*Rx*)	Various
Injection, solution: 500 mg and 1 g (*Rx*)	*Vancomycin hydrochloride* (Baxter)

Indications

Parenteral: Serious or severe infections not treatable with other antimicrobials, including the penicillins and cephalosporins.

Severe staphylococcal infections – Severe staphylococcal infections (including methicillin-resistant staphylococci) in patients who cannot receive or who have failed to respond to penicillins and cephalosporins, or who have infections with resistant staphylococci. Infections may include endocarditis, bone infections, lower respiratory tract infections, septicemia, and skin and skin structure infections.

Endocarditis –

Staphylococcal: Vancomycin is effective alone.

Streptococcal: Vancomycin is effective alone or in combination with an aminoglycoside for endocarditis caused by *S. viridans* or *S. bovis*. It is only effective in combination with an aminoglycoside for endocarditis caused by enterococci (eg, *S. faecalis*).

Diphtheroid: Vancomycin is effective for diphtheroid endocarditis, and has been used successfully with rifampin, an aminoglycoside, or both in early onset prosthetic valve endocarditis caused by *Staphylococcus epidermidis* or diphtheroids.

Pseudomembranous colitis/staphylococcal enterocolitis caused by Clostridium difficile – The parenteral form may be administered orally; parenteral use alone is unproven. The oral use of parenteral vancomycin is not effective for other infections.

Oral: Staphylococcal enterocolitis and antibiotic-associated pseudomembranous colitis produced by *C. difficile*. The parenteral product may also be given orally for these infections. Oral vancomycin is *not* effective for other types of infection.

Administration and Dosage

Complete full course of therapy; do not discontinue therapy without notifying physician.

Oral:

Adults – 500 mg to 2 g/day given in 3 or 4 divided doses for 7 to 10 days.

Children – 40 mg/kg/day in 3 or 4 divided doses for 7 to 10 days. Do not exceed 2 g/day.

Neonates – 10 to 15 mg/kg/day in divided doses.

Parenteral: Administer each dose over at least 60 minutes. Intermittent infusion is the preferred administration method. Concentrations of no more than 5 mg/mL and at rates of no more than 10 mg/min are recommended in adults. In selected patients in need of fluid restriction, a concentration of up to 10 mg/mL may be used.

Adults –

Endocarditis/Staphylococcal infections: 2 g IV divided as 500 mg every 6 hours or 1 g every 12 hours.

Pseudomembranous colitis/Staphylococcal enterocolitis: 500 mg to 2 g orally daily given in 3 or 4 divided doses for 7 to 10 days.

Children –

Endocarditis/Staphylococcal infections:

1 month of age and older – 10 mg/kg/dose given every 6 hours.

Infants younger than 1 month of age – Initial dose of 15 mg/kg, followed by 10 mg/kg every 12 hours for neonates in the first week of life and every 8 hours thereafter up to the age of 1 month.

Renal function impairment: Adjust dosage; check serum levels regularly. In premature infants and the elderly, dosage reduction may be necessary caused by decreasing renal function.

For most patients, if CrCl can be measured or estimated accurately, the dosage may be calculated by using the following table.

Vancomycin Dosage in Impaired Renal Function	
CrCl (mL/min)	Dose (mg/24 h)
100	1,545
90	1,390
80	1,235
70	1,080
60	925
50	770
40	620
30	465
20	310
10	155

In patients with marked renal impairment, it may be more convenient to give maintenance doses of 250 to 1,000 mg once every several days rather than administering the drug on a daily basis.

Initial dosage – The initial dose should be no less than 15 mg/kg, even in patients with mild to moderate renal insufficiency.

Alternative dosage –

Adults:

GFR more than 50 mL/min – 1 g every 12 to 24 h.

GFR 10 to 50 mL/min – 1 g every 24 to 96 h.

GFR less than 10 mL/min – 1 g every 4 to 7 days.

Hemodialysis/Peritoneal dialysis – 1 g every 4 to 7 days.

Continuous renal replacement therapy – 1 g every 12 to 24 h.

Children:

GFR 30 to 50 mL/min per 1.73 m^2 – 10 mg/kg every 12 h.

GFR 10 to 29 mL/min per 1.73 m^2 – 10 mg/kg every 18 to 24 h.

GFR less than 10 mL/min per 1.73 m^2 – 10 mg/kg as needed per serum concentration monitoring.

Hemodialysis – 10 mg/kg as needed per serum concentration monitoring.

Peritoneal dialysis – 10 mg/kg as needed per serum concentration monitoring or loading dose 500 mg/L and maintenance dose 30 mg/L.

Continuous renal replacement therapy – 10 mg/kg every 12 to 24 h as needed per serum concentration monitoring.

Anuria: 1,000 mg every 7 to 10 days is recommended.

Anephric patients: Initial dose of 15 mg/kg. The dose required to maintain stable concentrations is 1.9 mg/kg every 24 hours.

Elderly: Vancomycin dosage schedules should be adjusted in elderly patients. Greater dosage reductions than expected may be necessary because of decreased renal function.

Admixture compatibility:

Compatibility – The following diluents are physically and chemically compatible with vancomycin: dextrose 5% injection, dextrose 5% injection and sodium chloride 0.9% injection, Ringer's lactate injection, dextrose 5% and Ringer's lactate injection, *Normosol*-M and dextrose 5%, sodium chloride 0.9% injection, and *Isolyte E*.

Incompatibility – Mixtures of solutions of vancomycin and beta-lactam antibiotics have been shown to be physically incompatible.

Actions

Pharmacology: Vancomycin is a tricyclic glycopeptide antibiotic that inhibits cell-wall biosynthesis. It also alters bacterial-cell-membrane permeability and RNA synthesis.

Pharmacokinetics:

Absorption/Distribution – Systemic absorption of oral vancomycin is generally poor. Vancomycin is approximately 55% serum protein bound. Vancomycin does not readily diffuse across healthy meninges into the spinal fluid, but, when the meninges are inflamed, penetration into the spinal fluid occurs.

Metabolism/Excretion – In the first 24 hours, approximately 75% of a dose is excreted in urine by glomerular filtration. Elimination half-life is 4 to 6 hours in adults and 2 to 3 hours in children. Mean plasma clearance is about 0.058 L/kg/h, and mean renal clearance is about 0.048 L/kg/h. About 60% of an intraperitoneal dose administered during peritoneal dialysis is absorbed systemically in 6 hours. Accumulation occurs in renal failure. Serum half-life in anephric patients is approximately 7.5 days. Vancomycin is not significantly removed by hemodialysis or continuous ambulatory peritoneal dialysis, although there have been reports of increased clearance with hemoperfusion and hemofiltration.

Contraindications

Hypersensitivity to vancomycin; solutions containing dextrose may be contraindicated in patients with known allergy to corn or corn products (premixed *Galaxy* containers only).

Warnings/Precautions

C. difficile-associated diarrhea: C. *difficile*–associated diarrhea has been reported with nearly all antibacterial agents, including vancomycin, and may range in severity from mild diarrhea to fatal colitis.

Hypersensitivity reactions: During or soon after the rapid infusion of vancomycin, patients may develop anaphylactoid reactions, including dyspnea, hypotension, pruritus, urticaria, or wheezing. Rapid infusion may also cause flushing of the upper body ("red neck") or pain and muscle spasm of the chest and back. These reactions usually resolve within 20 minutes but may persist for several hours. Such reactions are infrequent if vancomycin is given by a slow infusion over 60 minutes.

Hypotension: Rapid bolus administration may be associated with exaggerated hypotension, including shock, and rarely, cardiac arrest. To avoid hypotension, administer in a dilute solution over 60 minutes or more. Stopping the infusion usually results in prompt cessation of these reactions.

Intraperitoneal and intrathecal routs: Reports have revealed that administration of sterile vancomycin by the intraperitoneal route during continuous ambulatory peritoneal dialysis (CAPD) has resulted in a syndrome of chemical peritonitis. This syndrome has ranged from a cloudy dialysate alone to a cloudy dialysate accompanied by variable degrees of abdominal pain and fever. This syndrome appears to be short-lived after discontinuation of intraperitoneal vancomycin.

Ototoxicity: Ototoxicity has occurred in patients receiving vancomycin. It may be transient or permanent. It has occurred mostly in patients who have been given excessive doses, who have an underlying hearing loss, or who are receiving concomitant therapy with another ototoxic agent.

Pseudomembranous colitis: In rare instances, pseudomembranous colitis has occurred because of C. *difficile* developing in patients who received IV vancomycin.

Reversible neutropenia: Reversible neutropenia has occurred in patients receiving vancomycin.

Superinfection: Prolonged use of vancomycin may result in the overgrowth of nonsusceptible organisms.

Systemic absorption: Clinically significant serum concentrations may occur in some patients who have taken multiple oral doses for active C. *difficile*-induced pseudomembranous colitis or who have inflammatory disorders of the intestinal mucosa; the risk is greater with the presence of renal impairment.

Tissue irritation: Vancomycin is irritating to tissue and must be given by a secure IV route of administration. Pain, tenderness, and necrosis occur with IM injection or inadvertent extravasation.

Renal function impairment: Use vancomycin with caution in patients with renal insufficiency because the risk of toxicity is appreciably increased by high, prolonged blood concentrations.

Pregnancy: Category C per manufacturer's prescribing information, *Category B* per Briggs' *Drugs in Pregnancy and Lactation.*

Lactation: Vancomycin is excreted in breast milk.

Children: In premature and full-term neonates it may be appropriate to confirm desired vancomycin serum concentrations.

Monitoring: Perform auditory function serial tests and monitor serum levels.

Periodically monitor the leukocyte count of patients who will undergo prolonged therapy with vancomycin or those who are receiving concomitant drugs that may cause neutropenia.

Maintain trough concentrations above 10 mg/L to avoid development of resistance. However, the minimum trough concentration should be higher (at least 15 mg/L) to generate a target AUC/MIC of 400 when the MIC is 1 mg/L. In complicated infections (eg, endocarditis, osteomyelitis, meningitis, hospital-acquired pneumonia related to *S. aureus*), higher serum trough concentrations (15 to 20 mg/L) are recommended to improve penetrations and optimize clinical outcomes.

ATS guidelines recommend trough levels of 15 to 20 mg/L for hospital-acquired pneumonia.

Drug Interactions

Drugs that may interact with vancomycin include aminoglycosides, anesthetics, indomethacin, methotrexate, neurotoxic/nephrotoxic agents, and nondepolarizing muscle relaxants.

Adverse Reactions

Adverse reactions may include renal impairment; hearing loss; neutropenia; anaphylaxis; drug fever; nausea; chills; eosinophilia; rashes; hypotension; wheezing; dyspnea; urticaria; inflammation at injection site; Red Man (or Redneck) syndrome; chemical peritonitis has been reported following intraperitoneal administration of vancomycin; pain and muscle spasms of the chest and back; pruritus; Stevens-Johnson syndrome, toxic epidermal necrolysis.

TELAVANCIN

Injection, lyophilized powder for solution: 250 and 750 mg (*Rx*) — *Vibativ* (Astellas)

Warning:

Fetal risk: Women of childbearing potential should have a serum pregnancy test prior to administration of telavancin.

Avoid use of telavancin during pregnancy unless the potential benefit to the patient outweighs the potential risk to the fetus.

Adverse developmental outcomes observed in 3 animal species at clinically relevant doses raise concerns about potential adverse developmental outcomes in humans.

Indications

Complicated skin and skin structure infections: For the treatment of adults with complicated skin and skin structure infections caused by susceptible isolates of the following gram-positive microorganisms: *Staphylococcus aureus* (including methicillin-susceptible and methicillin-resistant isolates), *Streptococcus pyogenes*, *Streptococcus agalactiae*, *Streptococcus anginosus* group (includes *S. anginosus*, *S. intermedius*, and *S. constellatus*), or *Enterococcus faecalis* (vancomycin-susceptible isolates only).

Combination therapy may be clinically indicated if the documented or presumed pathogens include gram-negative organisms.

Administration and Dosage

Adults:

Complicated skin and skin structure infections – 10 mg/kg administered by intravenous (IV) infusion over 60 minutes once every 24 hours for 7 to 14 days.

Renal function impairment:

Telavancin Dosage Adjustment in Adults With Renal Impairment	
CrCl[a] (mL/min)	Telavancin dosage regimen
> 50	10 mg/kg every 24 hours
30 to 50	7.5 mg/kg every 24 hours
10 to ≤ 30	10 mg/kg every 48 hours

[a] As calculated using the Cockcroft-Gault formula.

Administration: Administer by IV infusion over a period of 60 minutes.

Actions

Pharmacology: Telavancin is a semisynthetic lipoglycopeptide antibacterial that is a synthetic derivative of vancomycin. Telavancin inhibits bacterial cell wall synthesis by interfering with the polymerization and cross-linking of peptidoglycan. Telavancin binds to the bacterial membrane and disrupts membrane barrier function.

Pharmacokinetics:

Absorption – In healthy young adults, the pharmacokinetics of telavancin administered IV were linear following single doses. Steady-state concentrations were achieved by the third daily dose.

Distribution – Telavancin binds to human plasma proteins, primarily to serum albumin, in a concentration-independent manner. The mean binding is approximately 90% and is not affected by renal or hepatic impairment.

Metabolism – The metabolic pathway for telavancin has not been identified.

Excretion – Telavancin is primarily eliminated by the kidney.

Contraindications

None known.

Warnings/Precautions

Women of childbearing potential: If not already pregnant, instruct women of childbearing potential to use effective contraception during telavancin treatment.

Nephrotoxicity: Increases in serum creatinine to 1.5 times baseline occurred more frequently among telavancin-treated patients with normal baseline serum creatinine (15%) compared with vancomycin-treated patients with normal baseline serum creatinine (7%).

Infusion-related reactions: Administer over a period of 60 minutes to reduce the risk of infusion-related reactions. Rapid IV infusions of the glycopeptide class of antimicrobial agents can cause "red-man syndrome"–like reactions, including flushing of the upper body, urticaria, pruritus, or rash. Stopping or slowing the infusion may result in cessation of these reactions.

Clostridium difficile–associated diarrhea: *Clostridium difficile*–associated diarrhea has been reported with nearly all antibacterial agents and may range in severity from mild diarrhea to fatal colitis.

QTc prolongation: In a study involving healthy volunteers, doses of telavancin 7.5 and 15 mg/kg prolonged the QTc interval. Patients with congenital long QT syndrome, known prolongation of the QTc interval, uncompensated heart failure, or severe left ventricular hypertrophy were not included in clinical trials of telavancin. Avoid use of telavancin in patients with these conditions. Caution is warranted when prescribing telavancin to patients taking drugs known to prolong the QT interval.

Renal function impairment: The complicated skin and skin structure infections trials included patients with normal renal function and patients with varying degrees of renal impairment. Patients with underlying renal dysfunction or risk factors for renal dysfunction had a higher incidence of renal adverse events. Patients with creatinine clearance (CrCl) 50 mL/min or less also had lower clinical cure rates.

Superinfection: As with other antibacterial drugs, use of telavancin may result in overgrowth of nonsusceptible organisms, including fungi.

Pregnancy: Category C.

Pregnancy exposure registry – There is a pregnancy registry that monitors pregnancy outcomes in women exposed to telavancin during pregnancy. Health care providers are encouraged to register pregnant patients, or pregnant women may enroll themselves in the telavancin pregnancy registry by calling 1-888-658-4228.

Lactation: It is not known whether telavancin is excreted in human milk.

Children: The safety and effectiveness have not been studied.

Elderly: Telavancin is substantially excreted by the kidney, and the risk of adverse reactions may be greater in patients with impaired renal function. Because elderly patients are more likely to have decreased renal function, take care in dose selection in this age group.

Monitoring: Monitor renal function (ie, serum creatinine, CrCl) in all patients receiving telavancin.

Drug Interactions

QT prolongation: An additive effect of telavancin with other drugs that prolong the QT interval cannot be excluded.

Drugs that may interact with telavancin include drugs affecting kidney function and QT-prolonging drugs.

Adverse Reactions

Adverse reactions occurring in 3% or more of patients include decreased appetite, diarrhea, dizziness, foamy urine, generalized pruritus, infusion-site erythema, infusion-site pain, nausea, pruritus, rash, rigors, taste disturbance, and vomiting.

LINEZOLID

Tablets: 600 mg[a] (*Rx*)	Zyvox (Pfizer)
Powder for oral suspension: 100 mg per 5 mL[b] (*Rx*)	
Injection: 2 mg/mL[c] (*Rx*)	

[a] Sodium content is 2.92 mg per 600 mg tablet (0.1 mEq per tablet).
[b] Sodium content is 8.52 mg per 5 mL (0.4 mEq per 5 mL).
[c] Sodium content is 0.38 mg/mL (5 mEq per 300 mL bag, 3.3 mEq per 200 mL bag, 1.7 mEq per 100 mL bag).

Indications

Community-acquired pneumonia: For the treatment of community-acquired pneumonia caused by *Streptococcus pneumoniae* (including multidrug resistant strains), including cases with concurrent bacteremia, or *Staphylococcus aureus* (methicillin-susceptible strains only).

Complicated skin and skin structure infections: Complicated skin and skin structure infections, including diabetic foot infections, without concomitant osteomyelitis, caused by *S. aureus* (methicillin-susceptible and -resistant strains), *Streptococcus pyogenes*, or *Streptococcus agalactiae*.

Linezolid has not been studied in the treatment of decubitus ulcers.

Nosocomial pneumonia: For the treatment of nosocomial pneumonia caused by *S. aureus* (methicillin-susceptible and -resistant strains), or *S. pneumoniae* (including multidrug-resistant strains).

Uncomplicated SSSIs: For the treatment of uncomplicated SSSIs caused by *S. aureus* (methicillin-susceptible strains only) or *S. pyogenes*.

Vancomycin-resistant Enterococcus faecium infections: For the treatment of vancomycin-resistant *E. faecium* infections, including cases with concurrent bacteremia.

Because of concerns about inappropriate use of antibiotics leading to increase in resistant organisms, carefully consider alternatives before initiating treatment with linezolid in the outpatient setting.

Administration and Dosage

Administer without regard to meals. Large quantities of foods or beverages with high tyramine content should be avoided while taking linezolid.

Linezolid Dosage Guidelines

Infection[a]	Dosage and route of administration: Pediatric patients[b] (birth through 11 years of age)	Dosage and route of administration: Adults and adolescents (≥ 12 years of age)	Recommended duration of treatment (consecutive days)
Complicated SSSIs	10 mg/kg IV or oral[c] every 8 h	600 mg IV or oral[c] every 12 h	10 to 14
Community-acquired pneumonia, including concurrent bacteremia			
Nosocomial pneumonia			
Methicillin-resistant staphylococcal infections		600 mg[b] every 12 h	
Vancomycin-resistant *E. faecium* infections, including concurrent bacteremia	10 mg/kg IV or oral[c] every 8 h	600 mg IV or oral[c] every 12 h	14 to 28
Uncomplicated SSSIs	< 5 y: 10 mg/kg oral[c] every 8 h 5 to 11 y: 10 mg/kg oral[c] every 12 h	*Adults*: 400 mg oral[c] every 12 h *Adolescents*: 600 mg oral[c] every 12 h	10 to 14

[a] Due to the designated pathogens.
[b] Neonates younger than 7 days: most preterm neonates younger than 7 days of age (gestational age less than 34 weeks) have lower systemic linezolid clearance values and larger AUC values than many full-term neonates and older infants. Initiate these neonates with a dosing regimen of 10 mg/kg twice daily. Consider the use of 10 mg/kg 3 times daily regimen in neonates with a suboptimal clinical response. Give all neonatal patients 10 mg/kg 3 times daily by 7 days of life.
[c] Oral dosing using either linezolid tablets or linezolid for oral suspension.

Treat patients with methicillin-resistant S. *aureus* infection with linezolid 600 mg per 12 hours.

No dose adjustment is necessary when switching from IV to oral administration. Patients who are started on IV therapy may be switched to tablets or oral suspension when clinically indicated.

Renal function impairment:

Hemodialysis – Both linezolid and the 2 metabolites are eliminated by dialysis. Linezolid should be given after hemodialysis.

Patients receiving continuous renal replacement therapy or intermittent hemodialysis should receive the normal dosage regimen (ie, 600 mg IV every 12 hours).

IV administration: Administer over a period of 30 to 120 minutes. Do not use IV infusion bag in series connections. Do not introduce additives into this solution. Do not administer concomitantly with another drug; administer each drug separately.

Compatible IV solutions: 5% dextrose injection, 0.9% sodium chloride injection; lactated Ringer's injection.

Admixture incompatibilities: Physical incompatibilities resulted when linezolid IV injection was combined with the following drugs during simulated Y-site administration: amphotericin B, chlorpromazine hydrochloride, diazepam, pentamidine isothionate, erythromycin lactobionate, phenytoin sodium, and trimethoprim-sulfamethoxazole. Additionally, chemical incompatibility resulted when linezolid IV injection was combined with ceftriaxone sodium.

Actions

Pharmacology: Linezolid is a synthetic antibacterial agent of oxazolidinones. Linezolid binds to a site on the bacterial 23S ribosomal RNA of the 50S subunit and prevents the formation of a functional 70S initiation complex, which is an essential component of the bacterial translation process. The results of time-kill studies have shown linezolid to be bacteriostatic against enterococci and staphylococci. For streptococci, linezolid was found to be bactericidal for the majority of strains.

Pharmacokinetics:

Absorption – Linezolid is rapidly and extensively absorbed after oral dosing, with an absolute bioavailability of approximately 100%. The half-life is 4.4 to 5.5 hours. Peak concentrations are reached within 1 to 2 hours.

Distribution – The plasma protein binding of linezolid is approximately 31%. The volume of distribution at steady state averaged 40 to 50 L in healthy adult volunteers.

Metabolism – Linezolid is primarily metabolized by oxidation of the morpholine ring, which results in 2 inactive metabolites. Linezolid is minimally metabolized and may be mediated by human cytochrome P450 (CYP-450).

Excretion – Nonrenal clearance accounts for approximately 65% of the total clearance of linezolid. The renal clearance of linezolid is low and suggests net tubular reabsorption.

Contraindications

Known hypersensitivity to linezolid or any other product components; patients taking any medicinal product that inhibits monoamine oxidases A or B (eg, isocarboxazid, phenelzine) or within 2 weeks of taking any such medicinal product; uncontrolled hypertension, pheochromocytoma, thyrotoxicosis, and/or patients taking any of the following types of medications: directly and indirectly acting sympathomimetic agents (eg, pseudoephedrine), vasopressive agents (eg, epinephrine, norepinephrine), or dopaminergic agents (eg, dopamine, dobutamine), unless monitored for potential increase in blood pressure; carcinoid syndrome and/or patients taking any of the following medications: serotonin reuptake inhibitors, tricyclic antidepressants, serotonin 5-HT_1 receptor agonists (triptans), meperidine, or buspirone, unless carefully observed for signs and/or symptoms of serotonin syndrome.

Warnings/Precautions

Myelosuppression: Myelosuppression (including anemia, leukopenia, pancytopenia, and thrombocytopenia) has been reported in patients receiving linezolid. Monitor complete blood counts weekly in patients who receive linezolid, particularly in those who receive linezolid for more than 2 weeks, those with preexisting myelosuppression, those receiving concomitant drugs that produce bone marrow suppression, or those with a chronic infection who have received previous or concomitant antibiotic therapy.

Catheter-related infections: Linezolid is not approved and should not be used for the treatment of patients with catheter-related bloodstream infections or catheter-site infections.

Gram-negative infections: Linezolid has no clinical activity against gram-negative pathogens and is not indicated for the treatment of gram-negative infections.

Clostridium difficile–associated diarrhea: *Clostridium difficile*–associated diarrhea has been reported with nearly all antibacterial agents, including linezolid, and may range in severity from mild to life-threatening.

Duration of therapy: The safety and efficacy of linezolid formulations given for more than 28 days have not been evaluated in controlled clinical trials.

Phenylketonurics: Each 5 mL of the 100 mg per 5 mL oral suspension contains phenylalanine 20 mg. Advise patients to contact their physician or pharmacist.

Lactic acidosis: Lactic acidosis has been reported with the use of linezolid. In reported cases, patients experienced repeated episodes of nausea and vomiting. Patients who develop recurrent nausea or vomiting, unexplained acidosis, or a low bicarbonate level while receiving linezolid should receive immediate medical evaluation.

Serotonin syndrome: Spontaneous reports of serotonin syndrome associated with the coadministration of linezolid and serotonergic agents, including antidepressants such as selective serotonin reuptake inhibitors (SSRIs), have been reported.

Peripheral and optic neuropathy: Peripheral and optic neuropathy have been reported in patients treated with linezolid, primarily those patients treated for longer than the maximum recommended duration of 28 days.

Convulsions: Convulsions have been reported in patients when treated with linezolid.

Resistance: Prescribing linezolid in the absence of a proven or strongly suspected bacterial infection or a prophylactic indication is unlikely to provide benefit to the patient and increases the risk of the development of drug-resistant bacteria.

Renal function impairment: The 2 primary metabolites of linezolid may accumulate in patients with renal insufficiency, with the amount of accumulation increasing with the severity of renal dysfunction. The clinical significance of accumulation of these 2 metabolites has not been determined in patients with severe renal insufficiency.

Special risk: Linezolid has not been studied in patients with uncontrolled hypertension, pheochromocytoma, carcinoid syndrome, or untreated hyperthyroidism.

Superinfection: The use of antibiotics may promote the overgrowth of nonsusceptible organisms. If superinfection occurs during therapy, take appropriate measures.

Pregnancy: Category C.

Lactation: It is not known whether linezolid is excreted in human breast milk. Because many drugs are excreted in human milk, exercise caution when linezolid is administered to a breast-feeding woman.

Children: See Administration and Dosage.

Monitoring: Monitor complete blood cell counts weekly, particularly in those who receive linezolid for longer than 2 weeks, those with preexisting myelosuppression, those receiving concomitant drugs that produce bone marrow suppression, or those with a chronic infection who have received previous or concomitant antibiotic therapy.

Where administration of linezolid and concomitant serotonergic agents is clinically appropriate, closely observe patients for signs and symptoms of serotonin syndrome, such as cognitive dysfunction, hyperpyrexia, hyperreflexia, and incoordination.

Monitor visual function in all patients taking linezolid for extended periods (at least 3 months) and in all patients reporting new visual symptoms, regardless of length of therapy with linezolid.

Drug Interactions

Drugs that may affect linezolid include apraclonidine, ginseng, MAOIs, rifamycins, sibutramine, tetrabenazine, and tryptophan.

Drugs that may be affected by linezolid include atomoxetine, beta-2 agonists, bupropion, buspirone, COMT inhibitors (eg, entacapone), cyclobenzaprine, dopaminergic agents (eg, dobutamine) levodopa, MAOIs, meperidine, methylphenidate, propoxyphene, selective 5-HT_1 receptor agonists (eg, sumatriptan), serotonin reuptake inhibitors (eg, fluoxetine), sibutramine, sympathomimetic agents (eg, pseudoephedrine), tricyclic antidepressants (eg, amitryptyline), tryptophan, vasopressive agents (eg, epinephrine).

Drug/Food interactions: Large quantities of foods or beverages with high tyramine content should be avoided while taking linezolid. Quantities of tyramine consumed should be less than 100 mg per meal.

Adverse Reactions

Adverse reactions occurring in at least 3% of patients include abnormal AST and bilirubin, and platelet, white blood cell, and neutrophil count; anemia; diarrhea; dyspnea; fever; headache; injection site reaction; lab test abnormalities (hemoglobin, ALT, alkaline phosphatase, and lipase); nausea; rash; sepsis; thrombocytopenia; trauma; upper respiratory infection; vascular catheter site reaction; vomiting.

LINCOSAMIDES

CLINDAMYCIN	
Capsules: 75, 150, and 300 mg (as hydrochloride) (*Rx*)	Various, *Cleocin* (Pfizer)
Granules for oral solution: 75 mg (as palmitate)/5 mL (*Rx*)	*Cleocin Pediatric* (Pfizer)
Injection, solution, concentrate: 150 mg (as phosphate)/mL (*Rx*)	*Cleocin Phosphate* (Pharmacia)
Injection: 300, 600, and 900 mg (*Rx*)	*Cleocin Phosphate IV* (Upjohn)
LINCOMYCIN	
Injection: 300 mg/mL (as hydrochloride) (*Rx*)	*Lincocin* (Upjohn)

Warning:

Pseudomembranous colitis has been reported with nearly all antibacterial agents, including lincosamides, and may range in severity from mild to life-threatening. Therefore, it is important to consider this diagnosis in patients who present with diarrhea subsequent to the administration of antibacterial agents.

Because lincosamide therapy has been associated with severe colitis, which may end fatally, it should be reserved for serious infections for which less toxic antimicrobial agents are inappropriate. It should not be used in patients with nonbacterial infections such as most upper respiratory tract infections. Treatment with antibacterial agents alters the normal flora of the colon and may permit overgrowth of clostridia. Studies indicate that a toxin produced by *Clostridium difficile* is one primary cause of antibiotic-associated colitis.

After the diagnosis of pseudomembranous colitis has been established, initiate therapeutic measures. Mild cases of pseudomembranous colitis usually respond to drug discontinuation alone. In moderate to severe cases, consider management with fluids and electrolytes, protein supplementation, and treatment with an antibacterial drug clinically effective against C. *difficile* colitis.

Diarrhea, colitis, and pseudomembranous colitis have begun up to several weeks following cessation of therapy with lincosamides.

Indications

Clindamycin (oral):

Anaerobes – Serious respiratory tract infections such as empyema, anaerobic pneumonitis, and lung abscess; serious skin and soft tissue infections; septicemia, intra-abdominal infections such as peritonitis and intra-abdominal abscess (typically resulting from anaerobic organisms resident in the normal GI tract); infections of the female pelvis and genital tract such as endometritis, nongonococcal tubo-ovarian abscess, pelvic cellulitis, and postsurgical vaginal cuff infection.

Streptococci and staphylococci – Serious respiratory tract infections; serious skin and soft tissue infections.

Pneumococci – Serious respiratory tract infections.

Serious infections – Serious infections caused by susceptible strains of streptococci, pneumococci, staphylococci, and anaerobic bacteria.

Clindamycin (parenteral): For the treatment of serious infections caused by susceptible anaerobic bacteria.

Bone and joint infections – Acute hematogenous osteomyelitis.

Gynecological infections – Endometritis, nongonococcal tubo-ovarian abscess, pelvic cellulitis, and postsurgical vaginal cuff infections.

Intra-abdominal infections – Peritonitis and intra-abdominal abscess.

Lower respiratory tract infections – Pneumonia, empyema, and lung abscess.

Septicemia – Caused by S. *aureus*, streptococci, anaerobes.

Serious infections – For the treatment of serious infections caused by streptococci, pneumococci, and staphylococci.

Lincomycin (parenteral):

Serious infections – For the treatment of serious infections caused by susceptible strains of streptococci, pneumococci, and staphylococci. Its use should be reserved for penicillin-allergic patients or other patients for whom a penicillin is inappropriate. Before selecting lincomycin and because of the risk of antibiotic-associated pseudomembranous colitis, consider the nature of the infection and the suitability of less toxic alternatives (eg, erythromycin).

Administration and Dosage

CLINDAMYCIN:

Oral – Take with a full glass of water to avoid esophageal irritation. Clindamycin absorption is not affected by food.

Adults:

Serious infections – 150 to 300 mg every 6 hours.

More severe infections – 300 to 450 mg every 6 hours.

Children:

Clindamycin hydrochloride –

Serious infections: 8 to 16 mg/kg/day divided into 3 or 4 equal doses.

More severe infections: 16 to 20 mg/kg/day divided into 3 or 4 equal doses.

Clindamycin palmitate hydrochloride –

Serious infections: 8 to 12 mg/kg/day divided into 3 or 4 equal doses.

Severe infections: 13 to 25 mg/kg/day divided into 3 or 4 equal doses. In children weighing no more than 10 kg, administer 37.5 mg 3 times daily as the minimum dose.

Streptococcal infections: In cases of beta-hemolytic streptococcal infections, treatment should continue for at least 10 days.

Discontinuation of therapy: If significant diarrhea occurs during therapy, this antibiotic should be discontinued.

Parenteral – May be administered IM or IV. Single IM injections of more than 600 mg are not recommended.

Infusion rates should not exceed 30 mg/min. The usual infusion dilutions and rates are as follows:

Clindamycin Infusion Rates		
Dose	Volume diluent	Time
300 mg	50 mL	10 min
600 mg	50 mL	20 min
900 mg	50 to 100 mL	30 min
1,200 mg	100 mL	40 min

The following drugs are physically incompatible with clindamycin: ampicillin sodium, phenytoin sodium, barbiturates, aminophylline, calcium gluconate, and magnesium sulfate.

Adults:

Serious infections – Serious infections due to aerobic gram-positive cocci and the more sensitive anaerobes: 600 to 1200 mg/day in 2 to 4 equal doses IM or IV.

More severe infections – More severe infections, particularly those caused by *Bacteroides fragilis*, *Peptococcus* sp. or *Clostridium* sp. other than *C. perfringens*: 1.2 to 2.7 g/day in 2 to 4 equal doses IM or IV.

In life-threatening situations – In life-threatening situations caused by aerobes or anaerobes, doses of 4.8 g/day have been given IV to adults. Single IM injections greater than 600 mg are not recommended.

Children (older than 1 month of age): 20 to 40 mg/kg/day in 3 or 4 equal doses, depending on the severity of infection, administered IM or IV.

Alternatively, children may be dosed based on body surface area:

Serious infections – 350 mg/m^2/day; *more serious infections* – 450 mg/m^2/day.

Neonates (younger than 1 month of age): 15 to 20 mg/kg/day in 3 to 4 equal doses.

Maximum dose:

Adults – Doses of up to 4,800 mg daily IV have been given. Single IM doses of more than 600 mg are not recommended.

Children (at least 1 month of age) – 40 mg/kg/day or 450 mg/m^2/day.

Streptococcal infections: In cases of beta-hemolytic streptococcal infections, treatment should be continued for at least 10 days.

Discontinuation of therapy: If diarrhea occurs during therapy, this antibiotic should be discontinued.

LINCOMYCIN: If significant diarrhea occurs during therapy, this antibiotic should be discontinued.

IM –

Adults:

Serious infections – 600 mg every 24 hours.

More severe infections – 600 mg every 12 hours or more often.

Children older than 1 month of age:

Serious infections – 10 mg/kg (5 mg/lb) every 24 hours.

More severe infections – 10 mg/kg (5 mg/lb) every 12 hours or more often.

IV – Dilute to 1 g/100 mL (minimum) and infuse over 1 hour/1 g dose. Severe cardiopulmonary reactions have occurred when given at greater than the recommended concentration and rate.

Lincomycin Infusion Rates

Dose	Volume diluent	Time
600 mg	100 mL	1 h
1 g	100 mL	1 h
2 g	200 mL	2 h
3 g	300 mL	3 h
4 g	400 mL	4 h

Adults:

Serious infections – 600 mg to 1 g every 8 to 12 hours.

Severe to life-threatening situations – Doses of 8 g/day have been given.

Maximum recommended dose – 8 g/day.

Children older than 1 month of age: Infuse 10 to 20 mg/kg/day (5 to 10 mg/lb/day), depending on severity of infection, in divided doses as described above for adults.

Subconjunctival injection: 75 mg/0.25 mL injected subconjunctivally results in ocular fluid levels of antibiotic (lasting for 5 hours or more) with MICs sufficient for most susceptible pathogens.

Renal function impairment: When required, an appropriate dose is 25% to 30% of that recommended for patients with normal renal function.

IV admixture compatibilities:

Infusion solutions – Dextrose 5% injection, dextrose 10% injection, dextrose 5% and sodium chloride 0.9% injection, dextrose 10% and sodium chloride 0.9% injection, Ringer's injection, 1/6 M sodium lactate injection, *Travert* 10%-Electrolyte No. 1, and Dextran in Saline 6% w/v.

Vitamins in infusion solutions – B-complex and B-complex with ascorbic acid.

Antibiotics in infusion solutions – Penicillin G sodium (satisfactory for 4 hours), cephalothin, tetracycline, cephaloridine, colistimethate (satisfactory for 4 hours), ampicillin, methicillin, chloramphenicol, and polymyxin B sulfate.

Actions

Pharmacology: **Lincomycin** and **clindamycin**, known collectively as lincosamides, bind exclusively to the 50 S subunit of bacterial ribosomes and suppress protein synthesis. Cross-resistance has been demonstrated between these 2 agents.

Pharmacokinetics: Administration with food markedly impairs **lincomycin** (but not **clindamycin**) oral absorption.

Dialysis –

Select Pharmacokinetic Parameters of Lincosamides

Lincosamides	Bioavailability (%)	Mean peak serum level (mcg/mL)	Time to peak serum level (h)	Half-life (h)	Elimination (%)		
					Hepatic	Unchanged in urine (range)	Feces
Clindamycin[a]							
Oral	90	2.5	0.75				
IM		9 (adults) 6 (children)	3 (adults) 1 (children)	2.4	> 90	10	3.6
IV		11.9 (adults) 10 (children)					
Lincomycin							
IM		11.6	1	4.4 to 6.4	> 90	17.3 (2 to 25)	
IV		15.9	2			13.8 (5 to 30)	

[a] Clindamycin palmitate and phosphate are rapidly hydrolyzed to the base.

Contraindications

Hypersensitivity to lincosamides.

Warnings/Precautions

Pseudomembranous colitis: Pseudomembranous colitis has been reported with nearly all antibacterial agents, including lincosamides, and may range in severity from mild to life-threatening.

Also consider other causes of colitis. Make a careful inquiry concerning previous sensitivities to drugs or other allergens.

Meningitis: **Clindamycin** does not diffuse adequately into CSF; do not use for meningitis.

Benzyl alcohol: Some of these products contain benzyl alcohol, which has been associated with fatal "gasping syndrome" in premature infants.

Hypersensitivity reactions: Use with caution in patients with a history of asthma or significant allergies. Refer to Management of Acute Hypersensitivity Reactions.

Tartrazine sensitivity: Some of the products contain tartrazine, which may cause allergic-type reactions (including bronchial asthma) in susceptible individuals.

Renal function impairment: Cautiously give **clindamycin** to patients with severe renal or hepatic disease accompanied by severe metabolic aberrations. Use of **lincomycin** in pre-existing liver disease is not recommended unless special clinical circumstances so indicate.

Pregnancy:

Clindamycin – *Category B.*

Lincomycin – *Category C.*

Lactation: **Clindamycin** and **lincomycin** appear in breast milk. Because of the potential for serious adverse reactions in breast-feeding infants, decide whether to discontinue breast-feeding or the drug, taking into account the importance of the drug to the mother.

Children: Safety and effectiveness in children younger than 1 month of age have not been established for lincomycin. When **clindamycin** is administered to children (birth to 16 years of age), monitor organ system functions. Each mL of clindamycin and lincomycin injection contains benzyl alcohol 9.45 mg.

Elderly: Older patients with associated severe illness may not tolerate diarrhea well.

Monitoring: In prolonged therapy, perform liver/kidney function tests and blood counts. Monitor serum levels of lincosamides during high-dose therapy.

Drug Interactions

Drugs that may interact with lincosamides include erythromycin, kaolin-pectin, and neuromuscular blockers (nondepolarizing).

Adverse Reactions

Abscess, sterile; abdominal pain; agranulocytosis; aplastic anemia; azotemia; cardiopulmonary arrest; dermatitis (exfoliative and vesiculobullous); diarrhea; eosinophilia; esophagitis; glossitis; hypotension; induration; jaundice; leukopenia; liver function test abnormalities; metallic taste; nausea; neutropenia; oliguria; pain; pancytopenia; proteinuria; pruritus; pseudomembranous colitis; skin rashes; stomatitis; thrombocytopenia; thrombocytopenic purpura; thrombophlebitis; tinnitus; urticaria; vaginitis; vertigo; vomiting.

AMINOGLYCOSIDES, PARENTERAL

AMIKACIN SULFATE	
Injection: 250 mg/mL (*Rx*)	Various, *Amikin* (Apothecon)
Pediatric injection: 50 mg/mL (*Rx*)	Various, *Amikin* (Apothecon)
GENTAMICIN	
Injection: 2, 10, and 40 mg/mL (*Rx*)	Various, *Garamycin* (Schering)
KANAMYCIN SULFATE	
Injection: 500 mg and 1 g (*Rx*)	Various, *Kantrex* (Apothecon)
Pediatric injection: 75 mg (*Rx*)	Various, *Kantrex* (Apothecon)
STREPTOMYCIN SULFATE	
Injection: 400 mg/mL (*Rx*)	*Streptomycin Sulfate* (Pfizer)
TOBRAMYCIN SULFATE	
Pediatric injection: 10 and 40 mg/mL (*Rx*)	Various
Injection: 0.8, 1.2, and 10 mg/mL (as sulfate) (*Rx*)	Various
Powder for injection: 1.2 g (*Rx*)	Various
Nebulizer solution: 300 mg/5 mL (*Rx*)	*TOBI* (PathoGenesis)

Warning:

Toxicity: Aminoglycosides are associated with significant nephrotoxicity or ototoxicity. The serum half-life will be prolonged and significant accumulation will occur in patients with impaired renal function. Toxicity may develop even with conventional doses, particularly in patients with prerenal azotemia or impaired renal function.

Ototoxicity: Neurotoxicity, manifested as auditory (cochlear) and vestibular ototoxicity, can occur with any of these agents. Auditory changes are irreversible, usually bilateral and may be partial or total. Risk of hearing loss increases with the degree of exposure to high peak or high trough serum concentrations and continues to progress after drug withdrawal. The risk is higher in patients with renal function impairment and with preexisting hearing loss. High frequency deafness usually occurs first and can be detected by audiometric testing. Vestibular toxicity is more predominant with gentamicin and streptomycin; auditory toxicity is more common with kanamycin and amikacin. Tobramycin affects both functions equally. Relative ototoxicity is streptomycin = kanamycin > amikacin = gentamicin = tobramycin.

Renal toxicity: This may be characterized by decreased creatinine clearance (CrCl), cells or casts in the urine, decreased urine specific gravity, oliguria, proteinuria, or evidence of nitrogen retention (increasing blood urea nitrogen [BUN], nonprotein nitrogen [NPN], or serum creatinine). Renal damage usually is reversible. The relative nephrotoxicity of these agents is estimated to be kanamycin = amikacin = gentamicin > tobramycin > streptomycin.

Monitoring: Closely observe all patients treated with aminoglycosides. Monitoring renal and eighth cranial nerve function at onset of therapy is essential for patients with known or suspected renal function impairment and in those whose renal function initially is normal, but who develop signs of renal dysfunction. Evidence of renal function impairment or ototoxicity requires drug discontinuation or appropriate dosage adjustments. When feasible, monitor drug serum concentrations. Avoid concomitant use with other ototoxic, neurotoxic, or nephrotoxic drugs.

Indications

Reserve these drugs for treatment of infections caused by organisms not sensitive to less toxic agents. Safety for treatment periods longer than 14 days has not been established.

For approved indications, refer to the Administration and Dosage section.

Unlabeled uses:

Gentamicin – An alternative regimen for pelvic inflammatory disease is gentamicin plus clindamycin. Continue for at least 4 days and at least 48 hours after patient improves; then continue clindamycin 450 mg orally 4 times daily for 10 to 14 days total therapy.

Amikacin sulfate – Intrathecal/intraventricular administration has been suggested at 8 mg/24 hours.

Administration and Dosage

Synergism: In vitro studies indicate that aminoglycosides combined with penicillins or cephalosporins act synergistically against some strains of gram-negative organisms and enterococci (*Streptococcus faecalis*). Aminoglycosides may exhibit a synergistic effect when combined with ticarcillin for *Pseudomonas* infections.

AMIKACIN SULFATE:

Adults and children – Use the patient's ideal body weight for dosage calculation. Administer IM or IV. Administer 15 mg/kg/day divided into 2 or 3 equal doses at equally divided intervals. Treatment of heavier patients should not exceed 1.5 g/ day. In uncomplicated UTIs, use 250 mg twice daily.

Neonates: A loading dose of 10 mg/kg is recommended, followed by 7.5 mg/kg every 12 hours. Lower dosages may be safer during the first 2 weeks of life.

Renal function impairment – Adjust doses in patients with impaired renal function by administering normal doses at prolonged intervals or by administering reduced doses at a fixed interval.

Normal dosage at prolonged intervals: If the CrCl is not available and the patient's condition is stable, calculate a dosage interval (in hours) for the normal dose by multiplying the patient's serum creatinine by 9.

Reduced dosage at fixed time intervals: Measure serum concentration to ensure accurate administration and to avoid concentrations greater than 35 mcg/mL. Initiate therapy by administering a normal dose, 7.5 mg/kg, as a loading dose.

To determine maintenance doses administered every 12 hours, reduce the loading dose in proportion to the reduction in the patient's CrCl:

$$\text{Maintenance dose every 12 hours} = \frac{\text{observed Ccr (mL/min)}}{\text{normal Ccr (mL/min)}} \times \text{calculated loading dose (mg)}$$

Dialysis: Approximately half the normal mg/kg dose can be given after hemodialysis; in peritoneal dialysis, a parenteral dose of 7.5 mg/kg is given, and then amikacin is instilled in peritoneal dialysate at a concentration desired in serum.

GENTAMICIN:

Dosage – May be given IM or IV. For patients with serious infections and normal renal function, give 3 mg/kg/day in 3 equal doses every 8 hours. For patients with life-threatening infections, administer up to 5 mg/kg/day in 3 or 4 equal doses. Reduce dosage to 3 mg/kg/day as soon as clinically indicated.

Obese patients: Base dosage on an estimate of lean body mass.

Children: 6 to 7.5 mg/kg/day (2 to 2.5 mg/kg every 8 hours).

Infants and neonates: 7.5 mg/kg/day (2.5 mg/kg every 8 hours).

Premature or full term neonates (1 week of age or younger): 5 mg/kg/day (2.5 mg every 12 hours). A regimen of either 2.5 mg/kg every 18 hours or 3 mg/kg every 24 hours may also provide satisfactory peak and trough levels in preterm infants younger than 32 weeks gestational age.

Prevention of bacterial endocarditis –

In dental, oral, or upper respiratory tract procedures (alternate regimen): 1 to 2 g (50 mg/kg for children) ampicillin plus 1.5 mg/kg (2 mg/kg for children) gentamicin not to exceed 80 mg, both IM or IV ½ hour prior to procedure, followed by 1.5 g (25 mg/kg for children) amoxicillin 6 hours after initial dose or repeat parenteral dose 8 hours after initial dose.

GU or GI procedures (standard regimen): 2 g (50 mg/kg for children) ampicillin plus 1.5 mg/kg (2 mg/kg for children) gentamicin not to exceed 80 mg, both IM or IV ½ hour prior to procedure followed by 1.5 mg (25 mg/kg for children) amoxicillin.

Renal function impairment –

Rule of eights: Approximate the interval between doses (in hours) by multiplying the serum creatinine level (mg/dL) by 8. For example, a patient weighing 60 kg with a serum creatinine level of 2 mg/dL could be given 60 mg (1 mg/kg) every 16 hours (2 × 8).

IV – A 1 to 2 mg/kg loading dose may be used, followed by a maintenance dose.

Intrathecal – In general, the recommended dose for infants and children 3 months of age and older is 1 to 2 mg once a day. For adults, administer 4 to 8 mg once a day.

KANAMYCIN SULFATE: Do not exceed total 1.5 g/day by any route.

IM – For adults or children, 7.5 mg/kg every 12 hours (15 mg/kg/day). If continuously high blood levels are desired, give daily dose of 15 mg/kg in equally divided doses every 6 or 8 hours. Usual treatment duration is 7 to 10 days. Doses of 7.5 mg/kg give mean peak levels of 22 mcg/mL. At 8 hours after a 7.5 mg/kg dose, mean serum levels are 3.2 mcg/mL.

IV –

Adults: Do not exceed 15 mg/kg/day. Give slowly over 30 to 60 minutes. Divide daily doses into 2 to 3 equal doses.

Children: Use sufficient diluent to infuse drug over 30 to 60 minutes.

Renal failure – Calculate the dosage interval with the following formula: Serum creatinine (mg/dL) × 9 equals dosage interval (in hours).

Intraperitoneal (following exploration for peritonitis or after peritoneal contamination caused by fecal spill during surgery) – 500 mg in 20 mL sterile distilled water instilled through a polyethylene catheter into wound.

Aerosol treatment – 250 mg 2 to 4 times/day.

Other routes – Concentrations of 0.25% have been used as irrigating solutions in abscess cavities, pleural space, peritoneal and ventricular cavities.

STREPTOMYCIN SULFATE: Administer IM only.

Tuberculosis (TB) – The standard regimen for the treatment of drug-susceptible TB has been 2 months of INH, rifampin, and pyrazinamide followed by 4 months of INH and rifampin (patients with concomitant infection with tuberculosis and HIV may require treatment for a longer period). When streptomycin is added to this regimen because of suspected or proven drug resistance, the recommended dosing for streptomycin is as follows:

Streptomycin Dosing for TB			
	Daily	Twice weekly	Three times weekly
Children	20 to 40 mg/kg max 1 g	25 to 30 mg/kg max 1.5 g	25 to 30 mg/kg max 1.5 g
Adults	15 mg/kg max 1 g	25 to 30 mg/kg max 1.5 g	25 to 30 mg/kg max 1.5 g

Streptomycin usually is administered daily as a single IM injection. Give a total dose of less than 120 g over the course of therapy unless there are no other therapeutic options. In patients older than 60 years of age, use a reduced dosage. The total period of drug treatment for TB is a minimum of 1 year.

Tularemia – 1 to 2 g/day in divided doses for 7 to 14 days, or until afebrile 5 to 7 days.

Plague – 2 g daily in 2 divided doses for a minimum of 10 days.

Bacterial endocarditis –

Streptococcal: In penicillin-sensitive alpha and nonhemolytic streptococci, use streptomycin for 2 weeks with penicillin: 1 g twice daily for 1 week, 0.5 g twice daily for the second week. If patient is older than 60 years of age, give 0.5 g twice daily for the entire 2-week period.

Enterococcal: 1 g twice daily for 2 weeks and 0.5 g twice daily for 4 weeks in combination with penicillin.

Other susceptible infections –

Adults: 1 to 2 g in divided doses every 6 to 12 hours for moderate-to-severe infections. Doses should generally not exceed 2 g/day.

Children: 20 to 40 mg/kg/day in divided doses every 6 to 12 hours.

Renal function impairment – Reduce dosage.

TOBRAMYCIN SULFATE:

Dosage – Use the patient's ideal body weight for dosage calculation. Peak and trough serum concentrations should be measured. Avoid prolonged peak concentrations greater than 12 mcg/mL or troughs greater than 2 mcg/mL.

Adults with serious infections – Administer 3 mg/kg/day in 3 equal doses every 8 hours.

Life-threatening infections: Administer up to 5 mg/kg/day in 3 or 4 equal doses. Reduce dosage to 3 mg/kg/day as soon as clinically indicated.

Children – Administer 6 to 7.5 mg/kg/day in 3 or 4 equally divided doses (2 to 2.5 mg/kg every 8 hours or 1.5 to 1.9 mg/kg every 6 hours).

Premature or full-term infants (1 year of age or younger) – Administer up to 4 mg/kg/day in 2 equal doses every 12 hours. Preliminary data suggest that 2.5 mg/kg every 18 hours or 3 mg/kg every 24 hours may achieve safe and effective peak and trough serum concentrations in newborn infants weighing less than 1 kg at birth.

Renal function impairment – Following a loading dose of 1 mg/kg, adjust subsequent dosage, either with reduced doses administered at 8-hour intervals or with normal doses given at prolonged levels.

An alternative guide for determining reduced dosage at 8-hour intervals (for patients whose steady-state serum creatinine values are known) is to divide the normally recommended dose by the patient's serum creatinine.

Hemodialysis – Hemodialysis removes approximately 50% of a dose in 6 hours. In patients maintained by regular dialysis, the usual dose of 1.5 to 2 mg/kg given after every dialysis usually maintains therapeutic, nontoxic serum levels. In patients receiving intermittent peritoneal dialysis, patients dialyzed twice weekly should receive a 1.5 to 2 mg/kg loading dose followed by 1 mg/kg every 3 days. Where dialysis occurs every 2 days, a 1.5 mg/kg loading dose is given after the first dialysis and 0.75 mg/kg after each subsequent dialysis.

IV administration – The IV dose is the same as the IM dose. Infuse the diluted solution over a period of 20 to 60 minutes. Infusion periods of less than 20 minutes are not recommended because peak serum levels may exceed 20 mcg/mL.

Cystic fibrosis (nebulizer solution) – Recommended dosage for adults and children 6 years of age and older is 300 mg twice a day in repeating cycles of 28 days on drug/28 days off drug. Do not adjust dosage by age or weight. Take as close to 12 hours apart as possible; do not take less than 6 hours apart. Administer by inhalation over a 10- to 15-minute period, using a hand-held *PARI LC PLUS* reusable nebulizer with a *DeVilbiss Pulmo-Aide* compressor. Do not dilute or mix with dornase alfa in the nebulizer. Instruct patients on multiple therapies to take them first, followed by tobramycin. Bronchospasm, which can occur with inhalation of tobramycin, may be reduced if inhalation of tobramycin nebulization solution follows bronchodilator therapy.

Monitoring: In patients with normal renal function, serum tobramycin concentrations are approximately 1 mcg/mL 1 hour after dose administration. Monitoring of serum concentrations in patients with renal dysfunction or patients treated with concomitant parenteral tobramycin may reduce the risk of toxicity.

Actions

Pharmacology: The aminoglycosides are bactericidal antibiotics used primarily in the treatment of gram-negative infections.

Pharmacokinetics:

Absorption/Distribution – Absorption from IM injection is rapid, with peak blood levels achieved within 1 hour.

Excretion is by glomerular filtration, largely as unchanged drug; thus, high urine levels are attained. Aminoglycosides are removed by hemodialysis (4 to 6 hours removes approximately 50%) and peritoneal dialysis (range, removal of 23% in 8 hours to only 4% in 22 hours).

Serum levels – Because of the narrow range between therapeutic and toxic serum levels, careful attention to dosage calculations is essential, especially in patients with renal impairment, geriatric and female patients, those requiring high peak serum levels, patients on prolonged therapy (longer than 10 days), patients with unstable renal function or those undergoing dialysis, those with abnormal extracellular fluid volume, or with prior exposure to ototoxic or nephrotoxic drugs. Age markedly affects peak concentration in children; it is generally lower in young children and infants. Monitor drug serum levels. Peak levels indicate therapeutic levels. Trough serum level determinations (just before next dose) best indicate drug accumulation. Obtain serum levels within 48 hours of start of therapy and every 3 to 4 days assuming stable renal function; also, levels are indicated when dose is changed or in changing renal function. Generally, to measure peak levels, draw a serum sample about 30 minutes after IV infusion or 1 hour after an IM dose. For trough levels, obtain serum samples at 8 hours or just prior to the next dose.

Various Pharmacokinetic Parameters of the Aminoglycosides

Aminoglycoside	Half-life (h) Normal	Half-life (h) ESRD	Therapeutic serum levels (peak) (mcg/mL)	Toxic serum levels (mcg/mL) Peak[a]	Toxic serum levels (mcg/mL) Trough[b]	Dose (mg/kg/day) (normal CrCl)
Amikacin	2 to 3	24 to 60	16 to 32	> 35	> 10	15
Gentamicin	2	24 to 60	4 to 8	> 12	> 2	3 to 5
Kanamycin	2 to 3	24 to 60	15 to 40	> 35	> 10	15
Streptomycin	2.5	100	20 to 30	> 50	—	15
Tobramycin	2 to 2.5	24 to 60	4 to 8	> 12	> 2	3 to 5

[a] Measured 1 hour after IM administration.
[b] Measured immediately prior to next dose.

Microbiology:

Organisms Generally Susceptible to Aminoglycosides

	Organisms	Amikacin	Gentamicin	Kanamycin	Streptomycin	Tobramycin
Gram-positive	*Mycobacterium tuberculosis*	✓[a]			✓[b]	
	Staphylococci	✓[c]	✓[c]			✓
	Staphylococcus aureus	✓	✓	✓[c]		✓
	Staphylococcus epidermidis	✓		✓		
	Streptococci				✓[b]	
	Streptococcus faecalis		✓[b]		✓[b]	✓[b]

Organisms Generally Susceptible to Aminoglycosides

	Organisms	Amikacin	Gentamicin	Kanamycin	Streptomycin	Tobramycin
Gram-negative	*Acinetobacter* sp.	✓		✓		
	Brucella sp.				✓	
	Citrobacter sp.	✓	✓	✓	✓	✓
	Enterobacter sp.	✓	✓	✓	✓	✓
	Escherichia coli	✓	✓	✓	✓	✓
	Haemophilus influenzae	✓		✓	✓[b]	
	Haemophilus ducreyi				✓	
	Klebsiella sp.	✓	✓	✓	✓[b]	✓
	Morganella morganii					✓
	Neisseria sp.	✓		✓	✓	
	Proteus sp.	✓[d]	✓[d]	✓[d]	✓	✓[d]
	Providencia sp.	✓	✓	✓	✓	✓
	Pseudomonas sp.	✓				
	P. aeruginosa	✓	✓[b]		✓	✓
	Salmonella sp.	✓	✓	✓	✓	✓
	Serratia sp.	✓	✓	✓	✓	✓
	Shigella sp.	✓	✓	✓	✓	✓
	Yersinia (Pasteurella) pestis	✓	✓	✓	✓	✓

[a] ✓ = generally susceptible
[b] Usually used concomitantly with other anti-infectives.
[c] Penicillinase-producing and nonpenicillinase-producing.
[d] Indole-positive and indole-negative.

Contraindications

Previous reactions to these agents. With the exception of the use of streptomycin in tuberculosis, these agents generally are not indicated in long-term therapy because of the ototoxic and nephrotoxic hazards of extended administration.

Warnings/Precautions

Toxicity: See Warning Box.

Burn patients: In patients with extensive burns, altered pharmacokinetics may result in reduced serum concentrations of aminoglycosides.

Hypomagnesemia: Hypomagnesemia may occur in more than ⅓ of patients whose oral diet is restricted or who are eating poorly.

Neuromuscular blockade: Neurotoxicity can occur. Aminoglycosides may aggravate muscle weakness because of a potential curare-like effect on the neuromuscular junction.

Neuromuscular blockade resulting in respiratory paralysis has occurred with these agents, especially if given with or soon after anesthesia or muscle relaxants.

Nephrotoxicity: Nephrotoxicity may occur. Risk factors include the elderly, patients with a history of renal impairment who are treated for longer periods or with higher doses than those recommended, a recent course of aminoglycosides (within 6 weeks), concurrent use of other nephrotoxic agents, frequent dosing, potassium depletion, and decreased intravascular volume. Adverse renal effects can occur in patients with initially normal renal function. Of patients receiving an aminoglycoside for several days or more, approximately 8% to 26% will develop mild renal impairment that is generally reversible.

Hydration – These drugs reach high concentrations in the renal system; keep patients well hydrated to minimize chemical irritation of tubules.

Dosing interval: Preliminary evidence indicates that aminoglycosides may be administered on a once-daily basis without compromising efficacy and without increasing the potential for nephrotoxicity and ototoxicity. It is possible that the incidence of nephrotoxicity may even be decreased.

Intrathecal gentamicin: Use of excessive (40 to 160 mg) doses of intrathecal **gentamicin** has produced neuromuscular disturbances (eg, ataxia, paresis, incontinence).

Cross-allergenicity: Cross-allergenicity among the aminoglycosides has been demonstrated.

Monitoring: Monitor peak and trough serum concentrations periodically to ensure adequate levels and to avoid potentially toxic levels. Also monitor serum calcium, magnesium and sodium (see Adverse Reactions).

Eighth cranial nerve function testing – Serial audiometric tests are suggested, particularly when renal function is impaired or prolonged aminoglycoside therapy is required; also repeat such tests periodically after treatment if there is evidence of a hearing deficit or vestibular abnormality before or during therapy, or when consecutive or concomitant use of other potentially ototoxic drugs is unavoidable.

Syphilis: In the treatment of sexually transmitted disease, if concomitant syphilis is suspected, perform a darkfield examination before treatment is started. Perform monthly serologic tests for 4 months or more.

Topical use: Aminoglycosides are quickly and almost totally absorbed when applied topically in association with surgical procedures, except to the urinary bladder.

Pregnancy: *Category D* (amikacin, gentamicin, kanamycin, streptomycin, tobramycin).

Lactation: Small amounts of **streptomycin** and **kanamycin**are excreted in breast milk.

Children: Use with caution in premature infants and neonates because of their renal immaturity and the resulting prolongation of serum half-life of these drugs.

A syndrome of apparent CNS depression, characterized by stupor and flaccidity to coma and deep respiratory depression, has been reported in very young infants given **streptomycin** in doses higher than those recommended. Do not exceed recommended doses in infants.

Elderly: Elderly patients may have reduced renal function that is not evident in the results of routine screening tests, such as BUN or serum creatinine. A CrCl determination may be more useful.

Drug Interactions

Drugs that may affect aminoglycosides include cephalosporins, enflurane, methoxyflurane, vancomycin, indomethacin IV, loop diuretics, and penicillins.

Drugs that may be affected by aminoglycosides include depolarizing and nondepolarizing neuromuscular blockers and polypeptide antibiotics.

Adverse Reactions

Aminoglycoside Adverse Reactions (%)

	Adverse Reaction	Amikacin	Gentamicin	Kanamycin	Streptomycin	Tobramycin
Central/Peripheral nervous system	Headache	rare	✓[a]	rare		✓
	Confusion		✓			✓
	Fever		✓		✓	✓
	Lethargy		✓			✓
	Disorientation					✓
	Neuromuscular blockade[b]	✓		✓	✓	
	Paresthesia	rare		rare		
GI	Vomiting	rare	✓	rare	✓	✓
	Nausea	rare	✓	rare	✓	✓
	Diarrhea			rare		✓

Aminoglycoside Adverse Reactions (%)

	Adverse Reaction	Amikacin	Gentamicin	Kanamycin	Streptomycin	Tobramycin
Hematologic	Anemia	rare	✓			✓
	Eosinophilia	rare	✓		✓	✓
	Leukopenia		✓		✓	✓
	Thrombocytopenia		✓		✓	✓
Hypersensitivity	Rash	rare	✓	rare	✓	✓
	Urticaria		✓		✓	✓
	Itching		✓			✓
Special senses	Dizziness		✓			✓
	Tinnitus		✓			✓
	Vertigo		✓		✓	✓
	Hearing loss/deafness[c]	✓	✓	✓[c]	✓	✓
Renal[a]	Oliguria	✓	✓	✓		✓
	Proteinuria	✓	✓	✓		✓
	Rising serum creatinine[b]	✓	✓	✓		✓
	Casts	✓	✓			
	Rising BUN[b]		✓	✓		✓
	Red and white cells in urine	✓		✓		
	Azotemia	✓			✓	
Lab test abnormalities	Increased AST/ALT		✓			✓
	Increased bilirubin		✓			✓
Other	Apnea	✓	✓	✓	✓	✓
	Pain/Irritation at injection site		✓	✓		✓
	Hypotension	rare	✓			

[a] ✓ = Reported; no incidence given
[b] See Warnings
[c] Partially reversible to irreversible bilateral hearing loss.

AMINOGLYCOSIDES, ORAL

NEOMYCIN SULFATE	
Tablets: 500 mg (*Rx*)	Various, *Neo-Tabs* (Pharma-Tek)
Oral solution: 125 mg/5 mL (*Rx*)	*Mycifradin* (Pharmacia), *Neo-Fradin* (Pharma-Tek)
PAROMOMYCIN SULFATE	
Capsules: 250 mg (*Rx*)	Various, *Humatin* (Parke-Davis)

For complete information on the aminoglycosides, refer to the Aminoglycosides, Parenteral monograph.

Indications

Suppression of intestinal bacteria.

Hepatic coma.

Neomycin sulfate: Many studies have documented lipid-lowering efficacy of neomycin. Alone, it reduced LDL cholesterol levels by 24%. Combined with niacin, it reduced LDL cholesterol levels to below the 90th percentile in 92% of patients.

Administration and Dosage

NEOMYCIN SULFATE:

Preoperative prophylaxis for elective colorectal surgery –

Recommended Bowel Preparation Regimen (Proposed Surgery Time 8 am)[a]			
Therapy	Day 3 before surgery	Day 2 before surgery	Day 1 before surgery
Diet	Minimum residue or clear liquid	Minimum residue or clear liquid	Clear liquid
Bisacodyl, 1 oral cap	6 pm (-62 h)		
Magnesium sulfate, 30 mL of a 50% solution orally		10 am (−46 h). Repeat at 2 pm (−42 h) and 6 pm (−38 h)	10 am (−22 h). Repeat at 2 pm (−18 h).
Enema		7 pm (−37 h) and 8 pm (−36 h). Repeat hourly until no solid feces return with last enema	None
Supplemental IV fluids			As needed
Neomycin and erythromycin tablets, 1 g each, orally			1 pm (−19 h). Repeat at 2 pm (−18 h) and 11 pm (−9 h)

[a] On day of surgery, patient should evacuate rectum at 6:30 am (-1½ h) for 8 am procedure.

Hepatic coma (as adjunct) –

Adults: 4 to 12 g/day in divided doses.

Children: 50 to 100 mg/kg/day in divided doses. Continue treatment over a period of 5 to 6 days; during this time, return protein to the diet incrementally. Chronic hepatic insufficiency may require up to 4 g/day over an indefinite period.

PAROMOMYCIN SULFATE:

Intestinal amebiasis –

Adults and children: Usual dose is 25 to 35 mg/kg/day, in 3 doses with meals for 5 to 10 days.

Management of hepatic coma –

Adults: Usual dose: 4 g/day in divided doses at regular intervals for 5 to 6 days.

Paromomycin sulfate has been recommended for other parasitic infections — *Dientamoeba fragilis* (25 to 30 mg/kg/day in 3 doses for 7 days); *Diphyllobothrium latum, Taenia saginata, Taenia solium, Dipylidium caninum* (*adults:* 1 g every 15 minutes for 4 doses; *pediatric:* 11 mg/kg every 15 minutes for 4 doses); *Hymenolepis nana* (45 mg/kg/day for 5 to 7 days).

Actions

Pharmacokinetics: Oral aminoglycosides are poorly absorbed; therefore, use only for suppression of GI bacterial flora.

Contraindications

Presence of intestinal obstruction; hypersensitivity to aminoglycosides.

Warnings/Precautions

Increased absorption: Although negligible amounts are absorbed through intact mucosa, consider the possibility of increased absorption from ulcerated or denuded areas.

Nephrotoxicity/Ototoxicity: Because of reported cases of deafness and potential nephrotoxic effects, closely observe patients. Refer to the Warning Box in the Aminoglycosides, Parenteral monograph concerning aminoglycoside toxicity.

Muscular disorders: Use with caution in patients with muscular disorders such as myasthenia gravis or parkinsonism.

GI effects:

Neomycin – Orally administered neomycin increases fecal bile acid excretion and reduces intestinal lactase activity.

Paromomycin – Use with caution in individuals with ulcerative lesions of the bowel to avoid renal toxicity through inadvertent absorption.

Pregnancy:

Neomycin – Category D.

Lactation: It is not known whether **neomycin** is excreted in breast milk. Other aminoglycosides are excreted in breast milk.

Children: The safety and efficacy of oral **neomycin** in patients younger than 18 years of age have not been established. If treatment is necessary, use with caution; do not exceed a treatment period of 3 weeks because of absorption from the GI tract.

Drug Interactions

Drugs that may be affected by aminoglycosides include anticoagulants, digoxin, methotrexate, neuromuscular blockers (depolarizing and nondepolarizing).

Adverse Reactions

Nausea, vomiting, diarrhea (most common); "malabsorption syndrome" characterized by increased fecal fat, decreased serum carotene, and fall in xylose absorption. *Clostridium difficile*-associated colitis (following **neomycin** therapy); nephrotoxicity and ototoxicity (following prolonged and high-dosage therapy in hepatic coma).

METRONIDAZOLE

Tablets; oral: 250 mg and 500 mg (*Rx*)	Various, *Flagyl* (Kabivitrum)
Tablets, extended-release; oral: 750 mg (*Rx*)	Various, *Flagyl ER* (Kabivitrum)
Capsules; oral: 375 mg (*Rx*)	Various, *Flagyl* (Kabivitrum)
Injection, ready-to-use: 500 mg/100 mL (*Rx*)	Various, *Metro* (B. Braun)

Metronidazole also is available for topical and intravaginal use and also is used orally as an amebicide.

Warning:
Metronidazole is carcinogenic in rodents. Avoid unnecessary use.

Indications

Anaerobic infections: Treatment of serious infections caused by susceptible anaerobic bacteria. Effective in *Bacteroides fragilis* infections resistant to clindamycin, chloramphenicol, and penicillin.

Intra-abdominal infections – Peritonitis, intra-abdominal abscess, and liver abscess caused by *Bacteroides* sp. (*B. fragilis*, *B. distasonis*, *B. ovatus*, *B. thetaiotaomicron*, *B. vulgatus*), *Clostridium* sp., *Eubacterium* sp., *Peptostreptococcus* sp., and *Peptococcus* sp.

Skin and skin structure infections – Caused by *Bacteroides* sp. including the *B. fragilis* group, *Clostridium* sp., *Peptococcus* sp., *Peptostreptococcus niger*, and *Fusobacterium* sp.

Gynecologic infections – Endometritis, endomyometritis, tubo-ovarian abscess, and postsurgical vaginal cuff infection caused by *Bacteroides* sp. including the *B. fragilis* group, *Clostridium* sp., *Peptococcus niger*, and *Peptostreptococcus* sp.; bacterial vaginosis (*Flagyl ER* only).

Bacterial septicemia – Caused by *Bacteroides* sp. including the *B. fragilis* group and *Clostridium* sp.

Bone and joint infections – Caused by *Bacteroides* sp. including the *B. fragilis* group, as adjunctive therapy.

CNS infections – Meningitis and brain abscess caused by *Bacteroides* sp. including the *B. fragilis* group.

Lower respiratory tract infections – Pneumonia, empyema, and lung abscess caused by *Bacteroides* sp. including the *B. fragilis* group.

Endocarditis – Caused by *Bacteroides* sp. including the *B. fragilis* group.

Prophylaxis: Preoperative, intraoperative, and postoperative IV metronidazole may reduce the incidence of postoperative infection in patients undergoing elective colorectal surgery which is classified as contaminated or potentially contaminated.

Discontinue within 12 hours after surgery. If there are signs of infection, obtain specimens for cultures to identify the causative organisms.

Metronidazole also is indicated for amebiasis and trichomoniasis, intravaginally for bacterial vaginosis, and topically for acne rosacea.

Unlabeled uses: The CDC has recommended the use of oral metronidazole for bacterial vaginosis (500 mg twice daily for 7 days). Single-dose therapy for bacterial vaginosis (2 g) also appears to be as effective as multiple-dose therapy.

Administration and Dosage

Anaerobic bacterial infections: In the treatment of most serious anaerobic infections, metronidazole is usually administered IV initially.

IV –

Loading dose: 15 mg/kg infused over 1 hour (about 1 g for a 70 kg adult).

Maintenance dose: 7.5 mg/kg infused over 1 hour every 6 hours (about 500 mg for a 70 kg adult). Administer the first maintenance dose 6 hours following the initiation of loading dose. Do not exceed a maximum of 4 g in 24 hours.

Administer by slow IV drip infusion only, either as continuous or intermittent infusion. Do not use equipment containing aluminum (eg, needles, cannulae). If used with a primary IV fluid system, discontinue the primary solution during infusion. Do not give by direct IV bolus injection because of the low pH (0.5 to

2) of the reconstituted product. The drug must be further diluted and neutralized for infusion. Do not introduce additives into the solution.

Oral: Following IV therapy, use oral metronidazole when conditions warrant. The usual adult oral dosage is 7.5 mg/kg every 6 hours (about 500 mg for a 70 kg adult). Do not exceed a maximum of 4 g in 24 hours.

Duration: The usual duration of therapy is 7 to 10 days; however, infections of the bone and joints, lower respiratory tract, and endocardium may require longer treatment.

Bacterial vaginosis:

7-day course of treatment – 750 mg ER once daily by mouth for 7 consecutive days. Take *Flagyl ER* tablets under fasting conditions, at least 1 hour before or 2 hours after meals.

Prophylaxis: To prevent postoperative infection in contaminated or potentially contaminated colorectal surgery, the recommended adult dosage is 15 mg/kg infused over 30 to 60 minutes and completed about 1 hour before surgery; followed by 7.5 mg/kg infused over 30 to 60 minutes at 6 and 12 hours after the initial dose.

Complete administration of the initial preoperative dose about 1 hour before surgery so that adequate drug levels are present in the serum and tissues at the time of initial incision, and administer, if necessary, at 6-hour intervals to maintain effective drug levels. Limit prophylactic use to the day of surgery only.

Elderly: Dosage adjustment may be necessary; monitor serum levels.

Actions

Pharmacology: Metronidazole, a nitroimidazole, is active against various anaerobic bacteria and protozoa. It is believed to invoke cytotoxicity on the reduced nitro group in the bacterium cell. The liberated inactive end products are believed to target the RNA, DNA, or cellular proteins of the organisms.

Pharmacokinetics:

Absorption/Distribution – Metronidazole is well absorbed after oral administration. Peak serum levels occur at about 1 to 2 hours. Metronidazole appears in CSF, saliva, and breast milk in concentrations similar to those found in plasma. Less than 20% of the circulating metronidazole is bound to plasma proteins.

Metabolism – Unchanged metronidazole accounts for about 20% of the total.

Excretion – The major route of elimination of metronidazole and its metabolites is via the urine (60% to 80% of the dose); fecal excretion accounts for 6% to 15% of the dose. Metronidazole has an average elimination half-life in healthy subjects of 8 hours. Metronidazole and its metabolites are removed by hemodialysis.

Contraindications

Hypersensitivity to metronidazole or other nitroimidazole derivatives; pregnancy (first trimester in patients with trichomoniasis).

Warnings/Precautions

Neurologic effects: Seizures and peripheral neuropathy have occurred. Appearance of abnormal neurologic signs demands prompt discontinuation of therapy. Administer metronidazole with caution to patients with CNS diseases.

Crohn's disease: Crohn's disease patients are known to have an increased incidence of GI and certain extraintestinal cancers. There have been some reports in the medical literature of breast and colon cancer in Crohn's disease patients who have been treated with metronidazole at high doses for extended periods of time.

Candidiasis: Candidiasis may present more prominent symptoms during therapy and requires treatment with a candicidal agent.

Hematologic effects: Use with care in patients with evidence or history of blood dyscrasia. Mild leukopenia has been seen during administration. Perform total and differential leukocyte counts before and after therapy.

Renal function impairment: Do not specifically reduce the dose in anuric patients; accumulated metabolites may be rapidly removed by dialysis.

Hepatic function impairment: Patients with severe hepatic disease metabolize metronidazole slowly. Accumulation of the drug and its metabolites may occur.

Carcinogenesis: Metronidazole has shown evidence of carcinogenic activity with chronic oral administration in rodents.

Pregnancy: *Category B.* Do not administer to pregnant women during the first trimester. Restrict metronidazole for trichomoniasis in the second and third trimesters to those in whom local palliative treatment has been inadequate to control symptoms.

Lactation: Because of the potential for tumorigenicity, decide whether to discontinue nursing or to discontinue the drug, taking into account the importance of the drug to the mother. Metronidazole is secreted in breast milk in concentrations similar to those found in plasma.

Children: Safety and efficacy in children have not been established, except for the treatment of amebiasis. Newborns demonstrate a diminished capacity to eliminate metronidazole; half-life may be as high as 22 hours.

Elderly: Because the pharmacokinetics of metronidazole may be altered in the elderly, monitoring of serum levels may be necessary to adjust the dosage accordingly.

Drug Interactions

Drugs that may affect metronidazole include barbiturates and cimetidine. Drugs that may be affected by metronidazole include anticoagulants, disulfiram, ethanol, hydantoins, and lithium.

Drug/Lab test interactions: The drug may interfere with chemical analyses for AST, ALT, LDH, triglycerides, and hexokinase glucose.

Adverse Reactions

Adverse reactions may include dysuria; cystitis; polyuria; incontinence; proliferation of *Candida* in the vagina; dyspareunia; darkened urine; seizures and peripheral neuropathy; dizziness; vertigo; incoordination; ataxia; confusion; irritability; depression; weakness; insomnia; headache; syncope; nausea; diarrhea; epigastric distress; constipation; proctitis; glossitis; stomatitis; sharp, unpleasant metallic taste; urticaria; erythematous rash; flushing; nasal congestion; vaginitis; genital pruritus; abnormal urine; dysmenorrhea; upper respiratory tract infection; rhinitis; sinusitis; pharyngitis; bacterial infection; influenza-like symptoms; moniliasis; abnormal cramping; furry tongue; decreased libido; neutropenia; thrombocytopenia (rare); dryness of the mouth, vagina, or vulva; fever; thrombophlebitis (after IV infusion); abdominal pain. Flattening of the T-wave may be seen in ECG tracings.

RIFAXIMIN

Tablets; oral: 200 and 550 mg (*Rx*)	*Xifaxan* (Salix)

Indications

Hepatic encephalopathy (550 mg): For reduction in risk of overt hepatic encephalopathy recurrence in patients 18 years of age and older.

Rifaximin has not been studied in patients with Model for End-Stage Liver Disease (MELD) scores greater than 25, and only 8.6% of patients in the controlled trial had MELD scores over 19. There is increased systemic exposure in patients with more severe hepatic dysfunction.

Traveler's diarrhea (200 mg): For the treatment of patients 12 years of age and older with traveler's diarrhea caused by noninvasive strains of *Escherichia coli.*

Do not use rifaximin tablets in patients with diarrhea complicated by fever or blood in the stool or diarrhea due to pathogens other than *E. coli.*

Administration and Dosage

Adults:

Hepatic encephalopathy – 550 mg 2 times a day.

Traveler's diarrhea – 200 mg 3 times a day for 3 days.

Children:

Traveler's diarrhea –

12 years of age and older: 200 mg 3 times a day for 3 days.

Administration: Rifaximin tablets can be administered orally with or without food.

Actions

Pharmacology: Rifaximin is a nonaminoglycoside semisynthetic antibacterial derived from rifamycin SV. Rifaximin acts by binding to the beta-subunit of bacterial DNA-dependent RNA polymerase, resulting in inhibition of bacterial RNA synthesis.

For hepatic encephalopathy, rifaximin is thought to have an effect on the GI flora.

Pharmacokinetics:

Absorption –

Hepatic encephalopathy: After a single dose and multiple doses of rifaximin 550 mg in healthy subjects, the mean time to reach peak plasma concentrations was approximately 1 hour. When pharmacokinetic parameters were analyzed based on Child-Pugh class A, B, and C, the mean area under the curve (AUC_{tau}) was 10-, 13-, and 20-fold higher, respectively, compared with healthy subjects.

Traveler's diarrhea: Rifaximin plasma concentrations and exposures were low and variable. There was no evidence of accumulation of rifaximin following repeated administration for 3 days.

Distribution – Rifaximin is moderately bound (67.5%) to human plasma proteins.

Metabolism/Excretion – Absorbed rifaximin undergoes metabolism with minimal renal excretion of the unchanged drug. The enzymes responsible for metabolizing rifaximin are unknown.

Contraindications

Hypersensitivity to rifaximin, any of the rifamycin antimicrobial agents, or any of the components of rifaximin.

Warnings/Precautions

Traveler's diarrhea not caused by E. coli: Rifaximin tablets were not found to be effective in patients with diarrhea complicated by fever and/or blood in the stool or diarrhea due to pathogens other than *E. coli.*

Clostridium difficile–associated diarrhea: *C. difficile*–associated diarrhea has been reported with use of nearly all antibacterial agents, including rifaximin, and may range in severity from mild diarrhea to fatal colitis.

Resistance: Prescribing rifaximin for traveler's diarrhea in the absence of a proven or strongly suspected bacterial infection or a prophylactic indication is unlikely to provide benefit to the patient and increases the risk of development of drug-resistant bacteria.

Hypersensitivity reactions: Hypersensitivity reactions have included exfoliative dermatitis, angioneurotic edema, and anaphylaxis.

Hepatic function impairment: The systemic exposure of rifaximin was approximately 10-, 13-, and 20-fold higher in those patients with mild (Child-Pugh class A), moderate (Child-Pugh class B), and severe (Child-Pugh class C) hepatic impairment. No dosage adjustment is recommended because rifaximin is presumably acting locally. Exercise caution when rifaximin is administered to patients with severe hepatic impairment.

Pregnancy: Category C.

Lactation: It is not known whether rifaximin is excreted in human milk. Because many drugs are excreted in human milk and because of the potential for adverse reactions in breast-feeding infants from rifaximin, decide whether to discontinue breast-feeding or the drug, taking into account the importance of the drug to the mother.

Children: The safety and efficacy of rifaximin 200 mg in children with traveler's diarrhea younger than 12 years of age have not been established.

The safety and effectiveness of rifaximin 550 mg for hepatic encephalopathy have not been established in patients younger than 18 years of age.

Drug Interactions

None known.

Adverse Reactions

Abdominal distension, abdominal pain, abdominal pain upper, anemia, arthralgia, ascites, back pain, constipation, cough, defecation urgency, depression, dizziness, dyspnea, edema peripheral, fatigue, flatulence, headache, insomnia, muscle spasms, nasopharyngitis, nausea, pruritus, pyrexia, rash, rectal tenesmus.

NYSTATIN, ORAL

Tablets: 500,000 units (*Rx*)	Various, *Nystatin* (Major), *Mycostatin* (Apothecon)

Indications

Nonesophageal membrane GI candidiasis: Treatment of nonesophageal membrane GI candidiasis.

Administration and Dosage

500,000 to 1,000,000 units 3 times daily. Continue treatment for at least 48 hours after clinical cure to prevent relapse.

Actions

Pharmacology: A polyene antibiotic with antifungal activity. Nystatin probably acts by binding to sterols in the cell membrane of the fungus, with a resultant change in membrane permeability allowing leakage of intracellular components.

Pharmacokinetics: Sparingly absorbed after oral use.

Contraindications

Hypersensitivity to nystatin.

Adverse Reactions

Nystatin is virtually nontoxic and nonsensitizing and is well tolerated by all age groups including debilitated infants, even on prolonged administration.

MICONAZOLE

Tablet: 50 mg (*Rx*)	*Oravig* (Strativa Pharmaceuticals)

Indications

Oropharyngeal candidiasis: For the local treatment of oropharyngeal candidiasis in adults.

Administration and Dosage

Adults:

Oropharyngeal candidiasis – 50 mg (1 tablet) to the upper gum region (canine fossa) once daily for 14 days.

Children:

Oropharyngeal candidiasis –

16 years of age and older: See Adults for dosing.

Administration: Apply typically to the gum in the morning with dry hands, after brushing the teeth. Do not crush, chew, or swallow the tablet. Place the rounded side surface of the tablet against the upper gum just above the incisor tooth (canine fossa) and hold in place with slight pressure over the upper lip for 30 seconds to ensure adhesion. The tablet is round on one side for comfort, but either side of the tablet can be applied to the gum. Food and drink can be taken normally when the tablet is in place, but chewing gum should be avoided.

Subsequent applications should be made to alternate sides of the mouth. Before applying the next tablet, the patient should clear away any remaining tablet material.

If the tablet does not adhere or falls off within the first 6 hours, the same tablet should be repositioned immediately. If the tablet still does not adhere, a new tablet should be placed.

If the tablet is swallowed within the first 6 hours, the patient should drink a glass of water and a new tablet should be applied only once.

If the tablet falls off or is swallowed after it was in place for 6 hours or more, a new tablet should not be applied until the next regularly scheduled dose.

Actions

Pharmacology: Miconazole is an antifungal drug and inhibits the enzyme cytochrome P450 14-alpha-demethylase, which leads to inhibition of ergosterol synthesis, an essential component of the fungal cell membrane. Miconazole also affects the synthesis of triglycerides and fatty acids and inhibits oxidative and peroxidative enzymes, increasing the amount of reactive oxygen species within the cell.

Pharmacokinetics:

Absorption/Distribution –

Miconazole Pharmacokinetic Parameters in Saliva (N = 18)[a]	
Salivary pharmacokinetic parameters	Mean ± SD (min to max)
$AUC_{0\text{-}24h}$ (mcg•h/mL)	55.2 ± 35.1 (0.5 to 128.3)
C_{max} (mcg/mL)	15.1 ± 16.2 (0.5 to 64.8)
T_{max} (hour)	7[b] (2 to 24.1)

In healthy volunteers, the duration of buccal adhesion was on average 15 hours following a single dose application.

Metabolism/Excretion – Most of the absorbed miconazole is metabolized by the liver, with less than 1% of the administered dose found unchanged in urine. In healthy volunteers, the terminal half-life is 24 hours following systemic administration. There are no active metabolites of miconazole.

Contraindications

Known hypersensitivity (eg, anaphylaxis) to miconazole, milk protein concentrate, or any other component of the product.

Warnings/Precautions

Hypersensitivity reactions: Allergic reactions, including anaphylactic reactions and hypersensitivity, have been reported with the administration of miconazole products, including the buccal tablets. Discontinue miconazole immediately at the first sign of hypersensitivity.

Hepatic function impairment: Administer miconazole with caution in patients with hepatic impairment.

Pregnancy: Category C.

Lactation: It is not known whether this drug is excreted in human milk.

Children: Safety and effectiveness of miconazole in children younger than 16 years of age have not been established. The ability of children to comply with the application instructions has not been evaluated. Use in younger children is not recommended because of the potential risk of choking.

Monitoring: Monitor patients with a history of hypersensitivity to azoles.

Drug Interactions

Drugs that may interact with miconazole include phenytoin, glyburide, and warfarin.

Adverse Reactions

Adverse reactions occurring in at least 3% of patients include headache, diarrhea, nausea, vomiting, general disorders and administration-site conditions, infections and infestations, dysgeusia, and abdominal pain upper.

KETOCONAZOLE

Tablets: 200 mg (*Rx*)	Various

Warning:

Ketoconazole has been associated with hepatic toxicity, including some fatalities. Closely monitor patients and inform them of the risk.

Indications

Systemic fungal infections: Candidiasis, chronic mucocutaneous candidiasis, oral thrush, candiduria, blastomycosis, coccidioidomycosis, histoplasmosis, chromomycosis, and paracoccidioidomycosis.

Treatment of severe recalcitrant cutaneous dermatophyte infections not responding to topical therapy or oral griseofulvin or in patients unable to take griseofulvin.

Do not use ketoconazole for fungal meningitis because it penetrates poorly into the CSF.

Administration and Dosage

If antacids, anticholinergics, or H_2 blockers are needed, give at least 2 hours after administration. Take with food to alleviate GI disturbance.

Adults: Initially, 200 mg once daily. In very serious infections, or if clinical response is insufficient, increase dose to 400 mg once daily.

Children:

(Older than 2 years of age) – 3.3 to 6.6 mg/kg/day as a single daily dose.

(Younger than 2 years of age) – Daily dosage has not been established.

Minimum treatment is 1 or 2 weeks for candidiasis and 6 months for the other indicated systemic mycoses. Chronic mucocutaneous candidiasis usually requires maintenance therapy.

Minimum treatment of recalcitrant dermatophyte infections is 4 weeks in cases involving glabrous skin. Palmar and plantar infections may respond more slowly.

Actions

Pharmacology: Ketoconazole, an imidazole broad-spectrum antifungal agent, impairs the synthesis of ergosterol, the main sterol of fungal cell membranes, allowing increased permeability and leakage of cellular components.

Pharmacokinetics:

Absorption/Distribution – Bioavailability depends on an acidic pH for dissolution and absorption. In vitro, plasma protein binding is approximately 95% to 99%, mainly to albumin.

Metabolism/Excretion – The drug undergoes extensive hepatic metabolism to inactive metabolites. Plasma elimination is biphasic; half-life is 2 hours during the first 10 hours, and 8 hours thereafter. The major excretory route is enterohepatic. From 85% to 90% is excreted in bile and feces and 13% in urine.

Contraindications

Hypersensitivity to ketoconazole. Do not use ketoconazole for the treatment of fungal meningitis because it penetrates poorly into the CSF. Concomitant administration of ketoconazole with oral triazolam is contraindicated.

Warnings/Precautions

Hepatotoxicity: Hepatotoxicity, primarily of the hepatocellular type, has been associated with ketoconazole, including rare fatalities. Measure liver function before starting treatment and frequently during treatment. Monitor patients receiving ketoconazole concurrently with other potentially hepatotoxic drugs, particularly those patients requiring prolonged therapy or those with a history of liver disease. Transient minor elevations in liver enzymes have occurred.

Prostatic cancer: In clinical trials involving 350 patients with metastatic prostatic cancer, 11 deaths were reported within 2 weeks of starting high-dose ketoconazole (1200 mg/day). It is not known whether death was related to therapy. High ketoconazole doses are known to suppress adrenal corticosteroid secretion.

Hormone levels: Testosterone levels are impaired with doses of 800 mg/day and abolished by 1600 mg/day. It also decreases ACTH-induced corticosteroid serum levels at similar high doses.

Gastric acidity: Ketoconazole requires acidity for dissolution and absorption. In achlorhydria, dissolve each tablet in 4 mL aqueous solution of 0.2 N hydrochloride. Use a glass or plastic straw to avoid contact with teeth. Follow with a glass of water.

Hypersensitivity reactions: Anaphylaxis occurs rarely after the first dose. Hypersensitivity reactions, including urticaria, have been reported.

Pregnancy: Category C.

Lactation: Ketoconazole is excreted in breast milk. Administer to nursing mothers only if the potential benefits outweigh the potential risks to the infant.

Children: Safety for use in children younger than 2 years of age has not been established.

Drug Interactions

Ketoconazole is a potent inhibitor of the cytochrome P450 3A4 enzyme system. Coadministration of ketoconazole with other drugs metabolized by the same enzyme system may result in increased plasma concentrations of the drugs that could increase or prolong both therapeutic and adverse effects. Unless otherwise specified, dosage adjustment may be necessary.

Drugs that may affect ketoconazole include antacids, didanosine, histamine H_2 antagonists, isoniazid, sucralfate, proton pump inhibitors, and rifampin. Drugs that may be affected by ketoconazole include oral anticoagulants, corticosteroids, cyclosporine, protease inhibitors, tricyclic antidepressants, carbamazepine, quinidine, sulfonylureas, benzodiazepines, buspirone, oral contraceptives, donepezil, nisoldipine, tacrolimus, vinca alkaloids, zolpidem, and theophylline.

Adverse Reactions

Adverse reactions occurring in at least 3% of patients include nausea and vomiting.

AMPHOTERICIN B

Powder for injection: 50 mg (as desoxycholate) (*Rx*)	Various
Injection, suspension: 5 mg/mL (as lipid complex) (*Rx*)	*Abelcet* (Enzon)
Injection, lyophilized, powder for solution: 50 mg and 100 mg (as cholesteryl) (*Rx*)	*Amphotec* (Three Rivers Pharmaceuticals)
Injection, lyophilized, powder for suspension: 50 mg (*Rx*)	*AmBisome* (Astellas)

Warning:

Use primarily for treatment of patients with progressive and potentially fatal fungal infections. Do not use to treat noninvasive forms of fungal disease such as oral thrush, vaginal candidiasis, and esophageal candidiasis in patients with normal neutrophil counts.

Indications

Fungal infections, systemic:

Amphotericin B deoxycholate – Intended to treat the following potentially life-threatening invasive fungal infections: Aspergillosis; cryptococcosis (torulosis); North American blastomycosis; candidiasis; coccidioidomycosis; histoplasmosis; zygomycosis including mucormycosis caused by *Mucor*, *Rhizopus*, and *Absidia* sp.; infections caused by related susceptible species of *Conidiobolus* and *Basidiobolus*; sporotrichosis.

Lipid-based formulations – For use in patients refractory to conventional amphotericin B deoxycholate therapy or where renal impairment or unacceptable toxicity precludes the use of the deoxycholate formulation for the treatment of invasive fungal infections (lipid complex); for the treatment of invasive aspergillosis (cholesteryl); for the treatment of infections caused by *Aspergillus*, *Candida*, or *Cryptococcus* sp. (liposomal).

Fungal infections, empirical: For empirical treatment in febrile, neutropenic patients with presumed fungal infection (liposomal only).

Cryptococcal meningitis in HIV: Treatment of cryptococcal meningitis in HIV-infected patients (*AmBisome* only).

Leishmaniasis: For treatment of visceral leishmaniasis (liposomal only); treatment of American mucocutaneous leishmaniasis, but not as primary therapy (deoxycholate).

Unlabeled uses: Prophylaxis for fungal infection in patients with bone marrow transplantation (0.1 mg/kg/day).

Administration and Dosage

Amphotericin B cholesteryl (Amphotec):

Adults and children –

Aspergillosis, invasive: 3 to 4 mg/kg intravenously (IV) as required once a day.

A test dose is advisable (eg, 10 mL of final preparation containing between 1.6 to 8.3 mg infused over 15 to 30 min). The recommended dose is 3 to 4 mg/kg/day prepared as a 0.6 mg/mL (range, 0.16 to 0.83 mg/mL) infusion delivered at a rate of 1 mg/kg/h. Do not use an in-line filter.

Creatinine clearance of less than 10 mL/min – 3 to 6 mg/kg every 24 to 36 hours.

Amphotericin B lipid complex (Abelcet):

Fungal infections, systemic – The recommended dose is 5 mg/kg/day prepared as a 1 mg/mL infusion and delivered at a rate of 2.5 mg/kg/h. For children and patients with cardiovascular disease, the drug may be diluted to a final concentration of 2 mg/mL. If the infusion exceeds 2 hours, mix the contents by shaking the infusion bag every 2 hours. Do not use an in-line filter. Use with caution in patients with reduced renal function.

Amphotericin B liposome (AmBisome):

Cryptococcal meningitis in HIV – Administer 6 mg/kg/day.

Fungal infection, empirical – Administer 3 mg/kg/day.

Fungal infection, systemic – The recommended dose is 3 to 5 mg/kg/day.

Visceral leishmaniasis – Administer 3 mg/kg/day on days 1 through 5, 14, and 21 to immunocompetent patients; a repeat course of therapy may be useful if parasitic clearance is not achieved. Administer 4 mg/kg/day on days 1 through 5, 10, 17, 24, 31, and 38 to immunocompromised patients; seek expert advice regarding further therapy if parasitic clearance is not achieved or if relapse is experienced.

Dilution and administration – Prepare as a 1 to 2 mg/mL infusion. Lower infusion concentrations of 0.2 to 0.5 mg/mL may be appropriate for infants and small children to provide sufficient volume for infusion. Use a controlled infusion device over approximately 120 minutes; infusion time may be reduced to 60 minutes if well tolerated or increased if patient experiences discomfort. An in-line membrane filter of 1 micron or more mean pore diameter may be used.

Amphotericin B desoxycholate:

Life-threatening fungal infections – Maximum dose is 1.5 mg/kg/day. Overdoses can result in cardiorespiratory arrest. A single IV test dose (1 mg in 20 mL of dextrose 5% solution) administered over 20 to 30 minutes may be preferred. The patient's temperature, pulse, respiration, and blood pressure should be recorded every 30 minutes for 2 to 4 hours. In patients with good cardio-renal function and a well-tolerated test dose, therapy is usually initiated with a daily dose of 0.25 mg/kg of body weight. However, in those patients having severe and rapidly progressive fungal infection, therapy may be initiated with a daily dose of 0.3 mg/kg of body weight. In patients with impaired cardio-renal function or a severe reaction to the test dose, therapy should be initiated with smaller daily doses (ie, 5 to 10 mg). Depending on the patient's cardio-renal status, doses may gradually be increased by 5 to 10 mg/day to final daily dosage of 0.5 to 0.7 mg/kg. Total daily dosage may range up to 1 mg/kg/day or up to 1.5 mg/kg when given on alternate days. Whenever medication is interrupted for a period of more than 7 days, therapy should be resumed by starting with the lowest dosage level (eg, 0.25 mg/kg of body weight) and increased gradually.

Aspergillosis: Aspergillosis has been treated with amphotericin B IV for a period of up to 11 months, with a total dose of up to 3.6 g.

Rhinocerebral phycomycosis: A cumulative dose of at least amphotericin B 3 g is recommended. Although a total dose of 3 to 4 g will infrequently cause lasting renal impairment, this would seem a reasonable minimum where there is clinical evidence of invasion of deep tissue.

Sporotrichosis: Therapy with IV amphotericin B for sporotrichosis has ranged up to 9 months, with a total dose of up to 2.5 g.

Renal function impairment – In some patients, hydration and sodium repletion prior to amphotericin B administration may reduce the risk of developing nephrotoxicity.

For patients with creatinine clearance of less than 10 mL/min, the dosage should be 0.5 to 0.7 mg/kg every 24 to 48 hours.

Adults receiving continuous renal replacement therapy: A dosage of 0.5 to 1 mg/kg IV every 24 hours is recommended for patients receiving continuous venovenous hemofiltration, continuous venovenous hemodialysis, or continuous venovenous hemodialfiltration. This recommendation assumes ultrafiltration and dialysis flow rates of 1 to 2 L/h.

Adults receiving intermittent hemodialysis: 0.5 to 1 mg/kg IV every 24 hours administered after the dialysis session. This recommendation assumes the patient is receiving standard intermittent hemodialysis 3 times per week and completes the full dialysis sessions.

Unlabeled:

Amphotericin B cholesteryl –

Fungal infections, systemic (eg, Aspergillus sp, Candida sp, Cryptococcus sp) in patients intolerant of or refractory to conventional amphotericin B:

Children and adolescents – Usual dosage is 3 to 6 mg/kg/day. Maximum dose is 6 mg/kg/day. However, dosages as high as 7.5 mg/kg/day have been used.

Premature neonates – Usual dosage is 3 mg/kg/day on day 1, then 5 mg/kg/day thereafter. Maximum dose is 6 mg/kg/day. However, dosages as high as 7.5 mg/kg/day have been used.

Amphotericin B lipid complex –

Febrile neutropenia, empirical therapy:

Children 2 to 16 years of age – Usual dosage is 5 mg/kg/day. Maximum dose is 5 mg/kg/day. However, dosages as high as 6.5 to 13 mg/kg/day have been given.

Fungal infections, systemic therapy (Aspergillus sp, Candida sp, Cryptococcus sp):

Infants and children 2 to 17 years of age – Usual dosage is 2.5 to 5 mg/kg/day. Maximum dose is 5 mg/kg/day. However, dosages as high as 6.5 to 13 mg/kg/day have been given.

Neonates – Usual dosage is 2.5 to 5 mg/kg/day. One study administered up to 6.5 mg/kg/day. Maximum dose is 5 mg/kg/day. However, dosages as high as 6.5 to 13 mg/kg/day have been given.

Visceral leishmaniasis (refractory or intolerant to conventional amphotericin B):

Children – 1 to 3 mg/kg/day for 5 days.

Amphotericin B liposome –

Fungal infection, systemic:

Infants/Children/Adolescents – Usual dosage is 3 to 5 mg/kg/day. Dosages as high as 15 mg/kg/day have been used. Dosages as high as 10 mg/kg/day have been used in patients with *Aspergillus*.

Neonates (term and preterm) – 3 to 5 mg/kg/day. Dosages as high as 7 mg/kg/day have been reported.

Solid bone marrow transplant, prophylaxis and treatment:

Children and adolescents – 2 to 6 mg/kg/day IV over a mean of 25 days (range, 5 to 90 days). In hematopoietic stem cell transplant, 10 mg/kg/day once weekly may be useful for prophylaxis against fungal infections.

Visceral leishmaniasis:

Immunocompetent patients (children and adolescents) – 4 mg/kg IV on days 1 to 5 and on day 10. Mediterranean visceral leishmaniasis has been treated with 20 mg/kg administered as 4 mg/kg for 5 days or 10 mg/kg for 2 days.

Amphotericin B desoxycholate –

Bladder irrigation for candidal cystitis:

Continuous irrigation – Concentrations of 10 and 50 mg/L administered into the bladder continuously over 24 to 48 hours in patients with indwelling catheters. In one study, amphotericin B was administered into the bladder at a rate of 42 mL/h.

Intermittent irrigation – Doses of 20 to 40 mg or 5 to 200 mg/L administered into the bladder (and retained there for 90 minutes) every 8 hours for 3 days have been used.

Ocular aspergillosis:

Intraocular – 5 to 10 mcg per injection administered intaviterally or intracamerally, repeated in cases of ongoing infection at intervals of approximately 1 week after resolution of any local inflammatory response from the previous injection. The recommended volume for each injection is 0.1 mL.

Topical – Amphotericin B 0.15% to 0.2% drops applied topically every 30 to 60 minutes until symptoms resolve. Therapy usually continues for days to weeks.

Actions

Pharmacology: Amphotericin B is fungistatic or fungicidal, depending on the concentration obtained in body fluids and on the susceptibility of the fungus. It acts by binding to sterols in the fungal cell membrane with a resultant change in membrane permeability, allowing leakage of a variety of intracellular components.

Liposomal encapsulation or incorporation in a lipid complex can substantially affect a drug's functional properties relative to those of the unencapsulated or nonlipid-associated drug. Lipid-based formulations increase the circulation time and alter the biodistribution of associated amphotericin. Increasing drug levels at site of action and reducing levels in normal tissues offers 2 distinct clinical advantages: an increased therapeutic index and altered toxicity profile relative to free drug.

Different lipid-based formulations with a common active ingredient may vary from one another in the chemical composition (eg, phospholipid and cholesterol content) and physical form of the lipid component (eg, sphere, disc, ribbon). Such differences may affect functional properties of these drug products.

Pharmacokinetics:

Absorption/Distribution – Amphotericin B is highly protein bound (greater than 90%) and is poorly dialyzable.

Metabolism/Excretion – Amphotericin B has a relatively short initial serum half-life of 24 hours, followed by a second elimination phase with a half-life of approximately 15 days. The drug is slowly excreted by the kidneys, with 2% to 5% as the biologically active form.

The following table presents pharmacokinetic parameters at steady-state for lipid-based formulations of amphotericin B; the assay used to measure serum levels did not distinguish between free and complex amphotericin B.

Pharmacokinetic Parameters of Lipid-Based Amphotericin B Formulations[a]						
Parameter	*AmBisome* 1 mg/kg/day (n = 7)	*AmBisome* 2.5 mg/kg/day (n = 7)	*AmBisome* 5 mg/kg/day (n = 9)	*Amphotec* 3 mg/kg/day (predicted)[b]	*Amphotec* 4 mg/kg/day (predicted)[b]	*Abelcet* 5 mg/kg/day (n = varied)[c]
C_{max} (mcg/mL)	≈ 12.2	≈ 31.4	≈ 83	2.6	2.9	≈ 1.7
AUC (mcg/mL•h)	≈ 60	≈ 197	≈ 555	29	36	≈ 14
half—life (h)	≈ 7	≈ 6.3	≈ 6.8	27.5 (100 to 153)[d]	28.2 (100 to 153)[d]	≈ 173.4
Vss (L/kg)	≈ 0.14	≈ 0.16	≈ 0.1	3.8	4.1	≈ 131
CL (mL/h/kg)	≈ 17	≈ 22	≈ 11	105	112	≈ 436

[a] Data are pooled from separate studies and are not necessarily comparable; C_{max} = maximal plasma concentration; AUC = area under the curve; CL = confidence limit.

[b] Values based on the population model developed from 51 bone marrow transplant patients with systemic fungal infections given *Amphotec* 0.5 to 8 mg/kg/day.

[c] Data obtained from various studies in patients with mucocutaneous leishmaniasis or cancer with presumed or proven fungal infections.

[d] Based on total amphotericin B levels measured within a 24-hour dosing interval (or up to 49 days after dosing).

Contraindications

Hypersensitivity to amphotericin B, unless the condition requiring treatment is life-threatening and amenable only to amphotericin B therapy.

Warnings/Precautions

Fatal fungal diseases: Amphotericin B is frequently the only effective treatment for potentially fatal fungal diseases. Balance its possible lifesaving effect against its dangerous side effects.

Nephrotoxicity: Renal damage is a limiting factor for the use of amphotericin B. Renal dysfunction usually improves upon interruption of therapy, dose reduction, or increased dosing interval; however, some permanent impairment often occurs, especially in patients receiving large doses (greater than 5 g) or receiving other nephrotoxic agents. Decreased glomerular filtration rate and renal blood flow, increased serum creatinine, and renal tubular dysfunction are prominent. In some patients, hydration and sodium repletion prior to amphotericin B administration may reduce the risk of developing nephrotoxicity.

Lipid formulations of amphotericin B have been shown to reduce the severe kidney toxicity of amphotericin B and are indicated in patients with renal impairment or when unacceptable toxicity precludes the use of amphotericin B deoxycholate in effective doses.

Infusion reactions: Acute reactions including fever, shaking chills, hypotension, anorexia, vomiting, nausea, headache, and tachypnea are common 1 to 3 hours after starting an IV infusion. These reactions usually are more severe with the first few doses of amphotericin B and usually diminish with subsequent doses. Avoid rapid IV infusion because it has been associated with hypotension, hypokalemia, arrhythmias, bronchospasm, and shock.

Leukocyte transfusions: Since acute pulmonary reactions have been reported in patients given amphotericin B during or shortly after leukocyte transfusions, it is advisable to temporarily separate these infusions as far as possible and to monitor pulmonary function.

Leukoencephalopathy: This has been reported following use of amphotericin B. The literature has suggested that total body irradiation may be a predisposition.

Therapy interruption: Whenever medication is interrupted for more than 7 days, resume therapy with the lowest dosage level; increase gradually.

Hypersensitivity reactions: Anaphylaxis has been reported with amphotericin B. If severe respiratory distress occurs, discontinue the infusion immediately. Do not give further infusions. Have cardiopulmonary resuscitation facilities available during administration.

Renal function impairment: Amphotericin B should be used with care in patients with reduced renal function; frequent monitoring of renal function is recommended. In some patients, hydration and sodium repletion prior to amphotericin B administration may reduce the risk of developing nephrotoxicity. Supplemental alkali medication may decrease renal tubular acidosis complications.

Pregnancy: *Category B.*

Lactation: It is not known whether amphotericin B is excreted in breast milk; however, consider discontinuing breast-feeding.

Children: Safety and efficacy of amphotericin B desoxycholate in children have not been established. Systemic fungal infections have been successfully treated in children without reports of unusual side effects. Limit administration to the least amount compatible with an effective therapeutic regimen.

Children younger than 16 years of age (n = 97) with systemic fungal infections have been treated with amphotericin B cholesteryl at daily mg/kg doses similar to those given in adults and had significantly less renal toxicity than the desoxycholate formulation (12% vs 52%); 273 children 1 month to 16 years of age with presumed fungal infections, confirmed systemic fungal infections, or with visceral leishmaniasis have been successfully treated with liposomal amphotericin B (*AmBisome*); 111 children younger than 16 years of age, including 11 patients younger than 1 year of age, have been treated with amphotericin B lipid complex (*Abelcet*) at 5 mg/kg/day, and 5 children with hepatosplenic candidiasis were effectively treated with 2.5 mg/kg/day. Safety and efficacy in patients younger than 1 month of age have not been established.

Lab test abnormalities:

Serum electrolyte abnormalities – Hypomagnesemia, hyperkalemia, hypokalemia, hypercalcemia, hypocalcemia, hypophosphatemia.

Liver function test abnormalities – Increased AST, ALT, GGT, bilirubin, alkaline phosphatase, and LDH.

Renal function impairment – Increased BUN and serum creatinine.

Other test abnormalities – Acidosis, hyperamylasemia, hypoglycemia, hyperglycemia, hyperuricemia.

Monitoring: Monitor renal function frequently during amphotericin B therapy. It is also advisable to monitor liver function, serum electrolytes (particularly magnesium and potassium), blood counts, and hemoglobin concentrations on a regular basis. Use laboratory test results as a guide to subsequent dose adjustments. Monitor complete blood count and prothrombin time as medically indicated.

Record the patient's temperature, pulse, respiration, and blood pressure every 30 minutes for 2 to 4 hours after administration.

Drug Interactions

Drugs that may interact with amphotericin B include antineoplastic agents, azole antifungal agents, corticosteroids, cyclosporine, digitalis glycosides, flucytosine, foscarnet, leukocyte transfusions, other nephrotoxic agents, skeletal muscle relaxants, thiazides, and zidovudine.

Adverse Reactions

Adverse reactions may include abdominal pain; acidosis; anemia; anorexia; anxiety; apnea; asthenia; asthma; arrhythmias; azotemia; bilirubinemia; blood product transfusion reaction; chest/back pain; coagulation disorder; confusion; cough increased; cramping; decreased prothrombin time; depression; diarrhea; dizziness; dry mouth; dyspepsia; dyspnea; edema; epigastric pain; epistaxis; eye hemorrhage; face edema; fever (sometimes with shaking chills); generalized pain, including muscle and joint pains; GI hemorrhage; headache; heart arrest; hematemesis; hematuria; hemoptysis; hemorrhage; hypernatremia; hypertension; hyperventilation; hypokalemia; hypovolemia; hyposthenuria; hypotension; hypoxia; increased serum creatinine; infection; insomnia; jaundice; leukopenia; lung disorder; maculopapular rash; malaise; mucous membrane disorder; multiple organ failure; nausea; normochromic, normocytic anemia; pain; peripheral edema; pleural effusion; pneumonia; pruritus; rash; renal tubular acidosis and nephrocalcinosis; respiratory disorder; respiratory failure; rhinitis; sepsis; somnolence; stomatitis; sweating; tachycardia; tachypnea; thinking abnormal; thrombocytopenia; tremor; vomiting; venous pain at the injection site with phlebitis and thrombophlebitis; weight loss/gain.

Prevention of adverse reactions: Most patients will exhibit some intolerance, often at less than full therapeutic dosage. Severe reactions may be lessened by giving aspirin, antipyretics (eg, acetaminophen), antihistamines, and antiemetics before the infusion and by maintaining sodium balance. Administration on alternate days may decrease anorexia and phlebitis. Small doses of IV adrenal corticosteroids given prior to or during the infusion may decrease febrile reactions. Meperidine (25 to 50 mg IV) has been shown in some patients to decrease the duration of shaking chills and fever that may accompany infusion of amphotericin B.

VORICONAZOLE

Tablets: 50 and 200 mg (*Rx*) — *Vfend* (Roerig)
Powder for oral suspension: 45 g (40 mg/mL after reconstitution) (*Rx*)
Powder for injection, lyophilized: 200 mg (*Rx*)

Indications

Candidemia: For the treatment of candidemia in nonneutropenic patients and the following *Candida* infections: disseminated infections in skin and infections in abdomen, kidney, bladder wall, and wounds.

Esophageal candidiasis: For the treatment of esophageal candidiasis.

Invasive aspergillosis: For the treatment of invasive aspergillosis. In clinical trials, the majority of isolates recovered were *Aspergillus fumigatus*. There were a small number of cases of culture-proven disease caused by species of *Aspergillus* other than *A. fumigatus*.

Serious fungal infections: For the treatment of serious fungal infections caused by *Scedosporium apiospermum* (asexual form of *Pseudallescheria boydii*) and *Fusarium* sp. including *Fusarium solani*, in patients intolerant of, or refractory to, other therapy.

Administration and Dosage

Correct electrolyte disturbances (eg, hypokalemia, hypomagnesemia, hypocalcemia) prior to initiation of voriconazole therapy.

Use in adults:

Candidemia in nonneutropenic patients and other deep tissue Candida infections – See the following table. Patients should be treated for at least 14 days following resolution of symptoms or following last positive culture, whichever is longer.

Esophageal candidiasis – See the following table. Patients should be treated for a minimum of 14 days and for at least 7 days following resolution of symptoms.

Invasive aspergillosis and serious fungal infections caused by Fusarium spp. and S. apiospermum – For the treatment of adults with invasive aspergillosis and infections caused by *Fusarium* spp. and *S. apiospermum*, therapy must be initiated with the specified loading dose regimen of IV voriconazole to achieve plasma concentrations on day 1 that are close to steady state. On the basis of high oral bioavailability, switching between IV and oral administration is appropriate when clinically indicated. Once the patient can tolerate medication given by mouth, the oral tablet form or oral suspension form of voriconazole may be utilized.

The recommended dosing regimen of voriconazole is as follows:

Voriconazole Recommended Dosing Regimen

	Loading dosage	Maintenance dosage
Infection	IV	IV
Candidemia in nonneutropenic patients and other deep tissue *Candida* infections	6 mg/kg every 12 h for the first 24 h	3 to 4 mg/kg every 12 h[a]
Esophageal candidiasis	[b]	[b]
Invasive aspergillosis	6 mg/kg every 12 h for the first 24 h	4 mg/kg every 12 h
Scedosporiosis and fusariosis	6 mg/kg every 12 h for the first 24 h	4 mg/kg every 12 h

[a] In clinical trials, patients with candidemia received 3 mg/kg every 12 hours as primary therapy, while patients with other deep tissue *Candida* infections received 4 mg/kg as salvage therapy. Base appropriate dosage on the severity and nature of the infection.
[b] Not evaluated in patients with esophageal candidiasis.

Dosage adjustment – If patients are unable to tolerate 4 mg/kg IV, reduce the IV maintenance dosage to 3 mg/kg every 12 hours.

Coadministration with phenytoin: Phenytoin may be coadministered with voriconazole if the IV maintenance dosage of voriconazole is increased to 5 mg/kg every 12 hours.

Hepatic function impairment: No dose adjustment is necessary in patients with liver function tests less than or equal to 5 times the upper limit of normal. Continued monitoring of liver function tests for further elevations is recommended (see Warnings).

It is recommended that the standard loading dose regimens be used but that the maintenance dose be halved in patients with mild to moderate hepatic cirrhosis (Child-Pugh class A and B).

Renal function impairment: In patients with moderate or severe renal insufficiency (CrCl below 50 mL/min), accumulation of the IV vehicle, SBECD, occurs. Administer oral voriconazole to these patients, unless an assessment of the benefit/risk to the patient justifies the use of IV voriconazole. Closely monitor serum creatinine levels in these patients, and, if increases occur, consider changing to oral voriconazole therapy.

IV administration: Voriconazole IV for injection requires reconstitution to 10 mg/mL and subsequent dilution to 5 mg/mL or less prior to administration as an infusion. Infuse at a maximum rate of 3 mg/kg/h over 1 to 2 hours. Not for IV bolus injection.

Oral administration: Take voriconazole tablets or oral suspension at least 1 hour before or 1 hour following a meal.

Instructions for use – Shake the closed bottle of reconstituted suspension for approximately 10 seconds before each use. Administer the reconstituted oral suspension only using the oral dispenser supplied with each pack.

Actions

Pharmacology: Voriconazole is a triazole antifungal agent. The primary mode of action of voriconazole is the inhibition of fungal cytochrome P450-mediated 14 alpha-lanosterol demethylation, an essential step in fungal ergosterol biosynthesis. The accumulation of 14 alpha-methyl sterols correlates with the subsequent loss of ergosterol in the fungal cell wall and may be responsible for the antifungal activity of voriconazole. Voriconazole has been shown to be more selective for fungal cytochrome P450 enzymes than for various mammalian cytochrome P450 enzyme systems.

Pharmacokinetics:

Absorption – The pharmacokinetic properties of voriconazole are similar following administration by the IV and oral routes. The oral bioavailability of voriconazole is estimated to be 96% (CV 13%). Bioequivalence was established between the 200 mg tablet and the 40 mg/mL oral suspension when administered as a 400 mg loading dose every 12 hours followed by a 200 mg maintenance dose every 12 hours. Maximum plasma concentration (C_{max}) is achieved 1 to 2 hours after dosing.

The pharmacokinetics of voriconazole are nonlinear because of the saturation of its metabolism. The interindividual variability of voriconazole pharmacokinetics is high.

Steady-state trough plasma concentrations with voriconazole are achieved after approximately 5 days of oral or IV dosing without a loading dose regimen. However, when an IV loading dose regimen is used, steady-state trough plasma concentrations are achieved within 1 day.

Distribution – The volume of distribution at steady state for voriconazole is estimated to be 4.6 L/kg, suggesting extensive distribution into tissues. Plasma protein binding is estimated to be 58% and was shown to be independent of plasma concentrations achieved following single and multiple oral doses. Varying degrees of hepatic and renal insufficiency do not affect the protein binding of voriconazole.

Metabolism – In vitro studies showed that voriconazole is metabolized by the human hepatic cytochrome P450 enzymes CYP2C19, CYP2C9, and CYP3A4.

Excretion – Voriconazole is eliminated via hepatic metabolism with less than 2% of the dose excreted unchanged in the urine.

Special populations –

Race: CYP2C19 exhibits genetic polymorphism. For Caucasians and Blacks, the prevalence of poor metabolizers is 3% to 5%. Studies conducted in healthy Caucasian and Japanese subjects have shown that poor metabolizers have, on average, a 4-fold higher voriconazole exposure (AUC) than their homozygous extensive metabolizer counterparts. Subjects who are heterozygous extensive metabolizers have, on average, a 2-fold higher voriconazole exposure than their homozygous extensive metabolizer counterparts.

Renal function impairment: A pharmacokinetic study in subjects with renal failure undergoing hemodialysis showed that voriconazole is dialyzed with clearance of 121 mL/min. The IV vehicle, SBECD, is hemodialyzed with clearance of 55 mL/min. A 4-hour hemodialysis session does not remove a sufficient amount of voriconazole to warrant dose adjustment.

Microbiology: Voriconazole has demonstrated in vitro activity against *Aspergillus* sp. (*A. fumigatus*, *A. flavus*, *A. niger*, *A. terreus*), *Candida* sp. (*C. albicans*, *C. glabrata*, *C. krusei*), *Scedosporium apiospermum*, and *Fusarium* sp., including *F. solani.*

Cross-resistance – Fungal isolates exhibiting reduced susceptibility to fluconazole or itraconazole also may show reduced susceptibility to voriconazole, suggesting that cross-resistance can occur among these azoles.

Contraindications

Known hypersensitivity to voriconazole or its excipients. Use caution when prescribing voriconazole to patients with hypersensitivity to other azoles.

Coadministration of the CYP3A4 substrates, cisapride, pimozide, or quinidine with voriconazole is contraindicated because increased plasma concentrations of these drugs can lead to QT prolongation and rare occurrences of torsades de pointes.

Coadministration of voriconazole with sirolimus, rifampin, carbamazepine, long-acting barbiturates, rifabutin, ergot alkaloids (ergotamine and dihydroergotamine), ritonavir (400 mg every 12 hours), or efavirenz.

Warnings/Precautions

Visual disturbances: If treatment continues beyond 28 days, the effect of voriconazole on visual function is not known. If treatment continues beyond 28 days, monitor visual function including visual acuity, visual field, and color perception.

Hepatic toxicity: There have been uncommon cases of serious hepatic reactions during treatment with voriconazole (eg, clinical hepatitis, cholestasis, and fulminant hepatic failure, including fatalities). Liver dysfunction usually has been reversible on discontinuation of therapy.

Evaluate liver function tests at the start of and during the course of voriconazole therapy. Monitor patients who develop abnormal liver function tests during voriconazole therapy for the development of more severe hepatic injury. Discontinuation of voriconazole must be considered if clinical signs and symptoms consistent with liver disease develop that may be attributable to voriconazole.

Hepatic function impairment: It is recommended that the standard loading dose regimens be used but that the maintenance dose be halved in patients with mild to moderate hepatic cirrhosis (Child-Pugh class A and B) receiving voriconazole.

Renal function impairment: In patients with moderate to severe renal dysfunction (CrCl below 50 mL/min), accumulation of the IV vehicle, SBECD, occurs.

Galactose intolerance: Voriconazole tablets contain lactose and should not be given to patients with rare hereditary problems of galactose intolerance, Lapp lactase deficiency, or glucose-galactose malabsorption.

Arrhythmias and QT prolongation: Some azoles, including voriconazole, have been associated with prolongation of the QT interval on the electrocardiogram.

Infusion-related reactions: Anaphylactoid-type reactions, including flushing, fever, sweating, tachycardia, chest tightness, dyspnea, faintness, nausea, pruritus, and rash, have occurred uncommonly. Symptoms appeared immediately upon initiating the infusion.

Renal toxicity: Acute renal failure has been observed in severely ill patients undergoing treatment with voriconazole.

Dermatological reactions: Patients have rarely developed serious cutaneous reactions, such as Stevens-Johnson syndrome, during treatment with voriconazole.

Photosensitivity: Voriconazole has been infrequently associated with photosensitivity skin reaction, especially during long-term therapy. It is recommended that patients avoid strong, direct sunlight during voriconazole therapy.

Pregnancy: Category D.

Lactation: Voriconazole should not be used by nursing mothers unless the benefit clearly outweighs the risk.

Children: Safety and effectiveness in pediatric patients younger than 12 years of age have not been established.

Monitoring: Patient management should include laboratory evaluation of renal (particularly serum creatinine) and hepatic function (particularly liver function tests and bilirubin).

Drug Interactions

CYP450: Voriconazole is metabolized by CYP2C19, CYP2C9, and CYP3A4. The affinity of voriconazole is highest for CYP2C19, followed by CYP2C9, and is appreciably lower for CYP3A4. Inhibitors or inducers of these 3 enzymes may increase or decrease voriconazole systemic exposure (plasma concentrations), respectively.

Voriconazole inhibits the metabolic activity of CYP2C19, CYP2C9, and CYP3A4. The inhibition potency of voriconazole for CYP3A4 was significantly less than that of 2 other azoles, ketoconazole and itraconazole. The major metabolite of voriconazole, the voriconazole N-oxide, inhibits the metabolic activity of CYP2C9 and CYP3A4 to a greater extent than that of CYP2C19. There is potential for voriconazole and its major metabolite to increase the systemic exposure (plasma concentration) of other drugs metabolized by these CYP450 enzymes.

Drugs that affect voriconazole include the following: barbiturates (long acting), cimetidine, nonnucleoside reverse transcriptase inhibitors (NNRIs), phenytoin, protease inhibitors, proton pump inhibitors, rifampin, rifabutin.

Drugs affected by voriconazole include the following: benzodiazepines, calcium channel blockers, cisapride, coumarin anticoagulants, cyclosporine, ergot alkaloids, HMG-CoA reductase inhibitors, NNRTIs, phenytoin, protease inhibitors, pimozide, proton pump inhibitors, quinidine, prednisolone, rifabutin, sirolimus, sulfonylureas, tacrolimus, vinca alkaloids.

Adverse Reactions

The most frequently reported adverse events (all causalities) in the therapeutic trials were visual disturbances, fever, rash, vomiting, nausea, diarrhea, headache, sepsis, peripheral edema, abdominal pain, and respiratory disorder. The treatment-related adverse events that most often led to discontinuation of voriconazole therapy were elevated liver function tests, rash, and visual disturbances.

Adverse reactions occurring in at least 3% of patients included the following: abnormal vision, alkaline phosphatase increased, ALT/AST increased, chills, fever, hallucinations, headache, hepatic enzymes increased, liver function test abnormal, nausea, peripheral edema, photophobia, rash, vomiting.

POSACONAZOLE

Suspension, oral: 40 mg/mL (*Rx*)	*Noxafil* (Schering Corporation)

Indications

Oropharyngeal candidiasis: For the treatment of oropharyngeal candidiasis, including oropharyngeal candidiasis refractory to itraconazole and/or fluconazole.

Prophylaxis of invasive fungal infection: Prophylaxis of invasive *Aspergillus* and *Candida* infections in patients 13 years of age and older who are at high risk of developing these infections because of being severely immunocompromised, such as hematopoietic stem cell transplant (HSCT) recipients with graft-versus-host disease (GVHD) or patients with hematologic malignancies with prolonged neutropenia from chemotherapy.

Administration and Dosage

Dosage:

Posaconazole Dosing	
Indication	Dose and duration of therapy
Prophylaxis of invasive fungal infections	200 mg (5 mL) 3 times daily. The duration of therapy is based on recovery from neutropenia or immunosuppression.
Oropharyngeal candidiasis	Loading dose of 100 mg (2.5 mL) twice daily on the first day, then 100 mg (2.5 mL) once daily for 13 days.
Oropharyngeal candidiasis refractory to itraconazole and/or fluconazole	400 mg (10 mL) twice daily. Duration of therapy should be based on the severity of the patient's underlying disease and clinical response.

Actions

Pharmacology: Posaconazole is a triazole antifungal agent. It blocks the synthesis of ergosterol, a key component of the fungal cell membrane, through the inhibition of the enzyme lanosterol 14α-demethylase and accumulation of methylated sterol precursors.

Pharmacokinetics:

Absorption – Posaconazole is absorbed with a medium time to reach maximum drug concentration (T_{max}) of approximately 3 to 5 hours. Steady-state plasma concentrations are attained at 7 to 10 days following multiple-dose administration.

In order to ensure attainment of adequate plasma concentrations, administering posaconazole with food or a nutritional supplement is recommended.

Distribution – Posaconazole has an apparent volume of distribution of 1,774 L, suggesting extensive extravascular distribution and penetration into the body tissues. Posaconazole is highly protein bound (greater than 98%), predominantly to albumin.

Metabolism – Of the circulating metabolites, the majority are glucuronide conjugates formed via uridine diphosphate glucuronidation.

Excretion – Posaconazole is eliminated with a mean half-life of 35 hours (range, 20 to 66 hours). Posaconazole is predominantly eliminated in the feces, with the major component eliminated as parent drug.

Contraindications

Hypersensitivity to the active substance or to any of the excipients; coadministration with ergot alkaloids; coadministration with the CYP3A4 substrates terfenadine, astemizole, cisapride, pimozide, halofantrine, or quinidine because this may result in increased plasma concentrations of the drugs, leading to QTc prolongation and rare occurrence of torsades de pointes.

Warnings/Precautions

Hepatic toxicity: In clinical trials, there were infrequent cases of hepatic reactions (eg, mild to moderate elevations in ALT, AST, alkaline phosphatase, total bilirubin, and/or clinical hepatitis). The elevations in liver function tests were generally reversible upon discontinuation of therapy and, in some instances, these tests normalized without drug interruption and rarely required drug discontinuation.

Cardiac effects: Administer posaconazole with caution to patients with potentially proarrhythmic conditions; do not administer with drugs that are known to prolong the QTc interval and are metabolized through CYP3A4. Make rigorous attempts to correct potassium, magnesium, and calcium before starting posaconazole.

Hypersensitivity reactions: Use caution when prescribing posaconazole to patients with hypersensitivity to other azoles.

Pregnancy: Category C.

Lactation: Posaconazole is excreted in the milk of lactating rats. The excretion of posaconazole in human breast milk has not been investigated. Do not prescribe posaconazole to breast-feeding mothers unless the benefit clearly outweighs the potential risk to the infant.

Children: Safety and efficacy of posaconazole in children younger than 13 years of age have not been established.

Monitoring: Evaluate liver function tests at the start of and during the course of posaconazole therapy. Monitor for the development of more severe hepatic injury in patients who develop abnormal liver function tests during posaconazole therapy.

Closely monitor for breakthrough fungal infections in patients who have severe diarrhea or vomiting.

Make rigorous attempts to correct potassium, magnesium, and calcium before starting posaconazole therapy.

Closely monitor patients with severe renal function impairment for breakthrough invasive fungal infection.

Generally avoid coadministration of drugs that can decrease the plasma concentrations of posaconazole unless the benefit outweighs the risk. If such drugs are necessary, closely monitor patients for breakthrough fungal infections.

Drug Interactions

Drugs that may affect posaconazole include cimetidine, phenytoin, and rifabutin.

Drugs that may be affected by posaconazole include phenytoin, rifabutin, benzodiazepines, calcium channel blockers, CYP3A4 substrates, ergot alkaloids, HMG-CoA reductase inhibitors, immunosuppressants, and vinca alkaloids.

Adverse Reactions

Adverse reactions occurring in more than 10% of patients include abdominal pain, ALT increased, anemia, anorexia, anxiety, arthralgia, AST increased, back pain, bacteremia, bilirubinemia, constipation, coughing, cytomegalovirus, diarrhea, dizziness, dyspepsia, dyspnea, edema, epistaxis, fatigue, febrile neutropenia, fever, headache, hepatic enzymes increased, herpes simplex, hyperglycemia, hypertension, hypocalcemia, hypokalemia, hypomagnesemia, hypotension, insomnia, mucositis, musculoskeletal pain, nausea, neutropenia, petechiae, pharyngitis, pneumonia, pruritus, QT/QTc prolongation, rash, rigors, tachycardia, thrombocytopenia, upper respiratory tract infection, vaginal hemorrhage, vomiting, and weakness.

FLUCONAZOLE

Tablets: 50, 100, 150, and 200 mg (*Rx*)	Various, *Diflucan* (Roerig)
Powder for oral suspension: 10 and 40 mg/mL when reconstituted (*Rx*)	
Injection: 2 mg/mL (*Rx*)	

Indications

Candidiasis: Oropharyngeal and esophageal candidiasis.

Candidal urinary tract infections, peritonitis, and systemic candidal infections including candidemia, disseminated candidiasis and pneumonia.

Cryptococcal meningitis: Treatment of cryptococcal meningitis.

Prophylaxis: To decrease the incidence of candidiasis in patients undergoing bone marrow transplantation who receive cytotoxic chemotherapy or radiation therapy.

Vaginal candidiasis: Vaginal candidiasis (vaginal yeast infections caused by *Candida*).

Administration and Dosage

Single dose:

Vaginal candidiasis – 150 mg as a single oral dose.

Multiple dose: The daily dose of fluconazole is the same for oral and IV administration. In general, a loading dose of twice the daily dose is recommended on the first day of therapy to result in plasma levels close to steady state by the second day of therapy.

Patients with AIDS and cryptococcal meningitis or recurrent oropharyngeal candidiasis usually require maintenance therapy to prevent relapse.

Adults –

Oropharyngeal candidiasis: 200 mg on the first day, followed by 100 mg once daily. Continue treatment for at least 2 weeks to decrease the likelihood of relapse.

Esophageal candidiasis: 200 mg on the first day, followed by 100 mg once daily. Doses up to 400 mg/day may be used, based on the patient's response. Treat patients with esophageal candidiasis for a minimum of 3 weeks and for at least 2 weeks following resolution of symptoms.

Candidiasis, other: For candidal UTIs and peritonitis, 50 to 200 mg/day has been used. For systemic candidal infections (including candidemia, disseminated candidiasis, and pneumonia), optimal dosage and duration have not been determined, although doses up to 400 mg/day have been used.

Prevention of candidiasis in bone marrow transplant: 400 mg once daily. In patients who are anticipated to have severe granulocytopenia (less than 500 neutrophils/mm^3), start fluconazole prophylaxis several days before the anticipated onset of neutropenia, and continue for 7 days after the neutrophil count rises above 1000 cells/mm^3.

Cryptococcal meningitis: 400 mg on the first day, followed by 200 mg once daily. A dosage of 400 mg once daily may be used, based on the patient's response to therapy. The duration of treatment for initial therapy of cryptococcal meningitis is 10 to 12 weeks after the cerebrospinal fluid becomes culture negative. The dosage of fluconazole for suppression of relapse of cryptococcal meningitis in patients with AIDS is 200 mg once daily.

Children –

Fluconazole Dosage in Children

Pediatric Patients	Adults
3 mg/kg	100 mg
6 mg/kg	200 mg
12 mg/kg[a]	400 mg

[a] Some older children may have clearances similar to that of adults. Absolute doses greater than 600 mg/day are not recommended.

Neonates: Based on the prolonged half-life seen in premature newborns (gestational age 26 to 29 weeks), these children, in the first 2 weeks of life, should receive the same dosage (mg/kg) as older children, but administered every 72 hours. After the first 2 weeks, dose neonates once daily.

Oropharyngeal candidiasis: The recommended dosage is 6 mg/kg on the first day, followed by 3 mg/kg once daily. Administer treatment for at least 2 weeks.

Esophageal candidiasis: The recommended dosage is 6 mg/kg on the first day followed by 3 mg/kg once daily. Doses up to 12 mg/kg/day may be used based on medical judgment of the patient's response to therapy. Treat patients with esophageal candidiasis for a minimum of 3 weeks and for at least 2 weeks following the resolution of symptoms.

Systemic Candida infections: For the treatment of candidemia and disseminated *Candida* infections, daily doses of 6 to 12 mg/kg/day have been used.

Cryptococcal meningitis: The recommended dosage is 12 mg/kg on the first day, followed by 6 mg/kg once daily. A dosage of 12 mg/kg once daily may be used. The recommended duration of treatment for initial therapy of cryptococcal meningitis is 10 to 12 weeks after the CSF becomes culture negative. For suppression of relapse of cryptococcal meningitis in children with AIDS, the recommended dose is 6 mg/kg once daily.

Renal function impairment: There is no need to adjust single dose therapy for vaginal candidiasis in patients with impaired renal function. In patients with impaired renal function who will receive multiple doses, give an initial loading dose of 50 to 400 mg. After the loading dose, base the daily dose on the following table:

Fluconazole Dose in Impaired Renal Function	
CrCl (mL/min)	Percent of recommended dose
> 50	100%
≤ 50	50%
Patients receiving regular hemodialysis	One recommended dose after each dialysis

Injection: Fluconazole injection has been used safely for up to 14 days of IV therapy. Administer the IV infusion of fluconazole at a maximum rate of approximately 200 mg/h, given as a continuous infusion. Fluconazole injections are intended only for IV administration.

Actions

Pharmacology: Fluconazole, a synthetic broad spectrum bis-triazole antifungal agent, is a highly selective inhibitor of fungal cytochrome P450 and sterol C-14 alpha-demethylation.

Pharmacokinetics:

Absorption/Distribution – The pharmacokinetic properties of fluconazole are similar following administration by the IV or oral routes. In healthy volunteers, the bioavailability of oral fluconazole is more than 90% compared with IV administration.

Peak plasma concentrations (C_{max}) in fasted healthy volunteers occur between 1 and 2 hours with a terminal plasma elimination half-life of approximately 30 hours (range, 20 to 50 hours) after oral administration.

Steady-state concentrations are reached within 5 to 10 days following oral doses of 50 to 400 mg given once daily. The apparent volume of distribution approximates that of total body water. Plasma protein binding is low (11% to 12%).

Metabolism/Excretion – Fluconazole is cleared primarily by renal excretion, with approximately 80% of the dose appearing in the urine unchanged, approximately 11% as metabolites. The dose may need to be reduced in patients with impaired renal function. A 3-hour hemodialysis session decreases plasma concentrations by approximately 50%.

Contraindications

Hypersensitivity to fluconazole or to any excipients in the product. There is no information regarding cross-hypersensitivity between fluconazole and other azole antifungal agents; use with caution in patients with hypersensitivity to other azoles.

Warnings/Precautions

Hepatic injury: Fluconazole has been associated with rare cases of serious hepatic toxicity. Instances of fatal hepatic reactions occurred primarily in patients with serious underlying medical conditions (predominantly AIDS or malignancy) and often while taking multiple concomitant medications.

Anaphylaxis: In rare cases, anaphylaxis has occurred.

Dermatologic changes: Patients have rarely developed exfoliative skin disorders during treatment with fluconazole.

Vaginal candidiasis: Weigh the convenience and efficacy of the single-dose regimen for treatment of vaginal yeast infections against the acceptability of a higher incidence of adverse reactions with fluconazole (26%) vs intravaginal agents (16%).

Pregnancy: Category C.

Lactation: The use of fluconazole in nursing mothers is not recommended.

Children: Efficacy has not been established in children younger than 6 months of age, although a small number of patients ranging from day 1 to 6 months of age have been treated safely with fluconazole.

Drug Interactions

Fluconazole is an inhibitor of the cytochrome P450 3A4 and 2C9 enzyme systems. Coadministration of fluconazole with other drugs metabolized by the same enzyme system may result in increased plasma concentrations of the drugs, which could increase or prolong therapeutic and adverse effects. Unless otherwise specified, dosage adjustment may be necessary.

Drugs that may affect fluconazole include cimetidine, hydrochlorothiazide, and rifampin. Drugs that may be affected by fluconazole include alfentanil, benzodiazepines, buspirone, carbamazepine, cisapride, oral contraceptives, corticosteroids, cyclosporine, haloperidol, HMG-CoA reductase inhibitors, losartan, nisoldipine, phenytoin, protease inhibitors, rifabutin, sirolimus, sulfonylureas, tacrolimus, theophylline, tolterodine, tricyclic antidepressants, vinca alkaloids, warfarin, zidovudine, and zolpidem.

Adverse Reactions

Adverse reactions occurring in at least 3% of patients include headache, nausea, abdominal pain, and diarrhea.

ITRACONAZOLE

Capsules; oral: 100 mg (*Rx*)	Various, *Sporanox* (Janssen-Ortho)
Solution; oral: 10 mg/mL (*Rx*)	*Sporanox* (Ortho Biotech)

Warning:

CHF: Do not administer itraconazole for the treatment of onychomycosis in patients with evidence of ventricular dysfunction, such as CHF or a history of CHF. Discontinue if signs and symptoms of CHF occur during treatment. If signs and symptoms of CHF occur during treatment, reassess the continued use of itraconazole. When itraconazole was administered IV to dogs and healthy human volunteers, negative inotropic effects were seen.

Drug interactions: Coadministration of cisapride, pimozide, dofetilide, or quinidine with itraconazole is contraindicated. Itraconazole is a potent inhibitor of the cytochrome P450 3A4 isoenzyme system and may raise plasma concentrations of drugs metabolized by this pathway. Serious cardiovascular events, including QT prolongation, torsades de pointes, ventricular tachycardia, cardiac arrest, and/or sudden death have occurred in patients taking itraconazole concomitantly with cisapride, pimozide, or quinidine, which are inhibitors of the cytochrome P450 3A4 system.

Indications

Aspergillosis (capsules): Treatment of pulmonary and extrapulmonary aspergillosis in nonimmunocompromised or immunocompromised patients who are intolerant of or who are refractory to amphotericin B therapy.

Blastomycosis (capsules): Treatment of pulmonary and extrapulmonary blastomycosis in nonimmunocompromised or immunocompromised patients.

Febrile neutropenia, empiric (oral solution): For empiric therapy of febrile neutropenic (ETFN) patients with suspected fungal infections.

Histoplasmosis (capsules): Treatment of histoplasmosis, including chronic cavitary pulmonary disease and disseminated, nonmeningeal histoplasmosis in nonimmunocompromised or immunocompromised patients.

Onychomycosis (capsules only): Treatment of onychomycosis of the toenail with or without fingernail involvement and onychomycosis of the fingernail because of dermatophytes (*Tinea unguium*) in nonimmunocompromised patients.

Oropharyngeal/esophageal candidiasis (oral solution only): Treatment of oropharyngeal or esophageal candidiasis.

Administration and Dosage

When itraconazole therapy may be indicated, isolate and identify the type of organism responsible for the infection; however, therapy may be initiated prior to obtaining these results when clinically warranted.

Do not use capsules and oral solution interchangeably.

Capsules: Take with a full meal to ensure maximal absorption.

Aspergillosis – A daily dose of 200 to 400 mg is recommended.

Blastomycosis/histoplasmosis – 200 mg once daily. If there is no obvious improvement or there is evidence of progressive fungal disease, increase the dose in 100 mg increments to a maximum of 400 mg/day. Give doses above 200 mg/day in 2 divided doses.

Life-threatening situations – Although clinical studies did not provide for a loading dose, it is recommended, based on pharmacokinetic data, that a loading dose of 200 mg 3 times/day be given for the first 3 days of treatment.

Continue treatment for a minimum of 3 months and until clinical parameters and laboratory tests indicate that the active fungal infection has subsided. An inadequate period of treatment may lead to recurrence of active infection.

Treatment of onychomycosis (fingernails only) – Two treatment pulses, each consisting of 200 mg twice daily for 1 week. The pulses are separated by a 3-week period without itraconazole.

Treatment of onychomycosis (toenails with or without fingernail involvement) – 200 mg/day for 12 weeks.

Oral solution: Take without food, if possible.

Esophageal candidiasis – 100 mg/day for a minimum treatment of 3 weeks. Continue treatment for 2 weeks following resolution of symptoms. Doses up to 200 mg/day may be used based on medical judgment of the patient's response to therapy. Vigorously swish the solution in the mouth (10 mL at a time) for several seconds and swallow.

ETFN patients with suspected fungal infections – After approximately 14 days of IV therapy, continue treatment with oral solution 200 mg twice daily until resolution of clinically significant neutropenia. The safety and efficacy of itraconazole use exceeding 28 days in ETFN is not known.

Oropharyngeal candidiasis – 200 mg/day for 1 to 2 weeks. Vigorously swish the solution in the mouth (10 mL at a time) for several seconds and swallow. For patients with oropharyngeal candidiasis unresponsive/refractory to treatment with fluconazole tablets, the recommended dose of itraconazole is 100 mg twice daily. Expect clinical response in 2 to 4 weeks. Patients may be expected to relapse shortly after discontinuing therapy. Limited data on the safety of long-term use (more than 6 months) of the oral solution are available at this time.

Renal function impairment: Do not use in patients with CrCl below 30 mL/min.

Actions

Pharmacology: Itraconazole is a synthetic triazole antifungal agent. In vitro, itraconazole inhibits the cytochrome P450-dependent synthesis of ergosterol, which is a vital component of fungal cell membranes.

Pharmacokinetics:

Absorption/Distribution –

Oral solution: The oral bioavailability is maximal when itraconazole oral solution is taken without food. Steady state is reached after 1 to 2 weeks during chronic administration. Peak plasma levels are observed 2 hours (fasting) to 5 hours (with food) following oral administration. Steady-state plasma concentrations are approximately 25% lower when the oral solution is taken with food.

Capsules: The oral bioavailability of itraconazole is maximal when itraconazole capsules are taken with a full meal. Peak plasma levels are observed 3.3 hours (fasting) and 4 hours (with food) following capsule administration.

Plasma protein binding is 99.8%. It is extensively distributed into tissues that are prone to fungal invasion. Concentrations in the lung, kidney, liver, bone, stomach, spleen, and muscle were found to be 2 to 3 times higher than the corresponding plasma concentration. Following IV administration, the volume of distribution averaged 796 ± 185 L.

Metabolism/Excretion – Itraconazole is metabolized by the cytochrome P450 3A4 to several metabolites including the major metabolite hydroxyitraconazole. Fecal excretion of the parent drug varies between 3% and 18% of the dose. Renal excretion of the parent drug is less than 0.03% of the dose. Itraconazole is not removed by hemodialysis.

The estimated mean half-life at steady-state of itraconazole after IV infusion was 35.4 hours.

Contraindications

CHF: Do not administer itraconazole capsules for the treatment of onychomycosis or dermatomycoses in patients with evidence of ventricular dysfunction, such as CHF or a history of CHF.

Coadministration of pimozide, quinidine, dofetilide, cisapride, triazolam, or oral midazolam; HMG-CoA reductase inhibitors metabolized by the CYP3A4 enzyme system (eg, lovastatin, simvastatin), ergot alkaloid metabolized by CYP3A4, such as dihydroergotamine, ergotamine, ergonovine, and methylergonovine (see Warning Box and Drug Interactions); hypersensitivity to the drug or its excipients (there is no information regarding cross-hypersensitivity between itraconazole and other azole antifungal agents; use caution in prescribing to patients with hypersensitivity to other azoles).

Warnings/Precautions

Cystic fibrosis: If a patient with cystic fibrosis does not respond to itraconazole oral solution, consider switching to alternative therapy.

HIV infection: Because hypochlorhydria has been reported in HIV-infected patients, the absorption of itraconazole may be decreased in these patients. Administration with a cola beverage has been shown to increase itraconazole absorption in these patients.

Cardiac dysrhythmias: Life-threatening cardiac dysrhythmias or sudden death have occurred in patients using cisapride, pimozide, or quinidine concomitantly with itraconazole or other CYP3A4 inhibitors. Concomitant administration of these drugs with itraconazole is contraindicated.

Cardiac disease: Do not administer itraconazole for the treatment of onychomycosis in patients with evidence of ventricular dysfunction such as CHF or a history of CHF. Do not use itraconazole in patients with evidence of ventricular dysfunction unless the benefit clearly outweighs the risk.

Cases of CHF, peripheral edema, and pulmonary edema have been reported in the postmarketing period among patients being treated for onychomycosis and/or systemic fungal infections.

Hepatotoxicity: Itraconazole has been associated with rare cases of serious hepatotoxicity, including liver failure and death. Some of these cases had neither pre-existing liver disease, nor a serious underlying medical condition. If liver function tests are abnormal, discontinue treatment. In patients with raised liver enzymes or an active liver disease or who have experienced liver toxicity with other drugs, do not start treatment unless the expected benefit exceeds the risk of hepatic injury. In such cases, liver enzyme monitoring is necessary.

Interchangeability: Do not use itraconazole capsules and oral solution interchangeably. Drug exposure is greater with the oral solution than with the capsules when the same dose of drug is given. Additionally, the topical effects of mucosal exposure may be different between the two formulations.

Severely neutropenic patients: Itraconazole oral solution as treatment for oropharyngeal and/or esophageal candidiasis was not investigated in severely neutropenic patients. Because of its pharmacokinetic properties, itraconazole oral solution is not recommended for initiation of treatment in patients at immediate risk of systemic candidiasis.

Neuropathy: Discontinue if neuropathy occurs that may be attributable to itraconazole capsules or oral solution.

Decreased gastric acidity: Under fasted conditions, itraconazole absorption was decreased in the presence of decreased gastric acidity. The absorption of itraconazole may be decreased with coadministration of antacids or gastric acid secretion suppressors. Studies conducted under fasted conditions demonstrated that administration with 8 oz of a cola beverage resulted in increased absorption of itraconazole in AIDS patients with relative or absolute achlorhydria. This increase relative to the effects of a full meal is unknown.

Pregnancy: Category C. During postmarketing experience, cases of congenital abnormalities have been reported.

Women of childbearing potential – Do not administer itraconazole to women of childbearing potential for the treatment of onychomycosis unless they are using effective measures to prevent pregnancy and they begin therapy on the second or third day following the onset of menses. Continue effective contraception throughout itraconazole therapy and for 2 months following the end of treatment.

Lactation: Itraconazole is excreted in breast milk.

Children: Safety and efficacy have not been established. A small number of patients from 3 to 16 years of age have been treated with 100 mg/day for systemic fungal infections and no serious adverse effects have been reported. Itraconazole oral solution was given to 26 pediatric patients 6 months to 12 years of age. Itraconazole was dosed at 5 mg/kg once daily for 2 weeks, and no serious unexpected adverse events were reported.

Elderly: In general, use caution in dose selection for an elderly patient, reflecting the greater frequency of decreased hepatic, renal, or cardiac function, and of concomitant disease or other drug therapy.

Monitoring: Monitor liver function in patients with pre-existing hepatic function abnormalities or those who have experienced liver toxicity with other medications; consider monitoring in all patients. Stop treatment immediately and conduct liver function testing in patients who develop signs and symptoms suggestive of liver dysfunction.

Drug Interactions

Both itraconazole and its major metabolite, hydroxyitraconazole, are inhibitors of the cytochrome P450 3A4 enzyme system. Coadministration of itraconazole and drugs primarily metabolized by the cytochrome P450 3A4 enzyme system may result in increased plasma concentrations of the drugs that could increase or prolong therapeutic and adverse effects.

Drugs that may affect itraconazole include antacids, carbamazepine, didanosine, H_2 antagonists, hydantoins, macrolide antibiotics, nevirapine, phenobarbital, phenytoin, protease inhibitors, proton pump inhibitors, and rifamycins.

Drugs that may be affected by itraconazole include alfentanil, almotriptan, alprazolam, amphotericin B, aripiprazole, benzodiazepines, buspirone, busulfan, calcium blockers, carbamazepine, cilostazol, cisapride, corticosteroids, cyclosporine, digoxin, disopyramide, docetaxel, dofetilide, eletriptan, eplerenone, ergot alkaloids, haloperidol, HMG-CoA reductase inhibitors, hydantoins (phenytoin), hypoglycemic agents, oral midazolam, phosphodiesterase type 5 inhibitors, pimozide, polyenes, protease inhibitors, quinidine, rifamycins, sirolimus, tacrolimus, tolterodine, triazolam, trimetrexate, vinca alkaloids, warfarin, and zolpidem.

Adverse Reactions

Adverse reactions occurring in at least 3% of patients include the following: Nausea, vomiting, diarrhea, rash, hypokalemia, bilirubinemia, increased ALT, headache, pruritus, fever, fatigue, abnormal hepatic function, hypertension, asthenia, abdominal pain, dyspepsia, flatulence, cystitis, urinary tract infection, rhinitis, sinusitis, upper respiratory tract infection, myalgia, injury, anxiety, depression, malaise, constipation, gingivitis, ulcerative stomatitis, bursitis, pain, hypertriglyceridemia, increased serum creatinine, increased sweating, coughing, chest pain.

TERBINAFINE HYDROCHLORIDE

Tablets; oral: 250 mg (*Rx*)	Various, *Lamisil* (Novartis)
Granules; oral: 125 and 187.5 mg per packet (*Rx*)	*Lamisil* (Novartis)

Indications

Onychomycosis (tablets): Treatment of onychomycosis of the toenail or fingernail caused by dermatophytes.

Tinea capitis (oral granules): For the treatment of *T. capitis* in patients 4 years of age and older.

Administration and Dosage

Onychomycosis:

Fingernail – 250 mg/day for 6 weeks.

Toenail – 250 mg/day for 12 weeks.

The optimal clinical effect is seen some months after mycological cure and cessation of treatment. This is related to the period required for outgrowth of healthy nail.

T. capitis: Terbinafine oral granules should be taken once a day for 6 weeks based on body weight.

Terbinafine Oral Granules Dosage by Body Weight	
Body weight (kg)	Dosage
< 25 kg	125 mg/day
25 to 35 kg	187.5 mg/day
> 35 kg	250 mg/day

Administration – Sprinkle contents of each packet on a spoonful of pudding or other soft, nonacidic food, such as mashed potatoes, and swallow the entire spoonful without chewing. Do not use applesauce or fruit-based foods. Take with food.

Actions

Pharmacology: Terbinafine is a synthetic allylamine derivative that exerts its antifungal effect by inhibiting squalene epoxidase, a key enzyme in sterol biosynthesis in fungi. This action results in a deficiency in ergosterol and a corresponding accumulation of squalene within the fungal cell and causes fungal cell death.

Pharmacokinetics: Terbinafine is well absorbed (more than 70%). Bioavailability is approximately 40%. Peak plasma concentrations appear up to 2 hours after a single 250 mg dose. Terbinafine is more than 99% bound to plasma proteins, with a half-life of approximately 36 hours. A terminal half-life of 200 to 400 hours may represent the slow elimination of terbinafine from tissues.

Prior to excretion, terbinafine is extensively metabolized. No metabolites have been identified that have antifungal activity similar to terbinafine. Approximately 70% of the administered dose is eliminated in the urine.

Contraindications

Hypersensitivity to terbinafine or any component of the product.

Warnings/Precautions

Hepatic failure: Rare cases of liver failure, some leading to death or liver transplant, have occurred with the use of terbinafine for the treatment of onychomycosis in individuals with and without pre-existing liver disease.

The severity of hepatic events or their outcome may be worse in patients with active or chronic liver disease. Discontinue treatment with terbinafine if biochemical or clinical evidence of liver injury develops.

Ophthalmic: Changes in the ocular lens and retina have been reported following the use of terbinafine.

Hematologic effects:

Absolute lymphocyte counts – Transient decreases in absolute lymphocyte counts have been observed in controlled clinical trials. In patients with known or suspected immunodeficiency, consider monitoring complete blood cell counts (CBCs) if terbinafine therapy will exceed 6 weeks.

Neutropenia: Isolated cases of severe neutropenia have been reported but were reversible with discontinuation of treatment with or without supportive therapy. If the neutrophil count is 1,000 cells/mm^3 or less, discontinue treatment and start supportive management.

Dermatologic: There have been isolated reports of serious skin reactions (eg, Stevens-Johnson syndrome, toxic epidermal necrolysis).

Systemic lupus erythematosus: Precipitation and exacerbation of cutaneous and systemic lupus erythematosus have been reported infrequently.

Renal/Hepatic function impairment: In patients with renal impairment (creatinine clearance 50 mL/min or less) or chronic or active liver disease, the use of terbinafine is not recommended.

Pregnancy: *Category B.*

Lactation: After oral administration, terbinafine is present in breast milk. Use of terbinafine tablets is not recommended in breast-feeding mothers.

Monitoring:

Immunodeficiency – Monitor CBC in patients receiving treatment for longer than 6 weeks.

Hepatic – Pretreatment serum transaminase (ALT and AST) tests are advised for all patients before taking terbinafine.

Drug Interactions

Drugs that may interact with terbinafine include the following: cimetidine, fluconazole, and rifampin.

Drugs that may be affected by terbinafine include the following: antiarrhythmics class type 1C, beta-blockers, caffeine, cyclosporine, dextromethorphan, monoamine oxidase inhibitors type B, selective reuptake inhibitors, tricyclic antidepressants, and warfarin.

Adverse Reactions

Adverse reactions occurring in at least 3% of patients include the following: cough, diarrhea, dyspepsia, headache, liver enzyme abnormalities, nasopharyngitis, pyrexia, rash, upper abdominal pain, upper respiratory tract infection, and vomiting.

CASPOFUNGIN ACETATE

Injection, lyophilized powder for solution: 50 and 70 mg *Cancidas* (Merck)
(*Rx*)

Indications

Candidemia and other Candida infections: For the treatment of candidemia and the following *Candida* infections: intra-abdominal abscesses, peritonitis, and pleural space infections.

Esophageal candidiasis: For the treatment of esophageal candidiasis.

Fungal infections, empirical: For the treatment of presumed fungal infections in febrile, neutropenic patients.

Invasive aspergillosis: For the treatment of invasive aspergillosis in patients who are refractory to or intolerant of other therapies (ie, amphotericin B, lipid formulations of amphotericin B, itraconazole).

Administration and Dosage

Adults: Administer caspofungin by slow intravenous (IV) infusion over approximately 1 hour.

Candidemia and other Candida infections – Administer a single 70 mg loading dose on day 1, followed by 50 mg/day thereafter. In general, continue antifungal therapy for at least 14 days after the last positive culture.

Esophageal candidiasis – 50 mg/day. Because of the risk of relapse of oropharyngeal candidiasis in patients with HIV infections, consider suppressive oral therapy.

Fungal infections, empirical – Administer a single 70 mg loading dose on day 1, followed by 50 mg/day thereafter. Continue empirical therapy until resolution of neutropenia. Treat patients found to have a fungal infection for a minimum of 14 days; continue treatment for at least 7 days after neutropenia and clinical symptoms are resolved. If the 50 mg dose is well tolerated but does not provide an adequate clinical response, the daily dose can be increased to 70 mg.

Invasive aspergillosis – Administer a single 70 mg loading dose on day 1, followed by 50 mg/day thereafter.

Hepatic function impairment – For patients with moderate hepatic impairment (Child-Pugh score 7 to 9), caspofungin 35 mg/day is recommended. However, where recommended, still administer a 70 mg loading dose on day 1. There is no clinical experience in patients with severe hepatic impairment (Child-Pugh score greater than 9) and in children with any degree of hepatic function impairment.

Children 3 months to 17 years of age: Administer a single 70 mg/m^2 loading dose on day 1, followed by 50 mg/m^2 daily thereafter.

The maximum loading dose and the daily maintenance dose should not exceed 70 mg, regardless of the patient's calculated dose. Calculate the maintenance dose in mg as body surface area (BSA) (m^2 × 50 mg/m^2. Duration of treatment should be individualized to the indication. If the 50 mg/m^2 daily dose is well tolerated but does not provide an adequate clinical response, the daily dose can be increased to 70 mg/m^2 daily (not to exceed 70 mg).

Concomitant medication with inducers of drug clearance: Patients on rifampin should receive caspofungin 70 mg/day. Patients on nevirapine, efavirenz, carbamazepine, dexamethasone, or phenytoin may require an increase in dosage to caspofungin 70 mg/day. When caspofungin is coadministered to children with inducers of drug clearance, such as rifampin, efavirenz, nevirapine, phenytoin, dexamethasone, or carbamazepine, consider a caspofungin dose of 70 mg/m^2 IV infusion daily (not to exceed 70 mg).

Admixture incompatibilities: Do not mix or coinfuse caspofungin with other medications. Do not use diluents containing dextrose.

Actions

Pharmacology: Caspofungin is an echinocandin antifungal drug that inhibits the synthesis of beta (1,3)-D-glucan, an essential component of the cell wall of susceptible *Aspergillus* and *Candida* species.

Pharmacokinetics:

Distribution – Plasma concentrations of caspofungin decline in a polyphasic manner following single 1-hour IV infusions. A short alpha phase occurs immediately postinfusion, followed by a beta phase (half-life, 9 to 11 hours). Distribution, rather than excretion or biotransformation, is the dominant mechanism influencing plasma clearance. Caspofungin is bound extensively to albumin (approximately 97%), and distribution into red blood cells is minimal.

Metabolism – Caspofungin is metabolized slowly by hydrolysis and N-acetylation. Caspofungin also undergoes spontaneous chemical degradation to an open-ring peptide compound, L-747969.

Excretion – Excretion of caspofungin and its metabolites in humans was 35% in feces and 41% in urine. A small amount of caspofungin is excreted unchanged in urine (approximately 1.4% of dose). Renal clearance of parent drug is low (approximately 0.15 mL/min), and total clearance of caspofungin is 12 mL/min.

Special populations –

Renal function impairment: No dosage adjustment is necessary for patients with renal impairment. Caspofungin is not dialyzable, thus supplementary dosing is not required following hemodialysis.

Hepatic function impairment: For adults with moderate hepatic function impairment (Child-Pugh score, 7 to 9), caspofungin 35 mg daily is recommended based on pharmacokinetic data. However, where recommended, still administer a 70 mg loading dose on day 1. There is no clinical experience in adults with severe hepatic function impairment (Child-Pugh score, greater than 9) and in children with any degree of hepatic function impairment.

Contraindications

Hypersensitivity to any component of this product.

Warnings/Precautions

Concomitant use with cyclosporine: Only use caspofungin and cyclosporine concomitantly in patients for whom the potential benefit outweighs the potential risk. Monitor patients who develop abnormal liver function tests during concomitant therapy with cyclosporine, and evaluate the risk/benefit of continuing therapy.

Hepatic effects: Laboratory abnormalities in liver function tests have been seen in healthy volunteers and in adults and children treated with caspofungin. Monitor patients who develop abnormal liver function tests during caspofungin therapy for evidence of worsening hepatic function and evaluate them for the risks/benefits of continuing caspofungin therapy.

Pregnancy: Category C.

Lactation: Caspofungin was found in the milk of lactating, drug-treated rats. It is not known whether caspofungin is excreted in human milk.

Children: The efficacy and safety of caspofungin has not been adequately studied in prospective clinical trials involving neonates and infants younger than 3 months of age.

Elderly: No dose adjustment is recommended for elderly patients; however, greater sensitivity of some older individuals cannot be ruled out.

Monitoring: Monitor patients who develop abnormal liver function tests during concomitant therapy with cyclosporine, and evaluate the risk/benefit of continuing therapy.

Drug Interactions

Drugs that may interact with caspofungin include cyclosporine, inducers of drug clearance or mixed inducers/inhibitors, and tacrolimus.

Adverse Reactions

Adverse reactions occurring in at least 3% of adults include abdominal pain, anemia, chills, cough, diarrhea, edema peripheral, fever, headache, hypokalemia, nausea, phlebitis, pleural effusion, pneumonia, rales, rash, respiratory failure, septic shock, vascular disorders, and vomiting. Increases have occurred in ALT, AST, blood glucose, blood urea, direct serum bilirubin, serum alkaline phosphatase, serum creatinine, total serum bilirubin, urine red blood cell counts, and urine white blood cell (WBC) counts. Decreases have occurred in blood magnesium, hematocrit, hemoglobin, neutrophils, platelet count, WBC count, serum albumin, serum potassium, and total serum protein.

Adverse reactions occurring in at least 3% of children include abdominal pain, ALT increased, AST increased, back pain, blood potassium decreased, chills, cough, diarrhea, edema, erythema, headache, hypertension, hypokalemia, hypotension, immune system disorders, infections and infestations, investigations, mucosal inflammation, nausea, pruritus, pyrexia, rash, respiratory distress, tachycardia, vascular disorders, and vomiting.

MICAFUNGIN SODIUM

Powder for injection: 50 and 100 mg (*Rx*)	*Mycamine* (Astellas Pharma)

Indications

For the treatment of patients with esophageal candidiasis, prophylaxis of *Candida* infections in patients undergoing hematopoietic stem cell transplantation (HSCT), and for the treatment of patients with candidemia, acute disseminated candidiasis, *Candida* peritonitis, and abscesses.

Administration and Dosage

Micafungin Dosage	
Indication	Recommended dose
Treatment of candidemia, acute disseminated candidiasis, *Candida* peritonitis, and abscesses[a]	100 mg/day
Treatment of esophageal candidiasis[b]	150 mg/day
Prophylaxis of *Candida* infections in HSCT recipients[c]	50 mg/day

[a] In patients treated successfully for candidemia and other *Candida* infections, the mean duration of treatment was 15 days (range, 10 to 47 days).
[b] In patients treated successfully for esophageal candidiasis, the mean duration of treatment was 15 days (range, 10 to 30 days).
[c] In HSCT recipients who experienced success of prophylactic therapy, the mean duration of prophylaxis was 19 days (range, 6 to 51 days).

Administration: Administer micafungin by intravenous (IV) infusion over a period of 1 hour. More rapid infusions may result in more frequent histamine-mediated reactions.

Note: Flush an existing IV line with 0.9% sodium chloride injection prior to infusion of micafungin.

Admixture incompatibility: Do not mix or coinfuse micafungin with other medications. Micafungin has been shown to precipitate when mixed directly with a number of other commonly used medications.

Actions

Pharmacology: Micafungin is a semisynthetic lipopeptide (echinocandin) synthesized by a chemical modification of a fermentation product of *Coleophoma empetri* F-11899. Micafungin inhibits the synthesis of 1,3-β-D-glucan, an essential component of fungal cell walls, which is not present in mammalian cells.

Pharmacokinetics:

Absorption/Distribution –

Pharmacokinetic Parameters of Micafungin in Adult Patients						
			Pharmacokinetic parameters (Mean ± SD[a])			
Population	n	Dose	C_{max} (mcg/mL)	AUC_{0-24} (mcg•h/mL)	$t_{1/2}$ (h)	Cl (mL/min/kg)
Patients with candidemia or other *Candida* infections: steady state	20	100 mg	10.1 ± 4.4	97 ± 29	13.4 ± 2	0.298 ± 0.115
HIV-positive patients with EC[b] (day 14 or 21)	20	50 mg	5.1 ± 1	54 ± 13	15.6 ± 2.8	0.3 ± 0.063
	20	100 mg	10.1 ± 2.6	115 ± 25	16.9 ± 4.4	0.301 ± 0.086
	14	150 mg	16.4 ± 6.5	167 ± 40	15.2 ± 2.2	0.297 ± 0.081
HSCT recipients (day 7)	8	3 mg/kg	21.1 ± 2.84	234 ± 34	14 ± 1.4	0.214 ± 0.031
	10	4 mg/kg	29.2 ± 6.2	339 ± 72	14.2 ± 3.2	0.204 ± 0.036
	8	6 mg/kg	38.4 ± 6.9	479 ± 157	14.9 ± 2.6	0.224 ± 0.064
	8	8 mg/kg	60.8 ± 26.9	663 ± 212	17.2 ± 2.3	0.223 ± 0.081

[a] SD = standard deviation.
[b] EC = esophageal candidiasis.

The mean ± SD volume of distribution of micafungin at terminal phase was 0.39 ± 0.11 L/kg body weight when determined in adults with esophageal candidiasis at the dose range of 50 to 150 mg.

Micafungin is highly (more than 99%) protein bound in vitro, independent of plasma concentrations over the range of 10 to 100 mcg/mL. The primary binding protein is albumin; however, micafungin, at therapeutically relevant concentrations does not competitively displace bilirubin binding to albumin. Micafungin also binds to a lesser extent to $alpha_1$-acid-glycoprotein.

Metabolism – Micafungin is metabolized to M-1 (catechol form) by arylsulfatase, with further metabolism to M-2 (methoxy form) by catechol-O-methyltransferase. M-5 is formed by hydroxylation at the side chain (ω-1 position) of micafungin catalyzed by cytochrome P(CYP)-450 isozymes. Even though micafungin is a substrate for, and a weak inhibitor of, CYP3A in vitro, hydroxylation by CYP3A is not a major pathway for micafungin metabolism in vivo. Micafungin is neither a P-glycoprotein substrate nor an inhibitor in vitro.

Excretion – At 28 days after administration, mean urinary and fecal recovery of total radioactivity accounted for 82.5% (76.4 to 87.9%) of the administered dose. Fecal excretion is the major route of elimination (total radioactivity at 28 days was 71% of the administered dose).

Contraindications

Hypersensitivity to any component of this product.

Warnings/Precautions

Hematological effects: Isolated cases of significant hemolysis and hemolytic anemia have also been reported in patients treated with micafungin.

Hepatic effects: Laboratory abnormalities in liver function tests have been seen in healthy volunteers and patients treated with micafungin.

Renal effects: Elevations in serum urea nitrogen (BUN) and creatinine and isolated cases of significant renal dysfunction or acute renal failure have been reported in patients who received micafungin.

Hypersensitivity reactions: Isolated cases of serious hypersensitivity (anaphylaxis and anaphylactoid) reactions (including shock) have been reported in patients receiving micafungin. If these reactions occur, discontinue micafungin infusion and administer appropriate treatment.

Pregnancy: Category C.

Lactation: It is not known whether micafungin is excreted in human milk.

Monitoring: Monitor patients who develop abnormal liver function tests during micafungin therapy for evidence of worsening hepatic function, and evaluate them for the risk/benefit of continuing micafungin therapy. Closely monitor patients who develop clinical or laboratory evidence of hemolysis or hemolytic anemia during micafungin therapy for evidence of worsening of these conditions, and evaluate them for the risk/benefit of continuing micafungin therapy.

Drug Interactions

Micafungin may interact with cyclosporine, itraconazole, nifedipine, and sirolimus.

Adverse Reactions

Possible histamine-mediated symptoms have been reported with micafungin, including facial swelling, pruritus, rash, and vasodilation.

Injection-site reactions, including phlebitis and thrombophlebitis, have been reported at micafungin dosages of 50 to 150 mg/day. These reactions tended to occur more often in patients receiving micafungin via peripheral IV administration.

Delirium and rash were the most common drug-related adverse reactions resulting in micafungin discontinuation.

ANIDULAFUNGIN

Powder for injection, lyophilized: 50 and 100 mg (*Rx*) *Eraxis* (Roerig)

Indications

Candidemia and other Candida infections: For the treatment of candidemia and other forms of *Candida* infections (intra-abdominal abscess and peritonitis).

Esophageal candidiasis: For the treatment of esophageal candidiasis.

Administration and Dosage

Candidemia and other Candida infections: The recommended dosage is a single 200 mg loading dose on day 1, followed by 100 mg/day thereafter. Duration of treatment should be based on the patient's clinical response. In general, continue antifungal therapy for at least 14 days after the last positive culture.

Esophageal candidiasis: The recommended dosage is a single 100 mg loading dose on day 1, followed by 50 mg/day thereafter. Treat patients for a minimum of 14 days and for at least 7 days following resolution of symptoms. Duration of treatment should be based on the patient's clinical response.

Compatibilities/Incompatibilities: Prior to administration, anidulafungin for injection requires reconstitution with the companion diluent (20% [w/w] dehydrated alcohol in water for injection) and subsequent dilution with 5% dextrose injection or 0.9% sodium chloride injection (normal saline). Do not dilute with other solutions or co-infuse with other medications or electrolytes.

Actions

Pharmacology: Anidulafungin inhibits glucan synthase, an enzyme present in fungal, but not mammalian, cells. This results in inhibition of the formation of 1,3-β-D-glucan, an essential component of the fungal cell wall.

Pharmacokinetics:

Absorption – Systemic exposures of anidulafungin are dose-proportional.

Distribution – Characterized by a short distribution half-life (0.5 to 1 hour) and a volume of distribution of 30 to 50 L that is similar to total body fluid volume. Anidulafungin is extensively bound to plasma proteins in humans (99%).

Metabolism – Anidulafungin undergoes slow chemical degradation. The in vitro degradation half-life of anidulafungin under physiologic conditions is about 24 hours.

Excretion – The clearance of anidulafungin is about 1 L/hour, and anidulafungin has a terminal half-life of 40 to 50 hours.

Contraindications

Known hypersensitivity to anidulafungin, any component of anidulafungin, or other echinocandins.

Warnings/Precautions

Hepatic effects: Laboratory abnormalities in liver function tests (LFTs) have been seen in patients treated with anidulafungin. Monitor patients who develop abnormal LFTs during anidulafungin therapy for evidence of worsening hepatic function and evaluate for risk/benefit of continuing anidulafungin therapy.

Pregnancy: Category C.

Lactation: Administer to breast-feeding mothers only if the potential benefit justifies the risk. It is not known whether anidulafungin is excreted in human milk.

Children: Safety and efficacy of anidulafungin in children have not been established.

Monitoring: Monitor patients who develop abnormal LFTs during anidulafungin therapy for evidence of worsening hepatic failure.

Drug Interactions

Cyclosporine: Coadministration with cyclosporine slightly increased the steady-state area under the curve of anidulafungin by 22%.

Adverse Reactions

Adverse reactions occurring in at least 3% of patients included diarrhea and hypokalemia.

SULFADIAZINE

SULFADIAZINE
Tablets: 500 mg (*Rx*) Various

Indications

Sulfonamide Indications	
✔ – Labeled Indications	Sulfadiazine
Chancroid	✔
Inclusion conjunctivitis	✔
Malaria[a]	✔
Meningitis, *Haemophilus influenzae*[b]	✔
Meningitis, meningococcal[c]	✔
Nocardiosis	✔
Otitis media, acute[d]	✔
Rheumatic fever	✔
Toxoplasmosis[e]	✔
Trachoma	✔
Urinary tract infections[f] (pyelonephritis, cystitis)	✔

[a] As adjunctive therapy because of chloroquine-resistant strains of *Plasmodium falciparum*.
[b] As adjunctive therapy with parenteral streptomycin.
[c] When the organism is susceptible and for prophylaxis when sulfonamide-sensitive group A strains prevail.
[d] Caused by *H. influenzae* when used with penicillin or erythromycin.
[e] As adjunctive therapy with pyrimethamine.
[f] In the absence of obstructive uropathy or foreign bodies, when caused by *Escherichia coli, Klebsiella-Enterobacter, Staphylococcus aureus, Proteus mirabilis,* and *Proteus vulgaris.*

Administration and Dosage

SULFADIAZINE: Administer each dose of sulfadiazine with 237 mL (8 oz) of water and administer water at frequent intervals throughout the day.

Adults –

Loading dose: 2 to 4 g.

Maintenance dose: 4 to 8 g/day in 4 to 6 divided doses.

Children (older than 2 months of age) –

Loading dose: 75 mg/kg (or 2 g/m^2).

Maintenance dose: 150 mg/kg/day (4 g/m^2/day) in 4 to 6 divided doses every 24 hours.

Maximum dose: 6 g/day.

Rheumatic fever prophylaxis: Under 30 kg (66 lbs). 500 mg every 24 hours; over 30 kg (66 lbs), 1 g every 24 hours.

Infants (younger than 2 months of age) – Contraindicated, except as adjunctive therapy with pyrimethamine in the treatment of congenital toxoplasmosis.

Loading dose – 75 to 100 mg/kg.

Maintenance dose – 100 to 150 mg/kg/day in 4 divided doses.

Other recommended doses for toxoplasmosis (for 3 to 4 weeks) include –

Infants (younger than 2 months of age): 25 mg/kg/dose 4 times daily.

Children (older than 2 months of age): 25 to 50 mg/kg/dose 4 times daily.

Prevention of recurrent attacks of rheumatic fever (not for initial treatment of streptococcal infections) –

Patients more than 30 kg (more than 66 lbs): 1 g/day.

Patients less than 30 kg (less than 66 lbs): 0.5 g/day.

Actions

Pharmacology: Sulfonamides inhibit bacterial synthesis of dihydrofolic acid by preventing the condensation of the pteridine with aminobenzoic acid through competitive inhibition of the enzyme dihydropteroate synthase.

Pharmacokinetics:

Absorption/Distribution – The oral sulfonamides are readily absorbed from the GI tract. Protein binding of sulfadiazine is 38% to 48%.

Sulfadiazine diffuses into the cerebrospinal fluid; free drug reaches 32% to 65% of blood levels and total drug reaches 40% to 60%.

Excretion – Sulfadiazine is largely excreted in the urine.

Microbiology: Sulfonamides have a broad antibacterial spectrum that includes gram-positive and gram-negative organisms.

Contraindications

Hypersensitivity to sulfonamides; infants younger than 2 months of age (except as adjunctive therapy with pyrimethamine in the treatment of congenital toxoplasmosis); in pregnancy at term; during the breast-feeding period (sulfadiazine).

Warnings/Precautions

Death: Fatalities associated with the administration of sulfonamides, although rare, have occurred because of severe reactions, including Stevens-Johnson syndrome, toxic epidermal necrolysis, fulminant hepatic necrosis, agranulocytosis, aplastic anemia, and other blood dyscrasias.

Streptococcal infections: Do not use for the treatment of group A beta-hemolytic streptococcal infections.

Renal effects: The frequency of renal complications is considerably lower in patients receiving more soluble sulfonamides.

Asthma: Give sulfonamides with caution to patients with allergy.

Glucose-6-phosphate dehydrogenase (G6PD) deficiency: Hemolysis may occur in individuals deficient in G6PD. This reaction is dose-related.

Urinary tract infections: The frequency of organisms limits the usefulness of antibacterial agents, including the sulfonamides, as sole therapy in the treatment of urinary tract infections.

Dermatologic effects: Discontinue sulfonamides at the first appearance of skin rash or any signs of an adverse reaction. In rare instances, a skin rash may be followed by more severe reactions.

Respiratory effects: Cough, shortness of breath, and pulmonary infiltrates are hypersensitivity reactions of the respiratory tract that have been reported in association with sulfonamide treatment.

Hydration: Adequate fluid intake must be maintained in order to prevent crystalluria and stone formation.

Hypersensitivity reactions: Give sulfonamides with caution to patients with severe allergy.

Renal/Hepatic function impairment: Give sulfonamides with caution to patients with renal or hepatic function impairment.

Pregnancy: *Category* C; *Category D* if used near term.

Lactation: Sulfadiazine is contraindicated for use in breast-feeding women because sulfonamides are excreted in human milk and may cause kernicterus.

Children: Sulfonamides are contraindicated for use in infants younger than 2 months of age, except in the treatment of congenital toxoplasmosis as adjunctive therapy with pyrimethamine.

Monitoring: Measure blood levels in patients receiving sulfonamides at the higher recommended doses or patients being treated for serious infections. Free sulfonamide blood levels of 50 to 150 mcg/mL may be considered therapeutically effective for most infections, with optimal blood levels for serious infections of 120 to 150 mcg/mL. The maximum sulfonamide level should not exceed 200 mcg/mL. Perform complete blood cell counts frequently; discontinue sulfonamide if a significant reduction in the count of any formed blood element is noted. Perform urinalyses with careful microscopic examination and renal function tests during therapy, particularly for patients with renal function impairment.

Drug Interactions

Drugs that may be affected by sulfonamides include oral anticoagulants, cyclosporine, diuretics, hydantoins, methotrexate, sulfonylureas, thiopental, and uricosuric agents.

Drugs that may affect sulfonamides include indomethacin, probenecid, and salicylates.

Drug/Lab test interactions: Sulfonamides may produce false-positive **urinary glucose tests** when performed by Benedict's method..

Adverse Reactions

Abdominal pains; acute renal failure; agranulocytosis; allergic myocarditis; allergic reactions; anaphylactoid reactions; anemia; angioedema; anorexia; anxiety; apathy; aplastic anemia; arthralgia; arteritis; ataxia; chills; conjunctival and scleral injection; convulsions; cough; crystalluria; cyanosis; depression; diarrhea; disorientation; diuresis; dizziness; drowsiness; drug fever; edema (including periorbital); elevated creatinine; emesis; eosinophilia; exfoliative dermatitis; fatigue; flatulence; flushing; generalized skin eruptions; GI hemorrhage; glossitis; goiter production; hallucinations; headache; hearing loss; hematuria; hemolytic anemia; hepatitis; hepatocellular necrosis; hypofibrinogenemia; hypoglycemia; hypoprothrombinemia; insomnia; intracranial hypertension; jaundice; lassitude; leukopenia; liver enzymes elevated; lupus erythematous; melena; methemoglobinemia; myalgia; nausea; nephritis; palpitations; pancreatitis; paresthesia; periarteritis nodosu; peripheral neuritis; photosensitization; pneumonitis; pruritus; pseudomembranous colitis; psychosis; pulmonary infiltrates; purpura; pyrexia; rash; rigors; salivary gland enlargement; serum sickness; serum urea nitrogen (BUN) increased; shortness of breath; Stevens-Johnson–type erythema multiforme; stomatitis; stone formation; sulfhemoglobinemia; syncope; tachycardia; thrombocytopenia; tinnitus; toxic epidermal necrolysis; toxic nephrosis with oliguria and anuria; urinary retention; urticaria; vasculitis; vertigo; weakness.

NITROFURANTOIN

Capsules (as macrocrystals): 25, 50, 100 mg (*Rx*)	Various, *Macrodantin* (Procter & Gamble)
Capsules (as monohydrate/macrocrystals): 100 mg (*Rx*)	Various, *Macrobid* (Procter & Gamble)
Oral suspension: 25 mg per 5 mL (*Rx*)	*Furadantin* (First Horizon)

Indications

Urinary tract infections (UTIs): For the treatment of UTIs when caused by susceptible strains of *Escherichia coli*, enterococci, *Staphylococcus aureus*, and certain susceptible strains of *Klebsiella* and *Enterobacter* species.

Nitrofurantoin monohydrate/macrocrystals is indicated only for the treatment of acute uncomplicated UTIs (acute cystitis) caused by susceptible strains of *E. coli* or *Staphylococcus saprophyticus* in patients 12 years of age and older.

Administration and Dosage

Give nitrofurantoin with food to improve drug absorption and, in some patients, tolerance.

Adults: 50 to 100 mg 4 times a day (lower dosage level recommended for uncomplicated UTIs); 100 mg every 12 hours for 7 days for adults and children older than 12 years of age (monohydrate/macrocrystals only).

Long-term suppressive therapy – 50 to 100 mg at bedtime may be adequate.

Children (1 month of age and older): 5 to 7 mg/kg of body weight per 24 hours, given in 4 divided doses (contraindicated in infants younger than 1 month of age).

Continue therapy for 1 week or for at least 3 days after sterility of the urine is obtained.

For long-term suppressive therapy in pediatric patients, doses as low as 1 mg/kg per 24 hours, given in a single dose or in 2 divided doses, may be adequate.

Oral suspension (25 mg per 5 mL) –

Nitrofurantoin Dosage in Children Based on Body Weight		
Body weight		Dosage amount
Pounds	Kilograms	4 times daily
15 to 26	7 to 11	2.5 mL
27 to 46	12 to 21	5 mL
47 to 68	22 to 30	7.5 mL
69 to 91	31 to 41	10 mL

Actions

Pharmacology: Nitrofurantoin is bactericidal in urine at therapeutic doses. Nitrofurantoin is reduced by bacterial flavoproteins to reactive intermediates that inactivate or alter bacterial ribosomal proteins and other macromolecules.

Pharmacokinetics:

Absorption – Blood concentrations at therapeutic dosage are usually low.

Oral suspension: Oral nitrofurantoin is readily absorbed.

Macrocrystals, monohydrate/macrocrystals: The absorption of nitrofurantoin macrocrystals is slower when compared with nitrofurantoin oral suspension.

Distribution – When monohydrate/macrocrystals is administered with food, the bioavailability of nitrofurantoin is increased by approximately 40%.

Excretion – It is highly soluble in urine.

Oral suspension: Nitrofurantoin oral suspension is rapidly excreted in urine.

Macrocrystals, monohydrate/macrocrystals: Excretion for nitrofurantoin macrocrystals is somewhat less when compared with nitrofurantoin oral suspension.

Contraindications

Anuria, oliguria, or significant impairment of renal function (creatinine clearance [CrCl] less than 60 mL/min or clinically significant elevated serum creatinine); hypersensitivity to nitrofurantoin.

Because of the possibility of hemolytic anemia caused by immature erythrocyte enzyme systems (glutathione instability), the drug is contraindicated in pregnant patients at term (38 to 42 weeks gestation), during labor and delivery, or when the onset of labor is imminent; also contraindicated in neonates younger than 1 month of age.

Warnings/Precautions

Pulmonary reactions: Acute, subacute, or chronic pulmonary reactions have been observed in patients treated with nitrofurantoin.

Acute – Acute pulmonary reactions are commonly manifested by fever, chills, cough, chest pain, dyspnea, pulmonary infiltration with consolidation or pleural effusion on x-ray, and eosinophilia. Acute reactions usually occur within the first week of treatment.

Subacute – In subacute pulmonary reactions, fever and eosinophilia occur less often than in the acute form. Upon cessation of therapy, recovery may require several months.

Chronic – Chronic pulmonary reactions generally occur in patients who have received continuous treatment for 6 months or longer.

Peripheral neuropathy: Peripheral neuropathy, which may become severe or irreversible, has occurred.

Optic neuritis: Optic neuritis has been reported rarely.

Hematologic effects: Cases of hemolytic anemia of the primaquine-sensitivity type have been induced by nitrofurantoin.

Pseudomembranous colitis: Pseudomembranous colitis has been reported with nearly all antibacterial agents, including nitrofurantoin, and may range from mild to life-threatening.

Hepatic reactions: Hepatic reactions, including hepatitis, cholestatic jaundice, chronic active hepatitis, and hepatic necrosis, occur rarely.

Drug resistance: To reduce the development of drug-resistant bacteria and maintain the efficacy of nitrofurantoin and other antibacterial drugs, only use nitrofurantoin to treat or prevent infections that are proven or strongly suspected to be caused by bacteria.

Superinfection: As with other antimicrobial agents, superinfections caused by resistant organisms (eg, *Pseudomonas* or *Candida* species) can occur.

Fertility impairment: Dosages of 10 mg/kg/day or greater in healthy men may, in certain unpredictable instances, produce a slight to moderate spermatogenic arrest with a decrease in sperm count.

Pregnancy: Category B.

Labor and delivery – Because of the possibility of hemolytic anemia caused by immature erythrocyte enzyme systems (glutathione instability), the drug is contraindicated in pregnant patients at term (38 to 42 weeks gestation), during labor and delivery, or when the onset of labor is imminent.

Lactation: Nitrofurantoin has been detected in human breast milk in trace amounts. Because of the potential for serious adverse reactions from nitrofurantoin in nursing infants younger than 1 month of age, decide whether to discontinue breastfeeding or to discontinue the drug, taking into account the importance of the drug to the mother.

Children: Nitrofurantoin is contraindicated in infants younger than 1 month of age.

Safety and efficacy of nitrofurantoin monohydrate/macrocrystals in pediatric patients younger than 12 years of age have not been established.

Elderly: Spontaneous reports suggest a higher proportion of pulmonary reactions, including fatalities, in elderly patients.

In general, consider the greater frequency of decreased hepatic, renal, or cardiac function, and of concomitant disease or other drug therapy when prescribing nitrofurantoin. Anuria, oliguria, or significant impairment of renal function (CrCl less than 60 mL/min or clinically significant elevated serum creatinine) are contraindications.

Monitoring: Periodically monitor patients receiving long-term therapy for changes in renal and pulmonary function.

Drug Interactions

Drugs that may interact with nitrofurantoin include anticholinergics, magnesium salts, and uricosurics.

Drug/Lab test interactions: A false-positive reaction for glucose in the urine may occur. This has been observed with Benedict and Fehling solutions but not with the glucose enzymatic test.

Adverse Reactions

Cardiovascular: Benign intracranial hypertension (pseudotumor cerebri) has been reported rarely. Bulging fontanels, as a sign of benign intracranial hypertension in infants, have been reported rarely. Changes in electrocardiogram (eg, nonspecific ST/T wave changes, bundle branch block) have been reported in association with pulmonary reactions.

CNS: Asthenia, confusion, depression, dizziness, drowsiness, headache, nystagmus, peripheral neuropathy (see Warnings/Precautions), psychotic reactions, vertigo.

Dermatologic: Erythema multiforme (including Stevens-Johnson syndrome), exfoliative dermatitis (rare); transient alopecia.

GI: Abdominal pain, anorexia, diarrhea, emesis, nausea, pancreatitis, pseudomembranous colitis, sialadenitis.

Hepatic: Cholestatic jaundice, chronic active hepatitis, hepatic necrosis, hepatic reactions, hepatitis (rare).

Hypersensitivity: Anaphylaxis; angioedema; arthralgia; chills; drug fever; eczematous, erythematous, or maculopapular eruptions; lupus-like syndrome associated with pulmonary reactions; myalgia; pruritus; urticaria.

Lab test abnormalities: Agranulocytosis, decreased hemoglobin, eosinophilia, glucose-6-phosphate dehydrogenase deficiency anemia, granulocytopenia, hemolytic anemia, increased ALT, increased AST, increased serum phosphorus, leukopenia, megaloblastic anemia, thrombocytopenia. In most cases, these hematologic abnormalities resolved following cessation of therapy. Aplastic anemia (rare).

Respiratory: Chronic, subacute, or acute pulmonary hypersensitivity reactions may occur (see Warnings); cyanosis (rare).

Miscellaneous: Optic neuritis, superinfections caused by resistant organisms.

Monohydrate/macrocrystals: In clinical trials of monohydrate/macrocrystals, the most frequent adverse reactions that were reported as possibly or probably drug-related were nausea (8%), headache (6%), and flatulence (1.5%). Additional clinical adverse reactions reported as possibly or probably drug-related occurred in less than 1% of patients studied and are listed below:

CNS – Amblyopia, dizziness, drowsiness.
Dermatologic – Alopecia.
GI – Abdominal pain, constipation, diarrhea, dyspepsia, emesis.
Hypersensitivity – Pruritus, urticaria.
Respiratory – Acute pulmonary hypersensitivity reaction.
Miscellaneous – Chills, fever, malaise.

ANTITUBERCULOSIS DRUGS

Antituberculosis drugs have been described in terms of the following 3 areas of activity: Bactericidal activity, sterilizing activity, and drug resistance prevention.

Standard treatment regimens are divided into the following 2 phases: An initial phase, during which agents are used to kill rapidly multiplying populations of *Mycobacterium tuberculosis* and to prevent the emergence of drug resistance, followed by a continuation phase, during which sterilizing drugs kill the intermittently dividing populations.

The initial phase of the regimen must contain at least 3 of the following drugs: Isoniazid, rifampin, and pyrazinamide, along with either ethambutol or streptomycin if the local resistance pattern to isoniazid is not documented or is greater than 4%.

Directly observed therapy (DOT): Adherence to the treatment regimen can be achieved by DOT, the "gold standard." The health care provider watches the patient swallow each dose of medication. This allows for monitoring of the number of doses that an individual has taken. DOT may be given intermittently (2 to 3 times/week) or daily.

Recommended Drugs for the Treatment of Tuberculosis in Children and Adults[a]

Drug	Daily dose[b]		Maximum daily dose in children and adults	Twice weekly dose		3 times/week dose	
	Children	Adults		Children	Adults	Children	Adults
Initial treatment							
Isoniazid	10 to 20 mg/kg PO or IM	5 mg/kg PO or IM	300 mg	20 to 40 mg/kg max 900 mg	15 mg/kg max 900 mg	20 to 40 mg/kg max 900 mg	15 mg/kg max 900 mg
Rifampin	10 to 20 mg/kg PO	10 mg/kg PO	600 mg	10 to 20 mg/kg max 600 mg	10 mg/kg max 600 mg	10 to 20 mg/kg max 600 mg	10 mg/kg max 600 mg
Pyrazinamide	15 to 30 mg/kg PO	15 to 30 mg/kg PO	2 g	50 to 70 mg/kg max 4 g	50 to 70 mg/kg max 4 g	50 to 70 mg/kg max 3 g	50 to 70 mg/kg max 3 g
Streptomycin	20 to 40 mg/kg IM	15 mg/kg IM	1 g[c]	25 to 30 mg/kg IM max 1.5 g	25 to 30 mg/kg IM max 1.5 g	25 to 30 mg/kg max 1.5 g	25 to 30 mg/kg max 1.5 g
Ethambutol	15 to 25 mg/kg PO	15 to 25 mg/kg PO	—	50 mg/kg	50 mg/kg	25 to 30 mg/kg	25 to 30 mg/kg
Rifapentine	—	—	—	—	600 mg PO	—	—
Second-line treatment							
Cycloserine	15 to 20 mg/kg PO	15 to 20 mg/kg PO	1 g	—	—	—	—
Ethionamide	15 to 20 mg/kg PO	15 to 20 mg/kg PO	1 g	—	—	—	—
Capreomycin	15 to 30 mg/kg IM	15 to 30 mg/kg IM	1 g	—	—	—	—
Kanamycin	15 to 30 mg/kg IM or IV	15 to 30 mg/kg IM or IV	1 g	—	—	—	—
Ciprofloxacin	—	1000 to 1500 mg PO	1500 mg	—	—	—	—
Ofloxacin	—	800 mg PO	800 mg	—	—	—	—
Levofloxacin	—	500 to 750 mg PO	750 mg	—	—	—	—
Sparfloxacin	—	200 mg PO	200 mg	—	—	—	—

Recommended Drugs for the Treatment of Tuberculosis in Children and Adults[a]

Drug	Daily dose[b]		Maximum daily dose in children and adults	Twice weekly dose		3 times/week dose	
	Children	Adults		Children	Adults	Children	Adults
P-amino-salicy-clic acid	150 mg/kg PO	150 mg/kg PO	12 g	—	—	—	—
Rifabutin	—	300 to 450 mg PO	—	—	—	—	—

[a] For detailed dosing information and frequency, see individual monographs.
[b] Doses based on weight. Adjust as weight changes.
[c] In people ≥ 60 years of age, limit the daily dose of streptomycin to 0.5 g IM.

Treatment regimens: The CDC recommends at least a 3-drug regimen with rifampin, isoniazid, and pyrazinamide for a minimum of 2 months, followed by rifampin and isoniazid for 4 months in areas with a low incidence of tuberculosis. Administer streptomycin or ethambutol for the first 2 months in areas with a high incidence of tuberculosis.

Retreatment: Retreatment is necessary when treatment fails because of noncompliance or inadequate drug treatment. Retreatment regimens include at least 4 drugs; however, depending on disease progression and the bacteriostatic or bactericidal activity of the drug, no more than 7 drugs can be used. Retreatment drug regimens most commonly include the second-line agents of ethionamide, aminosalicylic acid, cycloserine, and capreomycin, as well as ofloxacin and ciprofloxacin.

Individualize treatment on the basis of the susceptibility pattern of the infecting organism when retreating patients known to be infected with drug-resistant isolates. Include in this regimen at least 3 new drugs to which the organism is susceptible. Continue therapy until sputum cultures convert to negative, and then continue therapy for an additional 12 months with 2 drugs. Treatment may be continued for 24 months after sputum culture conversion.

HIV: The initial phase of a 6-month tuberculosis regimen consists of isoniazid, rifabutin, pyrazinamide, and ethambutol for patients receiving therapy with protease inhibitors or nonnucleoside reverse transcriptase inhibitors. These drugs are administered a) daily for at least the first 2 weeks, followed by twice weekly dosing for 6 weeks or b) daily for 8 weeks to complete the 2-month induction phase. The second phase of treatment consists of rifabutin and isoniazid administered twice weekly or daily for 4 months.

Do not use tuberculosis regimens consisting of isoniazid, ethambutol, and pyrazinamide (ie, 3-drug regimens that do not contain a rifamycin, an aminoglycoside [eg, streptomycin, amikacin, kanamycin], or capreomycin) for the treatment of patients with HIV-related tuberculosis. The minimum duration of therapy is 18 months (or 12 months after documented culture conversion) if these regimens are used for the treatment of tuberculosis.

Administer pyridoxine (vitamin B_6) 25 to 50 mg daily or 50 to 100 mg twice weekly to all HIV-infected patients who are undergoing tuberculosis treatment with isoniazid to reduce the occurrence of isoniazid-induced side effects in the central and peripheral nervous system.

Because the *MMWR*'s most recent recommendations for the use of antiretroviral therapy strongly advise against interruptions of therapy, and because alternative tuberculosis treatments that do not contain rifampin are available, previous antituberculosis therapy options that involved stopping protease inhibitor therapy to allow the use of rifampin are no longer recommended.

Pregnancy: Do not delay treatment for suspected or confirmed tuberculosis during pregnancy. The best therapeutic choices with the least danger to the fetus appear to be combinations of isoniazid, ethambutol, and rifampin. Pyrazinamide and streptomycin are not recommended during pregnancy because of possible teratogenic effects. Administer pyridoxine to all pregnant women receiving tuberculosis treatment to prevent peripheral neuropathy as a result of taking isoniazid. In pregnant women, delay prophylaxis until after delivery.

Multidrug resistance: The most recent cultures should undergo susceptibility testing to all antituberculosis drugs if cultures remain positive after 3 to 4 months of treatment.

Chemoprophylaxis: Administer isoniazid to adults in a daily dose of 300 mg for 1 year. Administer 10 mg/kg to a maximum daily dose of 300 mg for 1 year to children.

ISONIAZID (Isonicotinic acid hydrazide; INH)

Tablets: 100 and 300 mg (*Rx*)	Various
Syrup: 50 mg/5 mL (*Rx*)	
Injection: 100 mg/mL (*Rx*)	Various, *Nydrazid* (Apothecon)

Warning:

Severe and sometimes fatal hepatitis associated with isoniazid therapy may occur or develop even after many months of treatment. The risk of developing hepatitis is age-related. Risk of hepatitis increases with daily alcohol consumption.

Carefully monitor and interview patients at monthly intervals. For people older than 35 years of age, in addition to a monthly symptom review, measure hepatic enzymes (specifically AST and ALT) prior to starting isoniazid therapy and periodically throughout treatment. Isoniazid-associated hepatitis usually occurs during the first 3 months of treatment. Enzyme levels generally return to normal despite continuance of the drug, but in some cases, progressive liver dysfunction occurs. Other factors associated with an increased risk of hepatitis include daily use of alcohol, chronic liver disease, and injection drug use. A report suggests an increased risk of fatal hepatitis associated with isoniazid among women, particularly black and Hispanic women. The risk also may be increased during the postpartum period. Consider more careful monitoring in these groups, possibly including more frequent laboratory monitoring. If abnormalities of liver function exceed 3 to 5 times the upper limit of normal, consider discontinuation of isoniazid. Liver function tests are not a substitute for a clinical evaluation at monthly intervals or for the prompt assessment of signs or symptoms of adverse reactions occurring between regularly scheduled evaluations. Instruct patients to report immediately signs or symptoms consistent with liver damage or other adverse effects. If these symptoms appear, or if signs suggestive of hepatic damage are detected, discontinue isoniazid promptly because continued use of the drug in such cases may cause a more severe form of liver damage.

Treat patients with tuberculosis who have hepatitis attributed to isoniazid with appropriate alternative drugs. Reinstitute isoniazid after symptoms and laboratory abnormalities have become normal. Restart the drug in very small doses; gradually increase doses and withdraw immediately if there is any indication of recurrent liver involvement.

Defer preventive treatment in people with acute hepatic diseases.

Indications

Used for all forms of tuberculosis in which organisms are susceptible.

Also recommended as preventive therapy (chemoprophylaxis) for specific situations.

IM administration is intended for use whenever oral is not possible.

Administration and Dosage

Treatment of tuberculosis: Use in conjunction with other effective antituberculosis agents.

Adults – 5 mg/kg/day (up to 300 mg total) in a single dose, or 15 mg/kg (less than or equal to 900 mg daily) 2 to 3 times weekly.

Children – 10 to 15 mg/kg (less than or equal to 300 mg daily) in a single dose, or 20 to 40 mg/kg (less than or equal to 900 mg/day) 2 to 3 times weekly.

Preventive treatment:

Adults (greater than 30 kg) – 300 mg/day in a single dose.

Infants and children – 10 mg/kg/day (up to 300 mg total) in a single dose.

Actions

Pharmacology: Isoniazid inhibits the synthesis of mycoloic acids, an essential component of the bacterial cell wall. At therapeutic levels, isoniazid is bacteriocidal against actively growing intracellular and extracellular *Mycobacterium tuberculosis* organisms.

Pyridoxine (vitamin B_6) deficiency sometimes is observed in adults taking high doses of INH and is probably caused by the drug's competition with pyridoxal phosphate for the enzyme apotryptophanase.

Pharmacokinetics:

Absorption – INH is rapidly and completely absorbed orally and parenterally and produces peak blood levels within 1 to 2 hours. However, the rate and extent of absorption is decreased by food.

Distribution – INH readily diffuses into all body fluids (including cerebrospinal, pleural, and ascitic), tissues, organs, and excreta (saliva, sputum, feces). It also passes through the placental barrier and into breast milk in concentrations comparable to those in plasma.

Metabolism – The half-life of INH is widely variable and dependent on acetylator status. Isoniazid is primarily acetylated by the liver; this process is genetically controlled. Fast acetylators metabolize the drug about 5 to 6 times faster than slow acetylators. Several minor metabolites have been identified, one or more of which may be "reactive" (monoacetylhydrazine is suspected), and responsible for liver damage. The rate of acetylation does not significantly alter the effectiveness of INH. However, slow acetylation may lead to higher blood levels of the drug, and thus to an increase in toxic reactions.

Excretion – Approximately 50% to 70% of a dose of isoniazid is excreted as unchanged drug and metabolites by the kidneys in 24 hours.

Contraindications

Previous isoniazid-associated hepatic injury or other severe adverse reactions.

Warnings/Precautions

Laboratory tests: Because there is a higher frequency of isoniazid-associated hepatitis among certain patient groups, obtain transaminase measurements prior to starting and monthly during preventative therapy, or more frequently as needed. If any of the values exceed 3 to 5 times the upper limit of normal, temporarily discontinue isoniazid and consider restarting therapy.

Periodic ophthalmologic examinations: Periodic ophthalmologic examinations during isoniazid therapy are recommended even when visual symptoms do not occur.

Pyridoxine administration: Pyridoxine administration is recommended in individuals likely to develop peripheral neuropathies secondary to INH therapy. Prophylactic doses of 10 to 25 mg of pyridoxine daily have been recommended.

Hypersensitivity reactions: Stop all drugs and evaluate at the first sign of a hypersensitivity reaction. If isoniazid must be reinstituted, give only after symptoms have cleared. Restart the drug in very small and gradually increasing doses and withdraw immediately if there is any indication of recurrent hypersensitivity reaction.

Renal/Hepatic function impairment: Monitor patients with active chronic liver disease or severe renal dysfunction.

Carcinogenesis: Isoniazid induces pulmonary tumors in a number of strains of mice.

Pregnancy: Category C.

Lactation: The small concentrations of isoniazid in breast milk do not produce toxicity in the nursing newborn; therefore, do not discourage breastfeeding. However, because levels of isoniazid are so low in breast milk, they cannot be relied upon for prophylaxis or therapy in nursing infants.

Drug Interactions

Drugs that may interact with isoniazid include acetaminophen, carbamazepine, chlorzoxazone, disulfiram, enflurane, hydantoins, ketoconazole, rifampin, and theophylline.

Drug/Food interactions: Rate and extent of INH absorption is decreased by food.

Adverse Reactions

Toxic effects are usually encountered with higher doses of isoniazid; the most frequent are those affecting the nervous system and the liver.

Adverse reactions include pyridoxine deficiency; hyperglycemia; gynecomastia; peripheral neuropathy; convulsions; optic neuritis and atrophy; memory impairment; toxic psychosis; nausea; vomiting; epigastric distress; elevated AST, ALT; bilirubinemia; jaundice; anorexia; fatigue; malaise; weakness; agranulocytosis; hemolytic, sideroblastic, or aplastic anemia; thrombocytopenia; eosinophilia; fever; skin eruptions; lymphadenopathy; vasculitis.

RIFAMPIN

Capsules: 150 and 300 mg (*Rx*)	Various, *Rifadin* (Aventis), *Rimactane* (Novartis)
Powder for injection: 600 mg (*Rx*)	Various, *Rifadin* (Aventis)

Indications

Tuberculosis:

Oral – Oral treatment is for all forms of tuberculosis. A 3-drug regimen consisting of rifampin, isoniazid, and pyrazinamide is recommended in the initial phase of short-course therapy that is usually continued for 2 months.

IV – Initial treatment and retreatment of tuberculosis when the drug cannot be taken by mouth.

Neisseria meningitidis carriers: Treatment of asymptomatic carriers of *N. meningitidis* to eliminate meningococci from the nasopharynx. Not indicated for treatment of meningococcal infection.

Administration and Dosage

Oral: Administer once daily, either 1 hour before or 2 hours after meals.

Data is not available to determine dosage for children younger than 5 years of age.

Oral and IV:

Tuberculosis: Adults – 10 mg/kg in a single daily administration not to exceed 600 mg once daily.

Children – 10 to 20 mg/kg, not to exceed 600 mg/day.

The 2-month regimen: According to the MMWR, the 2-month daily regimen of rifampin and pyrazinamide is recommended in HIV-infected people. However, the drug toxicities may be increased.

The 4-month regimen: According to the MMWR, rifampin given daily for 3 months has resulted in better protection than placebo in treatment of LTBI in non-HIV patients with silicosis in a randomized prospective trial. However, because the patients receiving rifampin had a high rate of active tuberculosis (4%), experts have concluded that a 4-month regimen would be more prudent when using rifampin alone. This option may be useful for patients who cannot tolerate isoniazid or pyrazinamide.

The 6-month regimen: Ordinarily this consists of an initial 2-month phase of rifampin, isoniazid, and pyrazinamide and, if clinically indicated, streptomycin or ethambutol, followed by 4 months of rifampin and isoniazid. Reassess the need for a fourth drug when the results of susceptibility testing are known. If community rates of INH resistance are currently less than 4%, an initial treatment regimen with less than

4 drugs may be considered. Continue treatment for more than 6 months if the patient is still sputum- or culture-positive, if resistant organisms are present, or if the patient is HIV positive.

Meningococcal carriers: Once daily for 4 consecutive days in the following doses:

Adults – 600 mg.

Children – 10 to 20 mg/kg, not to exceed 600 mg/day.

The following dosage has also been recommended –

Adults: 600 mg every 12 hours for 2 days.

Children (1 month of age and older): 10 mg/kg every 12 hours for 2 days.

Children (younger than 1 month of age): 5 mg/kg every 12 hours for 2 days.

Actions

Pharmacology: Rifampin inhibits DNA-dependent RNA polymerase activity in susceptible cells. Specifically, it interacts with bacterial RNA polymerase, but does not inhibit the mammalian enzyme. Cross-resistance has only been shown with other rifamycins. Rifampin at therapeutic levels has demonstrated bactericidal activity against intracellular and extracellular *Mycobacterium tuberculosis* organisms.

Pharmacokinetics:

Oral –

Absorption/Distribution: Rifampin is almost completely absorbed and achieves mean peak plasma levels within 1 to 4 hours. Absorption of rifampin is reduced by approximately 30% when the drug is ingested with food.

Metabolism: Rifampin is metabolized in the liver by deacetylation; the metabolite is still active against *Mycobacterium tuberculosis*. About 40% is excreted in bile and undergoes enterohepatic circulation; however, the deacetylated metabolite is poorly absorbed. The half-life is approximately 3 hours after a 600 mg oral dose, up to 5.1 after a 900 mg oral dose. With repeated administration, the half-life decreases and averages approximately 2 to 3 hours.

Excretion: Elimination occurs mainly through the bile and, to a much lesser extent, the urine. Dosage adjustment is not necessary in renal failure, but is with hepatic dysfunction. Rifampin is not significantly removed by hemodialysis.

Contraindications

Hypersensitivity to any rifamycin.

Warnings/Precautions

Hepatotoxicity: There have been fatalities associated with jaundice in patients with liver disease or patients receiving rifampin concomitantly with other hepatotoxic agents. Carefully monitor liver function, especially AST and ALT, prior to therapy and then every 2 to 4 weeks during therapy.

Hyperbilirubinemia: Hyperbilirubinemia, resulting from competition between rifampin and bilirubin for excretory pathways of the liver at the cell level, can occur in early days of treatment.

Porphyria: Isolated reports have associated porphyria exacerbation with rifampin administration.

Meningococci resistance: The possibility of rapid emergence of resistant meningococci restricts use to short-term treatment of asymptomatic carrier state. Not for treatment of meningococcal disease.

Intermittent therapy: Intermittent therapy may be used if the patient cannot or will not self-administer drugs on a daily basis. Closely monitor patients on intermittent therapy for compliance, and caution against intentional or accidental interruption of prescribed therapy because of increased risk of serious adverse reactions.

Urine, feces, saliva, sputum, sweat, and tears may be colored red-orange. Soft contact lenses may be permanently stained. Advise patients of these possibilities.

IV: For IV infusion only. Must not be administered by IM or subcutaneous route.

Thrombocytopenia: Thrombocytopenia has occurred, primarily with high dose intermittent therapy, but has also been noted after resumption of interrupted treatment.

Cerebral hemorrhage and fatalities have occurred when rifampin administration has continued or resumed after appearance of purpura.

Hypersensitivity reactions: Hypersensitivity reactions have occurred during intermittent therapy or when treatment was resumed following accidental or intentional interruption and were reversible with rifampin discontinuation and appropriate therapy.

Hepatic function impairment: Dosage adjustment is necessary.

Pregnancy: Category C.

Lactation: Rifampin is excreted in breast milk.

Monitoring: Perform baseline measurements of hepatic enzymes, bilirubin, serum creatinine, CBC, and platelet count (or estimate) in adults treated for tuberculosis with rifampin. Baseline tests are unnecessary in pediatric patients unless a complicating condition is known or clinically suspected.

Drug Interactions

Rifampin is known to induce the hepatic microsomal enzymes that metabolize various drugs such as acetaminophen, oral anticoagulants, barbiturates, benzodiazepines, beta blockers, chloramphenicol, clofibrate, oral contraceptives, corticosteroids, cyclosporine, disopyramide, estrogens, hydantoins, mexiletine, quinidine, sulfones, sulfonylureas, theophyllines, tocainide, verapamil, digoxin, enalapril, morphine, nifedipine, ondansetron, progestins, protease inhibitors, buspirone, delavirdine, doxycycline, fluoroquinolones, losartan, macrolides, sulfonylureas, tacrolimus, thyroid hormones, TCAs, zolpidem, zidovudine, and ketoconazole. The therapeutic effects of these drugs may be decreased.

Enzyme induction properties: Rifampin has enzyme induction properties that can enhance the metabolism of endogenous substrates including adrenal hormones, thyroid hormones, and vitamin D. Rifampin and isoniazid have been reported to alter vitamin D metabolism. In some cases, reduced levels of circulating 25-hydroxy vitamin D and 1,25-dihydroxy vitamin D have been accompanied by reduced serum calcium and phosphate, and elevated parathyroid hormone.

Drug/Lab test interactions: Therapeutic levels of rifampin inhibit standard assays for serum folate and vitamin B_{12}.

Transient abnormalities in liver function tests (eg, elevation in serum bilirubin, alkaline phosphatase, serum transaminases), and reduced biliary excretion of contrast media used for visualization of the gallbladder have also been observed.

Drug/Food interactions: Food interferes with the absorption of rifampin, possibly resulting in decreased peak plasma concentrations. Take on an empty stomach with a full glass of water.

Adverse Reactions

High doses of rifampin (greater than 600 mg) given once or twice weekly have resulted in a high incidence of adverse reactions including the following: "Flu-like" syndrome; hematopoietic reactions; cutaneous, GI, and hepatic reactions; shortness of breath; shock; renal failure; asymptomatic elevations of liver enzymes; rash.

RIFABUTIN

Capsules: 150 mg (*Rx*)	*Mycobutin* (Pharmacia)

Indications

Prevention of disseminated *Mycobacterium avium* complex (MAC) disease in patients with advanced HIV infection.

Administration and Dosage

Usual dose: 300 mg once daily. For those patients with propensity to nausea, vomiting, or other GI upset, administration of rifabutin at doses of 150 mg twice daily taken with food may be useful.

Actions

Pharmacology: Rifabutin, an antimycobacterial agent, is a semisynthetic ansamycin antibiotic derived from rifamycin S. It is not known whether rifabutin inhibits DNA-dependent RNA polymerase in *Mycobacterium avium* or in *Mycobacterium intracellulare* that comprise MAC.

Pharmacokinetics: Following a single oral dose of 300 mg to healthy adult volunteers, rifabutin was readily absorbed from the GI tract with mean peak plasma levels attained in 3.3 hours. Plasma concentrations post-C_{max} declined in an apparent biphasic manner. Rifabutin was slowly eliminated from plasma in healthy adult volunteers, presumably because of distribution-limited elimination, with a mean terminal half-life of 45 hours. Although the systemic levels of rifabutin following multiple dosing decreased by 38%, its terminal half-life remained unchanged. Estimates of apparent steady-state distribution volume (9.3 L/kg) in HIV-positive patients, following IV dosing, exceed total body water by approximately 15-fold. About 85% of the drug is bound in a concentration-independent manner to plasma proteins over a concentration range of 0.05 to 1 mcg/mL.

Mean systemic clearance in healthy adult volunteers following a single oral dose was 0.69 L/h/kg; renal and biliary clearance of unchanged drug each contribute approximately 5%. About 30% of the dose is excreted in the feces; 53% of the oral dose is excreted in the urine, primarily as metabolites. Of the five metabolites that have been identified, 25-O-desacetyl and 31-hydroxy are the most predominant, and show a plasma metabolite:parent AUC ratio of 0.1 and 0.07, respectively. The 25-O-desacetyl metabolite has an activity equal to the parent drug and contributes less than or equal to 10% to the total antimicrobial activity.

Absolute bioavailability assessed in HIV-positive patients averaged 20%. Somewhat reduced drug distribution and faster drug elimination in compromised renal function may result in decreased drug concentrations.

Contraindications

Hypersensitivity to this drug or to any other rifamycins.

Warnings/Precautions

Active tuberculosis: Rifabutin prophylaxis must not be administered to patients with active tuberculosis. HIV-positive patients are likely to have a nonreactive purified protein derivative (PPD) despite active disease. Chest X-ray, sputum culture, blood culture, urine culture, or biopsy of a suspicious lymph node may be useful in the diagnosis of tuberculosis in the HIV-positive patient.

There is no evidence that rifabutin is effective prophylaxis against M. *tuberculosis*. Patients requiring prophylaxis against both M. *tuberculosis* and M. *avium* complex may be given isoniazid and rifabutin concurrently.

Pregnancy: *Category B.*

Lactation: It is not known whether rifabutin is excreted in breast milk. Because of the potential for serious adverse reactions in nursing infants, decide whether to discontinue nursing or discontinue the drug, taking into account the importance of the drug to the mother.

Children: Safety and efficacy in children have not been established. Limited safety data are available from treatment use in 22 HIV-positive children with MAC who received rifabutin in combination with at least 2 other antimycobacterials for periods from 1 to 183 weeks. Mean doses (mg/kg) for these children were: 18.5 for infants 1 year of age; 8.6 for children 2 to 10 years of age; and 4 for adolescents 14 to 16 years of age. There is no evidence that doses greater than 5 mg/kg/day are useful.

Monitoring: Because rifabutin may be associated with neutropenia, and, more rarely, thrombocytopenia, consider obtaining hematologic studies periodically in patients receiving prophylaxis.

Drug Interactions

CYP450: Rifabutin has liver enzyme-inducing properties. The related drug, rifampin, is known to reduce the activity of a number of other drugs. Because of the structural similarity of rifabutin and rifampin, rifabutin may be expected to have similar interactions. However, unlike rifampin, rifabutin appears not to affect the acetylation of isoniazid. Rifabutin appears to be a less potent enzyme inducer than rifampin. The significance of this finding for clinical drug interactions is not known.

Drugs that may interact with rifabutin include the following: Anticoagulants, azole antifungal agents, benzodiazepines, beta blockers, buspirone, corticosteroids, cyclosporine, delavirdine, doxycycline, hydantoins, indinavir, rifamycins, losartan, macrolide antibiotics, methadone, morphine, nelfinavir, quinine, quinidine, theophylline, aminophylline, tricyclic antidepressants, and zolpidem.

Drug/Food interactions: High-fat meals slow the rate of absorption without influencing the extent.

Adverse Reactions

Rifabutin is generally well tolerated. Discontinuation of therapy because of an adverse event was required in 16% of patients receiving rifabutin vs 8% with placebo.

Adverse reactions occurring in at least 3% of patients include the following: Abdominal pain, headache, diarrhea, dyspepsia, eructation, nausea, vomiting, rash, taste perversion, discolored urine, increased AST and ALT, anemia, leukopenia, neutropenia, and thrombocytopenia.

ETHAMBUTOL

Tablets: 100 and 400 mg (*Rx*)	*Myambutol* (X-Gen)

Indications

Pulmonary tuberculosis: Use in conjunction with at least 1 other antituberculosis drug(s).

In patients who have received previous therapy, mycobacterial resistance to other drugs used in initial therapy is frequent. In retreatment patients, combine ethambutol with at least 1 of the second-line drug(s) not previously administered to the patient, and to which bacterial susceptibility has been indicated.

Administration and Dosage

Do not use ethambutol alone. Administer once every 24 hours only. Absorption is not significantly altered by administration with food. Continue therapy until bacteriological conversion has become permanent and maximal clinical improvement has occurred.

Initial treatment: In patients who have not received previous antituberculosis therapy, administer 15 mg/kg (7 mg/lb) as a single oral dose once every 24 hours. Isoniazid has been administered concurrently in a single, daily oral dose.

Retreatment: In patients who have received previous antituberculosis therapy, administer 25 mg/kg (11 mg/lb) as a single oral dose once every 24 hours. Concurrently administer at least 1 other antituberculosis drug(s) to which the organisms have been demonstrated to be susceptible by in vitro tests. Suitable drugs usually include those not previously used in the treatment of the patient. After 60 days of administration, decrease the dose to 15 mg/kg and administer as a single oral dose once every 24 hours.

Children: Not recommended for use in children younger than 13 years of age.

Actions

Pharmacology: Ethambutol diffuses into actively growing mycobacterium cells such as tubercle bacilli. It inhibits the synthesis of at least 1 metabolite, thus causing impairment of cell metabolism, arrest of multiplication, and cell death. No cross-resistance with other agents has been demonstrated.

Pharmacokinetics:

Absorption/Distribution – Ethambutol absorption is not influenced by food. Following a single oral dose of 15 to 25 mg/kg, ethambutol attains a peak of 2 to 5 mcg/mL in serum 2 to 4 hours after administration. Serum levels are similar after prolonged dosing. The serum level is undetectable 24 hours after the last dose except in some patients with abnormal renal function.

Metabolism – During the 24 hours following oral administration, approximately 20% of ethambutol is metabolized by the liver.

Excretion – Unchanged drug is excreted (approximately 50%) in the urine, 8% to 15% as metabolites and 20% to 22% unchanged in the feces. Marked accumulation may occur with renal insufficiency. Ethambutol is not significantly removed by hemodialysis.

Contraindications

Hypersensitivity to ethambutol; known optic neuritis, unless clinical judgment determines that it may be used.

Warnings/Precautions

Visual effects: This drug may have adverse effects on vision. The effects are generally reversible when the drug is discontinued promptly. Perform testing before beginning therapy and periodically during drug administration (monthly when a patient is receiving more than 15 mg/kg/day).

Advise patients to report promptly any change in visual acuity. If evaluation confirms visual change and fails to reveal other causes, discontinue drug and reevaluate patient at frequent intervals.

Renal function impairment: Patients with decreased renal function require reduced dosage (as determined by serum levels) because this drug is excreted by the kidneys.

Pregnancy: Category B.

Children: Not recommended for use in children younger than 13 years of age.

Monitoring: Perform periodic assessment of renal, hepatic, and hematopoietic systems during long-term therapy.

Drug Interactions

Aluminum salts: Aluminum salts may delay and reduce the absorption of ethambutol. Separate their administration by several hours.

Adverse Reactions

Adverse reactions may include anaphylactoid reactions, dermatitis, pruritus, decreases in visual acuity, anorexia, nausea, vomiting, GI upset, abdominal pain, fever, malaise, headache, dizziness, mental confusion, disorientation, possible hallucinations, peripheral neuritis, elevated serum uric acid levels, precipitation of acute gout, transient impairment of liver function, and joint pain.

PYRAZINAMIDE

Tablets; oral: 500 mg (*Rx*)	Various

Indications

Tuberculosis:

Drug-susceptible disease – Initial treatment of active tuberculosis in adults and children when combined with other antituberculosis agents.

The current CDC recommendation for drug-susceptible initial treatment of active tuberculosis disease is a 6-month regimen consisting of isoniazid, rifampin, and pyrazinamide given for 2 months, followed by isoniazid and rifampin for 4 months.

Drug-resistant disease – Treat patients with a drug-resistant disease with regimens individualized to their situation. Pyrazinamide frequently will be an important component of such therapy.

Treatment failure: After treatment failure with other primary drugs in any form of active tuberculosis.

Administration and Dosage

Administer pyrazinamide with other effective antituberculosis drugs. It is administered for the initial 2 months of a 6-month or longer treatment regimen for drug susceptible patients. Treat patients who are known or suspected to have drug-resistant disease with regimens individualized to their situation.

HIV infection: Patients with concomitant HIV infection may require longer courses of therapy. Be alert to any revised recommendations from CDC for this group of patients.

Usual dose: 15 to 30 mg/kg once daily. Do not exceed 3 g/day. The CDC recommendations do not exceed 2 g/day when given as a daily regimen.

Alternative dosing: Alternatively, a twice weekly dosing regimen (50 to 70 mg/kg twice weekly based on lean body weight) has been developed to promote patient compliance on an outpatient basis. In studies evaluating the twice weekly regimen, doses of pyrazinamide in excess of 3 g twice weekly have been administered without an increased incidence of adverse reactions.

Actions

Pharmacology: Pyrazinamide, the pyrazine analog of nicotinamide, may be bacteriostatic or bactericidal against *Mycobacterium tuberculosis* depending on the concentration of the drug attained at the site of infection. The mechanism of action is unknown.

Pharmacokinetics:

Absorption/Distribution – Pyrazinamide is well absorbed from the GI tract and attains peak plasma concentrations within 2 hours. It is widely distributed in body tissues and fluids including the liver, lungs, and cerebrospinal fluid. Pyrazinamide is approximately 10% bound to plasma proteins.

Metabolism/Excretion – The half-life is 9 to 10 hours; it may be prolonged in patients with impaired renal or hepatic function.

Approximately 70% of an oral dose is excreted in urine, mainly by glomerular filtration, within 24 hours. Pyrazinamide is significantly dialyzed and should be dosed after hemodialysis.

Contraindications

Severe hepatic damage; hypersensitivity; acute gout.

Warnings/Precautions

Combination therapy: Use only in conjunction with other effective antituberculosis agents.

Hyperuricemia: Pyrazinamide inhibits renal excretion of urates, frequently resulting in hyperuricemia that is usually asymptomatic. Patients started on pyrazinamide should have baseline serum uric acid determinations. Discontinue the drug and do not resume if signs of hyperuricemia accompanied by acute gouty arthritis appear.

HIV infection: In patients with concomitant HIV infection, be aware of current recommendations of CDC. It is possible these patients may require a longer course of treatment.

Diabetes mellitus: Use with caution in patients with a history of diabetes mellitus, as management may be more difficult.

Primary resistance of M. tuberculosis: Primary resistance of M. *tuberculosis* to pyrazinamide is uncommon. In cases with known or suspected drug resistance, perform in vitro susceptibility tests with recent cultures of M. *tuberculosis* against pyrazinamide and the usual primary drugs.

Renal function impairment: It does not appear that patients with impaired renal function require a reduction in dose. It may be prudent to select doses at the low end of the dosing range, however.

Hepatic function impairment: Closely follow those patients with pre-existing liver disease or those at increased risk for drug-related hepatitis. Discontinue pyrazinamide and do not resume if signs of hepatocellular damage appear.

Pregnancy: Category C.

Lactation: Pyrazinamide has been found in small amounts in breast milk. Therefore, it is advised that pyrazinamide be used with caution in nursing mothers, taking into account the risk-benefit of this therapy.

Children: Pyrazinamide appears to be well tolerated in children.

Elderly: In general, dose selection for an elderly patient should be cautious, usually starting at the low end of the dosing range, reflecting the greater frequency of decreased hepatic or renal function, and of concomitant disease or other drug therapy.

Monitoring: Determine baseline liver function studies (especially ALT and AST) and uric acid levels prior to therapy. Perform appropriate laboratory testing at periodic intervals and if any clinical signs or symptoms occur during therapy.

Drug Interactions

Drug/Lab test interactions: Pyrazinamide has been reported to interfere with *Acetest* and *Ketostix* urine tests to produce a pink-brown color.

Adverse Reactions

Adverse reactions may include the following: Fever; porphyria; dysuria; gout; hepatic reaction; nausea; vomiting; anorexia; thrombocytopenia and sideroblastic anemia with erythroid hyperplasia; vacuolation of erythrocytes; increased serum iron concentration; adverse effects on blood clotting mechanisms; mild arthralgia and myalgia; hypersensitivity reactions including rashes, urticaria, pruritus; acne; photosensitivity; interstitial nephritis.

AMINOSALICYLATE SODIUM (Para-Aminosalicylate Sodium)

Granules, delayed-release; oral: 4 g (*Rx*)	*Paser* (Jacobus Pharm.)

Refer to the general discussion in the Antituberculosal Agents introduction.

Indications

Tuberculosis: Treatment of tuberculosis in combination with other active agents. It is most commonly used in patients with multi-drug resistant tuberculosis (MDR-TB) or in situations when therapy with isoniazid and rifampin is not possible because of a combination of resistance and intolerance.

Administration and Dosage

Tuberculosis: The adult dosage of 4 g (1 packet) 3 times/day, or correspondingly smaller doses in children, is to be taken without chewing by sprinkling on applesauce or yogurt or by swirling in the glass to suspend the granules in an acidic drink such as tomato or orange juice or food such as applesauce or yogurt. The coating will last at least 2 hours.

Do not use if packet is swollen or the granules have lost their tan color, turning dark brown or purple.

Actions

Pharmacology: Aminosalicylic acid is bacteriostatic against *Mycobacterium tuberculosis*. It inhibits the onset of bacterial resistance to streptomycin and isoniazid. The mechanism of action has been postulated to be inhibition of folic acid synthesis (but without potentiation with antifolic compounds) or inhibition of synthesis of the cell wall component, mycobactin, thus reducing iron uptake by M. *tuberculosis*.

Pharmacokinetics:

Absorption/Distribution – In a single 4 g pharmacokinetic study with food in normal volunteers, the initial time to a 2 mcg/mL serum level was 2 hours; the median time to peak was 6 hours. Approximately 50% to 60% of aminosalicylic acid is protein-bound; binding is reported to be reduced 50% in kwashiorkor.

Excretion – 80% of aminosalicylic acid is excreted in the urine by glomerular filtration, with at least 50% of the dosage excreted in acetylated form.

Contraindications

Hypersensitivity to any component of this medication; severe renal disease.

Warnings/Precautions

Hepatitis: In 1 retrospective study of 7492 patients on rapidly absorbed aminosalicylic acid preparations, drug-induced hepatitis occurred in 38 patients (0.5%); in these 38, the first symptom usually appeared within 3 months of the start of therapy with a rash as the most common event followed by fever and much less frequently by GI disturbances of anorexia, nausea, or diarrhea.

Malabsorption syndrome: A malabsorption syndrome can develop in patients on aminosalicylic acid but usually is not complete.

Hypersensitivity reactions: Stop all drugs at the first sign suggesting a hypersensitivity reaction. They may be restarted one at a time in very small but gradually increasing doses to determine whether the manifestations are drug-induced and, if so, which drug is responsible.

Desensitization has been accomplished successfully.

Renal function impairment: Patients with severe renal disease will accumulate aminosalicylic acid and its acetyl metabolite but will continue to acetylate, thus leading exclusively to the inactive acetylated form; deacetylation, if any, is not significant. Patients with end-stage renal disease should not receive aminosalicylic acid.

Hepatic function impairment: Use with caution.

Pregnancy: Category C.

Lactation: Aminosalicylic acid is excreted in breast milk.

Lab test abnormalities: Aminosalicylic acid has been reported to interfere technically with the serum determinations of albumin by dye-binding AST by the azoene dye method and with qualitative urine tests for ketones, bilirubin, urobilinogen, or porphobilinogen.

Crystalluria may develop and can be prevented by the maintenance of urine at a neutral or alkaline pH.

Drug Interactions

Aminosalicylic acid may affect isoniazid, digoxin, and vitamin B_{12}.

Adverse Reactions

GI: The most common side effect is GI intolerance manifested by nausea, vomiting, diarrhea, and abdominal pain.

Hypersensitivity: Fever, skin eruptions of various types, including exfoliative dermatitis, infectious mononucleosis-like, or lymphoma-like syndrome, leukopenia, agranulocytosis, thrombocytopenia, Coombs' positive hemolytic anemia, jaundice, hepatitis, pericarditis, hypoglycemia, optic neuritis, encephalopathy, Leoffler's syndrome, vasculitis, and a reduction in prothrombin.

ETHIONAMIDE

Tablets; oral: 250 mg (*Rx*)	*Trecator* (Wyeth-Ayerst)

Indications

Recommended for any form of active tuberculosis when treatment with first-line drugs (isoniazid, rifampin) has failed. Use only with other effective antituberculosis agents.

Administration and Dosage

Administer with at least 1 other effective antituberculosis drug(s).

Average adult dose: 15 to 20 mg/kg/day taken once daily up to a maximum of 1 g/day.

Children: A dose of 10 to 20 mg/kg/day in 2 to 3 divided doses given after meals or 15 mg/kg/24 hours as a single daily dose has been recommended.

Concomitant administration of pyridoxine is recommended.

Actions

Pharmacology: Ethionamide may be bacteriostatic or bactericidal in action, depending on the concentration of the drug attained at the site of infection and the susceptibility of the infecting organism. The exact mechanism of action has not been fully explained, but the drug appears to inhibit peptide synthesis.

Pharmacokinetics:

Absorption/Distribution – Ethionamide is essentially completely absorbed following oral administration and is not subjected to any appreciable first pass metabolism.

The drug is approximately 30% bound to plasma proteins. Ethionamide is rapidly and widely distributed into body tissues and fluids, with concentrations in plasma and various organs being approximately equal. Significant concentrations also are present in cerebrospinal fluid.

Metabolism/Excretion – Ethionamide is extensively metabolized to active and inactive metabolites with less than 1% excreted as the free form in urine. Ethionamide has a plasma elimination half-life of approximately 2 hours after oral dosing.

Monitoring – Normal serum concentrations of 1 to 5 mcg/mL are usually seen 2 hours following doses of 250 to 500 mg and approximate the therapeutic range for this drug.

Contraindications

Severe hypersensitivity to ethionamide; severe hepatic damage.

Warnings/Precautions

Resistance: The use of ethionamide alone in the treatment of tuberculosis results in rapid development of resistance.

Compliance: It is recommended that directly observed therapy be practiced when patients are receiving antituberculosis medication.

Pregnancy: Category C.

Lactation: Because no information is available on the excretion of ethionamide in breast milk, administer to nursing mothers only if the benefits outweigh the risks.

Children: Investigations have been limited; do not use in pediatric patients younger than 12 years of age except when the organisms are definitely resistant to primary therapy and systemic dissemination of the disease, or other life-threatening complications of tuberculosis, is judged to be imminent.

Monitoring: Make determinations of serum transaminase (AST, ALT) prior to and monthly during therapy. Monitor blood glucose and thyroid function tests periodically.

Drug Interactions

Ethionamide may interact with isoniazid and cycloserine.

Adverse Reactions

Adverse reactions may include the following: Depression; drowsiness and asthenia; convulsions; peripheral neuritis and neuropathy; olfactory disturbances; blurred vision; diplopia; optic neuritis; dizziness; headache; restlessness; tremors; psychosis; anorexia; nausea and vomiting; diarrhea; metallic taste; hepatitis; jaundice; stomatitis; postural hypotension; skin rash; acne; alopecia; thrombocytopenia; pellagra-like syndrome; gynecomastia; impotence; menorrhagia; and increased difficulty managing diabetes mellitus.

CYCLOSERINE

Capsules; oral: 250 mg (*Rx*)	*Seromycin Pulvules* (Dura)

Indications

Treatment of active pulmonary and extrapulmonary tuberculosis (including renal disease) when organisms are susceptible, after failure of adequate treatment with the primary medications. Use in conjunction with other effective chemotherapy.

May be effective in the treatment of acute urinary tract infections caused by susceptible strains of gram-positive and gram-negative bacteria, especially *Enterobacter* sp. and *Escherichia coli*. It usually is less effective than other antimicrobial agents in the treatment of urinary tract infections caused by bacteria other than mycobacteria. Consider using only when the more conventional therapy has failed and when the organism has demonstrated sensitivity.

Administration and Dosage

Administer 500 mg to 1 g daily in divided doses monitored by blood levels. The usual initial dosage is 250 mg twice daily at 12-hour intervals for the first 2 weeks. Do not exceed 1 g/day.

Pyridoxine 200 to 300 mg/day may prevent the neurotoxic effects.

Actions

Pharmacology: Inhibits cell-wall synthesis in susceptible strains of gram-positive and gram-negative bacteria and in *Mycobacterium tuberculosis*.

Pharmacokinetics:

Absorption/Distribution – When given orally, cycloserine is rapidly absorbed, reaching peak plasma concentrations in 4 to 8 hours. It is widely distributed throughout body fluids and tissues; cerebrospinal fluid levels are similar to plasma.

Metabolism/Excretion – Approximately 35% of the drug is metabolized; 50% of a parenteral dose is excreted unchanged in the urine in the first 12 hours. About 65% of the drug is recoverable in 72 hours.

Contraindications

Hypersensitivity to cycloserine; epilepsy; depression; severe anxiety; psychosis; severe renal insufficiency; excessive concurrent use of alcohol.

Warnings/Precautions

CNS toxicity: Discontinue or reduce dosage if patient develops symptoms of CNS toxicity, such as convulsions, psychosis, somnolence, depression, confusion, hyperreflexia, headache, tremor, vertigo, paresis, or dysarthria. The risk of convulsions is increased in chronic alcoholics.

Allergic dermatitis: Discontinue the drug or reduce dosage if patient develops allergic dermatitis.

Toxicity: Toxicity is closely related to excessive blood levels (more than 30 mcg/mL) that are caused by high dosage or inadequate renal clearance. The therapeutic index in tuberculosis is small.

Obtain cultures: Obtain cultures and determine susceptibility before treatment.

Determine blood levels: Determine blood levels weekly for patients having reduced renal function, for individuals receiving more than 500 mg/day, and for those with symptoms of toxicity. Adjust dosage to maintain blood level less than 30 mcg/mL.

Anticonvulsant drugs or sedatives: Anticonvulsant drugs or sedatives may be effective in controlling symptoms of CNS toxicity, such as convulsions, anxiety, and tremor. Closely observe patients receiving more than 500 mg/day for such symptoms. Pyridoxine may prevent CNS toxicity, but its efficacy has not been proven.

Anemia: Administration has been associated in a few cases with vitamin B_{12} or folic acid deficiency, megaloblastic anemia, and sideroblastic anemia. If evidence of anemia develops, institute appropriate studies and therapy.

Renal function impairment: Patients will accumulate cycloserine and may develop toxicity if the dosage regimen is not modified. Patients with severe impairment should not receive the drug.

Pregnancy: Category C.

Lactation: Because of the potential for serious adverse reactions in nursing infants, decide whether to discontinue nursing or to discontinue the drug.

Children: Safety and dosage not established for pediatric use.

Monitoring: Monitor patients by hematologic, renal excretion, blood level, and liver function studies.

Drug Interactions

Drugs that may interact with cycloserine include alcohol, ethionamide, and isoniazid.

Adverse Reactions

Adverse reactions related to more than 500 mg/day may include the following: Convulsions; drowsiness and somnolence; headache; tremor; dysarthria; vertigo; confusion and disorientation with loss of memory; psychoses, possibly with suicidal tendencies, character changes, hyperirritability, aggression; paresis; hyperreflexia; paresthesias; major and minor (localized) clonic seizures; coma; sudden development of CHF; skin rash; and elevated transaminase.

CAPREOMYCIN

Powder for injection: 1 g (as sulfate)/10 mL vial (*Rx*) *Capastat Sulfate* (Dura)

Warning:

Undertake the use of capreomycin in patients with renal insufficiency or pre-existing auditory impairment with great caution. Weigh the risk of additional eighth nerve impairment or renal injury against benefits to be derived from therapy.

Because other parenteral antituberculosis agents (eg, streptomycin, viomycin) also have similar and sometimes irreversible toxic effects, particularly on eighth cranial nerve and renal function, simultaneous administration of these agents with capreomycin is not recommended. Use concurrent nonantituberculosis drugs (eg, polymyxin A sulfate, colistin sulfate, amikacin, gentamicin, tobramycin, vancomycin, kanamycin, neomycin) having ototoxic or nephrotoxic potential only with great caution.

Indications

Intended for use concomitantly with other antituberculosis agents in pulmonary infections caused by capreomycin-susceptible strains of *Mycobacterium tuberculosis*, when the primary agents (eg, isoniazid, rifampin) have been ineffective or cannot be used because of toxicity or the presence of resistant tubercle bacilli.

Administration and Dosage

May be administered IM or IV following reconstitution.

IV: For IV infusion, further dilute reconstituted capreomycin solution in 100 mL of 0.9% Sodium Chloride Injection and administer over 60 minutes.

IM: Give reconstituted capreomycin by deep IM injection into a large muscle mass; superficial injections may be associated with increased pain and sterile abscesses.

Usual dose: 1 g daily (not to exceed 20 mg/kg/day) given IM or IV for 60 to 120 days, followed by 1 g by either route 2 or 3 times weekly.

Renal function impairment: Reduce the dosage based on CrCl using the guidelines in the table. These dosages are designed to achieve a mean steady-state capreomycin level of 10 mcg/L.

Capreomycin Dosage in Renal Function Impairment

CrCl (mL/min)	Capreomycin clearance (L/kg/h×10^{-2})	Half-life (hours)	Dose[a](mg/kg) for the following dosing intervals		
			24 h	48 h	72 h
0	0.54	55.5	1.29	2.58	3.87
10	1.01	29.4	2.43	4.87	7.30
20	1.49	20.0	3.58	7.16	10.7
30	1.97	15.1	4.72	9.45	14.2
40	2.45	12.2	5.87	11.7	
50	2.92	10.2	7.01	14	
60	3.40	8.8	8.16		
80	4.35	6.8	10.4[b]		
100	5.31	5.6	12.7[b]		
110	5.78	5.2	13.9[b]		

[a] Initial maintenance dose estimates are given for optional dosing intervals; longer dosing intervals are expected to provide greater peak and lower trough serum capreomycin levels than shorter dosing intervals.

[b] The usual dosage for patients with normal renal function is 1 g daily, not to exceed 20 mg/kg/day, for 60 to 120 days, then 1 g 2 to 3 times weekly.

Actions

Pharmacology: A polypeptide antibiotic isolated from *Streptomyces capreolus*.

Pharmacokinetics:

Absorption – Capreomycin sulfate is not absorbed in significant quantities from the GI tract and must be administered parenterally. The AUC is similar for single-dose capreomycin (1 g) administered IM and by IV (over 1 hour) routes of administration. Capreomycin peak concentrations after IV infusion were approximately 30% higher than after IM administration.

Distribution – Peak serum concentrations following IM administration of 1 g are achieved in 1 to 2 hours. Low serum concentrations are present at 24 hours. Doses of 1 g daily for 30 days or longer produce no significant accumulation in subjects with normal renal function.

Excretion – Capreomycin is excreted essentially unaltered; 52% is excreted in the urine within 12 hours.

Contraindications

Hypersensitivity to capreomycin.

Warnings/Precautions

Neuromuscular blockade: A partial neuromuscular blockade was demonstrated after large IV doses of capreomycin. This action was enhanced by ether anesthesia (as has been reported for neomycin) and was antagonized by neostigmine.

Ototoxicity: Perform audiometric measurements and assessment of vestibular function prior to initiation of therapy and at regular intervals during treatment.

Nephrotoxicity: Perform regular tests of renal function throughout treatment, and reduce dose in patients with renal impairment. Renal injury with tubular necrosis, elevation of BUN or serum creatinine, and abnormal sediment have been noted. Reduce the dosage or withdraw the drug.

Hypokalemia: Hypokalemia may occur during therapy; therefore, determine serum potassium levels frequently.

Hypersensitivity reactions: Has occurred when capreomycin and other antituberculosis drugs were given concomitantly.

Renal function impairment: Dosage reduction is necessary. See Administration and Dosage.

Pregnancy: Category C.

Lactation: It is not known whether this drug is excreted in breast milk.

Children: Safety for use in infants and children has not been established.

Drug Interactions

Drugs that may interact with capreomycin include aminoglycosides and nondepolarizing neuromuscular blocking agents.

Adverse Reactions

Adverse reactions may include the following: Ototoxicity; tinnitus; vertigo; pain, induration, and excessive bleeding at the injection sites; sterile abscesses; leukocytosis; leukopenia; eosinophilia; abnormal results in liver function tests; urticaria; and maculopapular skin rashes.

RIFAPENTINE

Tablets: 150 mg (*Rx*)	*Priftin* (Aventis)

Indications

Tuberculosis: For the treatment of pulmonary tuberculosis (TB). Rifapentine must always be used in conjunction with at least 1 other antituberculosis drug(s) to which the isolate is susceptible.

Administration and Dosage

Do not use rifapentine alone. Concomitant administration of pyridoxine (vitamin B_6) is recommended in the malnourished, in those predisposed to neuropathy (eg, alcoholics, diabetics), and in adolescents.

Tuberculosis:

Intensive phase – 600 mg (four 150 mg tablets twice weekly) with an interval of 3 days or more (72 hours) between doses continued for 2 months. May be given with food if stomach upset, nausea, or vomiting occurs.

Continuation phase – Continue treatment with rifapentine once weekly for 4 months in combination with isoniazid or an appropriate agent for susceptible organisms. If the patient is still sputum-smear- or culture-positive, if resistant organisms are present, or if the patient is HIV-positive, follow ATS/CDC treatment guidelines.

The above recommendations apply to patients with drug-susceptible organisms. Patients with drug-resistant organisms may require longer duration treatment with other drug regimens.

CDC recommendations: Rifapentine may be used once weekly with isoniazid in the continuation phase of treatment for HIV-seronegative patients with noncavitary, drug-susceptible pulmonary tuberculosis who have negative sputum smears at completion of the initial phase of treatment. Continue this regimen for 4 months (total of 6 months of TB treatment). Have treatment for patients receiving isoniazid and rifapentine, and whose 2–month cultures are positive, extended by an additional 3 months (total of 9 months).

For adults, the maximum recommended dose is 10 mg/kg (600 mg), once weekly during the continuation phase. Data have suggested that a dose of 900 mg is well tolerated, but the clinical efficacy of this dose has not been established.

Actions

Pharmacology: Rifapentine is a rifamycin-derivative antibiotic and has a similar profile of microbiological activity to rifampin.

Pharmacokinetics:

Absorption/Distribution – The absolute bioavailability of rifapentine has not been determined. C_{max} is 15.05 mcg/mL and half-life is 13.19 hours. The estimated apparent volume of distribution is approximately 70 L. In healthy volunteers, rifapentine and 25-desacetyl rifapentine (active metabolite) were 97.7% and 93.2% bound to plasma proteins, respectively, mainly to albumin.

Metabolism/Excretion – Rifapentine is hydrolyzed by an esterase enzyme to form a microbiologically active 25-desacetyl rifapentine. Rifapentine and 25-desacetyl rifapentine account for 99% of total drug in plasma. Plasma AUC and C_{max} values of the 25-desacetyl rifapentine metabolite are 50% and 33% those of rifapentine, respectively. Eighty-seven percent of the total dose was recovered in the urine (17%) and feces (70%); more than 80% was excreted within 7 days.

Special populations –

Gender: The estimated apparent oral clearance of rifapentine for males and females was approximately 2.51 and 1.69 L/h, respectively. The clinical significance of the difference in the estimated apparent oral clearance is not known.

Contraindications

Hypersensitivity to any of the rifamycins (rifampin and rifabutin).

Warnings/Precautions

Compliance: Poor compliance with the dosage regimen, particularly daily administered nonrifamycin drugs in the intensive phase, was associated with late sputum conversion and a high relapse rate.

Hyperbilirubinemia: An isolated report showing a moderate rise in bilirubin or transaminase level is not an indication to interrupt treatment; rather, repeat tests, noting trends in the levels, and consider them in conjunction with the patient's clinical condition.

Pseudomembranous colitis: If suspected, stop rifapentine immediately and treat the patient with supportive and specific treatment without delay (eg, oral vancomycin). Products inhibiting peristalsis are contraindicated in this clinical situation.

HIV-infected patients: As with other antituberculosis treatments, when rifapentine is used in HIV-infected patients, employ a more aggressive regimen (eg, more frequent dosing). Once-weekly dosing during the continuation phase of treatment is not recommended at this time.

Porphyria: Do not use rifapentine in patients with porphyria.

Resistance: M. *tuberculosis* organisms resistant to other rifamycins are likely to be resistant to rifapentine. Cross-resistance does not appear between rifapentine and non-rifamycin antimycobacterial agents such as isoniazid and streptomycin.

Red discoloration of body fluids: Rifapentine may produce a predominately red-orange discoloration of body tissues or fluids (eg, skin, teeth, tongue, urine, feces, saliva, sputum, tears, sweat, cerebrospinal fluid). Contact lenses may become permanently stained.

Hepatic function impairment: Only give patients with abnormal liver tests or liver disease rifapentine in cases of necessity and then with caution and under strict medical supervision. In these patients, carefully monitor liver tests (especially serum transaminases) prior to therapy and then every 2 to 4 weeks during therapy. If signs of liver disease occur or worsen, discontinue rifapentine.

Pregnancy: *Category* C.

Lactation: Because of the potential for serious adverse reactions in nursing infants, decide whether to discontinue nursing or discontinue the drug, taking into account the importance of the drug to the mother.

Children: Safety and efficacy in children younger than 12 years of age have not been established.

Elderly: In general, use caution in dose selection for elderly patients, usually starting at the low end of the dosing range, reflecting the greater frequency of decreased hepatic, renal, or cardiac function and of concomitant disease or other drug therapy.

Monitoring: Obtain baseline measurements of hepatic enzymes, bilirubin, a CBC, and a platelet count (or estimate). Assess patients at least monthly during therapy. Routine laboratory monitoring for toxicity in people with normal baseline measurements is generally not necessary.

Drug Interactions

Use rifapentine with extreme caution, if at all, in patients who are also taking protease inhibitors (eg, indinavir).

Cytochrome P450: Rifapentine is an inducer of cytochromes P450 3A4 and P450 2C8/9 and may increase the metabolism of other coadministered drugs that are metabolized by these enzymes.

Note: Advise patients using oral or other systemic hormonal contraceptives to change to nonhormonal methods of birth control.

Antiarrhythmics (eg, disopyramide, mexiletine, quinidine, tocainide)
Antibiotics (eg, chloramphenicol, clarithromycin, dapsone, doxycycline, fluoroquinolones [such as ciprofloxacin])
Anticonvulsants (eg, phenytoin)
Antifungals (eg, fluconazole, itraconazole, ketoconazole)
Barbiturates
Benzodiazepines (eg, diazepam)
Beta blockers
Buspirone
Calcium channel blockers (eg, diltiazem, nifedipine, verapamil)
Cardiac glycoside preparations
Clofibrate
Corticosteroids
Estrogens
Haloperidol
HIV protease inhibitors (eg, indinavir, ritonavir, nelfinavir, saquinavir [see Rifapentine-indinavir interaction above])
HMG-CoA reductase inhibitors (eg, simvastatin)
Immunosuppressants (eg, cyclosporine, tacrolimus)
Lamotrigine
Levothyroxine
Meglitinides (eg, repaglinide)
Narcotic analgesics (eg, methadone)
Oral anticoagulants (eg, warfarin)

Oral hypoglycemic agents (eg, sulfonylureas)
Oral or other systemic hormonal contraceptives
Progestins
Quinine
Reverse transcriptase inhibitors (eg, delavirdine, zidovudine)
Sildenafil
Tamoxifen
Theophylline
Toremifene
Tricyclic antidepressants (eg, amitriptyline, nortriptyline)

Drug/Lab test interactions: Therapeutic concentrations of rifampin have been shown to inhibit standard microbiological assays for serum folate and vitamin B_{12}.

Drug/Food interactions: Food (850 total calories: 33 g protein, 55 g fat, and 58 g carbohydrate) increased AUC and C_{max} in healthy volunteers by 43% and 44%, respectively, and in asymptomatic HIV-infected volunteers by 51% and 53%, respectively.

Adverse Reactions

Adverse reactions occurring in 3% or more of patients receiving rifapentine combination therapy include the following: Rash; pyuria; proteinuria; hematuria; urinary casts; neutropenia; lymphopenia; hyperuricemia; and an increase in ALT and AST.

FOSCARNET SODIUM (Phosphonoformic acid)

Injection: 24 mg/mL (*Rx*) Various

Warning:

Renal impairment, the major toxicity, occurs to some degree in most patients. Continual assessment of a patient's risk and frequent monitoring of serum creatinine with dose adjustment for changes in renal function are imperative.

Seizures related to alterations in plasma minerals and electrolytes have been associated with foscarnet treatment. Therefore, patients must be carefully monitored for such changes and their potential sequelae. Mineral and electrolyte supplementation may be required.

Foscarnet causes alterations in plasma minerals and electrolytes that have led to seizures. Monitor patients frequently for such changes and their potential sequelae.

Indications

Cytomegalovirus (CMV) retinitis: Treatment of CMV retinitis in patients with AIDS.

Combination: Combination therapy with ganciclovir for patients who have relapsed after monotherapy with either drug.

Herpes simplex virus (HSV) infections: Treatment of acyclovir-resistant mucocutaneous HSV infections in immunocompromised patients.

Administration and Dosage

HSV infections: Foscarnet is not a cure for HSV infections. While complete healing may occur, relapse occurs in most patients.

Caution: Do not administer by rapid or bolus IV injection. Toxicity may be increased as a result of excessive plasma levels. An infusion pump must be used.

It is recommended that 750 to 1000 mL of normal saline or 5% dextrose solution be given prior to the first infusion of foscarnet to establish diuresis. With subsequent infusions, 750 to 1000 mL of hydration fluid should be given with 90 to 120 mg/kg of foscarnet, and 500 mL with 40 to 60 mg/kg of foscarnet. Hydration fluid may need to be decreased if clinically warranted. After the first dose, administer the hydration fluid concurrently with each infusion of foscarnet.

Induction treatment: The recommended initial dose for patients with normal renal function is 60 mg/kg, adjusted for individual patients' renal function, given IV at a constant rate over a minimum of 1 hour every 8 hours for 2 to 3 weeks, depending on clinical response.

Maintenance treatment: 90 to 120 mg/kg/day (individualized for renal function) as an IV infusion over 2 hours. It is recommended that most patients be started on maintenance treatment with 90 mg/kg/day. Escalation to 120 mg/kg/day may be considered should early reinduction be required because of retinitis progression.

Patients who experience progression of retinitis while receiving maintenance therapy may be retreated with the induction and maintenance regimens above.

Dose adjustment in renal impairment:

Foscarnet Dosing Guide Based on CrCl for Induction

	HSV: Equivalent to		CMV: Equivalent to
CrCl (mL/min/kg)	80 mg/kg/day	120 mg/kg/day	180 mg/kg/day
> 1.4	40 q 12 h	40 q 8 h	60 q 8 h
> 1 to 1.4	30 q 12 h	30 q 8 h	45 q 8 h
> 0.8 to 1	20 q 12 h	35 q 12 h	50 q 12 h
> 0.6 to 0.8	35 q 24 h	25 q 12 h	40 q 12 h
> 0.5 to 0.6	25 q 24 h	40 q 24 h	60 q 24 h
≥ 0.4 to 0.5	20 q 24 h	35 q 24 h	50 q 24 h
< 0.4	Not recommended	Not recommended	Not recommended

Foscarnet Dosing Guide Based on CrCl for Maintenance		
CrCl (mL/min/kg)	CMV: Equivalent to	
	90 mg/kg/day	120 mg/kg/day
> 1.4	90 q 24 h	120 q 24 h
> 1 to 2.4	70 q 24 h	90 q 24 h
> 0.8 to 1	50 q 24 h	65 q 24 h
> 0.6 to 0.8	80 q 48 h	105 q 48 h
> 0.5 to 0.6	60 q 48 h	30 q 48 h
≥ 0.4 to 0.5	50 q 48 h	65 q 48 h
< 0.4	Not recommended	Not recommended

Actions

Pharmacology: Foscarnet exerts its antiviral activity by a selective inhibition at the pyrophosphate binding site on virus-specific DNA polymerases and reverse transcriptases at concentrations that do not affect cellular DNA polymerases. CMV strains resistant to ganciclovir may be sensitive to foscarnet. Acyclovir- or ganciclovir-resistant mutants may be resistant to foscarnet.

Pharmacokinetics: Foscarnet is 14% to 17% bound to plasma protein at plasma drug concentrations of 1 to 1000 mcM.

Approximately 80% to 90% of IV foscarnet is excreted unchanged in the urine of patients with normal renal function. Both tubular secretion and glomerular filtration account for urinary elimination of foscarnet.

Plasma half-life increases with the severity of renal impairment. Half-lives of 2 to 8 hours occurred in patients having estimated or measured 24-hour CrCl of 44 to 90 mL/min.

The foscarnet terminal half-life determined by urinary excretion was 87.5 ± 41.8 hours, possibly because of release of foscarnet from bone. Postmortem data provide evidence that foscarnet does accumulate in bone in humans.

Variable penetration into cerebrospinal fluid (CSF) has been observed. Disease-related defects in the blood-brain barrier may be responsible for the variations seen.

Contraindications

Hypersensitivity to foscarnet.

Warnings/Precautions

Mineral and electrolyte imbalances: Foscarnet has been associated with changes in serum electrolytes including hypocalcemia (15%), hypophosphatemia (8%) and hyperphosphatemia (6%), hypomagnesemia (15%), and hypokalemia (16%). Foscarnet is associated with a transient, dose-related decrease in ionized serum calcium, which may not be reflected in total serum calcium.

Accidental exposure: Accidental skin and eye contact with foscarnet sodium solution may cause local irritation and burning sensation. Flush the exposed area with water.

Other CMV infections: Safety and efficacy have not been established for the treatment of other CMV infections (eg, pneumonitis, gastroenteritis); congenital or neonatal CMV disease; nonimmunocompromised individuals.

Neurotoxicity and seizures: Foscarnet was associated with seizures in AIDS patients.

Statistically significant risk factors associated with seizures were low baseline absolute neutrophil count (ANC), impaired baseline renal function, and low total serum calcium. Several cases of seizures were associated with death.

Diagnosis of CMV retinitis: Diagnosis of CMV retinitis should be established by an ophthalmologist familiar with the retinal presentation of these conditions.

Toxicity/Local irritation: The maximum single-dose administered was 120 mg/kg by IV infusion over 2 hours. It is likely that larger doses, or more rapid infusions, would result in increased toxicity. Infuse solutions containing foscarnet only into veins with adequate blood flow to permit rapid dilution and distribution, and avoid local irritation. Local irritation and ulcerations of penile epithelium have occurred in patients receiving foscarnet, possibly because of drug in urine. Adequate hydration with close attention to personal hygiene may minimize the occurrence of such events.

Anemia: Anemia occurred in 33% of patients. Granulocytopenia occurred in 17% of patients.

Renal function impairment: The major toxicity of foscarnet is renal impairment, which occurs to some degree in most patients. Approximately 33% of 189 patients with AIDS and CMV retinitis who received IV foscarnet in clinical studies developed significant impairment of renal function, manifested by a rise in serum creatinine concentration to 2 mg/dL or more.

Pregnancy: Category C.

Lactation: It is not known whether foscarnet is excreted in breast milk.

Children: The safety and efficacy of foscarnet in children have not been studied.

Elderly: Because these individuals frequently have reduced glomerular filtration, pay particular attention to assessing renal function before and during administration.

Monitoring: The majority of patients will experience some decrease in renal function due to foscarnet administration. Therefore, it is recommended that CrCl be determined at baseline, 2 to 3 times/week during induction therapy, and at least once every 1 to 2 weeks during maintenance therapy, with foscarnet dose adjusted accordingly. More frequent monitoring may be required for some patients. It also is recommended that a 24-hour CrCl be determined at baseline and periodically thereafter to ensure correct dosing. Discontinue if CrCl drops to less than 0.4 mL/min/kg.

Because of foscarnet's propensity to chelate divalent metal ions and alter levels of serum electrolytes, closely monitor patients for such changes. It is recommended that a schedule similar to that recommended for serum creatinine be used to monitor serum calcium, magnesium, potassium, and phosphorus.

Careful monitoring and appropriate management of creatinine are of particular importance in patients with conditions that may predispose them to seizures.

Drug Interactions

Drugs that may interact with foscarnet include nephrotoxic drugs (eg, aminoglycosides, amphotericin B, IV pentamidine), pentamidine, and zidovudine.

Foscarnet decreases serum levels of ionized calcium. Exercise particular caution when other drugs known to influence serum calcium levels are used concurrently.

Adverse Reactions

Adverse reactions occurring in at least 3% of patients include fever; nausea; anemia; diarrhea; abnormal renal function including acute renal failure, decreased CrCl and increased serum creatinine; vomiting; headache; seizure; death; marrow suppression; injection site pain or inflammation; paresthesia; dizziness; involuntary muscle contractions; hypoesthesia; neuropathy; sensory disturbances; influenza-like symptoms; bacterial/fungal infections; rectal hemorrhage; dry mouth; melena; flatulence; ulcerative stomatitis; pancreatitis; granulocytopenia; leukopenia; thrombocytopenia; platelet abnormalities; thrombosis; WBC abnormalities; lymphadenopathy; electrolyte abnormalities; neurotoxicity; renal impairment; decreased weight; increased alkaline phosphatase, LDH and BUN; acidosis; cachexia; thirst; depression; confusion; anxiety; aggressive reaction; hallucination; coughing; dyspnea; pneumonia; sinusitis; pharyngitis; rhinitis; respiratory disorders or insufficiency; pulmonary infiltration; stridor; pneumothorax; hemoptysis; bronchospasm; rash; increased sweating; pruritus; skin ulceration; seborrhea; erythematous rash; maculopapular rash; vision abnormalities; taste perversions; eye abnormalities; eye pain; conjunctivitis; hypertension; palpitations; ECG abnormalities.

GANCICLOVIR (DHPG)

Capsules: 250 and 500 mg (*Rx*)	Various
Powder for injection, lyophilized: 500 mg/vial ganciclovir (*Rx*)	Various, *Cytovene* (Genentech)

Warning:

The clinical toxicity of ganciclovir includes granulocytopenia, anemia, and thrombocytopenia. In animal studies, ganciclovir was carcinogenic, teratogenic, and caused aspermatogenesis.

Ganciclovir IV is indicated for use only in the treatment of cytomegalovirus (CMV) retinitis in immunocompromised patients and for the prevention of CMV disease in transplant patients at risk for CMV disease.

Ganciclovir capsules are indicated only for prevention of CMV disease in patients with advanced HIV infection at risk for CMV disease and for maintenance treatment of CMV retinitis in immunocompromised patients.

Because oral ganciclovir is associated with a risk of more rapid rate of CMV retinitis progression, use only in those patients for whom this risk is balanced by the benefit associated with avoiding daily IV infusions.

Indications

IV:

CMV retinitis – Treatment of CMV retinitis in immunocompromised patients, including patients with AIDS.

CMV disease – Prevention of CMV disease in transplant recipients at risk for CMV disease.

Oral:

CMV retinitis – Alternative to the IV formulation for maintenance treatment of CMV retinitis in immunocompromised patients, including patients with AIDS, in whom retinitis is stable following appropriate induction therapy and for whom the risk of more rapid progression is balanced by the benefit associated with avoiding daily IV infusions.

CMV disease – Prevention of CMV disease in individuals with advanced HIV infection at risk for developing CMV disease.

Administration and Dosage

IV: Do not administer by rapid or bolus IV injection. The toxicity may be increased as a result of excessive plasma levels. Do not exceed the recommended infusion rate. IM or subcutaneous injection of reconstituted ganciclovir may result in severe tissue irritation because of high pH.

CMV retinitis treatment (normal renal function):

Induction – Recommended initial dose is 5 mg/kg (given IV at a constant rate of 1 hour) every 12 hours for 14 to 21 days. Do not use oral ganciclovir for induction.

Maintenance –

IV: Following induction, the recommended maintenance dose is 5 mg/kg given as a constant rate IV infusion over 1 hour once per day 7 days per week, or 6 mg/kg once per day 5 days/week.

Oral: Following induction, the recommended maintenance dose of oral ganciclovir is 1,000 mg 3 times daily with food. Alternatively, the dosing regimen of 500 mg 6 times daily every 3 hours with food during waking hours may be used.

For patients who experience progression of CMV retinitis while receiving maintenance treatment with either formulation of ganciclovir, reinduction treatment is recommended.

Prevention of CMV disease in transplant recipients with normal renal function:

IV – The recommended initial dose of IV ganciclovir for patients with normal renal function is 5 mg/kg (given IV at a constant rate over 1 hour) every 12 hours for 7 to 14 days, followed by 5 mg/kg once daily 7 days/week or 6 mg/kg once daily 5 days/week.

Oral – The recommended prophylactic dosage is 1,000 mg 3 times daily with food.

The duration of treatment with ganciclovir in transplant recipients is dependent on the duration and degree of immunosuppression. In controlled clinical trials in bone marrow allograft recipients, IV ganciclovir treatment was continued until day 100 to 120 posttransplantation. CMV disease occurred in several patients who discontinued treatment with IV ganciclovir prematurely. In heart allograft recipients, the onset of newly diagnosed CMV disease occurred after treatment with IV ganciclovir was stopped at day 28 post-transplant, suggesting that continued dosing may be necessary to prevent late occurrence of CMV disease in this patient population.

Prevention of CMV disease in patients with advanced HIV infection and normal renal function: The recommended dose of ganciclovir capsules is 1,000 mg 3 times daily with food.

Renal function impairment:

IV – Refer to the table for recommended doses and adjust the dosing interval as indicated.

IV Ganciclovir Dose in Renal Impairment

CrCl (mL/min)	Ganciclovir induction dose (mg/kg)	Dosing interval (hours)	Ganciclovir maintenance dose (mg/kg)	Dosing interval (hours)
≥ 70	5	12	5	24
50 to 69	2.5	12	2.5	24
25 to 49	2.5	24	1.25	24
10 to 24	1.25	24	0.625	24
< 10	1.25	3 times/week following hemodialysis	0.625	3 times/week following hemodialysis

Hemodialysis: Dosing for patients undergoing hemodialysis should not exceed 1.25 mg/kg 3 times/week, following each hemodialysis session. Give shortly after completion of the hemodialysis session, since hemodialysis reduces plasma levels by approximately 50%.

Oral: In renal impairment, modify the dose of oral ganciclovir as follows:

Oral Ganciclovir Dose in Renal Impairment

CrCl (mL/min)	Ganciclovir doses
≥ 70	1,000 mg 3 times daily or 500 mg q 3 h, 6 times/day
50 to 69	1,500 mg daily or 500 mg 3 times daily
25 to 49	1,000 mg daily or 500 mg twice daily
10 to 24	500 mg daily
< 10	500 mg 3 times/week, following hemodialysis

Patient monitoring: Because of the frequency of granulocytopenia, anemia, and thrombocytopenia, it is recommended that CBCs and platelet counts be performed frequently, especially in patients in whom ganciclovir or other nucleoside analogs have previously resulted in cytopenia, or in whom neutrophil counts are less than 1,000/mcL at the beginning of treatment. Patients should have serum creatinine or CrCl values followed carefully to allow for dosage adjustment in renally impaired patients.

Reduction of dose: Dose reductions are required with IV therapy and should be considered with oral therapy for patients with renal impairment and for those with neutropenia, anemia, or thrombocytopenia. Do not administer in severe neutropenia (ANC less than 500/mcL) or severe thrombocytopenia (platelets less than 25,000/mcL).

Actions

Pharmacology: Ganciclovir, a synthetic guanine derivative active against CMV, is an acyclic nucleoside analog of 2'-deoxyguanosine that inhibits replication of herpes viruses both in vitro and in vivo. Sensitive human viruses include CMV, herpes simplex virus (HSV)-1 and -2, herpes virus type 6, Epstein-Barr virus, varicella-zoster virus, and hepatitis B virus.

Pharmacokinetics:

Absorption – Absolute bioavailability of oral ganciclovir under fasting conditions was approximately 5%; following food it was 6% to 9%. When given with a high-fat meal, steady-state AUC increased and there was a significant prolongation of time to peak serum concentrations.

At the end of a 1-hour IV infusion of 5 mg/kg, total AUC and C_{max} ranged between 22.1 and 26.8 mcg•h/mL and 8.27 and 9 mcg/mL, respectively.

Distribution – The steady-state volume of distribution after IV administration was 0.74 L/kg. Cerebrospinal fluid concentrations obtained 0.25 and 5.67 hours postdose in 3 patients who received 2.5 mg/kg ganciclovir IV every 8 or 12 hours ranged from 0.31 to 0.68 mcg/mL, representing 24% to 70% of the respective plasma concentrations. Binding to plasma proteins was 1% to 2% over ganciclovir concentrations of 0.5 and 51 mcg/mL.

Metabolism – Following oral administration of a single 1,000 mg dose, 86% of the administered dose was recovered in the feces and 5% was recovered in the urine.

Excretion – When administered IV, ganciclovir exhibits linear pharmacokinetics over the range of 1.6 to 5 mg/kg and when administered orally, it exhibits linear kinetics up to a total daily dose of 4 g/day. Renal excretion of unchanged drug by glomerular filtration and active tubular secretion is the major route of elimination. In patients with normal renal function, 91.3% of IV ganciclovir was recovered unmetabolized in the urine. After oral administration, steady state is achieved within 24 hours. Renal clearance following oral administration was 3.1 mL/min/kg. Half-life was 3.5 hours following IV administration and 4.8 following oral use.

Children: At an IV dose of 4 or 6 mg/kg in 27 neonates (2 to 49 days of age), the pharmacokinetic parameters were, respectively, C_{max} of 5.5 and 7 mcg/mL, systemic clearance of 3.14 and 3.56 mL/min/kg and half-life of 2.4 hours for both.

Contraindications

Hypersensitivity to ganciclovir or acyclovir.

Warnings/Precautions

CMV disease: Safety and efficacy have not been established for congenital or neonatal CMV disease, nor for the treatment of established CMV disease other than retinitis, nor for use in nonimmunocompromised individuals. The safety and efficacy of oral ganciclovir have not been established for treating any manifestation of CMV disease other than maintenance treatment of CMV retinitis.

Diagnosis of CMV retinitis: The diagnosis should be made by indirect ophthalmoscopy. Other conditions in the differential diagnosis of CMV retinitis include candidiasis, toxoplasmosis, histoplasmosis, retinal scars, and cotton wool spots, any of which may produce a retinal appearance similar to CMV. The diagnosis may be supported by a culture of CMV from urine, blood, or throat, but a negative CMV culture does not rule out CMV retinitis.

Retinal detachment: Retinal detachment has been observed in subjects with CMV retinitis both before and after initiation of therapy with ganciclovir. Its relationship to therapy is unknown. Patients with CMV retinitis should have frequent ophthalmologic evaluations to monitor the status of their retinitis and to detect any other retinal pathology.

Hematologic: Do not administer if the absolute neutrophil count is less than $500/mm^3$ or the platelet count is less than $25,000/mm^3$. Granulocytopenia (neutropenia), anemia, and thrombocytopenia have been observed in patients treated with ganciclovir. The frequency and severity of these events vary widely in different patient populations. Therefore, use with caution in patients with pre-existing cytopenias or with a history of cytopenic reactions to other drugs, chemicals, or irradiation.

Granulocytopenia usually occurs during the first or second week of treatment, but may occur at any time during treatment. Cell counts usually begin to recover within 3 to 7 days of discontinuing the drug. Colony-stimulating factors have increased neutrophil and WBC counts in patients receiving IV ganciclovir for CMV retinitis.

Large doses/rapid infusion: The maximum single dose administered was 6 mg/kg by IV infusion over 1 hour. Larger doses have resulted in increased toxicity. It is likely that more rapid infusions would also result in increased toxicity.

Phlebitis/Pain at injection site: Initially, reconstituted ganciclovir solutions have a high pH (pH 11). Despite further dilution in IV fluids, phlebitis or pain may occur at the site of IV infusion. Take care to infuse solutions containing ganciclovir only into veins with adequate blood flow to permit rapid dilution and distribution.

Hydration: Because ganciclovir is excreted by the kidneys and normal clearance depends on adequate renal function, administration of ganciclovir should be accompanied by adequate hydration.

Renal function impairment: Use ganciclovir with caution. Half-life and plasma/serum concentrations of ganciclovir will be increased because of reduced renal clearance (see Administration and Dosage).

If renal function is impaired, dosage adjustments are required for ganciclovir IV and should be considered for oral ganciclovir. Base such adjustments on measured or estimated CrCl values.

Hemodialysis reduces plasma levels of ganciclovir by approximately 50%.

Carcinogenesis: Consider ganciclovir a potential carcinogen.

Mutagenesis: Because of the mutagenic and teratogenic potential of ganciclovir, advise women of childbearing potential to use effective contraception during treatment. Similarly, advise men to practice barrier contraception during and for at least 90 days following treatment with ganciclovir.

Fertility impairment: Although data in humans have not been obtained regarding this effect, it is considered probable that ganciclovir, at recommended doses, causes temporary or permanent inhibition of spermatogenesis.

Pregnancy: Category C.

Lactation: It is not known whether ganciclovir is excreted in breast milk. The possibility of serious adverse reactions from ganciclovir in nursing infants is considered likely. Instruct mothers to discontinue nursing if they are receiving ganciclovir. The minimum interval before nursing can safely be resumed after the last dose of ganciclovir is unknown.

Children: Safety and efficacy in children have not been established. The use of ganciclovir in children warrants extreme caution to the probability of long-term carcinogenicity and reproductive toxicity. Administer to children only after careful evaluation and only if the potential benefits of treatment outweigh the risks. Oral ganciclovir has not been studied in children younger than 13 years of age.

There has been very limited clinical experience using ganciclovir for the treatment of CMV retinitis in patients younger than 12 years of age.

The spectrum of adverse reactions reported in 120 immunocompromised pediatric clinical trial participants with serious CMV infections receiving IV ganciclovir were similar to those reported in adults. Granulocytopenia (17%) and thrombocytopenia (10%) were most commonly reported.

Elderly: Pharmacokinetic profile in elderly patients is not established. Because elderly individuals frequently have a reduced glomerular filtration rate, pay particular attention to assessing renal function before and during ganciclovir therapy.

Monitoring: Because of the frequency of neutropenia, anemia, and thrombocytopenia in patients receiving ganciclovir, it is recommended that CBCs and platelet counts be performed frequently, especially in patients in whom ganciclovir or other nucleoside analogs have previously resulted in leukopenia, or in whom neutrophil counts are less than $1{,}000/mm^3$ at the beginning of treatment. Patients should also have serum creatinine or CrCl values followed carefully.

Drug Interactions

Drugs that may affect ganciclovir include imipenem-cilastatin, nephrotoxic drugs, probenecid, didanosine, and zidovudine. Drugs that may be affected by ganciclovir include cytotoxic drugs, didanosine, and zidovudine.

Adverse Reactions

Adverse reactions occurring in at least 3% of AIDS patients include fever; infection; chills; sepsis; diarrhea; anorexia; vomiting; leukopenia; anemia; thrombocytopenia; neuropathy; sweating; pruritus.

VALGANCICLOVIR

Tablets: 450 mg (*Rx*)	*Valcyte* (Roche)
Powder for solution, oral: 50 mg/mL (*Rx*)	*Valcyte* (Roche)

Warning:

The clinical toxicity of valganciclovir, which is metabolized to ganciclovir, includes granulocytopenia, anemia, and thrombocytopenia. In animal studies, ganciclovir was carcinogenic, teratogenic, and caused aspermatogenesis.

Indications

Cytomegalovirus (CMV) retinitis: For the treatment of CMV retinitis in patients with acquired immunodeficiency syndrome (AIDS).

CMV disease: For the prevention of CMV disease in kidney, heart, and kidney-pancreas transplant adult patients at high risk (Donor CMV seropositive/Recipient CMV seronegative [(D+/R−)]); for the prevetion of CMV disease in kidney and heart transplant pediatric patients (4 months to 16 years of age) at high risk.

Administration and Dosage

Strict adherence to dosage recommendations is essential to avoid overdose. Valganciclovir tablets cannot be substituted for ganciclovir capsules on a one-to-one basis.

Adults:

CMV retinitis (normal renal function) –

Active disease:

Initial dosage – 900 mg (two 450 mg tablets) twice daily for 21 days with food.

Maintenance dosage – Following initial treatment, or in patients with inactive CMV retinitis, the recommended dosage is 900 mg (two 450 mg tablets) once daily with food.

Prevention of CMV disease: 900 mg (two 450 mg tablets) once daily with food starting within 10 days of transplantation until 100 days posttransplantation.

Children –

Cytomegalovirus disease prevention:

4 months to 16 years of age –

Usual dosage: Dose is administered once daily starting within 10 days of transplantation until 100 days posttransplantation and is calculated using the following equation (BSA = body surface area; CrCl = creatinine clearance):

Dose (mg) = 7 × BSA × CrCl (calculated using a modified Schwartz formula) where

$$\text{BSA (m}^2\text{)} = \sqrt{\frac{\text{ht (cm)} \times \text{wt (kg)}}{3600}}$$

$$\text{CrCl (mL/min/1.73 m}^2\text{)} = K \times \frac{\text{body length or height (cm)}}{\text{serum creatinine (mg/dL)}}$$

Where K = 0.45 for patients younger than 1 year of age; K = 0.45 for patients 1 to younger than 2 years of age (note: K value is 0.45 instead of the typical value of 0.55); K = 0.55 for boys 2 to younger than 13 years of age and for girls 2 to 16 years of age; and K = 0.7 for boys 13 to 16 years of age.

All calculated doses should be rounded to the nearest 25 mg increment for the actual deliverable dose. If the calculated dose exceeds 900 mg, a maximum dose of 900 mg should be administered.

Maximum dose: 900 mg once daily.

Renal impairment: Monitor serum creatinine or CrCl levels carefully. Dosage adjustment is required according to CrCl, as shown in the table below. Increased monitoring for cytopenias may be warranted in patients with renal impairment.

Oral Valganciclovir in Renal Impairment

CrCl[a] (mL/min)	Initial dose	Maintenance/ prevention dose
≥ 60	900 mg twice daily	900 mg once daily
40 to 59	450 mg twice daily	450 mg once daily
25 to 39	450 mg once daily	450 mg every 2 days
10 to 24	450 mg every 2 days	450 mg twice weekly
< 10 (on hemodialysis[b])	Not recommended	Not recommended

[a] Estimated creatinine clearance.
[b] For patients on hemodialysis, it is recommended that ganciclovir be used rather than valganciclovir.

Administration: Adults should use valganciclovir tablets, not valganciclovir oral solution.

Children – Valganciclovir tablets may be used if the calculated doses are within 10% of the available tablet strength (450 mg).

Handling and disposal: Exercise caution in the handling of valganciclovir tablets. Do not break or crush tablets. Because valganciclovir is considered a potential teratogen and carcinogen in humans, observe caution in handling broken tablets, the powder for oral solution, and the constituted oral solution. Avoid direct contact of broken or crushed tablets, the powder for oral solution, and the constituted oral solution with skin or mucous membranes. If such contact occurs, wash thoroughly with soap and water, and rinse eyes thoroughly with plain water.

Because ganciclovir shares some of the properties of antitumor agents (ie, carcinogenicity and mutagenicity), consider handling and disposing according to guidelines issued for antineoplastic drugs.

Actions

Pharmacology: Valganciclovir is an L-valyl ester (prodrug) of ganciclovir. After oral administration, both diastereomers are rapidly converted to ganciclovir by intestinal and hepatic esterases. Ganciclovir is a synthetic analog of 2′-deoxyguanosine, which inhibits replication of human CMV.

Pharmacokinetics:

Absorption – Valganciclovir is well absorbed from the GI tract and rapidly metabolized in the intestinal wall and liver to ganciclovir. The absolute bioavailability of ganciclovir from valganciclovir tablets following administration with food was about 60%. Ganciclovir median T_{max} following administration of 450 to 2625 mg valganciclovir tablets ranged from 1 to 3 hours. Systemic exposure to the prodrug, valganciclovir, is transient and low, and the AUC_{24} and C_{max} values are about 1% and 3% of those of ganciclovir, respectively.

Distribution – Plasma protein binding of ganciclovir is 1% to 2%. When ganciclovir was administered IV, the steady-state volume of distribution of ganciclovir was about 0.703 L/kg (n = 69).

Metabolism – Valganciclovir is rapidly hydrolyzed to ganciclovir; no other metabolites have been detected.

Excretion – The major route of elimination of valganciclovir is by renal excretion as ganciclovir through glomerular filtration and active tubular secretion.

The terminal half-life of ganciclovir following oral administration of valganciclovir tablets to either healthy or HIV-positive/CMV-positive subjects was about 4.08 hours (n = 73), and that following administration of IV ganciclovir was about 3.81 hours (n = 69).

Contraindications

Hypersensitivity to valganciclovir, ganciclovir, or any component of the formulation.

Warnings/Precautions

Acute renal failure: Acute renal failure may occur in elderly patients with or without reduced renal function, patients receiving potential nephrotoxic drugs, and patients without adequate hydration.

Hematologic: Valganciclovir tablets should not be administered if the absolute neutrophil count is less than 500 cells/mm^3, the platelet count is less than 25,000/mm^3, or the hemoglobin is less than 8 g/dL.

Severe leukopenia, neutropenia, anemia, thrombocytopenia, pancytopenia, bone marrow depression, and aplastic anemia have been observed in patients treated with valganciclovir tablets (and ganciclovir) (see Precautions and Adverse Reactions).

Cytopenia may occur at any time during treatment and may increase with continued dosing. Cell counts usually begin to recover within 3 to 7 days of discontinuing drug.

Liver transplant patients: In liver transplant patients, there was a significantly higher incidence of tissue-invasive CMV disease in the valganciclovir-treated group compared with the oral ganciclovir group. Valganciclovir is not indicated for use in liver transplant patients.

Toxicity: The clinical toxicity of valganciclovir, which is metabolized to ganciclovir, includes granulocytopenia, anemia, and thrombocytopenia. In animal studies, ganciclovir was carcinogenic, teratogenic, and caused aspermatogenesis.

Renal function impairment: If renal function is impaired, dosage adjustments are required for valganciclovir.

For adult patients on hemodialysis (CrCl less than 10 mL/min), it is recommended that ganciclovir be used.

Fertility impairment: It is considered probable that in humans, valganciclovir at the recommended doses may cause temporary or permanent inhibition of spermatogenesis. Animal data also indicate that suppression of fertility in females may occur.

Because of the mutagenic and teratogenic potential of ganciclovir, advise women of childbearing potential to use effective contraception during treatment. Similarly, advise men to practice barrier contraception during and for at least 90 days following treatment with valganciclovir.

Pregnancy: Category C.

Lactation: It is not known whether ganciclovir or valganciclovir is excreted in human milk. Because of potential for serious adverse events in breast-feeding infants, decide whether to discontinue breast-feeding or the drug, taking into consideration the importance of the drug to the mother. The Centers for Disease Control and Prevention recommend that HIV-infected mothers not breast-feed their infants to avoid risking postnatal transmission of HIV.

Children: The safety and efficacy of valganciclovir for oral solution and tablets have not been established in children for prevention of CMV disease in liver transplant patients, solid organ transplants other than those indicated, pediatric solid organ transplant patients younger than 4 months of age, or for treatment of congenital CMV disease

Elderly: The pharmacokinetic characteristics of valganciclovir in elderly patients have not been established. Since elderly individuals frequently have a reduced glomerular filtration rate, pay particular attention to assessing renal function before and during administration of valganciclovir.

Monitoring: Because of the frequency of neutropenia, anemia, and thrombocytopenia in patients receiving valganciclovir tablets, it is recommended that complete blood counts and platelet counts be performed frequently, especially in patients in whom ganciclovir or other nucleoside analogs have previously resulted in leukopenia, or in whom neutrophil counts are less than 1000 cells/mm^3 at the beginning of treatment. Increased monitoring for cytopenias may be warranted if therapy with oral ganciclovir is changed to oral valganciclovir, because of increased plasma concentrations of ganciclovir after valganciclovir administration.

Increased serum creatinine levels have been observed in trials evaluating valganciclovir tablets. Patients should have serum creatinine or CrCl values monitored carefully to allow for dosage adjustments in renally impaired patients. The mechanism of impairment of renal function is not known.

Drug Interactions

No in vivo drug interaction studies were conducted with valganciclovir. However, because valganciclovir is rapidly and extensively converted to ganciclovir, interactions associated with ganciclovir will be expected for valganciclovir tablets (see Ganciclovir monograph).

Drugs that may affect valganciclovir include didanosine, mycophenolate mofetil, myelosuppressive drugs or irradiation, nephrotoxic drugs, probenecid, trimethoprim, and zidovudine. Drugs that may be affected by valganciclovir include didanosine, mycophenolate mofetil, myelosuppressive drugs or irradiation, and zidovudine.

Drug/Food interactions: When valganciclovir tablets were administered with a high-fat meal containing about 600 total calories (31.1 g fat, 51.6 g carbohydrates, and 22.2 g protein) at a dose of 875 mg once daily to 16 HIV-positive subjects, the steady-state ganciclovir AUC increased by 30% (95% CI 12% to 51%), and the C_{max} increased by 14% (95% CI −5% to 36%), without any prolongation in time to peak plasma concentrations (T_{max}). Administer valganciclovir tablets with food.

Adverse Reactions

Adverse reactions occurring in at least 3% of patients include the following: Abdominal pain, anemia, diarrhea, graft rejection, headache, hypertension, insomnia, leukopenia, nausea, neutropenia, paresthesia, peripheral neuropathy, pyrexia, retinal detachment, increased serum creatinine, thrombocytopenia, tremors, vomiting.

ACYCLOVIR (Acycloguanosine)

Tablets: 400 and 800 mg (*Rx*)	Various, *Zovirax* (GlaxoSmithKline)
Capsules: 200 mg (*Rx*)	
Suspension: 200 mg/5 mL (*Rx*)	
Injection: 50 mg/mL (*Rx*)	
Powder for injection: 500 mg/vial (as sodium) (*Rx*)	

Indications

Neonatal herpes simplex virus infection: Treatment of neonatal herpes infections.

Parenteral: Treatment of initial and recurrent mucosal and cutaneous herpes simplex virus (HSV)-1 and -2 and varicella-zoster virus (VZV/shingles) infections in immunocompromised patients.

Herpes simplex encephalitis.

Severe initial clinical episodes of genital herpes in patients who are not immunocompromised.

Oral: Treatment of initial episodes and management of recurrent episodes of genital herpes.

Administration and Dosage

Parenteral: For IV infusion only. Avoid rapid or bolus IV, IM, or subcutaneous injection. Administer over at least 1 hour to prevent renal tubular damage. Initiate therapy as soon as possible following onset of signs and symptoms.

IV Acyclovir Dosage/Management Guidelines		
	Dosage	
Indication	Adults	Children (< 12 years)
Mucosal and cutaneous HSV infections in immunocompromised patients	5 mg/kg infused at a constant rate over 1 hour every 8 hours (15 mg/kg/day) for 7 days[a]	10 mg/kg^2 infused at a constant rate over 1 hour every 8 hours for 7 days
Varicella-zoster infections (shingles) in immunocompromised patients[b]	10 mg/kg infused at a constant rate over 1 hour every 8 hours for 7 days[c]	20 mg/kg infused at a constant rate over at least 1 hour every 8 hours for 7 days
Herpes simplex encephalitis	10 mg/kg infused at a constant rate over at least 1 hour every 8 hours for 10 days	20 mg/kg infused at a constant rate over at least 1 hour every 8 hours for 10 days[c]
Neonatal HSV infections	NA	10 mg/kg infused at a constant rate over 1 hour every 8 hours for 10 days[d]

[a] For severe initial clinical episodes of herpes genitalis, use the same dose for 5 days.
[b] Base dosage for obese patients on ideal body weight (10 mg/kg).
[c] Children 3 months to 12 years of age.
[d] Children birth to 3 months. Doses of 15 or 20 mg/kg infused at a constant rate over 1 hour every 8 hours have been used; however, safety and efficacy of these doses are unknown.

CDC recommendations for neonatal herpes infections –

Disseminated and CNS disease: 20 mg/kg IV every 8 hours for 21 days.

Mucocutaneous disease: 20 mg/kg IV every 8 hours for 14 days.

Renal function impairment, acute or chronic –

Parenteral Acyclovir Dosage in Renal Function Impairment		
CrCl (mL/min/1.73 m^2)	Percent of recommended dose	Dosing interval (hours)
> 50	100%	8
25 to 50	100%	12
10 to 25	100%	24
0 to 10	50%	24

Hemodialysis – The mean plasma half-life of acyclovir during hemodialysis is approximately 5 hours; a 60% decrease in plasma concentrations follows a 6-hour dialysis period. Therefore, administer a dose after each dialysis.

Oral:

Herpes simplex – For severe disease that requires hospitalization (eg, disseminated infection, pneumonitis, hepatitis, meningitis, encephalitis) IV acyclovir therapy is recommended.

Initial genital herpes: 200 mg every 4 hours 5 times/day for 10 days.

Chronic suppressive therapy for recurrent disease: 400 mg 2 times/day for up to 12 months, followed by reevaluation. Reevaluate the frequency and severity of the patient's HSV after 1 year of therapy to assess the need for continuation of therapy.

Intermittent therapy: 200 mg every 4 hours 5 times daily for 5 days. Initiate therapy at the earliest sign or symptom (prodrome) of recurrence.

CDC guidelines recommend the following oral regimens –

First initial clinical episode of genital herpes: 400 mg 3 times/day for 7 to 10 days or 200 mg 5 times/day for 7 to 10 days.

Episodic therapy for recurrent genital herpes: 400 mg 3 times/day or 200 mg 5 times/day for 5 days.

Herpes zoster, acute treatment – 800 mg every 4 hours 5 times/day for 7 to 10 days.

Chickenpox – Initiate treatment at earliest sign or symptom. There are no data about the efficacy of therapy initiated more than 24 hours after onset of signs and symptoms.

Adults and children (greater than 40 kg): 800 mg 4 times daily for 5 days.

Children (2 years and older; 40 kg or less): 20 mg/kg 4 times daily for 5 days.

Renal impairment, acute or chronic –

Oral Acyclovir Dosage in Renal Function Impairment			
Normal dosage regimen (5× daily)	CrCl (mL/min/1.73 m^2)	Adjusted dosage regimen	
		Dose (mg)	Dosing interval
200 mg every 4 hours	> 10 0 to 10	200 200	Every 4 hours, 5× daily Every 12 hours
400 mg every 12 hours	> 10 0 to 10	400 200	Every 12 hours Every 12 hours
800 mg every 4 hours	> 25 10 to 25 0 to 10	800 800 800	Every 4 hours, 5× daily Every 8 hours Every 12 hours

Hemodialysis – For patients that require hemodialysis, adjust dosing schedule so that a dose is administered after each dialysis. No supplemental dose is necessary after peritoneal dialysis.

Bioequivalence: Acyclovir suspension was shown to be bioequivalent to acyclovir capsules, and one 800 mg acyclovir tablet was shown to be bioequivalent to four 200 mg acyclovir capsules.

Actions

Pharmacology: A synthetic purine nucleoside analog, acyclovir has in vitro and in vivo inhibitory activity against HSV-1, HSV-2, and VZV (shingles).

In vitro, acyclovir triphosphate stops replication of herpes viral DNA.

Drug resistance – Consider the possibility of viral resistance to acyclovir in patients who show poor clinical response during therapy.

Pharmacokinetics:

Absorption/Distribution – When acyclovir was administered to adults at 5 mg/kg by 1 hour infusions every 8 hours, mean steady-state peak and trough concentrations were 9.8 mcg/mL and 0.7 mcg/mL, respectively. When acyclovir was administered to adults at 10 mg/kg by 1 hour infusions every 8 hours, mean steady-state peak and trough concentrations were 22.9 mcg/mL and 1.9 mcg/mL, respectively. Absorption is unaffected by food. Bioavailability is between 10% and 20% and decreases with increasing doses. Concentrations achieved in CSF are approximately 50% of plasma values. Plasma protein binding is 9% to 33%. Acyclovir distributes widely in body fluids including vesicular fluid, aqueous humor, and cerebrospinal fluid. Acyclovir is concentrated in breast milk, amniotic fluid, and placenta.

Metabolism/Excretion – Renal excretion of unchanged drug following IV use accounts for 62% to 91% of the dose.

Half-life and total body clearance depend on renal function:

Acyclovir Half-Life and Total Body Clearance Based on Renal Function		
CrCl (mL/min/1.73 m^2)	Half-life (h)	Total body clearance (mL/min/1.73 m^2)
> 80	2.5	327
50 to 80	3	248
15 to 50	3.5	190
0 (Anuric)	19.5	29

Special populations –

Elderly: Acyclovir plasma concentrations are higher in elderly patients compared with younger adults. This may be in part because of age-related renal function changes.

Contraindications

Hypersensitivity to acyclovir or any component of the formulation.

Warnings/Precautions

Genital herpes: Acyclovir is not a cure for genital herpes. There are no data evaluating whether acyclovir will prevent transmission of infection to others. Avoid contact with lesions, or avoid intercourse when lesions and/or symptoms are present to prevent infecting partners. Genital herpes can also be transmitted in the absence of symptoms. Initiate therapy at the first sign or symptom of an episode.

Herpes zoster infections: There are no data on treatment initiated more than 72 hours after the onset of the rash. Initiate treatment as soon as possible after diagnosis. In clinical trials, treatment was most effective when started within the first 48 hours of rash onset.

Chickenpox: Although chickenpox in otherwise healthy children is usually a self-limited disease of mild to moderate severity, adolescents and adults tend to have more severe disease. Treatment was initiated within 24 hours of the typical chickenpox rash in the controlled studies, and there is no information regarding the effects of treatment begun later in the disease course. IV acyclovir is indicated for the treatment of varicella-zoster infections in immunocompromised patients.

Do not exceed: Do not exceed the recommended dosage, frequency, or length of treatment. Base dosage adjustments on estimated CrCl.

Renal function impairment: Renal failure, sometimes fatal, has been observed with acyclovir therapy. Dosage adjustment is recommended in patients with renal impairment (see Administration and Dosage). Use caution when coadministering acyclovir with other potentially nephrotoxic agents.

Precipitation of acyclovir crystals in renal tubules can occur if the drug is administered by bolus injection. Ensuing renal tubular damage can produce acute renal failure.

Occurrence of renal failure depends also on the patient's state of hydration, other treatments, and the rate of drug administration. Concomitant use of other nephrotoxic agents, pre-existing renal disease, and dehydration make further renal impairment with acyclovir more likely.

Thrombotic thrombocytopenic purpura/hemolytic uremic syndrome (TTP/HUS): TTP/HUS which has resulted in death, has occurred in immunocompromised patients receiving acyclovir therapy.

Hydration: Accompany IV infusion by adequate hydration.

Encephalopathic changes: Approximately 1% of patients receiving acyclovir IV have manifested encephalopathic changes characterized by either lethargy, obtundation, tremors, confusion, hallucinations, agitation, seizures, or coma. Use with caution in those patients who have underlying neurologic abnormalities; those with serious renal, hepatic, or electrolyte abnormalities or significant hypoxia.

Photosensitivity: Photosensitive rash may occur; therefore, caution patients to take protective measures (ie, sunscreens, protective clothing) against exposure to ultraviolet light or sunlight until tolerance is determined.

Pregnancy: *Category B.*

Lactation: Acyclovir concentrates in breast milk. Exercise caution when administering to a breastfeeding woman.

Children: Safety and efficacy of oral acyclovir in children younger than 2 years of age have not been established.

Drug Interactions

Drugs that may interact with acyclovir include hydantoins, probenecid, theophylline, valproic acid, and zidovudine.

Adverse Reactions

Adverse reactions (parenteral) occurring in at least 3% of patients include inflammation or phlebitis at injection site, transient elevations of serum creatinine or BUN, and nausea or vomiting.

Adverse reactions (oral) occurring in at least 3% of patients include diarrhea, malaise, and nausea.

FAMCICLOVIR

Tablets: 125, 250, and 500 mg (*Rx*) Various, *Famvir* (Novartis)

Indications

Herpes simplex infections: Treatment or suppression of recurrent genital herpes in immunocompetent patients; treatment of recurrent herpes labialis (cold sores) in immunocompetent patients; treatment of recurrent mucocutaneous herpes simplex infections in HIV-infected patients.

Herpes zoster: Treatment of acute herpes zoster (shingles).

Administration and Dosage

Herpes simplex infections:

Recurrent genital herpes – 1,000 mg twice daily for 1 day. Initiate therapy at the first sign or symptom if medical management of a genital herpes recurrence is indicated. The efficacy of famciclovir has not been established when treatment is initiated more than 6 hours after onset of symptoms or lesions.

Recurrent herpes labialis (cold sores) – 1,500 mg as a single dose. Initiate therapy at the earliest sign or symptom of a cold sore (eg, tingling, itching, burning).

Suppression of recurrent genital herpes – 250 mg twice daily for up to 1 year. The safety and efficacy of famciclovir therapy beyond 1 year of treatment have not been established.

Herpes zoster: 500 mg every 8 hours for 7 days. Therapy should be initiated as soon as herpes zoster is diagnosed. No data are available on the efficacy of treatment started more than 72 hours after rash onset.

HIV-infected patients: For recurrent orolabial or genital herpes simplex infection, the recommended dosage is 500 mg twice daily for 7 days.

Renal function impairment:

Famciclovir Dosage in Renal Function Impairment

Indication and normal dosage regimen	CrCl[a] (mL/min)	Adjusted dosage regimen dose (mg)	Dosing interval
Single-day dosing regimens			
Recurrent genital herpes			
1,000 mg every 12 hours for 1 day	≥ 60	1,000	every 12 hours for 1 day
	40 to 59	500	every 12 hours for 1 day
	20 to 39	500	single dose
	< 20	250	single dose
	HD[b]	250	single dose following dialysis
Recurrent herpes labialis			
1,500 mg single dose	≥ 60	1,500	single dose
	40 to 59	750	single dose
	20 to 39	500	single dose
	< 20	250	single dose
	HD[b]	250	single dose following dialysis

Famciclovir Dosage in Renal Function Impairment			
Indication and normal dosage regimen	CrCl[a] (mL/min)	Adjusted dosage regimen dose (mg)	Dosing interval
Multiple-day dosing regimens			
Herpes zoster			
500 mg every 8 hours	≥ 60	500	every 8 hours
	40 to 59	500	every 12 hours
	20 to 39	500	every 24 hours
	< 20	250	every 24 hours
	HD[b]	250	following each dialysis
Suppression of recurrent genital herpes			
250 mg every 12 hours	= 40	250	every 12 hours
	20 to 39	125	every 12 hours
	< 20	125	every 24 hours
	HD[b]	125	following each dialysis
Recurrent orolabial and genital herpes simplex infection in HIV-infected patients			
500 mg every 12 hours	= 40	500	every 12 hours
	20 to 39	500	every 24 hours
	< 20	250	every 24 hours
	HD[b]	250	following each dialysis

[a] CrCl = creatinine clearance.
[b] HD = hemodialysis.

Actions

Pharmacology: Famciclovir undergoes rapid biotransformation to the active antiviral compound penciclovir, which is converted to penciclovir triphosphate. Penciclovir triphosphate inhibits HSV-2 polymerase. Consequently, herpes viral DNA synthesis and, therefore, replication are selectively inhibited.

Pharmacokinetics:

Absorption – The absolute bioavailability of famciclovir is 77%. The area under the plasma concentration-time curve (AUC) was 8.6 mcg•h/mL. The maximum concentration (C_{max}) was 3.3 mcg/mL and the time to C_{max} (T_{max}) was 0.9 hours.

Penciclovir is less than 20% bound to plasma proteins. The blood/plasma ratio of penciclovir is approximately 1.

Metabolism – Famciclovir given orally is deacetylated and oxidized to form penciclovir. Cytochrome P450 does not play an important role in famciclovir metabolism.

Excretion – The plasma elimination half-life of penciclovir was 2 hours after IV penciclovir and 2.3 hours after 500 mg oral famciclovir.

Contraindications

Hypersensitivity to famciclovir.

Warnings/Precautions

Renal function impairment: Dosage adjustment is recommended in renal insufficiency (see Administration and Dosage).

Pregnancy: Category B.

Lactation: It is not known whether famciclovir is excreted in breast milk. Decide whether to discontinue breastfeeding or to discontinue the drug, taking into account the importance of the drug to the mother.

Children: Safety and efficacy in children younger than 18 years of age have not been established.

Elderly: Mean penciclovir AUC was 40% larger and penciclovir renal clearance was 22% lower after the oral administration of famciclovir in elderly volunteers compared with younger volunteers.

Drug Interactions

The conversion of 6-deoxy penciclovir to penciclovir is catalyzed by aldehyde oxidase. Interactions with other drugs metabolized by this enzyme could occur.

Concurrent use with probenecid or other drugs significantly eliminated by active renal tubular secretion may result in increased plasma concentrations of penciclovir.

Drug/Food interactions: When famciclovir was administered with food, penciclovir C_{max} decreased approximately 50%. Because the systemic availability of penciclovir (AUC) was not altered, it appears that famciclovir may be taken without regard to meals.

Adverse Reactions

Adverse reactions occurring in 3% or more of patients include dizziness, diarrhea, abdominal pain, dysmenorrhea, fatigue, fever, flatulence, headache, migraine, nausea, pruritus, rash, and vomiting.

Drug/Lab: Neutropenia (less than 0.8 × normal range low), ALT (more than 2 × normal range high), lipase (more than 1.5 × normal range high).

VALACYCLOVIR HYDROCHLORIDE

Caplets: 500 mg, 1 g (*Rx*)	Various, *Valtrex* (GlaxoSmithKline)

Indications

Herpes zoster: Treatment of herpes zoster (shingles).

Genital herpes: Treatment or suppression of genital herpes in immunocompetent individuals and for the suppression of recurrent genital herpes in HIV-infected individuals.

When valacyclovir is used as suppressive therapy in immunocompetent individuals with genital herpes, the risk of heterosexual transmission to susceptible partners is reduced. Instruct patients to use safer sex practices with suppressive therapy (see current Centers for Disease Control and Prevention *Sexually Transmitted Disease Treatment Guidelines*).

Herpes labialis: For the treatment of herpes labialis (cold sores).

Administration and Dosage

Valacyclovir may be given without regard to meals.

Herpes zoster: The recommended dosage is 1 g 3 times daily for 7 days. Initiate therapy at the earliest sign or symptom of herpes zoster; it is most effective when started within 48 hours of the onset of zoster rash. No data are available on efficacy of treatment started more than 72 hours after rash onset.

Genital herpes:

Initial episodes – The recommended dosage is 1 g twice daily for 10 days. There are no data on the effectiveness of treatment when initiated more than 72 hours after the onset of signs and symptoms. Therapy was most effective when administered within 48 hours of the onset of signs and symptoms.

Recurrent episodes – The recommended dosage is 500 mg twice daily for 3 days. Advise patients to initiate therapy at the first sign or symptom of an episode. There are no data on the efficacy of treatment started more than 24 hours after the onset of signs or symptoms.

Suppressive therapy – The recommended dosage for chronic suppressive therapy of recurrent genital herpes is 1 g once daily in immunocompetent patients. In patients with a history of 9 or fewer recurrences per year, an alternative dose is 500 mg once daily. The safety and efficacy of therapy with valacyclovir beyond 1 year have not been established.

Transmission – The recommended dosage of valacyclovir for reduction of transmission of genital herpes in patients with a history of 9 or fewer recurrences per year is 500 mg once daily for the source partner. Counsel patients to use safer sex practices in combination with suppressive therapy with valacyclovir. The efficacy of reducing transmission beyond 8 months in discordant couples has not been established.

HIV-infected patients: In HIV-infected patients with CD4 cell count at least 100 cells/mm^3, the recommended dosage of valacyclovir for chronic suppressive therapy of recurrent genital herpes is 500 mg twice daily. The safety and efficacy of therapy with valacyclovir beyond 6 months in patients with HIV infection have not been established.

Herpes labialis: The recommended dosage of valacyclovir for the treatment of cold sores is 2 g twice daily for 1 day taken approximately 12 hours apart. Initiate therapy at the earliest symptom of a cold sore (eg, tingling, itching, burning). There are no data on the effectiveness of treatment initiated after the development of clinical signs of a cold sore (eg, papule, vesicle, ulcer). Therapy beyond 1 day does not appear to provide additional clinical benefit.

Acute or chronic renal impairment:

Valacyclovir Dosage Adjustments for Renal Impairment

Indication	Normal dosage (CrCl ≥ 50)	CrCl (mL/min)		
		30 to 49	10 to 29	< 10
Herpes zoster	1 g q 8 h	1 g q 12 h	1 g q 24 h	500 mg q 24 h
Genital herpes				
Initial treatment	1 g q 12 h	No reduction	1 g q 24 h	500 mg q 24 h
Recurrent episodes	500 mg q 12 h	No reduction	500 mg q 24 h	500 mg q 24 h
Suppressive therapy	1 g q 24 h	No reduction	500 mg q 24 h	500 mg q 24 h
Suppressive therapy (≤ 9 recurrences/yr)	500 mg q 24 h	No reduction	500 mg q 48 h	500 mg q 48 h
Suppressive therapy in HIV-infected patients	500 mg q 12 h	No reduction	500 mg q 24 h	500 mg q 24 h
Herpes labialis (cold sores) (do not exceed 1 day of treatment)	Two 2 g doses taken ≈ 12 h apart	Two 1 g doses taken ≈ 12 h apart	Two 500 mg doses taken ≈ 12 h apart	500 mg single dose

Hemodialysis: During hemodialysis, the half-life of acyclovir after administration of valacyclovir is approximately 4 hours. Patients requiring hemodialysis should receive the recommended dose of valacyclovir after hemodialysis.

Peritoneal dialysis: Supplemental doses of valacyclovir should not be required following chronic ambulatory peritoneal dialysis (CAPD) or continuous arteriovenous hemofiltration/hemodialysis (CAVHD).

Actions

Pharmacology: Valacyclovir is the hydrochloride salt of L-valyl ester of the antiviral drug acyclovir. Valacyclovir is rapidly converted to acyclovir, which has in vitro and in vivo inhibitory activity against herpes simplex virus types I (HSV-1) and II (HSV-2), and varicella-zoster virus (VZV). In cell culture, acyclovir has the highest antiviral activity against HSV-1, followed by (in decreasing order of potency) HSV-2 and VZV.

In vitro, acyclovir triphosphate stops replication of herpes viral DNA in 3 ways: 1) Competitive inhibition of viral DNA polymerase; 2) incorporation and termination of the growing viral DNA chain; and 3) inactivation of the viral DNA polymerase.

Pharmacokinetics:

Absorption/Distribution – Valacyclovir is rapidly absorbed and is rapidly and nearly completely converted to acyclovir and L-valine by first-pass metabolism. The absolute bioavailability of acyclovir after administration of valacyclovir is 54.5%.

Metabolism – Neither valacyclovir nor acyclovir metabolism is metabolized by cytochrome P450 enzymes.

Excretion – Acyclovir accounted for 88.6% excreted in the urine. Renal clearance of acyclovir following the administration of a single 1 g valacyclovir dose to 12 healthy volunteers was approximately 255 mL/min, which represents 41.9% of total acyclovir apparent plasma clearance.

The plasma elimination half-life of acyclovir typically averaged 2.5 to 3.3 hours in volunteers with normal renal function.

Contraindications

Hypersensitivity or intolerance to valacyclovir, acyclovir, or any component of the formulation.

Warnings/Precautions

Thrombotic thrombocytopenic purpura/hemolytic uremic syndrome (TTP/HUS): TTP/HUS, in some cases resulting in death, has been reported in patients with advanced HIV disease and in bone marrow and renal transplant recipients.

Immunocompromised patients: The safety and efficacy of valacyclovir have not been established in immunocompromised patients, other than for the suppression of genital herpes in HIV-infected patients.

Transmission of genital herpes: The efficacy of valacyclovir for reducing transmission of genital herpes has not been established in individuals with multiple partners and non-heterosexual couples.

Cold sore treatment: Given the dosage recommendations for treatment of cold sores, pay special attention when prescribing valacyclovir for cold sores in patients who are elderly or who have impaired renal function. Treatment should not exceed 1 day (2 doses of 2 g in 24 hours).

Renal function impairment: Dosage reduction is recommended with renal impairment (see Administration and Dosage). Acute renal failure and CNS symptoms have been reported in patients with underlying renal disease who have received inappropriately high doses for their level of renal function. Exercise similar caution when administering valacyclovir to elderly patients and patients receiving potentially nephrotoxic agents.

Hepatic function impairment: Administration of valacyclovir to patients with moderate (biopsy-proven cirrhosis) or severe (with and without ascites and biopsy-proven cirrhosis) liver disease indicated that the rate but not the extent of conversion of valacyclovir to acyclovir was reduced, and the acyclovir half-life was not affected. Dosage modification is not recommended for patients with cirrhosis.

Pregnancy: Category B.

Lactation: Consider temporary discontinuation of nursing, as the safety of valacyclovir has not been established in infants.

Children: Safety and efficacy have not been established in prepubertal children.

Elderly: Dosage reduction may be required in geriatric patients, depending on the underlying renal status of the patient.

Drug Interactions

Drugs that may affect valacyclovir include cimetidine/probenecid.

Adverse Reactions

Adverse reactions occurring in 3% or more of patients include nausea, headache, vomiting, dizziness, abdominal pain, depression, AST abnormalities, dysmenorrhea, and arthralgia.

AMANTADINE HYDROCHLORIDE

Tablets: 100 mg (*Rx*)	Various, *Symmetrel* (Endo)
Capsules: 100 mg (*Rx*)	Various
Syrup: 50 mg/5 mL (*Rx*)	Various, *Symmetrel* (Endo)

Indications

Influenza A prophylaxis: For chemoprophylaxis against signs and symptoms of influenza A virus infection when early vaccination is not feasible or when the vaccine is contraindicated or not available.

Influenza A treatment: Treatment of uncomplicated respiratory tract illness caused by influenza A virus strains especially when administered early in the course of illness.

Parkinson disease: Treatment of idiopathic Parkinson's disease (paralysis agitans), postencephalitic parkinsonism, and symptomatic parkinsonism which may follow injury to the nervous system by carbon monoxide intoxication. It is indicated in those elderly patients believed to develop parkinsonism in association with cerebral arteriosclerosis.

Drug-induced extrapyramidal reactions: In the treatment of drug-induced extrapyramidal reactions.

Administration and Dosage

Influenza A virus illness:

Prophylaxis – Start in anticipation of contact or as soon as possible after exposure. Use daily for at least 10 days following a known exposure. The infectious period extends from shortly before onset of symptoms to up to 1 week after. Because amantadine does not appear to suppress antibody response, it can be used in conjunction with inactivated influenza A virus vaccine until protective antibody responses develop; administer for 2 to 4 weeks after vaccine has been given. When the vaccine is unavailable or contraindicated, give amantadine for the duration of known influenza A in the community because of repeated and unknown exposure.

Symptomatic management – Start as soon as possible after onset of symptoms and continue for 24 to 48 hours after symptoms disappear.

Parkinsonism: 100 mg twice a day when used alone.

The initial dose of amantadine hydrochloride is 100 mg daily for patients with serious associated medical illnesses or who are receiving high doses of other antiparkinsonism drugs. After 1 to several weeks, increase to 100 mg twice daily, if necessary.

Patients may benefit from an increase up to 400 mg daily in divided doses.

Dosage:

Amantadine Dosage by Patient Age and Renal Function

Renal function	Dosage
No recognized renal disease	
1 to 9 yrs[a]	4.4 to 8.8 mg/kg/day given once daily or divided twice daily, not to exceed 150 mg/day
9 to 12 yrs	100 mg twice daily
13 to 64 yrs	200 mg once daily or divided twice daily
≥ 65 yrs	100 mg once daily
Renal function impairment – CrCl (mL/min/1.73 m²)	
30 to 50	200 mg 1st day; 100 mg daily thereafter
15 to 29	200 mg 1st day; then 100 mg on alternate days
< 15	200 mg every 7 days
Hemodialysis patients	200 mg every 7 days

[a] Use in children younger than 1 year of age has not been evaluated adequately.

Dosage for concomitant therapy: Amantadine hydrochloride should be held constant at 100 mg daily or twice daily while the daily dose of levodopa is gradually increased to optimal benefit.

Alternative dosing: A 100 mg daily dose has also been shown in experimental challenge studies to be effective as prophylaxis in healthy adults who are not at high risk for influenza-related complications. The 100 mg dose is recommended for persons who have demonstrated intolerance to 200 mg of amantadine hydrochloride daily because of CNS or other toxicities.

Dosage adjustments: For adults younger than 65 years of age, if CNS effects develop in a once-daily dosage, a split dosage schedule may reduce such complaints.

Special risk patients: Dose may need reduction in patients with CHF, peripheral edema, orthostatic hypotension, or impaired renal function.

Actions

Pharmacology: Amantadine's antiviral activity is not completely understood. Its mode of action appears to be the prevention of the release of infectious viral nucleic acid into the host cell. Amantadine does not appear to interfere with the immunogenicity of inactivated influenza A virus vaccine.

Parkinson's disease – Data from animal studies have either shown or suggested amantadine hydrochloride to enhance extracellular concentrations of dopamine by increasing dopamine release or decreasing reuptake of dopamine into presynaptic neurons; to stimulate the dopamine receptor itself; or drive the postsynaptic dopaminergic system to a more dopamine-sensitive status.

Pharmacokinetics:

Absorption/Distribution – Clearance of amantadine is significantly reduced in adults with renal insufficiency. Elimination half-life increases 2- to 3-fold when CrCl is less than 40 mL/min/1.73 m^2 and averages 8 days in patients on chronic hemodialysis.

The time to peak concentration was 3.3 ± 1.5 hours. The half-life was 17 ± 4 hours (range, 10 to 25 hours). Across other studies, amantadine plasma half-life has averaged 16 ± 6 hours (range, 9 to 31 hours) in 19 healthy volunteers.

Amantadine is approximately 67% bound to plasma proteins.

Excretion – Amantadine is primarily excreted unchanged in the urine by glomerular filtration and tubular secretion.

Contraindications

Hypersensitivity to amantadine.

Warnings/Precautions

Deaths: Deaths have been reported from overdose with amantadine.

Suicide attempts: Suicide attempts, some of which have been fatal, have been reported in patients treated with amantadine, many of whom received short courses for influenza treatment or prophylaxis. Suicide attempts and suicidal ideation have been reported in patients with and without prior history of psychiatric illness. Amantadine can exacerbate mental problems in patients with a history of psychiatric disorders or substance abuse.

Seizures and other CNS effects: Closely observe patients with a history of seizures for increased seizure activity. Caution patients who note CNS effects or blurring of vision against driving or working in situations where alertness and adequate motor coordination are important.

CHF or peripheral edema: Closely follow patients with a history of CHF or peripheral edema as there are patients who developed CHF while receiving amantadine.

Parkinson disease: Patients with Parkinson disease improving on amantadine hydrochloride should resume normal activities gradually and cautiously, consistent with other medical considerations, such as the presence of osteoporosis or phlebothrombosis.

Glaucoma: Because amantadine has anticholinergic effects and may cause mydriasis, do not give to patients with untreated angle closure glaucoma.

Other: Exercise care when administering to patients with a history of recurrent eczematoid rash, or to patients with psychosis or severe psychoneurosis not controlled by chemotherapeutic agents.

Abrupt withdrawal: Do not discontinue amantadine abruptly in patients with Parkinson's disease. A few patients have experienced a parkinsonian crisis (a sudden marked clinical deterioration) when this medication was suddenly stopped. Abrupt discontinuation also may precipitate delirium, agitation, delusions, hallucinations, paranoid reaction, stupor, anxiety, depression, and slurred speech.

Bacterial infections: Serious bacterial infections may begin with influenza-like symptoms or may coexist with or occur as complications during the course of influenza.

Neuroleptic malignant syndrome (NMS): Sporadic cases of possible NMS have been reported in association with dose reduction or withdrawal of amantadine therapy. Observe patients carefully when the dosage of amantadine is reduced abruptly or discontinued, especially if the patient is receiving neuroleptics.

Renal function impairment: Reduce the dose in renal impairment.

Hepatic function impairment: Exercise care when administering amantadine hydrochloride to patients with liver disease.

Pregnancy: Category C.

Lactation: Amantadine is excreted in breast milk. Use is not recommended in nursing mothers.

Children: Safety and efficacy for use in neonates and infants younger than 1 year of age have not been established.

Elderly: Reduce dose in individuals 65 years of age and older.

Drug Interactions

Drugs that may affect amantadine include anticholinergic agents, triamterene and thiazide diuretics, quinidine, quinine, and trimethoprim/sulfamethoxazole.

Drugs that may be affected by amantadine include CNS stimulants.

Adverse Reactions

Adverse reactions occurring in at least 1% of patients include nausea; dizziness; lightheadedness; insomnia; depression; anxiety; irritability; hallucinations; confusion; anorexia; dry mouth; constipation; ataxia; livedo reticularis; peripheral edema; orthostatic hypotension; headache; somnolence; nervousness; dream abnormality; agitation; dry nose; diarrhea; fatigue.

RIBAVIRIN

Tablets; oral: 200 mg (*Rx*)	Various, *Copegus* (Roche), *Ribasphere* (Three Rivers)
400 and 600 mg (*Rx*)	*Ribasphere* (Three Rivers)
Capsules; oral: 200 mg (*Rx*)	Various, *Rebetol* (Schering), *Ribasphere* (Three Rivers)
Solution; oral: 40 mg/mL (*Rx*)	*Rebetol* (Schering)
Powder for solution, lyophilized; inhalation: 6 g (*Rx*)	*Virazole* (Valent)

Warning:

Capsules/Tablets/Oral solution: Ribavirin monotherapy is not effective for the treatment of chronic hepatitis C virus (HCV) infection and should not be used alone for this indication.

The primary toxicity of ribavirin is hemolytic anemia that may result in worsening of cardiac disease and lead to fatal and nonfatal myocardial infarctions (MIs). Do not treat patients with a history of significant or unstable cardiac disease with ribavirin.

Significant teratogenic or embryocidal effects have been demonstrated in all animal species exposed to ribavirin. In addition, ribavirin has a multiple-dose half-life of 12 days, and it may persist in nonplasma compartments for as long as 6 months. Therefore, ribavirin therapy is contraindicated in women who are pregnant and in the male partners of women who are pregnant. Extreme care must be taken to avoid pregnancy during therapy and for 6 months after completion of treatment in these individuals. At least 2 reliable forms of effective contraception must be used during treatment and during the 6-month posttreatment follow-up period.

continued on next page

Warning: (cont.)

Aerosol: Use of aerosolized ribavirin in patients requiring mechanical ventilator assistance should be undertaken only by health care providers and support staff familiar with the specific ventilator being used and this mode of administration of the drug. Pay strict attention to procedures that have been shown to minimize the accumulation of drug precipitate that can result in mechanical ventilator dysfunction and associated increased pulmonary pressures.

Sudden deterioration of respiratory function has been associated with initiation of aerosolized ribavirin use in infants. Carefully monitor respiratory function during treatment. If initiation of aerosolized ribavirin treatment appears to produce sudden deterioration of respiratory function, stop treatment and reinstitute only with extreme caution, continuous monitoring, and consideration of concomitant administration of bronchodilators.

Ribavirin aerosol is not indicated for use in adults. Health care providers and patients should be aware that ribavirin has been shown to produce testicular lesions in rodents and to be teratogenic in all animal species in which adequate studies have been conducted (rodents and rabbits).

Indications

Tablets:

Chronic hepatitis C virus – In combination with peginterferon alfa-2a for the treatment of adults with chronic HCV infection who have compensated liver disease and have not been previously treated with interferon alpha. Patients in whom efficacy was demonstrated included patients with compensated liver disease and histological evidence of cirrhosis (Child-Pugh class A). Efficacy of *Copegus* was also demonstrated in patients with HIV disease that is clinically stable.

Capsules/Oral solution:

Ribasphere – In combination with interferon alfa-2b for the treatment of chronic HCV in patients 18 years of age and older with compensated liver disease previously untreated with alpha interferon and in patients 18 years of age and older who have relapsed following alpha interferon therapy; in combination with peginterferon alfa-2b for the treatment of chronic HCV in patients with compensated liver disease who have not previously been treated with interferon alpha and are at least 18 years of age.

Rebetol – In combination with interferon alfa-2b (pegylated and nonpegylated) for the treatment of chronic HCV in patients 3 years of age and older with compensated liver disease.

Aerosol:

Severe lower respiratory tract infections – Treatment of hospitalized infants and young children with severe lower respiratory tract infections caused by respiratory syncytial virus (RSV).

Administration and Dosage

Chronic hepatic C virus infection:

Copegus or Ribasphere tablets/peginterferon alfa-2a – 800 to 1,200 mg administered orally in 2 divided doses. Individualize the dose to the patient, depending on baseline disease characteristics (eg, genotype), response to therapy, and tolerability of the regimen.

Copegus or Ribasphere Tablets/Peginterferon Alfa-2a Dosing Recommendations

Genotype[a]	Peginterferon alfa-2a dose	*Ribavirin* tablet dose[b]	Duration
Genotype 1, 4	180 mcg	< 75 kg = 1,000 mg	48 wk
		≥ 75 kg = 1,200 mg	48 wk
Genotype 2, 3	180 mcg	800 mg	24 wk

[a] Genotypes non-1 showed no increased response to treatment beyond 24 weeks. Data on genotypes 5 and 6 are insufficient for dosing recommendations.

[b] Administer in 2 divided doses.

Duration of therapy: 24 to 48 weeks for patients previously untreated with ribavirin and interferon.

Rebetol or Ribasphere capsules/interferon alfa-2b –

Usual dosage:

76 kg or more – 600 mg in the morning and 600 mg in the evening with interferon alfa-2b 3 million units 3 times weekly subcutaneously.

75 kg or less – 400 mg in the morning and 600 mg in the evening with interferon alfa-2b 3 million units 3 times weekly subcutaneously.

Duration of therapy: 24 to 48 weeks for patients previously untreated with interferon; 24 weeks for patients who relapsed following nonpegylated interferon monotherapy.

Ribasphere capsules/peginterferon alfa-2b – Ribasphere 800 mg/day in 2 divided doses (400 mg in the morning and 400 mg in the evening).

Rebetol/Peginterferon alfa-2b –

Usual dosage:

***Rebetol*/Peginterferon Alfa-2b Dosing Recommendations in Adults**					
Body weight	Peginterferon alfa-2b strength	Amount of peginterferon alfa-2b to administer	Volume[a] of peginterferon alfa-2b to administer	*Rebetol* daily dose	Number of *Rebetol* capsules
< 40 kg	50 mcg per 0.5 mL	50 mcg	0.5 mL	800 mg/day	2 × 200 mg capsules in the morning 2 × 200 mg capsules in the evening
40 to 50 kg	80 mcg per 0.5 mL	64 mcg	0.4 mL	800 mg/day	2 × 200 mg capsules in the morning 2 × 200 mg capsules in the evening
51 to 60 kg		80 mcg	0.5 mL	800 mg/day	2 × 200 mg capsules in the morning 2 × 200 mg capsules in the evening
61 to 65 kg	120 mcg per 0.5 mL	96 mcg	0.4 mL	800 mg/day	2 × 200 mg capsules in the morning 2 × 200 mg capsules in the evening
66 to 75 kg		96 mcg	0.4 mL	1,000 mg/day	2 × 200 mg capsules in the morning 3 × 200 mg capsules in the evening
76 to 80 kg		120 mcg	0.5 mL	1,000 mg/day	2 × 200 mg capsules in the morning 3 × 200 mg capsules in the evening
81 to 85 kg				1,200 mg/day	3 × 200 mg capsules in the morning 3 × 200 mg capsules in the evening

***Rebetol*/Peginterferon Alfa-2b Dosing Recommendations in Adults**					
Body weight	Peginterferon alfa-2b strength	Amount of peginterferon alfa-2b to administer	Volume[a] of peginterferon alfa-2b to administer	*Rebetol* daily dose	Number of *Rebetol* capsules
86 to 105 kg	150 mcg per 0.5 mL	150 mcg	0.5 mL	1,200 mg/day	3 × 200 mg capsules in the morning 3 × 200 mg capsules in the evening
> 105 kg	†[b]	†[b]	†[b]	1,400 mg/day	3 × 200 mg capsules in the morning 4 × 200 mg capsules in the evening

[a] When reconstituted as directed.

[b] For patients weighing > 105 kg, the peginterferon alfa-2b dosage of 1.5 mcg/kg/wk should be calculated based on the individual patient's weight. Two vials of peginterferon alfa-2b may be necessary to provide the dose.

Duration of therapy:

Interferon alpha–naive patients – 48 weeks for patients with genotype 1; 24 weeks for patients with genotypes 2 and 3.

Re-treatment with peginterferon alfa-2b of prior treatment failures – 48 weeks, regardless of HCV genotype.

Chronic hepatic C virus with HIV coinfection:

Copegus/Peginterferon alfa-2a –

Usual dosage: *Copegus* 800 mg/day and peginterferon alfa-2a 180 mcg subcutaneously once weekly.

Duration of therapy: 48 weeks regardless of genotype.

Children:

Chronic hepatic C virus infection –

Rebetol/Interferon alfa-2b:

Usual dosage –

76 kg or more: 600 mg in the morning and 600 mg in the evening with interferon alfa-2b 3 million units 3 times weekly subcutaneously.

62 to 75 kg: 400 mg in the morning and 600 mg in the evening with interferon alfa-2b 3 million units 3 times weekly subcutaneously.

25 to 61 kg: 15 mg/kg/day (divided dose in the morning and in the evening) with interferon alfa-2b 3 million units/m^2 3 times weekly subcutaneously.

Duration of therapy – 48 weeks for children with genotype 1; 24 weeks for children with genotype 2 and 3.

Rebetol/Peginterferon alfa-2b combination:

3 to 17 years of age –

Usual dosage:

Ribavirin[a] Dosing Guidelines in Children		
Body weight	Ribavirin daily dose	Number of ribavirin capsules
< 47 kg	15 mg/kg/day	Use oral solution[b]
47 to 59 kg	800 mg/kg	2 × 200 mg capsules in the morning 2 × 200 mg capsules in the evening
60 to 73 kg	1,000 mg/kg	2 × 200 mg capsules in the morning 3 × 200 mg capsules in the evening
> 73 kg	1,200 mg/day	3 × 200 mg capsules in the morning 3 × 200 mg capsules in the evening

[a] Ribavirin to be used in combination with peginterferon alfa-2b 60 mcg/m^2 weekly. Patients who reach their 18th birthday while receiving these medications should remain on the pediatric dosing regimen.

[b] Ribavirin solution may be used for any patient regardless of body weight.

Duration of therapy: 48 weeks for patients with genotype 1; 24 weeks for patients with genotypes 2 and 3.

Severe respiratory syncytial virus infection (aerosol) –

Infants and young children:

Usual dosage – 20 mg/mL as the starting solution in the drug reservoir of the small-particle aerosol generator (SPAG-2) unit, with continuous aerosol administration for 12 to 18 hours per day.

Duration of therapy – 3 to 7 days.

Renal function impairment: Do not use in patients with creatinine clearance (CrCl) less than 50 mL/min.

Hepatic function impairment: Discontinue therapy in patients who develop hepatic decompensation during treatment.

Dose modifications: If severe adverse reactions or laboratory abnormalities develop during combination therapy, modify or discontinue the dose, if appropriate, until the adverse reactions abate or decrease in severity. If intolerance persists after dose adjustment, discontinue combination therapy.

Ribavirin –

Adults:

Ribavirin Dosage Modification and Discontinuation Guidelines

Hb[a]	Reduce ribavirin dose to 600 mg/day[b] if:	Discontinue ribavirin tablets if:
Patients with no cardiac disease	Hb < 10 g/dL	Hb < 8.5 g/dL
Patients with history of stable cardiac disease	≥ 2 g/dL decrease in Hb during any 4-week treatment period	Hb < 12 g/dL despite 4 weeks at reduced dose

[a] Hb = hemoglobin.

[b] One 200 mg tablet in the morning and two 200 mg tablets in the evening.

Tablets – Once ribavirin has been withheld because of a laboratory abnormality or clinical manifestation, an attempt may be made to restart ribavirin at 600 mg/day and further increase the dosage to 800 mg/day. However, it is not recommended that ribavirin be increased to the original assigned dose (1,000 to 1,200 mg).

Children: Modify the recommended dose from the original starting dosages of 15 mg/kg daily in a 2-step process to 12 mg/kg/day, then to 8 mg/kg/day if needed.

Rebetol –

Dose Modification and Discontinuation of *Rebetol* Combination Therapy in Adults and Children

	Adults	Children		Adults	Children
Laboratory values	Peginterferon alfa-2b/ interferon alfa-2b	Peginterferon alfa-2b	Interferon alfa-2b	*Rebetol*	
Hb < 10 g/dL	For patients with cardiac disease, reduce by 50%[a]	See footnote[a]	See footnote[a]	Adjust dose[b]	1st reduction to 12 mg/kg/day 2nd reduction to 8 mg/kg/day
WBC[c] < 1.5×10^9/L	Adjust dose[d]	1st reduction to 40 mcg/m²/wk 2nd reduction to 20 mcg/m²/wk	Reduce by 50%	No dose change	No dose change
Neutrophils < 0.75×10^9/L					
Platelets < 50×10^9/L (adults) < 70×10^9/L (children)					

Dose Modification and Discontinuation of *Rebetol* Combination Therapy in Adults and Children

	Adults	Children		Adults	Children
Laboratory values	Peginterferon alfa-2b/ interferon alfa-2b	Peginterferon alfa-2b	Interferon alfa-2b	*Rebetol*	
Hb < 8.5 g/dL	Permanently discontinue	Permanently discontinue	Permanently discontinue	Permanently discontinue	Permanently discontinue
WBC < 1×10^9/L					
Neutrophils < 0.5×10^9/L					
Creatinine > 2 mg/dL (children)					
Platelets < 25×10^9/L (adults) < 50×10^9/L (children)					

[a] For adults with a history of stable cardiac disease receiving peginterferon alfa-2b or interferon alfa-2b in combination with ribavirin, the peginterferon alfa-2b or interferon alfa-2b dose should be reduced by half and the ribavirin dose by 200 mg/day if a > 2 g/dL decrease in Hb is observed during any 4-week period. Both peginterferon alfa-2b and ribavirin or interferon alfa-2b and ribavirin should be permanently discontinued if patients have Hb levels < 12 g/dL after this ribavirin dose reduction. Children who have preexisting cardiac conditions and experience a Hb decrease ≥ 2 g/dL during any 4-week period during treatment should have weekly evaluations and hematology testing.

[b] First dose reduction of ribavirin is by 200 mg/day, except in patients receiving the 1,400 mg dose it is by 400 mg/day; second dose reduction of ribavirin (if needed) is by an additional 200 mg/day.

[c] WBC = white blood cell count.

[d] For patients on ribavirin/peginterferon alfa-2b combination therapy: first dose reduction of peginterferon alfa-2b is to 1 mcg/kg/wk, second dose reduction (if needed) of peginterferon alfa-2b is to 0.5 mcg/kg/wk. For patients receiving ribavirin/interferon alfa-2b combination therapy, reduce interferon alfa-2b dose by 50%.

Discontinuation of therapy:

Ribavirin/Interferon alfa-2b – Treatment discontinuation should be considered in any patient who has not achieved an HCV-RNA below the limit of detection of the assay by 24 weeks.

Ribavirin/Peginterferon alfa-2a – Consider discontinuation in patients who do not achieve at least a 2 $\log_{10}$ drop from baseline in HCV-RNA at 12 weeks, or undetectable HCV-RNA levels after 24 weeks of therapy. Retreated patients who fail to achieve undetectable HCV-RNA at week 12 of therapy, or whose HCV-RNA remains detectable after 24 weeks of therapy, are highly unlikely to achieve sustained virologic response, and discontinuation of therapy should be considered. Discontinue ribavirin tablets in patients who develop hepatic decompensation during treatment.

Administration: Administer *Copegus*, *Rebetol*, and *Ribasphere* tablets with food.

Ribasphere capsules may be administered without regard to food but should be administered in a consistent manner with respect to food intake. Do not open, crush, or break the capsules.

Actions

Pharmacology: Ribavirin is a synthetic nucleoside analog. It has antiviral activity in vitro against RSV, influenza A and B viruses, and herpes simplex virus. The mechanism by which the combination of ribavirin and an interferon product exerts its effect against HCV has not been fully established.

Pharmacokinetics:

Absorption –

Tablets: The average time to reach maximum plasma concentration was 2 hours.

Capsules/Solution: Ribavirin was rapidly and extensively absorbed following oral administration. However, because of first-pass metabolism, the absolute bioavailability averaged 64%.

Aerosol: Ribavirin administered by aerosol is absorbed systemically.

Distribution –

Capsules/Solution: Extensive volume of distribution, but ribavirin does not bind to plasma proteins.

Aerosol: Bioavailability of the aerosol is unknown and may depend on mode of delivery.

Accumulation of drug or metabolites in red blood cells occurs, with plateauing in red cells in approximately 4 days. Accumulation gradually declines with an apparent half-life of 40 days.

Metabolism –

Tablets: Ribavirin is not a substrate of CYP-450 enzymes.

Capsules/Solution: Ribavirin is hepatically metabolized.

Excretion –

Tablets: The terminal half-life following a single dose administration is approximately 120 to 170 hours. The total apparent clearance is about 26 L/h.

Capsules/Solution: Ribavirin and its metabolites are excreted renally. Upon discontinuation of dosing, the mean half-life was 298 hours.

Aerosol: The plasma half-life was 9.5 hours.

Contraindications

Patients with hemoglobinopathies (eg, thalassemia major, sickle-cell anemia); women who are or who may become pregnant or in men whose female partners are pregnant because ribavirin may cause fetal harm when administered to a pregnant woman; autoimmune hepatitis; in cirrhotic chronic HCV monoinfected patients with hepatic decompensation (Child-Pugh score of more than 6; class B and C) before or during treatment, and in cirrhotic chronic HCV patients coinfected with HIV who have hepatic decompensation with a Child-Pugh score of 6 or more before or during treatment (in combination with peginterferon alfa-2a); known hypersensitivity reactions, such as Stevens-Johnson syndrome, toxic epidermal necrolysis, and erythema multiforme, to ribavirin or any component of the product; CrCl less than 50 mL/min; coadministration with didanosine.

Warnings/Precautions

Monotherapy:

Capsules/Tablets/Oral solution – Ribavirin monotherapy is not effective for the treatment of chronic HCV infection. The safety and efficacy of ribavirin capsules and oral solution have only been established when used together with interferon alfa-2b, recombinant as interferon alfa-2b/ribavirin capsule combination therapy, or with peginterferon alfa-2b injection.

Combination therapy adverse reactions:

Capsules/Tablets/Oral solution – There are significant adverse reactions caused by ribavirin capsules/interferon alfa-2b or peginterferon alfa-2b therapy, and ribavirin tablets/peginterferon alfa-2a therapy, including severe depression and suicidal ideation, hemolytic anemia, suppression of bone marrow function, autoimmune and infectious disorders, pulmonary dysfunction, pancreatitis, and diabetes.

Suicidal ideation (capsules/oral solution): Suicidal ideation or suicide attempts occurred more frequently among children, primarily adolescents, during treatment and off-therapy follow-up.

Hemolytic anemia:

Capsules/Tablets/Oral solution – The primary toxicity of ribavirin is hemolytic anemia, which occurs within 1 to 2 weeks of initiation of therapy.

Aerosol – Although anemia has not been reported with aerosol use, it occurs frequently with experimental oral and intravenous ribavirin. Cases of anemia, reticulocytosis, and hemolytic anemia associated with aerosolized ribavirin use have been reported in postmarketing reporting systems.

Cardiovascular effects:

Capsules/Tablets/Oral solution – Fatal and nonfatal MIs have been reported in patients with anemia caused by ribavirin.

Pulmonary effects:

Aerosol – Pulmonary function significantly deteriorated during aerosolized ribavirin treatment in 6 of 6 adults with chronic obstructive lung disease and in 4 of 6 asthmatic adults. Dyspnea and chest soreness were also reported. The role of ribavirin in these reactions is indeterminate.

Capsules/Tablets/Oral solution – Pulmonary symptoms, including dyspnea, pulmonary infiltrates, pneumonitis, and pneumonia have been reported during therapy with ribavirin and interferon. Occasional cases of fatal pneumonia have occurred. In addition, sarcoidosis or the exacerbation of sarcoidosis has been reported.

Ophthalmologic disorders: Decrease or loss of vision; retinopathy, including macular edema, retinal artery or vein, thrombosis, retinal hemorrhages, and cotton wool spots; optic neuritis; papilledema; and serous retinal detachment are induced or aggravated by treatment with alpha interferons. Give all patients an eye examination at baseline. Give patients with preexisting ophthalmologic disorders (eg, diabetic or hypertensive retinopathy) periodic ophthalmologic exams during combination therapy with alpha interferon treatment. Perform a prompt and complete eye examination in any patient who develops ocular symptoms. Discontinue combination therapy with alpha interferons in patients who develop new or worsening ophthalmologic disorders.

Dental and periodontal disorders: Dental and periodontal disorders have been reported in patients receiving ribavirin and interferon or peginterferon combination therapy.

Pancreatitis: Suspend ribavirin, interferon alfa-2b, peginterferon alfa-2b, or peginterferon alfa-2a therapy in patients with signs and symptoms of pancreatitis, and discontinue in patients with confirmed pancreatitis.

Organ transplant recipients: Safety and efficacy of interferon alfa-2b and peginterferon alfa-2b alone or in combination with ribavirin for the treatment of HCV in liver or other organ transplant recipients have not been established.

Other infections and conditions: The safety and efficacy of ribavirin and peginterferon alfa-2a, interferon alfa-2b, and peginterferon alfa-2b combination therapy for the treatment of HIV infection, hepatitis B coinfection, adenovirus, RSV, parainfluenza, or influenza infections have not been established. Do not use oral ribavirin for these indications.

The safety and efficacy of ribavirin and interferon alfa-2b or peginterferon alfa-2a combination therapy have not been established in patients with liver or other organ transplants, patients with decompensated liver disease due to HCV infection, or patients who are nonresponders to interferon therapy.

Copegus – The safety and efficacy of ribavirin and interferon alfa-2b or peginterferon alfa-2a combination therapy have not been established in patients coinfected with hepatitis B virus or HIV and a CD4+ cell count of less than 100 cells/mcL.

Use with mechanical ventilators:

Aerosol – Strict attention must be paid to procedures that have been shown to minimize the accumulation of drug precipitate, which can result in increases in pulmonary pressure. These procedures include the use of bacteria filters in series in the expiratory limb of the ventilator circuit with frequent changes (every 4 hours); water column pressure release valves to indicate elevated ventilator pressure; frequent monitoring of these devices; verification that ribavirin crystals have not accumulated within the ventilator circuitry; and frequent suctioning and monitoring of the patient.

Deaths:

Aerosol – Deaths during or shortly after treatment with aerosolized ribavirin have been reported. These were in infants who experienced worsening respiratory status related to bronchospasm while being treated with the drug. Several other cases have been attributed to mechanical ventilator malfunction in which ribavirin precipitation within the ventilator apparatus led to excessively high pulmonary pressures and diminished oxygenation.

Health care personnel:

Aerosol – Health care workers directly providing care to patients receiving aerosolized ribavirin should be aware that ribavirin is teratogenic in all animal species in which adequate studies have been conducted.

Health care workers who are pregnant should consider avoiding direct care of patients receiving aerosolized ribavirin. If close patient contact cannot be avoided, take precautions to limit exposure.

Hypersensitivity reactions: If an acute hypersensitivity reaction develops, discontinue ribavirin immediately and institute appropriate medical therapy.

Renal function impairment:

Capsules/Tablets/Oral solution – Do not treat patients with CrCl less than 50 mL/min with ribavirin.

Hepatic function impairment: Chronic HCV patients with cirrhosis may be at risk of hepatic decompensation and death when treated with alpha interferons, including peginterferon alfa-2a. Cirrhotic chronic HCV patients coinfected with HIV receiving highly active antiretroviral therapy and interferon alfa-2a, with or without ribavirin, appear to be at increased risk for the development of hepatic decompensation.

Carcinogenesis:

Aerosol – Chronic feeding of ribavirin to rats at doses of 16 to 100 mg/kg/day (estimated human equivalent of 2.3 to 14.3 mg/kg/day, based on body surface area adjustment for adults) suggest that ribavirin may induce benign mammary, pancreatic, pituitary, and adrenal tumors.

Mutagenesis:

Tablets – The in vitro mouse lymphoma assay demonstrated mutagenic activity.

Aerosol – An increased incidence of cell transformations and mutations was shown.

Fertility impairment:

Capsules/Tablets/Oral solution – Use ribavirin with caution in fertile men. Upon cessation of treatment, essentially total recovery from ribavirin-induced testicular toxicity was apparent within 1 or 2 spermatogenesis cycles.

Aerosol – Doses administered to mice between 35 and 150 mg/kg/day resulted in significant seminiferous tubule atrophy, decreased sperm concentrations, and increased numbers of sperm with abnormal morphology. Partial recovery of sperm production was apparent 3 to 6 months following dose cessation. Testicular lesions (tubular atrophy) in adult rats at oral dose levels as low as 16 mg/kg/day were shown.

Pregnancy: Category X.

Lactation:

Aerosol – Ribavirin is toxic to lactating animals and their offspring.

Capsules/Tablets/Oral solution – It is not known whether ribavirin is excreted in human milk. Because of the potential for serious adverse reactions from the drug in breast-feeding infants, decide whether to discontinue breast-feeding or to delay or discontinue ribavirin.

Children:

Tablets – Safety and efficacy of ribavirin tablets have not been established in children younger than 18 years of age.

Capsules/Oral solution – Suicidal ideation or attempts occurred more frequently among children, primarily adolescents, compared with adults during treatment and off-therapy follow-up. Safety and efficacy of ribavirin in combination with peginterferon alfa-2b has not been established in children.

During a 48-week course of therapy, there was a decrease in the rate of linear growth (mean percentile assignment decrease of 9%) and a decrease in the rate of weight gain (mean percentile assignment decrease of 13%). A general reversal of these trends was noted during the 24-week posttreatment period.

Elderly:

Capsules/Oral solution – In clinical trials, elderly subjects had a higher frequency of anemia than did younger patients.

In general, cautiously administer ribavirin capsules to elderly patients, starting at the lower end of the dosing range, reflecting the greater frequency of decreased hepatic, renal, or cardiac function, and of concomitant disease or other drug therapy. Do not use ribavirin in elderly patients with CrCl less than 50 mL/min.

Monitoring:

Capsules/Tablets/Oral solution – Assess patients for underlying cardiac disease before initiation of ribavirin therapy and appropriately monitor them during therapy. The following laboratory tests are recommended for all patients treated with ribavirin prior to beginning treatment and then periodically thereafter:

- Standard hematologic tests: Including hemoglobin (pretreatment, week 2 and week 4 of therapy, and as clinically appropriate), complete and differential white blood cell counts, and platelet count.
- Blood chemistries: Liver function tests and thyroid-stimulating hormone.
- Pregnancy: Including monthly monitoring for women of childbearing potential and for 6 months after discontinuing therapy.
- electrocardiogram.

Aerosol – Monitor respiratory function and fluid status during treatment.

Drug Interactions

Drugs that may interact with ribavirin and peginterferon alfa-2a include nucleoside reverse transcriptase inhibitors (eg, didanosine, lamivudine, stavudine, zidovudine). Drugs that may interact with ribavirin include thiopurines and warfarin.

Adverse Reactions

Aerosol: Adverse reactions may include anemia and hemolytic anemia; apnea; atelectasis; bacterial pneumonia; bigeminy; bradycardia; bronchospasm; cardiac arrest; conjunctivitis; cyanosis; digitalis toxicity; dyspnea; hypotension; hypoventilation; pneumothorax; pulmonary edema; rash; reticulocytosis; tachycardia; ventilator dependence; worsening of respiratory status.

Health care personnel – Headache (51%); conjunctivitis (32%); dizziness, lacrimation, pharyngitis, nausea, rash, rhinitis (10% to 20%).

Capsules/Tablets/Oral solution combination therapy: Adverse reactions occurring in at least 3% of patients include abdominal pain; agitation; alopecia; anemia; anorexia; anxiety/emotional lability/irritability; arthralgia; asthenia; back pain; blurred vision; chest pain; concentration impaired; conjunctivitis; constipation; coughing; depression; dermatitis; diarrhea; dizziness; dry mouth; dry skin; dyspepsia; dyspnea; eczema; fatigue; fever; flushing; fungal/viral infection; headache; hepatomegaly; hypothyroidism; increased sweating; influenza-like symptoms; injection-site inflammation; injection- site reaction; insomnia; irritability; leukopenia; lymphopenia; malaise; memory impairment; menstrual disorder; mood alteration; musculoskeletal pain; myalgia; nausea; nervousness; neutropenia; overall resistance mechanism disorders; pharyngitis; pruritus; rash; rhinitis; right upper quadrant pain; rigors; sinusitis; taste perversion; thrombocytopenia; vomiting; weight decrease.

RIMANTADINE HYDROCHLORIDE

Tablets: 100 mg (*Rx*)	Various, *Flumadine* (Caraco)

Indications

Adults: Prophylaxis/treatment of illness caused by various strains of influenza A virus.

Children: Prophylaxis against influenza A virus.

Administration and Dosage

Prophylaxis:

Adults and children 10 years of age and older – 100 mg twice daily. In patients with severe hepatic dysfunction or renal failure (CrCl less than or equal to 10 mL/min) and in elderly nursing home patients, a dose reduction to 100 mg daily is recommended.

Treatment:

Adults – 100 mg twice daily. In patients with severe hepatic dysfunction or renal failure (CrCl less than or equal to 10 mL/min) and in elderly nursing home patients, a dose reduction to 100 mg daily is recommended. Initiate therapy as soon as possible, preferably within 48 hours after onset of signs and symptoms of influenza A infection. Continue therapy for approximately 7 days from the initial onset of symptoms.

Children – The usual dosage is 5 mg/kg once daily, and the maximum dose is 150 mg for children 1 to 9 years of age.

Actions

Pharmacology: Rimantadine is a synthetic antiviral agent that appears to exert its inhibitory effect early in the viral replicative cycle, possibly inhibiting the uncoating of the virus.

Pharmacokinetics: The time to peak concentration was 6 hours in healthy adults. The single dose elimination half-life in this population was 25.4 hours. The single-dose elimination half-life in a group of healthy 71- to 79-year-old subjects was 32 hours.

The in vitro human plasma protein binding is approximately 40%.

Following oral administration, rimantadine is extensively metabolized in the liver with less than 25% of the dose excreted in the urine as unchanged drug. Three hydroxylated metabolites have been found in plasma. These metabolites, an additional conjugated metabolite and parent drug account for 74% of a single 200 mg dose excreted in urine over 72 hours.

Contraindications

Hypersensitivity to drugs of the adamantine class, including rimantadine and amantadine.

Warnings/Precautions

Seizures: An increased incidence of seizures has been reported in patients with a history of epilepsy who received the related drug amantadine. In clinical trials, the occurrence of seizure-like activity was observed in a small number of patients with a history of seizures who were not receiving anticonvulsant medication while taking rimantadine. If seizures develop, discontinue the drug.

Resistance: Consider transmission of rimantadine-resistant virus when treating patients whose contacts are at high risk for influenza A illness. Influenza A virus strains resistant to rimantadine can emerge during treatment and may be transmissible and cause typical influenza illness. Of patients with initially sensitive virus upon treatment with rimantadine, 10% to 30% shed rimantadine-resistant virus.

Bacterial infections: Serious bacterial infections may begin with influenza-like symptoms or may coexist with or occur as complications during the course influenza. Rimantidine has not been shown to prevent such complications.

Live vaccines: Do not administer the live, attenuated intranasal influenza vaccine 48 hours after cessation of rimantadine, and do not administer rimantadine until 2 weeks after the administration of the live, attenuated intranasal influenza vaccine unless medically indicated.

Renal/Hepatic function impairment: Because of the potential for accumulation of rimantadine and its metabolites in plasma, exercise caution when patients with renal or hepatic insufficiency are treated with rimantadine.

Pregnancy: Category C.

Lactation: Rimantadine should not be administered to nursing mothers because of the adverse affects noted in offspring of rats treated with rimantadine during the nursing period.

Children: The safety and effectiveness of rimantadine in the treatment of symptomatic influenza infection in children 1 to 16 years of age have not been established.

Monitoring: Monitor patients with any degree of renal or hepatic insufficiency for adverse reactions and adjust the dose as needed.

Drug Interactions

Drugs that may affect rimantadine include acetaminophen, aspirin, and cimetidine.

Adverse Reactions

Geriatric subjects who received 200 or 400 mg of rimantadine daily experienced considerably more CNS and GI adverse events than comparable geriatric subjects receiving placebo. CNS events, including dizziness, headache, anxiety, asthenia, and fatigue occurred up to 2 times more often with rimantadine than with placebo. GI symptoms, particularly nausea, vomiting, and abdominal pain occurred at least twice as frequently with rimantadine than with receiving placebo. The GI symptoms appeared to be dose-related.

ZANAMIVIR

Blisters of powder for inhalation: 5 mg (*Rx*)	*Relenza* (GlaxoSmithKline)

Indications

Influenza treatment: Treatment of uncomplicated acute illness caused by influenza A and B virus in adults and children 7 years of age and older who have been symptomatic for no more than 2 days.

Prophylaxis of influenza: In adults and children at least 5 years of age for prophylaxis of influenza.

Administration and Dosage

Treatment: The recommended dose of zanamivir in patients 7 years of age and older is 10 mg twice daily (about 12 hours apart) for 5 days. Two doses should be taken on the first day of treatment whenever possible, provided there is at least 2 hours between doses. On subsequent days, doses should be approximately 12 hours apart at approximately the same time each day.

Prophylaxis:

Household setting – For patients 5 years of age and older, 10 mg once daily for 10 days. The dose should be administered at approximately the same time each day. There are no data on the efficacy of prophylaxis in a household setting when initiated more than 1.5 days after the onset of signs or symptoms in the index case.

Community outbreaks – For patients 12 years of age and older, 10 mg once daily for 28 days. The dose should be administered at approximately the same time each day. There are no data on the efficacy of prophylaxis in a community outbreak when initiated more than 5 days after the outbreak was identified in the community.

Patients scheduled to use an inhaled bronchodilator at the same time as zanamivir should use their bronchodilator before taking zanamivir.

Actions

Pharmacology: Zanamivir is an antiviral drug and is an inhibitor of influenza virus neuraminidase, affecting release of viral particles.

Pharmacokinetics:

Absorption – Approximately 4% to 17% of the inhaled dose is systemically absorbed. Peak serum concentrations ranged from 17 to 142 ng/mL within 1 to 2 hours after a 10 mg dose.

Distribution – Zanamivir has limited plasma protein binding (less than 10%).

Metabolism – Zanamivir is renally excreted as unchanged drug. No metabolites have been detected.

Excretion – The serum half-life of zanamivir following oral inhalation ranges from 2.5 to 5.1 hours. It is excreted unchanged in the urine with excretion of a single dose completed within 24 hours. Total clearance ranges from 2.5 to 10.9 L/h. Unabsorbed drug is excreted in the feces.

Contraindications

Hypersensitivity to any component of the formulation, including lactose.

Warnings/Precautions

Underlying airway diseases: Zanamivir is not recommended for treatment or prophylaxis of influenza in individuals with underlying airway disease (eg, asthma, chronic obstructive pulmonary disease [COPD]).

Neuropsychiatric effects: Influenza can be associated with a variety of neurologic and behavioral symptoms, which can include reactions such as seizures, hallucinations, delirium, and abnormal behavior.

Bacterial infections: Serious bacterial infections may begin with influenza-like symptoms or may coexist with or occur as complications during the course of influenza. Zanamivir has not been shown to prevent such complications.

Hypersensitivity reactions: Allergic-like reactions, including oropharyngeal edema, serious skin rashes, and anaphylaxis have been reported in postmarketing experience with zanamivir. Stop zanamivir and institute appropriate treatment if an allergic reaction occurs or is suspected.

Pregnancy: Category C.

There are no adequate and well-controlled studies in pregnant women. Use during pregnancy only if the potential benefit justifies the potential risk to the fetus.

Lactation: It is not known whether zanamivir is excreted in human breast milk. Exercise caution when zanamivir is administered to a nursing mother.

Children: Safety and efficacy of zanamivir have not been established for the treatment of influenza in pediatric patients younger than 7 years of age and for the prophylaxis of influenza in children younger than 5 years of age.

Elderly: No overall differences in safety or efficacy were observed between these subjects and younger patients, and other reported clinical experience has not identified differences in responses between the elderly and younger patients; however, greater sensitivity of some older individuals cannot be ruled out.

Monitoring: Closely monitor patients with influenza for signs of abnormal behavior.

Drug Interactions

Do not administer live attenuated influenza vaccine within 2 weeks before or 48 hours after administration of zanamivir, unless medically indicated.

Adverse Reactions

Adverse reactions occurring in at least 3% of patients include anorexia/decreased or increased appetite, chills, cough, fatigue, fever, headache, malaise, muscle pain, musculoskeletal pain, nasal signs and symptoms, throat/tonsil discomfort and pain, viral respiratory infections.

Lab test abnormalities: Elevations of liver enzymes and CPK, lymphopenia, and neutropenia occurred. These were reported in similar proportions of zanamivir and lactose-vehicle placebo recipients with acute influenza-like illness.

OSELTAMIVIR

Capsules; oral: 30, 45, and 75 mg (30, 45, and 75 mg free base equivalent of the phosphate salt) (*Rx*) — *Tamiflu* (Roche)

Powder for oral suspension: 12 mg/mL after reconstitution (*Rx*)

Indications

Influenza infection:

Treatment – Treatment of uncomplicated acute illness caused by influenza infection in patients older than 1 year of age who have been symptomatic for no more than 2 days.

Prophylaxis – For prophylaxis of influenza in patients 1 year of age and older.

Administration and Dosage

Oseltamivir may be taken without regard to food. However, when taken with food, tolerability may be enhanced. Shake the oral suspension well before each use.

Treatment of influenza:

Adults and adolescents 13 years of age and older – 75 mg twice daily for 5 days. Begin treatment within 2 days of onset of symptoms of influenza.

Children – The recommended oral dose of oseltamivir oral suspension for children 1 year of age and older or adults who cannot swallow a capsule is in the following table.

Oseltamivir Dosing for the Treatment of Influenza in Children				
Body weight (kg)	Body weight (lb)	Recommended dose for 5 days	Number of bottles needed to obtain the recommended dose	Number of capsules needed to obtain the recommended dose for a 5-day regimen
≤ 15	≤ 33	30 mg twice daily	1	10 (30 mg)
> 15 to 23	> 33 to 51	45 mg twice daily	2	10 (45 mg)
> 23 to 40	> 51 to 88	60 mg twice daily	2	20 (30 mg)
> 40	> 88	75 mg twice daily	3	10 (75 mg)

Influenza prophylaxis: The recommended oral dose for influenza prophylaxis in adults and adolescents 13 years of age and older following close contact with an infected individual is 75 mg once daily for at least 10 days. Begin therapy within 2 days of exposure. The recommended dose for prophylaxis during a community outbreak of influenza is 75 mg once daily. Safety and efficacy have been demonstrated for up to 6 weeks. The duration of protection lasts for as long as dosing is continued.

Children (1 year of age and older) – Prophylaxis in children following close contact with an infected individual is recommended for 10 days. Prophylaxis in patients 1 to 12 years of age has not been evaluated for longer than 10 days' duration. Begin therapy within 2 days of exposure.

The recommended oral dosage of oral suspension for children 1 year of age and older following close contact with an infected individual is listed in the following table.

Oseltamivir Dosing in Influenza Prophylaxis in Children				
Body weight (kg)	Body weight (lbs)	Recommended dosage for 10 days	Number of bottles needed to obtain the recommended dose	Number of capsules needed to obtain the recommended dose for a 10-day regimen
≤ 15 kg	≤33 lbs	30 mg once daily	1	10 (30 mg)
> 15 to 23 kg	> 33 to 51 lbs	45 mg once daily	2	10 (45 mg)
> 23 to 40 kg	> 51 to 88 lbs	60 mg once daily	2	20 (30 mg)
> 40 kg	> 88 lbs	75 mg once daily	3	10 (75 mg)

Renal function impairment:

Influenza treatment – For patients with creatinine clearance between 10 and 30 mL/min receiving oseltamivir, it is recommended that the dose be reduced to 75 mg once daily for 5 days.

Influenza prophylaxis – For patients with creatinine clearance between 10 and 30 mL/min, it is recommended that the dose be reduced to 75 mg every other day or 30 mg every day.

Actions

Pharmacology: Oseltamivir is an ethyl ester prodrug requiring ester hydrolysis for conversion to the active form, oseltamivir carboxylate. The proposed mechanism of action of oseltamivir is via inhibition of influenza virus neuraminidase with the possibility of alteration of virus particle aggregation and release.

Pharmacokinetics:

Absorption – Oseltamivir phosphate is readily absorbed from the GI tract after oral administration.

Coadministration with food has no significant effect on the peak plasma concentration and the area under the plasma concentration time curve of oseltamivir carboxylate.

Distribution – The binding of oseltamivir carboxylate to human plasma protein is low (3%). The binding of oseltamivir to human plasma protein is 42%, which is insufficient to cause significant displacement-based drug interactions.

Metabolism – Oseltamivir is extensively converted to oseltamivir carboxylate by esterases located predominantly in the liver. Neither oseltamivir nor oseltamivir carboxylate is a substrate for, or inhibitor of, CYP-450 isoforms.

Excretion – Plasma concentrations of oseltamivir carboxylate declined with a half-life of 6 to 10 hours in most subjects. Oseltamivir carboxylate is eliminated entirely (more than 99%) by renal excretion. Renal clearance (18.8 L/h) exceeds glomerular filtration rate (7.5 L/h), indicating that tubular secretion occurs in addition to glomerular filtration. Less than 20% of an oral dose is eliminated in feces.

Contraindications

Hypersensitivity to any of the components of the product.

Warnings/Precautions

Bacterial infections: Serious bacterial infections may begin with influenza-like symptoms or may coexist with or occur as complications during the course of influenza.

Start of treatment: Efficacy of oseltamivir in patients who begin treatment after 40 hours of symptoms has not been established.

High-risk patients: Efficacy of oseltamivir in subjects with chronic cardiac disease or respiratory disease has not been established.

Neuropsychiatric reactions: Influenza can be associated with a variety of neurologic and behavioral symptoms, which can include events such as hallucinations, delirium, and abnormal behavior, in some cases resulting in fatal outcomes. These events may occur in the setting of encephalitis or encephalopathy, but can occur without obvious severe disease.

Repeated courses: Safety and efficacy of repeated treatment or prophylaxis courses have not been established.

Hypersensitivity reactions: Rare cases of anaphylaxis and serious skin reactions, including toxic epidermal necrolysis, Stevens-Johnson Syndrome, and erythema multiforme, have been reported in postmarketing experiences with oseltamivir. Stop oseltamivir and institute appropriate treatment if an allergic-like reaction occurs or is suspected.

Renal function impairment: Dose adjustment is recommended for patients with a serum creatinine clearance less than 30 mL/min.

Pregnancy: Category C.

Lactation: It is not known whether oseltamivir or oseltamivir carboxylate is excreted in human breast milk. Therefore, use oseltamivir only if the potential benefit for the breast-feeding mother justifies the potential risk to the breast-fed infant.

Children: The safety and efficacy in children less than 1 year of age have not been established.

Monitoring: Closely monitor patients with influenza for signs or unhealthy behavior throughout the treatment period.

Drug Interactions

Live, attenuated influenza vaccine: Do not administer intranasal live, attenuated influenza vaccine within 2 weeks before or 48 hours after administration of oseltamivir, unless medically indicated.

Probenecid: Coadministration of probenecid results in an approximate 2-fold increase in exposure to oseltamivir carboxylate because of a decrease in active anionic tubular secretion in the kidney.

Adverse Reactions

Adverse reactions occurring in at least 3% of patients include abdominal pain, asthma, cough, diarrhea, dizziness, epistaxis, fatigue, headache, nausea, otitis media, pneumonia, sinusitis, and vomiting.

ADEFOVIR

Tablets: 10 mg (*Rx*)	*Hepsera* (Gilead Sciences)

Warning:

Severe acute exacerbations of hepatitis have been reported in patients who have discontinued antihepatitis B therapy, including adefovir. Closely monitor hepatic function in patients who discontinue antihepatitis B therapy. If appropriate, resumption of antihepatitis B therapy may be warranted.

In patients at risk of or having renal dysfunction, chronic administration of adefovir may result in nephrotoxicity. Closely monitor for renal function and adjust dose as required.

HIV resistance may emerge in chronic hepatitis B patients with unrecognized or untreated HIV infection treated with antihepatitis B therapies, such as adefovir, that may have activity against HIV.

Lactic acidosis and severe hepatomegaly with steatosis, including fatal cases, have been reported with the use of nucleoside analogs alone or in combination with other antiretrovirals.

Indications

Chronic hepatitis B: Treatment of chronic hepatitis B in patients 12 years of age and older with active viral replication and either persistent elevations in serum aminotransferases (ALT or AST) or histologically active disease.

Administration and Dosage

The recommended dose in patients 12 years of age and older is 10 mg once daily without regard to food. Adefovir is not recommended for use in children younger than 12 years of age.

Renal function impairment:

Adefovir Dosage Adjustment in Renal Impairment

	CrCl (mL/min)			
	≥ 50	30 to 49	10 to 29	Hemodialysis patients
Recommended dose and dosing interval	10 mg every 24 h	10 mg every 48 h	10 mg every 72 h	10 mg every 7 days following dialysis

Actions

Pharmacology: Adefovir is an acyclic nucleotide analog of adenosine monophosphate.

Pharmacokinetics:

Absorption/Distribution – The oral bioavailability is 59%. Peak adefovir plasma concentration occurs between 0.58 and 4 hours (median, 1.75 hours) postdose.

Binding of adefovir to plasma or proteins is 4% or less.

Metabolism/Excretion – Elimination half-life is approximately 7.5 hours. Adefovir is renally excreted.

Special populations –

Renal impairment: In subjects with impaired renal function or with end-stage renal disease requiring hemodialysis, C_{max}, AUC, and $t_{1/2}$ were increased. It is recommended that the dosing interval of adefovir be modified in these patients.

Contraindications

Previously demonstrated hypersensitivity to any of the components of the product.

Warnings/Precautions

Exacerbations of hepatitis after discontinuation of treatment: Severe acute exacerbation of hepatitis has been reported in patients who have discontinued antihepatitis B therapy, including adefovir. Monitor patients who discontinue adefovir for hepatic function.

Nephrotoxicity: Nephrotoxicity characterized by a delayed onset of gradual increases in serum creatinine and decreases in serum phosphorus was shown to be the treatment-limiting toxicity of adefovir therapy at higher doses in HIV-infected patients (60 and 120 mg/day) and in chronic hepatitis B patients (30 mg/day). Chronic administration of adefovir (10 mg once daily) may result in nephrotoxicity. This is of special importance in patients at risk of or having renal dysfunction and patients taking concomitant nephrotoxic agents (eg, aminoglycosides, cyclosporine, nonsteroidal anti-inflammatory drugs, tacrolimus, vancomycin).

HIV resistance: Prior to initiating adefovir therapy, offer HIV antibody testing to all patients. Treatment with antihepatitis B therapies, such as adefovir, that have activity against HIV in a chronic hepatitis B patient with unrecognized or untreated HIV infection may result in emergence of HIV resistance.

Lactic acidosis/severe hepatomegaly with steatosis: Lactic acidosis and severe hepatomegaly with steatosis, including fatal cases, have been reported with nucleoside analogs alone or in combination with antiretrovirals.

Renal function impairment: It is recommended that the dosing interval for adefovir be modified in adults with baseline creatinine clearance less than 50 mL/min.

Pregnancy: Category C. To monitor fetal outcomes of pregnant women exposed to adefovir, a pregnancy registry has been established. Health care providers are encouraged to register patients by calling (800) 258-4263.

Lactation: It is not known whether adefovir is excreted in human milk. Decide whether to discontinue adefovir or breast-feeding, taking into account the importance of the drug to the mother.

Children: Adefovir is not recommended for use in children younger than 12 years of age.

Elderly: Exercise caution in elderly patients who may have a greater frequency of decreased renal or cardiac function caused by concomitant disease or other drug therapy.

Monitoring: Closely monitor hepatic function at repeated intervals with both clinical and laboratory follow-up for at least several months in patients who discontinue antihepatitis B therapy.

Drug coadministration – Closely monitor patients when adefovir is coadministered with drugs that are excreted renally or with other drugs known to affect renal function. Closely monitor renal function in all patients during therapy, especially patients at risk of having underlying renal function impairment or patients who develop renal function impairment during therapy with adefovir.

Drug Interactions

Coadministration of adefovir with drugs that reduce renal function or compete for active tubular secretion may increase serum concentrations of adefovir or these coadministered drugs.

Adverse Reactions

Adverse reactions occurring in patients may include abdominal pain, asthenia, diarrhea, dyspepsia, flatulence, headache, and nausea. Laboratory abnormalities may include hematuria, increased ALT or AST, increased amylase, increased creatine kinase, and increased serum creatinine.

ENTECAVIR

Tablets: 0.5 mg, 1 mg (*Rx*) — *Baraclude* (Bristol-Myers Squibb)
Oral solution: 0.05 mg/mL (*Rx*)

Warning:

Severe acute exacerbations of hepatitis B have been reported in patients who have discontinued antihepatitis B therapy, including entecavir. Closely monitor hepatic function with clinical and laboratory follow-up for at least several months in patients who discontinue antihepatitis B therapy. If appropriate, initiation of antihepatitis B therapy may be warranted.

Limited clinical experience suggests there is a potential for the development of resistance to HIV nucleoside reverse transcriptase inhibitors (NRTIs) if entecavir is used to treat chronic hepatitis B virus (HBV) infection in patients with HIV infection that is not being treated. Therapy with entecavir is not recommended for HIV/HBV co-infected patients who are not also receiving highly active antiretroviral therapy (HAART).

Lactic acidosis and severe hepatomegaly with steatosis, including fatal cases, have been reported with the use of nucleoside analogs alone or in combination with antiretrovirals.

Indications

Chronic hepatitis B: For the treatment of chronic hepatitis B virus (HBV) infection in adults with evidence of active viral replication and either evidence of persistent elevations in serum aminotransferases (ALT or AST) or histologically active disease.

Administration and Dosage

Administer entecavir on an empty stomach (at least 2 hours after a meal and 2 hours before the next meal).

Nucleoside-treatment-naive patients: The recommended dosage in adults and adolescents 16 years of age and older is 0.5 mg once daily.

Coadministration with lamivudine or lamivudine- or telbivudine-resistant patients: The recommended dosage in adults and adolescents 16 years of age and older is 1 mg once daily.

Renal function impairment:

Recommended Dosage of Entecavir in Patients with Renal Function Impairment

CrCl (mL/min)	Usual dose (0.5 mg) (nucleoside-naive)	Lamivudine-refractory (1 mg)
≥ 50	0.5 mg once daily	1 mg once daily
30 to < 50	0.25 mg once daily or 0.5 mg every 48 h	0.5 mg once daily or 1 mg every 48 h
10 to < 30	0.15 mg once daily or 0.5 mg every 72 h	0.3 mg once daily or 1 mg every 72 h
< 10; hemodialysis[a] or CAPD[b]	0.05 mg once daily or 0.5 mg every 7 days	0.1 mg once daily or 1 mg every 7 days

[a] Administer after hemodialysis.
[b] CAPD = continuous ambulatory peritoneal dialysis.

Duration of therapy: The optimal duration of treatment with entecavir for patients with chronic HBV infection and the relationship between treatment and long-term outcomes such as cirrhosis and hepatocellular carcinoma are unknown.

Actions

Pharmacology: Entecavir is a nucleoside analog with activity against HBV polymerase. Entecavir triphosphate functionally inhibits all 3 activities of HBV polymerase.

Pharmacokinetics:

Absorption/Distribution – Following oral administration, entecavir peak plasma concentrations occurred between 0.5 and 1.5 hours. Steady state was achieved after 6 to 10 days of once-daily administration. The bioavailability of the tablet was 100% relative to the oral solution. The oral solution and tablet may be used interchangeably.

Binding of entecavir to human serum proteins in vitro was approximately 13%.

Metabolism/Excretion – The terminal elimination half-life is approximately 128 to 149 hours.

Entecavir is predominantly eliminated by the kidney with urinary recovery of unchanged drug at steady state ranging from 62% to 73% of the administered dose. Entecavir undergoes both glomerular filtration and net tubular secretion.

Contraindications

Previously demonstrated hypersensitivity to entecavir or any component of the product.

Warnings/Precautions

Lactic acidosis/hepatomegaly: Lactic acidosis and severe hepatomegaly with steatosis, including fatal cases, have been reported with the use of nucleoside analog alone or in combination with antiretrovirals.

Patients coinfected with HIV and HBV: Therapy with entecavir is not recommended for HIV/HBV co-infected patients who are not also receiving HAART.

Posttreatment exacerbations of hepatitis: Severe acute exacerbations of hepatitis B have been reported in patients who have discontinued antihepatitis B therapy, including entecavir.

Renal function impairment: Dosage adjustment of entecavir is recommended for patients with a CrCl less than 50 mL/min, including patients on hemodialysis or CAPD.

Pregnancy: Category C. To monitor fetal outcomes of pregnant women exposed to entecavir, a pregnancy registry has been established. Health care providers are encouraged to register patients by calling 1-800-258-4263.

Lactation: It is not known whether this drug is excreted in human milk. Decide whether to discontinue breast-feeding or the drug.

Children: Safety and effectiveness in pediatric patients younger than 16 years of age have not been established.

Elderly: Because elderly patients are more likely to have decreased renal function, take care in dose selection, and monitor renal function.

Monitoring: Periodic monitoring of hepatic function is recommended during treatment and for at least several months after treatment in patients who discontinue antihepatitis B therapy. Monitor patients closely for adverse events when entecavir is coadministered with drugs that are renally eliminated or known to affect renal function. Monitor patients for signs/symptoms of lactic acidosis/hepatomegaly.

Liver transplant recipients – Safety and efficacy in liver transplant recipients are unknown. If entecavir treatment is necessary for a liver transplant recipient who has received or is receiving an immunosuppressant that may affect renal function (eg, cyclosporine, tacrolimus), renal function must be carefully monitored before and during treatment with entecavir.

Drug Interactions

Drugs affected by renal function impairment: Because entecavir primarily is eliminated by the kidneys, coadministration of entecavir with drugs that reduce renal function or compete for active tubular secretion may increase serum concentrations of either entecavir or the coadministered drug.

Drug/Food interactions: Oral administration of entecavir 0.5 mg with a standard high-fat meal or a light meal resulted in a delay in absorption, a decrease in C_{max}, and a decrease in AUC.

Adverse Reactions

Adverse reactions occurring in 3% or more of patients include fatigue, headache, and hyperglycemia. Lab test abnormalities included the following: ALT greater than 5 times the ULN; lipase greater than 2 times the ULN; total bilirubin greater than 2.5 g/dL; glycosuria; hematuria.

SAQUINAVIR

Tablets: 500 mg (as mesylate) (*Rx*)	*Invirase* (Genentech)
Capsules: 200 mg (as mesylate) (*Rx*)	

Indications

HIV infection: In combination with ritonavir and other antiretroviral agents is indicated for the treatment of HIV infection in adults (older than 16 years of age).

Administration and Dosage

Adults (older than 16 years of age): Saquinavir mesylate 1,000 mg twice daily (5 × 200 mg capsules or 2 × 500 mg tablets) in combination with ritonavir 100 mg twice daily.

Give saquinavir mesylate at the same time as ritonavir and within 2 hours after a meal.

Concomitant therapy with lopinavir/ritonavir: When administered with lopinavir 400 mg/ ritonavir 100 mg twice daily, the appropriate dosage of saquinavir mesylate is 1,000 mg twice daily (with no additional ritonavir).

Dose adjustment for combination therapy with saquinavir: For serious toxicities that may be associated with saquinavir mesylate, the drug should be interrupted. Saquinavir mesylate at doses less than 1,000 mg with ritonavir 100 mg twice daily are not recommended because lower doses have not shown antiviral activity. For recipients of combination therapy with saquinavir mesylate and ritonavir, dose adjustments may be necessary. These adjustments should be based on the known toxicity profile of the individual agent and the pharmacokinetic interaction between saquinavir and the coadministered drug. Refer the complete monographs for these drugs for comprehensive dose adjustment recommendations and drug-associated adverse reactions of nucleoside analogues.

Actions

Pharmacology: Saquinavir is an inhibitor of HIV protease, which cleaves viral polyprotein precursors to generate functional proteins in HIV-infected cells. The cleavage of viral polyprotein precursors is essential for maturation of infectious virus. Saquinavir is a synthetic peptide-like substrate analog that inhibits the activity of HIV protease and prevents the cleavage of viral polyproteins.

Pharmacokinetics:

Absorption/Distribution – Saquinavir exhibits a low absolute bioavailability of 4% following a single dose of *Invirase* after a high-fat breakfast (48 g protein, 60 g carbohydrate, 57 g fat, 1,006 kcal). This is considered to be the result of incomplete absorption and extensive first-pass metabolism.

Saquinavir 24-hour AUC and maximal plasma concentration (C_{max}) following the administration of a higher-calorie meal (943 kcal, 54 g fat) were on average 2 times higher than after a lower-calorie, lower-fat meal (355 kcal, 8 g fat).

The mean steady-state volume of distribution following 12 mg intravenous (IV) is 700 L, suggesting saquinavir partitions into tissues. Saquinavir is approximately 98% bound to plasma proteins. cerebrospinal fluid levels are negligible.

Metabolism/Excretion – In vitro, the metabolism of saquinavir is cytochrome P450 mediated with the specific isoenzyme, CYP3A4, responsible for more than 90% of the hepatic metabolism. In vitro, saquinavir is rapidly metabolized to a range of mono- and di-hydroxylated inactive compounds; 88% and 1% of the oral dose was recovered in feces and urine, respectively, within 5 days of dosing; 81% and 3% of an IV dose was recovered in feces and urine, respectively, within 5 days of dosing.

Systemic clearance of saquinavir was rapid: 1.14 L/h/kg after IV doses of 6, 36, and 72 mg. The mean residence time of saquinavir was 7 hours.

Contraindications

Congenital long QT syndrome; refractory hypokalemia or hypomagnesemia; complete atrioventricular (AV) block without implanted pacemakers, or patients who are at high risk of complete AV block; hypersensitivity (eg, anaphylactic reaction, Stevens-Johnson syndrome) to saquinavir, saquinavir mesylate, or any of the components contained in the capsule or tablet, or to ritonavir; severe hepatic impairment when coadministered with ritonavir; coadministration with drugs that both increase saquinavir plasma concentrations and prolong the QT interval; coadministration with CYP3A substrates (alfuzosin, amiodarone, bepridil, cisapride, dihydroergotamine, dofetilide, ergonovine, ergotamine, flecainide, lidocaine [systemic], lovastatin, methylergonavine, midazolam [orally administered], pimozide, propafenone, quinidine, rifampin, sildenafil [for the treatment of pulmonary arterial hypertension], simvastatin, trazodone, or triazolam).

Warnings/Precautions

Concomitant therapy: Saquinavir must be used in combination with ritonavir.

Toxicity: If a serious or severe toxicity occurs during treatment with saquinavir, interrupt therapy until the etiology of the event is identified or the toxicity resolves. At the time, resumption of treatment with full-dose saquinavir may be considered.

Cardiovascular effects:

PR interval prolongation – Saquinavir/ritonavir prolongs the PR interval in a dose-dependent fashion. Cases of second- or third-degree AV block have been reported rarely. Patients with underlying structural heart disease, pre-existing conduction system abnormalities, cardiomyopathies, and ischemic heart disease may be at increased risk for developing cardiac conduction abnormalities.

QT interval prolongation: Saquinavir/ritonavir causes dose-dependent QT prolongation. Avoid saquinavir/ritonavir in patients with long QT syndrome. Perform an electrocardiogram prior to initiation of treatment.

Diabetes mellitus and hyperglycemia: New-onset diabetes mellitus, exacerbation of pre-existing diabetes mellitus, and hyperglycemia have been reported in HIV-infected patients receiving protease inhibitors.

Hemophilia: There have been reports of spontaneous bleeding in patients with hemophilia A and B treated with protease inhibitors. In some patients, additional Factor VIII was required.

Fat redistribution: Redistribution/accumulation of body fat, including central obesity, dorsocervical fat enlargement (buffalo hump), facial wasting, peripheral wasting, breast enlargement, and "cushingoid appearance" have been observed in patients receiving protease inhibitors.

Immune reconstitution syndrome: Immune reconstitution syndrome has been reported in patients treated with combination antiretroviral therapy, including saquinavir mesylate. During the initial phase of combination antiretroviral treatment, patients whose immune systems respond may develop an inflammatory response to indolent or residual opportunistic infections, which may necessitate further evaluation and treatment.

Hyperlipidemia: Elevated cholesterol and/or triglyceride levels have been observed in some patients taking saquinavir in combination with ritonavir. Marked elevation in triglyceride levels is a risk factor for development of pancreatitis.

Resistance/cross-resistance: Varying degrees of cross-resistance among protease inhibitors have been observed. Continued administration of saquinavir mesylate therapy following loss of viral suppression may increase the likelihood of cross-resistance to other protease inhibitors.

Hepatic function impairment: In patients with underlying hepatitis B or C, cirrhosis, long-term alcoholism, and/or other underlying liver abnormalities, there have been reports of worsening liver disease.

Saquinavir in combination with ritonavir is contraindicated in patients with severe hepatic impairment.

Pregnancy: *Category B.*

Antiretroviral pregnancy registry – To monitor maternal-fetal outcomes of pregnant women exposed to antiretroviral medications, an antiretroviral pregnancy registry has been established. Health care providers are encouraged to register patients by calling 1-800-258-4263.

Lactation: It is not known whether saquinavir is excreted in breast milk. Because of the potential for serious adverse reactions in breast-feeding infants from saquinavir, decide whether to discontinue breast-feeding or the drug, taking into account the importance of saquinavir to the mother.

The Centers for Disease Control and Prevention advises HIV-infected women not to breast-feed to avoid postnatal transmission of HIV to a child who may not be infected.

Children: Safety and efficacy in HIV-infected children or adolescents younger than 16 years of age have not been established.

Monitoring: Perform clinical chemistry tests prior to initiating saquinavir therapy and at appropriate intervals thereafter. Periodically monitor triglyceride levels during therapy.

Drug Interactions

Drugs that may affect saquinavir/ritonavir include anticonvulsants, antimycobacterials, atazanavir, azole antifungals, clarithromycin, delavirdine, dexamethasone, efavirenz, erythromycin, fluoxetine, garlic, immunosuppressants, indinavir, loperamide, lopinavir/ritonavir, nevirapine, proton pump inhibitors, QT prolonging agents, St. John's wort, and tripranavir/ritonavir.

Drugs that may be affected by saquinavir/ritonavir include antiarrhythmics, anticonvulsants, antimycobacterials, antipsychotic agents, azole antifungals, benzodiazepines, bosentan, buspirone, calcium channel blockers, cabazitaxel, cisapride, clarithromycin, colchicine, contraceptives (oral), delavirdine, digoxin, docetaxel, efavirenz, eplerenone, ergot derivatives, erlotinib, erythromycin, eszopiclone, fluoxetine, fluticasone (inhaled/nasal), HMG-CoA reductase inhibitors, iloperidone, immunosuppressants, ixabepilone, loperamide, maraviroc, methadone, mTOR inhibitors, muscarinic receptor antagonists, nilotinib, opioid analgesics, PDE5 inhibitors, pimozide, proton pump inhibitors, QT prolonging agents, quinazolines, ranolazine, romidepsin, salmeterol, selective 5-HT_1 receptor agonists, thyroid hormones, trazodone, tricyclic antidepressants, tyrosine kinase inhibitors, vasopressin receptor antagonists, warfarin.

Cytochrome P-450 system: Because saquinavir is metabolized mainly by the CYP3A enzyme systems, substances known to inhibit these enzymes may decrease metabolism or increase bioavailability of saquinavir, as indicated by increased whole blood or plasma concentrations. Drugs known to induce these enzyme systems may result in an increased metabolism of saquinavir or decreased bioavailability, as indicated by decreased whole blood or plasma concentrations. Monitoring of blood concentrations and appropriate dosage adjustments are essential when such drugs are used concomitantly.

Adverse Reactions

Adverse reactions occurring in at least 3% of patients include abdominal pain, diarrhea, fatigue, fever, lipodystrophy, nausea, pneumonia, pruritus, rash, vomiting.

RITONAVIR

Tablets; oral: 100 mg (*Rx*) — *Norvir* (Abbott)
Capsules, soft gelatin, oral: 100 mg (*Rx*)
Solution, oral: 80 mg/mL (*Rx*)

Warning:

Coadministration of ritonavir with sedative hypnotics, antiarrhythmics, or ergot alkaloid preparations may result in potentially serious and/or life-threatening adverse reactions due to possible effects of ritonavir on the hepatic metabolism of certain drugs.

Indications

HIV infection: In combination with other antiretroviral agents for the treatment of HIV infection.

Administration and Dosage

Adults: The recommended dosage is 600 mg twice daily. Start ritonavir at 300 mg twice daily and increase at 2- to 3-day intervals by 100 mg twice daily.

Children: The recommended dosage of ritonavir in children 1 month of age and older is 350 to 400 mg/m² twice daily by mouth and should not exceed 600 mg twice daily. Ritonavir should be started at 250 mg/m² and increased at 2- to 3-day intervals by 50 mg/m² twice daily. Administer oral solution dose using a calibrated dosing syringe.

Dosage Guidelines for Ritonavir in Children

Body surface area[a] (m^2)	Twice-daily dose 250 mg/m²	Twice-daily dose 300 mg/m²	Twice-daily dose 350 mg/m²	Twice-daily dose 400 mg/m²
0.2	0.6 mL (50 mg)	0.75 mL (60 mg)	0.9 mL (70 mg)	1 mL (80 mg)
0.25	0.8 mL (62.5 mg)	0.9 mL (75 mg)	1.1 mL (87.5 mg)	1.25 mL (100 mg)
0.5	1.6 mL (125 mg)	1.9 mL (150 mg)	2.2 mL (175 mg)	2.5 mL (200 mg)
0.75	2.3 mL (187.5 mg)	2.8 mL (225 mg)	3.3 mL (262.5 mg)	3.75 mL (300 mg)
1	3.1 mL (250 mg)	3.75 mL (300 mg)	4.4 mL (350 mg)	5 mL (400 mg)
1.25	3.9 mL (312.5 mg)	4.7 mL (375 mg)	5.5 mL (437.5 mg)	6.25 mL (500 mg)
1.5	4.7 mL (375 mg)	5.6 mL (450 mg)	6.6 mL (525 mg)	7.5 mL (600 mg)

[a] Body surface area (m^2) can be calculated with the following equation: Multiply the square root of a patient's height in centimeters by the patient's weight in kilograms divided by 3,600.

Concomitant therapy with other protease inhibitors: Dose reduction of ritonavir is necessary when used with other protease inhibitors (eg, amprenavir, atazanavir, darunavir, fosamprenavir, saquinavir, tipranavir).

Conversion: Patients who take ritonavir capsules may experience more GI adverse reactions when switching from the capsule to the tablet because of greater maximum plasma concentration achieved with the tablet formulation relative to the capsule. These adverse reactions (GI or paresthesias) may diminish as therapy is continued.

Administration: Ritonavir is administered orally and should be taken with meals.

Tablets – Ritonavir tablets should be swallowed whole, and not chewed, broken, or crushed.

Solution – Shake well before each use. When possible, administer the dose using a calibrated dosing syringe. Patients may improve the taste of the solution by mixing with chocolate milk or enteral nutritional liquid therapy liquids (eg, *Advera, Ensure*) within 1 hour of dosing.

Actions

Pharmacology: Ritonavir is an inhibitor of the HIV-1 and HIV-2 proteases. Inhibition of HIV protease renders the enzyme incapable of processing the Gag-Pol polyprotein precursor, which leads to production of noninfectious immature HIV particles.

Pharmacokinetics: Peak concentrations of ritonavir were achieved approximately 2 and 4 hours after dosing under fasting and nonfasting conditions, respectively. The extent of absorption of ritonavir from the capsule formulation was 13% higher when administered with a meal. Ritonavir is almost 99% protein bound.

CYP-450 3A (CYP3A) is a major isoform involved in ritonavir metabolism, although CYP2D6 also contributes to the formation of M-2. Approximately 11.3% of the dose was excreted into the urine and 86.4% in the feces. Elimination half-life is 3 to 5 hours.

Contraindications

Coadministration with alfuzosin, amiodarone, bepridil, cisapride, dihydroergotamine, ergonovine, ergotamine, flecainide, lovastatin, methylergonovine, oral midazolam, pimozide, propafenone, quinidine, St. John's wort (*Hypericum perforatum*), and sildenafil (*Revatio*; only when used for the treatment of pulmonary arterial hypertension, simvastatin, triazolam, voriconazole; hypersensitivity to ritonavir or any of its ingredients.

Warnings/Precautions

Hepatic effects: Hepatic transaminase elevations exceeding 5 times the upper limit of normal, clinical hepatitis, and jaundice have occurred in patients receiving ritonavir alone or in combination with other antiretroviral drugs.

Pancreatitis: Pancreatitis has been observed in patients receiving ritonavir therapy, including those who developed hypertriglyceridemia. Patients with advanced HIV disease may be at increased risk of elevated triglycerides and pancreatitis.

Diabetes mellitus/Hyperglycemia: New-onset diabetes mellitus, exacerbation of pre-existing diabetes mellitus, diabetic ketoacidosis, and hyperglycemia have been reported in HIV-infected patients receiving protease inhibitors.

Resistance/Cross-resistance: Varying degrees of cross-resistance among protease inhibitors have been observed. Continued administration of ritonavir therapy following loss of viral suppression may increase the likelihood of cross-resistance to other protease inhibitors.

Hemophilia: There have been reports of increased bleeding, including spontaneous skin hematomas and hemarthrosis, in patients with hemophilia type A and B treated with protease inhibitors.

PR interval prolongation: Ritonavir prolongs the PR interval in some patients. Use ritonavir with caution in patients with underlying structural heart disease, preexisting conduction system abnormalities, ischemic heart disease, and cardiomyopathies.

Fat redistribution: Redistribution/accumulation of body fat, including central obesity, dorsocervical fat enlargement (buffalo hump), peripheral wasting, breast enlargement, and "cushingoid appearance," have been observed in patients receiving antiretroviral therapy.

Lipid disorders: Treatment with ritonavir alone or in combination with saquinavir has resulted in substantial increases in the concentration of total triglycerides and cholesterol.

Ritonavir has been shown to increase triglycerides, cholesterol, AST, ALT, gamma glutamyl transferase (GGT), creatine phosphokinase (CPK), and uric acid. Perform appropriate laboratory testing prior to initiating ritonavir therapy and at periodic intervals or if any clinical signs or symptoms occur during therapy.

Immune reconstitution syndrome: Immune reconstitution syndrome has been reported in HIV-infected patients treated with combination antiretroviral therapy, including ritonavir.

Hypersensitivity reactions: Allergic reactions, including urticaria, mild skin eruptions, bronchospasm, and angioedema, have been reported. Rare cases of anaphylaxis and Stevens-Johnson syndrome also have been reported.

Hepatic function impairment: Ritonavir is principally metabolized by the liver. Exercise caution when administering this drug to patients with impaired hepatic function.

Pregnancy: Category B.

Antiretroviral pregnancy registry – To monitor maternal-fetal outcomes of pregnant women exposed to ritonavir, an antiretroviral pregnancy registry has been established. Health care providers are encouraged to register patients by calling 1-800-258-4263.

Lactation: It is not known whether this drug is excreted in breast milk. The Centers for Disease Control and Prevention advises HIV-infected women not to breastfeed to avoid postnatal transmission of HIV to a child who may not be infected.

Elderly: In general, dose selection for an elderly patient should be cautious, usually starting at the low end of the dosing range, reflecting the greater frequency of decreased hepatic, renal, or cardiac function, and of concomitant disease or other drug therapy.

Monitoring: Consider increased AST/ALT monitoring in patients with hepatitis B or C, especially during the first 3 months of ritonavir treatment.

Ritonavir has been shown to increase triglycerides, cholesterol, AST, ALT, GGT, CPK, and uric acid. Monitor blood glucose levels closely.

Drug Interactions

Drugs that may affect ritonavir include aldesleukin, anticonvulsants, azole antifungals, clarithromycin, immunosuppressants, mefloquine, nonnucleoside reverse transcriptase inhibitors, rifamycins, selective serotonin reuptake inhibitors, and St. John's wort.

Drugs that may be affected by ritonavir include alfuzosin, antiarrhythmic agents, anticonvulsants, antidepressants, antineoplastic agents, antipsychotics, azole antifungals, atovaquone, benzodiazepines, beta blockers, bosentan, buspirone, calcium channel blockers, cisapride, colchicine, clarithromycin, conivaptan, contraceptives (hormonal), corticosteroids, deferasirox, didanosine, disulfiram, digoxin, dronabinol, dronedarone, eplerenone, ergot derivatives, eszopiclone, HMG-CoA reductase inhibitors, iloperidone, immunosuppressants, ixabepilone, levothyroxine, maraviroc, methamphetamine, metronidazole, muscarinic receptor antagonists, nilotinib, opioid analgesics, PDE5 inhibitors, protease inhibitors, quinine, ranolazine, rifamycins, salmeterol, selective 5-HT_1 receptor agonists, sulfamethoxazole, theophylline, trimethoprim, tyrosine kinase receptor inhibitors, warfarin, zidovudine, and zolpidem.

Drug/Food interactions: Grapefruit juice may increase the plasma concentrations and pharmacologic effects of ritonavir. If grapefruit juice cannot be avoided, close clinical monitoring is indicated. Adjust the ritonavir dose accordingly.

Adverse Reactions

Adverse reactions occurring in at least 3% of patients include abdominal pain, anorexia, asthenia, constipation, depression, diarrhea, dizziness, dyspepsia, fever, flatulence, headache, insomnia, malaise, nausea, pain (unspecified), paresthesia, paresthesia (circumoral), paresthesia (peripheral), rash, skin rash/allergy, sweating, taste perversion, vasodilation, vomiting.

INDINAVIR

Capsules: 100, 200, and 400 mg (*Rx*)	*Crixivan* (Merck)

Indications

HIV infection: Treatment of HIV infection in combination with other antiretroviral agents.

Administration and Dosage

Adults: The recommended dosage is 800 mg (two 400 mg capsules) orally every 8 hours.

For optimal absorption, administer without food, but with water, 1 hour before or 2 hours after a meal, or administer with other liquids, such as skim milk, juice, coffee or tea, or with a light meal.

Delavirdine: Consider dose reduction of indinavir to 600 mg every 8 hours when administering delavirdine 400 mg 3 times/day.

Didanosine: If indinavir and didanosine are administered concomitantly, administer them at least 1 hour apart on an empty stomach.

Itraconazole: Dose reduction of indinavir to 600 mg every 8 hours is recommended when concurrently administering itraconazole 200 mg twice daily.

Ketoconazole: Dose reduction of indinavir to 600 mg every 8 hours is recommended when concurrently administering ketoconazole.

Rifabutin: Dose reduction of rifabutin to half the standard dose and a dose increase of indinavir to 1,000 mg every 8 hours are recommended when rifabutin and indinavir are coadministered.

Cirrhosis: Reduce the dosage of indinavir to 600 mg every 8 hours in patients with mild to moderate hepatic insufficiency caused by cirrhosis.

Nephrolithiasis/Urolithiasis: In addition to adequate hydration, medical management in patients who experience nephrolithiasis/urolithiasis may include temporary interruption of therapy (eg, 1 to 3 days) or discontinuation of therapy.

Actions

Pharmacology: Indinavir is an inhibitor of the HIV protease. Indinavir binds to the protease active site and inhibits the activity of the enzyme. This inhibition prevents cleavage of the viral polyproteins, resulting in the formation of immature, noninfectious viral particles.

Pharmacokinetics:

Absorption/Distribution – Indinavir was rapidly absorbed in the fasted state with a time to peak plasma concentration (T_{max}) of 0.8 hours. Indinavir was approximately 60% bound to human plasma proteins.

Metabolism – Following a 400 mg dose of ^{14}C-indinavir, 83% and 19% of the total radioactivity was recovered in feces and urine, respectively. In vitro studies indicate that cytochrome P450 3A4 (CYP3A4) is the major enzyme responsible for formation of the oxidative metabolites.

Excretion – Indinavir is excreted (less than 20%) unchanged in the urine. Indinavir was rapidly eliminated with a half-life of 1.8 hours.

Contraindications

Hypersensitivity to any of the components of indinavir; coadministration with alfuzosin, amiodarone, dihydroergotamine, ergonovine, ergotamine, methylergonovine, cisapride, pimozide, oral midazolam, triazolam, alprazolam, and sildenafil (when used for the treatment of pulmonary arterial hypertension).

Warnings/Precautions

Nephrolithiasis/Urolithiasis: Nephrolithiasis/Urolithiasis has occurred with indinavir. The frequency of nephrolithiasis is substantially higher in pediatric patients (29%) than in adult patients (12.4%).

Hemolytic anemia: Short-term hemolytic anemia, including cases resulting in death, has been reported in patients treated with indinavir.

Hepatitis: Hepatitis, including cases resulting in hepatic failure and death, has been reported in patients treated with indinavir. Because the majority of these patients had confounding medical conditions and/or were receiving concomitant therapy(ies), a causal relationship between indinavir and these events has not been established. Hepatitis, including cases resulting in hepatic failure and death, has been reported in patients treated with indinavir.

Hyperglycemia: New-onset diabetes mellitus, exacerbation of pre-existing diabetes mellitus, and hyperglycemia have been reported during postmarketing surveillance in HIV-infected patients receiving protease inhibitor therapy.

Hyperbilirubinemia: Indirect hyperbilirubinemia has occurred frequently during treatment with indinavir and has infrequently been associated with increases in serum transaminases.

Immune reconstitution syndrome: Immune reconstitution syndrome has been reported in patients treated with combination antiretroviral therapy (CART), including indinavir.

Tubulointerstitial nephritis: Reports of tubulointerstitial nephritis with medullary calcification and cortical atrophy have been observed in patients with asymptomatic severe leukocyturia (greater than 100 cells/high power field).

Hemophilia: There have been reports of spontaneous bleeding in patients with hemophilia A and B treated with protease inhibitors.

Fat redistribution: Redistribution/accumulation of body fat, including central obesity, dorsocervical fat enlargement (buffalo hump), peripheral wasting, breast enlargement, and "cushingoid appearance," have been observed in patients receiving protease inhibitors.

Hepatic function impairment: Patients with hepatic insufficiency because of cirrhosis should have the dosage of indinavir lowered because of decreased metabolism.

Pregnancy: Category C.

Lactation: Although it is not known whether indinavir is excreted in breast milk, the potential for adverse effects from indinavir in nursing infants exists. Instruct mothers to discontinue nursing if they are receiving indinavir.

Children: The optimal dosing regimen for use of indinavir in children has not been established.

Elderly: In general, exercise caution in dose selection for an elderly patient, reflecting the greater frequency of decreased hepatic, renal, or cardiac function, and of concomitant disease or other drug therapy.

Monitoring: Monitor patients for signs or symptoms of nephrolithiasis/urolithiasis (including flank pain with or without hematuria or microscopic hematuria), consider temporary interruption (eg, 1 to 3 days) or discontinuation of therapy.

Monitor blood glucose levels closely; new-onset diabetes or exacerbation of preexisting diabetes has been associated with protease-inhibitor therapy. Closely follow patients with asymptomatic sever leukocyturia and frequently monitor with urinalysis.

Drug Interactions

Drugs that may affect indinavir include anticonvulsants, atazanavir, azole antifungals, clarithromycin, delavirdine, didanosine, efavirenz, esomeprazole, interleukins, lansoprazole, nelfinavir, nevirapine, omeprazole, pantoprazole, rifamycins, ritonavir, St. John's wort, and venlafaxine.

Drugs that may be affected by indinavir include amiodarone, antiarrhythmics, atazanavir, benzodiazepines, calcium channel blockers, cisapride, clarithromycin, conivaptan, corticosteroids (inhaled/nasal; eg, fluticasone), dihydropyridine, ergot alkaloids, fentanyl, HMG-CoA reductase inhibitors, immunosuppressant agents, ixabepilone, lapatinib, phosphodiesterase type 5 inhibitors, pimozide, ranolazine, rifamycins, ritonavir, saquinavir, and trazodone.

Drug/Food interactions: Administration of indinavir with a meal high in calories, fat, and protein (784 kcal, 48.6 g fat, 31.3 g protein) resulted in a 77% reduction in AUC and an 84% reduction in C_{max}. Administration with lighter meals resulted in little or no change in AUC, C_{max}, or trough concentration.

Adverse Reactions

Adverse reactions occurring in at least 3% of patients include abdominal pain; nausea; diarrhea; vomiting; headache; dizziness; pruritus; nephrolithiasis/urolithiasis; back pain; increased ALT, AST, and total serum bilirubin.

TIPRANAVIR

Capsules, oral: 250 mg (*Rx*)	*Aptivus* (Boehringer Ingelheim)
Solution, oral: 100 mg/mL[a]	

[a] Each mL of oral solution contains vitamin E 116 units.

Warning:

Hepatotoxicity: Clinical hepatitis and hepatic decompensation, including some fatalities, have been reported. Extra vigilance is warranted in patients with chronic hepatitis B or hepatitis C coinfection, as these patients have an increased risk of hepatotoxicity

Intracranial hemorrhage: Both fatal and nonfatal intracranial hemorrhage have been reported.

Indications

HIV infection: Tipranavir, coadministered with ritonavir, is indicated for combination antiretroviral treatment of HIV-1–infected adult patients who are treatment-experienced and have HIV-1 strains resistant to more than 1 protease inhibitor (PI).

Administration and Dosage

500 mg (two 250 mg capsules) coadministered with ritonavir 200 mg twice daily.

Take with food.

Children 2 to 18 years of age:

HIV-1 infection –

Usual doseage: Tipranavir 14 mg/kg with ritonavir 6 mg/kg twice daily. Alternatively, tipranavir 375 mg/m^2 coadministered with ritonavir 150 mg/m^2 twice daily.

Maximum dose: Tipranavir 500 mg coadministered with ritonavir 200 mg twice daily.

Dosage adjustment: For children who develop intolerance or toxicity and cannot continue with tipranavir 14 mg/kg with ritonavir 6 mg/kg, health care providers may consider decreasing the dose to tipranavir 12 mg/kg with ritonavir 5 mg/kg (or tipranavir 290 mg/m^2 coadministered with ritonavir 115 mg/m^2) taken twice daily, provided their virus is not resistant to multiple PIs.

Hepatic function impairment: Tipranavir/ritonavir is contraindicated in patients with moderate or severe (Child-Pugh class B and C, respectively) hepatic impairment.

Actions

Pharmacology: Tipranavir is a nonpeptidic HIV-1 PI that inhibits the virus-specific processing of the viral Gag and Gag-Pol polyproteins in HIV-1–infected cells, thus preventing formation of mature virions.

Pharmacokinetics:

Absorption – Steady state is attained in most subjects after 7 to 10 days of dosing.

Food effects: For tipranavir capsules or oral solution coadministered with ritonavir at steady state, no clinically significant changes in C_{max}, Cp12h, and AUC were observed under fed conditions (500 to 682 Kcal, 23% to 25% calories from fat) compared with fasted conditions. Tipranavir coadministered with ritonavir may be taken with or without food.

Distribution – Tipranavir is extensively bound to plasma proteins (more than 99.9%).

Metabolism – In vitro metabolism studies with human liver microsomes indicated that CYP3A4 is the predominant CYP enzyme involved in tipranavir metabolism.

Excretion – Administration of ^{14}C-tipranavir to subjects that received tipranavir 500 mg/ritonavir 200 mg dosed to steady state demonstrated that most radioactivity (median, 82.3%) was excreted in feces. The effective mean elimination half-life of tipranavir/ritonavir in healthy volunteers and HIV-infected adult patients was approximately 4.8 and 6 hours, respectively, at steady state.

Contraindications

Moderate or severe (Child-Pugh class B or C, respectively) hepatic impairment; coadministration of tipranavir/ritonavir with the following drugs that are highly dependent on CYP3A for clearance or are potent CYP3A inducers: alfuzosin, amiodarone, bepridil, cisapride, dihydroergotamine, ergonovine, ergotamine, flecainide, lovastatin, methylergonovine, midazolam (oral), pimozide, propafenone, quinidine, rifampin, sildenafil (Revatio for the treatment of pulmonary arterial hypertension, simvastatin, St. John's wort (Hypericum perforatum), and triazolam. Because of the need for coadministration of tipranavir with ritonavir, refer to the Ritonavir monograph for a description of ritonavir contraindications.

Warnings/Precautions

Coadministration with ritonavir: Tipranavir must be coadministered with ritonavir 200 mg to exert its therapeutic effect.

Diabetes mellitus/hyperglycemia: New-onset diabetes mellitus, exacerbation of preexisting diabetes mellitus, and hyperglycemia have been reported during postmarketing surveillance in HIV-1–infected patients receiving PI therapy.

Hepatic toxicity: Tipranavir coadministered with ritonavir 200 mg has been associated with reports of clinical hepatitis and hepatic decompensation, including some fatalities.

Intracranial hemorrhage: Tipranavir coadministered with ritonavir 200 mg has been associated with reports of both fatal and nonfatal intracranial hemorrhage. Routine measurement of coagulation parameters is not currently indicated in the management of patients on tipranavir.

Platelet aggregation inhibition: Tipranavir was observed to inhibit human platelet aggregation in in vitro experiments. Use tipranavir/ritonavir with caution in patients who may be at risk of increased bleeding from trauma, surgery, or other medical conditions, or who are receiving medications known to increase the risk of bleeding, such as antiplatelet agents or anticoagulants.

Sulfa allergy: Use tipranavir with caution in patients with a known sulfonamide allergy. Tipranavir contains a sulfonamide moiety.

Vitamin E: Advise patients taking tipranavir oral solution not to take supplemental vitamin E greater than a standard multivitamin because tipranavir oral solution contains vitamin E 116 units/mL, which is higher than the reference daily intake (adults, 30 units; children, approximately 10 units).

Rash: Mild to moderate rashes, including urticarial rash, maculopapular rash, and possible photosensitivity, have been reported in subjects receiving tipranavir/ritonavir.

Hemophilia: There have been reports of increased bleeding, including spontaneous skin hematomas and hemarthrosis, in patients with hemophilia type A and B treated with PIs.

Lipid elevations: Treatment with tipranavir coadministered with ritonavir 200 mg has resulted in large increases in the concentration of total cholesterol and triglycerides.

Fat redistribution: Redistribution/accumulation of body fat, including central obesity, dorsocervical fat enlargement (buffalo hump), peripheral wasting, facial wasting, breast enlargement, and "cushingoid appearance," have been observed in patients receiving antiretroviral therapy.

Immune reconstitution syndrome: Immune reconstitution syndrome has been reported in patients treated with combination antiretroviral therapy, including tipranavir.

Hepatic function impairment: Exercise caution when administering tipranavir/ritonavir to patients with mild hepatic impairment (Child-Pugh class A). Tipranavir is contraindicated in patients with moderate or severe (Child-Pugh class B or C, respectively) hepatic impairment.

Pregnancy: Category C.

Lactation: The Centers for Disease Control and Prevention recommend that HIV-infected mothers not breast-feed their infants to avoid risking postnatal transmission of HIV. Because of the potential for HIV transmission and possible adverse reactions of tipranavir, instruct mothers not to breast-feed if they are receiving tipranavir.

Children: The safety, pharmacokinetic profile, and virologic and immunologic responses of tipranavir oral solution and capsules were evaluated in HIV-1 infected children 2 to 18 years of age.

The most frequent adverse reactions (grades 2 to 4) were similar to those described in adults. However, rash was reported more frequently in children than in adults.

The risk-benefit has not been established in children younger than 2 years of age.

Elderly: In general, exercise caution in the administration and monitoring of tipranavir in elderly patients, reflecting the greater frequency of decreased hepatic, renal, or cardiac function, and of concomitant disease or other drug therapy.

Monitoring: Perform liver function tests prior to initiating therapy with tipranavir/ritonavir, and frequently throughout the duration of treatment.

Perform triglyceride and cholesterol testing prior to initiating tipranavir/ritonavir therapy and at periodic intervals during therapy. Manage lipid disorders as clinically appropriate.

Monitor patients for signs or symptoms of hepatitis (eg, acholic stools, anorexia, bilirubinuria, fatigue, hepatomegaly, jaundice, liver tenderness, malaise, nausea).

Drug Interactions

Drugs that may affect tipranavir include aluminum- and magnesium-based antacids, anticonvulsants (eg, carbamazepine, phenobarbital, phenytoin), azole antifungals, clarithromycin, delavirdine, efavirenz, loperamide, nevirapine, nucleoside reverse transcriptase inhibitors (NRTIs) (ie, didanosine, zidovudine), rifamycins (eg, rifampin), St. John's wort, tenofovir.

Drugs that may be affected by tipranavir include anticholinergic agents (eg, darifenacin, fesoterodine, solifenacin, tolterodine), anticonvulsants (eg, valproic acid), aripiprazole, azole antifungals, clarithromycin, colchicine, delavirdine, digoxin, dronedarone, eplerenone, erlotinib, eszopiclone, loperamide, NRTIs (eg, abacavir, didanosine, zidovudine), rifamycins (eg, rifabutin), rosuvastatin, tenofovir, antiarrhythmic agents (eg, amiodarone, bepridil, flecainide, propafenone, quinidine), benzodiazepines (eg, midazolam, triazolam), calcium channel blockers (eg, diltiazem, felodipine, nicardipine, nisoldipine, verapamil), cisapride, hormonal contraceptives (estrogen-containing), desipramine, disulfiram, metronidazole, ergot derivatives, fluticasone, HMG-CoA reductase inhibitors (ie, atorvastatin, lovastatin, rosuvastatin, simvastatin,), hypoglycemic agents (ie, glimepiride, glipizide, glyburide, tolbutamide, pioglitazone, repaglinide), immunosuppressants (ie, cyclosporine, sirolimus, tacrolimus), maraviroc, omeprazole, opioid analgesics (eg, meperidine, methadone), phosphodiesterase type 5 inhibitors (ie, sildenafil, tadalafil, vardenafil), pimozide, protease inhibitors (ie, amprenavir, lopinavir, saquinavir), protein-tyrosine kinase inhibitors (eg, dasatinib, lapatinib, pazopanib, sorafenib, sunitinib), quetiapine, ranolazine, selective serotonin reuptake inhibitors (ie, fluoxetine, paroxetine, sertraline), trazodone, vasopressin receptor antagonists (eg, conivaptan, tolvaptan), warfarin.

Adverse Reactions

The most frequent adverse reactions were diarrhea, fatigue, headache, nausea, and vomiting.

Other adverse effects occurring in 3% or more of patients receiving tipranavir/ritonavir include abdominal pain, pyrexia, weight decreased, anemia, hypertriglyceridemia, cough (5.5%), and rash (5.5%).

Lab test abnormalities: White blood cell count decrease; amylase; ALT; AST; ALT and/or AST; cholesterol; triglycerides.

DARUNAVIR

Tablets: 75, 150, 400, and 600 mg (as ethanolate) (*Rx*)	*Prezista* (Tibotec Therapeutics)

Indications

HIV infection: For the treatment of HIV-1 infection, coadministered with ritonavir and with other antiretroviral agents in adult patients and children 6 years of age and older.

Administration and Dosage

General dosing recommendations: Darunavir must be coadministered with ritonavir and food to exert its therapeutic effect. Failure to correctly coadminister darunavir with ritonavir will result in plasma levels of darunavir that will be insufficient to achieve the desired antiviral effect and will alter some drug interactions.

Adults:

Treatment-naive – 800 mg (two 400 mg tablets) taken with ritonavir 100 mg once daily and with food.

Treatment-experienced – 600 mg twice daily taken with ritonavir 100 mg twice daily and with food.

Children 6 years of age and older:

Darunavir/Ritonavir Recommended Dosage for Children		
Body weight		Dosage
(kg)	(lbs)	
≥ 20 kg to < 30 kg	≥ 44 lbs to < 66 lbs	Darunavir 375 mg/ritonavir 50 mg twice daily with food
≥ 30 kg to < 40 kg	≥ 66 lbs to < 88 lbs	Darunavir 450 mg/ritonavir 60 mg twice daily with food
≥ 40 kg	≥ 88 lbs	Darunavir 600 mg/ritonavir 100 mg twice daily with food

The maximum dosage is darunavir 600 mg/ritonavir 100 mg twice daily.

Administration: Administer with food. Before prescribing darunavir, children should be assessed for the ability to swallow tablets. If a child is unable to reliably swallow a tablet, the use of darunavir may not be appropriate. Do not use once-daily dosing in children or treatment-experience adults.

Hepatic impairment: Darunavir/Ritonavir is not recommended for use in patients with severe hepatic impairment.

Missed dose: If the patient misses a dose of darunavir or ritonavir by more than 12 hours, instruct the patient to wait and then take the next dose of darunavir and ritonavir at the regularly scheduled time. If the patient misses a dose of darunavir or ritonavir by less than 12 hours, instruct the patient to take darunavir and ritonavir immediately, and then take the next dose of darunavir and ritonavir at the regularly scheduled time. If a dose of darunavir or ritonavir is skipped, advise the patient not to double the next dose.

Actions

Pharmacology: It selectively inhibits the cleavage of HIV encoded Gag-Pol polyproteins in infected cells, thereby preventing the formation of mature virus particles.

Pharmacokinetics:

Absorption – Darunavir, coadministered with ritonavir 100 mg twice daily, was absorbed following oral administration with a time to maximum concentration of approximately 2.5 to 4 hours. The absolute oral bioavailability of a single darunavir 600 mg dose with ritonavir 100 mg twice daily was 82%.

Effects of food: When administered with food, the maximum effective plasma concentration (C_{max}) and area under the curve (AUC) of darunavir, coadministered with ritonavir, is approximately 30% higher relative to the fasting state. Therefore, always take darunavir tablets, coadministered with ritonavir, with food.

Distribution – Darunavir is approximately 95% bound to plasma proteins. Darunavir binds primarily to plasma alpha-1 acid glycoprotein.

Metabolism – Darunavir is extensively metabolized by CYP enzymes, primarily by CYP3A.

Excretion – The terminal elimination half-life of darunavir was approximately 15 hours when combined with ritonavir.

Contraindications

Coadministration with drugs that are highly dependent on CYP3A for clearance and drugs for which elevated plasma concentrations are associated with serious and/or life-threatening events (narrow therapeutic index) (eg, alfuzosin, ergot derivatives [dihydroergotamine, ergonovine, ergotamine, methylergonovine]; cisapride; pimozide; orally administered midazolam; triazolam; St. John's wort, lovastatin, simvastatin, rifampin).

PDE-5 (phosphodiesterase type 5) inhibitors (eg, sildenafil for treatment of pulmonary arterial hypertension) are contraindicated. A safe and effective dose for the treatment of pulmonary arterial hypertension has not been established. There is an increased potential for sildenafil-associated adverse events, which include visual disturbances, hypotension, prolonged erection, and syncope.

Warnings/Precautions

Dermatologic effects: During the clinical development program, severe skin rash, including erythema multiforme and Stevens-Johnson syndrome, has been reported. In some cases, fever and elevations of transaminases have also been reported. Discontinue treatment with darunavir if severe rash develops.

Sulfa allergy: Darunavir contains a sulfonamide moiety. Use darunavir with caution in patients with a known sulfonamide allergy.

Diabetes mellitus/hyperglycemia: New onset diabetes mellitus, exacerbation of preexisting diabetes mellitus, and hyperglycemia have been reported during postmarketing surveillance in HIV-infected patients receiving PI therapy.

Hemophilia: There have been reports of increased bleeding, including spontaneous skin hematomas and hemarthrosis, in patients with hemophilia type A and B treated with PIs. In some patients, additional factor VIII was given.

Hepatotoxicity: Drug-induced hepatitis (eg, acute hepatitis, cytolytic hepatitis) has been reported with darunavir/ritonavir. If there is evidence of new or worsening liver function impairment in patients on darunavir/ritonavir, interruption or discontinuation of treatment must be considered.

Fat redistribution: Redistribution/accumulation of body fat, including central obesity, dorsocervical fat enlargement (buffalo hump), peripheral wasting, facial wasting, breast enlargement, and "cushingoid appearance" have been observed in patients receiving antiretroviral therapy.

Immune reconstitution syndrome: During the initial phase of treatment, patients responding to antiretroviral therapy may develop an inflammatory response to indolent or residual opportunistic infections.

Resistance/Cross-resistance: Because the potential for HIV cross-resistance among protease inhibitors has not been fully explored in darunavir/ritonavir-treated patients.

Hepatic function impairment: Darunavir is primarily metabolized by the liver. Exercise caution when darunavir/ritonavir is given to patients with hepatic function impairment; increased plasma concentrations are expected in patients with hepatic function impairment.

Pregnancy: Category C.

Antiretroviral Pregnancy Registry – To monitor maternal-fetal outcomes of pregnant women exposed to darunavir, an antiretroviral pregnancy registry has been established. Patients can be registered by calling 1-800-258-4263.

Lactation: The Centers for Disease Control and Prevention recommend that HIV-infected mothers not breast-feed their infants in order to avoid risking postnatal transmission of HIV. Because of the potential for HIV transmission and the potential for serious adverse reactions in breast-feeding infants, instruct mothers not to breast-feed if they are receiving darunavir.

Children: The safety and efficacy of darunavir/ritonavir in children 3 to younger than 6 years of age have not been established.

Elderly: Exercise caution in the administration and monitoring of darunavir in elderly patients, reflecting the greater frequency of decreased hepatic function and of concomitant disease or other drug therapy.

Monitoring: Monitor liver function tests as clinically appropriate. Consider increased AST/ALT monitoring in patients with underlying chronic hepatitis, cirrhosis, or in patients who have pretreatment evaluations of transaminases, especially during the first several months of darunavir/ritonavir treatment.

Drug Interactions

Cytochrome P450 system: Darunavir and ritonavir are inhibitors of CYP3A and CYP2D6. Coadministration of darunavir and ritonavir with drugs that are primarily metabolized by CYP3A and CYP2D6 may result in increased plasma concentrations of such drugs, which could increase or prolong their therapeutic effect and adverse reactions.

Darunavir and ritonavir are metabolized by CYP3A. Drugs that induce CYP3A activity would be expected to increase the clearance of darunavir and ritonavir, resulting in lowered plasma concentrations of darunavir and ritonavir. Coadministration of darunavir and ritonavir and other drugs that inhibit CYP3A may decrease the clearance of darunavir and ritonavir and may result in increased plasma concentrations of darunavir and ritonavir.

Drugs that may affect darunavir include alpha-1 adrenoreceptor antagonists, anticonvulsants, azole antifungals, carbamazepine, corticosteroids, didanosine, efavirenz, indinavir, lopinavir/ritonavir, nonnucleoside reverse transcriptase inhibitors, rifamycins, saquinavir, and St. John's wort.

Drugs that may be affected by darunavir include antiarrhythmic agents, anipsychotics, anticonvulsants, azole antifungals, benzodiazepines, beta blockers, calcium channel blockers, carbamazepine, cisapride, clarithromycin, colchicine, contraceptives (hormonal), corticosteroids, desipramine, dextromethorphan, didanosine, digoxin, dronedarone, ergot derivatives, indinavir, HMG-CoA reductase inhibitors, immunosuppressants, iloperidone, lopinavir/ritonavir, maraviroc, methadone, nonnucleoside reverse transcriptase inhibitors, omeprazole, opioid analgesics, phosphodiesterase type 5 inhibitors, rifamycins, pimozide, quetiapine, selective serotonin reuptake inhibitors, tenofovir, trazodone, and warfarin.

Drug/Food interactions: Always take darunavir tablets coadministered with ritonavir with food.

Adverse Reactions The most common treatment-emergent adverse reactions (greater than 10%) were diarrhea, headache, nasopharyngitis, and nausea.

Adverse reactions occurring in 3% or more of patients include lab test abnormality increases in alanine aminotransferase, alkaline phosphatase, aspartate aminotransferase, bicarbonate, gamma-glutamyltransferase, hyperuricemia, hypoalbuminemia, pancreatic amylase, pancreatic lipase, partial thromboplastin time, plasma prothrombin time, total cholesterol, and triglycerides; and lab test abnormality decreases in lymphocytes, platelet count, absolute neutrophil count, and white blood cell count.

NELFINAVIR

Tablets: 250 and 625 mg (as base) (*Rx*) — *Viracept* (Agouron)
Powder: 50 mg/g (as base) (*Rx*)

Warning:
Nelfinavir is indicated for the treatment of human immunodeficiency virus (HIV) infection when antiretroviral therapy is warranted. At present, there are no results from controlled trials evaluating the effect of therapy with nelfinavir on clinical progression of HIV infection, such as survival or the incidence of opportunistic infections.

Indications
HIV: For the treatment of HIV infection when antiretroviral therapy is warranted.

Administration and Dosage
Take with a meal.

Adults: The recommended dose is 1250 mg (five 250 mg tablets or two 625 mg tablets) twice daily or 750 mg (three 250 mg tablets) 3 times/day.

Pediatric patients (2 to 13 years of age): 20 to 30 mg/kg/dose 3 times/day. Doses as high as 45 mg/kg every 8 hours have been used.

Pediatric Dose of Nelfinavir (administered 3 times/day)

Body weight		Number of level 1 g scoops	Number of level teaspoons	Number of 250 mg tablets
kg	lbs			
7 to < 8.5	15.5 to < 18.5	4	1	-
8.5 to < 10.5	18.5 to < 23	5	1¼	-
10.5 to < 12	23 to < 26.5	6	1½	-
12 to < 14	26.5 to < 31	7	1¾	-
14 to < 16	31 to < 35	8	2	-
16 to < 18	35 to < 39.5	9	2¼	-
18 to < 23	39.5 to < 50.5	10	2½	2
≥ 23	≥ 50.5	15	3¾	3

Oral powder – The oral powder may be mixed with a small amount of water, milk, formula, soy formula, soy milk, or dietary supplement; once mixed, the entire contents must be consumed in order to obtain the full dose. Acidic food or juice (eg, orange juice, apple juice, or apple sauce) are not recommended because of bitter taste. Do not reconstitute with water in its original container. Once mixed, store the oral powder for no more than 6 hours. May be refrigerated for up to 6 hours.

Actions
Pharmacology: Nelfinavir is an inhibitor of the HIV-1 protease. Inhibition of the viral protease prevents cleavage of the gagpol polyprotein resulting in the production of immature, noninfectious virus.

Pharmacokinetics:

Absorption – After multiple oral doses of 750 mg 3 times/day or 1,250 mg 2 times/day for 28 days (steady-state), peak plasma concentrations averaged 3 to 4 mg/mL, plasma concentrations prior to the morning dose were 1.4 to 2.2 mg/L, and prior to afternoon or evening dose were 0.7 to 1 mg/L.

Effect of food: Maximum plasma concentrations and area under the plasma concentration-time curve (AUC) were 2- to 3-fold higher under fed conditions compared with fasting.

Distribution – The apparent volume of distribution following oral administration of nelfinavir was 2 to 7 L/kg. Nelfinavir in serum is extensively protein-bound (greater than 98%).

Metabolism – Unchanged nelfinavir comprised 82% to 86% of the total plasma. In vitro multiple cytochrome P450 isoforms including CYP3A and CYP2C19 are responsible for metabolism of nelfinavir. One major and several minor oxidative metabolites were found in plasma. The major oxidative metabolite has in vitro antiviral activity comparable with the parent drug.

Excretion – The terminal half-life in plasma was typically 3.5 to 5 hours. The majority (87%) of an oral 750 mg dose was recovered in the feces, which consisted of numerous oxidative metabolites (78%) and unchanged nelfinavir (22%). Only 1% to 2% of the dose was recovered in the urine, of which unchanged nelfinavir was the major component.

Contraindications

Hypersensitivity to any component of the product. Coadministration of nelfinavir is contraindicated with drugs that are highly dependent on CYP3A for clearance and for which elevated plasma concentrations are associated with serious and/or life-threatening events (eg, amiodarone, quinidine, ergot derivatives, pimozide, midazolam, triazolam, lovastatin, simvastatin; see Drug Interactions).

Warnings/Precautions

Diabetes mellitus/hyperglycemia: New-onset diabetes mellitus, exacerbation of pre-existing diabetes mellitus and hyperglycemia have been reported during postmarketing surveillance in HIV-infected patients receiving protease inhibitor therapy. Some patients required either initiation or dose adjustments of insulin or oral hypoglycemic agents for treatment of these events. In some cases, diabetic ketoacidosis has occurred.

Phenylketonurics: Nelfinavir oral powder contains 11.2 mg phenylalanine per g of powder.

Fat redistribution: Redistribution/accumulation of body fat including central obesity, dorsocervical fat enlargement (buffalo hump), peripheral wasting, facial wasting, breast enlargement, and "cushingoid appearance" have been observed in patients receiving antiretroviral therapy.

Hemophilia: There have been reports of increased bleeding, including spontaneous skin hematomas and hemarthrosis, in patients with hemophilia type A and B treated with protease inhibitors.

Hepatic function impairment: Nelfinavir is principally metabolized by the liver. Exercise caution when administering this drug to patients with hepatic impairment.

Pregnancy: Category B.

Lactation: The US Public Health Service Centers for Disease Control and Prevention advises HIV-infected women not to breastfeed to avoid postnatal transmission of HIV to a child who may not yet be infected. It is not known whether nelfinavir is excreted in breast milk.

Children: A similar adverse event profile was seen during the pediatric clinical trial as in adult patients. The evaluation of the antiviral activity of nelfinavir in pediatric patients is ongoing.

The safety, efficacy, and pharmacokinetics of nelfinavir have not been evaluated in pediatric patients younger than 2 years of age.

Drug Interactions

CYP450: Nelfinavir is an inhibitor of CYP3A (cytochrome P450 3A). Coadministration of nelfinavir and drugs primarily metabolized by CYP3A may result in increased plasma concentrations of the other drug, which could increase or prolong its therapeutic and adverse effects.

Drugs that may affect nelfinavir include anticonvulsants, azithromycin, azole antifungals, efavirenz, delavirdine, HMG-CoA reductase inhibitors, indinavir, interleukins, nevirapine, rifabutin, rifampin, ritonavir, saquinavir, St. John's wort.

Drugs that may be affected by nelfinavir include amiodarone, antiarrhythmics (amiodarone, quinidine), azithromycin, benzodiazepines, efavirenz, ergot alkaloids, delavirdine, didanosine, fentanyl, indinavir, lamivudine; methadone, nonsedating antihistamines, oral contraceptives, phenytoin, pimozide, quinidine, rifabutin, saquinavir, sildenafil, sirolimus, tacrolimus, zidovudine.

Drug/Food interactions: Maximum plasma concentrations and AUC were 2- to 3-fold higher under fed conditions compared with fasting.

Adverse Reactions

Adverse effects occurring in at least 3% of patients include diarrhea, nausea, flatulence, hematologic abnormalities, rash, and increases in ALT, AST, and creatine kinase.

ATAZANAVIR

Capsules; oral: 100, 150, 200, and 300 mg (as base) (*Rx*) *Reyataz* (Bristol-Myers Squibb)

Indications

HIV infection: In combination with other antiretroviral agents for the treatment of HIV-1 infection.

Administration and Dosage

General dosing recommendations: Must be taken with food.

When coadministered with didanosine-buffered or enteric-coated formulations, give atazanavir (with food) 2 hours before or 1 hour after didanosine. When coadministered with H_2-receptor antagonists or proton pump inhibitors, dose separation may be required.

Safety and efficacy of atazanavir with ritonavir in dosages greater than 100 mg once daily have not been established. The use of higher ritonavir doses might alter the safety profile of atazanavir (eg, cardiac effects, hyperbilirubinemia) and, therefore, is not recommended.

Atazanavir without ritonavir is not recommended for treatment-experienced patients with prior virologic failure.

Adults:

Therapy-naive patients – 400 mg once daily with food.

For treatment-naive patients who are unable to tolerate ritonavir, the recommended dose is atazanavir 400 mg (without ritonavir) once daily, taken with food.

Concomitant therapy: Atazanavir 300 mg with ritonavir 100 mg once daily (all as a single dose with food) if combined with the following:

Tenofovir – Atazanavir 300 mg with ritonavir 100 mg once daily (all as a single dose with food) if combined with tenofovir.

Didanosine – When coadministered with didanosine-buffered or enteric-coated formulations, give atazanavir with food 2 hours before or 1 hour after didanosine.

H_2-receptor antagonist – The H_2-receptor antagonist dose should not exceed a dose comparable with famotidine 40 mg twice daily. Atazanavir 300 mg and ritonavir 100 mg should be administered simultaneously with, and/or at least 10 hours after, the dose of the H_2-receptor antagonist. For patients unable to tolerate ritonavir, atazanavir 400 mg once daily with food should be administered at least 2 hours before and at least 10 hours after the H_2-receptor antagonist. For these patients, no single dose of the H_2-receptor antagonist should exceed a dose comparable with famotidine 20 mg, and the total daily dose should not exceed a dose comparable with famotidine 40 mg.

Proton pump inhibitors – The proton pump inhibitor dose should not exceed a dose comparable with omeprazole 20 mg and must be taken approximately 12 hours prior to the atazanavir 300 mg and ritonavir 100 mg dose.

Efavirenz – If atazanavir is combined with efavirenz, atazanavir 400 mg (two 200 mg capsules) with ritonavir 100 mg should be administered once daily all as a single dose with food, and efavirenz should be administered on an empty stomach, preferably at bedtime.

Therapy-experienced patients – Atazanavir 300 mg with ritonavir 100 mg once daily (all as a single dose with food).

Concomitant therapy:

Didanosine – When coadministered with didanosine-buffered or enteric-coated formulations, give atazanavir (with food) 2 hours before or 1 hour after didanosine.

H_2-receptor antagonist – Whenever an H_2-receptor antagonist is given to a patient receiving atazanavir with ritonavir, the H_2-receptor antagonist dose should not exceed a dosage comparable with famotidine 20 mg twice daily, and the atazanavir and ritonavir doses should be administered simultaneously with, and/or at least 10 hours after, the dose of the H_2-receptor antagonist.

Atazanavir 300 mg with ritonavir 100 mg once daily should be given all as a single dose with food if taken with an H_2-receptor antagonist.

Tenofovir/H_2-receptor antagonist combination – Atazanavir 400 mg (two 200 mg capsules) with ritonavir 100 mg once daily should be given all as a single dose with food if taken with both tenofovir and an H_2-receptor antagonist.

Proton pump inhibitors – Proton pump inhibitors should not be used in treatment-experienced patients receiving atazanavir.

Efavirenz – Dosing recommendations for efavirenz and atazanavir in treatment-experienced patients have not been established.

Children: The recommended dosage of atazanavir for children is based on body weight and should not exceed the recommended adult dosage.

6 to younger than 18 years of age –

HIV infection, therapy-naive children:

Without ritonavir – For treatment-naive patients at least 13 years of age and weighing at least 39 kg who are unable to tolerate ritonavir, the recommended dosage is atazanavir 400 mg (without ritonavir) once daily with food. The data are insufficient to recommend dosing of atazanavir without ritonavir in patients younger than 13 years of age.

With ritonavir –

Atazanavir Dosage for Treatment-Naive Children

Body weight			
(kg)	(lb)	Atazanavir dose[a,b]	Ritonavir dose[b]
15 to < 25	33 to < 55	150 mg	80 mg[c]
25 to < 32	55 to < 70	200 mg	100 mg[d]
32 to < 39	70 to < 86	250 mg	100 mg[d]
≥ 39	≥ 86	300 mg	100 mg[d]

[a] The recommended dosage of atazanavir can be achieved using a combination of commercially available capsule strengths.
[b] The dosage of atazanavir and ritonavir was calculated as follows:

- 15 kg to < 20 kg: atazanavir 8.5 mg/kg with ritonavir 4 mg/kg once daily with food
- ≥ 20 kg: atazanavir 7 mg/kg with ritonavir 4 mg/kg once daily with food, not to exceed atazanavir 300 mg and ritonavir 100 mg.

[c] Ritonavir liquid.
[d] Ritonavir capsule or liquid.

HIV infection, therapy-experienced children: The data are insufficient to recommend dosing of treatment-experienced children weighing less than 25 kg.

Atazanavir Dosage for Treatment-Experienced Children

Body weight			
(kg)	(lb)	Atazanavir dose[a,b]	Ritonavir dose[b]
25 to < 32	55 to < 70	200 mg	100 mg[c]
32 to < 39	70 to < 86	250 mg	100 mg[c]
≥ 39	≥ 86	300 mg	100 mg[c]

[a] The recommended dosage of atazanavir can be achieved using a combination of commercially available capsule strengths.
[b] The dosage was calculated as atazanavir 7 mg/kg with ritonavir 4 mg/kg once daily with food, not to exceed atazanavir 300 mg and ritonavir 100 mg.
[c] Ritonavir capsule or liquid.

Younger than 6 years of age: The data are insufficient to recommend dosing of atazanavir for patients younger than 6 years of age or treatment-experienced children with body weight less than 25 kg. Do not administer atazanavir to children younger than 3 months of age because of the risk of kernicterus. The safety, activity, and pharmacokinetic profiles of atazanavir in children 3 months to younger than 6 years of age have not been established.

Renal function impairment: Treatment-naive patients with end-stage renal disease managed with hemodialysis should receive atazanavir 300 mg with ritonavir 100 mg. Atazanavir should not be administered to HIV-treatment–experienced patients with end-stage renal disease managed with hemodialysis.

Hepatic function impairment: For patients with moderate hepatic function impairment (Child-Pugh class B) who have not experienced prior virologic failure, consider a dosage reduction to 300 mg once daily. Do not use atazanavir in patients with severe hepatic function impairment (Child-Pugh class C).

Actions

Pharmacology: Atazanavir is an azapeptide HIV-1 protease inhibitor.

Pharmacokinetics:

Absorption/Distribution – Atazanavir is rapidly absorbed, with a T_{max} of approximately 2.5 hours in healthy subjects (2 hours in HIV-infected patients). Steady state is achieved between days 4 and 8. Atazanavir is 86% bound to human serum proteins.

Metabolism/Excretion – Atazanavir is extensively metabolized and eliminated primarily by the liver. In vitro studies using human liver microsomes suggested that atazanavir is metabolized by CYP3A. The mean elimination half-life of atazanavir is about 7.9 hours in healthy subjects and 6.5 hours in subjects with HIV infection.

Effect of food – Administration of atazanavir with food enhances bioavailability and reduces pharmacokinetic variability.

Contraindications

Known hypersensitivity (eg, Stevens-Johnson syndrome, erythema multiforme, toxic skin eruptions) to atazanavir or any of its ingredients; coadministration with the following drugs that are highly dependent on CYP3A or UGT1A1 for clearance and for which elevated plasma concentrations are associated with serious and/or life-threatening events: cisapride, dihydroergotamine, ergonovine, ergotamine, indinavir, irinotecan, lovastatin, methylergonovine, midazolam (orally administered), pimozide, rifampin, St. John's wort, simvastatin, and triazolam.

Warnings/Precautions

PR interval prolongation: Atazanavir has been shown to prolong the PR interval of the electrocardiogram (ECG) in some patients. In healthy volunteers and in patients, abnormalities in atrioventricular (AV) conduction were asymptomatic and generally limited to first-degree AV block. There have been rare reports of second-degree AV block and other conduction abnormalities.

Diabetes mellitus/Hyperglycemia: New-onset diabetes mellitus, exacerbation of preexisting diabetes mellitus, and hyperglycemia have been reported during postmarketing surveillance in HIV-infected patients receiving protease inhibitor therapy. Some patients required either initiation or dose adjustments of insulin or oral hypoglycemia agents for treatment of these events. In some cases, diabetic ketoacidosis has occurred.

Immune reconstitution syndrome: Reported in patients treated with combination antiretroviral therapy, including atazanavir. During the initial phase of combination antiretroviral treatment, patients whose immune systems respond may develop an inflammatory response to indolent or residual opportunistic infections (such as *Mycobacterium avium* infection, cytomegalovirus, *Pneumocystis jiroveci* pneumonia, or tuberculosis), which may necessitate further evaluation and treatment.

Hyperbilirubinemia: Most patients taking atazanavir experience asymptomatic elevations in indirect (unconjugated) bilirubin related to inhibition of UDP-glucuronosyl transferase. This hyperbilirubinemia is reversible upon discontinuation of atazanavir.

Nephrolithiasis: Cases of nephrolithiasis were reported during postmarketing surveillance in HIV-infected patients receiving atazanavir therapy.

Resistance/Cross-resistance: Various degrees of cross-resistance among protease inhibitors have been observed. Resistance to atazanavir may not preclude the subsequent use of other protease inhibitors.

Hemophilia: There have been reports of increased bleeding, including spontaneous skin hematomas and hemarthrosis in patients with hemophilia type A and B treated with protease inhibitors.

Fat redistribution: Redistribution/accumulation of body fat, including central obesity, dorsocervical fat enlargement (buffalo hump), peripheral wasting, facial wasting, breast enlargement, and cushingoid appearance, have been observed in patients receiving antiretroviral therapy.

Rash: In controlled clinical trials, rash occurred in 21% of patients treated with atazanavir. Discontinue atazanavir if severe rash develops. Cases of Stevens-Johnson syndrome and erythema multiforme have been reported in patients receiving atazanavir.

Immune reconstitution syndrome: Immune reconstitution syndrome has been reported in patients treated with combination antiretroviral therapy, including atazanavir.

Hepatic function impairment: Atazanavir is principally metabolized by the liver; exercise caution when administering this drug to patients with hepatic impairment because atazanavir concentrations may be increased.

Pregnancy: Category B.

Antiretroviral pregnancy registry – To monitor maternal-fetal outcomes of pregnant women exposed to atazanavir, an antiretroviral pregnancy registry has been established. Physicians are encouraged to register patients by calling 1-800-258-4263.

Lactation: It is not known whether atazanavir is secreted in human breast milk. Because of the potential for HIV transmission and the potential for serious adverse reactions in breast-feeding infants, instruct mothers not to breast-feed if they are receiving atazanavir.

Children: Do not administer atazanavir to children younger than 3 months of age because of the risk of kernicterus.

Elderly: In general, exercise appropriate caution in the administration and monitoring of atazanavir in elderly patients.

Monitoring: Monitor ECG at baseline and periodically during treatment. Monitor glucose, lipids, and liver function tests. Monitor CD4+ cell count and HIV RNA load.

Drug Interactions

Drugs that may be affected by atazanavir include the following: antiarrhythmics, benzodiazepines, calcium channel blockers, carbamazepine, cisapride, clarithromycin, corticosteroids, didanosine (enteric-coated), ergot derivatives, HMG-CoA reductase inhibitors, hormonal contraceptives, immunosuppressants, irinotecan, itraconazole, ixabepilone, ketoconazole, lapatinib, nevirapine, opioid analgesics, PDE5 inhibitors, pimozide, protease inhibitors, ranolazine, rifabutin, saquinavir, tenofovir, trazodone, tricyclic antidepressants, voriconazole, and warfarin.

Drugs that may affect atazanavir include the following: antacids and buffered medications, carbamazepine, clarithromycin, didanosine (buffered formulation only), H_2-receptor antagonists, itraconazole, ketoconazole, nonnucleoside reverse transcriptase inhibitors, protease inhibitors, proton pump inhibitors, rifampin, St. John's wort, tenofovir, voriconazole.

Adverse Reactions

Adverse reactions occurring in at least 3% of patients include the following: abdominal pain, diarrhea, headache, insomnia, jaundice/scleral icterus, myalgia, nausea, peripheral neurologic symptoms, rash, vomiting.

Lab test abnormalities: Amylase or lipase 2.1 × ULN or higher; AST, ALT, or creatine kinase 5.1 × ULN or higher; glucose 251 mg/dL or higher; hemoglobin less than

8 g/dL; neutrophils less than 750 cells/mm^3; platelets less than 50,000/mm^3; total bilirubin 2.6 × ULN or higher; total cholesterol 240 mg/dL or higher; triglycerides 751 mg/dL or higher.

LOPINAVIR/RITONAVIR

Tablets, oral: lopinavir 100 mg/ritonavir 25 mg and lopinavir 200 mg/ritonavir 50 mg (*Rx*) — *Kaletra* (Abbott)
Solution, oral: lopinavir 80 mg/ritonavir 20 mg/mL (*Rx*)

Indications

HIV infection: In combination with other antiretroviral agents for the treatment of HIV infection.

Administration and Dosage

Adults:

Therapy-naive patients – The recommended dosage is lopinavir 400 mg/ritonavir 100 mg (5 mL with food, or 2 lopinavir 200 mg/ritonavir 50 mg tablets with or without food) twice daily or lopinavir 800 mg/ritonavir 200 mg (10 mL with food, or four 200/50 mg tablets with or without food) once daily with less than 3 lopinavir resistance-associated substitutions.

Therapy-experienced patients – The recommended dosage is lopinavir 400 mg/ritonavir 100 mg (5 mL with food, or 2 lopinavir 200 mg/ritonavir 50 mg tablets with or without food) twice daily.

Concomitant therapy –

Anticonvulsants: Lopinavir/ritonavir should not be administered once daily in combination with carbamazepine, phenobarbital, or phenytoin.

Antiretrovirals: Lopinavir/ritonavir should not be administered as a once-daily regimen in combination with efavirenz, nevirapine, (fos)amprenavir, or nelfinavir.

Tablets – Lopinavir 500 mg/ritonavir 125 mg twice daily when used in combination with efavirenz, nevirapine, (fos)amprenavir, or nelfinavir.

Oral solution – Lopinavir 533 mg/ritonavir 133 mg (6.5 mL) twice daily taken with food when used in combination with efavirenz, nevirapine, (fos)amprenavir, or nelfinavir.

Children:

14 days to 6 months of age – The recommended dosage of lopinavir/ritonavir using the oral solution is lopinavir 16 mg/ritonavir 4 mg per kg or lopinavir 300 mg/ritonavir 75 mg per m^2 twice daily. Calculate the appropriate dose based on body weight or body surface area (BSA).

6 months to 18 years of age:

Without efavirenz, nevirapine, (fos)amprenavir, or nelfinavir concomitant therapy – In children 6 months to 18 years of age, the recommended dosage of lopinavir/ritonavir using lopinavir/ritonavir oral solution without concomitant efavirenz, nevirapine, (fos)amprenavir, or nelfinavir is lopinavir 230 mg/ritonavir 57.5 mg per m^2 given twice daily. If weight-based dosing is preferred, the recommended dosage of lopinavir/ritonavir for patients weighing less than 15 kg is lopinavir 12 mg/ritonavir 3 mg per kg given twice daily, and the dosage for patients weighing 15 to 40 kg is lopinavir 10 mg/ritonavir 2.5 mg per kg given twice daily with food.

Dosing Recommendations for Children 6 Months to 18 Years of Age for Lopinavir/Ritonavir Tablets Without Concomitant Efavirenz, Nevirapine, (Fos)amprenavir, or Nelfinavir

Body weight (kg)	BSA (m^2)[a]	Recommended number of lopinavir 100 mg/ritonavir 25 mg tablets twice daily
15 to 25	0.6 to < 0.9	2
> 25 to 35	0.9 to < 1.4	3

Dosing Recommendations for Children 6 Months to 18 Years of Age for Lopinavir/Ritonavir Tablets Without Concomitant Efavirenz, Nevirapine, (Fos)amprenavir, or Nelfinavir		
Body weight (kg)	BSA (m²)[a]	Recommended number of lopinavir 100 mg/ ritonavir 25 mg tablets twice daily
> 35	≥ 1.4	4 (or 2 lopinavir 200 mg/ ritonavir 50 mg tablets)

[a] Lopinavir/ritonavir oral solution is available for children with a BSA < 0.6 m^2 or those who are unable to reliably swallow a tablet.

The maximum dose is lopinavir 400 mg/ritonavir 100 mg twice daily.

Concomitant efavirenz, nevirapine, (fos)amprenavir, or nelfinavir therapy – Lopinavir 300 mg/ ritonavir 75 mg/m^2 twice daily. If dosing by body weight, lopinavir 13 mg/ritonavir 3.25 mg per kg given twice daily for patients weighing less than 15 kg and lopinavir 11 mg/ritonavir 2.75 mg per kg given twice daily for patients weighing 15 to 45 kg.

Dosing Recommendations for Children 6 Months to 18 Years of Age for Lopinavir/Ritonavir Tablets With Concomitant Efavirenz,[a] Nevirapine, (Fos)amprenavir,[a] or Nelfinavir[a]		
Body weight (kg)	BSA (m²)[b]	Recommended number of lopinavir 100 mg/ ritonavir 25 mg tablets twice daily
15 to 20	0.6 to < 0.8	2
> 20 to 30	0.8 to < 1.2	3
> 30 to 45	1.2 to < 1.7	4 (or 2 lopinavir 200 mg/ ritonavir 50 mg tablets)
> 45	≥ 1.7	4 or 6 (or 2 or 3 lopinavir 200 mg/ ritonavir 50 mg tablets)

[a] Refer to the individual product labels for appropriate dosing in children.
[b] Lopinavir/ritonavir oral solution is available for children with a BSA < 0.6 m^2 or those who are unable to reliably swallow a tablet.

Administration – Lopinavir/ritonavir tablets may be taken with or without food; oral solution must be taken with food. Tablets should be swallowed whole and not chewed, broken, or crushed. The dose of the oral solution should be administered using a calibrated syringe.

Actions

Pharmacology: Lopinavir, an HIV protease inhibitor, prevents cleavage of the Gag-Pol polyprotein, resulting in the production of immature, noninfectious viral particles. As coformulated in the lopinavir/ritonavir combination, ritonavir inhibits the CYP3A-mediated metabolism of lopinavir, providing increased lopinavir plasma levels.

Pharmacokinetics:

Absorption –

Tablets: No clinically significant changes in maximal drug concentrations (C_{max}) and area under the curve (AUC) were observed following administration of lopinavir/ritonavir tablets under fed conditions compared with fasted conditions. Therefore, lopinavir/ritonavir tablets may be taken with or without food.

Oral solution: Relative to fasting, administration of lopinavir/ritonavir oral solution with a moderate-fat meal increased lopinavir AUC and C_{max} by 80% and 54%, respectively. To enhance bioavailability and minimize pharmacokinetic variability, take lopinavir/ritonavir oral solution with food.

Distribution – Lopinavir is approximately 98% to 99% bound to plasma proteins.

Metabolism – Lopinavir is extensively metabolized by the hepatic CYP-450 system, almost exclusively by the CYP3A isozyme. Ritonavir is a potent CYP3A inhibitor that inhibits the metabolism of lopinavir and, therefore, increases plasma levels of lopinavir. Ritonavir has been shown to induce metabolic enzymes, resulting in the induction of its own metabolism.

Excretion – Less than 3% of the lopinavir dose is excreted unchanged in the urine. The half-life of lopinavir over a 12-hour dosing interval averaged 5 to 6 hours.

Contraindications

Hypersensitivity (eg, Stevens-Johnson syndrome, erythema multiforme) to any of the ingredients, including ritonavir; coadministration with drugs that are highly dependent on CYP3A for clearance; coadministration with potent CYP3A inducers; coadministration with alfuzosin, astemizole, cisapride, dihydroergotamine, ergonovine, ergotamine, lovastatin, methylergonovine, oral midazolam, pimozide, rifampin, sildenafil when used to treat pulmonary arterial hypertension, simvastatin, St. John's wort, and triazolam.

Warnings/Precautions

Pancreatitis: Pancreatitis has been observed in patients receiving lopinavir/ritonavir therapy, including those who developed marked triglyceride elevations. Fatalities have been observed. Although a causal relationship to lopinavir/ritonavir has not been established, marked triglyceride elevation is a risk factor for development of pancreatitis.

Hepatotoxicity: Patients with underlying hepatitis B or C or marked elevations in transaminase prior to treatment may be at increased risk for developing or worsening of transaminase elevations or hepatic decompensation with use of lopinavir/ritonavir.

Diabetes mellitus/hyperglycemia: New-onset diabetes mellitus, exacerbation of pre-existing diabetes mellitus, and hyperglycemia have been reported during postmarketing surveillance in HIV-infected patients receiving protease inhibitor therapy.

Cardiovascular effects:

PR interval prolongation – Lopinavir/ritonavir prolongs the PR interval in some patients. Cases of second or third degree atrioventricular block have been reported. Use lopinavir/ritonavir with caution in patients with underlying structural heart disease, preexisting conduction system abnormalities, ischemic heart disease, or cardiomyopathies.

QT interval prolongation – Postmarketing cases of QT interval prolongation and torsade de pointes have been reported. Avoid use in patients with congenital long QT syndrome, those with hypokalemia, and with other drugs that prolong the QT interval.

Immune reconstitution syndrome: Immune reconstitution syndrome has been reported in patients treated with combination antiretroviral therapy, including lopinavir/ritonavir.

Fat redistribution: Redistribution/accumulation of body fat, including central obesity, dorsocervical fat enlargement (buffalo hump), peripheral wasting, facial wasting, breast enlargement, and cushingoid appearance, have been observed in patients receiving antiretroviral therapy.

Lipid elevations: Treatment with lopinavir/ritonavir has resulted in large increases in the concentration of total cholesterol and triglycerides.

Hemophilia: There have been reports of increased bleeding, including spontaneous skin hematomas and hemarthrosis, in patients with hemophilia types A and B treated with protease inhibitors.

Hepatic function impairment: Lopinavir/ritonavir is principally metabolized by the liver; therefore, exercise caution when administering this drug to patients with hepatic function impairment because lopinavir concentrations may be increased.

Pregnancy: Category C. To monitor maternal-fetal outcomes of pregnant women exposed to lopinavir/ritonavir, an antiretroviral pregnancy registry has been established. Register patients by calling (800) 258-4263.

Lactation: The Centers for Disease Control and Prevention recommend that HIV-infected mothers not breast-feed their infants to avoid risking postnatal transmission of HIV.

Children: The safety, efficacy, and pharmacokinetic profiles of lopinavir/ritonavir in children younger than 14 days of age have not been established. Lopinavir/ritonavir once daily has not been evaluated in children.

Elderly: Exercise appropriate caution in the administration and monitoring of lopinavir/ritonavir in elderly patients, reflecting the greater frequency of decreased hepatic, renal, or cardiac function and of concomitant disease or other drug therapy.

Monitoring: Monitor patients for hepatic dysfunction prior to initiating treatment and closely during treatment. Consider increased AST/ALT monitoring in these patients, especially during the first several months of therapy.

Perform triglyceride and cholesterol testing prior to initiating lopinavir/ritonavir therapy and at periodic intervals during therapy.

Monitor blood glucose levels closely.

Drug Interactions

Drugs that might be affected by lopinavir/ritonavir include antiarrhythmics, anticonvulsants, aripiprazole, astemizole, atovaquone, benzodiazepines, beta-blockers, bosentan, bupropion, buspirone, calcium channel blockers, cisapride, clarithromycin, colchicine, conivaptan, contraceptives, hormonal, corticosteroids, darunavir, deferasirox, didanosine, digoxin, disulfiram, docetaxel, dronabinol, dronedarone, eletriptan, eplerenone, ergot derivatives, erlotinib, erythromycin, eszopiclone, fosamprenavir, HMG-CoA reductase inhibitors, iloperidone, immunosuppressants, indinavir, irinotecan, ixabepilone, levothyroxine, maraviroc, methamphetamine, mTOR inhibitors, muscarinic receptor antagonists, nefazodone, nilotinib, NRTIs, olanzapine, opioid analgesics, PDE5 inhibitors, phenothiazines, pimozide, prednisone, quetiapine, quinazolines, quinine, ranolazine, rifabutin and rifabutin metabolite, rifampin, risperidone, romidepsin, salmeterol, saquinavir, selective serotonin reuptake inhibitors, theophylline, trazodone, triamcinolone, triazolam, tricyclic antidepressants, tyrosine kinase receptor inhibitors, vasopressin receptor, vinblastine, vincristine, voriconazole, warfarin, and zolpidem.

Drugs that may affect lopinavir/ritonavir include aldesleukin (IL-2), anticonvulsants, azole antifungals, cat's claw, clarithromycin, corticosteroids, darunavir, delavirdine, efavirenz, evening primrose, fosamprenavir, nelfinavir, rifamycins, selective serotonin reuptake inhibitors, St. John's wort, and tipranavir.

Adverse Reactions

Adverse reactions occurring in at least 3% of patients include abdominal pain, amenorrhea, amylase, asthenia, calculated CrCl, creatine phosphokinase, diarrhea, dyspepsia, flatulence, headache, insomnia, lipase, nausea, rash, vasodilation, vomiting, and weight loss. Lab abnormalities include elevations of AST, ALT, GGT, glucose, neutrophils, total cholesterol, triglycerides, and uric acid.

Children – Lab abnormalities occurring in at least 3% of patients include total bilirubin, AST, ALT, amylase, sodium, total cholesterol, and platelet count.

TENOFOVIR (PMPA)

Tablets: 300 mg (equivalent to tenofovir disoproxil 245 mg) (*Rx*)	*Viread* (Gilead Sciences)

Warning:

Lactic acidosis and severe hepatomegaly with steatosis, including fatal cases, have been reported with the use of nucleoside analogs alone or in combination with other antiretrovirals.

Severe acute exacerbations of hepatitis have been reported in hepatitis B virus (HBV)infected patients who have discontinued anti-hepatitis B therapy, including tenofovir. Monitor hepatic function closely with both clinical and laboratory follow-up for at least several months in patients who discontinue anti-hepatitis B therapy, including tenofovir. If appropriate, resumption of anti-hepatitis B therapy may be warranted.

Indications

Chronic hepatitis B: For the treatment of chronic hepatitis B in adults.

HIV infection: In combination with other antiretroviral agents for the treatment of HIV-1 infection.

Administration and Dosage

300 mg once daily taken orally without regard to food.

Renal function impairment: Adjust the dosing interval of tenofovir in patients with baseline creatinine clearance (CrCl) less than 50 mL/min using the recommendations in the following table. The safety and effectiveness of these dosing interval recommendations have not been clinically evaluated; closely monitor clinical response to treatment and renal function in these patients.

Tenofovir Dosage Adjustment for Patients with Altered CrCl

	CrCl (mL/min)[a]			Hemodialysis patients
	≥ 50	30 to 49	10 to 29	
Recommended 300 mg dosing interval	Every 24 hours	Every 48 hours	Every 72 to 96 hours	Every 7 days or after a total of ≈ 12 hours of dialysis[b]

[a] Calculated using ideal (lean) body weight.
[b] Generally once weekly assuming 3 hemodialysis sessions/week of approximately 4-hours duration. Administer tenofovir following completion of dialysis.

The pharmacokinetics of tenofovir have not been evaluated in nonhemodialysis patients with CrCl less than 10 mL/min; therefore, no dosing recommendation is available for these patients.

Actions

Pharmacology: Tenofovir disoproxil, an acyclic nucleoside phosphonate diester analog of adenosine monophosphate, inhibits the activity of HIV reverse transcriptase.

Pharmacokinetics:

Absorption – The oral bioavailability of tenofovir in fasted patients is about 25%. Maximum serum concentrations (C_{max}) are achieved in about 1 hour.

Administration of tenofovir disoproxil following a high-fat meal increases the oral bioavailability with an increase in tenofovir $AUC_{0-\infty}$ of about 40% and an increase in C_{max} of about 14%. Food delays the time to C_{max} by approximately 1 hour.

Distribution – Binding of tenofovir to serum proteins is 7.2%. The volume of distribution at steady state is about 1.3 L/kg.

Metabolism/Excretion – Following a single oral dose of tenofovir, the terminal elimination half-life is approximately 17 hours. Tenofovir is eliminated by a combination of glomerular filtration and active tubular secretion.

Contraindications

Previously demonstrated hypersensitivity to any of the components of the product.

Warnings/Precautions

Coinfection: Because of the risk of development of HIV-1 resistance, only use tenofovir in HIV-1 and HBV coinfected patients as part of an appropriate antiretroviral combination regimen. Offer HIV-1 antibody testing to all HBV-infected patients before initiating therapy with tenofovir. It is recommended that all patients with HIV be tested for the presence of chronic HBV before initiating tenofovir.

Lactic acidosis/severe hepatomegaly with steatosis: Lactic acidosis and severe hepatomegaly with steatosis, including fatal cases, have been reported with the use of nucleoside analogs alone or in combination with other antiretrovirals. Exercise particular caution when administering nucleoside analogs to any patient with known risk factors for liver disease.

Fixed-dose combination emtricitabine/tenofovir: Do not use tenofovir in combination with the fixed-dose combination products emtricitabine/tenofovir or emtricitabine/efavirenz/tenofovir.

Bone effects: In HIV-infected patients treated with tenofovir, in study 903 through 144 weeks, decreases from baseline in bone mineral density (BMD) were seen at the lumbar spine and hip in both arms of the study

Fat redistribution: Redistribution and accumulation of body fat have been observed in patients receiving antiretroviral therapy.

Immune reconstitution syndrome: Immune reconstruction syndrome has been reported in HIV-infected patients treated with combination antiretroviral therapy.

Renal function impairment: Renal impairment, including cases of acute renal failure and Fanconi syndrome, has been reported in association with the use of tenofovir.

Avoid tenofovir with concurrent or recent use of a nephrotoxic agent.

Pregnancy: *Category B.*

Antiretroviral Pregnancy Registry – To monitor fetal outcomes of pregnant women exposed to tenofovir, an Antiretroviral Pregnancy Registry has been established. Health care providers are encouraged to register patients by calling (800) 258-4263.

Lactation: The Centers for Disease Control and Prevention recommend that HIV-infected mothers not breastfeed their infants to avoid risking postnatal transmission of HIV.

Children: Safety and efficacy have not been established.

Elderly: In general, dose selection for the elderly patient should be cautious, keeping in mind the greater frequency of decreased hepatic, renal, or cardiac function, and of concomitant disease or other drug therapy.

Monitoring: Consider bone monitoring for HIV-infected patients who have a history of pathologic bone fractures or are at risk for osteopenia. Monitor hepatic function closely with both clinical and laboratory follow-up for at least several months and discontinue tenofovir in patients coinfected with HIV and HBV that exhibit clinical or laboratory findings suggestive of lactic acidosis or hepatotoxicity. Monitor patients at risk for, or with a history of, renal function impairment and patients receiving concomitant nephrotoxic agents for changes in serum creatinine and phosphorus.

Drug Interactions

Drugs eliminated by the kidneys: Coadministration of tenofovir with drugs that are eliminated by active tubular secretion may increase serum concentrations of tenofovir and/or the coadministered drug. Some examples include, but are not limited to, acyclovir, adefovir dipivoxil, cidofovir, ganciclovir, valacyclovir, and valganciclovir. Drugs that decrease renal function also may increase serum concentrations of tenofovir.

Drugs that may affect tenofovir include atazanavir, indinavir, and lopinavir/ritonavir.

Drugs that may be affected by tenofovir include abacavir, atazanavir, didanosine (buffered formulation or enteric coated), indinavir, lamivudine, and saquinavir/ritonavir.

Adverse Reactions

Adverse reactions occurring in at least 3% of treatment-experienced and treatment-naive patients include abdominal pain, anorexia, anxiety, arthralgia, asthenia, back pain, chest pain, depression, diarrhea, dizziness, dyspepsia, fatigue, fever, flatulence, headache, insomnia, myalgia, nasopharyngitis, nausea, pain, peripheral neuropathy, pneumonia, rash event, sinusitis, sweating, upper respiratory tract infections, vomiting, and weight loss.

Lab test abnormalities include the following: ALT, AST, cholesterol, creatine kinase, hematuria, neutrophils, serum amylase, serum glucose, triglycerides, urine glucose.

DIDANOSINE (ddI; dideoxyinosine)

Capsules, delayed release (with enteric-coated beadlets): 125, 200, 250, and 400 mg (*Rx*)	Various, *Videx EC* (Bristol-Myers Squibb)
Powder for oral solution, buffered: 100 and 250 mg (*Rx*)	*Videx* (Bristol-Myers Squibb)
Powder for oral solution, pediatric: 2 and 4 g (*Rx*)	*Videx* (Bristol-Myers Squibb)

Warning:

Fatal and nonfatal pancreatitis has occurred during therapy with didanosine alone or in combination regimens in treatment-naive and treatment-experienced patients, regardless of degree of immunosuppression. Suspend didanosine in patients with suspected pancreatitis, and discontinue therapy in patients with confirmed pancreatitis (see Warnings).

Lactic acidosis and severe hepatomegaly with steatosis, including fatal cases, have been reported with the use of nucleoside analogs alone or in combination, including didanosine and other antiretrovirals. Fatal lactic acidosis has been reported in pregnant women who received the combination of didanosine and stavudine with other antiretroviral agents. The combination of didanosine and stavudine should be used with caution during pregnancy and is recommended only if the potential benefit clearly outweighs the potential risk (see Warnings).

Indications

HIV infection: For the treatment of HIV-1 infection in combination with other antiretroviral agents.

Administration and Dosage

All didanosine formulations should be administered on an empty stomach at least 30 minutes before or 2 hours after eating.

Adults:

HIV infection –

Delayed-release capsule:

60 kg or greater – 400 mg once daily.

25 kg to less than 60 kg – 250 mg once daily

20 kg to less than 25 kg – 200 mg once daily

Pediatric powder for oral solution:

60 kg or greater – 200 mg twice daily is preferred or 400 mg once daily.

Less than 60 kg – 125 mg twice daily is preferred or 250 mg once daily.

Children:

HIV infection –

Delayed-release capsule: See Adults for dosing.

Pediatric powder for oral solution:

Older than 8 months of age – 120 mg/m^2 twice daily.

2 weeks to 8 months of age – 120 mg/m^2 twice daily.

Renal function impairment:

Recommended Didanosine Dosage in Adults With Renal Impairment[a]				
	Patient weight ≥ 60 kg		Patient weight < 60 kg	
CrCl[b] (mL/min)	Delayed-release capsule (mg)	Pediatric powder for oral suspension (mg)	Delayed-release capsule (mg)	Pediatric powder for oral suspension (mg)
≥ 60	400 mg once daily	200 mg twice daily[c]	250 mg once daily	125 mg twice daily[c]
30 to 59	200 mg once daily	200 mg once daily or 100 mg twice daily	125 mg once daily	150 mg once daily or 75 mg twice daily
10 to 29	125 mg once daily	150 mg once daily	125 mg once daily	100 mg once daily
< 10	125 mg once daily	100 mg once daily	[d]	75 mg once daily

[a] Based on studies using a buffered formulation of didanosine.
[b] CrCl = creatinine clearance.
[c] 400 mg once daily (60 kg or greater) or 250 mg once daily (less than 60 kg) for patients whose management requires once-daily frequency of administration.
[d] Not suitable for use in patients < 60 kg with CrCl < 10 mg/mL. An alternative formulation of didanosine should be used.

Hemodialysis/Continuous ambulatory peritoneal dialysis – For patients requiring continuous ambulatory peritoneal dialysis (CAPD) or hemodialysis, follow dosing recommendations for patients with CrCl of less than 10 mL/min, as shown in the previous table. It is not necessary to administer a supplemental dose of didanosine following hemodialysis.

Pancreatitis: Clinical and laboratory signs suggestive of pancreatitis should prompt dose suspension and careful evaluation of the possibility of pancreatitis. Didanosine use should be discontinued in patients with confirmed pancreatitis.

Peripheral neuropathy: Based on data with buffered didanosine formulations, patients with symptoms of peripheral neuropathy may tolerate a reduced dose of didanosine after resolution of the symptoms of peripheral neuropathy upon drug interruption. If neuropathy recurs after resumption of didanosine, permanent discontinuation of didanosine should be considered.

Method of preparation:

Pediatric powder for oral solution – Prior to dispensing, the pharmacist must constitute dry powder with Purified Water, USP, to an initial concentration of 20 mg/mL and immediately mix the resulting solution with antacid to a final concentration of 10 mg/mL as follows:

20 mg/mL initial solution: Reconstitute the product to 20 mg/mL by adding 100 or 200 mL Purified Water, USP, to the 2 or 4 g of powder, respectively, in the product bottle. Prepare final admixture as described below.

10 mg/mL final admixture:

1.) Immediately mix 1 part of the 20 mg/mL initial solution with 1 part of either *Mylanta Double Strength Liquid*, *Extra Strength Maalox Plus Suspension*, or *Maalox TC Suspension* for a final dispensing concentration of 10 mg/mL. For patient home use, dispense the admixture in flint-glass or plastic bottles with child-resistant closures. This admixture is stable for 30 days under refrigeration at 2° to 8°C (36° to 46°F).

2.) Instruct the patient or caregiver to shake the admixture thoroughly prior to use and to store the tightly closed container in the refrigerator at 2° to 8°C (36° to 46°F) up to 30 days.

Actions

Pharmacology: Didanosine is a synthetic purine nucleoside analog of deoxyadenosine, in which the 3′-hydroxyl group is replaced by hydrogen. Intracellularly, it is converted by cellular enzymes to the active metabolite, dideoxyadenosine

5′-triphosphate. It inhibits the activity of HIV-1 reverse transcriptase by competing with the natural substrate, deoxyadenosine 5′-triphosphate, and by incorporating in viral DNA causing termination of viral DNA chain elongation.

Pharmacokinetics:

Effect of food on oral absorption – Didanosine C_{max} and AUC were decreased by approximately 55% when didanosine tablets were administered up to 2 hours after a meal. Administration of didanosine tablets up to 30 minutes before a meal did not result in any significant changes in bioavailability.

Enteric-coated capsules: In the presence of food, C_{max} and AUC for didanosine capsules were reduced by approximately 46% and 19%, respectively, compared with the fasting state. Take didanosine capsules on an empty stomach.

Pharmacokinetic Parameters of Didanosine in Adult and Pediatric Patients

Parameter	Adult patients[a]	Pediatric patients
Oral bioavailability	≈ 42%	≈ 25%
Apparent volume of distribution[b]	≈ 1.08 L/kg	≈ 28 L/m^2
CSF[c]-plasma ratio[d]	≈ 21%	46% (range, 12% to 85%)
Systemic clearance[b]	≈ 13 mL/min/kg	≈ 516 mL/min/m^2
Renal clearance[e]	≈ 5.5 mL/min/kg	≈ 240 mL/min/m^2
Elimination half-life[e]	≈ 1.5 h	≈ 0.8 h
Urine recovery of didanosine[e]	≈ 18%	≈ 18%

[a] Administered as buffered formulation.
[b] Following IV administration.
[c] CSF = cerebrospinal fluid.
[d] Following IV administration in adults and IV or oral administration in pediatric patients.
[e] Following oral administration.

Children – The pharmacokinetics of didanosine have been evaluated in HIV-exposed and HIV-infected children from birth to 19 years of age. Overall, the pharmacokinetics of didanosine in children are similar to those of didanosine in adults. Didanosine plasma concentrations increased in proportion to oral doses ranging from 25 to 120 mg/m^2 in children younger than 5 months of age and from 80 to 180 mg/m^2 in children older than 8 months of age.

Contraindications

Hypersensitivity to any of the components of the formulations.

Warnings/Precautions

Fat redistribution: Redistribution/accumulation of body fat, including central obesity, dorsocervical fat enlargement ("buffalo hump"), peripheral wasting, facial wasting, breast enlargement, and "cushingoid appearance," have been observed in patients receiving antiretroviral therapy.

Hyperuricemia: Didanosine has been associated with asymptomatic hyperuricemia; consider suspending treatment if clinical measures aimed at reducing uric acid levels fail.

Immune reconstitution syndrome: Immune reconstitution syndrome has been reported in patients treated with combination antiretroviral therapy, including didanosine. During the initial phase of combination antiretroviral treatment, patients whose immune systems respond may develop an inflammatory response to indolent or residual opportunistic infections (such as *Mycobacterium avium* infection, cytomegalovirus, *Pneumocystis jiroveci* pneumonia [PCP], or tuberculosis), which may necessitate further evaluation and treatment.

Lactic acidosis/Severe hepatomegaly with steatosis: Lactic acidosis and severe hepatomegaly with steatosis, including fatal cases, have been reported with the use of nucleoside analogs alone or in combination, including didanosine and other antiretrovirals. A majority of these cases have been in women. Obesity and prolonged nucleoside exposure may be risk factors (see Warning Box).

Pancreatitis: Fatal and nonfatal pancreatitis has occurred during didanosine therapy used alone or in combination regimens in treatment-naive and treatment-experienced patients regardless of degree of immunosuppression (see Warning Box).

Peripheral neuropathy: Peripheral neuropathy, manifested by numbness, tingling, or pain in the hands or feet, has been reported in patients receiving didanosine therapy.

Retinal changes and optic neuritis: Retinal changes and optic neuritis have been reported in adult and pediatric patients. Consider periodic retinal examinations for patients receiving didanosine.

Renal function impairment: Patients with renal impairment (serum creatinine greater than 1.5 mg/dL or CrCl less than 60 mL/min) may be at greater risk of toxicity from didanosine because of decreased drug clearance; consider a dose reduction. The magnesium hydroxide content of each buffered tablet (8.6 mEq) may present an excessive magnesium load to patients with significant renal impairment, particularly after prolonged dosing.

Hepatic function impairment: It is unknown if hepatic impairment significantly affects didanosine pharmacokinetics. Therefore, monitor these patients closely for evidence of didanosine toxicity.

Pregnancy: *Category B.*

To monitor maternal-fetal outcomes of pregnant women exposed to didanosine and other antiretroviral agents, an Antiretroviral Pregnancy Registry has been established. Physicians are encouraged to register patients by calling (800) 258-4263.

Lactation: It is not known whether didanosine is excreted in breast milk. Because of the potential for serious adverse reactions from didanosine in nursing infants, instruct mothers to discontinue nursing when taking didanosine; this is consistent with the CDC's recommendation that HIV-infected mothers not breastfeed their infants to avoid risking postnatal transmission of HIV infection.

Children: Use of didanosine in children from 2 weeks of age through adolescence is supported by evidence from adequate and well-controlled studies of didanosine in adults and pediatric patients.

Pediatric powder for oral solution – Dosing recommendations for didanosine in patients younger than 2 weeks of age cannot be made because the pharmacokinetics of didanosine in these children are too variable to determine an appropriate dose.

Delayed-release capsules – Additional pharmacokinetic studies in children support use in children who weigh at least 20 kg.

Elderly: In an expanded access program using a buffered formulation of didanosine for the treatment of advanced HIV infection, patients 65 years of age and older had a higher frequency of pancreatitis (10%) than younger patients (5%).

Drug Interactions

Drugs that may affect didanosine include allopurinol, ganciclovir, methadone, ribavirin, and tenofovir.

Drugs that may be affected by didanosine include ganciclovir, antacids, antifungal agents, antiretroviral drugs, fluoroquinolones, and stavudine.

Drug/Food interactions: Ingestion of didanosine with food reduces the absorption of didanosine by as much as 50%. Therefore, administer on an empty stomach, at least 30 minutes before or 2 hours after eating.

Adverse Reactions

A serious toxicity of didanosine is pancreatitis, which may be fatal (see Warnings). Other important toxicities include lactic acidosis/severe hepatomegaly with steatosis; retinal changes and optic neuritis; and peripheral neuropathy (see Warnings and Precautions).

When didanosine is used in combination with other agents with similar toxicities, the incidence of these toxicities may be higher than when didanosine is used alone. Thus, patients treated with didanosine in combination with stavudine, with or without hydroxyurea, may be at increased risk for pancreatitis and liver function abnormalities (see Warnings). Patients treated with didanosine in combination with stavudine may also be at increased risk for peripheral neuropathy (see Precautions).

Adverse reactions occurring in at least 3% of patients include diarrhea, neuropathy (all grades), rash/pruritus, abdominal pain, headache, pain, nausea/vomiting, pancreatitis, and laboratory abnormalities including amylase, ALT, AST, and uric acid.

TELBIVUDINE

Tablets: 600 mg (*Rx*) — *Tyzeka* (Idenix Pharmaceuticals)
Solution; oral: 100 mg per 5 mL

Warning:

Lactic acidosis and severe hepatomegaly with steatosis, including fatal cases, have been reported with the use of nucleoside analogs alone or in combination with antiretrovirals.

Severe acute exacerbations of hepatitis B have been reported in patients who have discontinued anti–hepatitis B therapy, including telbivudine. Closely monitor hepatic function with both clinical and laboratory follow-up for at least several months in patients who discontinue anti–hepatitis B therapy. If appropriate, resumption of anti–hepatitis B therapy may be warranted.

Indications

Chronic hepatitis B: For treatment of chronic hepatitis B in adult patients with evidence of viral replication and either evidence of persistent elevations in serum aminotransferases (ALT or AST) or histologically active disease.

Administration and Dosage

Adults and adolescents (16 years of age and older): 600 mg once daily, taken orally, with or without food.

Renal function impairment: Telbivudine should be administered after hemodialysis.

Telbivudine Dose Interval Adjustment in Patients With Renal Function Impairment

CrCl (mL/min)[a]	Telbivudine oral solution dose (5 mL = 100 mg)	Dose of telbivudine
≥ 50 mL/min	30 mL once daily	600 mg once daily
30 to 49 mL/min	20 mL once daily	600 mg once every 48 hours
< 30 mL/min (not requiring dialysis)	10 mL once daily	600 mg once every 72 hours
ESRD[b]	[c]	600 mg once every 96 hours

[a] CrCl = creatinine clearance.
[b] ESRD = end-stage renal disease; when administered on hemodialysis days, telbivudine should be administered after hemodialysis.
[c] Dosing recommendations for telbivudine oral solution in patients with ESRD have not been established.

Administration: Telbivudine oral solution (30 mL) may be considered for patients who have difficulty swallowing tablets.

Actions

Pharmacology: Telbivudine is a synthetic thymidine nucleoside analog with activity against hepatitis B virus (HBV) DNA polymerase, which inhibits HBV DNA polymerase (reverse transcriptase).

Pharmacokinetics:

Absorption – Steady state was achieved after approximately 5 to 7 days of once-daily administration with an effective half-life of approximately 15 hours.

Distribution – In vitro binding to human plasma proteins is low (3.3%).

Metabolism/Excretion – Telbivudine is not a substrate or inhibitor of the CYP-450 enzyme system.

After reaching the peak concentration, plasma concentrations of telbivudine declined with a terminal elimination half-life of 40 to 49 hours. Telbivudine is eliminated primarily by urinary excretion of unchanged drug. The renal clearance of telbivudine approaches normal glomerular filtration rate. Because renal excretion is the predominant route of elimination, patients with moderate to severe renal function impairment and those undergoing hemodialysis require a dose interval adjustment.

Contraindications

None known.

Warnings/Precautions

Lactic acidosis: Lactic acidosis and severe hepatomegaly with steatosis, including fatal cases, have been reported with the use of nucleoside analogs alone or in combination with antiretrovirals.

Skeletal muscle: Cases of myopathy have been reported with telbivudine use several weeks to months after starting therapy. Myopathy has also been reported with some other drugs in this class.

Peripheral neuropathy: Peripheral neuropathy has been reported with telbivudine alone or in combination with pegylated interferon alfa-2a and other interferons.

Exacerbations of hepatitis: Severe acute exacerbations of hepatitis B have been reported in patients who have discontinued anti-hepatitis B therapy. Closely monitor hepatic function with both clinical and laboratory follow-up for at least several months in patients who discontinue anti-hepatitis B therapy. If appropriate, initiation of anti-hepatitis B therapy may be warranted.

Resistance: There are no adequate and well-controlled studies for telbivudine treatment of patients with established lamivudine-resistant HBV infection.

Renal function impairment: Telbivudine is eliminated primarily by renal excretion, therefore, dose interval adjustment is recommended in patients with CrCl less than 50 mL/min, including patients on hemodialysis.

Hepatic function impairment: The safety and efficacy of telbivudine in liver transplant recipients are unknown. If telbivudine treatment is determined to be necessary for a liver transplant recipient who has received or is receiving an immunosuppressant that may affect renal function, monitor renal function before and during treatment with telbivudine.

Pregnancy: Category B.

Lactation: Instruct mothers not to breast-feed if they are receiving telbivudine.

Children: Safety and efficacy of telbivudine in children have not been established.

Elderly: In general, exercise caution when prescribing telbivudine to elderly patients, considering the greater frequency of decreased renal function because of concomitant disease or other drug therapy. Monitor renal function in elderly patients and institute dosage adjustments accordingly.

Monitoring: Closely monitor hepatic function with both clinical and laboratory follow-up for at least several months in patients who discontinue anti-hepatitis B therapy.

Monitor patients for any signs or symptoms of unexplained muscle pain, tenderness, or weakness, particularly during periods of upward dosage titration.

Monitor renal function in elderly patients and in patients taking drugs that may alter renal function (eg, cyclosporine, tacrolimus).

Drug Interactions

Drugs that alter renal function: Telbivudine is eliminated primarily by renal excretion; coadministration of telbivudine with drugs that alter renal function may alter plasma concentrations of telbivudine.

Pegylated interferon alfa-2a: A clinical trial investigating the combination of telbivudine 600 mg daily with pegylated interferon alfa-2a 180 mcg once weekly by subcutaneous administration indicates that this combination may be associated with an increased risk of peripheral neuropathy occurrence and severity, in comparison with telbivudine alone.

Adverse Reactions

Adverse reactions occurring in 3% or more of patients include abdominal distension, abdominal pain, ALT increased, arthralgia, back pain, creatine kinase increased, cough, diarrhea, dizziness, dyspepsia, fatigue, headache, increased ALT, insomnia, myalgia, nausea, pharyngolaryngeal pain, pyrexia, rash.

LAMIVUDINE (3TC)

Tablets: 100 mg (*Rx*)	*Epivir-HBV* (GlaxoSmithKline)
150 and 300 mg (*Rx*)	*Epivir* (GlaxoSmithKline)
Oral solution: 5 mg/mL (*Rx*)	*Epivir-HBV* (GlaxoSmithKline)
10 mg/mL (*Rx*)	*Epivir* (GlaxoSmithKline)

Warning:

Lactic acidosis and severe hepatomegaly with steatosis, including fatal cases, have been reported with the use of nucleoside analogs alone or in combination, including lamivudine and other antiretroviral agents (see Warnings). Suspend treatment with lamivudine in any patient who develops clinical or laboratory findings suggestive of lactic acidosis or pronounced hepatotoxicity.

Lamivudine tablets and oral solution (used to treat HIV infection) contain a higher dose of the active ingredient (lamivudine) than lamivudine-HBV tablets and oral solution (used to treat chronic hepatitis B). Patients with HIV infection should receive only dosing forms appropriate for the treatment of HIV (see Warnings and Precautions). The formulation and dosage of lamivudine-HBV are not appropriate for patients dually infected with HBV and HIV.

Offer HIV counseling and testing to patients before beginning lamivudine-HBV and periodically during treatment. Lamivudine-HBV tablets and oral solution contain a lower dose of the same active ingredient (lamivudine) as the lamivudine tablets and oral solution used to treat HIV infection. If treatment with lamivudine-HBV is prescribed for chronic hepatitis B for a patient with unrecognized or untreated HIV infection, rapid emergence of HIV resistance is likely because of subtherapeutic dose and inappropriate monotherapy.

Severe acute exacerbations of hepatitis B have been reported in patients who have discontinued anti-hepatitis B therapy (including lamivudine-HBV) or are coinfected with HBV and HIV and have discontinued lamivudine. Monitor hepatic function closely with both clinical and laboratory follow-up for at least several months in patients who discontinue anti-hepatitis B therapy or who discontinue lamivudine and are coinfected with HIV and HBV. If appropriate, initiation of anti-hepatitis B therapy may be warranted.

Indications

HIV infection (Epivir): in combination with other antiretroviral agents is indicated for the treatment of HIV infection.

Chronic hepatitis B (Epivir-HBV): Treatment of chronic hepatitis B associated with evidence of hepatitis B viral replication and active liver inflammation.

Administration and Dosage

HIV infection:

Adults – 300 mg/day, administered as either 150 mg twice daily or 300 mg once daily, in combination with other antiretroviral agents.

Children (3 months of age up to 16 years of age) – 4 mg/kg twice daily (up to a maximum of 150 mg twice a day) administered with other antiretroviral agents.

Lamivudine scored tablets: Lamivudine is also available as a scored tablet for HIV-infected children who weigh at least 14 kg and for whom a solid dosage form is appropriate. Before prescribing lamivudine tablets, children should be assessed for the ability to swallow tablets.

Dosing Recommendations for Lamivudine Tablets in Children

Weight (kg)	Dosage regimen using scored 150 mg tablets		Total daily dose
	AM dose	PM dose	
14 to 21	½ tablet (75 mg)	½ tablet (75 mg)	150 mg
> 21 to < 30	½ tablet (75 mg)	1 tablet (150 mg)	225 mg
≥ 30	1 tablet (150 mg)	1 tablet (150 mg)	300 mg

Renal function impairment – Adjust lamivudine dose in accordance with renal function. Insufficient data are available to recommend a dosage of lamivudine in dialysis.

Adjustment of Lamivudine Dosage in HIV-Infected Adult and Adolescent Patients with Renal Function Impairment

CrCl (mL/min)	Recommended lamivudine dosage
≥ 50	150 mg twice daily or 300 mg once daily
30 to 49	150 mg once daily
15 to 29	150 mg first dose, then 100 mg once daily
5 to 14	150 mg first dose, then 50 mg once daily
< 5	50 mg first dose, then 25 mg once daily

No additional dosing of lamivudine is required after routine (4-hour) hemodialysis or peritoneal dialysis.

In children with renal function impairment, a reduction in the dose and/or an increase in the dosing interval should be considered.

Chronic hepatitis B:

Adults – 100 mg once daily.

Children (2 to 17 years of age) – 3 mg/kg once daily up to a maximum daily dose of 100 mg.

Renal function impairment – Adjust the dose of lamivudine in accordance with renal function. No additional dosing of lamivudine is required after routine (4-hour) hemodialysis or peritoneal dialysis.

Adjustment of Lamivudine Dosage in Chronic Hepatitis B Adult Patients with Renal Function Impairment

CrCl (mL/min)	Recommended lamivudine dosage
≥ 50	100 mg once daily
30 to 49	100 mg first dose, then 50 mg once daily
15 to 29	100 mg first dose, then 25 mg once daily
5 to 14	35 mg first dose, then 15 mg once daily
< 5	35 mg first dose, then 10 mg once daily

Actions

Pharmacology: Lamivudine is a synthetic nucleoside analog with activity against HIV and hepatitis B virus (HBV). Lamivudine is phosphorylated to lamivudine 5′-triphosphate (L-TP). Incorporation of the monophosphate form into viral DNA results in DNA chain termination. L-TP also inhibits the RNA- and DNA-dependent DNA polymerase activities of HIV-1 reverse transcriptase.

Pharmacokinetics:

Absorption/Distribution – Lamivudine is rapidly absorbed after oral administration. Absolute bioavailability is 86% for the tablet and 87% for the oral solution. The solution and tablet may be used interchangeably. The apparent volume of distribution (V_d) is 1.3 L/kg. Binding of lamivudine to plasma proteins is less than 36% and independent of dose.

Metabolism/Excretion – Metabolism is a minor route of elimination. The mean elimination half-life of lamivudine ranges from 5 to 7 hours. The majority of the dose is eliminated in the urine as unchanged drug.

Contraindications

Hypersensitivity to any of the components of the products.

Warnings/Precautions

Pancreatitis: Pancreatitis has been reported in patients receiving lamivudine, particularly in HIV-infected children with prior nucleoside exposure.

Lactic acidosis/severe hepatomegaly with steatosis: Lactic acidosis and severe hepatomegaly with steatosis, including fatal cases, have occurred with the use of antiretroviral nucleoside analogs alone or in combination. A majority of these cases have been in women. Obesity and prolonged nucleoside exposure may be risk factors.

Differences between lamivudine-containing products/risk of emergence of resistant HIV: The formulation and dosage of lamivudine in *Epivir-HBV* are not appropriate for patients infected with both HBV and HIV. If treatment with *Epivir-HBV* is prescribed for chronic hepatitis B for a patient with unrecognized or untreated HIV infection, rapid emergence of HIV resistance is likely to result. If a decision is made to administer lamivudine to patients dually infected with HIV and HBV, use *Epivir* tablets or oral solution or *Combivir* tablets as a part of an appropriate combination regimen. Do not administer *Combivir* concomitantly with *Epivir*, *Epivir-HBV*, *Retrovir*, or *Trizivir*.

Posttreatment exacerbations of hepatitis: Clinical and laboratory evidence of exacerbations of hepatitis have occurred after discontinuation of lamivudine. Although most events appear to have been self-limited, fatalities have been reported in some cases. Closely monitor patients with clinical and laboratory follow-up for at least several months after stopping treatment.

Use with interferon- and ribavirin-based regimens: In vitro ribavirin can reduce the phosphorylation of pyrimidine nucleoside analogs, such as lamivudine. Hepatic decompensation (some fatal) has occurred in HIV/HCV coinfected patients receiving combination antiretroviral therapy for HIV and interferon alfa, with or without ribavirin. Closely monitor patients receiving interferon alfa, with or without ribavirin, and lamivudine for treatment-associated toxicities, especially hepatic decompensation.

HIV and HBV coinfection: The safety and efficacy of lamivudine have not been established for treatment of chronic hepatitis B in patients dually infected with HIV and HBV. In non-HIV infected patients treated with lamivudine for chronic hepatitis B, emergence of lamivudine-resistant HBV has been detected and has been associated with diminished treatment response. Emergence of HBV variants associated with resistance to lamivudine has also been reported in HIV-infected patients who have received lamivudine-containing antiretroviral regimens in the presence of concurrent infection with HBV. Posttreatment exacerbations of hepatitis have also been reported.

Immune reconstitution syndrome: Immune reconstitution syndrome has been reported in patients treated with combination antiretroviral therapy, including lamivudine.

Differences between dosing regimens: Trough levels of lamivudine in plasma and intracellular lamivudine triphosphate were lower with once-daily dosing than with twice-daily dosing. The clinical significance of this observation is not known.

Emergence of resistance-associated HBV mutations: Progression of hepatitis B, including death, has been reported in some patients with YMDD-mutant HBV, including patients from the liver transplant setting and from other clinical trials. Increased clinical and laboratory monitoring may aid in treatment decisions if emergence of viral mutants is suspected.

Fat redistribution: Redistribution/Accumulation of body fat, including central obesity, dorsocervical fat enlargement (buffalo hump), peripheral wasting, facial wasting, breast enlargement, and "cushingoid appearance," have been observed in patients receiving antiretroviral therapy.

Special risk: Safety and efficacy of *Epivir-HBV* have not been established in patients with decompensated liver disease or organ transplants; children younger than 2 years of age (use appropriate infant immunizations to prevent HBV); patients dually infected with HBV and HCV, hepatitis delta, or HIV; or other populations not included in the principal phase III controlled studies.

Pregnancy: *Category* C.

Lamivudine has not affected the transmission of HBV from mother to infant; immunize infants appropriately to prevent neonatal acquisition of HBV.

Antiretroviral pregnancy registry – To monitor maternal-fetal outcomes of women exposed to lamivudine, an Antiretroviral Pregnancy Registry has been established. Physicians are encouraged to register patients by calling (800) 258-4263.

Lactation: Lamivudine is excreted in human breast milk. Instruct mothers to discontinue breast-feeding if they are receiving lamivudine, which is consistent with the CDC recommendation that HIV-infected mothers not breast-feed their infants to avoid risking postnatal transmission of HIV infection.

Children:

Hepatitis B – Safety and efficacy in children younger than 2 years of age have not been established.

HIV infection – The safety and effectiveness of twice-daily lamivudine in combination with other antiretroviral agents have been established in children 3 months of age and older.

Elderly: Because elderly patients are more likely to have decreased renal function, monitor renal function and make dose adjustments accordingly.

Monitoring:

Epivir-HBV – Monitor patients regularly during treatment. The safety and efficacy of treatment with *Epivir-HBV* beyond 1 year have not been established. During treatment, combinations of reactions such as return of persistently elevated ALT, increasing levels of HBV DNA over time after an initial decline below assay limit, progression of clinical signs or symptoms of hepatic disease, and/or worsening of hepatic necroinflammatory findings may be considered as potentially reflecting loss of therapeutic response. Consider such observations when determining the advisability of continuing therapy.

Drug Interactions

Drugs that may affect lamivudine include interferon alpha, ribavirin, trimethoprim/sulfamethoxazole, and zalcitabine.

Drugs that may be affected by lamivudine include zalcitabine and zidovudine.

Adverse Reactions

HIV – Adverse reactions occurring in at least 5% of patients include abdominal pain/cramps, anorexia, arthralgia, chills, cough, depression, diarrhea, dizziness, dyspepsia, fatigue, fever, headache, insomnia, malaise, musculoskeletal pain, myalgia, nasal symptoms, nausea, neuropathy, skin rash, and vomiting. Lab abnormalities may include anemia, neutropenia, thrombocytopenia, and elevations in amylase, AST, ALT, and bilirubin.

Chronic hepatitis B – Adverse reactions occurring in at least 3% of patients include abdominal discomfort/pain; arthralgia; diarrhea; ear, nose, and throat infections; fever or chills; headache; malaise/fatigue; myalgia; nausea/vomiting; rash; sore throat. Lab abnormalities may include decreased platelets and elevations in ALT, CPK, and serum lipase.

Children – Adverse reactions in children are similar to adults and include abnormal breath sounds/wheezing, cough, diarrhea, ear signs or symptoms, fever, hepatomegaly, lymphadenopathy, nasal discharge or congestion, nausea and vomiting, pancreatitis, skin rashes, splenomegaly, and stomatitis. Lab abnormalities may include elevated lipase and amylase, and neutropenia.

STAVUDINE (d4T)

Capsules: 15, 20, 30, and 40 mg (*Rx*) — *Zerit* (BMS Virology)
Powder for oral solution: 1 mg/mL when reconstituted (*Rx*)

Warning:
Lactic acidosis and severe hepatomegaly with steatosis, including fatal cases, have been reported with the use of nucleoside analogs alone or in combination, including stavudine and other antiretrovirals (see Warnings). Fatal lactic acidosis has been reported in pregnant women who received the combination of stavudine and didanosine with other antiretroviral agents. Use the combination of stavudine and didanosine with caution during pregnancy; it is recommended only if the potential benefit clearly outweighs the potential risk (see Warnings).

Fatal and nonfatal pancreatitis have occurred during therapy when stavudine was part of a combination regimen that included didanosine, with or without hydroxyurea, in both treatment-naive and treatment-experienced patients, regardless of degree of immunosuppression (see Warnings).

Indications

Human immunodeficiency virus (HIV) infection: For the treatment of HIV-1 infection in combination with other antiretroviral agents.

Administration and Dosage

Stavudine immediate-release:

Adults – The recommended starting dose based on body weight is as follows:

Patients weighing 60 kg or greater: 40 mg every 12 hours.

Patients weighing less than 60 kg: 30 mg every 12 hours.

Stavudine may be taken without regard to meals.

Children – The recommended dose for newborns from birth to 13 days of age is 0.5 mg/kg/dose given every 12 hours. The recommended dose for pediatric patients at least 14 days of age and weighing less than 30 kg is 1 mg/kg/dose, given every 12 hours without regard to meals. Pediatric patients weighing 30 kg or greater should receive the recommended adult dosage.

Dosage adjustment in renal function impairment – Stavudine may be administered to adult patients with impaired renal function. The following schedule is recommended:

Stavudine Dosage in Renal Function Impairment

Creatinine clearance (mL/min)	Recommended stavudine dose by patient weight	
	≥ 60 kg	< 60 kg
> 50	40 mg every 12 hours	30 mg every 12 hours
26 to 50	20 mg every 12 hours	15 mg every 12 hours
10 to 25	20 mg every 24 hours	15 mg every 24 hours

Because urinary excretion is a major route of elimination of stavudine in pediatric patients, the clearance also may be altered in children with renal impairment. Although there are insufficient data to recommend a specific dose adjustment in this patient population, consider a reduction in the dose or an increase in the interval between doses.

Hemodialysis patients: The recommended dose is 20 mg every 24 hours (60 kg or more) or 15 mg every 24 hours (less than 60 kg) administered after the completion of hemodialysis and at the same time of day on nondialysis days.

Stavudine, extended-release:

Adults – The recommended daily dose is based on body weight and is administered in a once-daily schedule as follows:

Patients weighing 60 kg or more: 100 mg once daily.

Patients weighing less than 60 kg: 75 mg once daily

For patients who have difficulty swallowing intact capsules, the capsule can be carefully opened and the contents mixed with 30 mL of yogurt or applesauce. Patients should be cautioned not to chew or crush the beads while swallowing.

Children – Extended-release stavudine has not been studied in pediatric patients.

Renal impairment – Extended-release stavudine has not been studied in patients with renal impairment.

Dosage adjustment in peripheral neuropathy: Monitor patients for the development of peripheral neuropathy, which is usually characterized by numbness, tingling, or pain in the feet or hands. These symptoms may be difficult to detect in young children. If these symptoms develop, interrupt stavudine therapy. Symptoms may resolve if therapy is withdrawn promptly. In some cases, symptoms may worsen temporarily following discontinuation of therapy. Switching the patient to an alternate treatment regimen should be considered. If switching to an alternate regimen is not suitable and if symptoms resolve satisfactorily, resumption of treatment may be considered at 50% of the recommended dose using the following dosage schedule:

Patients weighing 60 kg or greater –

Immediate-release: 20 mg every 12 hours.

Extended-release: 50 mg once daily.

Patients weighing less than 60 kg –

Immediate-release: 15 mg every 12 hours.

Extended-release: 37.5 mg once daily.

If peripheral neuropathy recurs after resumption of stavudine, consider permanent discontinuation.

Actions

Pharmacology: Stavudine is a synthetic thymidine nucleoside analog active against HIV. It inhibits the replication of HIV in human cells in vitro.

Pharmacokinetics:

Absorption/Distribution – Following oral administration, stavudine is rapidly absorbed with peak plasma concentrations occurring within 1 hour after dosing. The systemic exposure to stavudine is the same following administration as capsules or solution. Binding to serum proteins was negligible. Oral bioavailability in adults is approximately 86%. The apparent oral volume of distribution is about 66 L.

Excretion – Renal elimination accounted for about 40% of the overall clearance regardless of the route of administration. The elimination half-life is about 1.4 hours.

Special populations –

Renal function impairment: Adjust dosage in patients with reduced CrCl and in patients receiving maintenance hemodialysis (see Administration and Dosage).

Contraindications

Hypersensitivity to stavudine or to any components of the formulation.

Warnings/Precautions

Lactic acidosis/severe hepatomegaly with steatosis/hepatic failure: Lactic acidosis and severe hepatomegaly with steatosis, including fatal cases, have been reported with the use of nucleoside analogs alone or in combination, including stavudine and other antiretrovirals. Female gender, obesity, and prolonged nucleoside exposure may be risk factors. Fatal lactic acidosis has been reported in pregnant women who received the combination of stavudine and didanosine with other antiretroviral agents. Use the combination of stavudine and didanosine with caution during pregnancy; it is recommended only if the potential benefit clearly outweighs the potential risk (see Pregnancy). Deaths attributed to hepatotoxicity have occurred in patients receiving the combination of stavudine, didanosine, and hydroxyurea. Exercise caution when administering stavudine to any patient with known risk factors for liver disease; however, cases also have been reported in patients with no known risk factors. Suspend treatment with stavudine in any patient who develops clinical or laboratory findings suggestive of lactic acidosis or pronounced hepatotoxicity (which may include hepatomegaly and steatosis even in the absence of marked transaminase elevations). An increased risk of hepatotoxicity, which may be fatal, may occur in patients treated with stavudine in combination with didanosine and hydroxyurea compared with when stavudine is used alone. Closely monitor patients treated with this combination for signs of liver toxicity.

Neurologic symptoms: Motor weakness has been reported rarely. Most of these cases occurred in the setting of lactic acidosis. The evolution of motor weakness may mimic the clinical presentation of Guillain-Barré syndrome (including respiratory failure). Symptoms may continue or worsen following discontinuation of therapy.

Stavudine therapy has been associated with peripheral neuropathy, which can be severe and is dose-related. Peripheral neuropathy has occurred more frequently in patients with advanced HIV disease, a history of neuropathy, or concurrent neurotoxic drug therapy, including didanosine (see Adverse Reactions).

Monitor patients for development of neuropathy. Stavudine-related peripheral neuropathy may resolve if therapy is withdrawn promptly. Symptoms may worsen temporarily following therapy discontinuation. If symptoms resolve completely, resumption of treatment may be considered at 50% of the dose (see Administration and Dosage). If stavudine must be given in this clinical setting, careful monitoring is essential. If neuropathy recurs after resumption of stavudine, consider permanent discontinuation.

Pancreatitis: Fatal and nonfatal pancreatitis have occurred during therapy when stavudine was part of a combination regimen that included didanosine, with or without hydroxyurea, in treatment-naive and treatment-experienced patients, regardless of degree of immunosuppression. In patients with suspected pancreatitis, suspend the combination of stavudine and didanosine (with or without hydroxyurea) and any other agents that are toxic to the pancreas. Reinstitution of stavudine after a confirmed diagnosis of pancreatitis should be undertaken with particular caution and close patient monitoring. The new regimen should not contain either didanosine or hydroxyurea.

Fat redistribution: Redistribution/accumulation of body fat including central obesity, dorsocervical fat enlargement (buffalo hump), peripheral wasting, facial wasting, breast enlargement, and "cushingoid appearance" have been observed in patients receiving antiretroviral therapy. The mechanism and long-term consequences of these events are currently unknown. A causal relationship has not been established.

Pregnancy: Category C.

To monitor maternal-fetal outcomes of pregnant women exposed to stavudine and other antiretroviral agents, an Antiretroviral Pregnancy Registry has been established. Physicians are encouraged to register patients by calling (800) 258-4263.

Fatal lactic acidosis has been reported in pregnant women who received the combination of stavudine and didanosine with other antiretroviral agents (see Warning Box).

Lactation: Because of the potential for adverse reactions in nursing infants, instruct mothers to discontinue nursing if they are receiving stavudine. To avoid risking postnatal transmission of HIV infection, instruct HIV-infected mothers not to breastfeed their infants; this is consistent with the CDC's recommendation.

Children: Use of stavudine in pediatric patients is supported by evidence from adequate and well-controlled studies of stavudine in adults with additional pharmacokinetic and safety data in pediatric patients.

Elderly: Clinical studies of stavudine did not include sufficient numbers of patients 65 years of age or older to determine whether they respond differently than younger patients. Closely monitor elderly patients for signs and symptoms of peripheral neuropathy. Because elderly patients are more likely to have decreased renal function, it may be useful to monitor renal function.

Drug Interactions

Drugs that may interact with stavudine include didanosine, doxorubicin, hydroxyurea, methadone, ribavirin, and zidovudine.

Adverse Reactions

When stavudine is used in combination with other agents with similar toxicities, the incidence of adverse events may be higher than when stavudine is used alone. Pancreatitis, peripheral neuropathy, and liver function abnormalities occur more frequently in patients treated with the combination of stavudine and didanosine, with or without hydroxyurea. Fatal pancreatitis and hepatotoxicity may occur more frequently in patients treated with stavudine in combination with didanosine and hydroxyurea (see Warnings).

Adverse reactions occurring in at least 3% of patients include headache, diarrhea, peripheral neurologic symptoms/neuropathy, rash, nausea, and vomiting. Lab abnormalities include elevations in AST, ALT, and amylase.

ZIDOVUDINE (Azidothymidine; AZT; Compound S)

Tablets; oral: 300 mg (*Rx*)	Various, *Retrovir* (GlaxoSmithKline)
Capsules; oral: 100 mg (*Rx*)	
Syrup; oral: 50 mg/5 mL (*Rx*)	
Injection, solution: 10 mg/mL (*Rx*)	*Retrovir* (GlaxoSmithKline)

Warning:

Zidovudine has been associated with hematologic toxicity, including neutropenia and severe anemia, particularly in patients with HIV (see Warnings). Prolonged use of zidovudine has been associated with symptomatic myopathy.

Lactic acidosis and severe hepatomegaly with steatosis, including fatal cases, have been reported with the use of nucleoside analogs alone or in combination, including zidovudine and other antiretrovirals (see Warnings).

Indications

HIV infection: In combination with other antiretroviral agents for the treatment of HIV infection.

Maternal-fetal HIV transmission – For the prevention of maternal-fetal HIV-1 transmission. The indication is based on a dosing regimen that included 3 components: antepartum therapy of HIV-1 infected mothers, intrapartum therapy of HIV-1 infected mothers, and postpartum therapy of HIV-1 exposed neonates.

Administration and Dosage

HIV infection:

Adults (oral) – 600 mg/day in divided doses in combination with other antiretroviral agents.

Adults (IV) – Recommended IV dose is 1 mg/kg infused over 1 hour. Administer this dose 5 to 6 times daily (5 to 6 mg/kg/day). Patients should receive zidovudine IV infusion only until oral therapy can be administered. The IV dosing regimen equivalent to the oral administration of 100 mg every 4 hours is approximately 1 mg/kg IV every 4 hours. Avoid rapid infusion or bolus injection. Do not give IM.

Children (oral) – The recommended dosage in children 6 weeks of age and older and weighing 4 kg or more is provided in the following table. Zidovudine syrup should be used to provide accurate dosage when whole tablets or capsules are not appropriate.

Zidovudine Pediatric Dosage (≥ 6 Weeks of Age)			
		Dosage regimen and dose	
Body weight (kg)	Total daily dose	Twice daily	3 times daily
4 to < 9	24 mg/kg/day	12 mg/kg	8 mg/kg
≥ 9 to < 30	18 mg/kg/day	9 mg/kg	6 mg/kg
≥ 30	600 mg/day	300 mg	200 mg

Alternatively, dosing of zidovudine can be based on body surface area (BSA) for each child. The recommended oral dose of zidovudine is 480 mg/m^2/day in divided doses (240 mg/m^2 twice daily or 160 mg/m^2 3 times daily). In some cases, the dose calculated by mg/kg will not be the same as that calculated by BSA.

Maternal-fetal HIV transmission: Recommended dosing regimen to pregnant women (greater than 14 weeks of pregnancy) and their neonates is as follows:

Maternal dosing (oral) – 100 mg orally 5 times per day until the start of labor.

Maternal dosing (IV) – During labor and delivery, administer IV zidovudine at 2 mg/kg (total body weight) over 1 hour followed by a continuous IV infusion of 1 mg/kg/h (total body weight) until clamping of the umbilical cord.

Neonatal dosing (oral) – 2 mg/kg orally every 6 hours, starting within 12 hours after birth and continuing through 6 weeks of age.

Neonatal dosing (IV) – Neonates unable to receive oral dosing may be given zidovudine IV at 1.5 mg/kg, infused over 30 minutes, every 6 hours.

Dose adjustment: Significant anemia (hemoglobin of less than 7.5 g/dL or reduction of greater than 25% from baseline) and/or significant neutropenia (granulocyte count of less than 750 cells/mm^3 or reduction of greater than 50% from baseline) may require a dose interruption until evidence of marrow recovery is observed. In patients who develop significant anemia, dose interruption does not necessarily eliminate the need for transfusion. If marrow recovery occurs following dose interruption, resumption in dose may be appropriate using adjunctive measures such as epoetin alfa at recommended doses, depending on hematologic indices such as serum erythropoietin level and patient tolerance.

Renal function impairment – In end-stage renal disease patients maintained on hemodialysis or peritoneal dialysis, the recommended dosage is 100 mg every 6 to 8 hours.

Hepatic function impairment – Because zidovudine is primarily eliminated by hepatic metabolism, a reduction in the daily dose may be necessary in these patients. Frequent monitoring for hematologic toxicities is advised.

Actions

Pharmacology: Zidovudine is a synthetic nucleoside analog of the naturally occurring nucleoside thymidine. The active metabolite, zidovudine 5′-triphosphate (AztTP), inhibits the activity of the HIV reverse transcriptase by competing for utilization with the natural substrate deoxythymidine 5′-triphosphate (dTTP) and by its incorporation into viral DNA.

Pharmacokinetics:

Adults – Following oral administration, zidovudine is rapidly absorbed and extensively distributed, with peak serum concentrations occurring within 0.5 to 1.5 hours. Zidovudine is primarily eliminated by hepatic metabolism.

Zidovudine Pharmacokinetic Parameters in Fasting Adult Patients	
Parameter	Mean value
Oral bioavailability (%)	Approximately 64
Apparent volume of distribution (L/kg)	Approximately 1.6
Plasma protein binding (%)	< 38
CSF:plasma ratio[a]	0.6 (0.04 to 2.62)
Systemic clearance (L/h/kg)	Approximately 1.6
Renal clearance (L/h/kg)	Approximately 0.34
Elimination half-life (h)[b]	0.5 to 3 (oral); 1.1 (IV)

[a] Median (range).
[b] Approximate range.

Adults with impaired renal function – A dose adjustment should not be necessary for patients with creatinine clearance (CrCl) greater than or equal to 15 mL/min.

Zidovudine Pharmacokinetics Parameters in Patients with Severe Renal Impairment		
Parameter	Control subjects (normal renal function) (n = 6)	Patients with renal impairment (n = 14)
CrCl (mL/min)	Approximately 120	Approximately 18
Zidovudine AUC (ng•h/mL)	Approximately 1,400	Approximately 3,100
Zidovudine half-life (h)	Approximately 1	Approximately 1.4

A dosage adjustment is recommended for patients undergoing hemodialysis or peritoneal dialysis.

Patients younger than 3 months of age – The half-life was about 13 hours. In neonates 14 days of age or younger, bioavailability was greater, total body clearance was slower, and half-life was longer than in pediatric patients more than 14 days of age.

Zidovudine Pharmacokinetic Parameters in Pediatric Patients			
Parameter	Birth to 14 days of age	14 days to 3 months of age	3 months to 12 years of age
Oral bioavailability (%)	Approximately 89	Approximately 61	Approximately 65
CSF:Plasma ratio	no data	no data	Approximately 0.68 (0.03 to 3.25)[a] (oral); approximately 0.26[a] (IV)
CL (L/h/kg)	Approximately 0.65	Approximately 1.14	Approximately 1.85
Elimination half-life (h)	Approximately 3.1	Approximately 1.9	Approximately 1.5

[a] Median (range).

Contraindications

Potentially life-threatening allergic reactions to any of the components of the product.

Warnings/Precautions

Bone marrow suppression: Use with extreme caution in patients who have bone marrow compromise evidenced by granulocyte count less than 1,000/mm^3 or hemoglobin less than 9.5 g/dL. Anemia and granulocytopenia are the most significant adverse events observed. Reversible pancytopenia has been reported.

Myopathy: Myopathy and myositis with pathological changes, similar to that produced by HIV disease, have been associated with prolonged use of zidovudine.

Lactic acidosis/severe hepatomegaly with steatosis: Rare occurrences of lactic acidosis in the absence of hypoxemia and severe hepatomegaly with steatosis have been reported with the use of antiretroviral nucleoside analogs, including zidovudine and zalcitabine, and are potentially fatal.

Immune reconstitution syndrome: Immune reconstitution syndrome has been reported in patients treated with combination antiretroviral therapy, including zidovudine.

Fat redistribution: Redistribution/accumulation of body fat, including central obesity, dorsocervical fat enlargement (buffalo hump), peripheral wasting, facial wasting, breast enlargement, and "cushingoid appearance," have been observed in patients receiving antiretroviral therapy.

Combination therapy: Lamivudine/zidovudine and abacavir/lamivudine/zidovudine are combination product tablets that contain zidovudine as one of their components. Do not administer zidovudine concomitantly with lamivudine/zidovudine or abacavir/lamivudine/zidovudine.

Renal/Hepatic function impairment: Zidovudine is eliminated from the body primarily by renal excretion following metabolism in the liver (glucuronidation). In patients with severely impaired renal function (CrCl less than 15 mL/min), dosage reduction is recommended. Although very little data are available, patients with severely impaired hepatic function may be at greater risk of toxicity.

Pregnancy: Category C.

Antiretroviral pregnancy registry – Health care providers are encouraged to register patients by calling (800) 258-4263.

Lactation: The Centers for Disease Control and Prevention recommend that HIV-infected women not breast-feed to avoid postnatal transmission of HIV.

Zidovudine is excreted in breast milk. Because of the potential for HIV transmission and for serious adverse reactions in breast-feeding infants, instruct mothers not to breast-feed if they are receiving zidovudine.

Children: Zidovudine has been studied in HIV-infected children over 3 months of age who had HIV-related symptoms or who were asymptomatic with abnormal laboratory values indicating significant HIV-related immunosuppression. Zidovudine also has been studied in neonates perinatally exposed to HIV.

Drug Interactions

Drugs that may affect zidovudine include acetaminophen, atovaquone, bone marrow suppressive/cytotoxic agents (eg, adriamycin, dapsone), clarithromycin, doxorubicin, fluconazole, ganciclovir, methadone, nelfinavir/ritonavir, phenytoin, probenecid, ribavirin, rifamycins, stavudine, trimethoprim, and valproic acid.

Drugs that may be affected by zidovudine include phenytoin.

Adverse Reactions

The frequency and severity of adverse reactions associated with the use of zidovudine are greater in patients with more advanced infection at the time of initiation of therapy.

The most frequent adverse reactions and abnormal laboratory values reported in the placebo-controlled clinical trial of oral zidovudine were anemia and granulocytopenia.

Adverse reactions occurring in at least 5% of patients with asymptomatic HIV infection include anorexia, asthenia, constipation, headache, malaise, nausea, and vomiting.

Other adverse reactions observed in clinical studies were abdominal cramps, abdominal pain, arthralgia, chills, dyspepsia, fatigue, hyperbilirubinemia, insomnia, musculoskeletal pain, myalgia, and neuropathy.

ABACAVIR SULFATE

Tablets: 300 mg (*Rx*) — *Ziagen* (GlaxoSmithKline)
Oral solution: 20 mg/mL (*Rx*)

Warning:

Hypersensitivity reactions: Serious and sometimes fatal hypersensitivity reactions have been associated with abacavir therapy. Hypersensitivity to abacavir is a multi-organ clinical syndrome usually characterized by a sign or symptom in 2 or more of the following groups:

- constitutional, including achiness, fatigue, or generalized malaise;
- fever;
- GI, including abdominal pain, diarrhea, nausea, or vomiting;
- rash;
- respiratory, including cough, dyspnea, or pharyngitis.

Discontinue abacavir as soon as a hypersensitivity reaction is suspected. Permanently discontinue abacavir if hypersensitivity cannot be ruled out, even when other diagnoses are possible.

continued on next page

Warning: (cont.)

Patients who carry the HLA-B*5701 allele are at high risk for experiencing a hypersensitivity reaction to abacavir. Prior to initiating therapy with abacavir, screening for the HLA-B*5701 allele is recommended; this approach has been found to decrease the risk of hypersensitivity reaction. Screening is also recommended prior to reinitiation of abacavir in patients of unknown HLA-B*5701 status who have previously tolerated abacavir. HLA-B*5701–negative patients may develop a suspected hypersensitivity reaction to abacavir; however, this occurs significantly less frequently than in HLA-B*5701–positive patients.

Regardless of HLA-B*5701 status, permanently discontinue abacavir if hypersensitivity cannot be ruled out, even when other diagnoses are possible.

Following a hypersensitivity reaction to abacavir, never restart abacavir or any abacavir-containing product because more severe symptoms can occur within hours and may include life-threatening hypotension and death.

Reintroduction of abacavir or any other abacavir-containing product, even in patients who have no identified history or unrecognized symptoms of hypersensitivity to abacavir therapy, can result in serious or fatal hypersensitivity reactions. Such reactions can occur within hours.

Lactic acidosis and severe hepatomegaly: Lactic acidosis and severe hepatomegaly with steatosis, including fatal cases, have been reported with the use of nucleoside analogs alone or in combination, including abacavir and other antiretrovirals.

Indications

HIV infection: In combination with other antiretroviral agents for the treatment of HIV-1 infection.

Administration and Dosage

Dispense Medication Guide and Warning Card that provide information about recognition of hypersensitivity reactions with each new prescription and refill.

Always use abacavir in combination with other antiretroviral agents. Do not add abacavir as a single agent when antiretroviral regimens are changed because of loss of virologic response.

Abacavir may be taken with or without food.

Adults: The recommended dose is 300 mg twice daily or 600 mg once daily in combination with other antiretroviral agents.

Children (3 months to up to 16 years of age): 8 mg/kg twice daily (up to a maximum of 300 mg twice daily) in combination with other antiretroviral agents.

Dose adjustment in hepatic impairment: The recommended dose of abacavir in patients with mild hepatic impairment (Child-Pugh score 5 to 6) is 200 mg twice daily. To enable dose reduction, use abacavir oral solution (10 mL twice daily) to treat these patients. The safety, efficacy, and pharmacokinetic properties of abacavir have not been established in patients with moderate to severe hepatic impairment; therefore, abacavir is contraindicated in these patients.

Actions

Pharmacology: Abacavir is a synthetic carbocyclic synthetic nucleoside analog with inhibitory activity against HIV. Abacavir has synergistic activity in combination with amprenavir, nevirapine, and zidovudine and additive activity in combination with didanosine, lamivudine, stavudine, and zalcitabine in vitro.

Pharmacokinetics:

Absorption – Abacavir was rapidly and extensively absorbed after oral administration with bioavailability at 83%. Systemic exposure to abacavir was comparable after administration of oral solution and tablets. Therefore, these products may be used interchangeably.

Distribution – The apparent volume of distribution after IV administration of abacavir was approximately 0.86 L/kg. Binding to human plasma proteins is approximately 50%.

Metabolism – Abacavir is not significantly metabolized by cytochrome P450 enzymes.

Excretion – Of the 99% of the total abacavir dose recovered, 1.2% was excreted unchanged in the urine as abacavir. Fecal elimination accounted for 16% of the dose. In single-dose studies, the observed elimination half-life was approximately 1.54 hours.

Contraindications

Hypersensitivity to any of the components of the product.

Moderate or severe hepatic impairment (Child-Pugh score greater than 6).

Warnings/Precautions

Lactic acidosis/severe hepatomegaly with steatosis: Lactic acidosis and severe hepatomegaly with steatosis, including fatal cases, have been reported with the use of nucleoside analogs alone or in combination, including abacavir and other antiretrovirals. Suspend treatment with abacavir in any patient who develops clinical or laboratory findings suggestive of lactic acidosis or pronounced hepatotoxicity (which may include hepatomegaly and steatosis even in the absence of marked transaminase elevations).

Immune reconstitution syndrome: Immune reconstitution syndrome has been reported in patients treated with combination antiretroviral therapy, including abacavir. During the initial phase of combination antiretroviral treatment, patients whose immune systems respond may develop an inflammatory response to indolent or residual opportunistic infections (such as *Mycobacterium avium* infection, cytomegalovirus, *Pneumocystis jirovecii* pneumonia, or tuberculosis), which may necessitate further evaluation and treatment.

Myocardial infarction: As a precaution, consider the underlying risk of coronary heart disease when prescribing antiretroviral therapies (including abacavir) and taking action to minimize all modifiable risk factors (eg, hypertension, hyperlipidemia, diabetes mellitus, smoking).

Cross-resistance: In clinical trials, patients with prolonged prior nucleoside reverse transcriptase inhibitor (NRTI) exposure or who had HIV-1 isolates that contained multiple mutations conferring resistance to NRTIs had limited response to abacavir. Consider the potential for cross-resistance between abacavir and other NRTIs when choosing new therapeutic regimens in therapy-experienced patients.

Fat redistribution – Redistribution/accumulation of body fat, including central obesity, dorsocervical fat enlargement (buffalo hump), peripheral wasting, facial wasting, breast enlargement, and "cushingoid appearance" have been observed in patients receiving antiretroviral therapy.

Hypersensitivity reactions: Serious and sometimes fatal hypersensitivity reactions have been associated with abacavir therapy. Patients who carry the HLA-B*5701 allele are at high risk for experiencing a hypersensitivity reaction to abacavir. Discontinue abacavir in patients developing signs or symptoms of hypersensitivity as soon as a hypersensitivity reaction is first suspected. Do not restart abacavir following a hypersensitivity reaction because more severe symptoms will recur within hours and may include life-threatening hypotension and death.

Abacavir hypersensitivity reaction registry – Physicians should register patients by calling (800) 270-0425.

Hepatic function impairment: The safety, efficacy, and pharmacokinetics of abacavir have not been studied in patients with moderate or severe hepatic function impairment, therefore abacavir is contraindicated in these patients.

Pregnancy: Category C.

Antiretroviral pregnancy registry – Physicians are encouraged to register patients by calling (800) 258-4263.

Lactation: The Centers for Disease Control and Prevention recommend that HIV-infected mothers not breastfeed their infants to avoid risking postnatal transmission of HIV infection.

Children: Use of abacavir in pediatric patients 3 months to 13 years of age is safe and effective.

Elderly: In general, use caution in dose selection for an elderly patient, reflecting the greater frequency of decreased hepatic, renal, or cardiac function, and of concomitant disease or other drug therapy.

Drug Interactions

Other antiretrovirals: Abacavir had synergistic activity in vitro in combination with amprenavir, nevirapine, and zidovudine, and additive activity in combination with didanosine, lamivudine, stavudine, tenofovir, and zalcitabine. Ribavirin had no effect on the in vitro anti-HIV-1 activity of abacavir.

Other NRTIs: Cross-resistance has been observed among NRTIs.

Methadone: Coadministration increased oral methadone clearance by 22%. An increased methadone dose may be required in a small number of patients.

Ethanol: Coadministration of ethanol and abacavir resulted in a 41% increase in abacavir AUC_{∞} and a 26% increase in abacavir half-life.

Adverse Reactions

Adverse effects occurring in at least 5% of patients include the following: abdominal pain/gastritis/GI signs and symptoms, anxiety, bronchitis, depressive disorders, diarrhea, dizziness, dreams/sleep disorders, drug hypersensitivity, ear/nose/throat infections, fatigue/malaise, fever and/or chills, headaches/migraine, musculoskeletal pain, nausea, rashes, viral respiratory infections, vomiting,

Hypersensitivity: Serious and sometimes fatal hypersensitivity reactions have been associated with abacavir therapy (see Warnings and Warning Box).

Lab test abnormalities: Liver function test abnormalities, CPK or creatinine elevations, lymphopenia, triglyceride elevations occurred in at least 3% of patients.

LAMIVUDINE/ZIDOVUDINE (3TC/ZDV, 3TC/AZT)

Tablets: 150 mg lamivudine/300 mg zidovudine (*Rx*)	*Combivir* (GlaxoSmithKline)

Consult the complete prescribing information for each agent, lamivudine and zidovudine, prior to administration of lamivudine/zidovudine combination tablets.

Warning:

Zidovudine has been associated with hematologic toxicity, including neutropenia and severe anemia, particularly in patients with advanced HIV disease. Prolonged use of zidovudine has been associated with symptomatic myopathy.

Lactic acidosis and severe hepatomegaly with steatosis, including fatal cases, have been reported with use of nucleoside analogs alone or in combination, including lamivudine, zidovudine, and other antiretrovirals.

Severe acute exacerbations of hepatitis B have been reported in patients who are coinfected with hepatitis B virus (HBV) and HIV and have discontinued lamivudine. Monitor hepatic function closely with both clinical and laboratory follow-up for at least several months in patients who discontinue lamivudine/zidovudine and are coinfected with HIV and HBV. If appropriate, initiation of hepatitis B therapy may be warranted.

Indications

HIV infection: In combination with other antiretrovirals for the treatment of HIV infection.

Administration and Dosage

Adults and children weighing more than 30 kg: One tablet (150 mg/300 mg) orally twice daily without regard to food.

Renal function impairment: Not recommended if CrCl is less than 50 mL/min.

Hepatic function impairment: Because lamivudine/zidovudine is a fixed-dose combination that cannot be adjusted for patients with impaired hepatic function or liver cirrhosis, it is not recommended.

Elderly: In general, use caution in dose selection for elderly patients, reflecting the greater frequency of decreased hepatic, renal, or cardiac function, and of concomitant disease or other drug therapy.

Actions

Pharmacology: Lamivudine/zidovudine combination tablets contain 2 synthetic nucleoside analog reverse transcriptase inhibitors with activity against HIV. Lamivudine in combination with zidovudine has exhibited synergistic antiretroviral activity.

Pharmacokinetics: One combination lamivudine/zidovudine (150/300 mg) tablet is bioequivalent to a 150 mg lamivudine tablet plus a 300 mg zidovudine tablet.

Select Pharmacokinetic Parameters for Lamivudine and Zidovudine[a]

	Bioavailability (%)	V_d (L/kg)	Plasma protein binding (%)	Clearance (L/h/kg)	Renal clearance (L/h/kg)	t½ (h)
Lamivudine	≈ 86	≈ 1.3	< 36	≈ 0.33	≈ 0.22	5 to 7
Zidovudine	≈ 64	≈ 1.6	< 38	≈ 1.6	≈ 0.34	0.5 to 3

[a] In adults.

Contraindications

Hypersensitivity to any of the components of this product.

Warnings/Precautions

Bone marrow suppression: Use lamivudine/zidovudine with caution in patients who have bone marrow compromise evidenced by granulocyte count less than 1000 cells/mm^3 or hemoglobin less than 9.5 g/dL.

Fat redistribution: Redistribution/accumulation of body fat, including central obesity, dorsocervical fat enlargement (buffalo hump), peripheral wasting, facial wasting, breast enlargement, and cushingoid appearance, has been observed in patients receiving antiretroviral therapy.

Immune reconstitution: Immune reconstitution syndrome has been reported in patients treated with combination antiretroviral therapy, including lamivudine/zidovudine. During the initial phase of combination antiretroviral treatment, patients whose immune systems respond may develop an inflammatory response to indolent or residual opportunistic infections, which may necessitate further evaluation and treatment.

Lactic acidosis/severe hepatomegaly with steatosis: Lactic acidosis and severe hepatomegaly with steatosis, including fatal cases, have been reported with the use of nucleoside analogs alone or in combination, including lamivudine, zidovudine, and other antiretrovirals. Suspend treatment with lamivudine/zidovudine in any patient who develops clinical or laboratory findings suggestive of lactic acidosis or pronounced hepatotoxicity (which may include hepatomegaly and steatosis even in the absence of marked transaminase elevations).

Myopathy: Myopathy and myositis, with pathological changes similar to that produced by HIV disease, have been associated with prolonged use of zidovudine, and, therefore, may occur with lamivudine/zidovudine therapy.

Pancreatitis: Use lamivudine/zidovudine with caution in patients with a history of pancreatitis or other significant risk factors for the development of pancreatitis. Stop treatment with lamivudine/zidovudine immediately if clinical signs, symptoms, or laboratory abnormalities suggestive of pancreatitis occur.

Pregnancy: Category C.

Antiretroviral pregnancy registry – To monitor maternal-fetal outcomes of pregnant women exposed to lamivudine/zidovudine and other antiretroviral agents, an antiretroviral pregnancy registry has been established. Register patients by calling 1-800-258-4263.

Lactation: The Centers for Disease Control and Prevention recommend that HIV-infected mothers not breast-feed their infants to avoid risking postnatal transmission of HIV infection.

Children: Lamivudine/zidovudine should not be administered to pediatric patients younger than 12 years of age because it is a fixed-dose combination that cannot be adjusted for this patient population.

Monitoring: Blood counts are recommended frequently for patients with advanced HIV disease and periodically for patients with asymptomatic or early HIV disease. Monitor hepatic function closely with clinical and laboratory follow-up for at least several months in patients who discontinue lamivudine/zidovudine and are coinfected with HIV and HBV.

Drug Interactions

Drugs that may affect lamivudine/zidovudine include acetaminophen, atovaquone, bone marrow suppressive/cytotoxic agents, clarithromycin, doxorubicin, fluconazole, methadone, nelfinavir, probenecid, ribavirin/interferon, rifamycins, ritonavir, stavudine, trimethoprim, trimethoprim/sulfamethoxazole, valproic acid, zalcitabine, didanosine.

Drugs that may be affected by lamivudine/zidovudine include zalcitabine and didanosine.

Adverse Reactions

Adverse reactions affecting at least 3% of patients include abdominal cramps/pain, abnormalities in ALT and amylase, anorexia and/or decreased appetite, arthralgia, chills, cough, depressive disorders, diarrhea, dizziness, dyspepsia, fatigue, fever, headache, insomnia and other sleep disorders, malaise, musculoskeletal pain, myalgia, nasal signs and symptoms, nausea, neutropenia, neuropathy, skin rashes, vomiting.

ABACAVIR SULFATE/LAMIVUDINE/ZIDOVUDINE

Tablets; oral: 300 mg abacavir sulfate/150 mg lamivudine/ 300 mg zidovudine (*Rx*)	*Trizivir* (GlaxoSmithKline)

Consult the complete prescribing information for each agent, abacavir, lamivudine, and zidovudine, prior to administration of abacavir/lamivudine/zidovudine combination tablets.

Warning:

This product contains 3 nucleoside analogs (ie, abacavir sulfate, lamivudine, zidovudine) and is intended only for patients whose regimen would otherwise include these 3 components.

Hypersensitivity reactions: Serious and sometimes fatal hypersensitivity reactions have been associated with abacavir sulfate, a component of abacavir/lamivudine/zidovudine. Hypersensitivity to abacavir is a multi-organ clinical syndrome usually characterized by a sign or symptom in 2 or more of the following groups: fever, rash, gastrointestinal, constitutional, respiratory.

Discontinue abacavir/lamivudine/zidovudine as soon as a hypersensitivity reaction is suspected.

continued on next page

Warning: (cont.)

Patients who carry the HLA-B*5701 allele are at high risk for experiencing a hypersensitivity reaction to abacavir. Prior to initiating therapy with abacavir, screening for HLA-B*5701 allele is recommended; this approach has been found to decrease the risk of hypersensitivity reaction. Screening is also recommended prior to reinitiation of abacavir in patients of unknown HLA-B*5701 status who have previously tolerated abacavir. HLA-B*5701–negative patients may develop a suspected hypersensitivity reaction to abacavir; however, this occurs significantly less frequently than in HLA-B*5701–positive patients.

Regardless of HLA-B*5701 status, permanently discontinue abacavir/lamivudine/zidovudine if hypersensitivity cannot be ruled out, even when other diagnoses are possible.

Following a hypersensitivity reaction to abacavir, never restart abacavir/lamivudine/zidovudine or any other abacavir-containing product because more severe symptoms can occur within hours and may include life-threatening hypotension and death.

Reintroduction of abacavir/lamivudine/zidovudine or any other abacavir-containing product, even in patients who have no identified history or unrecognized symptoms of hypersensitivity to abacavir therapy, can result in serious or fatal hypersensitivity reactions. Such reactions can occur within hours (see Warnings).

Hematologic toxicity: Zidovudine has been associated with hematologic toxicity including neutropenia and severe anemia, particularly in patients with advanced HIV disease (see Warnings). Prolonged use of zidovudine has been associated with symptomatic myopathy.

Lactic acidosis and severe hepatomegaly: Lactic acidosis and severe hepatomegaly with steatosis, including fatal cases, have been reported with the use of nucleoside analogs alone or in combination, including abacavir, lamivudine, zidovudine, and other antiretrovirals (see Warnings).

Exacerbations of hepatitis B: Severe acute exacerbations of hepatitis B have been reported in patients who are co-infected with hepatitis B virus (HBV) and HIV and have discontinued lamivudine, which is one component of abacavir/lamivudine/zidovudine. Hepatic function should be monitored closely with both clinical and laboratory follow-up for at least several months in patients who discontinue abacavir/lamivudine/zidovudine and are co-infected with HIV and HBV. If appropriate, initiation of anti-HBV therapy may be warranted (see Warnings).

Indications

HIV infection: Alone or in combination with other antiretroviral agents for the treatment of HIV-1 infection in patients weighing more than 40 kg.

Administration and Dosage

Dispense a Medication Guide and Warning Card that provide information about recognition of hypersensitivity reactions with each new prescription or refill. To facilitate reporting hypersensitivity reactions and collection of information on each case, an Abacavir Hypersensitivity Registry has been established. Physicians should register patients by calling (800) 270-0425.

Abacavir/lamivudine/zidovudine may be administered with or without food.

Adults and adolescents weighing 40 kg or more: 1 tablet twice daily. Not recommended in adults or adolescents who weigh less than 40 kg because it is a fixed-dose tablet.

Dose adjustment: Because it is a fixed-dose tablet, do not prescribe for patients requiring dosage adjustments such as those with CrCl less than 50 mL/min, patients with hepatic impairment, or those experiencing dose-limiting adverse events.

Actions

Pharmacology: The combination tablets contain the following 3 synthetic nucleoside analogs: Abacavir sulfate, lamivudine, and zidovudine. Abacavir is a carbocyclic synthetic nucleoside analog. Lamivudine and zidovudine are synthetic nucleoside analogs.

Pharmacokinetics: Following oral administration, abacavir, lamivudine, and zidovudine are rapidly absorbed and extensively distributed. Binding of abacavir to human plasma proteins is about 50%; binding of lamivudine and zidovudine to plasma proteins is low.

The pharmacokinetic properties of abacavir, lamivudine, and zidovudine in fasting patients are summarized below.

Pharmacokinetic Parameters for Abacavir, Lamivudine, and Zidovudine in Adults

Parameter	Abacavir	Lamivudine	Zidovudine
Oral bioavailability (%)	≈ 86	≈ 86	≈ 64
Apparent volume of distribution (L/kg)	≈ 0.86	≈ 1.3	≈ 1.6
Systemic clearance (L/h/kg)	≈ 0.8	≈ 0.33	≈ 1.6
Renal clearance (L/h/kg)	≈ 0.007	≈ 0.22	≈ 0.34
Elimination half-life (h)[a]	≈ 1.45	5 to 7	0.5 to 3

[a] Approximate range.

Contraindications

Previously demonstrated hypersensitivity to abacavir or to any other component of the product; hepatic impairment.

Following a hypersensitivity reaction to abacavir, never restart abacavir/lamivudine/zidovudine or any other abacavir-containing product.

Warnings/Precautions

Hypersensitivity reactions: Serious and sometimes fatal hypersensitivity reactions have been associated with abacavir/lamivudine/zidovudine and other abacavir-containing products. Permanently discontinue abacavir/lamivudine/zidovudine if hypersensitivity cannot be ruled out, even when other diagnoses are possible.

Lactic acidosis/severe hepatomegaly with steatosis: Lactic acidosis and severe hepatomegaly with steatosis, including fatal cases, have been reported with the use of nucleoside analogs alone or in combination and other antiretrovirals. A majority of these cases have been in women. Obesity and prolonged nucleoside exposure may be risk factors. Exercise particular caution when administering abacavir/lamivudine/zidovudine to any patient with known risk factors for liver disease; however, cases also have been reported in patients with no known risk factors.

Bone marrow suppression: Use with caution in patients who have bone marrow compromise evidenced by granulocyte count less than 1,000 cells/mm^3 or hemoglobin less than 9.5 g/dL.

Myopathy: Myopathy and myositis have been associated with prolonged use of zidovudine.

Posttreatment exacerbations of hepatitis: Evidence of exacerbations of hepatitis have occurred after discontinuation of lamivudine, detected primarily by serum ALT elevations in addition to re-emergence of HBV DNA.

Fixed-dose combination: Abacavir/lamivudine/zidovudine contains fixed doses of 3 nucleoside analogs: abacavir, lamivudine, and zidovudine and should not be administered concomitantly with abacavir, lamivudine, emtricitabine, or zidovudine. Do not administer abacavir/lamivudine/zidovudine concomitantly with the fixed-dose combination drugs: lamivudine/zidovudine, abacavir and lamivudine, or emtricitabine and tenofovir.

Because abacavir/lamivudine/zidovudine is a fixed-dose tablet, it should not be prescribed for adolescents who weigh less than 40 kg or other patients requiring dosage adjustment.

Therapy-experienced patients: Consider the potential for cross-resistance between abacavir and other NRTIs when choosing new therapeutic regimens in therapy-experienced patients.

HIV and HBV coinfection: Safety and efficacy of lamivudine have not been established for treatment of chronic hepatitis B in patients dually infected with HIV and HBV. In non-HIV-infected patients treated with lamivudine for chronic hepatitis B, emergence of lamivudine-resistant HBV has been detected and has been associated with diminished treatment response.

Immune reconstitution syndrome: Immune reconstitution syndrome has been reported in patients treated with combination antiretroviral therapy.

Myocardial infarction: As a precaution, consider the underlying risk of coronary heart disease when prescribing antiretroviral therapies, including abacavir, and take action to minimize all modifiable risk factors (eg, diabetes mellitus, hyperlipidemia, hypertension, smoking).

Fat redistribution: Redistribution/accumulation of body fat including central obesity, dorsocervical fat enlargement (buffalo hump), peripheral wasting, facial wasting, breast enlargement, and cushingoid appearance have been observed.

Renal function impairment: Patients with CrCl less than 50 mL/min should not receive abacavir/lamivudine/zidovudine.

Hepatic function impairment: Abacavir/lamivudine/zidovudine is contraindicated in patients with hepatic impairment.

Pregnancy: Category C.

Antiretroviral pregnancy registry – Physicians are encouraged to register patients by calling (800) 258-4263.

Lactation: The Centers for Disease Control and Prevention recommend that HIV-infected mothers not breast-feed their infants to avoid risking postnatal transmission of HIV infection.

Because of both the potential for HIV transmission and the potential for serious adverse reactions in nursing infants, instruct mothers not to breast-feed if they are receiving abacavir/lamivudine/zidovudine.

Children: Abacavir/lamivudine/zidovudine is not intended for use in pediatric patients. Abacavir/lamivudine/zidovudine should not be administered to adolescents who weigh less than 40 kg.

Elderly: In general, dose selection for an elderly patient should be cautious, reflecting the greater frequency of decreased hepatic, renal, or cardiac function, and of concomitant disease or other drug therapy. Abacavir/lamivudine/zidovudine is not recommended for patients with impaired renal function (ie, CrCl less than 50 mL/min).

Drug Interactions

Drugs that may be affected by abacavir sulfate/lamivudine/zidovudine include methadone, and phenytoin.

Drugs that may affect abacavir sulfate/lamivudine/zidovudine include acetaminophen, atovaquone, bone marrow suppressive/cytotoxic agents, clarithromycin, doxorubicin, ethanol, fluconazole, ganciclovir, methadone, nelfinavir/ritonavir, phenytoin, probenecid, ribavirin, ribavirin/interferon, rifamycins, stavudine, trimethoprim/sulfamethoxazole, and valproic acid.

Adverse Reactions

Adverse reactions occurring in 3% or more patients include the following: ALT (greater than 5 × ULN), anxiety, depressive disorders, diarrhea, ear/nose/throat infections, elevated CPK, fever and/or chills, headache, hypersensitivity reaction, malaise and fatigue, musculoskeletal pain, nausea, neutropenia, skin rashes, viral respiratory infections, vomiting.

EMTRICITABINE/TENOFOVIR DISOPROXIL FUMARATE

Tablets: 200 mg emtricitabine/300 mg tenofovir disoproxil fumarate (equivalent to 245 mg tenofovir disoproxil) (*Rx*)	*Truvada* (Gilead Sciences)

Consult the complete prescribing information for each agent prior to administration of emtricitabine/tenofovir disoproxil fumarate combination tablets.

Warning:

Lactic acidosis and severe hepatomegaly with steatosis, including fatal cases, have been reported with the use of nucleoside analogs, including tenofovir (a component of emtricitabine/tenofovir), in combination with other antiretrovirals.

Emtricitabine/tenofovir disoproxil fumarate is not approved for the treatment of long-term hepatitis B virus (HBV) infection; safety and efficacy have not been established in patients coinfected with HBV and HIV. Severe short-term exacerbations of hepatitis B have been reported in patients who are coinfected with HBV and HIV-1 who have discontinued emtricitabine or tenofovir disoproxil fumarate. Closely monitor hepatic function with clinical and laboratory follow-up for at least several months in patients who discontinue emtricitabine/tenofovir disoproxil fumarate and are coinfected with HIV and HBV. If appropriate, initiation of antihepatitis B therapy may be warranted (see Warnings).

Indications

HIV infection: In combination with other antiretroviral agents (such as nonnucleoside reverse transcriptase inhibitors or protease inhibitors) for the treatment of HIV-1 infection in adults.

Administration and Dosage

The dose of emtricitabine/tenofovir disoproxil fumarate is 1 tablet taken orally once daily with or without food.

Renal function impairment:

Dosage Adjustment for Patients with Altered CrCl			
CrCl (mL/min)[a]	≥ 50	30 to 49	< 30 (including patients requiring hemodialysis)
Recommended dosing interval	Every 24 hours	Every 48 hours	Not to be administered

[a] Calculated using ideal (lean) body weight.

Actions

Pharmacology: Refer to individual monographs for a complete explanation of mechanisms of action.

Pharmacokinetics:

Absorption/Distribution – Emtricitabine is rapidly absorbed, with C_{max} occurring at 1 to 2 hours. Binding of emtricitabine to human plasma proteins is less than 4%.

Following oral administration, maximum tenofovir serum concentrations are achieved in about 1 hour. Binding of tenofovir to human plasma proteins is less than 0.7%.

Metabolism/Excretion – Emtricitabine is eliminated by a combination of glomerular filtration and active tubular secretion. The plasma emtricitabine half-life is approximately 10 hours.

Tenofovir is eliminated by a combination of glomerular filtration and active tubular secretion. The terminal elimination half-life of tenofovir is approximately 17 hours.

Single Dose Pharmacokinetic Parameters for Emtricitabine and Tenofovir in Adults		
	Emtricitabine	Tenofovir
Fasted oral bioavailability[a] (%)	≈ 92	≈ 25
Plasma terminal elimination half-life[a] (h)	≈ 10	≈ 17

[a] Median (range).

Contraindications

Previously demonstrated hypersensitivity to any of the components of the product.

Warnings/Precautions

HIV-1 and hepatitis B coinfection: It is recommended that all patients with HIV-1 be tested for the presence of long-term HBV before initiating antiretroviral therapy.

Bone effects: Consider bone mineral density (BMD) monitoring for HIV-1–infected patients who have a history of pathologic bone fracture or are at risk for osteopenia. Although the effect of supplementation with calcium and vitamin D was not studied, such supplementation may be beneficial for all patients.

Fat redistribution: Redistribution/accumulation of body fat, including central obesity, dorsocervical fat enlargement (buffalo hump), peripheral wasting, facial wasting, breast enlargement, and "cushingoid appearance," have been observed in patients receiving antiretroviral therapy.

Immune reconstitution syndrome: Immune reconstitution syndrome has been reported in patients treated with combination antiretroviral therapy, including emtricitabine/tenofovir.

Early virologic failure: Clinical studies in HIV-infected patients have demonstrated that certain regimens that only contain 3 nucleoside reverse transcriptase inhibitors (NRTIs) are generally less effective than triple drug regimens containing 2 NRTIs in combination with either a non-NRTI or an HIV-1 protease inhibitor.

Lactic acidosis/severe hepatomegaly with steatosis: Lactic acidosis and severe hepatomegaly with steatosis, including fatal cases, have been reported with the use of nucleoside analogs alone or in combination with other antiretrovirals. A majority of these cases have been in women. Obesity and prolonged nucleoside exposure may be risk factors.

Renal function impairment: Dosing interval adjustment is recommended in all patients with CrCl 30 to 49 mL/min; do not administer the combination to patients with CrCl less than 30 mL/min or patients requiring hemodialysis.

Renal impairment, including cases of short-term renal failure and Fanconi syndrome (renal tubular injury with severe hypophosphatemia), has been reported in association with the use of tenofovir disoproxil fumarate.

Pregnancy: Category B.

Lactation: The Centers for Disease Control and Prevention recommend that HIV-infected mothers not breastfeed their infants to avoid risking postnatal transmission of HIV.

Children: Emtricitabine/tenofovir is not recommended for patients younger than 18 years of age because it is a fixed-dose combination tablet containing tenofovir, for which safety and efficacy have not been established in this age group.

Elderly: In general, use caution when selecting dosage for elderly patients, keeping in mind the greater frequency of decreased hepatic, renal, or cardiac function, and of concomitant disease or other drug therapy.

Monitoring: Monitor for signs of lactic acidosis. For at least several months, closely monitor hepatic function with clinical and laboratory follow-up in patients who discontinue emtricitabine/tenofovir and are coinfected with HIV and HBV.

Calculate CrCl in all patients prior to initiating therapy and as clinically appropriate during therapy with emtricitabine/tenofovir. Routinely monitor calculated CrCl and serum phosphorus in patients at risk for renal impairment. Consider BMD monitoring for HIV-1–infected patients who have a history of pathologic bone fracture or are at risk for osteopenia.

Carefully monitor patients on a therapy utilizing a triple nucleoside-only regimen, and consider them for treatment modification.

Drug Interactions

Fixed-dose combination: Emtricitabine/tenofovir is a fixed-dose combination of emtricitabine and tenofovir. Do not administer emtricitabine/tenofovir with efavirenz/emtricitabine/tenofovir, emtricitabine, or tenofovir.

Drugs that may affect emtricitabine/tenofovir include acyclovir, adefovir dipivoxil, atazanavir, cidofovir, ganciclovir, indinavir, loprinavir/ritonavir, nephrotoxic agents, tacrolymis, valacyclovir, and valgancyclovir.

Drugs that may be affected by emtricitabine/tenofovir include abacavir, acyclovir, adefovir dipivoxil, atazanavir, cidofovir, didanosine, entecavir, ganciclovir, indinavir, lamivudine, nephrotoxic agents, saquinavir/ritonavir, valacyclovir, valgancyclovir, and zidovudine.

Adverse Reactions

Adverse reactions occurring in at least 5% of patients include depression, diarrhea, dizziness, fatigue, headache, insomnia, nausea, nasopharyngitis, rash, sinusitis, and upper respiratory tract infection.

Other adverse reactions (5% or more): Abdominal pain, anxiety, arthralgia, back pain, cough increased, dyspepsia, fever, myalgia, pain, paresthesia, peripheral neuropathy (including peripheral neuritis and neuropathy), pneumonia, and rhinitis.

Lab test abnormalities: Fasting cholesterol (more than 240 mg/dL); creatine kinase (M: more than 990 units/L), (F: more than 845 units/L); serum amylase (more than 175 units/L); AST (M: more than 180 units/L) (F: more than 170 units/L); hematuria (more than 75 RBC/HPF); neutrophils (less than 750/mm^3); fasting triglycerides (more than 750 mg/dL).

Common adverse reactions (10% or more): The most common adverse reactions (incidence of at least 10%, any severity) occurring in study 934, an active-controlled clinical study of efavirenz, emtricitabine, and tenofovir, included abnormal dreams, depression, diarrhea, dizziness, fatigue, headache, insomnia, nausea and rash, Skin discoloration, manifested by hyperpigmentation on the palms and/or soles, was generally mild and asymptomatic. The mechanism and clinical significance are unknown.

ABACAVIR/LAMIVUDINE

Tablets: 600 mg abacavir (as sulfate)/300 mg lamivudine (*Rx*) *Epzicom* (GlaxoSmithKline)

Warning:

This product contains 2 nucleoside analogs (abacavir sulfate and lamivudine) and is intended only for patients whose regimen would otherwise include these 2 components.

Hypersensitivity reactions: Serious and sometimes fatal hypersensitivity reactions have been associated with abacavir, a component of *Epzicom*. Hypersensitivity to abacavir is a multiorgan clinical syndrome usually characterized by a sign or symptom in 2 or more of the following groups: fever, rash, GI (eg, nausea, vomiting, diarrhea, abdominal pain), constitutional (eg, generalized malaise, fatigue, achiness), and respiratory (eg, dyspnea, cough, pharyngitis). Discontinue abacavir/lamivudine as soon as a hypersensitivity reaction is suspected. Permanently discontinue abacavir/lamivudine if hypersensitivity cannot be ruled out, even when other diagnoses are possible.

continued on next page

Warning: (cont.)

Patients who carry the HLA-B*5701 allele are at high risk for experiencing a hypersensitivity reaction to abacavir. Prior to initiating therapy with abacavir, screening for the HLA-B*5701 allele is recommended; this approach has been found to decrease the risk of hypersensitivity reaction. Screening is also recommended prior to reinitiation of abacavir in patients of unknown HLA-B*5701 status who have previously tolerated abacavir. HLA-B*5701–negative patients may develop a suspected hypersensitivity reaction to abacavir; however, this occurs significantly less frequently than in HLA-B*5701–positive patients.

Following a hypersensitivity reaction to abacavir, never restart abacavir/lamivudine or any other abacavir-containing product because more severe symptoms can occur within hours and may include life-threatening hypotension and death.

Reintroduction of abacavir/lamivudine or any other abacavir-containing product, even in patients who have no identified history or unrecognized symptoms of hypersensitivity to abacavir therapy, can result in serious or fatal hypersensitivity reactions. Such reactions can occur within hours.

Lactic acidosis and severe hepatomegaly: Lactic acidosis and severe hepatomegaly with steatosis, including fatal cases, has been reported with the use of nucleoside analogs alone or in combination, including abacavir, lamivudine, and other antiretrovirals.

Exacerbations of hepatitis B: Severe acute exacerbations of hepatitis B have been reported in patients who are co-infected with hepatitis B virus (HBV) and human immunodeficiency virus (HIV) and have discontinued lamivudine, which is one component of abacavir/lamivudine. Closely monitor hepatic function with clinical and laboratory follow-up for at least several months in patients who discontinued abacavir/lamivudine and are co-infected with HIV and HBV. If appropriate, initiation of anti-hepatitis B therapy may be warranted.

Indications

HIV infection: For use in combination with other antiretroviral agents for the treatment of HIV-1 infection.

Administration and Dosage

A Medication Guide and Warning Card that provide information about recognition of hypersensitivity reactions should be dispensed with each new prescription and refill. Because it is a fixed-dose tablet, abacavir/lamivudine should not be prescribed to patients requiring dosage adjustment, such as those with a CrCl of less than 50 mL/min, those with hepatic impairment, or those experiencing dose-limiting adverse reactions. Use of lamivudine oral solution and abacavir oral solution may be considered.

Adults: 1 tablet daily, in combination with other antiretroviral agents. May be taken without regard to food.

Dose adjustment: Do not prescribe abacavir/lamivudine to patients requiring dosage adjustment such as those with CrCl less than 50 mL/min, those with hepatic impairment, or those experiencing dose-limiting adverse events.

Elderly: Dose selection for an elderly patient should be made with caution, reflecting the greater frequency of decreased hepatic, renal, or cardiac function, and of concomitant disease or other drug therapy.

Actions

Pharmacology: The combination tablets contain 2 synthetic nucleoside analogs, abacavir sulfate and lamivudine, with inhibitory activity against HIV.

Pharmacokinetics: Following oral administration, abacavir and lamivudine are absorbed rapidly and distributed extensively. Binding of abacavir to human plasma proteins is about 50%; binding of lamivudine to plasma proteins is low.

The pharmacokinetic properties of abacavir and lamivudine in fasting patients are summarized below.

Pharmacokinetic Parameters for Abacavir and Lamivudine in Adults		
Parameter	Abacavir	Lamivudine
Oral bioavailability (%)	≈ 86	≈ 86
Apparent volume of distribution (L/kg)	≈ 0.86	≈ 1.3
Systemic clearance (L/h/kg)	≈ 0.8	≈ 0.33
Renal clearance (L/h/kg)	≈ 0.007	≈ 0.22
Elimination half-life (h)	≈ 1.45	5 to 7[a]

[a] Approximate range.

Special populations –

Renal function impairment: Lamivudine requires dose adjustment in the presence of renal insufficiency; abacavir/lamivudine is not recommended for use in patients with CrCl less than 50 mL/min.

Liver function impairment: Abacavir is contraindicated in patients with moderate to severe hepatic impairment, and dose reduction is required in patients with mild hepatic impairment. Because abacavir/lamivudine is a fixed-dose combination and cannot be dose adjusted, abacavir/lamivudine is contraindicated for patients with hepatic impairment.

Contraindications

Hepatic impairment or a previously demonstrated hypersensitivity to abacavir or to any other component of the product.

Warnings/Precautions

Hypersensitivity reactions: To facilitate reporting of hypersensitivity reactions and collection of information on each case, an abacavir hypersensitivity registry has been established. Health care providers should register patients by calling 1-800-270-0425.

Lactic acidosis/severe hepatomegaly with steatosis: Lactic acidosis and severe hepatomegaly with steatosis, including fatal cases, have been reported with the use of nucleoside analogs alone or in combination, including abacavir and lamivudine and other antiretrovirals.

Posttreatment exacerbations of hepatitis: In clinical trials in non-HIV-infected patients treated with lamivudine for chronic HBV, clinical and laboratory evidence of exacerbations of hepatitis have occurred after discontinuation of lamivudine. These exacerbations have been detected primarily by serum ALT elevations in addition to re-emergence of HBV DNA. Although most events appear to have been self-limited, fatalities have been reported in some cases.

Immune reconstitution syndrome: Immune reconstitution syndrome has been reported in patients treated with combination antiretroviral therapy, including abacavir/lamivudine.

Fat redistribution: Redistribution/accumulation of body fat, including central obesity, dorsocervical fat enlargement (buffalo hump), peripheral wasting, facial wasting, breast enlargement, and cushingoid appearance, have been observed in patients receiving antiretroviral therapy.

Myocardial infarction: As a precaution, consider the underlying risk of coronary heart disease when prescribing antiretroviral therapies, including abacavir, and take action to minimize all modifiable risk factors (eg, hypertension, hyperlipidemia, diabetes mellitus, smoking).

Fixed-dose combination: This combination contains fixed doses of 2 nucleoside analogs, abacavir and lamivudine, and should not be administered concomitantly with other abacavir-containing and/or lamivudine-containing products.

Hypersensitivity reactions: Serious and sometimes fatal hypersensitivity reactions have been associated with abacavir/lamivudine and other abacavir-containing products.

Renal function impairment: Because abacavir/lamivudine is a fixed-dose tablet and the dosage of the individual components cannot be altered, patients with CrCl less than 50 mL/min should not receive abacavir/lamivudine.

Hepatic function impairment: Abacavir/lamivudine is contraindicated in patients with hepatic impairment because it is a fixed-dose tablet, and the dosage of the individual components cannot be altered.

Pregnancy: Category C.

Lactation: Because of the potential for HIV transmission and the potential for serious adverse reactions in nursing infants, instruct mothers not to breastfeed if they are receiving abacavir/lamivudine. Lamivudine is excreted in human breast milk.

ETRAVIRINE

Tablets; oral: 100 mg (*Rx*)	*Intelence* (Tibotec Therapeutics)

Indications

HIV infection: In combination with other antiretroviral agents for the treatment of type 1 HIV (HIV-1) infection in antiretroviral treatment-experienced adult patients who have evidence of viral replication and HIV-1 strains resistant to nonnucleoside reverse transcriptase inhibitors (NNRTIs) and other antiretroviral agents.

Administration and Dosage

Dose: 200 mg (two 100 mg tablets) taken twice daily following a meal.

Patients who are unable to swallow etravirine tablets whole may disperse the tablets in a glass of water. Once dispersed, patients should stir the dispersion well and drink it immediately. The glass should be rinsed with water several times and each rinse completely swallowed to ensure that the entire dose is consumed.

Actions

Pharmacology: Etravirine is an NNRTI of HIV-1. Etravirine binds directly to reverse transcriptase (RT) and blocks the RNA- and DNA-dependent DNA polymerase activities by causing a disruption of the enzyme's catalytic site. Etravirine does not inhibit the human DNA polymerases alpha, beta, and gamma.

Pharmacokinetics:

Absorption – Etravirine was absorbed with a time to maximum plasma concentration of approximately 2.5 to 4 hours.

Effect of food: The systemic exposure (AUC) to etravirine was decreased by approximately 50% when etravirine was administered under fasting conditions, compared with etravirine administration following a meal; therefore, always take etravirine following a meal.

Distribution – Etravirine is approximately 99.9% bound to plasma proteins.

Metabolism – In vitro experiments with human liver microsomes indicate that etravirine primarily undergoes metabolism by CYP3A4, CYP2C9, and CYP2C19 enzymes.

Excretion – The mean (± SD) terminal elimination half-life of etravirine was approximately 41 (± 20) hours.

Contraindications

None well documented.

Warnings/Precautions

Skin reactions: Severe and potentially life-threatening skin reactions have occurred in patients taking etravirine, including Stevens-Johnson syndrome, hypersensitivity reaction, and erythema multiforme.

Fat redistribution: Redistribution/accumulation of body fat, including central obesity, dorsocervical fat enlargement (buffalo hump), peripheral wasting, facial wasting, breast enlargement, and cushingoid appearance have been observed.

Immune reconstitution syndrome: Immune reconstitution syndrome has been reported in patients treated with combination antiretroviral therapy, including etravirine.

Renal/Hepatic function impairment: No dose adjustments are required in patients with renal function impairment or in patients with mild (Child-Pugh class A) or moderate (Child-Pugh class B) hepatic function impairment. The pharmacokinetics of etravirine have not been evaluated in patients with severe hepatic function impairment (Child-Pugh class C).

Pregnancy: *Category B.*

Lactation: The Centers for Disease Control and Prevention recommends that HIV-infected mothers do not breast-feed their infants to avoid risking postnatal transmission of HIV. It is not known whether etravirine is secreted in human milk.

Children: Safety and effectiveness in children have not been established.

Elderly: Dose selection for an elderly patient should be cautious, reflecting the greater frequency of decreased hepatic, renal, or cardiac function, and of concomitant disease or other drug therapy.

Drug Interactions

Etravirine is a substrate of CYP3A4, CYP2C9, and CYP2C19; therefore, coadministration of etravirine with drugs that induce or inhibit CYP3A4, CYP2C9, and CYP2C19 may alter the therapeutic effect or adverse reaction profile of etravirine. Etravirine is an inducer of CYP3A4 and inhibitor of CYP2C9 and CYP2C19; therefore, coadministration of drugs that are substrates of CYP3A4, CYP2C9, and CYP2C19 with etravirine may alter the therapeutic effect or adverse reaction profile of the coadministered drug(s).

Drugs that may affect etravirine include the following: anticonvulsants, antifungals, atazanavir/ritonavir, charcoal, darunavir/ritonavir, dexamethasone (systemic), lopinavir/ritonavir, NNRTIs, rifabutin, rifampin, rifapentine, ritonavir, saquinavir/ritonavir, St. John's wort, and tipranavir/ritonavir.

Drugs that may be affected by etravirine include the following: antifungals, atazanavir, antiarrhythmic agents, clarithromycin, diazepam, fosamprenavir/ritonavir, HMG-CoA reductase inhibitors, immunosuppressants, methadone, PDE-5 inhibitors, protease inhibitors, and warfarin.

Adverse Reactions

The following adverse reactions have occurred in at least 3% of patients treated with etravirine: abdominal pain, diarrhea, fatigue, nausea, rash (any type).

Lab test abnormalities: There have been reported increases in the following laboratory tests: pancreatic amylase, lipase, creatinine, total cholesterol, low-density lipoprotein, triglycerides, glucose, ALT, AST. There have been reported decreases in neutrophils.

NEVIRAPINE

Tablets: 200 mg (*Rx*) — *Viramune* (Boehringer Ingelheim)
Oral suspension: 50 mg/5 mL (as hemihydrate) (*Rx*)

Warning:

Hepatotoxicity: Severe, life-threatening, and, in some cases, fatal hepatotoxicity, particularly in the first 18 weeks, has been reported in patients treated with nevirapine. In some cases, patients presented with nonspecific prodromal signs or symptoms of hepatitis and progressed to hepatic failure. These events are often associated with rash. Women and patients with higher CD4+ cell counts at initiation of therapy are at increased risk. Women with CD4+ cell counts higher than 250 cells/mm^3, including pregnant women receiving nevirapine in combination with other antiretrovirals for treatment of HIV-1 infection, are at the greatest risk. However, hepatotoxicity associated with nevirapine use can occur in both genders, at all CD4+ cell counts, and at any time during treatment. Hepatic failure has also been reported in patients without HIV taking nevirapine for postexposure prophylaxis. Use of nevirapine for occupational and nonoccupational postexposure prophylaxis is contraindicated. Patients with signs or symptoms of hepatitis, or with increased transaminases combined with rash or other systemic symptoms, must discontinue nevirapine and seek medical evaluation immediately.

Skin reactions: Severe, life-threatening skin reactions, including fatal cases, have occurred in patients treated with nevirapine. These have included cases of Stevens-Johnson syndrome, toxic epidermal necrolysis, and hypersensitivity reactions characterized by rash, constitutional findings, and organ dysfunction. Patients developing signs or symptoms of severe skin reactions or hypersensitivity reactions must discontinue nevirapine and seek medical evaluation immediately. Check transaminase levels immediately for all patients who develop a rash in the first 18 weeks of treatment. The 14-day lead-in period with nevirapine daily dosing has been observed to decrease the incidence of rash and must be followed.

Monitoring: It is essential that patients be monitored intensively during the first 18 weeks of therapy with nevirapine to detect potentially life-threatening hepatotoxicity or skin reactions. Extra vigilance is warranted during the first 6 weeks of therapy, which is the period of greatest risk of these reactions. Do not restart nevirapine following severe hepatic, skin, or hypersensitivity reactions. In some cases, hepatic injury has progressed despite discontinuation of treatment.

Indications

Human immunodeficiency virus type 1 (HIV-1) infection: In combination with other antiretroviral agents for the treatment of HIV-1 infection.

Administration and Dosage

A patient experiencing mild to moderate rash without constitutional symptoms during the 14-day lead-in period should not have their nevirapine dose increased until the rash has resolved. The total duration of the once-daily lead-in dosing period should not exceed 28 days, at which point an alternative regimen should be sought.

Adults: The maximum dose is 400 mg daily.

Initial therapy – 200 mg tablet daily for 14 days. May administer with or without food.

Maintenance – 200 mg tablet twice daily in combination with other antiretroviral agents.

Children:

HIV infection –

15 days of age and older: 120 to 200 mg/m^2 twice daily. Children younger than 8 years of age may require higher dosages (eg, 200 mg/m^2 twice daily).

The maximum dose is 400 mg daily; 200 mg per dose.

The initial dose is 150 mg/m^2 once daily for 14 days; 120 mg/m^2 once daily for 14 days has also been used.

The maintenance dose is 150 mg/m^2 twice daily; 120 mg/m^2 twice daily has also been used.

Nevirapine Suspension for Dosing in Children Based on a Dose of 150 mg/m^2 of BSA[a]	
BSA range	Volume
0.06 to 0.12 m^2	1.25 mL
0.12 to 0.25 m^2	2.5 mL
0.25 to 0.42 m^2	5 mL
0.42 to 0.58 m^2	7.5 mL
0.58 to 0.75 m^2	10 mL
0.75 to 0.92 m^2	12.5 mL
0.92 to 1.08 m^2	15 mL
1.08 to 1.25 m^2	17.5 mL
> 1.25 m^2	20 mL

[a] BSA = body surface area.

Suspension – Shake nevirapine suspension gently prior to administration. Administer the entire measured dose of suspension by using an oral dosing syringe or dosing cup. If a dosing cup is used, thoroughly rinse with water and administer the rinse to the patient.

Missed doses: Patients who interrupt nevirapine dosing for more than 7 days should restart using 150 mg/m^2 per day for the first 14 days (lead-in) followed by 150 mg/m^2 twice daily.

Elderly: Use caution with dose selection, reflecting the greater frequency of decreased hepatic, renal, or cardiac function, and of concomitant disease or other drug therapy.

Dosage adjustment: Discontinue nevirapine if patients experience severe rash or a rash accompanied by constitutional findings.

If clinical (symptomatic) hepatitis occurs, permanently discontinue nevirapine and do not restart after recovery.

Renal function impairment: An additional nevirapine 200 mg dose following each dialysis treatment is indicated in patients requiring dialysis.

Hepatic function impairment: Contraindicated in patients with moderate or severe (Child-Pugh class B or C, respectively) hepatic impairment.

Missed doses: Patients who interrupt nevirapine dosing for more than 7 days should restart the recommended dosing, using one 200 mg tablet daily (150 mg/m^2) for the first 14 days (lead-in), followed by one 200 mg tablet twice daily (150 mg/m^2 twice daily, for children).

Actions

Pharmacology: Nevirapine is a nonnucleoside reverse transcriptase inhibitor (NNRTI) with activity against HIV-1.

Pharmacokinetics:

Absorption – Nevirapine is readily absorbed (more than 90%) after oral administration. Peak plasma nevirapine concentrations were attained within 4 hours following a single 200 mg dose. Nevirapine tablets and suspension have been shown to be comparably bioavailable and interchangeable at doses 200 mg or less.

Distribution – Nevirapine is highly lipophilic and is essentially nonionized at physiologic pH. Following IV administration to healthy adults, the volume of distribution of nevirapine was 1.21 L/kg. Nevirapine is approximately 60% bound to plasma proteins.

Metabolism/Excretion – Nevirapine is extensively biotransformed via cytochrome P450 (oxidative) metabolism to several hydroxylated metabolites.

Nevirapine has been shown to be an inducer of hepatic cytochrome P450 metabolic enzymes 3A4 and 2B6. The pharmacokinetics of autoinduction are characterized by an approximately 1.5- to 2-fold increase in the apparent oral clearance of nevirapine as treatment continues. Auto-induction also results in a corresponding decrease in the terminal phase half-life of nevirapine in plasma from approximately 45 hours (single dose) to approximately 25 to 30 hours following multiple dosing.

Contraindications

Moderate or severe (Child-Pugh class B or C, respectively) hepatic impairment; for use as part of occupational and nonoccupational postexposure prophylaxis regimens.

Warnings/Precautions

Skin reactions: Severe and life-threatening skin reactions, including fatal cases have been reported, occurring most frequently during the first 6 weeks of therapy. These have included Stevens-Johnson syndrome, toxic epidermal necrolysis, and hypersensitivity reactions characterized by rash, constitutional findings, and organ dysfunction. Discontinue nevirapine in patients developing a severe rash, accompanied by constitutional symptoms such as fever, fatigue, blistering, oral lesions, conjunctivitis, facial edema, and/or hepatitis, eosinophilia, granulocytopenia, lymphadenopathy, renal dysfunction, muscle or joint aches, or general malaise. Do not restart nevirapine following severe skin rash, skin rash combined with increased transaminases or other symptoms, or hypersensitivity reaction.

The majority of rashes associated with nevirapine occur within the first 6 weeks of initiation of therapy. Instruct patients not to increase the 200 mg/day (4 mg/kg/day in children) dosage if any rash occurs during the 2-week lead-in dosing period until the rash resolves.

Resistant virus: Resistant virus emerges rapidly and uniformly when nevirapine is administered as monotherapy. Therefore, always administer nevirapine in combination with other antiretroviral agents.

Fat redistribution: Redistribution/accumulation of body fat, including central obesity, dorsocervical fat enlargement (buffalo hump), peripheral wasting, facial wasting, breast enlargement, and "cushingoid appearance," has been observed in patients receiving antiretroviral therapy.

Immune reconstitution syndrome: Immune reconstitution syndrome has been reported in patients treated with combination antiretroviral therapy, including nevirapine.

Renal function impairment: See Administration and Dosage for more information.

Hepatic function impairment: See Contraindications for more information.

Hepatotoxicity – Severe, life-threatening, and in some cases fatal hepatotoxicity, including fulminant and cholestatic hepatitis, hepatic necrosis, and hepatic failure, have been reported in patients treated with nevirapine. The risk of hepatic events regardless of severity was greatest in the first 6 weeks of therapy; however, hepatic events may occur at any time during treatment. Discontinue nevirapine in patients with signs or symptoms of hepatitis.

Pregnancy: *Category B.*

Lactation: Nevirapine readily crosses the placenta and is found in breast milk. Instruct patients receiving nevirapine to discontinue nursing, consistent with the recommendation by the US Public Health Service Centers for Disease Control and Prevention that HIV-infected mothers not breastfeed their infants to avoid risking postnatal transmission of HIV.

Children: See Administration and Dosage for more information. See Averse Reactions for more information.

Elderly: Make dose selection with caution, reflecting the greater frequency of decreased hepatic, renal, or cardiac function, and of concomitant disease or other drug therapy.

Monitoring: The first 18 weeks of therapy with nevirapine are a critical period during which intensive patient monitoring is required to detect potentially life-threatening hepatic events and skin reactions. The optimal frequency of monitoring during this time period has not been established. After the initial 18-week period, continue frequent clinical and laboratory monitoring throughout treatment. Immediately perform liver function tests if a patient experiences signs or symptoms suggestive of hepatitis, hypersensitivity reaction, and/or rash.

Drug Interactions

Nevirapine induces hepatic CYP3A4 and 2B6. Coadministration of nevirapine and drugs primarily metabolized by CYP3A4 or CYP2B6 may result in decreased plasma concentrations of these drugs.

Drugs that may affect nevirapine include rifamycins (eg, rifampin, rifabutin), fluconazole, St. John's wort.

Drugs that may be affected by nevirapine include rifamycins, antiarrhythmics (eg, amiodarone, disopyramide, lidocaine), anticonvulsants (eg, carbamazepine, clonazepam, ethosuximide), cabazitaxel, calcium channel blockers (eg, diltiazem, nifedipine, verapamil), cisapride, clarithromycin, contraceptives hormonal, cyclophosphamide, efavirenz, ergot alkaloids (eg, ergotamine), exemestane, immunosuppressants (eg, cyclosporine, sirolimus, tacrolimus), itraconazole, ketoconazole, maraviroc, opioid analgesics (eg, fentanyl, methadone), protease inhibitors, tyrosine kinase receptor inhibitors (eg, lapatinib, nilotinib, pazopanib), warfarin, zidovudine.

Adverse Reactions

The most frequent adverse events related to nevirapine therapy are abnormal liver function tests, fatigue, headache, nausea, and rash.

Lab test abnormalities: Decreased hemoglobin and neutrophils. Increased ALT and AST.

Children – The most frequently reported adverse events related to nevirapine in children were similar to those observed in adults, with the exception of granulocytopenia, which was more commonly observed in children.

DELAVIRDINE MESYLATE

Tablets: 100 and 200 mg (*Rx*)	*Rescriptor* (Agouron)

Warning:

Delavirdine tablets are indicated for the treatment of HIV-1 infection in combination with appropriate antiretroviral agents when therapy is warranted. This indication is based on surrogate marker changes in clinical studies. Clinical benefit was not demonstrated for delavirdine based on survival or incidence of AIDS-defining clinical events in a completed trial comparing delavirdine plus didanosine with didanosine monotherapy.

Resistant virus emerges rapidly when delavirdine is administered as monotherapy. Therefore, always administer delavirdine in combination with appropriate antiretroviral therapy.

Indications

Human immunodeficiency virus-1 (HIV-1): For the treatment of HIV-1 infection in combination with appropriate antiretroviral agents when therapy is warranted.

Administration and Dosage

The recommended dosage for delavirdine is 400 mg (four 100 mg or two 200 mg tablets) 3 times daily. Use delavirdine in combination with appropriate other antiretroviral therapy. Consult the complete prescribing information for other antiretroviral agents for information on dosage and administration.

The 100 mg delavirdine tablets may be dispersed in water prior to consumption. To prepare a dispersion, add four 100 mg tablets to at least 3 ounces of water, allow to stand for a few minutes, and then stir until a uniform dispersion occurs. Consume the dispersion promptly. Rinse the glass and swallow the rinse to ensure the entire dose is consumed. Take the 200 mg tablets intact because they are not readily dispersed in water.

Administer delavirdine with or without food. Patients with achlorhydria should take delavirdine with an acidic beverage (eg, orange or cranberry juice). However, the effect of an acidic beverage on the absorption of delavirdine in patients with achlorhydria has not been investigated.

Actions

Pharmacology: Delavirdine is a nonnucleoside reverse transcriptase inhibitor (NNRTI) of HIV-1. Delavirdine binds directly to reverse transcriptase (RT) and blocks RNA-dependent and DNA-dependent DNA polymerase activities.

Cross-resistance – Rapid emergence of HIV strains that are cross-resistant to certain NNRTIs has been observed in vitro. Delavirdine may confer cross-resistance to other non-nucleoside reverse transcriptase inhibitors when used alone or in combination. The potential for cross-resistance between delavirdine and protease inhibitors and between NNRTIs and nucleoside analog RT inhibitors is low.

Pharmacokinetics:

Absorption – Delavirdine is rapidly absorbed following oral administration with peak plasma concentrations occurring at approximately 1 hour. The single-dose bioavailability of delavirdine tablets was increased by approximately 20% when a slurry of drug was prepared by allowing the tablets to disintegrate in water before administration.

Distribution – Delavirdine is extensively bound (approximately 98%) to plasma proteins, primarily albumin. CSF concentrations of delavirdine averaged 0.4% of the corresponding plasma delavirdine concentrations.

Metabolism/Excretion – Delavirdine is extensively converted to several inactive metabolites. Delavirdine is primarily metabolized by cytochrome P450 3A (CYP3A), but in vitro data suggest that delavirdine may also be metabolized by CYP2D6. The apparent plasma half-life of delavirdine increases with dose; mean half-life following 400 mg 3 times daily is 5.8 hours (range, 2 to 11 hours).

Delavirdine reduces CYP3A activity and inhibits its own metabolism. In vitro studies have also shown that delavirdine reduces CYP2C9 and CYP2C19 activity. Inhibition of CYP3A by delavirdine is reversible within 1 week after discontinuation of the drug.

Gender – Following administration of delavirdine (400 mg every 8 hours), median delavirdine AUC was 31% higher in female patients than in male patients.

Contraindications

Hypersensitivity to any of the components of the formulation.

Warnings/Precautions

Cytochrome P450 inhibition: Coadministration of delavirdine tablets with certain nonsedating antihistamines, sedative hypnotics, antiarrhythmics, calcium channel blockers, ergot alkaloid preparations, amphetamines, and cisapride may result in potentially serious or life-threatening adverse events caused by possible effects of delavirdine on the hepatic metabolism of certain drugs metabolized by CYP3A and CYP2C9.

Resistance/Cross-resistance: NNRTIs, when used alone or in combination, may confer cross-resistance to other NNRTIs.

Skin rash: Skin rash attributable to delavirdine has occurred in 18% of patients in combination regimens in clinical trials who received delavirdine 400 mg 3 times daily.

Hepatic function impairment: Delavirdine is metabolized primarily by the liver. Therefore, exercise caution when administering to patients with impaired hepatic function.

Pregnancy: Category C.

Lactation: The US Public Health Services Centers for Disease Control and Prevention advises HIV-infected women not to breastfeed to avoid postnatal transmission of HIV to a child who may not yet be infected.

Children: Safety and efficacy of delavirdine in combination with other antiretroviral agents has not been established in HIV-1-infected individuals younger than 16 years of age.

Monitoring: Monitor hepatocellular enzymes (ALT/AST) frequently if delavirdine is prescribed with saquinavir.

Drug Interactions

Drugs that may affect delavirdine include the following: Anticonvulsants, antacids, clarithromycin, didanosine, fluoxetine, histamine H_2 antagonists, ketoconazole, rifabutin, rifampin, and saquinavir.

Drugs that may be affected by delavirdine include the following: Clarithromycin, indinavir, amprenavir, benzodiazepines, cisapride, dihydropyridine calcium channel blockers, ergot derivatives, quinidine, sildenafil, warfarin, saquinavir, and didanosine.

Adverse Reactions

Adverse reactions occurring in at least 3% of patients include the following: Headache; fatigue; nausea; diarrhea; increased ALT and AST; rash; maculopapular rash; neutropenia; increased amylase; pruritus.

EFAVIRENZ

Tablets: 600 mg (*Rx*) **Capsules:** 50 and 200 mg (*Rx*)	*Sustiva* (Bristol-Myers Squibb Oncology/ Immunology)

Indications

Human immunodeficiency virus (HIV) infection: In combination with other antiretroviral agents for the treatment of HIV-1 infection.

Administration and Dosage

Adults: The recommended dosage is 600 mg once daily in combination with a protease inhibitor or nucleoside analog reverse transcriptase inhibitors (NRTIs). It is recommended that efavirenz be taken on an empty stomach, preferably at bedtime. The increased efavirenz concentration following administration of efavirenz with food may lead to an increase in adverse events.

To improve the tolerability of nervous system side effects, bedtime dosing is recommended during the first 2 to 4 weeks of therapy and in patients who continue to experience these symptoms.

Concomitant antiretroviral therapy: Efavirenz must be given in combination with other antiretroviral medications.

Children: It is recommended that efavirenz be taken on an empty stomach, preferably at bedtime. The following table describes the recommended dose for pediatric patients 3 years of age and older and weighing between 10 and 40 kg (22 and 88 lbs). The recommended dosage for pediatric patients weighing more than 40 kg (88 lbs) is 600 mg once daily.

Pediatric Dose of Efavirenz to be Administered Once Daily

Body weight		Efavirenz dose (mg)
kg	lbs	
10 to < 15	22 to < 33	200
15 to < 20	33 to < 44	250
20 to < 25	44 to < 55	300
25 to < 32.5	55 to < 71.5	350
32.5 to < 40	71.5 to < 88	400
≥ 40	≥ 88	600

Dosage adjustment: If efavirenz is coadministered with voriconazole, the voriconazole maintenance dosage should be increased to 400 mg every 12 hours, and the efavirenz dosage should be decreased to 300 mg once daily using the capsule formulation (three 100 mg capsules, or one 200 mg and one 100 mg capsule). Efavirenz tablets should not be broken.

Actions

Pharmacology: Efavirenz is a nonnucleoside reverse transcriptase inhibitor (NNRTI) of HIV-1. Its activity is mediated predominantly by noncompetitive inhibition of HIV-1 reverse transcriptase (RT). It does not inhibit HIV-2 RT and human cellular DNA polymerases alpha, beta, gamma, and delta.

Pharmacokinetics: Time-to-peak plasma concentrations were approximately 3 to 5 hours and steady-state plasma concentrations were reached in 6 to 10 days. Efavirenz is highly protein-bound (approximately 99.5% to 99.75%), predominantly to albumin. It is principally metabolized by the cytochrome P450 system (CYP3A4 and CYP2B6) to hydroxylated metabolites with subsequent glucuronidation of these hydroxylated metabolites. Efavirenz induces P450 enzymes, resulting in the induction of its own metabolism. It has a terminal half-life of 52 to 76 hours after single doses and 40 to 55 hours after multiple doses.

Contraindications

Hypersensitivity to efavirenz or any of its components; coadministration with astemizole, bepridil, cisapride, midazolam, pimozide, triazolam, or ergot derivatives; coadministration with standard doses of voriconazole.

Warnings/Precautions

Resistance: Resistant virus emerges rapidly when NNRTIs are administered as monotherapy. Therefore, efavirenz must not be used as a single agent to treat HIV or added on as a sole agent to a failing regimen. The choice of new antiretroviral agents to be used in combination with efavirenz should take into consideration the potential for viral cross-resistance.

Psychiatric symptoms: Serious psychiatric adverse experiences have been reported in patients treated with efavirenz. Patients with a history of psychiatric disorders appear to be at greater risk for serious psychiatric adverse experiences.

CNS symptoms: Inform patients that common symptoms were likely to improve with continued therapy and were not predictive of subsequent onset of the less frequent psychiatric symptoms. Dosing at bedtime improves the tolerability of these CNS symptoms. Alert patients to the potential for additive CNS effects when efavirenz is used concomitantly with alcohol or psychoactive drugs.

Skin rash: In controlled clinical trials, 26% of patients treated with 600 mg efavirenz experienced new onset skin rash compared with 17% of patients treated in control groups. Rash associated with blistering, moist desquamation, or ulceration occurred in 0.9% of patients treated with efavirenz. The incidence of Grade 4 rash in patients treated with efavirenz in all studies and expanded access was 0.1%. The median time to onset of rash in adults was 11 days and the median duration, 16 days. Appropriate antihistamines or corticosteroids may improve the tolerability and hasten the resolution of rash.

Rash was reported in 46% of children treated with efavirenz capsules. The median time to onset of rash in children was 8 days. Consider prophylaxis with appropriate antihistamines prior to initiating therapy in children.

Convulsions: Convulsions have been observed in patients receiving efavirenz, generally in the presence of known medical history of seizures. Caution must be taken in any patient with a history of seizures. Patients who are receiving concomitant anticonvulsant medications primarily metabolized by the liver, such as phenytoin and phenobarbital, may require periodic monitoring of plasma levels.

Fat redistribution: Redistribution/accumulation of body fat including central obesity, dorsocervical fat enlargement (buffalo hump), peripheral wasting, facial wasting, breast enlargement, and "cushingoid appearance" have been observed in patients receiving antiretroviral therapy.

Immune reconstitution syndrome: Immune reconstitution syndrome has been reported in patients treated with combination antiretroviral therapy, including efavirenz.

Hepatic function impairment: In patients with persistent elevations of serum transaminases to more than 5 times the upper limit of normal (ULN) range, the benefit of continued therapy with efavirenz needs to be weighed against the unknown risks of significant liver toxicity.

Hazardous tasks: Advise patients who experience CNS symptoms such as dizziness, impaired concentration, or drowsiness to avoid potentially hazardous tasks such as driving or operating machinery.

Pregnancy: *Category D.*

Lactation: Instruct mothers not to breast-feed during treatment.

Children: Efavirenz has not been studied in pediatric patients under 3 years of age or who weigh less than 13 kg (29 lbs).

Elderly: Use caution in dose selection for an elderly patient, reflecting the greater frequency of decreased hepatic, renal, or cardiac function, and of concomitant disease or other therapy.

Monitoring: Consider monitoring cholesterol and triglycerides in patients treated with efavirenz.

Hepatic enzymes – Monitor liver enzymes in patients with known or suspected history of hepatitis B or C infection and in patients treated with other medications associated with liver toxicity.

Drug Interactions

P450 system: Efavirenz induces CYP3A4 in vitro. Compounds that are substrates of CYP3A4 may have decreased plasma concentrations when coadministered with efavirenz. Drugs that induce CYP3A4 activity would be expected to increase the clearance of efavirenz, resulting in lowered plasma concentrations.

In vitro, efavirenz inhibits 2C9, 2C19, and 3A4 isozymes. Coadministration with drugs metabolized by these isozymes may result in altered plasma concentrations of the coadministered drug. Dose adjustments may be necessary for these drugs (see Administration and Dosage section for voriconazole dosing specifics).

Drugs that may affect efavirenz include carbamazepine, phenobarbital, phenytoin, rifamycins, ritonavir, and St. John's wort.

Drugs that may be affected by efavirenz include amprenavir, benzodiazepines, carbamazepine, clarithromycin, ethinyl estradiol, indinavir, itraconazole, ketoconazole, methadone, nelfinavir, phenobarbital, phenytoin, ritonavir, saquinavir, voriconazole, and warfarin.

Drug/Lab test interactions:

Cannabinoid test interaction – False-positive urine cannabinoid test results have been reported in uninfected volunteers who received efavirenz. False-positive test results have been observed only with the CEDIA DAU Multi-Level THC assay used for screening and have not been observed with tests used for confirmation of positive results. Efavirenz does not bind to cannabinoid receptors.

Drug/Food interactions: Food increases efavirenz concentrations and may increase the frequency of adverse events (see Administration and Dosage).

Adverse Reactions

The most significant adverse events with efavirenz are nervous system symptoms and rash. Of patients receiving efavirenz, 52% reported CNS and psychiatric symptoms.

Adverse events occurring in at least 3% of patients include dizziness, fatigue, headache, concentration impaired, insomnia, abnormal dreams, somnolence, depression, anxiety, pruritus, nervousness, rash, nausea, vomiting, diarrhea, dyspepsia, abdominal pain.

Skin rash – Rashes are usually mild to moderate maculopapular skin eruptions that occur within the first 2 weeks of initiating therapy. Rash is more common in children and more often of higher grade (ie, more severe). In most patients, rash resolves with continuing therapy within 1 month. Efavirenz can be reinitiated in patients interrupting therapy because of rash.

Lab test abnormalities: Increased hepatic enzymes, lipids, and serum amylase.

Miscellaneous:

Children – Clinical adverse experiences observed in 10% or more of pediatric patients 3 to 16 years of age who received efavirenz capsules were the following: Rash, diarrhea/loose stools, fever, cough, dizziness/lightheadedness/fainting; ache/pain/discomfort, nausea/vomiting, headache.

EFAVIRENZ/EMTRICITABINE/TENOFOVIR DISOPROXIL FUMARATE

Tablets: 600 mg efavirenz, 200 mg emtricitabine, 300 mg tenofovir disoproxil fumarate (equivalent to 245 mg tenofovir disoproxil) (*Rx*)	*Atripla* (Bristol-Myers Squibb/Gilead Sciences)

Warning:

Lactic acidosis and severe hepatomegaly with steatosis, including fatal cases, have been reported with the use of nucleoside analogs alone or in combination with other antiretrovirals.

Efavirenz/emtricitabine/tenofovir is not indicated for the treatment of chronic hepatitis B virus (HBV) infection, and the safety and efficacy of efavirenz/emtricitabine/tenofovir have not been established in patients coinfected with HBV and HIV. Severe acute exacerbations of hepatitis B have been reported in patients who have discontinued emtricitabine or tenofovir. Closely monitor hepatic function with both clinical and laboratory follow-up for at least several months in patients who discontinue efavirenz/emtricitabine/tenofovir and who are coinfected with HIV and HBV. If appropriate, initiation of anti-hepatitis B therapy may be warranted.

Indications

HIV infection: For use alone as a complete regimen or in combination with other antiretroviral agents for the treatment of HIV infection in adults.

Administration and Dosage

Adults: One tablet once daily taken orally on an empty stomach. Dosing at bedtime may improve the tolerability of nervous system symptoms.

Children: Not recommended for use in patients younger than 18 years of age.

Renal function impairment: Because efavirenz/emtricitabine/tenofovir is a fixed-dose combination, it should not be prescribed for patients requiring dosage adjustment, such as those with moderate or severe renal function impairment (creatinine clearance [CrCl] less than 50 mL/min).

Actions

Pharmacology:

Efavirenz – Efavirenz is a nonnucleoside reverse transcriptase inhibitor of HIV-1. Efavirenz activity is mediated predominantly by noncompetitive inhibition of HIV-1 reverse transcriptase (RT).

Emtricitabine – Emtricitabine is a synthetic nucleoside analog of cytidine. Emtricitabine 5'-triphosphate inhibits the activity of the HIV-1 RT by competing with the natural substrate deoxycytidine 5'-triphosphate and by being incorporated into nascent viral DNA, which results in chain termination.

Tenofovir – Tenofovir is an acyclic nucleoside phosphonate diester analog of adenosine monophosphate. Tenofovir inhibits the activity of HIV-1 RT by competing with the natural substrate deoxyadenosine 5'-triphosphate and, after incorporation into DNA, by DNA chain termination.

Pharmacokinetics:

Absorption/Distribution –

Efavirenz: Time to peak plasma concentrations was approximately 3 to 5 hours and steady-state plasma concentrations were reached in 6 to 10 days. Efavirenz is highly bound (approximately 99.5% to 99.75%) to human plasma proteins, predominantly albumin.

Emtricitabine: Following oral administration, emtricitabine is rapidly absorbed, with peak plasma concentrations occurring at 1 to 2 hours postdose. The mean absolute bioavailability of emtricitabine was 93%. In vitro binding of emtricitabine to human plasma proteins is less than 4%.

Tenofovir: Following oral administration of a single dose of tenofovir, C_{max} was achieved in 1 ± 0.4 hours The oral bioavailability of tenofovir in fasted patients is approximately 25%. In vitro binding of tenofovir to human plasma proteins is less than 0.7%.

Food effects: Efavirenz/emtricitabine/tenofovir has not been evaluated in the presence of food. Administration of efavirenz with a high-fat meal increased the mean AUC and C_{max}. Dosing of tenofovir and emtricitabine in combination with either a high-fat meal or a light meal increased the mean AUC and C_{max} of tenofovir without affecting emtricitabine exposures.

Metabolism/Excretion –

Efavirenz: In vitro studies suggest CYP3A4 and CYP2B6 are the major isozymes responsible for efavirenz metabolism. Efavirenz has been shown to induce P-450 enzymes, resulting in induction of its own metabolism. Efavirenz has a terminal half-life of 52 to 76 hours after single doses and 40 to 55 hours after multiple doses.

Emtricitabine: Emtricitabine is eliminated by a combination of glomerular filtration and active tubular secretion. Following a single oral dose, the plasma emtricitabine half-life is approximately 10 hours.

Tenofovir: Tenofovir is eliminated by a combination of glomerular filtration and active tubular secretion. Following a single oral dose, the terminal elimination half-life of tenofovir is approximately 17 hours.

Contraindications

Previously demonstrated hypersensitivity to any of the components of the product; coadministration with astemizole, bepridil, cisapride, ergot derivatives, midazolam, pimozide, triazolam, or voriconazole.

Warnings/Precautions

Lactic acidosis/severe hepatomegaly with steatosis: See the Warning box for more information.

Bone mineral density (BMD): Tenofovir was associated with significant increases in biochemical markers of bone metabolism, suggesting increased bone turnover. Serum parathyroid hormone levels and 1,25 vitamin D levels were also higher in patients receiving tenofovir. The effects of tenofovir-associated changes in BMD and biochemical markers on long-term bone health and future fracture risk are unknown.

CNS symptoms: Fifty-three percent of patients receiving efavirenz in controlled trials reported CNS symptoms compared with 25% of patients receiving control regimens. These symptoms included abnormal dreams, dizziness, hallucinations, impaired concentration, insomnia, and somnolence. These symptoms usually begin during the first or second day of therapy and generally resolve after the first 2 to 4 weeks of therapy. Dosing at bedtime may improve the tolerability of these nervous system symptoms.

Convulsions: Convulsions have been observed in patients receiving efavirenz, generally in those with a known medical history of seizures.

Fat redistribution: Redistribution/accumulation of body fat, including breast enlargement, central obesity, "cushingoid appearance," dorsocervical fat enlargement (buffalo hump), facial wasting, and peripheral wasting have been observed in patients receiving antiretroviral therapy.

Immune reconstitution syndrome: Immune reconstitution syndrome has been reported in patients treated with combination antiretroviral therapy, including the components of efavirenz/emtricitabine/tenofovir. During the initial phase of combination antiretroviral treatment, patients whose immune systems respond may develop an inflammatory response to indolent or residual opportunistic infections.

Psychiatric symptoms: Serious psychiatric adverse reactions have been reported in patients treated with efavirenz. Instruct patients with serious psychiatric adverse reactions to seek immediate medical evaluation.

Skin rash: Discontinue efavirenz/emtricitabine/tenofovir in patients developing severe rash associated with blistering, desquamation, fever, or mucosal involvement.

Renal function impairment: See Administration and Dosage for more information.

Renal function impairment, including cases of acute renal failure and Fanconi syndrome (renal tubular injury with severe hypophosphatemia), has been reported.

Hepatic function impairment: Because of the extensive CYP-450–mediated metabolism of efavirenz and limited clinical experience in patients with hepatic function impairment, exercise caution when administering efavirenz/emtricitabine/tenofovir to these patients.

Hazardous tasks: Patients who experience CNS symptoms, such as dizziness, drowsiness, and/or impaired concentration, should avoid potentially hazardous tasks such as driving or operating machinery.

Pregnancy: Category D.

Antiretroviral pregnancy registry – To monitor fetal outcomes of pregnant women, an antiretroviral pregnancy registry has been established. Health care providers are encouraged to register patients who become pregnant by calling 1-800-258-4263.

Lactation: The CDC recommend that HIV-infected mothers not breast-feed their infants in order to avoid risking postnatal transmission of HIV.

Because of both the potential for HIV transmission and the potential for serious adverse reactions in breast-feeding infants, instruct mothers not to breast-feed if they are receiving efavirenz/emtricitabine/tenofovir.

Children: Efavirenz/emtricitabine/tenofovir is not recommended for patients younger than 18 years of age.

Elderly: Use caution during dose selection for elderly patients, keeping in mind the greater frequency of decreased hepatic, renal, or cardiac function, and of concomitant disease or other drug therapy.

Monitoring: Monitor liver enzymes in patients with known or suspected history of hepatitis B or C infection and in patients treated with other medications associated with liver toxicity.

Consider bone monitoring for HIV-infected patients who have a history of pathologic bone fracture or are at risk for osteopenia.

Patients who are receiving concomitant anticonvulsant medications primarily metabolized by the liver, such as phenytoin and phenobarbital, may require periodic monitoring of plasma levels.

Drug Interactions

Drugs that may affect efavirenz/emtricitabine/tenofovir include atazanavir, carbamazepine, lopinavir/ritonavir, phenobarbital, phenytoin, rifabutin, rifampin, ritonavir, St. John's wort, and voriconazole. Drugs that may be affected by efavirenz/emtricitabine/tenofovir include amprenavir, atazanavir, atorvastatin, carbamazepine, cisapride, clarithromycin, didanosine, dihydroergotamine, ergonovine, ethinyl estradiol, fosamprenavir, indinavir, itraconazole, ketoconazole, lopinavir/ritonavir, methadone, midazolam, phenobarbital, phenytoin, pravastatin, rifabutin, ritonavir, saquinavir, sertraline, simvastatin, triazolam, voriconazole, and warfarin. Drugs that should not be coadministered with efavirenz/emtricitabine/tenofovir include abacavir/lamivudine, abacavir/lamivudine/zidovudine, astemizole, cisapride, ergot derivatives, efavirenz, emtricitabine, emtricitabine/tenofovir, lamivudine, lamivudine-HBV, lamivudine/zidovudine, midazolam, St. John's wort, tenofovir, triazolam, and voriconazole.

Adverse Reactions

Adverse reactions occurring in 3% or more of patients include abnormal dreams, depression, diarrhea, dizziness, fatigue, headache, insomnia, nausea, nasopharyngitis, rash, sinusitis, somnolence, and upper respiratory tract infections.

Significant laboratory abnormalities include any grade 3 or greater laboratory abnormality, AST, creatinine kinase, fasting cholesterol, fasting triglyceride, neutrophil, and serum amylase.

MARAVIROC

Tablets: 150 and 300 mg (*Rx*)	*Selzentry* (Pfizer)

Warning:

Hepatotoxicity has been reported with maraviroc use. Evidence of a systemic allergic reaction (eg, eosinophilia or elevated immunoglobulin E, pruritic rash) prior to the development of hepatotoxicity may occur. Immediately evaluate patients with signs or symptoms of hepatitis or allergic reactions following use of maraviroc.

Indications

HIV infection: In combination with other antiretroviral agents, for treatment of adult patients infected only with chemokine receptor 5 (CCR5)-tropic HIV-1.

Administration and Dosage

Adults: Maraviroc can be taken with or without food.

The recommended dosage of maraviroc varies based on concomitant medications because of drug interactions.

Maraviroc Recommended Dosing Regimens	
Concomitant medications	Maraviroc dose
CYP3A4 inhibitors (with or without a CYP3A inducer)	
Protease inhibitors (except tipranavir/ritonavir)	150 mg twice daily
Delavirdine	
Ketoconazole, itraconazole, clarithromycin	
Other strong CYP3A inhibitors (eg, nefazodone, telithromycin)	
Other concomitant medications, including tipranavir/ritonavir, nevirapine, raltegravir, all NRTIs[a], and enfuvirtide	300 mg twice daily

Maraviroc Recommended Dosing Regimens	
Concomitant medications	Maraviroc dose
CYP3A inducers (without a strong CYP3A inhibitor)	
Carbamazepine, phenobarbital, phenytoin	600 mg twice daily
Efavirenz	
Etravirine	
Rifampin	

[a] NRTIs = nucleoside reverse transcriptase inhibitors.

Children:

HIV infection –

16 years of age and older: See Adults for dosing.

Actions

Pharmacology: Maraviroc is an antiviral drug and a member of a therapeutic class called CCR5 coreceptor antagonists. Maraviroc selectively binds to the human chemokine receptor CCR5 present on the cell membrane, preventing the interaction of HIV-1 gp120 and CCR5 necessary for CCR5-tropic HIV-1 to enter cells.

Pharmacokinetics:

Absorption/Distribution – Peak plasma concentrations are attained 0.5 to 4 hours following single oral doses. The absolute bioavailability of a 100 mg dose is 23% and is predicted to be 33% at 300 mg.

Maraviroc is bound (approximately 76%) to human plasma proteins and shows moderate affinity for albumin and alpha-1 acid glycoprotein. The volume of distribution of maraviroc is approximately 194 L.

Metabolism/Excretion – Maraviroc is principally metabolized by the CYP-450 system to metabolites that are essentially inactive against HIV-1.

The terminal half-life of maraviroc following oral dosing to steady-state in healthy volunteers was 14 to 18 hours.

Contraindications

In patients with severe renal impairment or ESRD (CrCl < 30 mL/min) who are taking potent CYP3A inhibitors or inducers.

Warnings/Precautions

Hepatotoxicity: A case of possible maraviroc-induced hepatotoxicity with allergic features has been reported in a study of healthy volunteers. Consider discontinuation of maraviroc in any patient with signs or symptoms of hepatitis, or with increased liver transaminases combined with rash or other systemic symptoms.

Cardiovascular effects:

Myocardial ischemia/infarction – Use with caution in patients at increased risk of cardiovascular events.

Postural hypotension: Use caution when administering maraviroc in patients with a history of postural hypotension or on concomitant medication known to lower blood pressure.

Patients with impaired renal function may have cardiovascular comorbidities and could be at increased risk of cardiovascular adverse events triggered by postural hypotension. An increased risk of postural hypotension may occur in patients with severe renal insufficiency or in those with ESRD because of increased maraviroc exposure in some patients.

Immune reconstitution syndrome: Immune reconstitution syndrome has been reported in patients treated with combination antiretroviral therapy, including maraviroc.

Risk of infection: Maraviroc antagonizes the CCR5 coreceptor located on some immune cells, and therefore, could potentially increase the risk of developing infections.

Risk of malignancy: While no increase in malignancy has been observed with maraviroc, because of this drug's mechanism of action, it could affect immune surveillance and lead to an increased risk of malignancy.

Hazardous tasks: Instruct patients who experience dizziness while taking maraviroc to avoid driving or operating machinery.

Renal function impairment: If patients with severe renal impairment or ESRD not receiving a concomitant potent CYP3A inhibitor or inducer experience any symptoms of postural hypotension while taking maraviroc 300 mg twice daily, reduce the dose to 150 mg twice daily. No studies have been performed in patients with severe renal impairment or ESRD cotreated with potent CYP3A inhibitors or inducers. Hence, no dose of maraviroc can be recommended, and maraviroc is contraindicated for these patients.

Hepatic function impairment: Maraviroc is principally metabolized by the liver; therefore, exercise caution when administering this drug to patients with hepatic impairment because maraviroc concentrations may be increased. Maraviroc has not been studied in patients with severe hepatic impairment.

Pregnancy: *Category B.*

Lactation: Because of the potential for both HIV transmission and serious adverse reactions in breast-feeding infants, instruct mothers not to breast-feed if they are taking maraviroc.

Children: Do not use maraviroc in children younger than 16 years of age.

Elderly: Exercise caution when administering maraviroc in elderly patients; this reflects the greater frequency of decreased hepatic and renal function and of concomitant disease, and other drug therapy.

Monitoring: Monitor liver function tests at baseline and periodically during treatment. Monitor blood pressure in patients with a history of postural hypotension or those on antihypertensive agents. Monitor patients closely for signs of infection.

Drug Interactions

Drugs that may affect maraviroc include atazanavir, atazanavir/ritonavir, carbamazepine, clarithromycin, delavirdine, efavirenz, etravirine, itraconazole, ketoconazole, nefazodone, phenobarbital, phenytoin, protease inhibitors (except tipranavir/ritonavir), rifampin, St. John's wort, and telithromycin.

Adverse Reactions

Adverse reactions occurring in more than 3% of patients include vascular hypertensive disorders, depressive disorders, disturbances in consciousness, disturbances in initiating and maintaining sleep, dizziness/postural dizziness, paresthesias and dysesthesias, peripheral neuropathies, sensory abnormalities, apocrine and eccrine gland disorders, folliculitis, pruritus, rash, constipation, bladder and urethral symptoms, joint-related signs and symptoms, breathing abnormalities, bronchitis, coughing and associated symptoms, sinusitis, upper respiratory tract infection, herpes infection, anxiety symptoms, lipodystrophies, skin neoplasms benign, appetite disorders, urinary tract signs and symptoms, muscle pains, nasal congestion and inflammations, paranasal sinus disorders, upper respiratory tract signs and symptoms, pyrexia, AST, ALT, total bilirubin, amylase, lipase, absolute neutrophil count, memory loss (excluding dementia), acne, lipodystrophies, nail and nail bed conditions (excluding infections and infestations), flatulence, bloating, and distention, GI atonic and hypomotility disorders, GI signs and symptoms NEC, erection and ejaculation conditions and disorders, anemias NEC, neutropenias, lower respiratory tract and lung infections, bacterial infections NEC, body temperature perception, ear disorders NEC, herpes zoster/varicella, joint-related signs and symptoms, Neisseria infections, tinea infections, viral infections NEC, creatine kinase, pain and discomfort.

RALTEGRAVIR

Tablets; oral: 400 mg (*Rx*)	*Isentress* (Merck)

Indications

HIV infection: In combination with other antiretroviral agents for the treatment of HIV-1 infection in adult patients.

Administration and Dosage

HIV infection:

Adults –

Usual dosage: 400 mg administered orally twice daily, with or without food.

Concomitant therapy: During coadministration with rifampin, the recommended dosage of raltegravir is 800 mg twice daily.

Renal function impairment: Because the extent to which raltegravir may be dialyzable is unknown, dosing before a dialysis session should be avoided.

Actions

Pharmacology: Raltegravir inhibits the catalytic activity of HIV-1 integrase, an HIV-1 encoded enzyme that is required for viral replication.

Pharmacokinetics:

Absorption – Raltegravir is absorbed with a time of maximal concentration of approximately 3 hours. With twice-daily dosing, steady state is achieved within approximately the first 2 days of dosing.

Distribution – Raltegravir is approximately 83% bound to human plasma protein.

Metabolism/Excretion – The apparent terminal half-life of raltegravir is approximately 9 hours. Following administration of an oral dose of radiolabeled raltegravir, approximately 51% and 32% of the dose was excreted in feces and urine, respectively.

Warnings/Precautions

Immune reconstitution syndrome: During the initial phase of treatment, patients responding to antiretroviral therapy may develop an inflammatory response to indolent or residual opportunistic infections.

Pregnancy: Category C.

Antiretroviral pregnancy registry – To monitor maternal-fetal outcomes of pregnant patients exposed to raltegravir, an antiretroviral pregnancy registry has been established. Health care providers are encouraged to register patients by calling 1-800-258-4263.

Lactation: Breast-feeding is not recommended while taking raltegravir. In addition, it is recommended that HIV-infected mothers not breast-feed their infants to avoid risking postnatal transmission of HIV.

Children: The safety and effectiveness have not been established.

Elderly: In general, dose selection for an elderly patient should be cautious, reflecting the greater frequency of decreased hepatic, renal, or cardiac function, and of concomitant disease or other drug therapy.

Monitoring: Monitor CD4+ cell count and HIV RNA load.

Drug Interactions

Drugs that may interact with raltegravir include atazanavir, atazanavir/ritonavir, efavirenz, etravirine, omeprazole, rifampin, and tipranavir/ritonavir.

Adverse Reactions

Adverse reactions occurring in 3% or more of patients include absolute neutrophil count grade 2 and 3, ALT grade 2 and 3, AST grade 2 and 3, diarrhea, fasting (nonrandom) serum glucose test grade 2, headache, hemoglobin grade 2, insomnia, platelet count grade 2, serum creatine kinase grade 3, serum pancreatic amylase test grade 3, serum lipase test grade 2, and total serum bilirubin grade 2.

ENFUVIRTIDE

Powder for injection, lyophilized: 108 mg (≈ 90 mg/mL when reconstituted) (*Rx*)	*Fuzeon* (Hoffman-La Roche)

Indications

HIV-1 infection: In combination with other antiretroviral agents for the treatment of HIV-1 infection in treatment-experienced patients with evidence of HIV-1 replication despite ongoing antiretroviral therapy.

Administration and Dosage

Adults: 90 mg (1 mL) twice daily injected subcutaneously into the upper arm, anterior thigh, or abdomen.

Children: In pediatric patients 6 through 16 years of age, the recommended dosage is 2 mg/kg twice daily up to a maximum dose of 90 mg twice daily injected subcutaneously into the upper arm, anterior thigh, or abdomen. Monitor weight periodically and adjust the enfuvirtide dose accordingly.

Enfuvirtide Pediatric Dosing Guidelines

Weight		Dose per bid injection (mg/dose)	Injection volume (90 mg enfuvirtide per mL)
Kilograms (kg)	Pounds (lb)		
11 to 15.5	24 to 34	27	0.3 mL
15.6 to 20	> 34 to 44	36	0.4 mL
20.1 to 24.5	> 44 to 54	45	0.5 mL
24.6 to 29	> 54 to 64	54	0.6 mL
29.1 to 33.5	> 64 to 74	63	0.7 mL
33.6 to 38	> 74 to 84	72	0.8 mL
38.1 to 42.5	> 84 to 94	81	0.9 mL
≥ 42.6	> 94	90	1 mL

Administration: Give each injection at a site different from the preceding injection site, and only where there is no current injection site reaction from an earlier dose. Do not inject enfuvirtide into moles, scar tissue, bruises, or the navel.

Preparation for administration: Enfuvirtide must only be reconstituted with 1.1 mL of sterile water for injection.

Enfuvirtide contains no preservatives. Once reconstituted, inject enfuvirtide immediately or keep refrigerated in the original vial; use within 24 hours. The subsequent dose can be reconstituted in advance, stored in the refrigerator in the original vial, and used within 24 hours.

Actions

Pharmacology: Enfuvirtide is an inhibitor of the fusion of HIV-1 with CD4+ cells. Enfuvirtide interferes with the entry of HIV-1 into cells by inhibiting fusion of viral and cellular membranes.

Pharmacokinetics:

Absorption – The absolute bioavailability (using a 90 mg IV dose as a reference) was 84.3% ± 15.5%.

Distribution – The volume of distribution after IV administration of enfuvirtide is 5.5 ± 1.1 L.

Enfuvirtide is approximately 92% bound to plasma proteins in HIV-infected plasma over a concentration range of 2 to 10 mcg/mL.

Metabolism/Excretion – As a peptide, enfuvirtide is expected to undergo catabolism to its constituent amino acids, with subsequent recycling of the amino acids in the body pool.

Following a single 90 mg subcutaneous dose of enfuvirtide the mean ± SD elimination half-life of enfuvirtide is 3.8 ± 0.6 hours and the mean ± SD apparent clearance was 24.8 ± 4.1 mL/h/kg.

Contraindications

Enfuvirtide is contraindicated in patients with known hypersensitivity to enfuvirtide or any of its components (see Warnings).

Warnings/Precautions

Local injection site reactions: The most common adverse events associated with enfuvirtide use are local injection site reactions. Manifestations may include pain and discomfort, induration, erythema, nodules and cysts, pruritus, and ecchymosis.

Pneumonia: An increased rate of bacterial pneumonia was observed in subjects treated with enfuvirtide in the phase 3 clinical trials compared with the control arm.

Non-HIV infected individuals: There is a theoretical risk that enfuvirtide use may lead to the production of antienfuvirtide antibodies that cross react with HIV gp41. This could result in a false positive HIV test with an ELISA assay; a confirmatory western blot test would be expected to be negative. Enfuvirtide has not been studied in non-HIV infected individuals.

Hypersensitivity reactions: Hypersensitivity reactions have been associated with enfuvirtide therapy and may recur on rechallenge. Hypersensitivity reactions have included individually and in combination: Rash, fever, nausea and vomiting, chills, rigors, hypotension, and elevated serum liver transaminases. Other adverse events that may be immune mediated and have been reported in subjects receiving enfuvirtide include primary immune complex reaction, respiratory distress, glomerulonephritis, and Guillain-Barre syndrome.

Pregnancy: Category B.

Antiretroviral pregnancy registry – To monitor maternal-fetal outcomes of pregnant women exposed to enfuvirtide and other antiretroviral drugs, an antiretroviral pregnancy registry has been established. Physicians are encouraged to register patients by calling 1-800-258-4263.

Lactation: It is not known whether enfuvirtide is excreted in human milk. Because of the potential for HIV transmission and the potential for serious adverse reactions in nursing infants, mothers should be instructed not to breastfeed if they are receiving enfuvirtide.

Children: The safety and pharmacokinetics of enfuvirtide have not been established in pediatric subjects below 6 years of age.

Adverse Reactions

Local injection site reactions including pain/discomfort, induration, erythema, nodules and cysts, pruritus, and ecchymosis were the most frequent adverse events associated with the use of enfuvirtide.

Other frequently reported events in subjects receiving enfuvirtide plus background regimen were diarrhea, nausea, and fatigue.

Adverse reactions occurring in at least 3% of patients included the following: Upper abdominal pain, anxiety, appetite decrease, asthenia, constipation, cough, depression, herpes simplex, influenza, insomnia, myalgia, peripheral neuropathy, pruritus (not otherwise specified), sinusitis, skin papilloma, weight decreased.

EMTRICITABINE

Capsules: 200 mg (*Rx*)	*Emtriva* (Gilead Sciences)
Oral solution: 10 mg/mL (*Rx*)	

Warning:

Lactic acidosis and severe hepatomegaly with steatosis, including fatal cases, have been reported with the use of nucleoside analogs alone or in combination with other antiretrovirals.

continued on next page

Warning: (cont.)

Emtricitabine is not indicated for the treatment of chronic hepatitis B virus (HBV) infection, and the safety and efficacy of emtricitabine have not been established in patients coinfected with HBV and HIV. Severe acute exacerbations of hepatitis B have been reported in patients after the discontinuation of emtricitabine. Closely monitor hepatic function with clinical and laboratory follow-up for at least several months in patients who discontinue emtricitabine and are coinfected with HIV and HBV. If appropriate, initiation of antihepatitis B therapy may be warranted.

Indications

HIV infection: In combination with other antiretroviral agents for the treatment of HIV-1 infection.

Administration and Dosage

May be taken without regard to food.

Adults 18 years of age and older:

Capsules – 200 mg administered orally once daily.

Oral solution – 240 mg (24 mL) administered orally once daily.

Children 3 months through 17 years of age:

Capsules – For children weighing more than 33 kg who can swallow an intact capsule, one 200 mg capsule administered orally once daily.

Oral solution – 6 mg/kg, up to a maximum of 240 mg (24 mL), administered orally once daily.

Children 0 to 3 months of age:

Solution – 3 mg/kg once daily.

Renal function impairment:

Dose Adjustment in Adult Patients with Renal Impairment

Formulation	CrCl[a] (mL/min) ≥ 50	30 to 49	15 to 29	< 15 or on hemodialysis[b]
Capsule (200 mg)	200 mg every 24 hours	200 mg every 48 hours	200 mg every 72 hours	200 mg every 96 hours
Oral solution (10 mg/mL)	240 mg every 24 hours (24 mL)	120 mg every 24 hours (12 mL)	80 mg every 24 hours (8 mL)	60 mg every 24 hours (6 mL)

[a] CrCl = creatinine clearance.

[b] Hemodialysis patients: if dosing on day of dialysis, administer after dialysis.

Actions

Pharmacology: Emtricitabine is a synthetic nucleoside analog of cytosine. Emtricitabine inhibits the activity of the HIV-1 reverse transcriptase, which results in chain termination.

Pharmacokinetics:

Absorption – Emtricitabine is rapidly and extensively absorbed following oral administration, with peak plasma concentrations occurring at 1 to 2 hours postdose. The mean absolute bioavailability of emtricitabine was 93%, while the mean absolute bioavailability of emtricitabine oral solution was 75%.

Distribution – Binding of emtricitabine to human plasma proteins was less than 4%.

Metabolism/Excretion – Emtricitabine is not an inhibitor of human CYP-450 enzymes. Following administration of emtricitabine, complete recovery of the dose was achieved in urine (approximately 86%) and feces (approximately 14%). The plasma emtricitabine half-life is approximately 10 hours. The renal clearance of emtricitabine is greater than the estimated CrCl, suggesting elimination by both glomerular filtration and active tubular secretion.

Contraindications

Previously demonstrated hypersensitivity to any of the components of the products.

Warnings/Precautions

Coinfection with HIV and hepatitis B virus: It is recommended that all patients with HIV be tested for the presence of chronic HBV before initiating antiretroviral therapy.

Lactic acidosis/Severe hepatomegaly with steatosis: Lactic acidosis and severe hepatomegaly with steatosis, including fatal cases, have been reported with the use of nucleoside analogs alone or in combination, including emtricitabine and other antiretrovirals. Treatment with emtricitabine should be suspended in any patient who develops clinical or laboratory findings suggestive of lactic acidosis or pronounced hepatotoxicity.

Fat redistribution: Redistribution/accumulation of body fat, including central obesity, dorsocervical fat enlargement (buffalo hump), peripheral wasting, facial wasting, breast enlargement, and "cushingoid appearance," has been observed in patients receiving antiretroviral therapy.

Immune reconstitution syndrome: Immune reconstitution syndrome has been reported in patients treated with combination antiretroviral therapy.

Pregnancy: Category B.

Antiretroviral pregnancy registry – To monitor fetal outcomes of pregnant women exposed to emtricitabine, an antiretroviral pregnancy registry has been established. Health care providers are encouraged to register patients by calling (800) 258-4263.

Lactation: The Centers for Disease Control and Prevention recommend that HIV-infected mothers not breast-feed their infants to avoid risking postnatal transmission of HIV.

Children: Safety and efficacy in children younger than 3 months of age have not been established.

Elderly: Dose selection for elderly patients should be cautious, keeping in mind the greater frequency of decreased hepatic, renal, or cardiac function, and of concomitant disease or other drug therapy.

Monitoring: Closely monitor hepatic function for at least several months in patients who discontinue emtricitabine and are coinfected with HIV and HBV.

Adverse Reactions

Adults: Adverse reactions occurring in at least 3% of patients include the following: abdominal pain, abnormal dreams, asthenia, depressive disorders, diarrhea, dizziness, dyspepsia, headache, insomnia, lab test abnormalities (eg, ALT, AST, creatine kinase, neutrophils, serum amylase, serum glucose, triglycerides) nausea, neuropathy/peripheral neuritis, paresthesia, rash event, vomiting.

Children: Adverse reactions occurring in at least 3% of patients include the following: abdominal pain, anemia, diarrhea, fever, gastroenteritis, hyperpigmentation, increased cough, infection, otitis media, pneumonia, rash, rhinitis, vomiting.

FOSAMPRENAVIR CALCIUM

Tablets; oral: 700 mg (as fosamprenavir calcium; equiv. to amprenavir 600 mg) (*Rx*) **Suspension, oral:** 50 mg/mL (as fosamprenavir calcium; equiv. to amprenavir 43 mg/mL) (*Rx*)	*Lexiva* (GlaxoSmithKline)

Indications

HIV infection: In combination with other antiretroviral agents for the treatment of HIV infection in adults.

Administration and Dosage

Higher than approved dose combinations of fosamprenavir plus ritonavir are not recommended because of an increased risk of transaminase elevations.

Fosamprenavir tablets may be taken with or without food. Adults should take fosamprenavir oral suspension without food. Children should take fosamprenavir oral suspension with food. If emesis occurs within 30 minutes after dosing, redose fosamprenavir oral suspension.

Therapy-naive patients: Fosamprenavir 1,400 mg twice daily (without ritonavir); fosamprenavir 1,400 mg once daily plus ritonavir 200 mg once daily; fosamprenavir 1,400 mg once daily plus ritonavir 100 mg once daily; or fosamprenavir 700 mg twice daily plus ritonavir 100 mg twice daily.

PI-experienced patients: Fosamprenavir 700 mg twice daily plus ritonavir 100 mg twice daily.

Children 2 to 18 years of age:

Therapy-naive patients 2 to 5 years of age – Fosamprenavir 30 mg/kg oral suspension twice daily, not to exceed the adult dose of fosamprenavir 1,400 mg twice daily.

Therapy-naive patients 6 years of age and older – Either fosamprenavir 30 mg/kg oral suspension twice daily, not to exceed the adult dose of fosamprenavir 1,400 mg twice daily, or fosamprenavir 18 mg/kg oral suspension plus ritonavir 3 mg/kg twice daily, not to exceed the adult dose of fosamprenavir 700 mg plus ritonavir 100 mg twice daily.

Therapy-experienced patients 6 years of age and older – Fosamprenavir 18 mg/kg oral suspension plus ritonavir 3 mg/kg administered twice daily, not to exceed the adult dose of fosamprenavir 700 mg plus ritonavir 100 mg twice daily.

When administered without ritonavir, the adult regimen of fosamprenavir 1,400 mg tablets twice daily may be used for children weighing at least 47 kg.

When administered in combination with ritonavir, fosamprenavir tablets may be used for children weighing at least 39 kg; ritonavir capsules may be used for children weighing at least 33 kg.

Hepatic function impairment:

Mild hepatic function impairment (Child-Pugh score from 5 to 6) – 700 mg twice daily without ritonavir (therapy-naive patients) or 700 mg twice daily plus ritonavir 100 mg once daily (therapy-naive or PI-experienced patients)

Moderate hepatic function impairment (Child-Pugh score from 7 to 9) – 700 mg twice daily (therapy-naive patients) without ritonavir or 450 mg twice daily plus ritonavir 100 mg once daily (therapy-naive or PI-experienced patients)

Severe hepatic function impairment (Child-Pugh score from 10 to 15) – 350 mg twice daily without ritonavir (therapy-naive patients) or 300 mg twice daily plus ritonavir 100 mg once daily (therapy-naive or protease inhibitor-experienced patients.

Actions

Pharmacology: Fosamprenavir is a prodrug of amprenavir, an inhibitor of HIV-1 protease.

Pharmacokinetics:

Absorption/Distribution – Fosamprenavir is a prodrug that is rapidly hydrolyzed to amprenavir. After administration of a single dose of fosamprenavir to HIV-1-infected patients, the time to peak amprenavir concentration (T_{max}) occurred between 1.5 and 4 hours (median, 2.5 hours).

Amprenavir is approximately 90% bound to plasma proteins, primarily to $alpha_1$-acid glycoprotein.

Metabolism/Excretion – Fosamprenavir is rapidly and almost completely hydrolyzed to amprenavir. Amprenavir is metabolized in the liver by the CYP-450 3A4 (CYP3A4) enzyme system.

The plasma elimination half-life of amprenavir is approximately 7.7 hours.

Contraindications

Hypersensitivity to any of the components of this product or to amprenavir; coadministration with cisapride, delavirdine, dihydroergotamine, ergonovine, ergotamine, lovastatin, methylergonovine, midazolam, pimozide, rifampin, simvastatin, St. John's wort, or triazolam.

If fosamprenavir is coadministered with ritonavir, the antiarrhythmic agents flecainide and propafenone also are contraindicated.

Warnings/Precautions

Skin reactions: Severe or life-threatening skin reactions, including Stevens-Johnson syndrome, were reported in patients treated with fosamprenavir in the clinical studies. Discontinue treatment with fosamprenavir for severe or life-threatening rashes and moderate rashes accompanied by systemic symptoms.

Hemolytic anemia: Acute hemolytic anemia has been reported.

Diabetes mellitus/hyperglycemia: New-onset diabetes mellitus, exacerbation of preexisting diabetes mellitus, and hyperglycemia have been reported during postmarketing surveillance in HIV-infected patients receiving PI therapy.

Hemophilia: There have been reports of spontaneous bleeding in patients with hemophilia A and B treated with PI.

Hepatic toxicity: Patients with underlying hepatitis B or C, or marked elevations in transaminases prior to treatment may be at increased risk for developing or worsening transaminase elevations.

Immune reconstitution syndrome: Immune reconstitution syndrome has been reported in patients treated with combination antiretroviral therapy, including fosamprenavir.

Fat redistribution: Redistribution/accumulation of body fat has been observed in patients receiving antiretroviral therapy, including fosamprenavir.

Lipid elevations: Treatment with fosamprenavir plus ritonavir has resulted in increases in the concentration of triglycerides and cholesterol.

Nephrolithiasis: Cases of nephrolithiasis were reported during postmarketing surveillance in HIV-infected patients receiving fosamprenavir.

Resistance/Cross-resistance: Because the potential for HIV cross-resistance among PI has not been fully explored, it is unknown what effect therapy with fosamprenavir will have on the activity of subsequently administered PI.

Hypersensitivity reactions: Use fosamprenavir with caution in patients with a known sulfonamide allergy. Fosamprenavir contains a sulfonamide moiety.

Hepatic function impairment: Exercise caution when administering fosamprenavir to patients with hepatic function impairment. Patients with hepatic function impairment receiving fosamprenavir without concurrent ritonavir may require dose reduction.

Pregnancy: Category C.

Antiretroviral pregnancy registry – To monitor maternal-fetal outcomes of pregnant women exposed to fosamprenavir, an Antiretroviral Pregnancy Registry has been established. Physicians are encouraged to register patients by calling 1-800-258-4263.

Lactation: The Centers for Disease Control and Prevention recommend that HIV-infected mothers not breast-feed their infants to avoid risking postnatal transmission of HIV.

Children: The safety, pharmacokinetic profile, and virologic response of fosamprenavir oral suspension and tablets were evaluated in children 2 to 18 years of age in 2 open-label studies. No data are available for children younger than 2 years of age.

Elderly: In general, dose selection for an elderly patient should be cautious, reflecting the greater frequency of decreased hepatic, renal, or cardiac function, and of concomitant disease or other drug therapy.

Monitoring: Perform triglyceride and cholesterol testing prior to initiating therapy with fosamprenavir and at periodic intervals during therapy. Monitor liver function tests prior to initiating therapy and periodically thereafter.

Drug Interactions

Drugs that may be affected by fosamprenavir include antiarrhythmics; anticholinergic agents; aripiprazole; atazanavir; azole antifungals; benzodiazepines; calcium channel blockers; carbamazepine; cisapride; colchicine, contraceptives, hormonal; corticosteroids; delavirdine; dronedarone; eplerenone; ergot derivatives; erythromycin; esomeprazole; esopiclone; HMG-CoA reductase inhibitors; immunosuppressants; indinavir; ixabepilone; lopinavir plus ritonavir; maraviroc; methadone; mammalian target of rapamycin inhibitors; nevirapine; nilotinib; opioid analgesics; PDE5 inhibitors; paroxetine; phenytoin, pimozide; protein-tyrosine kinase inhibitors; quetiapine; ranolazine; rifabutin; trazodone; tricyclic antidepressants; vasopressin receptor antagonists; warfarin; zidovudine.

Drugs that may affect fosamprenavir include anticonvulsants; azole antifungals; contraceptives, hormonal; CYP-450 3A4 inhibitors; delavirdine; dexamethasone; efavirenz; efavirenz/ritonavir; histamine H_2 receptor antagonists; HMG-CoA reductase inhibitors; indinavir; lopinavir plus ritonavir; methadone; nevirapine; rifabutin; rifampin; saquinavir; St. John's wort; zidovudine.

Fosamprenavir plus ritonavir may interact with flecainide, propafenone, efavirenz plus ritonavir, and lopinavir plus ritonavir. Efavirenz may affect fosamprenavir with or without ritonavir.

Drug/Food interactions: Administration of a single dose of fosamprenavir 1,400 mg oral suspension in the fed state compared with the fasted state was associated with a 46% reduction in C_{max}, a 0.72-hour delay in T_{max}, and a 28% reduction in amprenavir $AUC_{0-\infty}$. Grapefruit juice may increase plasma concentrations of amprenavir. If grapefruit juice cannot be avoided, closely monitor the patient and adjust the fosamprenavir dose as needed. Garlic ingestion may reduce amprenavir plasma concentrations, decreasing the pharmacologic effects. Avoid garlic ingestion.

Adverse Reactions

Adverse reactions occurring in at least 3% of patients include the following: ALT more than 5 times the upper limit of normal (ULN), AST greater than 5 times ULN, diarrhea, fatigue, headache, hypertriglyceridemia (more than 750 mg/dL), nausea, neutropenia (less than 750 cells/mm^3), rash, serum lipase more than 2 times ULN, vomiting.

TRIMETHOPRIM AND SULFAMETHOXAZOLE (Co-Trimoxazole; TMP-SMZ)

Tablets; oral: 80 mg trimethoprim and 400 mg sulfamethoxazole (*Rx*)	Various, *Bactrim* (AR Scientific), *Septra* (Monarch)
Tablets, double strength; oral: 160 mg trimethoprim and 800 mg sulfamethoxazole (*Rx*)	Various, *Bactrim DS* (AR Scientific), *Septra DS* (Monarch)
Suspension; oral: 40 mg trimethoprim and 200 mg sulfamethoxazole/5 mL (*Rx*)	Various, *Sulfatrim* (Activis MidAtlantic)
Injection: sulfamethoxazole 80 mg and trimethoprim 16 mg per mL (*Rx*)	Various

Indications

Sulfamethoxazole and Trimethoprim Indications[a]

Indication	Adults	Children	Organism
FDA-approved uses			
Acute exacerbations of chronic bronchitis	X		*Haemophilus influenzae, Streptococcus pneumoniae*
Acute otitis media[b]		X	*H. influenzae, S. pneumoniae*
Enteritis[c]	X	X	*Shigella flexneri, Shigella sonnei*
PCP prophylaxis[d]	X	X	*P. carinii*
PCP treatment[c]	X	X	*P. carinii*
Traveler's diarrhea	X		Enterotoxigenic *Escherichia coli*
UTIs[c,e]	X	X	*E. coli, Klebsiella* and *Enterobacter* species, *Morganella morganii, Proteus mirabilis, Proteus vulgaris*
Off-label uses[f]			
Acute and chronic bacterial prostatitis	X		
Cholera and salmonella-type infections and nocardiosis[c]	X		*Vibrio cholerae, Salmonella* sp., *Nocardia* sp.
Prevention of recurrent UTIs in women	X		
Skin and soft-tissue infections[c]	X	X	Methicillin-sensitive *S. aureus* or methicillin-resistant *S. aureus*

[a] FDA = Food and Drug Administration; PCP = *Pneumocystis carinii* pneumonia; UTI = urinary tract infection.
[b] Not indicated for prophylactic or prolonged administration in otitis media at any age.
[c] Parenteral indications.
[d] Prophylaxis against PCP in individuals who are immunosuppressed and considered to be at increased risk.
[e] Treat initial uncomplicated UTIs with a single antibacterial agent. Parenteral therapy is indicated in severe or complicated infections when oral therapy is not feasible.
[f] Low-dose sulfamethoxazole and trimethoprim has been studied in the prophylaxis of neutropenic patients with *P. carinii* infections or leukemia patients to reduce the incidence of gram-negative rod bacteremia. Prophylaxis with sulfamethoxazole 1,600 mg and trimethoprim 320 mg per day appears beneficial in reducing the incidence of bacterial infection following renal transplant and may provide protection against PCP.

Administration and Dosage

Administration and Dosage of Sulfamethoxazole/Trimethoprim

Organisms/Infections	Dosage
Urinary tract infections, enteritis, and acute otitis media:	
Adults:	Sulfamethoxazole 800 mg and trimethoprim 160 mg every 12 hours for 10 to 14 days (5 days for enteritis).

Administration and Dosage of Sulfamethoxazole/Trimethoprim

Organisms/Infections	Dosage
Children (≥ 2 months of age):	Sulfamethoxazole 40 mg/kg and trimethoprim 8 mg/kg per day given in 2 divided doses every 12 hours for 10 days (5 days for enteritis).
Guideline for proper dosage:	Dose every 12 hours:
Weight (kg)	Suspension / Tablets
10	5 mL / -
20	10 mL / 1
30	15 mL / 1½
40	20 mL / 2 (or 1 double strength tablet)
IV: Adults and children > 2 months with normal renal function for severe UTIs and enteritis.	8 to 10 mg/kg/day (based on trimethoprim) in 2 to 4 divided doses every 6, 8 or 12 hours for up to 14 days for severe UTIs and 5 days for enteritis.
Travelers' diarrhea in adults:	Sulfamethoxazole 800 mg and trimethoprim 160 mg every 12 h for 5 days.
Acute exacerbations of chronic bronchitis in adults:	Sulfamethoxazole 800 mg and trimethoprim 160 mg every 12 h for 14 days.
Pneumocystis carinii pneumonia:	
Treatment:	Sulfamethoxazole 75 to 100 mg/kg and trimethoprim 15 to 20 mg/kg per day in divided doses every 6 hours for 14 to 21 days.
Guideline for proper dosage in children	Dose every 6 hours:
Weight (kg)	Suspension / Tablets
8	5 mL / -
16	10 mL / 1
24	15 mL / 1½
32	20 mL / 2 (or 1 double strength tablet)
IV for adults and children > 2 months:	15 to 20 mg/kg/day (based on trimethoprim) in 3 or 4 divided doses every 6 to 8 hours for up to 14 days.
Prophylaxis:	
Adults:	Trimethoprim 160 mg and sulfamethoxazole 800 mg given orally every 24 hours.
Children:	Trimethoprim 150 mg/m² and sulfamethoxazole 750 mg/m² per day given orally in equally divided doses twice a day, on 3 consecutive days per week. The total daily dose should not exceed trimethoprim 320 mg and sulfamethoxazole 1,600 mg.
Guideline for proper dosage in children	Dose every 12 hours
Body surface area (m²)	Suspension / Tablets
0.26	2.5 mL / -
0.53	5 mL / ½
1.06	10 mL / 1
Patients with impaired renal function CrCl (mL/min):	Recommended dosage regimen:
> 30	Usual regimen
15 to 30	½ usual regimen
< 15	Not recommended
Off-label dosing:	
Acute and chronic bacterial prostatitis in adults:	Sulfamethoxazole 800 mg and trimethoprim 160 mg twice daily up to 12 weeks.
Nocardiosis in adults:	15 mg/kg/day (based on trimethoprim) in 2 to 4 divided doses for 3 to 4 weeks, then decrease dosage to 10 mg/kg/day (based on trimethoprim) in 2 to 4 divided doses for 3 to 6 months.

Administration and Dosage of Sulfamethoxazole/Trimethoprim	
Organisms/Infections	Dosage
P. carinii pneumonia:	
Adult prophylactic dosage:	Sulfamethoxazole 400 mg and trimethoprim 80 mg orally every 24 hours or sulfamethoxazole 800 mg and trimethoprim 160 mg orally 3 times per week
Pediatric prophylactic dosage:	Sulfamethoxazole 750 mg/m^2 and trimethoprim 150 mg/m^2 per day in a single daily dose for 3 consecutive days per week; Sulfamethoxazole 750 mg/m^2 and trimethoprim 150 mg/m^2 per day in equally divided doses twice a day; or Sulfamethoxazole 750 mg/m^2 and trimethoprim 150 mg/m^2 per day in equally divided doses twice a day 3 times per week on alternate days.
Prevention of recurrent urinary tract infections in adult women:	Sulfamethoxazole 200 mg and trimethoprim 40 mg daily at bedtime a minimum of 3 times weekly or postcoitally
Skin and soft tissue infections:	
Adults	Sulfamethoxazole 800 to 1,600 mg and trimethoprim 160 to 320 mg orally twice daily.
Children	8 to 12 mg/kg (based on the trimethoprim component) in equally divided doses every 12 hours.

Parenteral:

IV – Administer over 60 to 90 minutes. Avoid rapid infusion or bolus injection. Do not give IM.

Actions

Pharmacology: Sulfamethoxazole inhibits bacterial synthesis of dihydrofolic acid by competing with para-aminobenzoic acid. Trimethoprim blocks the production of tetrahydrofolic acid by inhibiting the enzyme dihydrofolate reductase.

Pharmacokinetics:

Absorption/Distribution – Sulfamethoxazole/trimethoprim is rapidly and completely absorbed following oral administration. Approximately 44% of trimethoprim and 70% of sulfamethoxazole are protein bound. Following oral administration, the half-lives of trimethoprim (8 to 11 hours) and sulfamethoxazole (10 to 12 hours) are similar. Following IV administration, the mean plasma half-life was 11.3 hours for trimethoprim and 12.8 hours for sulfamethoxazole.

Metabolism/Excretion – Sulfamethoxazole undergoes biotransformation to inactive compounds; trimethoprim is metabolized to a small extent.

Urine concentrations are considerably higher than serum concentrations.

Contraindications

Hypersensitivity to sulfamethoxazole or trimethoprim; megaloblastic anemia caused by folate deficiency; pregnancy at term and lactation; infants younger than 2 months of age.

The sulfonamides are chemically similar to some goitrogens, diuretics (acetazolamide and the thiazides), and oral hypoglycemic agents. Goiter production, diuresis, and hypoglycemia occur rarely in patients receiving sulfonamides. Cross-sensitivity may exist with these agents.

Warnings/Precautions

Sever reactions: Fatalities associated with the administration of sulfonamides, although rare, have occurred because of severe reactions, including agranulocytosis, aplastic anemia, fulminant hepatic necrosis, Stevens-Johnson syndrome, toxic epidermal necrolysis, and other blood dyscrasias.

Respiratory effects: Cough, pulmonary infiltrates, and shortness of breath are hypersensitivity reactions of the respiratory tract that have been reported in association with sulfonamide treatment.

Group A beta-hemolytic streptococci: Do not use sulfamethoxazole and trimethoprim for the treatment of group A beta-hemolytic streptococcal infections.

Clostridium difficile-associated diarrhea: C. *difficile*-associated diarrhea has been reported with use of nearly all antibacterial agents, including sulfamethoxazole and trimethoprim, and may range in severity from mild diarrhea to fatal colitis.

Hematologic effects: Sulfonamide-associated deaths, although rare, have occurred from hypersensitivity of the respiratory tract, Stevens-Johnson syndrome, toxic epidermal necrolysis, fulminant hepatic necrosis, agranulocytosis, aplastic anemia, and other blood dyscrasias.

IV use at high doses or for extended periods of time may cause bone marrow depression manifested as thrombocytopenia, leukopenia, or megaloblastic anemia.

Hyperkalemia: A high dosage of trimethoprim, as used in patients with PCP, induces a progressive but reversible increase of serum potassium concentrations in a substantial number of patients.

Hypoglycemia: Cases of hypoglycemia in nondiabetic patients treated with sulfamethoxazole and trimethoprim are seen rarely, usually occurring after a few days of therapy.

Phenylketonuria: Trimethoprim has been noted to impair phenylalanine metabolism, but this is if no significance in phenylketonuric patients on appropriate dietary restriction.

Pneumocystis carinii pneumonia in patients with AIDS: AIDS patients may not tolerate or respond to sulfamethoxazole and trimethoprim.

Renal/Hepatic function impairment: Use with caution. Maintain adequate fluid intake to prevent crystalluria and stone formation. Patients with severely impaired renal function exhibit an increase in the half-lives of both sulfamethoxazole and trimethoprim, requiring dosage regimen adjustment.

Special risk: Use with caution in patients with possible folate deficiency, severe allergy, or bronchial asthma. In G-6-PD deficient individuals, hemolysis may occur; it is frequently dose-related.

Pregnancy: *Category* C.

Lactation: Sulfamethoxazole and trimethoprim is not recommended in the breastfeeding period because sulfonamides are excreted in breast milk and may cause kernicterus. Premature infants and infants with hyperbilirubinemia or G-6-PD deficiency are also at risk for adverse effects.

Children: Not recommended for infants younger than 2 months of age.

Elderly: There may be an increased risk of severe adverse reactions, particularly when complicating conditions exist.

Drug Interactions

Drugs that may be affected by sulfamethoxazole and trimethoprim include ACE inhibitors, diuretics, indomethacin, methenamine, sulfones, and tretinoin. Drugs that may affect sulfamethoxazole and trimethoprim include ACE inhibitors, amantadine, cyclosporin, digoxin, diuretics, dofetilide, ethanol, hydantoins, meglitinides, methotrexate, procainamide, pyrimethamine, sulfones, sulfonylureas, thiazolidinediones, and tretinoin.

Adverse Reactions

Adverse reactions may include agranulocytosis; allergic myocarditis; allergic skin reactions; anaphylactoid reactions; angioedema; anorexia; apathy; aplastic, hemolytic, or megaloblastic anemia; arthralgia; ataxia; BUN and serum creatinine elevation; chills; convulsions; crystalluria; drug fever; elevation of serum transaminase and bilirubin; eosinophilia; erythema multiforme; exfoliative dermatitis; fatigue; GI disturbances; generalized allergic reactions; glossitis; hallucinations; headache; hyperkalemia; hyponatremia; hypoprothrombinemia; insomnia; interstitial nephritis; leukopenia; mental depression; methemoglobinemia; myalgia ; nervousness; neutropenia; pancreatitis; peripheral neuritis; photosensitization; pruritus; rash; renal failure; skin eruptions, generalized; Stevens-Johnson syndrome; stomatitis; systemic lupus erythematosus; thrombocytopenia; tinnitus; toxic epidermal necrolysis; toxic nephrosis with oliguria and anuria; urticaria; vertigo; weakness.

ERYTHROMYCIN ETHYLSUCCINATE AND SULFISOXAZOLE

Suspension, granules; oral: Erythromycin ethylsuccinate (equivalent to 200 mg erythromycin activity) and sulfisoxazole acetyl (equivalent to 600 mg sulfisoxazole)/5 mL when reconstituted (*Rx*)	Various

Indications

Children: Acute otitis media caused by susceptible strains of *Haemophilus influenzae.*

Administration and Dosage

Do not administer to infants younger than 2 months of age; systemic sulfonamides are contraindicated in this age group.

Acute otitis media: 50 mg/kg/day erythromycin and 150 mg/kg/day (to a maximum of 6 g/day) sulfisoxazole. Give in equally divided doses 4 times daily for 10 days. Administer without regard to meals.

Erythromycin/Sulfisoxazole Dosage Based on Weight		
Weight		
kg	lb	Dose (every 6 hours)
< 8	< 18	Adjust dosage by body weight
8	18	2.5 mL
16	35	5 mL
24	53	7.5 mL
> 45	> 100	10 mL

PENTAMIDINE ISETHIONATE

Injection: 300 mg (*Rx*)	*Pentam 300* (Lyphomed), *Pentacarinat* (Armour)
Powder for injection, lyophilized: 300 mg (*Rx*)	*Pentamidine Isethionate* (Abbott)
Aerosol: 300 mg (*Rx*)	*NebuPent* (Lyphomed)

Indications

Injection: Treatment of *Pneumocystis carinii* pneumonia (PCP).

Inhalation: Prevention of PCP in high-risk, HIV-infected patients defined by one or both of the following criteria: History of 1 or more episodes of PCP; a peripheral CD4+ (T4 helper/inducer) lymphocyte count less than or equal to 200 mm^3.

Administration and Dosage

Injection:

Adults and children – 4 mg/kg once a day for 14 days administered deep IM or IV only. The benefits and risks of therapy for longer than 14 days are not well defined. Dosage in renal failure should be patient-specific. If necessary, reduce dosage, use a longer infusion time or extend the dosing interval.

Preparation of solution:

IM – Dissolve the contents of 1 vial in 3 mL of Sterile Water for Injection.

IV – Dissolve the contents of 1 vial in 3 to 5 mL of Sterile Water for Injection or 5% Dextrose Injection. Further dilute the calculated dose in 50 to 250 mL of 5% Dextrose solution.

Infuse the diluted IV solution over 60 minutes.

Aerosol:

Prevention of PCP – 300 mg once every 4 weeks administered via the *Respirgard* II nebulizer by Marquest.

Deliver the dose until the nebulizer chamber is empty (approximately 30 to 45 minutes). The flow rate should be 5 to 7 L/min from a 40 to 50 lbs/in^2 (PSI) air or oxygen source. Alternatively, a 40 to 50 PSI air compressor can be used with flow limited by setting the flowmeter at 5 to 7 L/min or by setting the pressure at 22 to 25 PSI. Do not use low pressure (less than 20 PSI) compressors.

Reconstitution – The contents of 1 vial must be dissolved in 6 mL Sterile Water for Injection, USP. It is important to use *only* sterile water; saline solution will cause the drug to precipitate. Place the entire reconstituted contents of the vial into the

Respirgard II nebulizer reservoir for administration. Do not mix the pentamidine solution with any other drugs.

Actions

Pharmacology: Pentamidine isethionate, an aromatic diamidine antiprotozoal agent, has activity against *P. carinii*. In vitro studies indicate that the drug interferes with nuclear metabolism and inhibits the synthesis of DNA, RNA, phospholipids, and protein synthesis.

Pharmacokinetics:

Absorption/Distribution – Pentamidine is well absorbed after IM administration.

Metabolism/Excretion – Pentamidine may accumulate in renal failure.

Plasma concentrations after aerosol administration are substantially lower than those observed after a comparable IV dose. The extent of pentamidine accumulation and distribution following chronic inhalation therapy are not known.

Contraindications

Injection: Once the diagnosis of PCP has been established, there are no absolute contraindications to the use of pentamidine.

Inhalation: Patients with a history of an anaphylactic reaction to inhaled or parenteral pentamidine isethionate.

Warnings/Precautions

Development of acute PCP: Development of acute PCP still exists in patients receiving pentamidine prophylaxis. The use of pentamidine may alter the clinical and radiographic features of PCP and could result in an atypical presentation, including but not limited to mild diseases or focal infection.

Prior to initiating pentamidine prophylaxis, evaluate symptomatic patients to exclude the presence of PCP. The recommended dose for the prevention of PCP is insufficient to treat acute PCP.

Fatalities: Fatalities caused by severe hypotension, hypoglycemia, and cardiac arrhythmias have been reported, both by the IM and IV routes. Severe hypotension may result after a single dose. Limit administration of the drug to patients in whom *P. carinii* has been demonstrated.

Use with caution: Use with caution in patients with hypertension, hypotension, hypoglycemia, hyperglycemia, hypocalcemia, leukopenia, thrombocytopenia, anemia, hepatic or renal dysfunction, ventricular tachycardia, pancreatitis, and Stevens-Johnson syndrome.

Hypotension: Patients may develop sudden, severe hypotension after a single dose, whether given IV or IM. Therefore, patients receiving the drug should be supine; monitor blood pressure closely during drug administration and several times thereafter until the blood pressure is stable. Have equipment for emergency resuscitation readily available. If pentamidine is administered IV, infuse over 60 minutes.

Hypoglycemia: Pentamidine-induced hypoglycemia has been associated with pancreatic islet cell necrosis and inappropriately high plasma insulin concentrations. Hyperglycemia and diabetes mellitus, with or without preceding hypoglycemia, also have occurred, sometimes several months after therapy. Therefore, monitor blood glucose levels daily during therapy and several times thereafter.

Pulmonary: Inhalation of pentamidine isethionate may induce bronchospasm or cough, particularly in patients who have a history of smoking or asthma. In patients who experience bronchospasm or cough, administration of an inhaled bronchodilator prior to giving each pentamidine dose may minimize recurrence of the symptoms.

Extrapulmonary infection with *P. carinii* has been reported infrequently with inhalation use.

Laboratory tests – Laboratory tests to perform before, during, and after therapy:

1.) Daily BUN, serum creatinine and blood glucose.
2.) Complete blood count and platelet counts.
3.) Liver function test, including bilirubin, alkaline phosphatase, AST, and ALT.

4.) Serum calcium.
5.) ECG at regular intervals.

Pregnancy: Category C.

Lactation: It is not known whether pentamidine is excreted in breast milk. Because of the potential for serious adverse reactions in nursing infants, decide whether to discontinue nursing or to discontinue the drug, taking into account the importance of the drug to the mother.

Children: Safety and efficacy of inhalation solution have not been established.

Adverse Reactions

Injection – 244 of 424 (57.5%) patients treated with pentamidine injection developed some adverse reaction. Most of the patients had acquired immunodeficiency syndrome (AIDS). In the following, "severe" refers to life-threatening reactions or reactions that required immediate corrective measures and led to discontinuation of pentamidine.

Severe – Leukopenia (less than 1000/mm^3) 2.8%; hypoglycemia (less than 25 mg/dL) 2.4%; thrombocytopenia (less than 20,000/mm^3) 1.7%; hypotension (less than 60 mm Hg systolic) 0.9%; acute renal failure (serum creatinine greater than 6 mg/dL) 0.5%; hypocalcemia (0.2%); Stevens-Johnson syndrome and ventricular tachycardia (0.2%); fatalities caused by severe hypotension, hypoglycemia, and cardiac arrhythmias.

Adverse reactions occurring in at least 3% of patients include elevated serum creatinine; sterile abscess, pain, or induration at the IM injection site; elevated liver function tests; leukopenia; nausea; anorexia; hypotension; fever; hypoglycemia; rash; bad taste in mouth; shortness of breath; dizziness; cough; pharyngitis; chest pain/congestion; night sweats; chills; vomiting; bronchospasm; pneumothorax; diarrhea; headache; anemia (generally associated with zidovudine use), myalgia; abdominal pain; edema.

Adverse reactions may also include tachycardia; hypertension; palpitations; syncope; cerebrovascular accident; vasodilation; vasculitis; gingivitis; dyspepsia; oral ulcer/abscess; gastritis; gastric ulcer; hypersalivation; dry mouth; splenomegaly; melena; hematochezia; esophagitis; colitis; pancreatitis; pancytopenia; neutropenia; eosinophilia; thrombocytopenia; hepatitis; hepatomegaly; hepatic dysfunction; renal failure; flank pain; nephritis; tremors; confusion; anxiety; memory loss; seizure; neuropathy; paresthesia; insomnia; hypesthesia; drowsiness; emotional lability; vertigo; paranoia; neuralgia; hallucination; depression; unsteady gait; rhinitis; laryngitis; pneumonitis; pleuritis; cyanosis; tachypnea; rales; pruritus; erythema; dry skin; desquamation; urticaria; eye discomfort; conjunctivitis; blurred vision; blepharitis; loss of taste and smell; incontinence; miscarriage; arthralgia; allergic reactions; extrapulmonary pneumocystosis.

TINIDAZOLE

Tablets; oral: 250 and 500 mg (*Rx*)	*Tindamax* (Mission Pharmacal)

Warning:

Carcinogenicity has been seen in mice and rats treated chronically with metronidazole; the 2 drugs are structurally related and have similar biologic effects. Although such data have not been reported for tinidazole, avoid unnecessary use. Reserve tinidazole use for the conditions described in Indications.

Indications

Amebiasis: For the treatment of intestinal amebiasis and amebic liver abscess caused by *Entamoeba histolytica* in adults and children older than 3 years of age.

Bacterial vaginosis: For the treatment of bacterial vaginosis (formerly referred to as *Haemophilus* vaginitis, *Gardnerella* vaginitis, nonspecific vaginitis, or anaerobic vaginosis) in nonpregnant women.

Giardiasis: For the treatment of giardiasis caused by *Giardia duodenalis* (also termed *Giardia lamblia*) in adults and children older than 3 years of age.

Trichomoniasis: For the treatment of trichomoniasis caused by *Trichomonas vaginalis* in female and male patients. Because trichomoniasis is a sexually transmitted disease with potentially serious sequelae, partners of infected patients should be treated simultaneously in order to prevent reinfection.

Administration and Dosage

Take tinidazole with food to minimize the incidence of epigastric discomfort and other GI side effects.

Tinidazole Dosing Regimens

Indication	Adult dose	Pediatric dose (≥ 3 years of age)	Duration of therapy
Amebiasis			
Amebic liver abscess	2 g/day	50 mg/kg/day (up to 2 g)	3 to 5 days
Intestinal	2 g/day	50 mg/kg/day (up to 2 g)	3 days
Giardiasis	2 g	50 mg/kg (up to 2 g)	Single dose
Trichomoniasis	2 g	—	Single dose
Bacterial vaginosis	2 g/day	—	2 days
	1 g/day	—	5 days

Dosing in hemodialysis patients: If tinidazole is administered on a day when dialysis is performed, administer an additional dose of tinidazole equivalent to one half the recommended dose after the end of the hemodialysis.

Extemporaneous oral suspension: Grind four 500 mg oral tablets to a fine powder with a mortar and pestle. Add approximately 10 mL of cherry syrup to the powder and mix until smooth. Transfer the suspension to a graduated amber container. Use several small rinses of cherry syrup to transfer any remaining drug in the mortar to the final suspension for a final volume of 30 mL. The suspension of crushed tablets in artificial cherry syrup (*Humco*) is stable for 7 days at room temperature. When this suspension is used, shake well before each administration.

Actions

Pharmacology:

Mechanism of action – Tinidazole is an antiprotozoal agent.

Pharmacokinetics:

Absorption – After oral administration, tinidazole is rapidly and completely absorbed. Steady-state conditions are reached in 2½ to 3 days of multi-day dosing. Administration of tinidazole tablets with food resulted in a delay in time to maximum plasma concentration of approximately 2 hours and a decline in maximum plasma concentration of approximately 10% compared with fasted conditions. Administration of tinidazole with food did not affect area under the curve or half-life in this study.

Distribution – Tinidazole is distributed into virtually all tissues and body fluids and crosses the blood-brain barrier. The apparent volume of distribution is approximately 50 L. Plasma protein binding of tinidazole is 12%. Tinidazole crosses the placental barrier and is secreted in breast milk.

Metabolism – Tinidazole is partly metabolized by oxidation, hydroxylation, and conjugation. Tinidazole is biotransformed mainly by CYP3A4.

Excretion – The plasma half-life of tinidazole is approximately 12 to 14 hours. Tinidazole is excreted by the liver and the kidneys.

During hemodialysis, clearance of tinidazole is significantly increased; the half-life is reduced from 12 to 4.9 hours.

Contraindications

Hypersensitivity to tinidazole, any component of the tablet, or other nitroimidazole derivatives; during the first trimester of pregnancy.

Warnings/Precautions

Neurologic effects: Convulsive seizures and peripheral neuropathy, the latter characterized mainly by numbness or paresthesia of an extremity, have been reported in patients treated with nitroimidazole drugs including tinidazole and metronidazole. The appearance of abnormal neurologic signs demands the prompt discontinuation of tinidazole therapy. Administer tinidazole with caution to patients with central nervous system diseases.

Vaginal candidiasis: The use of tinidazole may result in *Candida* vaginitis.

Hematologic effects: Use with caution in patients with evidence of or history of blood dyscrasia. Tinidazole may produce transient leukopenia and neutropenia. Total and differential leukocyte counts are recommended if retreatment is necessary.

Drug resistance: Prescribing tinidazole in the absence of a proven or strongly suspected bacterial infection or a prophylactic indication is unlikely to provide benefit to the patient and increases the risk of the development of drug-resistant bacteria.

Hepatic function impairment: Patients with severe hepatic disease metabolize nitroimidazoles slowly, with resultant accumulation of parent drug in the plasma. For patients with hepatic dysfunction, cautiously administer the usual recommended doses of tinidazole.

Pregnancy: Category C.

Lactation: Tinidazole is excreted in breast milk in concentrations similar to those seen in serum. Tinidazole can be detected in breast milk for up to 72 hours following administration. Interruption of breast-feeding is recommended during tinidazole therapy and for 3 days following the last dose.

Children: Other than for use in the treatment of giardiasis and amebiasis in children older than 3 years of age, safety and efficacy of tinidazole in children have not been established.

Elderly: In general, dose selection for an elderly patient should be cautious, reflecting the greater frequency of decreased hepatic, renal, or cardiac function, and of concomitant disease or other drug therapy.

Drug Interactions

The following drug interactions were reported for metronidazole, a chemically related nitroimidazole. Therefore, these drug interactions may occur with tinidazole. Drugs that may affect tinidazole include cholestyramine, CYP3A4 inducers and inhibitors, and oxytetracycline. Drugs that may be affected by tinidazole include alcohols, anticoagulants, cyclosporine, tacrolimus, disulfiram, fluorouracil, hydantoins, and lithium.

Drug/Lab test interactions: Tinidazole may interfere with certain serum chemistry values, such as aspartate aminotransferase AST, ALT, lactate dehydrogenase, triglycerides, and hexokinase glucose.

Adverse Reactions

Adverse reactions occurring in at least 3% of patients include the following: metallic/bitter taste and nausea.

ATOVAQUONE

Suspension: 750 mg per 5 mL (*Rx*)	*Mepron* (GlaxoSmithKline)

Indications

Pneumocystis carinii pneumonia (PCP): Prevention of PCP in patients who are intolerant to trimethoprim-sulfamethoxazole (TMP-SMZ).

Acute oral treatment of mild to moderate PCP in patients who are intolerant to TMP-SMZ.

Administration and Dosage

Prevention of PCP:

Adults and adolescents 13 to 16 years of age – 1500 mg once daily with a meal.

Treatment of mild to moderate PCP:

Adults and adolescents 13 to 16 years of age – 750 mg administered with food twice daily for 21 days (total daily dose 1500 mg).

Failure to administer with food may result in lower atovaquone plasma concentrations and may limit response to therapy.

Actions

Pharmacology: Atovaquone, an analog of ubiquinone, is an antiprotozoal with antipneumocystis activity.

Pharmacokinetics: Absorption is enhanced approximately 2-fold when given with food. Atovaquone is extensively bound to plasma proteins (greater than 99.9%). CSF concentratons are less than 1% of plasma concentrations. Half-life ranged from 67 to 77.6 hours following the suspension. The long half-life is caused by presumed enterohepatic cycling and eventual fecal elimination. There is indirect evidence that atovaquone may undergo limited metabolism; however, a specific metabolite has not been identified.

Contraindications

Development or history of potentially life-threatening allergic reactions to any of the components of the formulation.

Warnings/Precautions

Severe PCP: Clinical experience has been limited to patients with mild to moderate PCP. Treatment of more severe episodes of PCP has not been systematically studied. Atovaquone efficacy in patients who are failing therapy with TMP-SMZ has not been systematically studied.

Absorption: Absorption of atovaquone is limited but can be significantly increased when the drug is taken with food. Plasma concentrations correlate with the likelihood of successful treatment and survival. GI disorders may limit absorption of orally administered drugs. Patients with these disorders also may not achieve plasma concentrations of atovaquone associated with response to therapy in controlled trials.

Concurrent pulmonary conditions: Atovaquone is not effective therapy for concurrent pulmonary conditions such as bacterial, viral, or fungal pneumonia or mycobacterial diseases. Clinical deterioration in patients may be due to infections with other pathogens, as well as progressive PCP.

Hepatic function impairment: Use caution in patients with severe hepatic impairment, and closely monitor administration.

Pregnancy: Category C.

Lactation: It is not known whether atovaquone is excreted into breast milk.

Children: Safety and efficacy have not been established. Preliminary analysis suggests that the pharmacokinetics are age-dependent.

Elderly: Dose selection for an elderly patient should be cautious. Exercise caution when treating elderly patients reflecting the greater frequency of decreased hepatic, renal, and cardiac function.

Drug Interactions

Use caution when administering atovaquone concurrently with other highly plasma protein bound drugs with narrow therapeutic indices as competition for binding sites may occur.

Drugs that may interact include rifamycins, TMP-SMZ, and zidovudine.

Drug/Food interactions: Administering atovaquone with food enhances its absorption by approximately 2-fold.

Adverse Reactions

Adverse reactions occurring in at least 3% of patients include rash (including maculopapular), nausea, diarrhea, headache, vomiting, fever, cough, insomnia, asthenia, pruritus, monilia (oral), abdominal pain, constipation, dizziness, anemia, neutropenia, elevated ALT and AST, elevated alkaline phosphatase, elevated amylase, hyponatremia, pain, sweating, anxiety, anorexia, sinusitis, dyspepsia, rhinitis, and taste perversion.

ANTHELMINTICS

The following table lists the major parasitic infections, causative organisms, and drugs of choice for treatment.

Major Parasite Infections

	Infection (common name)	Organism	Drug(s) of Choice
Intestinal Nematodes	Ascariasis[a] (Roundworm)	*Ascaris lumbricoides*	Mebendazole, Pyrantel pamoate, or Diethylcarbamazine
	Uncinariasis (Hookworm)	*Ancylostoma duodenale* *Necator americanus*	Mebendazole or Pyrantel pamoate[b]
	Strongyloidiasis (Threadworm)	*Strongyloides stercoralis*	Thiabendazole
	Trichuriasis (Whipworm)	*Trichuris trichiura*	Mebendazole
	Enterobiasis[c] (Pinworm)	*Enterobius vermicularis*	Mebendazole, Pyrantel pamoate, or Albendazole
	Capillariasis	*Capillaria philippinensis*	Mebendazole or Thiabendazole
Tissue Nematodes	Trichinosis	*Trichinella spiralis*	Steroids for severe symptoms plus Thiabendazole, Albendazole, Flubendazole,[d] or Mebendazole[b]
	Cutaneous larva migrans (creeping eruption)	*Ancylostoma braziliense* and others	Thiabendazole, Albendazole, or Ivermectin[e]
	Onchocerciasis (River blindness)	*Onchocerca volvulus*	Suramin,[f] Diethylcarbamazine, or Ivermectin[e]
	Dracontiasis (guinea worm)	*Dracunculus medinensis*	Thiabendazole or Mebendazole
	Angiostrongyliasis (rat lungworm)	*Angiostrongylus cantonensis*	Thiabendazole or Mebendazole
	Loiasis	*Loa loa*	Diethylcarbamazine
Cestodes	Taeniasis (Beef tapeworm)	*Taenia saginata*	Praziquantel[b] or Niclosamide
	(Pork tapeworm)	*Taenia solium*	Praziquantel,[b] Niclosamide, or Albendazole
	Diphyllobothriasis (Fish tapeworm)	*Diphyllobothrium latum*	Praziquantel[b] or Niclosamide
	Dog tapeworm	*Dipylidium caninum*	Praziquantel[b]
	Hymenolepiasis (Dwarf tapeworm)	*Hymenolepis nana*	Praziquantel[b] or Niclosamide[d]
	Hydatid cysts	*Echinococcus granulosus*	Albendazole or Praziquantel
Trematodes	Schistosomiasis	*Schistosoma mansoni*	Praziquantel or Oxamniquine
		Schistosoma japonicum	Praziquantel
		Schistosoma haematobium	Praziquantel
		Schistosoma mekongi	Praziquantel
	Hermaphroditic Flukes Fasciolopsiasis (Intestinal fluke)	*Fasciolopsis buski*	Praziquantel
		Heterophyes heterophyes *Metagonimus yokogawai*	Praziquantel
	Clonorchiasis (Chinese liver fluke)	*Clonorchis sinensis*	Praziquantel
	Fascioliasis (Sheep liver fluke)	*Fasciola hepatica*	Praziquantel or Bithionol[e]
	Opisthorchiasis (Liver fluke)	*Opisthorchis viverrini*	Praziquantel
	Paragonimiasis (Lung fluke)	*Paragonimus westermani*	Praziquantel or Bithionol[e] (alternate)

[a] The following drugs also are indicated in *Ascariasis*: Piperazine citrate (if intestinal or biliary obstruction); thiabendazole.

[b] Unlabeled use.

[c] The following drugs also are indicated in *Enterobiasis*: Piperazine and thiabendazole.

[d] Not available in the US.

[e] Available from the CDC.

[f] Available from the CDC, although generally not recommended.

Chapter 10

BIOLOGIC AND IMMUNOLOGIC AGENTS

DENOSUMAB

Injection, solution: 60 mg/mL (*Rx*)	*Prolia* (Amgen)
70 mg/mL (*Rx*)	*Xgeva* (Amgen)

Indications

Bone metastasis from solid tumors (Xgeva only): For the prevention of skeletal-related events in patients with bone metastases from solid tumors.

Osteoporosis (Prolia only): For the treatment of postmenopausal women with osteoporosis at high risk for fracture, defined as a history of osteoporotic fracture, or multiple risk factors for fracture; or patients who have failed or are intolerant to other available osteoporosis therapies.

Administration and Dosage

Individuals sensitive to latex should not handle the gray needle cap on the single-use prefilled syringe, which contains dry natural rubber (a derivative of latex).

Bone metastasis from solid tumors (Xgeva only): The usual dosage is 120 mg subcutaneously every 4 weeks. Administer with calcium and vitamin D as necessary to treat or prevent hypocalcemia.

Osteoporosis (Prolia only): The usual dosage is 60 mg subcutaneously once every 6 months. All patients should receive 1,000 mg of calcium daily and at least 400 units of vitamin D daily.

Missed dose – If a dose of denosumab is missed, administer the injection as soon as the patient is available. Thereafter, schedule injections every 6 months from the date of the last injection.

Actions

Pharmacology: Denosumab binds to receptor activator of nuclear factor kappa-B ligand (RANKL), a transmembrane or soluble protein essential for the formation, function, and survival of osteoclasts, the cells responsible for bone resorption.

Pharmacokinetics:

Absorption – Following a single subcutaneous dose of denosumab 60 mg after fasting (for at least 12 hours), the mean maximum denosumab concentration (C_{max}) was 6.75 mcg/mL (standard deviation [SD], 1.89 mcg/mL). The median time to denosumab C_{max} was 10 days (range, 3 to 21 days). After C_{max}, serum denosumab concentrations declined over a period of 4 to 5 months. The mean denosumab area under the curve up to 16 weeks ($AUC_{0\text{-}16\ weeks}$) was 316 mcg•day/mL (SD, 101 mcg•day/mL).

Excretion – Denosumab has a mean half-life of 25.4 days (SD, 8.5 days; n = 46).

Contraindications

Hypocalcemia.

Warnings/Precautions

Hypocalcemia and mineral metabolism: Hypocalcemia may be exacerbated by the use of denosumab. Preexisting hypocalcemia must be corrected prior to initiating therapy with denosumab.

Hypocalcemia following denosumab administration is a significant risk in patients with severe renal impairment (CrCl less than 30 mL/min) or receiving dialysis.

Adequately supplement all patients with calcium and vitamin D.

Serious infections: In a clinical trial of women with postmenopausal osteoporosis, serious infections leading to hospitalization were reported more frequently in the denosumab group than in the placebo group. Serious skin infections, as well as infections of the abdomen, urinary tract, and ear, and endocarditis were more frequent in patients treated with denosumab.

Patients on concomitant immunosuppressant agents or with impaired immune systems may be at increased risk for serious infections.

Dermatologic effects: In a clinical trial of women with postmenopausal osteoporosis, epidermal and dermal adverse reactions, such as dermatitis, eczema, and rashes, occurred at a significantly higher rate in the denosumab group.

Osteonecrosis of the jaw: Osteonecrosis of the jaw, which can occur spontaneously, is generally associated with tooth extraction and/or local infection with delayed healing.

Long-term use: In clinical trials in women with postmenopausal osteoporosis, treatment with denosumab resulted in significant suppression of bone remodeling as evidenced by markers of bone turnover and bone histomorphometry.

Immunogenicity: Denosumab is a human monoclonal antibody. As with all therapeutic proteins, there is potential for immunogenicity.

Renal function impairment: In clinical studies, patients with severe renal impairment (CrCl less than 30 mL/min) or receiving dialysis were at greater risk of developing hypocalcemia.

Pregnancy: Category C.

Pregnancy registry – Women who become pregnant during denosumab treatment are encouraged to enroll in the manufacturer's Pregnancy Surveillance Program. Patients or their health care provider should call 1-800-772-6436 to enroll.

Lactation: It is not known whether denosumab is excreted into human milk.

Children: Denosumab is not recommended in children.

Monitoring: Monitor patients for the development of infections. Monitor patients in long-term therapy for the development of osteonecrosis of the jaw, atypical fractures, and delayed fracture healing.

Drug Interactions

None well documented.

Adverse Reactions

Adverse reactions occurring in 3% or more of people include the following: abdominal pain (upper), anemia, back pain, bone pain, cystitis, edema (peripheral), hypercholesterolemia, insomnia, musculoskeletal pain, pain in extremity, pneumonia, sciatica, upper respiratory tract infection, vertigo.

AZATHIOPRINE

Tablets; oral: 50 mg (*Rx*)	Various, *Imuran* (Prometheus)
75 and 100 mg (*Rx*)	*Azasan* (aaiPharma)
Injection: 100 mg (as sodium)/vial (*Rx*)	Various, *Imuran* (GlaxoSmithKline)

Warning:

Chronic immunosuppression with azathioprine increases the risk of neoplasia. Physicians using this drug should be familiar with this risk as well as with the mutagenic potential to men and women and with possible hematologic toxicities.

Indications

Renal homotransplantation: As an adjunct for the prevention of rejection in renal homotransplantation.

Rheumatoid arthritis: Indicated only in adult patients meeting criteria for classic or definite rheumatoid arthritis as specified by the American Rheumatism Association. Restrict use to patients with severe, active, and erosive disease not responsive to conventional management.

Administration and Dosage

Renal homotransplantation: Initial dose is usually 3 to 5 mg/kg/day, given as a single daily dose on the day of transplantation, and in a minority of cases, 1 to 3 days before transplantation. It is often initiated IV, with subsequent use of tablets (at the same dose level) after the postoperative period. Reserve IV administration for patients unable to tolerate oral medications. Maintenance levels are 1 to 3 mg/kg/day.

Children – An initial dose of 3 to 5 mg/kg/day IV or orally followed by a maintenance dose of 1 to 3 mg/kg/day has been recommended.

Rheumatoid arthritis: Initial dose is approximately 1 mg/kg (50 to 100 mg) given as a single dose or twice daily. The dose may be increased, beginning at 6 to 8 weeks and thereafter by steps at 4-week intervals, if there are no serious toxicities and if initial response is unsatisfactory. Use dose increments of 0.5 mg/kg/day, up to a maximum dose of 2.5 mg/kg/day.

Use the lowest effective dose for maintenance therapy; lower decrementally with changes of 0.5 mg/kg or approximately 25 mg/day every 4 weeks while other therapy is kept constant.

Renal function impairment: Relatively oliguric patients, especially those with tubular necrosis in the immediate postcadaveric transplant period, may have delayed clearance of azathioprine or its metabolites.

Use with allopurinol: Reduce dose of azathioprine to approximately 25% to 33% of the usual dose.

Actions

Pharmacology: Azathioprine, an imidazoyl derivative of 6-mercaptopurine (6-MP), has many biological effects similar to those of the parent compound.

Homograft survival – Although the use of azathioprine for inhibition of renal homograft rejection is well established, the mechanism(s) for this action are obscure.

Immuno-inflammatory response – The severity of adjuvant arthritis is reduced by azathioprine. The mechanisms whereby it affects autoimmune diseases are not known.

Pharmacokinetics: Azathioprine is well absorbed following oral administration. Blood levels are of little value for therapy because the magnitude and duration of clinical effects correlate with thiopurine nucleotide levels in tissues rather than with plasma drug levels.

Contraindications

Hypersensitivity to azathioprine; pregnancy in rheumatoid arthritis patients.

Warnings/Precautions

Hematologic effects: Severe leukopenia or thrombocytopenia, macrocytic anemia, severe bone marrow depression, and selective erythrocyte aplasia may occur in patients on azathioprine. Hematologic toxicities are dose-related, may occur late in the course of therapy, and may be more severe in renal transplant patients whose homograft is undergoing rejection. Perform complete blood counts, including platelet counts, weekly during the first month, twice monthly for the second and third months of treatment, then monthly or more frequently if dosage alterations or other therapy changes are necessary.

Infections: Serious infections are a constant hazard for patients on chronic immunosuppression, especially for homograft recipients. The incidence of infection in renal homotransplantation is 30 to 60 times that in rheumatoid arthritis. Fungal, viral, bacterial, and protozoal infections may be fatal and should be treated vigorously.

GI toxicity: A GI hypersensitivity reaction characterized by severe nausea and vomiting has been reported. These symptoms also may be accompanied by diarrhea, rash, fever, malaise, myalgias, elevations in liver enzymes, and, occasionally, hypotension.

Hepatotoxicity: Hepatotoxicity with elevated serum alkaline phosphatase and bilirubin may occur primarily in allograft recipients. Periodically measure serum transaminases, alkaline phosphatase and bilirubin for early detection of hepatotoxicity.

Carcinogenesis: Azathioprine is carcinogenic in animals and may increase the patient's risk of neoplasia.

Mutagenesis: Azathioprine is mutagenic in animals and humans.

Pregnancy: Category D.

Lactation: Use of azathioprine in nursing mothers is not recommended.

Children: Safety and efficacy in children have not been established. However, azathioprine has been used in children.

Drug Interactions

Drugs that may affect azathioprine include ACE inhibitors, allopurinol, and methotrexate.

Drugs that may be affected by azathioprine include anticoagulants, cyclosporine, and nondepolarizing neuromuscular blockers.

Adverse Reactions

The principal and potentially serious toxic effects are hematologic and GI. Adverse reactions may include leukopenia, infections, and neoplasia.

TACROLIMUS (FK506)

Capsules; oral: 0.5, 1, and 5 mg (*Rx*)	Various, *Prograf* (Astellas)
Injection: 5 mg/mL (*Rx*)	*Prograf* (Astellas)

Tacrolimus also is available as a cream for moderate to severe atopic dermatitis; refer to the Dermatologics chapter.

Warning:

Increased susceptibility to infection and the possible development of lymphoma may result from immunosuppression. Manage patients receiving the drug in facilities equipped and staffed with adequate laboratory and supportive medical resources.

Indications

Organ rejection prophylaxis: Prophylaxis of organ rejection in patients receiving allogeneic liver, heart, or kidney transplants. It is recommended that tacrolimus be used concomitantly with adrenal corticosteroids. In heart and kidney transplant recipients, it is recommended that tacrolimus be used in conjunction with azathioprine or mycophenolate mofetil. Because of the risk of anaphylaxis, reserve the injection for patients unable to take the capsules orally.

Unlabeled uses:

Crohn disease – According to an American Gastroenterological Association position statement, the potential toxicities of tacrolimus make it appropriate for use in the treatment of Crohn disease only in patients with complex perianal fistulas who have failed multiple other treatments. Although some studies have enrolled children, the majority of reported experience is in patients 12 years of age and older

Pyoderma gangrenosum – A limited number of individual case reports suggest oral tacrolimus may be an effective treatment for pyoderma gangrenosum.

Administration and Dosage

Injection: For intravenous (IV) infusion only.

In patients unable to take the capsules, therapy may be initiated with the injection. Administer the initial dose no sooner than 6 hours after transplantation. The recommended starting dose for kidney and liver transplant in adults and children is 0.03 to 0.05 mg/kg/day as a continuous IV infusion and for heart transplant in adults is 0.01 mg/kg/day as a continuous IV infusion. Give adult patients doses at the lower end of the dosing range. Concomitant adrenal corticosteroid therapy is recommended early posttransplantation. Proceed with continuous IV infusion only until the patient can tolerate oral administration.

Oral:

Tacrolimus Oral Dose Recommendations and Typical Whole Blood Trough Concentrations

Patient population	Recommended initial oral dose[a]	Typical whole blood trough concentrations
Adult kidney transplant patients	0.2 mg/kg/day	Month 1 through 3: 7 to 20 ng/mL Month 4 through 12: 5 to 15 ng/mL
Adult liver transplant patients	0.1 to 0.15 mg/kg/day	Month 1 through 12: 5 to 20 ng/mL
Pediatric liver transplant patients	0.15 to 0.2 mg/kg/day	Month 1 to 12: 5 to 20 ng/mL
Adult heart transplant patients	0.075 mg/kg/day	Month 1 through 3: 10 to 20 ng/mL Month ≥ 4: 5 to 15 ng/mL

[a] Two divided doses every 12 hours.

Heart transplantation – The recommended starting oral dose is 0.075 mg/kg/day administered every 12 hours in 2 divided doses. If possible, initiating oral therapy with tacrolimus capsules is recommended. If IV therapy is necessary, conversion from IV to oral tacrolimus is recommended as soon as oral therapy can be tolerated. This usually occurs within 2 to 3 days. The initial dose of tacrolimus should be administered no sooner than 6 hours after transplantation. In a patient receiving an IV infusion, the first dose of oral therapy should be given 8 to 12 hours after discontinuing the IV infusion.

Dosing should be titrated based on clinical assessments of rejection and tolerability. Lower tacrolimus dosages may be sufficient as maintenance therapy. Adjunct therapy with adrenal corticosteroids is recommended early posttransplant.

Kidney transplantation – The initial dose is 0.2 mg/kg/day in combination with azathioprine or 0.1 mg/kg/day when used in combination with mycophenolate mofetil and interleukin-2 receptor antagonist. Administer in 2 divided doses, given every 12 hours. It is recommended that tacrolimus be used in conjunction with azathioprine or mycophenolate mofetil and interleukin-2 receptor antagonist. The initial dose of tacrolimus may be administered within 24 hours of transplantation, but should be delayed until renal function has recovered (as indicated, for example, by a serum creatinine of 4 mg/dL or less). Black patients may require higher doses to achieve comparable blood concentrations.

The data in kidney transplant patients indicate that the black patients required a higher dose to attain comparable trough concentrations compared with white patients.

Tacrolimus Dosing Recommendations by Race				
	White (n = 114)		Black (n = 56)	
Time after transplant	Dose (mg/kg)	Trough concentrations (ng/mL)	Dose (mg/kg)	Trough concentrations (ng/mL)
Day 7	0.18	12	0.23	10.9
Month 1	0.17	12.8	0.26	12.9
Month 6	0.14	11.8	0.24	11.5
Month 12	0.13	10.1	0.19	11

Liver transplant – The initial dose is 0.1 to 0.15 mg/kg/day administered in 2 divided daily doses every 12 hours. The initial dose should be administered no sooner than 6 hours after transplantation. In a patient receiving an IV infusion, the first dose of oral therapy should be given 8 to 12 hours after discontinuing the IV infusion.

Dosing should be titrated based on clinical assessments of rejection and tolerability. Lower tacrolimus dosages may be sufficient as maintenance therapy. Adjunct therapy with adrenal corticosteroids is recommended early posttransplant.

If IV therapy is necessary, conversion from IV to oral tacrolimus is recommended as soon as oral therapy can be tolerated. This usually occurs within 2 to 3 days.

Children (under 12 years of age): It is recommended that therapy be initiated in children at the high end of the recommended adult IV and oral dosing ranges (0.0.3 to 0.05 mg/kg/day IV and 0.15 to 0.2 mg/kg/day oral).

Hepatic/Renal function impairment – Because of the reduced clearance and prolonged half-life, patients with severe hepatic impairment (Child-Pugh score of 10 or more) may require lower doses of tacrolimus. Close monitoring of blood concentrations is warranted.

Because of the potential for nephrotoxicity, give patients with renal or hepatic impairment doses at the lowest value of the recommended IV and oral dosing ranges. Therapy may need to be delayed by up to 48 hours or longer in patients with postoperative oliguria.

Conversion from one immunosuppressive regimen to another – Do not use tacrolimus simultaneously with cyclosporine. Discontinue either agent at least 24 hours before initiating the other.

Unlabeled dosing:

Crohn disease – Tacrolimus 0.1 mg/kg orally twice daily, adjusted to maintain serum concentrations of 10 to 20 ng/mL, or 1 g topically twice daily. Therapy can continue until maximal benefit is achieved and then be discontinued, or it may be continued long term for maintenance therapy.

Pyoderma gangrenosum – 0.1 mg/kg/day for 3 months as adjunctive therapy or monotherapy (range, 0.1 to 0.3 mg/kg/day in divided doses for 1 month to 2 years).

Actions

Pharmacology: Tacrolimus is a macrolide immunosuppressant that prolongs the survival of the host and transplanted graft and inhibits T-lymphocyte activation, although the exact mechanism of action is not known.

Pharmacokinetics:

Pharmacokinetic Parameters of Tacrolimus[a]

Population	n	Route (dose)	C_{max} (ng/mL)	T_{max} (h)	AUC (ng•h/mL)	t½ (h)	Clearance (L/h/kg)	Volume (L/kg)
Healthy volunteers	8	IV (0.025 mg/kg/4 h)	—[b]	—	≈ 598[c] ± 125	≈ 34.2 ± 7.7	≈ 0.04 ± 0.009	≈ 1.91 ± 0.31
	16	Orally (5 mg)	≈ 29.7 ± 7.2	≈ 1.6 ± 0.7	≈ 243[d] ± 73	≈ 34.8 ± 11.4	≈ 0.041[e] ± 0.008	≈ 1.94[e] ± 0.53
Kidney transplant patients	26	IV (0.02 mg/kg/12 h)	—	—	≈ 294[f] ± 262	≈ 18.8 ± 16.7	≈ 0.083 ± 0.050	1.41 ± 0.66
		Orally (0.2 mg/kg/day)	≈ 19.2 ± 10.3	3	≈ 203[f] ± 42	NA[g]	NA	NA
		Orally (0.3 mg/kg/day)	≈ 24.2 ± 15.8	1.5	≈ 288[f] ± 93	NA	NA	NA
Liver transplant patients	17	IV (0.05 mg/kg/12 h)	—	—	≈ 3,300[f] ± 2,130	≈ 11.7 ± 3.9	≈ 0.053 ± 0.017	≈ 0.85 ± 0.30
		Orally (0.3 mg/kg/day)	≈ 68.5 ± 30.00	≈ 2.3 ± 1.5	≈ 519[f] ± 179	NA	NA	NA
Heart transplant patients	11	IV (0.01 mg/kg/day as a continuous infusion)	—	—	954[h] ± 334	23.6 ± 9.22	0.051 ± 0.015	NA
	11	Orally (0.075mg/kg/day)[i]	14.7 ± 7.79	2.1 [0.5 -6.0][j]	82.7[k] ± 63.2	—	NA	NA
	14	Orally (0.15mg/kg/day)[i]	24.5 ± 13.7	1.5 [0.4 -4.0][j]	142[k] ± 116	—	NA	NA

[a] C_{max} = maximal plasma concentration; T_{max} = time to maximal plasma concentration; AUC = area under the curve; t½ = half-life.
[b] — = Not applicable
[c] AUC_{0-120}
[d] AUC_{0-72}
[e] Corrected for individual bioavailability.
[f] $AUC_{0-\infty}$
[g] NA = not available
[h] AUC_{0-t}
[i] Determined after the first dose
[j] Median [range]
[k] AUC_{0-12}

The plasma protein binding of tacrolimus is approximately 99%. Tacrolimus is bound mainly to albumin and alpha-1 acid glycoprotein and has a high level of association with erythrocytes. It is extensively metabolized by the mixed-function oxidase system, primarily the cytochrome P450 system (CYP3A). The disposition of tacrolimus from whole blood was biphasic, with a terminal elimination half-life of 11.7 hours in liver transplant patients.

Contraindications

Hypersensitivity to tacrolimus.

Warnings/Precautions

Insulin-dependent posttransplant diabetes mellitus: Insulin-dependent posttransplant diabetes mellitus (PTDM) was reported in 20% of tacrolimus-treated kidney patients without pretransplant history of diabetes mellitus in the phase 3 study. The median time to onset of PTDM was 68 days. Insulin dependence was reversible in 15% of these PTDM patients at 1 year and in 50% at 2 years posttransplant. Black and Hispanic kidney transplant patients were at an increased risk of development of PTDM.

Nephrotoxicity: Tacrolimus can cause nephrotoxicity, particularly when used in high doses. Nephrotoxicity has been noted in approximately 52% of kidney transplantation patients and in 40% and 36% of liver transplantation patients receiving the drug in the United States and Europe, respectively.

Hyperkalemia: Mild to severe hyperkalemia has been noted with tacrolimus and may require treatment.

Neurotoxicity: Neurotoxicity, including tremor, headache, and other changes in motor function, mental status, and sensory function occurred in approximately 55% of liver transplant recipients. Tremor occurred more often in tacrolimus-treated kidney transplant patients (54%) compared with cyclosporine-treated patients. Tremor and headache have been associated with high whole-blood concentrations of tacrolimus and may respond to dosage adjustment. Seizures have occurred in adults and children. Coma and delirium also have been associated with high plasma concentrations of tacrolimus.

Lymphomas: As with other immunosuppressants, patients receiving tacrolimus are at increased risk of developing lymphomas and other malignancies, particularly of the skin.

Infections: A lymphoproliferative disorder related to Epstein-Barr virus (EBV) infection has been reported in immunosuppressed organ transplant recipients. The risk of lymphoproliferative disorder appears greatest in young children who are at risk for primary EBV infection while immunosuppressed or who are switched to tacrolimus following long-term immunosuppression therapy.

Latent viral infections – Immunosuppressed patients are at increased risk for opportunistic infections, including activation of latent viral infections.

Tacrolimus in combination with sirolimus: The use of full-dose tacrolimus with sirolimus (2 mg/day) in heart transplant recipients was associated with an increased risk of wound healing complications, renal impairment, and insulin-dependent posttransplant diabetes mellitus and is not recommended.

Hypertension: Hypertension is a common adverse effect of tacrolimus therapy. Mild or moderate hypertension is reported more frequently than severe hypertension.

Myocardial hypertrophy: Myocardial hypertrophy has been reported in association with the administration of tacrolimus and generally is manifested by echocardiographically demonstrated concentric increases in left ventricular posterior wall and interventricular septum thickness. Hypertrophy has been observed in infants, children, and adults. This condition appears reversible in most cases following dose reduction or discontinuance of therapy.

Hypersensitivity reactions: A few patients receiving the injection have experienced anaphylactic reactions. Although the exact cause of these reactions is not known, other drugs with castor oil derivatives in the formulation have been associated with anaphylaxis in a small percentage of patients.

Continuously observe patients receiving the injection for at least the first 30 minutes following the start of the infusion and at frequent intervals thereafter.

Renal/Hepatic function impairment: The use of tacrolimus in liver transplant recipients experiencing posttransplant hepatic impairment may be associated with increased risk of developing renal insufficiency related to high whole-blood levels of tacrolimus.

Photosensitivity: As with other immunosuppressive agents, owing to the potential risk of malignant skin changes, patients should limit their exposure to sunlight and ultraviolet light by wearing protective clothing and using a sunscreen with a high sun protection factor.

Carcinogenesis: An increased incidence of malignancy is a recognized complication of immunosuppression in recipients of organ transplants.

Pregnancy: Category C. The use of tacrolimus during pregnancy has been associated with neonatal hyperkalemia and renal dysfunction.

Lactation: Tacrolimus is excreted in breast milk; avoid breast-feeding.

Children: Experience with tacrolimus in pediatric kidney and heart transplant patients is limited. Successful liver transplants have been performed in children (up to 16 years of age) using tacrolimus. Children generally required higher doses of tacrolimus to maintain blood trough concentrations of tacrolimus similar to those of adult patients.

Monitoring: Regularly assess serum creatinine and potassium. Perform routine monitoring of metabolic and hematologic systems as clinically warranted.

Drug Interactions

Drugs that may affect tacrolimus include nephrotoxic agents (aminoglycosides, amphotericin B, cisplatin, cyclosporine), antifungals, bromocriptine, calcium channel blockers, carbamazepine, chloramphenicol, cimetidine, cisapride, clarithromycin, danazol, diltiazem, erythromycin, fosphenytoin, macrolide antibiotics, methylprednisolone, metoclopramide, metronidazole, nefazodone, omeprazole, phenobarbital, phenytoin, protease inhibitors, rifamycins, and St. John's wort.

Drugs that may be affected by tacrolimus include mycophenolate mofetil and vaccines.

Because tacrolimus is metabolized mainly by the cytochrome P450 3A enzyme systems, substances known to inhibit or induce these enzymes may affect the metabolism of tacrolimus with resultant increases or decreases in whole blood or plasma levels.

Drug/Food interactions: The presence of food reduced the absorption of tacrolimus (decrease in AUC and C_{max} and increase in T_{max}). The relative oral bioavailability (whole blood) was reduced by 27% compared with the fasting state.

Coadministered grapefruit juice has been reported to increase tacrolimus blood trough concentrations in liver transplant patients.

Adverse Reactions

The principal adverse reactions of tacrolimus are diarrhea, headache, hypertension, nausea, renal dysfunction, and tremor. Other reactions may include abdomen enlarged, abdominal pain, abnormal dreams, abnormal thinking, abnormal vision, agitation, alopecia, anemia, anorexia, anxiety, arthralgia, ascites, asthenia, asthma, back pain, bronchitis, chest pain, chills, coagulation disorder, confusion, constipation, convulsion, cough increased, depression, diabetes mellitus, dizziness, dyspnea, ecchymosis, fever, flatulence, generalized spasm, GI hemorrhage, GI perforation, hallucinations, hematuria, hepatitis, hirsutism, hyperglycemia, hyperlipemia, hyperphosphatemia, hyperuricemia, hypocalcemia, hyponatremia, hypophosphatemia, hypotension, incoordination, increased appetite, insomnia, jaundice, leg cramps, leukocytosis, leukopenia, liver damage, myalgia, nervousness, oral moniliasis, paresthesia, peripheral edema, peritonitis, pharyngitis, photosensitivity reaction, prothrombin decreased, pruritus, pulmonary edema, rash, rhinitis, sinusitis, somnolence, sweating, tachycardia, thrombocytopenia, tinnitus, voice alteration, vomiting.

SIROLIMUS

Tablets; oral: 1 and 2 mg (*Rx*)	*Rapamune* (Wyeth)
Solution; oral: 1 mg/mL (*Rx*)	

Warning:

Immunosuppression: Increased susceptibility to infection and the possible development of lymphoma may result from immunosuppression. Only health care providers experienced in immunosuppressive therapy and management of renal transplant patients should use sirolimus. Manage patients receiving the drug in facilities equipped and staffed with adequate laboratory and supportive medical resources. The health care provider responsible for maintenance therapy should have complete information requisite for the follow-up of the patient.

Liver transplantation:

Excess mortality, graft loss, and hepatic artery thrombosis – The use of sirolimus in combination with tacrolimus was associated with excess mortality and graft loss in a study in de novo liver transplant recipients. Many of these patients had evidence of infection at or near the time of death.

In this and another study in de novo liver transplant recipients, the use of sirolimus in combination with cyclosporine or tacrolimus was associated with an increase in hepatic artery thrombosis (HAT); most cases of HAT occurred within 30 days posttransplantation, and most led to graft loss or death. The safety and efficacy of sirolimus as immunosuppressive therapy have not been established in liver transplant patients; therefore, use is not recommended in these patients.

Lung transplantation:

Bronchial anastomotic dehiscence – Cases of bronchial anastomotic dehiscence, most fatal, have been reported in de novo lung transplant patients when sirolimus has been used as part of an immunosuppressive regimen. The safety and efficacy of sirolimus as immunosuppressive therapy have not been established in lung transplant patients; therefore, use is not recommended in these patients.

Indications

Renal transplant: For the prophylaxis of organ rejection in patients 13 years of age and older receiving renal transplants. Therapeutic drug monitoring is recommended for all patients receiving sirolimus.

Administration and Dosage

Sirolimus is to be administered orally once daily consistently with or without food. It is recommended that sirolimus be taken 4 hours after administration of cyclosporine (modified).

Timing of cyclosporine: The initial dose of sirolimus should be administered as soon as possible after transplantation. It is recommended that sirolimus be taken 4 hours after administration of cyclosporine oral solution (modified) and/or cyclosporine capsules (modified).

Low to moderate immunologic risk:

Sirolimus and cyclosporine combination therapy – Administer the initial dose as soon as possible after transplantation. A daily maintenance dose of 2 mg is recommended for use in renal transplant patients, with a 6 mg loading dose.

Sirolimus following cyclosporine withdrawal – At 2 to 4 months following transplantation, progressively discontinue cyclosporine over 4 to 8 weeks and adjust the sirolimus dose to obtain whole blood trough concentrations within the range of 12 to 24 ng/mL.

Once sirolimus maintenance dose is adjusted, retain patients on the new maintenance dose for at least 7 to 14 days before further dosage adjustment. In most patients dose adjustments can be based on simple proportion: new sirolimus dose = current dose × (target concentration/current concentration). Consider a loading dose in addition to a new maintenance dose when it is necessary to considerably increase sirolimus trough concentration: sirolimus loading dose = 3 × (new maintenance dose - current maintenance dose). The maximum sirolimus dose administered on any day should not exceed 40 mg. If an estimated daily dose exceeds 40 mg because of the addition of a loading dose, administer the loading dose over 2 days.

High immunologic risk: In patients with high immunologic risk, it is recommended that sirolimus be used in combination with cyclosporine and corticosteroids for the first 12 months following transplantation.

Initiate with a loading dose of up to 15 mg on day 1 posttransplantation. Beginning on day 2, an initial maintenance dosage of 5 mg/day should be given. A trough level should be obtained between days 5 and 7.

The starting dosage of cyclosporine should be up to 7 mg/kg/day in divided doses. Prednisone should be administered at a minimum of 5 mg/day.

Antibody induction therapy may be used.

Maximum dose: The maximum dose on any day should not exceed 40 mg.

Dosage adjustment: Frequent sirolimus dosage adjustments based on non–steady-state sirolimus concentrations can lead to overdosing or underdosing because sirolimus has a long half-life. Once the sirolimus maintenance dosage is adjusted, patients should continue on the new maintenance dosage for at least 7 to 14 days before further dosage adjustment with concentration monitoring. In most patients, dosage adjustments can be based on a simple proportion: new sirolimus dose = current dose × (target concentration/current concentration). A loading dose should be considered in addition to a new maintenance dosage when it is necessary to increase sirolimus trough concentrations: sirolimus loading dose = 3 × (new maintenance dose − current maintenance dose). The maximum sirolimus dose administered on any day should not exceed 40 mg. If an estimated daily dose exceeds 40 mg because of the addition of a loading dose, the loading dose should be administered over 2 days. Sirolimus trough concentrations should be monitored at least 3 to 4 days after a loading dose(s).

Children:

Low to moderate immunologic risk –

13 years of age and older: The maximum dose is 40 mg daily. For patients weighing 40 kg or more, the loading dose is 6 mg and maintenance dosage is 2 mg. For patients weighing less than 40 kg, the loading dose is 3 mg/m^2 and the maintenance dosage is 1 mg/m^2.

Hepatic function impairment: Reduce the maintenance dose of sirolimus by approximately 33% in patients with hepatic function impairment.

Bioequivalence: 2 mg of oral solution has been demonstrated to be clinically equivalent to 2 mg oral tablets, making them interchangeable on a milligram-to-milligram basis. However, it is not known if higher doses of oral solution are clinically equivalent to higher doses of tablets on a milligram-to-milligram basis. Patients receiving 2 mg/day oral solution demonstrated an overall better safety profile than did patients receiving 5 mg/day oral solution.

Therapeutic drug monitoring: Monitoring of sirolimus trough concentrations is recommended for all patients, especially in those patients likely to have altered drug metabolism, in patients 13 years of age and older who weigh less than 40 kg, in patients with hepatic function impairment, and during coadministration of strong CYP3A4 inducers and inhibitors.

Following cyclosporine withdrawal in transplant patients at low to moderate immunologic risk, the target sirolimus trough concentrations should be 16 to 24 ng/mL for the first year following transplantation. Thereafter, the target sirolimus concentrations should be 12 to 20 ng/mL.

Administration:

Dilution and administration of sirolimus oral solution – The amber oral dose syringe should be used to withdraw the prescribed amount of sirolimus oral solution from the bottle.

Empty the correct amount of sirolimus from the syringe into only a glass or plastic container holding at least 2 ounces (¼ cup, 60 mL) of water or orange juice. No other liquids, especially grapefruit juice, should be used for dilution. Stir vigorously and drink at once. Refill the container with an additional volume (minimum of 4 ounces [½ cup, 120 mL]) of water or orange juice, stir vigorously, and drink at once.

Sirolimus oral solution contains polysorbate 80, which is known to increase the rate of di-(2-ethylhexyl)phthalate extraction from polyvinyl chloride. It is important that the recommendations for administration be followed closely.

Tablets – Tablets should not be crushed, chewed, or split.

Actions

Pharmacology: Sirolimus, a macrolide immunosuppressive agent, inhibits both T-lymphocyte activation and proliferation that occurs in response to antigenic and cytokine (interleukin-2, -4, and -15) stimulation and also inhibits antibody production. In cells, sirolimus binds to the immunophilin, FK binding protein-12 (FKBP-12), to generate an immunosuppressive complex.

Pharmacokinetics:

Absorption – Sirolimus is rapidly absorbed following oral administration, with a mean time-to-peak concentration of approximately 1 hour after a single dose in healthy subjects and approximately 2 hours after multiple oral doses in renal transplant recipients. The systemic bioavailability of sirolimus was estimated to be approximately 14%. The mean bioavailability of sirolimus after administration of the tablet is approximately 27% higher relative to the solution. A loading dose of 3 times the maintenance dose will provide near steady-state concentrations within 1 day in most patients.

Distribution – Sirolimus is extensively bound (approximately 92%) to human plasma proteins. The binding of sirolimus was shown mainly to be associated with serum albumin (97%). Sirolimus also is distributed in high concentrations to the heart, intestines, kidneys, liver, lungs, muscle, spleen, and testes.

Metabolism – Sirolimus is a substrate for both cytochrome P450 IIIA4 (CYP3A4) and P-glycoprotein. Metabolites are detectable in plasma, fecal, and urine samples.

Excretion – After a single dose of sirolimus in healthy volunteers, 91% was recovered from the feces and 2.2% was excreted in urine. The mean half-life of sirolimus after multiple dosing was about 62 ± 16 hours.

Contraindications

Hypersensitivity to sirolimus.

Warnings/Precautions

Infection/Lymphoma/Other malignancies: Increased susceptibility to infection and the possible development of lymphoma and other malignancies, particularly of the skin, may result from immunosuppression. Oversuppression of the immune system can also increase susceptibility to infections, including opportunistic infections, fatal infections, and sepsis.

Liver transplantation: The safety and efficacy of sirolimus as immunosuppressive therapy have not been established in liver transplant patients; therefore, such use is not recommended.

Lung transplantation: The safety and efficacy of sirolimus as immunosuppressive therapy have not been established in lung transplant patients; therefore, such use is not recommended.

Angioedema: Sirolimus has been associated with the development of angioedema. The concomitant use of sirolimus with other drugs known to cause angioedema may increase the risk of developing angioedema.

Wound healing: There have been reports of impaired or delayed wound healing in patients receiving sirolimus.

Fluid accumulation: There have been reports of fluid accumulation, including peripheral edema, lymphedema, pleural effusion, and pericardial effusions in patients receiving sirolimus.

Lipids: Increased serum cholesterol and triglycerides that may require treatment occurred more frequently in patients treated with sirolimus compared with azathioprine or placebo controls.

Proteinuria: Periodic quantitative monitoring of urinary protein excretion is recommended.

Latent viral infections: Immunosuppressed patients are at increased risk for opportunistic infections, including activation of latent viral infections.

Interstitial lung disease: Cases of interstitial lung disease (including pneumonitis, bronchiolitis obliterans organizing pneumonia, and pulmonary fibrosis), some fatal, have occurred in patients receiving immunosuppressive regiments, including sirolimus. In some cases, the interstitial lung disease has resolved upon discontinuation of sirolimus.

De novo use without cyclosporine: The safety and efficacy of de novo use of sirolimus without cyclosporine have not been established in renal transplant patients.

Calcineurin inhibitor–induced reactions: The concomitant use of sirolimus with a calcineurin inhibitor (eg, cyclosporine, tacrolimus) may increase the risk of calcineurin inhibitor–induced hemolytic uremic syndrome/thrombotic thrombocytopenic purpura/thrombotic microangiopathy.

Antimicrobial prophylaxis: Cases of *Pneumocystis carinii* pneumonia (PCP) have been reported in patients not receiving antimicrobial prophylaxis. Therefore, administer antimicrobial prophylaxis for PCP for 1 year following transplantation. Cytomegalovirus (CMV) prophylaxis is recommended for 3 months after transplantation, particularly for patients at increased risk for CMV disease.

Skin cancer events: Patients on immunosuppressive therapy are at increased risk for skin cancer and should limit exposure to sunlight and ultraviolet (UV) light by wearing protective clothing and using a sunscreen with a high protective factor.

Vaccines: Vaccination may be less effective in patients during treatment with sirolimus. Avoid live vaccines.

Hypersensitivity reactions: Hypersensitivity reactions, including anaphylactic/anaphylactoid reactions, angioedema, exfoliative dermatitis, and hypersensitivity vasculitis, have been associated with the administration of sirolimus.

Renal function impairment: The rate of decline in renal function was greater in patients receiving sirolimus and cyclosporine compared with control therapies.

Hepatic function impairment: Reduce the maintenance dose of sirolimus in patients with hepatic function impairment.

Pregnancy: Category C.

Lactation: It is not known whether sirolimus is excreted in human breast milk. The pharmacokinetic and safety profiles of sirolimus in infants are not known. Because of the potential for adverse reactions in breast-feeding infants from sirolimus, decide whether to discontinue breast-feeding or the drug, taking into account the importance of the drug to the mother.

Children: The safety and efficacy of sirolimus in children younger than 13 years of age or in pediatric renal transplant patients younger than 18 years of age considered at high immunologic risk have not been established.

Elderly: In general, dose selection for an elderly patient should be cautious, usually starting at the low end of the dosing range, reflecting the greater frequency of decreased hepatic or cardiac function and of concomitant disease or other drug therapy.

Monitoring: Monitoring of sirolimus trough concentrations is recommended for all patients, especially in those patients likely to have altered drug metabolism, in patients 13 years of age or older who weigh less than 40 kg, in patients with hepatic function impairment, and during coadministration of strong CYP3A4 inducers and inhibitors.

During sirolimus therapy with cyclosporine, monitor patients administered an HMG-CoA reductase inhibitor and/or fibrate for the possible development of rhabdomyolysis and other adverse reactions as described in the respective monographs for these agents.

Closely monitor renal function during the administration of sirolimus in combination with cyclosporine.

Monitor all patients for hyperlipidemia and infections.

Periodic quantitative monitoring of urinary protein excretion is recommended.

Drug Interactions

Drugs that may affect sirolimus include amiodarone, cyclosporine, CYP3A4 and/or P-gp strong inhibitors, CYP3A4 and/or P-gp strong inducers, CYP3A4 inducers, CYP3A4 inhibitors, diltiazem, erythromycin, sirolimus, St. John's wort, streptogramins, and verapamil.

Drugs that may be affected by sirolimus include angiotensin-converting enzyme inhibitors, calcineurin inhibitors, disulfiram, erythromycin, furazolidone, metronidazole, mycophenolate, tacrolimus, and verapamil.

Drug/Food interactions: Grapefruit juice reduced CYP3A4-mediated metabolism of sirolimus and must not be used for dilution.

Adverse Reactions

Adverse reactions occurring in 3% or more of patients include abdominal pain, acne, anemia, arthralgia, constipation, diarrhea, edema, fever, headache, hypercholesterolemia, hypertension, hypertriglyceridemia, increased serum creatinine, nausea, pain, peripheral edema, rash, thrombocytopenia, and urinary tract infection.

MYCOPHENOLATE

Tablets; oral: 500 mg (as mofetil) (*Rx*)	*CellCept* (Roche)
Tablets, delayed release; oral: 180 and 360 mg (as sodium) (*Rx*)	*Myfortic* (Novartis)
Capsules; oral: 250 mg (as mofetil) (*Rx*)	Various, *CellCept* (Roche)
Powder for suspension; oral: 200 mg/mL (reconstituted, as mofetil) (*Rx*)	*CellCept* (Roche)
Injection, lyophilized powder for solution: 500 mg (as mofetil) (*Rx*)	*CellCept* (Roche)

Warning:

Increased susceptibility to infection and the possible development of lymphoma and other neoplasms may result from immunosuppression. Only health care providers experienced in immunosuppressive therapy and management of organ transplant patients should use mycophenolate. Manage patients receiving the drug in facilities equipped and staffed with adequate laboratory and supportive medical resources. The health care provider responsible for maintenance therapy should have complete information requisite for the follow-up of the patient.

Women of childbearing potential must use contraception. Use of mycophenolate mofetil during pregnancy is associated with increased risk of miscarriage and congenital malformations.

Indications

Renal, cardiac, and hepatic transplant: Mycophenolate is indicated for the prophylaxis of organ rejection in patients receiving allogeneic renal, cardiac, or hepatic transplants. Use mycophenolate concomitantly with cyclosporine and corticosteroids.

Administer mycophenolate IV within 24 hours following transplantation. Mycophenolate IV can be administered for up to 14 days; switch patients to oral mycophenolate as soon as they can tolerate oral medication.

Administration and Dosage

Give the initial oral dose as soon as possible following renal, cardiac, or hepatic transplantation. It is recommended that mycophenolate be administered on an empty stomach. In stable renal transplant patients, mycophenolate may be administered with food if necessary.

Note: If required, mycophenolate oral suspension can be administered via a nasogastric tube with a minimum size of 8 French (minimum 1.7 mm interior diameter).

Capsules/Tablets/Oral suspension:

Adults –

Renal transplantation: 1 g administered orally twice a day (daily dosage of 2 g) for renal transplant patients.

Cardiac transplantation: 1.5 g twice a day administered orally (daily dosage of 3 g) in adults.

Hepatic transplantation: 1.5 g twice a day administered orally (daily dosage of 3 g) in adults.

Children 3 months to 18 years of age – 600 mg/m^2 administered twice a day (up to a maximum daily dosage of 2 g per 10 mL oral suspension). Patients with a body surface area (BSA) of 1.25 to 1.5 m^2 may be dosed with capsules at a dosage of 750 mg twice a day (1.5 g daily dosage). Patients with a BSA greater than 1.5 m^2 may be dosed with capsules or tablets at a dosage of 1 g twice a day (2 g daily dosage).

Elderly – 1 g twice a day for renal transplant patients, 1.5 g twice a day for cardiac transplant patients, and 1.5 g twice a day in hepatic transplant patients.

Neutropenia – If neutropenia develops (absolute neutrophil count [ANC] less than 1.3 × 10^3/mcL), interrupt dosing or reduce the dosage.

Handling and disposal – Mycophenolate has demonstrated teratogenic effects in rats and rabbits. Do not crush mycophenolate tablets, and do not open or crush mycophenolate capsules. Avoid inhalation or direct contact with skin or mucous membranes of the powder contained in mycophenolate capsules and mycophenolate oral suspension (before or after constitution). If such contact occurs, wash thoroughly with soap and water; rinse eyes with plain water. If a spill occurs, wipe up using paper towels wetted with water to remove spilled powder or suspension.

Tablets, delayed-release: Mycophenolic acid delayed-release tablets and mycophenolate mofetil tablets and capsules should not be used interchangeably without physician supervision because the rate of absorption following the administration of these 2 products is not equivalent.

Do not crush, chew, or cut tablets prior to ingesting. Swallow the tablets whole in order to maintain the integrity of the enteric coating.

Renal transplantation –

Adults: 720 mg administered twice daily (1,440 mg total daily dose) on an empty stomach, 1 hour before or 2 hours after food intake.

Children: 400 mg/m^2 BSA administered twice daily (up to a maximum dose of 720 mg administered twice daily). Patients with a BSA of 1.19 to 1.58 m^2 may be dosed either with 3 mycophenolic acid 180 mg tablets or one 180 mg tablet plus one 360 mg tablet twice daily (1,080 mg daily dose). Patients with a BSA of greater than 1.58 m^2 may be dosed either with 4 mycophenolic acid 180 mg tablets or 2 mycophenolic acid 360 mg tablets twice daily (1,440 mg daily dose). Pediatric doses for patients with BSA less than 1.19 m^2 cannot be accurately administered using currently available formulations of mycophenolic acid tablets.

Elderly: 720 mg administered twice daily.

Renal function impairment – Carefully follow patients with severe chronic renal impairment (GFR less than 25 mL/min/1.73 m^2 BSA) for potential adverse reactions due to increase in free mycophenolic acid and total mycophenolic acid glucuronide concentrations.

Injection:

Adults –

Renal transplantation: 1 g administered IV (over no less than 2 hours) twice a day (daily dosage of 2 g).

Cardiac transplantation: 1.5 g twice a day administered IV (over no less than 2 hours).

Hepatic transplantation: 1 g twice a day administered IV (over no less than 2 hours).

Elderly – 1 g IV twice a day for renal transplant patients, 1.5 g IV twice a day for cardiac transplant patients, and 1 g IV twice a day in hepatic transplant patients.

Compatibility – Mycophenolate IV is incompatible with other IV infusion solutions. Following reconstitution, administer mycophenolate IV by slow IV infusion over a period of no less than 2 hours by either peripheral or central vein.

Do not administer mycophenolate IV or coadminister via the same infusion catheter with other IV drugs or infusion admixtures.

Caution: Never administer mycophenolate IV solution by rapid or bolus IV injection.

Dosage adjustments – In renal transplant patients with severe chronic renal impairment (GFR less than 25 mL/min per 1.73 m^2) outside the immediate posttransplant period, avoid dosages of mycophenolate greater than 1 g administered twice a day.

No data are available for cardiac or hepatic transplant patients with severe chronic renal impairment. Mycophenolate may be used for cardiac or hepatic transplant patients with severe chronic renal impairment if the potential benefits outweigh the potential risks.

Neutropenia: If neutropenia develops (ANC less than 1.3 × 10^3/mcL), interrupt dosing or reduce the dosage of mycophenolate, perform appropriate diagnostic tests, and manage the patient appropriately.

Handling and disposal – Exercise caution in the handling and preparation of solutions of mycophenolate IV. Avoid direct contact of the prepared solution of mycophenolate IV with skin or mucous membranes. If such contact occurs, wash thoroughly with soap and water; rinse eyes with plain water.

Actions

Pharmacology: Mycophenolate mofetil prolongs the survival of allogeneic transplants in animals (eg, bone marrow, heart, intestine, kidney, limb, liver, pancreatic islets, small bowel). It also reverses ongoing acute rejection. Mycophenolate was used alone or with other immunosuppressive agents in these studies. The drug inhibits immunologically mediated inflammatory responses in animal models, inhibits tumor development, and prolongs survival in murine tumor transplant models.

Pharmacokinetics:

Absorption/Distribution – Following oral and IV administration, mycophenolate undergoes rapid and complete absorption and complete hydrolysis to mycophenolic acid, the active metabolite. T_{max} ranges from 0.8 to 1.5 hours.

The mean absolute bioavailability of oral mycophenolate relative to IV mycophenolate was 94%.

The mean apparent volume of distribution of mycophenolic acid was approximately 3.6 and 4 L/kg following IV and oral administration, respectively. Mycophenolic acid is 97% bound to plasma albumin.

Metabolism/Excretion – Negligible amount of drug is excreted as mycophenolic acid (less than 1% of dose) in the urine. Oral administration resulted in complete recovery of the administered dose; 93% was recovered in the urine and 6% recovered in feces. Mean apparent half-life of mycophenolic acid is about 17.9 hours following oral administration.

Hemodialysis usually does not remove mycophenolic acid or mycophenolic acid glucuronate.

Renal transplant patients –

Mycophenolic Acid Pharmacokinetic Parameters in Renal Transplant Patients[a]

Study patient	Mycophenolate dosing	n	Dose (mg)	T_{max}[b] (h)	C_{max} (mcg/mL)	$AUC_{0\text{-}12\ h}$ (mcg•h/mL)
Adult	Single	24	720	2 (0.8 to 8)	26.1 ± 12	66.5 ± 22.6[c]
Children[d]	Single	10	450/m^2	2.5 (1.5 to 24)	36.3 ± 20.9	74.3 ± 22.5[c]
Adult	Multiple × 6 days, twice daily	10	720	2 (1.5 to 3)	37 ± 13.3	67.9 ± 20.3
Adult	Multiple × 28 days, twice daily	36	720	2.5 (1.5 to 8)	31.2 ± 18.1	71.2 ± 26.3
Chronic, multiple dose, twice daily						
Adult	2 weeks posttransplant	12	720	1.8 (1 to 5.3)	15 ± 10.7	28.6 ± 11.5
	3 months posttransplant	12	720	2 (0.5 to 2.5)	26.2 ± 12.7	52.3 ± 17.4
	6 months posttransplant	12	720	2 (0 to 3)	24.1 ± 9.6	57.2 ± 15.3
Adult	Chronic, multiple dose, twice daily	18	720	1.5 (0 to 6)	18.9 ± 7.9	57.4 ± 15

[a] Renal transplant patients on modified cyclosporin-based immunosuppression.
[b] Median (range).
[c] $AUC_{0\text{-}\infty}$
[d] Age range, 5 to 16 years.

Contraindications

Hypersensitivity to the drug, mycophenolic acid, or any component of the drug product; people with a sensitivity to polysorbate 80 (*Tween*) (IV only).

Warnings/Precautions

Lymphomas/Malignancies: Patients receiving immunosuppressive regimens involving combinations of drugs, including mycophenolate, as part of an immunosuppressive regimen are at increased risk of developing lymphomas and other malignancies, particularly of the skin.

Instruct patients to limit exposure to sunlight and UV light by wearing protective clothing and using a sunscreen with a high SPF.

Infection/Sepsis: Fatal infection/sepsis has occurred in approximately 2% of renal and cardiac patients and in 5% of hepatic patients.

Neutropenia: Up to 2% of renal transplant patients, up to 3.6% of hepatic transplant patients, and up to 2.8% of cardiac transplant patients receiving mycophenolate developed severe neutropenia. Neutropenia has been observed most frequently in the period from 31 to 180 days posttransplant in patients treated for prevention of rejection.

Progressive multifocal leukoencephalopathy (PML): Cases of PML, sometimes fatal, have been reported in patients treated with mycophenolate mofetil. Hemiparesis, apathy, confusion, cognitive deficiencies, and ataxia were the most frequent clinical features observed.

GI hemorrhage: GI bleeding has been observed in approximately 3% of renal transplants, 5.4% of hepatic transplants, and 1.7% of cardiac transplants treated with mycophenolate 3 g/day.

Delayed graft function: In patients with delayed graft function posttransplant, mean MPA AUC was comparable, but MPAG AUC was 2- to 3-fold higher, compared to that seen in posttransplant patients without delayed graft function. No dose adjustment is recommended for these patients; however, they should be carefully observed.

Rare hereditary deficiency: Avoid in patients with rare hereditary deficiency of hypoxanthine-guanine phosphoribosyl-transferase (HGPRT), such as Lesch-Nyhan and Kelley-Seegmiller syndromes.

Live, attenuated vaccines: During treatment with mycophenolate, avoid the use of live, attenuated vaccines and advise patients that vaccinations may be less effective.

Phenylketonuria: Mycophenolate oral suspension contains aspartame, a source of phenylalanine (0.56 mg phenylalanine/mL suspension).

Renal function impairment: Avoid doses greater than 1 g administered twice a day and carefully observe patients.

No data are available for cardiac or hepatic transplant patients with severe chronic renal impairment. Mycophenolate may be used for cardiac or hepatic transplant patients with severe chronic renal impairment if the potential benefits outweigh the potential risks.

Pregnancy: Category C.

Lactation: It is not known whether this drug is excreted in human milk. Because of the potential for serious adverse reactions in nursing infants from mycophenolate, decide whether to discontinue nursing or discontinue the drug, taking into account the importance of the drug to the mother.

Children: Safety and efficacy in patients receiving allogeneic cardiac or hepatic transplants have not been established.

Elderly: Use cautious dosage selection for an elderly patient, reflecting the greater frequency of decreased hepatic, renal, or cardiac function and of concomitant or other drug therapy. Elderly patients may be at an increased risk of adverse reactions compared with younger individuals.

Monitoring: Perform CBCs weekly during the first month of treatment, twice monthly for the second and third months, then monthly through the first year.

Drug Interactions

Drugs that alter the GI flora: Drugs that alter the GI flora may interact with mycophenolate by leading to less MPA available for absorption.

Drugs that may be affected by mycophenolate include acyclovir, ganciclovir, live attenuated vaccines, oral contraceptives, phenytoin, and theophylline.

Drugs that may affect mycophenolate include acyclovir, antacids, azathioprine, bile acid sequestrants, charcoal (activated), cholestyramine, ganciclovir, immunosuppressives, iron salts, rifamycins, probenecid, and salicylates.

Drug/Food interactions: MPA C_{max} was decreased by 40% in the presence of food.

Adverse Reactions

The principal adverse reactions associated with mycophenolate include diarrhea, leukopenia, sepsis, and vomiting, and there is evidence of a higher frequency of certain types of infections.

Adverse reactions occurring in at least 20% of patients include the following: abdominal pain; anemia; anorexia; anxiety; ascites; asthenia; back pain; BUN increased; cardiovascular disorder; chest pain; constipation; cough increased; creatinine increased; diarrhea; dizziness; dyspepsia; dyspnea; edema; fever; headache; hypercholesterolemia; hyperglycemia; hyperkalemia; hypertension; hypocalcemia; hypochromic anemia; hypokalemia; hypomagnesemia; hypotension; infection; insomnia; kidney function abnormal; LDH increased; leukocytosis; leukopenia; liver function tests abnormal; lung disorder; nausea; pain; paresthesia; peripheral edema; pleural effusion; rash; sepsis; sinusitis; tachycardia; thrombocytopenia; tremor; urinary tract infection; vomiting.

CYCLOSPORINE (Cyclosporin A)

Capsules; oral: 25 and 100 mg (*Rx*)	*Gengraf* (Abbott)
Capsules, soft gelatin; oral: 25 and 50 mg (*Rx*)	Various, *Sandimmune* (Novartis)
Capsules, soft gelatin for microemulsion; oral: 25 and 100 mg (*Rx*)	*Neoral* (Novartis)
Solution; oral: 100 mg/mL (*Rx*)	*Gengraf* (Abbott), *Sandimmune* (Novartis)
Solution for microemulsion; oral: 100 mg/mL (*Rx*)	*Neoral* (Novartis)
Injection: 50 mg/mL (*Rx*)	Various, *Sandimmune* (Novartis)

Warning:

Only physicians experienced in the management of systemic immunosuppressive therapy for the indicated disease should prescribe cyclosporine. Patients receiving the drug should be managed in facilities equipped and staffed with adequate laboratory and supportive medical resources. The physician responsible for maintenance therapy should have complete information requisite for the follow-up of the patient.

Administer *Sandimmune* with adrenal corticosteroids but not with other immunosuppressive agents. Increased susceptibility to infection and other possible development of lymphoma may result from immunosuppression.

Neoral and *Gengraf* may increase the susceptibility to infection and the development of neoplasia. In kidney, liver, and heart transplant patients, *Gengraf* and *Neoral* may be administered with other immunosuppressive agents. Increased susceptibility to infection and the possible development of lymphoma and other neoplasms may result from the increase in the degree of immunosuppression in transplant patients.

The absorption of *Sandimmune* during chronic administration was found to be erratic. It is recommended that patients taking *Sandimmune* over a period of time be monitored at repeated intervals to avoid toxicity from high levels and possible organ rejection from low absorption. This is of special importance in liver transplants.

Sandimmune capsules and oral solution have decreased bioavailability in comparison with *Neoral* capsules, *Neoral* oral solution, *Gengraf* capsules, and *Gengraf* oral solution. *Gengraf* and *Neoral* are not bioequivalent to *Sandimmune* and cannot be used interchangeably without physician supervision. For given trough concentrations, cyclosporine exposure will be greater with *Neoral* and *Gengraf* than with *Sandimmune*. If a patient receiving exceptionally high doses of *Sandimmune* is converted to *Neoral* or *Gengraf*, exercise particular caution. Monitor cyclosporine blood levels in transplant and rheumatoid arthritis (RA) patients taking *Gengraf* and *Neoral* to minimize possible organ rejection due to high concentrations. Make dose adjustments in transplant patients to minimize possible organ rejection due to low concentrations. Comparison of blood concentrations in the published literature with blood concentrations obtained using current assays must be done with detailed knowledge of the assay methods employed.

Psoriasis patients previously treated with PUVA and to a lesser extent, methotrexate or other immunosuppressive agents, UVB, coal tar, or radiation therapy, are at an increased risk of developing skin malignancies when taking *Neoral* or *Gengraf*.

Cyclosporine, in recommended doses, can cause systemic hypertension and nephrotoxicity. The risk increases with increasing dose and duration of cyclosporine therapy. Renal dysfunction, including structural kidney damage, is a potential consequence of cyclosporine, and therefore, renal function must be monitored during therapy.

Indications

Allogeneic transplants: For prophylaxis of organ rejection in kidney, liver, and heart allogeneic transplants. *Gengraf* and *Neoral* have been used in combination with azathioprine and corticosteroids. *Sandimmune* always is to be used with adrenal corticosteroids. *Sandimmune* also may be used in the treatment of chronic rejection in patients previously treated with other immunosuppressive agents. Because of the risk of anaphylaxis, reserve *Sandimmune* injection for patients who are unable to take the soft gelatin capsule or oral solution.

Psoriasis: *Neoral* and *Gengraf* are indicated for the treatment of adult, nonimmunocompromised patients with severe (ie, extensive and/or disabling), recalcitrant, plaque psoriasis who have failed to respond to at least 1 systemic therapy (eg, PUVA, retinoids, methotrexate) or in patients for whom other systemic therapies are contraindicated or cannot be tolerated. While rebound rarely occurs, most patients will experience relapse with *Neoral* or *Gengraf* as with other therapies upon cessation of treatment.

RA: *Neoral* and *Gengraf* are indicated for the treatment of patients with severe, active, RA where the disease has not adequately responded to methotrexate. *Neoral* and *Gengraf* can be used in combination with methotrexate in RA patients who do not respond adequately to methotrexate alone.

Administration and Dosage

Bioequivalency: *Sandimmune* capsules and oral solution have decreased bioavailability in comparison with *Neoral* capsules, *Neoral* oral solution, *Gengraf* capsules, and *Gengraf* oral solution. *Gengraf* and *Neoral* are not bioequivalent to *Sandimmune* and cannot be used interchangeably without physician supervision.

Adjunct therapy: Adjunct therapy with adrenal corticosteroids is recommended.

Sandimmune:

Initial – 15 mg/kg/day 4 to 12 hours prior to transplantation. There is a trend toward use of even lower initial doses for renal transplantation in the ranges of 10 to 14 mg/kg/day. Continue dose postoperatively for 1 to 2 weeks, then taper by 5% per week to a maintenance level of 5 to 10 mg/kg/day. Some centers successfully tapered the dose to as low as 3 mg/kg/day in selected renal transplant patients without an apparent rise in rejection rate.

Parenteral – For infusion only. Patients unable to take the oral solution or capsules preoperatively or postoperatively may be given the IV concentrate. Use the IV form at ⅓ the oral dose.

Initial dose: 5 to 6 mg/kg/day given 4 to 12 hours prior to transplantation as a single IV dose. Continue this daily single dose postoperatively until the patient can tolerate the oral doseforms. Switch patients to oral therapy as soon as possible.

Children – May use same dose and dosing regimen, but higher doses may be required.

Neoral and Gengraf: Always give the daily dosage of *Neoral* and *Gengraf* in 2 divided doses (twice daily) on a consistent schedule with regard to time of day and relation to meals.

Initial dose – The initial dose of *Neoral* and *Gengraf* can be given 4 to 12 hours prior to transplantation or postoperatively. In newly transplanted patients, the initial dose of *Neoral* and *Gengraf* are the same as the initial oral dose of *Sandimmune*. The mean doses were 9 mg/kg/day for heart transplant patients, 8 mg/kg/day for liver transplant patients and 7 mg/kg/day for heart transplant patients. Divide total daily dose into 2 equal daily doses. The *Neoral* or *Gengraf* dose is subsequently adjusted to achieve a predefined cyclosporine blood concentration. If cyclosporine trough blood concentrations are used, the target range is the same for *Neoral*or *Gengraf* as for *Sandimmune*. Using the same trough concentration target range as for *Sandimmune* results in greater cyclosporine exposure when *Neoral* is administered. Titrate dosing based on clinical assessments of rejection and tolerability. Lower *Neoral* or *Gengraf* doses may be sufficient as maintenance therapy.

Conversion from Sandimmune – In transplanted patients who are considered for conversion to *Neoral* or *Gengraf* from *Sandimmune*, start *Neoral* or *Gengraf* with the same daily dose as was previously used with *Sandimmune* (1:1 dose conversion). Subsequently adjust *Neoral* or *Gengraf* to attain the preconversion cyclosporine blood trough concentration. Using the same trough concentration target range for *Neoral* or *Gengraf* as for *Sandimmune* results in greater cyclosporine exposure when *Neoral* or *Gengraf* is administered. Monitor blood trough concentration every 4 to 7 days until preconversion value is obtained.

Poor Sandimmune absorption – Patients with lower than expected cyclosporine blood trough concentrations in relation to the oral dose of *Sandimmune* may have poor or inconsistent absorption. After conversion to *Neoral* or *Gengraf*, patients tend to have higher cyclosporine concentrations. Because of the increase in bioavailability following conversion to *Neoral* or *Gengraf*, the cyclosporine blood trough concentration may exceed the target range. Exercise particular caution when converting patients to *Neoral* at doses more than 10 mg/kg/day. Individually titrate *Neoral* or *Gengraf* dose based on cyclosporine trough concentrations, tolerability, and clinical response. Measure cyclosporine blood trough concentration more frequently, at least twice a week (daily, if initial dose exceeds 10 mg/kg/day) until concentration stabilizes within desired range.

Rheumatoid arthritis (Neoral or Gengraf only) – Initial dose of *Neoral* or *Gengraf* is 2.5 mg/kg/day, taken twice daily as a divided oral dose. Salicylates, NSAIDs and oral corticosteroids may be continued. Onset of action generally occurs between 4 and 8 weeks. If insufficient benefit is seen and tolerability is good (including serum creatinine less than 30% above baseline), the dose may be increased by 0.5 to 0.75 mg/kg/day after 8 weeks and again after 12 weeks to a maximum of 4 mg/kg/day. If no benefit is seen by 16 weeks of therapy, discontinue. There is limited long-term treatment data. Recurrence of disease activity is generally apparent within 4 weeks after stopping cyclosporine.

With methotrexate: Use the same initial dose and dosage range if *Neoral* is combined with the recommended dose of methotrexate. Most patients can be treated with *Neoral* doses of 3 mg/kg/day or less when combined with methotrexate doses of 15 mg/week or less.

Psoriasis (Neoral or Gengraf only) – The initial dose of *Neoral* or *Gengraf* is 2.5 mg/kg/day. Take *Neoral* or *Gengraf* twice daily, as a 1.25 mg/kg oral dose. Keep patients at that dose for 4 weeks or more, barring adverse events. If significant clinical improvement has not occurred in patients by that time, increase the patient's dosage at 2-week intervals. Based on patient response, make dose increases of approximately 0.5 mg/kg/day to a maximum of 4 mg/kg/day.

Patients generally show some improvement in the clinical manifestations of psoriasis in 2 weeks. Satisfactory control and stabilization of the disease may take 12 to 16 weeks to achieve. Discontinue treatment if satisfactory response cannot be achieved after 6 weeks at 4 mg/kg/day or the patient's maximum tolerated dose. Once a patient is adequately controlled and appears stable, lower the dose.

Upon stopping treatment with cyclosporine, relapse will occur in approximately 6 weeks (50% of patients) to 16 weeks (75% of patients). In the majority of patients, rebound does not occur after cessation of treatment with cyclosporine. Continuous treatment for extended periods longer than 1 year is not recommended. Consider alternation with other forms of treatment in the long-term management of patients with this disease.

Admixture compatibility/incompatibility:

Magnesium sulfate – Magnesium sulfate and cyclosporine in 5% dextrose stored in glass bottles at room temperature is stable for 6 hours.

Actions

Pharmacology: Cyclosporine is a potent immunosuppressive agent that in animals prolongs survival of allogenic transplants involving skin, kidney, liver, heart, pancreas, bone marrow, small intestine, and lung. Cyclosporine has been demonstrated to suppress some humoral immunity and to a greater extent, cell-mediated immune reactions such as allograft rejection, delayed hypersensitivity, experimental allergic encephalomyelitis, Freund's adjuvant arthritis, and graft vs host disease in many animal species for a variety of organs.

The effectiveness of cyclosporine results from specific and reversible inhibition of immunocompetent lymphocytes in the G_0 and G_1-phase of the cell cycle. T-lymphocytes are preferentially inhibited. The T-helper cell is the main target, although the T-suppressor cell also may be suppressed. Cyclosporine also inhibits lymphokine production and release including interleukin-2.

Pharmacokinetics:

Absorption –

Select Pharmacokinetic Parameters of Cyclosporine Formulations				
	Absolute bioavailability (%)	T_{max} (hours)	C_{max} (ng/mL/mg of dose)	t½ (hours)
Conventional: *Sandimmune*	30[a]	3.5	≈ 1 (2.7 to 1.4)[b]	19 (10 to 27)
Lipid microemulsion: *Neoral*	ND	1.5 to 2	↑ (40% to 106%)[c]	8.4 (5 to 18)
Gengraf	ND	1.5 to 2	↑ (40% to 106%)[c]	8.4 (5 to 18)

[a] < 10% in liver transplant and approximately 89% in renal transplant patients.
[b] Blood levels for low to high doses, respectively.
[c] In renal transplant patients treated with *Neoral* or *Gengraf*, peak levels were 40% to 106% greater than those following *Sandimmune* administration.

Absorption from the GI tract is incomplete and variable. There is very little difference in absorption between *Gengraf* and *Neoral*.

Distribution – Largely outside the blood volume; approximately 33% to 47% is in plasma, 4% to 9% in lymphocytes, 5% to 12% in granulocytes and 41% to 58% in erythrocytes. In plasma, approximately 90% is bound to proteins, primarily lipoproteins. Blood level monitoring is useful in patient management.

Metabolism – Cyclosporine is metabolized by the cytochrome P-450 3A4 hepatic enzyme system.

Excretion – Primarily biliary. Only 6% of the dose is excreted in urine.

Contraindications

Hypersensitivity to polyoxyethylated castor oil (injection only; see Warnings and Administration and Dosage), cyclosporine, or any component of the products; *Gengraf* and *Neoral* in psoriasis or RA patients with abnormal renal function, uncontrolled hypertension, or malignancies; *Gengraf* and *Neoral* concomitantly with PUVA or UVB, methotrexate or other immunosuppressive agents, coal tar or radiation therapy in psoriasis patients.

Warnings/Precautions

Nephrotoxicity: Nephrotoxicity has been noted in 25% of cases of renal transplantation, 38% of cases of cardiac transplantation, and 37% of cases of liver transplantation. Mild nephrotoxicity was generally noted 2 to 3 months after transplant and consisted of an arrest in the fall of the preoperative elevations of BUN and creatinine at a range of 35 to 45 mg/dL and 2 to 2.5 mg/dL, respectively. These elevations are often responsive to dosage reductions. More overt nephrotoxicity was seen early after transplantation and was characterized by a rapidly rising BUN and creatinine. Because these events are similar to rejection episodes, care must be taken to differentiate between them. This form of toxicity is usually responsive to cyclosporine dosage reduction.

Hepatotoxicity: Hepatotoxicity has been noted in 4%, 7%, and 4% of renal, cardiac, and liver transplantation cases, respectively. This usually occurred during the first month of therapy when high doses were used, and consisted of elevated hepatic enzymes and bilirubin.

Glomerular capillary thrombosis: Glomerular capillary thrombosis, which may result in graft failure, occasionally develops.

Convulsions: Convulsions have occurred in adult and pediatric patients receiving cyclosporine, particularly in combination with high-dose methylprednisolone.

Bioequivalency: *Sandimmune* is not bioequivalent to *Neoral* or *Gengraf*.

Thrombocytopenia and microangiopathic hemolytic anemia: Occasionally patients have developed a syndrome of thrombocytopenia and microangiopathic hemolytic anemia that may result in graft failure.

Hyperkalemia: Significant hyperkalemia (sometimes associated with hyperchloremic metabolic acidosis) and hyperuricemia have been seen occasionally in individual patients.

Encephalopathy: Encephalopathy has been described in postmarketing reports and in the literature. Manifestations include impaired consciousness, convulsions, visual disturbances (including blindness), loss of motor function, movement disorders, and psychiatric disturbances.

Hypomagnesemia: Hypomagnesemia has been reported in some, but not all, patients exhibiting convulsions while on cyclosporine therapy.

Vaccination: During treatment with cyclosporine, vaccination may be less effective; avoid the use of live attenuated vaccines.

Nephrotoxic drugs: Care should be taken in using cyclosporine with nephrotoxic drugs.

Elderly: Patients at least 65 years of age are more likely to develop systolic hypertension on therapy, and more likely to show serum creatinine rises greater than or equal to 50% above the baseline after 3 to 4 months of therapy. Monitor elderly patients with particular care, because decreases in renal function also occur with age. If patients are not properly monitored and dosages are not properly adjusted, cyclosporine therapy can cause structural kidney damage and persistent renal dysfunction.

Elevated BUN and serum creatinine: It is not unusual for serum creatinine and BUN levels to be elevated during cyclosporine therapy. These elevations in renal transplant patients do not necessarily indicate rejection, and each patient must be fully evaluated before dosage adjustment is indicated. These increases reflect a reduction in the glomerular filtration rate. Impaired renal function at any time requires close monitoring, and frequent dosage adjustments may be indicated. The frequency and severity of serum creatinine elevations increase with dose and duration of cyclosporine therapy. These elevations are likely to become more pronounced without dose reduction or discontinuation.

Malabsorption: Patients with malabsorption may have difficulty achieving therapeutic levels with oral *Sandimmune* use.

Hypertension: Hypertension is a fairly common side effect. Mild or moderate hypertension, which may occur in approximately 50% of patients following renal transplantation and in most cardiac transplant patients, is more frequently encountered than severe hypertension and the incidence decreases over time. Control of blood pressure can be accomplished with any of the common antihypertensive agents. Because cyclosporine may cause hyperkalemia, do not use potassium-sparing diuretics. While calcium antagonists can be effective agents in treating cyclosporine-associated hypertension, use care because interference with cyclosporine metabolism may require a dosage adjustment.

Hypersensitivity reactions: Anaphylactic reactions are rare (approximately 1 in 1,000) in patients on cyclosporine injection. Continuously observe patients on IV cyclosporine for at least the first 30 minutes after start of infusion and frequently thereafter. If anaphylaxis occurs, stop infusion.

Renal function impairment: Requires close monitoring and possibly frequent dosage adjustment. In patients with persistent high elevations of BUN and creatinine who are unresponsive to dosage adjustments, consider switching to other immunosuppressive therapy.

Carcinogenesis: The risk of malignancies in cyclosporine recipients is higher than in the healthy population but similar to that in patients receiving other immunosuppressive therapies.

With cyclosporine, some patients have developed a lymphoproliferative disorder, which regresses when the drug is discontinued. Patients receiving cyclosporine are at increased risk for development of lymphomas and other malignancies, particularly those of the skin. The increased risk appears related to the intensity and duration of immunosuppression rather than to the use of specific agents. Because of the danger of oversuppression of the immune system, which can also increase susceptibility to infection, do not give *Sandimmune* with other immunosuppressive agents except adrenal corticosteroids. Because of the danger of oversuppression of the immune system resulting in increased risk of infection or malignancy caused by *Neoral*, use a treatment regimen containing multiple immunosuppressants with caution.

Pregnancy: Category C.

Lactation: Avoid nursing; cyclosporine is excreted in breast milk.

Children: Patients as young as 6 months of age have received *Sandimmune* with no unusual adverse effects. Transplant recipients as young as 1 year of age have received *Neoral* or *Gengraf* with no unusual adverse effects. The safety and efficacy of *Neoral* or *Gengraf* treatment in children younger than 18 years of age with juvenile rheumatoid arthritis or psoriasis have not been established.

Monitoring:

Blood levels – Blood level monitoring of cyclosporine is a useful and essential component in patient management. While no fixed relationships have been established, blood concentration monitoring may assist in the clinical evaluation of rejection and toxicity, dose adjustments, and the assessment of compliance.

Of major importance to blood level analysis are the type of assay used, the transplanted organ, and the other immunosuppressant agents being administered.

While several assays and assay matrices are available, there is a consensus that parent-compound-specific assays correlate best with clinical events. Of these, HPLC is the standard reference, but the monoclonal antibody RIAs and the monoclonal antibody FPIA offer sensitivity, reproducibility, and convenience.

Repeatedly assess renal and liver functions by measurement of BUN, serum creatinine, serum bilirubin, and liver enzymes.

Drug Interactions

P-450 system: Monitoring of circulating cyclosporine levels and appropriate dosage adjustment are essential when drugs that affect hepatic microsomal enzymes, particularly the cytochrome P-450 3A enzymes, are used concomitantly (eg, HIV protease inhibitors, anticonvulsants, azole antifungals).

Nephrotoxic drugs: Use with caution in patients receiving cyclosporine. The following drugs may potentiate renal dysfunction: *antibiotics*: gentamicin, tobramycin, vancomycin, TMP-SMZ; *antineoplastics*: melphalan; *antifungals*: amphotericin B, ketoconazole; *anti-inflammatory drugs*: diclofenac, naproxen, sulindac; *GI agents*: cimetidine, ranitidine; *immunosuppressives*: tacrolimus.

Drugs that may affect cyclosporine include: allopurinol, amiodarone, androgens (eg, danazol, methyltestosterone), anticonvulsants (eg, carbamazepine, phenobarbital, phenytoin), azole antifungals (eg, fluconazole, ketoconazole), beta-blockers, bosentan, bromocriptine, calcium channel blockers, colchicine, oral contraceptives, corticosteroids, fluoroquinolones (eg, ciprofloxacin), foscarnet, HMG-CoA reductase inhibitors, imipenem-cilastatin, macrolide antibiotics, methotrexate, metoclopramide, nafcillin, nefazodone, orlistat, potassium-sparing diuretics, probucol, rifamycins (rifampin, rifabutin), serotonin reuptake inhibitors (SSRIs; eg, fluoxetine, sertraline), sirolimus, St. John's wort, sulfamethoxazole/trimethoprim, terbinafine, and ticlopidine.

Drugs that may be affected by cyclosporine include bosentan, digoxin, etopisode, and HMG-CoA reductase inhibitors, methotrexate, potassium-sparing diuretics, and sirolimus.

Drug/Food interactions: Administration of food with *Neoral* decreases the AUC and C_{max} of cyclosporine. A high-fat meal consumed within 30 minutes of *Neoral* administration decreased the AUC by 13% and C_{max} by 33%. The effects of a low-fat meal were similar. In addition, do not take cyclosporine simultaneously with grapefruit juice unless specifically instructed to do so; trough cyclosporine concentrations may be increased.

Adverse Reactions

Adverse reactions may include renal dysfunction; tremor; infectious complications; hirsutism; hypertension; gum hyperplasia; cramps; acne; convulsions; paresthesia.

METHOTREXATE

Tablets; oral: 2.5 mg (*Rx*)	Various, *Rheumatrex Dose Pack* (STADA)
5, 7.5, 10, and 15 mg (*Rx*)	*Trexall* (Barr)
Injection: 25 mg/mL (as base) (*Rx*)	Various, *Methotrexate LPF Sodium* (Xanodyne)
Injection, lyophilized powder for solution: 20 mg and 1 g (as base) (*Rx*)	Various

Warning:

Methotrexate should be used only by physicians whose knowledge and experience include the use of antimetabolite therapy.

Severe reactions: Because of the possibility of severe toxic reactions (which can be fatal), fully inform patients of the risks involved and assure constant supervision.

Deaths: Use methotrexate only in life-threatening neoplastic diseases, or in patients with psoriasis or rheumatoid arthritis (RA) with severe, recalcitrant, disabling disease that is not adequately responsive to other forms of therapy. Deaths have occurred with the use of methotrexate in malignancy, psoriasis, and RA. Closely monitor patients for bone marrow, liver, lung, and kidney toxicities.

Marked bone marrow depression may occur with resultant anemia, leukopenia, or thrombocytopenia.

Unexpectedly severe (sometimes fatal) bone marrow suppression, aplastic anemia, and GI toxicity have occurred with coadministration of methotrexate (usually in high dosage) along with some NSAIDs (see Precautions, Drug Interactions).

Monitoring: Periodic monitoring for toxicity, including CBC with differential and platelet counts, and liver and renal function testing is mandatory. Periodic liver biopsies may be indicated in some situations. Monitor patients at increased risk for impaired methotrexate elimination (eg, renal dysfunction, pleural effusions, ascites) more frequently (see Precautions).

Liver: Methotrexate causes hepatotoxicity, fibrosis, and cirrhosis, but generally only after prolonged use. Acutely, liver enzyme elevations are frequent, usually transient and asymptomatic, and also do not appear predictive of subsequent hepatic disease. Liver biopsy after sustained use often shows histologic changes, and fibrosis and cirrhosis have occurred; these latter lesions often are not preceded by symptoms or abnormal liver function tests (see Precautions). For this reason, periodic liver biopsies are usually recommended for psoriatic patients who are under long-term treatment. Persistent abnormalities in liver function tests may precede appearance of fibrosis or cirrhosis in the RA population.

continued on next page

Warning: (cont.)

Methotrexate-induced lung disease: Methotrexate-induced lung disease is a potentially dangerous lesion that may occur acutely at any time during therapy and has occurred at doses as low as 7.5 mg/week. It is not always fully reversible. Pulmonary symptoms (especially a dry, nonproductive cough) may require interruption of treatment and careful investigation.

Pregnancy: Fetal death and/or congenital anomalies have occurred; do not use in women of childbearing potential unless benefits outweigh possible risks. Pregnant women with psoriasis or RA should not receive methotrexate (see Contraindications).

Renal use: Use methotrexate in patients with impaired renal function with extreme caution, and at reduced dosages, because renal dysfunction will prolong elimination.

GI: Diarrhea and ulcerative stomatitis require interruption of therapy; hemorrhagic enteritis and death from intestinal perforation may occur.

Diluents: Do not use methotrexate formulations and diluents containing preservatives for intrathecal or high-dose methotrexate therapy.

Malignant lymphomas: Malignant lymphomas, which may regress following withdrawal of methotrexate, may occur in patients receiving low-dose methotrexate and, thus, may not require cytotoxic treatment. Discontinue methotrexate first and, if the lymphoma does not regress, institute appropriate treatment.

Tumor lysis syndrome: Like other cytotoxic drugs, methotrexate may induce tumor lysis syndrome in patients with rapidly growing tumors.

Skin reactions: Severe, occasionally fatal skin reactions have been reported following single or multiple doses of methotrexate. Reactions have occurred within days of oral, IM, IV, or intrathecal methotrexate administration. Recovery has been reported with discontinuation of therapy.

Potentially fatal opportunistic infections: Potentially fatal opportunistic infections, especially *Pneumocystis carinii* pneumonia, may occur with methotrexate therapy.

Radiotherapy: Methotrexate given concomitantly with radiotherapy may increase the risk of soft tissue necrosis and osteonecrosis.

Indications

Severe, active, classical or definite adult RA: (ACR criteria) in selected adults who have had an insufficient therapeutic response to, or are intolerant of, an adequate trial of first-line therapy including full-dose NSAIDs.

Polyarticular-course juvenile rheumatoid arthritis (JRA): Management of children with active polyarticular-course JRA who have had an insufficient therapeutic response to, or are intolerant of, an adequate trial of first-line therapy including full-dose NSAIDs.

Psoriasis: Symptomatic control of severe, recalcitrant, disabling psoriasis that is not adequately responsive to other forms of therapy.

Other: Methotrexate also is indicated as an antineoplastic chemotherapy in various types of cancers and acute lymphocytic leukemia.

Administration and Dosage

Arthritis: Therapeutic response for adult RA and polyarticular-course JRA usually begins within 3 to 6 weeks and the patient may continue to improve for another 12 weeks or more.

Adult RA –

Starting dose: Single oral doses of 7.5 mg/week or divided oral dosages of 2.5 mg at 12-hour intervals for 3 doses given as a course once weekly.

Polyarticular-course JRA –

Starting dose: 10 mg/m^2 given once weekly.

Dose adjustment – Dosages may be adjusted gradually to achieve an optimal response. Limited experience shows a significant increase in the incidence and severity of serious toxic reactions, especially bone marrow suppression, at doses greater than 20 mg/week in adults. Although there is experience with doses up to 30 mg/m^2/week in children, there are too few published data to assess how doses over 20 mg/m^2/week might affect the risk of serious toxicity in children. Experience suggests that children receiving 20 to 30 mg/m^2/week (0.65 to 1 mg/kg/week) may have better absorption and fewer GI side effects if methotrexate is administered either IM or subcutaneously.

Duration of therapy – Optimal duration of therapy is unknown. Limited data from long-term studies in adults indicate that initial clinical improvement is maintained at least 2 years with continued therapy. When methotrexate is discontinued, the arthritis usually worsens within 3 to 6 weeks.

Weekly therapy may be instituted with the *Rheumatrex Dose Packs*, which are designed to provide doses over a range of 5 to 15 mg administered as a single weekly dose. The dose packs are not recommended for weekly doses greater than 15 mg. Tailor schedules to the individual patient. An initial test dose may be given prior to the regular dosing schedule to detect any extreme sensitivity to adverse effects. Maximal myelosuppression usually occurs in 7 to 10 days.

Concomitant therapy – Aspirin, NSAIDs, and/or low-dose steroids may be continued, although the possibility of increased toxicity with concomitant use of NSAIDs, including salicylates, has not been fully explored. Steroids may be reduced gradually in patients who respond to methotrexate. Combined use of methotrexate with gold, penicillamine, hydroxychloroquine, sulfasalazine, or cytotoxic agents has not been studied and may increase the incidence of adverse effects. Note that the doses used in RA (7.5 to 15 mg/week) are somewhat lower than those used in psoriasis and that larger doses could lead to toxicity. Rest and physiotherapy as indicated should be continued.

Psoriasis:

Weekly single oral, IM, or IV dose schedule – 10 to 25 mg/week until adequate response is achieved. Do not exceed 30 mg/week.

Divided oral dose schedule – 2.5 mg at 12-hour intervals for 3 doses.

Dosages in each schedule may be gradually adjusted to achieve optimal clinical response; do not exceed 30 mg/week.

Once optimal clinical response has been achieved, reduce each schedule to the lowest possible amount of drug and to the longest possible rest period. The use of methotrexate may permit the return to conventional topical therapy, which should be encouraged.

Assess hematologic, hepatic, renal, and pulmonary function before beginning, periodically during, and before reinstituting therapy.

Actions

Pharmacology: The mechanism of action in RA is unknown; it may affect immune function. Methotrexate inhibits dihydrofolic acid reductase and interferes with DNA synthesis, repair, and cellular replication.

Pharmacokinetics:

Absorption – Peak serum levels are reached within 1 to 2 hours. The mean bioavailability is approximately 60%. Food delayed absorption and reduced peak concentration.

Distribution – Methotrexate is approximately 50% protein bound.

Metabolism – Methotrexate undergoes hepatic and intracellular metabolism. The terminal half-life reported is approximately 3 to 10 for patients receiving treatment for psoriasis, RA, or low-dose antineoplastic therapy (less than 30 mg/m^2).

Excretion – Renal excretion is the primary route of elimination and is dependent upon dosage and route of administration.

Contraindications

Hypersensitivity to the drug.

Patients with psoriasis or RA who have any of the following: alcoholism, alcoholic liver disease, or other chronic liver disease; overt or laboratory evidence of immunodeficiency syndromes; preexisting blood dyscrasias (eg, bone marrow hypoplasia, leukopenia, thrombocytopenia, significant anemia).

Pregnancy: Methotrexate can cause fetal death or teratogenic effects when administered to a pregnant woman. Methotrexate is contraindicated in pregnant women with psoriasis or RA and should be used in the treatment of neoplastic diseases only when the potential benefit outweighs the risk to the fetus. Women of childbearing potential should not be started on methotrexate until pregnancy is excluded and should be fully counseled on the serious risk to the fetus should they become pregnant while undergoing treatment. Pregnancy should be avoided if either partner is receiving methotrexate; during and for a minimum of 3 months after therapy for male patients, and during and for at least 1 ovulatory cycle after therapy for female patients.

Lactation – Because of the potential for serious adverse reactions from methotrexate in breastfed infants, it is contraindicated in nursing mothers.

Warnings/Precautions

Toxic effects: Toxic effects, potentially serious, may be related in frequency and severity to dose or frequency of administration, but have been seen at all doses. These effects can occur at any time during therapy; follow patients closely. Most adverse reactions are reversible if detected early. When reactions occur, reduce dosage or discontinue drug and take appropriate corrective measures; this could include use of leucovorin calcium. Use caution if therapy is reinstituted.

Weekly dose: Physicians and pharmacists should emphasize that the dose is taken weekly. Mistaken daily use has led to fatal toxicity. Encourage patients to read the Patient Instructions in the Dose Pack. Do not write or refill prescriptions on a PRN basis.

Organ system toxicity:

GI – If vomiting, diarrhea, or stomatitis occur, which may result in dehydration, discontinue methotrexate until recovery occurs. Use with extreme caution in the presence of peptic ulcer disease or ulcerative colitis.

Hematologic – Methotrexate can suppress hematopoiesis and cause anemia, aplastic anemia, pancytopenia, leukopenia, neutropenia, and/or thrombocytopenia. Use with caution, if at all, in patients with malignancy and preexisting hematopoietic impairment.

In psoriasis and RA, stop methotrexate immediately if there is a significant drop in blood counts.

Hepatic – Methotrexate has the potential for acute (elevated transaminases) and chronic (fibrosis and cirrhosis) hepatotoxicity. Chronic toxicity is potentially fatal; it generally occurs after prolonged use (generally 2 years or more) and after a total dose of at least 1.5 g.

Periodically perform liver function tests, including serum albumin, prior to dosing.

Psoriasis: The usual recommendation is to obtain a liver biopsy at 1) pretherapy or shortly after initiation of therapy (2 to 4 months), 2) a total cumulative dose of 1.5 g, and 3) after each additional 1 to 1.5 g. Moderate fibrosis or any cirrhosis normally leads to discontinuation of the drug; mild fibrosis normally suggests a repeat biopsy in 6 months.

RA: In RA, first use of methotrexate and duration of therapy have been reported as risk factors for hepatotoxicity. Persistent abnormalities in liver function tests may precede appearance of fibrosis or cirrhosis in this population.

Infection or immunologic states – Use with extreme caution in the presence of active infection.

Potentially fatal opportunistic infections, especially *P. carinii* pneumonia may occur with methotrexate therapy.

Neurologic – A transient acute neurologic syndrome has been observed in patients treated with high-dosage regimens. Manifestations of this stroke-like encephalopathy may include confusion, hemiparesis, transient blindness, seizures, and coma.

Pulmonary – Pulmonary symptoms (especially a dry, nonproductive cough) or a nonspecific pneumonitis indicate a potentially dangerous lesion and require interruption of treatment and careful investigation. The typical patient presents with fever, cough, dyspnea, hypoxemia, and an infiltrate on chest x-ray.

Renal – Methotrexate may cause renal damage that may lead to acute renal failure. Close attention to renal function including adequate hydration, urine alkalinization and measurement of serum methotrexate and creatinine levels are essential for safe administration.

Skin – Severe, occasionally fatal dermatologic reactions, including toxic epidermal necrolysis, Stevens-Johnson syndrome, exfoliative dermatitis, skin necrosis, and erythema multiforme, have been reported within days of methotrexate administration.

Vaccines: Immunization may be ineffective when given during methotrexate therapy. Immunization with live virus vaccines is generally not recommended. Disseminated vaccinia infections after smallpox immunization have occurred in patients receiving methotrexate.

Debility: Use with extreme caution in the presence of debility.

Pleural effusions or ascites: In patients with significant third space accumulations, evacuate the fluid before treatment and monitor plasma methotrexate levels.

Psoriasis lesions: Lesions of psoriasis may be aggravated by concomitant exposure to ultraviolet radiation. Radiation dermatitis and sunburn may be "recalled" by the use of methotrexate.

Folate deficiency: Folate deficiency states may increase methotrexate toxicity.

Benzyl alcohol: Methotrexate sodium for injection contains the preservative benzyl alcohol and is not recommended for use in neonates.

Renal function impairment: See Precautions.

Fertility impairment: Impairment of fertility, oligospermia, and menstrual dysfunction in humans has been reported during and for a short period after cessation of therapy.

Pregnancy: Category X. Avoid pregnancy if either partner is receiving methotrexate: During and for a minimum of 3 months after therapy for male patients, and during and for at least one ovulatory cycle after therapy for female patients.

Lactation: Methotrexate has been detected in human breast milk. Methotrexate is contraindicated in nursing mothers.

Children: Safety and efficacy in children have been established only in cancer chemotherapy and in polyarticular-course JRA.

Monitoring: Monitor hematology at least monthly, and liver and renal function every 1 to 2 months during therapy. During initial or changing doses, or periods of increased risk of elevated methotrexate blood levels (eg, dehydration), more frequent monitoring may be indicated. Stop methotrexate immediately if there is a significant drop in blood counts.

Transient liver function test abnormalities are observed frequently after methotrexate administration and are usually not cause for modification of therapy. Persistent liver function test abnormalities and/or depression of serum albumin may be indicators of serious liver toxicity and require evaluation.

Drug Interactions

Drugs that may affect methotrexate include oral aminoglycosides, charcoal, chloramphenicol, folic acid, NSAIDs, PCNs, probenecid, salicylates, sulfonamides, TCN, trimethoprim.

Drugs that may be affected by methotrexate include sulfonamides, digoxin, phenytoin, theophylline, and thiopurines (eg, azathioprine).

Drug/Food interactions: Food may delay the absorption and reduce the peak concentration of methotrexate.

Adverse Reactions

The most common adverse reactions include the following: Abdominal distress, chills, decreased resistance to infection, dizziness, fatigue, fever, leukopenia, malaise, nausea, ulcerative stomatitis.

Adult RA: Alopecia, diarrhea, dizziness, elevated liver function tests, leukopenia (WBC below 3,000/mm^3), nausea/vomiting, pancytopenia, rash/pruritus/dermatitis, stomatitis, thrombocytopenia (platelet count below 100,000/mm^3).

Polyarticular-course JRA: Virtually all patients were receiving concomitant NSAIDs, and some also were taking low doses of corticosteroids. Elevated liver function tests, GI reactions (eg, diarrhea, nausea, vomiting).

Psoriasis: Alopecia, photosensitivity, "burning of skin" lesions.

PEGINTERFERON ALFA-2A

Injection: 180 mcg (*Rx*) *Pegasys* (Roche)

Warning:

Alpha interferons, including peginterferon alfa-2a, may cause or aggravate fatal or life-threatening neuropsychiatric, autoimmune, ischemic, and infectious disorders. Closely monitor patients with periodic clinical and laboratory evaluations. Patients with persistently severe or worsening signs or symptoms of these conditions should be withdrawn from therapy. In many, but not all cases, these disorders resolve after stopping peginterferon alfa-2a (see Warnings and Adverse Reactions).

Use with ribavirin: Ribavirin may cause birth defects and/or death of the fetus. Extreme care must be taken to avoid pregnancy in female patients and in female partners of male patients. Ribavirin causes hemolytic anemia. The anemia associated with ribavirin therapy may result in a worsening of cardiac disease. Ribavirin is genotoxic and mutagenic and should be considered a potential carcinogen.

Indications

Chronic hepatitis B: For the treatment of adult patients with HBeAg-positive and HBeAG-negative chronic hepatitis B virus (HBV) infection who have compensated liver disease and evidence of viral replication and liver inflammation.

Chronic hepatitis C: Alone or in combination with ribavirin tablets for the treatment of adults with chronic hepatitis C virus (HCV) who have compensated liver disease and have not been treated previously with interferon alfa.

Administration and Dosage

Chronic HBV or HCV monoinfection:

Monotherapy – The recommended dose of peginterferon alfa-2a is 180 mcg (1 mL or 0.5 mL prefilled syringe) once weekly for 48 weeks by subcutaneous administration in the abdomen or thigh.

There are no safety and efficacy data on treatment of chronic HBV or HCV for longer than 48 weeks. For patients with HCV, consider discontinuing therapy after 12 to 24 weeks of therapy if the patient has failed to demonstrate an early virologic response, defined as undetectable HCV RNA or at least a $2\log_{10}$ reduction from baseline in HCV RNA titer by 12 weeks of therapy.

A patient should self-inject peginterferon alfa-2a only if the physician determines that it is appropriate, the patient agrees to medical follow-up as necessary, and training in proper injection technique has been provided.

Combination therapy with ribavirin (chronic HCV monoinfection) – The recommended dose of peginterferon alfa-2a when used in combination with ribavirin tablets is 180 mcg (1 mL vial or 0.5 mL prefilled syringe) subcutaneously once weekly. The recommended dose of ribavirin and duration for the peginterferon alfa-2a/ribavirin tablet combination therapy is based on viral genotype.

The daily dose of ribavirin tablets is 800 to 1,200 mg administered orally in 2 divided doses. Individualize the dose depending on baseline disease characteristics (eg, genotype), response to therapy, and tolerability of the regimen.

Because ribavirin tablet absorption increases when administered with a meal, advise patients to take the tablet with food.

Peginterferon Alfa-2a/Ribavirin Tablet Combination Dosing Recommendations

Genotype	Peginterferon alfa-2a dose	Ribavirin tablet dose	Duration
Genotype 1, 4	180 mcg	< 75 kg = 1000 mg	48 weeks
		≥ 75 kg = 1200 mg	48 weeks

Peginterferon Alfa-2a/Ribavirin Tablet Combination Dosing Recommendations			
Genotype	Peginterferon alfa-2a dose	Ribavirin tablet dose	Duration
Genotype 2, 3	180 mcg	800 mg	24 weeks

Chronic HCV with HIV coinfection:

Monotherapy – 180 mcg (1 mL vial or 0.5 mL prefilled syringe) once weekly for 48 weeks by subcutaneous administration in the abdomen or thigh.

Combination therapy with ribavirin – 180 mcg subcutaneously once weekly and ribavirin 800 mg daily given orally in 2 divided doses for a total of 48 weeks, regardless of genotype. Because ribavirin absorption increases when administered with a meal, patients are advised to take ribavirin with food.

Dose reduction: When dose modification is required for moderate to severe adverse reactions (clinical or laboratory), initial dose reduction to 135 mcg (0.75 mL) is generally adequate. However, in some cases, dose reduction to 90 mcg (0.5 mL) may be needed. Following improvement of the adverse reaction, re-escalation of the dose may be considered. If intolerance persists after dose adjustment, discontinue therapy.

Hematologic toxicity –

Peginterferon alfa-2a:

Peginterferon Alfa-2a Hematological Dose Modification Guidelines		
Laboratory values	Peginterferon alfa-2a dose	Discontinue peginterferon alfa-2a
ANC[a] ≥ 750/mm^3	Maintain 180 mcg	ANC < 500/mm^3, suspend treatment until ANC values return to more than 1,000/mm^3; reinstitute at 90 mcg and monitor ANC.
ANC < 750/mm^3	Reduce to 135 mcg	
Platelet ≥ 50,000/mm^3	Maintain 180 mcg	Platelet count < 25,000/mm^3
Platelet < 50,000/mm^3	Reduce to 90 mcg	

[a] ANC = absolute neutrophil count.

Ribavirin tablets: If severe adverse reactions or laboratory abnormalities develop during combination ribavirin tablet/peginterferon alfa-2a therapy, the dose should be modified or discontinued, if appropriate, until the adverse reactions abate. If intolerance persists after dose adjustment, ribavirin tablet/peginterferon alfa-2a therapy should be discontinued.

Ribavirin Tablet Dosage Modification Guidelines		
Laboratory values	Reduce only ribavirin tablet dose to 600 mg/day[a] if:	Discontinue ribavirin tablet if:
Hemoglobin in patients with no cardiac disease	< 10 g/dL	< 8.5 g/dL
Hemoglobin in patients with history of stable cardiac disease	≥ 2 g/dL decrease in hemoglobin during any 4-week period treatment	< 12 g/dL despite 4 weeks at reduced dose.

[a] One 200 mg tablet in the morning and two 200 mg tablets in the evening.

Once the ribavirin tablet has been withheld because of a laboratory abnormality or clinical manifestation, an attempt may be made to restart the ribavirin tablet at 600 mg/day and further increase the dose to 800 mg/day depending upon the physician's judgment. However, it is not recommended that the ribavirin tablet be increased to the original dose (1,000 or 1,200 mg).

Psychiatric depression –

Guidelines for Modification or Discontinuation of Peginterferon alfa-2a and for Scheduling Visits for Patients with Depression					
	Initial management (4 to 8 weeks)		Depression		
Depression severity	Dose modification	Visit schedule	Remains stable	Improves	Worsens
Mild	No change	Evaluate once weekly by visit and/or phone	Continue weekly visit schedule	Resume normal visit schedule	(see moderate or severe depression)
Moderate	Decrease peginterferon alfa-2a dose to 135 mcg (in some cases dose reduction to 90 mcg may be needed)	Evaluate once weekly (office visit at least every other week)	Consider psychiatric consultation. Continue reduced dosing	If symptoms improve and are stable for 4 weeks, may resume normal visit schedule. Continue reduced dosing or return to normal dose.	(see severe depression)
Severe	Discontinue peginterferon alfa-2a permanently	Obtain immediate psychiatric consultation	Psychiatric therapy necessary.		

Renal function impairment – In patients with end-stage renal disease requiring hemodialysis, dose reduction to 135 mcg peginterferon alfa-2a is recommended. Closely monitor for signs and symptoms of interferon toxicity. Do not use ribavirin in patients with creatinine clearance less than 50 mL/min.

Hepatic function impairment – In patients with progressive ALT increases above baseline values, reduce the dose of peginterferon alfa-2a to 135 mcg. Immediately discontinue therapy if ALT increases are progressive despite dose reduction or are accompanied by increased bilirubin or evidence of hepatic decompensation.

Chronic HBV: In chronic HBV patients with elevations in ALT (greater than 5 times the upper limit of normal [ULN]), perform more frequent monitoring of liver function and consider either reducing the dose of peginterferon alfa-2a to 135 mcg or temporarily discontinuing treatment. After peginterferon alfa-2a dose reduction or withholding, therapy can be resumed after ALT flares subside.

Chronic HCV: In chronic HCV patients with progressive ALT increases above baseline values, reduce the dose of peginterferon alfa-2a to 135 mcg and perform more frequent monitoring of liver function. After peginterferon alfa-2a dose reduction or withholding, therapy can be resumed after ALT flares subside.

Actions

Pharmacology: Interferons bind to specific receptors on the cell surface, initiating intracellular signaling via a complex cascade of protein-protein interactions and leading to rapid activation of gene transcription. Interferon-stimulated genes modulate many biological effects, including the inhibition of viral replication in infected cells, inhibition of cell proliferation, and immunomodulation. Peginterferon alfa-2a stimulates the production of effector proteins such as serum neopterin and 2′,5′-oligoadenylate synthetase.

Pharmacokinetics:

Absorption/Distribution – Maximal serum concentrations (C_{max}) occur between 72 to 96 hours postdose. Steady-state serum levels are reached within 5 to 8 weeks of once-weekly dosing. The peak-to-trough ratio at week 48 is approximately 2.

Metabolism/Excretion – The mean systemic clearance in healthy subjects given peginterferon alfa-2a was 94 mL/h. The mean terminal half-life after subcutaneous dosing in patients with chronic hepatitis C was 80 hours (range, 50 to 140 hours).

Gender – Similar pharmacokinetics in healthy male and female subjects.

Special populations –

Elderly: The AUC was increased from 1295 to 1663 ng•h/mL in subjects older than 62 years of age taking 180 mcg peginterferon alfa-2a, but peak concentrations were similar (9 vs 10 ng/mL) in those older and younger than 62 years of age.

Renal impairment: In patients with end-stage renal disease undergoing hemodialysis, there is a 25% to 45% reduction in clearance.

Contraindications

Hypersensitivity to peginterferon alfa-2a or any of its components; autoimmune hepatitis; hepatic decompensation (Child-Pugh score greater than 6 [class B and C]) in cirrhotic patients before or during treatment; hepatic decompensation with Child-Pugh score greater than or equal to 6 in cirrhotic chronic HCV patients coinfected with HIV before or during treatment; in neonates and infants because it contains benzyl alcohol. Benzyl alcohol is associated with an increased incidence of neurologic and other complications that are sometimes fatal in neonates and infants.

Combination therapy with ribavirin: Hypersensitivity to ribavirin or any component of the tablet; women who are pregnant; men whose female partners are pregnant; patients with hemoglobinopathies (eg, thalassemia major, sickle cell anemia).

Warnings/Precautions

Autoimmune disorders: Development or exacerbation of autoimmune disorders, including myositis, hepatitis, idiopathic thrombocytopenic purpura, psoriasis, rheumatoid arthritis, interstitial nephritis, thyroiditis, and systemic lupus erythematosus have been reported in patients receiving alpha interferon.

Benzyl alcohol: Peginterferon alfa-2a is contraindicated in neonates and infants because it contains benzyl alcohol.

Bone marrow toxicity: Peginterferon alfa-2a suppresses bone marrow function and may result in severe cytopenias. Ribavirin may potentiate the neutropenia and lymphopenia induced by alpha interferons including peginterferon alfa-2a. Alpha interferons may be associated with aplastic anemia very rarely.

Cardiovascular events: Hypertension, supraventricular arrhythmias, chest pain, and MI have been observed in patients treated with peginterferon alfa-2a.

Fatal and nonfatal MIs have been reported in patients with anemia caused by ribavirin.

Colitis: Ulcerative and hemorrhagic/ischemic colitis, sometimes fatal, has been observed within 12 weeks of starting alpha interferon treatment. Abdominal pain, bloody diarrhea, and fever are the typical manifestations of colitis.

Hepatitis exacerbations: Exacerbations of hepatitis during hepatitis B therapy are not uncommon and are characterized by transient and potentially severe increases in serum ALT.

Endocrine disorders: Peginterferon alfa-2a causes or aggravates hypothyroidism and hyperthyroidism. Hyperglycemia, hypoglycemia, and diabetes mellitus have developed in patients treated with peginterferon alfa-2a.

Hemolytic anemia: The primary toxicity of ribavirin is hemolytic anemia. The anemia associated with ribavirin tablets occurs within 1 to 2 weeks of initiation of therapy with maximum drop in hemoglobin observed during the first 8 weeks.

Infections: Serious and severe bacterial infections, some fatal, have been observed in patients treated with alfa interferons including peginterferon alfa-2a.

Neuropsychiatric events: Life-threatening or fatal neuropsychiatric reactions may manifest in patients receiving therapy with peginterferon alfa-2a. Depression, suicidal ideation, suicide, relapse of drug addiction, and drug overdose may occur in patients with and without previous psychiatric illness. Use peginterferon alfa-2a with extreme caution in patients who report a history of depression.

Ophthalmologic disorders: Decrease or loss of vision, retinopathy (including macular edema, retinal artery or vein thrombosis), retinal hemorrhages and cotton wool spots, optic neuritis, and papilledema are induced or aggravated by treatment with peginterferon alfa-2a or other alpha interferons. All patients should receive an eye examination at baseline.

Pancreatitis: Pancreatitis, sometimes fatal, has occurred during alpha interferon and ribavirin treatment.

Pulmonary disorders: Dyspnea, pulmonary infiltrates, pneumonia, bronchiolitis obliterans, interstitial pneumonitis, and sarcoidosis, some resulting in respiratory failure and/or patient deaths, may be induced or aggravated by peginterferon alfa-2a or alpha interferon therapy.

Fever: While fever is commonly caused by peginterferon alfa-2a therapy, other causes of persistent fever must be ruled out, particularly in patients with neutropenia.

Clinical study criteria: The following entrance criteria used for the clinical studies of peginterferon alfa-2a may be considered as a guideline to acceptable baseline values for initiation of treatment:

- platelet count greater than or equal to 90,000 cells/mm^3 (as low as 75,000 cells/mm^3 in HCV patients with cirrhosis or 70,000 cells/mm^3 in patients with chronic HCV and HIV)
- ANC greater than or equal to 1,500 cells/mm^3
- serum creatinine concentration less than 1.5 times the ULN
- TSH and thyroxine (T_4) within normal limits or adequately controlled thyroid function
- CD4+ cell count at least 200 cells/mcL or CD4+ cell count at least 100 cells/mcL but less than 200 cells/mcL and HIV-1 RNA less than 5,000 copies/mL in patients coinfected with HIV
- Hgb at least 12 g/dL for women and at least 13 g/dL for men in chronic HCV monoinfected patients
- Hgb at least 11 g/dL for women and at least 12 g/dL for men in patients with chronic HCV and HIV

Immunogenicity: Nine percent of patients treated with peginterferon alfa-2a with or without ribavirin tablets developed binding antibodies to interferon alfa-2a, as assessed by an ELISA assay. The clinical and pathological significance of the appearance of serum neutralizing antibodies is unknown.

Hypersensitivity reactions: Severe acute hypersensitivity reactions (eg, urticaria, angioedema, bronchoconstriction, anaphylaxis) have been rarely observed during alpha interferon and ribavirin therapy.

Renal function impairment: A 25% to 45% higher exposure to peginterferon alfa-2a is seen in subjects undergoing hemodialysis. In patients with impaired renal function, closely monitor for signs and symptoms of interferon toxicity. Use peginterferon alfa-2a with caution in patients with creatinine clearance less than 50 mL/min.

Hepatic function impairment: Chronic hepatitis C patients with cirrhosis may be at risk of hepatic decompensation and death when treated with alfa interferons, including peginterferon alfa-2a. Cirrhotic chronic hepatitis C patients coinfected with HIV receiving highly active antiretroviral therapy (HAART) and interferon alfa-2a with or without ribavirin appear to be at increased risk for the development of hepatic decompensation, compared with patients not receiving HAART.

Hazardous tasks: Caution patients who develop dizziness, confusion, somnolence, and fatigue to avoid driving or operating machinery.

Fertility impairment: Peginterferon alfa-2a may impair fertility in women.

Pregnancy: Category C.

Use with ribavirin – Category X.

If pregnancy occurs in a patient or partner of a patient during treatment or during the 6 months after treatment cessation, such cases should be reported to the ribavirin tablet Pregnancy Registry at (800) 526-6367.

Lactation: It is not known whether peginterferon alfa-2a or ribavirin or its components are excreted in breast milk.

Children: The safety and efficacy in children below 18 years of age have not been established.

Elderly: Younger patients have higher virologic response rates than older patients. Because elderly patients are more likely to have decreased renal function, take care in dose selection; it may be useful to monitor renal function.

Lab test abnormalities: Peginterferon alfa-2a treatment was associated with decreases in WBC, ANC, lymphocytes, and platelet counts, often starting within the first 2 weeks of treatment.

Transient elevations in ALT (2- to 5-fold above baseline) were observed in some patients receiving peginterferon alfa-2a and were not associated with deterioration of other liver function tests.

Immunogenicity –

Chronic HBV: Twenty-nine percent (42/143) of hepatitis B patients treated with peginterferon alfa-2a for 24 weeks developed binding antibodies to interferon alfa-, as assessed by an enzyme-linked immunosorbent assay (ELISA).

Chronic HCV: Nine percent (71/834) of patients treated with peginterferon alfa-2a with or without ribavirin developed binding antibodies to interferon alfa-2a, as assessed by an ELISA.

Monitoring: Before beginning peginterferon alfa-2a or peginterferon/ribavirin tablet combination therapy, standard hematological and biochemical laboratory tests are recommended for all patients. Pregnancy screening for women of childbearing potential must be performed. After initiation of therapy, perform hematological tests at 2 and 4 weeks and biochemical tests at 4 weeks. Periodically perform additional testing during therapy.

Drug Interactions

Drugs that may be affected by peginterferon alfa-2a include theophylline, methadone, and NRTIs (eg, didanosine, zidovudine, stavudine).

Adverse Reactions

The most common life-threatening or fatal events induced or aggravated by peginterferon alfa-2a and ribavirin tablets were depression, suicide, relapse of drug abuse/overdose, and bacterial infections; each occurred at a frequency of less than 1%. The most commonly reported adverse reactions were psychiatric reactions, including anxiety, depression, irritability, and flu-like symptoms such as fatigue, headache, myalgia, pyrexia, and rigors.

Peginterferon alfa-2a dose was reduced in 12% of patients receiving 1,000 to 1,200 mg ribavirin tablets for 48 weeks and in 7% of patients receiving 800 mg ribavirin tablets for 24 weeks. Ribavirin tablet dose was reduced in 21% of patients receiving 1,000 to 1,200 mg ribavirin tablets for 48 weeks and 12% in patients receiving 800 mg ribavirin tablets for 24 weeks.

Adverse reactions occurring in at least 3% of patients include the following: Abdominal pain, alopecia, anemia, anorexia, arthralgia, back pain, concentration impairment, cough, depression, dermatitis, diarrhea, dizziness, dry mouth, dry skin, dyspnea, fatigue/asthenia, headache, hypothyroidism, injection-site reaction, insomnia, irritability/anxiety/nervousness, lymphopenia, memory impairment, mood alteration, myalgia, nausea/vomiting, neutropenia, pain, pruritus, pyrexia, rash, overall resistance mechanism disorders, rigors, sweating increased, thrombocytopenia, vision blurred, weight decrease.

PEGINTERFERON ALFA-2B

Injection, lyophilized powder for solution: 50, 80, 120, 150 mcg/0.5 mL (*Rx*)	*PEG-Intron*[a] (Schering)

[a] Effective October 22, 2001, *PEG-Intron* only will be made available through the *PEG-Intron* Access Assurance program. Pharmacists must obtain an order authorization number prior to placing an order with their wholesaler. To obtain this number, call (888) 437-2608 to provide the patient's Access Assurance ID# and the quantity to be dispensed (maximum 4 units). Patients without an Access Assurance ID# also may call this number to enroll. Next, contact the wholesaler and provide the authorization number and order information.

Warning:

Alpha interferons, including peginterferon alfa-2b, cause or aggravate fatal or life-threatening neuropsychiatric, autoimmune, ischemic, and infectious disorders. Closely monitor patients with periodic clinical and laboratory evaluations. Withdraw from therapy patients with persistently severe or worsening signs or symptoms of these conditions. In many but not all cases, these disorders resolve after stopping peginterferon alfa-2b therapy.

Ribavirin use: Ribavirin may cause birth defects and/or death of the unborn child. Take extreme care to avoid pregnancy in female patients and in female partners of male patients. Ribavirin causes hemolytic anemia. The anemia associated with ribavirin therapy may result in a worsening of cardiac disease. Ribavirin is genotoxic and mutagenic; consider it a potential carcinogen (see Ribavirin monograph for additional information and warnings).

Indications

Chronic hepatitis C: For use alone or in combination with ribavirin capsules for the treatment of chronic hepatitis C in patients with compensated liver disease who have not been previously treated with interferon alpha and are at least 18 years of age.

When used in combination with ribavirin, refer to ribavirin monograph for additional prescribing information.

Administration and Dosage

Patients should self-inject only if the physician determines that it is appropriate and patients agree to medical follow-up as necessary and receive training in proper injection technique.

Monotherapy: 1 mcg/kg/week subcutaneously for 1 year. Administer the dose on the same day of the week. Base initial dosing on the patient's weight as described in the following table.

Recommended Dosing of Peginterferon Alfa-2b

Redipen or vial strength to use (mcg/0.5 mL)	Body weight (kg)	Amount of peginterferon alfa-2b to administer (mcg)	Volume[a] of peginterferon alfa-2b to administer (mL)
50	≤ 45	40	0.4
	46 to 56	50	0.5
80	57 to 72	64	0.4
	73 to 88	80	0.5
120	89 to 106	96	0.4
	107 to 136	120	0.5
150	137 to 160	150	0.5

[a] When reconstituted as directed.

Peginterferon alfa-2b/Ribavirin capsules combination therapy: When administered in combination with ribavirin capsules, the recommended dose of peginterferon alfa-2b is 1.5 mcg/kg/week. The volume of peginterferon alfa-2b to be injected depends on the strength of peginterferon alfa-2b and the patient's body weight.

Recommended Peginterferon Alfa-2b Combination Therapy Dosing			
Redipen or vial strength to use (mcg/0.5 mL)	Body weight (kg)	Amount of peginterferon alfa-2b to administer (mcg)	Volume[a] of peginterferon alfa-2b to administer (mL)
50	< 40	50	0.5
80	40 to 50	64	0.4
	51 to 60	80	0.5
120	61 to 75	96	0.4
	76 to 85	120	0.5
150	> 85	150	0.5

[a] When reconstituted as directed.

The recommended dose of ribavirin capsules is 800 mg/day in 2 divided doses; 2 capsules (400 mg) with breakfast and 2 capsules (400 mg) with dinner. Do not use ribavirin capsules in patients with CrCl less than 50 mL/min.

Discontinuation: It is recommended that patients receiving peginterferon alfa-2b alone or in combination with ribavirin be discontinued from therapy if hepatitis C virus (HCV) viral levels remain high after 6 months of therapy.

Dose reduction: If a serious adverse reaction develops during the course of treatment (see Warnings, Precautions), discontinue or modify the dosage of peginterferon alfa-2b and/or ribavirin capsules until the adverse reaction abates or decreases in severity. If persistent or recurrent serious adverse reactions develop despite adequate dosage adjustment, discontinue treatment. Decreases in hemoglobin, neutrophils, and platelets may require dose reduction or permanent discontinuation from therapy. For guidelines for dose modifications and discontinuation based on laboratory parameters, see the tables below.

Guidelines for Modification or Discontinuation of Peginterferon Alfa-2b or Peginterferon Alfa-2b/Ribavirin Capsules and for Scheduling Visits for Patients with Depression

	Initial management (4 to 8 weeks)		Depression		
Depression severity[a]	Dose modification	Visit schedule	Remains stable	Improves	Worsens
Mild	No change.	Evaluate once/week by visit or phone.	Continue weekly visit schedule.	Resume normal visit schedule.	(See moderate or severe depression.)
Moderate	Decrease IFN dose 50%.	Evaluate once/week (office visit at least every other week).	Consider psychiatric consultation. Continue reduced dosing.	If symptoms improve and are stable for 4 weeks, may resume normal visit schedule. Continue reduced dosing or return to normal dose.	(See severe depression.)
Severe	Discontinue IFN/R permanently.	Obtain immediate psychiatric consultation.	Psychiatric therapy necessary.		

[a] See DSM-IV for definitions.

Guidelines for Dose Modification and Discontinuation of Peginterferon Alfa-2b or Peginterferon Alfa-2b/Ribavirin Capsules for Hematologic Toxicity			
Laboratory values		Peginterferon alfa-2b	Ribavirin capsules
Hemoglobin[a]	< 10 g/dL	—	Decrease by 200 mg/day
	< 8.5 g/dL	Permanently discontinue	Permanently discontinue
WBC	$< 1.5 \times 10^9$/L	Reduce dose by 50%	—
	$< 1 \times 10^9$/L	Permanently discontinue	Permanently discontinue
Neutrophils	$< 0.75 \times 10^9$/L	Reduce dose by 50%	—
	$< 0.5 \times 10^9$/L	Permanently discontinue	Permanently discontinue
Platelets	$< 80 \times 10^9$/L	Reduce dose by 50%	—
	$< 50 \times 10^9$/L	Permanently discontinue	Permanently discontinue

[a] For patients with a history of stable cardiac disease receiving peginterferon alfa-2b in combination with ribavirin capsules, reduce the peginterferon alfa-2b dose by half and the ribavirin capsule dose by 200 mg/day if a more than 2 g/dL decrease in hemoglobin is observed during any 4-week period. Permanently discontinue peginterferon alfa-2b and ribavirin capsules if patient has hemoglobin levels less than 12 g/dL after this ribavirin dose reduction.

Reconstitution:

Redipen – To reconstitute the lyophilized peginterferon alfa-2b in the *Redipen*, hold the *Redipen* upright (dose button down) and press the two halves of the pen together until there is an audible click. Gently invert the pen to mix the solution. Do not shake. Keeping the pen upright, attach the supplied needle and select the appropriate peginterferon alfa-2b dose by pulling back on the dosing button until the dark bands are visible and turning the button until the dark band is aligned with the correct dose. The *Redipen* is for single use only.

Vials – Reconstitute the peginterferon alfa-2b lyophilized product with only 0.7 mL of supplied diluent (sterile water for injection). The diluent vial is for single use only. Discard the remaining diluent. Do not add any other medication to solutions containing peginterferon alfa-2b, and do not reconstitute peginterferon alfa-2b with other diluents. Swirl gently to hasten complete dissolution of the powder.

Actions

Pharmacology: The biological activity of peginterferon alfa-2b is derived from its interferon alfa-2b moiety. Interferons exert their cellular activities by binding to specific membrane receptors on the cell surface and initiate a complex sequence of intracellular events.

Pharmacokinetics:

Absorption/Distribution – Maximal serum concentrations (C_{max}) occur between 15 and 44 hours postdose and are sustained for up to 48 to 72 hours.

Metabolism/Excretion – The mean peginterferon alfa-2b elimination half-life is approximately 40 hours (range, 22 to 60 hours) in patients with HCV infection. The apparent clearance of peginterferon alfa-2b is estimated to be approximately 22 mL/h•kg. Renal elimination accounts for 30% of the clearance.

Pegylation of interferon alfa-2b produces a product (peginterferon alfa-2b) whose clearance is lower than that of nonpegylated interferon alfa-2b. When compared to interferon alfa-2b, peginterferon alfa-2b (1 mcg/kg) has an approximately 7-fold lower mean apparent clearance and a 5-fold greater mean half life permitting a reduced dosing frequency.

Contraindications

Peginterferon alfa-2b: Hypersensitivity to peginterferon alfa-2b or any component of the product; autoimmune hepatitis; decompensated liver disease.

Peginterferon alfa-2b/Ribavirin capsules combination: Hypersensitivity to ribavirin capsules or any other component of the product; pregnant women; men whose female partners are pregnant; patients with hemoglobinopathies (eg, thalassemia major, sickle-cell anemia).

Warnings/Precautions

Neuropsychiatric events: Life-threatening or fatal neuropsychiatric events, including suicide, suicidal and homicidal ideation, depression, relapse of drug addiction/overdose, and aggressive behavior have occurred in patients with and without a previous psychiatric disorder during peginterferon alfa-2b treatment and follow-up. Psychoses, hallucinations, bipolar disorders, and mania have been observed in patients treated with alpha interferons.

Bone marrow toxicity: Peginterferon alfa-2b suppresses bone marrow function, sometimes resulting in severe cytopenias. Ribavirin may potentiate the neutropenia induced by interferon alpha. Very rarely, alpha interferons may be associated with aplastic anemia.

Colitis: Fatal and nonfatal ulcerative or hemorrhagic/ischemic colitis have been observed within 12 weeks of the start of alpha interferon treatment. Abdominal pain, bloody diarrhea, and fever are the typical manifestations.

Pancreatitis: Fatal and nonfatal pancreatitis have been observed in patients treated with alpha interferons.

Pulmonary disorders: Dyspnea, pulmonary infiltrates, pneumonia, bronchiolitis obliterans, interstitial pneumonitis, and sarcoidosis, some resulting in respiratory failure and/or patient deaths, may be induced or aggravated by peginterferon alfa-2b or alpha-interferon therapy.

Endocrine disorders: Peginterferon alfa-2b causes or aggravates hypothyroidism and hyperthyroidism. Hyperglycemia has been observed in patients treated with peginterferon alfa-2b. Diabetes mellitus has been observed in patients treated with alpha interferons.

Cardiovascular events: Cardiovascular events, including hypotension, arrhythmia, tachycardia, cardiomyopathy, angina pectoris, and MI have been observed in patients treated with peginterferon alfa-2b.

Autoimmune disorders: Development or exacerbation of autoimmune disorders (eg, thyroiditis, thrombocytopenia, rheumatoid arthritis, interstitial nephritis, systemic lupus erythematosus, psoriasis) has been observed in patients receiving peginterferon alfa-2b.

Ophthalmologic disorders: Decrease or loss of vision, retinopathy (including macular edema), retinal artery or vein thrombosis, retinal hemorrhages and cotton wool spots, optic neuritis, and papilledema may be induced or aggravated by treatment with peginterferon alfa-2b or other alpha interferons. All patients should receive an eye examination at baseline.

Anemia: Ribavirin caused hemolytic anemia in 10% of peginterferon alfa-2b/ribavirin capsule-treated patients within 1 to 4 weeks of initiation of therapy. Obtain complete blood counts pretreatment and at weeks 2 and 4 of therapy or more frequently if clinically indicated.

Immunogenicity: Approximately 2% of patients receiving peginterferon alfa-2b or interferon alfa-2b with or without ribavirin capsules developed low-titer (160 or less) neutralizing antibodies to peginterferon alfa-2b or interferon alfa-2b.

HIV or HBV coinfections: The safety and efficacy of peginterferon alfa-2b/ribavirin capsules for the treatment of patients with HCV coinfected with HIV or HBV have not been established.

Organ transplants: The safety and efficacy of peginterferon alfa-2b alone or in combination with ribavirin capsules for the treatment of hepatitis C in patients who have received liver or other organ transplants have not been studied. Preliminary data indicate that interferon alpha therapy may be associated with an increased rate of kidney graft rejection. Liver graft rejection also has been reported, but a causal association to interferon alpha therapy has not been established.

Triglycerides: Elevated triglyceride levels have been observed in patients treated with interferons, including peginterferon alfa-2b therapy. Manage elevated triglyceride levels as clinically appropriate. Hypertriglyceridemia may result in pancreatitis. Consider discontinuation of peginterferon alfa-2b therapy for patients with persistently elevated triglycerides (ie, triglycerides greater than 1000 mg/dL) associated with symptoms of potential pancreatitis, such as abdominal pain, nausea, or vomiting.

Hypersensitivity reactions: Serious, acute hypersensitivity reactions (eg, urticaria, angioedema, bronchoconstriction, anaphylaxis) have been rarely observed during alpha interferon therapy.

Renal function impairment: Closely monitor patients with impairment of renal function for signs and symptoms of interferon toxicity and adjust doses of peginterferon alfa-2b accordingly. Use peginterferon alfa-2b with caution in patients with CrCl less than 50 mL/min.

Pregnancy: Category C (Category X if used with ribavirin). Peginterferon alfa-2b should be assumed to have abortifacient potential. Use during pregnancy only if the potential benefit justifies the potential risk to the fetus. Therefore, peginterferon alfa-2b is recommended for use in fertile women only when they are using effective contraception during the treatment period.

Lactation: It is not known whether the components of interferon alfa-2b are excreted in human milk.

Children: Safety and efficacy in pediatric patients younger than 18 years of age have not been established.

Elderly: Treatment with alpha interferons, including peginterferon alfa-2b, is associated with CNS, cardiac, and systemic (flu-like) adverse effects. Because these adverse reactions may be more severe in the elderly, exercise caution in the use of interferon alfa-2b in this population.

Lab test abnormalities: Peginterferon alfa-2b alone or in combination with ribavirin capsules may cause severe decreases in neutrophil and platelet counts and abnormality of TSH. In 10% of patients treated with peginterferon alfa-2b, ALT levels rose 2- to 5-fold above baseline. The elevations were transient and were not associated with deterioration of other liver functions.

Monitoring: Patients on peginterferon alfa-2b or peginterferon alfa-2b/ribavirin capsules combination therapy should have hematology and blood chemistry testing before the start of treatment and then periodically thereafter. Measure HCV RNA at 6 months of treatment. Discontinue peginterferon alfa-2b or peginterferon alfa-2b/ribavirin capsules combination therapy in patients with persistent high viral levels. Administer an ECG to patients who have preexisting cardiac abnormalities before treatment with peginterferon alfa-2b/ribavirin capsules.

Adverse Reactions

Adverse reactions occurring in at least 3% of patients include the following: Abdominal pain; agitation; alopecia; anemia; anorexia; anxiety/emotional lability/irritability; arthralgia; asthenia; blurred vision; chest pain; concentration impaired; conjunctivitis; constipation; coughing; depression; diarrhea; dizziness; dry mouth; dry skin; dyspepsia; dyspnea; fatigue; fever; flushing; headache; hepatomegaly; hypothyroidism; injection site inflammation/reaction; insomnia; leukopenia; malaise; menstrual disorder; musculoskeletal pain; myalgia; nausea; nervousness; neutropenia; pharyngitis; pruritus; rash; rhinitis; right upper quadrant pain; rigors; sinusitis; sweating increased; taste perversion; thrombocytopenia; viral/fungal infection; vomiting; weight decrease.

INTERFERON GAMMA-1B

Injection, solution: 100 mcg (2 million units) per 0.5 mL (*Rx*)	*Actimmune* (InterMune)

Indications

Chronic granulomatous disease (GCD): For reducing the frequency and severity of serious infections associated with chronic granulomatous disease.

Malignant osteopetrosis: For delaying time to disease progression in patients with severe, malignant osteopetrosis.

Administration and Dosage

Recommended dose: 50 mcg/m^2 (1 million $units/m^2$) for patients whose body surface area (BSA) is more than 0.5 m^2, and 1.5 mcg/kg/dose for patients whose BSA is 0.5 m^2 or less. Injections should be administered subcutaneously 3 times a week (ie, Monday, Wednesday, Friday).

Note that the above activity is expressed in international units (1 million units per 50 mcg). This is equivalent to what was previously expressed as units (1.5 million units per 50 mcg).

Higher doses are not recommended. Safety and efficacy have not been established for interferon gamma-1b given in doses more than or less than the recommended dose of 50 mcg/m^2. The minimum effective dose of interferon gamma-1b has not been established.

Dose reduction: If a severe reaction occurs, the dosage should be reduced by 50% or therapy should be discontinued until the adverse reaction abates.

Administration: Avoid excessive or vigorous agitation. Interferon gamma-1b may be administered using either sterilized glass or plastic disposable syringes. Interferon gamma-1b should not be mixed with other drugs in the same syringe. The optimal sites of injection are the right and left deltoid and anterior thigh.

The formulation does not contain a preservative. A vial of interferon gamma-1b is suitable for a single dose only. The unused portion of any vial should be discarded.

Actions

Pharmacology: Interferons bind to specific cell surface receptors and initiate a sequence of intracellular events that lead to the transcription of interferon-stimulated genes. The 3 major groups of interferons (ie, alpha, beta, gamma) have partially overlapping biological activities that include immunoregulation, such as increased resistance to microbial pathogens and inhibition of cell proliferation.

Pharmacokinetics: After IM or subcutaneous injection, the apparent fraction of dose absorbed was greater than 89%. The mean elimination half-life after IV administration was 38 minutes. The mean elimination half-lives for IM and subcutaneous dosing were 2.9 and 5.9 hours, respectively. Peak plasma concentrations occurred approximately 4 hours after IM dosing and 7 hours after subcutaneous dosing.

Contraindications

Hypersensitivity to interferon gamma, *Escherichia coli* derived products, or any component of the product.

Warnings/Precautions

CNS disorders: CNS adverse reactions including decreased mental status, gait disturbance, and dizziness have been observed, particularly in patients receiving doses greater than 250 mcg/m^2/day. Most of these abnormalities were mild and reversible within a few days upon dose reduction or discontinuation of therapy. Exercise caution in patients with seizure disorders and compromised CNS function.

Cardiac disease: Acute and transient "flu-like" symptoms, such as fever and chills induced by interferon gamma-1b at doses of 250 mcg/m^2/day (more than 10 times the weekly recommended dose) or higher may exacerbate preexisting cardiac conditions. Use with caution in patients with pre-existing cardiac disease, including symptoms of ischemia, CHF, or arrhythmia.

Hematologic effects: Exercise caution when administering to patients with myelosuppression.

Hepatic effects: Elevations of AST and/or ALT (25-fold or less) have been observed during interferon gamma-1b therapy.

Hypersensitivity reactions: Isolated cases of acute serious hypersensitivity reactions have been observed in patients receiving interferon gamma-1b. If such an acute reaction develops, discontinue the drug immediately and institute appropriate medical therapy.

Pregnancy: Category C.

Lactation: It is not known whether interferon gamma is excreted in breast milk.

Monitoring: The following laboratory tests are recommended prior to the beginning of, and at 3-month intervals during, treatment: hematologic tests, including complete blood counts, differential and platelet counts; blood chemistries, including renal and liver function tests; and urinalysis. In patients younger than 1 year of age, measure liver function tests monthly.

Drug Interactions

Exercise caution when administering interferon gamma in combination with other potentially myelosuppressive agents. Possible depression of CYP450 hepatic metabolism of drugs.

Adverse Reactions

Adverse reactions may include fever, headache, rash, chills, injection site erythema or tenderness, fatigue, diarrhea, vomiting, nausea, abdominal pain, myalgia, and depression.

INTERFERON BETA

INTERFERON BETA-1a	
Injection: 8.8 mcg per 0.2 mL (2.4 million units), 22 mcg per 0.5 mL (6 million units), and 44 mcg per 0.5 mL (12 million units) (*Rx*)	*Rebif* (Serono)
Injection, lyophilized powder for solution: 33 mcg (6.6 milliunits) (*Rx*)	*Avonex* (Biogen Idec)
Prefilled syringe: 30 mcg/0.5 mL (*Rx*)	
INTERFERON BETA-1b	
Injection, lyophilized powder for solution: 0.3 mg (*Rx*)	*Betaseron* (Bayer)

Indications

Interferon beta-1a:

Multiple sclerosis (MS) – For the treatment of relapsing forms of MS to slow the accumulation of physical disability and decrease the frequency of clinical exacerbations.

Interferon beta-1b:

MS – For use in ambulatory patients with relapsing forms of MS to reduce the frequency of clinical exacerbations.

Administration and Dosage

Interferon beta-1a:

Avonex – 30 mcg IM once/week in the thigh or upper arm.

Do not substitute subcutaneous administration of *Avonex* for IM administration.

Rebif – Administer subcutaneously 3 times per week at the same time (preferably in the late afternoon or evening) on the same 3 days at least 48 hours apart each week. Generally, start patients at 20% of the prescribed dose 3 times per week and increase over a 4-week period to the targeted dose, either 22 or 44 mcg 3 times per week, as shown in the following table.

Rebif Schedule for Patient Titration				
	Recommended titration	Titration dose for *Rebif* 22 mcg	Titration dose for *Rebif* 44 mcg	Injection volume
Weeks 1 to 2	20%	4.4 mcg	8.8 mcg	0.1 mL
Weeks 3 to 4	50%	11 mcg	22 mcg	0.25 mL
Weeks 5+	100%	22 mcg	44 mcg	0.5 mL

Leukopenia or elevated liver function tests may necessitate dose reductions of 20% to 50% until toxicity is resolved.

Interferon beta-1b:

Relapsing/Remitting MS – 0.25 mg injected subcutaneously every other day. Patients should be started at 0.0625 mg (0.25 mL) subcutaneously every other day and increased over a 6-week period to 0.25 mg (1 mL) every other day, as shown in the following table.

Interferon Beta-1b Schedule for Dose Titration			
	Recommended titration	Interferon beta-1b dose	Volume
Weeks 1 to 2	25%	0.0625 mg	0.25 mL
Weeks 3 to 4	50%	0.125 mg	0.50 mL
Weeks 5 to 6	75%	0.1875 mg	0.75 mL
Weeks 7+	100%	0.25 mg	1 mL

Administration: Sites for self-injection include arms, abdomen, hips, and thighs.

Actions

Pharmacology: Interferon beta-1a and beta-1b have antiviral, antiproliferative, and immunoregulatory activities. The mechanisms by which they exert their actions in MS are not clearly understood.

Pharmacokinetics:

Interferon beta-1a – Biological response marker levels increase within 12 hours of dosing and remain elevated for at least 4 days. Peak biological response marker levels typically are observed 48 hours after dosing.

Interferon Beta-1a Pharmacokinetic Parameters[a]				
Route	Mean C_{max} (IU/mL)	T_{max} (h)	Mean AUC (IU•h/mL)	$t_{1/2}$ (h)
IM	4.9	3 to 15	65	10
Subcutaneous[b]	5.1	16 (median)	294	69

[a] Data are pooled from different studies and are not necessarily comparable.
[b] Based on a single dose of 60 mcg.

Interferon beta-1b – Peak serum concentrations occurred between 1 and 8 hours. Bioavailability, based on a total dose of 0.5 mg given as 2 subcutaneous injections at different sites, was approximately 50%.

Mean serum clearance values ranged from 9.4 to 28.9 mL/min/kg and were independent of dose. Mean terminal elimination half-life values ranged from 8 minutes to 4.3 hours and mean steady-state volume of distribution values ranged from 0.25 to 2.88 L/kg. IV dosing 3 times/week for 2 weeks resulted in no accumulation of interferon beta-1a or beta-1b in the serum of patients.

Contraindications

Hypersensitivity to natural or recombinant interferon beta, albumin human, or any other component of the formulation.

Warnings/Precautions

Chronic progressive MS: The safety and efficacy of interferon beta in chronic progressive MS have not been evaluated.

Depression: Use interferon beta with caution in patients with depression or other mood disorders, conditions that are common with MS. Depression and suicide have been reported in patients receiving interferon compounds. Advise patients treated with interferon beta to immediately report any symptoms of depression or suicidal ideation.

Injection-site necrosis (ISN): ISN has been reported. Typically, ISN occurs within the first 4 months of therapy. Periodically re-evaluate patient understanding and use of aseptic self-injection techniques, particularly if ISN has occurred.

Anaphylaxis: Anaphylaxis has been reported as a rare complication of interferon beta use.

Decreased peripheral blood counts: Decreased peripheral blood counts in all cell lines, including rare pancytopenia and thrombocytopenia, have been reported from postmarketing experience.

Albumin (human): Some of these products contain albumin, a derivative of human blood. Based on effective donor screening and product manufacturing processes, it carries an extremely remote risk for transmission of viral diseases.

Special risk patients: Exercise caution when administering **interferon beta-1a** to patients with pre-existing seizure disorders. Seizures have been associated with the use of beta interferons.

Cardiac disease: Closely monitor patients with cardiac disease, such as angina, CHF, or arrhythmia, for worsening of their clinical condition during initiation and continued treatment.

Self-administration: Instruct patients in injection techniques to ensure the safe self-administration of interferon beta.

Flu-like symptoms complex: Flu-like symptoms, including headache, fever, fatigue, rigors, chest pain, back pain, and myalgia, have been commonly reported with interferon beta therapy. Symptoms usually occur 4 hours after injection and subside within 24 hours. Acetaminophen or NSAIDs prior to and/or following injection may help to prevent or treat these symptoms.

Autoimmune disorders: Autoimmune disorders of multiple target organs have been reported postmarketing, including idiopathic thrombocytopenia, hyper- and hypothyroidism, and rare cases of autoimmune hepatitis.

Hepatic injury: Hepatic injury, including elevated serum hepatic enzyme levels and hepatitis, some of which have been severe, has been reported postmarketing. Monitor patients for signs of hepatic injury and exercise caution when interferons are used concomitantly with other drugs associated with hepatic injury.

Immunogenicity: As with all therapeutic proteins, there is a potential for immunogenicity.

Latex sensitivity: Administer with caution to patients with a possible history of latex sensitivity; packaging may contain dry natural rubber.

Hepatic function impairment: Severe liver dysfunction, leading to hepatic failure requiring liver transplantation, has been reported very rarely in patients taking interferon beta.

Photosensitivity: Photosensitization (photoallergy or phototoxicity) may occur.

Fertility impairment: Menstrual irregularities were observed in monkeys administered **interferon beta-1a** at a dose 100 times the recommended weekly human dose.

Pregnancy: Category C.

Lactation: It is not known whether interferon beta is excreted in breast milk.

Children: Safety and efficacy in children under 18 years of age have not been established.

Monitoring: In addition to the laboratory tests normally required for monitoring patients with MS, blood cell counts and liver function tests are recommended at baseline and regular intervals (1, 3, and 6 months) and then periodically thereafter in the absence of clinical symptoms. Thyroid function tests are recommended every 6 months in patients with a history of thyroid dysfunction or as clinically indicated. Patients with myelosuppression may require more intensive monitoring of complete blood cell counts, with differential and platelet counts.

Adverse Reactions

Adverse reactions occurring in at least 3% of patients may include injection site reaction, headache, fever, flu-like symptoms, pain, asthenia, chills, infection, abdominal pain, chest pain, malaise, generalized edema, pelvic pain, injection site necrosis/inflammation, cyst/ovarian cyst, suicide attempt, hypersensitivity reaction, migraine, palpitation, hypertension, tachycardia, peripheral vascular disorder, hemorrhage, syncope, vasodilation, lymphocytes less than 1500/mm^3, ANC less than 3000/mm^3, lymphadenopathy, anemia, eosinophils at least 10%, HCT (%) up to 37, sinusitis, upper respiratory tract infection, dyspnea, laryngitis, myalgia, myasthenia, arthralgia, nausea, diarrhea, constipation, vomiting, dyspepsia, anorexia, GI disorder, ALT more than 5 times baseline, glucose less than 55 mg/dL, total bilirubin more than 2.5 times baseline, urine protein more than 1+, AST more than 5 times baseline, weight gain/loss, AST at least 3 times the upper limit of normal, mental symptoms, hypertonia, sleep difficulty, dizziness, muscle spasm, somnolence, speech disorder, convulsion, sweating, urticaria, alopecia, nevus, herpes zoster, conjunctivitis, abnormal vision, otitis media, hearing decreased, dysmenorrhea, menstrual disorder, metrorrhagia, cystitis, breast pain, menorrhagia, urinary urgency, vaginitis, fibrocystic breast.

ANAKINRA

Injection: 100 mg per 0.67 mL (*Rx*)	*Kineret* (Amgen)

Indications

Rheumatoid arthritis (RA): For the reduction in signs and symptoms and slowing the progression of structural damage in moderately to severely active RA in patients 18 years of age and older who have failed 1 or more disease-modifying antirheumatic drugs (DMARDs). Anakinra can be used alone or in combination with DMARDs other than tumor necrosis factor (TNF)-blocking agents.

Administration and Dosage

The recommended dose of anakinra is 100 mg/day administered at approximately the same time daily by subcutaneous injection. Higher doses did not result in a higher response. Administer the dose at approximately the same time every day.

Actions

Pharmacology: Anakinra is a recombinant, nonglycosylated form of the human interleukin-1 receptor antagonist (IL-1Ra). Anakinra differs from native human IL-1Ra in that it has a single methionine residue at its amino terminus. It is produced by recombinant DNA technology using an *Escherichia coli* bacterial expression system.

Anakinra blocks the biologic activity of IL-1 by competitively inhibiting IL-1 binding to the interleukin-1 type I receptor (IL-1RI), which is expressed in a wide variety of tissues and organs.

Pharmacokinetics: The absolute bioavailability after a 70 mg subcutaneous bolus injection in healthy subjects (n = 11) is 95%. In subjects with RA, maximum plasma concentrations occurred 3 to 7 hours after subcutaneous administration of anakinra at clinically relevant doses (1 to 2 mg/kg; n = 18); the terminal half-life ranged from 4 to 6 hours. In RA patients, no unexpected accumulation was observed after daily subcutaneous doses for up to 24 weeks. The estimated clearance increased with increasing CrCl and body weight.

Special populations –

Renal function impairment: The mean plasma clearance decreased 70% to 75% in normal subjects with severe or end-stage renal disease (CrCl less than 30 mL/min).

Contraindications

Patients with known hypersensitivity to *E. coli*-derived proteins, anakinra, or any component of the product.

Warnings/Precautions

Infections: Anakinra has been associated with an increased incidence of serious infections (2%) vs placebo (less than 1%). Discontinue administration if a patient develops a serious infection. Do not initiate treatment with anakinra in patients with active infections. The safety and efficacy of anakinra in immunocompromised patients or in patients with chronic infections have not been evaluated. Coadministration of anakinra and etanercept has not demonstrated increased clinical benefit. Carefully monitor patients when considering initiation of anakinra therapy concurrently with etanercept therapy.

Immunosuppression: The impact of treatment with anakinra on active and/or chronic infections and the development of malignancies is not known.

Vaccinations: Do not give live vaccines concurrently with anakinra. No data are available on the secondary transmission of infections by live vaccines in patients receiving anakinra. Because anakinra interferes with normal immune response mechanisms to new antigens such as vaccines, vaccination may not be effective in patients receiving anakinra.

Hematologic events: Patients may experience a decrease in neutrophil counts.

Immunogenicity: In 2 studies, 26% of patients tested positive for anti-anakinra antibodies at month 12 in a highly sensitive, anakinra-binding biosensor assay. Of the 1,318 subjects with available data at week 12 or later, 1% were seropositive in a cell-based bioassay for antibodies capable of neutralizing the biologic effects of anakinra. Two of the 15 of these subjects were positive for neutralizing antibodies at more than 1 time point up to the week 52 visit and 4 were positive at week 52. No correlation between antibody development and clinical response or adverse events was observed. The long-term immunogenicity of anakinra is unknown.

Hypersensitivity reactions: Hypersensitivity reactions associated with anakinra administration are rare. If a severe hypersensitivity reaction occurs, discontinue anakinra administration and initiate appropriate therapy.

Renal function impairment: This drug is known to be substantially excreted by the kidney, and the risk of toxic reactions to this drug may be greater in patients with impaired renal function.

Pregnancy: *Category B.*

Lactation: It is not known whether anakinra is secreted in human milk. Because many drugs are secreted in human milk, exercise caution if anakinra is administered to nursing women.

Children: Safety and efficacy in patients with juvenile RA have not been established.

Elderly: Because there is a higher incidence of infections in the elderly population in general, use caution in treating the elderly.

Monitoring: Assess neutrophil counts prior to initiating anakinra treatment, and while receiving anakinra, monthly for 3 months, and thereafter quarterly for a period up to 1 year.

Adverse Reactions

The most serious adverse reactions were serious infection and neutropenia, particularly when used in combination with TNF-blocking agents. The most common adverse reaction with anakinra is injection site reactions, the majority of which were reported as mild. These typically lasted for 14 to 28 days and were characterized by 1 or more of the following reactions: Erythema, ecchymosis, inflammation, and pain.

Adverse reactions occurring in at least 5% of RA patients include injection site reaction, worsening of RA, infection (eg, upper respiratory infection, sinusitis, influenza-like symptoms, other infections), headache, nausea, diarrhea, sinusitis, arthralgia, and abdominal pain.

FINGOLIMOD

Capsules; oral: 0.5 mg	*Gilenya* (Novartis)

Indications

Multiple sclerosis: For the treatment of patients with relapsing forms of multiple sclerosis (MS).

Administration and Dosage

General dosing considerations: Observe patients for 6 hours after the first dose to monitor for signs and symptoms of bradycardia.

Adults:

Multiple sclerosis – 0.5 mg once daily.

Hepatic function: Closely monitor patients with severe hepatic impairment because adverse reactions may be greater.

Administration: Administer with or without food.

Actions

Pharmacology: Fingolimod-phosphate blocks the capacity of lymphocytes to egress from lymph nodes, reducing the number of lymphocytes in peripheral blood. The mechanism by which fingolimod exerts therapeutic effects in MS is unknown, but may involve reduction of lymphocyte migration into the central nervous system.

Pharmacodynamics –

Electrophysiology:

Heart rate and rhythm – Fingolimod causes a transient reduction in heart rate and atrioventricular (AV) conduction at treatment initiation. The maximal decline of heart rate is seen in the first 6 hours postdose.

Potential to prolong the QT interval – In a thorough QT interval study, fingolimod treatment resulted in a prolongation of QTc, with the upper bound of the 90% confidence interval (CI) of 14.0 ms.

Immune system:

Immune cell numbers – In a study in which 12 subjects received fingolimod 0.5 mg daily, the lymphocyte count decreased to approximately 60% of baseline within 4 to 6 hours after the first dose. With continued daily dosing, the lymphocyte count continued to decrease over a 2-week period, reaching a nadir count of approximately 30% of baseline.

Pharmacokinetics:

Absorption – The time to maximum concentration (T_{max}) of fingolimod is 12 to 16 hours. The apparent absolute oral bioavailability is 93%.

Steady-state blood concentrations are reached within 1 to 2 months following once-daily administration.

Distribution – Fingolimod is more than 99.7% protein bound.

Metabolism – Fingolimod is primarily metabolized via human CYP4F2, with a minor contribution of CYP2D6, 2E1, 3A4, and 4F12.

Excretion – Fingolimod has an average apparent terminal half-life of 6 to 9 days. After oral administration, approximately 81% of the dose is slowly excreted in the urine as inactive metabolites.

Contraindications

None well documented.

Warnings/Precautions

Cardiovascular effects:

Bradycardia – Initiation of fingolimod treatment results in a decrease in heart rate. Observe all patients for a period of 6 hours for signs and symptoms of bradycardia.

Atrioventricular blocks – Initiation of fingolimod treatment has resulted in transient AV conduction delays.

Re-initiation of therapy following discontinuation – If fingolimod therapy is discontinued for more than 2 weeks, the effects on heart rate and AV conduction may recur upon reintroduction of fingolimod treatment, and the same precautions as for initial dosing should apply.

Blood pressure effects – In MS clinical trials, patients treated with fingolimod 0.5 mg had an average increase of approximately 2 mm Hg in systolic pressure and approximately 1 mm Hg in diastolic pressure, first detected after approximately 2 months of treatment initiation.

Infections: Fingolimod causes a dose-dependent reduction in peripheral lymphocyte count; therefore, fingolimod may increase the risk of infections, some serious in nature.

Varicella zoster virus antibody testing/vaccination – Before initiating therapy, test patients without a history of chickenpox or without vaccination against varicella zoster virus (VZV) for antibodies to VZV. Consider VZV vaccination of antibody-negative patients prior to commencing treatment, following which postpone the initiation of treatment for 1 month to allow the full effect of vaccination to occur.

Vaccines – Vaccination may be less effective during and for up to 2 months after discontinuing fingolimod. Avoid live attenuated vaccine administration during this period.

Immune system effects following discontinuation – Fingolimod remains in the blood and has pharmacodynamic effects, including decreased lymphocyte counts, for up to 2 months following the last dose. Initiating other drugs during this period warrants the same considerations needed for coadministration (eg, risk of additive immunosuppressant effects).

Macular edema: In patients receiving fingolimod 0.5 mg, macular edema occurred in 0.4% of patients. Perform an adequate ophthalmologic evaluation at baseline and 3 to 4 months after treatment initiation.

Respiratory effects: Dose-dependent reductions in FEV-1 and diffusing lung capacity for carbon monoxide (DL_{CO}) were observed in patients as early as 1 month after treatment initiation.

Hepatic effects: Elevations of liver enzymes may occur in patients receiving fingolimod.

Renal function impairment: The blood level of some fingolimod metabolites is increased (up to 13-fold) in patients with severe renal impairment. The toxicity of these metabolites has not been fully explored.

Hepatic function impairment: Because fingolimod, but not fingolimod-phosphate, exposure is doubled in patients with severe hepatic impairment, closely monitor patients with severe hepatic impairment. Patients with preexisting liver disease may be at increased risk of developing elevated liver enzymes.

Pregnancy: Category C.

Lactation: It is not known whether this drug is excreted in human milk.

Children: The safety and effectiveness of fingolimod in children with MS younger than 18 years of age have not been established.

Elderly: Use fingolimod with caution in patients 65 years of age and older, reflecting the greater frequency of decreased hepatic or renal function, and of concomitant disease or other drug therapy.

Monitoring: Perform an adequate ophthalmologic evaluation at baseline and 3 to 4 months after treatment initiation. Ensure that MS patients with diabetes mellitus or a history of uveitis undergo an ophthalmologic evaluation prior to initiating fingolimod therapy and have regular follow-up ophthalmologic evaluations.

Spirometric evaluation of respiratory function and evaluation of DL_{CO} should be performed during therapy with fingolimod if clinically indicated.

Ensure that recent (ie, within last 6 months) transaminase and bilirubin levels are available before initiation of fingolimod therapy. Monitor liver enzymes in patients who develop symptoms suggestive of hepatic dysfunction.

Observe all patients for a period of 6 hours after the first dose for signs and symptoms of bradycardia. If a recent electrocardiograph (within 6 hours) is not available, obtain one in patients using antiarrhythmics, those with cardiac risk factors, and those who have a slow or irregular heartbeat prior to starting fingolimod. Monitor blood pressure during treatment with fingolimod.

Before initiating treatment, ensure that a recent complete blood cell count (CBC) (ie, within 6 months) is available. Monitor patients for infection during treatment and for at least 2 months after discontinuation.

Drug Interactions

QT prolongation: An additive effect of fingolimod with other drugs that prolong the QT interval cannot be excluded. The following drugs may prolong the QT interval and increase the risk of life-threatening agents (eg, amiodarone, bretylium, disopyramide, dofetilide, procainamide, quinidine, sotalol), arsenic trioxide, chlorpromazine, cisapride, dolasetron, droperidol, gatifloxacin, halofantrine, levomethadyl, mefloquine, mesoridazine, moxifloxacin, pentamidine, pimozide, probucol, sparfloxacin, thioridazine, and ziprasidone.

Drugs that may affect fingolimod include antineoplastics, beta-blockers (eg, atenolol), class Ia (eg, procainamide, quinidine) and class III (eg, amiodarone, sotalol), diltiazem, immune modulating therapies, immunosuppressives, ketoconazole (oral).

Drugs that may be affected by fingolimod include beta-blockers (eg, atenolol), diltiazem, ketoconazole (oral).

Drug/Lab test interactions: Because fingolimod reduces blood lymphocyte counts, peripheral blood lymphocyte counts cannot be used to evaluate the lymphocyte subset status. Ensure that a recent CBC is available before starting fingolimod treatment.

Adverse Reactions

Adverse reactions occurring in at least 3% of patients include the following:

Cardiovascular: Bradycardia, hypertension.

CNS: Asthenia, depression, dizziness, headache, migraine, paresthesia.

Dermatologic: Alopecia, eczema, pruritus.

GI: Diarrhea, gastroenteritis.

Hematologic: Leukopenia, lymphopenia.

Lab test abnormalities: ALT/AST increased, blood triglycerides increased, gamma glutamyl transferase increased.

Respiratory: Bronchitis, cough, dyspnea, sinusitis.

Special senses: Eye pain, vision blurred.

Miscellaneous: Back pain, herpes viral infections, influenza viral infections, tinea infections, weight decreased.

INFLIXIMAB

Injection, lyophilized powder for solution: 100 mg (*Rx*) *Remicade* (Centocor)

Warning:

Tuberculosis (TB) (frequently disseminated or extrapulmonary at clinical presentation), invasive fungal infections, and other opportunistic infections have been observed in patients receiving infliximab. Some of these infections have been fatal (see Warnings).

Risk of serious infections: Patients treated with infliximab are at an increased risk for developing serious infections that may lead to hospitalization or death. Most patients who developed these infections were taking concomitant immunosuppressants such as methotrexate or corticosteroids.

continued on next page

Warning: (cont.)

Discontinue infliximab if a patient develops a serious infection or sepsis. Reported infections include:

- Active TB, including reactivation of latent TB. Patients with TB have frequently presented with disseminated or extrapulmonary disease. Test patients for latent TB before infliximab use and during therapy. Initiate treatment for latent infection prior to infliximab use.
- Invasive fungal infections, including histoplasmosis, coccidioidomycosis, candidiasis, aspergillosis, blastomycosis, and pneumocystosis. Patients with histoplasmosis or other invasive fungal infections may present with disseminated, rather than localized, disease. Antigen and antibody testing for histoplasmosis may be negative in some patients with active infection. Empiric antifungal therapy should be considered in patients who develop severe systemic illness.
- Bacterial, viral, and other infections caused by opportunistic pathogens.

Evaluate patients for latent tuberculosis infection with a tuberculin skin test. Initiate treatment of latent tuberculosis infection prior to therapy with infliximab.

Malignancy: Lymphoma and other malignancies, some fatal, have been reported in children and adolescent patients treated with tumor necrosis factor (TNF) blockers, including infliximab.

Hepatosplenic T-cell lymphomas: Postmarketing cases of hepatosplenic T-cell lymphoma, a rare type of T-cell lymphoma, have been reported in patients treated with TNF blockers, including infliximab. These cases had a very aggressive disease course and have been fatal. All reported infliximab cases have occurred in patients with Crohn disease or ulcerative colitis, and the majority were in adolescent and young adult males. All of these patients received treatment with azathioprine or 6-mercaptopurine concomitantly with infliximab at or prior to diagnosis.

Indications

Ankylosing spondylitis: For reducing signs and symptoms in patients with active ankylosing spondylitis.

Crohn disease: For reducing signs and symptoms and inducing and maintaining clinical remission in patients with moderately to severely active Crohn disease who have had an inadequate response to conventional therapy.

Crohn disease, fistulizing – For reducing the number of draining enterocutaneous and rectovaginal fistulas and maintaining fistula closure.

Plaque psoriasis: For treatment of adult patients with chronic, severe (ie, extensive and/or disabling) plaque psoriasis who are candidates for systemic therapy and when other systemic therapies are medically less appropriate. Only administer infliximab to patients who will be closely monitored and have regular follow-up visits with a health care provider.

Psoriatic arthritis: For reducing signs and symptoms of active arthritis, inhibiting the progression of structural damage, and improving physical function in patients with psoriatic arthritis.

Rheumatoid arthritis (RA), moderate to severe: In combination with methotrexate for reducing the signs and symptoms and inhibiting the progression of structural damage and improving physical function in patients with moderately to severely active RA who have had an inadequate response to methotrexate.

Ulcerative colitis: For reducing signs and symptoms, achieving clinical remission and mucosal healing, and eliminating corticosteroid use in patients with moderately to severely active ulcerative colitis who have had an inadequate response to conventional therapy.

Administration and Dosage

Ankylosing spondylitis: 5 mg/kg given as an intravenous (IV) infusion, followed by similar doses at 2 and 6 weeks after the first infusion, then every 6 weeks thereafter.

Crohn disease or fistulizing Crohn disease:

Adults – 5 mg/kg given as an induction regimen at 0, 2, and 6 weeks followed by a maintenance regimen of 5 mg/kg every 8 weeks thereafter. For patients who respond and then lose their response, consider treatment with 10 mg/kg. Patients who do not respond by week 14 are unlikely to respond with continued dosing; consider discontinuing infliximab in these patients.

Children – 5 mg/kg given as an IV induction regimen at 0, 2, and 6 weeks followed by a maintenance regimen of 5 mg/kg every 8 weeks.

Plaque psoriasis: 5 mg/kg given as an IV infusion followed by additional doses at 2 and 6 weeks after the first infusion, then every 8 weeks thereafter.

Psoriatic arthritis: 5 mg/kg given as an IV infusion, followed by similar doses at 2 and 6 weeks after the first infusion, and every 8 weeks thereafter. Infliximab can be used with or without methotrexate.

RA: 3 mg/kg given as an IV infusion followed with similar doses at 2 and 6 weeks after the first infusion, then every 8 weeks thereafter. Give infliximab in combination with methotrexate. For patients who have an incomplete response, consider adjusting the dose up to 10 mg/kg or treating as often as every 4 weeks.

Ulcerative colitis: 5 mg/kg given as an induction regimen at 0, 2, and 6 weeks, followed by a maintenance regimen of 5 mg/kg every 8 weeks.

Actions

Pharmacology: Infliximab neutralizes the biological activity of tumor necrosis factor alpha (TNFα) by binding to its soluble and transmembrane forms and inhibits TNFα receptor binding. Infliximab does not neutralize TNFβ (lymphotoxin α), a related cytokine that uses the same receptors as TNFα.

Pharmacokinetics: A study of single IV infusions of 3 to 20 mg/kg in Crohn disease or RA patients showed a linear relationship between the dose and the maximum serum concentration. The volume of distribution at steady state was independent of dose and indicated that infliximab was distributed primarily within the vascular compartment. The median terminal half-life of infliximab ranged between 8 to 9.5 days.

No systemic accumulation of infliximab occurred upon continued repeated administration. Development of antibodies to infliximab increased infliximab clearance.

Contraindications

Do not administer doses of infliximab greater than 5 mg/kg to patients with moderate to severe heart failure (New York Heart Association class III/IV) (see Warnings).

Hypersensitivity to any murine proteins or other components of the product.

Warnings/Precautions

Risk of serious infections: Serious and sometimes fatal infections caused by bacterial, mycobacterial, invasive fungal, viral, or other opportunistic pathogens have been reported in patients receiving TNF-blocking agents. Among opportunistic infections, TB, histoplasmosis, aspergillosis, candidiasis, coccidioidomycosis, listeriosis, and pneumocystosis were the most commonly reported. Patients have frequently presented with disseminated rather than localized disease, and are often taking concomitant immunosuppressants, such as methotrexate or corticosteroids, with infliximab.

Treatment with infliximab should not be initiated in patients with an active infection, including clinically important localized infections. Consider the risks and benefits of treatment prior to initiating therapy in patients with long-term or recurrent infection; who have been exposed to TB; who have resided or traveled in areas of endemic TB or endemic mycoses, such as histoplasmosis, coccidioidomycosis, or blastomycosis; or with underlying conditions that may predispose them to infection.

Cases of reactivation of TB or new TB infections have been observed in patients receiving infliximab, including patients who have previously received treatment for latent or active TB. Evaluate patients for TB risk factors and test for latent infection prior to initiating infliximab and periodically during therapy.

Malignancies: Malignancies, some fatal, have been reported among children, adolescents and young adults who received treatment with TNF-blocking agents (initiation of therapy, 18 years of age or younger), including infliximab. Approximately half of these cases were lymphomas, including Hodgkin and non-Hodgkin lymphomas. The other cases represented a variety of malignancies, including rare malignancies that are usually associated with immunosuppression and malignancies that are not usually observed in children and adolescents. The malignancies occurred after a median of 30 months (range, 1 to 84 months) after the first dose of TNF blocker therapy. Most of the patients were receiving concomitant immunosuppressants. These cases were reported postmarketing and were derived from a variety of sources, including registries and spontaneous postmarketing reports.

Postmarketing cases of hepatosplenic T-cell lymphomas, a rare type of T-cell lymphoma, have been reported in patients treated with TNF blockers, including infliximab. These cases have had a very aggressive disease course and have been fatal. All reported infliximab cases have occurred in patients with Crohn disease or ulcerative colitis, and the majority were in adolescent and young adult males. All of these patients had received treatment with the immunosuppressants azathioprine or 6-mercaptopurine concomitantly with infliximab at or prior to diagnosis. It is uncertain whether the occurrence of hepatosplenic T-cell lymphomas is related to infliximab or infliximab in combination with these other immunosuppressants.

Hepatitis B virus (HBV) reactivation: Use of TNF blockers, including infliximab, has been associated with reactivation of HBV in patients who are chronic carriers of this virus.

Hepatotoxicity: Severe hepatic reactions, including acute liver failure, jaundice, hepatitis, and cholestasis, have been reported rarely in postmarketing data in patients receiving infliximab. Autoimmune hepatitis has been diagnosed in some of these cases. Severe hepatic reactions occurred between 2 weeks to more than a year after initiation of infliximab; elevations in hepatic aminotransferase levels were not noted prior to discovery of the liver injury in many of these cases. Some of these cases were fatal or necessitated liver transplantation.

Heart failure: Infliximab has been associated with adverse outcomes in patients with heart failure; use in patients with heart failure only after consideration of other treatment options.

Hematologic events: Cases of leukopenia, neutropenia, thrombocytopenia, and pancytopenia, some with a fatal outcome, have been reported in patients receiving infliximab. Advise all patients to seek immediate medical attention if they develop signs and symptoms suggestive of blood dyscrasias or infection (eg, persistent fever) while on infliximab. Consider discontinuation of infliximab therapy in patients who develop significant hematologic abnormalities.

CNS effects: Infliximab and other agents that inhibit TNF have been associated in rare cases with optic neuritis, seizure, and new onset or exacerbation of clinical symptoms and/or radiographic evidence of CNS-demyelinating disorders, including multiple sclerosis and CNS manifestations of systemic vasculitis and peripheral demyelinating disorders, including Guillain-Barré syndrome. Exercise caution when considering the use of infliximab in patients with preexisting or recent onset of CNS-demyelinating or seizure disorders.

Autoimmunity: Treatment with infliximab therapy may result in the formation of autoantibodies and, rarely, in the development of a lupus-like syndrome. Discontinue treatment if a patient develops symptoms suggestive of a lupus-like syndrome following treatment with infliximab.

Vaccinations: No data are available on the response to vaccination with live vaccines or on the secondary transmission of infection by live vaccines in patients receiving anti-TNF therapy. It is recommended that live vaccines not be given concurrently.

Immunogenicity: Treatment with infliximab can be associated with the development of antibodies to infliximab. Approximately 10% of patients were antibody-positive. The majority of antibody-positive patients had low titers. Patients who were antibody-positive were more likely to have a higher rate of clearance, reduced efficacy and experience an infusion reaction.

Hypersensitivity reactions: Infliximab has been associated with hypersensitivity reactions that vary in their time of onset and required hospitalization in some cases. Urticaria, dyspnea, and hypotension have occurred during or within 2 hours of infliximab infusion. However, in some cases, serum sickness-like reactions have been observed in Crohn disease patients 3 to 12 days after infliximab therapy was reinstituted following an extended period without infliximab treatment. Symptoms associated with these reactions include the following: fever, rash, headache, sore throat, myalgias, polyarthralgias, hand and facial edema, dysphagia. These reactions were associated with a marked increase in antibodies to infliximab, loss of detectable serum concentrations of infliximab, and possible loss of drug efficacy. Discontinue infliximab if severe reactions occur.

Pregnancy: *Category B.*

Lactation: It is not known whether infliximab is excreted in human breast milk or absorbed systemically after ingestion.

Children: Infliximab has not been studied in children with Crohn disease younger than 6 years of age. The longer-term (more than 1 year) safety and efficacy of infliximab in children with Crohn disease have not been established in clinical trials.

Safety and efficacy of infliximab in patients with juvenile RA and children with ulcerative colitis and plaque psoriasis have not been established.

Elderly: Because there is a higher incidence of infections in the elderly population in general, use caution when treating the elderly.

Monitoring: Monitor for signs and symptoms of infection during and after treatment with infliximab. Closely monitor new infections. If a serious infection develops, discontinue therapy. Evaluate and monitor chronic carriers of hepatitis B prior to the initiation of and during treatment with infliximab. Monitor patients closely who develop new or worsening symptoms of heart failure.

Drug Interactions

Concurrent administration of etanercept (another TNFα-blocking agent) and anakinra (an interleukin-1 antagonist) has been associated with an increased risk of serious infections, and increased risk of neutropenia and no additional benefit compared with these medicinal products alone. Other TNFα-blocking agents (including infliximab) used in combination with anakinra also may result in similar toxicities. Therefore, the combination of infliximab and anakinra is not recommended.

Vaccinations: No data are available on the response to vaccination or on the secondary transmission of infection by live vaccines in patients receiving anti-TNF therapy. Do not administer live vaccines concurrently.

Adverse Reactions

The most common reasons for discontinuation of treatment were infusion-related reactions (ie, dyspnea, flushing, headache, rash).

Adverse reactions occurring in 5% or more of patients receiving 4 or more infusions include the following: abdominal pain, arthralgia, back pain, bronchitis, chills, coughing, diarrhea, dyspepsia, fatigue, fever, flu syndrome, headache, hypertension, moniliasis, nausea, pain, pharyngitis, pruritus, rash, rhinitis, sinusitis, upper respiratory tract infection, urinary tract infection.

MITOXANTRONE

Injection: 2 mg mitoxantrone free base/mL (*Rx*) — Various, *Novantrone* (Serono)

Warning:

Mitoxantrone should be administered under the supervision of a health care provider experienced in the use of cytotoxic chemotherapy agents.

Mitoxantrone should be given slowly into a freely flowing intravenous (IV) infusion. It must never be given subcutaneously, intramuscularly (IM), or intra-arterially. Severe local tissue damage may occur if there is extravasation during administration.

Not for intrathecal use. Severe injury with permanent sequelae can result from intrathecal administration.

Except for the treatment of acute nonlymphocytic leukemia, mitoxantrone therapy generally should not be given to patients with baseline neutrophil counts of less than 1,500 cells/mm^3. In order to monitor the occurrence of bone marrow suppression, primarily neutropenia, which may be severe and result in infection, it is recommended that frequent peripheral blood cell counts be performed on all patients receiving mitoxantrone.

Cardiotoxicity: Congestive heart failure (CHF), potentially fatal, may occur during therapy with mitoxantrone or months to years after termination of therapy. Cardiotoxicity risk increases with cumulative mitoxantrone dose and may occur whether or not cardiac risk factors are present. Presence or history of cardiovascular disease, radiotherapy to the mediastinal/pericardial area, previous therapy with other anthracyclines or anthracenediones, or use of other cardiotoxic drugs may increase this risk. In cancer patients, the risk of symptomatic CHF was estimated to be 2.6% for patients receiving up to a cumulative dose of 140 mg/m^2. To mitigate the cardiotoxicity risk with mitoxantrone, consider the following:

- All patients should be assessed for cardiac signs and symptoms by history, physical examination, and electrocardiogram (ECG) prior to start of mitoxantrone therapy.
- All patients should have baseline quantitative evaluation of left ventricular ejection fraction (LVEF) using appropriate methodology (eg, echocardiogram, multigated radionuclide angiography [MUGA], or magnetic resonance imaging [MRI])
- Multiple sclerosis (MS) patients with a baseline LVEF below the lower limit of normal should not be treated with mitoxantrone.
- MS patients should be assessed for cardiac signs and symptoms by history, physical examination, and ECG prior to each dose.
- MS patients should undergo quantitative reevaluation of LVEF prior to each dose using the same methodology that was used to assess baseline LVEF. Additional doses of mitoxantrone should not be administered to MS patients who have experienced either a drop in LVEF to below the lower limit of normal or a clinically significant reduction in LVEF during mitoxantrone therapy.
- MS patients should not receive a cumulative mitoxantrone dose higher than 140 mg/m^2.
- MS patients should undergo yearly quantitative LVEF evaluation after stopping mitoxantrone to monitor for late-occurring cardiotoxicity.

continued on next page

Warning: (cont.)

Secondary acute myelogenous leukemia: Secondary acute myelogenous leukemia (AML) has been reported in MS and cancer patients treated with mitoxantrone. In a cohort of mitoxantrone-treated MS patients followed for varying periods of time, an elevated leukemia risk of 0.25% (2/802) has been observed. Postmarketing cases of secondary AML have also been reported. In 1,774 patients with breast cancer who received mitoxantrone concomitantly with other cytotoxic agents and radiotherapy, the cumulative risk of developing treatment-related AML was estimated as 1.1% and 1.6% at 5 and 10 years, respectively. Secondary AML has been reported in cancer patients treated with anthracyclines. Mitoxantrone is an anthracenedione, a related drug.

The occurrence of refractory secondary leukemia is more common when anthracyclines are given in combination with DNA-damaging antineoplastic agents, when patients have been heavily pretreated with cytotoxic drugs, or when doses of anthracyclines have been escalated.

Indications

Acute nonlymphocytic leukemia: In the initial therapy of acute nonlymphocytic leukemia (ANLL) in adults in combination with other approved drug(s).

MS: For reducing neurologic disability and/or the frequency of clinical relapses in patients with secondary (chronic) progressive, progressive relapsing, or worsening relapsing-remitting MS (ie, patients whose neurologic status is significantly abnormal between relapses). Mitoxantrone is not indicated in the treatment of patients with primary progressive MS.

Prostate cancer: As initial chemotherapy for the treatment of patients with pain related to advanced hormone-refractory prostate cancer in combination with corticosteroids.

Administration and Dosage

Except for the treatment of acute nonlymphocytic leukemia, mitoxantrone generally should not be administered to patients with neutrophil counts less than 1,500 cells/mm^3.

Acute nonlymphocytic leukemia:

Induction therapy – 12 mg/m^2 daily on days 1 through 3 given as an IV infusion, and 100 mg/m^2 of cytarabine for 7 days given as a continuous 24-hour infusion on days 1 through 7. In the event of an incomplete antileukemic response, a second induction course may be given. Mitoxantrone should be given for 2 days and cytarabine for 5 days using the same daily dosage levels.

Consolidation therapy – 12 mg/m^2 IV infusion daily on days 1 and 2 and cytarabine 100 mg/m^2 for 5 days given as a continuous 24-hour infusion on days 1 through 5. The first course was given approximately 6 weeks after the final induction course; the second was generally administered 4 weeks after the first.

MS: 12 mg/m^2 given as a short (approximately 5 to 15 minutes) IV infusion every 3 months.

Do not administer mitoxantrone to MS patients who have received a cumulative lifetime dose of 140 mg/m^2 or more.

Prostate cancer: 12 to 14 mg/m^2 given as a short IV infusion every 21 days.

Hepatic function impairment: Ordinarily, do not treat patients with MS who have hepatic impairment with mitoxantrone. Administer mitoxantrone with caution to other patients with hepatic impairment; dosage adjustment may be required.

Administration: Infuse slowly through a freely running IV infusion of 0.9% sodium chloride injection or 5% dextrose injection over a period of not less than 3 minutes. Avoid veins over joints or in extremities with compromised venous or lymphatic drainage. Mitoxantrone should not be administered subcutaneously.

Avoid contact of mitoxantrone with the skin, mucous membranes, or eyes.

Extravasation: If any signs or symptoms of extravasation have occurred, including burning, pain, pruritus, erythema, swelling, blue discoloration, or ulceration, the injection or infusion should be immediately terminated and restarted in another vein. If known or suspected subcutaneous extravasation has occurred, it is recommended that intermittent ice packs be placed over the area of extravasation and that the affected extremity be elevated. Because of the progressive nature of extravasation reactions, the area of injection should be frequently examined and surgery consultation obtained early if there is any sign of a local reaction.

IV incompatibility: Do not mix in the same infusion as heparin. Mitoxantrone not be mixed in the same infusion with other drugs.

Women with MS who are biologically capable of becoming pregnant, even if they are using birth control, should have a pregnancy test, and the results must be known before receiving each dose of mitoxantrone.

Actions

Pharmacology: Mitoxantrone is a synthetic antineoplastic anthracenedione.

It has a cytocidal effect on both proliferating and nonproliferating cultured human cells, suggesting lack of cell cycle phase specificity.

Pharmacokinetics:

Absorption/Distribution – Distribution to tissues is extensive: Steady-state volume of distribution exceeds 1000 L/m^2. Mitoxantrone is 78% bound to plasma proteins.

Metabolism/Excretion – The mean alpha half-life of mitoxantrone is 6 to 12 minutes, the mean beta half-life is 1.1 to 3.1 hours, and the mean gamma (terminal or elimination) half-life is 23 to 215 hours. Mitoxantrone is excreted in urine and feces as either unchanged drug or as inactive metabolites.

Contraindications

Hypersensitivity to mitoxantrone.

Warnings/Precautions

Myelosuppression: High doses of mitoxantrone (more than 14 mg/m^2/day for 3 days) will cause severe myelosuppression. Assure full hematologic recovery before undertaking consolidation therapy and monitor patients closely during this phase.

Patients with preexisting myelosuppression as the result of prior drug therapy should not receive mitoxantrone unless the possible benefit warrants the risk of further suppression.

Administration: Safety for use by routes other than IV administration has not been established. Mitoxantrone is not indicated for subcutaneous, IM, or intra-arterial injection. Mitoxantrone must not be given by intrathecal injection.

Cardiac: Functional cardiac changes including decreases in LVEF and irreversible CHF can occur with mitoxantrone. Cardiac toxicity may be more common in patients with prior treatment with anthracyclines, prior mediastinal radiotherapy, or with preexisting cardiovascular disease. Such patients should have regular cardiac monitoring of LVEF from the initiation of therapy.

Multiple sclerosis – Changes in cardiac function may occur in patients with MS treated with mitoxantrone. MS patients should be assessed for cardiac signs and symptoms by history, physical examination, ECG, and quantitative LVEF evaluation using appropriate methodology (eg, echocardiogram, MRI, MUGA) prior to the start of mitoxantrone therapy.

Secondary leukemia: Secondary leukemia has been reported in cancer patients treated with mitoxantrone.

Acute leukemia/myelodysplasia: Topoisomerase II inhibitors, including mitoxantrone, have been associated with the development of acute leukemia and myelodysplasia.

Systemic infections: Treat concomitantly with or just before starting mitoxantrone.

Hepatic function impairment: Do not ordinarily treat patients with MS who have hepatic impairment with mitoxantrone. Administer mitoxantrone with caution to other patients with hepatic impairment.

Pregnancy: Category D.

Lactation: Mitoxantrone is excreted in breast milk. Because of the potential for serious adverse reactions in infants, discontinue breastfeeding before starting treatment.

Children: Safety and efficacy for use in children have not been established.

Monitoring: Frequently observe the patient and monitor hematologic and chemical laboratory parameters. Obtain a complete blood count, including platelets, prior to each course of mitoxantrone and in the event that signs and symptoms of infection develop. Liver function tests should also be performed prior to each course of therapy.

Women with MS who are biologically capable of becoming pregnant, even if they are using birth control, should have a pregnancy test and the results should be known before receiving each dose of mitoxantrone (see Warnings).

In patients with MS, LVEF should be evaluated by echocardiogram or MUGA prior to administration of the initial dose of mitoxantrone and all subsequent doses. In addition, LVEF evaluations are recommended if signs or symptoms of CHF develop at any time during treatment with mitoxantrone. Mitoxantrone should not be administered to MS patients with an LVEF less than 50% or with a clinically significant reduction in LVEF.

Hyperuricemia – Monitor serum uric acid levels and institute hypouricemic therapy prior to the initiation of antileukemic therapy.

Adverse Reactions

Adverse drug reactions occurring in at least 3% of patients include the following: abdominal pain, alkaline phosphatase, alopecia, amenorrhea, ANC low, anemia, anxiety/depression, aphthosis, arrythmia, AST and ALT increased, asthenia, back pain, blood urea nitrogen, blurred vision, cardiac ischemia, CHF, chills, conjunctivitis, constipation, cough, creatinine, cutaneous mycosis, decreased LVEF, diarrhea, dyspepsia, dyspnea, ECG abnormal, edema, fatigue, fever, fungal infections, gamma-GT increased, gastralgia/stomach burn/epigastric pain, GI bleeding, glucose high, granulocytopenia, headache, hematuria, hemoglobin low, hypertension, hypocalcemia, hypokalemia, hyponatremia, impotence/libido, infections, jaundice, leukopenia, lymphocytes low, malaise, menorrhagia, menstrual disorder, mucositis, myalgias/arthralgias, nail bed changes, nausea/vomiting, neurologic/mood, neurologic/motor, other endocrine problems, other kidney or bladder problems, other liver problems, other neurologic problems, other pulmonary problems, pain, petechiae/ecchymoses/bleeding, pharyngitis/throat disorder, platelets low, pneumonia, potassium low, proteinuria, renal failure, rhinitis, seizures, sepsis, sinusitis, skin infection, sterility, stomatitis, transaminase, upper respiratory tract infection, urine abnormal, urinary tract infection, weight gain, weight loss.

HYDROXYCHLOROQUINE

Tablets; oral: 200 mg (equiv. to 155 mg base) (*Rx*)	Various, *Plaquenil* (Sanofi Synthelabo)

Warning:

Physicians should completely familiarize themselves with the complete contents of the package insert before prescribing hydroxychloroquine.

Indications

Lupus erythematosus: For the treatment of chronic discoid and systemic lupus erythematosus (SLE) in patients who have not responded satisfactorily to drugs with less potential for serious side effects.

Malaria: For the suppressive treatment and treatment of acute attacks of malaria caused by *Plasmodium vivax*, *P. malariae*, *P. ovale*, and susceptible strains of *P. falciparum*.

Rheumatoid arthritis (RA): For the treatment of acute or chronic RA in patients who have not responded satisfactorily to drugs with less potential for serious side effects.

Administration and Dosage

Lupus erythematosus: Initially, 400 mg once or twice daily in adults, continued for several weeks or months depending on response. For prolonged maintenance therapy, 200 to 400 mg daily frequently will suffice.

RA: Initially, 400 to 600 mg daily, taken with a meal or a glass of milk. Side effects may require temporary reduction. Later (usually from 5 to 10 days), dose may be increased gradually to optimum response level. For maintenance therapy, when a good response is obtained (usually in 4 to 12 weeks), reduce dosage by 50% and continue at a level of 200 to 400 mg daily.

Maximum effects may not be obtained for several months. If objective improvement (reduced joint swelling, increased mobility) does not occur within 6 months, discontinue the drug.

If relapse occurs after drug withdrawal, resume therapy or continue on an intermittent schedule if there are no ocular contraindications.

Corticosteroids and salicylates may be used with this compound; generally they can be decreased gradually or eliminated after hydroxychloroquine has been used for several weeks.

Actions

Pharmacology: The precise mechanism of action is not known.

Pharmacokinetics:

Absorption/Distribution – Hydroxychloroquine is absorbed very rapidly and almost completely after oral administration. Hydroxychloroquine is distributed widely into body tissues and concentrates in the spleen, liver, kidney, melanin-containing tissues, and lungs. It has a large apparent volume of distribution (more than 100 L/kg). It is bound approximately 60% to plasma proteins.

Contraindications

Retinal or visual field changes attributable to any 4-aminoquinoline compound; hypersensitivity to 4-aminoquinoline compounds; long-term therapy in children.

Warnings/Precautions

Psoriasis: Use in patients with psoriasis may precipitate a severe attack. Porphyria may be exacerbated. Do not use unless the benefit to the patient outweighs possible risks.

Ophthalmic effects: Irreversible retinal damage has been observed in some patients who had received long-term or high-dosage 4-aminoquinoline therapy for discoid and SLE or RA. When prolonged therapy is contemplated, perform initial (baseline) and periodic (every 3 months) ophthalmologic examinations (including visual acuity, expert slit-lamp, funduscopic, and visual field tests).

Retinal changes – Retinal changes and visual disturbances may progress even after cessation of therapy.

Muscular weakness: Examine patients on long-term therapy periodically, and test knee and ankle reflexes to detect evidence of muscular weakness. If weakness occurs, discontinue drug.

RA: In RA, discontinue if objective improvement does not occur within 6 months.

Hepatic disease: Use with caution in patients with hepatic disease or in conjunction with hepatotoxic drugs.

Alcoholism: Use with caution in patients with alcoholism.

Dermatologic reactions: Dermatologic reactions may occur; exercise care when given to any patient receiving a drug with significant tendency to produce dermatitis.

Toxic symptoms: If serious toxic symptoms occur, administer ammonium chloride (8 g daily in divided doses for adults) 3 or 4 days a week for several months after therapy has been stopped; acidification of the urine increases renal excretion by 20% to 90%. Exercise caution in renal function impairment and/or metabolic acidosis.

Renal/Hepatic function impairment: Use with caution.

Pregnancy: According to *Drugs in Pregnancy and Lactation* by Briggs, the pregnancy risk factor is a *Category* C. The Centers for Disease Control and Prevention recommends use for prophylaxis in pregnant women who are traveling to areas with chloroquine-sensitive *P. falciparum* malaria.

Avoid use during pregnancy, except in the suppression of malaria when the benefit outweighs the possible hazard.

Lactation: The drug has been detected in breast milk from 2 mothers receiving 400 mg daily doses for SLE or RA.

Children: Children are especially sensitive to 4-aminoquinolines. Safe use of the drug in the treatment of JRA and SLE has not been established.

Monitoring: Perform periodic blood cell counts during prolonged therapy. If a severe blood disorder appears, consider discontinuation. Use caution in glucose-6-phosphate dehydrogenase (G-6-PD) deficiency.

Drug Interactions

Drugs that may affect hydroxychloroquine include cimetidine. Drugs that may be affected by hydroxychloroquine include beta blockers, cyclosporine, digoxin, magnesium salts, and mefloquine.

Adverse Reactions

The following have occurred with 1 or more of the 4-aminoquinoline compounds.

CNS: Ataxia; convulsions; dizziness; emotional changes; headache; irritability; nerve deafness; nervousness; nightmares; nystagmus; psychosis; tinnitus; vertigo.

Dermatologic: Alopecia; bleaching of hair; photosensitivity; precipitation of nonlight-sensitive psoriasis; pruritus; skin and mucosal pigmentation; skin eruptions (urticarial, morbilliform, lichenoid, maculopapular, purpuric, erythema annulare centrifugum, Stevens-Johnson syndrome, acute generalized exanthematous pustulosis, and exfoliative dermatitis).

GI: Abdominal cramps; anorexia; diarrhea; nausea; vomiting.

Hematologic: Agranulocytosis; aplastic anemia; hemolysis in individuals with G-6-PD deficiency; leukopenia; thrombocytopenia.

Musculoskeletal: Skeletal muscle palsies, myopathy, or neuromyopathy leading to progressive weakness and atrophy of proximal muscle groups, depression of tendon reflexes, and abnormal nerve conduction.

Ophthalmic:

Ciliary body – See Warnings. Disturbance of accommodation with blurred vision. This reaction is dose-related and reversible with cessation of therapy.

Cornea – Decreased corneal sensitivity; punctate to lineal opacities; transient edema.

Retina – Abnormal pigmentation (mild pigment stippling to a "bull's eye" appearance); atrophy; edema; elevated retinal threshold to red light in macular, paramacular, and peripheral retinal areas; increased macular recovery time following exposure to a bright light (photo-stress test); loss of foveal reflex.

Retinopathy – Reading and seeing difficulties (ie, words, letters, or parts of objects missing); photophobia; blurred distance vision; missing or blacked out areas in the central or peripheral visual field; light flashes and streaks.

Other fundus changes – Attenuation of retinal arterioles; fine granular pigmentary disturbances in the peripheral retina; optic disc pallor and atrophy; prominent choroidal patterns in advanced stage.

Visual field defects – Central scotoma with decreased visual acuity; field constriction (rare); pericentral or paracentral scotoma.

Miscellaneous: Weight loss; lassitude; exacerbation or precipitation of porphyria.

Chapter 11
DERMATOLOGICAL AGENTS

ISOTRETINOIN (13-cis-Retinoic Acid)

Capsules; oral: 10, 20, 30, and 40 mg (*Rx*)	*Amnesteem* (Mylan), *Claravis* (Barr)
Capsules, soft gel; oral: 10, 20, 30, and 40 mg (*Rx*)	*Sotret* (Ranbaxy)

Warning:

Isotretinoin must not be used by women and adolescents who are pregnant or who may become pregnant. There is an extremely high risk that severe birth defects can result if pregnancy occurs while taking isotretinoin in any amount, even for short periods of time. Potentially, any fetus exposed during pregnancy can be affected. There are no accurate means of determining whether an exposed fetus has been affected.

Birth defects that have been documented following isotretinoin exposure include abnormalities of the face, eyes, ears, skull, CNS, cardiovascular system, and thymus and parathyroid glands. Cases of intelligence quotient (IQ) scores less than 85 with or without other abnormalities have been reported. There is an increased risk of spontaneous abortion, and premature births have been reported.

Documented external abnormalities include skull abnormality; ear abnormalities (including anotia, micropinna, small or absent external auditory canals); eye abnormalities (including microphthalmia); facial dymorphia; cleft palate. Documented internal abnormalities include CNS abnormalities (including cerebral abnormalities, cerebellar malformation, hydrocephalus, microcephaly, cranial nerve deficit); cardiovascular abnormalities; thymus gland abnormality; parathyroid hormone deficiency. In some cases, death has occurred with some of the abnormalities previously noted.

If pregnancy does occur during treatment of a female patient who is taking isotretinoin, isotretinoin must be discontinued immediately and she should be referred to an obstetrician-gynecologist experienced in reproductive toxicity for further evaluation and counseling.

Special prescribing requirements: Because of isotretinoin's teratogenicity and to minimize fetal exposure, isotretinoin is approved for marketing only under a special restricted distribution program approved by the Food and Drug Administration. This program is called iPLEDGE. Isotretinoin must only be prescribed by prescribers who are registered and activated with the iPLEDGE program. Isotretinoin must only be dispensed by a pharmacy registered and activated with iPLEDGE, and must only be dispensed to patients who are registered and meet all the requirements of iPLEDGE.

Information for pharmacist: Access the iPLEDGE system via the internet (http://www.ipledgeprogram.com) or telephone (1-866-495-0654) to obtain an authorization and the "do not dispense to patient after" date. Isotretinoin must only be dispensed in no more than a 30-day supply.

Refills require a new prescription and a new authorization from the iPLEDGE system.

An isotretinoin Medication Guide must be given to the patient each time isotretinoin is dispensed, as required by law. This isotretinoin Medication Guide is an important part of the risk management program for the patient.

Indications

Severe recalcitrant nodular acne: For the treatment of severe recalcitrant nodular acne.

Administration and Dosage

Recommended course of therapy: The recommended dose is 0.5 to 1 mg/kg/day divided into 2 doses for 15 to 20 weeks. Administer isotretinoin with food. Adult patients whose disease is very severe with scarring or is primarily manifested on the trunk may require up to the maximum recommended dose, 2 mg/kg/day, as tolerated. Failure to take isotretinoin with food will significantly decrease absorption. Before upward dose adjustments are made, question patients about their compliance with food instructions. Once-daily dosing is not recommended. If the total nodule count decreases by more than 70% prior to completing 15 to 20 weeks of treatment, the drug may be discontinued. After 2 months or more off therapy, and if warranted by persistent or recurring severe nodular acne, a second course of therapy may be initiated.

Isotretinoin Dosing by Body Weight

Body weight		Total mg/day		
kg	lbs	0.5 mg/kg	1 mg/kg	2 mg/kg[a]
40	88	20	40	80
50	110	25	50	100
60	132	30	60	120
70	154	35	70	140
80	176	40	80	160
90	198	45	90	180
100	220	50	100	200

[a] The recommended dosage range is 0.5 to 1 mg/kg/day.

Actions

Pharmacology: Isotretinoin is a retinoid that, when administered in pharmacologic dosages of 0.5 to 1 mg/kg/day, inhibits sebaceous gland function and keratinization. The exact mechanism of action of isotretinoin is unknown.

Clinical improvement in nodular acne occurs in association with a reduction in sebum secretion. The decrease in sebum secretion is temporary, is related to the dose and duration of treatment with isotretinoin, and reflects a reduction in sebaceous gland size and an inhibition of sebaceous gland differentiation.

Pharmacokinetics:

Absorption – Because of its high lipophilicity, oral absorption of isotretinoin is enhanced when given with a high-fat meal.

Pharmacokinetic Parameters of Isotretinoin Mean (%CV), N = 74

Isotretinoin 2 × 40 mg capsules	$AUC_{(0-\infty)}$ (ng•h/mL)	C_{max} (ng/mL)	T_{max} (h)	t½ (h)
Fed[a]	10,004 (22%)	862 (22%)	5.3 (77%)	21 (39%)
Fasted	3,703 (46%)	301 (63%)	3.2 (56%)	21 (30%)

[a] Eating a standardized high-fat meal.

Distribution – Isotretinoin is more than 99.9% bound to plasma proteins, primarily albumin.

Metabolism – Following oral administration of isotretinoin, at least 3 metabolites have been identified in human plasma.

In vitro studies indicated that the primary P450 isoforms involved in isotretinoin metabolism are 2C8, 2C9, 3A4, and 2B6. Isotretinoin and its metabolites are further metabolized into conjugates, which are then excreted in urine and feces.

Excretion – Following oral administration of an 80 mg dose of ^{14}C-isotretinoin as a liquid suspension, ^{14}C-activity in blood declined with a half-life of 90 hours. After a single 80 mg oral dose of isotretinoin under fed conditions, the mean elimination half-lives of isotretinoin and 4-*oxo*-isotretinoin were approximately 21 and 24 hours, respectively.

Contraindications

Pregnancy (see Warning Box); hypersensitivity to this medication or any of its components; hypersensitivity to parabens (used as a preservative in the formulation).

Warnings/Precautions

Psychiatric disorders: Isotretinoin may cause depression, psychosis, and rarely, suicidal ideation, suicide attempts, suicide, and aggressive or violent behavior. Discontinuation of isotretinoin therapy may be insufficient; further evaluation may be necessary. No mechanism of action has been established for these events.

Pseudotumor cerebri (benign intracranial hypertension): Isotretinoin use has been associated with a number of cases of pseudotumor cerebri, some of which involved concomitant use of tetracyclines. Therefore, avoid concomitant treatment with tetracyclines. Early signs and symptoms include papilledema, headache, nausea, vomiting, and visual disturbances. Screen patients with these symptoms for papilledema; if present, discontinue drug immediately and consult a neurologist.

Pancreatitis: Acute pancreatitis has been reported in patients with elevated or normal serum triglyceride levels. In rare instances, fatal hemorrhagic pancreatitis has been reported. Stop isotretinoin if hypertriglyceridemia cannot be controlled at an acceptable level or if symptoms of pancreatitis occur.

Visual impairment: Carefully monitor visual problems. If visual difficulties occur, discontinue the drug and have an ophthalmological examination.

Corneal opacities – These have appeared in patients receiving isotretinoin for acne and more frequently in patients on higher dosages for keratinization disorders. Corneal opacities have either completely resolved or were resolving at followup 6 to 7 weeks after discontinuation.

Decreased night vision – Decreased night vision has occurred during therapy and in some cases persisted after therapy was discontinued. Because the onset in some patients was sudden, advise patients of this potential problem and warn them to be cautious when driving or operating any vehicle at night.

iPLEDGE program: Isotretinoin must only be prescribed by health care providers who are registered and activated with the iPLEDGE program. Isotretinoin must only be dispensed by a pharmacy registered and activated with iPLEDGE and must only be dispensed to patients who are registered and meet all the requirements of iPLEDGE. Registered and activated pharmacies must receive isotretinoin only from wholesalers registered with iPLEDGE.

Prescribers – To prescribe isotretinoin, the health care provider must access the iPLEDGE system via the internet (http://www.ipledgeprogram.com) or telephone (1-866-495-0654) to:

1.) Register each patient in the iPLEDGE program.
2.) Confirm monthly that each patient has received counseling and education.

For female patients of childbearing potential –

- Enter patient's 2 chosen forms of contraception each month.
- Enter monthly result from CLIA-certified laboratory conducted pregnancy test.

Pharmacists – To dispense isotretinoin, the pharmacist must:

1.) Be trained by the responsible site pharmacist concerning the iPLEDGE program requirements.
2.) Obtain authorization from the iPLEDGE program via the internet (http://www.ipledgeprogram.com) or telephone (1-866-495-0654) for every isotretinoin prescription. Authorization signifies that the patient has met all program requirements and is qualified to receive isotretinoin.
3.) Write the Risk Management Authorization (RMA) number on the prescription.

Isotretinoin must be dispensed only:

- in no more than a 30-day supply
- with an isotretinoin Medication Guide
- after authorization from the iPLEDGE program
- prior to the "do not dispense to patient after" date provided by the iPLEDGE system (within 7 days of the office visit)
- with a new prescription for refills and another authorization from the iPLEDGE program (no automatic refills allowed).

Elevated creatine phosphokinase (CPK): Some patients undergoing vigorous physical activity have experienced elevated CPK levels.

Inflammatory bowel disease: Inflammatory bowel disease, including regional ileitis, has been associated with isotretinoin in patients without a history of intestinal disorders. In some instances, symptoms have been reported to persist after isotretinoin therapy has been stopped. Discontinue treatment immediately if abdominal pain, rectal bleeding, or severe diarrhea occurs.

Hypertriglyceridemia: Hypertriglyceridemia in excess of 800 mg/dL occurred in approximately 25% of patients; approximately 15% developed a decrease in high density lipoproteins (HDL) and approximately 7% showed an increase in cholesterol levels. Perform blood lipid determinations before isotretinoin is given and then at intervals until the lipid response to isotretinoin is established, which usually occurs within 4 weeks.

Musculoskeletal effects: Spontaneous reports of osteoporosis, osteopenia, bone fractures, and delayed healing of bone fractures have been seen in the isotretinoin population. It is important that isotretinoin be given at the recommended doses for no longer than the recommended duration.

Hyperostosis – A high prevalence of skeletal hyperostosis was noted in clinical trials for disorders of keratinization

Premature epiphyseal closure – There are spontaneous reports of premature epiphyseal closure in acne patients receiving recommended doses of isotretinoin.

Hepatotoxicity: Clinical hepatitis possibly or probably related to isotretinoin therapy has been reported. Additionally, mild to moderate elevations of liver enzymes have been seen in approximately 15% of patients, some of whom normalized with dosage reduction or continued administration of the drug. If normalization does not readily occur, or if hepatitis is suspected, stop the drug and further investigate etiology.

Hearing impairment: Impaired hearing has been reported in patients taking isotretinoin; in some cases, the hearing impairment has been reported to persist after therapy has been discontinued. Patients who experience tinnitus or hearing impairment should discontinue isotretinoin treatment and be referred to specialized care for further evaluation.

Diabetes: Certain patients have experienced problems in the control of their blood sugar. In addition, new cases of diabetes have been diagnosed during therapy, although no causal relationship has been established.

Hypersensitivity reactions: Anaphylactic reactions and other allergic reactions have been reported. Cutaneous allergic reactions and serious cases of allergic vasculitis, often with purpura (bruises and red patches), of the extremities and extracutaneous involvement (including renal) have been reported. Severe allergic reaction necessitates discontinuation of therapy and appropriate medical management.

Special risk: Use caution when prescribing isotretinoin to patients with a genetic predisposition for age-related osteoporosis, a history of childhood osteoporosis conditions, osteomalacia, or other disorders of bone metabolism. This would include patients diagnosed with anorexia nervosa and those who are on chronic drug therapy that causes drug-induced osteoporosis/osteomalacia and/or affects vitamin D metabolism, such as systemic corticosteroids and any anticonvulsant.

Patients may be at increased risk when participating in sports with repetitive impact where the risks of spondylolisthesis with and without pars fractures and hip growth plate injuries in early and late adolescence are known.

Photosensitivity: Photosensitization (photoallergy or phototoxicity) may occur; caution patients to take protective measures (eg, sunscreens, protective clothing) against exposure to ultraviolet light or sunlight until tolerance is determined.

Pregnancy: Category X (see Warning Box).

Lactation: It is not known whether this drug is excreted in breast milk. Because of the potential for adverse effects, do not give to a nursing mother.

Children: The use of isotretinoin in pediatric patients less than 12 years of age has not been studied. Carefully consider isotretinoin use in pediatric patients 12 to 17 years of age, especially for those patients in whom a known metabolic or structural bone disease exists.

Adverse reactions reported in children were similar to those described in adults except for the increased incidence of back pain and arthralgia (both of which were sometimes severe) and myalgia in children.

Monitoring:

Pregnancy test – Female patients of childbearing potential must have negative results from 2 urine or serum pregnancy tests with a sensitivity of at least 25 milliunit/mL before receiving the initial isotretinoin prescription. The first test is obtained by the prescriber when the decision is made to pursue qualification of the patient for isotretinoin (a screening test). The second pregnancy test (a confirmation test) must be done in a CLIA-certified laboratory. The interval between the 2 tests must be at least 19 days.

For patients with regular menstrual cycles, the second pregnancy test must be done during the first 5 days of the menstrual period and within 7 days following the office visit, immediately preceding the beginning of isotretinoin therapy, and after the patient has used 2 forms of contraception for 1 month.

For patients with amenorrhea or irregular cycles, or for those using a contraceptive method that precludes withdrawal bleeding, the second pregnancy test must be done within 7 days following the office visit, immediately preceding the beginning of isotretinoin therapy, and after the patient has used 2 forms of contraception for 1 month.

Each month of therapy, the patient must have a negative result from a urine or serum pregnancy test. A pregnancy test must be repeated each month, in a CLIA-certified laboratory, prior to the female patient receiving each prescription.

Vision impairment – Carefully monitor visual problems. All isotretinoin patients experiencing visual difficulties should discontinue isotretinoin treatment and have an ophthalmological examination.

Lipids – Obtain pretreatment and followup blood lipids under fasting conditions. After consumption of alcohol, at least 36 hours should elapse before these determinations are made. It is recommended that these tests be performed at weekly or biweekly intervals until the lipid response to isotretinoin is established.

Liver function tests – Perform pretreatment and followup liver function tests at weekly or biweekly intervals until the response to isotretinoin has been established.

Drug Interactions

Drugs that may affect isotretinoin include systemic corticosteroids, tetracycline, vitamin A, and phenytoin.

Drugs that may be affected by isotretinoin include systemic corticosteroids, phenytoin, and vitamin A.

Drug/Food interactions: Because of its high lipophilicity, oral absorption of isotretinoin is enhanced when given with a high-fat meal.

Adverse Reactions

Dose relationship: Cheilitis and hypertriglyceridemia are usually dose related. Most adverse reactions reported in clinical trials were reversible when therapy was discontinued; however, some persisted after cessation of therapy.

Cardiovascular – Palpitation, stroke, tachycardia, vascular thrombotic disease.

CNS – Aggression, depression, dizziness, drowsiness, emotional instability, headache, insomnia, lethargy, malaise, nervousness, paresthesias, pseudotumor cerebri, psychosis, seizures, stroke, suicidal ideation, suicide, suicide attempts, syncope, violent behaviors, weakness.

Of the patients reporting depression, some reported that the depression subsided with discontinuation of therapy and recurred with reinstitution of therapy.

Dermatologic – Abnormal wound healing (delayed healing or exuberant granulation tissue with crusting), acne fulminans, alopecia (which in some cases persists), bruising, cheilitis (dry lips), dry mouth, dry nose, dry skin, epistaxis, eruptive xanthomas, flushing, fragility of skin, hair abnormalities, hirsutism, hyperpigmentation and hypopigmentation, infections (including disseminated herpes simplex), nail dystrophy, paronychia, peeling of palms and soles, photoallergic/photosensitizing reactions, pruritus, pyogenic granuloma, rash (including eczema, facial erythema, and seborrhea), sunburn susceptibility increased, sweating, urticaria, vasculitis (including Wegener granulomatosis).

Endocrine – Alterations in blood sugar levels, hypertriglyceridemia.

GI – Bleeding and inflammation of the gums, colitis, esophageal ulceration, esophagitis, hepatitis, ileitis, inflammatory bowel disease, nausea, pancreatitis, other nonspecific GI symptoms.

GU – Abnormal menses, glomerulonephritis, microscopic or gross hematuria, nonspecific urogenital findings, proteinuria, white cells in the urine.

Lab test abnormalities – Decrease in serum HDL levels, elevation of plasma triglycerides, elevations of serum cholesterol during treatment.

Increased alkaline phosphatase, ALT, AST, gamma-glutamyl transpeptidase (GGTP), or lactate dehydrogenase (LDH).

Elevation of CPK, elevations of fasting blood sugar, hyperuricemia.

Decreases in red blood cell parameters, decreases in white blood cell counts (including severe neutropenia and rare reports of agranulocytosis), elevated platelet counts, elevated sedimentation rates, thrombocytopenia.

Microscopic or gross hematuria, proteinuria, white cells in the urine.

Musculoskeletal – Arthritis, calcification of tendons and ligaments, decreases in BMD, elevations of CPK/rare reports of rhabdomyolysis, musculoskeletal symptoms (sometimes severe) including arthralgia, back pain, and myalgia, other types of bone abnormalities, premature epiphyseal closure, skeletal hyperostosis, tendonitis, transient pain in the chest.

Ophthalmic – Cataracts, color vision disorder, conjunctivitis, corneal opacities, decreased night vision that may persist, dry eyes, eyelid inflammation, keratitis, optic neuritis, photophobia, visual disturbances.

Respiratory – Bronchospasms (with or without a history of asthma), respiratory tract infection, voice alteration.

Special senses – Hearing impairment, tinnitus.

Miscellaneous – Allergic reactions including systemic hypersensitivity and vasculitis, edema, fatigue, lymphadenopathy, weight loss.

CORTICOSTEROIDS, TOPICAL

ACLOMETASONE DIPROPIONATE	
Ointment: 0.05% (*Rx*)	Various, *Aclovate* (Pharmaderm)
Cream: 0.05% (*Rx*)	
AMCINONIDE	
Ointment: 0.1% (*Rx*)	Various
Cream: 0.1% (*Rx*)	
Lotion: 0.1% (*Rx*)	
AUGMENTED BETAMETHASONE DIPROPIONATE	
Ointment: 0.05% (*Rx*)	*Diprolene* (Schering)
Cream: 0.05% (*Rx*)	*Diprolene AF* (Schering)
Lotion: 0.05% (*Rx*)	*Diprolene* (Schering)
Gel: 0.05% (*Rx*)	*Diprolene* (Schering)
BETAMETHASONE BENZOATE	
Cream: 0.025% (*Rx*)	*Uticort* (Parke-Davis)
Lotion: 0.025% (*Rx*)	
Gel: 0.025% (*Rx*)	
BETAMETHASONE DIPROPIONATE	
Ointment: 0.05% (*Rx*)	Various
Cream: 0.05% (*Rx*)	
Lotion: 0.05% (*Rx*)	
BETAMETHASONE VALERATE	
Ointment: 0.1% (*Rx*)	Various
Cream: 0.1% (*Rx*)	Various
Lotion: 0.1% (*Rx*)	Various
Foam: 0.12% (*Rx*)	*Luxiq* (GlaxoSmithKline)
CLOBETASOL PROPIONATE	
Ointment: 0.05% (*Rx*)	Various, *Temovate* (Pharmaderm)
Cream: 0.05% (*Rx*)	Various, *Cormax* (Watson), *Temovate* (Pharmaderm)
Lotion: 0.05% (*Rx*)	*Clobex* (Galderma)
Solution: 0.05% (*Rx*)	*Clobetasol Propionate* (Taro), *Cormax* (Watson)
Scalp application: 0.05% (*Rx*)	*Temovate* (Pharmaderm)
Shampoo: 0.05% (*Rx*)	*Clobex* (Gladerma)
Gel: 0.05% (*Rx*)	Various, *Temovate* (Pharmaderm)
Spray: 0.05% (*Rx*)	*Clobex* (Gladerma)
Foam: 0.05% (*Rx*)	Various, *Olux*, *Olux-E* (Stiefel Labs)
CLOCORTOLONE PIVALATE	
Cream: 0.1% (*Rx*)	*Cloderm* (Hermal)
DESONIDE	
Ointment: 0.05% (*Rx*)	Various, *DesOwen* (Owen/Galderma)
Cream: 0.05% (*Rx*)	
Lotion: 0.05% (*Rx*)	Various, *DesOwen* (Owen/Galderma), *LoKara* (PharmaDerm)
Gel: 0.05% (*Rx*)	*Desonate* (SkinMedica)
Foam: 0.05% (*Rx*)	*Verdeso* (Connetics)
DESOXIMETASONE	
Ointment: 0.25% (*Rx*)	Various, *Topicort* (Taro)
Cream: 0.05%, 0.25% (*Rx*)	Various, *Topicort* (Taro)
Gel: 0.05% (*Rx*)	Various, *Topicort* (Taro)
DEXAMETHASONE SODIUM PHOSPHATE	
Aerosol: 0.01%, 0.04% (*Rx*)	*Aeroseb-Dex* (Herbert)
DIFLORASONE DIACETATE	
Ointment: 0.05% (*Rx*)	*Maxiflor* (Herbert)
Cream: 0.05% (*Rx*)	*Psorcon* (Dermik)

FLUOCINOLONE ACETONIDE	
Ointment: 0.025% (*Rx*)	Various
Cream: 0.01%, 0.025%, 0.2% (*Rx*)	
Solution: 0.01% (*Rx*)	
Shampoo: 0.01% (*Rx*)	*FS Shampoo* (Hill), *Capex* (Galderma)
Oil: 0.01% (*Rx*)	*Derma-Smoothe/FS* (Hill)
FLUOCINONIDE	
Cream: 0.05%, 0.1% (*Rx*)	Various, *Fluonex* (ICN), *Lidex* (Syntex), *Vanos* (Medicis)
Ointment: 0.05% (*Rx*)	Various, *Lidex* (Syntex)
Solution: 0.05% (*Rx*)	
Gel: 0.05% (*Rx*)	
FLURANDRENOLIDE	
Ointment: 0.05% (*Rx*)	*Cordran* (Oclassen)
Cream: 0.05% (*Rx*)	*Cordran SP* (Oclassen)
Lotion: 0.05% (*Rx*)	Various, *Cordran* (Oclassen)
Tape: 4 mcg/cm^2 (*Rx*)	*Cordran* (Oclassen)
FLUTICASONE PROPIONATE	
Ointment: 0.005% (*Rx*)	*Cutivate* (Pharmaderm)
Cream: 0.05% (*Rx*)	
Lotion: 0.05% (Rx)	
HALCINONIDE	
Ointment: 0.1% (*Rx*)	*Halog* (Ranbaxy)
Cream: 0.025%, 0.1% (*Rx*)	*Halog* (Ranbaxy), *Halog-E* (Ranbaxy)
Solution: 0.1% (*Rx*)	*Halog* (Ranbaxy)
HALOBETASOL PROPIONATE	
Ointment: 0.05% (*Rx*)	Various, *Ultravate* (Ranbaxy)
Cream: 0.05% (*Rx*)	
HYDROCORTISONE	
Ointment: 0.5%, 1%, 2.5% (*Rx/otc*)	Various, *Cortizone•10* (Chattem Consumer)
Cream: 0.5%, 1%, 2.5% (*Rx/otc*)	Various, *Anusol-HC* (Salix), *Aveeno Anti-itch Maximum Strength* (Johnson & Johnson Consumer), *Caldecort* (Insight), *Cortaid Advanced 12 Hour* (Johnson & Johnson Consumer), *Cortaid Intensive Therapy* (Johnson & Johnson Consumer), *Cortaid Maximum Strength* (Johnson & Johnson Consumer), *KeriCort 10* (Ciba-Geigy), *Monistat Soothing Care* (Johnson & Johnson Healthcare), *Noble Formula HC* (Ontos), *Preparation H Hydrocortisone* (Wyeth Consumer), *proctoCream•HC 2.5%* (Alaven), *Proctocort* (Salix), *Procto-Pak* (Rising Pharm), *Proctosol HC* (Ranbaxy), *Proctozone-HC* (Rising Pharma)
Enema: 100 mg per 60 mL (*Rx*)	Various, *Colocort* (Paddock)
Lotion: 0.25%, 0.5%, 1%, 2%, 2.5% (*Rx/otc*)	Various, *Ala-Scalp* (Del-Ray), *Aquanil HC* (Person and Covey), *Cortizone•10 Eczema* (Chattem Consumer), *Itch-X* (B.F. Ascher and Co.), *Sarnol-HC* (GlaxoSmithKline), *Theracort* (Harmony)
Foam: 1% (*otc*)	*Itch-X* (B.F. Ascher and Co.)
Gel: 1%, 2%, 10% (*Rx/otc*)	*Corticool* (Tec Laboratories), *Cortizone•10* (Chattem Consumer), *First-Hydrocortisone* (Cutis Pharma), *Instacort 10* (Altaire)
Solution: 1% and 2.5% (*Rx*)	*Cortaid Intensive Therapy* (Johnson & Johnson Consumer), *Noble Formula HC* (Ontos), *Scalpicin Maximum Strength* (Combe), *Texacort* (JSJ Pharm)
HYDROCORTISONE ACETATE	
Ointment: 0.5%, 1% (*otc*)	*Cortaid Maximum Strength* (Johnson & Johnson Consumer), *Tucks Anti-itch* (Johnson & Johnson Healthcare)
Lotion: 2% (*Rx*)	Various, *Nucort* (Gentex)

Cream: 0.5%, 1% (*Rx/otc*)	Various, *Demarest Dricort* (Del), *Gynecort 10* (Combe), *Lanacort-10* (Combe), *U-Cort* (Thames)
Foam: 90 mg (*Rx*)	*Cortifoam* (Alaven)
HYDROCORTISONE/ALOE VERA	
Cream: 0.5%, 1% (*otc*)	Various, *Cortizone-10 Intensive Healing*, *Cortizone 10/Aloe*, *Cortizone-10 Plus* (Chattem Consumer)
Liquid: 1% (*otc*)	*Cortizone 10/Aloe* (Chattem Consumer)
Ointment: 1% (*otc*)	Various
HYDROCORTISONE ACETATE/ALOE VERA	
Gel: 2% (*Rx*)	Various, *CortAlo* (Aletheia), *NuZon* (Wraser)
Cream: 0.5% (*Rx*)	Various
HYDROCORTISONE BUTYRATE	
Ointment: 0.1% (*Rx*)	Various, *Locoid* (Triax)
Cream: 0.1% (*Rx*)	
Lotion; topical: 0.1% (*Rx*)	
Solution: 0.1% (*Rx*)	
Cream: 0.1% (hydrophilic lipo base) (*Rx*)	*Locoid Lipocream* (Triax)
HYDROCORTISONE PROBUTATE	
Cream: 0.1% (*Rx*)	*Pandel* (Pharmaderm)
HYDROCORTISONE SODIUM SUCCINATE	
Solution, reconstituted: 100, 250, 500, 1,000 mg (*Rx*)	*Solu-CORTEF* (Kabivitrum)
HYDROCORTISONE VALERATE	
Ointment: 0.2% (*Rx*)	Various
Cream: 0.2% (*Rx*)	Various, *Westcort* (Westwood-Squibb)
MOMETASONE FUROATE	
Ointment: 0.1% (*Rx*)	Various, *Elocon* (Schering)
Cream: 0.1% (*Rx*)	
Lotion: 0.1% (*Rx*)	
PREDNICARBATE	
Cream: 0.1% (*Rx*)	Various, *Dermatop* (Aventis)
TRIAMCINOLONE ACETONIDE	
Ointment: 0.025%, 0.1%, 0.5% (*Rx*)	Various
Cream: 0.025%, 0.1%, 0.5% (*Rx*)	Various, *Kenonel* (Marnel), *Triderm* (Del-Ray)
Lotion: 0.025% and 0.1% (*Rx*)	Various
Aerosol: (2 sec. spray) (*Rx*)	*Kenalog* (Ranbaxy)

Indications

Pruritus:

Relief of inflammatory and pruritic manifestations of corticosteroid-responsive dermatoses – Contact dermatitis, atopic dermatitis, nummular eczema, stasis eczema, asteatotic eczema, lichen planus, lichen simplex chronicus, insect and arthropod bite reactions, first- and second-degree localized burns, and sunburns.

Alternative/Adjunctive treatment: Psoriasis, seborrheic dermatitis, severe diaper rash, dishidrosis, nodular prurigo, chronic discoid lupus erythematosus, alopecia areata, lymphocytic infiltration of the skin, mycosis fungoides, and familial benign pemphigus of Hailey-Hailey.

Possibly effective: Possibly effective in the following conditions: Bullous pemphigoid, cutaneous mastocytosis, lichen sclerosus et atrophicus, and vitiligo.

Nonprescription hydrocortisone preparations: Temporary relief of itching associated with minor skin irritations, inflammation, and rashes caused by eczema, insect bites, poison ivy, poison oak, poison sumac, soaps, detergents, cosmetics, jewelry, seborrheic dermatitis, psoriasis, and external genital and anal itching.

Administration and Dosage

Usual dose: Apply sparingly to affected areas 1 to 4 times/day.

Actions

Pharmacology: The primary therapeutic effects of the topical corticosteroids are caused by their antiinflammatory activity, which is nonspecific (ie, they act against most causes of inflammation including mechanical, chemical, microbiological, and immunological).

Pharmacokinetics: The amount of corticosteroid absorbed from the skin depends on the intrinsic properties of the drug itself, the vehicle used, the duration of exposure, and the surface area and condition of the skin to which it is applied.

Vehicles – Ointments are more occlusive and are preferred for dry scaly lesions. Use creams on oozing lesions or in intertriginous areas where the occlusive effects of ointments may cause maceration and folliculitis.

Relative potency – The relative potency of a product depends on several factors including the characteristics and concentration of the drug and the vehicle used.

Topical corticosteroids are ranked into several classes according to their potency based on vasoconstrictor activity; Group I has the highest potency and highest potential for localized as well as systemic side effects. The percent of the corticosteroid agent is NOT an indication of potency. Use high potency agents for very short periods of time for acute exacerbations and only on areas that are lichenified; avoid use of these agents on facial areas, skin folds, and on infants. Intermediate and lower potency agents can be used for longer durations and to treat chronic symptoms on areas of the torso and extremities.

Relative Potency of Selected Topical Corticosteroid Products

	Drug	Dosage Form	Strength
I.	***Very high potency***		
	Augmented betamethasone dipropionate	Ointment	0.05%
	Clobetasol propionate	Cream, Ointment	0.05%
	Diflorasone diacetate	Ointment	0.05%
	Halobetasol propionate	Cream, Ointment	0.05%
II.	***High potency***		
	Amcinonide	Cream, Lotion, Ointment	0.1%
	Augmented betamethasone dipropionate	Cream	0.05%
	Betamethasone dipropionate	Cream, Ointment	0.05%
	Betamethasone valerate	Ointment	0.1%
	Desoximetasone	Cream, Ointment	0.25%
		Gel	0.05%
	Diflorasone diacetate	Cream, Ointment (emollient base)	0.05%
	Fluocinolone acetonide	Cream	0.2%
	Fluocinonide	Cream, Ointment, Gel	0.05%
	Halcinonide	Cream, Ointment	0.1%
	Triamcinolone acetonide	Cream, Ointment	0.5%
III.	***Medium potency***		
	Betamethasone benzoate	Cream, Gel, Lotion	0.025%
	Betamethasone dipropionate	Lotion	0.05%
	Betamethasone valerate	Cream	0.1%
	Clocortolone pivalate	Cream	0.1%
	Desoximetasone	Cream	0.05%
	Fluocinolone acetonide	Cream, Ointment	0.025%
	Flurandrenolide	Cream, Ointment	0.025%
		Cream, Ointment, Lotion	0.05%
		Tape	4 mcg/cm^2
	Fluticasone propionate	Cream	0.05%
		Ointment	0.005%
	Hydrocortisone butyrate	Ointment, Solution	0.1%
	Hydrocortisone valerate	Cream, Ointment	0.2%
	Mometasone furoate	Cream, Ointment, Lotion	0.1%
	Triamcinolone acetonide	Cream, Ointment, Lotion	0.025%
		Cream, Ointment, Lotion	0.1%

Relative Potency of Selected Topical Corticosteroid Products			
Drug		Dosage Form	Strength
IV.	***Low potency***		
	Aclometasone dipropionate	Cream, Ointment	0.05%
	Desonide	Cream	0.05%
	Dexamethasone	Aerosol	0.01%
		Aerosol	0.04%
	Dexamethasone sodium phosphate	Cream	0.1%
	Fluocinolone acetonide	Cream, Solution	0.01%
	Hydrocortisone	Lotion	0.25%
		Cream, Ointment, Lotion, Aerosol	0.5%
		Cream, Ointment, Lotion, Solution	1%
		Cream, Ointment, Lotion	2.5%
	Hydrocortisone acetate	Cream, Ointment	0.5%
		Cream, Ointment	1%

Contraindications

Hypersensitivity to any component; monotherapy in primary bacterial infections such as impetigo, paronychia, erysipelas, cellulitis, angular cheilitis, erythrasma (clobetasol), treatment of rosacea, perioral dermatitis, or acne; use on the face, groin, or axilla (very high or high potency agents); ophthalmic use.

Warnings/Precautions

Systemic effects: Systemic absorption of topical corticosteroids has produced reversible HPA axis suppression, Cushing syndrome, hyperglycemia, and glycosuria.

As a general rule, little effect on the HPA axis will occur with a potent topical corticosteroid in amounts of less than 50 g weekly for an adult and 15 g weekly for a small child, without occlusion. To cover the adult body 1 time requires 12 to 26 g.

Local irritation: If local irritation develops, discontinue use and institute appropriate therapy.

Psoriasis: Do not use topical corticosteroids as sole therapy in widespread plaque psoriasis.

Atrophic changes: Skin atrophy is common and may be clinically significant in 3 to 4 weeks with potent preparations. Certain areas of the body, such as the face, groin, and axillae, are more prone to atrophic changes than other areas of the body following treatment with corticosteroids.

Infections: Treating skin infections with topical corticosteroids can extensively worsen the infection.

Occlusive therapy: Occlusive dressings such as a plastic wrap increase skin penetration by 10-fold. Discontinue the use of occlusive dressings if infection develops and institute appropriate antimicrobial therapy.

Do not use occlusive dressings in augmented betamethasone dipropionate, betamethasone dipropionate, clobetasol, halobetasol propionate, and mometasone treatment regimens.

Pregnancy: Category C.

Lactation: It is not known whether topical corticosteroids could result in sufficient systemic absorption to produce detectable quantities in breast milk.

Children: Children may be more susceptible to topical corticosteroid-induced hypothalamic-pituitary-adrenal (HPA) axis suppression and Cushing syndrome than adults because of a larger skin surface area to body weight ratio.

Adverse Reactions

Adverse reactions may include burning; itching; irritation; erythema; dryness; folliculitis; hypertrichosis; pruritus; acneiform eruptions; hypopigmentation; perioral dermatitis; allergic contact dermatitis; numbness of fingers; stinging and cracking/tightening of skin; maceration of the skin; secondary infection; skin atrophy; striae; miliaria; telangiectasia. These may occur more frequently with occlusive dressings.

DICLOFENAC

Gel; topical: 1%[a] and 3%[b] (*Rx*)	*Solaraze* (Pharmaderm), *Voltaren* (Novartis)
Patch; transdermal: 1.3%[c] (*Rx*)	*Flector* (Alpharma)

[a] 1 g contains diclofenac sodium 10 mg.
[b] 1 g contains diclofenac sodium 30 mg.
[c] 180 mg per patch.

Warning:

Cardiovascular and GI risk (Voltaren only):

Cardiovascular risk – Nonsteroidal anti-inflammatory drugs (NSAIDs) may cause an increased risk of serious cardiovascular thrombotic events, myocardial infarction, and stroke, which can be fatal. This risk may increase with duration of use. Patients with cardiovascular disease or risk factors for cardiovascular disease may be at greater risk.

Diclofenac is contraindicated for the treatment of perioperative pain in the setting of coronary artery bypass graft (CABG) surgery.

GI risk – NSAIDs cause an increased risk of serious GI adverse reactions, including bleeding, ulceration, and perforation of the stomach or intestines, which can be fatal. These reactions can occur at any time during use and without warning symptoms. Elderly patients are at greater risk for serious GI reactions.

Indications

Actinic keratoses (Solaraze only): For the topical treatment of actinic keratoses (AK). Sun avoidance is indicated during therapy.

Osteoarthritis (Voltaren only): For the relief of the pain of osteoarthritis of joints, such as the knees and joints of the hands. Diclofenac gel has not been evaluated for use on the spine, hip, or shoulder.

Administration and Dosage

Solaraze: Apply gel to lesion areas twice daily. It is to be smoothed onto the affected skin gently. Normally, 0.5 g of gel is used on each 5 cm × 5 cm lesion site. The recommended duration of therapy is from 60 to 90 days. Complete healing may not be evident for up to 30 days following cessation of therapy.

Voltaren:

Lower extremities, including the knees, ankles, and feet – Apply 4 g to the affected foot, knee, or ankle 4 times daily. Massage into the skin, ensuring application to the entire affected foot, knee, or ankle. Do not apply more than 16 g daily to any single joint of the lower extremities.

Upper extremities, including the elbows, wrists, and hands – Apply 2 g to the affected hand, elbow, or wrist 4 times daily. Gently massage into the skin, ensuring application to the entire affected hand, elbow, or wrist. Do not apply more than 8 g/day to any single joint of the upper extremities.

Total dose should not exceed 32 g per day, over all affected joints.

Administration: The proper amount should be measured using the dosing cards supplied in the drug product carton. One dosing card should be used for each application of drug product. The dosing card can be used to apply the gel.

Actions

Pharmacokinetics:

Absorption – Systemic absorption of diclofenac is much lower than that occurring after oral daily dosing of diclofenac sodium.

Distribution – Diclofenac binds tightly to serum albumin.

Metabolism – Metabolism following topical administration is thought to be similar to that after oral administration.

Excretion – The terminal plasma half-life is 1 to 2 hours.

Contraindications

Patients with a known hypersensitivity to diclofenac, benzyl alcohol, polyethylene glycol monomethyl ether 350, or hyaluronate sodium.

Warnings/Precautions

Hypersensitivity reactions: As with other NSAIDs, anaphylactoid reactions may occur in patients without prior exposure to diclofenac. Administer diclofenac with caution to patients with the aspirin triad.

Special risk: Use diclofenac gel with caution in patients with active GI ulceration or bleeding and severe renal or hepatic impairments. Do not apply to open skin wounds, infections, or exfoliative dermatitis.

Pregnancy: Category B.

Lactation: Because of the potential for serious adverse reactions in breast-feeding infants, a decision should be made whether to discontinue breast-feeding or to discontinue the drug, taking into account the importance of the drug to the mother.

Children: AK is not a condition seen within the pediatric population; do not use diclofenac gel in children.

Drug Interactions

NSAIDs: Minimize concomitant oral administration of other NSAIDs, such as aspirin, at anti-inflammatory/analgesic doses.

Adverse Reactions

Adverse reactions occurring in at least 3% of patients include accidental injury, acne, application-site reaction, AST increased, back pain, conjunctivitis, contact dermatitis, dry skin, dyspepsia, edema, exfoliation, flu syndrome, hyperesthesia, infection, myalgia, pain, paresthesia, pharyngitis, photosensitivity reaction, pruritus, rash, skin carcinoma, and vesiculobullous rash.

TRETINOIN (trans-Retinoic Acid; Vitamin A Acid)

Cream: 0.02% (*Rx*)	*Renova* (Ortho Dermatological)
0.025% (*Rx*)	*Tretinoin* (Various), *Avita* (Bertek), *Retin-A* (Ortho)
0.05% (*Rx*)	*Tretinoin* (Spear Dermatology), *Renova* (Ortho Dermatological), *Retin-A* (Ortho)
0.1% (*Rx*)	*Tretinoin* (Spear Dermatology), *Retin-A* (Ortho)
Gel: 0.01% (*Rx*)	*Tretinoin* (Spear Dermatology), *Retin-A* (Ortho)
0.025% (*Rx*)	*Tretinoin* (Spear Dermatology), *Avita* (Bertek), *Retin-A* (Ortho)
0.04% and 0.1% (*Rx*)	*Retin-A Micro* (Ortho)

Indications

Acne (except Renova): Topical treatment of acne vulgaris.

Renova:

Dermatologic conditions –

0.02% cream: Adjunctive agent for use in the mitigation (palliation) of fine wrinkles in patients who use comprehensive skin care and sun avoidance programs.

0.05% cream: Adjunctive agent for use in the mitigation (palliation) of fine wrinkles, mottled hyperpigmentation, and tactile roughness of facial skin in patients who do not achieve such palliation using comprehensive skin care and sun avoidance programs alone.

Administration and Dosage

Acne treatment: Apply once a day before bedtime or in the evening. Cover the entire affected area lightly.

Closely monitor alterations of vehicle, drug concentration, or dose frequency. During the early weeks of therapy, an apparent exacerbation of inflammatory lesions may occur due to the action of the medication on deep, previously undetected lesions; this is not a reason to discontinue therapy.

Therapeutic results should be seen after 2 to 3 weeks, but may not be optimal until after 6 weeks. Once lesions have responded satisfactorily, maintain therapy with less frequent applications or other dosage forms.

Patients may use cosmetics, but thoroughly cleanse area to be treated before applying medication.

Gel: Excessive application results in "pilling" of the gel, which minimizes the likelihood of overapplication by the patient.

Renova: Gently wash face with a mild soap, pat the skin dry, and wait 20 to 30 minutes before applying. Apply tretinoin to the face once a day in the evening, using only enough to cover the entire affected area lightly. Apply a pea-sized amount of cream to cover the entire face. Take caution to avoid contact with eyes, ears, nostrils, and mouth.

For best results, do not apply another skin care product or cosmetic for at least 1 hour after applying tretinoin.

Do not wash face for at least 1 hour after applying tretinoin.

Application of tretinoin may cause a transitory feeling of warmth or slight stinging.

Mitigation (palliation) of fine facial wrinkling, mottled hyperpigmentation, and tactile roughness may occur gradually over the course of therapy. Up to 6 months of therapy may be required before the effects are seen. Most of the improvement noted with tretinoin is seen during the first 24 weeks of therapy. Thereafter, therapy primarily maintains the improvement noticed during the first 24 weeks.

Patients treated with tretinoin may use cosmetics, but the areas to be treated should be cleansed thoroughly before the medication is applied.

Actions

Pharmacology: Tretinoin is a retinoid metabolite of vitamin A. Although the exact mode of action of tretinoin is unknown, current evidence suggests that topical tretinoin decreases cohesiveness of follicular epithelial cells with decreased microcomedo formation. Additionally, tretinoin stimulates mitotic activity and increases turnover of follicular epithelial cells, causing extrusion of the comedones.

Pharmacokinetics: The transdermal absorption of tretinoin from various topical formulations ranged from 1% to 31% of applied dose, depending on whether it was applied to healthy skin or dermatitic skin.

In vitro and in vivo pharmacokinetic studies with tretinoin cream and gel indicated that less than 0.3% of the topically applied dose is bioavailable. Circulating plasma levels of tretinoin are only slightly elevated above those found in healthy normal controls. Estimates of in vivo bioavailability of *Retin-A Micro* following single and multiple daily applications, for a period of 28 days with the 0.1% gel, were approximately 0.82% and 1.41%, respectively. When percutaneous absorption of *Renova* was assessed in healthy male subjects (n = 14) after a single application, as well as after repeated daily applications for 28 days, the absorption of tretinoin was less than 2% and endogenous concentrations of tretinoin and its major metabolites were unaltered.

Contraindications

Hypersensitivity to any component of the product (discontinue if hypersensitivity to any ingredient is noted).

Warnings/Precautions

For external use only: Keep tretinoin away from the eyes, mouth, angles of the nose, and mucous membranes.

Renova:

Mitigating effects – Tretinoin has shown no mitigating effects on significant signs of chronic sun exposure (eg, coarse or deep wrinkling, skin yellowing, lentigines, telangiectasia, skin laxity, keratinocytic atypia, melanocytic atypia, dermal elastosis).

Tretinoin 0.02% cream has shown no mitigating effects on tactile roughness or mottled hyperpigmentation.

Tretinoin does not eliminate wrinkles, repair sun damaged skin, reverse photoaging, or restore a more youthful or younger dermal histologic pattern.

Many patients achieve desired palliative effect on fine wrinkling, mottled hyperpigmentation, and tactile roughness of facial skin with the use of comprehensive skin care and sun avoidance programs including sunscreens, protective clothing, and nonprescription emollient creams.

Long-term use – Tretinoin is a dermal irritant, and the results of continued irritation of the skin for greater than 48 weeks are not known. There is evidence of atypical changes in melanocytes and keratinocytes and of increased dermal elastosis in some patients treated with tretinoin 0.05% for longer than 52 weeks.

Irritation: Tretinoin may induce severe local erythema, pruritus, burning, stinging, and peeling at the application site. If the degree of local irritation warrants, use medication less frequently or discontinue use temporarily or completely. Tretinoin may cause severe irritation to eczematous skin; use with caution in patients with this condition.

Photosensitivity: It is advisable to "rest" a patient's skin until effects of keratolytic agents subside before beginning tretinoin. Minimize exposure to sunlight and sunlamps, and advise patients with sunburn not to use tretinoin until fully recovered because of heightened susceptibility to sunlight as a result of tretinoin use. Patients who undergo considerable sun exposure due to occupation and those with inherent sun sensitivity should exercise particular caution. Use sunscreen products and wear protective clothing over treated areas. Weather extremes, such as wind and cold, also may irritate treated areas.

Pregnancy: Category C.

Lactation: It is not known whether this drug is excreted in breast milk. Exercise caution when tretinoin is administered to a nursing mother.

Children:

Renova – Safety and efficacy in patients less than 18 years of age have not been established.

Drug Interactions

Sulfur, resorcinol, benzoyl peroxide, or salicylic acid: Cautiously use concomitant topical medications because of possible interactions with tretinoin. Significant skin irritation may result. It also is advisable to "rest" a patient's skin until the effects of such preparations subside before use of tretinoin is begun.

Topical preparations: Cautiously use medicated or abrasive soaps and cleansers, soaps, and cosmetics that have a strong drying effect, and products with high concentrations of alcohol, astringents, spices, or lime, permanent wave solutions, electrolysis, hair depilatories or waxes, and products that may irritate the skin in patients being treated with tretinoin because they may increase irritation.

Photosensitizers: Do not use tretinoin if the patient also is taking drugs known to be photosensitizers (eg, thiazides, tetracyclines, fluoroquinolones, phenothiazines, sulfonamides) because of the possibility of augmented phototoxicity.

Adverse Reactions

Almost all patients reported 1 or more local reactions such as peeling, dry skin, burning, stinging, erythema, and pruritus during therapy with tretinoin.

Sensitive skin may become excessively red, edematous, blistered, or crusted. If these effects occur, discontinue medication until skin integrity is restored or adjust to a tolerable level. True contact allergy is rare.

Temporary hyperpigmentation or hypopigmentation has been reported with repeated application. Some individuals have a heightened susceptibility to sunlight while under treatment.

All adverse effects have been reversible upon discontinuation.

CAPSAICIN

Cream: 0.025% (*otc*)	Various, *Pain Doctor* (Fougera), *Zostrix* (Health Care Products)
0.035% (*otc*)	*Capzasin•P* (Chattem)
0.075% (*otc*)	Various, *Rid•a•Pain•HP* (Pfeiffer), *Zostrix Maximum Strength, Zostrix Diabetic Foot Pain, Zostrix-HP* (Health Care Products)
0.1% (*otc*)	*Capzasin•HP* (Chattem)
0.25% (*otc*)	*Axasain* (Rodlen Labs)
Lotion: 0.025% and 0.075% (*otc*)	*Capsin* (Fleming)
Roll-on: 0.075% (*otc*)	*No pain-HP* (Young Again Products)
Patch, topical: 0.025% (*otc*)	*Icy Hot PM* (Chattem)
8% (*Rx*)	*Qutenza* (NeurogesX)

Indications

OTC:

Muscle/Joint pain – For the temporary relief of minor aches and pains of muscles and joints associated with backache, strains, sprains, arthritis, rheumatoid arthritis, and osteoarthritis. For use in treating neuralgias, consult a health care provider.

Rx: For the management of neuropathic pain associated with postherpetic neuralgia.

Administration and Dosage

OTC:

Muscle/Joint pain – Apply a thin film of capsaicin to affected area 3 to 4 times daily. Application schedules of less than 3 to 4 times a day or for less than 2 weeks may not provide optimum pain relief. Unless treating hands, wash hands thoroughly after each application.

Rx: Only physicians, or health care providers under the close supervision of physicians, are to administer capsaicin. Use only nitrile gloves when handling capsaicin.

Adults – Apply a single, 60-minute application of up to 4 patches. May repeat every 3 months or as warranted by the return of pain (not more frequently than every 3 months).

Preparation for administration: Use only nitrile gloves when handling capsaicin and when cleansing capsaicin residue from the skin. Do not use latex gloves because they do not provide adequate protection.

The treatment area (painful area including area of hypersensitivity and allodynia) must be identified by a health care provider and marked on the skin. If necessary, clip hair (do not shave) in and around the identified treatment area to promote patch adherence. Gently wash the treatment area with mild soap and water and dry thoroughly. Use capsaicin only on dry, intact (unbroken) skin.

Pretreat with a topical anesthetic to reduce discomfort associated with the application of capsaicin. Apply topical anesthetic to the entire treatment area and surrounding 1 to 2 cm, and keep the local anesthetic in place until the skin is anesthetized prior to the application of the capsaicin patch. Remove the topical anesthetic with a dry wipe. Gently wash the treatment area with mild soap and water and dry thoroughly.

Administration: Apply the capsaicin patch within 2 hours of opening the pouch. Capsaicin can be cut to match the size and shape of the treatment area. Cut capsaicin before removing the protective release liner. The diagonal cut in the release liner is to aid in its removal. Peel a small section of the release liner back, and place the adhesive side of the patch on the treatment area. While slowly peeling back the release liner from under the patch with one hand, use the other hand to smooth the patch down on to the skin. Once capsaicin is applied, leave in place for 60 minutes. To ensure capsaicin maintains contact with the treatment area, a dressing, such as rolled gauze, may be used. Instruct the patient not to touch the patch or treatment area. Remove capsaicin patches by gently and slowly rolling them inward.

After removal of capsaicin, generously apply cleansing gel to the treatment area and leave on for at least 1 minute. Remove cleansing gel with a dry wipe and gently wash the area with mild soap and water and dry thoroughly.

Inform patients that the treated area may be sensitive to heat for a few days (eg, hot showers/baths, direct sunlight, vigorous exercise).

Handling and disposal: The prescription capsaicin patch contains capsaicin capable of producing severe irritation of eyes, skin, respiratory tract, and mucous membranes. Do not dispense the prescription capsaicin patch to patients for self-administration. It is critical that health care providers who administer the prescription capsaicin patch have completely familiarized themselves with proper dosing, handling, and disposal procedures before handling the prescription capsaicin patch to avoid accidental or inadvertent capsaicin exposure to themselves or others.

Actions

Pharmacology: Capsaicin is a natural chemical derived from plants. Although the precise mechanism of action is not fully understood, evidence suggests that the drug renders skin and joints insensitive to pain by depleting and preventing reaccumulation of substance P in peripheral sensory neurons.

Warnings/Precautions

OTC: OTC capsaicin is for external use only. It should not be applied to wounds or to damaged or irritated skin. It should not be wrapped tightly.

Capsaicin should not come in contact with mucous membranes, eyes, or contact lenses. If this occurs, the affected area should be rinsed thoroughly with water.

This product should be discontinued and a health care provider consulted if condition worsens or does not improve after regular use, if blistering occurs, or if severe burning persists.

Heat should not be applied to the treated area immediately before or after applications, because this may increase the burning sensation.

Rx:

Eye and mucous membrane exposure – Do not apply prescription capsaicin to the face or scalp to avoid risk of exposure to the eyes or mucous membranes.

Aerosolization – Aerosolization of capsaicin can occur upon rapid removal of prescription capsaicin patches. Therefore, remove capsaicin patches gently and slowly by rolling the adhesive side inward.

Application pain – Even following use of a local anesthetic prior to administration of prescription capsaicin patches, patients may experience substantial procedural pain.

Hypertension – In clinical trials, increases in blood pressure occurred during or shortly after exposure to prescription capsaicin patches. Increases in blood pressure were unrelated to the pretreatment blood pressure but were related to treatment-related increases in pain.

Pregnancy: *Category* C (OTC); *Category B* (Rx).

Lactation: It is unknown whether capsaicin is excreted in human breast milk.

Children: Consult a health care provider before using in patients younger than 18 years of age.

Monitoring:

Rx – Monitor blood pressure periodically during treatment.

Drug Interactions

Angiotensin-converting enzyme inhibitors: Capsaicin, including topical use, may cause or exacerbate coughing associated with angiotensin-converting enzyme (ACE) inhibitor treatment and vice versa.

Adverse Reactions

OTC: Adverse reactions include burning; stinging; erythema; cough; respiratory tract irritation.

Rx: Application site edema, application site erythema, application site pain, application site papules, application site pruritus, nasopharyngitis, nausea, sinusitis, vomiting.

ACYCLOVIR (Acycloguanosine)

Ointment: 5% (50 mg/g) (*Rx*) *Zovirax* (Biovail)
Cream: 5% (50 mg/g) (*Rx*)

Indications

Ointment: Management of initial episodes of herpes genitalis and in limited non-life-threatening mucocutaneous herpes simplex virus infections in immunocompromised patients.

Cream: Treatment of recurrent herpes labialis (cold sores) in adults and adolescents (12 years of age and older).

Administration and Dosage

Initiate therapy as early as possible following onset of signs and symptoms.

Ointment: Apply sufficient quantity to adequately cover all lesions every 3 hours 6 times daily for 7 days. Use approximately a one-half inch ribbon of ointment per 4 square inches of surface area. Use a finger cot or rubber glove when applying acyclovir to prevent autoinoculation of other body sites and transmission of infection to other people.

Cream: Apply 5 times/day for 4 days. For adolescents 12 years of age and older the dosage is the same as in adults.

Actions

Pharmacokinetics:

Ointment – Systemic absorption of acyclovir after topical application is minimal.
Cream – Systemic absorption of acyclovir from the cream is minimal in adults.

Warnings/Precautions

For cutaneous use only: Do not use in eyes, nose, or mouth.

Pregnancy: Category B.

Lactation: Systemic exposure following topical administration is minimal.

Adverse Reactions

Mild pain with transient burning/stinging; pruritus.

Post-marketing events: Edema and/or pain at application site; rash (ointment). Angioedema, anaphylaxis, contact dermatitis, eczema, and application site reactions including inflammation (cream).

PENCICLOVIR

Cream: 10 mg/kg (*Rx*) *Denavir* (GlaxoSmithKline)

Indications

Herpes labialis: For the treatment of recurrent herpes labialis (cold sores) in adults.

Administration and Dosage

Apply penciclovir every 2 hours while awake for 4 days. Start treatment as early as possible (eg, during the prodrome or when lesions appear).

Actions

Pharmacology: Penciclovir is an antiviral agent active against herpes viruses. It has in vitro inhibitory activity against herpes simplex virus types 1 (HSV-1) and 2 (HSV-2).

Pharmacokinetics: Measurable penciclovir concentrations were not detected in plasma or urine of healthy male volunteers following single or repeat application of the 1% cream at a dose of 180 mg penciclovir daily (about 67 times the estimated usual clinical dose).

Contraindications

Hypersensitivity to the product or any of its components.

Warnings/Precautions

Mucous membranes: Use penciclovir on herpes labialis on the lips and face only. Application to human mucous membranes is not recommended. Avoid application in or near the eyes because it may cause irritation.

Immunocompromised patients: Penciclovir's effect in immunocompromised patients has not been established.

Pregnancy: Category B.

Lactation: There is no information on whether penciclovir is excreted in breast milk after topical administration.

Children: Safety and efficacy in pediatric patients have not been established.

Adverse Reactions

Adverse reactions occurring in at least 3% of patients include headache.

ALUMINUM CHLORIDE (HEXAHYDRATE)

Solution: 20% in 88.5% SD alcohol 40-2 (*Rx*)	*Aluminum Chloride Hexahydrate* (Glades)
20% in 93% SD alcohol 40 (*Rx*)	*Drysol* (Person & Covey)

Indications

An astringent used as an aid in the management of hyperhidrosis.

Administration and Dosage

Apply to the affected area once daily, only at bedtime. To help prevent irritation, completely dry area prior to application. Do not apply to broken, irritated, or recently shaved skin.

For maximum effect, cover the treated area with plastic wrap, held in place by a snug fitting T-shirt or body shirt, mitten, or sock (never hold plastic wrap in place with tape). Wash the treated area the following morning. Excessive sweating may stop after 2 or more treatments. Thereafter, apply once or twice weekly or as needed.

Warnings/Precautions

For external use only: Avoid contact with the eyes.

Discontinue use: If irritation or sensitization occurs, discontinue use.

Metals/Fabrics: Aluminum chloride (hexahydrate) may be harmful to certain metals and fabrics.

Adverse Reactions

Burning or prickling sensation may occur.

FORMALDEHYDE

Liquid: 10% (*Rx*)	*Formalaz* (River's Edge)
Spray: 10% (*Rx*)	*Formaldehyde-10* (Pedinol)
Solution: 10% (*Rx*)	*Lazer Formaldehyde* (Pedinol)

Indications

Drying agent for presurgical and postsurgical removal of warts or for *Histofreezer* treatment of warts where dryness is required. Safeguards against offensive odor and dries excessive moisture of feet.

Administration and Dosage

Apply once daily to affected areas as directed.

Contraindications

Hypersensitivity to any ingredients of the product.

Warnings/Precautions

For external use only: Avoid contact with and keep away from face, eyes, nose, and mucous membranes.

Irritation/Sensitivity: May be irritating and sensitizing to the skin of some patients; check skin for sensitivity prior to application. If redness or irritation persists, consult physician.

COLLAGENASE

Ointment: 250 units collagenase enzyme/g (*Rx*)	*Collagenase Santyl* (Ross)

Indications

For debriding chronic dermal ulcers and severely burned areas.

Administration and Dosage

Apply once daily (or more frequently if the dressing becomes soiled, as from incontinence). When clinically indicated, crosshatching thick eschar with a No. 10 blade allows collagenase more surface contact with necrotic debris. It also is more desirable to remove, with forceps and scissors, as much loosened detritus as can be done readily.

Instructions for use:

1.) Prior to application, cleanse the wound of debris and digested material by gently rubbing with a gauze pad saturated with normal saline solution, or with the desired cleansing agent compatible with collagenase, followed by a normal saline solution rinse.
2.) Whenever infection is present, it is desirable to use an appropriate topical antibiotic powder. Apply the antibiotic to the wound prior to the application of collagenase ointment. If the infection does not respond, discontinue therapy with collagenase until remission of the infection.
3.) Collagenase may be applied directly to the wound or to a sterile gauze pad, which is applied to the wound and secured.
4.) Terminate use of collagenase when debridement of necrotic tissue is completed and granulation tissue is well established.

Actions

Pharmacology: Because collagen accounts for 75% of the dry weight of skin tissue, the ability of collagenase to digest collagen in the physiological pH and temperature range makes it particularly effective in the removal of detritus. Collagenase thus contributes toward the formation of granulation tissue and subsequent epithelization of dermal ulcers and severely burned areas. Collagen in healthy tissue or in newly formed granulation tissue is not attacked.

Contraindications

Local or systemic hypersensitivity to collagenase.

Warnings/Precautions

For external use only: Avoid contact with the eyes.

Optimal pH range: The optimal pH range of collagenase is 6 to 8. Higher or lower pH conditions will decrease the enzyme's activity; take appropriate precautions. The enzymatic activity also is adversely affected by certain detergents and heavy metal ions, such as mercury and silver, which are used in some antiseptics. When it is suspected that such materials have been used, carefully cleanse the site by repeatedly washing with normal saline before collagenase is applied. Avoid soaks containing metal ions or acidic solutions because of the metal ion and low pH. Cleansing materials such as hydrogen peroxide, Dakin's solution, and normal saline are compatible with the collagenase ointment.

Systemic bacterial infections: Closely monitor debilitated patients for systemic bacterial infections because of the theoretical possibility that debriding enzymes may increase the risk of bacteremia.

Erythema: Slight transient erythema has been noted in the surrounding tissue, particularly when collagenase was not confined to the wound. Therefore, apply carefully within the wound area.

Children: Safety and efficacy in children are not established.

Adverse Reactions

Hypersensitivity: One case of systemic manifestations of hypersensitivity to collagenase occurred with treatment of more than 1 year with both collagenase and cortisone.

ENZYME COMBINATIONS, TOPICAL

Aerosol: 0.1 mg trypsin, 72.5 mg balsam peru, and 650 mg castor oil per 0.82 mL (*Rx*)	*Granul-Derm* (Qualitest)
0.12 mg trypsin, 87 mg balsam peru, and 788 mg castor oil per g (*Rx*)	*Granulex* (Bertek)
Ointment: 90 units trypsin, 87 mg balsam peru, and 788 mg castor oil (*Rx*)	*Allanderm-T* (Allan), *Xenaderm* (Healthpoint)
1.1×10^6 units papain and 100 mg urea per g (*Rx*)	*Ethezyme* (Ethex)
6.5×10^5 units papain and 10% urea per g	*Kovia 6.5* (Stratus)
8.3×10^5 units papain and 100 mg urea per g (*Rx*)	*Accuzyme* (Healthpoint), *Ethezyme 830* (Ethex), *Gladase* (Smith & Nephew) *Pap-Urea* (Cypress)
≥ 405,900 units papain, 10% urea, 0.5% chlorophyllin copper complex sodium per g (*Rx*)	*Ziox 405* (Stratus)
≥ 521,700 units papain, 10% urea, 0.5% chlorophyllin copper complex sodium per g (*Rx*)	*Papain-Urea-Chlorophyllin* (Cypress), *Gladase-C* (Healthpoint), *Panafil* (Healthpoint)
Spray: ≥ 405,900 units papain, 10% urea, 0.5% chllorophyllin copper complex sodium per g (*Rx*)	*AllanfillEnzyme* (Allan), *Panafil SE* (Healthpoint)
≥ 521,700 units papain, 10% urea, 0.5% chlorophyllin copper complex sodium per g (*Rx*)	*Panafil* (Healthpoint)
6.5×10^5 units papain and 10% urea per g (*Rx*)	*Accuzyme SE* (Healthpoint), *AllanEnzyme* (Allan)
8.3×10^5 units papain and 10% urea per g (*Rx*)	*Accuzyme* (Healthpoint)

Indications

For debridement of necrotic tissue and liquefication of slough in acute and chronic lesions such as pressure ulcers, varicose, diabetic, and decubitus ulcers, burns, postoperative wounds, pilonidal cyst wounds, carbuncles, and miscellaneous traumatic or infected wounds. Also stimulates vascular bed activity to improve epithelization.

Administration and Dosage

Cleanse the wound prior to application with wound cleanser or saline. For papain-containing products, avoid cleansing with hydrogen peroxide solution.

Aerosol: Shake well. Hold upright and approximately 12 inches from the area to be treated. Press valve and coat wound rapidly. Wound may be left unbandaged or a wet dressing may be applied. Apply 2 to 3 times daily, or as often as necessary. To remove, wash gently with water.

Ointment: Apply ointment directly to the wound, cover with appropriate dressing, and secure into place. Daily or twice daily applications are preferred. Irrigate the wound at each redressing to remove any accumulation of liquefied necrotic material.

Longer intervals between redressings (2 or 3 days) have proved satisfactory, and ointment may be applied under pressure dressings.

Spray: Shake well. Begin initial use by holding spray upright directly over the wound, and prime the pump 6 to 8 times.

Hold the spray bottle approximately 2 to 3 inches from the wound and use even, firm, and consistent pressure to dispense product. When sprayed from the appropriate distance, the spray should appear in a nickel-sized diameter.

Completely cover the wound site with spray. Cover wound with appropriate dressing of choice (eg, saline-moistened gauze, semi-occlusive dressings), and secure into place.

Contraindications

Sensitivity to papain or any other components of these preparations.

Warnings/Precautions

Arterial clots: Do not spray aerosol products on fresh arterial clots.

For external use only: Avoid contact with the eyes.

Transient burning: Transient burning may occur upon application.

Papain: Papain may be inactivated by the salts of heavy metals such as lead, silver, and mercury. Avoid contact with medications containing these metals.

Adverse Reactions

Generally well-tolerated and nonirritating. A transient burning sensation may be experienced by a small percentage of patients upon application. Occasionally, the profuse exudate from enzymatic digestion may irritate the skin. In such cases, more frequent dressing changes will alleviate discomfort until exudate decreases.

IMIQUIMOD

Cream: 5% (*Rx*)	*Aldara* (Graceway Pharmaceuticals)
Cream; topical: 5%	*Imiquimod* (Fougera)
Cream; topical: 3.75%	*Zyclara* (Graceway Pharmaceuticals)

Indications

Actinic keratosis: For the topical treatment of clinically typical, nonhyperkeratotic, nonhypertrophic, visible or palpable actinic keratoses on the face or scalp in immunocompetent adults.

Genital and perianal warts (5% cream only): Treatment of external genital and perianal warts/condyloma acuminata in patients 12 years of age and older.

Superficial basal cell carcinoma (5% cream only): For the topical treatment of biopsy-confirmed, primary superficial basal cell carcinoma (sBCC) in immunocompetent adults, with a maximum tumor diameter of 2 cm, located on the trunk (excluding anogenital skin), neck, or extremities (excluding hands and feet), only when surgical methods are medically less appropriate and patient follow-up can be reasonably assured.

Administration and Dosage

Adults:

Actinic keratosis – Apply 2 times per week (eg, Monday and Thursday or Tuesday and Friday) prior to sleeping hours for 16 weeks to a defined treatment area on the face or scalp (but not both concurrently).

3.75% cream:

Usual dosage – Apply a thin film once daily before bedtime to the skin of the affected area (either the face or balding scalp). Leave on the skin for 8 hours, then remove with mild soap and water.

Maximum dose – Up to 2 packets of the cream may be applied to the treatment area at each application.

Duration of therapy – Treat for two 2-week treatment cycles separated by a 2-week no-treatment period.

Treatment should continue for the full treatment course even if all actinic keratoses appear to be gone.

5% cream:

Usual dosage – Leave on the skin for approximately 8 hours, then remove with mild soap and water.

Maximum dose – No more than one packet of cream should be applied to the contiguous treatment area at each application.

Genital and perianal warts – Apply a thin layer 3 times per week to external genital/perianal warts, prior to normal sleeping hours, and leave on the skin for 6 to 10 hours. Remove by washing with mild soap and water. Continue imiquimod treatment until there is total clearance of the genital/perianal warts or for a maximum of 16 weeks.

Superficial basal cell carcinoma – Apply 5 times per week prior to bedtime, for 6 weeks. Leave on the skin for approximately 8 hours. Remove with mild soap and water. The treatment area should include a 1 cm margin of skin around the tumor. Continue treatment for 6 weeks.

Amount of Imiquimod for Administration

Target tumor diameter	Size of cream droplet (diameter)	Approximate amount of cream
0.5 to < 1 cm	4 mm	10 mg
≥ 1 to < 1.5 cm	5 mm	25 mg
≥ 1.5 to 2 cm	7 mm	40 mg

Children:

Genital and perianal warts (5% cream only) –

12 years of age and older: See Adults for dosing.

Administration: Avoid contact with the lips, nostrils, and in or near the eyes.

Actinic keratosis –

5% cream: Before applying the cream, wash the treatment area with mild soap and water and allow the area to dry thoroughly (at least 10 minutes).

Superficial basal cell carcinoma – Before applying the cream, wash the treatment area with mild soap and water, and allow the area to dry thoroughly.

Local skin reactions: Local skin reactions at the treatment site are common. A rest period of several days may be taken if required by the patient's discomfort or severity of the local skin reaction. Treatment may resume once the reaction subsides.

Actions

Pharmacology: Imiquimod is an immune response modifier. The mechanism of action of imiquimod is unknown.

Pharmacokinetics:

Absorption/Distribution –

3.75% cream: Following dosing with 2 packets once daily (imiquimod 18.75 mg/day), the median time to maximal concentrations occurred at 9 hours after dosing. Based on the plasma half-life of imiquimod observed at the end of the study, 29.3±17 hours, steady-state concentrations can be anticipated to occur by day 7 with once-daily dosing.

Metabolism/Excretion – The apparent half-life was approximately 10 times greater with topical dosing than the 2-hour apparent half-life seen following subcutaneous dosing, suggesting prolonged retention of drug in the skin.

Contraindications

None well documented.

Warnings/Precautions

Human papilloma viral disease: Imiquimod 5% cream has not been evaluated for the treatment of urethral, intravaginal, cervical, rectal, or intra-anal human papilloma viral disease.

Other types of basal cell carcinomas: Safety and efficacy of imiquimod cream have not been established for other types of basal cell carcinomas, including nodular, morpheaform (fibrosing or sclerosing) types, and it is not recommended for treatment of BCC subtypes other than the superficial variant (sBCC). Patients with sBCC treated with imiquimod cream are recommended to have regular follow-up of the treatment site.

Superficial basal cell carcinoma – The safety and efficacy of treating sBCC lesions on the face, head, and anogenital area with imiquimod 5% have not been established.

Basal cell nevus syndrome or xeroderma pigmentosum – The efficacy and safety of imiquimod cream have not been established for patients with basal cell nevus syndrome or xeroderma pigmentosum.

Immunosuppressed patients: The safety and efficacy of imiquimod cream in immunosuppressed patients have not been established.

Previous drug or surgical treatment: Imiquimod cream administration is not recommended until the skin is completely healed from any previous drug or surgical treatment.

Local inflammatory reactions: Intense local inflammatory reactions, including skin weeping or erosion, can occur after few applications of imiquimod and may require an interruption of dosing. Imiquimod has the potential to exacerbate inflammatory conditions of the skin, including long-term graft versus host disease.

Imiquimod has the potential to exacerbate inflammatory conditions of the skin.

Systemic reactions: Flu-like signs and symptoms may accompany, or even precede, local inflammatory reactions and may include malaise, fever, nausea, myalgias, and rigors. Consider an interruption of dosing and an assessment of the patient.

Actinic keratosis: Safety and efficacy have not been established for imiquimod 5% cream in the treatment of actinic keratosis with repeated use (more than 1 treatment course) in the same 25 cm^2 area.

Photosensitivity: Avoid exposure to sunlight (including sunlamps) or minimize it during use of imiquimod cream because of concern for heightened sunburn susceptibility.

Pregnancy: Category C.

Lactation: It is not known whether imiquimod is excreted in breast milk.

Children: Safety and efficacy of imiquimod 5% cream in patients younger than 12 years of age have not been established.

Elderly: No overall differences in safety or efficacy were observed between these patients and younger patients. No other clinical experience has identified differences in responses between the elderly and younger patients, but greater sensitivity of some older individuals cannot be ruled out.

Monitoring: Periodically assess response to therapy. Monitor for local skin reactions (eg, erythema, erosion, edema) to the application site and surrounding areas.

Adverse Reactions

Actinic keratosis: Application site reactions include bleeding, burning, itching, pain, and stinging.

Local skin reactions include edema, erosion/ulceration, erythema, flaking/scaling/dryness, scabbing/crusting, vesicles, and weeping/exudate.

3.75% cream (at least 2%) – Anorexia, application site pruritus, dizziness, fatigue, headache, herpes simplex, nausea, pain, pyrexia.

5% cream (more than 1%) – Carcinoma squamous, diarrhea, sinusitis, upper respiratory tract infection.

Superficial basal cell carcinoma: The adverse reactions with an incidence of at least 3% include application site reaction (burning, itching, and pain), back pain, edema, erosion, erythema, flaking/scaling, headache, induration, scabbing/crusting, ulceration, upper respiratory tract infection, and vesicles.

5% cream (more than 1%) – Back pain, lymphadenopathy, rhinitis.

External genital warts: The adverse reactions with an incidence of at least 3% include burning, edema, erosion, erythema, excoriation, flaking, fungal infection, headache, induration, influenza-like symptoms, itching, local pain, scabbing, soreness, ulceration, and vesicles.

5% cream (local skin reactions) – Excoriation, fungal infection, influenza-like symptoms, soreness.

TACROLIMUS

Ointment: 0.03%, 0.1% (*Rx*)	*Protopic* (Astellas Pharma)

Warning:

Long-term safety of topical calcineurin inhibitors has not been established.

Although a causal relationship has not been established, rare cases of malignancy (ie, skin cancer and lymphoma) have been reported in patients treated with topical calcineurin inhibitors, including tacrolimus ointment.

Therefore:

- Avoid continuous long-term use of topical calcineurin inhibitors, including tacrolimus ointment, in any age group, and limit application to areas of involvement with atopic dermatitis.
- Tacrolimus ointment is not indicated for use in children younger than 2 years of age. Only tacrolimus 0.03% ointment is indicated for use in children 2 to 15 years of age.

Indications

Moderate to severe atopic dermatitis: Tacrolimus ointment, 0.03% and 0.1% for adults, and 0.03% for children 2 to 15 years of age, is indicated as second-line therapy for the short-term and noncontinuous chronic treatment of moderate to severe atopic dermatitis in nonimmunocompromised adults and children who have failed to respond adequately to other topical prescription treatments for atopic dermatitis, or when those treatments are not advisable.

Administration and Dosage

Adults:

0.03% and 0.1% – Apply a thin layer to the affected skin areas twice daily. Use the minimum amount to control signs and symptoms. Stop using when signs and symptoms resolve.

Children:

0.03% – Apply a thin layer to the affected skin areas twice daily. Use the minimum amount to control signs and symptoms. Stop using when signs and symptoms resolve.

Long-term use: See Warning Box.

Re-examine patients to confirm diagnosis if signs and symptoms do not improve within 6 weeks (adults and children).

Tacrolimus 0.03% and 0.1% ointment should not be used with occlusive dressings.

Actions

Pharmacology: The mechanism of action of tacrolimus in atopic dermatitis is not known.

Pharmacokinetics:

Absorption – Tacrolimus is minimally absorbed after the topical application of tacrolimus ointment. The absolute bioavailability of tacrolimus in atopic dermatitis patients is approximately 0.5%.

Distribution – The plasma protein binding of tacrolimus is approximately 99%.

Metabolism – Tacrolimus is extensively metabolized by the cytochrome P-450 system (CYP3A).

Contraindications

History of hypersensitivity to tacrolimus or any other component of the preparation.

Warnings/Precautions

Infections/Lymphomas/Skin Malignancies: Rare cases of skin malignancy and lymphoma have been reported in patients treated with topical calcineurin inhibitors, including tacrolimus ointment.

Immunocompromised patients: Do not use tacrolimus ointment in immunocompromised adults and children.

Long-term use: If signs and symptoms of atopic dermatitis do not improve within 6 weeks, reexamine the patient and confirm the diagnosis.

Renal effects: Rare postmarketing cases of acute renal failure have been reported in patients treated with tacrolimus ointment.

Premalignant/Malignant skin conditions: Avoid the use of tacrolimus ointment on premalignant and malignant skin conditions.

Lymphadenopathy: Patients who develop lymphadenopathy should have the lymphadenopathy investigated. In the absence of a clear etiology, or in the presence of acute infectious mononucleosis, consider discontinuation of tacrolimus ointment. Monitor patients who develop lymphadenopathy to ensure that the lymphadenopathy resolves.

Netherton syndrome: The use of tacrolimus ointment in patients with Netherton syndrome or other skin diseases in which there is the potential for increased systemic absorption of tacrolimus is not recommended. The safety of tacrolimus ointment has not been established in patients with generalized erythroderma.

Local symptoms: The use of tacrolimus ointment may cause local symptoms such as skin burning (burning sensation, stinging, soreness) or pruritus.

Bacterial and viral skin infections: Before treatment with tacrolimus ointment, cutaneous bacterial or viral infections at treatment sites should be resolved.

Treatment with tacrolimus ointment may be independently associated with an increased risk of varicella zoster virus infection (chickenpox or shingles), herpes simplex virus infection, or eczema herpeticum.

Photosensitivity: Patients should minimize or avoid natural or artificial sunlight exposure, even while tacrolimus is not on the skin.

Pregnancy: *Category* C.

Lactation: Tacrolimus is excreted in human milk. Decide whether to discontinue nursing or to discontinue the drug, taking into account the importance of the drug to the mother.

Children: Tacrolimus 0.03% ointment may be used in children 2 years of age and older. Tacrolimus ointment is not indicated for children younger than 2 years of age.

Only the lower concentration, 0.03%, of tacrolimus ointment is recommended for use as a second-line therapy for short-term and noncontinuous chronic treatment of moderate to severe atopic dermatitis in nonimmunocompromised children 2 to 15 years of age who have failed to respond adequately to other topical prescription treatments for atopic dermatitis, or when those treatments are not advisable.

Drug Interactions

Drugs that may interact with tacrolimus include CYP3A4 inhibitors (eg, calcium channel blockers, cimetidine, erythromycin, itraconazole, ketoconazole, fluconazole) and alcohol.

Adverse Reactions

Adverse events that occurred in at least 3% of patients include the following: abdominal pain, accidental injury, acne, alcohol intolerance, allergic reaction, arthralgia, asthenia, asthma, back pain, bronchitis, conjunctivitis, contact dermatitis, cough increased, cyst, dry skin, dysmenorrhea, dyspepsia, exfoliative dermatitis, diarrhea, fever, flu-like symptoms, folliculitis, fungal dermatitis, gastroenteritis, headache, herpes simplex, hyperesthesia, infection, insomnia, lack of drug effect, lymphadenopathy, myalgia, nausea, otitis media, paresthesia, peripheral edema, pharyngitis, pneumonia, pruritus, pustular rash, rash, rhinitis, sinusitis, skin burning, skin disorder, skin erythema, skin infection, skin tingling, urticaria, varicella zoster/herpes zoster, vesiculobullous rash, vomiting.

Chapter 12

OPHTHALMIC AND OTIC AGENTS

TOPICAL OPHTHALMICS

General considerations in topical ophthalmic drug therapy: Proper administration is essential to optimal therapeutic response. In many instances, health professionals may be too casual when instructing patients on proper use of ophthalmics. The administration technique used often determines drug safety and efficacy.

- The normal eye retains approximately 10 mcL of fluid (adjusted for blinking). The average dropper delivers 25 to 50 mcL/drop. The value of more than 1 drop is questionable.
- Minimize systemic absorption of ophthalmic drops by compressing lacrimal sac for 3 to 5 minutes after instillation. This retards passage of drops via nasolacrimal duct into areas of potential absorption such as nasal and pharyngeal mucosa.
- Because of rapid lacrimal drainage and limited eye capacity, if multiple drop therapy is indicated, the best interval between drops is 5 minutes. This ensures the first drop is not flushed away by the second or the second is not diluted by the first.
- Topical anesthesia will increase the bioavailability of ophthalmic agents by decreasing the blink reflex and the production and turnover of tears.
- Factors that may increase absorption from ophthalmic dosage forms include lax eyelids of some patients, usually the elderly, which creates a greater reservoir for retention of drops, and hyperemic or diseased eyes.
- Eyecup use is discouraged because of the risk of contamination and spreading disease.
- Ophthalmic suspensions mix with tears less rapidly and remain in the cul-de-sac longer than solutions.
- Ophthalmic ointments maintain contact between the drug and ocular tissues by slowing the clearance rate to as little as 0.5%/min. Ophthalmic ointments provide maximum contact between drug and external ocular tissues.
- Ophthalmic ointments may impede delivery of other ophthalmic drugs to the affected side by serving as a barrier to contact.
- Ointments may blur vision during waking hours. Use with caution in conditions where visual clarity is critical (eg, operating motor equipment, reading).
- Monitor expiration dates closely. Do not use outdated medication.
- Solutions and ointments are frequently misused. Do not assume that patients know how to maximize safe and effective use of these agents. Combine appropriate patient education and counseling with prescribing and dispensing of ophthalmics.

Topical application is the most common route of administration for ophthalmic drugs. Advantages include convenience, simplicity, noninvasive nature, and the ability of the patient to self-administer. Because of blood and aqueous losses of drug, topical medications typically do not penetrate in useful concentrations to posterior ocular structures and therefore are of no therapeutic benefit for diseases of the retina, optic nerve, and other posterior segment structures.

Medications:

Solutions and suspensions – Most topical ocular preparations are commercially available as solutions or suspensions that are applied directly to the eye from the bottle, which serves as the eye dropper. Avoid touching the dropper tip to the eye because this can lead to contamination of the medication and also may cause ocular injury. Resuspend suspensions (notably, many ocular steroids) by shaking to provide an accurate dosage of drug.

Recommended procedures for administration of solutions or suspensions –

- Wash hands thoroughly before administration.
- Tilt head backward or lie down and gaze upward.
- Gently grasp lower eyelid below eyelashes and pull the eyelid away from the eye to form a pouch.
- Place dropper directly over eye. Avoid contact of the dropper with the eye, finger or any surface.
- Look upward just before applying a drop.

- After instilling the drop, look downward for several seconds.
- Release the lid slowly.
- With eyes closed, apply gentle pressure with fingers to the inside corner of eye for 3 to 5 minutes. This retards drainage of solution from intended solution.
- Do not rub the eye. Minimize blinking.
- Do not rinse the dropper.
- Do not use eye drops that have changed color.
- If more than 1 type of ophthalmic drop is used, wait at least 5 minutes before administering the second agent.
- When the instillation of eye drops is difficult (eg, pediatric patients, adults with particularly strong blink reflex), the close-eye method may be used. This involves lying down, placing the prescribed number of drops on the eyelid in the inner corner of the eye, then opening eye so that drops will fall into the eye by gravity.

Ointments – The primary purpose for an ophthalmic ointment vehicle is to prolong drug contact time with the external ocular surface. This is particularly useful for treating children, who may "cry out" topically applied solutions, and for medicating ocular injuries, such as corneal abrasions, when the eye is to be patched. Administer solutions before ointments. Ointments preclude entry of subsequent drops.

Recommended procedures for administration of ointments –

- Wash hands thoroughly before administration.
- Holding the ointment tube in the hand for a few minutes will warm the ointment and facilitate flow.
- When opening the ointment tube for the first time, squeeze out and discard the first 0.25 inch of ointment as it may be too dry.
- Tilt head backward or lie down and gaze upward.
- Gently pull down the lower lid to form a pouch.
- Place 0.25 to 0.5 inch of ointment with a sweeping motion inside the lower lid by squeezing the tube gently.
- Close the eye for 1 to 2 minutes and roll the eyeball in all directions.
- Temporary blurring of vision may occur. Avoid activities requiring visual acuity until blurring clears.
- Remove excessive ointment around the eye or ointment tube tip with a tissue.
- If using more than 1 kind of ointment, wait about 10 minutes before applying the second drug.

AGENTS FOR GLAUCOMA

Glaucoma is a condition of the eye in which an elevation of the intraocular pressure (IOP) leads to progressive cupping and atrophy of the optic nerve head, deterioration of the visual fields, and, ultimately, to blindness. Primary open-angle glaucoma is the most common type of glaucoma. Angle-closure glaucoma and congenital glaucoma are treated primarily by surgical methods, although short-term drug therapy is used to decrease IOP prior to surgery.

Drugs used in the therapy of primary open-angle glaucoma include a variety of agents with different mechanisms of action. The therapeutic goal in treating glaucoma is reducing the elevated IOP, a major risk factor in the pathogenesis of glaucomatous visual field loss. The higher the level of IOP, the greater the likelihood of glaucomatous visual field loss and optic nerve damage. Reduction of IOP may be accomplished by: 1) Decreasing the rate of production of aqueous humor or 2) increasing the rate of outflow (drainage) of aqueous humor from the anterior chamber of the eye.

The 5 groups of agents used in therapy of primary open-angle glaucoma are listed in the table, which summarizes their mechanism of decreasing IOP, effects on pupil size and ciliary muscle and duration of action.

Agents for Glaucoma

Drug	Strength	Duration (h)	Decrease aqueous production	Increase aqueous outflow	Effect on pupil	Effect on ciliary muscle
Sympathomimetics						
Apraclonidine[a]	0.5 to 1%	7 to 12	+++	NR	NR	NR
Brimonidine	0.2%	12	++	++	NR	NR
Dipivefrin	0.1%	12	+	++	mydriasis	NR
Epinephrine	0.1% to 2%	12 to 24	+	++	mydriasis	NR
Beta blockers						
Betaxolol	0.25% to 0.5%	12	+++	NR	NR	NR
Carteolol	1%	12	+++	nd	NR	NR
Levobunolol	0.25% to 0.5%	12 to 24	+++	NR	NR	NR
Metipranolol	0.3%	12 to 24	+++	+	NR	NR
Timolol	0.25% to 0.5%	12 to 24	+++	+	NR	NR
Miotics, direct-acting						
Acetylcholine[b]	1%	10 to 20 min	NR	+++	miosis	accommodation
Carbachol[b]	0.75% to 3%	6 to 8	NR	+++	miosis	accommodation
Pilocarpine[c]	0.25% to 10%	4 to 8	NR	+++	miosis	accommodation
Miotics, cholinesterase inhibitors						
Echothiophate	0.03% to 0.25%	days/wks	NR	+++	miosis	accommodation
Physostigmine	0.25% to 0.5%	12 to 36	NR	+++	miosis	accommodation
Carbonic anhydrase inhibitors						
Acetazolamide[d]	125 to 500 mg	8 to 12	+++	NR	NR	NR
Brinzolamide[e]	1%	≈ 8	+++	NR	NR	NR
Dichlorphenamide[d]	50 mg	6 to 12	+++	NR	NR	NR
Dorzolamide[e]	2%	≈ 8	+++	NR	NR	NR
Methazolamide[d]	25 to 50 mg	10 to 18	+++	NR	NR	NR

Agents for Glaucoma						
Drug	Strength	Duration (h)	Decrease aqueous production	Increase aqueous outflow	Effect on pupil	Effect on ciliary muscle
Prostaglandin analogs						
Bimatoprost	0.03%	≈ 24	NR	+++	NR	NR
Latanoprost	0.0005%	24	NR	+++	NR	NR
Travoprost	0.004%	≈ 24	NR	+++	NR	NR

+++ = significant activity ++ = moderate activity + = some activity NR = no activity reported
nd = No data available
[a] 1% used only to decrease IOP in surgery.
[b] Intraocular administration only for miosis during surgery; carbachol also available as a topical agent.
[c] Also available as a gel and an insert; the duration of these doseforms is longer (18 to 24 hours and 1 week, respectively) than the solution.
[d] Systemic agents; for detailed information, see group monograph in Cardiovascular section.
[e] Topical ophthalmic agent.

Prostaglandin analogs: Prostaglandin analogs increase uveoscleral outflow through a new mechanism of action; selective prostanoid receptor agonism. Latanoprost, currently the only agent available in this class, can be used concurrently with other topical ophthalmic drug products to reduce IOP.

BRIMONIDINE

Solution: 0.1%, 0.15% (*Rx*) *Alphagan, Alphagan-P* (Allergan)

Indications

Intraocular pressure (IOP): To lower IOP in patients with open-angle glaucoma or ocular hypertension.

Administration and Dosage

The recommended dose is 1 drop of brimonidine tartrate in the affected eye(s) 3 times daily, approximately 8 hours apart.

Actions

Pharmacology: Brimonidine is an alpha-2 adrenergic receptor agonist. It has a peak ocular hypotensive effect occurring at 2 hours postdose. Brimonidine has a dual mechanism of action; it reduces aqueous humor production and increases uveoscleral outflow.

Pharmacokinetics: After ocular administration of a 0.1% or 0.2% solution, plasma concentrations peaked within 0.5 to 2.5 hours and declined with a systemic half-life of approximately 2 hours.

Brimonidine is metabolized primarily by the liver. Urinary excretion is the major route of elimination of the drug and its metabolites. Approximately 87% of an orally administered radioactive dose was eliminated within 120 hours, with 74% found in the urine.

Contraindications

Hypersensitivity to brimonidine tartrate or any component of this medication; patients receiving monoamine oxidase inhibitor (MAOI) therapy.

Warnings/Precautions

Soft contact lenses: The preservative in brimonidine, benzalkonium chloride, may be absorbed by soft contact lenses. Instruct patients wearing soft contact lenses to wait at least 15 minutes after instilling brimonidine to insert soft contact lenses.

Cardiovascular disease: Exercise caution in treating patients with severe cardiovascular disease.

Use with caution: Use with caution in patients with depression, cerebral or coronary insufficiency, Raynaud phenomenon, orthostatic hypotension, or thromboangiitis obliterans.

Loss of effect: Loss of effect in some patients may occur. The IOP-lowering efficacy observed with brimonidine during the first month of therapy may not always reflect the long-term level of IOP reduction. Therefore, routinely monitor IOP.

Renal/Hepatic function impairment: Use caution when treating patients with hepatic or renal impairment.

Pregnancy: Category B.

Lactation: It is not known whether brimonidine is excreted in breast milk.

Children: Safety and efficacy in pediatric patients have not been established.

Drug Interactions

Drugs that may be affected by brimonidine include CNS depressants, beta-blockers, antihypertensives, MAOIs, and cardiac glycosides.

Drugs that may affect brimonidine include tricyclic antidepressants.

Adverse Reactions

Adverse events occurring in 10% to 30% of patients in descending order include oral dryness, ocular hyperemia, burning and stinging, headache, blurring, foreign body sensation, fatigue/drowsiness, conjunctival follicles, ocular allergic reactions, and ocular pruritus.

Adverse events occurring in 3% to 9% in descending order include corneal staining/erosion, photophobia, eyelid erythema, ocular ache/pain, ocular dryness, tearing, upper respiratory symptoms, eyelid edema, conjunctival edema, dizziness, blepharitis, ocular irritation, GI symptoms, asthenia, conjunctival blanching, abnormal vision, and muscular pain.

APRACLONIDINE

Solution: 0.5% and 0.01% (*Rx*)	*Iopidine* (Alcon)

Indications

1%: To control or prevent postsurgical elevations in IOP that occur in patients after argon laser trabeculoplasty or iridotomy.

0.5%: Short-term adjunctive therapy in patients on maximally tolerated medical therapy who require additional IOP reduction.

Administration and Dosage

0.5%: Instill 1 to 2 drops in the affected eye(s) 3 times daily. Because apraclonidine 0.5% will be used with other ocular glaucoma therapies, use an approximate 5-minute interval between instillation of each medication to prevent washout of the previous dose. Not for injection into the eye.

1%: Instill 1 drop in scheduled operative eye 1 hour before initiating anterior segment laser surgery. Instill second drop into same eye immediately upon completion of surgery.

Actions

Pharmacology: Apraclonidine hydrochloride is a relatively selective α-adrenergic agonist. When instilled into the eyes, apraclonidine reduces intraocular pressure (IOP) and has minimal effect on cardiovascular parameters.

Pharmacokinetics: Topical use of apraclonidine 0.5% leads to systemic absorption. The onset of action is usually within 1 hour and the maximum IOP reduction occurs 3 to 5 hours after application of a single dose.

Contraindications

Hypersensitivity to any component of this medication or to clonidine; concurrent monamine oxidase inhibitor therapy.

Warnings/Precautions

Concomitant therapy: The addition of 0.5% apraclonidine to patients already using 2 aqueous suppressing drugs (eg, beta blocker plus carbonic anhydrase inhibitor) as part of their maximally tolerated medical therapy may not provide additional benefit.

Tachyphylaxis: The IOP-lowering efficacy of 0.5% apraclonidine diminishes over time in some patients. The benefit for most patients is less than 1 month.

IOP reduction: Because apraclonidine is a potent depressor of IOP, closely monitor patients who develop exaggerated reductions in IOP.

Cardiovascular disease: Acute administration of 2 drops of apraclonidine has had minimal effect on heart rate or blood pressure; however, observe caution in treating patients with severe cardiovascular disease, including hypertension.

Use 0.5% apraclonidine with caution in patients with coronary insufficiency, recent MI, cerebrovascular disease, chronic renal failure, Raynaud disease, or thromboangiitis obliterans.

Depression: Use caution and monitor depressed patients because apraclonidine has been infrequently associated with depression.

Hypersensitivity reactions: Apraclonidine can lead to an allergic-like reaction characterized wholly or in part by the symptoms of hyperemia, pruritus, discomfort, tearing, foreign body sensation, and edema of the lids and conjunctiva. If ocular allergic-like symptoms occur, discontinue therapy.

Renal/Hepatic function impairment: Although the topical use of apraclonidine has not been studied in renal failure patients, structurally related clonidine undergoes a significant increase in half-life in patients with severe renal impairment. Close monitoring of cardiovascular parameters in patients with impaired renal function is advised if they are candidates for topical apraclonidine therapy. Close monitoring of cardiovascular parameters in patients with impaired liver function is also advised as the systemic dosage form of clonidine is partly metabolized in the liver.

Pregnancy: Category C.

Lactation: Consider discontinuing nursing for the day on which apraclonidine is used.

Children: Safety and efficacy for use in children have not been established.

Monitoring: Glaucoma patients on maximally tolerated medical therapy who are treated with 0.5% apraclonidine to delay surgery should have their visual fields monitored periodically. Discontinue treatment if IOP rises significantly.

Drug Interactions

Drugs that may interact include cardiovascular agents and MAOIs.

Adverse Reactions

Adverse reactions from 1% solution may include upper lid elevation; conjunctival blanching; mydriasis; burning; discomfort; foreign body sensation; dryness; itching; hypotony; blurred or dimmed vision; allergic response; conjunctival microhemorrhage; dry mouth; bradycardia; vasovagal attack; palpitations; orthostatic episode; headache; taste abnormalities; nasal burning or head-cold sensation; shortness of breath.

Adverse reactions from 0.5% solution may include hyperemia; pruritus; discomfort; tearing; taste perversion; use can lead to an allergic-type reaction.

BETA-ADRENERGIC BLOCKING AGENTS

BETAXOLOL HYDROCHLORIDE	
Solution: 5.6 mg (equiv. to 5 mg base) per mL (0.5%) (*Rx*)	Various
Suspension: 2.8 mg (equiv. to 2.5 mg base) per mL (0.25%) (*Rx*)	*Betoptic* S (Alcon)
CARTEOLOL HYDROCHLORIDE	
Solution: 1% (*Rx*)	Various
LEVOBUNOLOL HYDROCHLORIDE	
Solution: 0.25% and 0.5% (*Rx*)	Various, *AKBeta* (Akorn), *Betagan Liquifilm* (Allergan)
METIPRANOLOL HYDROCHLORIDE	
Solution: 0.3% (*Rx*)	*OptiPranolol* (Bausch & Lomb)

TIMOLOL MALEATE	
Solution: 0.25% and 0.5% (*Rx*)	Various, *Timoptic* (Merck) *Istalol* (Bausch & Lomb)
Solution, gel-forming: 0.25% and 0.5% (*Rx*)	Various, *Timoptic-XE* (Merck)

Indications

Glaucoma: Lowering intraocular pressure (IOP) in patients with chronic open-angle glaucoma and intraocular hypertension.

Administration and Dosage

BETAXOLOL HYDROCHLORIDE: Instill 1 to 2 drops twice daily.

CARTEOLOL HYDROCHLORIDE: One drop in the affected eye(s) twice daily.

LEVOBUNOLOL HYDROCHLORIDE:

0.5% – 1 to 2 drops in the affected eye(s) once daily.

0.25% – 1 to 2 drops in the affected eye(s) twice daily.

In patients with more severe or uncontrolled glaucoma, the 0.5% solution can be administered twice daily.

METIPRANOLOL HYDROCHLORIDE: One drop in the affected eye(s) twice a day. If the patient's IOP is not at a satisfactory level on this regimen, more frequent administration or a larger dose is not known to be of benefit.

TIMOLOL MALEATE:

Solution –

Initial therapy: 1 drop of 0.25% or 0.5% twice daily. If clinical response is not adequate, change the dosage to 1 drop of 0.5% solution twice a day. If the IOP is maintained at satisfactory levels, change the dosage to 1 drop once a day.

Gel – Administer other ophthalmics at least 10 minutes before the gel. Dose is 1 drop (0.25% or 0.5%) once daily. Dosages more than 1 drop of 0.5% have not been studied. Consider concomitant therapy if IOP is not at a satisfactory level.

Actions

Pharmacology: The exact mechanism of ocular antihypertensive action is not established, but it appears to be a reduction of aqueous production. However, some studies show a slight increase in outflow facility with **timolol** and **metipranolol**.

Pharmacokinetics:

Pharmacokinetics of Ophthalmic β-Adrenergic Blocking Agents

Drug	β-receptor selectivity	Onset (min)	Maximum effect (h)	Duration (h)
Carteolol	β_1 and β_2	nd[a]	2	12
Betaxolol	β_1	≤ 30	2	12
Levobunolol	β_1 and β_2	< 60	2 to 6	≤ 24
Metipranolol	β_1 and β_2	≤ 30	≈ 2	24
Timolol	β_1 and β_2	≤ 30	1 to 2	≤ 24

[a] nd = No data

Contraindications

Bronchial asthma, a history of bronchial asthma, or severe chronic obstructive pulmonary disease; sinus bradycardia; second- and third-degree AV block; overt cardiac failure; cardiogenic shock; hypersensitivity to any component of the products.

Warnings/Precautions

Systemic absorption: These agents may be absorbed systemically. The same adverse reactions found with systemic β-blockers may occur with topical use.

Cardiovascular: These agents can decrease resting and maximal exercise heart rate, even in healthy subjects.

Cardiac failure: Sympathetic stimulation may be essential for circulation support in diminished myocardial contractility; its inhibition by β-receptor blockade may precipitate more severe failure.

Bronchospasm: Nonallergic bronchospasm patients or patients with a history of chronic bronchitis, emphysema, etc., should receive β-blockers with caution; they may block bronchodilation produced by catecholamine stimulation of β_2-receptors.

Diabetes mellitus: Administer with caution to patients subject to spontaneous hypoglycemia or to diabetic patients (especially labile diabetics). Beta-blocking agents may mask signs and symptoms of acute hypoglycemia.

Thyroid: Beta-adrenergic blocking agents may mask clinical signs of hyperthyroidism (eg, tachycardia).

Cerebrovascular insufficiency: Because of potential effects of β-blockers on blood pressure and pulse, use with caution in patients with cerebrovascular insufficiency.

Angle-closure glaucoma: The immediate objective is to reopen the angle, requiring constriction of the pupil with a miotic. These agents have little or no effect on the pupil.

Muscle weakness: Beta-blockade may potentiate muscle weakness consistent with certain myasthenic symptoms (eg, diplopia, ptosis, generalized weakness).

Long-term therapy: In long-term studies (2 and 3 years), no significant differences in mean IOP were observed after initial stabilization.

Pregnancy: Category C.

Lactation: It is not known whether these agents are excreted in human breast milk.

Children: Safety and efficacy for use in children have not been established.

Drug Interactions

Ophthalmic beta blockers may affect oral beta blockers, catecholamine-depleting drugs, calcium antagonists, digitalis, and phenothiazines.

Drugs that may affect ophthalmic beta blockers include catecholamine-depleting drugs, digitalis, and quinidine.

Other drugs that may interact with systemic β-adrenergic blocking agents also may interact with ophthalmic agents.

Adverse Reactions

Adverse reactions may include headache; depression; arrhythmia; syncope; heart block; cerebral vascular accident; cerebral ischemia; CHF; palpitation; nausea; hypersensitivity, including localized and generalized rash; bronchospasm; respiratory failure; eratitis; blepharoptosis; visual disturbances including refractive changes; diplopia; ptosis.

Systemic β-adrenergic blocker-associated reactions – Consider potential effects with ophthalmic use.

The following adverse reactions have occurred with each individual agent::

Carteolol:

Ophthalmic – Transient irritation, burning, tearing, conjunctival hyperemia, edema (approximately 25%).

Betaxolol:

Ophthalmic – Brief discomfort (more than 25%); occasional tearing (5%).

Metipranolol:

Ophthalmic – Transient local discomfort; conjunctivitis; eyelid dermatitis; blepharitis; blurred vision; tearing; browache; abnormal vision; photophobia; edema; uveitis.

Levobunolol:

Ophthalmic – Transient burning/stinging (up to 33%); blepharoconjunctivitis (up to 5%).

Timolol:

Ophthalmic – Ocular irritation including conjunctivitis; blepharitis; keratitis; blepharoptosis; decreased corneal sensitivity; visual disturbances including refractive changes; diplopia; ptosis.

MIOTICS, DIRECT-ACTING

ACETYLCHOLINE CHLORIDE, INTRAOCULAR	
Solution: 1:100 acetylcholine chloride when reconstituted (*Rx*)	*Miochol-E* (Novartis Ophthalmic)
CARBACHOL, INTRAOCULAR	
Solution: 0.01% (*Rx*)	*Miostat* (Alcon)
CARBACHOL, TOPICAL	
Solution: 1.5% and 3% (*Rx*)	*Isopto Carbachol* (Alcon)
PILOCARPINE HYDROCHLORIDE	
Solution: 0.5%, 1%, 2%, 4%, and 6% (*Rx*)	Various, *Isopto Carpine* (Alcon)
Gel: 4% (*Rx*)	*Pilopine HS* (Alcon)
PILOCARPINE NITRATE	
Solution: 1%, 2%, and 4% (*Rx*)	*Pilagan* (Allergan)

Indications

Carbachol, topical; pilocarpine:

Glaucoma – To decrease elevated intraocular pressure (IOP) in glaucoma.

Acetylcholine; carbachol, intraocular:

Miosis – To induce miosis during surgery.

Administration and Dosage

ACETYLCHOLINE CHLORIDE, INTRAOCULAR:

Solution – 0.5 to 2 mL produces satisfactory miosis. Solution need not be flushed from the chamber after miosis occurs.

CARBACHOL, INTRAOCULAR: Gently instill no more than 0.5 mL into the anterior chamber before or after securing sutures. Miosis is usually maximal 2 to 5 minutes after application.

CARBACHOL, TOPICAL: Instill 2 drops into eye(s) up to 3 times daily.

PILOCARPINE:

Solution –

Initial: 1 or 2 drops 3 to 4 times daily. Individuals with heavily pigmented irides may require higher strengths.

Gel – Apply a 0.5 inch ribbon in the lower conjunctival sac of affected eye(s) once daily at bedtime.

PILOCARPINE NITRATE:

Glaucoma – 1 to 2 drops 2 to 4 times daily.

Emergency miosis – 1 to 2 drops of higher concentrations.

Reversal of mydriasis – Dosage and strength required are dependent on the cycloplegic used.

Actions

Pharmacology: Direct-acting miotics are parasympathomimetic (cholinergic) drugs which duplicate the muscarinic effects of **acetylcholine**. When applied topically, these drugs produce pupillary constriction, stimulate ciliary muscles, and increase aqueous humor outflow facility. With the increase in outflow facility, there is a decrease in IOP. Topical ophthalmic instillation of acetylcholine causes no discernible response, as cholinesterase destroys the molecule more rapidly than it can penetrate the cornea; therefore, acetylcholine only is used intraocularly.

Pharmacokinetics:

Miosis Induction of Direct-Acting Miotics

Miotic	Onset	Peak	Duration
Acetylcholine, intraocular	seconds	—	10 min
Carbachol			
Intraocular	seconds	2 to 5 min	1 to 2 days
Topical	10 to 20 min	—	4 to 8 hours
Pilocarpine, topical	10 to 30 min	—	4 to 8 hours

Contraindications

Hypersensitivity to any component of the formulation; where constriction is undesirable (eg, acute iritis, acute or anterior uveitis, some forms of secondary glaucoma, pupillary block glaucoma, acute inflammatory disease of the anterior chamber).

Warnings/Precautions

Corneal abrasion: Use carbachol with caution in the presence of corneal abrasion to avoid excessive penetration.

Systemic reactions: Caution is advised in patients with acute cardiac failure, bronchial asthma, peptic ulcer, hyperthyroidism, GI spasm, urinary tract obstruction, Parkinson's disease, recent MI, hypertension, or hypotension.

Retinal detachment: Retinal detachment has been caused by miotics in susceptible individuals, in individuals with pre-existing retinal disease, or in those who are predisposed to retinal tears.

Miosis: Miosis usually causes difficulty in dark adaptation. Advise patients to use caution while night driving or performing hazardous tasks in poor light.

Angle-closure: Although withdrawal of the peripheral iris from the anterior chamber angle by miosis may reduce the tendency for narrow-angle closure, miotics occasionally can precipitate angle closure by increasing resistance to aqueous flow from posterior to anterior chamber.

Pregnancy: Category C (carbachol, pilocarpine).

Lactation: It is not known whether these drugs are excreted in breast milk.

Children: Safety and efficacy for use in children have not been established.

Adverse Reactions

Acetylcholine:

Ophthalmic – Corneal edema; corneal clouding; corneal decompensation.

Systemic – Bradycardia; hypotension; flushing; breathing difficulties; sweating.

Carbachol:

Ophthalmic – Transient stinging and burning; corneal clouding; persistent bullous keratopathy; retinal detachment; transient ciliary and conjunctival injection; ciliary spasm with resultant temporary decrease of visual acuity.

Systemic – Headache; salivation; GI cramps; vomiting; diarrhea; asthma; syncope; cardiac arrhythmia; flushing; sweating; epigastric distress; tightness in bladder; hypotension; frequent urge to urinate.

Pilocarpine:

Ophthalmic – Transient stinging and burning; tearing; ciliary spasm; conjunctival vascular congestion; temporal, peri-, or supra-orbital headache; superficial keratitis-induced myopia; blurred vision; poor dark adaptation; reduced visual acuity in poor illumination in older individuals and in individuals with lens opacity.

MIOTICS, CHOLINESTERASE INHIBITORS

PHYSOSTIGMINE (Eserine)

Ointment: 0.25% (as sulfate) (*Rx*)	*Eserine Sulfate* (Novartis Ophthalmic)

Indications

Glaucoma: Therapy of open-angle glaucoma.

Administration and Dosage

PHYSOSTIGMINE (ESERINE):

Ointment – Apply small quantity to lower fornix, up to 3 times daily.

Actions

Pharmacology: Topical application to the eye produces intense miosis and muscle contraction. IOP is reduced by a decreased resistance to aqueous outflow.

Cholinesterase-Inhibiting Miotics					
	Miosis		IOP reduction		
Miotics	Onset (minutes)	Duration	Onset (h)	Peak (h)	Duration
Reversible					
Physostigmine	20 to 30	12 to 36 h	—	2 to 6	12 to 36 h

Contraindications

Hypersensitivity to cholinesterase inhibitors or any component of the formulation; active uveal inflammation or any inflammatory disease of the iris or ciliary body; glaucoma associated with iridocyclitis.

Warnings/Precautions

Surgery: In patients receiving cholinesterase inhibitors, administer succinylcholine with extreme caution before and during general anesthesia. Use prior to ophthalmic surgery only as a considered risk because of the possible occurrence of hyphema.

Concomitant therapy: Cholinesterase inhibitors may be used in combination with adrenergic agents, β-blockers, carbonic anhydrase inhibitors, or hyperosmotic agents.

Narrow-angle glaucoma: Use with caution in patients with chronic angle-closure (narrow-angle) glaucoma or in patients with narrow angles, because of the possibility of producing pupillary block and increasing angle blockage. Temporarily discontinue if cardiac irregularities occur.

Ophthalmic ointments: Ophthalmic ointments may retard corneal healing.

Miosis: Miosis usually causes difficulty in dark adaptation. Use caution while driving at night or performing hazardous tasks in poor light.

Gonioscopy: Use only when shorter-acting miotics have proven inadequate. Gonioscopy is recommended prior to use of medication.

Concomitant ocular conditions: When an intraocular inflammatory process is present, breakdown of the blood-aqueous barrier from anticholinesterase therapy requires abstention from, or cautious use of, these drugs. Use with great caution where there is a history of quiescent uveitis.

Systemic effects: Repeated administration may cause depression of the concentration of cholinesterase in the serum and erythrocytes, with resultant systemic effects.

Iris cysts: Iris cysts may form, enlarge, and obscure vision (more frequent in children).

Special risk: Use caution in patients with marked vagotonia, bronchial asthma, spastic GI disturbances, peptic ulcer, pronounced bradycardia/hypotension, recent MI, epilepsy, parkinsonism, and other disorders that may respond adversely to vagotonic effects.

Pregnancy: *Category C.*

Lactation: It is not known whether these drugs are excreted in breast milk.

Children: The occurrence of iris cysts is more frequent in children. Safety and efficacy for use of **physostigmine** have not been established.

Drug Interactions

Drugs that may interact with cholinesterase inhibitors include carbamate/organophosphate insecticides and pesticides, succinylcholine, and systemic anticholinesterases.

Adverse Reactions

Ophthalmic: Iris cysts; burning; lacrimation; lid muscle twitching; conjunctival and ciliary redness; browache; headache; activation of latent iritis or uveitis; induced myopia with visual blurring.

Systemic: Nausea; vomiting; abdominal cramps; diarrhea; urinary incontinence; fainting; sweating; salivation; difficulty in breathing; cardiac irregularities.

CARBONIC ANHYDRASE INHIBITORS

BRINZOLAMIDE	
Suspension: 1% (*Rx*)	*Azopt* (Alcon)
DORZOLAMIDE	
Solution: 2% (*Rx*)	Various, *Trusopt* (Merck)

Indications

Elevated intraocular pressure (IOP): Treatment of elevated IOP in patients with ocular hypertension or open-angle glaucoma.

Administration and Dosage

Dosage: One drop in the affected eye(s) 3 times daily.

Concomitant therapy: If more than one ophthalmic drug is being used, administer the drugs at least 10 minutes apart.

Actions

Pharmacology: **Brinzolamide** and **dorzolamide** are carbonic anhydrase inhibitors formulated for topical ophthalmic use.

Pharmacokinetics: Topical **brinzolamide** and **dorzolamide** reach the systemic circulation and accumulate in RBCs. Extensive distribution into RBCs yields a long half-life (3.5 to 4 months). The drugs primarily are excreted unchanged in the urine and the metabolite also is excreted in urine.

Contraindications

Hypersensitivity to any component of this product.

Warnings/Precautions

Systemic effects: These agents are sulfonamides and, although administered topically, are absorbed systemically. Therefore, the same types of adverse reactions attributable to sulfonamides may occur with topical administration of **brinzolamide** and **dorzolamide**.

Corneal endothelium effects: The effect of continued administration of **brinzolamide** and **dorzolamide** on the corneal endothelium has not been fully evaluated.

Acute angle-closure glaucoma: The management of patients with acute angle-closure glaucoma requires therapeutic interventions in addition to ocular hypotensive agents. These agents have not been studied in patients with acute angle-closure glaucoma.

Ocular effects: Local ocular adverse effects, primarily conjunctivitis and lid reactions, were reported with chronic administration.

Concomitant oral carbonic anhydrase inhibitors: There is a potential for an additive effect of the known systemic effects of carbonic anhydrase (CA) inhibition in patients receiving an oral and ophthalmic CA inhibitor. The concomitant administration of ocular and oral CA inhibitors is not recommended.

Contact lenses: The preservative in these products, benzalkonium chloride, may be absorbed by soft contact lenses. Do not administer these agents while wearing soft contact lenses; reinsert lenses 15 minutes or more after drug administration.

Renal function impairment: These agents have not been studied in patients with severe renal impairment (CrCl less than 30 mL/min). However, because the drugs and their metabolites are excreted predominantly by the kidney, these agents are not recommended in such patients.

Pregnancy: Category C.

Lactation: It is not known whether these drugs are excreted in breast milk.

Children: Safety and efficacy in children have not been established.

Drug Interactions

Although acid-base and electrolyte disturbances were not reported in the clinical trials, these disturbances have been reported with oral CA inhibitors and have, in some instances, resulted in drug interactions (eg, toxicity associated with high-dose salicylate therapy).

Adverse Reactions

Adverse reactions occurring in at least 3% of patients include ocular burning, stinging, or discomfort immediately following administration; bitter taste following administration; superficial punctate keratitis; signs and symptoms of ocular allergic reaction; blurred vision; tearing; dryness; photophobia; blepharitis; dermatitis, foreign body sensation, hyperemia, ocular discharge/keratitis/pain/pruritus; rhinitis.

PROSTAGLANDIN AGONISTS

BIMATOPROST	
Solution: 0.03% (*Rx*)	*Lumigan, Latisse* (Allergan)
LATANOPROST	
Solution: 0.005% (50 mcg/mL) (*Rx*)	*Xalatan* (Pfizer)
TRAVOPROST	
Solution: 0.004% (*Rx*)	*Travatanz* (Alcon)

Indications

Elevated intraocular pressure (IOP) (Lumigan): For reduction of elevated IOP in patients with open-angle glaucoma and ocular hypertension who are intolerant of other IOP-lowering medications or insufficiently responsive to another IOP-lowering medication.

Hypotrichosis of the eyelashes (Latisse): For the treatment of hypotrichosis of the eyelashes by increasing their growth, including length, thickness, and darkness.

Administration and Dosage

Intraocular pressure:

BIMATOPROST, LATANOPROST, TRAVOPROST – The recommended dosage is 1 drop in the affected eye(s) once daily in the evening. Do not exceed once-daily dosage because it has been shown that more frequent administration may decrease the IOP-lowering effect.

Bimatoprost, **latanoprost**, and **travoprost** may be used concomitantly with other topical ophthalmic drug products to lower IOP. If more than 1 topical ophthalmic drug is being used, administer the drugs at least 5 minutes apart.

Hypotrichosis: Advise patients to ensure their face is clean and that makeup and contact lenses are removed. Once nightly, patients should place 1 drop of bimatoprost 0.03% ophthalmic solution on the disposable sterile applicator supplied with the package and apply evenly along the skin of the upper eyelid margin at the base of the eyelashes. Bimatoprost should not be applied to the lower eyelash line. The upper lid margin in the area of lash growth should feel lightly moist without run-off. Any excess solution runoff outside the upper eyelid margin should be blotted with a tissue or other absorbent cloth. The applicator should be disposed of after one use. This procedure should be repeated for the opposite eyelid margin using a new sterile applicator.

Actions

Pharmacology: Prostanoid selective receptor agonists are believed to reduce IOP by increasing the outflow of aqueous humor.

Contraindications

Hypersensitivity to any component of these products, including benzalkonium chloride. **Travoprost** may interfere with the maintenance of pregnancy and should not be used by women during pregnancy or by women attempting to become pregnant.

Warnings/Precautions

Eye pigment changes: Prostaglandin agonists may gradually change eye color, increasing the amount of brown pigment in the iris by increasing the number of melanosomas (pigment granules) in melanocytes.

Eyelid skin darkening: Eyelid skin darkening, which may be reversible upon discontinuation of treatment, has been reported in association with the use of bimatoprost.

Hair growth: There is a potential for hair growth to occur in areas where bimatoprost solution comes in repeated contact with the skin surface.

Other forms of glaucoma: There is limited experience with latanoprost in the treatment of angle closure, inflammatory or neovascular glaucoma.

Bacterial keratitis: There have been reports of bacterial keratitis associated with the use of multiple-dose containers of topical ophthalmic products. These containers had been inadvertently contaminated by patients who, in most cases, had a concurrent corneal disease or a disruption of the ocular epithelial surface.

Contact lenses: Remove contact lenses prior to the administration of latanoprost, and reinsert 15 minutes after administration.

Macular edema: Macular edema, including cystoid edema, has been reported during treatment with prostaglandin agonists.

Active intraocular inflammation: Use **bimatoprost** and **latanoprost** with caution in patients with active intraocular inflammation (eg, uveitis).

Pregnancy: Category C.

Lactation: It is not known whether these drugs or their metabolites are excreted in breast milk.

Children: Safety and efficacy in children have not been established.

Monitoring: Prostaglandin agonists may gradually increase the pigmentation of the iris. These patients should be regularly examined and, depending on the clinical situation, treatment may be stopped if increased pigmentation ensues.

Drug Interactions

In vitro studies have shown that precipitation occurs when eye drops containing thimerosal are mixed with **latanoprost**. If such drugs are used, administer with an interval of at least 5 minutes between applications.

Adverse Reactions

Prostaglandin agonists:

Systemic – The most common systemic adverse events seen with prostaglandin agonists were upper respiratory tract infection/cold/flu (4% to 10%).

Bimatoprost:

Ophthalmic – Bimatoprost-associated ocular adverse events that occurred in 3% to 10% of patients, in descending order of incidence, included the following: Ocular dryness, visual disturbances, ocular burning, foreign body sensation, eye pain, pigmentation of the periocular skin, blepharitis, cataract, superficial punctate keratitis, eyelid erythema, ocular irritation, eyelash darkening.

Latanoprost:

Ophthalmic – Latanoprost-associated ocular adverse events reported at an incidence of 5% to 15% included the following: Blurred vision, burning and stinging, conjunctival hyperemia, foreign body sensation, itching, increased pigmentation of the iris, punctate epithelial keratopathy.

Travoprost:

Ophthalmic – Travoprost-associated ocular adverse events reported at an incidence of 5% to 15% included the following: Decreased visual acuity, eye discomfort, foreign body sensation, pain, pruritus.

CORTICOSTEROIDS

DEXAMETHASONE	
Solution; ophthalmic: 0.1% dexamethasone phosphate (*Rx*)	Various
Suspension; ophthalmic: 0.1% (*Rx*)	*Maxidex* (Alcon)
DIFLUPREDNATE	
Emulsion; ophthalmic: 0.05%	*Durezol* (Sirion)
FLUOCINOLONE ACETONIDE	
Implant, ophthalmic: 0.59 mg (*Rx*)	*Retisert* (Bausch & Lomb)
FLUOROMETHOLONE	
Suspension; ophthalmic: 0.1% and 0.25% (*Rx*)	Various, *FML* (Allergan), *FML Forte* (Allergan)
0.1% fluorometholone acetate (*Rx*)	*Flarex* (Alcon)
Ointment; ophthalmic: 0.1% (*Rx*)	*FML S.O.P.* (Allergan)
LOTEPREDNOL ETABONATE	
Suspension; ophthalmic: 0.5% (*Rx*)	*Lotemax* (Bausch & Lomb)
0.2% (*Rx*)	*Alrex* (Bausch & Lomb)
PREDNISOLONE	
Suspension; ophthalmic: 0.12%, 1% prednisolone acetate (*Rx*)	Various, *Pred Mild* (Allergan), *Pred Forte* (Allergan)
Solution; ophthalmic: 1% prednisolone sodium phosphate (*Rx*)	Various
RIMEXOLONE	
Suspension; ophthalmic: 1% (*Rx*)	*Vexol* (Alcon)

Indications

Inflammatory conditions: Treatment of steroid-responsive inflammatory conditions of the palpebral and bulbar conjunctiva, lid, sclera, cornea, and anterior segment of the globe, such as: allergic conjunctivitis; acne rosacea; superficial punctate keratitis; herpes zoster keratitis; iritis; cyclitis; and selected infective conjunctivitis (when the inherent hazard of steroid use is accepted to obtain an advisable diminution in edema and inflammation [prednisolone]); vernal conjunctivitis; episcleritis; epinephrine sensitivity; anterior uveitis; and chronic, noninfectious uveitis affecting the posterior segment of the eye.

Mild to moderate – For the treatment of mild to moderate noninfectious allergic and inflammatory disorders of the lid, conjunctiva, cornea, and sclera (including chemical and thermal burns) (**prednisolone**).

Moderate to severe – Use higher strengths for moderate to severe inflammations. In difficult cases of anterior segment eye disease, systemic therapy may be required. When deeper ocular structures are involved, use systemic therapy (**prednisolone**).

Ocular surgery: For treatment of postoperative inflammation and pain following ocular surgery.

Corneal injury: For corneal injury from chemical, radiation, or thermal burns, or from penetration of foreign bodies.

Administration and Dosage

Treatment duration varies with type of lesion and may extend from a few days to several weeks, depending on therapeutic response. If signs and symptoms fail to improve after 2 days, reevaluate the patient. Relapse may occur if therapy is reduced too rapidly; taper over several days. Relapses, more common in chronic active lesions than in self-limited conditions, usually respond to retreatment.

DEXAMETHASONE:

Solutions – Instill 1 to 2 drops into the conjunctival sac every hour during the day and every 2 hours during the night as initial therapy. When a favorable response is observed, reduce dosage to 1 drop every 4 hours. Further reduction in dosage to 1 drop 3 or 4 times daily may suffice to control symptoms.

Suspension – Shake well before using. Instill 1 or 2 drops in the conjunctival sac(s). In severe disease, drops may be used hourly, tapering to discontinuation as inflammation subsides. In mild disease, drops may be used up to 4 to 6 times daily.

DIFLUPREDNATE: Instill 1 drop into the conjunctival sac of the affected eye(s) 4 times daily beginning 24 hours after surgery and continuing throughout the first 2 weeks of the postoperative period, followed by 2 times daily for 1 week, and then a taper based on the response.

FLUOCINOLONE ACETONIDE: Fluocinolone is implanted surgically into the posterior segment of the affected eye through a pars plana incision. The implant contains 1 tablet of fluocinolone 0.59 mg. The implant is designed to release fluocinolone at a nominal initial rate of 0.6 mcg/day, decreasing over the first month to a steady state between 0.3 to 0.4 mcg/day within approximately 30 months. Following depletion of fluocinolone from the implant as evidenced by recurrence of uveitis, the fluocinolone implant may be replaced.

FLUOROMETHALONE: Consult a health care provider if there is no improvement after 2 days. Do not discontinue therapy prematurely. In chronic conditions, withdraw treatment by gradually decreasing the frequency of applications.

Suspension – Instill 1 drop into the conjunctival sac 2 to 4 times daily. During the initial 24 to 48 hours, the dosage may be increased to 1 drop every 4 hours.

Suspension (acetate form) – Shake well before using. Instill 1 to 2 drops into the conjunctival sac(s) 2 to 4 times daily. During the initial 24 to 48 hours, the dosage may be increased to 2 drops every 2 hours. If there is no improvement after 2 weeks, advise patients to consult their health care provider.

Ointment – Apply a small amount (about a ½ inch ribbon) of ointment to the conjunctival sac 1 to 3 times daily. During the first 24 to 48 hours, the dosing frequency may be increased to 1 application every 4 hours.

LOTEPREDNOL ETABONATE: Shake well before using.

Seasonal allergic conjunctivitis – Instill 1 drop into the affected eye(s) 4 times daily.

Steroid responsive disease – Instill 1 to 2 drops into the conjunctival sac of the affected eye(s) 4 times daily. During the initial treatment within the first week, the dosing may be increased up to 1 drop every hour. Advise patients not to discontinue therapy prematurely. If signs and symptoms fail to improve after 2 days, reevaluate the patient.

Postoperative inflammation – Instill 1 to 2 drops into the conjunctival sac of the operated eye(s) 4 times daily beginning 24 hours after surgery and continuing throughout the first 2 weeks of the postoperative period.

PREDNISOLONE:

Solutions – Depending on the severity of inflammation, instill 1 or 2 drops of solution into the conjunctival sac up to every hour during the day and every 2 hours during the night as necessary as initial therapy.

When a favorable response is observed, reduce dosage to 1 drop every 4 hours. Further reduction in dosage to 1 drop 3 to 4 times daily may suffice to control symptoms.

Suspensions – Shake well before using. Instill 2 drops in the eye(s) 4 times daily. For *Pred Mild* or *Pred Forte*, instill 1 to 2 drops in the conjunctival sac 2 to 4 times daily; during the initial 24 to 48 hours, the dosing frequency may be increased, if necessary.

In cases of bacterial infections, concomitant use of anti-infective agents is mandatory.

If signs and symptoms do not improve after 2 days, reevaluate the patient.

Dosing may be reduced, but advise patients not to discontinue therapy prematurely. In chronic conditions, withdraw treatment by gradually decreasing the frequency of applications.

RIMEXOLONE: Shake well before using.

Postoperative inflammation – Instill 1 to 2 drops into the conjunctival sac of the affected eye(s) 4 times daily beginning 24 hours after surgery and continuing throughout the first 2 weeks of the postoperative period.

Anterior uveitis – Apply 1 to 2 drops into the conjunctival sac of the affected eye every hour during waking hours for the first week, 1 drop every 2 hours during waking hours of the second week, and then taper until uveitis is resolved.

Actions

Pharmacology: Ocular corticosteroids are thought to act by the induction of phospholipase A_2 inhibitory proteins, collectively called lipocortins. It is postulated that these proteins control the biosynthesis of potent mediators of inflammation such as prostaglandins and leukotrienes by inhibiting the release of their common precursor arachidonic acid. Arachidonic acid is released from membrane phospholipids by phospholipase A_2. Ocular corticosteroids are capable of producing a rise in intraocular pressure.

Contraindications

Most viral diseases of the cornea and conjuctiva, including acute epithelial herpes simplex keratitis (dendritic keratitis), vaccinia, and varicella; mycobacterial infections of the eye and fungal disease of ocular structures; tuberculosis of the eye; acute, purulent untreated eye infections; known or suspected hypersensitivity to any of the ingredients in these preparations or to other corticosteroids.

Warnings/Precautions

Moderate to severe inflammation: Use higher strengths for moderate to severe inflammations. In difficult cases of anterior segment eye disease, systemic therapy may be required. When deeper ocular structures are involved, use systemic therapy.

Prolonged use: Prolonged use may result in glaucoma with damage to the optic nerve, defects in visual acuity and fields of vision, corneal and scleral thinning, and posterior subcapsular cataract formation. Prolonged use may suppress the host response and thus increase the hazard of secondary ocular infections.

Glaucoma: Use with caution in the presence of glaucoma.

Visual acuity: Following the implantation of fluocinolone, nearly all patients will experience an immediate and temporary decrease in visual acuity in the implanted eye, which lasts for approximately 1 to 4 weeks postoperatively.

Perforation: In diseases causing thinning of the cornea or sclera, perforations have been known to occur with the use of topical steroids.

Cataract surgery: The use of steroids after cataract surgery may delay healing and increase the incidence of bleb formation.

Infections: Prolonged use may result in secondary ocular infections caused by suppression of host response. Acute, purulent, untreated eye infections may be masked or activity enhanced by steroids. Fungal infections of the cornea have been reported with long-term local steroid applications.

Fungal infection: Fungal infections of the cornea are particularly prone to develop coincidentally with long-term local steroid application. Consider fungal invasion in any persistent corneal ulceration where a steroid has been or is currently used. Take fungal cultures when appropriate.

Corneal healing: Ophthalmic ointments may retard corneal healing.

Bilateral implantation: In order to limit the potential for bilateral postoperative infection, do not carry out simultaneous bilateral implantation.

Benzalkonium chloride: Benzalkonium chloride is a preservative used in some of these products that may be absorbed by soft contact lenses. Instruct patients wearing soft contact lenses to wait at least 15 minutes after instilling products containing this preservative before inserting their lenses.

Sulfite sensitivity: Dexamethasone sodium phosphate and prednisolone acetate contain sodium bisulfate, which may cause allergic type reactions in susceptible people.

Pregnancy: Category C.

Lactation: It is not known whether topical steroids are excreted in breast milk.

Children: Safety and efficacy have not been established in children. Safety and efficacy of fluocinolone in children younger than 12 years of age have not been established. Safety and efficacy of fluorometholone in infants younger than 2 years of age have not been established.

Monitoring: Monitor patients for increased intraocular pressure. If signs and symptoms fail to improve after 2 days, reevaluate the patient.

Adverse Reactions

Glaucoma (elevated IOP) with optic nerve damage, loss of visual acuity, and field defects; posterior subcapsular cataract formation; delayed wound healing; secondary ocular infection from pathogens, including herpes simplex and fungi liberated from ocular tissues; acute uveitis; perforation of globe where there is corneal or scleral thinning; exacerbation of viral, bacterial, and fungal corneal infections; transient stinging or burning; chemosis; dry eyes; epiphora; photophobia; keratitis; conjunctivitis; corneal ulcers; mydriasis; ptosis; blurred vision, discharge, discomfort, ocular pain, foreign body sensation, hyperemia, and pruritus (**rimexolone**).

Systemic: Systemic adverse reactions may occur with extensive use.

LODOXAMIDE

Solution: 0.1% (*Rx*)	*Alomide* (Alcon)

Indications

Treatment of the ocular disorders referred to by the terms vernal keratoconjunctivitis, vernal conjunctivitis, and vernal keratitis.

Administration and Dosage

Adults and children older than 2 years of age: 1 to 2 drops in each affected eye 4 times daily for up to 3 months.

Actions

Pharmacology: Lodoxamide is a mast cell stabilizer that inhibits the in vivo Type I immediate hypersensitivity reaction. Although lodoxamide's precise mechanism of action is unknown, the drug may prevent calcium influx into mast cells upon antigen stimulation.

Pharmacokinetics: The disposition of lodoxamide was studied in 6 healthy adult volunteers receiving a 3 mg oral dose. Urinary excretion was the major route of elimination. The elimination half-life was 8.5 hours in urine. In a study in 12 healthy adult volunteers, topical administration of 1 drop in each eye 4 times/day for 10 days did not result in any measurable lodoxamide plasma levels at a detection limit of 2.5 ng/mL.

Contraindications

Hypersensitivity to any component of this product.

Warnings/Precautions

For ophthalmic use only. Not for injection.

Contact lenses: As with all ophthalmic preparations containing benzalkonium chloride, instruct patients not to wear soft contact lenses during treatment with lodoxamide.

Burning/Stinging: Patients may experience a transient burning or stinging upon instillation of lodoxamide. Should these symptoms persist, advise patients to contact their physicians.

Pregnancy: Category B.

Lactation: It is not known whether lodoxamide is excreted in breast milk.

Children: Safety and efficacy in children younger than 2 years of age have not been established.

Adverse Reactions

Adverse reactions occurring in at least 3% of patients include transient burning, stinging or discomfort upon instillation; ocular itching/pruritus; blurred vision; dry eye; tearing/discharge; hyperemia; crystalline deposits; and foreign body sensation.

ANTIBIOTICS

AZITHROMYCIN	
Solution; ophthalmic: 1% (*Rx*)	*AzaSite* (Inspire)
BACITRACIN	
Ointment: 500 units/g (*Rx*)	Various
BESIFLOXACIN	
Suspension, ophthalmic: 0.6% (*Rx*)	*Besivance* (Bausch & Lomb)
CIPROFLOXACIN	
Solution: 3.5 mg/mL (equivalent to 3 mg base) (*Rx*)	Various, *Ciloxan* (Alcon)
Ointment: 3.33 mg/g (equivalent to 3 mg base) (*Rx*)	*Ciloxan* (Alcon)
ERYTHROMYCIN	
Ointment: 0.5% (*Rx*)	Various
GATIFLOXACIN	
Solution: 0.3% (3 mg/mL) (*Rx*)	*Zymar* (Allergan)
GENTAMICIN SULFATE	
Ointment: 3 mg/g (*Rx*)	Various, *Gentak* (Akorn)
Solution: 3 mg/mL (*Rx*)	Various
LEVOFLOXACIN	
Solution: 0.5% (*Rx*)	*Quixin* (Vistakon Pharmaceuticals)
1.5% (*Rx*)	*Iquix* (Vistakon Pharmaceuticals)
MOXIFLOXACIN HYDROCHLORIDE	
Solution: 0.5% (5 mg/mL) (*Rx*)	*Vigamox* (Alcon)
OFLOXACIN	
Solution: 3 mg/mL (*Rx*)	Various, *Ocuflox* (Allergan)
TOBRAMYCIN	
Ointment: 3 mg/g (*Rx*)	*Tobrex* (Alcon)
Solution: 0.3% (*Rx*)	Various, *AKTob* (Akorn), *Tobrex* (Alcon)

Indications

Infections: Treatment of superficial ocular infections involving the conjunctiva or cornea (eg, conjunctivitis, keratitis, keratoconjunctivitis, corneal ulcers, blepharitis, blepharoconjunctivitis, acute meibomianitis, dacryocystitis) caused by strains of microorganisms susceptible to antibiotics.

Azithromycin, besifloxacin:

Bacterial conjunctivitis – For the treatment of bacterial conjunctivitis caused by susceptible isolates of the following microorganisms: Centers for Disease Control and Prevention coryneform group G (efficacy studied in fewer than 10 infections), *Haemophilus influenzae*, *Staphylococcus aureus*, *Streptococcus mitis* group, and *Streptococcus pneumoniae*.

Tetracycline and erythromycin: Tetracycline and erythromycin also are indicated for the prophylaxis of ophthalmia neonatorum caused by *Neisseria gonorrhoeae* or *Chlamydia trachomatis*.

Topical Ophthalmic Antibiotic Preparations

		Miscellaneous					Quinolones						Aminoglycosides			Tetracyclines			Sulfonamides	
	Organism/Infection	Azithromycin	Bacitracin	Erythromycin	Gramicidin	Trimethoprim	Besifloxacin	Ciprofloxacin	Gatifloxacin	Levofloxacin	Moxifloxacin	Ofloxacin	Gentamicin	Neomycin	Tobramycin	Chlortetracycline	Oxytetracycline	Tetracycline	Sodium sulfacetamide	Sulfisoxazole
Gram-Positive	*Staphylococcus* sp.		✓		✓			✓		✓		✓	✓		✓					
	S. aureus	✓	✓	✓	✓	✓	✓	✓	✓	✓	✓	✓	✓	✓	✓	✓		✓	✓	
	S. epidermidis						✓		✓		✓									
	S. hominis						✓				✓									
	S. warneri										✓[a]									
	Streptococcus sp.		✓		✓		✓	✓		✓		✓			✓			✓	✓	
	S. mitis	✓					✓		✓[a]											
	S. pneumoniae	✓	✓	✓	✓	✓	✓	✓	✓	✓	✓	✓	✓[b]		✓			✓		
	α-hemolytic streptococci (viridans group)			✓						✓	✓									
	β-hemolytic streptococci		✓										✓[b]		✓					
	S. pyogenes		✓	✓		✓		✓				✓	✓			✓				
	Corynebacterium sp.		✓	✓	✓		✓		✓		✓[a]		✓	✓	✓					
	Micrococcus luteus										✓[a]									
Gram-Negative	*Escherichia coli*					✓		✓				✓	✓	✓	✓	✓	✓	✓	✓	✓
	Haemophilus aegyptius					✓							✓		✓				✓	✓
	H. ducreyi							✓					✓		✓	✓	✓			
	H. influenzae	✓		✓		✓		✓	✓	✓	✓	✓	✓	✓	✓	✓	✓			
	H. parainfluenzae										✓[a]									
	Klebsiella sp.							✓				✓		✓			✓			
	K. pneumoniae					✓		✓				✓	✓		✓	✓				
	Neisseria sp.		✓					✓					✓	✓	✓			✓		
	N. gonorrhoeae		✓	✓[c]				✓				✓	✓			✓		✓[c]	✓	
	Proteus sp.					✓		✓				✓	✓	✓	✓					
	Acinetobacter calcoaceticus							✓				✓	✓		✓					
	A. lwoffi									✓	✓[a]									
	Enterobacter aerogenes					✓		✓					✓	✓	✓		✓			
	Enterobacter sp.							✓				✓	✓	✓	✓					
	Serratia marcescens							✓		✓		✓	✓		✓					
	Moraxella sp.						✓					✓	✓		✓					
	Chlamydia trachomatis			✓[c]				✓			✓	✓				✓[d]		✓[d]	✓[e]	✓
	Pasteurella tularensis															✓	✓			
	Pseudomonas aeruginosa							✓				✓	✓[e]		✓					
	Bartonella bacilliformis																✓			
	Bacteroides sp.			✓												✓	✓	✓		
	Vibrio sp.							✓					✓		✓		✓			
	Yersinia pestis															✓	✓			

[a] Efficacy for this organism was studied in fewer than 10 infections.
[b] Increasing resistance has been seen.
[c] For prophylaxis.
[d] In conjunction with oral therapy.
[e] Adjunct in systemic sulfonamide therapy.

Administration and Dosage

Administration and dosage varies for the individual products. Refer to individual manufacturer inserts.

Contraindications

Hypersensitivity to any component of these products; epithelial herpes simplex keratitis (dendritic keratitis); vaccinia; varicella; mycobacterial infections of the eye; fungal diseases of the ocular structure; use of steroid combinations after uncomplicated removal of a corneal foreign body.

Warnings/Precautions

Sensitization: Sensitization from the topical use of an antibiotic may contraindicate the drug's later systemic use in serious infections.

Cross-sensitivity: Allergic cross-reactions may occur that could prevent future use of any or all of these antibiotics– kanamycin, neomycin, paromomycin, streptomycin, and possibly, gentamicin.

Superinfection: Do not use topical antibiotics in deep-seated ocular infections or in those that are likely to become systemic.

Systemic antibiotics – In all except very superficial infections, supplement the topical use of antibiotics with appropriate systemic medication.

Crystalline precipitate – A white crystalline precipitate located in the superficial portion of the corneal defect was observed in about 17% of patients on **ciprofloxacin**.

Pregnancy: *Category* B (tobramycin); *Category* C (gentamicin, ciprofloxacin, ofloxacin).

Lactation: It is not known whether **ciprofloxacin** or **ofloxacin** appear in breast milk following ophthalmic use. Exercise caution when administering ciprofloxacin to a breast-feeding mother.

Children: **Tobramycin** is safe and effective in children. Safety and efficacy of **ciprofloxacin** in children younger than 12 years of age and **ofloxacin** in infants younger than 1 year of age have not been established.

Adverse Reactions

Sensitivity reactions such as angioneurotic edema, burning, inflammation, itching, stinging, transient irritation, urticaria, and vesicular and maculopapular dermatitis have occurred in some patients.

Ciprofloxacin: Allergic reactions, bad taste in mouth, conjunctival hyperemia, corneal infiltrates, corneal staining, crystals/scales, decreased vision, foreign body sensation, itching, keratopathy/keratitis, lid edema, lid margin crusting, nausea, photophobia, tearing, white crystalline precipitates.

NATAMYCIN

Suspension: 5% (*Rx*)	*Natacyn* (Alcon)

Indications

Fungal infections: Fungal blepharitis, conjunctivitis, and keratitis caused by susceptible organisms. Natamycin is the initial drug of choice in Fusarium solani keratitis.

Administration and Dosage

Fungal keratitis: Instill 1 drop into the conjunctival sac at 1 or 2 hour intervals. The frequency of application can usually be reduced to 1 drop 6 to 8 times daily after the first 3 to 4 days. Generally, continue therapy for 14 to 21 days, or until there is resolution of active fungal keratitis. In many cases, it may help to reduce the dosage gradually at 4 to 7 day intervals to ensure that the organism has been eliminated.

Fungal blepharitis and conjunctivitis: 4 to 6 daily applications may be sufficient.

Actions

Pharmacology: Natamycin, a tetraene polyene antibiotic, is derived from *Streptomyces natalensis*.

It possesses in vitro activity against a variety of yeast and filamentous fungi, including *Candida, Aspergillus, Cephalosporium, Fusarium,* and *Penicillium*. The mechanism of action appears to be through binding of the molecule to the fungal cell membrane. The polyenesterol complex alters membrane permeability, depleting essential cellular constituents. Although activity against fungi is dose-related, natamycin is predominantly fungicidal.

Pharmacokinetics: Topical administration appears to produce effective concentrations within the corneal stroma, but not in intraocular fluid. Absorption from the GI tract is very poor. Systemic absorption should not occur after topical administration.

Contraindications

Hypersensitivity to any component of the formulation.

Warnings/Precautions

For topical use only: Not for injection.

Fungal endophthalmitis: The effectiveness of topical natamycin as a single agent in fungal endophthalmitis has not been established.

Resistance: Failure of keratitis to improve following 7 to 10 days of administration suggests that the infection may be caused by a microorganism not susceptible to natamycin. Base continuation of therapy on clinical reevaluation and additional laboratory studies.

Toxicity: Adherence of the suspension to areas of epithelial ulceration or retention in the fornices occurs regularly. Should suspicion of drug toxicity occur, discontinue the drug.

Diagnosis/Monitoring: Determine initial and sustained therapy of fungal keratitis by the clinical diagnosis (laboratory diagnosis by smear and culture of corneal scrapings) and by response to the drug. Whenever possible, determine the in vitro activity of natamycin against the responsible fungus. Monitor tolerance to natamycin at least twice weekly.

Pregnancy: Safety for use during pregnancy has not been established.

Adverse Reactions

One case of conjunctival chemosis and hyperemia, thought to be allergic in nature, was reported.

TOPICAL OPHTHALMIC ANTIVIRAL PREPARATIONS

The topical ophthalmic antiviral preparations appear to interfere with viral reproduction by altering DNA synthesis. Trifluridine is effective treatment for herpes simplex infections of the conjunctiva and cornea. Ganciclovir is indicated for use in immunocompromised patients with cytomegalovirus (CMV) retinitis and for prevention of CMV retinitis in transplant patients. Foscarnet is indicated for use only in AIDS patients with CMV retinitis.

The trifluridine monograph follows this introduction. Prescribing information for foscarnet and ganciclovir appear in the Antivirals section of the Anti-Infectives chapter.

Viral infection, especially epidemic keratoconjunctivitis (EKC), more often is associated with a follicular conjunctivitis, a serous conjunctival discharge, and preuricular lymphadenopathy. The exceptionally contagious organism causing EKC is not susceptible to antiviral therapy at this time.

TRIFLURIDINE (Trifluorothymidine)

Ophthalmic solution: 1% (*Rx*)	*Viroptic* (Burroughs Wellcome)

Indications

Primary keratoconjunctivitis and recurrent epithelial keratitis caused by herpes simplex virus types 1 and 2.

Epithelial keratitis that has not responded clinically to topical idoxuridine, or when ocular toxicity or hypersensitivity to idoxuridine has occurred. In a smaller number of patients resistant to topical vidarabine, trifluridine was also effective.

Administration and Dosage

Instill 1 drop onto the cornea of the affected eye(s) every 2 hours while awake for a maximum daily dosage of 9 drops until the corneal ulcer has completely re-epithelialized. Following re-epithelialization, treat for an additional 7 days with 1 drop every 4 hours while awake for a minimum daily dosage of 5 drops.

If there are no signs of improvement after 7 days, or if complete re-epithelialization has not occurred after 14 days, consider other forms of therapy. Avoid continuous administration for periods exceeding 21 days because of potential ocular toxicity.

Actions

Pharmacology: A fluorinated pyrimidine nucleoside with in vitro and in vivo activity against herpes simplex virus types 1 and 2, and vaccinia virus. Some strains of adenovirus are also inhibited in vitro. Its antiviral mechanism of action is not completely known.

Pharmacokinetics:

Absorption – Intraocular penetration occurs after topical instillation. Decreased corneal integrity or stromal or uveal inflammation may enhance the penetration into the aqueous humor. Systemic absorption following therapeutic dosing appears negligible.

Contraindications

Hypersensitivity reactions or chemical intolerance to trifluridine.

Warnings/Precautions

Efficacy in other conditions: The clinical efficacy in the treatment of stromal keratitis and uveitis caused by herpes simplex or ophthalmic infections caused by vaccinia virus and adenovirus, or in the prophylaxis of herpes simplex virus keratoconjunctivitis and epithelial keratitis has not been established by well-controlled clinical trials. Not effective against bacterial, fungal, or chlamydial infections of the cornea or trophic lesions.

Dosage/Frequency: Do not exceed the recommended dosage or frequency of administration.

Viral resistance: Viral resistance, although documented in vitro, has not been reported following multiple exposure to trifluridine; this possibility may exist.

Pregnancy: Safety for use during pregnancy has not been established.

Lactation: Safety and efficacy have not been established.

Adverse Reactions

Adverse reactions may include mild, transient burning or stinging upon instillation; palpebral edema; superficial punctate keratopathy; epithelial keratopathy; hypersensitivity reaction; stromal edema; irritation; keratitis sicca; hyperemia and increased intraocular pressure.

GANCICLOVIR

Gel, ophthalmic: 0.15% (*Rx*) — *Zirgan* (Sirion Therapeutics Inc)

Indications

Herpetic keratitis: For the treatment of acute herpetic keratitis (dendritic ulcers).

Administration and Dosage

Adults and children 2 years of age and older:

Herpetic keratitis –

Initial dosage: 1 drop in the affected eye 5 times per day (approximately every 3 hours while awake) until the corneal ulcer heals.

Maintenance dosage: 1 drop 3 times per day for 7 days.

Actions

Pharmacology: Ganciclovir is a guanosine derivative that inhibits DNA replication by herpes simplex viruses (HSV).

Pharmacokinetics: The ophthalmically administered daily dose is approximately 0.04% and 0.1% of the oral dose and IV doses, respectively; thus, minimal systemic exposure is expected.

Contraindications

None known.

Warnings/Precautions

Contact lenses: Instruct patients not to wear contact lenses if they have signs or symptoms of herpetic keratitis or during the course of therapy with ganciclovir.

Pregnancy: Category C.

Lactation: It is not known whether ophthalmic administration could produce detectable quantities in breast milk. Exercise caution when ganciclovir is administered to breast-feeding mothers.

Children: Safety and efficacy in children younger than 2 years of age have not been established.

Drug Interactions

None known.

Adverse Reactions

Common adverse reactions: Most common adverse reactions reported in patients were blurred vision (60%), eye irritation (20%), punctuate keratitis (5%), and conjunctival hyperemia (5%).

CYCLOSPORINE

Emulsion, ophthalmic: 0.05% (*Rx*)	*Restasis* (Allergan)

Indications

Increased tear production: To increase tear production in patients whose tear production is presumed to be suppressed due to ocular inflammation associated with keratoconjunctivitis sicca.

Administration and Dosage

Invert the unit dose vial a few times to obtain a uniform, white, opaque emulsion before using. Instill 1 drop twice a day in each eye, approximately 12 hours apart. Cyclosporine can be used concomitantly with artificial tears, allowing a 15-minute interval between products. Discard vial immediately after use.

Actions

Pharmacology: Cyclosporine is an immunosuppressive agent when administered systemically.

Pharmacokinetics:

Absorption – Blood concentrations of cyclosporine after topical administration of cyclosporine ophthalmic suspension were below the quantitation limit of 0.1 ng/mL. There was no detectable accumulation in blood during 12 months of treatment.

Contraindications

In patients with active ocular infections; in patients with known or suspected hypersensitivity to any of the ingredients in the formulation.

Warnings/Precautions

Administration: Cyclosporine ophthalmic emulsion is for ophthalmic use only.

Herpes keratitis: Cyclosporine ophthalmic emulsion has not been studied in patients with a history of herpes keratitis.

Pregnancy: Category C.

Lactation: Cyclosporine is known to be excreted in human milk following systemic administration, but excretion in human milk after topical treatment has not been investigated. Caution should be exercised when cyclosporine ophthalmic emulsion is administered to a nursing woman.

Children: The safety and efficacy of cyclosporine ophthalmic emulsion have not been established in pediatric patients below 16 years of age.

Adverse Reactions

The most common adverse reaction following the use of cyclosporine ophthalmic emulsion was ocular burning (17%).

Other events reported in 1% to 5% of patients included conjunctival hyperemia, discharge, epiphora, eye pain, foreign body sensation, pruritus, stinging, and visual disturbance (most often blurring).

OFLOXACIN

Solution; otic: 0.3% (3 mg/mL) (*Rx*) Various, *Floxin Otic* (Daiichi)

Indications

For the treatment of infections caused by susceptible isolates of the designated microorganisms in the following specific conditions.

Acute otitis media: In children 1 year of age and older with tympanostomy tubes due to *Staphylococcus aureus*, *Streptococcus pneumoniae*, *Haemophilus influenzae*, *Moraxella catarrhalis*, and *Pseudomonas aeruginosa*.

Chronic suppurative otitis media: In patients 12 years of age and older with perforated tympanic membranes caused by *Proteus mirabilis*, *P. aeruginosa*, and *S. aureus*.

Otitis externa: In adults and children 6 months of age and older, caused by *Escherichia coli*, *P. aeruginosa*, and *S. aureus*.

Administration and Dosage

Dosage:

Acute otitis media in children with tympanostomy tubes –

Children 1 to 12 years of age: 5 drops (0.25 mL, ofloxacin 0.75 mg) instilled into the affected ear twice daily for 10 days.

Chronic suppurative otitis media with perforated tympanic membranes –

Patients 12 years of age and older: 10 drops (0.5 mL, ofloxacin 1.5 mg) instilled into the affected ear twice daily for 14 days.

Otitis externa –

Children 6 months to 13 years of age: 5 drops (0.25 mL, ofloxacin 0.75 mL) instilled into the affected ear once daily for 7 days.

Patients 13 years of age and older: 10 drops (0.5 mL, ofloxacin 1.5 mg) instilled into the affected ear once daily for 7 days.

Administration:

Acute otitis media and chronic suppurative otitis media – The solution should be warmed by holding the bottle in the hand for 1 or 2 minutes to avoid dizziness that may result from the instillation of a cold solution. The patient should lie with the affected ear upward, and then the drops should be instilled. The tragus should then be pumped 4 times by pushing inward to facilitate penetration of the drops into the middle ear. This position should be maintained for 5 minutes. Repeat, if necessary, for the opposite ear.

Otitis externa – The solution should be warmed by holding the bottle in the hand for 1 or 2 minutes to avoid dizziness that may result from the instillation of a cold solution. The patient should lie with the affected ear upward, and then the drops should be instilled. This position should be maintained for 5 minutes to facilitate penetration of the drops in the ear canal. Repeat, if necessary, for the opposite ear.

Actions

Pharmacology: Ofloxacin has in vitro activity against a wide range of gram-negative and gram-positive microorganisms.

Pharmacokinetics: Drug concentrations in serum (in subjects with tympanostomy tubes and perforated tympanic membranes), in otorrhea, and in mucosa of the middle ear (in subjects with perforated tympanic membranes) were determined following otic administration of ofloxacin solution.

Warnings/Precautions

Administration: Ofloxacin otic solution is not for ophthalmic use or injection.

Arthropathy: The systemic administration of quinolones, including ofloxacin, at doses much higher than given or absorbed by the otic route, has led to lesions or erosions of the cartilage in weight-bearing joints and other signs of arthropathy in immature animals of various species.

Hypersensitivity reactions: Serious and occasionally fatal hypersensitivity (anaphylactic) reactions, some following the first dose, have been reported in patients receiving systemic quinolones, including ofloxacin. Some reactions were accompanied by cardiovascular collapse, loss of consciousness, angioedema (including laryngeal, pharyngeal, or facial edema), airway obstruction, dyspnea, urticaria, and itching. If an allergic reaction to ofloxacin is suspected, stop the drug. Serious acute hypersensitivity reactions may require immediate emergency treatment. Oxygen and airway management, including intubation, should be administered as clinically indicated.

Superinfection: As with other anti-infective preparations, prolonged use may result in overgrowth of nonsusceptible organisms, including fungi. If the infection is not improved after 1 week, cultures should be obtained to guide further treatment. If otorrhea persists after a full course of therapy, or if 2 or more episodes of otorrhea occur within 6 months, further evaluation is recommended to exclude an underlying condition such as cholesteatoma, foreign body, or a tumor.

Pregnancy: Category C.

Lactation: It is not known whether ofloxacin is excreted in human milk following topical otic administration.

Children: Although safety and efficacy have been demonstrated in children 1 year of age and older, safety and efficacy in infants younger than 1 year of age have not been established.

Adverse Reactions

Subjects with otitis externa: Adverse reactions occurring in 3% or more of patients include application site reaction and pruritus.

Subjects with acute otitis media with tympanostomy tubes and subjects with chronic suppurative otitis media with perforated tympanic membranes: Adverse reactions occurring in 3% or more of patients include taste perversion.

CIPROFLOXACIN

Solution; otic: 0.2% (*Rx*)	*Cetraxal* (WraSer Pharmaceuticals)

Indications

Otitis externa: For the treatment of acute otitis externa caused by susceptible isolates of *Pseudomonas aeruginosa* or *Staphylococcus aureus*.

Administration and Dosage

Otitis externa:

Adults and children (1 year of age and older) – Instill the contents of 1 single-use container (deliverable volume: 0.25 mL) into the affected ear twice daily (approximately 12 hours apart) for 7 days.

Administration: Wash hands before use. The solution should be warmed by holding the container in the hands for at least 1 minute to minimize the dizziness that may result from the instillation of a cold solution into the ear canal. The patient should lie with the affected ear upward and then the solution should be instilled. This position should be maintained for at least 1 minute to facilitate penetration of the drops into the ear. Repeat, if necessary, for the opposite ear.

Actions

Pharmacology: Ciprofloxacin is a fluoroquinolone antimicrobial. The bactericidal action of ciprofloxacin results from interference with the enzyme DNA gyrase, which is needed for the synthesis of bacterial DNA. Bacterial resistance to quinolones can develop through chromosomally or plasmid-mediated mechanisms.

Pharmacokinetics:

Absorption – The maximum plasma concentration of ciprofloxacin is anticipated to be less than 5 ng/mL.

Microbiology: Ciprofloxacin has been shown to be active against most isolates of the following bacteria, both in vitro and in clinical infections of acute otitis externa.

Aerobes, gram-positive – *S. aureus*.

Aerobes, gram-negative – *P. aeruginosa*.

Contraindications

Hypersensitivity to ciprofloxacin.

Warnings/Precautions

Administration: Ciprofloxacin is for otic use only. It should not be used for injection, for inhalation, or for topical ophthalmic use.

Arthropathy: There is no evidence that the otic administration of quinolones has any effect on weight bearing joints, even though systemic administration of some quinolones has been shown to cause arthropathy in immature animals.

Lack of clinical response: If the infection is not improved after one week of therapy, cultures may help guide further treatment.

Hypersensitivity reactions: Discontinue ciprofloxacin at the first appearance of a skin rash or any other sign of hypersensitivity.

Superinfection: As with other anti-infectives, use of ciprofloxacin may result in overgrowth of nonsusceptible organisms, including yeast and fungi. If super-infection occurs, discontinue use and institute alternative therapy.

Pregnancy: Category C.

Lactation: Ciprofloxacin is excreted in human milk with systemic use. It is not known whether ciprofloxacin is excreted in human milk following otic use.

Children: The safety and effectiveness of ciprofloxacin in infants younger than 1 year of age have not been established.

Adverse Reactions

Adverse reactions occurring in at least 3% of people include application site pain, ear pruritus, fungal ear superinfection, headache.

APPENDIX

FDA PREGNANCY CATEGORIES

The rational use of any medication requires a risk versus benefit assessment. Among the myriad of risk factors that complicate this assessment, pregnancy is one of the most perplexing.

The FDA has established five categories to indicate the potential of a systemically absorbed drug for causing birth defects. The key differentiation among the categories rests upon the degree (reliability) of documentation and the risk versus benefit ratio. Pregnancy *Category* X is particularly notable in that if any data exists that may implicate a drug as a teratogen and the risk versus benefit ratio does not support use of the drug, the drug is contraindicated during pregnancy. These categories are summarized below:

FDA Pregnancy Categories

Pregnancy Category	Definition
A	Controlled studies show no risk. Adequate, well-controlled studies in pregnant women have failed to demonstrate risk to the fetus.
B	No evidence of risk in humans. Either animal findings show risk, but human findings do not; or if no adequate human studies have been done, animal findings are negative.
C	Risk cannot be ruled out. Human studies are lacking, and animal studies are either positive for fetal risk or lacking. However, potential benefits may justify the potential risks.
D	Positive evidence of risk. Investigational or post-marketing data show risk to the fetus. Nevertheless, potential benefits may outweigh the potential risks. If needed in a life-threatening situation or a serious disease, the drug may be acceptable if safer drugs cannot be used or are ineffective.
X	Contraindicated in pregnancy. Studies in animals or human, or investigational or post-marketing reports have shown fetal risk which clearly outweighs any possible benefit to the patient.

Regardless of the designated pregnancy category or presumed safety, no drug should be administered during pregnancy unless it is clearly needed and potential benefits outweigh potential hazards to the fetus.

CONTROLLED SUBSTANCES

The Controlled Substances Act of 1970 regulates the manufacturing, distribution and dispensing of drugs that have abuse potential. The Drug Enforcement Administration (DEA) within the US Department of Justice is the chief federal agency responsible for enforcing the act.

DEA schedules: Drugs under jurisdiction of the Controlled Substances Act are divided into five schedules based on their potential for abuse and physical and psychological dependence. All controlled substances listed in *Drug Facts and Comparisons®* are identified by schedule as follows:

Schedule I (*c-i*) – High abuse potential and no accepted medical use (eg, heroin, marijuana, LSD).

Schedule II (*c-ii*) – High abuse potential with severe dependence liability (eg, narcotics, amphetamines, dronabinol, some barbiturates).

Schedule III (*c-iii*) – Less abuse potential than schedule II drugs and moderate dependence liability (eg, nonbarbiturate sedatives, nonamphetamine stimulants, limited amounts of certain narcotics).

Schedule IV (*c-iv*) – Less abuse potential than schedule III drugs and limited dependence liability (eg, some sedatives, antianxiety agents, nonnarcotic analgesics).

Schedule V (*c-v*) – Limited abuse potential. Primarily small amounts of narcotics (codeine) used as antitussives or antidiarrheals. Under federal law, limited quantities of certain *c-v* drugs may be purchased without a prescription directly from a pharmacist if allowed under state statutes. The purchaser must be at least 18 years of age and must furnish suitable identification. All such transactions must be recorded by the dispensing pharmacist.

Registration: Prescribing physicians and dispensing pharmacies must be registered with the DEA, PO Box 28083, Central Station, Washington, DC 20005.

Inventory: Separate records must be kept of purchases and dispensing of controlled substances. An inventory of controlled substances must be made every 2 years.

Prescriptions: Prescriptions for controlled substances must be written in ink and include the following: Date; name and address of the patient; name, address, and DEA number of the physician. Oral prescriptions must be promptly committed to writing. Controlled substance prescriptions may not be dispensed or refilled more than 6 months after the date issued or be refilled more than 5 times. A written prescription signed by the physician is required for schedule II drugs. In case of emergency, oral prescriptions for schedule II substances may be filled; however, the physician must provide a signed prescription within 72 hours. Schedule II prescriptions cannot be refilled. A triplicate order form is necessary for the transfer of controlled substances in schedule II. Forms are available for the individual prescriber at no charge from the DEA.

State laws: In many cases, state laws are more restrictive than federal laws and therefore impose additional requirements (eg, triplicate prescription forms).

MANAGEMENT OF ACUTE HYPERSENSITIVITY REACTIONS

Type I hypersensitivity reactions (immediate hypersensitivity or anaphylaxis) are immunologic responses to a foreign antigen to which a patient has been previously sensitized. Anaphylactoid reactions are not immunoogically mediated; however, symptoms and treatment are similar.

Signs and Symptoms

Acute hypersensitivity reactions typically begin within 1 to 30 minutes of exposure to the offending antigen. Tingling sensations and a generalized flush may proceed to a fullness in the throat, chest tightness, or a "feeling of impending doom." Generalized urticaria and sweating are common. *Severe* reactions include life-threatening involvement of the airway and cardiovascular system.

Treatment

Appropriate and immediate treatment is imperative. The following general measures are commonly employed:

Epinephrine: 1:1,000, 0.2 to 0.5 mg (0.2 to 0.5 mL) subcutaneously is the primary treatment. In children, administer 0.01 mg/kg or 0.1 mg. Doses may be repeated every 5 to 15 minutes if needed. A succession of small doses is more effective and less dangerous than a single large dose. Additionally, 0.1 mg may be introduced into an injection site where the offending drug was administered. If appropriate, the use of a tourniquet above the site of injection of the causative agent may slow its absorption and distribution. However, remove or loosen the tourniquet every 10 to 15 minutes to maintain circulation.

Epinephrine IV (generally indicated in the presence of hypotension) is often recommended in a 1:10,000 dilution, 0.3 to 0.5 mg over 5 minutes; repeat every 15 minutes, if necessary. In children, inject 0.1 to 0.2 mg or 0.01 mg/kg/dose over 5 minutes; repeat every 30 minutes.

A conservative IV epinephrine protocol includes 0.1 mg of a 1:100,000 dilution (0.1 mg of a 1:1,000 dilution mixed in 10 mL normal saline) given over 5 to 10 minutes. If an IV infusion is necessary, administer at a rate of 1 to 4 mcg/min. In children, infuse 0.1 to 1.5 (maximum) mcg/kg/min.

Dilute epinephrine 1:10,000 may be administered through an endotracheal tube, if no other parenteral access is available, directly into the bronchial tree. It is rapidly absorbed there from the capillary bed of the lung.

Airway: Ensure a patent airway via endotracheal intubation or cricothyrotomy (ie, inferior laryngotomy, used prior to tracheotomy) and administer oxygen. Severe respiratory difficulty may respond to IV aminophylline or to other bronchodilators.

Hypotension: The patient should be recumbent with feet elevated. Depending upon the severity, consider the following measures:

- Establish a patent IV catheter in a suitable vein.
- Administer IV fluids (eg, normal saline, lactated Ringer's).
- Administer plasma expanders.

- Administer cardioactive agents (see group and individual monographs). Commonly recommended agents include dopamine, dobutamine, norepinephrine, and phenylephrine.

Adjunctive therapy: Adjunctive therapy does not alter acute reactions, but may modify an ongoing or slow-onset process and shorten the course of the reaction.

- *Antihistamines: Diphenhydramine* – 50 to 100 mg IM or IV, continued orally at 5 mg/kg/day or 50 mg every 6 hours for 1 to 2 days. For children, give 5 mg/kg/day, maximum 300 mg/day.

  Chlorpheniramine – (adults, 10 to 20 mg; children, 5 to 10 mg) IM or slowly IV.

  Hydroxyzine – 10 to 25 mg orally or 25 to 50 mg IM 3 to 4 times daily.
- *Corticosteroids*, eg, hydrocortisone IV 100 to 1000 mg or equivalent, followed by 7 mg/kg/day IV or oral for 1 to 2 days. The role of corticosteroids is controversial.
- H_2 *antagonists: Cimetidine – Children*, 25 to 30 mg/kg/day IV in 6 divided doses; *adults*, 300 mg every 6 hours.

  Ranitidine – 50 mg IV over 3 to 5 minutes. May be of value in addition to H_1 antihistamines, although this opinion is not universally shared.

DRUG-INDUCED PROLONGATION OF THE QT INTERVAL AND TORSADES DE POINTES

The QT interval is the period between the beginning of the QRS complex and the end of the T wave. Thus, it is the estimate of the time interval between the earliest ventricular depolarization and the latest ventricular repolarization. Since the QT interval is affected by changes in the heart rate, corrections are usually made to the QT interval for these changes (QTc). There is no commonly accepted definition of a normal or prolonged QTc interval. The Committee for Proprietary Medicinal Products has suggested ranges for normal (ie, men less than 430 msec, women less than 450 msec), borderline (ie, men 430 to 450 msec, women 450 to 470 msec), and prolonged (ie, men greater than 450 msec, women greater than 470 msec) QTc intervals. Moderate and clinically important increases in the QT interval over baseline have been considered to be 15% and 25% increases, respectively.

Numerous drugs, representing a wide range of pharmacologic classes, have been implicated in prolonging the QT interval. Concern about serious and possibly fatal consequences of drug combinations that may cause prolongation of the QT interval has led to contraindicating the use of many drug pairs, even though coadministration may not have been studied. The potential of bepridil (*Vascor*), astemizole (*Hismanal*), grepafloxacin (*Raxar*), and terfenadine (*Seldane*) to prolong the QT interval played an important role in their removal from the market.

The precise mechanism by which QT interval prolongation (ie, long QT syndrome [LQTS]) occurs is unknown; however, it appears to be related to ion exchange (eg, outward repolarizing potassium current, inward depolarizing calcium or sodium current). Class III antiarrhythmic agents prolong the QT interval by blocking potassium flow. A prolonged QT interval may be congenital (eg, genetic) or acquired (eg, drug-induced). In some instances, patients may have an underlying predisposition toward a prolonged QT interval (eg, longer than normal QT interval before drug administration).

Drug-induced prolongation of the QT interval may be suspected if there are dose-related changes in the QT interval, the same drug causes QT prolongation in a number of patients, or prolonged QT interval recurs when a patient is rechallenged. Drug-induced QT prolongation may be prevented by 1) not exceeding the recommended drug dose; 2) limiting use of the drug in patients with preexisting heart disease; 3) avoiding coadministration of agents that increase plasma levels of the drug in question; 4) avoiding concurrent use of other medications that prolong the QT interval; and 5) identification and correction of risk factors (eg, hypokalemia) before giving a drug known to prolong the QT interval.

A great deal of attention has been focused on drug-induced prolongation of the QT interval and association of the prolongation with life-threatening ventricular arrhythmias, especially torsades de pointes. Torsades de pointes, meaning twisting of points, refers to a ventricular arrhythmia in which the QRS complexes change amplitude and contour, appearing to twist around the isoelectric line on the electrocardiogram (ECG). In patients who develop drug-induced torsades de pointes, the QT interval measured prior to drug exposure tends to be longer than in patients who receive the drug safely. In patients with drug-induced torsades de pointes, ventricular repolarization is prolonged and characterized by marked prolongation of the QT interval (greater than 500 msec) and QTc interval (greater than 470 msec) of the ECG. In individuals with a drug-induced increase in the QTc interval of more than 65 msec above normal (ie, greater than 500 msec), the risk of torsades de pointes may be greater than 3%. This risk of torsades de pointes increases greatly when the QT interval exceeds 600 msec. In the presence of a prolonged QT interval, women are at greater risk than men of developing torsades de pointes.

Amiodarone (eg, *Cordarone*) prolongs the QT interval but rarely causes torsades de pointes. However, class I antiarrhythmic agents (eg, procainamide [eg, *Procanbid*]) are more likely to cause torsades de pointes but have a moderate effect on the QT interval. Drug interactions may further prolong the QT interval and increase the risk of life-threatening cardiac arrhythmias, including torsades de pointes. Thus, administration of cisapride (eg, *Propulsid*), which prolongs the QT interval, with an inhibitor of cytochrome P450 (CYP) 3A4 (eg, grapefruit products, erythromycin) may increase cisapride plasma levels and the risk of life-threatening cardiac arrhythmias.

Identification and correction of risk factors (eg, hypokalemia) before giving a drug known to prolong the QT interval or cause torsades de pointes are important in preventing drug-induced torsades de pointes. Agents that prolong the QT interval are contraindicated in patients with a history of drug-induced torsades de pointes.

Summary: Numerous drugs from a wide range of pharmacologic classes can prolong the QT interval and precipitate torsades de pointes. However, the consequences of QT interval prolongation and the occurrence of torsades de pointes can be minimized or prevented by identification and correction of risk factors. Use of drugs that prolong the QT interval is contraindicated in patients with a history of torsades de pointes.

Drugs Reported to Prolong the QT Interval	
Analgesics	***Anticonvulsants***
Celecoxib (*Celebrex*)[a]	Felbamate (*Felbatol*)[a]
Methadone (eg, *Dolophine*)[a]	Fosphenytoin (*Cerebyx*)
Anesthetic agents	***Antiemetics***
Enflurane (eg, *Ethrane*)	Dolasetron (*Anzemet*)[c]
Isoflurane (eg, *Forane*)	Droperidol (eg, *Inapsine*)[a,c]
Halothane	Ondansetron (*Zofran*)
Antiarrhythmic agents	***Antihistamines***
Class IA	Desloratadine (*Clarinex*)[c] (overdose)
Disopyramide (eg, *Norpace*)[a]	Diphenhydramine (eg, *Benadryl*)[a]
Procainamide (eg, *Procanbid*)[a]	Fexofenadine (*Allegra*)
Quinidine[a]	Hydroxyzine (eg, *Vistaril*)
Class IC	***Anti-infectives***
Flecainide (eg, *Tambocor*)[a,b]	Amantadine (eg, *Symmetrel*)[a]
Propafenone (eg, *Rythmol*)[a,c]	Antimalarials
Class III	Mefloquine (eg, *Lariam*)[c]
Amiodarone (eg, *Cordarone*)[a,c]	Quinine[a]
Bretylium[a]	Antivirals
Dofetilide (*Tikosyn*)[a,c]	Efavirenz (*Sustiva*)[a]
Ibutilide (*Corvert*)[a,c]	
Sotalol (eg, *Betapace*)[a,c]	

Drugs Reported to Prolong the QT Interval

- Azole antifungal agents
  - Fluconazole (eg, *Diflucan*)[a,c]
  - Itraconazole (eg, *Sporanox*)
  - Ketoconazole (eg, *Nizoral*)
  - Voriconazole (*Vfend*)[a,c]
- Chloroquine (eg, *Aralen*)[a]
- Clindamycin (eg, *Cleocin*)
- Foscarnet (*Foscavir*)
- Macrolides and related antibiotics
  - Azithromycin (eg, *Zithromax*)
  - Clarithromycin (eg, *Biaxin*)[a,c]
  - Erythromycin (eg, *Ery-Tab*)[a,c]
  - Telithromycin (*Ketek*)[c]
  - Troleandomycin
- Pentamidine (eg, *Pentam 300*)[a]
- Quinolones
  - Gatifloxacin[a,c]
  - Levofloxacin (eg, *Levaquin*)[a-c]
  - Moxifloxacin (eg, *Avelox*)[c]
  - Ofloxacin (eg, *Floxin*)[a,c]
- Trimethoprim/sulfamethoxazole (eg, *Bactrim*)[a]

Antineoplastics
- Arsenic trioxide (*Trisenox*)[a,c]
- Doxorubicin (eg, *Adriamycin*)
- Tamoxifen (eg, *Nolvadex*)

Bronchodilators
- Albuterol (eg, *Proventil*)[c]
- Formoterol (*Foradil*)[c]
- Isoproterenol (eg, *Isuprel*)
- Salmeterol (*Serevent*)[c]
- Terbutaline (eg, *Brethine*)[c]

Calcium channel blockers
- Isradipine (*DynaCirc*)
- Nicardipine (eg, *Cardene*)

Contrast media
- Ionic contrast media[a]
- Non-ionic contrast media
  - Iohexol (*Omnipaque*)

Corticosteroids
- Prednisolone (eg, *Prelone*)
- Prednisone (eg, *Deltasone*)[a]

Diuretics
- Furosemide (eg, *Lasix*)
- Indapamide (eg, *Lozol*)

GI agents
- Cisapride (*Propulsid*)[a,c]
- Famotidine (eg, *Pepcid*)[a]

Immunosuppressants
- Tacrolimus (*Protopic*)[a,c] (postmarketing)

Miscellaneous
- Levomethadyl
- Moexipril/Hydrochlorothiazide (*Uniretic*)
- Octreotide (*Sandostatin*)[c]
- Oxytocin (eg, *Pitocin*; IV bolus)
- Papaverine (eg, *Pavaden TD*)[a]
- Probucol[a]
- Vasopressin (eg, *Pitressin*)[a]

Psychotropics
- Droperidol (eg, *Inapsine*)[a]
- Haloperidol (eg, *Haldol*)[a]
- Lithium (eg, *Eskalith*)[a]
- Maprotiline[a]
- Phenothiazines
  - Chlorpromazine (eg, *Thorazine*)[a]
  - Fluphenazine (eg, *Prolixin*)[a]
  - Perphenazine
  - Thioridazine[a,c]
  - Trifluoperazine
- Pimozide (*Orap*)[a,c]
- Quetiapine (*Seroquel*)[c]
- Risperidone (*Risperdal*)[c] (overdose)
- SSRIs
  - Citalopram (eg, *Celexa*)[a]
  - Fluoxetine (eg, *Prozac*)[a,b]
  - Paroxetine (eg, *Paxil*)[a]
  - Sertraline (*Zoloft*)[a-c] (postmarketing)
  - Venlafaxine (*Effexor*)[c] (postmarketing)
- Trazodone (eg, *Desyrel*)
- Tricyclic antidepressants
  - Amitriptyline[a]
  - Clomipramine (eg, *Anafranil*)
  - Desipramine (eg, *Norpramin*)[a]
  - Doxepin (eg, *Sinequan*)[a]
  - Imipramine (eg, *Tofranil*)[a]
  - Nortriptyline (eg, *Pamelor*)
- Ziprasidone (*Geodon*)[c]

Serotonin 5-HT$_1$ agonists
- Naratriptan (*Amerge*)
- Sumatriptan (*Imitrex*)[c]
- Zolmitriptan (*Zomig*)[c]

Skeletal muscle relaxants
- Tizanidine (eg, *Zanaflex*)[c] (animals)

[a] Drugs for which torsades de pointes has also been reported.
[b] Association unclear.
[c] QT, QTc, and/or torsades de pointes association listed in FDA approved product labeling.

Factors that increase the risk of torsades de pointes:

- Administration of drugs that prolong the QT interval
- Altered nutritional states (eg, anorexia nervosa, liquid protein diet)
- Baseline QTc interval greater than 460 msec
- Coadministration of certain drugs that prolong QT interval with drugs metabolized by CYP3A4
- Congenital LQT syndrome
- Female gender
- Electrolyte imbalance (eg, hypokalemia, hypomagnesemia)
- Liver disease
- Hypothyroidism
- Nervous system injury (eg, stroke, subarachnoid hemorrhage)
- Preexisting cardiac disease (eg, congestive heart failure, heart failure, ventricular hypertrophy)
- Renal disease
- Slow heart rate (ie, bradyarrhythmia)

CALCULATIONS

To calculate milliequivalent weight: $\text{mEq} = \dfrac{\text{gram molecular weight/valence}}{1000}$

$\text{mEq} = \dfrac{\text{mg}}{\text{eq wt}}$ equivalent weight or eq wt = $\dfrac{\text{gram molecular weight}}{\text{valence}}$

Commonly used mEq weights			
Chloride	35.5 mg = 1 mEq	Magnesium	12 mg = 1 mEq
Sodium	23 mg = 1 mEq	Potassium	39 mg = 1 mEq
Calcium	20 mg = 1 mEq		

To convert temperature °C ↔ °F: $\dfrac{°C}{°F - 32} = \dfrac{5}{9}$ *or* $°C = \dfrac{5}{9}(°F - 32)$

$°F = 32 + \dfrac{9}{5}\,°C$

To calculate creatinine clearance (Ccr) from serum creatinine:

Male: $\text{Ccr} = \dfrac{\text{weight (kg)} \times (140 - \text{age})}{72 \times \text{serum creatinine (mg/dL)}}$ Female: Ccr = 0.85 × calculation for males

To calculate ideal body weight (kg):

Male = 50 kg + 2.3 kg (each inch > 5 ft) Female = 45.5 kg + 2.3 kg (each inch > 5 ft)

To calculate body surface area (BSA) in adults and children:

1) *Dubois method:*

$\text{SA (cm}^2) = \text{wt (kg)}^{0.425} \times \text{ht (cm)}^{0.725} \times 71.84$

$\text{SA (m}^2) = K \times \sqrt[3]{\text{wt}^2\text{ (kg)}}$ (common K value 0.1 for toddlers, 0.103 for neonates)

2) *Simplified method:*

$\text{BSA (m}^2) = \sqrt{\dfrac{\text{ht (cm)} \times \text{wt (kg)}}{3600}}$

To approximate surface area (m²) of children from weight (kg):

Weight range (kg)	≈ Surface area (m^2)
1 to 5	(0.05 x kg) + 0.05
6 to 10	(0.04 x kg) + 0.10
11 to 20	(0.03 x kg) + 0.20
21 to 40	(0.02 x kg) + 0.40

Suggested Weights for Adults

Height*	Weight in pounds†
4'10"	91-119
4'11"	94-124
5'0"	97-128
5'1"	101-132
5'2"	104-137
5'3"	107-141
5'4"	111-146
5'5"	114-150
5'6"	118-155
5'7"	121-160
5'8"	125-164
5'9"	129-169
5'10"	132-174
5'11"	136-179
6'0"	140-184
6'1"	144-189
6'2"	148-195
6'3"	152-200
6'4"	156-205
6'5"	160-211
6'6"	164-216

* Without shoes. † Without clothes.

The higher weights in the ranges generally apply to people with more muscle and bone. Source: Nutrition and Your Health: Dietary Guidelines for Americans, 4th ed, 1995. US Department of Agriculture, US Department of Health and Human Services. At press time, these new guidelines had not been officially released. It is possible some changes to this chart will occur.

NORMAL LABORATORY VALUES

In the following tables, normal reference values for commonly requested laboratory tests are listed in traditional units and in SI units. The tables are a guideline only. Values are method dependent and "normal values" may vary between laboratories.

Blood, Plasma, or Serum

Determination	Reference Value: Conventional units	Reference Value: SI units
Alpha-fetoprotein	*Adult:* < 15 ng/mL *Pregnant (16-18 weeks):* 38-45 ng/mL	*Adult:* < 15 mcg/mL *Pregnant (16-18 weeks):* 38-45 mcg/L
Ammonia (NH_3) – diffusion	20-120 mcg/dL	12-70 mcmol/L
Ammonia nitrogen	15–45 mcg/dL	11–32 mcmol/L
Amylase	35-118 IU/L	0.58-1.97 mckat/L
Anion gap (Na^+–[Cl^-+HCO_3^-]) (P)	7–16 mEq/L	7–16 mmol/L
Antithrombin III (AT III)	80-120 units/dL	800-1200 units/L
Bicarbonate: Arterial	21–28 mEq/L	21–28 mmol/L
Venous	22–29 mEq/L	22–29 mmol/L
Bilirubin: Conjugated (direct)	≤ 0.2 mg/dL	≤ 4 mcmol/L
Total	0.1-1 mg/dL	2-18 mcmol/L
Calcitonin	< 100 pg/mL	< 100 ng/L
Calcium: Total	8.6-10.3 mg/dL	2.2-2.74 mmol/L
Ionized	4.4-5.1 mg/dL	1-1.3 mmol/L
Carbon dioxide content (plasma)	21-32 mmol/L	21-32 mmol/L
Carcinoembryonic antigen	< 3 ng/mL	< 3 mcg/L
Chloride	95-110 mEq/L	95-110 mmol/L
Coagulation screen:		
Bleeding time	3-9.5 min	180-570 sec
Prothrombin time	10-13 sec	10-13 sec
Partial thromboplastin time (activated)	22-37 sec	22-37 sec
Protein C	70%-140%	0.70-1.40
Protein S	70%-140%	0.70-1.40
Copper, total	70-160 mcg/dL	11-25 mcmol/L
Corticotropin (ACTH adrenocorticotropic hormone) – 0800 hr	< 60 pg/mL	< 13.2 pmol/L
Cortisol: 0800 hr	5-30 mcg/dL	138-810 nmol/L
1800 hr	2-15 mcg/dL	50-410 nmol/L
2000 hr	≤ 50% of 0800 hr	≤ 50% of 0800 hr
Creatine kinase: Female	20-170 units/L	0.33-2.83 mckat/L
Male	30-220 units/L	0.5-3.67 mckat/L
Creatine kinase isoenzymes, MB fraction	0-12 units/L	0-0.2 mckat/L
Creatinine	0.5-1.7 mg/dL	44-150 mcmol/L
Fibrinogen (coagulation factor I)	150-360 mg/dL	1.5-3.6 g/L
Follicle-stimulating hormone (FSH):		
Female	2-13 milliunits/mL	2-13 units/L
Midcycle	5-22 milliunits/mL	5-22 units/L
Male	1-8 milliunits/mL	1-8 units/L
Glucose, fasting	65-115 mg/dL	3.6-6.3 mmol/L
Glucose tolerance test (oral)	mg/dL Normal / Diabetic	mmol/L Normal / Diabetic
Fasting	70-105 / > 140	3.9-5.8 / > 7.8
60 min	120-170 / ≥ 200	6.7-9.4 / ≥11.1
90 min	100-140 / ≥ 200	5.6-7.8 / ≥ 11.1
120 min	70-120 / ≥ 140	3.9-6.7 / ≥ 7.8
Gamma - glutamyltransferase (GGT): Male	9-50 units/L	9-50 units/L
Female	8-40 units/L	8-40 units/L

Blood, Plasma, or Serum		
	Reference Value	
Determination	Conventional units	SI units
Haptoglobin	44-303 mg/dL	0.44-3.03 g/L
Hematologic tests:		
Fibrinogen	200-400 mg/dL	2-4 g/L
Hematocrit (Hct), Female	36%-44.6%	0.36-0.446 fraction of 1
Male	40.7%-50.3%	0.4-0.503 fraction of 1
Hemoglobin A_{1C}	5.3%-7.5% of total Hgb	0.053-0.075
Hemoglobin (Hb), Female	12.1-15.3 g/dL	121-153 g/L
Male	13.8-17.5 g/dL	138-175 g/L
Leukocyte count (WBC)	3,800-9,800/mcL	3.8-9.8 x 10^9/L
Erythrocyte count (RBC), Female	3.5-5 × 10^6/mcL	3.5-5 x 10^{12}/L
Male	4.3-5.9 × 10^6/mcL	4.3-5.9 x 10^{12}/L
Mean corpuscular volume (MCV)	80-97.6 mcm^3	80-97.6 fl
Mean corpuscular hemoglobin (MCH)	27-33 pg/cell	1.66-2.09 fmol/cell
Mean corpuscular hemoglobin concentrate (MCHC)	33-36 g/dL	20.3-22 mmol/L
Erythrocyte sedimentation rate (sedrate, ESR)	≤ 30 mm/hr	≤ 30 mm/hr
Erythrocyte enzymes: Glucose-6-phosphate dehydrogenase (G-6-PD)	250-5,000 units/10^6 cells	250-5,000 mcunits/cell
Ferritin	10-383 ng/mL	23-862 pmol/L
Folic acid: normal	> 3.1-12.4 ng/mL	7-28.1 nmol/L
Platelet count	150-450 × 10^3/mcL	150-450 × 10^9/L
Reticulocytes	0.5%-1.5% of erythrocytes	0.005-0.015
Vitamin B_{12}	223-1132 pg/mL	165-835 pmol/L
Iron: Female	30-160 mcg/dL	5.4-31.3 mcmol/L
Male	45-160 mcg/dL	8.1-31.3 mcmol/L
Iron binding capacity	220-420 mcg/dL	39.4-75.2 mcmol/L
Isocitrate dehydrogenase	1.2-7 units/L	1.2-7 units/L
Isoenzymes		
Fraction 1	14%-26% of total	0.14-0.26 fraction of total
Fraction 2	29%-39% of total	0.29-0.39 fraction of total
Fraction 3	20%-26% of total	0.20-0.26 fraction of total
Fraction 4	8%-16% of total	0.08-0.16 fraction of total
Fraction 5	6%-16% of total	0.06-0.16 fraction of total
Lactate dehydrogenase	100-250 units/L	1.67-4.17 mckat/L
Lactic acid (lactate)	6-19 mg/dL	0.7-2.1 mmol/L
Lead	≤ 50 mcg/dL	≤ 2.41 mcmol/L
Lipase	10-150 units/L	10-150 units/L

Blood, Plasma, or Serum		
Determination	Reference Value	
	Conventional units	SI units
Lipids:		
Total cholesterol		
Desirable	< 200 mg/dL	< 5.2 mmol/L
Borderline-high	200-239 mg/dL	< 5.2-6.2 mmol/L
High	> 239 mg/dL	> 6.2 mmol/L
LDL		
Desirable	< 130 mg/dL	< 3.36 mmol/L
Borderline-high	130-159 mg/dL	3.36-4.11 mmol/L
High	> 159 mg/dL	> 4.11 mmol/L
HDL		
Low	< 40 mg/dL	
Desirable	≥ 60 mg/dL	
Triglycerides		
Desirable	< 150 mg/dL	
Borderline-high	150-199 mg/dL	
High	200-499 mg/dL	
Very high	> 500 mg/dL	
Magnesium	1.3-2.2 mEq/L	0.65-1.1 mmol/L
Osmolality	280-300 mOsm/kg	280-300 mmol/kg
Oxygen saturation (arterial)	94%-100%	0.94 fraction of 1
PCO_2, arterial	35-45 mm Hg	4.7-6 kPa
pH, arterial	7.35-7.45	7.35-7.45
PO_2, arterial: Breathing room air[a]	80-105 mm Hg	10.6-14 kPa
On 100% O_2	> 500 mm Hg	
Phosphatase (acid), total at 37°C	0.13-0.63 IU/L	2.2-10.5 units/L or 2.2-10.5 mckat/L
Phosphatase alkaline[b]	20-130 IU/L	20-130 IU/L or 0.33-2.17 mckat/L
Phosphorus, inorganic[c] (phosphate)	2.5-5 mg/dL	0.8-1.6 mmol/L
Potassium	3.5-5 mEq/L	3.5-5 mmol/L
Progesterone		
Female	0.1-1.5 ng/mL	0.32-4.8 nmol/L
Follicular phase	0.1-1.5 ng/mL	0.32-4.8 nmol/L
Luteal phase	2.5-28 ng/mL	8-89 nmol/L
Male	< 0.5 ng/mL	< 1.6 nmol/L
Prolactin	1.4-24.2 ng/mL	1.4-24.2 mcg/L
Prostate specific antigen	0-4 ng/mL	0-4 ng/mL
Protein: Total	6-8 g/dL	60-80 g/L
Albumin	3.6-5 g/dL	36-50 g/L
Globulin	2.3-3.5 g/dL	23-35 g/L
Rheumatoid factor	< 60 units/mL	< 60 kilounits/L
Sodium	135-147 mEq/L	135-147 mmol/L
Testosterone: Female	6-86 ng/dL	0.21-3 nmol/L
Male	270-1,070 ng/dL	9.3-37 nmol/L
Thyroid hormone function tests:		
Thyroid-stimulating hormone (TSH)	0.35-6.2 mcunits/mL	0.35-6.2 munits/L
Thyroxine-binding globulin capacity	10-26 mcg/dL	100-260 mcg/L
Total triiodothyronine (T_3)	75-220 ng/dL	1.2-3.4 nmol/L
Total thyroxine by RIA (T_4)	4-11 mcg/dL	51-142 nmol/L
T_3 resin uptake	25%-38%	0.25-0.38 fraction of 1

Blood, Plasma, or Serum		
	Reference Value	
Determination	Conventional units	SI units
Transaminase, AST (aspartate aminotransferase, SGOT)	11-47 units/L	0.18-0.78 mckat/L
Transaminase, ALT (alanine aminotransferase, SGPT)	7-53 units/L	0.12-0.88 mckat/L
Transferrin	220-400 mg/dL	2.20-4 g/L
Urea nitrogen (BUN)	8-25 mg/dL	2.9-8.9 mmol/L
Uric acid	3-8 mg/dL	179-476 mcmol/L
Vitamin A (retinol)	15-60 mcg/dL	0.52-2.09 mcmol/L
Zinc	50-150 mcg/dL	7.7-23 mcmol/L

[a] Age dependent [b] Infants and adolescents up to 104 units/L [c] Infants in the first year up to 6 mg/dL

Urine		
	Reference value	
Determination	Conventional units	SI units
Calcium[a]	50-250 mcg/day	1.25-6.25 mmol/day
Catecholamines: Epinephrine	< 20 mcg/day	< 109 nmol/day
Norepinephrine	< 100 mcg/day	< 590 nmol/day
Catecholamines, 24-hr	< 110 mcg	< 650 nmol
Copper[a]	15-60 mcg/day	0.24-0.95 mcmol/day
Creatinine: Child	8-22 mg/kg	71-195 μmol/kg
Adolescent	8-30 mg/kg	71-265 μmol/kg
Female	0.6-1.5 g/day	5.3-13.3 mmol/day
Male	0.8-1.8 g/day	7.1-15.9 mmol/day
pH	4.5-8	4.5-8
Phosphate[a]	0.9-1.3 g/day	29-42 mmol/day
Potassium[a]	25-100 mEq/day	25-100 mmol/day
Protein		
Total	1-14 mg/dL	10-140 mg/L
At rest	50-80 mg/day	50-80 mg/day
Protein, quantitative	< 150 mg/day	< 0.15 g/day
Sodium[a]	100-250 mEq/day	100-250 mmol/day
Specific gravity, random	1.002-1.030	1.002-1.030
Uric acid, 24-hr	250-750 mg	1.48-4.43 mmol

[a] Diet dependent

Drug Levels†			
		Reference value	
Drug determination		Conventional units	SI units
Aminoglycosides	Amikacin		
	(trough)	1-8 mcg/mL	1.7-13.7 mcmol/L
	(peak)	20-30 mcg/mL	34-51 mcmol/L
	Gentamicin		
	(trough)	0.5-2 mcg/mL	1-4.2 mcmol/L
	(peak)	6-10 mcg/mL	12.5-20.9 mcmol/L
	Kanamycin		
	(trough)	5-10 mcg/mL	nd[a]
	(peak)	20-25 mcg/mL	nd
	Netilmicin		
	(trough)	0.5-2 mcg/mL	nd
	(peak)	6-10 mcg/mL	nd
	Streptomycin		
	(trough)	< 5 mcg/mL	nd
	(peak)	5-20 mcg/mL	nd
	Tobramycin		
	(trough)	0.5-2 mcg/mL	1.1-4.3 mcmol/L
	(peak)	5-20 mcg/mL	12.8-21.8 mcmol/L

Drug Levels[†]

	Drug determination	Reference value: Conventional units	Reference value: SI units
Antiarrhythmics	Amiodarone	0.5-2.5 mcg/mL	1.5-4 mcmol/L
	Bretylium	0.5-1.5 mcg/mL	nd
	Digitoxin	9-25 mcg/L	11.8-32.8 nmol/L
	Digoxin	0.8-2 ng/mL	0.9-2.5 nmol/L
	Disopyramide	2-8 mcg/mL	6-18 mcmol/L
	Flecainide	0.2-1 mcg/mL	nd
	Lidocaine	1.5-6 mcg/mL	4.5-21.5 mcmol/L
	Mexiletine	0.5-2 mcg/mL	nd
	Procainamide	4-8 mcg/mL	17-34 mcmol/mL
	Propranolol	50-200 ng/mL	190-770 nmol/L
	Quinidine	2-6 mcg/mL	4.6-9.2 mcmol/L
	Tocainide	4-10 mcg/mL	nd
	Verapamil	0.08-0.3 mcg/mL	nd
Anti-convulsants	Carbamazepine	4-12 mcg/mL	17-51 mcmol/L
	Phenobarbital	10-40 mcg/mL	43-172 mcmol/L
	Phenytoin	10-20 mcg/mL	40-80 mcmol/L
	Primidone	4-12 mcg/mL	18-55 mcmol/L
	Valproic acid	40-100 mcg/mL	280-700 mcmol/L
Antidepressants	Amitriptyline	110-250 ng/mL[b]	500-900 nmol/L
	Amoxapine	200-500 ng/mL	nd
	Bupropion	25-100 ng/mL	nd
	Clomipramine	80-100 ng/mL	nd
	Desipramine	115-300 ng/mL	nd
	Doxepin	110-250 ng/mL[b]	nd
	Imipramine	225-350 ng/mL[b]	nd
	Maprotiline	200-300 ng/mL	nd
	Nortriptyline	50-150 ng/mL	nd
	Protriptyline	70-250 ng/mL	nd
	Trazodone	800-1600 ng/mL	nd
Antipsychotics	Chlorpromazine	50-300 ng/mL	150-950 nmol/L
	Fluphenazine	0.13-2.8 ng/mL	nd
	Haloperidol	5-20 ng/mL	nd
	Perphenazine	0.8-1.2 ng/mL	nd
	Thiothixene	2-57 ng/mL	nd
Miscellaneous	Amantadine	300 ng/mL	nd
	Amrinone	3.7 mcg/mL	nd
	Chloramphenicol	10-20 mcg/mL	31-62 mcmol/L
	Cyclosporine[c]	250-800 ng/mL (whole blood, RIA) 50-300 ng/mL (plasma, RIA)	nd nd
	Ethanol[d]	0 mg/dL	0 mmol/L
	Hydralazine	100 ng/mL	nd
	Lithium	0.6-1.2 mEq/L	0.6-1.2 mmol/L
	Salicylate	100-300 mg/L	724-2,172 mcmol/L
	Sulfonamide	5-15 mg/dL	nd
	Terbutaline	0.5-4.1 ng/mL	nd
	Theophylline	10-20 mcg/mL	55-110 mcmol/L
	Vancomycin		
	(trough)	5-15 ng/mL	nd
	(peak)	20-40 mcg/mL	nd

[†] The values given are generally accepted as desirable for treatment without toxicity for most patients. However, exceptions are not uncommon.

[a] nd – no data available

[b] Parent drug plus N-desmethyl metabolite

[c] 24 hour trough values

[d] Toxic: 50-100 mg/dL (10.9-21.7 mmol/L)

Classification of Blood Pressure*

Category	Reference Value		
	Systolic (mm Hg)		Diastolic (mm Hg)
Normal	< 120	and	< 80
Prehypertension	120-139	or	80-89
Stage 1 hypertension	140-159	or	90-99
Stage 2 hypertension	≥ 160	or	≥ 100

Adapted from the Seventh Report of the Joint National Committee on Prevention, Detection, Evaluation, and Treatment of High Blood Pressure, National Institutes of Health. JAMA. 2003;289(19):2560-2571.

* For adults age 18 and older who are not taking antihypertensive drugs and not acutely ill. When systolic and diastolic blood pressures fall into different categories, the higher category should be selected to classify the individual's blood pressure status.

The classification is based on the average of 2 or more readings properly measured taken at each of 2 or more visits after an initial reading.

GENERAL MANAGEMENT OF ACUTE OVERDOSAGE

Rapid intervention is essential to minimize morbidity and mortality in an acute toxic ingestion. Institute measures to prevent absorption and hasten elimination as soon as possible; however, symptomatic and supportive care takes precedence over other therapy. It is assumed that basic life support measures, (eg, cardiopulmonary resuscitation [CPR]) have been instituted. Specific antidotes are discussed in the overdosage section of individual or group monographs. The discussion below outlines procedures used in the management of acute overdosage of orally ingested systemic drugs.

Advanced Life Support Measures

Adequate Airway: Adequate airway must be established and maintained, generally via oropharyngeal or endotracheal airways, cricothyrotomy, or tracheostomy.

Ventilation: Ventilation may then be performed via mouth-to-mouth insufflation, hand-operated bag (ambu bag) or by mechanical ventilator.

Circulation: Circulation must be maintained.

- *Hypotension:* If hypotension/hypoperfusion occurs, place the patient in shock position (head lowered, feet elevated); specific therapy may include:
  Establish IV access and initiate IV fluids (eg, 0.9% or 0.45% saline, lactated Ringer's, dextrose). A maintenance flow rate is generally 100 to 200 mL/hour; individualize as necessary.
  Plasma, plasma protein fractions, whole blood or plasma expanders may be required.
  Severe hypotension may require judicious use of cardiovascular active agents. The most commonly recommended agents are dopamine, dobutamine and norepinephrine.
- *Arrhythmia* treatment is dictated by the offending drug.
- *Hypertension*, sometimes severe, may occur. (See Nitroprusside and Diazoxide, Parenteral in the Agents for Hypertensive Emergencies section.)

Seizures: Simple isolated seizures may require only observation and supportive care. Repetitive seizures or status epilepticus require therapy. Give IV diazepam or lorazepam followed by fosphenytoin and/or phenobarbital. Pancuronium may also be considered.

Reduction of Absorption

Gastric emptying is generally recommended as soon as possible; however, this is generally not very effective unless employed within the first 1 to 2 hours after ingestion. Syrup of ipecac and gastric lavage are the two most commonly employed methods for gastric emptying.

- *Syrup of ipecac* is the method of choice outside the hospital. Do not induce vomiting if the medication is caustic or a petroleum or if the patient is in a coma or having seizures. Syrup of ipecac takes 20 to 30 minutes to work. Consider gastric lavage if response is needed immediately.

  6 months to 1 year – 10 mL
  1 year to 12 years – 15 mL
  > *12 years* – 30 mL

May be followed by a glass of water. A second dose may be given if results do not occur within 20 to 30 minutes.

- *Gastric lavage* is indicated in the comatose patient or for those in whom syrup of ipecac fails to produce emesis. Gastric lavage is immediate and does not have a delay reaction, and is preferred over forced emesis. Airway protection via endotracheal intubation is appropriate for the patient without a gag reflex or comatose patients. Position the patient on left side, face down and use a large bore tube. Instill warm water or saline 300 to 360 mL for adults. Avoid water for infants and children; use warm saline or 5% to 6% polyethylene glycol solution. Give until lavage solution becomes clear. Add charcoal before removing the tube.

Adsorption: Adsorption, using activated charcoal alone or after completion of emesis or lavage, is indicated for virtually all significant toxic ingestions. It adsorbs a wide variety of toxins and there are no contraindications. However, it adsorbs many orally administered antidotes as well, so space dosage properly. Give an adult 50 to 100 g of activated charcoal mixed in 240 mL of water; the pediatric dose is 1 g/kg, or 25 to 50 g in 120 mL of water.

Cathartics: Cathartics increase the elimination of charcoal-poison complex. Generally using a saline or osmotic cathartic (eg, magnesium sulfate or citrate or sorbitol) with 3 mL/kg of a 35% to 75% solution of sorbitol has the most rapid effect.

Whole bowel irrigation (WBI): Whole bowel irrigation utilizes rapid administration of large volumes of lavage solutions, such as PEG. The dose is 4 to 6 L over 1 to 2 hours for adults and 0.5 L/hr for children. It may be most useful to remove iron tablets, sustained-release capsules or cocaine-containing condoms or balloons.

Elimination of Absorbed Drug

Interruption of enterohepatic circulation: Interruption of enterohepatic circulation by "gastric dialysis" uses scheduled doses of activated charcoal for 1 to 2 days. Gastric dialysis not only interrupts the enterohepatic cycle of some drugs, but also creates an osmotic gradient, drawing drug from the plasma back into the gastrointestinal lumen where it is bound by the charcoal and excreted in the feces.

Diuresis: Diuresis may be effective as identified in the individual drug monographs.

- *Forced diuresis* is occasionally useful. It may cause volume overload or electrolyte disturbances. Forced diuresis is useful for phenobarbital, bromides, lithium, salicylate, or amphetamines overdoses. Do not use for tricyclic antidepressants, sedative-hypnotics, or highly protein-bound medications. The most common agents employed are furosemide and osmotic diuretics with mannitol.
- *Alkaline diuresis* promotes elimination of weak acids (eg, barbiturates, salicylates) and is accomplished by the administration of IV sodium bicarbonate.
- *Acid diuresis* may be indicated in overdoses with weak bases (eg, amphetamines, fenfluramine, quinine), but use with caution in patients with renal

or liver disease. It is usually accomplished with oral or IV ascorbic acid or ammonium chloride.

Dialysis: Dialysis is indicated in a minority of severe overdose cases. Drug factors that alter dialysis effectiveness include volume of distribution, drug compartmentalization, protein binding and lipid/water solubility.

- *Hemodialysis* may be used after an overdose and when the patient is having complications (eg, severe metabolic acidosis, electrolyte imbalances, renal failure).
- *Peritoneal dialysis* is even less effective than hemodialysis.
- *Charcoal hemoperfusion* is useful when a drug can be adsorbed by charcoal (eg, theophylline, barbiturates).

Poison Control Centers

The American Association of Poison Control Centers (AAPCC) has established a national toll-free poison center hotline. Now everyone in the United States can call

1-800-222-1222

to reach the local poison center. Poison center services are available 24 hours a day, 7 days a week.

The phone number can be used for a poison emergency or questions about poisons and poison prevention.

Regardless of where the call is placed, the hotline automatically connects callers to the closest poison control center. Existing local poison center numbers will still connect callers to their poison centers.

Callers who use a TTY/TDD and non-English speaking callers also can use this hotline. A Web site has been established for further nonemergency information: http://www.aapcc.org/.

INDEX

B

D

E

F

G

J

K

L

M

N

S

T

U

V